Infectious Diseases

DONALD ARMSTRONG
JONATHAN COHEN

Volume One

DEDICATION

We dedicate this book to those who have taught us so much – our patients, our fellows in training and our families, all of whom learned to live with infections and infectious disease physicians.

Infectious Diseases

Donald Armstrong

Emeritus Chief, Infectious Disease Service, Memorial-Sloan Kettering Cancer Center; Professor of Medicine, Cornell University Medical College, New York, New York, USA

Jonathan Cohen

Chairman, Department of Infectious Diseases and Microbiology, Imperial College School of Medicine; Honorary Consultant Physician, Hammersmith Hospital, London, UK

Seth F Berkley
President, International AIDS Vaccine Initiative, New York, New York, USA

Claude J Carbon
Professor of Internal Medicine, Service de Médecine Interne, CHU Bichat-Claude Bernard, Paris, France

Nathan Clumeck
Professor of Medicine and Infectious Diseases, Department of Infectious Diseases and Internal Medicine, St Pierre University Hospital, Brussels, Belgium

David T Durack
Vice President, Medical Affairs, Becton Dickinson Biosciences, Baltimore, Maryland; Consulting Professor of Medicine, Duke University, Durham, North Carolina, USA

Roger G Finch
Professor of Infectious Diseases, Department of Microbiology and Infectious Diseases, Nottingham City Hospital, Nottingham, UK

Timothy E Kiehn
Chief, Microbiology Service, Department of Clinical Laboratories, Memorial Sloan-Kettering Cancer Center, New York, New York, USA

Donald B Louria
Professor and Chairman, Department of Preventive Medicine and Community Health, New Jersey Medical School – University of Medicine and Dentistry of New Jersey, Newark, New Jersey, USA

Keith P W J McAdam
Wellcome Professor of Tropical Medicine, London School of Hygiene and Tropical Medicine; Director of Medical Research Council Laboratories, Fajara, The Gambia, West Africa

S Ragnar Norrby
Professor and Chairman, Department of Infectious Diseases, Lund University Hospital, Lund, Sweden

Steven M Opal
Professor of Medicine, Infectious Disease Division, Brown University School of Medicine, Memorial Hospital of Rhode Island, Pawtucket, Rhode Island, USA

Bruce W Polsky
Chief, Division of Infectious Diseases, Department of Medicine; Medical Director, Clinical Virology Laboratory, Department of Pathology and Laboratory Medicine, St Luke's–Roosevelt Hospital Center, New York, New York, USA

Paul G Quie
Regents' Professor of Pediatrics, Pediatric Infectious Diseases, University of Minnesota Medical School, Minneapolis, Minnesota, USA

Allan R Ronald
Infectious Diseases Consultant, St Boniface General Hospital; Associate Dean, Research Faculty of Medicine, University of Manitoba, Winnipeg, Manitoba, Canada

Claus O Solberg
Professor of Medicine and Infectious Diseases; Chairman, Medical Department, Bergen University Hospital, Bergen, Norway

Jan Verhoef
Professor of Medical Microbiology; Director, Eijkman-Winkler Institute for Microbiology, Infectious Diseases and Inflammation, University Medical Centre, Utrecht, The Netherlands

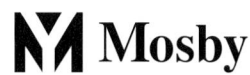

London   Philadelphia   St Louis   Sydney   Tokyo

MOSBY An imprint of Harcourt Publishers Ltd
© Harcourt Publishers Ltd 1999

 is a registered trademark of Harcourt Publishers Ltd

The right of D. Armstrong and J. Cohen to be identified as authors of this work has been asserted by them in accordance with the Copyright, Designs and Patents Act 1988

First published 1999

ISBN: 0 7234 2328 8

Typeset in Times, legends set in NewsGothic

Produced by Bantam Prospect, Basildon, Essex
Printed and bound by Grafos, SA Arte Sobre papel, Barcelona, Spain

Library of Congress Cataloging in Publication data
A catalog record for this book is available from the Library of Congress

British Library Cataloguing in Publication data
A catalogue record for this book is available from the British Library

Note
Medical knowledge is constantly changing. As new information becomes available, changes in treatment, procedures, equipment and the use of drugs become necessary. The editors/authors/contributors and the publishers have, as far as it is possible, taken care to ensure that the information given in this text is accurate and up-to-date. However, readers are strongly advised to confirm that the information, especially with regard to drug usage, complies with the latest legislation and standards of practice.

Publisher:	Richard Furn
Development Editor:	Richard Foulsham
Managing Editor:	Alison Whitehouse
Publishers' Assistant:	Christine Fryer
Project Manager:	Susan Rana
Senior Project Manager:	Katie Pattullo
Designer:	Pete Wilder
Design and Illustration:	Marie McNestry
	Richard Prime
	Danny Pyne
	Ian Spick
	Mick Ruddy
	Deborah Gyan
Proofreader:	Andy Baker
Copyeditor:	Robert Whittle
	Lindy van den Berghe
Production:	Mark Sanderson
	Siobhan Egan
Index:	Janine Ross

Preface

Infectious diseases are the world's greatest killers. Many infectious diseases can be treated and cured and many are readily preventable. Moreover, infection pervades virtually every medical discipline, and as the field becomes more and more complex the challenge to practitioners has become increasingly demanding. This book has been written to meet that challenge.

Several excellent text-reference books in infectious diseases already exist, but these are aimed largely at the specialist. Our goals in devising this all-new book were clear: we wanted to create a book for both specialist and non-specialist practitioners that would give clear, practical advice on the prevention, diagnosis and treatment of infection. It had to be accessible and take advantage of the extraordinary developments in publishing that would allow us to make full use of high-quality image reproduction. Extensive color illustration has been used throughout, along with a clear page design, to make it simple to navigate through the many interlocking areas of infectious disease. Uniform chapter templates avoid repetition and maintain consistency within Sections, making it easy to find your way. For the first time in a book of this type we have been able to include radiographs, pathology, and full-color tables and figures alongside the text in a way which both complements the understanding of disease and also provides a high-quality resource for teaching and learning. Nowadays, textbooks are just one way of accessing information; on the accompanying CD-ROM you will find not only all these photographs and artworks in an easily downloadable format, but a gateway to an extensive compilation of Internet websites dealing with infection.

In order to provide complete coverage of the entire field of infectious diseases we have divided the book into sections that focus on different aspects of the speciality. There is a systematic and complete review of infections by body system, and detailed sections on infection in immunocompromised hosts, HIV and AIDS and special problems in infectious disease practice, such as fever of unknown origin. Throughout, we have kept in mind the need to provide a complete differential diagnosis of both infectious and non-infectious diseases.

Infectious diseases are a global threat. The greatest toll is taken in the developing world but with wars, disasters, poor nutrition and constant traveling the edges between the developed and developing world are becoming blurred. Most larger cities in the developed world have pockets of a developing world within them. For the first time in a major infectious diseases textbook, we have included a complete section on geographic and travel-related medicine, written by authors from throughout the world who have first-hand experience of their subject.

Understanding microbiology is key to the practice of infectious diseases, and an extensive section on clinical microbiology provides in-depth discussion on how micro-organisms are identified, the problems associated with susceptibility testing and the use of antibiotics and, critically, the field of pathogenicity and how these organisms cause disease.

We know from our own experience that the answers to the clinical problems faced by practitioners are sometimes difficult to identify in reference texts. Often, large textbooks will not 'come off the fence' and give specific advice. To respond to this, we have included Practice Points – topics suggested by colleagues both junior and senior – which address these difficult subjects concisely and include specific expert answers and recommendations.

One of the joys of infectious disease practice is bringing together different disciplines – internal medicine, pediatrics, microbiology, and immunology – to solve patients' problems. Another is that most infectious diseases are curable when diagnosed accurately and early. There is no other area in the practice of medicine that is as challenging or as rewarding.

The aim of this text then is to help the practitioner in the care of the patient, to be an instructive source for teaching infectious diseases, and to stimulate research in this fascinating area of medicine and biology.

This book has been a very ambitious undertaking, and its success has depended on many people. One of our key objectives has been the firm intention to seek expertise from around the world. Working together with the Section Editors, internationally-renowned experts in their field, we have assembled a truly extraordinary group of contributors from many countries and many different backgrounds to ensure both a modern and an authoritative approach. Equally important has been the help and support from the publishers, in particular Richard Furn, whose enthusiasm and drive has been an inspiration. His colleagues Richard Foulsham, Alison Whitehouse, Susan Rana, Katie Pattullo and many others have turned our ideas into reality, and we are enormously grateful.

Donald Armstrong
Jonathan Cohen

User Guide

VOLUMES, SECTIONS AND COLOR-CODING

Infectious Diseases is divided into two volumes. The book is organized into eight sections, which are color-coded as follows for reference:

VOLUME 1

SECTION **1**	Introduction to Infectious Diseases
SECTION **2**	Syndromes by Body System
SECTION **3**	Special Problems in Infectious Disease Practice
SECTION **4**	Infections in the Immunocompromised Host

VOLUME 2

SECTION **5**	HIV and AIDS
SECTION **6**	Geographic and Travel Medicine
SECTION **7**	Anti-infective Therapy
SECTION **8**	Clinical Microbiology

Sections 1-4 appear in Volume One, and Sections 5-8 appear in Volume Two.

FINDING CHAPTERS AND PAGES

Within each section the chapters are numbered consecutively, with each chapter paginated and beginning on page 1. Each page gives the chapter and page number. An example is shown below. This example is page 4 of chapter 3 in section 5, page 5.3.4.

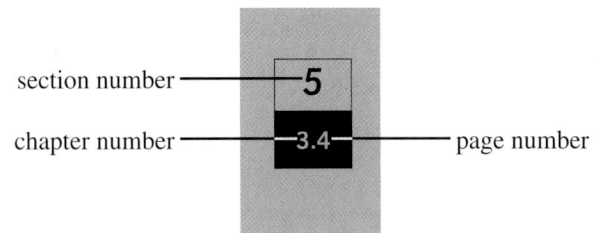

section number ⎯⎯ 5

chapter number ⎯⎯ 3.4 ⎯⎯ page number

To find a chapter turn to the purple section (Section 5), find chapter 3 and then turn to page 4.

A comprehensive subject index covering the entire book appears in the back of both volumes of *Infectious Diseases*.

FINDING PRACTICE POINTS

Practice Points are grouped together into Practice Point chapters; the pages are numbered consecutively throughout these chapters. To find a Practice Point find the chapter in which it appears and turn to the first page. On this page you will find a mini-contents page for that chapter which will give you the exact page number on which the Practice Point appears. Practice Points are colored in a gray tint in the Contents list.

INFECTIOUS DISEASES WEBSITES

A list of infectious disease related websites can be found at the back of Volume Two, just before the index. These same websites can be accessed using the CD-ROM on the inside front cover of Volume One.

Contents

Volume 1

SECTION 1 **INTRODUCTION TO INFECTIOUS DISEASES**   Donald B Louria & Claude J Carbon

SECTION 2 **SYNDROMES BY BODY SYSTEM**   David T Durack, Roger G Finch & Allan R Ronald

SECTION 3   **SPECIAL PROBLEMS IN INFECTIOUS DISEASE PRACTICE** Jonathan Cohen & Steven M Opal

Volume 2

SECTION 6 GEOGRAPHIC AND TRAVEL MEDICINE Keith PWJ McAdam & Seth F Berkley

---

SECTION 7   ANTI-INFECTIVE THERAPY   Donald Armstrong & S Ragnar Norrby

Contributors

ROBERT D ACTON
Medical Fellow, Department of Surgery, University of
Minnesota, Minneapolis, Minnesota, USA

KJELL ALESTIG
Professor of Infectious Diseases, Department of
Infectious Diseases, Sahlgrensuu University Hospital,
Ostra, Sweden

UPTON ALLEN
Infectious Diseases Consultant, Division of Infectious
Disease; Associate Professor of Pediatrics, University of
Toronto, Hospital for Sick Children, Toronto, Ontario,
Canada

ANTOINE ANDREMONT
Professor de Bactériologie-Virologie-Hygiene,
Laboratoire de Bactériologie, Group Hospitalier Bichat-
Claude Bernard, Paris, France

ROBERTO C ARDUINO
Assistant Professor of Medicine, Division of Infectious
Diseases, The University of Texas, Houston, Texas, USA

PAUL M ARGUIN
Epidemic Intelligence Service Officer, Rabies Section,
Centers for Disease Control and Prevention, Atlanta,
Georgia, USA

WENDY ARMSTRONG
Infectious Diseases Division, University Michigan
Medical Center, Ann Arbor, Michigan, USA

OM P ARYA
Emeritus Consultant Physician and Senior Research
Fellow Department of Medical Microbiology and
Genitourinary Medicine, University of Liverpool,
Liverpool, UK

EDWIN J ASTURIAS
Research Scientist, Center for Studies and Disease
Control – Guatamala; Department of International
Health, Johns Hopkins School of Public Health,
Baltimore, Maryland, USA

JOHN C ATHERTON
Senior Lecturer; MRC Clinician Scientist, School of
Medical and Surgical Sciences, Division of
Gastroenterology and Institute of Infections and
Immunity, University of Nottingham, Nottingham, UK

ROBIN BAILEY
Senior Lecturer, London School of Hygiene and Tropical
Medicine; Physician, Hospital for Tropical Disease,
London, UK

J WENDI BAILEY
Principal Experimental Officer, Diagnostic Laboratory,
Division of Tropical Medicine, Liverpool School of
Tropical Medicine, Liverpool, UK

GUY BAILY
Consultant Physician, Infections and Immunity Clinical
Group, The Royal London Hospital, London, UK

DAVID R BALDWIN
Consultant Respiratory Physician and Clinical Teacher,
Department of Respiratory Medicine, Nottingham City
Hospital, Nottingham, UK

PETER BALL
Honorary Senior Lecturer, School of Biological and
Medical Sciences, University of St Andrews, Fife,
Scotland, UK

BARBARA A BANNISTER
Consultant in Infectious and Tropical Diseases, Royal
Free Hospital, Department of Infectious and Tropical
Diseases, Coppetts Wood Hospital, London, UK

DAVID J BARILLO
Associate Professor of Surgery; Chief, Division of
Plastic Surgery and Adult Burn Center, Medical
University of South Carolina, Charleston; Former Chief,
Clinical Division, US Army Institiute of Surgical
Research, Fort Sam, Texas, USA

AMANDA J BARNES
Acting Consultant Microbiologist, Public Health
Laboratory, Manchester, UK

MICHAEL BARZA
Professor of Medicine, Tufts University School of
Medicine, Director of Medicine, Carney Hospital,
Boston, Massachusetts, USA

ROGER BAYSTON
Research Fellow Head, Biomaterials-Related Infection
Group, University Nottingham, Medical School Division
of Microbiology and Infectious Diseases, City Hospital,
Nottingham, UK

NICHOLAS J BEECHING
Senior Lecturer in Infectious Diseases, Division of
Tropical Medicine, Liverpool School of Tropical
Medicine, Liverpool, UK

RODOLFO E BEGUE
Professor of Pediatrics, Division of Infectious Diseases,
Louisiana State University, New Orleans; Director,
Infectious Diseases, Children's Hospital, New Orleans,
Louisiana, USA

CONSTANCE A BENSON
Professor of Medicine, Division of Infectious Diseases,
University of Colorado Health Sciences Center, Denver,
Colorado, USA

ANTHONY R BERENDT
Consultant Physician-in-Charge, Bone Infection Unit,
Nuffield Orthopaedic Centre, Oxford, UK

EUGENIE BERGOGNE-BÉRÉZIN
Consultant Microbiology-Pharmacology, Department of
Microbiology, Bichat-Claude Bernard Hospital, Paris,
France

VERKA BERIC
Specialist Registrar, Department of Imaging,
Hammersmith Hospital, London, UK

EDWARD M BERNARD
Research Associate, Infectious Diseases, Department of
Medicine, Memorial Sloan-Kettering Cancer Center,
New York, New York, USA

ALAN L BISNO
Professor and Vice Chairman, Department of Medicine,
University of Miami School of Medicine; Chief, Medical
Service, Miami Veterans Affairs Medical Center, Miami,
Florida, USA

ROBERT BJERKNES
Professor of Pediatrics, Department of Pediatrics,
University of Bergen, Bergen, Norway

FINN T BLACK
Professor of Infectious Diseases and Tropical Medicine,
Department of Infectious Diseases, University Hospital
of Aårhus, Aårhus, Denmark

GERALD P BODEY
Emeritus Professor of Medicine, Section of Infectious
Diseases, University of Texas, Anderson Cancer Center,
Houston, Texas, USA

ROBERT BORTOLUSSI
Professor of Pediatrics, Professor of Microbiology,
Dalhousie University; Chief of Research, IWK Grace
Health Centre, Halifax, Nova Scotia, Canada

CHARLES AB BOUCHER
Associate Professor, Department of Virology, Eijkman-
Winkler Institute, University Medical Centre, Utrecht,
The Netherlands

EMILIO BOUZA
Chief, Clinical Microbiology and Infectious Diseases,
Hospital General Universitario 'Gregorio Marañon';
Professor of Medicine, University of Madrid, Madrid,
Spain

RALEIGH A BOWDEN
Medical Director, Providence Seattle Cancer Program;
Affiliate Associate Member, FHCRC; Clinical Associate
Professor of Medicine and Pediatrics, University of
Washington School of Medicine, Seattle, Washington,
USA

WILLIAM R BOWIE
Professor of Medicine, Division of Infectious Diseases,
University of British Columbia, Vancouver, British
Columbia, Canada

BO BRISMAR
Associate Professor, Department of Surgery, Huddinge
University Hospital, Huddinge, Sweden

WARWICK J BRITTON
Associate Professor of Medicine, Department of Clinical
Immunology, Royal Prince Alfred Hospital and
Department of Medicine, University of Sydney, Sydney,
New South Wales, Australia

KENNETH BROMBERG
Vice Chairman of Pediatrics; Associate Professor of
Pediatrics, Medicine and Microbiology/Immunology,
State University of New York, Health Science Center at
Brooklyn, Brooklyn, New York, USA

ITZHAK BROOK
Professor of Pediatrics, Georgetown University,
Georgetown University School of Medicine, Washington
DC, USA

DAVID BROWN
Director, Enteric and Respiratory Virus Laboratory,
Central Public Health Laboratory, London, UK

FRANÇOISE BRUN-VÉZINET
Professor of Microbiology, Laboratoire de Virologie,
Hopital Bichat-Claude Bernard, Paris, France

ØYSTEIN BRUSERUD
Professor of Hematology, Medical Department, Bergen,
Norway

R MARK L BULLER
Associate Professor, Department of Microbiology, St
Louis University School of Medicine, St Louis,
Missouri, USA

WILLIAM CAMERON
Professor of Medicine, Division of Infectious Diseases,
University of Ottawa at Ottawa Hospital, Ottawa,
Ontario, Canada

MICHEL CARAËL
Team Leader, Prevention, Department of Policy, Strategy
and Research, UNAIDS, Geneva, Switzerland

JEAN CARLET
Head, Intensive Care Unit, Foundation Hôpital Saint-
Joseph, Paris, France

RICHARD A CASH
Fellow, Harvard Institute for International Development,
Cambridge, Massachusetts, USA; Lecturer, Harvard
School of Public Health, Department of Population and
International Health, Boston, Massachusetts, USA

KEVIN A CASSADY
Assistant Professor, University of Alabama at
Birmingham, Birmingham, Alabama, USA

RICHARD E CHAISSON
Professor of Medicine, Epidemiology and International
Health, Johns Hopkins University, Baltimore, Maryland,
USA

STEPHEN T CHAMBERS
Associate Professor of Pathology, Christchurch School
of Medicine, Department of Infectious Diseases,
Christchurch Hospital, Christchurch, New Zealand

JOHN S CHEESBROUGH
Consultant Microbiologist, Public Health Laboratory,
Royal Preston Hospital, Preston, UK; Honorary
Research Fellow, University Department of Medical
Microbiology and Genitourinary Medicine, The
University of Liverpool, Liverpool, UK

PETER L CHIODINI
Consultant Parasitologist, The Hospital for Tropical
Diseases, London, UK

LOLITA E CHIU
Infectious Diseases Division, Brown University School
of Medicine, Providence, Rhode Island, USA

JOHN C CHRISTENSON
Professor of Pediatrics, Department of Pediatrics,
Division of Infectious Diseases and Geographic
Medicine, University of Utah School of Medicine, Salt
Lake City, Utah, USA

ANTHONY C CHU
Head of the Section of Dermatology, Imperial College of
Science Technology; and Medicine Senior
Lecturer/Consultant Dermatologist, Hammersmith
Hospital, London, UK

LORRAINE M CLARKE
Director of Quality Assurance, New York State
Department of Health, Wadsworth Center, Albany, New
York, USA; Clinical Associate Professor of Pathology,
State University of New York Health Science Center,
Brooklyn, New York, USA

GRAHAM M CLEATOR
Reader in Medical Virology, Division of Virology,
Department of Pathological Sciences, Manchester Royal
Infirmary, Manchester, UK

DENNIS A CLEMENTS
Associate Professor of Pediatrics and Infectious
Diseases; Assistant Professor of Internal Medicine, Duke
Children's Hospital, Durham, North Carolina, USA

CLAY J COCKERELL
Professor of Dermatopathology and Pathology; Director,
HIV Associate Skin Disease Clinic, Parkland Hospital,
Dallas, Texas, USA

MYRON S COHEN
Director, UNC Center for Infectious Diseases; Chief,
Division of Infectious Diseases; Professor of Medicine,
Microbiology and Immunology, The University of North
Carolina at Chapel Hill, Chapel Hill, North Carolina,
USA

JAMES WT COHEN STUART
University Hospital Utrecht, Department of Virology,
Utrecht, The Netherlands

JOHN COLLINGE
Professor of Neurogenetics, Department of
Neurogenetics, Imperial College School of Medicine at
St Mary's, London, UK

JOHN A COLLINS
Professor of Obstetrics and Gynecology and Clinical
Epidemiology and Biostatistics, McMaster University,
Hamilton, Ontario, Canada

HILDE COLPIN
Pedagogical Sciences, Sexologist, Division of Infectious
Diseases, Bruxelles, Belgium

CHRISTOPHER P CONLON
Consultant Physician, Infectious Disease Unit, Nuffield
Department of Medicine, Oxford Radcliffe Hospital,
Oxford, UK

G RALPH COREY
Professor of Infectious Diseases, Duke University
Medical Center, Durham, North Carolina, USA

GEORGE COWAN
Postgraduate Medical and Dental Education, London,
UK

JOHN H CROSS
Professor, Tropical Public Health Department of
Preventive Medicine/Biometric Uniformed Services,
University of the Health Sciences, Bethesda, Maryland,
USA

GINA DALLABETTA
Director of Technical Support HIV/AIDS Prevention and
Care Department Family Health International, Arlington,
Virginia, USA

DAVID AB DANCE
Director and Consultant Medical Microbiologist, Public
Health Laboratory, Plymouth, Devon, UK

JACOB DANKERT
Professor of Medical Microbiology, Department of
Medical Microbiology, Academic Medical Centre,
Amsterdam, The Netherlands

ROBERT N DAVIDSON
Consultant Physician, Department of Infection and
Tropical Medicine Lister Unit, Northwick Park Hospital,
Harrow, Middlesex, UK

MARTIN DEDICOAT
Specialist Registrar, Department of Infection, Heartlands
Hospital, Birmingham, UK

DAVID T DENNIS
Chief, Bacterial Zoonoses Branch Division of Vector-
Borne Infectious Diseases, Centers for Disease Control
and Prevention, Fort Collins, Colorado, USA

STÉPHANE DE WIT
Senior Resident, St Pierre University Hospital, Division
of Infectious Diseases, Brussels, Belgium

GORDON M DICKINSON
Professor of Medicine and Interim Chief, Division of
Infectious Diseases, University of Miami School of
Medicine; Clinical Director, Special Immunology
Section, Miami Veterans Affairs Medical Center, Miami,
Florida, USA

TOM DOHERTY
Clinical Scientist, Malaria Programme, MRC
Laboratories, The Gambia, Africa

DOMINIQUE DORMONT
Chief of Neurovirology, Department Service de
Neuroviorologie, CEA/CRSSA/DSV/DRM, France

HARMINDER S DUA
Chair and Professor of Ophthalmology University of
Nottingham Queen's Medical Centre, University
Hospital, Nottingham, UK

MICHAEL P DUBÉ
Associate Professor of Clinical Medicine, Department of
Medicine, Division of Infectious Diseases, University of
Southern California School of Medicine, Los Angeles,
California, USA

JAY S DUKER
Vice-Chairman, Department of Ophthalmology;
Director, Vitreo-Retinal Service, New England Eye
Center, Boston, Massachusetts, USA

DAVID L DUNN
Professor and Chairman, Department of Surgery;
Director, Division of Surgical Infectious Disease,
University of Minnesota, Minneapolis, Minnesota, USA

HERBERT L DUPONT
Clinical Professor of Medicine, Baylor College of
Medicine and the University of Texas, Houston; Chief,
Internal Medicine St Luke's Episcopal Hospital,
Houston, Texas, USA

ANDROULLA EFSTRATIOU
Head, PHLS/WHO Streptococcus and Diphtheria
Reference Unit Respiratory and Systemic Infection
Laboratory, PHLS Central Public Health Laboratory,
London, UK

MARTHA ESPINOSA-CANTELLANO
Professor, Department of Experimental Pathology,
Center for Research and Advanced Studies, Mexico City,
Mexico

MICHAEL JG FARTHING
Professor of Gastroenterology Digestive Diseases
Research Centre, St Bartholomew's and The Royal
London School of Medicine and Dentistry, London, UK

ROBERT J FASS
Professor of Infectious Diseases; Professor of Internal
Medicine and Microbiology and Immunology; Director,
Division of Infectious Diseases, The Ohio State
University College of Medicine, Columbus, Ohio, USA

PATRICIA E FAST
Associate Director, Clinical Research, Aviron, Mountain
View, California, USA

MARY LYN FIELD
Technical Officer, Family Health International,
Arlington, Virginia, USA

SUSAN FISHER-HOCH
Directeur, Laboratoire Jean Mereieux de haute securite, Fondation marcel Merieux, Lyon, France

CHARLES W FLEXNER
Associate Professor of Medicine, Pharmacology and Molecular Sciences, and International Health, Johns Hopkins University, Baltimore, Maryland, USA

MARCO FLORIDIA
Researcher Laboratory of Virology, Retrovirus Department Istituto Superiore di Sanità, Rome, Italy

AD C FLUIT
Eijkman-Winkler Institute, University Hospital, Utrecht, The Netherlands

E LEE FORD-JONES
Associate Professor of Pediatrics, The Hospital for Sick Children, Toronto, Ontario, Canada

KIMBERLEY K FOX
Assistant Professor of Medicine and Epidemiology, University of North Carolina, Chapel Hill, North Carolina; Division of STD Prevention, Centers for Disease Control and Prevention, Atlanta, Georgia, USA

JON S FRIEDLAND
Senior Lecturer and Honorary Consultant, Department of Infectious Diseases, Imperial College of Science, Technology and Medicine, Hammersmith Hospital, London, UK

THOMAS R FRITSCHE
Head, Clinical Microbiology Division, Department of Laboratory Medicine, University of Washington Medical Center, Seattle, Washington, USA

KENNETH L GAGE
Plague Section Chief, Centers for Disease Control and Prevention, Fort Collins, Colorado, USA

NELSON M GANTZ
Chairman, Department of Medicine; Chief, Division of Infectious Diseases, Pinnacle Health Hospitals; Clinical Professor of Medicine, MCP Hahnemann School of Medicine, College of Medicine Pinnacle Health Systems, Harrisburg, Pennsylvania, USA

LYNNE S GARCIA
Manager, Clinical Microbiology, Department Pathology and Laboratory Medicine, UCLA Medical Center, Los Angeles, California, USA

MAÏTÉ GARROUSTE-ORGEAS
Réanimation Polyvalente Hôpital, Paris, France

ARTURO S GASTAÑADUY
Assistant Professor of Pediatrics, Division of Ambulatory Pediatrics, Louisiana State University, New Orleans, Louisiana, USA

BRUCE GELLIN
Staff Director, The Vaccine Initiative, Infectious Diseases Society of America/Pediatric Infectious Diseases Society; Assistant Professor, Department of Preventative Medicine, Vanderbilt University Medicial Center, Nashville, Tennessee, USA

ROBERT C GEORGE
Director, Respiratory and Systemic Infection Laboratory, Central Public Health Laboratory, London, UK

STEPHEN GILLESPIE
Reader and Honorary Consultant, Academic Department of Medical Microbiology, Royal Free and University College Medical School, London, UK

PIERRE-MARIE GIRARD
Service des Maladies Infectieuses et Tropicales Hôpital Rothschild, Centre Hospitalier Universitaire Saint-Antoine, Université Paris, Paris, France

JOHN W GNANN JR
Associate Professor of Medicine, Department of Medicine, Division of Infectious Diseases, University of Alabama at Birmingham School of Medicine, Birmingham, Alabama, USA

DIANE GOADE
Assistant Professor, Department of Medicine Division of Infectious Diseases, The University of New Mexico School of Medicine, Albuquerque, New Mexico, USA

ANDREW F GODDARD
School of Medical and Surgical Science, Division of Gastroenterology, University of Nottingham, Nottingham, UK

BRUNO GOTTSTEIN
Director, The Institute of Parasitology, Faculty of Medicine and Faculty of Veterinary Medicine; Professor of Parasitology, University of Berne, Berne, Switzerland

JOHN M GRANGE
Reader in Clinical Microbiology, Imperial College School of Medicine, London, UK; Visiting Professor, Royal Free and University College London Medical School, London, UK

GEORGE E GRIFFIN
Professor of Infectious Diseases and Medicine, Department of Infectious Diseases, St George's Hospital Medical School, Tooting, London, UK

DAVID E GRIFFITH
Professor of Medicine, University of Texas Health Center, Center for Pulmonary Infectious Disease Control, Tyler, Texas, USA

HANS-PETER GRUNERT
Senior Scientist, Department of Virology, Institute of Infectious Disease Medicine, University Hospital Benjamin Franklin, Free University of Berlin Hindenburgdamm, Berlin, Germany

ANUR R GUHAN
Specialist Registrar in Respiratory Medicine, Respiratory Medicine Unit, Nottingham City Hospital NHS Trust, Nottingham, UK

ADITYA K GUPTA
Associate Professor, Division of Dermatology, Department of Medicine, Sunnybrook Health Science Centre and the University of Toronto, Toronto, Ontario, Canada

KOK-ANN GWEE
Senior Lecturer, Department of Pharmacology, National University of Singapore, Singapore

SCOTT B HALSTEAD
Scientific Director of Infectious Diseases, Naval Medical Research and Development Command, Bethesda, Maryland, USA

DAVIDSON H HAMER
Director, Traveler's Health Service, New England Medical Center; Assistant Professor of Medicine, Tufts University School of Medicine; Project Scientist, ARCH Project, Harvard Institute for International Development, New England Medical Center, Boston, Massachusetts, USA

SAJEEV HANDA
Director, Academic Medical Center Internal Medicine Inpatient Service, Division of General Internal Medicine, Rhode Island Hospital and The Miriam Hospital, Providence, Rhode Island, USA

ANTHONY D HARRIES
Professor of Medicine, Malawi c/o British High Commission, Lilongwe, Malawi, Africa

BARRY J HARTMAN
Clinical Professor of Medicine, Division of Infectious Diseases, Weill Medical College of Cornell University, New York, New York, USA

PETER L HAVENS
Professor of Pediatrics and Epidemiology, Medical College of Wisconsin; Director, Wisconsin HIV Primary Care Support Network, Children's Hospital of Wisconsin, Milwaukee, Wisconsin, USA

RODERICK J HAY
Professor of Cutaneous Medicine, Guy's, King's and St Thomas' Schools of Medicine, St John's Institute of Dermatology, London, UK

DAVID K HENDERSON
Deputy Director for Clinical Care, Warren G Magnuson Clinical Center, National Institutes of Health, Bethesda, Maryland, USA

KELLY J HENNING
Clinical Assistant Professor of Medicine, University of Pennsylvania, Philadelphia, Pennsylvania, USA

LUKE HERBERT
Specialist Registrar in Ophthalmology, Moorfields Eye Hospital, London, UK

HARRY R HILL
Professor of Pathology, Pediatrics and Medicine, Department of Pathology, Division of Clinical Pathology and Clinical Immunology, University of Utah School of Medicine, Salt Lake City, Utah, USA

DAVID R HILL
Director, International Traveler's Medical Service, Division of Infectious Diseases; Associate Professor of Medicine, University of Connecticut Health Center, Farmington, Connecticut, USA

JOHN D HINZE
Fellow in Pulmonary Critical Care Medicine, Texas A & M College of Medicine, Temple, Texas, USA

BERNARD HIRSCHEL
Associate Professor; Chief, HIV/AIDS Division Division des maladies infectieuses, Hôpital Cantonal Universitaire, Geneve, Switzerland

LAWRENCE HIRST
Professor of Ophthalmology, Princess Alexandra Hospital, Woolloongabba, Queensland, Australia

ANDY IM HOEPELMAN
Head, Division of Infectious Diseases and AIDS, Department of Medicine and Eijkman-Winkler Institute for Clinical and Medical Microbiology, University Hospital, Utrecht, The Netherlands

STIG E HOLM
Professor of Clinical Bacteriology, Department of Clinical Bacteriology, University Hospital of Umeå, Umeå, Sweden

WILLEM NM HUSTINX
Department of Internal Medicine, Diakonessen Hospital, Utrecht, The Netherlands

CLARK B INDERLIED
Director of Clinical and Molecular Microbiology, Department of Pathology and Laboratory Medicine, Childrens Hospital, Los Angeles, California, USA; Professor of Pathology and Laboratory Medicine, University of Southern California, Los Angeles, California, USA

JENIFER LEAF JAEGER
Pediatrics Infectious Diseases, Rhode Island Hospital, Providence, Rhode Island, USA

JAMES R JOHNSON
Associate Professor of Medicine, University of
Minnesota Department of Medicine and Infectious
Diseases, Minneapolis; VA Medical Center,
Minneapolis, USA

ERIK K JOHNSON
Fellow, Division of International Medicine and
Infectious Diseases, Cornell University Medical
College, New York, New York, USA

THOMAS C JONES
Clinical Research Consultant; Infectious Diseases
Specialist; Medical Adviser, WHO; Adjunct Professor,
Cornell Medical School, Basle, Switzerland

MUNKOLENKOLE C KAMENGA
Technical Officer, HIV/AIDS Prevention and Care
Department, Family Health International, Arlington,
Virginia, USA

CHRISTINE KATLAMA
Professor of Infectious Diseases, Department of
Infectious Diseases, Tropical Medicine and Public
Health Centre, Hospitalier Pité Salpêtriere, Paris, France

POWEL KAZANJIAN
Director, HIV/AIDS Program, Infectious Diseases
Division; Associate Professor of Medicine, University
Michigan Medical Center, Ann Arbor, Michigan, USA

PATRICK J KELLY
University of Zimbabwe Veterinary School, Harare,
Zimbabwe

JASON S KENDLER
Division of International Medicine and Infectious
Diseases, Cornell University Medical College, New
York, New York, USA

WILLIAM A KENNEDY
Assistant Professor of Pediatrics, Division of Pediatric
Infectious Diseases, Harbor-UCLA Medical Center,
UCLA School of Medicine, Torrance, California, USA

GERALD T KEUSCH
Director, Fogarty International Center; Associate
Director for International Research, National Institutes
of Health, Bethesda, Maryland, USA

GEORGE R KINGHORN
Clinical Director, Directorate of Communicable
Diseases; Consultant Physician in Genitourinary
Medicine, Royal Hallamshire Hospital, Sheffield, UK

PAUL E KLAPPER
Principal Clinical Scientist, Clinical Virology,
Manchester Royal Infirmary, Manchester, UK

MENNO KOK
Microbiologist, Department of Genetics and
Microbiology, Faculty of Medicine, University of
Geneva Medical School, Geneva, Switzerland

JOHN N KRIEGER
Chief of Urology, Department of Urology, V.A. Puget
Sound Health Care System, University of Washington,
Seattle, Washington, USA

SIBYLLE KRISTENSEN
Gorgas Memorial Institute Fellow, Epidemiology and
Tropical Medicine Department of Medicine, University
of Alabama at Birmingham, Alabama, USA

BART-JAN KULLBERG
Associate Professor of Medicine, Catholic University
Nijmegen, Department of Internal Medicine, University
Hospital Nijmegen, Nijmegen, The Netherlands

DANIEL R KURITZKES
Associate Professor of Medicine and Microbiology,
University of Colorado, Health Sciences Center, Denver,
Colorado, USA

SANDRA L KWEDER
Deputy Director, Office of Drug Evaluation IV, Center
for Drug Evaluation and Research, US Food and Drug
Administration; Assistant Professor, Uniformed Services
University of Health Sciences, FE Herbert School of
Medicine, Department of Medicine, Bethesda,
Maryland, USA

DIDIER M LAMBERT
Associate Professor of Medical Chemistry, Unité de
Chimie Pharmeceutique et Radiopharmacie, Brussels,
Belgium

HAROLD LAMBERT
Emeritus Professor of Microbial Diseases,
St George's Hospital Medical School; Visiting Professor,
London School of Hygiene and Tropical Medicine,
London, UK

STEPHEN L LEIB
Attending Physician, Infectious Diseases, Institute for
Medical Microbiology, University of Berne, Berne,
Switzerland

ITZCHAK LEVI
Infectious Disease Unit, Sheba Medical Center, Tel Aviv
University, School of Medicine, Tel-Hashomer Ramat
Gan, Israel

XUGUANG LI
Research Associate, McGill University AIDS Centre,
Jewish General Hospital, Montreal, Quebec, Canada

WEI-SHEN LIM
Specialist Registrar, Respiratory Medicine Unit, City
Hospital Nottingham, Nottingham, UK

MIRIAM M LIPOVSKY
Department of Internal Medicine, Division of Infectious
Diseases and AIDS, University Hospital Utrecht,
Utrecht, The Netherlands

GRAHAM LLOYD
Head, Diagnosis and Reference, Centre of Applied
Microbiology and Research, Porton Down, Salisbury,
UK

WILLIAM A LYNN
Consultant Physician, Department of Infectious
Diseases, Infection and Immunity Unit, Ealing Hospital,
London, UK

JOHN T MACFARLANE
Consultant Physician and Clinical Teacher, University of
Nottingham Medical School, Respiratory Medicine Unit,
City Hospital, Nottingham, UK

ANDREW D MACKAY
Consultant Microbioloist, Department of Microbiology,
Greenwich District General Hospital, Vanburgh Hill,
Greenwich, London, UK

PHILIP A MACKOWIAK
Professor and Vice Chairman, Department of Medicine,
University of Maryland, School of Medicine; Director,
Medical Care Clinical Center, VA Maryland Health Care
System, Baltimore, Maryland, USA

KIM MAEDER
Infection Control Program Harbor, UCLA Medical
Center, Los Angeles, California, USA

JANINE R MAENZA
Assistant Professor of Medicine, Division of Infectious
Diseases, Johns Hopkins University School of Medicine,
Baltimore, Maryland, USA

ADEL AF MAHMOUD
Executive Vice President, Merck Vaccines, Whitehouse
Station, New Jersey, USA

JANICE MAIN
Senior Lecturer in Infectious Diseases and Medicine,
Department of Medicine, Imperial College School of
Medicine, London, UK

JULIE E MANGINO
Assistant Professor of Clinical Internal Medicine,
Division of Infectious Diseases, The Ohio State
University College of Medicine; Medical Director,
Hospital Epidemiology, The Ohio State University
College of Medicine, Columbus, Ohio, USA

PER-ANDERS MÅRDH
Professor of Clinical Bacteriology, Department of
Obstetrics and Gynaecology, University Hospital Lund,
Sweden

KIEREN A MARR
Research Associate, Program in Infectious Diseases,
Fred Hutchinson Cancer Research Center; Acting
Instructor, Division of Allergy and Infectious Disease,
University of Washington, Seattle, Washington, USA

PABLO MARTÍN-RABADÁN
Consultant, Clinical Microbiology and Infectious
Diseases, Hospital General Universitario 'Gregorio
Marañon', Madrid, Spain

AUGUSTO JULIO MARTINEZ
Professor of Pathology, Department of Pathology
(Neuropathology), University of Pittsburgh School of
Medicine, Pittsburgh, Pennsylvania, USA

ADOLFO MARTÍNEZ-PALOMO
Director General, Center for Research and Advanced
Studies México, México City, México

ELLEN M MASCINI
Eijkman-Winkler Institute, Department of Medical
Microbiology, University Hospital, Utrecht, The
Netherlands

PETER R MASON
Director General; Professor of Microbiology Biomedical
Research and Training Institute, Harare, Zimbabwe

JOSEPH B MCCORMICK
Director, Epidemiology Platform Pasteur Merieux
Connaught, Lyon, France

MICHAEL W MCKENDRICK
Consultant Physician, Department of Infection and
Tropical Medicine, Royal Hallamshire Hospital,
Sheffield, UK

ALBERT T MCMANUS
Senior Scientist; Chief, Laboratory Division US Army
Institute of Surgical Research, San Antonio, Texas, USA

JAMES G MCNAMARA
Chief, Pediatric Medicine Branch Division of AIDS
National Institute for Allegery and Infectious Diseases,
Bethesda, Maryland, USA

FRANCIS MÉGRAUD
Professor of Bacteriology, Hôpitae Pellegrin and
Universite Victor Segalen Bordeaux, Bordeaux, France

GREGORY MERTZ
Professor of Internal Medicine; Chief, Division of
Infectious Diseases; Department of Internal Medicine,
University of New Mexico, Albuquerque, New Mexico,
USA

MICHAEL A MILES
Pathogen Molecular Biology and Biochemistry Unit,
Department of Infectious Diseases and Tropical
Diseases, London School of Hygiene and Tropical
Medicine, London, UK

ALASTAIR MILLER
Consultant Physician and Clinical Director, Kidderminster General Hospital, Kidderminster UK; Hon. Senior Lecturer, Department of Infection, Birmingham University, Birmingham, UK

MARIE-PAULE MINGEOT-LACLERCQ
Chercheur Qualifié of the Belgian Fonds National de la Recherche Scientifique; Associate Professor of Pharmacology, Unité de Pharmacologie Cellulaire et Moleculaire, Brussels, Belgium

THOMAS G MITCHELL
Department of Microbiology, Duke University Medical Center, Durham, North Carolina, USA

PIERRE MOINE
Department d'Anesthesie Reanimation, Centre Hospitalier Universitaire de Bicêtre, Le Kremlin-Bicêtre, France

DAVID H MOLYNEUX
Director, Liverpool School of Medicine; Professor of Tropical Health Sciences, University of Liverpool, Liverpool, UK

JULIO SG MONTANER
Chair of AIDS Research; Professor of Medicine, St Paul's Hospital, Vancouver, British Columbia, Canada

VALENTINA MONTESSORI
Canadian HIV Trials Network, British Columbia Center for Excellence in HIV/AIDS, AIDS Research Program, St Paul's Hospital, University of British Columbia, Vancouver, British Columbia, Canada

JOHN Z MONTGOMERIE
Division of Infectious Diseases, Rancho los Amigos Medical Center, Downey, California; Professor Emeritus, Department of Medicine, USC School of Medicine, Los Angeles, California, USA

PHILIPPE MOREILLON
Laboratory of Infectious Diseases, Department of Internal Medicine, Centre Hospitalier Universitaire Vaudois (CHUV), Lausanne, Switzerland

PETER J MOSS
Honorary Lecturer, Liverpool School of Tropical Medicine, Liverpool, UK

PETER MORGAN-CAPNER
Honorary Professor of Clinical Virology, Public Health Laboratory Service North West, Preston, UK

MAURICE E MURPHY
Consultant Physician, Infection and Immunity Clinical Group, St Bartholomew's Hospital, London; Honorary Senior Lecturer, Department of Immunology, St Bartholomew's and the Royal London School of Medicine and Dentistry, Queen Mary and Westfield College, University of London, London, UK

ROBERT L MURRAY
Director, HIV Treatment Unit; Associate Professor of Medicine, Northwestern University Medical School, Chicago, Illinois, USA

ANDREW R MURRY
Clinical Assistant Professor of Internal Medicine, Division of Infectious Diseases, The Ohio State University College of Medicine, Columbus, Ohio, USA

KURT G NABER
Professor of Urology and Head of Department of Urology, Department of Urology, St. Elisabeth Hospital, Straubing, Germany

NAIEL N NASSAR
University of California, Davis, California, USA

W GARRETT NICHOLS
Fellow, Infectious Diseases, University of Washington, Seattle, Washington, USA

LINDSAY E NICOLLE
H.E. Sellers Professor and Chair, Department of Internal Medicine, University of Manitoba, Winnipeg, Manitoba, Canada

CHARLES H NIGHTINGALE
Vice President for Research, Hartford Hospital, Hartford, Connecticut, USA; Research Professor, University of Connecticut School of Pharmacy Storrs, CT Department of Medical Research, Hartford Hospital, Hartford, Connecticut, USA

CARL ERIK NORD
Professor of Microbiology; Chairman, Department of Immunology, Microbiology, Pathology and Infectious Diseases, Huddinge University Hospital, Huddinge, Sweden

CARL W NORDEN
Professor of Medicine; Head, Division of Infectious Diseases Cooper Hospital/University Medical Center, Camden, New Jersey, USA

EDMUND L ONG
Consultant Physician and Senior Lecturer, Department of Infection and Tropical Medicine, University of Newcastle Medical School, Newcastle General Hospital, Newcastle upon Tyne, UK

MICHELLE ONORATO
Assistant Professor, The University of Texas Medical Branch, Galveston, Texas, USA

DOUGLAS R OSMON
Assistant Professor of Medicine, Division of Infectious Diseases, Department of Internal Medicine, Mayo Clinic, Rochester, Minneapolis, USA

ERIC A OTTESEN
Coordinator, Lymphatic Filariasis Elimination, Communicable Disease Eradication and Elimination, World Health Organisation, Geneva, Switzerland

GIUSEPPE PANTALEO
Professor and Head, Laboratory of AIDS Immunopathogenisis, Department of Medicine, Division of Infectious Diseases, Centre Hospitalier Universitaire Vaudois (CHUV), Lausanne, Switzerland

ELDRYD HO PARRY
Department of Infectious and Tropical Diseases, London School of Hygiene and Tropical Medicine, London, UK

GEOFFREY PASVOL
Professor of Infection and Tropical Medicine, Imperial College School of Medicine, Morthwick Park and St Mark's Hospital, London, UK

NICHOLAS IJ PATON
Consultant Physician, Department of Infectious Diseases, Communicable Disease Centre, Tan Tock Seng Hospital, Singapore

ANDREW T PAVIA
Director for Clinical Research, University AIDS Center, Division of Pediatric Infectious Diseases and Geograhic Medicine; Associate Professor of Pediatrics and Medicine, University of Utah, Salt Lake City, Utah, USA

JEAN-CLAUDE PECHÈRE
Départment de Génétique and Microbiologie, Centre Médical Universitaire Geneva, Geneva, Switzerland

STEPHEN I PELTON
Professor of Pediatrics, Maxwell Finland Laboratory for Infectious Diseases at the Boston Medical Center, Boston, Massachusetts, USA

WALLACE PETERS
Emeritus Professor of Medical Parasitology, Pulridge House East, Little Gaddesen, Berkhamstead, Hertfordshire, UK

LINSEY PHILIP
Medical Director, SSTAR of RI; Attending Physician, Charlton Memorial Hospital, Fall River, Massachusetts, USA

ROBERT W PINNER
Director, Office of Surveillance, National Center for Infectious Diseases, Centers for Diseases Control and Prevention, Atlanta, Georgia, USA

PETER PIOT
Executive Director, UNAIDS, Geneva, Switzerland

STEPHEN C PISCITELLI
Coordinator, Clinical Center Pharmacy, Department Clinical Pharmacokinetics, Research Laboratory, Bethesda, Maryland, USA

RICHARD B POLLARD
Professor of Internal Medicine, Microbiology, Immunology and Pathology, The University of Texas, Medical Branch, Galveston, Texas, USA

BEATRIZ H PORRAS
Fellow in Dermatology, University of Texas, Southwestern Medical Center, Dallas, Texas, USA

WILLIAM G POWDERLY
Professor of Medicine; Director, Division of Infectious Diseases, Washington University School of Medicine, St. Louis, Missouri, USA

NICK PRICE
Medical Research Council Fellow, Department of Infectious Diseases and Microbiology, Hammersmith Hospital, London, UK

THOMAS C QUINN
Professor of Medicine, Division of Infectious Diseases, The Johns Hopkins University, Baltimore, Maryland, USA

RICHARD QUINTILIANI
Director, Anti-Infective Research and Pharmacoeconomic Studies, Hartford Hospital, Hartford, Connecticut, USA; Professor of Medicine, University of Connecticut School of Medicine, Farmington, Connecticut, USA

RICHARD QUINTILIANI JR
Adjunct Assistant Professor, Department of Microbiology and Immunology, Georgetown University Medical Center, Washington DC, USA

JUSTIN D RADOLF
Director, Center for Microbial Pathogenesis, UCONN Health Center School of Medicine, Farmington, Connecticut, USA

HABEEB RAHMAN
Fellow Infectious Diseases, St Michael's Medical Center, Newark, New Jersey, USA

DANIEL W RAHN
Professor of Medicine; Chief, Section of General Medicine; Vice Dean for Clinical Affairs, Medical College of Georgia, Augusta, Georgia, USA

ROBERT C READ
Honorary Consultant Physician, Central Sheffield University Hospital; Senior Lecturer in Infectious Diseases, University of Sheffield Medical School, Sheffield, UK

PETER REISS
Deputy Director, National AIDS Therapy Evaluation Center; Associate Professor of Medicine, Department of Infectious Diseases, Tropical Medicine and AIDS, Academic Medical Center, University of Amsterdam, Amsterdam, The Netherlands

MALCOLM D RICHARDSON
Specialist in Clinical Mycology, Department of Bacteriology and Immunology, Haartman Institute, University of Helsinki, Helsinki, Finland

JOHN RICHENS
Clinical Lecturer Department of Sexually Transmitted Diseases/ Div. of Pathology and Infectious Diseases, Royal Free and University College Medical School, London, UK

RENÉE RIDZON
Medical Epidemiologist, Division of Tuberculosis Elimination, Centers for Disease Control and Prevention, Atlanta, Georgia, USA

G PAOLO RIZZARDI
Assistant Laboratory of AIDS Immunopathogenesis, Department of Medicine, Division of Infectious Diseases, Centre Hospitalier Universitaire Vaudois (CHUV), Lausanne, Switzerland

KENNETH VI ROLSTON
Professor of Medicine; Chief, Section of Infectious Diseases, University of Texas M.D. Anderson Cancer Center, Houston, Texas, USA

RODRIGO LC ROMULO
Assistant Professor, Section of Infectious and Tropical Diseases, Department of Medicine, University of Santo Tomas Faculty of Medicine and Surgery, Manila, Philippines

NANCY E ROSENSTEIN
Medical Epidemiologist. Meningitis and Special Pathogens Branch, Division of Bacterial and Mycotic Diseases, National Center for Infectious Diseases, Centers for Disease Control and Prevention, Atlanta, Georgia, USA

VIRGINIA R ROTH
Fellow of Infectious Disease, Section of Infectious Diseases, University of Ottawa at Ottawa General Hospital, Ottawa, Ontario, Canada

MAJA ROZENBERG-ARSKA
Associate Professor, Eijkman-Winkler Institute for Microbiology, Infectious Diseases and Inflammation, Division of Clinical Microbiology, University Medical Center, Utrecht, The Netherlands

BINA RUBINOVITCH
Infectious Disease Unit Sheba Medical Center, Tel Aviv University, School of Medicine, Tel-Hashomer Ramat Gan, Israel

ETHAN RUBINSTEIN
Professor of Medicine, Infectious Diseases Unit, Sheba Medical Centre, Tel Aviv University, School of Medicine, Tel-Hashomer, Israel

CHARLES E RUPPRECHT
Rabies Section, Centers for Diseases Control and Prevention, Atlanta, Georgia, USA

GREG RYAN
Assistant Professor, Department of Obstetrics and Gynecology, Division of Maternal Fetal Medicine, Mount Sinai Hospital, Toronto, Ontario, Canada

STEPHEN D RYDER
Consultant Hepatologist and Physician, Queen's Medical Centre, Nottingham, UK

PEKKA A SAIKKU
Research Professor, Chlamydia Laboratory KTL, Department in Oulu, Oulu, Finland

ARIF R SARWARI
Assistant Professor and Consultant in Infectious Diseases, Department of Medicine, Aga Khan University, Karachi, Pakistan

FRED R SATTLER
Professor of Medicine, University of Southern California School of Medicine, Los Angeles, California, USA

FRANZ-JOSEF SCHMITZ
Assistant Professor, Institute for Medical Microbiology and Virology, Universitätsklinik Düsseldorf, Düsseldorf, Germany

BERNHARD SCHWARTLÄNDER
Team Leader, EPI Geneva, Switzerland

EUAN M SCRIMGEOUR
Associate Professor in Infectious and Tropical Diseases, Department of Medicine, Infectious Disease Service, Sultan Qaboos University Muscat, Al Khod, Sultanate of Oman

JOHN W SELLORS
Professor of Family Medicine and Clinical Epidemiology and Biostatistics, McMaster University HSV-2V7, McMaster University Hamilton, Ontario, Canada

KENT A SEPKOWITZ
Infectious Disease Specialist; Associate Chairman, Clinical Affairs, Department of Medicine, Infectious Disease Service, Memorial Sloan-Kettering Cancer Center, New York, New York, USA

GRAHAM R SERJEANT
Director, MRC Laboratories (Jamaica), University of West Indies, Kingston, Jamaica

BEVERLY E SHA
Associate Professor of Medicine, Section of Infectious Diseases, Rush-Presbyterian-St Luke's Medical Center, Chicago, Illinois, USA

KEERTI V SHAH
Professor, Department of Molecular Microbiology and Immunology, School of Public Health, Johns Hopkins University, Baltimore, Maryland, USA

FRANÇOIS SIMON
Laboratore de Virologie, Hopital Bichat-Claude Bernard, Paris, France

SVANTE SJÖSTEDT
Associate Professor, Department of Surgery, Nyköping Hospital, Nyköping, Sweden

MARY PE SLACK
University Lecturer in Bacteriology, Nuffield Department of Pathology and Bacteriology, University of Oxford; Director, Public Health Laboratory Service Haemophilus Reference Unit; Honorary Consultant Microbiologist, Oxford Radcliffe Hospital, John Radcliffe Hospital, Headington, Oxford, UK

DAVID H SMITH
Head Division of Tropical Medicine; Honorary Consultant Physician Tropical Medicine, Liverpool School of Tropical Medicine, Liverpool, UK

LEON SMITH
Director of Medicine, Chief of Infectious Diseases, Department of Medicine, St Michael's Medical Center; Professor of Medicine and Preventative Medicine, New Jersey Medical School, Newark, New Jersey, USA

MARIA L SMITH
Coordinator, Fogarty International Center Fellowship Program, Division of Geographic Medicine, Department of Medicine, University of Alabama at Birmingham, Birmingham, Alabama, USA

ROSEMARY SOAVE
Associate Professor of Medicine and Public Health, Cornell University Medical College, New York, New York, USA

JACK D SOBEL
Professor of Medicine; Chief, Division of Infectious Diseases, Department of Internal Medicine, Detroit Medical Center, Wayne State University School of Medicine, Detroit, Michigan, USA

SHIRANEE SRISKANDAN
Clinician Scientist, Department of Infectious Diseases, Imperial College School of Medicine at Hammersmith Hospital, London, UK

JAMES M STECKELBERG
Professor of Medicine, Mayo Medical School; Director, Infectious Diseases Research Laboratory; Consultant, Department of Internal Medicine and of Infectious Diseases, Rochester, Minneapolis, USA

JAMES H STEELE
Professor Emeritus of Public Health, Center for Infectious Diseases, The University of Texas Houston, School of Public Health, Houston, Texas, USA

MOLLY STENZEL
Infectious Disease Division, Brown University School of Medicine, Providence, Rhode Island, USA

DAVID S STEPHENS
Professor of Medicine; Professor of Microbiology and Immunology, Division of Infectious Diseases Department of Medicine, Emory University School of Medicine, Atlanta, Georgia, USA

IAIN STEPHENSON
Specialist Registrar in Infectious Diseases, Department of Infection and Tropical Medicine, Leicester Royal Infirmary, Leicester, UK

DENNIS L STEVENS
Professor of Medicine, University of Washington School of Medicine, Seattle, Washington, USA; Chief, Infectious Diseases Section, Veterans Affairs Medical Center, Boise, Idaho, USA

ATHENA STOUPIS
Internal Medicine In-Patient Service, Rhode Island Hospital/Jane Brown, Providence, Rhode Island, USA

MARC J STRUELENS
Professor of Microbiology and Hospital Infection Control, Universite Libre de Bruxelles; Head, Service de Microbiologie, Hopital Erasme, Brussels, Belgium

KHUNYING A SUKONTHAMAN
Chulalongkorn University, Bangkok, Thailand

RICHARD C SUMMERBELL
Mycologist, Laboratories Branch Ontario Ministry of Health, and Assistant Professor, Department of Laboratory Medicine and Pathobiology, University of Toronto, Toronto, Ontario, Canada

MARC A TACK
Infectious Diseases Consultant, Medical Associates of the Hudson Valley, P.C., The Kingston Hospital, The Benedictine Hospital, Kingston, USA

MARTIN G TÄUBER
Professor of Medicine, Chief, Infectious Diseases, and Co-Director Institute for Medical Microbiology, University of Berne, Berne, Switzerland

GLENN C TELLING
Programme Leader, MRC Prion Unit, Imperial College School of Medicine at St Mary's, London, UK

MARLEEN TEMMERMAN
Head of Department of Obstetrics, Director, The International Centre for Reproductive Health, State University of Ghent, Ghent, Belgium

STEVEN FT THIJSEN
Eijkman-Winkler Institute for Microbiology, Infectious Diseases and Inflammation, Utrecht, The Netherlands

ALAN D TICE
Practitioner, Infections Limited, PS and Clinical Associate Professor University of Washington, Tacoma, Washington, USA

JEAN-FRANÇOIS TIMSIT
Réanimation Polyvalente, Hôpital Saint-Joseph, Paris, France

UMBERTO TIRELLI
Professor of Oncology Director, Division of Medical Oncology and AIDS, Centron di Riferimento Oncologico, Aviano, Italy

WTA TODD
Consultant Physician Honorary Senior Clinical Lecturer (Glasgow), Monklands Hospital, Airdrie, Lanarkshire, UK

GREGORY C TOWNSEND
Associate Director, Infectious Diseases Clinic; Assistant Professor of Medicine Division of Infectious Diseases, University of Virginia Health Sciences Center, Charlottesville, Virginia, USA

PAUL M TULKENS
Professor of Pharmacology, Unité de Pharmacologie Cellulaire et Moleculaire, Brussels, Belgium

MARK TYNDALL
Program Director, Epidemiology, British Columbia Centre for Excellence in HIV/AIDS, Assistant Professor of Medicine, University of British Columbia, Division of Invfectious Diseases, St Pauls Hospital, Vancouver, British Columbia, Canada

EMANUELA VACCHER
Division of Medical Oncology and AIDS, Centro di Riferimento Oncologico, Aviano (PN), Italy

FRANÇOISE VAN BAMBEKE
Chargé de Recherches of the Belgian Fonds National de la Recherche Scientifique, Unité de Pharmacologie Cellulaire et Moléculaire, Brussels, Belgium

JOS WM VAN DER MEER
Professor of Medicine, Catholic University Nijmegen, Department of Internal Medicine, University Hospital Nijmegen, Nijmegen, The Netherlands

ANTON M VAN LOON
Head Department of Virology, Eijkman-Winkler Institute for Microbiology, Infectious Diseases and Inflammation, University Medical Center, Utrecht, The Netherlands

FREDERIK PL VAN LOON
Visiting Scientist, National Immunization Program, Centers for Disease Control and Prevention, Atlanta, Georgia, USA

ANDREW M VEITCH
Research Fellow in Gastroenterology Digestive Diseases Research Centre, St Bartholomew's and The Royal London School of Medicine and Dentistry, Whitechapel, London, UK

STEFANO VELLA
Director Retrovirus Department, Chair, National HIV Clinical Research Program, Instituto Superiore di Sanita', Rome, Italy

STEN H VERMUND
Professor and Chairman, Department of Epidemiology; Director, Divison of Geographic Medicine, Department of Medicine University of Alabama at Birmingham, Birmingham, Alabama, USA

MAARTEN R VISSER
Eykman-Winkler Institute for Microbiology, Infectious Diseases and Inflammation, University Hospital Utrecht, Utrecht, The Netherlands

GOVINDA S VISVESVARA
Research Microbiologist, Division of Parasitic Diseases, Centers for Disease Control and Prevention, Atlanta, Georgia, USA

MARK A WAINBERG
Professor of Microbiology and Medicine; Director, McGill University AIDS Centre, Jewish General Hospital, Montreal, Quebec, Canada

DAVID W WARNOCK
Consultant Clinical Scientist and Head, Mycology Reference Laboratory, Public Health Laboratory Service, Bristol; Senior Clinical Lecturer, Department of Pathology and Microbiology, University of Bristol, Bristol, UK

DAVID A WARRELL
Professor of Tropical Medicine and Infectious Diseases; Director, Centre for Tropical Medicine University of Oxford, John Radcliffe Hospital, Oxford, UK

MARY J WARRELL
Centre for Tropical Medicine, John Radcliffe Hospital, Oxford, UK

RAINER WEBER
Acting Head, Division of Infectious Diseases and Hospital Epidemiology, Department of Medicine Assistant Professor of Infectious Diseases, University Hospital, Zurich, Switzerland

WOLFGANG WEIDNER
Professor of Urology; Head of Urologic Clinic Medical Centre for Surgery, Anesthesiology and Urology, Giessen, Germany

PETER F WELLER
Professor of Medicine, Harvard Medical School; Co-Chief, Infectious Diseases Division; Chief, Allergy and Inflammation Division, Beth Israel Deaconess Medical Center, Boston, Massachusetts, USA

MICHAEL WHITBY
Director, Department of Infectious Diseases and Infection Control, Princess Alexandra Hospital, Brisbane, Australia

MARY H WHITE
Assistant Attending Physician, Infectious Disease Service Memorial Sloan-Kettering Cancer Center, New York, New York, USA

RICHARD J WHITLEY
Eminent Scholar Chair in Pediatrics; Professor of Pediatrics, Medicine and Microbiology Microbiology and Medicine, The University of Alabama at Birmingham, Birmingham, Alabama, USA

HILTON WHITTLE
MRC Laboratories, Fajara, The Gambia

RODNEY E WILLOUGHBY JR
Director, Clinical Infectious Diseases, Department of Pediatrics, Johns Hopkins Hospital, Baltimore, Maryland, USA

MARY E WILSON
Chief of Infectious Diseases, Mount Auburn Hospital; Assistant Clinical Professor, Harvard Medical School, Cambridge, Massachusetts, USA

RICHARD E WINN
Divison Director of Pulmonary Medicine, Infectious Diseases Staff, Scott and White Clinic; Professor of Internal Medicine, Texas A&M College of Medicine Texas A&M College of Medicine, Temple, Texas, USA

MARTIN WISELKA
Consultant and Senior Lecturer, Department of Infection and Tropical Medicine, Leicester Royal Infirmary, Leicester, UK

MARTIN J WOOD
Consultant Physician, Department of Infection and Tropical Medicine, Heartlands Hospital, Birmingham, UK

JAMES R YANKASKAS
Co-Director, Adult Cystic Fibrosis Center; Director, Critical Care Medicine Program, Division of Pulmonary and Critical Care Medicine; Professor of Medicine, The University of North Carolina, Chapel Hill, North Carolina, USA

RICHARD YU
Infectious Disease Division, Brown University School of Medicine, Providence, Rhode Island, USA

HEINZ ZEICHHARDT
Professor of Virology, Department of Virology, Institute of Infectious Diseases Medicine, University Hospital Bejamin Franklin, Free University of Berlin, Berlin, Germany

JONATHAN M ZENILMAN
Associate Professor of Medicine, Division of Infectious Diseases, Johns Hopkins University, Baltimore, Maryland, USA

GEORGE ZHANEL
Departments of Medical Microbiology and Infectious Diseases and Faculty of Pharmacy, University of Manitoba, Department of Medicine, Health Sciences Centre, Manitoba, Canada

ARIE J ZUCKERMAN
Professor of Medical Microbiology in the University of London; Principal and Dean, Royal Free and University College Medical School, University College London, London, UK

JANE N ZUCKERMAN
Senior Lecturer and Honorary Consultant and Head Academic Unit of Travel Medicine and Vaccines, Director of the Royal Free Travel Health Centre, Royal Free and University College Medical School, London, UK

ALIMUDDIN ZUMLA
Physician, Windeyer Institute of Medical Sciences, Royal Free and University College London Medical School, London, UK; Visiting Professor, Department of Medicine, University of Zambia School of Medicine, Lusaka, Zambia

Introduction to Infectious Diseases

Donald B Louria & Claude J Carbon

1

Nature and Pathogenicity of Micro-organisms

Menno Kok & Jean-Claude Pechère

In our daily life we are surrounded by a wealth of micro-organisms, the majority of which are inoffensive. Human existence would be impossible without these micro-organisms, which play critical roles in processes as diverse as photosynthesis, nitrogen fixation, production of vitamins in the human intestine and decomposition of organic matter. They are the sole, true 'recyclers' of our planet. Micro-organisms are also the major driving force behind the evolution of life. They evolved photosynthesis and respiration, which have since been acquired by present-day eukaryotes, and they mediate complex genome rearrangements in infected host cells.

In a rather simplified view, micro-organisms may be considered to be no more than 'little machines that multiply'. In fact, this is what they do best. We are starting to understand some of the strategies micro-organisms have developed to stay alive, grow and reproduce. The lifestyle of a micro-organism is intimately related to its environment, whether that environment is the human body or a polluted riverbed. Some highly specialized micro-organisms have adapted to the harsh conditions of hot ocean vents, oil tanks, or nuclear reactors; others prosper on waste dumps. Still others have been tempted by the abundant resources provided by higher organisms, such as plant root colonizing bacteria and our own intestinal flora. In this chapter we shall examine the lifestyle of pathogenic micro-organisms and how they infect us, reproduce and cause disease. We shall use the word 'pathogenicity' to indicate the capacity to cause disease (or damage). Although the word 'virulence' is often used in the same sense, it refers more specifically to transmissibility or infectiousness of micro-organisms.

The world of pathogenic microbiology is immensely diverse, ranging from prion proteins to worms. A better understanding of the behavior of these infectious agents will help us to design strategies for disease prevention and treatment.

DEFINITION AND COMPARISON OF INFECTIOUS AGENTS

The definition of an 'infectious agent' was proposed by J Henle in 1840 and put to the test by the German physician, Robert Koch. In 1876, Koch reported experiments on mice with *Bacillus anthracis*. He was able to show that a single micro-organism could be isolated from all animals suffering from anthrax, that the disease could be reproduced in an experimental host by infection with a pure culture of this bacterium, and that the same micro-organism could subsequently be re-isolated from the experimental host.

We shall divide infectious agents into four groups, presented in the order of increasing complexity, even though this is clearly an oversimplification.

PRIONS

Prions are the simplest infectious agents. They consist of a single protein molecule (PrP). The infectious particle is an abnormal form of the ubiquitous cellular protein PrP, known as PrP^{Sc}. This molecule has the following characteristics:
- the prion disease spongiform encephalopathy is transmissible between sheep and goats (see Chapter 2.19);
- even with the most advanced analytic techniques, no nucleic acid

could be detected in infective prion species; therefore, prions do not carry the genetic code for their own de-novo synthesis;
- the PrP^{Sc} protein catalyzes the conformational change of PrP into PrP^{Sc}, which is remarkably resistant to chemical and physical agents, making it difficult to 'disinfect' contaminated material; and
- prions induce the conversion of an endogenous protein, and their ability to produce disease is therefore host-dependent.

For a fuller description of the biology of prions see Chapter 8.12.

VIRUSES

Viruses contain at least two types of macromolecules: nucleic acid and protein. They share the following characteristics:
- they are small – the largest known virions are produced by poxvirus (approximately 230×270nm), and most viruses of medical importance are smaller than 200nm in diameter;
- they contain only one species of nucleic acid, either DNA or RNA, whereas bacteria always have both species;
- they attach to their host cell with a specific receptor-binding protein;
- they cannot replicate autonomously; in order to reproduce the information stored in its genome a virus requires the assistance of a living eukaryotic or prokaryotic cell; and
- when a virus infects a cell, information contained in the viral genome is used to divert the cellular machinery towards the production of new viral particles.

'Defective' and 'simplified' viruses

Some infective agents share many features of viruses but seem even more primitive. Some very small viruses require the assistance of another virus in the same host cell for their replication. The non-pathogenic dependoviruses owe their name to their dependence on an adenovirus or, occasionally, a herpesvirus to assist in their replication. The delta agent, also referred to as hepatitis D virus, is too small to code for even a single capsid protein, and needs help from hepatitis B virus for transmission. Hepatitis B and D are often cotransmitted. Viroids are ssRNA molecules that do not code for any protein species. As the delta agent, they are likely to replicate by using the cellular RNA polymerase.

BACTERIA AND ARCHAEA

Bacteria (eubacteria) and archaea (archaeabacteria) have long been united under the name 'prokaryotes'. Today, this terminology ('everything that is not eukaryote') is considered inadequate.[1] The main characteristics of prokaryotes, compared with eukaryotes, are given in Figure 1.1. Bacteria and archaea invariably have a DNA genome which, unlike the eukaryotic genome, is not physically separated from the rest of the cell contents by a membrane. Neither size (mycoplasmas are as small as viruses, about 200nm in diameter), nor obligatory reproduction in eukaryotic cells supply a definitive criterion to separate bacteria and archaea from viruses. However, in contrast to viruses, prokaryotes always contain both DNA and RNA. Even obligate intracellular bacteria, like *Chlamydia* spp. and *Rickettsia* spp., which appear to have adopted a virus-like lifestyle, remain enclosed within their own cell envelope throughout their lifecycle.

INTRODUCTION TO INFECTIOUS DISEASES

COMPARISON OF PROKARYOTES AND EUKARYOTES

Feature	Prokaryotes	Eukaryotes
Chromosome	Single, circular	Multiple
Gene organization	Operon-polycistronic mRNA	Single genes and block of genes
Nucleosomes	No	Yes
Nuclear membrane	No	Yes
Mitosis	No	Yes
Introns in genes	No	Yes
Transcription	Coupled with translation	Separate from translation
mRNA	No terminal polyadenylation (except archaeobacteria); polygenic	Terminal polyadenylation; usually monogenic
First amino acid	Unstable formylmethionine (except archaeobacteria)	Methionine
Ribosome	70S (30S + 50S)	80S (40S + 60S)
Cell wall	Presence of muramic acid, D-amino acids, peptidoglycan (except archaeobacteria and mycoplasma)	No muramic acid, D-amino acids, or peptidoglycan
Membrane	No sterols or phosphatidyl-choline (except mycoplasma)	Sterols and phosphotidyl-choline
Endoplasmic reticulum	No	Yes
Mitochondria	No	Yes
Lysosomes and peroxysomes	No	Yes
Movement	By flagella, composed of a single fiber	Ameboid, by cilia, or cilia-like flagella

Fig. 1.1 Comparison of prokaryotes and eukaryotes.

COMPARISON OF BACTERIA AND FUNGI

Characteristics	Bacteria	Fungi
Cell volume (μm^3)	0.6–5.0	Yeast: 20–50; molds: greater than yeast
Nucleus	No membrane	Membrane
Mitochondria	No	Yes
Endoplasmic reticulum	No	Yes
Sterol in cytoplasmic membrane	No (except for mycoplasma grown on sterols)	Yes
Cell wall components	Muramic acids and teichoic acids; no chitin, glucans, or mannans	Chitin, glucans, and mannans; no muramic acids or teichoic acids
Metabolism	Autotrophic or heterotrophic	Heterotrophic
Sensitivity to polyenes	No	Yes

Fig. 1.2 Comparison of bacteria and fungi.
Adapted from Kobayashi, 1990.[2]

Based on extensive nucleotide sequence data, it has been suggested that archaea are more closely related to eukaryotes than to bacteria. Indeed, these micro-organisms, which seem to have a particular preference for hostile environments seeded with toxic chemicals, deep-sea hydrothermal vents and oil deposits, share with eukaryotes at least one feature that is absent from bacteria – their genes frequently bear introns. Archaea do not play any role in human medicine.

In contrast, eubacteria include the hundreds of bacterial species that are commensal or pathogenic for humans. Bacteria come in various shapes and sizes (typically in the range of 1–2μm diameter). With the exception of *Mycoplasma* spp., bacteria characteristically have a rigid cell wall.

EUKARYOTES
Eukaryotes have subcellular compartimentalization. DNA transcription, photosynthesis, respiration and protein modification are physically restricted to specific organelles: the nucleus, chloroplasts, mitochondria and the Golgi system.

Fungi
Fungi and bacteria play similar roles in the biosphere, share the capacity to produce infectious disease and both have rigid cell walls, but their

THE FOUR MAJOR CLASSES OF FUNGI

Class	Representative genera
Phycomycetes	*Rhizopus, Mucor*
Ascomycetes	*Neurospora, Penicillinium, Aspergillus*
Basidiomycetes	Mushrooms, rusts, smuts
Denteromycetes (or fungi imperfecti)	Most human pathogens

Fig. 1.3 The four major classes of fungi.

cellular architecture is completely different (Fig. 1.2). Pathogenic fungi occur in two forms: the molds, which are filamentous, and the unicellular yeasts. There are four major classes of fungi (Fig. 1.3). *Pneumocystis carinii*, which causes severe pneumonia in immunosuppressed hosts, was long considered to be a protozoan. However, its ribosomal RNA, which was recently sequenced, showed greater similarity to that of fungi than to protozoa.[3]

1

1.2

Fig. 1.4 Protozoa that are important in humans.

IMPORTANT PROTOZOA IN HUMANS			
Category	Species	Disease	Estimated worldwide prevalence of human infections
Protozoa	*Toxoplasma gondii*	Toxoplasmosis	1–2 billion
	Entamoeba histolytica	Amebiasis	200–400 million
	Trichomonas vaginalis	Trichomoniasis	15% of women
	Plasmodium spp.	Malaria	200–300 million
	Giardia lamblia	Giardiasis	200 million
	Trypanosoma cruzi, T. brucei	Chagas' disease; African sleeping sickness	15–20 million
	Leishmania donovani, L. tropica	Leishmaniasis	1–2 million
Helminths	*Ascaris lumbricoides*	Ascariasis	1 billion
	Necator americanus	Hookworm disease	800–900 million
	Schistosoma mansoni	Schistosomiasis	200–300 million
	Wuchereria bancrofti	Lymphatic filiasis	200 million
	Enterobius vermicularis	Pinworm infection	60–100 million
	Strongyloides stercoralis	Strongyloidiasis	50–80 million
	Onchocerca volvulus	Onchocerciasis	50 million

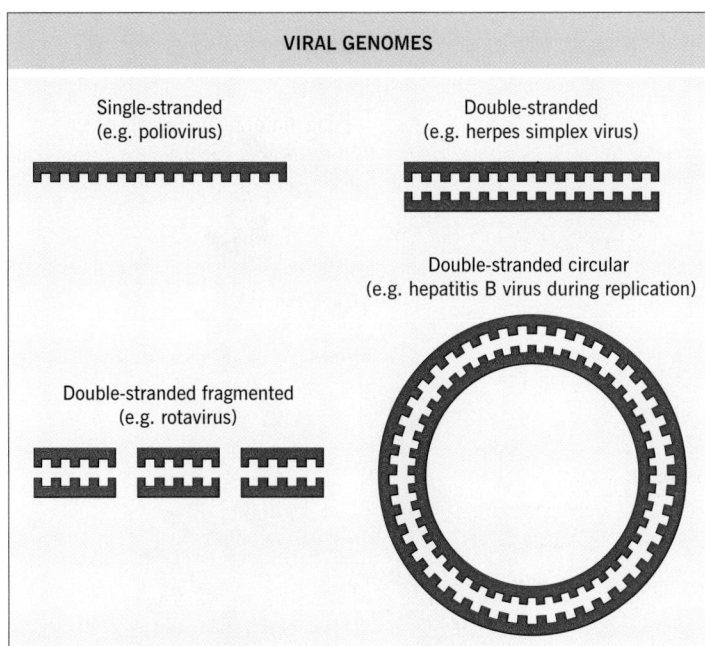

Fig. 1.5 Viral genomes.

Protozoa

Protozoa (Fig. 1.4) are unicellular eukaryotes. In contrast to fungi, they have a flexible cell membrane. Their movements can be ameboid or by cilia or cilia-like flagella. Pathogenic protozoa often have a complex lifecycle with both intrahuman and extrahuman stages. The sources of parasites in the environment are called reservoirs, which include other animals or free forms of the parasite found in the external environment (e.g. food contaminated with *Toxoplasma gondii* oocysts from cat feces).

Some protozoa that are pathogenic for humans, such as the malaria parasite, trypanosomes, and *Leishmania* spp., and *Toxoplasma* spp., invade deep tissues and reside inside host cells, at least during part of their lifecycle. These protozoa do not survive for long in the external environment, and they are often transmitted by living vectors such as flies and mosquitoes. Other protozoa are extracellular (e.g. the agents of amebiasis and giardiasis) and possess vegetative and resistant forms. The trophozoite produces the active disease and allows vegetative growth and

multiplication, whereas the highly resistant cyst form, which is able to survive in hostile environments, assures transmission between hosts.

Parasitic worms

Helminths are the largest parasites that infect humans. They are multicellular organisms ranging from 1cm to 10m in size. They usually are encased by an outer membrane or cuticle that protects internal differentiated organ systems. Helminths (or worms) are classified into three groups, generally distinguishable by their shape:
• nematodes (or roundworms),
• cestodes (or tapeworms), and
• trematodes (or flukes).
Some helminths have complex antigenic structures and lifecycles, which may include successive animal reservoirs and insect vectors.

GENERAL PROPERTIES AND CLASSIFICATION OF VIRUSES

STRUCTURE OF VIRUSES

The whole virus particle, the virion, is designed to offer protection to the viral genome and to mediate both the migration of the virus and the invasion of the target host cell. The viral genome can be packaged in a nucleocapsid, which in some virus families can contain a number of enzymes required for the early stages of virus multiplication. The capsid may in turn be surrounded by an outer membrane.

The genome

The genome is made up of either DNA or RNA, associated with proteins or polyamines. The size of nucleic acid per virion ranges from 3–300kb. There may be only one gene in the smallest virions, whereas the largest genomes, such as vaccinia, may encode hundreds of proteins. The *Parvoviridae*, which include the virus that causes erythema infectiosum, have a 5.5kb DNA genome, which codes for only three polypeptides. This may explain why these viruses need help from a larger virus, i.e. adenovirus, for their replication.

The nucleic acid may be either double stranded or single stranded (Fig. 1.5). The nucleic acid of all DNA viruses except parvoviruses is double stranded. In contrast, the nucleic acid of all RNA viruses except the reoviruses (e.g. influenza, bunya and arenaviruses) is single stranded. The genome may be linear or circular, and nonsegmented or segmented. Genome segmentation, a general feature of reoviruses,

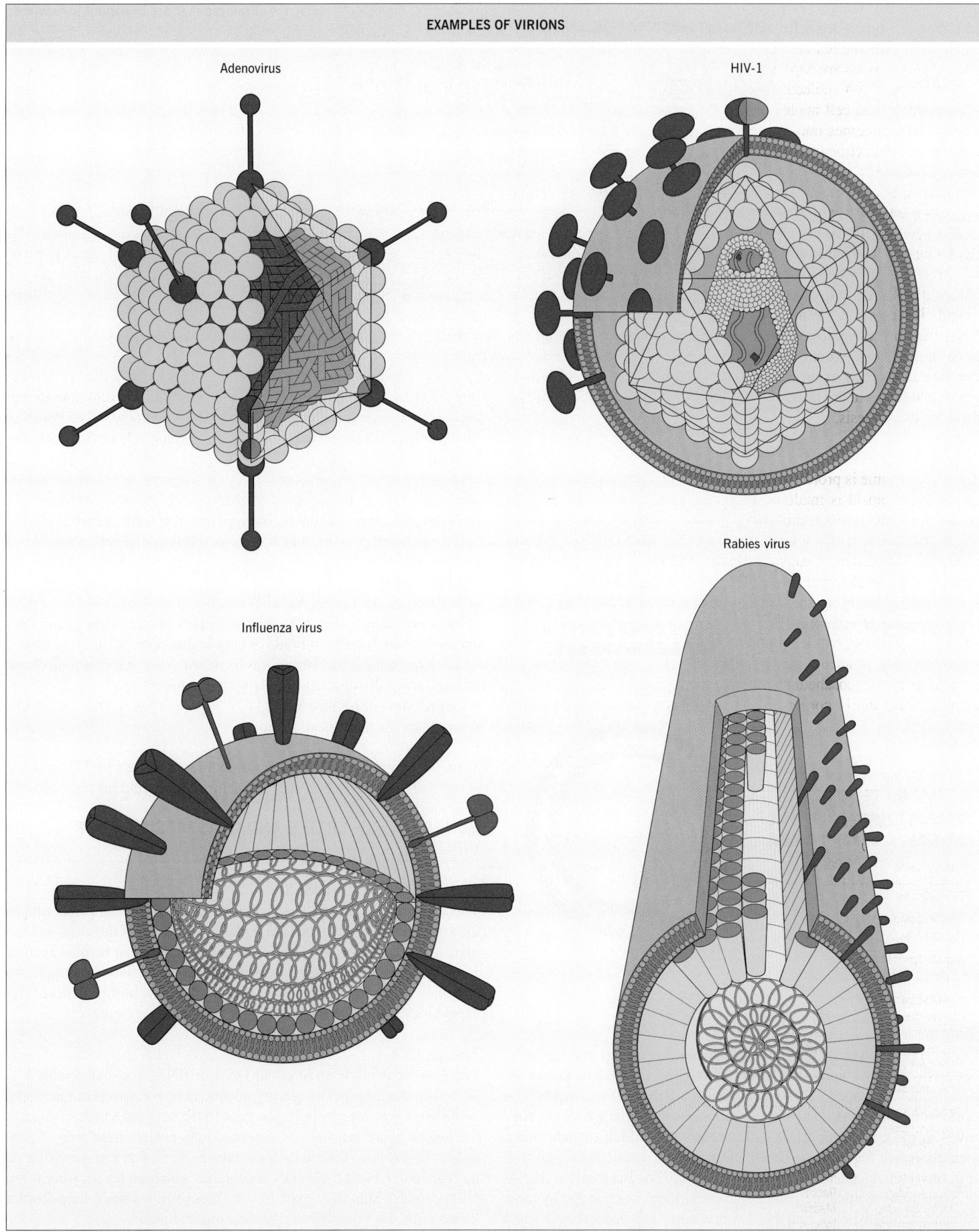

EXAMPLES OF VIRIONS

Adenovirus

HIV-1

Influenza virus

Rabies virus

Fig. 1.6 Examples of virions. Adenovirus is an icosahedral DNA virus without an envelope; fibers extend from the 12 points of the icosahedral coat; DNA forms a ribbon-like molecule. Approximate size: 80nm. HIV-1; glycoprotein (GP) molecules protrude through the lipid membrane; the icosahedral capsid encloses a vase-shape nucleocapsid, in which the diploid RNA is enclosed. Approximate size: 100nm. Influenza virus is an enveloped RNA virus, containing nucleocapsid of helical symmetry; spikes of hemagglutinin and neuraminidase protrude from the lipid bilayer. Approximate size: 100–200nm. Rabies virus is a helical RNA nucleocapsid with a bullet-shaped lipoprotein envelope, in which approximately 200 GPs are embedded. Approximate size: 150nm. (The diagram is not to relative scale.) Adapted from Collier L by permission of Oxford University Press.[4]

favors gene exchange between co-infecting virions. RNA virus genomes change at high frequency through point limitations and manage to evade the human immune response. With the exception of retroviruses, virions are haploid.

Some viral DNA molecules may contain alternative nucleotides, which inhibit host cell nucleases and thus protect the viral genome. Linear DNA genomes may contain terminal redundancies, allowing incomplete replication products to recombine, or they may carry proteins at both ends, and these proteins play a role in priming of DNA replication. Some viral DNA is flanked by repeat sequences, which suggests relatedness with transposable elements.

Most human RNA viruses have single-stranded genomes. The RNA molecule can have two polarities. The positive-strand RNAs can act directly as messengers for protein synthesis; they may resemble eukaroytic RNAs, with a cap at the 5' end and a poly-A chain at the 3' end. The negative-strand RNAs need to be transcribed by a viral RNA transcriptase into an mRNA. Negative-strand RNA genomes have neither a cap structure nor a poly-A tail. Retroviruses first synthesize a DNA copy of the positive-strand RNA genome, which integrates into the cellular DNA and may subsequently serve as a template for mRNA synthesis.

The capsid

The viral genome is protected by a protein coat, the capsid or nucleocapsid. The capsid is made of knob-like structures known as capsomeres, which consist entirely of proteins coded by the viral genome. The capsid accounts for a large portion of the viral mass. Poliovirus produces four different capsid proteins, but more complex viruses may encode a much larger variety. On the other hand, viruses with very small genomes only synthesize a limited number of different capsid proteins, sometimes only one. Different nucleocapsid morphologies have been observed by electron microscopy (Fig. 1.6)

Picornaviruses, adenoviruses and papovaviruses have a nucleocapsid structure with icosahedral symmetry. The capsid consists of 20 triangular facets and 12 corners or apices. Influenza, measles and rabies virus form capsids with helical symmetry. The central core is formed by the nucleic acid genome, around which the nucleocapsid proteins are arranged like the steps of a spiral staircase, forming long cylinders.

More complex virion morphologies also exist. Bacteriophages, which use bacteria as hosts, have additional attachment structures fixed to the capsid. The nucleocapsid of orthopoxviruses, such as variola and vaccinia virus, consists of a network of tubules, sometimes surrounded by an envelope, forming a brick-shaped virion.

The envelope

In some viruses the nucleocapsid is surrounded by an outer envelope. Enveloped viruses can contain nucleocapsids of icosahedral (e.g. herpesviruses and togavirus, which causes rubella) or helical symmetry (e.g. influenza virus). The outer envelope consists of a lipid bilayer, derived from the host cell membrane, in which the viral glycoproteins are embedded. The viral matrix proteins (M proteins) are firmly associated with the envelope. Matrix proteins play an important role in the structural organization of the virion and are thought to connect the capsid to the viral glycoprotein inserted in the lipid bilayer. Besides oligosaccharide residues, the glycoproteins contain a membrane anchor and, in many cases, one or two molecules of fatty acid. Glycoproteins play a key role in the attachment of virions to the cell surface and penetration into the cell. Some viruses, such as the influenza virus, have glycoproteins with neuraminidase activity; this promotes the release of newly formed viral particles from the host cell membrane. Once released from the host cell, virions are metabolically inert. The virus only comes 'alive' after entry into a suitable host cell and activation of its genome.

CLASSIFICATION OF VIRUSES

Viruses are classified into families, subfamilies and genera. The most important families are summarized in Figure 1.7. Classification criteria include the nucleic acid species, the number and polarity of the nucleic acid strands, the presence or absence of a lipid envelope, and the symmetry (icosahedral, helical, or complex) of the nucleocapsid.

Fig. 1.7 Classification of viruses.

CLASSIFICATION OF VIRUSES				
Family name	Example	Genome size (kb) and polarity (+ or −)	Morphology	Envelope
DNA viruses				
Single-stranded				
Parvoviridae	Human parvovirus B19	5 (±)	Icosahedral	No
Mixed-stranded				
Hepadnaviridae	Hepatitis B	3 (±)	Icosahedral	Yes
Double-stranded				
Papovaviridae	Wart virus	8 (±)	Icosahedral	No
Adenoviridae	Adenovirus	36–38 (±)	Icosahedral	No
Herpesviridae	Herpes simplex	120–220 (±)	Icosahedral	Yes
Poxviridae	Vaccinia	120–280 (±)	Complex	Yes
RNA viruses				
Single-stranded				
Picornaviridae	Poliovirus	7.2–8.4 (+)	Icosahedral	No
Togaviridae	Rubella	12 (+)	Icosahedral	Yes
Flaviviridae	Yellow fever	10 (+)	Icosahedral	Yes
Coronaviridae	Infectious bronchitis	16–21 (+)	Helical	Yes
Rhabdoviridae	Rabies	13–16 (−)	Helical	Yes
Paramyxoviridae	Measles	16–20 (−)	Helical	Yes
Ozthomyxoviridae	Influenza	14 (−)	Helical	Yes
Bunyaviridae	California encephalitis	13–21 (−)	Helical	Yes
Arenaviridae	Lassa fever	10–14 (−)	Helical	Yes
Retroviridae	HIV-1	3–9 (+)	Icosahedral	Yes
Filoviridae	Marburg, ebola	19 (−)	Helical	Yes
Double-stranded				
Reoviridae	Rotavirus	16–27 (±)	Icosahedral	No

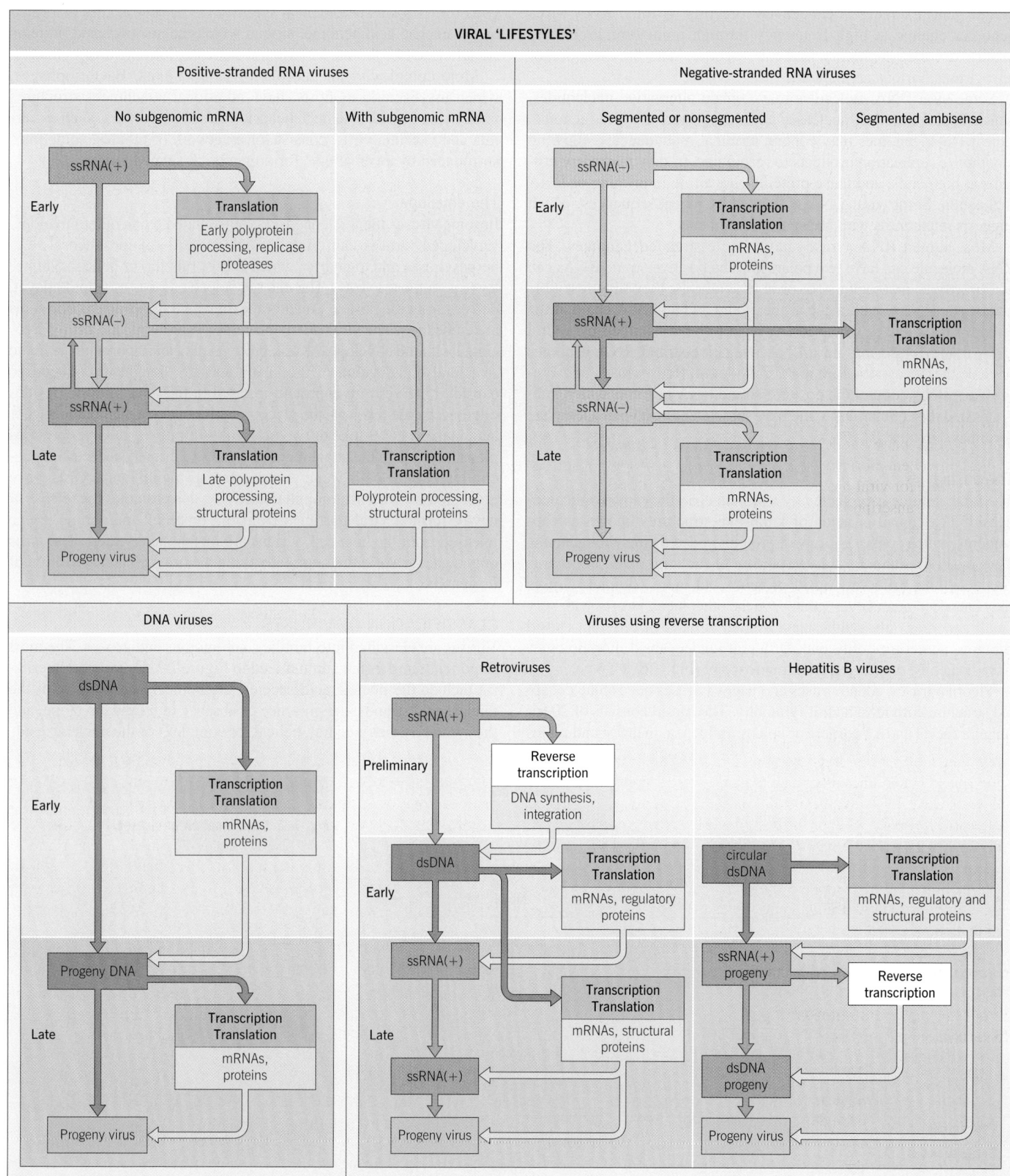

VIRAL 'LIFESTYLES'

Fig. 1.8 Viral 'lifestyles'.

VIRAL GENE EXPRESSION STRATEGIES

Viral infection can be separated in two phases. In the early phase of viral infection, the proper cell environment required for viral genome replication is established, and the viral DNA or RNA polymerase is produced. In the late phase, the viral genome is amplified and the structural components of the virion accumulate. At this point a considerable part of the cellular metabolism is committed to viral reproduction. Eventually the virion is assembled from its components and leaves the cell. Four viral replication strategies can be distinguished (Fig. 1.8).

Positive-strand RNA viruses

In positive-strand RNA viruses, the viral genome has the right polarity to serve immediately as an mRNA. The first step in viral infection consists of a complete translation of the genome to produce a polyprotein, which is sequentially processed into smaller polypeptides. Enzymatic cleavage of the composite protein is at least partially autocatalytic. In the early phase, processing preferentially produces proteases and the RNA-dependant polymerase.

In the late phase of infection, processing is reoriented towards the production of the structural proteins. This scheme applies to picornaviruses, flaviviruses and hepatitis C viruses.

For other virus families (e.g. togaviruses, coronaviruses, caliciviruses and hepatitis E viruses), the incoming genome is only partially translated to produce the proteases and the RNA polymerase. The portion of the genetic information that encodes the structural proteins is expressed from a transcript derived from the RNA intermediate in genome replication.

Negative-strand RNA viruses

The early phase is characterized by 'primary transcription' of the infecting genome by an RNA-dependant RNA polymerase. Primary transcription generates a positive-strand-RNA species, which can act as an mRNA for viral protein synthesis. In the late phase of genome replication, transcription and viral protein synthesis are simultaneously amplified.

In the case of the ambisense viruses, such as arenaviruses and some members of the bunyaviruses, the situation is somewhat more complex. The intermediate in genome-replication, positive-strand-RNA species also acts as a template for mRNA synthesis. This transcription strategy does not, however, result in the synthesis of complementary mRNA, because half of the genome is transcribed in one polarity and the other half in the opposite polarity.

DNA viruses

In the early phase, the virus 'takes the decision' whether or not to pursue exponential replication of its genome. If the cellular physiology favors virus amplification, the early phase is used to create the conditions that allow efficient DNA synthesis, and the cellular S phase is induced. Alternatively, viral gene expression is confined to the functions that prevent the efficient genome synthesis and the virus remains in a latent form.

In the case of ssDNA viruses (e.g. parvoviruses), the incoming genome is first used to express proteins that permit the synthesis of the complementary DNA strand. Double-stranded DNA is an obligatory replication intermediate.

The late phase is devoted to the accumulation of the structural components of the virion.

Viruses using reverse transcription

In the case of the retroviruses, genome synthesis takes place in two distinct steps:

- In a preliminary step, the viral RNA genome enters the cell together with the viral reverse transcriptase, which was synthesized and packaged in the virion during the previous infection cycle.
- The RNA genome is converted to a dsDNA-copy by reverse transcriptase and integrates into the cellular chromosome as a proviral genome. This remains in the 'dormant state' as long as the cells are quiescent, which represent conditions that do not favour virus multiplication.

In the case of the more complex retroviruses (e.g. spumaviruses, lentiviruses), transcription by the cellular RNA polymerase II of the integrated viral DNA first produces multispliced mRNAs, which direct the synthesis of regulatory proteins. As a consequence of the accumulation of certain regulatory proteins, the processing of the viral transcripts changes, and becomes oriented towards the production of unspliced or simply spliced mRNAs representing the viral genomes and serving the synthesis of the structural proteins.

GENERAL PROPERTIES AND CLASSIFICATION OF BACTERIA

Bacteria are small (0.6–4.0μm) unicellular organisms – 1×10^{12} bacteria weigh in the order of 1g. Under optimal physiologic conditions, a bacterium may divide between two and three times per hour. This means that in one day nearly 300g of bacterial mass can be produced from a single bacterial cell. Such small organisms profit from a favorable cell surface-to-volume ratio, which allows metabolic fluxes largely superior to those attained by the larger eukaryotic cells. Bacteria react very quickly to environmental changes, using regulation at the level of gene transcription to adapt their physiology.

Bacteria were probably the first cells to appear on earth more than 3.5 billion years ago. They have since developed into an overwhelming diversity representing the bulk of the world's biomass today. Evolution has not favored bacteria to become multicellular organisms. Yet bacteria are capable of cell-to-cell communication.[5] By using low-molecular-weight compounds, bacteria have found a way to 'see' how dense their local population is, and decide whether or not to activate developmental programs such as plasmid conjugation, light production (in association with deep-sea fish), or virulence gene expression.

Different cell morphologies can be observed with light microscopy (e.g. spherical cocci, rod-shape bacilli, curved vibrios). Electron microscopy unveils a distinctive cell wall, a simple nuclear body without a nuclear membrane, and the presence in the cytoplasm of ribosomes and mesosomes, sometimes granules of reserve material, but no endoplasmic reticulum and no organelles such as mitochondria or chloroplasts.

BACTERIAL DICHOTOMY REVEALED BY A SIMPLE STAINING TECHNIQUE

In 1884, the Danish bacteriologist Hans-Christian Gram developed a simple staining technique that distinguishes two types of bacteria – the Gram-positive and the Gram-negative bacteria. The distinction is based on the ability of one group of bacteria, the Gram positives, to retain a crystal-violet–iodine dye in the presence of alcohol or acetone. Gram-negatives lose the dye and can be counterstained with other dyes such as fuchsin. This simple observation turned out to reflect distinctive structures. Gram-positive bacteria characteristically have a thick wall made up mainly of a vast molecule of peptidoglycan, with protruding chains of teichoic acids. Gram-negative bacteria have an additional membrane (the outer membrane) surrounding the peptidoglycan skeleton in the periplasm (Fig. 1.9). *Escherichia coli* is an example of a Gram-negative bacterium; it is rod-shaped, and growing cells are between 2 and 4μm long.

The rigid cell wall determines the shape of bacteria and allows them to resist the osmotic pressure caused by the large difference in solute concentration between the cytoplasm and the environment. *Mycoplasma* spp. lack peptidoglycan, and thus have neither a rigid wall nor a defined shape.

ORGANIZATION OF THE BACTERIAL CELL

The bacterial cytoplasm does not contain physically separated compartments. Thus DNA replication, transcription, protein synthesis, central metabolism and respiration all take place in the same environment. Complex biochemical processes may nonetheless be spatially organized in the cell. Transcription of DNA into mRNA and translation of the mRNA into protein are coupled processes. This means that polysomes are linked to the DNA, via the enzyme RNA polymerase (Fig. 1.10). The cytoplasmic membrane not only contains numerous metabolite transport systems, but it also is the site of intense enzymatic activity. Like eukaryotic cells, bacteria possess active efflux systems that allow them to expel unwanted substances from the cytoplasm into the environment.

The genetic information is usually stored in a single chromosome, which is continuously replicated during growth. Bacterial chromosomes vary considerably in size. The *Haemophilus influenzae* chromosome, the first completely sequenced genome of a cellular life form, is

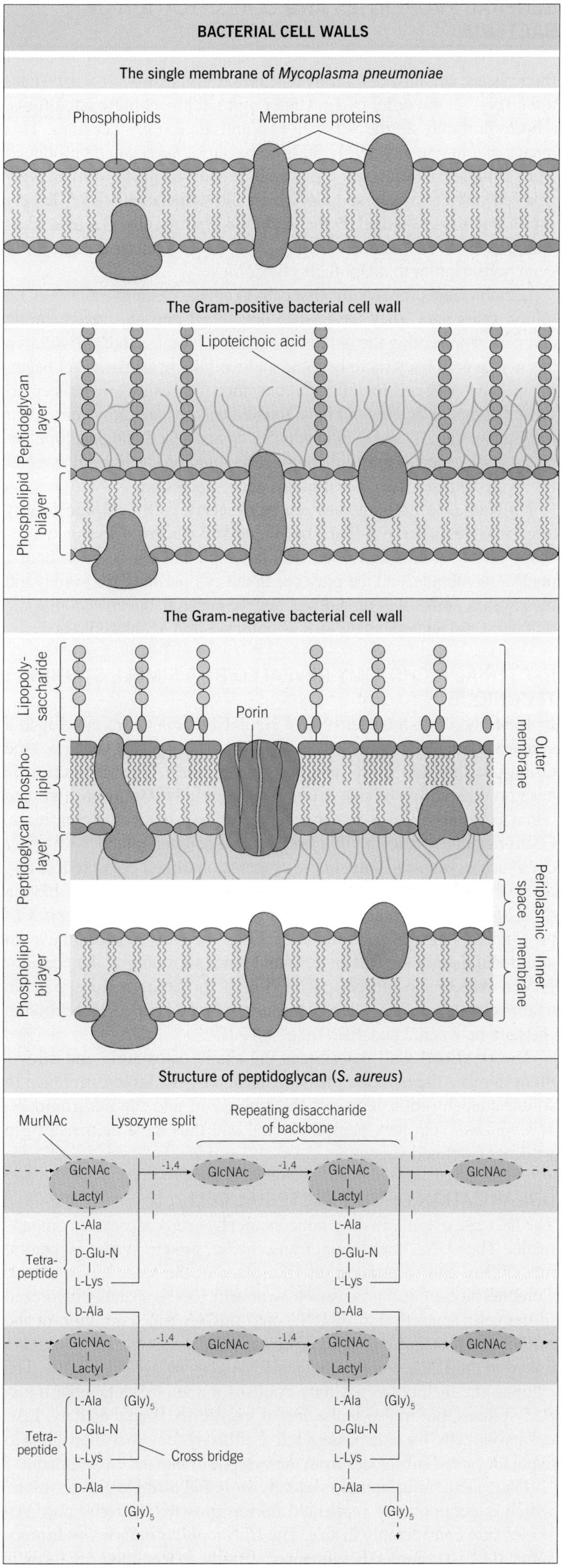

BACTERIAL CELL WALLS

The single membrane of *Mycoplasma pneumoniae*

Phospholipids

Membrane proteins

The Gram-positive bacterial cell wall

Lipoteichoic acid

Peptidoglycan layer

Phospholipid bilayer

The Gram-negative bacterial cell wall

Lipopolysaccharide

Porin

Peptidoglycan layer

Phospholipid

Phospholipid bilayer

Outer membrane

Periplasmic space

Inner membrane

Structure of peptidoglycan (*S. aureus*)

MurNAc

Lysozyme split

Repeating disaccharide of backbone

| GlcNAc | | GlcNAc | | GlcNAc | | GlcNAc |

Lactyl

-1,4

GlcNAc

Lactyl

-1,4

GlcNAc

Lactyl

GlcNAc

Tetrapeptide:
L-Ala
D-Glu-N
L-Lys
D-Ala

L-Ala
D-Glu-N
L-Lys
D-Ala

GlcNAc
Lactyl
-1,4
GlcNAc
-1,4
GlcNAc
Lactyl
GlcNAc

Tetrapeptide:
L-Ala (Gly)₅
D-Glu-N
L-Lys
D-Ala

Cross bridge

L-Ala (Gly)₅
D-Glu-N
L-Lys
D-Ala

(Gly)₅

(Gly)₅

1

1.8

Fig. 1.9 Bacterial cell walls. (a) *Mycoplasma pneumoniae* has a single membrane, made up of phospholipids and membrane proteins. (b) In Gram-positive organisms the cytoplasmic membrane is covered with a thick layer of peptidoglycan; chains of lipoteichoic acid protrude outside. (c) The cell wall of a Gram-negative rod is more complex. The layers are: the cytoplasmic membrane; the periplasmic space; a layer of peptidoglycan, which is thinner than that in Gram-positive bacteria; and an asymmetric outer membrane. The inner leaflet of the outer membrane is made of phospholipids. The outer leaflet has lipopolysaccharides as its principal lipids; porins, which are channel-forming proteins often organized as trimers, allow the penetration of hydrophilic molecules through the outer membrane. (d) The peptidoglycan of *Staphylococcus aureus* has polysaccharide chains ('backbone') that are alternating residues of *N*-acetylglucosamine (GlcNAc) and *N*-acetylmuramic acid (MurNAc). Tetrapeptides are attached to MurNAc and are linked together by pentaglycins bridging the L-lysin of each tetrapeptide chain to the D-alamine of the neighboring one.

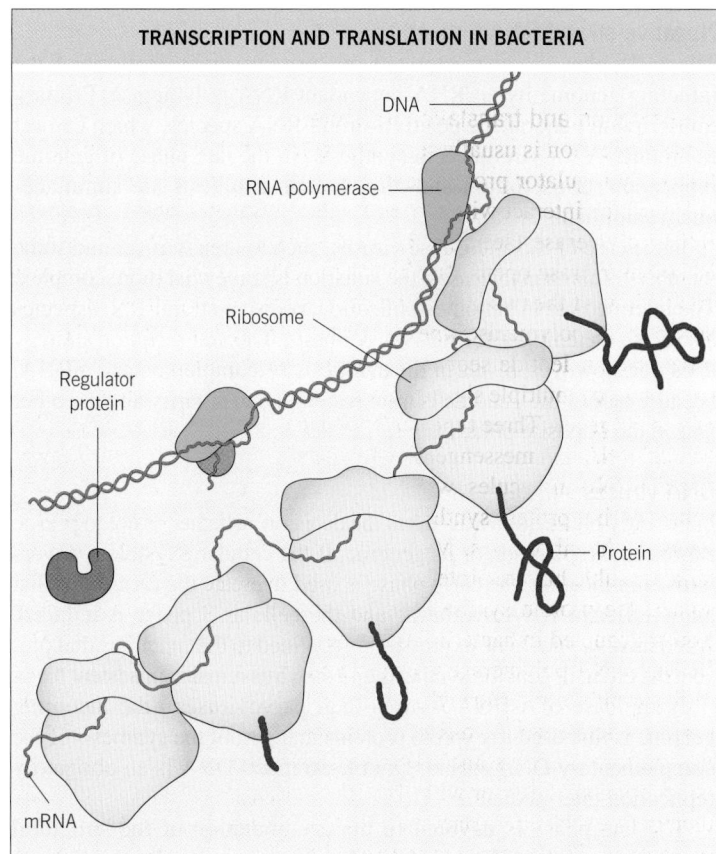

TRANSCRIPTION AND TRANSLATION IN BACTERIA

DNA

RNA polymerase

Ribosome

Regulator protein

Protein

mRNA

Fig. 1.10 Transcription and translation in bacteria (*Escherichia coli*).

1.83 millions of base pairs (Mbp) long and encodes 1703 putative proteins.[7] The chromosome of *Escherichia coli* is approximately 2.5 times bigger (5Mbp) – though still rather small if compared with the 30Mbp *Bacillus megaterium* genome – and is more than 500 times the length of the cell (Fig. 1.11). The bacterial chromosome codes for polypeptides; for example, *E. coli* probably contains well over 1500 different polypeptides with a variety of functions, such as maintenance of membrane structure; transport; respiration; degradation of nutrients; synthesis of amino acids, sugars, nucleotides, lipids and vitamins; and production of polymers such as DNA, RNA, proteins and polysaccharides. Mobile genetic elements, such as plasmids, bacteriophages, and transposable elements, are important sources of genetic variation. They supply genes that are not essential for bacterial growth but that may offer a selective advantage under specific conditions. Virulence factors and antibiotic resistance elements are frequently associated with these mobile DNA structures.

GENETIC INFORMATION IN BACTERIA (*E. COLI*)

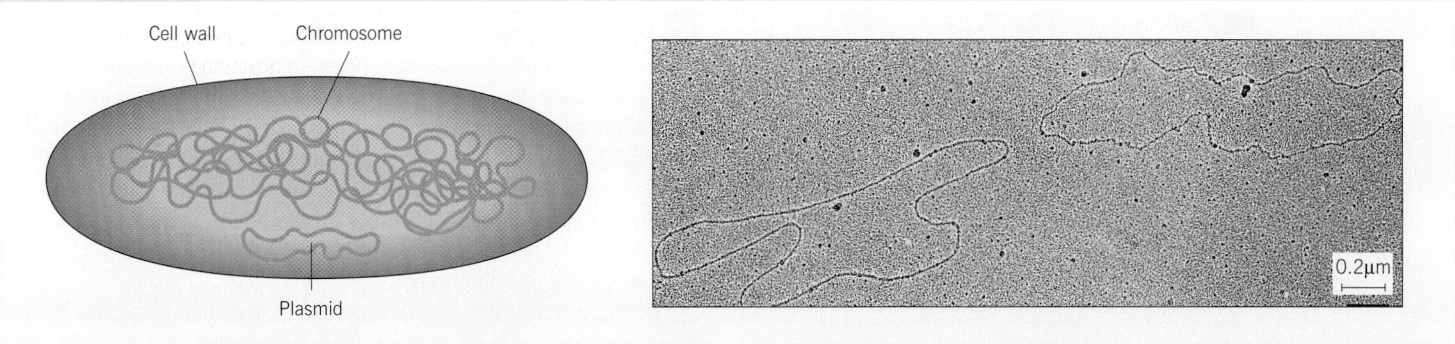

Fig. 1.11 Genetic information in bacteria. This example is *Escherichia coli*. Additional genetic information may be supplied by extrachromosomal elements such as plasmids or bacteriophages. Bacteria may carry a variety of these 'mobile genetic elements', which may transfer readily from one cell to another. The electron micrograph shows an 8.65kb *E. coli* plasmid that confers sulfonamide and streptomycin resistance (left) and a single stranded derivative of the plasmid (right).

Transcription and translation in bacteria

Gene expression is usually regulated at the level of transcription initiation by regulator proteins and occasionally by small RNA molecules, which interact with the 'promoter DNA' and with the enzyme RNA polymerase (see Fig. 1.10). The promoter is the site where RNA polymerase opens ('melts') the dsDNA to synthesize an RNA copy of one of the two DNA strands. A sigma factor transiently interacts with the polymerase when it binds the promoter DNA, and determines the nucleotide sequence specificity of the enzyme. Bacterial cells produce multiple sigma factors, each controlling the expression of a set of genes. Three types of RNA are produced: regulatory RNA, 'stable' RNA and messenger RNA (mRNA). Stable RNAs include the transfer RNA molecules, which position the amino acids on the ribosomes during protein synthesis and are important structural components of the ribosomes. Messenger RNA molecules are generally quite unstable but are protected from premature degradation by ribosomes, the protein synthesis machines.[6] Transcription and translation are coupled in bacteria; ribosomes bind the mRNA as soon as it 'leaves' RNA polymerase and start protein synthesis by coupling the initiator amino acid (formyl-methionine) to the second amino acid in decoding sequence. As mRNA elongation proceeds, more ribosomes bind to form a 'polysome'. The polypeptides that are produced fold either spontaneously or with the help of molecular chaperones in to their native structures. Bacterial mRNAs generally encode more than one protein. The bacterial protein synthesis machinery is an important target for antibiotics.

MOTILITY

Many bacterial species are equipped with a sophisticated detection system – 'chemotaxis' – which allows them to detect very small variations in concentrations of either valuable, or harmful substances in the surrounding environment.[8] Flagella are the effectors of chemotaxis (Fig. 1.12). By changing the direction of flagellar rotation, micro-organisms swim towards sites favorable to survival and growth. Amino acids and sugars are powerful chemoattractants. Although many pathogenic species are flagellated, a role for motility in virulence has not been established in all cases.

PATHOGENESIS OF INFECTIOUS DISEASE

The key microbial factors involved in the onset and spread of microbial infection can be identified by carefully analyzing the interaction of the micro-organism with its host (Fig. 1.13). Molecular techniques have contributed considerably to our present understanding of microbial pathogenesis. Insight into the intimate relationship between host and pathogen will help us find the answers to the all-important questions: how can we eliminate the cause of disease and how can we reduce its harmful effects on the human body?

Each pathogen has its own infection strategy, resulting in the development of a disease pattern with distinct symptoms. In the following sections we shall examine the lifestyles of some pathogenic species.

CONTAMINATION

In the developed areas of the world, the majority of human infections are caused by pathogens belonging to the normal microflora of the host (so-called endogenous infections), whereas those caused by exogenous micro-organisms have steadily declined over the past century. In contrast, exogenous infections are still prevalent in poorer areas.

Endogenous infections and normal microbial flora of the human host

The fetus *in utero* is normally sterile, but right after birth it starts building up its indigenous microflora, which will quickly outnumber its own cell content – a normal adult carries more than 10^{14} bacteria, which represents roughly 10 bacteria for each eukaryotic cell. In addition to bacteria, we may provide hospitality to an estimated 150 viral species, to fungi, protozoa and worms. The indigenous flora, or 'normal flora', is found in any part of the body exposed to the outside environment – the mouth, nose and the oropharynx, the anterior part of urethra, and the vagina and other moist areas of the skin (Fig. 1.14). The human microbial population is especially dense in the large intestine; it has been estimated that each gram of stool specimen contains about 10^{12} bacteria. The normal flora is well adapted to its niche, and may multiply rapidly under favorable nutritional conditions such as those found in the colon. Although the host's age and physical condition, and especially antibiotic treatment, may induce more or less important variations, the microbial population of the gastrointestinal tract seems to be stable, consisting of more than 99% of obligate anaerobic species. Facultative anaerobes such as *E. coli*, which are frequently used as markers for environmental pollution with human feces, represent less then 1% of the normal flora.

Transient micro-organisms, ingested with food or water, will normally pass through the high-flow-rate, central region of the gastrointestinal tract without being able to penetrate the mucous gel that overlays the intestinal epithelium or to reach the epithelial surface, which is densely populated with the indigenous flora. The top two-thirds of the ileum are less densely populated by the normal flora, probably owing to a combination of high motility and the acidity of the stomach contents. Population levels of the different areas of the gastrointestinal tract are controlled mainly at the level of metabolic

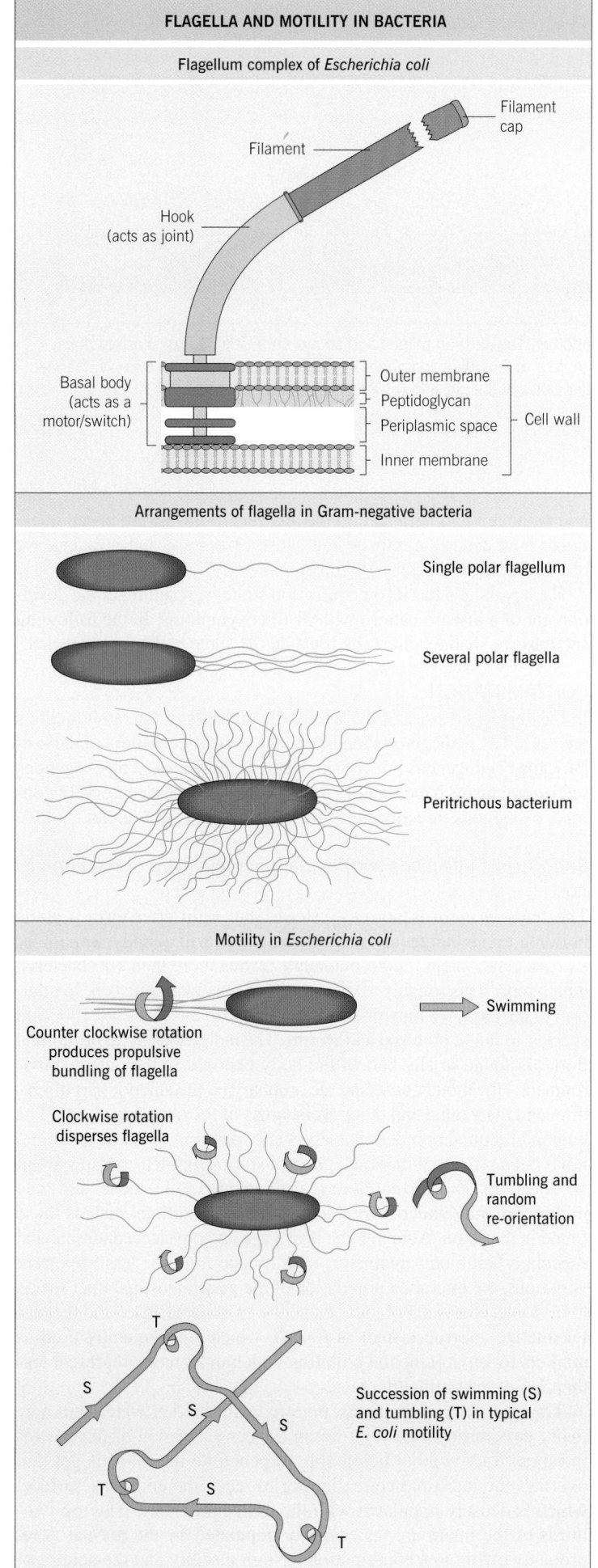

FLAGELLA AND MOTILITY IN BACTERIA

Flagellum complex of *Escherichia coli*

Filament cap

Filament

Hook (acts as joint)

Basal body (acts as a motor/switch)

Outer membrane
Peptidoglycan
Periplasmic space
Inner membrane
Cell wall

Arrangements of flagella in Gram-negative bacteria

Single polar flagellum

Several polar flagella

Peritrichous bacterium

Motility in *Escherichia coli*

Counter clockwise rotation produces propulsive bundling of flagella

Swimming

Clockwise rotation disperses flagella

Tumbling and random re-orientation

Succession of swimming (S) and tumbling (T) in typical *E. coli* motility

Fig. 1.12 Flagella and motility in bacteria.

competition, the normal flora being well adapted to the low oxidation reduction potentials, and tightly adherent to the mucosal epithelium. Pathogens that use the gastrointestinal tract as a portal of entry must find ways of dealing with the fierce microbial competition.

The skin is much less densely populated by the indigenous flora. In comparison with the gastrointestinal tract, it supplies a considerably less stable microenvironment and one that is often devoid of water. Although impermeable to bacteria, a number of parasites, among them *Schistosoma mansoni*, which poses a major health threat in developing countries, can penetrate the intact human skin. Moreover, skin disruptions due to lacerations or insect bites may allow entry of pathogenic microbes into the body.

The large majority of micro-organisms that belong to the human flora reside on the body surface without creating any damage. This peaceful cohabitation can be called symbiotic if in a 'both-sides-win' relationship; it is beneficial for both the host and the microbes. Some bacteria find shelter and food in the intestine and, in turn, supply vitamins or digest cellulose. However, symbiotic relationships are rather uncommon. More frequently, the micro-organisms, rather than the host, derive benefit from the association. These inhabitants of our body are called commensals. True commensals do not invade the host and, therefore, do not elicit an immune response. Parasitism constitutes a third category, where the micro-organisms, after invading the host, cause an infection.

The separation between parasitism, commensalism and symbiosis is not always clearly defined, and the condition of the host may make a big difference. Some micro-organisms, referred to as opportunistic pathogens, are commensals in the majority of people but cause disease in an immunocompromised host. With the progress of medicine, more and more highly immunocompromised hosts are able to be saved from a premature death, but this is creating at the same time a growing human reservoir for opportunistic pathogens.

The host and its indigenous microflora maintain a delicately balanced relationship that, when disrupted, may lead to the development of infectious disease.

An inevitable consequence of antibiotic treatment is the (local) elimination of susceptible bacteria, which, owing to fierce competition, are quickly replaced by antibiotic resistant species. This phenomenon can cause diseases such as candidiasis, pseudomembranous colitis, or severe enterococcal superinfection.

Any rupture of the body surface may favor the development of an infection. *Staphylococcus aureus* on our hands will become an invader and cause an infection as soon as we neglect a local wound. Dirty wounds containing soil particles are readily infected. Organisms with less pronounced pathogenic potential, such as *Staphylococcus epidermidis*, may also be involved.

The case of opportunistic infections in the immunocompromised host, already discussed, is another example of endogenous infection promoted by a rupture of the balance between the host and its microflora.

Probiotics (live micro-organisms) may help to restore the natural flora. For example, *Saccharomyces boulardii* may be used to treat colitis associated with *Clostridium difficile*.

IMPORTANT STEPS IN MICROBIAL PATHOGENESIS

- Encounter
- Attachment to host cells
- Local or general spread in the body (invasion)
- Cell and tissue damage
- Evasion of host defenses
- Shedding from the body

Fig. 1.13 Important steps in microbial pathogenesis.

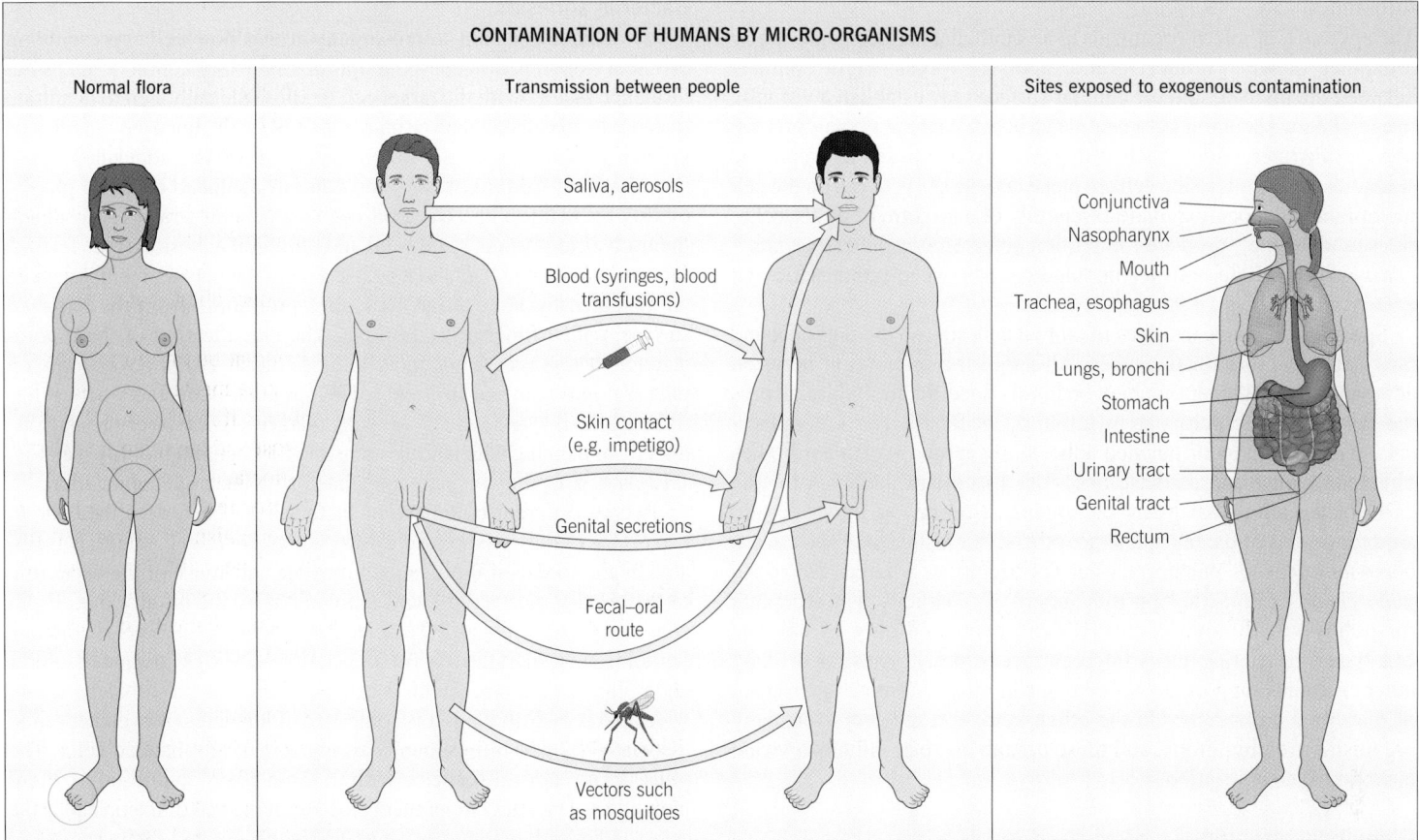

CONTAMINATION OF HUMANS BY MICRO-ORGANISMS

Normal flora | Transmission between people | Sites exposed to exogenous contamination

Saliva, aerosols

Blood (syringes, blood transfusions)

Skin contact (e.g. impetigo)

Genital secretions

Fecal–oral route

Vectors such as mosquitoes

Conjunctiva
Nasopharynx
Mouth
Trachea, esophagus
Skin
Lungs, bronchi
Stomach
Intestine
Urinary tract
Genital tract
Rectum

Fig. 1.14 Contamination of humans by micro-organisms. Many parts of the body are colonized by normal flora, which can be the source of endogenous infection. Large numbers of micro-organisms are found in moist areas of the skin (e.g. the groin, between the toes), the upper respiratory tract, the digestive tract (e.g. the mouth, the nasopharynx), the ileum and large intestine, the anterior parts of the urethra and the vagina. Other routes are interhuman transmission of infections and exposure to exogenous contamination.

Exogenous infections

Exogenous infections occur after a direct contamination from microbial populations in the environment:
- in air, soil and water,
- in live animals,
- in other people with infections, and
- in healthy people who are carriers.

Humans are continuously in intimate contact with the large exogenous microbial populations in the air, soil, and water, which all harbor highly pathogenic bacteria such as *Clostridium tetani* and *Bacillus anthracis*. Important pathogenic species, such as *Staphylococcus aureus*, *Clostridium perfringens* and *Clostridium botulinum*, may be present in our alimentation, and cause food poisoning.

Live animals represent another important source of exogenous micro-organisms. Infectious diseases of animals that may be transmitted to humans – the so-called zoonoses – include brucellosis, tularemia, plague, toxoplasmosis and rabies. In addition, microbial pathogens can be transmitted from animals to humans by insect vectors like flies, mosquitoes and ticks.

The most important source of exogenous infections are probably humans themselves (see Fig. 1.14). Well-known examples of human-to-human transmission include the common cold, AIDS, (other) sexually transmitted diseases, measles, diphtheria, tuberculosis and typhoid fever. Cross-infection in hospitals poses enormous problems, especially in intensive care units. Several regions of the body may be exposed to exogenous contamination (see Fig. 1.14). Healthy people may be carriers if they harbor and excrete potentially disease-producing micro-organisms. For instance, people recovering from typhoid fever may retain *Salmonella typhi* in the gallbladder and continue to excrete the pathogen in the feces long after recovery from the disease. These people are chronic carriers, even though they usually have mounted a protective immune response against the bacterium.

Exogenous infections, predominant in the past, have dramatically declined in the developed world thanks to improved hygiene, vaccination programs and infection control programs. They are, however, still prevalent in areas with limited resources. Community-acquired pneumonia, diarrheal diseases, malaria and tuberculosis are the main causes of over-mortality in developing countries.

THE INFECTION PROCESS

Three stages in the infection process may be functionally distinguished:
- attachment of the micro-organism to the target cell(s) and, for intracellular pathogens, entry into the host cell;
- development of the infection, local multiplication of the pathogen, and spread of the micro-organism to distant sites; and
- shedding of the organism and transfer to a new host.

Attachment to host cells

Only a few pathogens have the capacity to penetrate our body directly through the skin. Examples include the cercariae of various schistosome species, which can invade the skin with the help of their glandular secretions, and pathogens that enter the body after a bite (e.g. *Simulium* blackfly bite for *Onchocercus volvulus*, anopheles mosquito bite for malaria), intramuscular or intravenous injection, blood transfusion, or after injury of the body surface.

Although 'free' micro-organisms exist (for instance in the lumen of the intestine or in the saliva) most members of the human flora need to be attached to a cellular surface to avoid being swept away by the biologic fluxes such as urine or the passage of the alimentary bolus. For many microbial pathogens, adherence to the epithelial surface of the respiratory, digestive, or reproductive mucosa is a compulsory step in pathogenesis.

Adherence

The approach of micro-organisms to an epithelial surface is guided by a balance between attractive and repulsive forces. Tight contacts between the microbe and the cellular surface may establish a virtually irreversible association between the two. Such contacts may involve nonspecific interactions, such as those between exposed hydrophobic structures on the microbial cell envelope and lipophilic areas on the cell membrane. Glycocalyx, made essentially of a mixture of polysaccharides, and 'slime', produced in particular by *Staphylococcus epidermidis*, may mediate nonspecific adherence between prokaryotic and eukaryotic cells.

Specific adherence involves microbial adhesins on the one side, and host cell receptors on the other. Although the interaction between adhesins and cell receptors may be highly specific, this is not always the case. The specificity can be tested by artificially blocking adherence with an excess of purified adhesin, receptor, or with antibodies directed against one of these two. The specificity accounts for the early observation that many pathogens distinctively infect certain areas or organs of the body, and not others. For instance *Streptococcus pneumonia* causes pneumonia but not urethritis, whereas *Neisseria gonorrhoae* exhibits the opposite pattern of specificity. The receptors for poliovirus, rhinovirus and HIV are expressed only by specific cell types, restricting virus infection accordingly. These and many other examples support the notion that adhesins determine the tropism of microbial pathogens. On the other hand, cell receptors for many organisms are ubiquitous, and these organisms (e.g. influenza virus) have no tissue restriction.

Ubiquitous receptors

Fibrinogen, fibronectin, collagen and heparin-related polysaccharides are major components of the extracellular matrix (ECM), which coats the mucosal surface of epithelial cells. Members of the integrin family are involved in the interaction between the ECM and the underlying epithelium. A number of components of the ECM are used as receptors for microbial adhesins. Fibronectin specifically binds fibronectin-binding factors on the cell envelopes of *Staphylococcus aureus*, *Streptococcus pyogenes*, *Treponema pallidum* and *Mycobacterium* spp.; fibrinogen binds groups A, C and G streptococci, and a member of the integrin family binds the major invasion factor of *Yersinia pseudotuberculosis*. Their abundance and structural conservation among mammalian species makes ECM components ideal targets for bacterial adhesins.

Bacterial adhesins

Close contact between micro-organism and host cell represents an essential step in pathogenesis. It optimizes the interaction of microbial virulence factors with the target cell to allow the pathogen to penetrate or cause local cell damage, or both. Other possible functions of adhesins include modulation of the inflammatory response, adhesin-directed degranulation from mast cells and adhesin-mediated bacterial phagocytosis by neutrophils. Bacteria use two general strategies to attach themselves to host cells: fimbrial and afimbrial adhesion (Fig. 1.15).[10]

Pili and fibrillae. Attachment of bacteria to the plasma membrane can be mediated by filamentous structures protruding from the bacterial surface, called fimbriae or fibrillae. The classification of these colonization factors is based on morphologic criteria. Fimbriae (or common pili) are rigid hair-like structures with a regular diameter, whereas fibrillae are flexible and have an irregular diameter. These structures are distinct from flagella, which are responsible for bacterial motility (see Fig. 1.12), and sex pili, which are associated with bacterial conjugation.

Twenty different colonization factors have been described for *E. coli*.[11] One of these, expressed by uropathogenic E. coli strains, is mediated by the so-called P-pili, which mediate adherence of the bacterium to the urinary mucosa to avoid elimination by the urinary flux. P-pili consists of a long and rigid base section attached to an outer membrane scaffold, and a short flexible tip (Fig. 1.16).[12] The rigid section measures about 7nm in diameter, with a central channel approximately 1.5nm wide, and is 1–2μm long. It is composed of hundreds of pyelonephritis-associated (PapA) pilin subunits arranged in a right-handed helix. The pilus tip is 2nm in diameter with a 15nm pitch composed of PapE monomers. The PapG monomer is located at the end of the tip and is the actual adhesin. It recognizes the glycolipid receptor globobiose (α-1–4 linked di-galactose) on the host cell surface. During pilus formation, the tip is assembled and exported first, followed by the addition of the pilin subunits forming the shaft. The assembly of pili requires periplasmic chaperones, which assist in protein folding and assembly but never become part of the pili structure.

Afimbrial adhesins. Afimbrial adhesins, such as lectins (carbohydrate-binding proteins), also mediate tight binding between the bacteria and the host cell but, unlike pili, they do not form supramolecular structures. Similar adhesins exist in viruses, fungi and protozoa. Afimbrial binding has been extensively studied in Streptococcus pyogenes (Fig. 1.17). Two surface components are believed to be critical in the colonization of an epithelial surface: lipoteichoic acid and fibronectin binding protein.

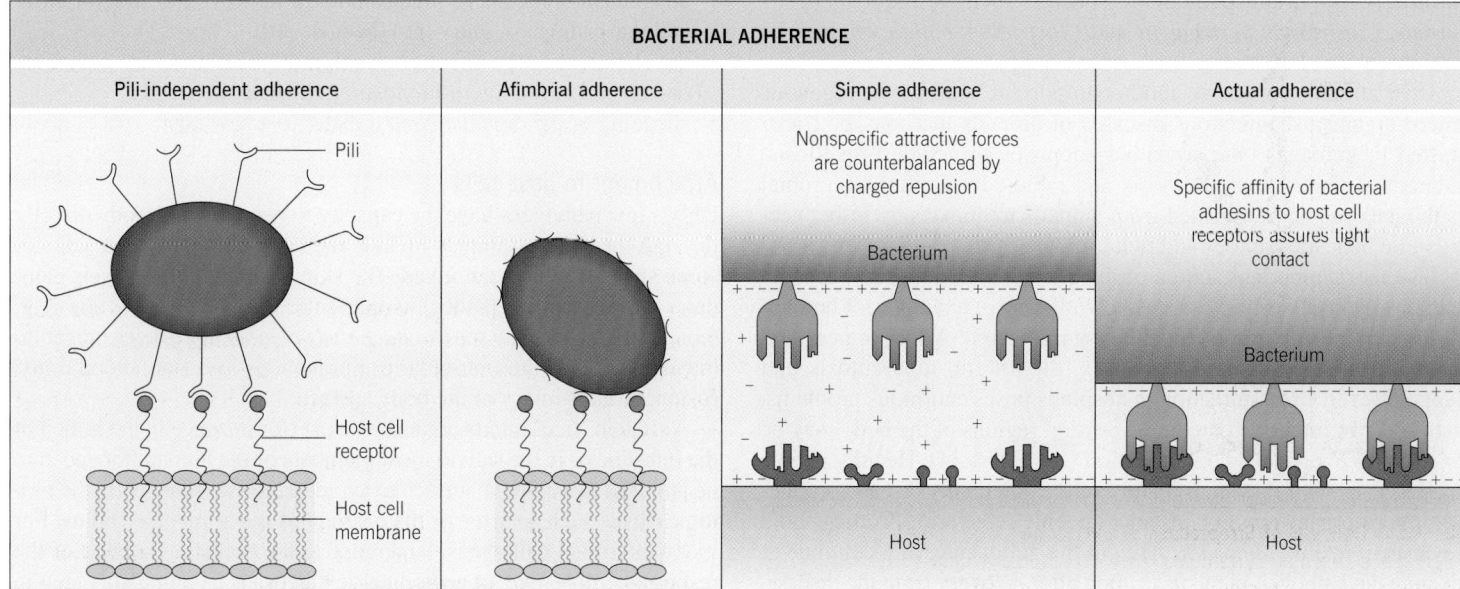

Fig. 1.15 Bacterial adherence.

Purified lipoteichoic acid binds to fibronectin and inhibits the binding of *S. pyogenes* to oral epithelial cells. The binding properties are confined to the lipid moiety of lipotechoic acid. Similarly, artificially added fibronectin-binding protein inhibits adhesion of *S. pyogenes* to epithelial cells even after the streptococci have been depleted of lipotechoic acid.

The complex surface of this micro-organism also includes the M protein.[14] This protein is a major virulence factor, but it does not seem

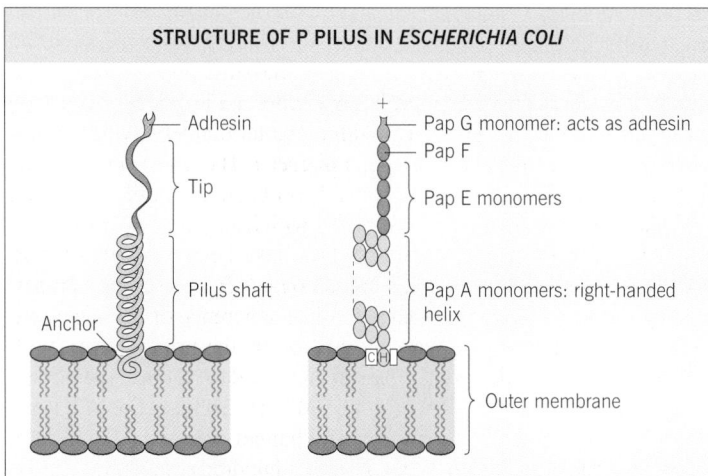

Fig. 1.16 Structure of P pilus in *Escherichia coli*.

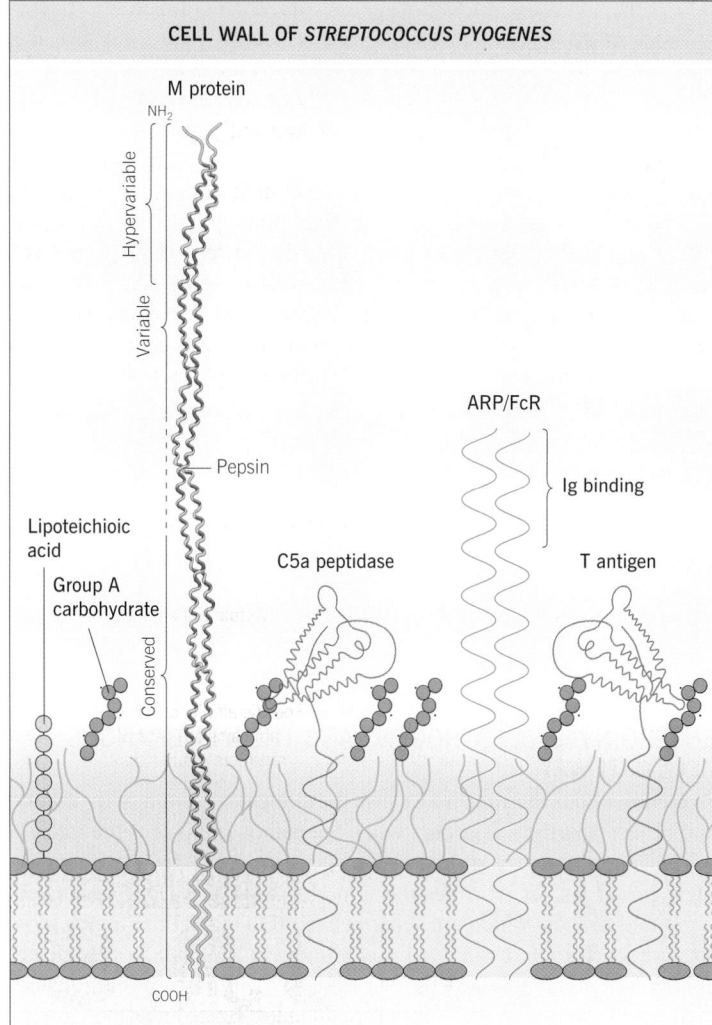

Fig. 1.17 Cell wall of *Streptococcus pyogenes*. The proposed model of the M protein is based on current sequence and structural data. ARP, immunoglobulin A receptor protein; FcR, receptor for the Fc portions of immunoglobulin. Adapted from Kehoe, 1991.[13]

to be involved in adherence to epithelial cells as was previously assumed. However, the M protein binds fibrinogen in a stoichiometric fashion and exerts an antiphagocytic effect, which may partially explain its key role in virulence.

Viral adhesion

Viral adhesion and invasion are generally mediated by the same set of viral proteins, and they may be considered as a single event. Initial attachment represents the first in a series of steps that ultimately leads to the delivery of the viral genome to its site of replication. Non-enveloped viruses appear to pass or slide through the plasma membrane directly. Enveloped viruses, such as measles and mumps virus, enter the cell after fusion with the plasma membrane.[15] These virions have a fusion protein that initiates the contact between the two membranes. Virus internalization may be mediated by a protein called clathrin, which forms membrane invaginations containing the virion. Once in the cytoplasm, the virus escapes from the clathrin-coated pits to reach the cytosol. The low pH inside the vacuole seems to trigger escape of the virion.

Cell specificity is determined by receptor availability. It may thus be rather relaxed for viruses that use ubiquitous receptors, and, on the other hand, be strongly restricted for viruses that simultaneously use two or more cellular receptors. An example of the latter is HIV; it requires co-expression of CD4 and chemokine receptors for efficient adhesion and invasion of the target cell. Herpes simplex virus 1 has an enveloped icosahedral capsid. The envelope contains at least 12 glycoproteins, of which two (glycoproteins B and C) interact with heparin sulfate on the plasma membrane. A second, specific interaction is probably required between glycoprotein D and an as yet unidentified cellular receptor to trigger fusion of the viral envelope and the plasma membrane. Following fusion, the capsid is released in the cytosol and is transported to the nuclear membrane. Herpes simplex virus first infects epithelial cells of the skin and mucosal membranes, where the initial replication cycles take place. It subsequently infects axon termini of neurons, the ultimate infection site.

Viral adherence and invasion may be blocked by neutralizing antibodies, which specifically bind the active site(s) of the adhesin(s). Many viruses have hidden this region in a protein pocket (or 'canyon'), making it physically inaccessible to potentially neutralizing antibodies.

INVASION

INVASIVE AND NONINVASIVE MICRO-ORGANISMS

Many micro-organisms, including those of the natural flora, remain at the epithelial surface without invading the underlying tissue (Fig. 1.18). This type of colonization is usually harmless, although it may, in some cases, induce damage to adjacent cells through the production of toxins, or elicit a local inflammatory or allergic response. Nonpenetrating micro-organisms include *Streptococcus pyogenes* and *Corynebacterium diphtheriae*, which cause pharyngitis, *Mycoplasma pneumoniae*, which causes atypical pneumonia, and *Trichomonas vaginalis*, a cause of vaginitis.

Other micro-organisms gain access to deeper tissues only after a physical or chemical injury of the epithelial barrier. *Staphylococcus aureus*, which is commonly found on the human skin, usually does not cause disease unless skin injury occurs. After penetration of the skin, *S. aureus* may become a dangerous toxin-producing pathogen.

Invasive micro-organisms exhibit the capacity to penetrate the target tissue to which they adhere without the need for local disruption of the protective epithelium. Invasive bacteria enter host cells, which are not naturally phagocytic. Penetration into these 'nonprofessional' phagocytes is achieved by:
- specific attachment to the host cell; and
- induction of local rearrangements of the cytoskeleton, through polymerization and depolymerization of actin.

This results in the formation of pseudopod-like structures, which

INTERACTION OF MICRO-ORGANISMS WITH EPITHELIAL CELLS			
	Order	Micro-organism	Disease
Generally confined to epithelial surfaces	Bacteria	*Bordetella pertussis* *Chlamydia trachomatis* *Corynebacterium diphtheriae* *Streptococcus pyogenes*	Pertussis Trachoma, urethritis Diphtheria Uncomplicated pharyngitis
	Viruses	Coronaviruses Rhinoviruses Rotaviruses	Common cold Common cold Diarrhea
	Fungi	*Candida albicans* *Trichophyton* spp.	Thrush Athlete's foot
	Protoza	*Giardia lamblia* *Trichomonas vaginalis*	Diarrhea Vaginitis
Enter through the epithelium	Bacteria	*Mycobacterium tuberculosis* *Brucella melitensis* *Neisseria meningitidis* *Salmonella typhi* *Treponema pallidum* *Yersinia pestis*	Tuberculosis Brucellosis Meningitis Typhoid fever Syphilis Plague
	Viruses	Measles virus Rubella virus Varicella Poliovirus	Measles Rubella Chickenpox Poliomyelitis
	Fungi	*Cryptococcus* spp. *Histoplasma* spp.	Cryptococcosis Histoplasmosis
	Protozoa	*Toxoplasma gondii* *Entamoeba histolytica*	Toxoplasmosis Liver abscess

Fig. 1.18 Interaction of micro-organisms with epithelial cells.

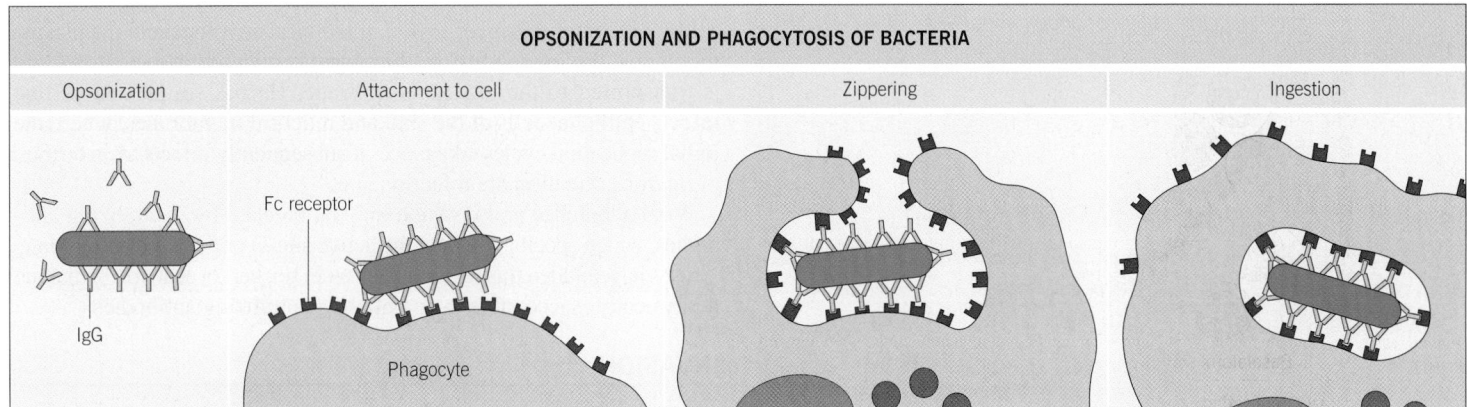

OPSONIZATION AND PHAGOCYTOSIS OF BACTERIA			
Opsonization	Attachment to cell	Zippering	Ingestion

Fig. 1.19 **Opsonization and phagocytosis of bacteria.** Bacteria are covered with IgG, specific for surface antigens. Bound IgG interacts with the phagocyte Fcγ-receptor, and pseudopods are formed, engulfing the bacterium into the host cell.

eventually engulf the pathogen into the host cell (Fig. 1.19). In order to induce ingestion by the host cell, the pathogens produce surface proteins called invasins.

In some cases infection remains confined to the epithelial surface (see Fig. 1.18), but in others the micro-organism may be transported across the superficial epithelium to be released into subepithelial space. This process is called transcytosis and involves the host cell actin network (see below). After transcytosis, the underlying tissues may be invaded and infected, and the infection may eventually spread all over the body (e.g. *Neisseria meningitidis* may get across the pharyngeal epithelium and cause meningitis, and *Salmonella typhi* may cross the intestinal epithelium and cause typhoid fever). For a more detailed analysis of the mechanisms of invasion, we shall use the example of enteroinvasive pathogens.

ENTEROINVASIVE PATHOGENS AND THE MEMBRANOUS CELL GATEWAY

Acute infectious diarrhea may cause the clinical spectrum of dysentery and bloody diarrhea. It occurs when the pathogen invades the intestinal mucosa and causes structural damage to the intestine. The immunologic protection of the intestine is performed by the gut-associated lymphoid tissues, which are separated from the intestinal lumen by a specialized follicle-associated epithelium. In the follicle-associated epithelium, membranous cells (M cells) play a prominent role because they are specialized in the transport of antigens. Enteroinvasive viruses, protozoa and bacteria exploit the transport facilities provided by M cells to invade the host. Entry (and passage) of M cells by these pathogens is preceded by adherence, in the case of reovirus type 1 through the specific adhesins σ1 or μ1 of the outer capsid.

Enteroinvasive bacteria such as *Salmonella*, *Shigella* and *Yersinia* spp. appear to distinguish between different subsets of M cells. Membranous cells produce glycocalyx, which contains a distinctive profile of lectin binding sites. Diversity in lectin-binding sites between different locations of the gut may account for the tropism of enteric pathogens, such as the preferential colonization of colonic mucosa for *Shigella* spp. versus that of *Salmonella* spp., which are more commonly found at the end of the ileum. Following adherence, the interactions with the M cells vary according to the pathogen (Fig. 1.20). Enteroadherent *E. coli* is not internalized and hence is not invasive. *Vibrio cholerae* is taken up and transported by the M cells but rapidly killed thereafter. It is considered to be invasive at the cellular level but not at the clinical level.

Detailed molecular analyses of virulence factors produced by enteroinvasive *Shigella* spp. has revealed that all virulent species harbor a 220kb plasmid, of which a 31kb fragment, encoding 32 genes, is both necessary and sufficient for invasion of epithelial cells.[17] The four invasion plasmid antigens (IpaA, B, C and D) encoded by this fragment are key players in the invasion process. Secretion of the 'Ipa complex' is induced by contact with the target cells and is accomplished by a specialized entry-associated secretion apparatus encoded by a set of genes (*mxi*, *spa*) located in the same region as the virulence plasmid. The *Salmonella* spp. entry functions are clustered in a 35–40kb region of the chromosome at centisome 63.[18] Such clustering of virulence genes is a typical example of a genetic 'pathogenicity island'.[19] These pathogenicity islands are often transmissible from one microbial species to another as a single DNA fragment by way of mobile genetic elements such as plasmids, transposons or bacteriophages.

The *Salmonella* and *Shigella* spp. genes involved in invasion of the eukaryotic host cell are homologous and have been remarkably well

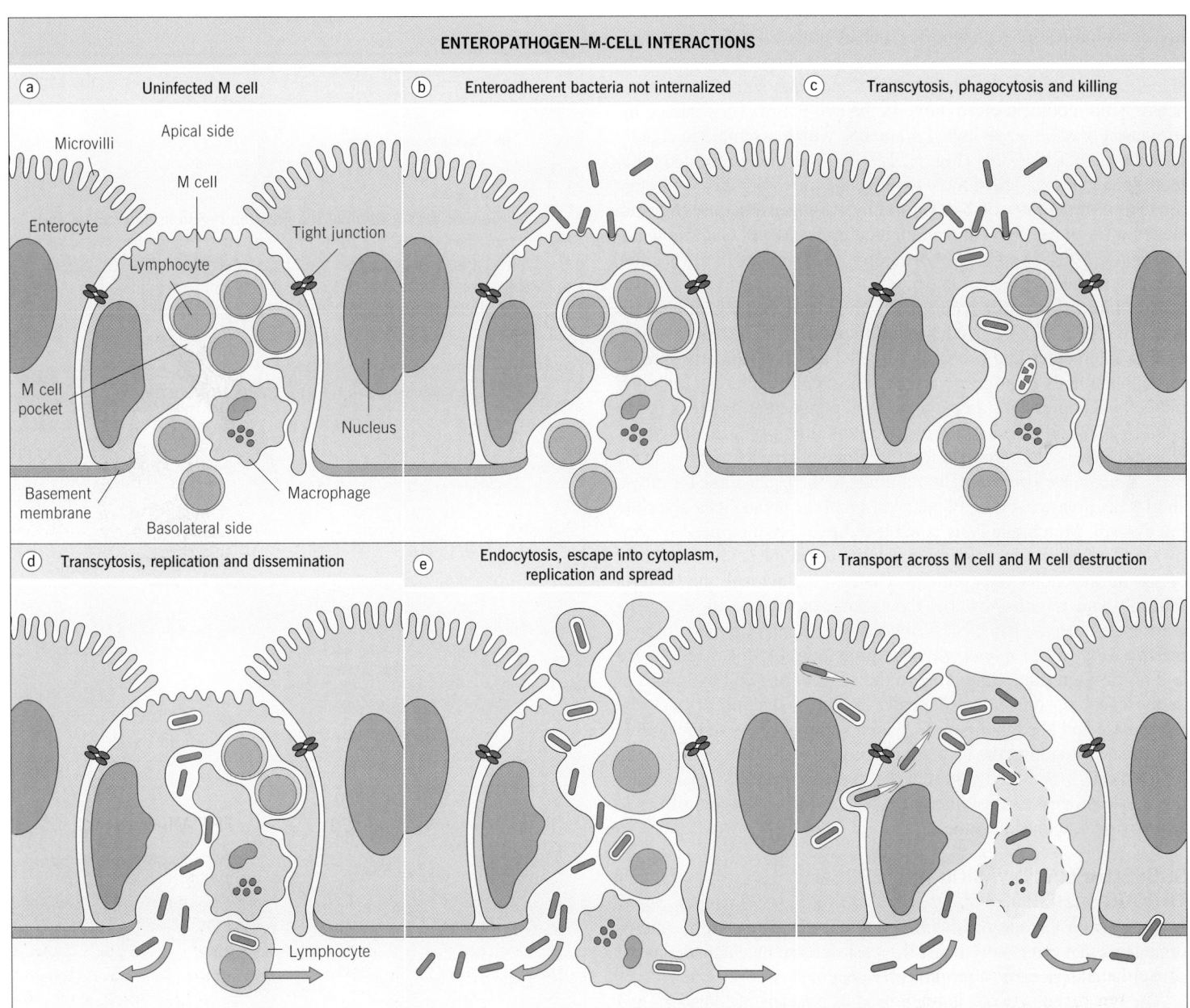

Fig. 1.20 Enteropathogen–M-cell interactions. (a) An uninfected M cell, enclosed between two adjacent enterocytes. The basolateral side forms a pocket where lymphocytes and macrophages are located. (b) Enteroadherent *Escherichia coli* forms microcolonies at the M cell surface, but is not internalized. (c) *Vibrio cholerae* undergoes transcytosis but is efficiently phagocytosed in the submucosa. (d) *Campylobacter jejuni* and *Yersinia* spp. undergo transcytosis, replicate in the submucosa and disseminate. (e) *Salmonella* spp. are transported across M cell, leading to destruction of the M cell. (f) *Shigella flexneri* is endocytosed by M cells, escapes into the cytoplasm, replicates, is propelled by actin tails and spreads to adjacent enterocytes. Adapted from Siebers and Finlay, 1996.[16]

conserved both with respect to the individual coding sequences and to their genetic organization (Fig. 1.21).[20] Yet the interplay between target cell and bacteria during the invasion processes of these two genera is different. Another important difference between the pathogenic lifestyles of these two bacterial species involves the intracellular fate of the bacteria. Both *Salmonella typhi* and *Shigella* spp. enter the cell by similar, although apparently nonidentical, architectural changes in the cellular cytoskeleton at the site of bacterial adhesion. Once internalized, the bacteria find themselves enclosed by a host cell membrane in an endocytic vesicle, and so are deprived of their nutrients. In professional phagocytes, such as macrophages and Langerhans cells, these endosomes are programmed to fuse to a prelysosome, releasing the hydrolytic enzymes required for the destruction of the bacterial cell. *Salmonella* spp. do not readily escape from the endosome into the nutritious cytoplasm, but *Shigella* spp. do so soon after entry into the cell.

ACTIN-BASED INTRACELLULAR MOTILITY OF MICROBIAL PATHOGENS

Enteroinvasive micro-organisms use passive actin modification to invade nonprofessional phagocytes such as epithelial cells. Local modification of the cytoskeleton is induced by the pathogen by diverting the signaling pathways of the host cells. In addition some bacteria use active actin modification to move in the cytoplasm. They induce the formation of actin cross-linked filaments, which assemble in characteristics 'comet-like tails' (Fig. 1.22).[21,22] Elongation of the actin filaments generates sufficient force to move the micro-organisms through the cytoplasm at rates of 2–100μm/min. Pathogens that use the actin skeleton for intracellular spread include bacteria (e.g. *Listeria monocytogenes*, *Shigella* spp., *Rickettsia* spp.) and viruses (e.g. vaccinia, measles, rabies).

The intracellular lifecycle of *L. monocytogenes* illustrates this strategy (Fig. 1.23).[23,24] Under natural conditions, *Listeria* first penetrates enterocytes and probably M cells, and subsequently spreads through the body to infect a variety of host cells, including endothelial cells, Kuppfer cells, hepatocytes and phagocytes. Entry is facilitated by the products encoded by the internalin (*inl*) family of genes, which seem to confer tropism for different cell-types. Once inside the cell, *L. monocytogenes* remains confined to the phagosome for only a short time. Following lysis of the endosomal membrane it escapes into the cytosol. Membrane lysis is achieved by a production of lysteriolysin-O, which attains maximum activity under the acidic conditions of the intravacuolar environment. Once in the cytosol, the bacteria multiply and migrate towards the plasma membrane by using the actin-based mechanism as described above. Actin polymerization is mediated by the *L. monocytogenes* protein ActA, localized at one end of the bacterium. Spreading to the neighboring cell by means of actin-dependant movement depends on the production of bacterial lecithinase and phospholipase C, which stimulate lysis of the double membrane separating the bacterium from the cytoplasm of the newly infected cell. Interestingly, most of the virulence genes associated with the whole process as described are clustered in one region of the *L. monocytogenes* chromosome.

SUBEPITHELIAL INVASION AND SPREAD THROUGH THE BODY

Invasion from the site of infection can only be achieved by micro-organisms that effectively resist the host defense mechanisms in the subepithelial space, most prominently phagocytosis.

The lymphatic network is often used as a means of transport, and successful micro-organisms may rapidly reach the nearest local lymph nodes, which have an important filtering function. In the lymph nodes, resident macrophages and polymorphonuclear cells will actively fight the invaders. As a result the first line of lymph nodes are often inflamed. If the invading micro-organism is sufficiently virulent or present in sufficiently large numbers, it may pass into efferent lymphatic vessels to

be conducted to the bloodstream. The result is primary bacteremia or viremia. Some microbes can enter directly into the blood vessels via an injury. A typical example is provided by viridians streptococci, which enter the bloodstream during dental extraction, enabling them to infect a cardiac valve and produce endocarditis. Insect bites (malaria and arthropod-borne viruses) or damage to the blood vessel wall inflicted by hemorrhagenic viruses are alternative ways to circumvent the body's first line of defense: the mucosal immune system.

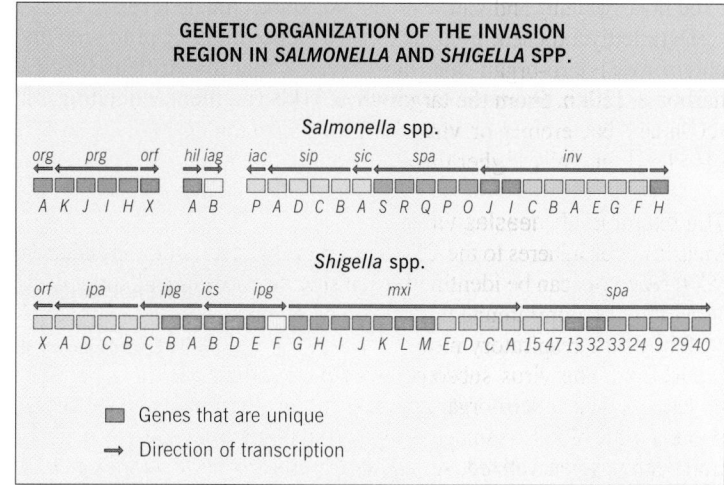

Fig. 1.21 Genetic organisation of the invasion region in *Salmonella* and *Shigella* spp. Identical patterns indicate topologically conserved blocks of genes. Each genus has genes that are unique. Despite remarkable genetic similarities, the invasion strategies of the two bacteria are quite different (see Fig. 1.20). Adapted from Galan, 1996.[18]

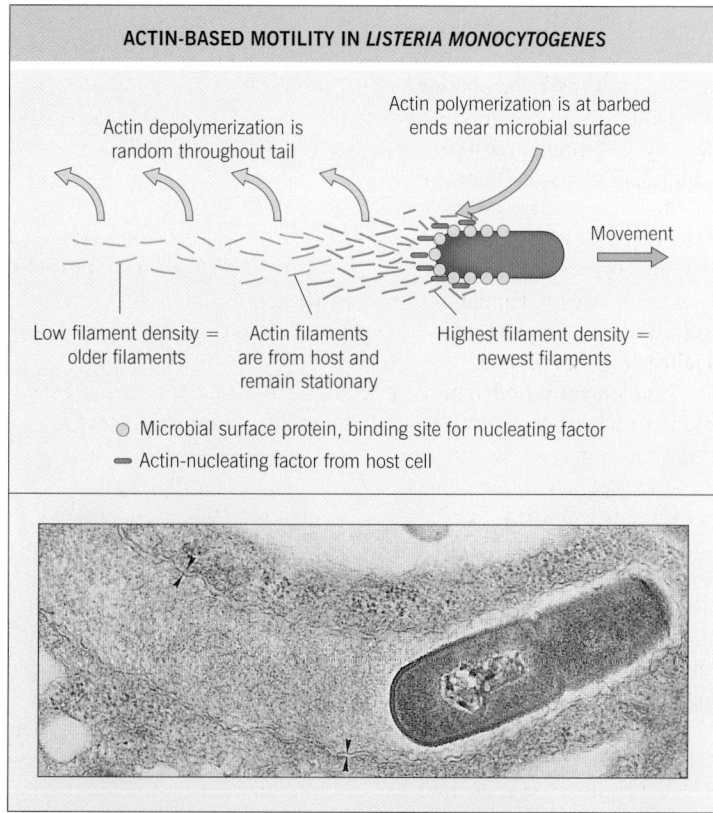

Fig. 1.22 Actin-based motility in *Listeria monocytogenes*. The bacterium moves forwards at the rate of actin-filament growth behind the pathogen. Adapted from Sanders MC & Theriot JA, 1996.[21] The EM shows a section of a CaCo-2 cell infected with *Listeria monocytogenes*; the bacterium protrudes into the cytoplasm of an adjacent cell; protrusion is limited by a double membrane (arrowheads).

Once in the bloodstream, the micro-organisms may circulate either as an extracellular or as an intracellular species. Pathogens have been found in polymorphonuclear cells (staphylococci), in lymphocytes (HIV), in macrophages (*Mycobacterium tuberculosis*), and even in red blood cells (*Plasmodium* spp.), which provide protection against potent humoral factors in the serum, such as complement.

Infection of distant target organs

Transported by the bloodstream, the invasive micro-organisms can reach distant target organs and create infective metastases throughout the body. Almost any tissue can be reached, but the organs containing abundant capillary and sinusoid networks (e.g. lungs, liver, kidneys) are especially exposed, because blood flows slowly at these sites and transported micro-organisms get the opportunity to adhere and establish an infection. From the target organs, the invaders may produce a secondary bacteremia or viremia, in which microbial counts in the blood are generally higher than during primary infections.

The example of measles virus

Measles virus adheres to the CD46 receptor.[25] Cluster of differentiation (CD) receptors can be identified using specific monoclonal antibodies. Infection of a nonimmune host proceeds by invasion of the epithelial surface of the respiratory mucosa, where the virus undergoes limited replication. The virus subsequently migrates to the regional lymph nodes, and those micro-organisms that survive local macrophage attack will enter the bloodstream, causing a primary viremia. When the infection becomes generalized, several target areas are affected, including the lungs, the skin, and the central nervous system. At this stage, the virus undergoes further replication in the leukocytes (causing leukopenia) as well as in the lymphoid tissues and in the target organs. The result is secondary viremia and fever. Rash appears later and is due to the destruction of infected cells by cytotoxic T lymphocytes rather than to a direct cytopathic effect of the virus on skin cells.

These pathogenic steps correspond to different clinical periods. During the initial encounter with the virus, the viral spread to target organs and the primary viremia there are no clinical symptoms; this corresponds to the incubation period, which lasts for about 10 days. After this, disease develops, and about 4 days later (i.e. typically 14 days after contamination) the skin rash occurs, corresponding to local inflammation and cellular immunity.

Serum resistance in *Neisseria gonorrhoeae* and *Salmonella* spp.

Immunocompetent hosts contracting gonorrhea usually do not develop a systemic disease. Human serum contains a variety of humoral factors, including the complement system, which provide effective protection against *N. gonorrhoeae*.

Complement is both a major effector of specific humoral immunity and a participant in natural (innate) immunity. The complement system involves some 30 serum proteins and is aimed at extracellular pathogens. The complement system may be activated by one of two convergent pathways. The 'classical pathway' is activated by specific binding of either two IgG or one IgM molecule to a circulating target. The first component of the complement system (C1) binds in a co-operative fashion to two adjacent Fc fragments of the immunoglobulin attached to the target, and initiates a proteolytic activation cascade, culminating in the erection of a multiprotein complex that strongly stimulates phagocytosis. The complement system may directly induce cytolytic activity through the membrane-attack complex anchored on the microbial envelope. The 'alternative pathway' does not depend on the availability of specific immune globulins and is initiated directly by fixation of complement proteins to specifically recognized structures on the target surface. The outcome of both pathways is in many respects similar.

The ability to resist complement killing contributes to virulence of *Salmonella* spp. Complement resistance can be provided by very long O-side chains in the *Salmonella* LPS. In addition, the outer membrane

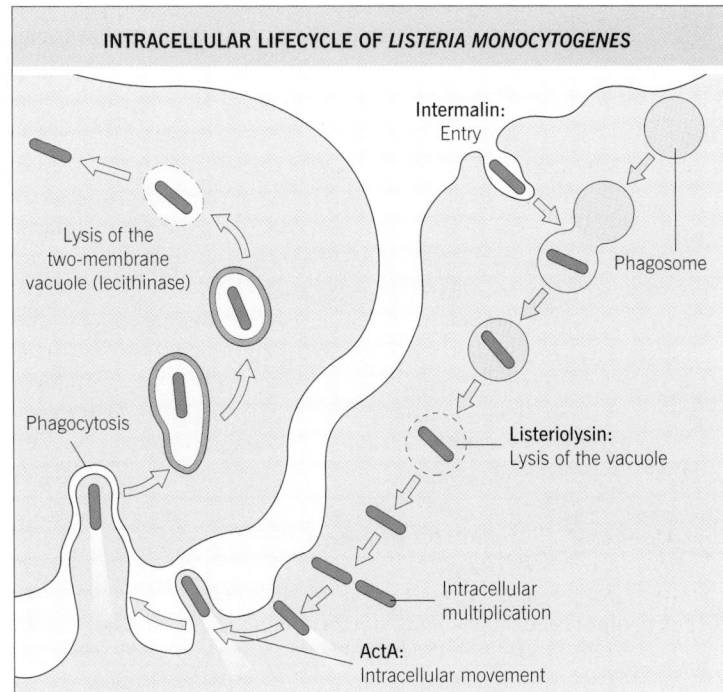

Fig. 1.23 Intracellular lifecycle of *Listeria monocytogenes*.

INTRACELLULAR LIFECYCLE OF *LISTERIA MONOCYTOGENES*

Intermalin: Entry

Phagosome

Lysis of the two-membrane vacuole (lecithinase)

Phagocytosis

Listeriolysin: Lysis of the vacuole

Intracellular multiplication

ActA: Intracellular movement

protein Rck (resistance to complement killing) may provide protection of the bacterium against complement mediated killing. The last step in the assembly of the membrane attack complex onto the bacterial membrane (insertion of polymerized C9 into the outer membrane) is prevented by Rck. The *rck* gene is located on the large virulence plasmids of *Salmonella dublin* and *Salmonella typhimurium*.

Some strains of *N. gonorrhoeae* are serum resistant and do cause disseminated infection in normal hosts. These strains are protected against complement by changes in the carbohydrate portion of their lipo-oligosaccharide. In some of the resistant strains, a galactose residue of LPS covalently binds an activated form of sialic acid from human blood, thus abolishing complement activation.[26] In addition, individuals with genetic defects in the terminal complement components (C6–C9) are unable to assemble the membrane attack complex. They are more susceptible to disseminated neisserial infections although there is a lower case mortality.

CELL AND TISSUE DAMAGE INDUCED BY MICRO-ORGANISMS

Infectious disease is often characterized by cell and tissue damage. Paralysis in poliomyelitis, exanthem in varicella, gastroduodenal ulcers in *Helicobacter pylori* infections and bloody diarrhea in shigellosis all result from damage caused directly or indirectly by micro-organisms. Cell damage can be generated by a variety of different mechanisms (Fig. 1.24).

BACTERIAL TOXINS

Bacteria produce a large diversity of toxins, which have been classified according to their mode of action (Figs 1.25 & 1.26). Traditionally, exotoxins (or excreted toxins) are distinguished from endotoxin (equivalent to the lipopolysaccharide of the outer membrane of Gram-negative bacteria). However, some of the so-called exotoxins are actually intracellular, and are released into the environment only after cell lysis. The pneumolysin of *Streptococcus pneumoniae*, for example, is cytoplasmic, the adenylate cyclase of *Bordetella pertussis* is associated with the cytoplasmic membrane, and the heat-labile toxin I (LT-I) from *E. coli* is periplasmic. The genetic information that encodes bacterial toxins is frequently carried on mobile DNA elements, which may readily pass from one microbial host to another. The toxins associated with diphtheria, botulism and

MECHANISMS OF CELL AND TISSUE DAMAGE PRODUCED BY MICRO-ORGANISMS		
	Mechanism	Examples
Direct damage by micro-organisms	Production of toxins	See Figure 1.25
	Production of enzymes	Proteases, coagulase, DNAses produced by *Staphylococcus aureus*
	Apoptosis	HIV (CD4$^+$ T lymphocytes); *Shigella flexneri* (macrophages)
	Virus-induced cytopathic effects: Cell lysis	Cytomegalovirus
	Formation of syncytium	Respiratory syncytial virus
	Inclusion bodies Intracytoplasmic Nuclear	Rabies Herpesviruses
	Transformation	Human papillomaviruses type 16
Damage via the host immune response	Cytotoxic T lymphocytes and natural killer lymphocytes	Production of the measles rash
	Autoimmunity	Acute rheumatic fever
	Immediate hypersensitivity	Rashes associated with helminthic infections
	Cytotoxic hypersensitivity	Cell necrosis induced by hepatitis B
	Immune complexes	Glomerulonephritis in malaria
	Delayed type hypersensitivity	Tuberculous granuloma

Fig. 1.24 Mechanisms of cell and tissue damage produced by micro-organisms.

Fig. 1.25 Examples of bacterial toxins.

EXAMPLES OF BACTERIAL TOXINS					
Toxin type	Example of sources	Toxin	Targets	Mechanisms	Effects
Endotoxin (LPS, lipid A)	Gram-negative bacteria	Endotoxin	Macrophages, neutrophils, lymphocytes, plasma components	Activation of target cells, complement; release of IL-1, TNF, kinins	Septic shock
Membrane-disrupting toxins	*Staphylococcus aureus*	α-Toxin	Many cell types	Formation of pores	Tissue necrosis
	Listeria monocytogenes	Listeriolysin	Many cell types	Formation of pores at acidic pH	Escape from the phagosome
	Clostridium perfringens	Perfringolysin-0	Many cell types	Phospholipase (removes polar head groups from phospholipids)	Gas gangrene
A–B-type toxins	*Clostridium tetani*	Tetanospasmin	Synaptic transmission	Inhibits release of inhibitory neurotransmitters	Spastic paralysis
	Clostridium diphtheriae	Diphtheria toxin	Many cell types	ADP ribosylation of EF-2	Paralysis
	Vibrio cholerae	Cholera toxin	Intestinal cells	ADP ribosylation of adenylate cyclase, leading to rise in cyclic AMP	Profuse watery diarrhea
Superantigen	*Streptococcus pyogenes*	Streptococcal pyogenic exotoxin	T lymphocytes, macrophages	T lymphocyte stimulation, release of IL-1, IL-2, TNF; possible enhancement of LPS activities	Fever, eruption, toxic shock-like syndrome
	Staphylococcus aureus	Toxic shock toxin	T lymphocytes, macrophages	Same as streptococcal pyrogenic toxin	Toxic shock syndrome

scarlet fever, as well as Shiga-like toxin in *E. coli*, are encoded by temperate bacteriophages. Genes for LT-I and methanol-susceptible heat-stable toxin (Sta) of *E. coli* are carried on plasmids.

Toxins deregulate the physiology of the host cell before or during bacterial adhesion and invasion. The bacteria may profit from the induced damage, which compromises the cellular defense against the intruder and may release nutrients from the cytosol.

The diphtheria toxin as example of an A–B toxin

Diphtheria toxin belongs to the so-called A–B toxins (Fig. 1.27). These toxins are bifunctional molecules. Portion A mediates the enzymatic activity responsible for the toxicity after internalization into the target cell, but cannot penetrate by itself. Portion B is not toxic but binds to a cell receptor localized on the cell surface and mediates the translocation of the A chain into the cytosol. Portion B accounts for the cell specificity of the A–B toxins. The receptor recognized by the B chain of diphtheria toxin is a heparin-binding precursor of epidermal growth factor. Epidermal growth factor is an important hormone for growth and differentiation of many different cell types.

Uptake of diphtheria toxin proceeds via receptor-mediated endocytosis. Acidification of the endocytic vesicle induces a conformational change in the enclosed holotoxin, enabling the A subunit to traverse the membrane and reach its cytoplasmic target. The A subunit of diphtheria toxin catalyzes ADP-ribosylation of the elongation factor-2 (EF-2). After attachment of the ADP-ribosyl group, EF-2 becomes inactive, causing the death of the target cell.

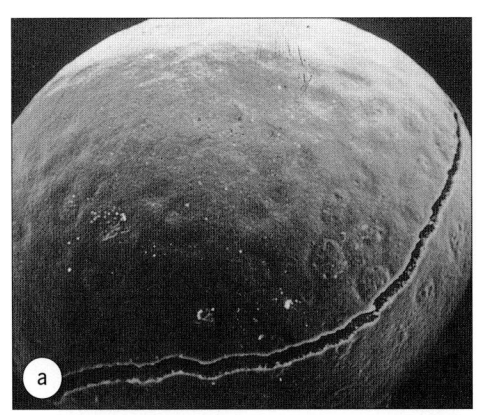
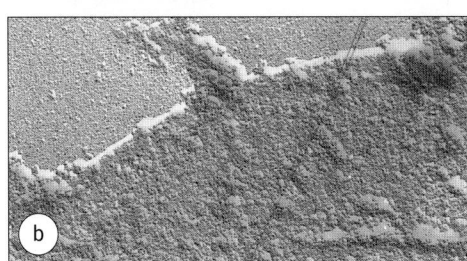

Fig. 1.26 Action of bacterial toxins. (a) *Xenopus* oocyte treated with the cytolytic delta toxin (perfringolysin) of *Clostridium perfringens*. (b) Rabbit erythrocyte exposed to a very small quantity of streptolysin-O, produced by *Streptococcus* A,C,G. Hemoglobin escapes from sites of membrane rupture. Courtesy of Dr J Alouf.

Only *Corynebacterium* lysogenic for temperate bacteriophage carrying the *tox* gene produce the toxin. The *tox* gene is under the control of the repressor protein DtxR, which forms a complex with iron, DtxR–Fe (Fig. 1.28). DtxR–Fe, but not DtxR, can bind DNA and repress *tox* expression. Thus diphtheria toxin is produced under low iron conditions, suggesting that it may be produced to stimulate iron-release from the target cell. Interestingly the *Pseudomonas aeruginosa* exotoxin A has a very similar structure, but uses a different cell receptor: the α-2 macroglobin low-density lipoprotein receptor. Like diphtheria toxin, exotoxin enters the cell via receptor-mediated endocytosis, but the toxin is released only after passage through the Golgi system.

Hydrolysing enzymes

Microbial pathogens often secrete hydrolysing enzymes, such as proteases, hyaluronidases, coagulases and nucleases. As such these enzymes cannot harm the host cells, and they are therefore not considered to be toxins. However, in the context of an ongoing infection they are assumed to facilitate colonization of host tissues by a variety of mechanisms, such as proteolysis of IgA; fluidification of pus; induction of plasma clotting, which may hinder the influx of phagocytes into the focus of infection; and a general disorganization of the host tissue structure. The release of hydrolytic enzymes by phagocytes damaged by a bacterial toxin may have similar effects.

Apoptosis

Apoptosis is a process in which the cell activates an intrinsic suicide program. It plays key roles in processes like organ development and tissue repair, both of which critically depend on the generation of a self-limiting organized structure through addition of new cells and elimination of 'old' cells. The morphologic changes associated with apoptotic death are a reduction of the volume of the cytosol and nuclear condensation (Fig. 1.29). The genome is fractionated by an induced endonuclease activity, which cuts the DNA into multiples of 180–200.[27] Finally, the cell corpse is removed by phagocytosis.

Apoptosis is distinct from necrosis. In necrosis, which may, for example, be induced by a bacterial toxin, the cell does not participate actively in its own death. Another important difference between apoptosis and necrosis is that the former does not induce the host cell inflammatory response that usually accompanies necrosis.

Many viruses trigger apoptotic death of the infected host cell. For instance, apoptosis seems to contribute to the depletion of CD4+ T lymphocytes, both in cell culture and in HIV-infected people.[28] Apoptotic

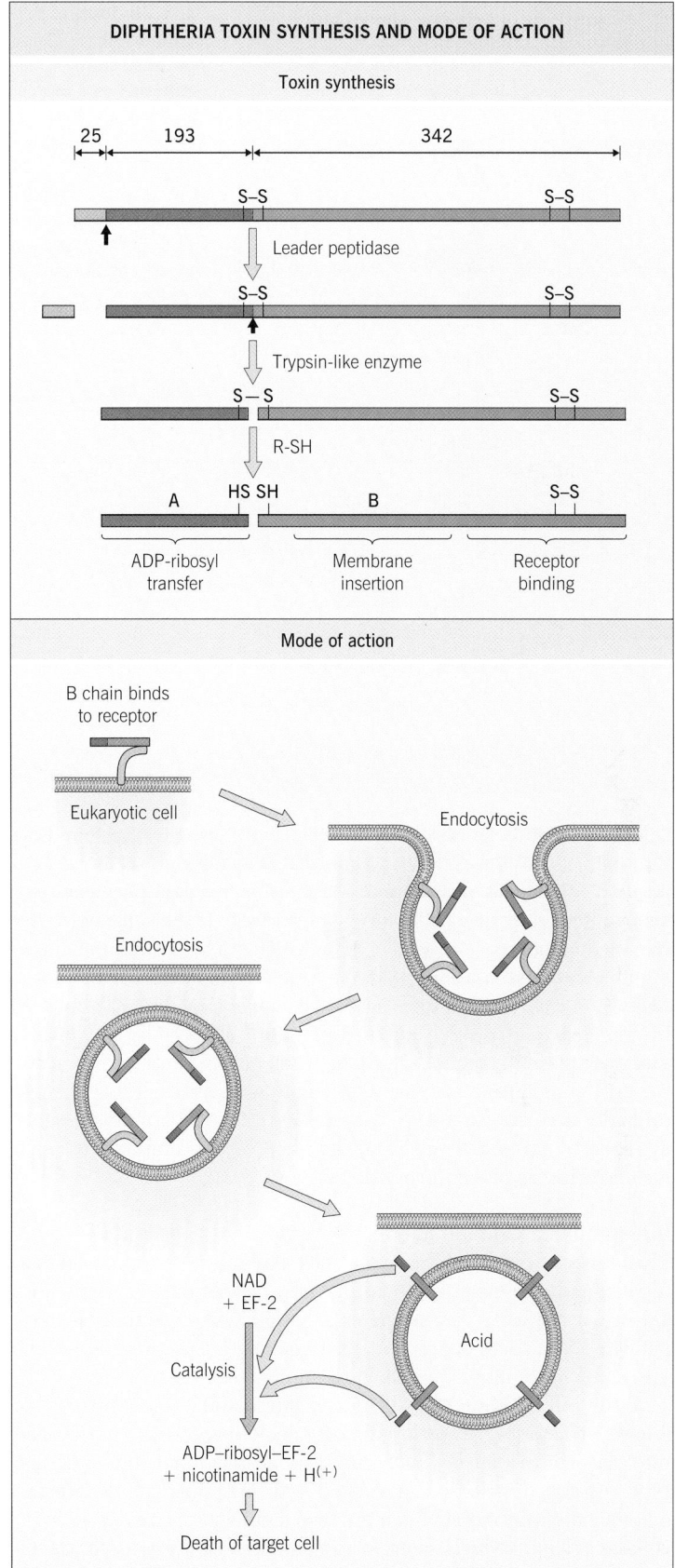

Fig. 1.27 Diphtheria toxin synthesis and mode of action. (Top) The 25-residue leader sequence is cleaved off by the bacterial leader peptidase; the A and B subunits are generated from the precursor protein by a 'trypsin-like enzyme'. Once in the cytoplasm of a targeted eukaryotic cell, the A chain, responsible for ADP-ribosyl transfer, is disconnected from the B chain, responsible for receptor binding and membrane insertion. (Bottom) The B chain binds to a specific receptor on the eukaryotic cell. After endocytosis, acidification in the endosome induces insertion of the B chain into the endosomal membrane and translocation of subunit A into the cytosol, where it catalyzes the ADP ribosylation of EF-2. As a result, protein synthesis is inhibited, and the targeted cell dies.

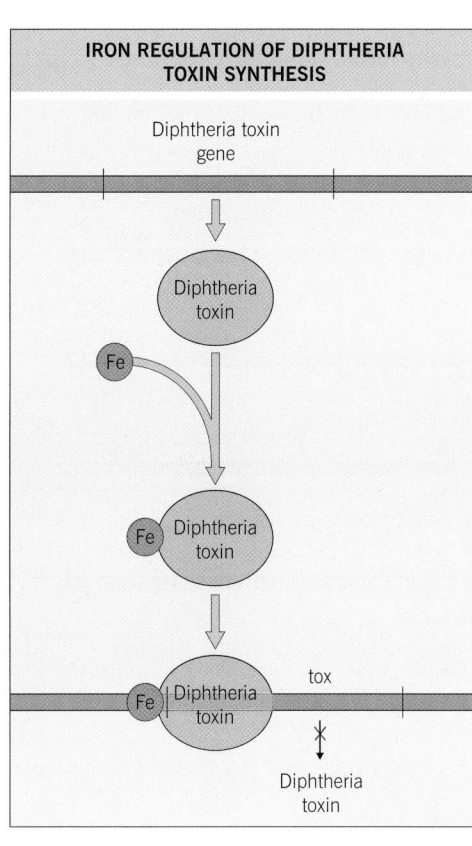

IRON REGULATION OF DIPHTHERIA TOXIN SYNTHESIS

Diphtheria toxin gene

Diphtheria toxin

Fe

Fe + Diphtheria toxin

Fe + Diphtheria toxin — tox

Diphtheria toxin

Fig. 1.28 Iron regulation of diphtheria toxin synthesis. High iron concentrations in the environment repress the synthesis of diphtheria toxin: when bound to iron DtxR–Fe acts as a transcriptional repressor of the *tox* gene.

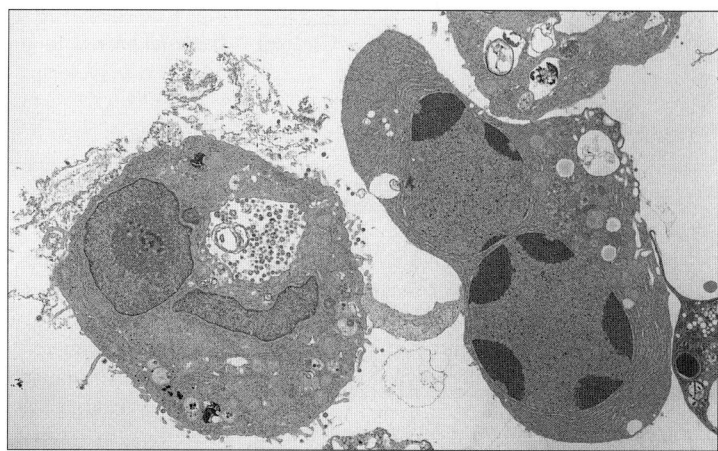

Fig. 1.29 Apoptosis induced by Sendai virus. Morphologic changes in the apoptotic Sendai infected cell (left), include the typical fragmentation of chromosomal DNA. No stigma of apoptosis is seen in the uninfected cell (right). Courtesy of Dr Dick Compans and Dr Kiyoshi Tanebayashi.

cells have also been observed in infections caused by Epstein–Barr virus and adenoviruses. Bacteria can also induce apoptosis. *Bordetella pertussis*, the agent of whooping cough, triggers macrophage apoptosis by interfering with cellular regulation at the level of the cytoplasmic second messenger cyclic AMP (cAMP).[29] The bacterium induces high levels of cytoplasmic cAMP, favoring the induction of apoptosis. *Shigella flexneri*, the etiologic agent of dysentery, can kill macrophages by apoptosis. Cell death is induced by IpaB,[30] encoded by the *Shigella* virulence plasmid (see Fig. 1.21). Invasion plasmid antigen B binds to the host cytoplasmic enzyme interleukin-1β converting enzyme and probably activates it.[31] This enzyme activates the proinflammatory cytokine by proteolytic cleavage, and hydrolyzes a number of other host proteins involved in later stages of apoptosis.

Virus-induced cytopathic effect

Most viruses severely damage the cells they infect, sometimes inducing distinctive cytopathic effects that may be useful in diagnosis (Fig. 1.30). A large variety of mechanisms may be involved in these cytopathic effects, some being direct consequences of the presence of the virus, others resulting from the host immune response.

Virus infection may result in the intracellular accumulation or release of a number of small molecules, including reactive oxygen and nitrogen intermediates, which may play an important role in certain types of cell destruction, particularly in macrophages. Rotavirus, cytomegalovirus and HIV can produce significant increases in intracellular calcium, which seems to be a common pathway for the development of irreversible cell injury.

In addition to cell lysis, other cytopathic effects exist. Paramyxoviruses such as respiratory syncytial virus, parainfluenza viruses, and measles virus, as well as herpesvirus and some retroviruses, cause the formation of multinucleated giant cells. The formation of these giant cells (syncytia) is mediated by virus-encoded fusion proteins. Viral infection can also produce eosinophilic or basophilic inclusion bodies, which appear in the cytoplasm or the nucleus. Inclusion bodies may represent aggregations of mature virions, areas of altered staining at sites of viral growth, or simply degenerative changes.

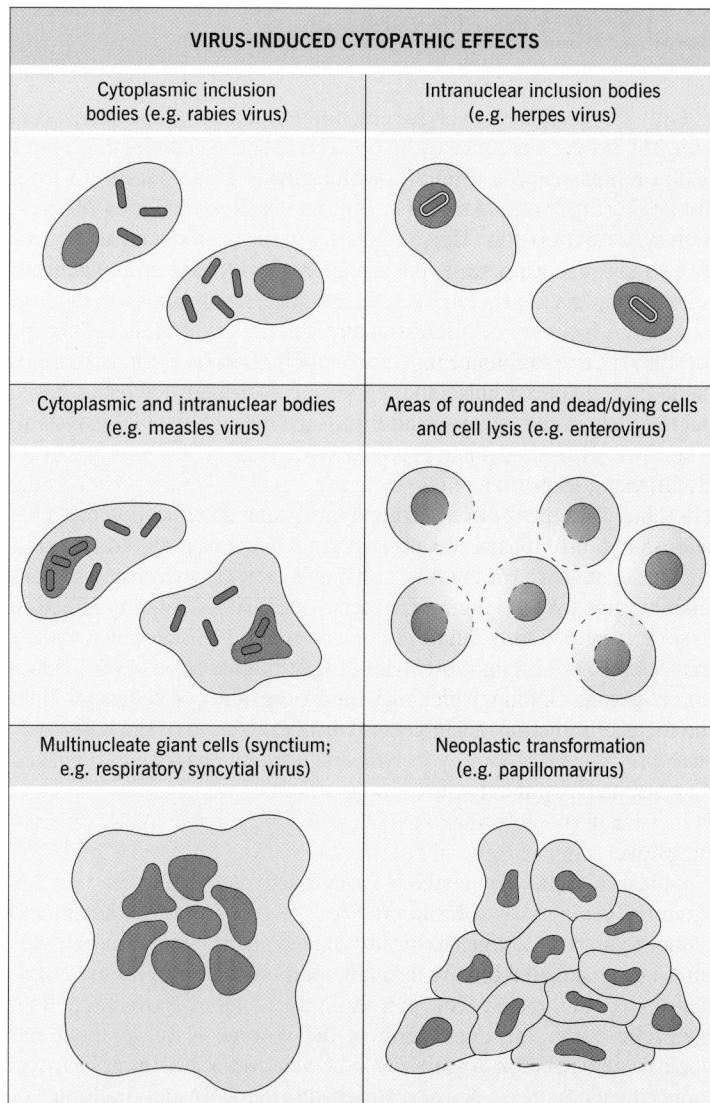

VIRUS-INDUCED CYTOPATHIC EFFECTS

Cytoplasmic inclusion bodies (e.g. rabies virus)	Intranuclear inclusion bodies (e.g. herpes virus)
Cytoplasmic and intranuclear bodies (e.g. measles virus)	Areas of rounded and dead/dying cells and cell lysis (e.g. enterovirus)
Multinucleate giant cells (synctium; e.g. respiratory syncytial virus)	Neoplastic transformation (e.g. papillomavirus)

Fig. 1.30 Virus-induced cytopathic effects.

Host cell transformation by viruses results in increased cellular multiplication rates and disorderly growth. It may be caused by DNA viruses (for instance Burkitt's lymphoma associated with Epstein–Barr virus), or retroviruses (adult T-cell leukemia caused by human T-cell lymphotropic virus type 1). Malignancy is induced by the expression of viral oncogenes, which closely resemble their cellular homologs.

Damage resulting from cytotoxic lymphocytes

The most effective host defense mechanism against most viral infections is mediated by the CD8+ cytotoxic T lymphocytes (CTLs). The CTLs recognize, attack and lyse virus-infected cells that present viral antigens on their surface in the context of MHC class I molecules. In addition to CTLs, natural killer lymphocytes similarly kill virus infected cells. The cytotoxic reaction contributes to the pathologic and the clinical picture of many viral diseases. The characteristic measles rash is produced after the attack of CTLs on skin cells infected by the measles virus. This explains why children with defects in cell-mediated immunity do not develop a rash during measles infection. In this disease, rash indeed represents a good immune response by the host, whereas its absence may signal uncontrolled viral growth. It is also believed that lymphocyte-induced cytotoxicity contributes to the pathology associated with persistent virus infections, such as the subacute sclerosing panencephalitis caused by a defective measles virus.

HARMFUL IMMUNE RESPONSES

The destructive potential of the immune system is considerable. It can damage the host in a variety of ways.

Autoimmunity

Autoimmune reactions break the rules of the 'self-versus-nonself' dichotomy. Autoimmune reactions, directed against 'self-proteins', may result from partial identity of antigenic determinants of the host and an infective agent, or from alterations of self-components caused by infection. Acute rheumatic fever occurring after group A streptococcal pharyngitis has been associated with antigens found in the cell wall of the streptococcus. These antigens cross-react with components of the heart muscle and the joint synovial membrane molecules, and thus induce an autoimmune response. Heat-shock proteins, which are omnipresent and remarkably conserved proteins in nature, are often associated with autoimmunity. Mycobacterial infection may give rise to antibodies and T lymphocytes that are reactive to both the microbial (nonself) and the host (self) heat-shock proteins.

Autoimmune reactions that follow an infection may also result from the release of self-components that are normally sequestered in a compartment that is relatively inaccessible to the immune system. Multiple sclerosis might provide an example of this type of autoimmune disease, although this is hypothetical because correlation of the disease with a microbial infection has as yet to be established.

Hypersensitivity reactions

Hypersensitivity reactions occur if the host immune system seemingly over-reacts to microbial infection. Hypersensitivity reactions have been classified by Gell and Coombs into four types.

Type I or immediate hypersensitivity. Type I hypersensitivity occurs within minutes of antigen exposure. It results from antigen binding to mast-cell-associated IgE. Vasoactive amines are released and anaphylactic reactions may develop. Certain forms of rash after helminth infections seem to be due to this type of hypersensitivity.

Type II or cytotoxic hypersensitivity . Type II hypersensitivity is consequence of the binding of specific antibodies to cell-surface-associated antigens. Antibody binding mediates cytoxicity via complement activation or natural killer cells. Thus cells bearing microbial antigens may be lyzed via an antibody-dependent mechanism. Such a mechanism has been suggested to account for liver cell necrosis during hepatitis B infection.

Type III or immune-complex-mediated hypersensitivity. Type III hypersensitivity is induced by classical complement activation, caused by extracellular antibody–antigen complexes. This causes inflammation

and changes in vascular permeability, and it attracts neutrophils to tissues where the immune complexes are deposited, including the kidneys, joints and small vessels of the skin. Glomerulonephritis in malaria is probably due to this mechanism.

Type IV or delayed-type hypersensitivity. Type IV hypersensitivity typically occurs at least 48 hours after exposure to an antigen. It involves activated T lymphocytes, which release cytokines, macrophages attracted by these cytokines, and cytotoxic CD8+ T lymphocytes.

Prolonged antigen exposure. During prolonged antigen exposure, such as in chronic infections, granuloma can be formed. Delayed-type hypersensitivity and granuloma play a major role in tissue damage observed during infections with slow-growing intracellular organisms, such as *Mycobacterium tuberculosis* (tuberculosis) and *Mycobacterium leprae* (leprosy), and histoplasmosis. Many of the clinical manifestations of chlamydial disease, in particular trachoma, seems to result from a delayed-type hypersensitivity triggered by chlamydial heat-shock proteins. In spite of the involvement of bacterial heat-shock proteins, this is not an autoimmune phenomenon, because the unique rather than the conserved portions of these proteins seem to be implicated here.

Superantigens and bacterial components associated with toxic and septic shock

Toxic shock and septic shock are exceptionally impressive syndromes associated with a variety of infectious diseases. Severe hypotension, multiple organ failure and intravascular disseminated coagulopathy occur in the most severe cases. Pathogenesis of these syndromes is complex. Various bacterial components, including lipopolysaccharides, peptidoglycan, lipoteichoic acid and (in some cases) toxins acting as superantigens (see Fig. 1.25) trigger an intense, potentially lethal host response. In the cascade of events leading to this condition, some cells (e.g. macrophages or T lymphocytes) play important roles (see Chapters 2.3 & 2.47) as well as releasing high levels of inflammatory response mediators, notably tumor necrosis factor and interleukin-1.

HOW MICRO-ORGANISMS ESCAPE HOST DEFENSE

In spite of the efficacy of host defense mechanisms, microbial pathogens can still infect humans and cause disease. This is in part due to the very potent weapons micro-organisms have – a single millilitre of botulinum toxin might kill more than 1 million people – but it is also due to intricate strategies that micro-organisms use to evade host defenses (Fig. 1.31).

SURVIVING THE PHAGOCYTE AND COMPLEMENT ATTACK

Immediately after passage of the epithelial surface, the invading micro-organism encounters the most powerful actors of host defense: phagocytes. Two main types of phagocytes are involved, the polymorphonuclear neutrophils (PMNs) and the macrophages. 'Professional' phagocytes can bind micro-organisms with a variety of receptors, some of which specifically interact with bacterial lipopolysaccharide or with antibodies bound to the microbial surface (opsonized micro-organisms). The micro-organisms usually pass into the cell via phagocytosis or pinocytosis, although some (especially viruses) may enter the cytosol directly.

Bacteria invariably go through an endosomal stage, in which they will be exposed to a multitude of macrophage defense mechanisms such as acidification, exposure to reactive oxygen species, bacteriocidic peptides and hydrolytic enzymes released after endosome–prolysosome fusion. In addition, in the endosomal pathway, micro-organisms are deprived of the nutritional wealth of the cytosol. Finally, the pathogens are killed and degraded, and the microbial antigens may be presented to lymphocytes. However, micro-organisms have developed strategies to avoid, mislead, deregulate, or even profit from phagocytes.[32]

EVASION OF HOST DEFENSES

Mechanism	Examples
Surviving the phagocyte and complement attack	
Inhibition of chemotaxis	C5a Peptidase by *Streptococcus pyogenes*
Killing the phagocyte before ingestion	α-Toxin and leukocidin by *Staphylococus aureus*
Avoiding ingestion	Bacterial capsules (e.g. *Streptococcus pneumoniae*)
	LPS O antigen in Gram-negative rods
	Coating with IgA antibodies (*Neisseria meningitidis*)
	M protein (*Streptococcus pyogenes*)
Surviving within phagocytes	Inhibition of phagolysosome fusion (*Chlamydia trachomatis*)
	Escape from phagolysosome (*Listeria monocytogenes*)
	Resistance to lysosomial products (*Salmonella typhimurium*)
	Inhibition of early host gene expression (*Mycobacterium tuberculosis*)
Antigenic variations	Shift and drift in influenza A virus
Tolerance	Prenatal infections
Immunosuppression	
Destroying lymphocytes	Depletion of CD4[+] lymphocytes by HIV
Proteolysis of antibodies	IgA protease by *Haemophilus influenzae*
Presence in inaccessible sites	Latent infection in dorsal root ganglia (herpes simplex virus)

Fig. 1.31 Evasion of host defenses.

Inhibition of the mobilization of phagocytes

Extracellular micro-organisms can avoid phagocytes by inhibiting chemotaxis or complement activation (see below). A bacterial enzyme that degrades complement protein C5a, a main chemoattractant for phagocytes, has been discovered recently in *Streptococcus pyogenes*. Pertussis toxin catalyzes ADP-ribolysation in neutrophils, which causes a rise in intracellular cAMP levels and ultimately impairs chemotaxis. Other examples of toxins that are directed against phagocytes include α-toxins produced by *Staphylococcus aureus*, streptolysins produced by *Streptococcus pyogenes*, and the γ-toxin of *Clostridium perfringens*.

Killing the phagocytes before being ingested

Many soluble products excreted by bacteria are potentially toxic for phagocytes entering the foci of infection. Streptolysin O binds to cholesterol in cell membranes, which results in rapid lysis of PMNs. In the process, the lysosomes are also disrupted and release their toxic contents, which may have deleterious effects on the neighboring cells. *Staphylococcus aureus* produces α, β and γ hemolysins, as well as leucocidin, which can kill and lyze the PMNs. Several toxins from *Clostridium perfringens* produce similar effects. Indeed, pus sampled from gas gangrene may contain numerous Gram-positive rods without any visible PMNs.

'Professional' phagocytes as vectors

Legionella pneumophila provokes entry in mononuclear phagocytes by accumulating complement factor C3bi on the envelope of the organism. This complement factor is a ligand for the phagocyte receptor CR3, and enhances phagocytosis. Following uptake, *Legionella* remains in the endosomes, which do not fuse with prelysosomes and

thus provide protection. Alveolar macrophages are host cells for *Mycobacterium tuberculosis*.[33] Like *Legionella*, phagocytosed *Mycobacterium* prevents fusion to the prelysosome and assumes a latent lifestyle. Many years after initial infection, resident *Mycobacterium* may be reactivated and cause acute disease.

Avoiding ingestion

The surface of numerous pathogenic bacteria is covered with a loose network of polymers, which constitute the bacterial capsule.[34] Capsular material may be very thin, visible only by electron microscopy, as is the case with the hyaluronate capsule of *Streptococcus pyogenes*. In some species (*Streptococcus pneumoniae*, *Klebsiella pneumoniae*) capsule material is abundant, easily visible with a light microscope and responsible for a mucoid aspect of the bacterial colonies. Most of the capsules are composed of polysaccharides, others are made of proteins or a combination of carbohydrate and protein. Some capsule contents mimic host polysaccharides and are thus recognized as 'self' by the host immune system. Examples are the capsules of *Neisseria meningitidis*, which contain sialic acid, and the capsules of *Streptococcus pyogenes*, which contain hyaluronic acid.

Capsules may protect bacteria from complement activation.[26] As a result, capsulated bacteria are not immediately recognized as invaders by the phagocytes. Capsulated *Streptococcus pneumoniae* resist engulfment by macrophages and PMNs and are virulent; however, noncapsulated strains are easily phagocytosed and are avirulent.[35] There are more than 80 distinct capsular serotypes, with different contributions to virulence, ranging from the highly virulent pneumococci of serotype 3 to the low virulent serotype 37.

The outer membrane of Gram-negative bacteria is covered with lipopolysaccharide (LPS), which serves as an attachment site for the complement fragments C3b (required for the triggering of the alternative pathway) and C5b. The polysaccharide chain of LPS (the O antigen) may contain sialic acid, which prevents formation of C3 convertase. It has also been shown that very long O antigen chains prevent the bacterial killing by the membrane attack complex (which is made from C5b, C6, C7, C8 and C9, and forms pores in the outer membrane of Gram-negative bacteria).

Meningococci circulating in the blood are coated with IgA, which is not an activator of the complement cascade. *Schistosoma mansoni* incorporates decay accelerating factors in its membrane; these are host plasma proteins that inhibit deposition of C3 onto host cell membranes. Activation of complement in the blood is thus avoided by the parasite.

Matrix proteins, which form fibrillae (see Fig. 1.17), are considered to be the primary virulence determinants of *Streptococcus pyogenes*. Matrix protein renders the bacteria resistant to phagocytosis by human neutrophils. Matrix fibrillae are approximately 50–60nm in length and exhibit a seven-residue periodicity. They exist as stable dimers, arranged in a coiled coil configuration, with the carboxyl-terminal portion closely associated with the cell wall (see Fig. 1.17). Streptococci that express M proteins on their surface are poorly opsonized by the alternate pathway and resist PMN phagocytosis. In contrast, streptococci that fail to express M protein are readily opsonized and phagocytosed. Resistance to phagocytosis can be overcome by antibodies directed against type-specific M epitopes. The mechanism of antiphagocytic activity of M proteins is still unclear. According to one hypothesis, fibrinogen, known to bind to M protein, may hinder access to complement-binding sites on the bacterial surface, disguising the pathogen as 'self'. In another hypothesis, a complement control protein (protein H), which also binds M, may be responsible for the observed complement resistance of virulent *Streptococcus pyogenes*.

Survival within phagocytes

Once ingested by the phagocyte, the pathogen may survive and grow using a variety of strategies (Fig. 1.32). Some microbes prevent exposure to hydrolytic enzymes by inhibiting the fusion of the endosome with the prolysosome, others are capable of surviving within the

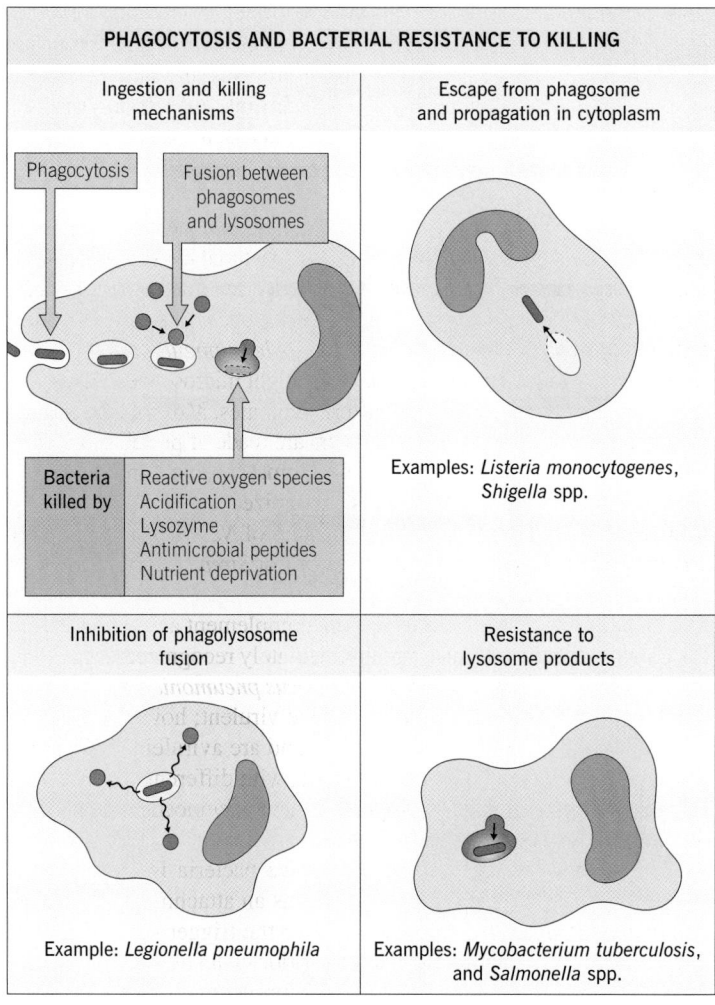

Fig. 1.32 Phagocytosis and bacterial resistance to killing.

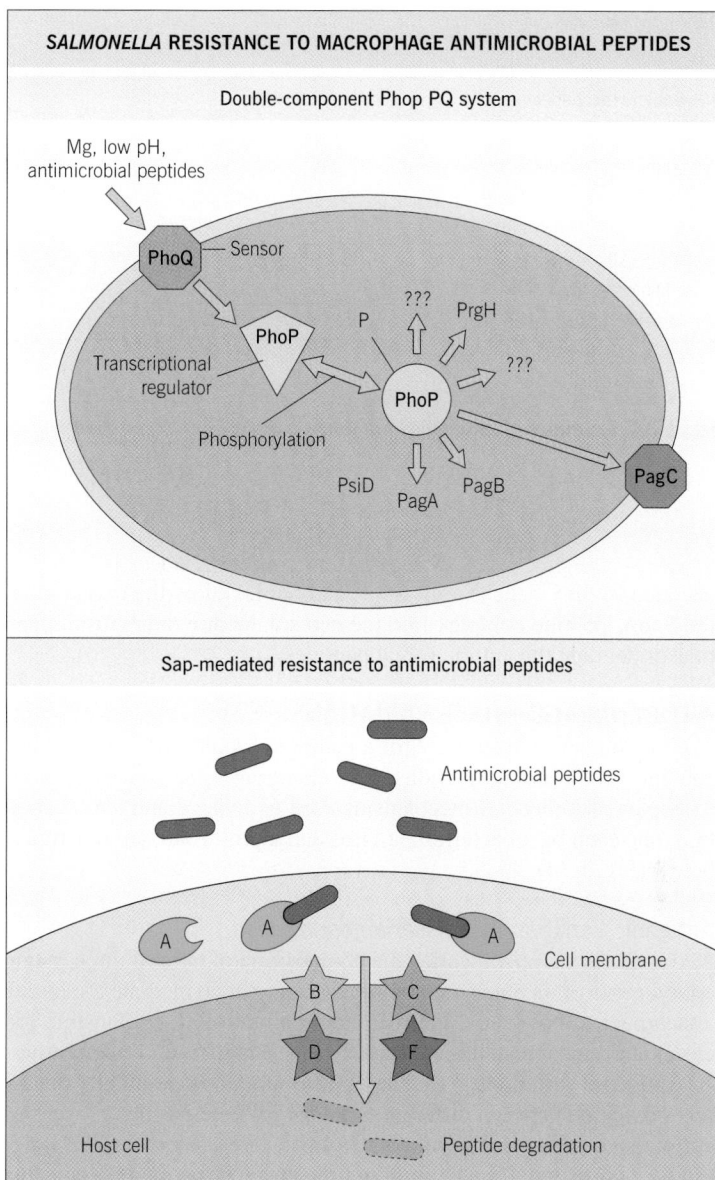

Fig. 1.33 Mechanisms of resistance to macrophage antimicrobial peptides by *Salmonella* spp. *Salmonella* produces the SapA (A) peptide, which complexes with host cell antimicrobial peptides. Other proteins encoded by the *sap* locus (SapB, SapC and SapD) are required for the transport of the SapA-antimicrobial peptide complex into the cytosol where the antimicrobial peptide is degraded. The other mechanism is the double component Phop PQ system: a sensor, PhoQ, located in the cytoplasmic membrane, is stimulated by antimicrobial peptides, activating PhoP, a transcriptional regulator, by phosphorylation. As a consequence, a series of genes are activated (*pag* genes) or repressed (*prg* genes), providing protection against antimicrobial peptides.

phagolysosome because they resist enzymatic degradation or neutralize lysosomal toxic products. Certain types of bacteria rapidly escape from the phagolysome and propagate in the cytoplasm, as described above for *Listeria monocytogenes*. Recent studies suggest that intracellular pathogens, notably *Mycobacterium tuberculosis*, may inhibit the early host response at the level of host gene expression.

Inhibition of phagolysomal fusion

Salmonella spp. have developed several strategies to survive and propagate in macrophages; *Salmonella* spp. that lack this capacity to survive in macrophages are avirulent. Several hours after infection *in vitro*, two distinct *Salmonella* populations can be seen in the macrophage. One consists of rapidly dividing bacteria located in large unfused phagosomes. This population may rapidly grow and kill the macrophage, leading to the liberation of intracellular bacteria.[36] *In vivo*, this population may be responsible for the acute stage of salmonellosis.

The second population of *Salmonella* consists of nondividing organisms located in phagolysosomes. This population resists the toxic effect of lysosomal products, and are believed to account for the prolonged survival of *Salmonella* spp. in the body. Long-living stromal macrophages of the bone marrow may act as long-term *Salmonella* carriers and be responsible for the very late relapses of salmonellosis that are seen in some patients. The dormant phase represents a well-regulated physiologic condition associated with nutrient deprivation *in vitro*.

Inactivation of reactive oxygen species

Reactive oxygen species damage DNA and inhibit the bacterial oxidative phosphorylation. *Salmonella* spp. produce superoxide dismutase (SOD) and catalase, two enzymes that might eliminate the reactive

oxygen species. In addition, the damage to DNA is efficiently repaired through a RecA-dependent pathway. This pathway seems to be more important than the production of SOD and catalase because mutants that produce neither SOD nor catalase remain virulent, whereas *rec*A mutants are avirulent.

Resistance to antimicrobial peptides

Several cationic peptides are produced within the lysosomal granules and are believed to kill intracellular pathogens by forming channels in the bacterial cell wall. *Salmonella* spp. resists these antimicrobial peptides by at least two mechanisms (Fig. 1.33), one of which, encoded by the *sap* locus, is characterized in some detail. It seems that the SapA protein forms a complex with the antimicrobial peptides, reducing the deleterious effect on the bacterial membranes. Other proteins

EXAMPLES OF ANTIGENIC VARIATIONS

Generic mechanisms	Examples
Recombination between different copies of pilin genes	Pili in *Neisseria gonorrhoeae*
Phase variation – turning expression of an antigen on or off ('flip-flop')	Flagella in *Salmonella*; pili in *Neisseria gonorrhoeae*
Gene reassortment between two strains infecting the same cell	Influenza virus type A
Mutation of surface antigens	Influenza virus type A, B and C
Gene switch leading to surface glycoprotein changes	*Trypanosoma brucei*

Fig. 1.34 Examples of antigenic variations.

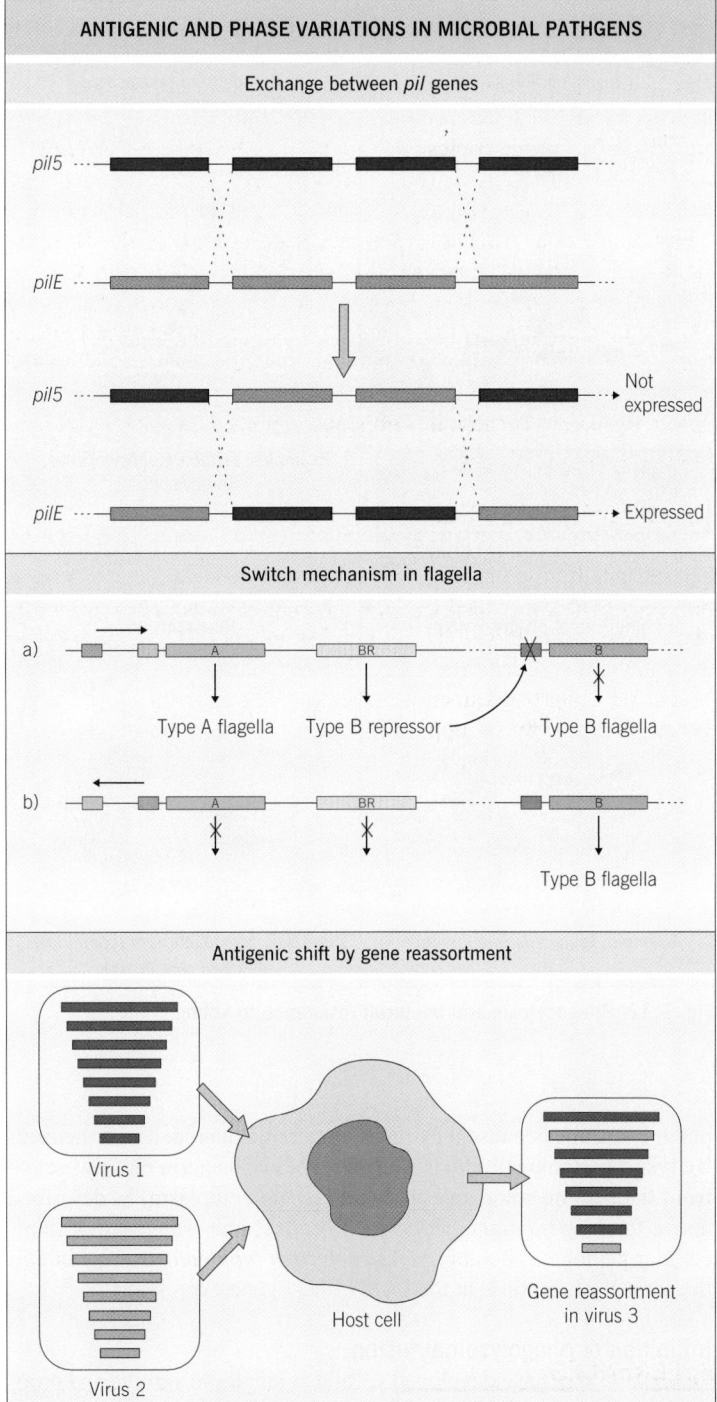

encoded by *sap* locus (SapB, SapC and SapD) allow the transport of the SapA–peptide complex into the cytosol. Within the cytosol, peptidases degrade the antimicrobial peptides.

ANTIGENIC AND PHASE VARIATIONS

A powerful survival strategy for a pathogen would be to mislead the specific host immune response by 'changing appearances'. Three examples of molecular mechanisms used to achieve antigenic variation, one each by a bacterium, a virus and a protozoan, are illustrated below (Fig. 1.34).

Antigenic variation in *Neisseria gonorrhoeae*

Neisseria gonorrhoeae varies the composition of at least three major components of its outer membrane: the pili, which mediate the initial attachment to host cells; the membrane protein P.II, responsible for closer attachment resulting in phagocytosis; and LPS, described earlier.

Antigenic variations in the major pilin subunit is essentially due to recombination between different copies of *pil* genes scattered over the chromosome (Fig. 1.35). Only one or two of these are expressed (*pilE* – E for 'expressed') at any point in time, but an array of antigenically distinct pili may be produced in response to an antibody challenge. In addition to this mechanism, pili are subject to phase variation (i.e. switches between *pil*-positive and *pil*-negative variants). Phase variation is controlled at the transcriptional level.

The P.II protein is similarly subject to genetic variation. As a consequence, the specific immune response never quite catches up with genetic variation in the bacterial population. The combination of this mechanism, LPS sialylation (see above) and IgA protease production makes *Neisseria gonorrhoeae* a very recalcitrant pathogen.

Shift and drift in influenza A viruses

Nearly every year, during the recurrent influenza epidemics, vaccination programs are confronted with the problem of antigenic variation. Two different mechanisms account for genetic variation of influenza virus. Antigenic shift results from the infection of a single cell by two different influenza strains. 'New' genomes may be assembled from the available genetic information, leading to gene exchange between the two parent strains. Antigenic shift may result in dramatic changes in the antigenic composition of the surface hemagglutinin (which binds the host cell receptor) or the neuraminidase (which modifies these receptors), and cause devastating epidemics in immunologically unprepared populations. Antigenic drift results from high mutation rates associated with RNA viruses. In influenza viruses A, B and C, mutants with antigenic changes tend to have a selective advantage over the nonmutant viral population. Therefore, new strains are continually being selected, as exemplified by the 1997 outbreak of 'chicken flu' in Hong Kong.

Fig. 1.35 Antigenic and phase variations in microbial pathogens. Three mechanisms are shown. (Top) Exchange of DNA between nonexpressed copies of *pilS* and the expressed gene *pilE* in *Neisseria gonorrhoeae* can change the expressed antigen. (Middle) A switch mechanism is responsible for the (mutually exclusive) production of type A and type B flagella in *Salmonella typhimurium*. Phase variation depends on the orientation of a DNA fragment adjacent to the type A flagella gene. When A is expressed (a) from the promoter in the invertable fragment, the repressor for the type B flagella is expressed at the same time. As a consequence the type B flagella gene is repressed. Inversion of the DNA fragment abolishes expression of the A-repressor gene and the B-repressor gene (b). In this situation type B flagella are produced. (Bottom) Antigenic shift by gene reassortment results from infection of a single cell by two different virions.

Antigenic variations in *Trypanosoma brucei*

African trypanosomes (*Trypanosoma brucei*) are flagellated protozoa, transmitted to humans by several species of *Glossina* (tsetse). The parasite survives in mammalian body fluids thanks to antigenic variation of the variant surface glycoprotein (VSG), which forms a 15nm thick monolayer covering most of the parasite surface.[37] Within a single generation, most or all of the 10^7 VSG molecules may be replaced by an unrelated species, stemming from a repertoire of an estimated 1000 genomic copies of the gene. The VSG gene is invariably expressed from a polycistronic transcription unit, in the so-called telomeric expression site adjacent to the telomeric repeats. During chronic infection, patients experience successive episodes of parasitemia, each episode coinciding with the expression of a new VSG on the surface of the parasite. With this strategy, trypanosomes avoid complete eradication by the specific immune response, while maintaining the pathogenic burden at sublethal levels. The closely related *T. brucei brucei*, which causes the bovine disease nagana, does not spread to humans because it is sensitive to high-density lipoprotein in human serum.

IMMUNOSUPPRESSION

The most illustrative example of immunosuppression induced by microbial infection is provided by HIV. Human immunodeficiency virus circulating in the blood stream readily infects CD4+ lymphocytes, macrophages and dendritic cells. The destruction of CD4+ T-helper cells is particularly detrimental to the host and accounts for the emergence of a variety of opportunistic infections as soon as the T-lymphocyte counts drops below a critical level.

Other viruses may produce immunosuppression in a more subtle fashion. Measles virus infects both B lymphocytes and T lymphocytes, interfering with the immunocompetence of the host. As a consequence, in areas with a high prevalence of tuberculosis, measles epidemics may be followed by outbreaks of tuberculosis. Gonococci, meningococci, and *Haemophilus influenzae* produce proteases that hydrolyse secretory IgA1 antibodies. Protease negative mutants of these bacterial strains are less virulent, suggesting a role for mucosal IgA1 antibodies in host defense against these pathogens.

CONCLUSION

Throughout evolution, man, like all mammalian species, has maintained an intimate relationship with the microbial world. We have survived thanks to the efficient defense mechanisms we have developed against potentially dangerous micro-organisms. Pathogenic micro-organisms are still here because they have found ways of avoiding elimination by their host or by the microbial competition. 'Successful' pathogens have developed strategies to enter the body and reach and colonize their favorite niche, while defying the powerful human immune system.

In this chapter we have looked into microbial survival strategies. Although some of these have been analyzed in 'molecular detail', a lot remains to be discovered. Future remedies for infectious diseases are likely to be aimed at specific molecular interactions between the pathogenic micro-organism and its host.

REFERENCES

1. Woese CR. There must be a prokaryote somewhere: microbiology's search for itself. Microbiol Rev 1994;58:1–9.
2. Kobayashi GS. Fungi. In: Davies BD, Dulbecco R, Elsen HN, Ginsberg HS, eds. Microbiology, 4th ed. Philadelphia: JB Lippincott; 1990:737–65.
3. Stringer JR. *Pneumocystis carinii*: what it is exactly? Clin Microbiol Rev 1996;9:489–98
4. Collier L, Oxford J. Human virology. Oxford: Oxford University Press; 1990:8–10.
5. Wirth R, Muscholl A, Wanner G. The role of pheromones in bacterial interactions. Trends Microbiol 1996;4:96–104.
6. Frank J, Zhu J, Ponczek P, *et al*. A model of protein synthesis based on cryo-electron microscopy of the *E. coli* ribosome. Nature 1995;376:441–4.
7. Freishmann RD, Adams MD, White O, *et al*. Whole genome random sequencing and assembly of *Haemophilus influenzae* Rd. Science 1995;269:496–512.
8. Macnab RM. Flagella and motility. In: Neidhardt FC, ed. *Escherichia coli* and *Salmonella* cellular and molecular biology, 2nd ed. Washington DC: ASM Press; 1996:123–57.

9. Pechère JC. Stratégies du microbe. In: Pechère JC, Acar J, Armengaud M, *et al*, eds. Les infections, 3rd ed. Quebec: Edisem; 1991:3–20.
10. Hultgren SJ, Abraham S, Caparon M, *et al*. Pilus and nonpilus bacterial adhesions: assembly and function in cell recognition. Cell 1993:73:887–901.
11. Gaastra W, Svennerholm A-M. Colonization factors of human enterotoxigenic *Escherichia coli* (ETEC). Trends Microbiol 1996;4:444–52.
12. Hultgren SL, Normark S, Abraham SN. Chaperone-assisted assembly and molecular architecture of adhesive pili. Annu Rev Microbiol 1991;43:383–415.
13. Kehoe MA. Group A streptococcal antigens and vaccine potential. Vaccine 1991;9:797–806.
14. Fishetti VA. Streptococcal M protein: molecular design and biological behavior. Clin Microbiol Rev 1989;2:285–314.
15. White JM. Membrane fusion. Science 1992;258:917–24.
16. Siebers A, Finlay BB. M cells and the pathogenesis of microsal and systemic infections. Trends Microbiol 1996;4:22–8.

17. Ménard R, Dehio C, Sansonetti PJ. Bacterial entry into epithelial cells: the paradigm of *Shigella*. Trends Microbiol 1996;4:220–6.
18. Galan JE. Molecular genetic basis of *Salmonella* entry into host cells. Mol Microbiol 1996;20:263–71.
19. Hacker J, Blum-Oehler G, Mühldorfer I, Tschäpe H. Pathogenicity islands of virulent bacteria: structure, function and impact on microbial evolution. Mol Microbiol 1997;23:1089–97.
20. Hermant D, Ménard R, Arricau N, Parsot C, Popoff MY. Functional conservation of the *Salmonella* and *Shigella* effectors of entry in epithelial cells. Mol Microbiol 1995;17:785–9.
21. Sanders MC, Theriot JA. Tails from the hall of infection: actin-based motility of pathogens. Trends Microbiol 1996;4:211–3.
22. Kocks C, Marchaud J-B, Gouin E, *et al*. The unrelated proteins ActA of *Listeria monocytogenes* and LcsA of *Shigella flexneri* are sufficient to confer actin-based motility on *Listeria innocua* and *Escherichia coli* respectively. Mol Microbiol 1995;18:413–23.

23. Dramsi S, Lebrun M, Cossart P. Molecular and genetic determinants involved in invasion of mammalian cells by *Listeria monocytogenes*. Curr Top Microbiol Immunol 1995;209:61–78.

24. Mounier J, Ryter A, Coquis-Rondon M, Sansonetti P. Intracellular and cell-to-cell spread of *Listeria monocytogenes* involves interaction with F-actin in enterocytelike cell line Caco-2. Infect Immun 1990;58:1048–58.

25. Döring RE, Marcil A, Chopra A, Richardson CD. The human CD46 molecule is a receptor for measles virus (Edmonston strain). Cell 1993;75:295–305.

26. Horstmann RD. Target recognition failure by the nonspecific defense system: surface constituents of pathogens interfere with the alternative pathway of complement activation. Infect Immun 1992;60:721–7.

27. Martin SJ, Green DR. Protease activation during apoptosis death by a thousand cuts? Cell 1995;82:349–52.

28. Laurent-Crawford AG, Krust GB, Muller S, *et al*. The cytopathic effect of HIV is associated with apoptosis. Virology 1991;185:829–39.

29. Khelef N, Zychlinsky A, Guiso N. *Bordetella pertussis* induces apoptosis in macrophages: role of adenylate cyclase hemolysis. Infect Immun 1993;61:4064–71.

30. Zychinsky A, Kenny B, Ménard R, *et al*. IpaB mediates macrophage apoptosis induced by *Shigella flexneri*. Mol Microbiol 1994;11:619–27.

31. Chen Y, Smith MR, Thizumalai K, Zychlinsky A. A bacterial invasion induces macrophage apoptosis by binding directly to ICE. EMBO J 1996;15:3853–60.

32. Russel DG. Of microbes and macrophages: entry, survival and persistence. Curr Opin Immunol 1995;7:479–84.

33. Clemens DL. Characterization of the *Mycobacterium tuberculosis* phagosome. Trends Microbiol 1996;4:113–8.

34. Gross A. The biological significance of bacterial encapsulation. Curr Top Microbiol Immunol 1990;150:87–95.

35. Bruyn GAW, Zeyers, BJM, van Furth R. Mechanisms of host defense against infection with *Streptococcus pneumoniae*. Clin Infect Dis 1992;14:251–62.

36. Radman M, Sjaastad MD, Falkow S. Acidification of phagosomes containing *Salmonella typhimurium* in murine macrophages. Infect Immun 1996;64:2765–73.

37. Pays E, Vanhamme L, Berberoff M. Genetic controls for the expression of surface antigens in African trypanosomes. Annu Rev Microbiol 1994;48:25–52.

Host Responses to Infection

Gerald T Keusch

INTRODUCTION

The need for parasitism, as for evil, has never been satisfactorily explained. In its less severe manifestations – for example, competitive interactions within the food chain – parasitism could have led to the classic 'fight or flight' response because the ability to withstand an 'eat or be eaten' situation would have obvious survival value. However, when competing organisms are placed within a balanced ecosystem they do not require overly aggressive parasitism for survival. The hallmark of such ecosystems is that the individual organisms within it consume no more than they need for survival, for to do so would perturb the whole system.

As the new millennium approaches we are increasingly becoming aware of the reality that our lives are permeated by the effects of inter-related systems, and, as a result, we are all beginning to think ecologically. This readily extends to clinical microbiology and infectious diseases, in which ecologic niches and ecosystems determine the nature and components of the microbial flora living on us humans, as well as their impact on health and disease.

In this sense, the 'normal flora' can be considered as an example of 'ecoparasitism', which implies a balanced system that sustains multiple microbial species, each occupying a particular niche. If this is so, then the development of specific host defenses to normal flora might be not only unnecessary but even detrimental if there is a 'cost' resulting from the diversion of metabolic resources from functions of growth or maintenance to the synthesis of unneeded immunologically active cells and their products. However, host defenses have evolved in a complex and functionally overlapping manner, suggesting that true parasitism has always been a serious threat to survival and that evolution of pathogens and host defenses are linked by selection pressures.

It is important at the outset to understand that host defenses are not limited to the immune response, defined as an induced cellular or humoral defense mechanism that is specific for the challenging agents or their cell-free antigens.[1] The simple presence of an intact integument, normal gastric acid secretion, peristalsis or mucin production may exert profound protective effects for the host in the context of host–pathogen interactions. In addition, many metabolic and physiologic events are initiated in the course of infections, and these must be understood as being part of the host response to microbial challenge. The context is even broader, for these events are not restricted to infection but are part of a stereotyped response to other processes that activate the inflammatory response, including trauma and surgery, vasculitis, and connective tissue diseases such as rheumatoid arthritis. Nonantigen-specific metabolic events are also triggered by inflammation of any etiology; their relationship to host response is discussed first in this chapter because they are the least appreciated events in host defense, appear to be of survival value and are as dependent on molecular signaling as are the antigen-specific responses.

GENERAL SIGNS, SYMPTOMS AND CONSEQUENCES OF THE HOST RESPONSE TO INFECTION

The classic peripheral signs and symptoms of inflammation (rubor, calor, dolor and tumor – redness, heat, pain and swelling) commonly go hand in hand with general systemic signs and symptoms such as fever, chills, myalgias, headache and anorexia (Fig. 2.1). This relationship between peripheral and systemic responses is one consequence of the common mechanisms that initiate and mediate these events (see Fig. 2.2). With progression of the underlying process involved in the activation of inflammation, a clinically recognizable syndrome, the systemic inflammatory response syndrome, may become manifest. When the systemic inflammatory response syndrome is caused by infection it is called sepsis, which, if uncontrolled, can evolve further into the sepsis syndrome with its life-threatening consequences of septic shock and multiple-organ dysfunction syndrome (see Fig. 2.3; Chapter 2.47). If these events are viewed in evolutionary terms, there must be a range within which they are beneficial to the host in response to the inflammatory stimulus or for combating an infection, but when they occur in excess and are uncontrolled they may prove to be harmful or even

CONSEQUENCES OF THE GENERAL CLINICAL RESPONSES TO INFECTION AND INFLAMMATION		
Sign/ symptom	Metabolic effect	Benefit for host
Fever	Increased energy consumption is required to cause and maintain body temperature above normal Enzyme reactions are accelerated	Beneficial effect on survival at moderate increases [102–104°F (39–40°C)]. May be detrimental with more marked increases [e.g. >107°F (>42°C)]
Anorexia	Decreased nutrient intake requires catabolism of body stores for new protein synthesis Amino acids are converted to glucose by way of hepatic gluconeogenesis	No apparent benefit in infection May permit survival during the healing process after trauma
Lethargy	Decreased voluntary activity reduces energy needs	Benefits of rest documented in some infections (poliovirus, Coxsackie B4 virus) in which exercise increases severity of clinical manifestations Allows metabolic support to be directed to host defense responses
Myalgia	Result of muscle activity and muscle catabolism to breakdown muscle protein releases amino acids into the circulation	Generates heat to elevate body temperature Provides source of amino acids for increased protein synthesis of host defense molecules and cells

Fig. 2.1 Consequences of the general symptom responses to infection and inflammation.

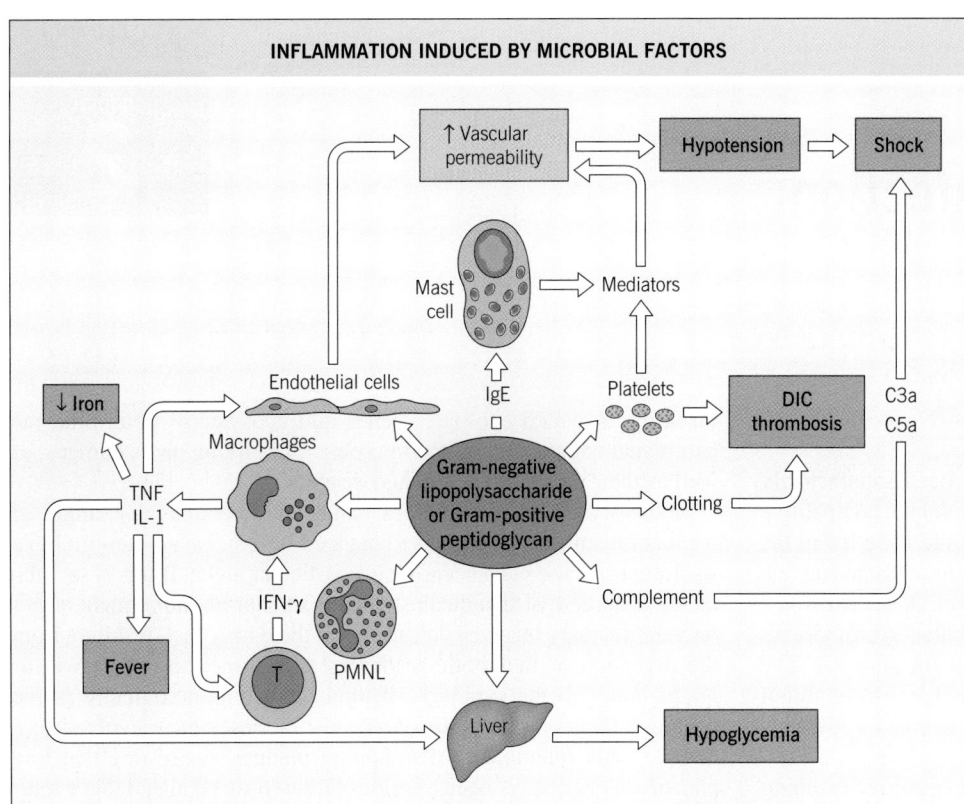

Fig. 2.2 Pathways of inflammation induced by microbial factors. Components of Gram-negative organisms (lipopolysaccharide) and Gram-positive bacteria (peptidoglycan) can activate similar pathogens. C3a, biologically active soluble cleavage product of the activation of complement factor 3; C5a, biologically active soluble cleavage product of the activation of complement factor 5; DIC, disseminated intravascular coagulation; IFN, interferon; IL, interleukin; PMNL, polymorphonuclear leukocyte; TNF, tumor necrosis factor.

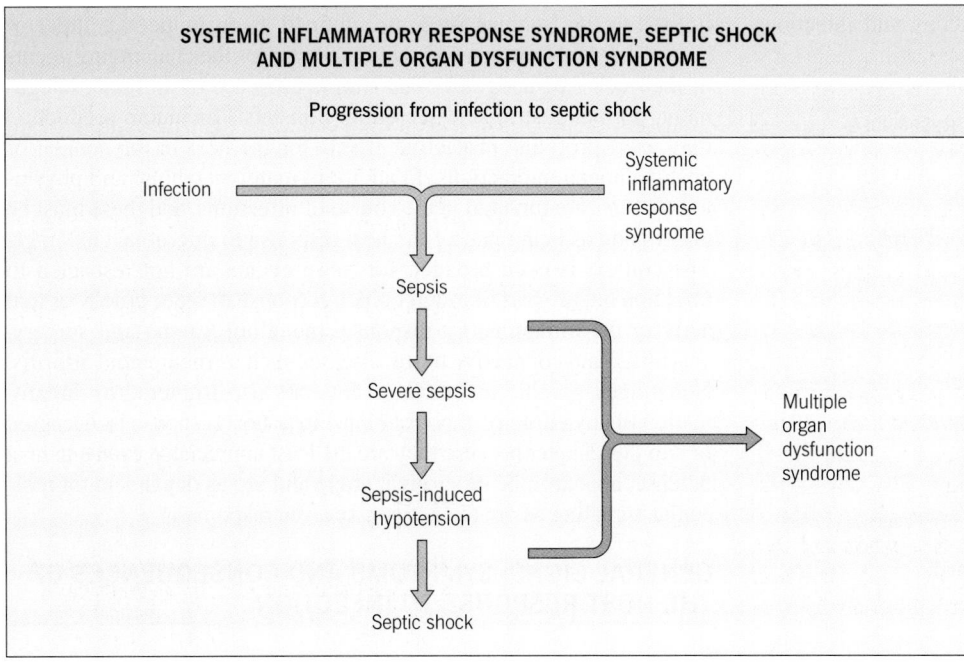

Fig. 2.3 Systemic inflammatory response syndrome, septic shock and multiple organ dysfunction syndrome.

lethal. It is not always clear, however, what the beneficial effect may be, or where the threshold for adverse effects begins.

FEVER

This most readily recognized manifestation of inflammation has no doubt been known since the first parent touched her or his hand to the forehead of a sick child. The importance of fever as a marker of clinical status and the need for the body to control temperature in response to contagion were also recognized long before the instruments of clinical thermometry were introduced into common use for quantifying body temperature (Chapter 3.1).[2]

Fever is now understood as an elevation in body core temperature resulting from a resetting of the thermostatic regulatory system. Fever usually follows the same diurnal variation in core temperature exhibited in health, but with exaggerations in the slope and height of the peaks, often returning to normal levels between fever spikes. Temperature may also be continuously elevated, without returning to a normal baseline. These various fever patterns occur because fever is a regulated process in which alterations in the thermostatic control mechanisms in the hypothalamus of the brain are used to regulate heat production and heat loss in response to the new thermostatic set point to achieve the new temperature. Because there are important individual variations in the fever response to a given stimulus as well as variations in the response to different stimuli and in the effects of light–dark cycles and hormonal controls on body temperature, graphs of fever plotted against time have not proved to have much diagnostic

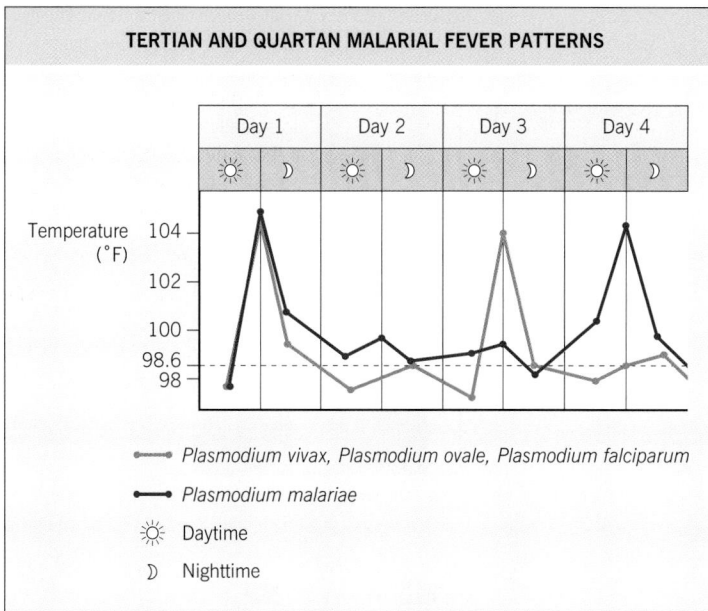

Fig. 2.4 **Tertian and quartan malarial fever patterns.**

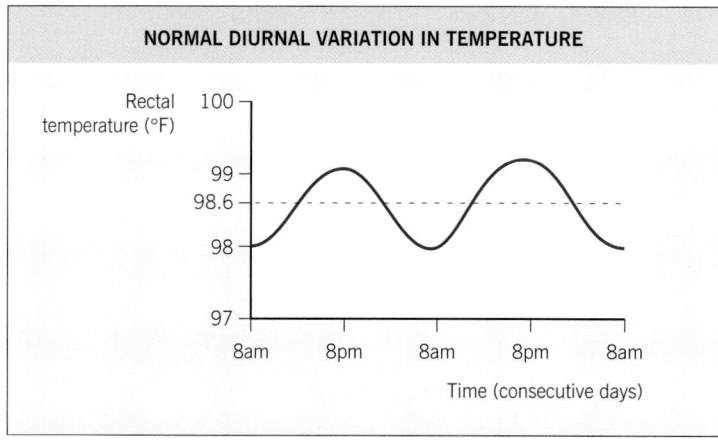

Fig. 2.5 **Normal diurnal variation in temperature.** These data are from 8 healthy volunteers (see Chapter 3.1).

PHYSIOLOGY AND MECHANISMS OF THERMOREGULATION			
Process		Mechanism and clinical manifestations	Physiologic regulation
Heat generation	Metabolic heat production	Involuntary muscle activity generating heat without work; manifested by shivering	Yes, by way of hypothalamic thermoregulatory centers; highly efficient
	Heat retention	Peripheral vasoconstriction lowers skin temperature and reduces heat loss by all mechanisms listed below	Yes, by way of vasomotor responses
Heat loss	Conduction	Heat transfer by direct contact of skin and another surface at a lower temperature; no clinical manifestations	Indirectly, by way of vasomotor responses; inefficient and limited because temperature equilibration rapidly occurs
	Convection	Heat transfer from skin to ambient air, facilitated by moving air; cooling of skin may induce shivering and vasoconstriction	Indirectly, by way of vasomotor responses
	Radiation	Heat transfer to another surface at a lower temperature without direct contact; no clinical manifestations	Indirectly, by way of vasomotor responses
	Sweating	Activation of sweat secretions consumes energy and releases heat through evaporation of sweat	Directly, by control of sweat glands by the hypothalamic thermoregulatory centers Indirectly, by vasomotor responses

Fig. 2.6 **Physiology and mechanisms of thermoregulation.**

significance (as was once believed when little else of specific diagnostic value was available – for example, tertian and quartan fever patterns were once thought useful for the presumptive etiologic diagnosis of malaria but are rarely observed) (Fig. 2.4).

Normal body temperature is 98.6°F (37°C) ± 1.8°F (1°C) (95% CI); it is lowest in the early morning and highest in the evening (Fig. 2.5). This is one reason why there is no single definition of the lower limit of fever. However, as body temperature cools below 96.8°F (36°C), metabolic processes slow, brain function may become impaired, respiration slows and metabolic needs decline. Controlled hypothermia, as in cardiac surgery, or hypothermia induced by immersion in cold water may, for a while, protect vital organs. As the period of hypothermia becomes longer and the temperature continues to drop, however, metabolism becomes increasingly anaerobic, resulting in acidosis and ultimately in fatal cardiac arrhythmias.

The principal mechanism for generating heat is muscle activity, which burns energy and produces work, with heat as a byproduct. In the development of a febrile response, involuntary muscle activity is controlled by the central nervous system (CNS), resulting in the shivering and rigors that occur as the temperature begins to climb. The slope of the rise and the ultimate peak of the temperature are also regulated by heat-loss mechanisms, and it is the combination of heat production and heat loss that results in the clinical temperature curve (Fig. 2.6). Heat loss occurs via four principal mechanisms under physiologic control:
• conduction,
• convection,
• radiation, and
• sweating.

Conduction is the direct transfer of heat between two surfaces in direct contact, from the higher to the lower temperature surface, until the temperature at the interface is equalized.

Convection is the removal of heat from a solid body to air at a cooler temperature, and it is facilitated by moving air across the convecting body, as by the use of a fan.

Radiation is the transfer of heat from one surface to another at a lower temperature across a distance. Black surfaces can absorb this radiated heat whereas white surfaces may reflect it; thus the nature as well as the temperature of the surface receiving radiated heat determines the efficiency of the process. Each of these mechanisms depends on temperature at the skin surface, and this is physiologically controlled by vasodilatation, which brings warmed blood to the skin and warms the skin surface.

Sweating is an important and effective mechanism of heat loss, as any one who has defervesced after taking aspirin will attest, because profuse sweating accompanies the rapid decline in body temperature towards the normal range.

The sequential engagement of these mechanisms results in shaking chills as muscle activity and peripheral vasoconstriction are called into play. This is followed by a sensation of fever as vasodilatation occurs to bring heat to the surface for conductive, convective and radiative loss of heat in order to blunt the rise in core temperature. This is followed by profuse sweating as core temperature is rapidly brought to a lower level before the next fever spike initiates the entire sequence again.

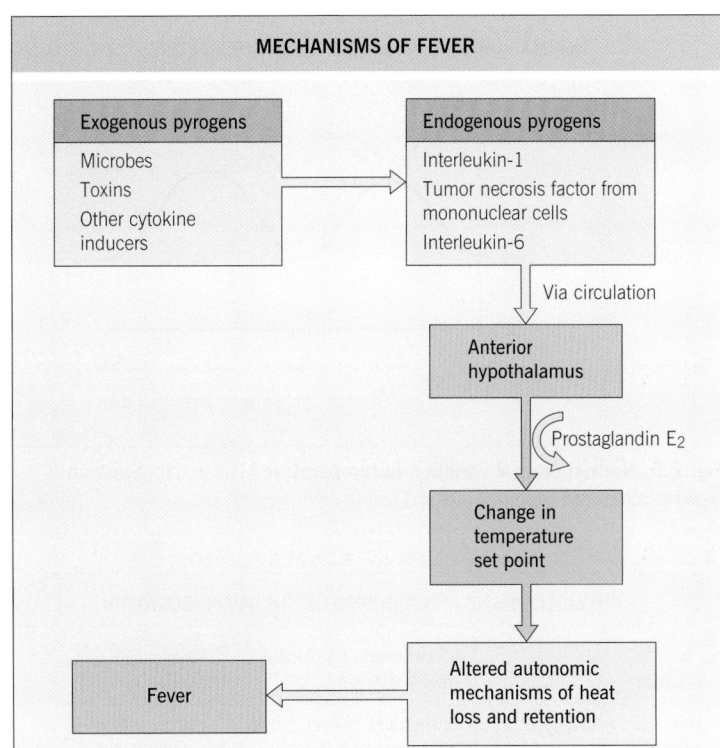

Fig. 2.7 Mechanisms of fever. Fever may be induced either by exogenous pyrogens, such as microbes or their toxins, or by endogenous pyrogens.

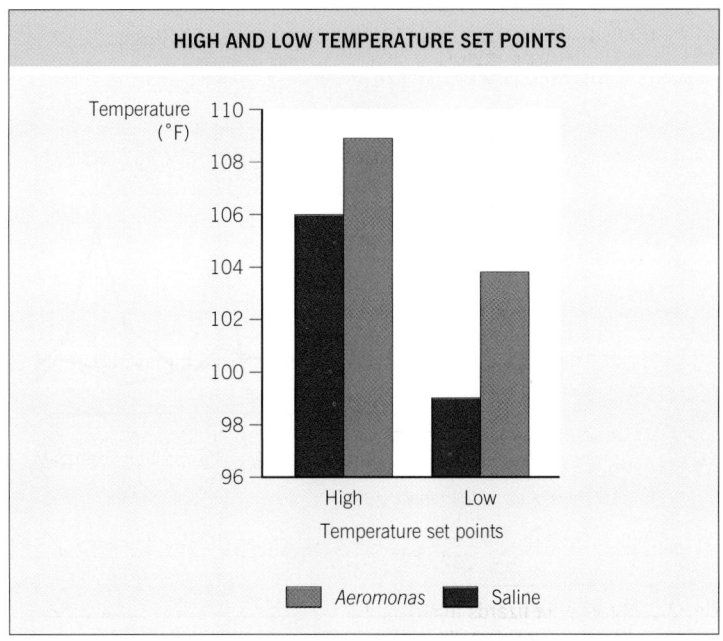

Fig. 2.8 High and low temperature set points. The temperature set point is the temperature at which the animal modifies temperature by moving in the temperature gradient chamber. The increased high and low setpoints in the animals challenged with *Aeromonas hydrophila* results in higher than normal temperature. The data were measured 3–6 hours after injection with saline or *Aeromonas hydrophila*. Data from Vaughan LK et al.[10]

Fever also has an upper limit, with temperatures above 106–108°F (41–42°C) rarely if ever noted.[3] At sustained temperatures above this range, as may occur during heat stroke, biologic abnormalities occur; these abnormalities include:
- acid–base changes due to hyperventilation and respiratory alkalosis,
- hypokalemia,
- hypernatremia and other electrolyte abnormalities,
- circulatory failure,
- shock, and
- disseminated intravascular coagulation, with cell swelling and damage in the brain, kidneys and liver, along with widespread hemorrhages.

Biologic alterations also occur, any one of which carries the potential of death; these changes include:[4]
- hypoxia and mitochondrial damage,
- energy depletion,
- protein denaturation,
- protein phosphorylation,
- ribosomal dysfunction,
- diminished protein synthesis,
- lysosomal enzyme release,
- changes in cytoskeletal and structural proteins,
- altered cell membrane fluidity owing to altered cholesterol and phospholipid content, and
- degradation or damage of DNA.

Temperature is regulated by warm- and cold-sensitive neurons in the CNS located in the preoptic region, anterior hypothalamus and adjacent septal areas.[5] Direct temperature alterations induced in these regions of the brain lead to all of the behavioral and physiologic events involved in normal thermoregulatory responses. The preoptic region and the anterior hypothalamus are strategically located near the organum vasculosum of the lamina terminalis (OVLT), the site of transfer of cytokines from blood to brain. This is significant because some cytokines [e.g. interleukin (IL)-1β and tumor necrosis factor (TNF)-α, and possibly IL-6 and interferon (IFN)-γ] are the principal peripheral signals to the brain to reset the normal temperature set point to cause fever (Fig. 2.7).[6] This signaling is mediated through the production of prostaglandin E₁, and is regulated by a number of possible endogenous

antipyretic mediators, such as arginine vasopressin, α-melanocyte-stimulating hormone, catechols, glucocorticoids and their inducers (which block the upregulation of cytokine genes), lipocortin (which is a mediator of glucocorticoid function), and natural cytokine inhibitors and soluble cytokine receptors.

Is there any benefit from the fever response? If the results of a set of truly brilliant investigations using the cold-blooded lizard, *Dipsosaurus dorsalis*, can be extrapolated to humans, then fever is a true determinant of the outcome of infection.[7-9] *Dipsosaurus dorsalis* is a typical poikilotherm and it lacks the physiologic mechanisms for temperature regulation. Nonetheless, in common with other cold-blooded animals, it regulates body temperature as much as possible through the use of behavioral modifications rather than physiologic mechanisms. Thus, it will move between sun and shade as necessary to maintain a constant temperature during the daytime. When placed within an environmental chamber that is able to maintain a gradient of temperature, the animal migrates to the area that allows its core temperature to approximate 101.3°F (38.5°C). However, when the lizards are injected with lipopolysaccharide (LPS) endotoxin or infected with a natural bacterial pathogen, *Aeromonas hydrophila*, the high and low temperature setpoints triggering migration are both increased (Fig. 2.8) and they migrate in the chamber in order to increase their core temperature by 2–4°F (1–2°C) in the first 24 hours and by another 2–4°F (1–2°C) in the second 24 hours. If the temperature rise is prohibited by keeping the lizards in a chamber with a set temperature or by injecting salicylate, both the incidence of bacteremia and the mortality rate increase (Fig. 2.9). When body temperature is, in a similar manner, fixed at over 107.6°F (42°C), mortality increases further and affects both infected and uninfected lizards.

These data clearly show that fever is protective, and that there is an upper limit beyond which the increased temperature is itself detrimental. There are no clearer demonstrations of the selective advantage of moderate elevations of temperature in host responses than these classic studies of the 1970s. Since then, no convincing mechanism by which this survival advantage is mediated has been demonstrated, in *D. dorsalis* or, if it pertains, in the higher mammals, including humans. Nonetheless, some investigators have concluded that it is unwise to

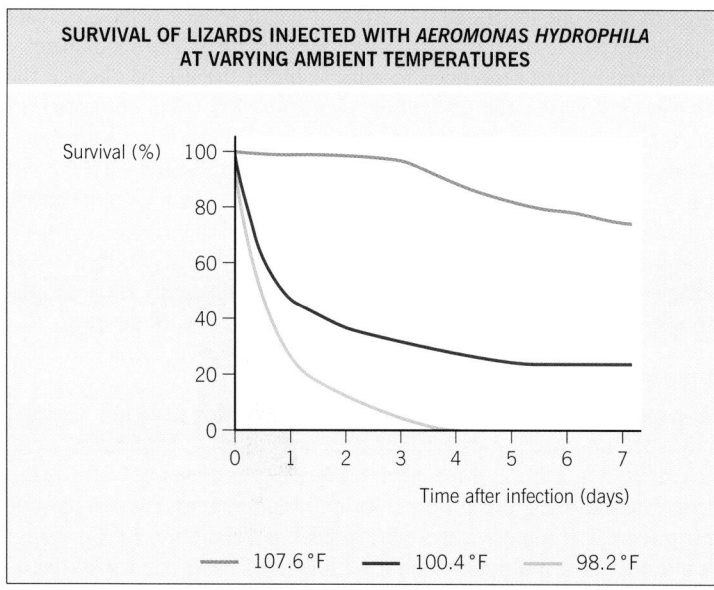

Fig. 2.9 **Survival of lizards injected with *Aeromonas hydrophila* at varying ambient temperatures.** Data from Kluger *et al.*[7]

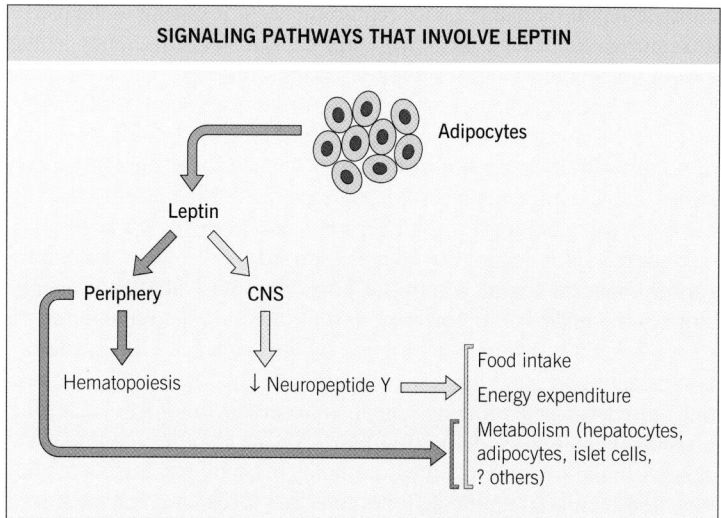

Fig. 2.10 **Signaling pathways that involve leptin.** ?, possibility of other effects.

modify the fever response to infection by the use of antipyretics such as salicylates.[11]

There are consequences of fever other than death that affect the benefit–risk ratio of this classic host response. One of these is an increase in energy requirements. This increase occurs, in part, because of the biophysical temperature coefficient effect, by which there is an approximately 10% increase in the rate of enzymatic reactions with an increase in reaction temperature of 1°C (Q_{10}). The Q_{10} effect occurs regardless of the cause of the increased temperature; infection triggers this effect as well as artificially increasing the temperature within a heat chamber.

Although this may speed up reactions that yield products of benefit to the host in fighting infection (e.g. the enzymes that result in bactericidal reactive oxygen intermediates such as hydrogen peroxide, superoxide or hydroxyl radicals), the Q_{10} effect also means that increased energy is required to drive the reactions. This increase in energy needs is not restricted to reactions that benefit the host; all enzyme reactions are affected. Secondly, the metabolic activity underlying the muscular activity that generates heat in order to raise the core temperature necessitates increased energy expenditures. Thirdly, energy is consumed in the increased metabolic activity needed for the synthesis of the large amounts of new proteins and new cells needed to combat the infection. In fact, energy requirements in humans with sepsis are 35–40% above basal needs.[12]

ANOREXIA

Loss of appetite is an early manifestation of infection. It is regulated in the CNS, where satiety or hunger is perceived and the appropriate feeding behaviors are triggered. Experiments in which cytokines such as IL-1β or TNF-α have been systemically administered to various species of animals have demonstrated the ability of these cytokines to induce a sharp diminution in food intake.[13–15] Such experiments suggest that the same cytokines that result in the fever response may also act to alter appetite and food consumption. Principles of 'conservation' of responses may be operative here, for the same response occurs with trauma. Although totally speculative, it is possible that in trauma the injured host may be better served by resting and allowing healing to begin than by foraging for food, and therefore anorexia may make it easier for the injured animal to remain quiescent. In support of this idea, it is striking that IL-1β induces slow-wave sleep patterns in the brain,[16] which explains why fatigue usually accompanies fever and anorexia in infection, and is a part of the teleologic interpretation of these events. Sleep also serves to

reduce substrate requirements over and above basal needs, by reducing physical activity and muscle metabolism.

The underlying mechanisms that regulate appetite and food intake are currently being defined, at least in the setting of obesity and hormonal disorders such as diabetes mellitus. A recently described cytokine-like peptide mediator produced by adipocytes, leptin, is one factor that appears to be involved (Fig. 2.10).[17] Genetically determined obesity disorders in experimental animals have played an essential role in the identification of leptin and the leptin receptor, and it is already clear that defects in either the ligand or the receptor may be responsible for some animal feeding disorders that underlie obesity. Administration of leptin to experimental animals leads to reduced food intake and body weight,[18] and when administered directly into the lateral ventricle the effect on food intake occurs within 30 minutes.[19] Leptin appears to act by inhibiting the release of neuropeptide Y in the hypothalamus,[20] which may be the proximate regulator of food-seeking behavior, hyperphagia and energy homeostasis in response to reductions in body energy stores.[21]

Leptin may also be one of a group of proteins whose production is markedly accelerated in the course of an acute inflammatory reaction under the influence of IL-6 (see Fig. 2.11).[22] Such proteins are collectively called acute phase proteins, and it is presumed that they serve some specific role in host response to the acute injury. However, as with fever, the extent of the acute phase response may determine whether the effect is beneficial with respect to the host's response to the initiating stimulus or whether it has harmful consequences (see Fig. 2.12). It is often difficult to sort this out *in vivo*, because there typically are multiple events occurring at the same time, many of which have overlapping functional impact.

METABOLIC HOST RESPONSES TO INFECTION

Infection results in marked changes in host metabolism, characterized by a dramatic increase in metabolic activity and altered priorities of synthesis. These involve all components of metabolic activity, including energy, protein, vitamins and minerals. What is even more remarkable is the way in which these changes are interrelated and supportive of the host defense needs for an effective response.

ENERGY METABOLISM

Because of increased metabolic demands in the infected host, it does not make any immediate sense for appetite and food intake to diminish as much as they do in infection; if anything, appetite should be ravenous in order to provide for the increased substrate needs without constricting basal maintenance requirements or resorting to the use of host stores. Yet nature has apparently chosen self-sufficiency as the guiding principle for this situation, and the infected patient reduces voluntary activity and begins to use his or her own sources of energy. Initially the energy store consumed consists primarily of liver glycogen, but within hours this resource is depleted. Because glycogen stores are not sufficient to serve as much more than a buffer for energy needs between feedings it soon becomes necessary to find an alternative source. This is the dilemma of reduced food intake: the energy source must be found within the host. The most abundant energy store in the body is fat; however, during infection, and in contrast to starvation, fat utilization is inhibited by the same cytokine mediators that initiate fever and other host responses. This means that the host must turn to muscle protein as the main reservoir for energy, requiring proteolysis and conversion of amino acids to glucose via gluconeogenesis in the liver. Direct measurements in septic patients have documented increased amino acid turnover in muscle and conversion of amino acids to glucose in the liver.[23] The same events have been shown to occur in patients in whom the inflammatory response is triggered by trauma or surgery.

At the same time, glucose turnover and blood glucose levels are elevated and glucose oxidation is increased; these changes are associated with hyperinsulinemia, hyperglucagonemia and increases in plasma growth hormone levels. In this array of characteristic responses, carbohydrate metabolism in sepsis resembles a state of 'pseudodiabetes'. Peripheral insulin resistance in muscle limits the use of glucose for energy and drives the utilization instead of branched-chain amino acids for energy. Thus, the local proteolytic events in muscle are made more efficient because branched chain amino acids are released and can be used *in situ*. As the complexities of the changes induced by infection and inflammation become better characterized, the more intricate they appear and the more co-ordinated they seem; the overall efficiency of the process becomes increasingly apparent. The response to infection is not a patchwork quilt; rather, it is a work of art.

VITAMIN METABOLISM

Previous studies of vitamin metabolism in infection have not revealed any striking changes that either support the host response or contribute to a metabolic imbalance. Some vitamins are lost in the urine in greater amounts than normal during inflammation, but this has not been seen as clinically important, at least in the short term. Certainly, individual and multiple vitamin deficiencies have been well documented as exerting influences on the host immune system but, with the exception of vitamin A deficiency, the setting of acute infection or inflammation does not itself significantly alter vitamin status. The exception, vitamin A deficiency, has long been known to progress rapidly during infection, and the early changes in the eye that occur in vitamin A deficiency can rapidly progress to blinding keratomalacia with an acute diarrheal or respiratory infection or, as so commonly seen in developing countries, measles.

However, a growing body of data indicates that vitamin A is also an acute phase reactant, being removed from the circulation during infection or acute inflammation. Where the vitamin goes, in what form, how, and what it does there is not known in detail. However, it is reasonable to presume that this, like other acute phase responses, has evolved through selection and therefore has functional significance in the host response to infection. Vitamin A is commonly known for its role in vision, and for too many students of medicine and biology this is its only recognized role. However, vitamin A and its metabolic products function as transcriptional regulators of many genes, many of which have obvious immunologic functions.[24,25] Thus, the movement of retinol from plasma to tissue during infection has the potential for transcriptionally activating genes that are critical to host responses. In the mammalian host, this may be an example of a global regulatory pathway that is activated by cytokines released during the response to infection or inflammation.

Vitamin C has received considerable public attention, at least as much for the prominence of some its proponents as for the evidence that it is an acute phase reactant with a physiologic role in the host response to infection. Indeed, whether increased vitamin C intake alters the course of infection is still controversial.

Another antioxidant vitamin, α-tocopherol or vitamin E, appears to play a more definitive role in host defense, and a number of vitamin E supplementation trials, especially in older persons, have demonstrated that additional vitamin E enhances immune responses and, by this effect, may decrease infection morbidity.[26,27] If this is true, whether supplementation is correcting a functional deficiency or not has yet to be determined. This is, however, a different issue from that of acute host responses altering vitamin distribution during infection, as occurs with vitamin A.

MINERALS

Acute reductions in plasma iron and zinc and an increase in plasma copper have long been known to accompany acute infection and inflammation (Fig. 2.13). The physiologic interpretation of the rapid development of hypoferremia and hypozincemia at the onset of infection has been that of an acute deficiency state. In the case of iron, this has also been interpreted to be of survival value, because the sequestration of iron should reduce the amount available for micro-organisms

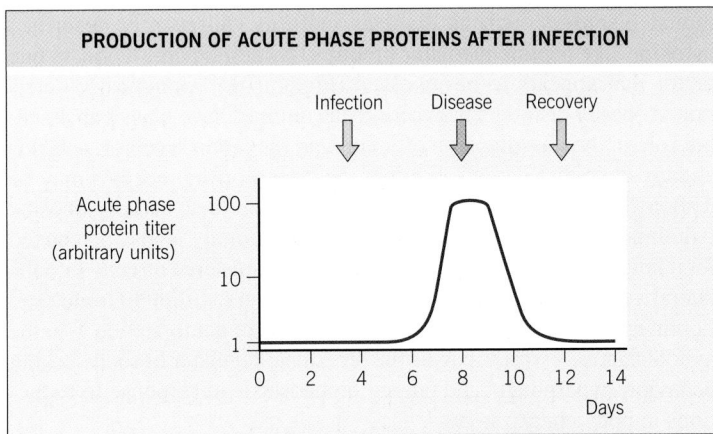

Fig. 2.11 Production of acute phase proteins after infection. Infection causes a rapid increase in the production of these proteins.

ACUTE PHASE PROTEINS PRODUCED IN RESPONSE TO INFECTION IN HUMANS		
Acute phase reactant		**Role**
Dramatic increases in concentration	C-reactive protein	Fixes complement, opsonizes
	Mannose-binding protein	Fixes complement, opsonizes
	α_1-acid glycoprotein	Acts as transport protein
	Serum amyloid A protein	Uncertain
Moderate increases in concentration	α_1-proteinase inhibitors	Inhibits bacterial proteases
	α_1-antichymotrypsin	Inhibits bacterial proteases
	C3, C9, factor B	Increase complement function
	Ceruloplasmin	Oxygen scavenger
	Fibrinogen	Coagulation
	Angiotensin	Elevates blood pressure
	Haptoglobin	Binds hemoglobin
	Fibronectin	Cell attachment

Fig. 2.12 Acute phase proteins produced in response to infection in humans.

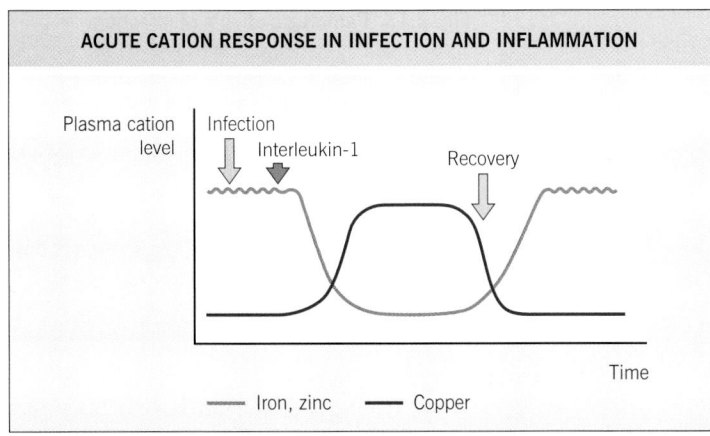

Fig. 2.13 Acute cation response in infection and inflammation.

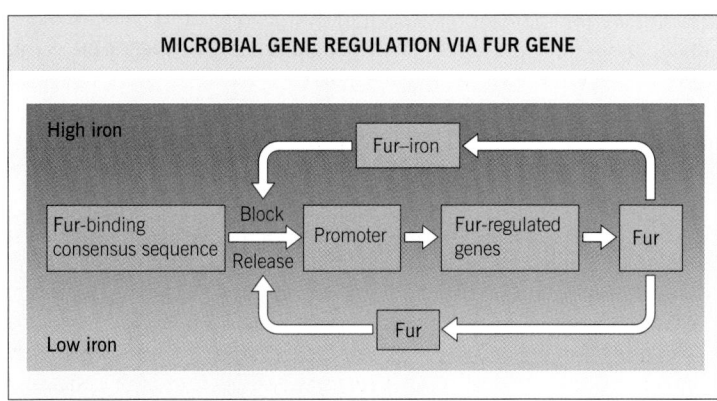

Fig. 2.14 Microbial gene regulation via Fur gene.

that require iron for survival, growth and replication. This putative host defense has been termed 'nutritional immunity'. There are many reasons to believe that nutritional immunity may not be physiologically relevant, principally because most bacteria and higher organisms have highly evolved iron acquisition systems that enable the microbes to compete for iron with protein-bound iron in the host. Indeed, many micro-organisms use low concentrations of free iron as a signal to activate genes involved in virulence or resistance to host defenses. Low free iron is also used to signal transcriptional activation of the genes involved in microbial iron binding and uptake. In one commonly used microbial regulatory gene, ferric uptake regulator (*fur*), the gene product, Fur, is an iron binding protein that, in the iron-replete form, recognizes a palindromic sequence in the promoter region of iron-regulated genes and blocks transcription (Fig. 2.14). In a low iron environment, Fur does not interact with its DNA binding site and transcription proceeds.[28,29]

Infection also activates host genes involved in production of the iron-binding protein ferritin, which results in iron uptake into cells, at the same time reducing synthesis of transferrin, the soluble circulating iron-binding protein that transfers iron from the circulation to an intracellular compartment.[30,31] Similarly, infection activates the synthesis of metallothienene, the intracellular zinc binding protein, resulting in the sequestration of zinc within cells. These responses are triggered by certain cytokines produced in the inflammatory response (e.g. IL-1β and TNF-α). In this manner, inflammation, whether due to infection or trauma, induces hypoferremia and hypozincemia. Because IL-1 is so important in the activation of immune host responses, coregulation of the metabolic response and immune activation suggests that the two are, in some way, functionally linked. This view also belies the characterization of infection-mediated hypoferremia and hypozincemia as acute deficiency states.

If the shift of iron and zinc from one host compartment to another is not designed by nature to inhibit microbial growth, what then is its purpose? Both iron and zinc serve as important active centers in metalloenzymes and transcription factors, many of which are involved in DNA synthesis and cell replication, such as occurs in response to infectious or inflammatory challenges. In fact, it is not possible for the host to make a response involving cell division without iron metalloenzymes and zinc-finger transcription factors. Because the activation of the humoral and cellular limbs of the immune response is a direct reflection of clonal selection and amplification of lymphoid cells, the production of macrophage antigen-presenting cells, and increased generation of polymorphonuclear phagocytic cells, the efficient utilization of iron and zinc in support of DNA synthesis and cell division is a prerequisite for the full host response. It appears that a mechanism to promote this has become a part of the acute host response to infection, and the same set of mediators is involved in the catabolic and anabolic events.

ANTIMICROBIAL HOST RESPONSES TO INFECTION

GENERAL PRINCIPLES OF MICROBIAL PATHOGENESIS

If the host response to infection is geared to host defense, then these events should relate to the mechanisms of disease pathogenesis caused by infectious agents. With few exceptions, microbial pathogens act directly on or in the host. The exceptions are limited; they include, for example, micro-organisms that may produce toxic molecules outside the host that can cause disease without infection, such as the *Staphylococcus aureus* enterotoxins involved in food poisoning. However, even these may have profound effects on the immune system in their role as superantigens. Pathogenic organisms typically interact directly with the host, and are capable of finding a niche in which the organism is able to grow, possibly invade across the skin or the mucous membranes and then disseminate, evade host defenses and cause changes in host physiology that translate into symptoms of the illness. Pathogens may produce specific metabolic products that directly cause damage to the host, or they may produce antigens that elicit immunologic responses, which at times may themselves be mechanisms of disease pathogenesis (see Fig. 2.15). There are at least four separate stages of the host–pathogen interaction that lead to possible pathology or pathophysiologic responses (see Fig. 2.16):

- colonization,
- invasion,
- multiplication, and
- dissemination.

Colonization

The initial encounter with the host is generally followed by multiplication of the organism. If this occurs on a mucous membrane it is considered colonization. Pathogens must have some means of establishing themselves in their preferred niche. Often these involve the production of specific colonization factors that allow the organisms both to identify their niche and to attach in a way that allows them to overcome host measures aimed at dislodging them. This is obvious in the gastrointestinal tract (see Fig. 2.17), in which the host produces liters of protease-rich wash fluids in the succus entericus as well as sticky mucins, and then propels these through the gut by means of peristalsis. Without an attachment strategy, potential pathogens may be washed through, explaining why the most efficient pathogens have developed molecular attachment strategies utilizing cell-bound colonization antigens. Typically these are proteins that recognize and bind to specific host glycoconjugates. They are present on the microbial cell surface, often on specialized structures that extend out from the cell surface, such as pili or fimbriae,[32] or sometimes on specialized microbial organelles.[33] This suggests the utility of a host strategy to resist this attachment not only in a nonspecific manner but also by developing anti-attachment mechanisms (e.g. by producing specific carbohydrate receptor blocking macromolecules or antibodies).

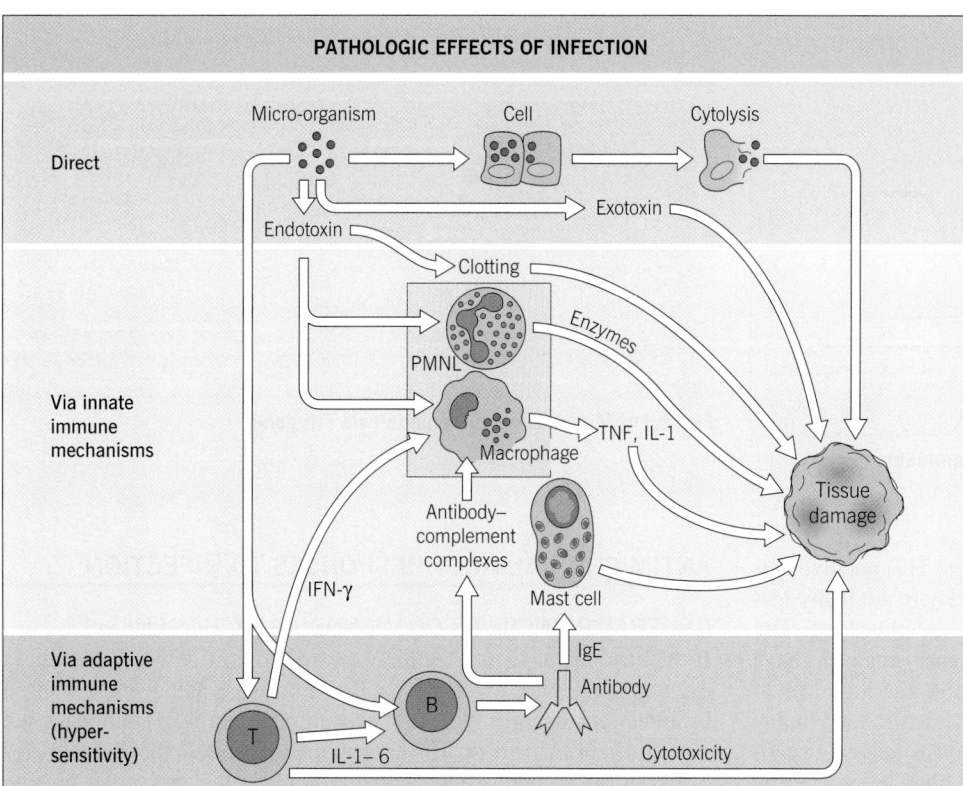

PATHOLOGIC EFFECTS OF INFECTION

Fig. 2.15 Pathologic effects of infection. B, B derived lymphocytes; IFN, interferon; IL, interleukin; PMNL, polymorphonuclear leukocyte; T, T lymphocytes; TNF, tumor necrosis factor.

Stage	Mechanism	Utility to pathogen
Colonization	Ligand-specific adherence to host receptors, commonly by way of specific sugar–protein interactions	Provides initial niche for the pathogen to establish and initiate adverse effects on the host
Invasion	Penetration of skin, mucosa or other epithelial membranes to reach the circulation or specific target organ or cell type	Provides entry of pathogen to the host; may also enter immunologic sanctuary, where it is sequestered and protected from host immune responses
Multiplication	Depends on preferred niche of the organism and its growth rate; multiplication may be slow or rapid, intracellular or extracellular	Organism increases in number and may be better able to survive host defenses
Dissemination	Organisms may spread locally or disseminate widely, depending on biologic attributes	Organism infects multiple sites, where it may cause added disease symptoms and survive indefinitely

STAGES IN HOST–PATHOGEN INTERACTIONS

Fig. 2.16 Stages in host–pathogen interactions.

Micro-organism	Disease	Attachment site	Mechanism
Vibrio cholerae	Cholera	Intestinal epithelium	Specific bacterial molecule (adhesin) binds to oligosaccharide receptor on cell
Escherichia coli (certain strains)	Diarrhea	Intestinal epithelium	
Salmonella typhi	Enteric fever		
Shigella spp.	Dysentery	Colonic epithelium	Bacteria induce epithelial cells to engulf them
Giardia lamblia	Diarrhea	Duodenal, jejunal epithelium	Protozoa bind to mannose-6 phosphate on host cell; also have mechanical sucker
Entamoeba histolytica	Dysentery	Colonic epithelium	Lectin on surface of amebae binds to asialofetuin on host cell
Poliovirus	Poliomyelitis	Intestinal epithelium	Viral capsid protein reacts with specific receptor on cell
Rotavirus	Diarrhea	Intestinal epithelium	Viral outer capsid protein binds to glycolipid receptor on cell

MICROBIAL ATTACHMENT IN THE INTESTINAL TRACT

Fig. 2.17 Microbial attachment in the intestinal tract.

Invasion

Attachment may lead to colonization on the mucosal surface but it may also lead to invasion across the epithelial cell layer. Microbial invasion is a complex process resulting from the sequential interaction of microbial products with the host cell.[34] These interactions are often cell signaling events, and host responses include:[35]

• the activation of protein kinases,
• protein phosphorylations and
• major rearrangements of the cellular cytoskeleton.

An example is the initial interaction of *Salmonella typhimurium* and the host cell, which results in an active, kinetic 'ruffling' of the cell surface, reminiscent of the effect of growth factors;[36] this is associated with the uptake of the bacteria within host membrane-delimited vesicles. Noninvasive organisms in the vicinity can also be swept up into these

vesicles and enter the host cell cytoplasm in a process known as 'passive entry', (Fig. 2.18).[37] The importance of this passive entry depends on the subsequent fate of the ingested organisms, which results from the ability of the organism to resist the microbicidal reactions of the inflammatory response.

Recent studies of the invasion mechanism of *Shigella flexneri* have revealed a different aspect of the role of the host inflammatory response (Chapters 2.35 & 8.17).[38] Firstly, *Shigella* spp. do not appear to invade across the luminal epithelial cell membrane, as previously thought. Rather, when intestinal epithelial cells are mounted on collagen-coated filters and allowed to form tight junctions, the bacteria are invasive

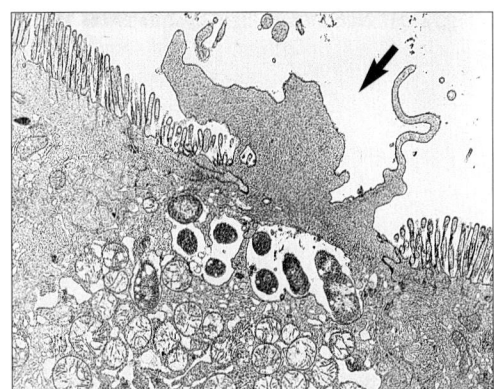

Fig. 2.18 Showing membrane ruffle (arrow) during microbial invasion. Note the presence of multiple intracellular bacteria already within vesicles beneath the region of membrane ruffling. Courtesy of Stanley Falkow.

VARIOUS MECHANISMS ADOPTED BY MICRO-ORGANISMS TO AVOID HOST CELL MICROBICIDAL MECHANISMS DURING PHAGOCYTOSIS

Inhibition of phagolysosome fusion

Fusion of phagosome and lysosome somehow inhibited by organism (e.g. *Mycobacterium tuberculosis, M. leprae, Toxoplasma* spp., *Chlamydia* spp.)

or

Escape into the cytoplasm

Organism escapes from the phagolysosome into the cytoplasm and replicates within the phagocyte (e.g. *Leishmania* spp., *Trypanosoma cruzi*)

or

Resistance to killing

Organism resists killing by producing antioxidants (e.g. by catalase in staphylococci) or by unknown mechanisms (e.g. mycobacteria, brucella, *Salmonella typhi*)

Fig. 2.20 Various mechanisms adopted by micro-organisms to avoid phagocytosis.

only from the basal surface. Nonetheless, when *S. flexneri* are placed within a loop of intestine in an *in-vivo* experiment in animals, the organisms invade, cause inflammation and result in fluid production. The interesting aspect of this is that if the inflammatory response is prevented by the administration of IL-1 antagonists or if the ability of polymorphonuclear leukocytes (PMNLs) to migrate is blocked by the administration of antibodies to PMNL surface antigens involved in locomotion (such as CD18). If neutrophil chemotaxis is blocked, *Shigella* spp. invasion is markedly reduced and no symptoms of disease ensue.

These findings demonstrate that the initial microbe–host interaction triggers an influx of PMNLs that is necessary for the subsequent, more massive invasion of organisms across the mucosa (Fig. 2.19). These results have changed the paradigm for the sequence of inflammatory responses in shigellosis from that of a reaction to invasion to an integral and essential part of invasion. In other words, infection with *Shigella* spp. is a clear example of host-mediated pathogenesis. This also demonstrates the ingenious nature of microbes in host–pathogen interactions, and the ability of pathogenic micro-organisms to take advantage of and subvert host defense systems for their own welfare. A better-known example of this is the use by HIV of the lymphocyte and macrophage cell surface differentiation antigen, CD4, together with host cell chemokine receptors to enter the target cells,[39] where the virus replicates, thereby initiating the destruction of immunologically active cells in the process, and leading, ultimately, to AIDS.

Multiplication and dissemination

These examples of colonization and invasion also highlight two other aspects of microbial pathogenesis: multiplication and, in some instances, dissemination. Multiplication may occur on mucosal surfaces, in tissues (e.g. in an abscess) or within cells. Some micro-organisms have become adapted to survival and multiplication within

the phagocytic cells, using a number of strategies to evade the host's microbicidal mechanisms (Fig. 2.20). Because of their ability to survive and multiply within these professional host defense cells, such micro-organisms are referred to as 'facultative intracellular pathogens'; they include *Salmonella typhi, Legionella pneumophila, Mycobacterium tuberculosis, Leishmania donovani* and *Toxoplasma gondii*. These organisms are able to avoid harmful effects of host defenses by a variety of measures. For example, some prevent the fusion of phagocytic vesicles with lysosomes, some block the acidification response within the vesicle by escaping to the cytoplasm, and others just resist everything the macrophage can throw at them.[40]

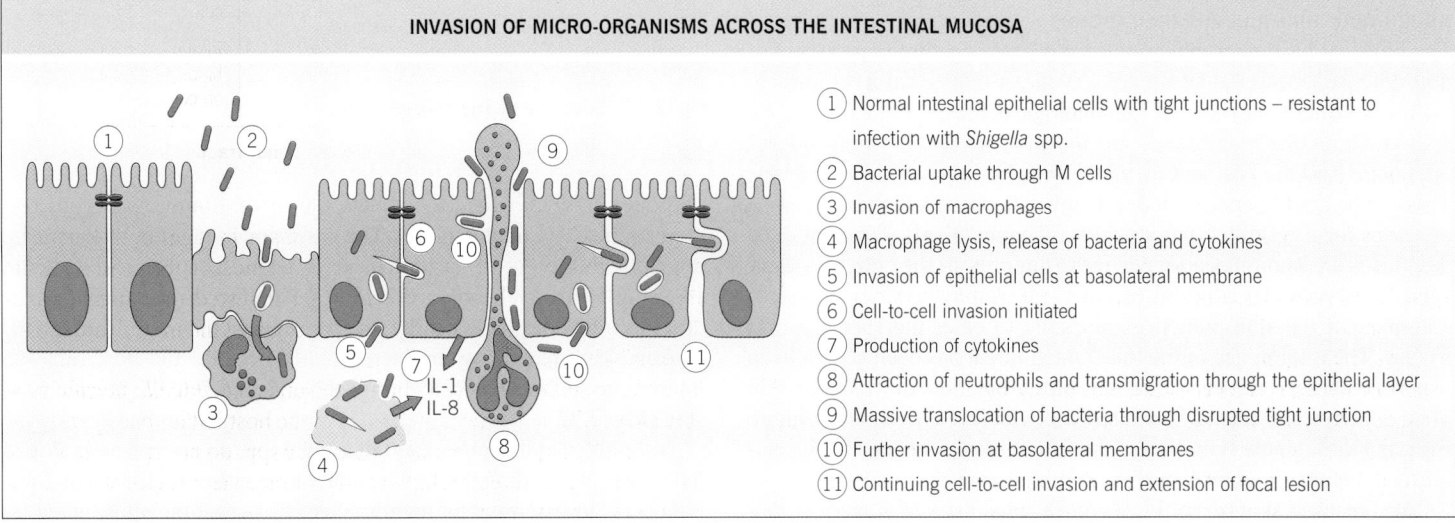

INVASION OF MICRO-ORGANISMS ACROSS THE INTESTINAL MUCOSA

1. Normal intestinal epithelial cells with tight junctions – resistant to infection with *Shigella* spp.
2. Bacterial uptake through M cells
3. Invasion of macrophages
4. Macrophage lysis, release of bacteria and cytokines
5. Invasion of epithelial cells at basolateral membrane
6. Cell-to-cell invasion initiated
7. Production of cytokines
8. Attraction of neutrophils and transmigration through the epithelial layer
9. Massive translocation of bacteria through disrupted tight junction
10. Further invasion at basolateral membranes
11. Continuing cell-to-cell invasion and extension of focal lesion

IL-1
IL-8

Fig. 2.19 Invasion of micro-organisms across the intestinal mucosa.

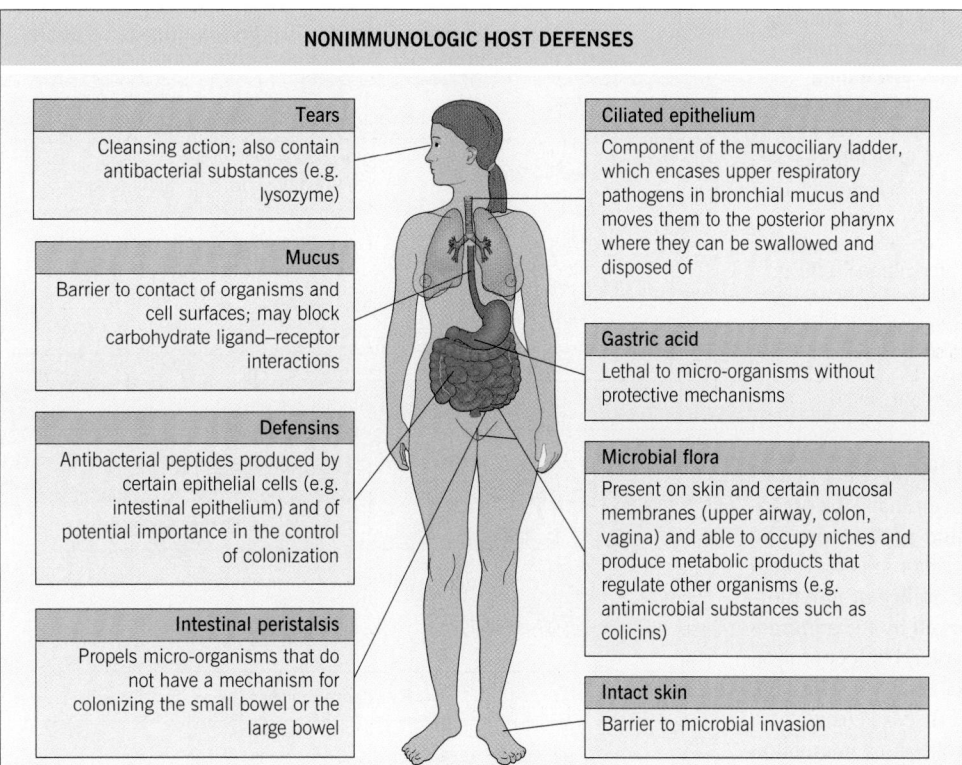

Fig. 2.21 Nonimmunologic host defenses.

NONIMMUNOLOGIC HOST DEFENSES

Tears Cleansing action; also contain antibacterial substances (e.g. lysozyme)	**Ciliated epithelium** Component of the mucociliary ladder, which encases upper respiratory pathogens in bronchial mucus and moves them to the posterior pharynx where they can be swallowed and disposed of
Mucus Barrier to contact of organisms and cell surfaces; may block carbohydrate ligand–receptor interactions	**Gastric acid** Lethal to micro-organisms without protective mechanisms
Defensins Antibacterial peptides produced by certain epithelial cells (e.g. intestinal epithelium) and of potential importance in the control of colonization	**Microbial flora** Present on skin and certain mucosal membranes (upper airway, colon, vagina) and able to occupy niches and produce metabolic products that regulate other organisms (e.g. antimicrobial substances such as colicins)
Intestinal peristalsis Propels micro-organisms that do not have a mechanism for colonizing the small bowel or the large bowel	**Intact skin** Barrier to microbial invasion

Whereas systemic dissemination of micro-organisms is generally associated with systemic manifestations of illness, such manifestations can occur in the absence of dissemination. For example, in diphtheria, the organisms colonize and multiply on the mucous membranes of the upper airway, but they produce a protein toxin that is transported systemically and leads to clinical illness owing to its ability to inhibit mammalian cell protein synthesis and cause tissue damage. Systemic invasion may also occur by devious means. For example, the gonococcus can attach to sperm and ride upstream through the female genital tract to the fallopian tubes, where the organism can cause acute salpingitis.[41]

NONIMMUNOLOGIC HOST DEFENSES

There are a number of important nonantigen-specific host defenses that are important components of the host barrier to infection (Fig. 2.21). These may be altered by genetics, disease or drugs, and, in the altered state, can predispose the host to certain groups of infectious agents. It is often possible to improve the resistance of the host by modifying these defenses (if they are recognized and known to the physician and if there are intervention strategies available).

Integument and mucous membranes

The physical barriers to infectious organisms constitute one aspect of host defense; because they are not specific or induced as a response to microbial stimuli, they are not immunologic defenses. For example, the skin and mucous membranes are the first contact between micro-organisms and the host and they are of major importance as barriers. This can be readily appreciated: ask any nail-biter how often he or she develops local cellulitis (paronychia). The most likely answer will be that this is a common occurrence if the integrity of the cuticle is damaged. This provides a portal of entry for *Staphylococcus aureus*, a colonizer of the skin, which is then able to enter the subcutaneous tissues. The importance of the intact integument has been shown in an experimental reproduction of the nail-biting situation, in which the skin of an experimental animal is painted with viable *S. aureus* and a suture is placed through the skin. Where the suture breaks the intact skin, cellulitis develops; in unbroken skin, nothing happens.

The breached skin barrier is, of course, a hallmark of surgery. A natural example of this also occurs in transmission of the protozoan

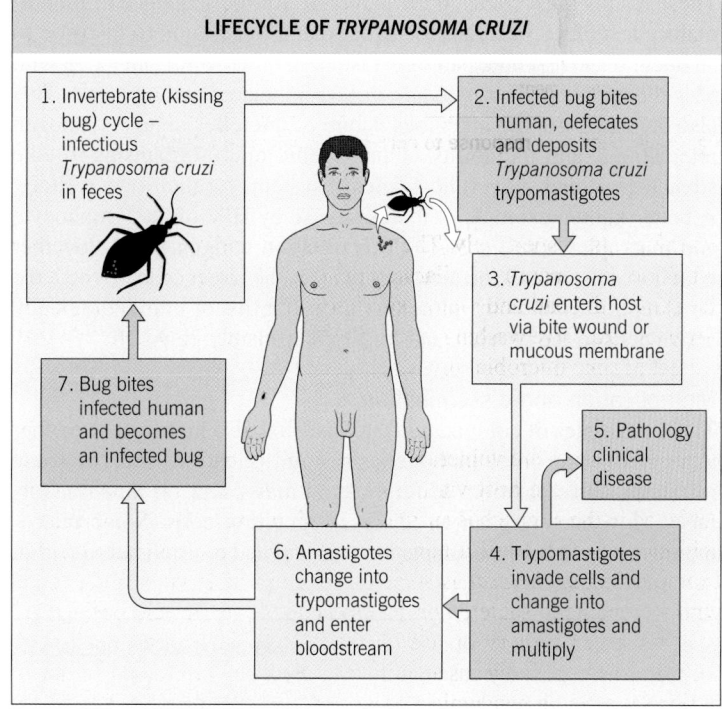

Fig. 2.22 Lifecycle of *Trypanosoma cruzi*.

pathogen *Trypanosoma cruzi*, the cause of South American trypanosomiasis (Chapter 6.33). The infectious stage of this parasite develops in the gut of an insect vector from the species of reduviid ('kissing') bugs. When the insect bites a host to take a blood meal, it deposits infectious feces nearby; the parasite can now enter through the broken skin created by the bite, usually because the host rubs the injured site and mechanically brings the organism into the breach in the skin (Fig. 2.22).

It should also be appreciated that many pathogens have developed the means of invading through an intact integument (often via hair follicles) or across mucous membranes after reaching these sites by means of ingestion, inhalation or insertion, as in the gut, respiratory or

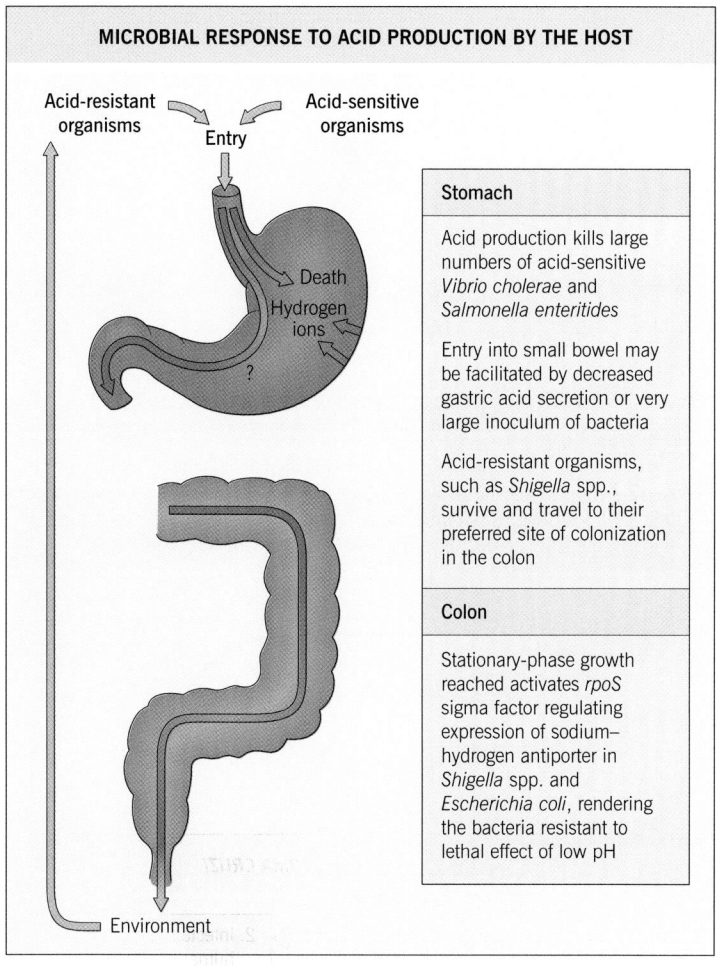

MICROBIAL RESPONSE TO ACID PRODUCTION BY THE HOST

Acid-resistant organisms — Entry — Acid-sensitive organisms

Death
Hydrogen ions
?

Environment

Stomach

Acid production kills large numbers of acid-sensitive *Vibrio cholerae* and *Salmonella enteritides*

Entry into small bowel may be facilitated by decreased gastric acid secretion or very large inoculum of bacteria

Acid-resistant organisms, such as *Shigella* spp., survive and travel to their preferred site of colonization in the colon

Colon

Stationary-phase growth reached activates *rpoS* sigma factor regulating expression of sodium–hydrogen antiporter in *Shigella* spp. and *Escherichia coli*, rendering the bacteria resistant to lethal effect of low pH

Fig. 2.23 Microbial response to acid production by the host.

genital tracts, respectively. The mechanisms employed may differ in detail but are generally similar in principle.[42] To some extent, washing the skin with soap and water can reduce the surface pathogen load; however, excessive washing can remove beneficial lipids from skin that protect against microbial invasion.

Gastric acid

Micro-organisms are vulnerable to extremes of pH, and for many that normally enter the host via the oral route, the low pH that may be achieved in the stomach is sufficient to kill them. In this sense, gastric acid can be considered a nonspecific host defense mechanism. For example, *Vibrio cholerae* is very sensitive to acid *in vitro*, and people who are unable to secrete normal amounts of gastric acid because of gastritis, ulcer surgery or use of antacids or drugs that block acid secretion are especially susceptible to clinical cholera. This was noted during the seventh pandemic spread of cholera in Europe and Israel in the 1970s, when clinical cases were observed to occur preferentially in hypochlorhydric people. Although acid killing may not be a specific mechanism, certain micro-organisms seem to be able to resist acid-mediated damage by means of genetically controlled properties. Thus, the acid resistance of *Shigella* spp. is associated with the activation of acid resistance genes, which are growth-cycle regulated as the micro-organisms enter the stationary growth phase. This is a very functional response on the part of the micro-organism because the acid-resistant phenotype is achieved just as the bacterium is excreted into the environment, and thus occurs before it infects a new susceptible host (Fig. 2.23). In this manner, *Shigella* spp. are prepared in advance to survive passage through the stomach of the potential new victim. Their ability to resist acid is one reason why so few *Shigella* organisms are needed to cause clinical illness in humans, that is because of their likely safe passage through the stomach (Chapter 2.35).

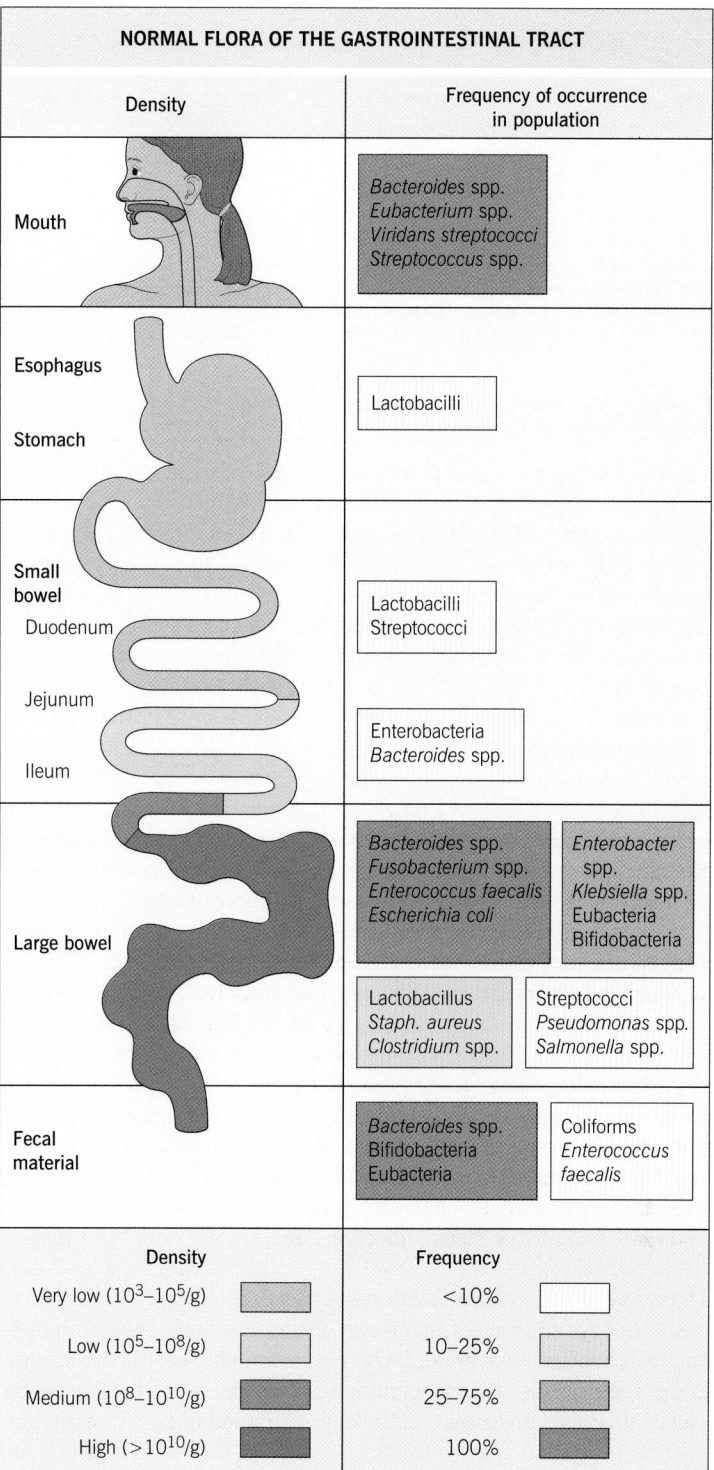

NORMAL FLORA OF THE GASTROINTESTINAL TRACT

Density		Frequency of occurrence in population
Mouth		*Bacteroides* spp. *Eubacterium* spp. *Viridans streptococci* *Streptococcus* spp.
Esophagus Stomach		Lactobacilli
Small bowel Duodenum Jejunum Ileum		Lactobacilli Streptococci Enterobacteria *Bacteroides* spp.
Large bowel		*Bacteroides* spp. *Enterobacter* spp. *Fusobacterium* spp. *Klebsiella* spp. *Enterococcus faecalis* Eubacteria *Escherichia coli* Bifidobacteria Lactobacillus Streptococci *Staph. aureus* *Pseudomonas* spp. *Clostridium* spp. *Salmonella* spp.
Fecal material		*Bacteroides* spp. Coliforms Bifidobacteria *Enterococcus* Eubacteria *faecalis*

Density		Frequency	
Very low (10^3–10^5/g)		<10%	
Low (10^5–10^8/g)		10–25%	
Medium (10^8–10^{10}/g)		25–75%	
High (>10^{10}/g)		100%	

Fig. 2.24 Normal flora of the gastrointestinal tract.

Nonspecific defense at the mucosal surface

Mucosal surfaces represent an enormous surface area and carry a huge burden of micro-organisms as normal (or abnormal) flora, especially at the upper and lower ends of the gastrointestinal tract (Fig. 2.24). There, the number of indigenous established micro-organisms, the majority of which are strictly anaerobic bacteria, exceeds the total number of cells that make up the whole host. Whereas many of these organisms are incapable of surviving in the body because they are so susceptible to host defense mechanisms, others become pathogens if they are able to breach the mucosal barrier. Therefore, a healthy mucosal barrier is an important component of host defense. One way of appreciating this is to examine the consequences of altering mucosal cell turnover and replacement by the use of cytotoxic cancer chemotherapeutic agents. These agents often lead to ulcerations of

INTERFERENCE WITH CILIARY ACTIVITY IN RESPIRATORY INFECTIONS		
Cause	Mechanisms	Importance
Infecting bacteria (*Bordetella pertussis*, *Haemophilus influenzae*, *Pseudomonas aeruginosa*, *Mycoplasma pneumoniae*)	Production of ciliostatic substance (tracheal cytotoxin from *Bordetella pertussis*, at least two substances from *Haemophilus influenzae*, at least seven substances from *Pseudomonas aeruginosa*)	++
Viral infection	Ciliated cell dysfunction or destruction by influenza viruses or measles virus	+++

Fig. 2.25 Interference with ciliary activity in respiratory infections.

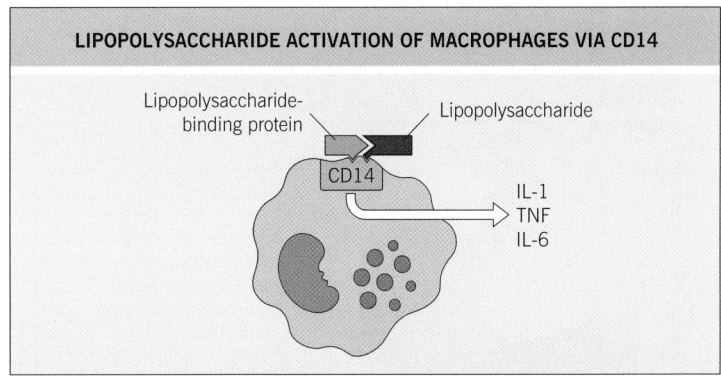

Fig. 2.26 Lipopolysaccharide activation of macrophages via CD14. IL, interleukin; TNF, tumor necrosis factor. TLR proteins are now recognized as coreceptors.[75]

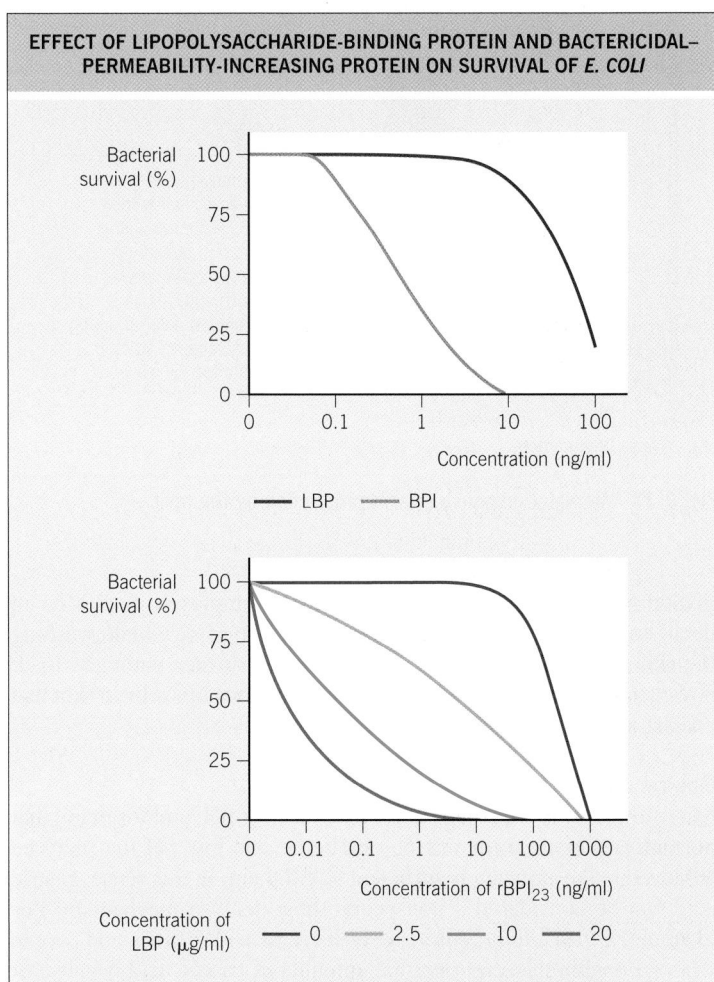

Fig. 2.27 Effect of lipopolysaccharide-binding protein (LBP) and bactericidal–permeability-increasing protein (BPI) on survival of *E. coli*. (Top) Survival of *E. coli* in the presence of increasing concentrations of LBP or BPI. (Bottom) Synergistic effect on *E. coli* survival of lipopolysaccharide-binding protein and a recombinant 23kDa *N*-terminal fragment of bactericidal–permeability-increasing protein (rBPI$_{23}$). Data from Horwitz AH *et al*.[49]

the mucous membranes and increase the risk of systemic invasion by facultative Gram-negative bacilli that normally live in the gastro-intestinal tract without causing harm, even in neutropenic patients.

Mucous membranes use several mechanisms to prevent microbial translocation. Some mucous membranes are the site of secretion of antibacterial proteins such as lysozyme, which hydrolyzes peptido-glycan and leads to the debility and death by lysis of Gram-positive organisms. The functional integrity of ciliated cells and mucus-secreting cells is another general mucosal host defense. Microbes can become embedded in balls of mucus, which are propelled to exit via a stoma by cilia in the upper respiratory tract or by peristalsis in the intestinal tract. Diseases that affect the function of cilia (e.g. viral infections) or the composition of mucus (e.g. cystic fibrosis) diminish the efficiency of this clearance mechanism and predispose to a variety of infections that a normal host would readily resist (Fig. 2.25).

Mucus itself is more interesting than its appearance as a slick and slippery substance. It is composed of a number of complex glycoconjugates expressing different antigenic epitopes, many of which may mimic receptors or microbial constituents and, by interacting with the host or pathogen surface, block the specific host–pathogen interaction that initiates infection. The mechanism by which breast milk protects the nursing infant from infection may depend on mimicry by the natural glycoconjugates present in colostrum and milk. By the same token, some micro-organisms use these interactions to establish colonization within the slime layers that overlay cells and use this niche to launch a more potent attack on host defenses, leading to systemic infectious diseases.

Initiation of the inflammatory response

Local and systemic manifestations of illness can be initiated by numerous mechanisms (Chapter 2.47). For example, the LPS of Gram-negative organisms and the peptidoglycans of Gram-positive organisms can initiate the production and release of proinflammatory cytokines such as IL-1β and TNF-α. In the case of LPS, the biologic effects are mediated by the lipid A portion of the molecule, a hydrophobic domain in the outer monolayer of the outer microbial cell membrane.[43] To be active, however, LPS must bind to LPS-binding protein (LBP), which is an acute phase protein of 456 amino acids that is derived from the host hepatocytes.[44] It is the LPS–LBP complex that binds to macrophages via the CD14 LPS receptor and initiates and markedly potentiates the cytokine response (Fig. 2.26).[45] Although they are not as well characterized as this, Gram-positive bacterial cell walls exert a similar effect, apparently by way of peptidoglycan, the major constituent of the cell wall, which has LPS-like properties on host cells,[46] through shared binding to CD14 on peripheral blood monocytes (Chapter 2.47).[47] CD14 is a GPI (glycerolphosphatidylinositol)-linked receptor which has no intracellular domain. Very recently it has been learnt that members of the Toll family of proteins, in particular TLR (Toll-like receptors 2 and 4) are the coreceptors which when activated by LPS result in signal transduction and intracellular signalling (see Yang *et al*.[75])

There is another host protein in the PMNL composed of 456 amino acids, bactericidal–permeability-increasing protein (BPI), which plays

a different role in the host response to LPS.[48] Bactericidal–permeability-increasing protein is a very cationic protein, representing approximately 1% of the total protein of the PMNL. It is produced only by immature PMNLs and it is stored in the primary granules of the cell; it is released when the cells are activated to degranulate, for example by LPS. Bactericidal–permeability-increasing protein acts by forming complexes with LPS in the outer membrane of living Gram-negative organisms, resulting in the very rapid cessation of microbial replication. With time, BPI damages the inner membrane, resulting in a loss of viability of the organism (Fig. 2.27). Extracellular complexing of BPI and LPS inhibits the further cell signaling that is mediated by the LPS.

SPECIFICITY AND REDUNDANCY IN HOST DEFENSES					
		Type of immune mechanism involved and effect on susceptibility to infection			
Pathogen		Phagocytosis	T lymphocytes	Complement	Antibody
Bacteria	*Staphylococcus aureus*	Increased	Not increased	Increased	Increased
	Enterobacteriaceae	Increased	Not increased	Increased	Some increase
	Haemophilus influenzae	Not increased	Not increased	Some increase	Increased
	Mycobacterium tuberculosis	Not increased	Increased	Not increased	Not increased
Viruses	Herpesviruses	Not increased	Increased	Not increased	Not increased
	Enteroviruses	Not increased	Some increase	Not increased	Increased
Fungi	*Candida albicans*	Increased	Increased	Not increased	Not increased
	Aspergillus spp.	Increased	Not increased	Not increased	Not increased
	Cryptococcus spp.	Not increased	Increased	Not increased	Not increased
Protozoa	*Pneumocystis carinii*	Not increased	Increased	Not increased	Not increased
	Cryptosporidium spp.	Not increased	Increased	Not increased	Possibly increased
	Malaria	Not increased	Not increased	Not increased	Possibly increased

Fig. 2.28 Specificity and redundancy in host defenses. Infectious complications of congenital immunodeficiency syndromes that affect various host defense mechanisms.

Antibodies to BPI block the microbicidal activity of PMN lysates and inflammatory secretions against Gram-negative bacteria, which suggest that BPI plays a role in PMNL mediated killing of these organisms. The *N*-terminal 199-amino-acid fragment of BPI is fully active *in vitro* and protects animals against lethal doses of LPS or Gram-negative bacteria. These properties have suggested a potential therapeutic use of this natural antimicrobial agent derived from the human host, and early clinical trials are currently being conducted.[50] It is interesting to note that the host is prepared to deal with Gram-negative bacteria by way of LBP and BPI, two related, small peptides: LBP binds LPS and allows it to transduce signals to phagocytic cells, resulting in degranulation and release of BPI. BPI can complex with and neutralize the effects of LPS and bind to and ultimately kill the infecting organisms, thereby releasing the LPS, which again initiates the whole process. This is another example of the exquisite orchestration of host responses to micro-organisms. However, in the cat-and-mouse-like relationship between host defenses and microbial virulence, it is perhaps inevitable that some organisms will have become adept at turning this inflammatory response to their own benefit, as in the case of *Shigella* spp. described above.

SPECIFIC ELICITED (IMMUNOLOGIC) RESPONSES

Immunologic responses may be defined as those in which microbial antigens elicit a host response that is specific for the structure that initiates the response. The regulation of these responses is rather complex and appears to be ever more complex as more factors involved in regulation are discovered. These factors include:[51]

- cells and secreted products, such as growth factors and signal-transducing mediators;
- soluble immune proteins that may be produced in the course of an immune response, such as antibody; and
- activation of reaction cascades involving circulating proteins, which result in protein–protein complex formation and the production of hydrolytic products with biologic activity, as occurs during the activation of the complement system.

Cells may interact with cells or proteins, or both, and proteins may interact with other proteins or nonprotein constituents such as oligosaccharides or complex carbohydrates. The hallmark of immunologic reactions is specificity for the eliciting antigen of the pathogen, although nonspecific or 'bystander' effects can occur and affect organisms other than the pathogen to which the response is directed (see below).

When the antimicrobial functions of these reactions is examined, they are often found to be redundant for certain organisms, to require interactions to be active against other organisms, and to be unique for other organisms. The fascination of this biologic system has never been greater than today, even though we know more about it than ever before, because the answer to one question is the genesis of a whole set of new questions. It is this deepening biologic complexity – along with the ingenuity and genetic plasticity of microbial pathogens, which leads to changes in virulence mechanisms and new ways of interacting with the host – that makes infectious diseases one of the most vibrant of the disciplines of modern medicine, pediatrics and surgery.

Redundancy of defenses

If there were a single defense mechanism for each class of micro-organism, people with congenital defects in specific limbs of the immune system would be subject to disease with all possible classes of pathogens. This is not the case, and this fact is a major reason to believe that alternative defense mechanisms exist (Fig. 2.28). For example, if we consider congenital defects in the four major limbs of the immune system (phagocytic cells, T lymphocytes, complement and antibody), it is clear that only certain pathogens commonly become problems for the affected host (Chapter 4.2):

- defects in phagocytic cells diminish host defenses to certain bacteria and fungi, but not to viruses or protozoa;
- defects in T lymphocyte impair cell-mediated immunity to mycobacteria and facultative intracellular bacteria, such as *Salmonella typhi*, *Listeria monocytogenes* and *Legionella pneumophila*, certain fungi, certain viruses and some protozoa, but not to pyogenic bacteria such as *S. aureus*;
- defects in complement may impair host defenses to encapsulated micro-organisms but not to fungi or viruses; and
- defects in antibody may impair host responses to encapsulated Gram-negative and Gram-positive bacterial pathogens but do not alter the host response to most viruses and fungi.

At the same time, vigorous immune responses may convey no protection at all and merely be a smoke screen response elicited by pathogens that are wholly unaffected. Such is the case with malaria or infection with *Leishmania* spp., which elicit a polyclonal antibody response to antigens that do not mediate immune protection but none the less consumes energy and amino acid substrates but offers little or no protection. Some micro-organisms, such as *Schistosome* spp., shed their outer coats as antibodies are produced, thus evading immune recognition. Indeed, it seems that the higher the organism is in the evolutionary tree, the more elaborate its means of avoiding immune destruction. This is not to say that more primitive organisms, despite the relatively limited size of their genome, cannot possess intricate invasive properties. The foremost example of an eloquent evasion of host defences is HIV with its attack on host immune regulatory cells bearing the CD4 determinant (Fig. 2.29). However, in biologic terms, this is a 'simple' mechanism, although it certainly leads to very complicated results because it disrupts the role of these cells as conductors of the immunologic orchestra (Chapter 5.6).

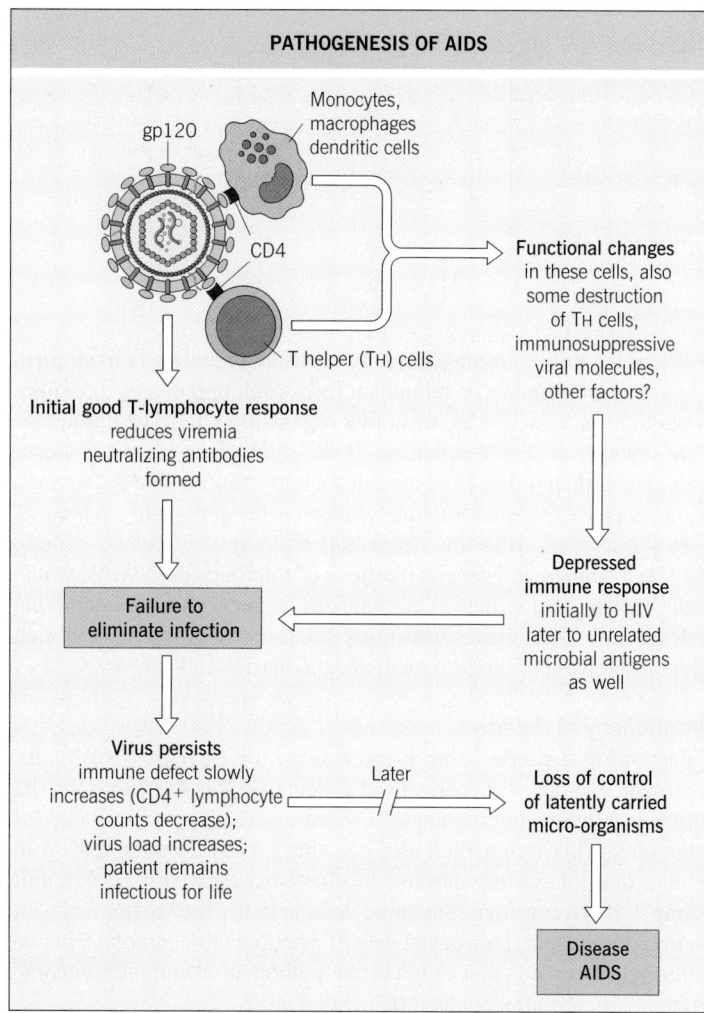

Fig. 2.29 Pathogenesis of AIDS. The pathogenesis begins with the binding of HIV binding to CD4 receptors on the regulatory cells of the immune system.

Phagocytosis

Although micro-organisms can invade epithelial cells by inducing a process that appears very similar to phagocytosis, it is the PMNLs and the cells of the monocyte–macrophage line that, by and large, carry out the host function of microbial ingestion and destruction (Fig. 2.30). However, these cells are not very adept at phagocytosis and microbial killing unless they are instructed to do so (Fig. 2.31). This instruction often comes in the form of messages from activated T lymphocytes or macrophage antigen-presenting cells, or in the form of soluble proteins derived from complement or immunoglobulin that are able to signal the phagocyte to ingest and kill. Eosinophils are ordinarily considered to be largely restricted to their role in allergy, but they may also ingest very large macroscopic multiple-cell pathogens such as worms.[52]

Phagocytosis by PMNLs and the activation of intracellular microbicidal reactions is a multifactorial process that is dependent, in the first instance, on the deposition of activated complement fragments or immunoglobulin on the surface of the organism, which renders them recognizable by receptors on the surface of the PMNL for C3b and the Fc fragment of immunoglobulin (Fig. 2.32). Subsequent ingestion requires complex signaling via protein phosphorylations that result in the rearrangement of the cytoskeleton, the ingestion of the organism within a vacuole made of host plasma membrane, and the subsequent fusion with primary and secondary granules to form phagolysosomes.[53] These granules contain a number of microbicidal proteins (e.g. BPI) and enzyme systems that are capable of generating reactive oxygen intermediates with microbicidal properties.[54]

To be effective, PMNLs must reach the site of infection. Chemical signals to attract these cells (chemotactic factors or chemoattractants) are produced during the initial host–pathogen interaction (Fig. 2.33). The ability of host defense cells to reach an infected area involves the regulated and co-ordinated expression or activation of both leukocyte adhesion molecules and endothelial cell adhesion molecules, which are called selectins (Fig. 2.34).[55] These adhesins mediate the cell–cell interactions that allow the initial sticking of PMNLs to the capillary endothelium and their subsequent migration across the capillary wall to the site of the infection (Fig. 2.35).[56] The importance of mechanisms of adherence and migration can be appreciated by considering the clinical problems experienced by people with the hyperimmunoglobulin E syndrome (also known as Job's syndrome).[57] Polymorphonuclear leukocytes can accumulate in subcutaneous tissues of these patients in response to microbial challenge, but their further migration is delayed and quantitatively diminished. Although the response is sufficient to prevent systemic spread of *S. aureus* from the skin, it is inadequate to prevent or clear the local subcutaneous lesions. These patients also have a deficiency in IgG and IgA antistaphylococcal antibodies and an excess of IgE, often with demonstrable specificity for *S. aureus* cell walls that, unfortunately, have little clinical importance. It is this finding, probably a reflection of lymphocyte abnormalities in the regulation of IgE production, that gives the syndrome its name.

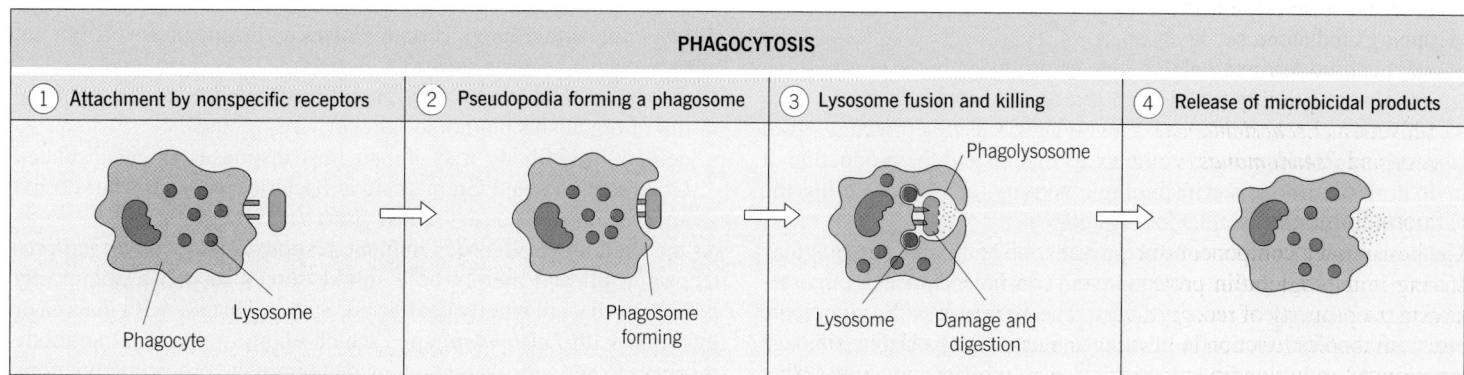

Fig. 2.30 The process of phagocytosis.

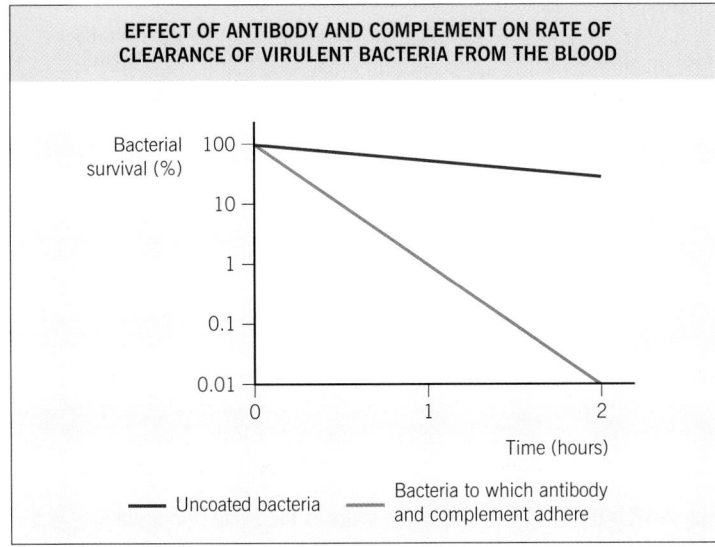

Fig. 2.31 Effect of antibody and complement on rate of clearance of virulent bacteria from the blood. Phagocytosis is greatly potentiated if the microbes are coated with antibody and complement.

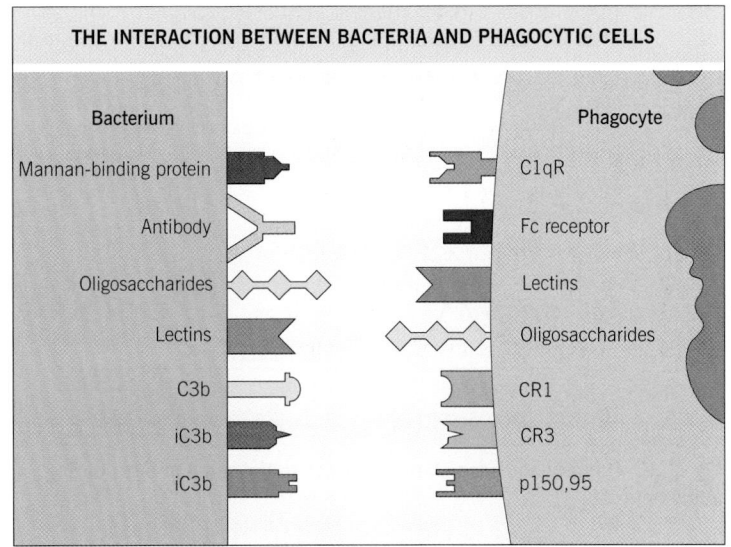

Fig. 2.32 The interaction between bacteria and phagocytic cells. This is facilitated by a variety of molecules, the precise nature of which may determine whether uptake occurs and whether killing mechanisms are triggered.

CHEMOTACTIC MOLECULES

Factor	Characteristic	Source	Action on
C5a	77 amino-acid peptide	N-terminus of C5 α chain	Neutrophils, eosinophils, macrophages
f.Met–Leu–Phe	Tripeptide with blocked N-terminus	Prokaryotes	Neutrophils, eosinophils, macrophages
Leukotriene B₄	Arachidonic acid metabolite via lipoxygenase pathway	Mast cells, basophils, macrophages	Neutrophils, eosinophils, macrophages
Various low-molecular weight chemokines	10kDa proteins	Different leukocyte populations	Selective actions on different leukocyte populations

Fig. 2.33 Chemotactic molecules.

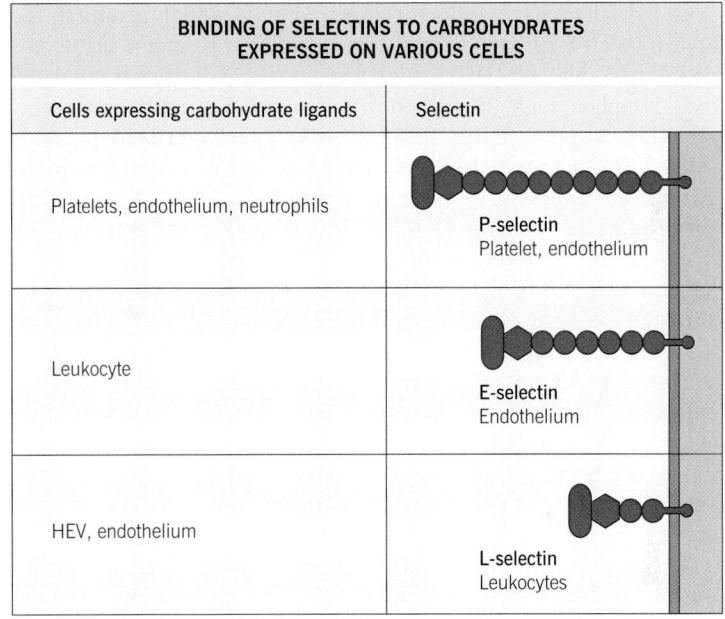

Fig. 2.34 Binding of selectins to carbohydrates expressed on various cells. HEV, high endothelial venules.

Several genetic defects in PMNL function (Chapter 4.2) confirm the importance of these cells for the defense against frequent staphylococcal infection. These genetic defects include:

- chronic granulomatous disease, a defect in production of microbicidal reactive oxygen intermediates,[58] which renders the host susceptible to infection with *S. aureus* and to a lesser extent with *Aspergillus* spp. and *Candida* spp., *Chromobacterium violaceum*, *Burkholderia cepacia* and various Gram-negative Enterobacteriaceae; and
- Chédiak–Higashi syndrome, a defect in degranulation of lysosomes[59] with abnormal early kinetics for killing of ingested *S. aureus*.

Cyclic neutropenia results in periodic severe neutropenia that exposes the host to the same set of infections that occur in secondary neutropenia caused, for example, by cancer chemotherapy. The result is increased susceptibility to infection with *S. aureus* and Gram-negative bacilli such as *Escherichia coli*, *Klebsiella pneumoniae*, *Enterobacter cloacae* and *Pseudomonas aeruginosa*.

Humoral immunity

The best-known component of humoral immunity is antibody, comprising immunoglobulin proteins produced by B lymphocytes and having the property of recognizing unique antigenic molecular structures. Antibodies function in host defense against infection when they are directed to antigenic components of micro-organisms, whether these antigenic components are free in the tissues or present on

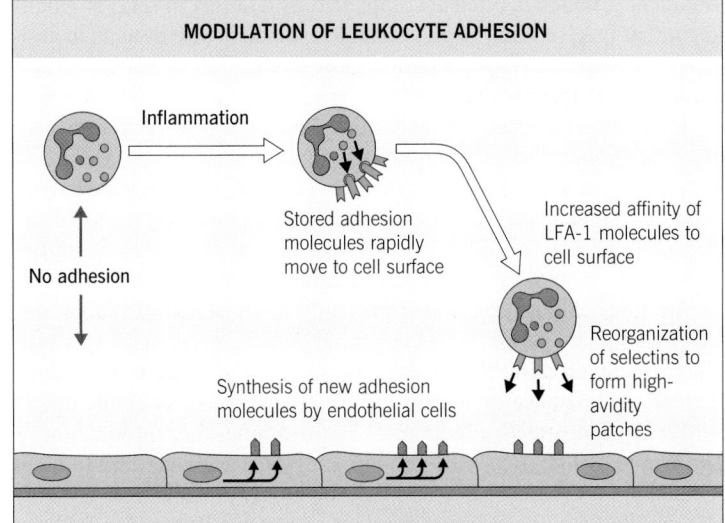

Fig. 2.35 Modulation of leukocyte adhesion. There are four ways in which leukocyte binding to endothelium can be enhanced. LFA-1, lymphocyte function associated antigen-1.

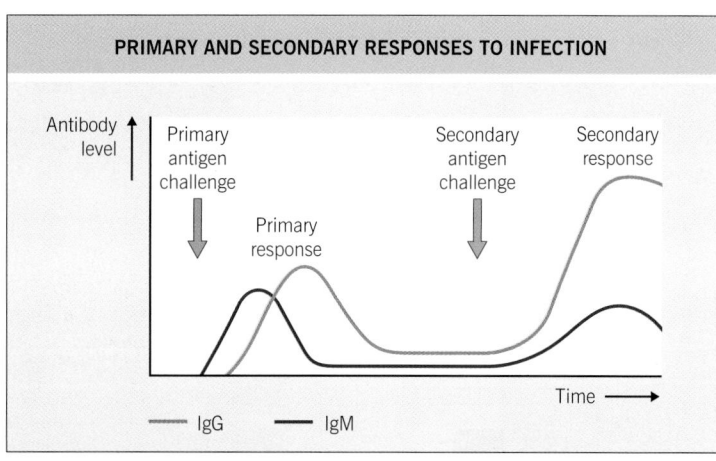

Fig. 2.36 **Primary and secondary responses to the same antigen during infection.**

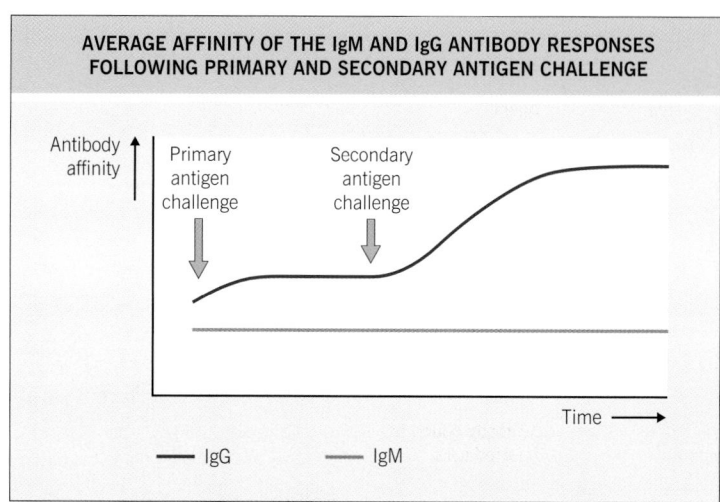

Fig. 2.37 **Affinity of the antibody responses following primary and secondary antigen challenge.**

whole organisms or on the surface of infected cells. For most infectious diseases, the host response depends on the processing of antigens by macrophage antigen-presenting cells, which results in the appearance of antigenic fragments in relation to major histocompatibility complex (MHC) locus determinants, and which is regulated by T lymphocytes.[60] The repertoire of circulating antibodies generally shifts from an initial IgM to a subsequent IgG predominance (Fig. 2.36), associated with a change from low-affinity to high-affinity antibodies against specific antigens (Fig. 2.37); this is sometimes referred to as an increase in the 'quality' of the antibody response (or 'antibody maturation'). The IgM response seems to have its value in being a rapid response to an infectious challenge, although the large size of the IgM molecule largely restricts its activity to the intravascular compartment. Immunoglobulin M is able to activate complement and generate the active byproducts of the classic pathway C3a (which acts as an opsonin) and C5a (which acts as an anaphylotoxin) in order to facilitate phagocytosis via the C3a receptor of the phagocytic cell and to enhance leukocyte migration to the site of infection. In contrast, the IgG response is more specific and may be more effective as well as wider in distribution, assuming the host has survived the initial challenge. By binding to microorganisms at the antibody combining site, IgG also acts as an opsonin because the phagocytes have receptors for the Fc portion of the immunoglobulin molecule. To some extent, IgG subclass antibodies act preferentially in certain infections. Thus, congenital IgG$_2$ subclass deficiency, which is often accompanied by a defect in IgG$_4$ or a deficiency in IgA, or both, is particularly associated with deficits in antibody to bacterial polysaccharide capsules and recurrent infections with encapsulated organisms.[61]

In addition to circulating antibodies, the secretory IgA system produces a special dimeric form of IgA, in which the dimers are linked together by a joining peptide, the J piece, with an associated carrier peptide, the secretory component, which facilitates transport of the complete secretory IgA molecule across mucosal surfaces. Secretory IgA is able to act locally to impair microbial colonization and invasion at the mucosal surface, and it probably has many more functions. Although many people with congenital defects in secretory IgA production remain clinically healthy, presumably because of the robust redundant response of various alternative defense systems, others suffer from repeated infections.[62] For example, the introduction of the *Haemophilus influenzae* protein–polysaccharide vaccine to elicit circulating IgG anticapsular antibodies not only protects from invasive *Haemophilus influenzae* type b infection but has shown that IgG can function on a mucosal surface as this has resulted in a marked decrease in upper airway colonization by the organism, which must be related to an effect of the antibody at the nasopharyngeal mucosal surface.[63]

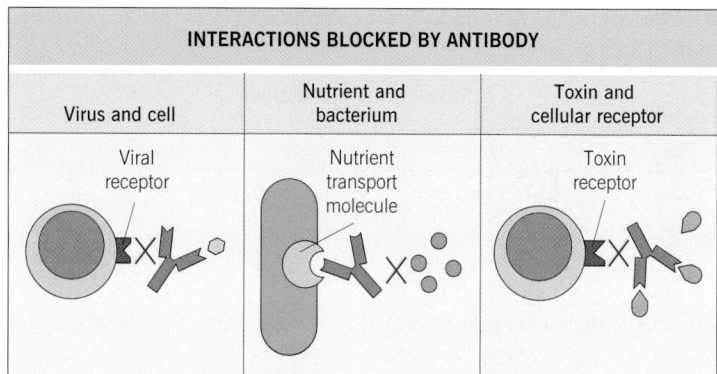

Fig. 2.38 **Examples of host-pathogen interactions blocked by antibody.**

Interestingly, protein-energy malnutrition has a marked inhibitory effect on the secretory IgA response, and this is one likely reason why mucosal infections are so prominent in affected children, with respiratory disease predominating among the very young, and diarrheal diseases among those who are older.

Antibodies have highly specific very discrete functions, for example the neutralization of biologic products produced by the microorganism (Fig. 2.38). The oldest and best-known example is the antitoxin response to bacterial toxins, which was used to develop protective bacterial vaccines consisting of biologically inactivated but antigenic toxoids of tetanus and diphtheria toxins. This approach produced spectacular results, even though the natural infection may not lead to significant protection, presumably because so little toxin antigen is produced. It is now known that toxins are often synthesized as heterodimers, with separate A and B subunits mediating the enzyme action of the toxin and its binding specificity, respectively. Antibody to either the A subunit or the B subunit can be protective, particularly when it is present before the toxin is introduced. Therefore, antitoxin antibody may be useful when it is elicited by a vaccine, although it may not be clinically effective when initiated during infection (as is the case with pertussis), because the pathophysiologic events elicited by the toxin have already occurred by the time the response is mature and antibodies are detectable *in situ*.

Antibody to viral antigens can also be an effective host defense (Fig. 2.39). These antibodies may develop during the course of the infection and play a prominent role in the control of infection and clearance of the circulating virus. This occurs in infection with poliovirus and influenza A virus, in both of which virus-neutralizing antibodies develop. Killed parenteral polio vaccine or influenza A vaccine also elicit virus-neutralizing antibodies which provide significant protection. How these antibodies work is not always clear,

ANTIVIRAL EFFECTS OF ANTIBODY

Target	Agent	Mechanism
Free virus	Antibody alone	Blocks binding to cell
		Blocks entry into cell
		Blocks uncoating of virus
	Antibody + complement	Damage to virus envelope
		Blockade of virus receptor
Virus-infected cells	Antibody + complement	Lysis of infected cell
		Opsonization of coated virus or infected cells for phagocytosis
	Antibody bound to infected cells	Antibody-dependent cell-mediated cytotoxicity by natural killer cells, macrophages and neutrophils

Fig. 2.39 Antiviral effects of antibody. Antibody acts to neutralize virus or kill virally infected cells.

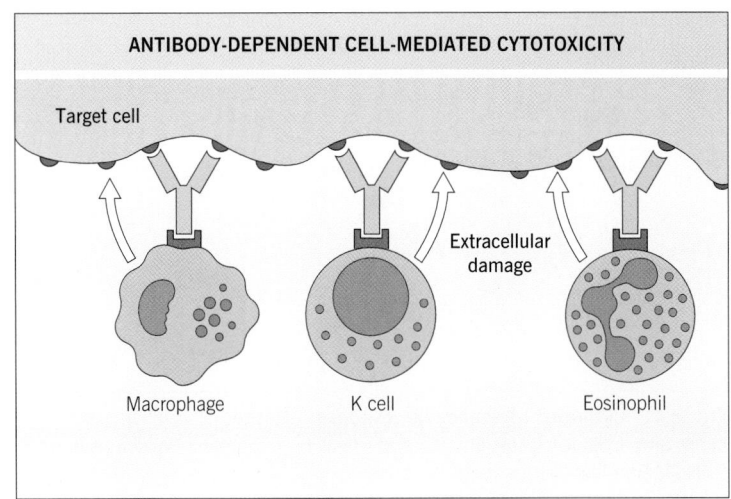

Fig. 2.40 Antibody-dependent cell-mediated cytotoxicity. Different effector cells bind to the surface of the target cell via their receptor for antibody.

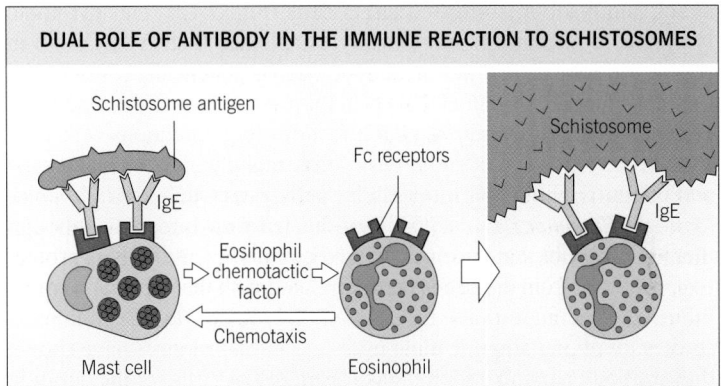

Fig. 2.41 Dual role of antibody in the immune reaction to schistosomes. Following contact with the schistosome antigen, mast cells sensitized with antischistosome IgE release chemotactic factor, which attracts eosinophils. When the eosinophils arrive they are able to bind to the antibody-coated worm via their Fc receptors and damage the parasite.

and there may be several different mechanisms involved at any one time. Protection may:

- be related to antibody-induced changes in viral surface charge or shape;
- be due to aggregation and rapid clearance of virus released from cells, preventing viral replication; or
- result in the lysis of infected cells, thus interrupting the life cycle of the virus.

The importance and specificity of antiviral antibody in the host response is shown by the predilection for some, but not all, viral infections in patients with congenital forms of agammaglobulinemia. The infections to which these patients are prone include poliovirus, echovirus and hepatitis B virus infection; the infections to which they are not unusually prone include measles and rubella. The difference between these groups of viruses may relate to the extent to which cell-mediated immunity contributes to host defense.

Antibody can also function in a co-operative host defense mechanism: antibody-dependent cellular cytotoxicity (ADCC) (Fig. 2.40). This is mediated by natural killer lymphocytes (NK cells), which possess high-affinity receptors for the Fc portion of the immunoglobulin molecule but lack markers of either T lymphocytes or B lymphocytes. As a result, they are capable of binding antibody by way of an interaction between the Fc portion of IgG molecule and the Fc receptor. Antibody-dependent cellular cytotoxicity is distinguished from other cellular cytotoxicity responses by the fact that antigenic specificity is provided by the specificity of the antibody, rather than the cellular effector, and it is not restricted by the MHC locus.[64] In-vitro, this mechanism occurs at physiologic concentrations of antibody, and therefore it could be expressed *in vivo*, especially at sites that are poor in complement activity, such as mucosal surfaces. However, there is as yet no convincing evidence for a role for ADCC in host defense against infection. A variant mechanism of ADCC involving eosinophils has also been described *in vitro* as a possible host defense to helminths.[65] These studies demonstrate that eosinophils, which are increased in number by many worm infections, adhere to and damage helminth larvae that have been coated with IgG, resulting in larval death (Fig. 2.41). This form of ADCC has been shown for *Schistosoma mansoni*, *Trichinella spiralis*, *Wuchereria bancrofti* and *Onchocerca volvulus*.

Cell-mediated host immunity

In contrast to humoral immunity resulting from the direct action of soluble host response molecules, such as antibody, cell-mediated immunity requires the action of intact cells of the mononuclear lineage, including macrophages or T lymphocytes, or both. This mechanism is dependent on specifically sensitized T lymphocytes, which have been activated by antigens of the micro-organism; indeed, in inbred mice, immunity can be adoptively transferred by injecting isolated cells from the spleen into a previously normal, uninfected animal. It is this phenomenon that led to the characterization of the immune response as cell-mediated, in contrast to immunity to pneumococci, which can be transferred by serum antibody alone. Tuberculosis is a particularly well-studied example of cell-mediated immunity (Chapter 2.30),[66] in which infection induces clonal expansion of specific mycobacterial antigen-sensitized T lymphocytes, which in turn activate the mycobactericidal mechanisms of the macrophage. This event depends on the production and release of soluble mediators from the T lymphocytes, and it is enhanced by activation of cytokine production from the macrophage, for example IFN-γ. Tuberculosis is also a classic example of granuloma formation, a cell-mediated response in which the organism is contained within a collection of macrophages surrounded by activated T lymphocytes. The granuloma is a recognizable pathologic unit that is present wherever the organism has spread (e.g. in lung or liver). It is granuloma formation that is initiated by the injection of tuberculin into the skin; indeed, the palpable reaction that characterizes a positive test is a focal granuloma induced by the injection of the antigen, which recruits macrophages and T lymphocytes to the site.

Granulomas also characterize the host response in schistosomiasis. It is the granulomatous response that results in the pathology of the infection. Measures that limit granuloma formation protect the host from the damage that results from the production by the granuloma of fibrogenic factors that induce the characteristic scarring of this disease.[67]

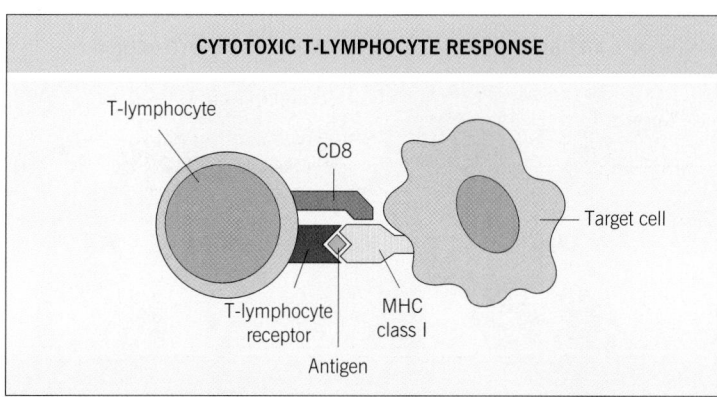

Fig. 2.42 Cytotoxic T-lymphocyte response. Cytotoxic T lymphocytes expressing CD8 recognize antigen and major histocompatibility complex (MHC), enabling them to bind target cells.

	Interferon-α	Interferon-ß	Interferon-γ
Alternative name	'Leukocyte' interferon	'Fibroblast' interferon	'Immune' interferon
Principal source	All cells	All cells	T lymphocytes
Inducing agent	Viral infection (or double-stranded RNA)	Viral infection (or double-stranded RNA)	Antigen (or mitogen)
Number of species	22	1	1
Chromosomal location of gene(s)	9	9	12
Antiviral activity	+++	+++	+
Immunoregulalory activity: Macrophage action	–	–	++
MHC class I upregulation	+	+	+
MHC class II upregulation	–	–	+

HUMAN INTERFERONS

Fig. 2.43 Human interferons. MHC, major histocompatibility complex.

Another manifestation of cell-mediated immunity is represented by the ability of cytotoxic subpopulations of CD8⁺ T lymphocytes to attack and lyse virus-infected target cells (Fig. 2.42). This cytotoxic lymphocyte response is more firmly established than ADCC, and in contrast to ADCC, requires no antibody and is genetically restricted by the MHC locus. Congenital defects in this system lead to increased susceptibility to and severity of viral infections (e.g. infections with varicella-zoster virus and other herpesviruses, including cytomegalovirus) and infection with other intracellular pathogens (such as *M. tuberculosis* and *Pneumocystis carinii*). In influenza virus infection, although there is no doubt that vaccine-induced circulating antibody is protective, recovery from disease is best correlated with the appearance of an influenza-specific response by cytotoxic T lymphocytes. Experimental studies involving athymic nude mice and influenza virus have shown that antibody administration blocks shedding of virus for the duration of the treatment, whereas adoptive transfer of virus specific cytotoxic T lymphocytes clears the virus from the lungs and cures the infection.[68,69] These findings suggest that the two forms of specific immune response may work together in the response to influenza and presumably to other infections as well.

Natural killer cells

Although they were originally defined as a class of naturally occurring tumoricidal cells, natural killer (NK) cells have since been shown to be involved in the response to infection, especially virus infection. Natural killer cells are distinctive cells that are characterized as relatively large, low-density, granular cells lacking the T-lymphocyte receptor and surface immunoglobulin, although they do express a number of cell surface receptors that are either unique or shared with other immunologically active cells.[70] Natural killer cells do not require prior activation to function; however, their action is modulated by MHC class I determinants.[71]

The best evidence for the function of NK cells in host defense is in viral infections. Animal models have been extensively used for this purpose, and by depleting and adoptively transferring NK cells, a role in host defense against herpes simplex virus, murine cytomegalovirus and Coxsackie B4 virus infection has been shown, whereas there is no apparent effect of NK cells on lymphocytic choriomeningitis virus. The role of NK cells in humans remains to be clearly shown.

Interferons

It is now 40 years since the first IFN was described as a host-derived antiviral protein. The IFNs are now known to be a family of proteins, which – rather than being simply antiviral substances – are intimately involved in the regulation of the immune system and play an important role in tumor control.[72] There are, in fact, three classes of IFNs (Fig. 2.43):
- α- (or leukocyte) IFN,
- β- (or fibroblast) IFN, and
- γ- (or immune) IFN.

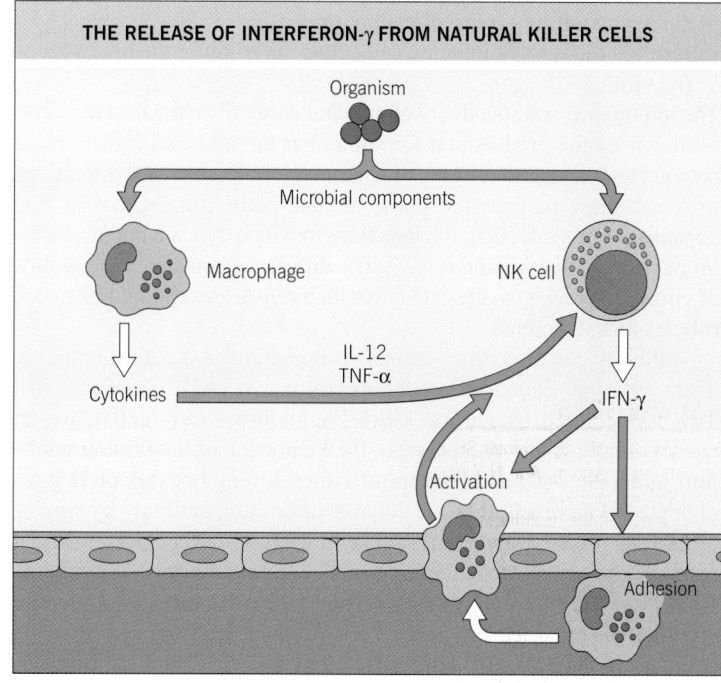

Fig. 2.44 The release of interferon (IFN)-γ from natural killer (NK) cells. IL, interleukin; TNF, tumor necrosis factor.

Interferons α and β are acid stable proteins produced in response to viral infections and dsRNA and related polyanions; each of these interferons is an antiviral protein. In contrast, IFN-γ, an acid-labile protein, is made during antigen or mitogen activation of T lymphocytes and NK cells, primarily in response to IL-12 released from macrophages (Fig. 2.44).[73] Interferon-γ, in turn, feeds back on macrophages to upregulate the expression of TNF-α, which, together with IFN-γ increases the expression of IL-12 and further drives the production of IFN-γ. Interleukin-12 together with IFN-γ favors the development of the T-helper-1 lymphocyte response, which:[74]
- activates macrophages to produce reactive oxygen intermediates such as superoxide and nitric oxide, and to express MHC and type II and Fc receptors;
- augments T-lymphocyte-mediated cytotoxicity; and
- induces NK cells.

In some intracellular infections of mononuclear cells, IFN-γ production is reduced due to increased IL-10 production from activated TH2 lymphocytes (e.g. in tuberculosis, leprosy and leishmaniasis), and this may be a major reason for the progression of these infections (Fig. 2.45). Successful therapy is associated with restoration of IGN-γ production. Low levels of IFN-γ are due to one of three abnormalities:

- abnormal IL-10 and/or IL-12 production,
- a deficiency of CD4+ T-lymphocytes, or
- a deficiency of IFN-γ receptors.

Deficiency of IFN-γ receptors has been identified in a small number of patients, and these patients have a prominent susceptibility to nontuberculous mycobacterial infection but not to other infections, suggesting a unique function specificity for IFN-γ in this infection.

Recently, a novel cytokine IL-18 (interferon gamma releasing factor) has been identified which appears to have an upstream regulatory role in IFN-γ regulation. The precise physiological or pathological role of IL-18 remains to be determined.

Interferon-γ has been used with success in chronic granulomatous disease, for which it is licensed by the US Food and Drug Administration (FDA), and in the treatment of lepromatous leprosy, visceral and diffuse cutaneous leishmaniasis and disseminated mycobacterial infections. The FDA has also approved the use of IFN-α for the treatment of hairy cell leukemia, condyloma acuminatum, Kaposi's sarcoma and hepatitis B and C virus infection. It is likely that the utility of IFN therapy will increase as the number of

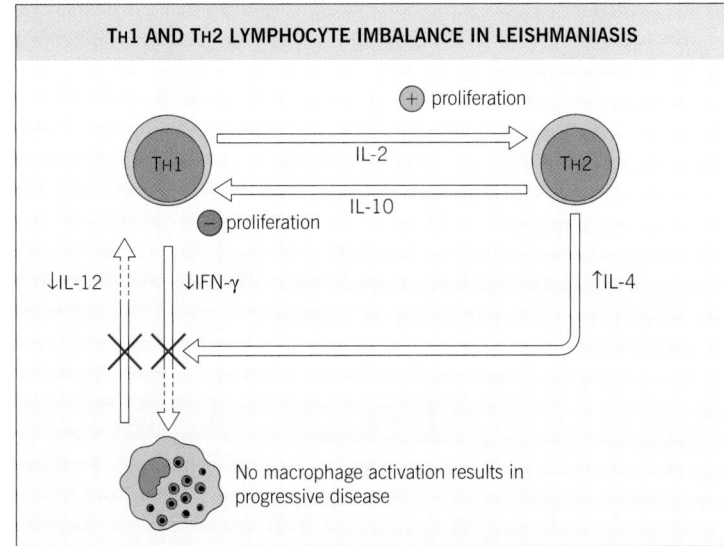

Fig. 2.45 T-helper (TH)1 and TH2 lymphocyte imbalance in leishmaniasis. Leishmaniasis is characterized by deficient interferon (IFN)-γ production and inhibition of its action. IL, interleukin.

disease indications in which it has an impact also increases, and the importance of providing the correct cosignal at the right time becomes better known.

REFERENCES

1. Marchalonis JJ, Schluter SF. Development of an immune system. Ann N Y Acad Sci 1994;712:1–12.
2. Galen. On the usefulness of the parts of the body [reprinted]. Icatha, New York, USA: Cornell University Press; 1968.
3. DuBois EF. Why are fever temperatures over 106°C rare? Am J Med Sci 1949;217:361–8.
4. Yatvin MB, Cramp WA. Role of cellular membranes in hyperthermia: some observations and theories reviewed. Int J Hyperthermia 1993;9:165–85.
5. Mackowiak PA, Boulant JA. Fever's glass ceiling. Clin Infect Dis 1995;22:525–36.
6. Dinarello CA. Endogenous pyrogens: the role of cytokines in the pathogenesis of fever. In: Mackowiak PA, ed. Fever: basic mechanisms and managements. New York: Raven; 1991:23–47.
7. Kluger MJ, Ringler DH, Anver MR. Fever and survival. Science 1975;188:166–8.
8. Bernheim HA, Kluger MJ. Fever: effect of drug-induced antipyresis on survival. Science 1976;193:237–9.
9. Bernheim HA, Bodel PT, Askenase PW, Atkins E. Effects of fever on host defense mechanisms after infection in the lizard Dipsosaurus dorsalis. Br J Exp Pathol 1978:59:76–84.
10. Vaughn LK, Bernheim HA, Kluger M. Fever in the lizard Dypsosaurus dorsalis. Nature 1974;252:473–4.
11. Kluger MJ, Kozak W, Conn CA, Leon LR, Soszynski D. The adaptive value of fever. Infect Dis Clin North Am 1996;10:1–20.
12. Kreyman G, Grossers S, Buggisch P, Gottschall C, Matthaei S, Greten H. Oxygen consumption and resting metabolic rate in sepsis, sepsis syndrome, and septic shock. Crit Care Med 1993;21:1012–9.
13. Tracey KJ, Cerami A. Tumor necrosis factor and regulation of metabolism in infection: role of systemic vs local levels. Proc Soc Exp Biol Med 1992;200:233–9.
14. Tracey KJ, Cerami A. Tumor necrosis factor: a pleiotropic cytokine and therapeutic target. Ann Rev Med 1994;45:491–503.
15. Dinarello CA, Endres S, Meydani SN, Meydani M, Hellerstein MK. Interleukin-1, anorexia, and dietary fatty acids. Ann N Y Acad Sci 1990;587:332–8.
16. Shoham S, Davenne D, Cady AB, Dinarello CA, Krueger JM. Recombinant tumor necrosis factor and interleukin-1 enhance slow wave sleep. Am J Physiol 1987;253:R142–9.
17. Zhang Y, Proenca R, Maffei M, Barone M, Leopold L, Friedman JM. Positional cloning of the mouse ob gene and its human homologue. Nature 1994;372:425–32.
18. Halaas J, Gajiwala KS, Maffei M, et al. Weight reducing effects of the plasma protein encoded by the obese gene. Science 1995;269:543–6.
19. Campfield LA, Smith FJ, Guisez Y, Devos R, Burn P. Recombinant mouse OB protein: evidence for a peripheral signal linking adiposity and central neural networks. Science 1995;269:546–9.
20. Stephens TW, Basinski M, Bristow PK, et al. The role of neuropeptide Y in the antiobesity action of the obese gene product. Nature 1995;377:530–2.
21. Tomaszuk A, Simpson C, Williams G. Neuropeptide Y, the hypothalamus and the regulation of energy homeostasis. Horm Res 1996;46:53–8.
22. Sarraf P, Frederich RC, Turner EM, et al. Multiple cytokines and acute inflammation raise mouse leptin levels: potential role in inflammatory anorexia. J Exp Med 1997;185:171–5.
23. Shaw JH, Klein S, Wolfe RR. Assessment of alanine, urea and glucose interrelationships in normal subjects and in patients with sepsis with stable isotopic tracers. Surgery 1985;97:557–68.
24. Cantorna MT, Nashold FE, Chun TY, Hayes CE. Vitamin A down regulation of IFN-gamma synthesis in cloned mouse Th1 lymphocytes depends on the CD28 costimulatory pathway. J Immunol 1996;156:2674–9.
25. Olson JA. Hypovitaminosis A: contemporary scientific issues. J Nutr 1994;124(suppl 8):1461–6.
26. Meydani SN, Meydani M, Blumberg JB, et al. Vitamin E supplentation and in vivo immune response in healthy elderly subjects. A randomized clinical trial. JAMA 1997;277:1380–6.
27. Meydani SN. Vitamin/mineral supplementation, the aging immune response, and risk of infection. Nutr Rev 1993;51:106–9.
28. Litwin CM, Calderwood SB. Role of iron in regulation of virulence genes. Clin Microbiol Rev 1993;6:137–49.
29. de Lorenzo V, Giovannini F, Herrero M, Neilands JB. Metal ion regulation of gene expression. Fur repressor–operator interaction at the promoter region of the aerobactin system of pColV-K30. J Molec Biol 1988;203:875–84.
30. de Silva DM, Askwith CC, Kaplin J. Molecular mechanisms of iron uptake in eukaryotes. Physiol Rev 1996;76:31–47.

31. Konihn AM. Iron metabolism in inflammation. Baillieres Clin Haematol 1994;7:829–49.

32. Hultgren SJ, Abraham S, Caparon M, Falk P, St Geme JW 3rd, Normark S. Pilus and non-pilus bacterial adhesins: assembly and function in cell recognition. Cell 1993;73:887–901.

33. Stevens MK, Krause DC. *Mycoplasma pneumoniae* cytadherence phase variable protein HMW3 is a component of the attachment organelle. J Bacteriol 1992;174:4265–74.

34. Finlay BB. Cell adhesion and invasion mechanisms in microbial pathogenesis. Curr Opin Cell Biol 1990;2:815–20.

35. Bliska JB, Galan JE, Falkow S. Signal transduction in the mammalian cell during bacterial attachment and entry. Cell 1993;73:903–20.

36. Jones BD, Patterson HF, Hall A, Falkow S. *Salmonella typhimurium* induces membrane ruffling by a growth factor-receptor-independent mechanism. Proc Natl Acad Sci U S A 1993;90:10390–4.

37. Francis CL, Ryan RA, Jones BD, Smith SJ, Falkow S. Ruffles induced by *Salmonella* and other stimuli direct macropinocytosis of bacteria. Nature 1993;364:639–42.

38. Parsot C, Sansonetti PJ. Invasion and the pathogenesis of *Shigella* infections. Curr Topics Microbiol Immunol 1996;209:25–42.

39. Dragic T, Litwin V, Allaway GP, *et al*. HIV-1 entry into CD4(+) cells is mediated by the chemokine receptor CC-CKR-5. Nature 1996;381:667–73.

40. Moors MA, Portnoy DA. Identification of bacterial genes that contribute to survival and growth in an intracellular environment. Trends Microbiol 1995;3:83–5.

41. Sparling PF. Bacterial virulence and pathogenesis: an overview. Rev Infect Dis 1983;5(Suppl 4):637–46.

42. Finlay BB, Falkow S. Common themes in microbial pathogenicity. Microbiol Rev 1989;53:210–30.

43. Raetz CRH. Bacterial endotoxins: extraordinary lipids that activate eucaryotic signal transduction. J Bacteriol 1993;175:5745–53.

44. Ulevitch RJ. Recognition of bacterial endotoxins by receptor-dependent mechanisms. Adv Immunol 1993;53:267–89.

45. Hailman E, Lichenstein HS, Wurfel MM *et al*. Lipopolysaccharide (LPS)-binding protein accelerates the binding of LPS to CD14. J Exp Med 1994;179:269–77.

46. Schwab JH. Phlogistic properties of peptidoglycan–polysaccharide polymers from cell walls of pathogenic and normal flora bacteria which colonize humans. Infect Immun 1993;61:4535–9.

47. Rabin RL, Bieber MM, Teng NN. Lipopolysaccharide and peptidoglycan share binding sites on human peripheral blood monocytes. J Infect Dis 1993;168:135–42.

48. Elsbach P. Bactericidal permeability-increasing protein in host defense against Gram-negative bacteria and endotoxin. Ciba Found Symp 1994;186:176–87.

49. Horwitz AH, Williams RE, Nowakowski G. Human lipopolysaccharide-binding protein potentiates bactericidal activity of human bactericidal/permeability increasing protein. Infect Immun 1995;63:522–7.

50. Elsbach P, Weiss J. Prospects for the use of recombinant BPI in the treatment of Gram negative bacterial infections. Infect Agents Dis 1995;4:102–9.

51. Henderson B, Poole S, Wilson M. Microbial/host interactions in health and disease: who controls the cyotkine network? Immunopharmacology 1996;35:1–21.

52. Gleich GJ, Adolphson CR, Leiferman KM. The biology of the eosinophilic leukocyte. Annu Rev Med 1993;44:85–101.

53. Baggiolini M, Boulay F, Badwey JA, Curnette JT. Activation of neutrophil leukocytes: chemoattractant receptors and respiratory burst. FASEB J 1993;7:1004–20.

54. Moncada S, Higgs A. The L-arginine–nitric oxide pathway. N Engl J Med 1993;329:2002–12.

55. Bevilaqua MP, Nelson RM. Selectins. J Clin Invest 1993;91:379–87.

56. Nourshargh S. Mechanisms of neutrophil and eosinophil accumulation in vivo. Am Rev Respir Dis 1993;148(suppl):60–4.

57. Dreskin SC, Goldsmith, PK, Gallin JI. Immunoglobulins in the hyperimmunoglobulin E and recurrent infection (Job's) syndrome: deficiency of anti-*Staphylococcus aureus* immunoglobulin. J Clin Invest 1985;75:26–34.

58. Curnutte JT. Chronic granulomatous disease: the solving of a clinical riddle at the molecular level. Clin Immunol Immunopathol 1993;67(suppl):2–15.

59. Root RK, Rosenthal AS, Balestra DJ. Abnormal bactericidal, metabolic, and lysosomal functions of Chediak–Higashi syndrome leukocytes. J Clin Invest 1972;51:649–65.

60. Berek C, Ziegner M. The maturation of the immune response. Immunol Today 1993;14:400–4.

61. Kuijpers TW, Weening RS, Out TA. IgG subclass deficiencies and recurrent pyogenic infections; unresponsiveness against bacterial polysaccharide antigens. Allergy Immunopathol 1992;20:28–34.

62. Neutra MR, Krahenbuhl JP. The role of transepithelial transport by M cells in microbial invasion and host defense. J Cell Sci 1993;17:209–15.

63. Barbour ML. Conjugate vaccines and the carriage of *Haemophilus influenzae* type b. Emerging Infectious Diseases 1966;2:176–82.

64. Sissons JGP, Oldstone MBA. Antibody-mediated destruction of virus-infected cells. Adv Immunol 1980;29:209–60.

65. Elsas PX, Elsas MI, Dessein AJ. Eosinophil cytotoxicity enhancing factor: purification, characterization and immunocytochemical localization on the monocyte surface. Eur J Immunol 1990;20:1143–51.

66. Dunlap NE, Briles DE. Immunology of tuberculosis. Med Clin North Am 1993;77:1235–51.

67. Wyler DJ. Why does liver fibrosis occur in schistosomiasis? Parasitol Today 1992;8:277–9.

68. Bender BS, Small PA Jr. Influenza: pathogenesis and host defense. Semin Respir Infect 1992;7:38–45.

69. Kuwano K, Scott M, Young JF, Ennis FA. HA2 subunit of influenza A H1 and H2 subtype viruses induces a protective cross-reactive cytotoxic T lymphocyte response. J Immunol 1988;140:1264–8.

70. Lanier LL, Phillips JH. Natural killer cells. Curr Opin Immunol 1992;4:38–42.

71. Bancroft GJ. The role of natural killer cells in innate resistance to infection. Curr Opin Immunol 1993;5:503–10.

72. Itri LM. The interferons. Cancer 1992;70:940–5.

73. Trinchieri G. Interleukin-12: a proinflammatory cytokine with immunoregulatory functions that bridge innate resistance and antigen-specific adaptive immunity. Annu Rev Immunol 1995;13:251–76.

74. Koziel MJ, Walker BD. Viruses, chemotherapy and immunity. Parasitology 1992;105:S85–92.

75. Yang RB, Mark MR, Gray A, *et al*. Toll-like receptor-2 mediates lipopolysaccharide-induced cellular signalling. Nature 1998;395:284–8.

The Past, Present and Future of the Clinical Microbiology Laboratory

Antoine Andremont

INTRODUCTION

Clinical microbiology as a medical science is a century old. Its practice began with Pasteur's discoveries and it has evolved with the advancement of laboratory techniques and the evolution of the clinical spectrum of infectious diseases. Today, clinical microbiology is a fully integrated part of medical practice, both for hospitalized patients and for outpatients. In addition, the results obtained in the clinical microbiology laboratory are important not only for medical decisions about the management of individual patients but also for the description of the epidemiology of transmissible diseases; thus, they are the grounds on which many public health policies are founded.

The practice of clinical microbiology is at a turning point in its history (Fig. 3.1). It is usually said that, until the beginning of the 1980s, clinical microbiologists working in hospitals had been using the same basic techniques for 50 or 70 years.

This generally accepted assumption has to be moderated, however, by two major changes that were introduced in the 1950s and 1960s. The first was the introduction of commercially available blood culture systems.[1] These systems have great advantages over locally prepared flasks. They are subjected to rigorous quality-control procedures and are much easier for both medical and paramedical personnel to use. In addition, they are specifically designed to reduce the number of contaminated samples. The availability of these systems has led to dramatic results: before their availability the sampling of blood for culture was performed on a relatively small scale, whereas now it is one of the most widely used tests and is performed in all febrile patients.

The second major change in the practice of medical microbiology introduced in the 1960s was the systematic determination of antibiotic susceptibility patterns in clinically significant isolates.[2,3] Because this determination profoundly influences the care of the patient, it has become the focus around which the relationship between clinicians and microbiologists has been built.

Profound technologic changes have been introduced into the everyday life of clinical microbiologists within the past 15 years, in contrast with the relatively stable preceding period (Fig. 3.2). Examples of these changes are:
- the general use of computers to acquire data and transmit results to clinicians;[4]
- the introduction of automation for some techniques, such as bacterial identification;[5]
- far more sophisticated antibiotic susceptibility testing;[6]
- the detection of blood culture positivity;[1] and
- the use of commercially available kits based on molecular biology techniques, which may even bypass the need for pure culture isolation of micro-organisms for identification.[7,8]

Recently, the combination of computer analysis and molecular techniques for typing micro-organisms has allowed in-depth review of the epidemiology and modes of transmission of several bacterial diseases, particularly nosocomial infections.[9] In the very near future, new advances in DNA and computer technology will again profoundly modify our approaches to microbiologic diagnosis.[10]

During the same period of time, the hospital environment in which clinical microbiologists work has also been greatly transformed, owing to:
- the rising concern about the control of nosocomial infections;[11]
- the increased susceptibility of patients to opportunistic infections following chemotherapy, retrovirus infections and intensive care procedures; and
- the introduction of concepts of health economy,[12] quality management[13] and medical care evaluation[13,14] in every day hospital life (see Fig. 3.3).

This chapter focuses on the net benefits resulting from the combination of all these changes for the role of the clinical microbiologist, with regard to everyday patient care as well the control of public health problems. It analyses the natural history of a microbiologic specimen – sampling, transporting, processing and reporting of results – and it deals with the organizational aspects that allow the clinical microbiologist to be actively involved in the decision-making process for day-to-day patient care and for collective epidemiologic measures aimed at the control of infections inside (and eventually outside) the hospital setting.

THE NATURAL HISTORY OF BACTERIOLOGIC SPECIMENS

Laboratory personnel must involve themselves in all aspects of specimen management, and not just the process of microbiologic analysis (see Fig. 3.4). Producing, revising and implementing guidelines are the core processes that determine the effectiveness of the laboratory (see Fig. 3.5) and the quality of the results provided to clinicians.

THE THREE PERIODS OF CLINICAL MICROBIOLOGY HISTORY	
First period (from Pasteur's discoveries to the 1950s)	Use of classic techniques for isolation and identification of micro-organisms
Second period (from the 1950s to the 1980s)	Development of better sampling techniques Development of susceptibility testing
Third period (from the 1980s to today)	Development of molecular biology Incorporation of molecular based epidemiology

Fig. 3.1 The three periods of clinical microbiology history.

AUTOMATION IN THE MICROBIOLOGY LABORATORY: AN IRREVERSIBLE TREND	
1980	Analysis of blood cultures Serologic assays (ELISA and others) Identification of bacteria and antibiotic susceptibility testing (first generation of automates)
1990	Identification of bacteria and antibiotic susceptibility testing (second generation of automates using expert system analysis) DNA fingerprinting Automated PCR and hybridization technologies
2000	DNA chip technology Fully automated sample processing (possibly)

Fig. 3.2 Automation in the microbiology laboratory: an irreversible trend.

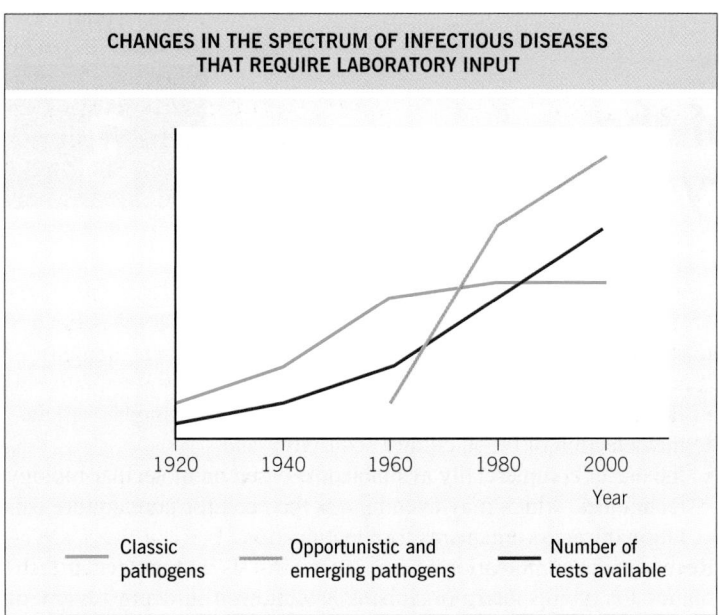

Fig. 3.3 Changes in the spectrum of infectious diseases that require laboratory work.

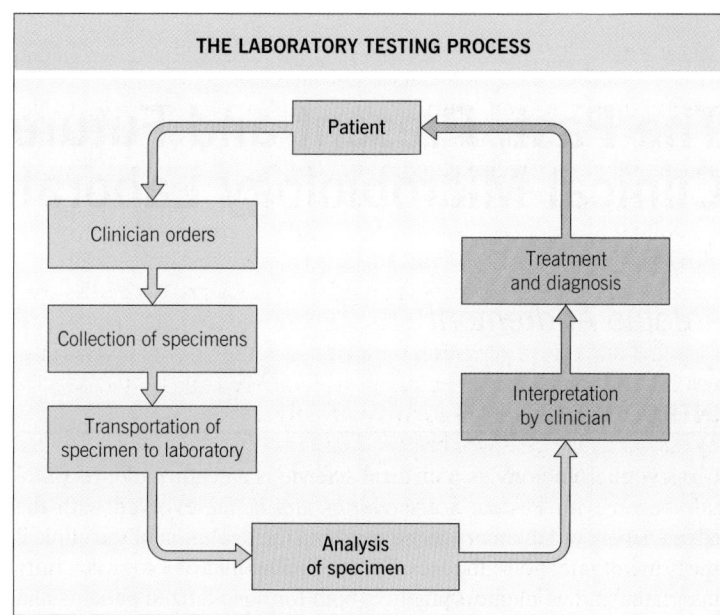

Fig. 3.4 The laboratory testing process.

SAMPLING

Clearly, the effectiveness of the laboratory largely depends on the quality of sampling procedures as well as on the medical rationales behind the ordering of microbiologic tests.

Quality at the time of sampling

High sample quality can only be achieved by implementing strict guidelines in the hospital wards. These guidelines must be discussed in joint meetings of the clinicians and the laboratory personnel. In a specific hospital, these guidelines should be based on the published guidelines[15] of the various national microbiology societies and adapted to the specific needs of each ward. Particular care must be made not to introduce modifications or simplifications that could result in decreased effectiveness of the test. The guidelines must be in written form. The supervisor of each ward must ensure that all personnel – including new members of staff – have read them. The guidelines must be regularly updated and constantly at hand (for example, in a clearly identified book in the nurses' room).

Number of samples

Controlling the number of samples that arrive in the laboratory is important in maintaining good laboratory performance. If inadequate and unnecessary samples overload the laboratory, a decrease in the quality of the technical work will ensue.[13,16] Because working on inadequate samples is not rewarding, the laboratory technicians will gradually lose faith in their work and become less motivated; this in turn will result in a further decrease in the overall quality of their work.

For all these reasons, it is the role of the clinical laboratory manager to keep their clinical colleagues aware of the volume of tests ordered from each ward and to alert them promptly when an unexplained change in that volume occurs. When such an increase corresponds to a new medical need, the microbiologists and clinicians must search together for ways to adapt the resources of the laboratory. Successful implementation of the necessary changes may require the use of a convenient computerized system; by introducing such a system the microbiologists aim both to keep their own laboratories on the correct ethical and economic tracks and to help their clinical colleagues to reduce the inappropriate ordering of microbiology tests, particularly when new and inexperienced doctors begin work in the hospital.

Assessing sample quality when they arrive in the laboratory

In addition to regulating the number of samples that arrive in the laboratory, the clinical microbiologist should also set up a system of specimen quality control, to which all samples must be submitted on arrival at the

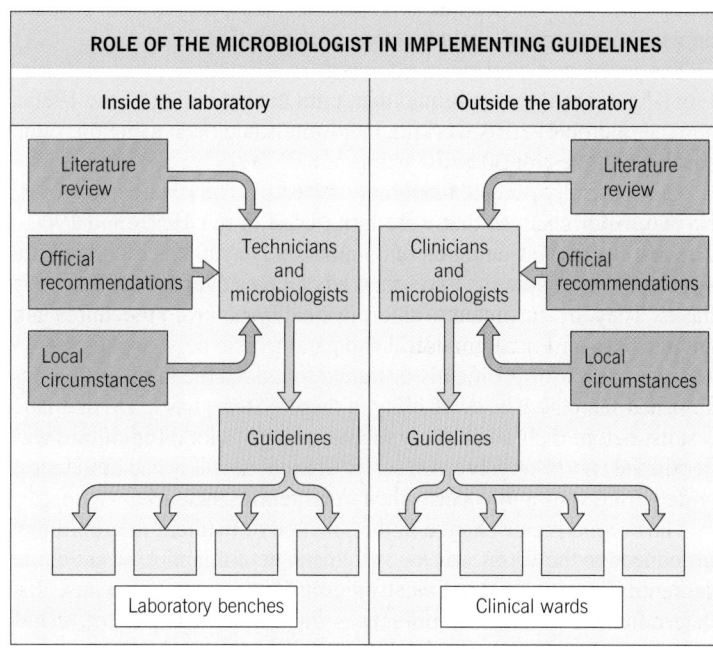

Fig. 3.5 Role of the microbiologist in the implementation of guidelines inside and outside the microbiology laboratory.

laboratory. The implementation of such a quality control system can lead to difficulties between laboratory staff and clinical staff. In order to ensure that it is accepted by everyone, this system must be based on guidelines[15] that have been discussed and approved by clinicians' representatives. It should include only accepted criteria that are based on those described in the literature and adapted to the local conditions. Rejection criteria[17–19] for inadequate clinical samples are designed to prevent microbiologists from producing misleading results. Indeed, testing inadequate samples is expensive and economically detrimental to the hospital community. It is also possibly detrimental to patient care in that it may lead to unwise decisions and wrong treatments.

Microbiologists should try to help clinicians by providing easy-to-consult documents in which the recommendations for sampling and transporting specimens are clearly described; these documents should include all practical information, such as the names of the people in charge of each type of test and how to reach them when necessary. Conversely, before rejecting specimens of borderline quality the microbiologist should bear in mind that these may have been collected in difficult clinical situations.

Providing clinical information

As for some other medical specialists,[20] one of the most frequent problems for clinical microbiologists and technicians is the lack of clinical information provided with the samples they have to examine. Pragmatic considerations have led most microbiologists to abandon the idea of obtaining precise clinical information with every sample sent to the laboratory. Nevertheless, some information is definitely needed for nonsterile specimens, such as feces, vaginal samples, urethral samples and throat samples, for which the techniques involved are very different depending on the clinical diagnosis and the presumed etiology.

Clinicians tend to provide information to the laboratory only when they feel that this information is needed to obtain adequate and rapid results. The compliance of clinicians with microbiologists' requests for clinical information is linked to the quality of the reporting of results by the microbiologists (see below). Clinicians should be aware that laboratory techniques can be performed adequately only if some clinical information is provided. Some laboratories organize periodic 'open-door' visits for medical and paramedical nonlaboratory personnel; these help to publicize the technical and practical aspects of the work performed in the laboratory.

TRANSPORT OF SAMPLES

Ideally, clinical specimens should be inoculated on culture media at the bedside of the patient immediately after sampling. This is the best way of obtaining a precise qualitative and quantitative representation of the micro-organisms present at the site of the suspected infection. Immediate inoculation minimizes both bacterial death, which can lead to false-negative results, and bacterial multiplication, which can lead to false-positive results. However, except for blood samples and sometimes for urine samples, immediate inoculation is usually not possible because nurses and doctors do not have adequate technical skills or time to perform it. Therefore, samples have to be transported to the laboratory for examination. Two aspects have to be examined concerning the transport of specimens – their physical transport to the laboratory and the transport medium used.

Physical transport

The clinical microbiologist should alert the hospital administration that rapid transport of the specimens to the laboratory is of primary importance because delay will result in a rapid decrease in quality.[21] Transport systems vary considerably from one hospital to another; they are largely dependent on the architecture of the hospital buildings. Mechanical or pneumatic transport systems were introduced a number of years ago, but they suffered from difficulties linked to the relatively primitive nature of the electronic systems that controlled their technology. With the huge development of programming and hospital computerization these problems are largely solved and mechanical transport systems are nowadays effective, rapid and reliable, and are used for the transport of specimens to many laboratories,[22,23] although their use may be associated with new and specific problems.[24] The choice between pneumatic and strictly mechanical transport of specimens is largely dependent on architectural and financial considerations, and most often the choice is that of the hospital administration. However, the clinical microbiologist should insist on being part of the discussion if a new system has to be implemented, both to discuss the speed with which different types of specimen must be transported and to alert the administration on the safety and security questions linked to the transport of infectious materials.

In many hospitals the transport of specimens is still made by specially assigned personnel. This has the advantage of some flexibility but the system is often very slow because the collection routes are organized to enable the collection of specimens from all wards in the hospital before reaching the laboratory. Also, in cases of emergency, personnel are often difficult to find.

For these reasons, more automatic systems for the transport of specimens should be advocated. Two major systems are currently used. The first one is pneumatic and the second is electromechanical. Both ensure rapid transport of specimens but, in both cases, microbiologists have to

ensure that problems linked to the possible deterioration of samples and packaging during transport should not endanger personnel by disseminating infectious agents or result in cross-contamination of specimens. The perfect transport system does not exist and probably never will. Therefore, with this limit in mind, each microbiologist must optimize the transport system by taking into account the specific design and organization of his or her particular institution.

Transport media

Several transport media can be used to decrease the death of micro-organisms in clinical specimens. These media are widely described in the microbiologic literature and their performances are compared.[15,25] It is the clinical microbiologist's responsibility to provide each clinical ward and outpatient clinic with adequate, institution-specific guidelines for specimen storage and transport.

The question often arises as to whether transport media should be ordered by the microbiologist and given upon request to clinicians. This procedure has the advantage in theory of ensuring that the transport media are stored in suitable conditions and that the proper ones are used for each type of specimen. However, because of its complexity, this system has a major practical disadvantage in that transport media are often not used correctly because they are not readily available when needed. Storage of transport media on the wards solves most of these problems, provided that the choice of media is made in agreement with the microbiologist and that the storage conditions are adequately controlled.

Quality control of transport

The time between specimen collection and arrival in the laboratory must be recorded for tracability and quality management of specimens. Clinicians and microbiologists must work at either end of the transport process to ensure that this is done. This information is easier to obtain when computerized transport systems are in use, because these systems usually allow automatic recording and allow all movements to be traced.

PROCESSING OF SAMPLES

The processing of adequate specimens is at the heart of the microbiologist's work. Laboratory work on each assay should follow published procedures and adhere to the recommendations for good laboratory practices.[13] Specimens should be processed promptly after arrival and the techniques used should be fully documented in order to ensure minimal variations between technicians. Techniques should be documented in accordance with agreements reached in working sessions organized periodically in each laboratory. It is the responsibility of the laboratory supervisor to ensure that all techniques used are properly documented and updated and that all quality control procedures, both external and internal, are implemented. All documented techniques should be further checked by the clinical microbiologists, who will ultimately decide which changes could, or should, eventually be implemented.

New techniques and rapid diagnosis

As mentioned above, the techniques used for processing specimens are changing rapidly. Rapid diagnosis is discussed in the literature.[26–28] There are two objectives in the use of rapid diagnosis. The major objective is to obtain a better outcome for the patient through an increase in the speed at which results are made available for clinical decisions. As a general rule, the microbial load at the site of infection increases as the infection develops. The rationale behind this objective is, therefore, that the efficacy of antimicrobial treatments is better and the risk of selection of resistant micro-organisms is lower early in the evolution of the infection, when the number of micro-organisms is relatively low.

The secondary objective in the use of rapid diagnosis is to decrease the duration of technical work and the costs associated with laboratory tests. Microbiologists often have to decide whether they should stick to classic techniques or to adopt new ones, particularly those based on molecular technology. Obviously, microbiologists decisions vary with each new technique, but it must be emphasized that the introduction of a new laboratory technique is not an isolated event. The time gained in using a new laboratory technique must be compared with the time that could be saved by optimizing transport of the specimens, reporting of results and decision making. However, it is possible to follow some general rules before making a decision about the introduction of a new technique:

- never adopt a new technique before its results have compared favorably with those of the classic techniques in trials performed by at least two different groups, both of which are independent of the company that sells the technique;
- do not rely for a decision on small-size, comparative trials performed at the request of the company that sells the new technique;
- compare thoroughly the financial factors of using the old and the new technique;
- favor techniques that will speed up communication of results to the clinician, but always make sure that this increased communication will modify the way the patient is treated; and
- try to evaluate how often (for instance, in terms of number of patients per year) results obtained using the new test will lead to a medical decision, or taken earlier, than with the old technique. Try to compare the benefit of these medical changes with financial changes resulting from the introduction of the new technique.

The application of these rules is difficult but it is the only way for the microbiologist to make proper decisions about the techniques used in the microbiology laboratory. It is useless to decrease the technical time needed to process a specimen by a few hours if the time of reporting is not modify accordingly. The results of these choices also depend on the size and scientific objectives of the individual laboratory.

The work of technicians versus the work of microbiologists

The division of labor between technicians and microbiologists is a major factor in laboratory efficiency. The generally accepted opinion is that microbiologists should be aware of and able to perform all the tasks that are performed by technicians, but that they should not perform them on a routine basis. Indeed, the specific tasks of microbiologists is to control the results of the technical work. In contrast, this means that the microbiologists should always be the first to perform a technique newly introduced into the laboratory, both to verify that it is acceptable in practice and that the changes that this new technique will introduce to the flow of work in the laboratory are well controlled. The absence of this precaution often leads to an unexpected 'chain-reaction' that disturbs and sometimes jeopardizes the whole organization of the laboratory.

REPORTING

Reporting of results is a major task for clinical microbiologists. The recent literature on the matter is relatively sparse.[29,30] Two aspects of reporting must be considered: what to report and how to report it.

What to report

The raw data obtained by the technicians should be transformed into a form that is immediately useful for medical decision making before being reported to clinicians The best example of such a transformation is the reporting of antibiotic susceptibility testing. Indeed, whatever technique is used, the data obtained by the technicians are always quantitative (e.g. inhibition zones measured in millimeters, MICs). By contrast, clinicians need qualitative answers as to whether a bacterium is 'susceptible', 'intermediate' or 'resistant' to a specific antibiotic.

This production of qualitative results from quantitative data is, by nature, interpretative. Microbiologists should perform such interpretation with care and make sure that the interpretation rules that they are using are up to date and in accordance with all the advances in knowledge reported in the literature. They should always be ready to explain the interpretation rules to clinicians. Because expert systems and computers are more and more in use, it is now possible to pinpoint automatically on the report the rationales behind each interpretation made by the microbiologist.[31–33]

How to report

Separate versus cumulative results. Several modes of reporting have been experimented with over the years, either alone or in combination.[34,35]

In individual reporting systems, results from each sample are reported and transmitted separately to the clinicians after having been controlled and signed by the microbiologist. This way of reporting has the major drawback of separating results from different assays on a single patient, making it difficult to link together the various results for a given patient. Not only may this cause someone to forgot an important piece of information but also, more frequently, it prevents the various results of a given patient being considered together. One of the best examples of this is positive results from several blood cultures for coagulase-negative staphylococci; each one is somewhat meaningless by itself but, taken together, they strongly support the diagnosis of true bacteremia.

The development of cumulative reporting of microbiologic results has been a major advance in clinical microbiology (Fig. 3.6). It has been used in a some centers for over 20 years. Cumulative reporting solves most of the problems caused by individual reporting. First, it helps the technicians and microbiologists to have a comprehensive view of results obtained in other parts of the laboratory. Therefore, when receiving a sample, the technicians can adapt their practice to the results of the tests that have been previously been done for that patient. When signing cumulative results, the microbiologist can detect discrepancies in results between different samples from a given patient. Furthermore, such discrepancies may occur with a particular frequency in the results of antibiotic susceptibility testing. In this sense, the use of cumulative reporting plays a major role in the quality control in the laboratory.

Means of reporting results. Paper is the classic means of reporting results. The microbiologist signs the report and can add written comments when necessary. Even before computers were in use, the simplest way of realizing cumulative reporting was to copy the results manually on a cumulative report form on which all the results concerning a given patient had been previously reported. Then a copy of this form was made and sent to the clinician with the new result underlined, signed and dated.

Such a system provided a comprehensive view of the patient's microbiologic results. However, reporting on paper, even of cumulative results, is very inadequate for epidemiologic reporting of results and for clinical research because the data can only be accessed via the patient's identification. This drawback can be overcome by the use of computerized results. Reporting on paper also necessitates the physical transport of the results, either by hand or mechanically, to the wards, a time-consuming process.

Using fax transmission bypasses the need of the physical transport of results and thus appeared at first to be an efficient means of reporting. It is fast and the results accumulate in the wards in a single place, and clinicians know that they will be available quickly after having been produced in the laboratory. However, because fax machines are relatively slow, fax transmission is not used very much for transmission of results. Its use is generally limited to the transmission of only a small fraction of results in order to overcome the slowness of physical transmission in specific circumstances (e.g. for results obtained in an emergency or for results for specific wards or outpatient clinics).

The telephone is often used for the transmission of results because it combines speed with the possibility of the microbiologist commenting on the results directly to the clinician. However, because of the lack of traceability of the transmission, the use of the telephone is best avoided. Certainly, it should never be used without the call being entered in a log book in the laboratory and immediately complemented by a written and signed report.

The use of computer and electronic networks is the best contemporary way to report results.[4,36,37] It is fast and flexible. Cumulative or individual results can be sent either immediately after having been produced or at fixed periods during the day. Electronic transmission has only two technical drawbacks. The first drawback is

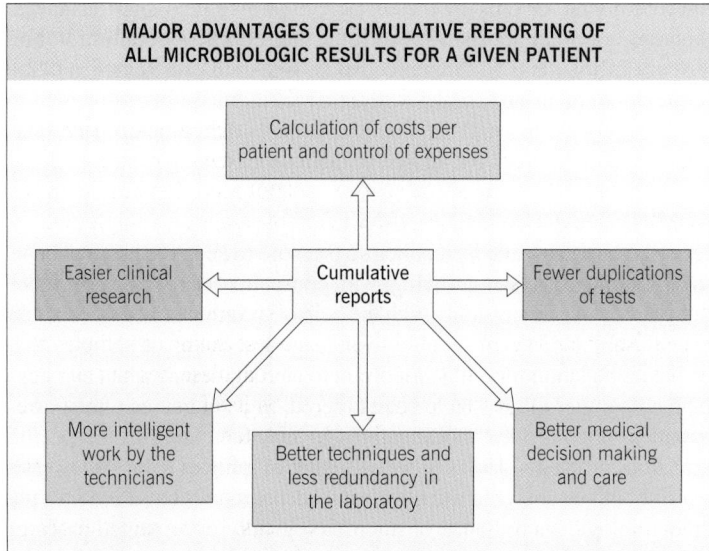

MAJOR ADVANTAGES OF CUMULATIVE REPORTING OF
ALL MICROBIOLOGIC RESULTS FOR A GIVEN PATIENT

Fig. 3.6 Major advantages of cumulative reporting of all microbiologic results for a given patient.

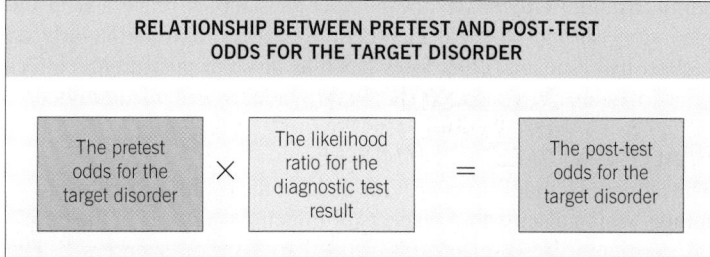

RELATIONSHIP BETWEEN PRETEST AND POST-TEST
ODDS FOR THE TARGET DISORDER

Fig. 3.7 Relationship between pre-test and post-test odds for the target disorder. *This is a major component in medical decision making and laboratory work.*

that the microbiologist cannot sign the results; the second is the lack of confidentiality of the network. The microbiologist should be aware of these two points and make sure that adequate technical solutions are provided by the hospital administration.

Electronic transmission of results provides a unique opportunity for clinicians and microbiologists to reorganize their common work. For instance, specific alerts can be automatically forwarded to the ward in given circumstances. An example is provided by the use of electronic networks within to alert a ward automatically when a patient colonized by a potential pathogen is transported from one ward to another or has to be moved for investigation procedures such as radiography or endoscopy.[38]

THE ROLE OF THE CLINICIAN IN GUIDING THE LABORATORY

The clinician has a major role in keeping the clinical microbiologist's work efficient. Clinicians must follow a number of rules when performing tests to be sent to the laboratory.

Perform tests only in appropriately chosen patients

There is a mathematical link between the predictive value of the results of laboratory tests for a given diagnosis and the pretest probability that a specific patient suffers from the disease (Fig. 3.7). This means that, even if using tests with both high sensitivities and specificities, the results of the tests will be of little clinical help if the suspicion of the disease is not high enough before the tests are performed. Moreover, when tests are performed in groups of patients with a low pretest probability of suffering from the disease in question, positive results correspond more often to false positivity. This can lead to unnecessary and costly treatments with potential side effects. In addition, it can turn the clinician's attention away from the correct diagnosis.

Determinations of the predictive values of the results obtained in the laboratory cannot be calculated by the microbiologist alone because they are dependent on the clinical characteristics of each individual patient for whom the tests are requested. Thus, it is mandatory that the clinician guides the laboratory work by giving some indications concerning the clinical presentation of the patients for whom the tests are requested. On the other hand, it is the role of the microbiologist to inform the clinician of the intrinsic sensitivities and specificities of the tests used in the laboratory.

Assist in the proper transport and storage of specimens

Clinicians should alert the laboratory whenever a specimen of particular value is sent to the laboratory. They should also always try to avoid delay in transportation by ensuring that the specimen leaves the ward promptly after collection. If a specimen must be kept frozen in a

clinical ward, the clinician must work together with the biologist to ensure that samples kept frozen in the ward are processed according to good laboratory practices.

Monitor the clinical use of test results

Monitoring the use of test results for medical decisions may be the best indicator of health outcomes. For instance, it can enable adequate comparison of the cost-effectiveness of conventional methods with rapid methods of analyzing and reporting. Special emphasis should be put on actions aimed at reducing the delay between the ordering of tests and the integration of the results in the therapeutic decision-making process (see Fig. 3.8).

INTERACTION WITH OTHERS WITHIN THE HOSPITAL

The effectiveness of the microbiologist largely depends on how he or she organizes the interactions with others inside and outside the hospital (see Fig. 3.9).

USE OF RESULTS IN DAY-TO-DAY PATIENT CARE

This is the classic way to use results. In order to obtain maximum efficiency, the microbiologist must visit the wards on a daily basis to discuss the significance of results with clinicians. Usually it will be necessary to select those areas where the infection-related problems are most difficult, for instance, the intensive care, meonatal or burns units.

Day-to-day patient care should also be influenced in a more collective way of using microbiologic results. For instance, many antibiotic treatments are empiric (i.e. they are administered before microbiologic results become available). Thus, the microbiologist must provide clinicians with up-to-date epidemiologic results of bacterial susceptibility from each individual ward.[39] At best, this epidemiologic information should be discussed in specific meetings and their trends over time analyzed. It is the role of the microbiologist to make sure that such epidemiologic information is available to, and is used by, all clinicians.

INFECTION CONTROL COMMITTEE

The results obtained by the microbiology laboratory are of major importance for the proper functioning of this committee. Several types of results should be provided. First, global and ward-specific epidemiologic data should be provided on a regular basis. When these data are obtained more or less manually, a yearly periodicity is often all that can be provided. The use of computers may enable the committee to be provided with up-to-date results for each of its meetings (usually monthly or every second month).[40,41]

In addition to providing data on trends, the results obtained in the laboratory will also identify epidemics and clusters of nosocomial infections. Although microbiologically documented cases of nosocomial infections are only a fraction of the total cases, several indices describing specific aspects of nosocomial infections can be produced by computerized laboratory databases. Rates of bacteremia and of bacteriuria are among the most commonly used. The number of patients discharged or the number of days of hospitalization should be used as denominators for these rates when they can be obtained from the hospital administration. Otherwise, the number of samples processed in the laboratory should be used. In specific instances, and particularly on request by clinicians, other rates (such as those of postsurgical infections) may also be generated and made available for the committee.

HEALTH AND SAFETY COMMITTEE

The laboratory should also provide data for the health and safety committee, which discusses all aspects of infectious hazards in the hospital, particularly those hazards related to hospital workers.[42] The laboratory may be requested to perform specific tests, for instance to control the safety of food products or of the environment. Because the regulations on the qualifications of the personnel who perform such tests vary from one country to another and are often different from those required for clinical microbiology, it is the role of the microbiologist to make sure that the laboratory personnel who perform these tests are adequately qualified.

CLINICAL RESEARCH

Laboratory data are an important source of clinical research. Some general rules should be followed in order to use the data in the most effective manner. When a project that is initiated by a microbiologist includes information about patients, the microbiologist should always inform the clinician of the results, because these may influence patient care. When the project is initiated by a clinician, the microbiologist should make access to the data easy. Furthermore, the clinical microbiology laboratory should be open to clinicians seeking laboratory experience and expertise. Microbiologists in teaching hospitals should try to promote collaborative research projects in which the clinicians are strongly involved.

DRUGS AND THERAPEUTICS (FORMULARY) COMMITTEES

Most hospitals have some means of regulating the introduction of new drugs, for financial reasons if no other. In the case of antimicrobial agents, there is the additional, and very important responsibility of regulating the use of these drugs in order to try and reduce the burden of inappropriate antibiotic consumption and so limit the development of resistance. Microbiologists have a critical role here in advising the committee, but there is often a fine line between excessive restriction and profligate use. It is usually unnecessary, for example, to have more than one drug in each class available on the formulary, but it will be difficult to resist the introduction of major new drugs with no other competitor. A compromise can sometimes be reached which allows the use of new (usually very expensive) drugs after discussion with the

microbiologist, or only in certain agreed and defined circumstances. Another common approach is to limit the reporting of antimicrobial susceptibility data; for instance, only first-line antibiotics will be reported out on urine samples with other antibiotic information held in the laboratory. This will then be available to the clinician if he telephones the laboratory for advice in difficult cases.

ADMINISTRATION AND FINANCES

Over the past 10 years, the economic pressure to keep the hospital costs to a minimum has been growing, with consequent burdens on the laboratory.[12,43,44] Again, it is only with the help of a computerized system that the microbiologist will be able to manage the fluxes of samples that arrive in the laboratory. It is important to alert clinicians when an unexplained number of tests have been ordered. Such increases often correspond to uncontrolled modifications in practices and not to specific infectious problems. Thus, the total number of samples requested in each ward should be analyzed using the same techniques as those used for the epidemiologic surveillance of microbiologically documented cases of infections. Each unexpected increase should be analyzed to determine its cause. This kind of surveillance data will, in addition, help the laboratory to discuss its budget with the hospital administration by enabling the activity of the laboratory to be forecast on solid grounds.

INTERACTION WITH OTHERS OUTSIDE THE HOSPITAL

GENERAL PRACTITIONERS

Increasingly, microbiology laboratories are providing diagnostic facilities for general practitioners and family doctors in the community. Specimen delivery services allow community physicians to send samples into the laboratory for examination, with results being returned by phone (for urgent samples), fax or local e-mail networks. The choice

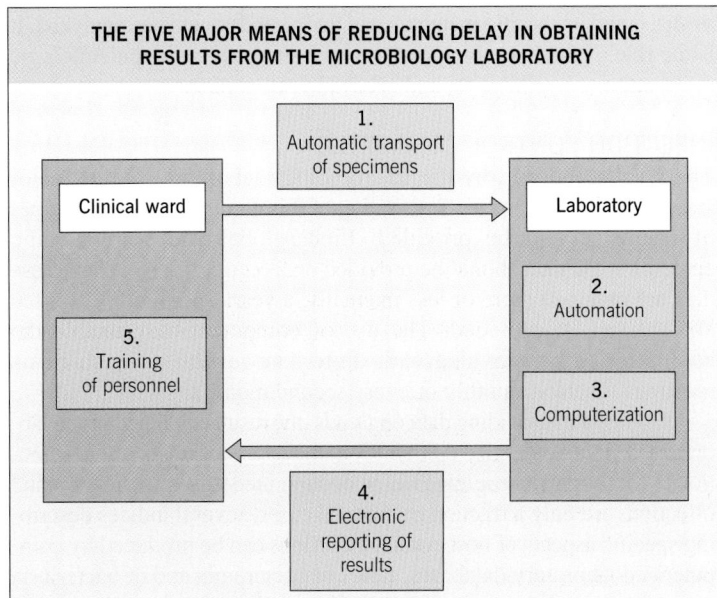

Fig. 3.8 The five major means of reducing delay in obtaining results from the microbiology laboratory.

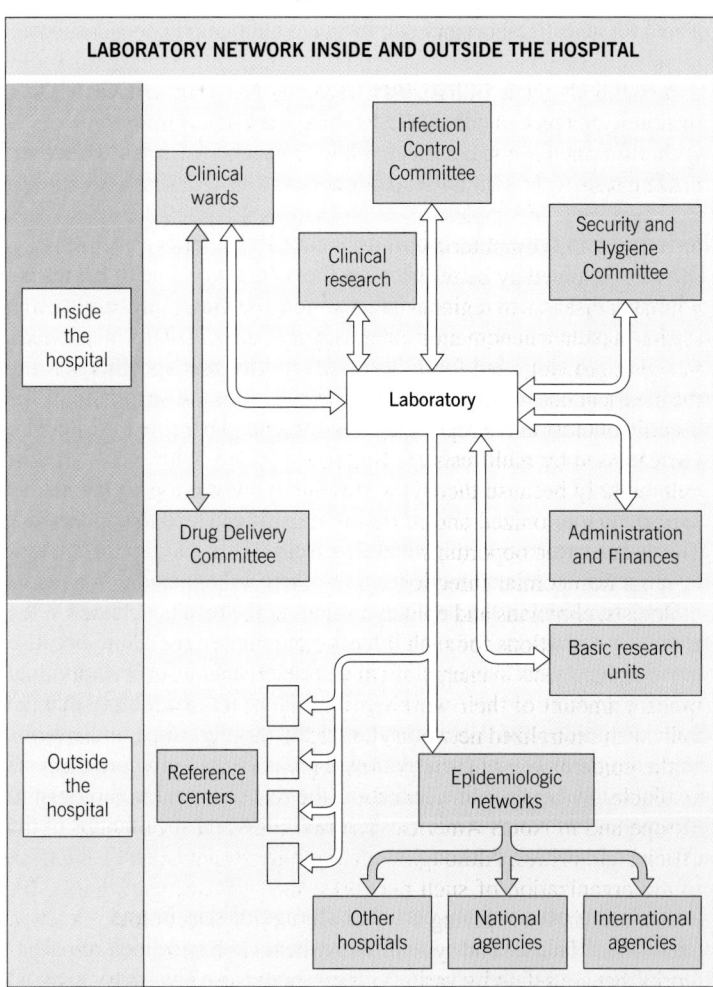

Fig. 3.9 Laboratory network inside and outside the hospital.

of antimicrobial susceptibility data provided in these reports has an important influence on drug use, and hence resistance pressure. Microbiologists are also an important source of clinical advice to colleagues in the community, and this is becoming an even greater part of their clinical workload.

OTHER LABORATORIES AND REFERENCE CENTERS

Given the increased complexity of microbiologic diagnosis, no single laboratory is able to perform all the possible tests that can be requested by clinicians. Thus, some samples will have to be sent to other laboratories. This is particularly true for tests that are not often requested in a given hospital. The procedure to be followed in such instances, and the choice of the corresponding laboratories, should be agreed between the clinicians and the microbiologists. The samples should always be addressed to the local laboratory by the clinician before being sent outside the hospital. It is the responsibility of the microbiologist to ensure that proper transport procedures are followed. Similarly, the results should be sent back to the local laboratory, which will enter them in the database together with other results from the patient before sending them to the clinician. For good practice, a specific note on the report should indicate where the result was obtained, and a copy of the original report form should also be sent to the clinician. The original should be archived.

EPIDEMIOLOGIC NETWORKS AND LOCAL AND NATIONAL AGENCIES

The clinical microbiology laboratory must interact with epidemiologic networks and with local and national agencies, both for long-term epidemiologic surveillance and for alerting relevant people in cases of epidemics or outbreaks of infection. Public health policies are occupying a growing place in the control of infectious diseases. In order to be effective, public health policies must be based on data obtained from surveillance systems that include figures from hospitalized patients. Thus, the clinical laboratory of each hospital must be integrated within organized networks in order to allow the results from each institution to be promptly taken into account in regional and national statistics, as well as in the process of public health decision making.[45]

Indeed, such a system has long been in place for a short list of notifiable diseases. It is noteworthy, however, that the reporting of notifiable diseases is incomplete in most instances. It may be that the present increase in the computerization of results in clinical laboratories will soon be followed by better transmission of complete data about these notifiable diseases to regional and national agencies. In addition, owing to the present phenomenon of emerging and re-emerging diseases, there is a growing need for notification of other diseases that are not on the classical lists of the notifiable diseases. For instance, there is now specific interest in the reporting of nosocomial infections, particularly those caused by multiresistant bacteria.[46] Such reporting is still difficult, notably because there is a thin line between cases in which the patients are colonized and those in which they are actually infected. This is due to the opportunistic nature of the infectious agents involved in most nosocomial infections. Only the combined work of microbiologists, clinicians and epidemiologists will allow simple and workable case definitions for such infections to be developed.

Microbiologists in charge of clinical laboratories should spend a significant amount of their working time trying to ensure that effective links with centralized networks devoted to the reporting and analyzing of the epidemiology of such emerging and re-emerging diseases are available. Two types of networks are currently functioning, both in Europe and in North America. The first type is that proposed by the official authorities. Although there are differences between countries in the organization of such networks, they are always more or less pyramidal, aiming at giving a global picture of epidemiologic situations and trends. The second type of network includes the numerous networks that are set up by various groups of professionals, such as medical societies or the pharmaceutic industries. These networks are often redundant, but their existence is exciting if it is seen as the mark of the interest that microbiologists and infectious diseases specialists are devoting to the epidemiologic approach to the control of infectious diseases. Great care should be taken, however, to prevent the development of loosely controlled figures and data. Conflicts of interest may also occur between private and public health efforts, particularly when the networks are supported by private funding from industry.

The second major interest in including the results from microbiology laboratories in networks is that it will allow each participant to benefit promptly from the information obtained by others. This is particularly important when epidemic phenomena begin to emerge because specific laboratory techniques often need to be implemented to detect cases of such emerging infections. The rapid alert given through effective governmental or nongovernmental networks is a key factor in controlling the spread of emerging pathogens.

RESEARCH UNITS

Because of the rapid development of new techniques, particularly molecular ones, for the diagnosis of microbiologic diseases, it is important for laboratory personnel, both technicians and microbiologists, to keep aware of new methodologies at the research level. If the laboratory is not linked directly to a research unit, then continuing education programs in the field of these new technologies should be implemented. The lack of such a program quickly creates a large conceptual gap between techniques that are well controlled by the laboratory personnel and those that are proposed by commercial interests. This is particularly important with regard to the new automatic machines that are currently proposed[5] or that will soon be proposed[10] for microbial identification and susceptibility testing, which do not use classic enzymatic technologies or the usual identification algorithms and antibiogram interpretation rules.

MANAGEMENT OF QUALITY AND AUDIT IN CLINICAL MICROBIOLOGY

The practice of quality control management is a key step in the functioning of the clinical microbiology laboratory in order to produce high-quality results while keeping the budget within limits.[13] Ideally, quality management has to be exercised at the various stages in which microbiologists are involved, including structure, process and outcome.

The structure consists of the buildings, personnel, standards, equipment and reimbursement that ensure the basic capability of providing quality care. The process is the action taken by all health care personnel in the course of providing patient care. The outcome is the

---

INDICATORS OF USE OF LABORATORY RESOURCES AND BENEFIT TO PATIENT CARE

- Physician ordering
- Transcription of order
- Specimen collection and transport
- Evaluation of quality of specimens
- Sources of poor-quality specimens
- Self-assessment of accuracy of smear interpretation
- Detection of contaminated specimens based on culture
- Cost of repeat collection of poor-quality specimens
- Intralaboratory processing:
    Errors in processing
    Monitoring of performance of personnel, equipment and reagents
    Revision of reports
    Time allowed for returning results
    Reports rendered on or after discharge of patient
    Placement of reports in the medical record
- Continuing education
- Clinical use of reported information

Fig. 3.10 Indicators of use of laboratory resources and benefit to patient care.

ultimate benefit derived by the patient from exposure to the health care system. Process monitoring is the classic part of quality control. Quality management in clinical microbiology began in the 1960s in the USA when both professional societies and the government introduced programs for proficiency testing and laboratory inspection and accreditation. A similar movement is currently being undertaken in most other countries. The initial emphasis of quality management was placed on the intralaboratory process. Later, attention was shifted to physician ordering, specimen collection, reporting and use of information. Quality management in the laboratory depends in large part on the monitoring of indicators that provide some evidence of how laboratory resources are being used and how the information benefits patient care (see Fig. 3.10).

Audit is an essential component of quality management. Laboratories need to put in place a regular program of audit to review the effectiveness of their procedures, and to ensure that they maintain the level of service that is required. For audit to be useful, it is important that deficiencies, if identified, are corrected and then subject to regular review, the process of 'closing the audit loop'.

CONCLUSION

The potential of the clinical microbiology laboratories has been renewed over the past few years, owing to the introduction of molecular biology techniques, computers and automated machines, the combination of which leads to previously unknown possibilities in terms of rapid diagnosis, reporting of everyday results and analysis of epidemiologic trends. Because the technologies involved are more complex than before, the laboratory work must be subjected to precise quality control procedures involving ordering of tests, transport, intralaboratory processes and clinical use of results. At the same time, the emergence of new infections and the re-emergence of older ones, together with generalized trends towards increased resistance of bacteria to antibiotics, have led to circumstances in which the use of classic microbiologic techniques do not allow the proper diagnosis of infecting micro-organisms. This is why, now more than ever, the work of the microbiologist and the development of the laboratory are dependent on the network of relationships within the hospital (with clinicians, epidemiologists and hospital administrators) and outside the hospital (with centralized agencies and research units).

REFERENCES

1. Reimer LG, Wilson ML, Weinstein MP. Update on detection of bacteremia and fungemia. Clin Microbiol Rev 1997;10:444–65.
2. Chabbert YA. L'antibiogramme. Paris: Éditions de la Tourelle; 1963.
3. Bauer AW, Kirby WMM, Sherris JC, Turk M. Antibiotic susceptibility testing by a standardized single disk method. Am J Clin Pathol 1966;45:493–6.
4. Stokes KJ, Morris DJ, Klapper PE, Semple AD, Crosdale E, Corbitt G. Computer network for a diagnostic virology laboratory. J Virol Methods 1993;45:277–89.
5. O'Hara CM, Tenover FC, Miller JM. Parallel comparison of accuracy of API 20E, Vitek GNI, MicroScan Walk/Away Rapid ID, and Becton Dickinson Cobas Micro ID-E/NF for identification of members of the family Enterobacteriaceae and common Gram-negative, non-glucose-fermenting bacilli. J Clin Microbiol 1993;31:3165–9.
6. Courvalin P, Goldstein F, Philippon A, Sirot J. L'antibiogramme. Paris: MPC-Videom, 1985.
7. Jungkind D, Direnzo S, Beavis KG, Silverman NS. Evaluation of automated Cobas Amplicor PCR system for detection of several infectious agents and its impact on laboratory management. J Clin Microbiol 1996;34:2778–83.
8. Glupczynski Y. La biologie moléculaire dans le diagnostic des maladies infectieuses. Rev Med Brux 1995;16:119–24.
9. Van Belkum A. DNA fingerprinting of medically important microorganisms by use of PCR. Clin Microbiol Rev 1994;7:174–84.
10. Christen R, Mabilat C. Applications des puces à ADN en bactériologie. Bull Soc Fr Microbiol 1998;13:10–7.
11. Emori TG, Gaynes RP. An overview of nosocomial infections, including the role of the microbiology laboratory. Clin Microbiol Rev 1993;6:428–42.
12. Staneck JL. Impact of technological developments and organizational strategies on clinical laboratory cost reduction. Diagn Microbiol Infect Dis 1995;23:61–73.
13. Bartlett RC, Mazens-Sullivan M, Tetreault JZ, Lobel S, Nivard J. Evolving approaches to management of quality in clinical microbiology. Clin Microbiol Rev 1994;7:55–88.
14. Baron EJ. Quality management and the clinical microbiology laboratory. Diagn Microbiol Infect Dis 1995;23:23–4.
15. Ellis CJ. The use and abuse of blood cultures. Infect Dis Newslett 1991;10:27–30.
16. Miller JM. A guide to specimen management in clinical microbiology. Washington, DC: ASM Press; 1996.

17. Fan K, Morris AJ, Reller LB. Application of rejection criteria for stool cultures for bacterial enteric pathogens. J Clin Microbiol 1993;31:2233–5.
18. Morris AJ, Smith LK, Mirrett S, Reller LB. Cost and time savings following introduction of rejection criteria for clinical specimens. J Clin Microbiol 1996;34:355–7.
19. Zaidi AK, Reller LB. Rejection criteria for endotracheal aspirates from pediatric patients. J Clin Microbiol 1996;34:352–4.
20. Gelford GJ. How to get clinical histories in a community general hospital, without losing rapport with the medical staff. Radiology 1975;117:487–8.
21. Jefferson H, Dalton HP, Escobar MR, Allison MJ. Transportation delay and the microbiological quality of clinical specimens. Am J Clin Pathol 1975;64:689–93.
22. Pragay DA, Fan P, Brinkley S, Chilcote ME. A computer directed pneumatic tube system: its effect on specimens. Clin Biochem 1980;13:259–61
23. Hardin G, Quick G, Ladd DJ. Emergency transport of AS-1 red cell units by pneumatic tube system. J Trauma 1990;30:346–8.
24. Astles JR, Lubarsky D, Loun B, Sedor FA, Toffaletti JG. Pneumatic transport exacerbates interference of room air contamination in blood gas samples. Arch Pathol Lab Med 1996;120:642–7.
25. Miller JM, Holmes HT. Specimen collection, transport, and storage. In: Murray PR, Baron EJ, Pfaller MA, Tenover FC, Yolken RH, eds. Manual of clinical microbiology, 6th ed. Washington, DC: ASM Press; 1995:19–32.
26. Doern GV. Clinically expedient reporting of rapid diagnostic test information. Diagn Microbiol Infect Dis 1986;4(3 Suppl):151S–156S.
27. Doern GV, Vautour R, Gaudet M, Levy B. Clinical impact of rapid in vitro susceptibility testing and bacterial identification. J Clin Microbiol 1994;32:1757–62.
28. Koontz FP. Clinician utilization of rapid antibiotic susceptibility data – a prospective study. J Assoc Rapid Methods Automat Microbiol 1991;4:69–75.
29. Jorgensen JH. Laboratory issues in the detection and reporting of antibacterial resistance. Infect Dis Clin North Am 1997;11:785–802.
30. Schifman RB, Pindur A, Bryan JA. Laboratory practices for reporting bacterial susceptibility tests that affect antibiotic therapy. Arch Pathol Lab Med 1997;121:1168–70.
31. Peyret M, Flandrois JP, Carret G, Pichat C. Interpretative reading and quality control of an antibiotic sensitivity test using an expert system. Application to the API ATB system and Enterobacteriaceae. Pathol Biol 1989;37:624–8.
32. Flandrois JP, Peyret M, Zindel J Influence of the culture medium (Isosensitest or Mueller–Hinton) on

the results of antibiotics susceptibility testing, its interpretation. Pathol Biol 1991;39:455–60.
33. Vedel G, Peyret M, Gayral JP, Millot P. Evaluation of an expert system linked to a rapid antibiotic susceptibility testing system for the detection of beta-lactam resistance phenotypes. Res Microbiol 1996;147:297–309.
34. Lupovitch A, Memminger JJ III, Corr RM. Manual, computerized cumulative reporting systems for the clinical microbiology laboratory. Am J Clin Pathol 1979;72:841–7.
35. Eggert AA, Smulka G, Walker L, Brandt G. Coordinated computer reporting of clinical microbiology data. Am J Clin Pathol 1981;76:43–9.
36. Cahill BP, Holmen JR, Bartleson PL. Mayo Foundation electronic results inquiry, the HL7 connection. Proc Annu Symp Comput Appl Med Care 1991:516–20.
37. Moritz VA, McMaster R, Dillon T, Mayall B. Selection, implementation of a laboratory computer system. Pathology 1995;27:260–7.
38. Pittet D, Safran E, Harbarth S, et al. Automatic alerts for methicillin-resistant Staphylococcus aureus surveillance, control: role of a hospital information system. Infect Control Hosp Epidemiol 1996;17:496–502.
39. Evangelista AT. The clinical impact of automated susceptibility reporting using a computer interface. Adv Exp Med Biol 1990;263:131–42.
40. Steed SA, Sheretz RJ, Reagan DR. Computers in hospitals epidemiology. In: Mayhall CG, ed. Hospital epidemiology, and infection control. Baltimore: Williams and Wilkins; 1996:115–22.
41. Clarseu DC, Pestotnick SL. The computer-based patient record: an essential technology for hospital epidemiology. In: Mayhall CG, ed. Hospital Epidemiology, and Infection Control. Baltimore: Williams and Wilkins; 1996:123–38.
42. Epidemiology, prevention of nosocomial infections in health care workers. In: Mayhall CG, ed. Hospital epidemiology, and infection control. Baltimore: Williams and Wilkins; 1996:825–912.
43. Scott DR. Influence of managed care, health maintenance organizations on the clinical microbiology laboratory. Diagn Microbiol Infect Dis 1995;23:17–21.
44. Wilson ML. Clinically relevant, cost-effective clinical microbiology. Strategies to decrease unnecessary testing. Am J Clin Pathol 1997;107:154–67.
45. Grant AD, Eke B. Application of information technology to the laboratory reporting of communicable disease in England and Wales. Community Dis Rep Rev 1993;3:R75–8.
46. Stelling JM, O'Brien TF. Surveillance of antimicrobial resistance: the WHONET program. Clin Infect Dis 1997;24(Suppl 1):157–68.

Prevention and Chemoprophylaxis

Bruce Gellin

Throughout history, human beings have used their contemporary understanding of the forces of nature to try to exercise some degree of control. Even without knowing the precise etiology of a disease, epidemiologic methods have successfully identified risk factors that have provided footholds for intervention. John Snow's investigation of cholera in London that led to the removal of the water pump handle is but one of many such prevention interventions.[1] However, it was the emergence of the germ theory of disease and the growing understanding of the microbial etiology of disease that provided a rationale for the prevention, treatment and control of infectious diseases. The maturation of epidemiologic methods and public health has grown in parallel with medicine itself. As we improve our understanding of the etiology of disease we can develop ever new approaches to prevention, treatment, control and possibly elimination of some diseases.

Following the discovery of the power and effectiveness of antibiotics in the treatment of infectious diseases, confidence in the science of medicine created a spirit that the war over infectious disease had been won. The sobering events that followed – highlighted recently by the AIDS pandemic and the rapid evolution of antibiotic-resistant organisms – reflect our concern that, despite the advances of modern medicine, the biomedical sciences, and epidemiology, the development and application of interventions that prevent infectious diseases will continue to require a combination of fundamental biomedical research, novel applications of research results, surveillance and a continual reevaluation of current strategies. In order to take full advantage of the applications of research the infrastructure that facilitates the practice of prevention will need to be strengthened.[2] The World Health Organization's 1997 World Health Report makes is clear that the problems of infectious diseases persist. At the same time, there is also tremendous hope that the effective interventions will have a significant impact (Fig. 4.1).[3]

Despite the increasing complexity and sophistication of modern society and the appropriate concerns about the threats of emerging infectious diseases, providing access to clean water and sanitation will have the most significant global impact on infectious diseases. The World Bank estimates that 1.3 billion of the poorest people in developing countries do not have access to safe water and that nearly 2 billion people do not have adequate sanitation services (Figs 4.2 & 4.3).[4,5] In addition, outdoor and indoor air pollution are growing public health problems. Indeed, indoor air pollution has been identified as one of the four most critical global environmental problems and as an important contributor to acute and chronic respiratory disease. Pneumonia is one of the leading causes of morbidity and mortality in young children in developing countries, accounting for almost 10% of the total disease burden. It is estimated that reducing indoor air pollution has the potential of halving the incidence of acute respiratory infections in children.[4,6]

HOST–MICROBE–ENVIRONMENT INTERACTIONS

Infectious diseases are the consequence of interaction of the infectious agent and the host. The environmental setting affects the likelihood that such an interaction will occur. Therefore, prevention efforts can be focused on each or any of these components, depending on the

THE CONTINUING PROBLEM OF INFECTIOUS DISEASES AND THE PROMISE OF PREVENTION
The problem today
Infectious and parasitic diseases account for 43% of the annual 40 million deaths in developing countries
The leading killer among infectious diseases in 1996 was acute lower respiratory infection, which killed 3.9 million people
Tuberculosis killed 3 million people in 1996
Diarrheal diseases killed 2.5 million people in 1996
Malaria killed between 1.5 million and 2.7 million people in 1996
About 1.5 million people died of HIV–AIDS in 1996
By the end of 1996, a cumulative total of 29.4 million children and adults had been infected with HIV
Worldwide, 75–85% of HIV infections in adults have been transmitted through unprotected sexual intercourse, with heterosexual intercourse accounting for more than 70%
The promise of prevention
Leprosy prevalence fell from 2.3 to 1.7 per 10,000 between 1995 and 1996, and the problem has been reduced by 82% worldwide in the past 11 years
The Onchocerciasis Control Programme, which began in West Africa in 1974, has now protected an estimated 36 million people from the disease
More than 120 million children under 5 years old in India were immunized against poliomyelitis in a single day in 1996
Field trials in Africa in 1996 showed that insecticide-treated bed nets can reduce childhood deaths from malaria by up to 35%

Fig. 4.1 The continuing problem of infectious diseases and the promise of prevention. From the 1997 World Health Report.[3]

disease in question and on the availability of appropriate intervention tools and tactics.

The specific characteristics of the host that increase the likelihood of exposure to an infectious agent or that predispose to infection, and the severity of the clinical course are discussed in detail elsewhere in this book. However, there are several general features of the host that, alone or together, can influence the ultimate clinical response and may offer the potential for intervention (Fig. 4.4). Similarly, features of the infectious organism can also affect the likelihood that it will establish an infection in humans and subsequently develop into a clinical illness (Fig. 4.5).[7]

The interplay of these factors can affect infectious diseases in many ways. For instance, although breast-feeding has been shown to protect against diarrhea,[8] recent evidence suggests that the protective effect of breast-feeding on respiratory tract infections in children in the first year of life is strongest among children who are exposed to tobacco smoke.[9,10]

Severe malnutrition can precipitate a downward spiral. Weight loss and stunted growth may be the outward manifestations of underlying mucosal damage that exacerbates the state of malnutritional through malabsorption. The weakened mucosal barrier may also increase the success of invading micro-organisms and result in a blunted mucosal

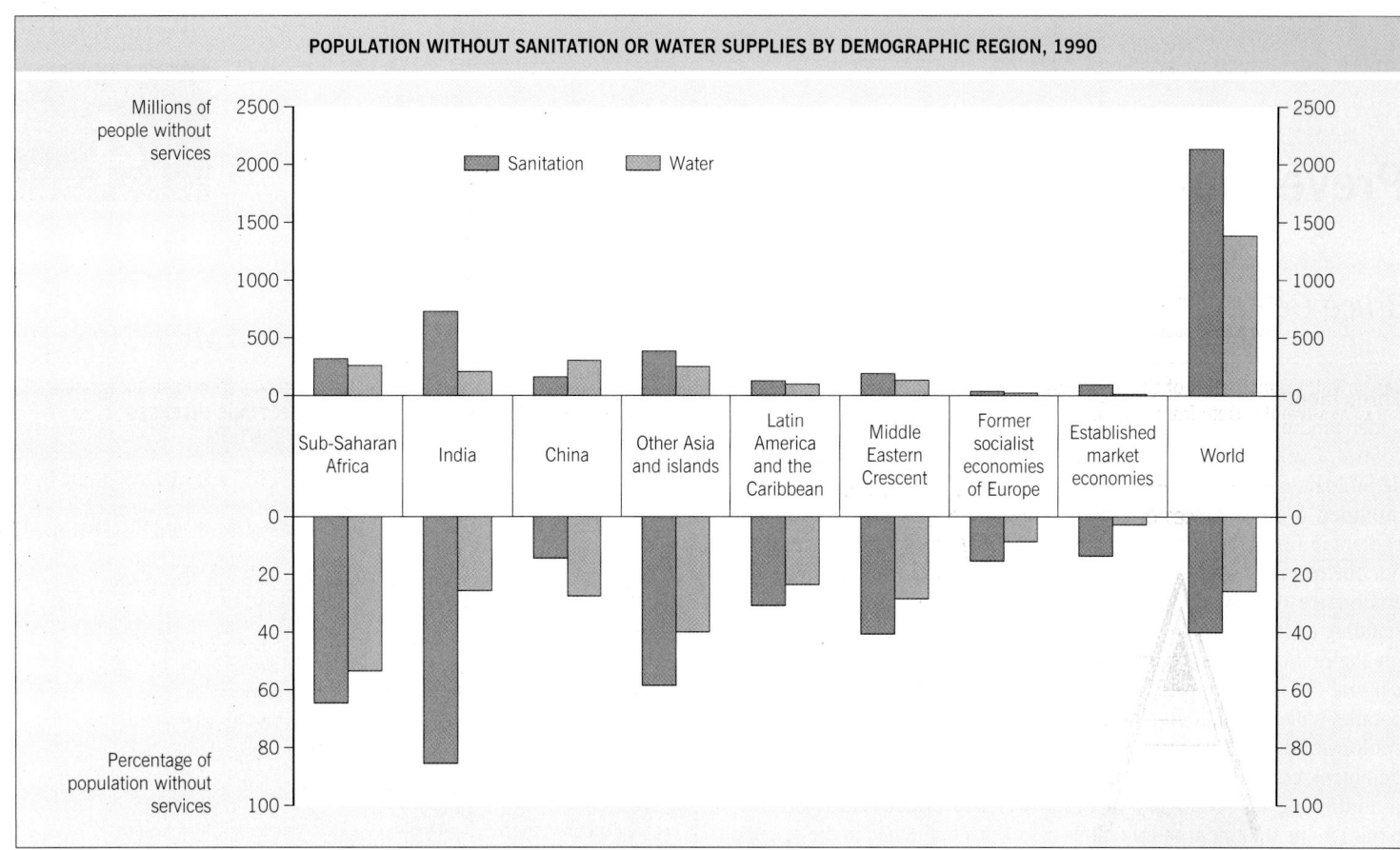

Fig. 4.2 Population without sanitation or water supply services. The figures are for 1990 and are given by demographic region. Coverage is defined in accordance with local standards. Modified from the World Bank's World Development Report.[4]

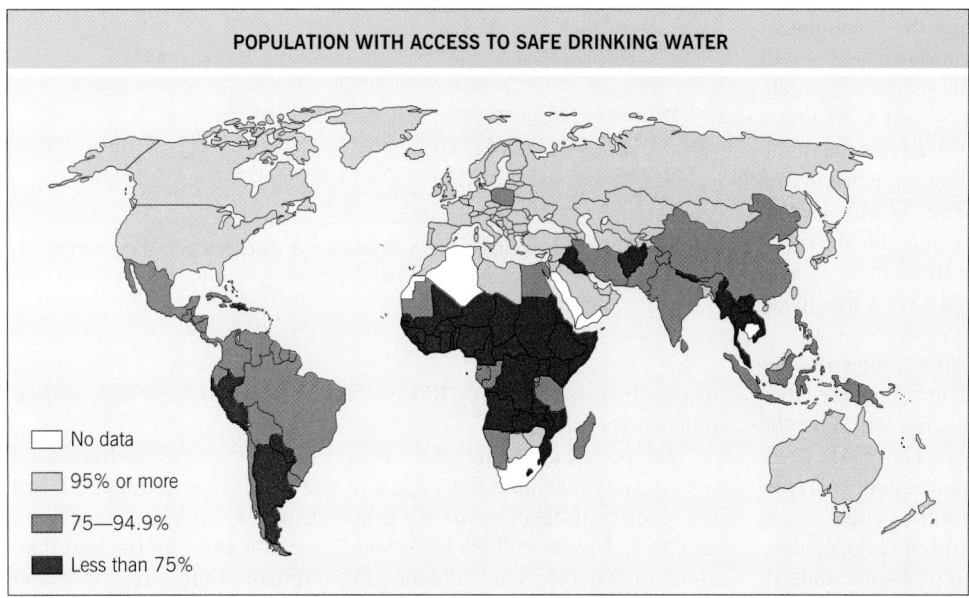

Fig. 4.3 Population without access to safe drinking water. Modified from Doyle.[5]

immune response. This can result in an increase in the incidence of disease in the population and an increase in the severity of disease in the affected individual.

In addition to the effects of severe malnutrition, a growing body of evidence suggests that micronutrients such as vitamin A may also have substantial effects on immunity. This effect has been most striking among young children in developing countries when affected with the measles virus. It is estimated that nearly half of the world's children have an inadequate intake of vitamin A, putting them at a 23% higher risk of death from common diseases (Fig. 4.6).[11] This recognition has led to the addition of vitamin A supplementation in infant immunization programs in many developing countries.[11–14]

There is also preliminary evidence that micronutrient supplementation with trace minerals such as zinc and selenium may also have a protective effect against infections in malnourished children,[15] institutionalized older people[16] and immunocompromised patients.[17,18] The mechanism that underlies this effect is thought to be related, in part, to an enhanced interferon response.[19]

PREVENTION

VECTOR CONTROL
By reducing the source of transmission, vector control efforts have had a substantial impact on disease incidence. It is estimated that 3% of the

CHARACTERISTICS OF THE HOST THAT INFLUENCE CLINICAL RESPONSE TO AN INFECTIOUS AGENT
• Age • Genetic determinants of immunity • Pre-existing level of immunity • Nutritional status • Underlying conditions and disease • Behavior (e.g. personal hygiene, exercise and activities that affect likelihood of exposure) • Psychologic factors (e.g. attitude and motivation)

Fig. 4.4 **Characteristics of the host that influence clinical response to infectious agents.** Data from Evans.[7]

CHARACTERISTICS OF INFECTIOUS AGENTS THAT INFLUENCE THEIR ABILITY TO CAUSE INFECTION AND CLINICAL ILLNESS
• Can it survive in the environment? • Is it effectively transmitted in the environment? • Is it transmitted by a vector? • Is there an animal reservoir or an intermediate host? • Can it attach to, invade and multiply in host cells? • Can it evade host immune response? • Can it evade antimicrobial therapy? • Can it be effectively transmitted from person to person?

Fig. 4.5 **Characteristics of infectious agents that influence their ability to cause infection and clinical illness.** Data from Evans.[7]

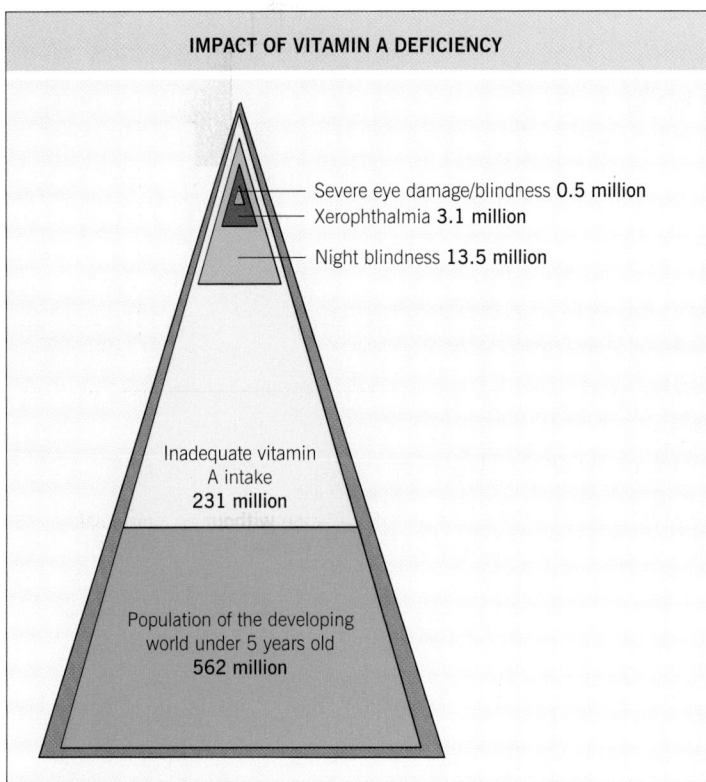

Fig. 4.6 **Impact of vitamin A deficiency.** The estimated impact of vitamin A deficiency on the population aged under 5 years in the developing world. A person with an inadequate intake of vitamin A has a 23% higher risk of death from common diseases than a person with an adequate intake. Modified from UNICEF.[11]

PREVENTION GUIDELINES	
HIV-related guidelines	USPHS/IDSA guidelines for the prevention of opportunistic infections in persons infected with HIV: Part I. Prevention of exposure[23]
	USPHS/IDSA guidelines for the prevention of opportunistic infections in persons infected with HIV: disease-specific recommendations[24]
	Preventing *Pneumocystis carinii* pneumonia in HIV-infected children: new guidelines for prophylaxis[25]
Institution-related guidelines (hospitals, day care centers, nursing homes)	Guidelines for the prevention of antimicrobial resistance in hospitals[26]
	Prevention of infections in child day care centers[27]
	Infection prevention and control in the long-term care facility[28]
	Guidelines for prevention of nosocomial pneumonia[29]
	Interim guidelines for prevention and control of staphylococcal infection associated with reduced susceptibility to vancomycin[30]
	APIC guideline for selection and use of disinfectants[31]
General clinical guidelines	Guidelines for the prevention and treatment of infection in patients with an absent or dysfunctional spleen[32]
	Guidelines on the control of methicillin-resistant *Staphylococcus aureus* in the community[33]
	Prevention of urinary tract infection[34]
	Recommendations for the prevention of bacterial endocarditis[35]
	Guidelines for use of hepatitis A vaccine and immune globulin[36]
	Guidelines for treatment of sexually transmitted diseases[37]
	Prevention of community-acquired and nosocomial pneumonia[38]
Guidelines relating to international travel	Prevention of malaria for travelers[39]
	Blood transfusion guidelines for international travelers[40]
	Protection from mosquitoes and other arthropod vectors[40]
	Prevention and treatment of 'traveler's diarrhea'[40]

Fig. 4.7 **Prevention guidelines.** A partial list of the many guidelines that are now available. APIC, Association for Professionals in Infection Control; IDSA, Infectious Diseases Society of America; USPHS, United States Public Health Service. For additional information see website: http://www.cdc.gov

global burden of disease is attributed to vector-borne diseases.[4,20] Novel, cost-effective approaches for vector control have included the use of impregnated bed nets to reduce the exposure to night-feeding anopheline mosquitoes and hence to reduce the risk of malaria transmission;[21] community-based *Aedes aegypti* larval control programs to reduce the breeding success of the mosquitoes that transmit dengue virus;[22] and the application of polystyrene beads to pit latrines has disturbed the breeding ground for *Culex* mosquitoes and reduced the transmission of filariasis.[4]

PREVENTION GUIDELINES

Beyond clean water, clean air, and available sanitation, our enhanced understanding of microbial pathogenesis, disease transmission, and host immunity now provide a number of options for intervention. This has resulted in an increasing number of prevention guidelines that are periodically updated as new information becomes available. These guidelines represent both primary prevention (a decrease in the likelihood of exposure and infection) and secondary prevention (a decrease in the likelihood of disease, given exposure). The details of each of the

many guidelines that are available are far too encompassing to include in a single chapter on prevention; however, a partial list of such guidelines is provided in Figure 4.7.

A series of recommended preventive and prophylactic strategies have also been developed. These focus on the clinical setting, the potential exposure, and the infectious agent (Figs 4.8a,b & 4.9).[35,41,42]

SYSTEMIC PROPHYLAXIS AND EPIDEMIOLOGIC TREATMENT WITH ANTIMICROBIAL AGENTS

Disease and circumstance		Treatment: agent, dosage, route, duration	Comments
Viral	**Hepatitis C** Postrenal transplant and induction chemotherapy	Although interferon and ribavirin is now approved for reduction of chronic hepatitis C , no data on use as post-exposure prohpylaxis. IG not effective	
	Hepatitis B Prevent re-infection after transplantation for hepatitis B-induced cirrhosis	Lamivudine 100mg q24h starting 4 weeks before tranplant and continuing for 12 months after transplant	Based on one uncontrolled study with impressive results; resistance to lamivudine developed in one patient
	HIV: occupational exposure (percutaneous) Blood at highest risk: both larger blood volume and blood containing a high HIV titer or any exposure to concentrated HIV (e.g. in a research laboratory or production facility)	Recommend: ZDV 200mg q8h + 3TC 150mg q12h + (IDV 800mg q8h or nelfinavir 750mg q8h) All po every 4 weeks	Can give ZDV + 3TC q12h in combination tablet that contains 300mg ZDV and 150mg 3TC
	Blood at increased risk: either exposure to larger blood volume or blood with high HIV titer	ZDV 200mg q8h + 3TC 150mg q12h + (IDV or nelfinavir). All po for 4 weeks	Can give ZDV + 3TC q12h in combination tablet that contains 300mg ZDV and 150mg 3TC
	Blood at no increased risk: neither exposure to large volume nor to blood with high HIV titer	Offer: ZDV 200mg q8h and 3TC 150mg q12h. All po for 4 weeks	
	Bloody fluid (e.g. semen, vaginal secretions, CSF, synovial or pleural fluid) or tissue	ZDV 200mg q8h + 3TC 150mg q12h + (IDV or nelfinavir). All po for 4 weeks	Can give ZDV + 3TC q12h in combination tablet that contains 300mg ZDV and 150mg 3TC
	Other body fluid (e.g. urine)	Do not offer	
	HIV: occupational exposure (mucous membrane, e.g. mouth, conjunctivae) Blood	Offer: ZDV 200mg q8h + 3TC 150mg q12h ± IDV 800mg q8h. All po for 4 weeks	Can give ZDV + 3TC q12h in combination tablet that contains 300mg ZDV and 150mg 3TC
	Fluid containing visible blood or other potential infectious fluid (e.g. semen, vaginal secretions, CSF/synoval/pleural, tissue)	Offer: ZDV 200mg q8h + 3TC 150mg q12h. All po for 4 weeks	Can give ZDV + 3TC q12h in combination tablet that contains 300mg ZDV and 150mg 3TC
	Other body fluid (e.g. urine)	Do not offer	
	HIV: occupational exposure (skin contact) Blood at increased risk (e.g. exposures involving high HIV titer, prolonged contact, large skin area or damaged skin: applies to all)	Offer: ZDV 200mg q8h and 3TC 150mg q12h ± IDV 800mg q8h. All po for 4 weeks	
	Fluid containing blood or other potential infectious fluid (e.g. semen, vaginal secretions, CSF, synovial or pleural fluid) or tissue	Offer: ZDV 200mg q8h and 3TC 150mg q12h. All po for 4 weeks	
	Other body fluid (e.g. urine)	Do not offer	
	HIV: sexual exposure Unprotected receptive and insertive anal and vaginal intercourse with a partner who is or is likely to be HIV-infected	Recommended: ZDV 300mg +3TC 150mg + (IDV 800mg q8h or nelfinavir 750mg q8h). All po for 4 weeks	Can give ZDV + 3TC q12h in combination tablet that contains 300mg ZDV and 150mg 3TC
	Receptive fellatio with ejaculation	Offered: ZDV 300mg +3TC 150mg + (IDV 800mg q8h or nelfinavir 750mg q8h). All po for 4 weeks	Can give ZDV + 3TC q12h in combination tablet that contains 300mg ZDV and 150mg 3TC
	Other sexual exposures, i.e. cunnilingus, receptive fellatio without ejaculation	Not recommended	
	Influenza type A	Amantadine or rimantadine 200mg q24h po	Continue until vaccine-induced immunity is accomplished, usually 6 weeks; adjust dose for renal function
	Respiratory synctial virus **Prevention:** Children < 24 months old with bronchopulmonary dysplasia requiring supplemental oxygen; possibly premature infants (<32 weeks' gestation) and <6 months old at start of RSV season	RSV immunoglobulin 750mg/kg iv once monthly between November and April (Northern hemisphere). First year of life for premature infants; perhaps up to 60 months of age for patients with bronchopulmonary dysplasia	Very expensive – estimated cost per infusion is US$1175

Fig. 4.8a Systemic prophylaxis and epidemiologic treatment with antimicrobial agents. AM–SB, ampicillin sulbactam; FQ,: fluoroquinolones – ciprofloxacin is FDA-approved for gastrointestinal uses in USA, norfloxacin is widely used in Europe but is not FDA-approved for this indication in USA; IP–TZ, piperacillin–tazobactam; MRSA, methicillin-resistant *Staphylococcus aureus*; PEP, postexposure prophylaxis; P Ceph 1, 2, first- or second-generation parenteral cephalosporin; SDD: selective decontamination of the digestive tract; TC–CL, ticarcillin–clavulanate; TMP–SMX, trimethoprim–sulfamethoxazole.

SYSTEMIC PROPHYLAXIS AND EPIDEMIOLOGIC TREATMENT WITH ANTIMICROBIAL AGENTS (continued)		
Disease and circumstance	Treatment: agent, dosage, route, duration	Comments
Bacterial Bacterial endocarditis prophylaxis	See tabulation at end of table for types of cardiac lesions, procedures, and recommendations (see Fig. 4.9)	
Gram-negative aerobic bacillary pneumonia in intubated ventilated patients	Selective decontamination of the digestive tract (SDD) regimens tried. CDC Hospital Infection Control Practices Advisory Committee makes no recommendation for SDD but if not contraindicated, elevate head of bed to 30–45º	
Haemophilus influenzae (meningitis) type b Household and/or day care contact: residing with index case or ≥4 hours. Day care contact: same day care as index case for 5–7 days before onset	Rifampin 20 mg/kg po (not to exceed 600 mg) q6h for 4 doses	Household: If there is one unvaccinated contact ≤4 yrs in the household, rifampin recommended for all household contacts except pregnant women. Child-care facilities: With 1 case, if attended by unvaccinated children ≤2 yrs, consider prophylaxis + vaccinate susceptibles. If all contacts >2 yrs: no prophylaxis. If ≥2 cases in 60 days and unvaccinated children attend, prophylaxis recommended for children and personnel
Methicillin-resistant *Staphylococcus aureus* (MRSA) colonization	Mupirocin 2% ointment to nares q12h for 5 days and to wounds q24h for 2 weeks	MRSA eliminated in 95% by 1 week but 40% recurrence (on maintenance treatment). 11% are mupirocin-resistant strains
Neisseria meningitidis exposure (close contact)	Rifampin 600mg q12h for 4 doses po. (Children 10mg/kg po q12h for 4 doses) or ciprofloxacin (adults) 500mg po single dose or ceftriaxone 250mg im for 1 dose (child <15 yrs, 125mg im for 1 dose) Spiramycin 500 mg q6h for 5 days po. Children 10 mg/kg po q6h for 5 days	*Nesseria meningitidis* spread by respiratory droplets, not aerosols, hence close contact required. Greater risk if close contact for at least 4 hours during week before illness onset (e.g. housemates, day care contacts, cellmates) or exposure to patient's nasopharyngeal secretions (e.g. via kissing, mouth-to-mouth resuscitation, intubation, nasotracheal suctioning). Azithro 500mg for 1 dose as effective as RIF 600mg q12h for 2 days Primary prophylactic regimen in many European countries
Neonatal Group B streptococcal disease Pregnant women – intrapartum antimicrobial prophylaxis. Two approaches: <ul><li>Prenatal screening cultures from vagina and rectum by swab at 35–37 weeks' gestation. Transport in Amies medium (survive at room temperature for up to 96 hours)</li><li>Risk factor approach – Treat if any of the following are present: (a) previously delivered infant with invasive GBS infection; (b) GBS bacteriuria during this pregnancy; (c) delivery at <37 weeks' gestation; (d) duration of ruptured membranes ≥18 hours; (e) intrapartum temperature ≥100.4°F (≥38.0°C)</li></ul>		If culture positive or risk factors dictate prophylaxis treat mother during labor with penicillin G 5MU iv (load) then 2.5MU iv q4h until delivery. Alternative treatment: Ampicillin 2g iv (load) then give q4h iv until delivery. Penicillin-allergic: Clindamycin 900 mg iv q8h until delivery or erythromycin 500mg iv q6h until delivery
Neonate delivered from mother who received prophylaxis	Careful observation of signs and symptoms	
Preterm, premature rupture of the membranes in Group B strep-negative women	(Ampicillin 2g q6h iv+ erythromycin 250 mg q8h iv) for 48h followed by amoxicillin 250 mg q8h po + erythromycin base 333mg q8h po for 5 days. Effective in decreasing infant morbidity	Antibiotic treatment reduced infant respiratory distress syndrome (50.6–40.8%, p=0.03), necrotizing enterocolitis (5.8–2.3%, p =0.03) and prolonged pregnancy (2.9–6.1 days, p<0.001) versus placebo
Streptococcal (Groups A, C, G) cellulitis complicating congenital (Milroy's) or acquired lymphedema	Benzathine penicillin G, 1.2MU im every 4 weeks [of minimal benefit in reducing recurrences in patients with underlying predisposing conditions	Indicated only if patient is having frequent episodes of cellulitis. Penicillin V 250mg q12h po should be effective but not aware of clinical trials. In penicillin-allergic patients: erythromycin 500 mg q24h po, azithro 250mg q24h po, or clarithro 500mg q24h po
Disease/ condition Afebrile neutropenic patients, e.g. post-chemotherapy	IDSA guidelines for afebrile neutropenic patients: Routine prophylaxis should be avoided, even though TMP/SMX 2 double strength tablets q12h po, or FQ (norfloxacin 400mg q12h po, ofloxacin 400mg q12h po, or ciprofloxacin 500mg q12h po) have been shown to reduce febrile episodes. No reduction in mortality and increase resistance prompt this recommendation	TMP/SMX (>30 studies) reduces infection rates (versus placebo) with fewer adverse effects. In a meta-analysis of 19 randomized studies, quinolone use reduced Gram-negative bacteremia (OR= 0.09) but not Gram-positive bacteremia (OR=1.05). Addition of penicillin, vancomycin, macrolide or rifampin reduced Gram-positive bacteremia (OR=0.46) but had no impact on fever-related morbidity (OR=0.83) or infection-related mortality (OR= 0.74). Oral fluconazole or parenteral amphotericin B prophylaxis not effective. Use of selective bowel decontamination did not reduce overall infection rate following liver transplant
Otitis media, recurrent acute. Likely agents: Pneumococci, *H. influenzae, M. catarrhalis,* Staph. aureus, Group A streptococcus	Sulfisoxazole 50 mg/kg po at bedtime or Amoxicillin 20mg/kg q24h po or Azithromycin 10mg/kg every week	Consider if ≥3 episodes in previous 6 months or ≥4 episodes in a yearr; or in infant, ≤6 months, 1 episode and family history of ear infections. Treat daily for 6 months during winter/spring. Use of antibiotics to prevent otitis media is a major contributor to emergence of antibiotic-resistant S. pneumococcus!
Peritonitis, spontaneous bacterial, in patients with cirrhosis and ascites	TMP/SMX-DS, 1 tablet 5 days per week po	Reduction in peritonitis or spontaneous bacteremia from 27–3%. Norfloxacin 400mg q24h po lowers the risk of spontaneous bacterial peritonitis and bacteremia caused by Gram-negative bacilli but increases the risk of severe staphylococcal infections and high-level resistance to antibiotics

Fig. 4.8a Systemic prophylaxis and epidemiologic treatment with antimicrobial agents continued.

SYSTEMIC PROPHYLAXIS AND EPIDEMIOLOGIC TREATMENT WITH ANTIMICROBIAL AGENTS (continued)		
Disease and circumstance	Treatment: agent, dosage, route, duration	Comments
Disease/ condition (continued) — **Post-splenectomy bacteremia.** Likely agents: Pneumococci, meningococci, *H. influenzae* type b (also at increase risk of fatal malaria, severe babesiosis) (immunization important, see Comments)	Penicillin V: Children <5 years 125mg q12h po, >5 years 250mg q12h po; Adults: 250mg q12h po. (Alternatives: Amoxicillin, TMP/SMX). NOTE: Repeat pneumococcal vaccine every 6 years	Daily antimicrobial prophylaxis effective with sickle-cell disease, but should be considered for asplenic children <5 years. Also recommended in children and adolescents for 3 years post splenectomy. Adjunct measures for all ages: meningococcal A and C, pneumococcal and Hib vaccines before elective splenectomy. Some authorities prescribe AM/CL for self-administration with onset of any fever for all ages.
Prosthetic joint infections: dental-induced	No prophylactic antibiotics recommended for dental procedures with exception of the following immuno-com-promised patients: (1) inflammatory arthropathies: rheumatoid arthritis, systemic lupus erythematosus; (2) disease-, drug- or radiation-induced immunosuppression; (3) insulin-dependent (type 1) diabetes; (4) 1st 2 years following joint placement; (5) previous prosthetic joint infections; (6) malnourishment; (7) hemophilia. Dosing regimens (all doses given 1 hour prior to dental procedure): Patients not allergic to penicillin: cephalexin, cephradine or amoxicillin 2g po; Patients not allergic to penicillin and unable to take oral medications: Cefazolin 1g or ampicillin 2g im or iv; Patients allergic to penicillin: Clindamycin 600mg po; Patients allergic to penicillin and unable to take oral medications: Clindamycin 600mg iv. No second doses are recommended for any of these dosing regimens.	
Rheumatic fever: post-Group A strepto-coccal pharyngitis Primary prophylaxis	Benzathine penicillin G 1.2MU im (see Pharyngitis)	Penicillin for 10 days, prevents rheumatic fever even when started 7–9 days after onset of illness.
Secondary prophylaxis (previous documented rheumatic fever)	Benzathine penicillin G 1.2MU im every 4 weeks (In South Africa, 1.2MU every 3 weeks recommended	Alternative: Penicillin V 250mg q12h po or sulfadiazine (sulfisoxazole) 1.0g q24h po or erythro 250mg q12h po. Duration of 2° prophylaxis varies: with carditis continue 10 years or until 25 years of age, without carditis continue 5 years or until 18 years of age
Sexual assault victim	Ceftriaxone 125mg im + doxycycline 100mg q12h po for 7 days + metronidazole 2gm po single dose	Perform bimanual pelvic exam. Examine wet mount for motile sperm, *T. vaginalis*. Culture for gonococci, chlamydia (if available), syphilis and HIV antibody test. Pregnancy test. Follow-up exam at 2 weeks. Repeat STS and serology for HIV at 12 weeks
Sexual contacts, likely agents: *N. gonorrhoeae, C. trachomatis*	[(Ceftriaxone 125mg im) + (doxycycline 100mg q12h po for 7 days)] or [(cefixime 400mg po) + (azithromycin 1.0g po), each as single dose]	Be sure to check for syphilis since all regimens may not eradicate incubating syphilis. If patient has been exposed to syphilis, treat within 3 months. Make effort to diagnose syphilis
Sickle-cell disease. Likely agent: *S. pneumoniae*	3 months to 5 years: Amoxicillin 125mg q12h po. >5 years, Penicillin V 250mg q12h po	Start prophylaxis before age 4 months. Children with SCD should receive vaccines: DTP, OPV, MMR, Hep B, Hib, pneumococcus, influenza ± meningococcal. Treat febrile episodes with ceftriaxone (50 mg/kg iv)
Transplantation Bone marrow	Regimens continue to evolve. Current 'standard' regimens include drugs active versus bacteria, fungi, pneumocystis, herpes simplex and CMV (see Comment).	Details of specific drugs and timing of administration vary from one transplant center to another. Similar regimen for solid organ transplants
Solid organ transplants: liver, kidney, heart, lung	Range of opportunistic infections and variability in prophylaxis protocols is greater than in bone marrow recipients. Many use TMP/SMX 1 single-strength tablet q24h po for 4–12 months. Special concern for CMV infections (see Comment)	Hard to define best regimens, as unethical to use placebo control. Ganciclovir better than acyclovir in prevention of CMV
Traveler's diarrhea	Not routinely indicated. Current recommendation is to take FQ + Imodium with first loose stool	Use in first 2 weeks only if activities are essential. Options: Bismuth sub-salicylate (Pepto-Bismol) 2 tablets (262mg) q24h po, or FQ-ciproflox 500mg q24h po, norflox 400mg q24h po
Urinary tract infection, child ≤5 years old, grade III–IV reflux	TMP/SMX (2mg TMP/10mg SMX/kg) q24h po or nitrofurantoin 2mg/kg q24h po	
Wegener's granulomatosis	TMP/SMX 800/160 tablet q12h po	Reduced relapses of patients in remission [18% (TMP/SMX) versus 40% (placebo)] over 24 months

Fig. 4.8a Systemic prophylaxis and epidemiologic treatment with antimicrobial agents continued. Adapted from Sanford JP *et al.*[41]

SURGICAL ANTIBIOTIC PROPHYLAXIS

Type of surgery	Treatment: agent, dosage, route, duration	Comments (to be optimally effective, antibiotics must be started in the interval: 2 hours before time of surgical incision)
Head and neck surgery	Cefazolin 2g iv (single dose) or clindamycin 600–900mg iv (single dose) ± gentamicin 1.5 mg/kg iv	Antimicrobial prophylaxis in head and neck surgery appears efficacious only for procedures involving oral/pharyngeal mucosa (i.e., laryngeal or pharyngeal tumor). Uncontaminated head and neck surgery does not require prophylaxis
Obstetric/gynecologic surgery Vaginal or abdominal hysterectomy	Cefazolin 1–2g or cefoxitin 1–2 gm or cefotetan 1–2g or cefuroxime 1.5g all iv 30 minutes before surgery	1 study found cefotetan superior to cefazolin. For prolonged procedures, doses can be repeated q4–8h for duration of procedure. NOTE: Also approved is trovafloxacin 200mg iv/po 30 minutes to 4 hours preoperative
Cesarean section for premature rupture of membranes or active labor	Cefazolin, administer iv as soon as umbilical cord clamped	
Abortion	First trimester: high-risk only (see Comments) aqueous penicillin G 2MU iv or doxycycline 300mg po. Second trimester: Cefazolin 1g iv	High-risk: Patients with previous pelvic inflammatory disease, gonorrhea or multiple sexual partners
Gastric, biliary and colonic surgery Gastroduodenal, includes percutaneous endoscopic gastrostomy (high-risk only; see Comments)	Cefazolin or cefoxitin or cefotetan or ceftizoxime or cefuroxime 1.5g iv single dose (some give additional doses q12h for 2–3 days). Dosage as C-section, above, except ceftizoxime 1g iv, repeat at 12–24 hours	Gastroduodenal: High-risk is marked obesity, obstruction, low gastric acid or low GI motility
Biliary, includes laparoscopic cholecystectomy (high-risk only; see Comments)		Biliary: Cephalosporins not active vs enterococci yet clinically effective as prophylaxis in biliary surgery. Cholangitis: treat as infection, not prophylaxis: TC/CL 3.1g iv or PIP/TZ 3.375g iv or AM/SB 3.0g iv, all q4–6h. Biliary high-risk: age >70 years, acute cholecystitis, non-functioning gallbladder, obstructive jaundice or common duct stones
Endoscopic retrograde cholangio-pancreatography	No rx without obstruction. If obstruction: Ciprofloxacin 500mg–1g po 2 hour prior to procedure. Ceftizoxime 1.5g iv 1 hour prior to procedure. Piperacillin 4g iv 1 hour prior to procedure	Most studies show that achieving adequate drainage will prevent postprocedural cholangitis or sepsis and no further benefit from prophylactic antibiotics. With inadequate drainage antibiotics may be of value. American Society for GI Endoscopy recommends use for known or suspected biliary obstruction. Oral cipro as effective as cephalosporins in 2 studies and less expensive
Colorectal, includes appendectomy Elective surgery	Neomycin + erythromycin po (see Comment for dose)	Elective colorectal prep: Pre-op day: (1) 10:00am 4 L polyethylene glycol electrolyte solution (Colyte) po over 2 hours. (2) Clear liquid diet only. (3) 1:00pm, 2:00pm and 10:00pm, neomycin 1g + erythro base 1g po. (4) NPO after midnight. There are alternative regimens which have been less well studied; GoLYTELY 1–6 pm, then neomycin 2g po + metronidazole 2.0g po at 7:00pm and 11:00pm. Oral regimen as effective as parenteral; parenteral in addition to oral not required. For emergency colorectal surgery, use parenteral
Elective surgery	[Cefazolin 1–2g iv + metronidazole 0.5g iv (single dose)] or cefoxitin or cefotetan 1–2g iv	
Ruptured viscus	Cefoxitin 2.0g iv, then 1.0g iv q8h for ≥5 days (base on clinical signs) or (clindamycin 600mg iv q6h + gentamicin 1.5mg/kg iv q8h) for ≥5 days	
Cardiovascular surgery Antibiotic prophylaxis in cardiovascular surgery has been proven beneficial only in the following procedures: • Reconstruction of abdominal aorta • Procedures on the leg that involve a groin incision • Any vascular procedure that inserts prosthesis/foreign body • Lower extremity amputation for ischemia • Cardiac surgery	Cefazolin 1.0g iv as a single dose or q8h for 1–2 days or cefuroxime 1.5g iv as a single dose or q8h for 1–2 days or vancomycin 1.0g iv as single initial dose or followed by 1.0g q12h or 0.5g q6h for 2 days	Single injection just before surgery probably as effective as multiple doses. Not recommended for cardiac catheterization. For prosthetic heart valves, customary to stop prophylaxis either after removal of retrosternal drainage catheters or just a second dose after coming off bypass. Vancomycin may be preferable in hospitals with higher frequency of MRSA but no coverage for Gram-negative bacilli, therefore would add cefazolin for groin incisions
Orthopedic surgery Hip arthroplasty, spinal fusion Total joint replacement (other than hip)	Same as cardiac Cefazolin 1–2g iv pre-op (± 2nd dose) or vancomycin 1.0g iv on call to operating room	Customarily stopped after 'Hemovac' removed Post-op: some would give no further treatment
Open reduction of closed fracture with internal fixation	Ceftriaxone 2g iv or im for 1 dose	8.3% versus 3.6% (for placebo) reduction found in Dutch trauma trial
Urologic surgery/procedures	Recommended antibiotic to patients with pre-operative bacteriuria: Cefazolin 1g iv q8h for 1–3 doses peri-operatively, followed by oral antibiotics (nitrofurantoin or TMP/SMX) until catheter is removed or for 10 days	Antimicrobials not recommended in patients with sterile urine. Patients with pre-operative bacteriuria should be treated
Transrectal prostate biopsy	Ciprofloxacin 500mg po 12 hours prior to biopsy and repeated 12 hours after biopsy (levo, norflox should work)	Ciprofloxacin reduced bacteremia from 37% (in gentamicin-rx group) to 7%
Neurosurgical procedures Clean, non-implant e.g., craniotomy	Cefazolin 1g iv (single dose). Or else: vancomycin 1g iv (single dose)	
Clean, contaminated (cross sinuses, or naso/oropharynx) CSF shunt surgery: controversial	Clindamycin 900mg iv (single dose) Vancomycin 10mg into cerebral ventricles + gentamicin 3mg into cerebral ventricles	British recommend amoxicillin/clavulanate 1.2g iv or (cefuroxime 1.5g iv + metronidazole 0.5g iv) Efficacy when infection rate >15%. Alternative: TMP (160mg) + SMX (800mg) iv pre-operative and q12h for 3 doses
Others Breast surgery, herniorrhaphy Traumatic (non-bite) wound	P Ceph 1,2, dosage (as C-section above) Either cefazolin 1g iv q8h or ceftriaxone 2g iv q24h for ≥5 days (base on clinical signs)	

Fig. 4.8b Surgical antibiotic prophylaxis. Operations in which antibiotic treatment decreases incisional infection include elective operations in which the gastrointestinal tract is opened; high-risk biliary surgery; abdominal and lower-extremity reconstruction; vaginal hysterectomy; cesarean section; hip nailing for fracture or spinal fusion; coronary artery bypass grafting; and cardiac pacemaker implantation. Adapted from Sanford JP et al.[41]

ANTIBIOTIC PROPHYLAXIS FOR THE PREVENTION OF BACTERIAL ENDOCARDITIS IN PATIENTS WITH UNDERLYING CARDIAC CONDITIONS

Endocarditis prophylaxis recommended	Endocarditis prophylaxis not recommended

Cardiac conditions associated with endocarditis
High-risk conditions:*
    Prosthetic valves – both bioprosthetic and homograft
    Previous bacterial endocarditis
    Complex cyanotic congenital heart disease (CHD), e.g. single
    ventricle, transposition,
        tetralogy of Fallot
    Surgically constructed systemic pulmonic shunts or conduits
Moderate-risk conditions:
    Most other CHD; hypertrophic cardiac myopathy; mitral prolapse with
    regurgitation
	Negligible-risk (same as general population):
	Atrial septal defect or repaired atrial septal defect/ventricular septal defect, or patent
	ductus arteriosus (beyond 6 months)
	Previous CABG; mitral prolapse without MI
	Physiologic, functional or innocent heart murmurs
	Previous Kawasaki or rheumatic fever without valve dysfunction
	Cardiac pacemakers (all) and implanted defibrillators

Dental and other procedures where prophylaxis is considered for patients with moderate- or high-risk cardiac conditions
Dental: Extractions, periodontal procedures*
    Implants, root canal, subgingival antibiotic fibers/strips
    Initial orthodontic bands (not brackets); intraligamentary local anesthetic
    Cleaning of teeth/implants if bleeding anticipated
Respiratory: T&A, surgery on respiratory mucosa, rigid bronchoscopy
GI: Sclerotherapy of esophageal varices; dilation of esophageal stricture; endoscopic
    retrograde cholangiography with biliary obstruction
    Biliary tract surgery; surgery on/through intestinal mucosa
GU: Prostate surgery; cystoscopy; urethral dilatation
	Dental: Filling cavities with local anesthetic
	    Rubber dams, suture removal, orthodontic removal
	    Orthodontic adjustments, dental radiographs
	    Shedding of primary teeth
	Respiratory: Intubation, flexible bronchoscopy§, tympanostomy tube
	GI: Transesophageal cardiac ECHO§, esophagogastroduodenostomy without
	    biopsy§
	GU: Vaginal hysterectomy§, vaginal delivery§, Cesarean-section
	    If uninfected, Foley catheter, uterine dilation and curettage, therapeutic
	    abortion, tubal ligation, insert/remove IUD
	Other: Cardiac cath, balloon angioplasty, implanted pacemaker, defibrillators,
	    coronary stents
	    Skin biopsy, circumcision

Situation	Agent	Regimen
Prophylactic regimens for dental, oral, respiratory tract or esophageal procedures Standard general prophylaxis	Amoxicillin	Adults 2.0g; children 50mg/kg orally 1 hour before procedure
Unable to take oral medications	Ampicillin	Adults 2.0g im or iv; children 50mg/kg im or iv within 30 minutes before procedure
Allergic to penicillin	Clindamycin, or	Adults 600mg; children 20mg/kg orally 1 hour before procedure
	Cephalexin** or cefadroxil**, or	Adults 2.0g; children 50mg/kg orally 1 hour before procedure
	Azithromycin or clarithromycin	Adults 500mg; children 15mg/kg orally 1 hour before procedure
Allergic to penicillin and unable to take oral medications	Clindamycin, or	Adults 600mg; children 20mg/kg iv within 30 minutes before procedure
	Cefazolin**	Adults 1.0g; children 25mg/kg im or iv within 30 minutes before procedure
Prophylactic regimens for genitourinary/gastro-intestinal (excluding esophageal) procedures High-risk patients	Ampicillin + gentamicin†	Adults: ampicillin 2.0g im or iv + gentamicin 1.5mg/kg (not to exceed 120mg) within 30 minutes of starting the procedure; 6 hr later, ampicillin 1g im/iv or amoxicillin 1g orally Children: ampicillin 50mg/kg im or iv (not to exceed 2.0g) + gentamicin 1.5mg/kg within 30 minutes of starting the procedure; 6 hours later, ampicillin 25mg/kg im/iv or amoxicillin 25mg/kg orally
High-risk patients allergic to ampicillin/amoxicillin	Vancomycin† + gentamicin†	Adults: vancomycin 1.0g iv over 1–2 hours + gentamicin 1.5mg/kg iv/im (not to exceed 120mg); complete injection/infusion within 30 minutes of starting the procedure Children: vancomycin 20mg/kg iv over 1–2 hours + gentamicin 1.5mg/kg iv/im; complete injection/infusion within 30 mins of starting the procedure
Moderate-risk patients	Amoxicillin or ampicillin	Adults: amoxicillin 2.0g orally 1 hour before procedure, or ampicillin 2.0g im/iv within 30 minutes of starting the procedure Children: amoxicillin 50mg/kg orally 1 hour before procedure, or ampicillin 50mg/kg im/iv within 30 minutes of starting the procedure
Moderate-risk patients allergic to ampicillin/amoxicillin	Vancomycin†	Adults: vancomycin 1.0g iv over 1–2 hours; complete infusion within 30 minutes of starting the procedure Children: vancomycin 20mg/kg iv over 1–2 hours; complete infusion within 30 minutes of starting the procedure

Fig. 4.9 Antimicrobial prophylaxis for the prevention of bacterial endocarditis in patients with underlying cardiac conditions. *Some now recommend that prophylaxis prior to dental procedures should only be used for extractions and gingival surgery (including implant replacement) and only for patients with prosthetic cardiac valves or previous endocarditis. If any of these four conditions exist then the American Heart Association recommends prophylactic antibiotics. † No second dose of vancomycin or gentamicin is recommended. § Prophylaxis optional for high-risk patients. **Cephalosporins should not be used in individuals with immediate-type hypersensitivity reaction to penicillins. Adapted from Sanford JP et al.[41]

GUIDE TO TETANUS PROPHYLAXIS IN ROUTINE WOUND MANAGEMENT

History of adsorbed tetanus toxoid	Clean, minor wounds		All other wounds	
	Tetanus, diphtheria	Tetanus immunoglobulin	Tetanus, diphtheria	Tetanus immunoglobulin
Unknown or fewer than three doses	Yes	No	Yes	Yes
Three or more doses	No (unless >10 years since last dose)	No	No (unless >5 years since last dose)	No

Fig. 4.10 Guide to tetanus prophylaxis in routine wound management. Wounds that are not clean or minor include wounds contaminated with dirt, feces, soil and saliva; puncture wounds; avulsions; and wounds resulting from missiles, crushing, burns and frostbite. For children <7 years of age, diphtheria–tetanus–pertussis vaccine (or diphtheria–tetanus if pertussis vaccine is contraindicated) is preferred to tetanus toxoid alone. For persons ≥ 7 years of age, tetanus–diphtheria is preferred to tetanus toxoid alone. If only three doses of fluid toxoid have been received, then a fourth dose of toxoid, preferably an adsorbed toxoid, should be given. From CDC.[43]

HEPATITIS B IMMUNOPROPHYLAXIS

Recommended schedule of hepatitis B immunoprophylaxis to prevent perinatal transmission

	Vaccine dose	Age of infant
Infant born to mother known to be HBsAg positive	First	Birth (within 12 hours)
	HBIG (0.5ml im, at a site different from that used for vaccine)	Birth (within 12 hours)
	Second	1 month
	Third	6 months*
Infant born to mother not screened for HBsAg	First	Birth (within 12 hours)
	HBIG (0.5ml im, at a site different from that used for vaccine)	If mother is found to be HBsAg positive, administer dose to infant as soon as possible, and not later than 1 week after birth
	Second	1–2 months
	Third	6 months*

Recommended schedule of hepatitis B vaccination for infants born to HBsAg-negative mothers

	Hepatitis B vaccine	Age of infant
Option 1	Dose 1	Birth or before hospital discharge
	Dose 2	1–2 months
	Dose 3	6–18 months
Option 2	Dose 1	1–2 months
	Dose 2	4 months
	Dose 3	6–18 months

Recommendations for heptatitis B prophylaxis following percutaneous exposure

Status of exposed person	Treatment when source is found to be HBsAg positive	Treatment when source is found to be HBsAg negative	Unknown or not tested
Unvaccinated	Administer HBIG once (0.06ml/kg im) and initiate hepatitis B vaccine	Initiate hepatitis B vaccine	Initiate hepatitis B vaccine
Previously vaccinated; known responder	Test exposed person for anti-HBs; if adequate (≥ 10mIU), no treatment; if inadequate, hepatitis B vaccine booster dose	No treatment	No treatment
Previously vaccinated; known nonresponder	HBIG twice, or HBIG once plus hepatitis B vaccine once	No treatment	If known high-risk source, may treat as if source were HBsAg positive
Previously vaccinated, response unknown	Test exposed person for anti-HB; if inadequate, HBIG once plus hepatitis B vaccine booster dose; if adequate, no treatment	No treatment	Test exposed person for anti-HBs; if inadequate (≤ 10mIU), hepatitis B vaccine booster dose; if adequate, no treatment

Fig. 4.11 Hepatitis B immunoprophylaxis. Recommended schedule of hepatitis B immunoprophylaxis to prevent perinatal transmission of hepatitis B virus infection, recommended schedule of hepatitis B vaccine for infants born to HbsAg-negative mothers and recommendations for hepatitis B prophylaxis following percutaneous exposure. *, if four dose (Energix-B) is used the third dose is administered at 2 months of age and the fourth dose at 12–18 months. HBIG, hepatitis B immunoglobulin; HBsAg, hepatitis B surface antigen; anti-HB, anti-hepatitis B antibody; anti-HBs, anti-hepatitis B surface antibody. From CDC.[45]

In addition, there are several circumstances in which postexposure prophylactic protocols have been established – following potential exposure to tetanus, rabies (see Chapter 8.8), and hepatitis B (Figs 4.10 & 4.11).[43–45]

MEASURING THE IMPACT OF PREVENTION – SURVEILLANCE
The systematic collection, analysis and interpretation of health information data is critical to prevention efforts. Surveillance data are used to establish priorities of disease control and also to create baselines by which the effectiveness of interventions can be measured. Concerns over the threat of emerging and re-emerging infectious diseases has placed a renewed emphasis on this key component of a public health system.

COST-EFFECTIVENESS OF PREVENTION
In the setting of health care reform around the globe, prevention of infections often translates into cost savings. The growing body of evidence that prevention is cost-effective offers renewed hope that investments in prevention will provide the payoff that they have long promised. With the goal of setting priorities for investments in preventive interventions, the World Health Organization and the World Bank developed the concept of 'disability-adjusted life years' (DALY) to provide a better means of assessing the global burden of disease that accounts for the impact of morbidity and mortality throughout life (Fig. 4.12).[4]

The DALY combines losses from premature death (defined as the difference between the actual age at death and the life expectancy at that age) with the loss of healthy life that results from the disease process and subsequent disability; it therefore incorporates both the severity and the duration of the condition. Although cost-effectiveness studies are not the sole determinant of health policies and priorities, they have become important considerations in decision making. A number of recent studies have documented the cost-effectiveness of prevention of a variety of infectious diseases.[46–49]

VACCINATION

DISEASES THAT CAN BE PREVENTED BY VACCINATION
The development and application of vaccines is the only factor that has had an impact on health and well-being that approaches the impact that access to safe water and sanitation has had. Prevention of infectious diseases and their complications is the goal of immunization programs; however, analysis of the level of use of vaccines in the population ('coverage') is often used as surrogate for disease reduction, especially in regions where disease surveillance systems are unreliable. The successful campaign that led to the eradication of smallpox by 1977 demonstrated the power of vaccines when coupled with appropriate strategies. That example set the stage for the goal of polio eradication by the year 2000 (Fig. 4.13).[50]

DISTRIBUTION OF DALY LOSS BY CAUSE AND DEMOGRAPHIC REGION 1990									
Cause	World	Sub-Saharan Africa	India	China	Rest of Asia	Latin America and the Caribbean	Middle East	Former socialist economies of Europe	Established market economies
Population (millions)	5267	510	850	1134	683	444	503	346	798
Communicable diseases (%)	45.8	71.3	50.5	25.3	48.5	42.2	51.0	8.6	9.7
Tuberculosis (%)	3.4	4.7	3.7	2.9	5.1	2.5	2.8	0.6	0.2
Sexually transmitted diseases and HIV (%)	3.8	8.8	2.7	1.7	1.5	6.6	0.7	1.2	3.4
Diarrhea (%)	7.3	10.4	9.6	2.1	8.3	5.7	10.7	0.4	0.3
Vaccine-preventable childhood infections (%)	5.0	9.6	6.7	0.9	4.5	1.6	6.0	0.1	0.1
Malaria (%)	2.6	10.8	0.3	< 0.05	1.4	0.4	0.2	< 0.05	< 0.05
Worm infections (%)	1.8	1.8	0.9	3.4	3.4	2.5	0.4	< 0.05	< 0.05
Respiratory infections (%)	9.0	10.8	10.9	6.4	11.1	6.2	11.5	2.6	2.6
Maternal causes (%)	2.2	2.7	2.7	1.2	2.5	1.7	2.9	0.8	0.6
Perinatal causes (%)	7.3	7.1	9.1	5.2	7.4	9.1	10.9	2.4	2.2
Other (%)	3.5	4.6	4.0	1.4	3.3	5.8	4.9	0.6	0.5
Noncommunicable diseases (%)	42.2	19.4	40.4	58.0	40.1	42.8	36.0	74.8	78.4
Cancer (%)	5.8	1.5	4.1	9.2	4.4	5.2	3.4	14.8	19.1
Nutritional deficiencies (%)	3.9	2.8	6.2	3.3	4.6	4.6	3.7	1.4	1.7
Neuropsychiatric disease (%)	6.8	3.3	6.1	8.0	7.0	8.0	5.6	11.1	15.0
Cerebrovascular disease (%)	3.2	1.5	2.1	6.3	2.1	2.6	2.4	8.9	5.3
Ischemic heart disease (%)	3.1	0.4	2.8	2.1	3.5	2.7	1.8	13.7	10.0
Pulmonary obstruction (%)	1.3	0.2	0.6	5.5	0.5	0.7	0.5	1.6	1.7
Other (%)	18.0	9.7	18.5	23.6	17.9	19.1	18.7	23.4	25.6
Injuries (%)	11.9	9.3	9.1	16.7	11.3	15.0	13.0	16.6	11.9
Motor vehicle accidents (%)	2.3	1.3	1.1	2.3	2.3	5.7	3.3	3.7	3.5
Intentional deaths (%)	3.7	4.2	1.2	5.1	3.2	4.3	5.2	4.8	4.0
Other (%)	5.9	3.9	6.8	9.3	5.8	5.0	4.6	8.1	4.3
DALYs (millions)	1362	293	292	201	177	103	144	58	94
Equivalent infant deaths (millions)	42.0	9.0	9.0	6.2	5.5	3.2	4.4	1.8	2.9
DALYs per 1000 population	259	575	344	178	260	233	286	168	117

Fig. 4.12 Distribution of DALY loss by cause and demographic region 1990. DALY, disability-adjusted life years. From the World Bank's World Development Report.[4]

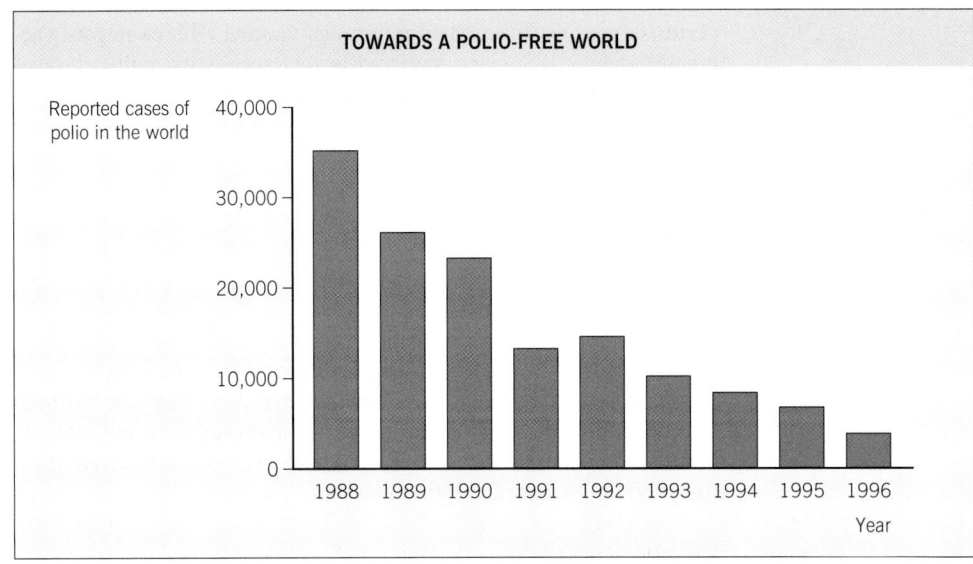

Fig. 4.13 **Towards a polio-free world.** Reported cases of poliomyelitis worldwide, 1988–1996. Modified from the World Health Organization's Vaccine and Immunization News.[50]

Disease	Maximum number of reported cases during the prevaccine era	Reported number of cases during 1997	Percentage change in morbidity
Diphtheria	206,939	5	−99.99
Measles	984,134	138	−99.98
Mumps	152,209	612	−99.60
Pertussis	265,269	5519	−97.92
Polio (paralytic)	21,269	0	−100.00
Rubella	57,686	161	−99.72
Congenital rubella syndrome	20,000	4	−99.98
Tetanus	1560	43	−97.24
Haemophilus influenzae type b/unknown (<5 years)	20,000	165	−99.18

REDUCTION IN VACCINE-PREVENTABLE DISEASES IN THE USA

Fig. 4.14 **Reduction in vaccine-preventable diseases in the USA.** The figures are for 1997 and the maximum number of reported cases during the prevaccine era is estimated for invasive congenital rubella syndrome and polio. Modified from CDC.[51]

In the USA, the 1996 coverage goal – the attainment of at least 90% of 2-year olds – was achieved and in some cases exceeded: 95% of 2-year olds received three doses of diphtheria, tetanus and pertussis (DPT) vaccine; 90% of 2-year olds received three doses of oral polio vaccine (OPV); 92% of 2-year olds received three doses of *Haemophilus influenzae* type b (Hib) vaccine; and 91% of children received a vaccine against measles. The 1996 goal for hepatitis B vaccine, the vaccine that had been most recently introduced into the childhood immunization schedule, was 70%, yet the actual coverage among 2-year olds was 82%. Overall, the coverage for the most common series (four doses of DPT vaccine, three doses of OPV and one dose of a measles-containing vaccine) was 78%, the highest coverage level ever recorded in the USA (Fig. 4.14).[51]

Technologic advances in genetics, chemistry and immunology have ushered in waves of new vaccines. As we approach the 21st century, novel approaches for vaccine development include DNA vaccines and mucosal vaccines, including the prospect of 'edible' vaccines produced in transgenic plants and vaccines that can be administered by aerosol spray. In a recent report from the US National Institute of Allergy and Infectious Diseases, there are approximately 350 vaccine candidates in some stage of development.[52] Although it is unlikely that all of these vaccines will become licensed products, the list of vaccines, immunoglobulins and antitoxins licensed in the USA continues to grow (Figs 4.15 & 4.16).[52,53]

The growing number of available vaccines has made the process of immunization increasingly complex. The current childhood immunization schedule in the USA (Fig. 4.17) demonstrates the number of vaccines and immunizations required in the first years of life.[54]

NEW VACCINES FOR DEVELOPING COUNTRIES – THE CHILDREN'S VACCINE INITIATIVE
In contrast to the vast possibilities that modern technologies offer for vaccine development, the World Health Organization's Expanded Program of Immunizations (EPI) has a more limited armamentarium. This program reaches children in the first 9 months of life and has achieved 80% coverage with vaccines that protect against tuberculosis (BCG vaccine), poliomyelitis [oral polio vaccine, (OPV)], diphtheria, pertussis and tetanus (DPT vaccine), and measles (measles vaccine) (Fig. 4.18).[11] Efforts to bring new vaccines into the EPI are the goal of the Children's Vaccine Initiative, a global coalition founded in 1990 and dedicated to the development and utilization of safe, effective, easy-to-deliver and widely available vaccines.

The 1997 Strategic Plan of the Children's Vaccine Initiative highlights a number of major vaccination targets by setting priorities for vaccine use and development based on the burden of disease, the cost of treatment, and the feasibility and cost of vaccine development and immunization programs (Fig. 4.19).[55]

VACCINES AND IMMUNIZATIONS: DEFINITIONS, PRINCIPLES, LOGISTICS AND USE
Because vaccines are biological agents that have their effect on the immune system, they are characterized as immunobiologics, a larger grouping that includes antigenic substances (vaccines and toxoids) and antibody-containing products (globulins and antitoxins). The receipt of preformed antibody is referred to as passive immunization; active immunization is the process whereby a vaccine induces an immunologic response in the recipient.

- Adenovirus vaccine, live oral, type 4
- Adenovirus vaccine, live oral, type 7
- Anthrax vaccine, adsorbed
- BCG, live
- Botulinum toxin type A
- Cholera vaccine
- Diphtheria and tetanus toxoids and acellular pertussis vaccine, adsorbed
- Diphtheria and tetanus toxoids and pertussis vaccine, adsorbed and *Haemophilus influenzae* type B, conjugate vaccine
- Diphtheria and tetanus toxoids, adsorbed
- *Haemophilus influenzae* type b, conjugate vaccine
- Hepatitis A vaccine, inactivated
- Hepatitis B vaccine, recombinant
- Influenza virus vaccine, inactivated
- Japanese encephalitis virus vaccine, inactivated
- Lyme vaccine, subunit vaccine
- Measles, mumps and rubella virus vaccine, live
- Measles and mumps virus vaccine, live
- Measles and rubella virus vaccine, live
- Measles vaccine, live
- Meningococcal polysaccharide vaccine group A
- Meningococcal polysaccharide vaccine group C
- Meningococcal polysaccharide vaccine groups A and C, combined
- Meningococcal polysaccharide vaccine groups A, C, Y and W-135, combined
- Mumps vaccine, live
- Pertussis vaccine, adsorbed
- Plague vaccine
- Pneumococcal vaccine (23-valent)
- Poliovirus vaccine, inactivated
- Poliovirus vaccine, live oral
- Rabies vaccine
- Rotavirus vaccine, live oral reassortant vaccine
- Rubella and mumps vaccine, live
- Rubella vaccine, live
- Tetanus and diphtheria toxoids, adsorbed (for adult use)
- Typhoid vaccine, live oral Ty21a
- Typhoid Vi polysaccharide vaccine
- Varicella vaccine, live
- Yellow fever vaccine

Fig. 4.15 Licensed vaccines in the USA 1998. Modified from National Institute of Allergy and Infectious Diseases' Jordan Report (National Institutes of Health).[52]

Vaccine components

In addition to the vaccine antigen that provides the target for the immune response, vaccines may also contain other ingredients, including suspending fluids (e.g. sterile water, saline, or fluids derived from the biologic system in which the vaccine is produced); preservatives, stabilizers and antibiotics to prevent bacterial contamination and to protect the antigen from degradation; and adjuvants (substances that enhance the immunologic response). In a patient with known allergies and sensitivities, each of these components should be considered before administration of any vaccine.

Vaccine storage and handling

Each vaccine has its own specific storage and handling requirements. For example, OPV and yellow fever vaccine are sensitive to heat and rapidly lose their potency at warm temperatures. In contrast, many vaccines are sensitive to freezing. These include diphtheria and tetanus toxoids, pertussis vaccine, inactivated poliovirus vaccine, Hib conjugate vaccines, hepatitis B vaccine, pneumococcal vaccine and influenza vaccine.[53] Maintaining the proper temperature of vaccines from their point of production to the vaccine recipient is referred to as the 'cold chain'. Because it may be difficult to distinguish a potent vaccine from one that has not been strictly maintained at the proper temperature, most vaccines are packed with temperature monitors during shipment.

Route of administration

The route of administration is specific to each vaccine. Because the process of development and testing vaccines for safety and efficacy is based on a specific route of administration, vaccines should only be administered as recommended. In general, vaccines that contain immune-stimulating adjuvants should be administered into muscle, because subcutaneous or intradermal administration can cause local irritation, induration and inflammation.

Vaccine schedules

Vaccines may not be effective in very young children with developing immune systems, or they may require several doses to be fully effective. Therefore, the timing sequence of immunizations effects the immune response. The administration of new vaccines is becoming increasingly complex; therefore, guidelines have been established for the spacing of vaccines and immune globulin preparations (Figs 4.20 & 4.21).[51,53] Because some children may not receive vaccines at the proper time in early childhood, special schedules have also been constructed to suit these purposes (Figs 4.22 & 4.23).[53]

VACCINE CONTRAINDICATIONS AND PRECAUTIONS

There are several contraindications and precautions to vaccination (Fig. 4.24).[53] With the exception of a moderate or severe underlying illness, contraindications are specific to the vaccine. Among the factors to consider before administering a vaccine are:
- underlying allergies to animal proteins (eggs or chicken embryo), antibiotics (streptomycin or neomycin) or one of the stabilizers;
- altered immunity; and
- pregnancy.

Because some vaccines are prepared in eggs, persons who are able to eat eggs or egg products without developing allergy should have no difficulty with the receipt of vaccines prepared in eggs or chicken embryos.

ADVERSE EVENTS FOLLOWING VACCINATION

No pharmaceutical product, when used broadly in the population, will be free of all side effects. The paradox of vaccine effectiveness is the growing concern over vaccine safety. Not only has the increase in vaccine coverage rates increased the number of doses of vaccines and the number of people who receive vaccines, but as the threat of disease disappears in a community, the risks, real and perceived, attributed to vaccines may achieve increased prominence.

In many countries, concern over vaccine safety that was focused on the whole-cell pertussis vaccine led to an erosion in confidence and a decline in the use of vaccines. Without vaccine-induced protective immunity the enlarging pool of susceptible people led to pertussis epidemics.[56]

In the USA, similar concerns led to the creation of the National Childhood Vaccine Injury Act of 1986 and established a compensation program for persons injured by vaccines.[51] This Act also established a scientific review process by the Institute of Medicine to examine the strength of the evidence linking childhood vaccinations to the adverse events that followed (Fig 4.25).[51,57-60] These examinations were the basis of the creation of a table of compensatable injuries to childhood vaccines, whether they are administered by private physicians or in public clinics. The vaccines currently included are DTP, measles, mumps, rubella, polio, hepatitis B, Hib and varicella vaccines.[61]

IMMUNE GLOBULINS AND ANTITOXINS AVAILABLE IN THE USA

Immunobiologic	Type	Indication(s)
Botulinum antitoxin	Specific equine antibodies	Treatment of botulism
Cytomegalovirus intravenous immune globulin	Specific human antibodies	Prophylaxis for bone marrow and kidney transplant recipients
Diphtheria antitoxin	Specific equine antibodies	Treatment of respiratory diphtheria
Immune globulin	Pooled human antibodies	Hepatitis A pre-exposure and postexposure prophylaxis; measles postexposure prophylaxis
Intravenous immune globulin	Pooled human antibodies	Replacement therapy for antibody deficiency disorders; immune thrombocytopenic purpura; hypogammaglobulinemia in chronic lymphocytic leukemia; Kawasaki disease
Hepatitis B immune globulin	Specific human antibodies	Hepatitis B postexposure prophylaxis
Human rabies immune globulin	Specific human antibodies	Rabies postexposure management of people not previously immunized with rabies vaccine
Tetanus immune globulin	Specific human antibodies	Treatment of tetanus; postexposure prophylaxis of people not adequately immunized with tetanus toxoid
Vaccinia immune globulin	Specific human antibodies	Treatment of eczema vaccinatum, vaccinia necrosum and ocular vaccinia
Varicella-zoster immune globulin	Specific human antibodies	Postexposure prophylaxis of susceptible immunocompromised people, certain susceptible pregnant women and perinatally exposed newborn infants

Fig. 4.16 Immune globulins and antitoxins available in the USA. The type and the indications for use are shown. Immune globulin preparations and antitoxins are administered intramuscularly unless otherwise indicated; and human rabies immune globulin is administered around the wounds in addition to the intramuscular injection. From CDC.[53]

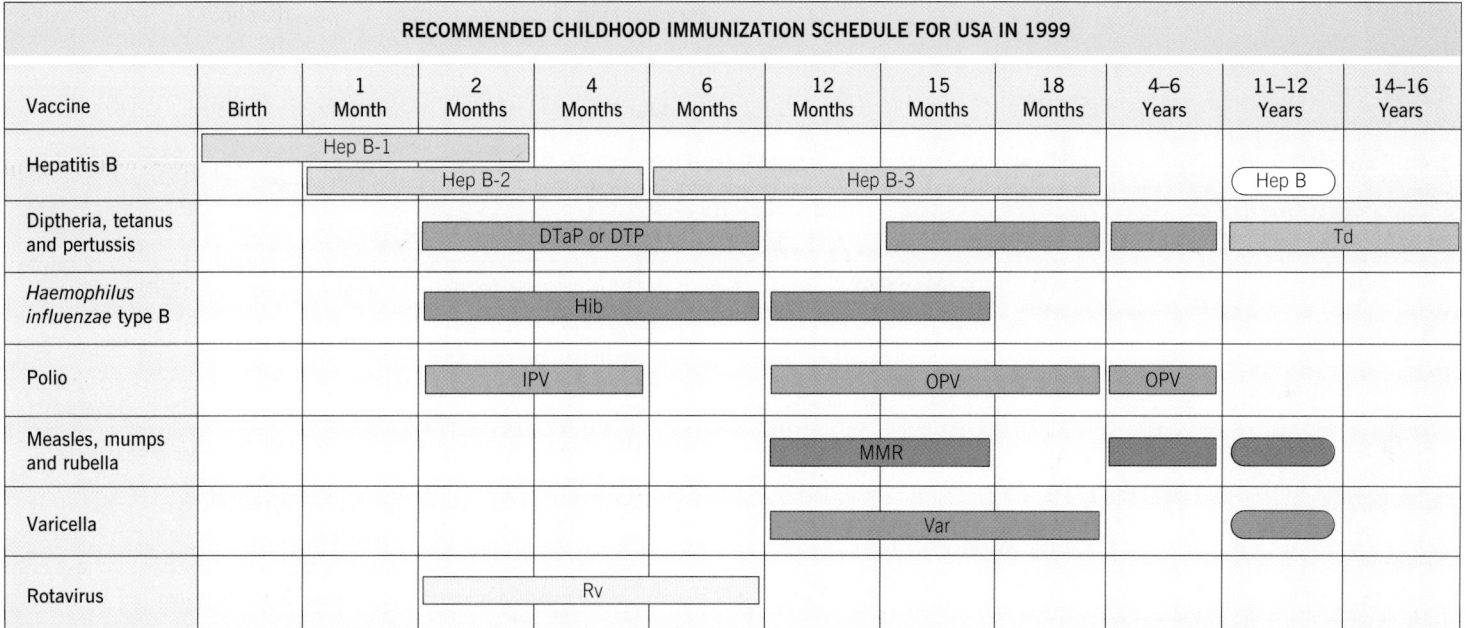

Fig. 4.17 Recommended childhood immunization schedule for USA in 1999

Vaccine	Birth	1 Month	2 Months	4 Months	6 Months	12 Months	15 Months	18 Months	4–6 Years	11–12 Years	14–16 Years
Hepatitis B		Hep B-1		Hep B-2		Hep B-3				Hep B	
Diptheria, tetanus and pertussis			DTaP or DTP							Td	
Haemophilus influenzae type B			Hib								
Polio			IPV			OPV			OPV		
Measles, mumps and rubella						MMR					
Varicella						Var					
Rotavirus			Rv								

Fig. 4.17 Recommended childhood immunization schedule for the USA in 1999. Vaccines are shown under the routinely recommended ages, and the range of acceptable ages for immunization is indicated. Catch-up immunization should be done during any visit when feasible. Oval-shaped areas indicate vaccines to be assessed and given if necessary during the early adolescent visit. Special efforts should be made to immunize children who were born in or whose parents were born in areas of the world with moderate or high endemicity of hepatitis B virus infection. Diphtheria and tetanus toxoids and a cellular pertussis vaccine (DTaP) is the preferred vaccine for all doses in the vaccination series, including completion of the series in children who have received one or more doses of whole-cell diphtheria, tetanus and pertussis (DTP) vaccine. Whole-cell DTP is an acceptable alternative to DTaP. The fourth dose (DTP or DTaP) may be administered as early as 12 months of age if 6 months have elapsed since the third dose and if the child is unlikely to return at 15–18 months of age. Tetanus and diphtheria toxoids (Td) are recommended at 11–12 years of age if at least 5 years have elapsed since the last dose of DTP, DTaP, or DT. Subsequent routine Td boosters are recommended every 10 years. Two poliovirus vaccines are currently licensed in the USA: inactivated poliovirus vaccine (IPV) and oral poliovirus vaccine

(OPV). The Advisory Committee on Immunization Practices recommends two doses of IPV at 2 months and 4 months of age, followed by two doses of OPV at 12–18 months and 4–6 years. Use of IPV for all doses is also acceptable and recommended for immunocompromised people and their household contacts. The second dose of measles, mumps and rubella vaccine is recommended routinely at 4–6 years of age, but it may be administered during any visit, provided that at least 1 month has elapsed since the first dose and that the first dose is administered at or after 12 months of age. Those who have not previously received their second dose should complete the schedule no later than the 11–12 year visit. Susceptible children may receive varicella vaccine at any visit after their first birthday, and those who lack a reliable history of chickenpox should be immunized during the 11–12 year visit. Susceptible children aged 13 years or older should receive two doses at least 1 month apart. The rotavirus vaccine (Rv) is a new vaccine and healthcare workers may require time and resources to incorporate it into practice. The first dose of of Rv vaccine should not be administered before 6 weeks of age, and the minimum interval between doses is 3 weeks. The Rv vaccine should not be initiated at 7 months of age or older, and all doses should be completed by the first birthday.[54]

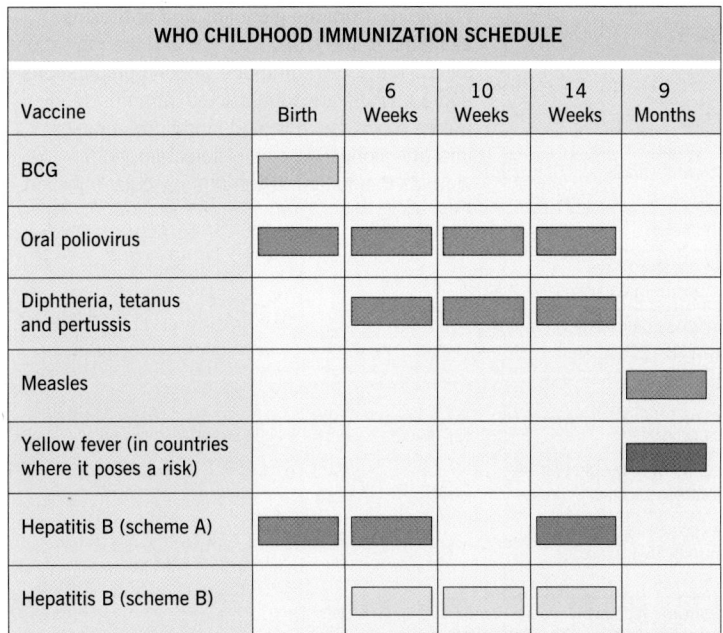

WHO CHILDHOOD IMMUNIZATION SCHEDULE

Vaccine	Birth	6 Weeks	10 Weeks	14 Weeks	9 Months
BCG	▨				
Oral poliovirus	▨	▨	▨	▨	
Diphtheria, tetanus and pertussis		▨	▨	▨	
Measles					▨
Yellow fever (in countries where it poses a risk)					▨
Hepatitis B (scheme A)	▨	▨		▨	
Hepatitis B (scheme B)		▨	▨	▨	

Fig. 4.18 Immunization schedule for infants recommended by the World Health Organization Expanded Programme on Immunization. Scheme A is recommended in countries where perinatal transmission of hepatitis B virus is frequent (e.g. in South East Asia). Scheme B may be used in countries where perinatal transmission is less frequent (e.g. in sub-Saharan Africa). From UNICEF.[11]

Unfortunately, inappropriate caution can lead to missed opportunities for vaccine administration. Therefore, it is important to distinguish the true contraindications to vaccinations as described in each products package insert, from conditions and circumstances in which immunization is not contraindicated (Fig. 4.26).[53]

ADOLESCENT AND ADULT IMMUNIZATION

The focus on reducing the vaccine-preventable diseases of children has been a success around the world as vaccines have become one of the foundations of routine pediatric care. However, despite the availability of safe and effective vaccines, approximately 50,000–70,000 adults die each year in the USA from complications of infections with *Streptococcus pneumoniae*, influenza and hepatitis B, infections for which vaccines are routinely recommended for many adults and the elderly. In contrast to the coverage rates of childhood vaccines in the USA (and around the world), current utilization in the USA of these vaccines in target adult populations for which these vaccines are recommended is estimated to be 55% for an annual influenza vaccine, 30% for pneumococcal vaccine and just 10% for hepatitis B vaccine. If used as recommended, these vaccines would have substantial impact on the health of younger and older adults (Fig. 4.27).[62]

As new vaccines become available for adolescents and adults, it will be increasingly important to develop delivery systems that can efficiently and effectively administer the vaccines as recommended. It has been suggested that this can be accomplished in part by integrating adolescent and adult vaccinations with other routine preventive services (Fig. 4.28).[63]

MAJOR VACCINATION TARGETS				
Goal	Burden of target disease	Direct medical cost of disease (US$)	Resources needed (US$; annual except where otherwise noted)	Comments
Application by existing tools: broader implementation, new strategies or wider introduction (to 80% or above wherever needed) by 2005				
Polio eradication	40,000–50,000 new cases of severe disability per year		2.7 billion total for years remaining to completion of eradication (of which 800 million – 1.0 billion is needed from external sources for endemic countries)	1.5 billion annual savings, following cessation of vaccination
Measles control improved worldwide (as a prerequisite for eradication after 2010)	700,000–1,500,000 child deaths	>900 million (>66% in high income countries)	250 million to achieve 90% coverage with two doses; estimated 4.5 billion required for all years to eradication	Eventual savings after cessation of vaccination program to be calculated
Hepatitis B vaccine (wider use)	800,000 deaths among adults, mostly from infections in early childhood	Calculation planned	Estimated 20 million annually to support low-income countries; calculation of incremental cost for global use planned	
Haemophilus influenzae type b vaccine (wider use)	400,000–700,000 child deaths	>750 million (80% spent in high middle- and high-income countries)	1 billion worldwide from all sources	Cost of prevention dependent on vaccine cost and number of doses
Rubella vaccine (wider use)	Approximately 300,000 severe congenital malformations	Calculation planned	Calculation planned	Disease burden estimates need to be improved
Selected regional or endemic disease vaccines				
Yellow fever vaccine use in high risk countries	Up to 30,000 deaths, all ages	Calculation planned	4.6 million for routine program in high-risk countries; estimated 17 million to provide catch-up immunization on once-only time basis	Outbreak control costly; precise disease burden difficult to calculate
Japanese encephalitis virus vaccine	10,000–12,000 deaths, all ages, one-third of cases with neurologic sequelae	Calculation in progress		Utility of existing vaccines for wider use needs to be assessed

Fig. 4.19 Major vaccination targets. The goals, burden of disease, medical costs and estimated costs of prevention are listed. DTaP, diphtheria, tetanus and acellular Pertussis vaccine; DTP, diphtheria, tetanus and pertussis vaccine. From Children's Vaccine Initiative.[55]

Goal	Burden of target disease	Direct medical cost of disease	Resources needed (US$) (annual except where otherwise noted)	Comments
MAJOR VACCINATION TARGETS (continued)				
Selected regional or endemic disease vaccines (continued)				
Meningococcal meningitis (polysaccharide vaccine)	20,000 to 30,000 deaths average, higher in epidemics	Calculation in progress	Calculation in progress	Utility of existing vaccines for wider use needs to be assessed; epidemic control costly
Use, in selected countries, of other new and combination vaccines, including typhoid, Hepatitis A, DTP–Hepatitis B, DTaP, varicella and vaccines against tick-borne encephalitis	Dependent on target	Dependent on target	Calculation planned	Wider public or private sector use of existing vaccines in high risk countries to be further considered
B.1 Completing development, licensing and introduction of imminent vaccines: by 2000–2002 effectiveness trials in developing countries completed; by 2005–2007, introduction occurring widely if successful				
Rotavirus vaccine	400,000–800,000 child deaths	Calculation in progress	Calculation in progress	Current vaccine has unknown efficacy in high endemicity countries
Pneumococcal conjugate vaccine	Approximately 1,200,000 child deaths	Calculation in progress	Calculation in progress	
Meningococcal conjugate vaccine	20,000–30,000 deaths average, higher in epidemics	Calculation in progress	Calculation in progress	Epidemic control costly
Cholera vaccine, improved	Approximately 120,000 deaths, all ages	Calculation planned	Calculation planned	For older children and adults
B.2 Medium-term development needs: between 2000 and 2005 efficacy and effectiveness trials anticipated; by 2010 introduction occurring wherever needed if successful				
Respiratory syncytial virus vaccine	400,000–500,000 child deaths	Calculation planned later	Calculation planned later	Disease burden estimates uncertain, need to be improved
Dengue and Japanese encephalitis vaccine (improved) vaccines for high risk countries	Dengue, up to 30,000 deaths; Japanese encephalitis virus, 10,000–12,000 deaths; all ages	Calculation planned later	Calculation planned later	
Bacterial diarrheas and typhoid (improved), for high-risk countries	2 million deaths (mostly children)	Calculation planned later	Calculation planned later	*Shigella* and *Escherichia coli* vaccines are main diarrheal vaccine candidates
Malaria vaccine	2.1 million deaths (including 1.2 million children, mainly in Africa)	Calculation planned	Calculation planned	
Influenza vaccine, improved	Periodic pandemics; disease burden uncertain	Calculation planned later	Calculation planned later	No vaccine delivery system in most of world for adults
HIV–AIDS vaccine	3.0 million new infections annually (mostly in young adults, likely to result in premature death)	Calculation planned later	Calculation planned later	Future annual new infections and deaths difficult to estimate
B.3 Priority targets for longer term research and development: promising candidates in efficacy and/or effectiveness trials in developing countries by 2005–2010				
Influenza vaccine, improved	Periodic pandemics; disease burden uncertain	Calculation planned later	Calculation planned later	No vaccine delivery system in most of world for adults
Tuberculosis vaccine, improved	3.0 million deaths all ages	Calculation planned later	Calculation planned later	
Other sexually transmitted disease vaccines (*Chlamydia*, *Neisseria gonorrhea* spp.)	200,000 deaths (congenital syphilis) and millions of cases of infertility	Calculation planned later	Calculation planned later	
Vaccines against other parasitic diseases, including leishmaniasis and schistosomiasis	1 million deaths; high prevalence and chronic morbidity	Calculation planned later	Calculation planned later	Numerous causes; suitability of vaccine prevention versus other options needs consideration

Fig. 4.19 Major vaccination targets continued.

SPECIAL POPULATIONS AND CIRCUMSTANCES

Although general recommendations can be made for routine vaccination, several groups and circumstances merit additional consideration. This includes an assessment of a person's host factors (e.g. pregnancy or immunocompromising condition) and exposure factors (e.g. known contact with a person with a vaccine-preventable disease, persons living in chronic care facilities, and occupations or behaviors that increase the chances of exposure to a vaccine preventable disease). In general, persons who are immunocompromised should receive special consideration before immunization.[64,65] Figures 4.29, 4.30 and 4.31 summarize the immunization recommendations for immunocompromised persons.

Immunization in pregnancy
Even though all vaccines may be administered safely to children of pregnant women and to breast-feeding mothers, because of the theoretic risk of vaccination during pregnancy, many health practitioners are understandably cautious when assessing the need for an immunization for pregnant women or women likely to become pregnant during the first 3 months after immunization. The combined tetanus and diphtheria toxoids (Td) are the only vaccines that are routinely recommended for pregnant women, if they have not received a Td booster within the previous 10 years. Before the administration of hepatitis B vaccine or influenza vaccine, a realistic consideration of the risk of disease often determines the decision to vaccinate. Live virus vaccines are generally not recommended for women who are pregnant, unless there are situations in which the threat of infection and its consequences outweighs concern over a potential adverse event to the developing fetus. Figure 4.32 provides a summary of recommendations for vaccination during pregnancy.[64]

GUIDELINES FOR SPACING IMMUNE GLOBULIN PREPARATIONS AND VACCINES CONTAINING LIVE MEASLES, MUMPS OR RUBELLA				
Simultaneous administration		Nonsimultaneous administration		
Immunobiologic combination	Recommended minimum time interval between doses	Immunobiologic administered		Recommended minimum time interval between doses
		First	Second	
Immune globulin and vaccine	Should generally not be administered simultaneously; if simultaneous administration of measles, mumps, and rubella vaccine, measles and rubella vaccine, and monovalent measles vaccine is unavoidable, administer at different sites and revaccinate or test for seroconversion after the recommended interval	Immune globulin	Vaccine	Dose related
		Vaccine	Immune globulin	2 weeks

Fig. 4.20 Guidelines for spacing immune globulin preparations and vaccines containing live measles, mumps or rubella. Immune globulin preparations include blood products containing large amounts of immune globulin, such as serum immune globulin, specific immune globulins (e.g. tetanus immune globulin and hepatitis B immune globulin), intravenous immune globulin, whole blood, packed red cells, plasma and platelet products. From CDC.[51]

SUGGESTED INTERVALS BETWEEN ADMINISTRATION OF VARIOUS IMMUNE GLOBULIN PREPARATIONS AND VACCINES CONTAINING LIVE MEASLES VIRUS		
Indication	Dose (including mg IgG/kg)	Time interval (months) before measles vaccination
Tetanus prophylaxis (immune globulin)	250U (10mg IgG/kg) im	3

Hepatitis A prophylaxis (immune globulin)
  Contact prophylaxis
  International travel
	
	0.02ml/kg (3.3mg IgG/kg) im
	0.06ml/kg (10mg Ig/kg) Im
		
		3
		3

Hepatitis B prophylaxis (immune globulin)	0.06ml/kg (10mg IgG/kg) im	3
Human rabies immune globulin	20IU/kg (22mg IgG/kg) im	4
Varicella prophylaxis (immune globulin)	125U/10kg (20–40mg IgG/kg) im (maximum 625U)	5

Measles prophylaxis (immune globulin)
  Standard (i.e. nonimmunocompromised contact)
  Immunocompromised contact
	
	0.25ml/kg (40mg IgG/kg) im
	0.50ml/kg (80mg IgG/kg) im
		
		5
		6

Blood transfusion
  Red blood cells, washed
  Red blood cells, adenine-saline added
  Packed red blood cells (hematocrit 65%)
  Whole blood cells (hematocrit 35–50%)
  Plasma and platelet products
	
	10ml/kg (negligible IgG/kg) iv
	10ml/kg (10mg IgG/kg) iv
	10ml/kg (60mg IgG/kg) iv
	10ml/kg (80–100mg IgG/kg)
	10ml/kg (160mg IgG/kg) iv
		
		0
		3
		6
		6
		7

Replacement therapy for immune deficiencies	300–400mg/kg iv (as iv immune globulin)	8
Immune thrombocytopenic purpura	400mg/kg iv (as iv immune globulin) daily for five consecutive days, or	8
	1000mg/kg iv (as iv immune globulin) daily for one or two consecutive days	10
Kawasaki disease	2g/kg iv (as iv immune globulin)	11

Fig. 4.21 Suggested intervals between administration of various immune globulin preparations and vaccines containing live measles virus. This table is not intended for determining the correct use of immune globulin preparations. Unvaccinated people may not be fully protected against measles during the entire suggested time interval, and additional doses of immune globulin, measles vaccine, or both may be indicated after exposure to measles. From CDC.[51]

RECOMMENDED ACCELERATED CHILDHOOD IMMUNIZATION SCHEDULE							
Visit number	1	2	3	4	5	6	7
Vaccine / Timing	≥4 months of age	1 month after visit 1	1 month after visit 2	6 weeks after visit 3	≥6 months after visit 3	Age 4–6 years	Age 14–16 years
Diphtheria, tetanus and (acellular) pertussis	DTP	DTP	DTP		DTP or DTaP		
Oral poliovirus (live, trivalent)	▉		▉	▉		▉	
Haemophilus influenzae type B	▉	▉	▉		▉		
Hepatitis B	▉	▉			▉		
Measles, mumps and rubella	▉					▉	
Tetanus and diphtheria toxoids (for use in persons aged ≥7 years)							▉

Fig. 4.22 Accelerated immunization schedule for infants and children for whom compliance cannot be assured. These recommendations are for infants and children under 7 years of age who start the series late or who are more than 1 month behind in the immunization schedule (i.e. children for whom compliance with scheduled return visits cannot be assured). If the schedule is initiated in the first year of life, administer diphtheria, tetanus and pertussis (DTP) vaccine doses 1, 2 and 3 and the oral poliovirus vaccine doses 1, 2 and 3 according to this schedule; administer measles, mumps and rubella vaccine when the child reaches 12–15 months of age. Diphtheria, tetanus and acellular pertussis (DTaP) preparations are currently recommended only for use as the fourth or fifth doses of the DTP series among children aged 15 months to 6 years. DTP and DTaP should not be used on or after the seventh birthday. The first additional visit (at age 4–6 years) should preferably be at or before school entry. Tetanus and diphtheria toxoids administration (first given at the visit at age 14–16 years) should be repeated every 10 years throughout life. The recommendations for *Haemophilus influenzae* type B (Hib) vaccines vary by manufacturer. Children beginning the HiIB vaccine series at age 2–6 months should receive a primary series of three doses of HbOC, or a licensed DTP–Hib combination vaccine; or two doses of PRP–OMP. An additional booster dose of any Hib conjugate vaccine should be administered at 12–15 months of age and at least 2 months after the previous dose. Children beginning the Hib vaccine series at 7–11 months of age should receive a primary series of two doses of an HbOC, PRP-T, or PRP–OMP-containing vaccine. An additional booster dose of any Hib conjugate vaccine should be administered at 12–18 months of age and at least 2 months after the previous dose. Children beginning the Hib vaccine series at ages 12–14 months should receive a primary series of one dose of an HbOC, PRP-T, or PRP–OMP-containing vaccine. An additional booster dose of any Hib conjugate vaccine should be administered 2 months after the previous dose. Children beginning the Hib vaccine series at ages 15–59 months should receive one dose of any licensed Hib vaccine. *Haemophilus influenzae* type b vaccine should not be administered after the fifth birthday except for special circumstances as noted in the specific recommendations for the use of Hib vaccine. HbOC, Hib conjugate vaccine, diphtheria CRM 197 protein conjugate; PRP-OMP, Hib conjugate vaccine, meningococcus protein conjugate; PRP-T, Hib conjugate vaccine, tetanus conjugate. From CDC.[51]

IMMUNIZATION SCHEDULE FOR CHILDREN NOT VACCINATED AT THE RECOMMENDED TIME IN EARLY INFANCY				
Visit number	1	2	3	4
Vaccine / Timing	1st visit	6–8 weeks after visit 1	6 months after visit 2	Additional visits
Tetanus and diphtheria toxoids (for use in persons aged ≥7 years)	▉	▉	▉	▉
Oral poliovirus (live, trivalent)	▉	▉	▉	
Measles, mumps and rubella	▉	▉		
Hepatitis B	▉	▉	▉	

Fig. 4.23 Immunization schedule for children not vaccinated at the recommended time in early infancy. These recommendations are for people aged over 7 years who were not vaccinated at the recommended time in early infancy. The diphtharia tetanus and pertussis diptheria, tetanus and acellular pertussis vaccine doses administered to children aged under 7 years who remain incompletely vaccinated at age 7 years or over should be counted as prior exposure to tetanus and diphtheria toxoids. When polio vaccine is administered to previously unvaccinated person aged 18 years or more, inactivated poliovirus vaccine is preferred to the live oral vaccine.

People born before 1957 can generally be considered to be immune to measles and mumps and need not be vaccinated. Rubella (or measles, mumps and rubella) vaccine can be administered to persons of any age, particularly to nonpregnant women of childbearing age. Selected high-risk groups for whom vaccination against hepatitis B is recommended include persons with occupational risk, such as health care and public safety workers who have occupational exposure to blood; clients and staff of institutions for the developmentally disabled; hemodialysis patients; recipients of certain blood products (e.g. clotting factor concentrates); household contacts and sexual partners of carriers of the hepatitis B virus; injecting drug users, sexually active homosexual and bisexual men; certain sexually active heterosexual men and women; inmates of long-term correctional facilities; certain international travelers; and families of hepatitis B surface antigen-positive adopted children from countries where hepatitis B is endemic. Because risk factors are often not identified directly among adolescents, universal hepatitis B vaccination of teenagers should be implemented in communities where injecting drug use, pregnancy among teenagers, or sexually transmitted diseases are common. A second dose of measles-containing vaccine (preferably measles, mumps and rubella to ensure immunity to mumps and rubella) for certain groups. Children with no documentation of live measles vaccination after their first birthday should receive two doses of live measles-containing vaccine not less than 1 month apart. In addition, the following persons born in 1957 or later should have documentation of measles immunity (i.e. two doses of measles-containing vaccine, at least one of which should be MMR), physician-diagnosed measles, or laboratory evidence of measles immunity: those entering post-high-school education; those beginning employment in health care settings who will have direct patient contact; and travelers to areas with endemic measles. From CDC.[53]

VACCINATION CONTRAINDICATIONS AND PRECAUTIONS

		True contraindications and precautions	Not contraindications (vaccines may be adminstered)
General for all vaccines (DTP, DTaP; OPV, IPV, MMR, HIB, hepatitis B)	Contraindications	Anaphylactic reaction to a vaccine contraindicates further doses of that vaccine Anaphylactic reaction to a vaccine constituent contraindicates the use of vaccines containing that substance Moderate or severe illnesses with or without a fever	Mild to moderate local reaction (soreness, redness, swelling) following a dose of an injectable antigen Mild acute illness with or without low-grade fever Current antimicrobial therapy Convalescent phase of illnesses Prematurity (same dosage and indications as for normal, full-term infants) Recent exposure to an infectious disease History of penicillin or other nonspecific allergies or family history of such allergies
DTP/DTaP	Contraindications	Encephalopathy within 7 days of administration of previous dose of DTP	Temperature of <105°F (40.5°C) following a previous dose of DTP Family history of convulsions Family history of sudden infant death syndrome Family history of an adverse event following DTP administration
	Precautions	Fever of ≥105°F (40.5°C) within 48 hours after vaccination with a prior dose of DTP Collapse or shock-like state (hypotonic–hyporesponsive episode) within 48 hours of receiving a prior dose of DTP Seizures within 3 days of receiving a prior dose of DTP Persistent, inconsolable crying lasting ≥3 hours within 48 hours of receiving a prior dose of DTP	
OPV	Contraindications	Infection with HIV or a household contact with HIV Known altered immunodeficiency (hematologic and solid tumors; congenital immunodeficiency; and long-term immunosuppressive therapy) Immunodeficient household contact	Breast-feeding Current antimicrobial therapy Diarrhea
	Precaution	Pregnancy	
IPV	Contraindication	Anaphylactic reaction to neomycin or streptomycin	
	Precaution	Pregnancy	
MMR	Contraindications	Anaphylactic reactions to egg ingestion or to neomycin Pregnancy Known altered immunodeficiency (hematologic and solid tumors; congenital immunodeficiency; and long-term immunosuppressive therapy)	Tuberculosis or positive purified protein derivative skin test Simultaneous TB skin testing Breast-feeding Pregnancy of mother of recipient Immunodeficient family member or household contact Infection with HIV Nonanaphylactic reactions to eggs or neomycin
	Precaution	Recent immunoglobulin administration	
HIB	Contraindication	None identified	History of HIB disease
Hepatitis B	Contraindication	Anaphylactic reaction to common baker's yeast	Pregnancy

Fig. 4.24 Vaccination contraindications and precautions. Note that acetaminophen given before administering DTP and thereafter q4h for 24 hours should be considered for children with a personal or family history of convulsions in siblings or parents. Acetaminophen given before administering DTP and thereafter every 4 hours should be considered for children with a personal or family history of convulsions in siblings or parents. DTP, diphtheria, tetanus, pertussis; DTaP, diphtheria, tetanus, acellular pertussis; OPV, oral poliovirus vaccine; IPV, inactivated poliovirus vaccine; MMR, measles, mumps and rubella; Hib, *Haemophilus influenzae* type B. From CDC.[53]

Health care workers

Given the potential for health care workers to be exposed to infectious diseases through contact with patients and clinical specimens, and the potential for health care workers to transmit infection to susceptible patients, maintaining immunity is an integral component of prevention and control of infectious diseases in health care settings. Recommendations for the immunization of health care workers has been established; these also take into account the immunization needs of health care workers with special conditions, such as pregnancy, immunosuppression, HIV infection, diabetes, alcoholism and cirrhosis, and renal failure (Figs 4.33 & 4.34).[66]

EVIDENCE OF POSSIBLE ASSOCIATION BETWEEN ADVERSE EFFECTS AND CHILDHOOD VACCINES						
	DT, Td, tetanus toxoid	Measles vaccine	Mumps vaccine	Oral poliovirus vaccine, inactivated poliovirus vaccine	Hepatitis B vaccine	*Haemophilus influenzae* type b vaccine
No evidence was available to establish a causal relationship	None	None	Neuropathy Residual seizure disorder	Transverse myelitis (IPV) Thrombocytopenia (IPV) Anaphylaxis (IPV)	None	None
Inadequate evidence to accept or reject a causal relationship	Residual seizure disorder other than infantile spasms Demyelinating diseases of the CNS Mononeuropathy Arthritis Erythema multiforme	Encephalopathy Subacute sclerosing panencephalitis Residual seizure disorder Sensorineural deafness (MMR) Optic neuritis Transverse myelitis Guillain–Barré syndrome Thrombocytopenia Insulin-dependent diabetes mellitus	Encephalopathy Aseptic meningitis Sensorineural deafness (MMR) Insulin-dependent diabetes mellitus Sterility Thrombocytopenia Anaphylaxis	Transverse myelitis (OPV) Guillain–Barré syndrome (IPV) Death from sudden infant death syndrome	Guillain–Barré syndrome Demyelinating diseases of the CNS Arthritis Death from sudden infant death syndrome	Guillain–Barré syndrome Transverse myelitis Thrombocytopenia Anaphylaxis Death from sudden infant death syndrome
Evidence favored rejection of a causal relationship	Encephalopathy Infantile spasms (DT only) Death from sudden infant death syndrome (DT only)	None	None	None	None	Early onset Hib disease (conjugate vaccines)
Evidence favored acceptance of a causal relationship	Guillain–Barré syndrome Brachial neuritis	Anaphylaxis	None	Guillain–Barré syndrome (OPV)	None	Early onset Hib disease in children aged ≥18 months whose first Hib vaccination was with unconjugated Hib vaccine
Evidence established a causal relationship	Anaphylaxis	Thrombocytopenia (MMR) Anaphylaxis (MMR) Death from measles-vaccine-strain viral infection	None	Poliomyelitis in recipient or contact (OPV) Death from polio-vaccine-strain viral infection	Anaphylaxis	None

Fig. 4.25 Evidence of possible association between adverse effects and childhood vaccines. In the cases of measles and mumps vaccines, if the data derived from studies of a monovalent preparation, then the causal relationship also extended to multivalent preparations. If the data derived exclusively from studies of the measles, mumps and rubella (MMR) vaccine, this is noted in parentheses. In the absence of data concerning the monovalent preparation, the causal relationship determined for the multivalent preparations did not extend to the monovalent components. Death from measles vaccine-strain viral infection occurred primarily in persons known to be immuno-compromised. In the case of the polio vaccines, assessment was made of the causal relationship between some adverse events and only one of the vaccines [oral poliovirus vaccine (i.e. OPV) for the adverse event of poliomyelitis; inactivated poliovirus vaccine (IPV) for the adverse events of anaphylaxis and thrombocytopenia]. If the conclusions for the two vaccines differed for the other adverse events, the vaccine to which the adverse event applied is specified in parentheses. DT, diphtheria and tetanus toxoids for pediatric use; Td, diphtheria and tetanus toxoids for adult use. From CDC.[51]

MISCONCEPTIONS CONCERNING CONTRAINDICATIONS TO DIPHTHERIA, TETANUS AND PERTUSSIS VACCINATION

- Soreness, redness, or swelling at the vaccination site or temperature of <105°F (<40.5°C)

- Mild, acute illness with low-grade fever or mild diarrheal illness affecting an otherwise healthy child

- Current antimicrobial therapy or the convalescent phase of an acute illness

- Recent exposure to an infectious disease

- Prematurity: the appropriate age for initiating vaccination in a premature infant is the usual chronologic age from birth; full doses should be used

- History of allergies or relatives with allergies

- Family history of convulsions

- Family history of sudden infant death syndrome

- Family history of an adverse event following vaccination

Fig. 4.26 Misconceptions concerning contraindications to diphtheria, tetanus and pertussis vaccination. From CDC.[53]

ESTIMATED EFFECT OF FULL USE OF VACCINES CURRENTLY RECOMMENDED FOR ADULTS

Disease	Estimated annual deaths (number)	Estimated vaccine efficacy in healthy adults (%)	Current vaccine utilization (%)	Additional preventable deaths per year (number)
Influenza	20,000	70	55	6300
Pneumococcal infection	20,000–40,000	60	30	8400–16,300
Hepatitis B	6000	90	10	4860
Tetanus and diphtheria	<25	99	40	<15
Measles, mumps and rubella	<30	95	variable	<30
Travelers' disease (cholera, typhoid, Japanese encephalitis, yellow fever, poliomyelitis and rabies)	<10	variable	unknown	<10

Fig. 4.27 Estimated effect of full use of vaccines currently recommended for adults. Additional preventable deaths per year are calculated as 'potential additional vaccine utilization' × 'estimated vaccine efficacy' × 'estimated annual deaths'. Modified from National Vaccine Advisory Committee.[62]

RECOMMENDED SCHEDULE OF VACCINATIONS FOR ADOLESCENTS

Immunobiologic	Indications	Dose	Frequency	Route
Hepatitis A vaccine	Increased risk of hepatitis A infection or its complications	720 EL U/0.5ml (HAVRIX)	A total of two doses at 0 and 6–12 months	im
		25U/0.5ml (VAQTA)	A total of two doses at 0 and 6–18 months	im
Hepatitis B vaccine	Not vaccinated previously for hepatitis B	5µg/0.5ml (Recombivax-HB)	A total of three doses at 0, 1–2 and 4–6 months	im
		10µg/0.5ml (Engerix-B)	A total of three doses at 0, 1–2 and 4–6 months	im
Influenza vaccine	Increased risk for complications caused by influenza or contact with persons at increased risk for these complications	0.5ml	Annually (September–December)	im
Measles, mumps and rubella vaccine	Not vaccinated previously with two doses of measles vaccine at ≥ 12 months of age	0.5ml	One dose	sc
Pneumococcal polysaccharide vaccine	Increased risk for pneumococcal disease or its complications	0.5ml	One dose	im or sc
Tetanus and diphtheria toxoids	Not vaccinated within the previous 5 years	0.5ml	Every 10 years	im
Varicella virus vaccine	Not vaccinated previously and no reliable history of chickenpox	0.5ml	One dose	sc

Fig. 4.28 Recommended schedule of vaccinations for adolescents. For the upper regimen for hepatitis A vaccine: an alternative dosage and schedule is 360 EL U/0.5ml, and a total of three doses administered at 0, 1 and 6–12 months. 0 Months represents timing of the initial dose, and subsequent numbers represent months after the initial dose. For varicella virus vaccine adolescents ≥ 13 years of age should be administered a total of two doses (0.5ml/dose) subcutaneously at 0 and 4–8 weeks. These recommendations apply to people aged 11–12 years. EL, Enzyme-linked immunosorbent assay (ELISA) units. From CDC.[63]

RECOMMENDATIONS FOR IMMUNIZATION OF IMMUNOCOMPROMISED INFANTS AND CHILDREN

	Vaccine	Routine (not immunocompromised)	HIV–AIDS	Severely immunocompromised (non-HIV related)	Asplenia	Renal failure	Diabetes
Routine infant immunizations	DTP, DT, T, Td						
	OPV						
	eIPV						
	MMR, MR, M, R						
	HIB						
	Hepatitis B						
Other childhood immunizations	Pneumococcal						
	Influenza						

Recommended Contraindicated Use if indicated Recommended/considered

Fig. 4.29 Recommendations for immunization of immunocompromised infants and children. Summary of the recommendations from the Advisory Committee on Immunization Practices. Pneumococcal vaccine is recommended for those aged 2 years or more. Influenza vaccine is not recommended for children under 6 months of age. D, diphtheria; T, tetanus; P, pertussis; Td, tetanus and diphtheria toxoids; OPV, oral poliovirus vaccine; eIPV, enhanced-potency, inactivated poliovirus vaccine; MMR, measles, mumps and rubella; Hib, Haemophilus influenzae type b. From CDC.[64]

RECOMMENDATIONS FOR IMMUNIZATION OF IMMUNOCOMPROMISED ADULTS

Vaccine	Routine (not immunocompromised)	HIV–AIDS	Severely immunocompromised (non-HIV related)	Post-solid organ transplant on chronic immunosuppressive therapy	Asplenia	Renal failure	Diabetes	Alcoholism and alcoholic cirrhosis
Tetanus, diphtheria								
Measles, mumps and rubella (MR/M/R)								
Hepatitis B								
Haemophilus influenzae type b								
Pneumococcal								
Meningococcal								
Influenza								

Recommended Contraindicated Use if indicated Recommended/considered Not recommended

Fig. 4.30 Recommendations for immunization of immunocompromised adults. Summary of the recommendations from the Advisory Committee on Immunization Practices. Pneumococcal and influenza vaccines are recommended for those aged 65 years or over. From CDC.[64]

RECOMMENDATIONS FOR THE USE OF IMMUNE GLOBULINS IN IMMUNOCOMPROMISED PERSONS			
Immune globulin	Not immunocompromised	HIV infected	Severely immunocompromised
Immune globulin	Recommended for infants and adults with contraindication to measles vaccine if exposed to measles	Recommended for symptomatic patients exposed to measles regardless of immunization status Recommended for persons with exposure to hepatitis A virus or who will travel to endemic areas	Recommended for patients exposed to measles regardless of immunization status
Varicella-zoster	Recommended for newborns of mothers who develop chickenpox within 5 days before and 48 hours after delivery Recommended for exposed newborns (≥28 weeks gestation) of susceptible mothers Recommended for exposed preterm (<28 weeks or <1000g body weight) May be used for exposed, susceptible adults, exposed pregnant women, and infants <28 days	Recommended for susceptible infants and adults after significant exposure to varicella-zoster	Recommended for susceptible infants and adults after significant exposure to varicella-zoster
Tetanus	Recommended for those with serious wounds who have received fewer than three doses of tetanus toxoid	Same as for not immunocompromised	Same as for not immunocompromised
Hepatitis B	Recommended for prophylaxis of infants born to hepatitis B surface antigen-positive mothers and susceptible persons with percutaneous, sexual, or mucosal exposure to hepatitis B virus	Same as for not immunocompromised	Same as for not immunocompromised
Human rabies	Recommended for postexposure prophylaxis of persons not previously vaccinated against rabies	Same as for not immunocompromised	Same as for not immunocompromised

Fig. 4.31 Recommendations for the use of immune globulins in immunocompromised persons. Summary of the recommendations from the Advisory Committee on Immunization Practices. From CDC.[64]

VACCINATION DURING PREGNANCY			
		Vaccine	Indications for vaccination during pregnancy
Live virus vaccine	Measles Mumps Rubella	Live-attenuated	Contraindicated
	Yellow fever	Live-attenuated	Contraindicated except if exposure to yellow fever virus is unavoidable
	Poliomyelitis	Trivalent live-attenuated (oral poliomyelitis vaccine)	Persons at substantial risk of exposure to polio
Inactivated virus vaccines	Hepatitis A	Killed virus	Data on safety in pregnancy are not available. Should weigh the theoretic risk of vaccination against the risk of disease
	Hepatitis B	Recombinant produced, purified hepatitis B surface antigen	Not contraindicated
	Influenza	Inactivated type A and type B virus vaccines	Recommended for women in 2nd and 3rd trimester of pregnancy during the influenza season
	Japanese encephalitis	Killed virus	Should reflect actual risks of disease and probable benefits of vaccine
	Poliomyelitis	Killed virus (inactivated poliovirus vaccine)	Oral poliovirus vaccine preferred when immediate protection of pregnant females is needed; however, inactivated poliovirus vaccine is an alternative if complete vaccination series can be administered before exposure
	Rabies	Killed virus Rabies immunoglobulin	Should reflect actual risks of disease and probable benefits of vaccine
Live bacterial vaccines	Typhoid (Ty21a)	Live bacterial	Substantial risk of exposure
Inactivated bacterial vaccines	Cholera Typhoid	Killed bacterial	Should reflect actual risks of disease and probable benefits of vaccine
	Plague	Killed bacterial	Selective vaccination of exposed persons
	Meningococcal	Polysaccharide	Only in unusual outbreak situations
	Pneumococcal	Polysaccharide	Only for high-risk persons
	Haemophilus influenzae type B	Polysaccharide–protein conjugate	Only for high-risk persons
Toxoids	Tetanus-diphtheria	Combined tetanus–diphtheria toxoids (adult formulation)	Lack of primary series, or no booster within past 10 years
Immune globulins, pooled or hyperimmune		Immunoglobulin or specific globulin preparations	Exposure or anticipated unavoidable exposure to measles, hepatitis A, hepatitis B, rabies, or tetanus

Fig. 4.32 Vaccination during pregnancy. From CDC.[64]

\multicolumn{5}{c}{IMMUNIZING AGENTS AND IMMUNIZATION SCHEDULES FOR HEALTH CARE WORKERS}

Generic name	Primary schedule and booster(s)	Indications	Major precautions and contraindications	Special considerations
Hepatitis A vaccine	Two doses of vaccine either 6–12 months apart or 6 months apart	Not routinely indicated in USA; recommended in those working with infected primates or with a laboratory researching hepatitis A virus	History of anaphylactic hypersensitivity to alum or 2-phenoxyethanol. The safety of the vaccine in pregnant women has not been determined – the risk associated with vaccination should be weighed against the risk for hepatitis A in women who may be at a high risk of exposure	
Meningococcal polysaccharide vaccine (tetravalent A, C, W135 and Y)	One dose in volume and by route specified by manufacturer; need for boosters unknown	Not routinely indicated in USA	The safety of the vaccine in pregnant women has not been evaluated; it should not be administered during pregnancy unless the risk of infection is high	
Typhoid vaccine, im, sc, and po	im: one 0.5ml dose, booster 0.5ml every 2 years; sc: two 0.5ml doses, ≥4 weeks apart, booster 0.5ml sc or 0.1ml id every 3 years if exposure continues; po: four doses on alternate days. The manufacturer recommends revaccination with the entire four-dose series every 5 years	Workers in microbiology laboratories who frequently work with *Salmonella typhi*	Severe local or systemic reactions to a previous dose. Ty21a (oral) vaccine should not be administered to immunocompromised persons or to persons receiving antimicrobial agents	Vaccination should not be considered an alternative to the use of proper procedures when handling specimens and cultures in the laboratory
Vaccinia vaccine (smallpox)	One dose administered with a bifurcated needle; boosters administered every 10 years	Laboratory workers who directly handle cultures with vaccinia, recombinant vaccinia viruses, or orthopox viruses that infect humans	Contraindicated in pregnancy, in persons with eczema or a history of eczema, and in immunocompromised persons and their household contacts	Vaccination may be considered for those who have direct contact with contaminated dressings or other infectious material from volunteers in clinical studies involving recombinant vaccinia virus
\multicolumn{5}{l}{Other vaccine-preventable diseases}
Tetanus and diphtheria toxoids	Two im doses 4 weeks apart; third dose 6–12 months after second dose; booster every 10 years	All adults	Except in the first trimester, pregnancy is not a precaution. History of a neurologic reaction or immediate hypersensitivity reaction after a previous dose History of severe local (arthus-type) reaction after a previous dose – these people should not receive further routine or emergency doses for 10 years	
Pneumococcal polysaccharide vaccine (23-valent)	One dose, 0.5ml, im or sc; revaccination recommended for those at highest risk 5 or more years after the first dose	Adults who are at increased risk of pneumococcal disease and its complications because of underlying health conditions; older adults, especially those who are aged 65 years or older and who are healthy	The safety of vaccine in pregnant women has not been evaluated; it should not be administered during pregnancy unless the risk of infection is high	Previous recipients of any type of pneumococcal polysaccharide vaccine who are at highest risk of fatal infection or antibody loss may be revaccinated 5 years or more after the first dose
Rubella live-virus vaccine	One dose sc; no booster	Indicated for both men and women with no documentation of prior vaccination on or after their first birthday or laboratory evidence of immunity; people born before 1957, except women who can become pregnant, can be considered immune	Pregnancy Immunocompromised persons Those with a history of anaphylactic reaction after administration of neomycin	The risk for rubella vaccine-associated malformations in the offspring of women pregnant when vaccinated or who become pregnant within 3 months after vaccination is negligible; such women should be counseled about the theoretic basis of concern for the fetus Measles, mumps and rubella vaccine is the vaccine of choice if recipients are likely to be susceptible to measles or mumps as well as to rubella
Varicella-zoster live-virus vaccine	Two 0.5ml doses sc 4–8 weeks apart if 13 years of age or older	Indicated if no reliable history of varicella or no serologic evidence of immunity	Pregnancy Immunocompromised persons History of anaphylactic reaction following receipt of neomycin or gelatin Avoid salicylate use for 6 weeks after vaccination	Vaccine is available from the manufacturer for certain patients with acute lymphocytic leukemia in remission Because 71–93% of persons without a history of varicella are immune, serologic testing before vaccination is likely to be cost-effective

1

4.23

Fig. 4.33 Immunizing agents and immunization schedules for health care workers. From CDC.[66]

IMMUNIZING AGENTS AND IMMUNIZATION SCHEDULES FOR HEALTH CARE WORKERS (continued)				
Generic name	Primary schedule and booster(s)	Indications	Major precautions and contraindications	Special considerations
Other vaccine-preventable diseases (continued)				
Varicella-zoster immune globulin	If <50kg: 125U/10kg im; if ≥50kg: 625U	Indicated for those known or likely to be susceptible if at high risk of complications, (e.g. pregnant women) following close and prolonged exposure		Serologic testing may help in assessing whether to administer; If use prevents varicella disease, patient should be vaccinated subsequently
BCG	One percutaneous dose of 0.3ml; no booster dose recommended	Consider only when drug-resistant tuberculosis is prevalent, infection likely and tuberculosis control efforts less than optimal	Should not be administered to immunocompromised persons, pregnant women	In the USA, tuberculosis-control efforts are directed towards early identification, treatment of cases and preventive therapy
Other immunobiologics that are or may be indicated for health care workers				
Immunoglobulin (hepatitis A)	Postexposure: one im dose of 0.02ml/kg given 2 weeks or sooner after exposure	Indicated for those exposed to feces of infectious patients	Contraindicated in persons with IgA deficiency; do not administer within 2 weeks after measles, mumps and rubella vaccine, or 3 weeks after varicella vaccine. Delay administration of mumps, measles and rubella vaccine for 3 months or more and varicella vaccine for 5 months or more	Administer in large muscle mass (deltoid, gluteal)
Immunizing agents strongly recommended for health care workers				
Hepatitis B recombinant vaccine	Two doses im 4 weeks apart; third dose 5 months after second; no booster	Those at risk of exposure to blood or body fluids	On the basis of limited data, no risk of adverse effects to developing fetuses is apparent. Pregnancy should not be considered a contraindication to vaccination of women. Previous anaphylactic reaction to common baker's yeast is a contraindication to vaccination	Prevaccination serologic screening is not indicated for persons being vaccinated because of occupational risk. Those who have contact with patients or blood should be tested 1–2 months after vaccination to determine serologic response
Hepatitis B immune globulin	0.06ml/kg im as soon as possible, but no later than 7 days after exposure; a second dose should be administered 1 month later if the hepatitis B vaccine series has not been started	For persons exposed to blood or body fluids containing hepatitis B surface antigen and who are not immune to HBV infection		
Influenza vaccine (inactivated whole-virus and split-virus vaccines)	Annual im vaccination with current vaccine	Those who have contact with patients at high risk for influenza or its complications; those who work in chronic care facilities; those with high-risk medical conditions; those aged 65 years or more	History of anaphylactic hypersensitivity to egg ingestion	No evidence exists of risk to mother or fetus when the vaccine is administered to a pregnant woman with an underlying high-risk condition, influenza vaccination is recommended during second and third trimesters of pregnancy
Measles live-virus vaccine	One dose sc; second dose at least 1 month later	For persons born after 1957 without documentation of physician-diagnosed measles, serologic evidence of immunity or receipt of two doses of live-attenuated vaccine on or after the first birthday. Consider immunization for all health care workers without proof of immunity, even if born before 1957	Pregnancy. Immunocompromised persons, including HIV-infected persons who have evidence of severe immunosuppression, anaphylaxis after gelatin ingestion or administration of neomycin. Recent administration of immunoglobulin	Measles, mumps and rubella vaccine is the vaccine of choice if recipients are likely to be susceptible to rubella or mumps as well as to measles. Persons vaccinated during 1963–1967 with a killed measles vaccine alone, killed vaccine followed by live vaccine, or with a vaccine of unknown type should be revaccinated with two doses of live measles virus vaccine
Mumps live-virus vaccine	One dose sc; no booster	Those believed to be susceptible can be vaccinated; those born before 1957 can be considered immune	Pregnancy. Immunocompromised persons. History of anaphylactic reaction after gelatin ingestion or administration of neomycin	Measles, mumps and rubella vaccine is the vaccine of choice if recipients are likely to be susceptible to measles and rubella as well as to mumps

Fig. 4.33 **Immunizing agents and immunization schedules for health care workers continued.**

RECOMMENDATIONS FOR IMMUNIZATION OF HEALTH CARE WORKERS WITH SPECIAL NEEDS

Vacccine	Pregnancy	HIV infection	Severe immunosuppression	Asplenia	Renal failure	Diabetes	Alcoholism and alcoholic cirrhosis
BCG	Contraindicated	Contraindicated	Contraindicated	Use if indicated	Use if indicated	Use if indicated	Use if indicated
Hepatitis A	Use if indicated	Use if indicated	Use if indicated	Use if indicated	Use if indicated	Use if indicated	Recommended
Hepatitis B	Recommended	Recommended	Recommended	Recommended	Recommended	Recommended	Recommended
Influenza	Recommended	Recommended	Recommended	Recommended	Recommended	Recommended	Recommended
Measles, mumps and rubella	Contraindicated	Recommended	Contraindicated	Recommended	Recommended	Recommended	Recommended
Meningococcus	Use if indicated	Use if indicated	Use if indicated	Recommended	Use if indicated	Use if indicated	Use if indicated
Poliovirus vaccine (inactivated)	Use if indicated	Use if indicated	Use if indicated	Use if indicated	Use if indicated	Use if indicated	Use if indicated
Poliovirus vaccine (live, oral)	Use if indicated	Contraindicated	Contraindicated	Use if indicated	Use if indicated	Use if indicated	Use if indicated
Pneumococcus	Use if indicated	Recommended	Recommended	Recommended	Recommended	Recommended	Recommended
Rabies	Use if indicated	Use if indicated	Use if indicated	Use if indicated	Use if indicated	Use if indicated	Use if indicated
Tetanus and diphtheria	Recommended	Recommended	Recommended	Recommended	Recommended	Recommended	Recommended
Typhoid (inactivated and Vi)	Use if indicated	Use if indicated	Use if indicated	Use if indicated	Use if indicated	Use if indicated	Use if indicated
Typhoid (Ty21a)	Use if indicated	Contraindicated	Contraindicated	Use if indicated	Use if indicated	Use if indicated	Use if indicated
Varicella	Contraindicated	Contraindicated	Contraindicated	Recommended	Recommended	Recommended	Recommended
Vaccinia	Contraindicated	Contraindicated	Contraindicated	Use if indicated	Use if indicated	Use if indicated	Use if indicated

Fig. 4.34 Recommendations for immunization of health care workers with special needs. Summary of the recommendations from the Advisory Committee on Immunization Practices. The recommendations for pneumococcus vaccine is based on the person's underlying condition rather than the occupation. Influenza vaccine is recommended for pregnant women who will be in the second or third trimester during the influenza season. Measles, mumps and rubella vaccination is contraindicated in HIV-infected persons who have evidence of severe immunosuppression. Polio vaccination is recommended for unvaccinated health care workers who have close contact with patients who may be excreting wild polioviruses. Primary vaccination with inactivated poliovirus vaccine (IPV) is recommended because the risk for vaccine-associated paralysis after administration of oral, live poliovirus vaccine (OPV) is higher among adults than among children. Health care workers who have had a primary series of OPV or IPV and who are directly involved in the provision of care to patients who may be excreting poliovirus may receive another dose of either OPV or IPV. Any suspected case of poliomyelitis should be investigated immediately. If evidence suggests transmission of wild poliovirus, control measures to prevent further transmission should be instituted immediately, including an OPV vaccination campaign. Modified from CDC.[66]

REFERENCES

1. Snow J. On the mode of transmission of cholera, 2nd edition. London: Churchill; 1855; reprinted New York: Commonwealth Fund; 1936.
2. Institute of Medicine. Emerging Infections: Microbial threats to health in the United States. Washington DC: National Academy Press; 1992.
3. World Health Organization. World Health Report. Geneva: World Health Organization; 1997.
4. World Bank. World Development Report 1993: Investing in Health. New York: Oxford University Press; 1993.
5. Doyle R. Access to safe drinking water. Sci Am 1997;277:38.
6. O'Dempsy TJ, McArdle TF, Morris J, et al. A study of risk factors for pneumococcal disease among children in a rural area of West Africa. Int J Epidemiol 1996;25:885–93.
7. Evans AS. Epidemiologic concepts and methods. In: Evans AS, ed. Viral infections of humans: epidemiology and control, 3rd ed. New York: Plenum Publishing 1991:3–50.
8. Golding J, Emmet PM, Rogers IS. Does breast-feeding protect against non-gastric infections? Early Hum Dev 1997;49(Suppl):105–20.
9. Nafstad P, Jaakola JJ, Hagen JA, et al. Breast-feeding, maternal smoking and lower respiratory tract infections. Eur Respir J 1996;9:2623–9.
10. English RM, Badcock JC, Giay T, et al. Effect of nutrition improvement project on morbidity from infectious diseases in preschool children in Vietnam: comparison with control commune. Br Med J 1997;15:1122–5.
11. UNICEF. The State of the World's Children 1995. Oxford and New York: Oxford University Press; 1995.
12. Semba RD, Akib A, Beeler J, et al. Effect of vitamin A supplementation on measles vaccination in nine-month-old infants. Public Health 1997;111:245–7.
13. Rosales FJ, Kjolhede C, Goodman S. Efficacy of a single oral dose of 200,000 IU of oil-soluble vitamin A in measles-associated morbidity. Am J Epidemiol 1996;143:413–22.
14. Coutsoudis A, Kiepiela P, Coovadia H, Broughton M. Vitamin A supplementation enhances specific IgG antibody levels and total lymphocyte numbers while improving morbidity in measles. Pediatr Infect Dis J 1992;11:203–9.
15. Roy SK, Tomkins AM, Akramuzzaman SM, et al. Randomized control trial of zinc supplementation in malnourished Bangladeshi children with acute diarrhea. Arch Dis Child 1997;77:196–200.

16. Johnson MA, Porter KH. Micronutrient supplementation and infection in institutionalized elders. Nutr Rev 1997;55:400–4.

17. Baum MK, Shor-Posner G, Lai H, et al. High risk of HIV-related mortality is associated with selenium deficiency. J Acquir Immune Defic Syndr Hum Retrovirol 1997;15:370–4.

18. Tang AM, Graham NM, Saah AJ. Effects of micronutrient intake on survival in human immunodeficiency virus type 1 infection. Am J Epidemiol 1996;143:1244–56.

19. Cakman I, Kirchner H, Rink L. Zinc supplementation reconstitutes the production of interferon-alpha by leukocytes from elderly persons. J Interferon Cytokine Res 1997;17:469–72.

20. Lehane MJ. Vector insects and their control. Ciba Found Symp 1996;200:8–16; discussion 16–21,46–7.

21. Muller O, Cham K, Jaffar S, Greenwood B. The Gambian National Impregnated Bednet Programme: evaluation of the 1994 cost recovery trial. Soc Science Med 1997;44:1903–9.

22. Gubler DJ, Clark GG. Community involvement in the control of Aedes aegypti. Acta Trop 1996;61:169–79.

23. Infectious Diseases Society of America/United States Public Health Service. 1997 USPHS/IDSA guidelines for the prevention of opportunistic infections in persons infected with HIV: Part I. Prevention of exposure. US Department of Health and Human Services, Public Health Service, Centers for Disease Control and Prevention. Am Fam Physician 1997;56:823–34.

24. Infectious Diseases Society of America/United States Public Health Service. 1997 USPHS/IDSA guidelines for the prevention of opportunistic infections in persons infected with human immunodeficiency virus: disease-specific recommendations. USPHS/IDSA Prevention of Opportunistic Infections Working Group. MMWR Morb Mortal Wkly Rep 1997;46(RR-12):1–46.

25. Grubman S, Simonds RJ. Preventing Pneumocystis carinii pneumonia in human immunodeficiency virus-infected children: new guidelines for prophylaxis. CDC, US Public Health Service, and the Infectious Diseases Society of America. Pediatr Infect Dis J 1996;15:165–8.

26. Shlaaes DM, Gerding DN, John JF Jr, et al. Society for Healthcare Epidemiology of America and Infectious Diseases Society of America Joint Committee on the Prevention of Antimicrobial Resistance: Guidelines for use of of antimicrobial resistance in hospitals. Clin Infect Dis 1997;25:584–99.

27. Lafontaine G, Bedard L. The prevention of infections in child daycare centers: potential influential factors. Can J Public Health 1997;88:250–4.

28. Smith PW, Rusnak PG. Infection prevention and control in the long-term-care facility. SHEA Long-Term-Care Committee and APIC Guidelines Committee. Am J Infect Control 1997;25:488–512.

29. Centers for Disease Control and Prevention. Guidelines for prevention of nosocomial pneumonia. MMWR Morb Mortal Wkly Rep 1997;46(RR-1):1–79.

30. Centers for Disease Control and Prevention. Interim guidelines for prevention and control of staphylococcal infection associated with reduced susceptibility to vancomycin. MMWR Morb Mortal Wkly Rep 1997;46:626–8.

31. Rutala WA. APIC guideline for selection and use of disinfectants. 1994, 1995, and 1996 APIC Guidelines Committee. Association for Professionals in Infection Control and Epidemiology, Inc. Am J Infect Control 1996;24:313–42.

32. Working Party of the British Committee for Standards in Haematology Clinical Haematology Task Force, UK. Guidelines for the prevention and treatment of infection in patients with an absent or dysfunctional spleen. Br Med J 1996;312:430–4.

33. Working Party of the British Society for Antimicrobial Chemotherapy and the Hospital Infection Society. Guidelines on the control of methicillin-resistant Staphylococcus aureus in the community. Report of a combined working party. J Hosp Infect 1995;31:1–12.

34. Stapleton A, Stamm WE. Prevention of urinary tract infection. Infect Dis Clin North Am 1997;11:719–33.

35. Dajani AS, Taubert KA, Wilson W, et al. Prevention of bacterial endocarditis. Recommendations by the American Heart Association. JAMA 1997;277:1794–801.

36. American Academy of Pediatrics. Prevention of hepatitis A infections: Guidelines for use of hepatitis A vaccine and immune globulin. American Academy of Pediatrics Committee on Infectious Diseases. Pediatrics 1996;98:1207–15.

37. Centers for Disease Control and Prevention. 1998 Guidelines for treatment of sexually transmitted diseases. Centers for Disease Control and Prevention. MMWR Morb Mortal Wkly Rep 1998;47(RR-1):1–111.

38. Simberkoff MS, Santos MR. Prevention of community-acquired and nosocomial pneumonia. Curr Opin Pulm Med 1996;2:228–35.

39. Lobel HO, Kozarsky PE. Update on prevention of malaria for travelers. JAMA 1997;278:1767–71.

40. Centers for Disease Control and Prevention. Health information for international travel. 1996–1997. Atlanta, GA; US Department of Health and Human Services, Public Health Service; 1997.

41. Sanford JP, Gilbert DN, Moellering RC Jr, Sande MA. Systemic preventive (prophylaxis) and epidemiologic treatment with antimicrobial agents. In: Sanford JP, Gilbert DN, Mollering RC Jr, Sande MA, eds. The Sanford guide to antimicrobial therapy 1999. Vienna, Virginia: Antimicrobial Therapy Inc; 1999.

42. Dajani AS, Bisno AL. Chung KJ, et al. Prevention of bacterial endocarditis. Recommendations by the American Heart Association. JAMA 1990;264:2919–22.

43. Centers for Disease Control and Prevention. Diphtheria, tetanus and pertussis: Recommendations for vaccine use and other preventive measures. MMWR Morb Mortal Wkly Rep 1991;40(RR-10):1–28.

44. Centers for Disease Control and Prevention. Rabies prevention, United States, 1991. Recommendations of the Advisory Committee on Immunization Practices. MMWR Morb Mortal Wkly Rep 1991;40(RR-3):1–19.

45. Centers for Disease Control and Prevention. Protection against viral hepatitis. Recommendations of the Advisory Committee on Immunization Practices. MMWR Morb Mortal Wkly Rep 1990;39(RR-2):1–26.

46. Fernandez AM, Herruzo CR, Gomez-Sancha F, Nieto S, Ray CJ. Economical saving due to prophylaxis in the treatment of a surgical wound infection. Eur J Epidemiol 1996;12:455–9.

47. Hatziandreu EJ, Brown RE. A cost benefit analysis of the Haemophilus influenzae type b (Hib) vaccine. Arlington, Virginia: Batelle; 1995.

48. Lieu TA, Cochi SL, Black SB, et al. Cost-effectiveness of a routine varicella vaccination program for US children. JAMA 1994;271:375–81.

49. Nichol KL, Margolis KL, Wuorenma J, et al. The efficacy and cost-effectiveness of vaccination against influenza among elderly persons living in the community. N Engl J Med 1994:331:778–84.

50. World Health Organization. Vaccine and immunization news. Newsletter of the Global Programme on Vaccines and Immunizations. November 1997.

51. Centers for Disease Control and Prevention. Update: vaccine side effects, adverse reactions, contraindications, and precautions. Recommendations of the Advisory Committee on Immunization Practices. MMWR Morb Mortal Wkly Rep; 1997.

52. National Institute of Allergy and Infectious Diseases. The Jordan Report 1998: accelerated vaccine development. Washington DC; 1998.

53. Centers for Disease Control and Prevention. General recommendations on immunization. Recommendations of the Advisory Committee on Immunization Practices (ACIP). 1994;43(RR-1).

54. Centers for Disease Control and Prevention. Recommended childhood immunization schedule, US, January–December 1999.

55. Children's Vaccine Initiative. The CVI Strategic Plan: Managing Opportunity and Change – A vision of vaccination for the 21st century. Children's Vaccine Initiative, Geneva, 1997.

56. Gangarosa EJ, Galazka AM, Wolfe CR et al. Impact of anti-vaccine movements on pertussis control: the untold story. Lancet 1998;351:356–61.

57. Howson CP, Howe CJ, Fineberg NV. Institute of Medicine. Adverse effects of pertussis and rubella vaccines. Washington DC: National Academy Press; 1991.

58. Stratton KR, Howe CJ, Johnston RB. Institute of Medicine. Adverse events associate with childhood vaccines: evidence bearing on causality. Washington DC: National Academy Press; 1994.

59. Institute of Medicine. DPT vaccine and chronic nervous system dysfunction: a new analysis. Washington, DC: National Academy Press; 1994.

60. Institute of Medicine. Research strategies for assessing adverse events associated with vaccines: a workshop summary. Washington DC: National Academy Press; 1994.

61. Peter G. 1997 Red Book: Report of the Committee on Infectious Diseases, 24th ed. American Academy of Paediatrics, 1997:682–8.

62. National Vaccine Advisory Committee. Adult immunizations. Washington DC; 1994.

63. Centers for Disease Control and Prevention. Immunization of adolescents. Recommendations of the Advisory Committee on Immunization Practices, the American Academy of Pediatrics, the American Academy of Family Physicians, and the American Medical Association. MMWR Morb Mortal Wkly Rep 1996;45(RR-13):1–16.

64. Centers for Disease Control and Prevention. Use of vaccines and immune globulins in persons with altered immunocompetance. Recommendations of the Advisory Committee on Immunization Practices. MMWR Morb Mortal Wkly Rep 1993;42(RR-4).

65. American College of Physicians Task Force on Adult Immunization and Infectious Diseases Society of America. Guide for adult immunization. Philadelphia: American College of Physicians; 1994.

66. Centers for Disease Control and Prevention. Immunization of health care workers: Recommendations of the Advisory Committee on Immunization Practices and the Hospital Infection Control Practices Advisory Committee. MMWR Morb Mortal Wkly Rep 1997;46(RR-16):1–42.

chapter

5

Emerging and Re-emerging Pathogens and Diseases

Donald B Louria & Claude Carbon

Humans have lived with emerging and re-emerging pathogens since before the dawn of civilization. Is the situation worse now than in past decades or centuries? The answer is probably yes because there are billions more of us and some of our activities allow such infections to appear and flourish. Additionally, our mobility within and between countries is conducive to the rapid spread of micro-organisms. Similar observations hold true for animals and plants, with frequent consequences for human health.

For the purpose of this chapter, we have arbitrarily divided emerging and re-emerging infections into five categories (Fig. 5.1).

CATEGORIES OF EMERGING AND RE-EMERGING PATHOGENS

DISEASES RELATED TO 'NEW' MICRO-ORGANISMS

AIDS, caused by HIV infection, is the most dramatic example of disease resulting from an apparently new micro-organism. The existence of the virus was not known until 1981 but since then it has infected more than 24 million individuals worldwide, with an expected cumulative figure of 40 million by the year 2000. The origin of the virus is still unknown but there is some evidence that it is related to viruses causing illnesses in monkeys in Central Africa.

In reality, there are only a few emerging infections that are truly new. More often, what appears to be a novel micro-organism is in fact a micro-organism that has been in existence for a long time but has only now been recognized. Similarly, as techniques develop, our ability to identify microbes suspected of causing disease increases. A number of etiologic agents and infectious diseases in humans and/or animals have been recognized in the past 25 years (Figs 5.2 & 5.3).

RE-EMERGING INFECTIONS

Several infectious diseases have re-emerged within past decades, and there are a variety of reasons for this. As they re-emerge, some diseases also spread to new geographic areas, thanks to the rapidity of travel. The diseases in question involve all the major modes of transmission (Fig. 5.4) and many types of micro-organisms (Fig. 5.5). Many factors

---

CATEGORIES OF EMERGING AND RE-EMERGING PATHOGENS

- Apparently new micro-organisms

- Re-emerging pathogens/infections

- Newly identified micro-organisms responsible for established infectious diseases (opportunistic/non-opportunistic)

- Diseases newly designated as infectious

- Organisms emerging because of high antimicrobial resistance

Fig. 5.1 Categories of emerging and re-emerging pathogens.

EXAMPLES OF ETIOLOGIC AGENTS AND INFECTIOUS DISEASES RECOGNIZED SINCE 1973

Year	Agent	Type	Disease/comments
1973	Rotavirus	Virus	Major cause of infantile diarrhea worldwide
1975	Parvovirus B19	Virus	Aplastic crisis in chronic hemolytic anemia
1976	*Cryptosporidium parvum*	Parasite	Acute and chronic diarrhea
1977	Ebola virus	Virus	Ebola hemorrhagic fever
1977	*Legionella pneumophila*	Bacterium	Legionnaires' disease
1977	Hantaan virus	Virus	Hemorrhagic fever with renal syndrome (HFRS)
1977	*Campylobacter jejuni*	Bacterium	Enteric pathogen distributed globally
1980	Human T-lympho-tropic virus 1 (HTLV-1)	Virus	T-cell lymphoma-leukemia
1981	Toxin-producing strains of *Staphylococcus aureus*	Bacterium	Toxic shock syndrome
1982	*Escherichia coli* O157:H7	Bacterium	Hemorrhagic colitis; hemolytic uremic syndrome
1982	HTLV-2	Virus	Associated with hairy cell leukemia, in drug use
1982	*Borrelia burgdorferi*	Bacterium	Lyme disease
1983	HIV	Virus	AIDS
1983	*Helicobacter pylori*	Bacterium	Peptic ulcer disease
1985	*Enterocytozoon bieneusi*	Parasite	Persistent diarrhea
1986	*Cylospora cayetanensis*	Parasite	Persistent diarrhea
1986	Bovine spongiform encephalopathy agent?	Non-conventional agent	Bovine spongiform encephalopathy in cattle
1988	Human herpesvirus 6 (HHV-6)	Virus	Exanthem subitum
1988	Hepatitis E virus	Virus	Enterically transmitted non-A, non-B hepatitis
1989	*Ehrlichia chaffeensis*	Bacterium	Human ehrlichiosis
1989	Hepatitis C virus	Virus	Parenterally transmitted non-A, non-B hepatitis
1991	Guanarito virus	Virus	Venezuelan hemorrhagic fever
1991	*Encephalitozoon hellem*	Parasite	Conjunctivitis, disseminated disease
1991	New species of *Babesia*	Parasite	Atypical babesiosis
1992	*Vibrio cholera* O139	Bacterium	New strain associated with epidemic cholera
1992	*Bartonella henselae*	Bacterium	Cat-scratch disease; bacillary angiomatosis
1993	Sin nombre virus	Virus	Hantavirus pulmonary syndrome
1993	*Encephalitozoon cuniculi*	Parasite	Disseminated disease
1994	Sabia virus	Virus	Brazilian hemorrhagic fever
1995	Human herpesvirus 8	Virus	Associated with Kaposi's sarcoma

Fig. 5.2 Examples of etiologic agents and infectious diseases recognized since 1973.[1]

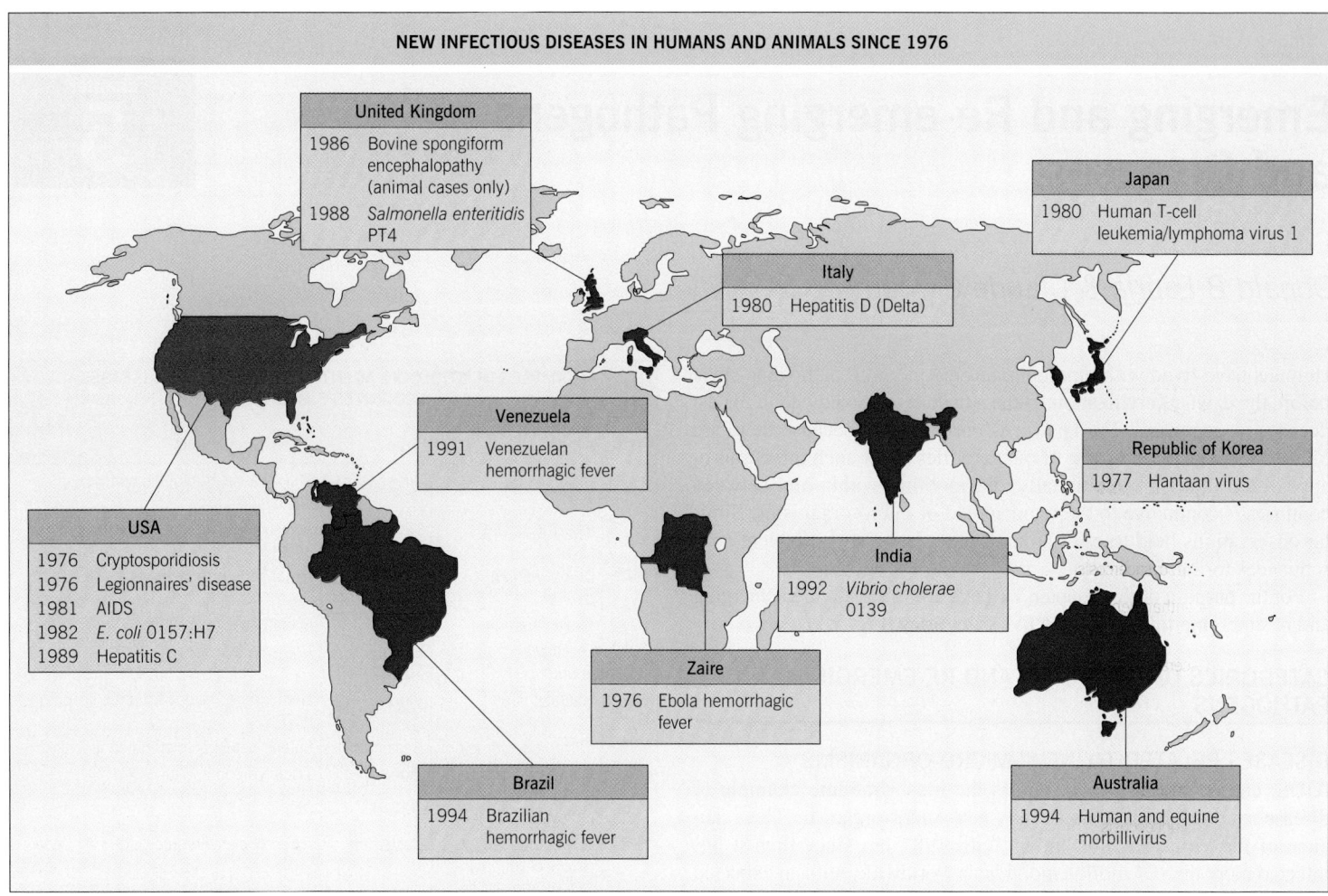

NEW INFECTIOUS DISEASES IN HUMANS AND ANIMALS SINCE 1976

United Kingdom

| 1986 | Bovine spongiform encephalopathy (animal cases only) |
| 1988 | *Salmonella enteritidis* PT4 |

Japan

| 1980 | Human T-cell leukemia/lymphoma virus 1 |

Italy

| 1980 | Hepatitis D (Delta) |

Venezuela

| 1991 | Venezuelan hemorrhagic fever |

Republic of Korea

| 1977 | Hantaan virus |

USA

1976	Cryptosporidiosis
1976	Legionnaires' disease
1981	AIDS
1982	*E. coli* 0157:H7
1989	Hepatitis C

India

| 1992 | *Vibrio cholerae* 0139 |

Zaire

| 1976 | Ebola hemorrhagic fever |

Brazil

| 1994 | Brazilian hemorrhagic fever |

Australia

| 1994 | Human and equine morbillivirus |

Fig. 5.3 New infectious disease in humans and animals since 1976. Countries in which cases first appeared or were first identified.[1]

contribute to re-emergence (Fig. 5.6), including the evolution of new variants or strains that have increased virulence or encounter highly susceptible individuals among human populations.

Despite historic predictions that infectious diseases would wane in countries such as the USA, a report published in 1996 on trends in US mortality caused by infectious diseases indicated that the death rate had increased by more than 50% since 1980; age-adjusted infectious disease mortality had increased by 39%.[3] Infectious diseases were the third leading cause of death in the USA in 1992. Death as a result of respiratory tract infections, HIV and sepsis accounted for most of the increase. Examples of emerging and re-emerging infection outbreaks in a recent year and the countries involved are illustrated in Figure 5.7.

DISEASES RELATED TO NEWLY IDENTIFIED MICRO-ORGANISMS PRODUCING HUMAN PATHOLOGY

This group includes a number of pathogens responsible for opportunistic and non-opportunistic infections in humans that have been identified through the development of new technology. Also included are agents previously known in animals, plants or the environment and only now recognized as causing infections in humans, especially in the immunocompromised host. Such agents are referred to as 'opportunistic' as they are poorly pathogenic in normal hosts.

A number of syndromes exist in which an infectious etiology is likely but the pathogen escapes the current methods of identification. New techniques in molecular biology, such as representational difference analysis, consensus sequence-based polymerase chain reaction and complementary DNA library screening, have allowed the identification of previously unculturable infectious agents.[4] These methods rely upon the identification of subgenomic fragments from the suspected agent. Once such a fragment has been isolated from tissues, it can be sequenced and used as a probe to identify additional infected tissues or to obtain extended portions of the agent's genome. These techniques must be applied in conjunction with epidemiologic procedures, in order to establish that a new pathogen is central to the disease process.

MODES OF TRANSMISSION OF INFECTIOUS DISEASES

- Air
- Food
- Water
- Vectors
- Blood product transfusions
- Human contacts

Fig. 5.4 Modes of transmission of infectious diseases.

RE-EMERGING INFECTIONS DURING THE PAST TWO DECADES AND CONTRIBUTING FACTORS		
Disease or agent		**Factors in re-emergence**
Viral	Rabies	Breakdown in public health measures, changes in land use, travel
	Dengue	Transportation, travel and migration, urbanization
	Yellow fever	Favorable conditions for mosquito vector
	Ebola	Lack of modern facilities, emergence of a new strain (Ivory Coast)
Parasitic	Malaria	Drug and insecticide resistance, civil strife, lack of economic resources
	Schistosomiasis	Dam construction, improved irrigation and ecologic changes favoring the snail host
	Neurocysticercosis	Immigration
	Acanthamoebiasis	Introduction of soft contact lenses, AIDS
	Visceral leishmaniasis	War, population displacement, immigration, habitat changes favorable to the insect vector, and increase in immunocompromised human hosts
	Giardiasis	Increased use of child-care facilities
	Echinococcosis	Ecologic changes that affect the habitats of the intermediate (animal) hosts
	Cryptosporidium spp.	Poor water quality
Bacterial	Group A *Streptococcus* spp.	Uncertain
	E. coli (O157:H7; O103:H2)	Acquisition of bacteriophages encoding for shiga-like toxin
	Trench fever	Breakdown of public health measures
	Plague	Economic development, land use
	Diphtheria	Interruption of immunization program because of political changes, population disruptions
	Tuberculosis	Human demographics and behavior, industry and technology, international commerce and travel, breakdown of public health measures, microbial adaptation
	Pertussis toxin	Refusal to vaccinate in some parts of the world because of the belief that injections or vaccines are not safe
	Salmonella spp.	Industry and technology, human demographics and behavior, microbial adaptation, food changes
	Pneumococcus	Human demographics, microbial adaptation, international travel and commerce, misuse and overuse of antibiotics
	Cholera	Travel, evolution of a new strain (O139)

Fig. 5.5 Re-emerging infections over the past two decades and contributing factors. Adapted from Lorber.[2]

Advances in the treatment of malignant diseases, aggressive therapy of some connective tissue diseases by immunosuppressive agents and the extension of the AIDS epidemic have created a significant population of immunocompromised patients. Consequently, a multiplicity of organisms that had previously only been identified in nonhuman pathology or in the environment are able to infect such individuals and cause disease. In the investigation of febrile episodes in immunocompromised patients who have unusual presentations, the potential role of new opportunistic pathogens must be investigated. Conversely, patients presenting with unusual infections should be investigated for the possibility of an underlying malignancy or immunosuppressive illness.

DISEASES RECENTLY RECOGNIZED AS INFECTIONS

Progress in the identification of micro-organisms in cells and tissues and the development of new methods in genetics and epidemiology have led to the discovery that transmissible agents may be responsible for diseases that were never suspected of being infectious in origin. Figure 5.8 outlines some of the non-neoplastic diseases associated with transmissible agents. These observations have provided evidence for the huge complexity of human–micro-organism interactions.[2] The mechanisms by which a micro-organism may cause the development of a nonclassic infectious disease are highly variable; in some cases, the agent is a direct cause, in others, it appears to act as a precipitating factor or a risk factor.

In some diseases the role of infectious organisms remains hypothetical but strongly suggestive, either because of the indirect demonstration of the beneficial effects of antimicrobials on the course of the disease, or from preliminary information on a possible causal relationship between the presence of organisms in tissues and responsibility for the pathophysiology of the disease (Fig. 5.9).

Approximately 10 million new cases of cancer were diagnosed in 1995. Up to 84% of cases of some cancers are attributable to viruses, parasites or bacteria (Fig. 5.10). The World Health Organization estimates that 15% of the new cases occurring each year could be avoided by preventing the infectious disease associated with them. The relative impact of infections on the overall cancer burden is more important in those populations in which communicable diseases are the leading cause of morbidity.[1]

Epidemiologic and molecular biology studies have shown that some micro-organisms are involved as cofactors in the multiple step process of carcinogenesis. Viral DNA probes or antibodies against viral proteins can prove to be useful tools for diagnosis [human T-cell leukemia/lymphoma virus (HTLV) Epstein–Barr virus, hepatitis B virus, hepatitis C virus] or prognosis (human papillomavirus) of the related cancer. The potential preventive intervention with vaccines – other than for hepatitis B – is still a matter of research.

FACTORS THAT CONTRIBUTE TO THE RE-EMERGENCE OF INFECTIOUS DISEASES
• Socio-economic changes
• Health care technologies
• Food production and processing
• Human behavior
• Environmental changes
• Inadequacy of public health infrastructure
• Microbial adaptation and changes

Fig. 5.6 Factors that contribute to the re-emergence of infectious diseases.

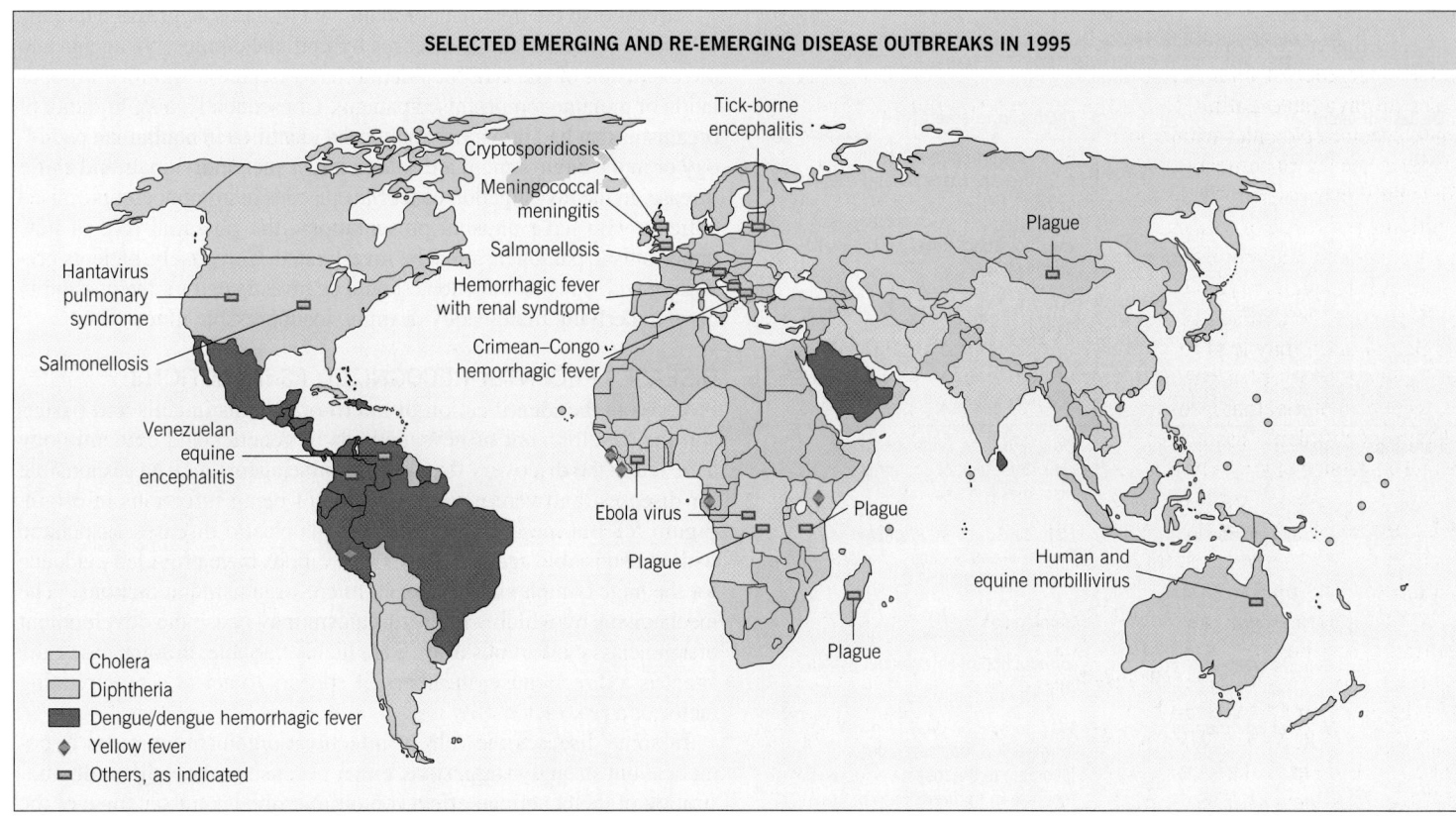

Fig. 5.7 Selected emerging and re-emerging disease outbreaks in 1995.[1]

NON-NEOPLASTIC DISEASES ASSOCIATED WITH INFECTIOUS AGENTS		
Disease/syndrome		**Agent**
Gastrointestinal disorders	Chronic gastritis	*Helicobacter pylori*
	Peptic ulcer	*Helicobacter pylori*
	Crohn's disease	*Tropheryma whippelii*
Neurologic disorders	Guillain–Barré syndrome	*Campylobacter jejuni*
	Bell's palsy	*Borrelia burgdorferi*, Herpes simplex virus
	Tropical spastic paraparesis	HTLV-1
Renal disorders	Hemolytic uremic syndrome	*Escherichia coli* O157:H7
	Thrombotic thrombocytopenic purpura	*Escherichia coli* O157:H7
Vascular disorders	Polyarteritis nodosa	Hepatitis B virus
	Mixed cryoglobulinemia	Hepatitis C virus
Insulin-dependent diabetes mellitus		Enterovirus
Coronary atherosclerosis		*Chlamydia pneumoniae*, cytomegalovirus
Arthritis	Reactive arthritis	*Salmonella* spp., *Yersinia* spp., *Chlamydia trachomatis*

Fig. 5.8 Non-neoplastic diseases associated with infectious agents.
Adapted from Lorber.[2]

RESISTANT MICRO-ORGANISMS AND THE ROLE OF ANTIMICROBIAL THERAPY

The multidrug-resistance of transmissible micro-organisms is a major health problem worldwide. Some infections have become virtually untreatable, both in hospitals and in the community.[5]

Physicians overprescribe antibiotics and the public demands their overutilization. In the USA more than 100 million courses of antibiotics are prescribed each year. Various studies indicate that perhaps 30% (range 15–65%) of these of treatment courses are unnecessary or inappropriate.[6,7] Additionally, in many countries antimicrobials are available in pharmacies without a prescription. A Chilean study found that 44% of antibiotic sales in 54 urban pharmacies were made without prescriptions.[8] If the definition of ideal antimicrobial therapy is use of the smallest amount of a single agent or the fewest number of agents (when

DISEASES SUSPECTED TO BE OF INFECTIOUS ORIGIN	
Disease	**Suspected agent**
Alzheimer's disease	Herpesvirus 1
Paget's disease	Paramyxovirus
Multiple sclerosis	Herpesviruses?
Depression	Bornavirus
Wegener's granulomatosis	[Response to trimethoprim–sulfamethoxazole (co-trimoxazole)]
Rheumatoid arthritis	(Response to tetracycline)

Fig. 5.9 Diseases suspected to be of infectious origin.

more than one antimicrobial is indicated) necessary to effect a cure, then it is clear that there is massive overusage. In turn, this overusage leads to the emergence of micro-organisms highly resistant to many, sometimes all, available antibiotics and consequently the infections they cause become epidemics within hospitals and communities. The increasing resistance of pneumococci to penicillins and alternative agents, the frequently extraordinary resistance of *Enterococcus faecium* and the multidrug resistance of *Salmonella typhi* are all examples of major problems created by the promiscuous use of antibiotics. There is no reason to believe this pattern will abate; indeed, it is likely to accelerate.

Bacteria have a remarkable propensity to overcome antibiotics. A single mutation may lead to resistance without altering the virulence and pathogenicity of a bacterial strain. Also, bacteria may acquire exogenous material that leads to antimicrobial resistance.[9] A selection of current problems associated with antimicrobial drugs for some bacterial groups is given in Figure 5.11. The link between antimicrobial drug resistance and the extent of antimicrobial use has been documented in many studies.[10,11] Some usage pattern characteristics such as daily dose and treatment duration appear to be involved in antibiotic selection pressures.[12]

Multidrug resistance may have an important impact on morbidity, mortality and health costs. Two examples may help illustrate the consequences of multidrug resistance among bacteria. Among patients who have bacteremia caused by vancomycin-resistant enterococci, a majority of whom had serious underlying diseases, the mortality directly related to the bacteremia was reported to approach 50%.[13] Several factors appeared to be associated with the acquisition of multi-resistant enterococci: the length of hospital stay, underlying conditions, antibiotic exposure (mainly oral and parenteral vancomycin)[9] and the use of glycopeptides in veterinary medicine and animal feeding.

The prevalence of primary multidrug resistance in *Mycobacterium tuberculosis*, defined as resistance to both isoniazid and rifampin (rifampicin), was 2% in the USA with a median prevalence of 1.4% (range 0–14.4%) in 33 countries studied between 1994 and 1997.[14] Several reports have emphasized the high mortality rate and low cure rate seen with such strains. In immunocompetent patients infected with multidrug-resistant *M. tuberculosis*, the overall survival rate was 61% and the median survival time was greater than 120 months. In patients who had AIDS, the mean duration of survival was 6.8 months.[15]

Reports on emergence of resistance among *Candida* spp. to various antifungal azoles agree that the prolonged use of low doses of drugs favors the selection of resistant strains.[16]

Malaria represents an interesting example of a double resistance problem: *Plasmodium* parasites are resistant to antiparasitic drugs and *Anopheles* mosquitoes are resistant to insecticides. The number of antimalarial compounds remains limited. The emergence of resistance among *Plasmodium falciparum* strains has been attributed in most areas of the world to inadequate therapeutic regimens and poor drug supply. Multidrug resistance is now common in areas such as Southeast Asia. Many mosquitoes are already resistant to the three classes of insecticides available for public health use.

Resistance of viruses to antiviral drugs represents a major issue in patient management. Herpesviruses and cytomegalovirus have been reported to develop resistance to aciclovir and ganciclovir, respectively.[17]

The first generation of agents prescribed to treat HIV were drugs that inhibited the reverse transcriptase enzyme of the virus (nucleoside or non-nucleoside analogs). The effects of these drugs appeared time limited, particularly when used as monotherapy, because of the development of resistance mediated by various mutations in the reverse transcriptase gene. Although thus far reported only in a small number of patients, exposure to some protease inhibitors can lead to the rapid emergence of drug-resistant variants *in vivo*. This resistance may extend to other structurally related protease inhibitors.[18]

Clearly, the emergence of resistance to chemotherapy among a large variety of micro-organisms should lead to the rational use of anti-infective agents and the development and application of various measures in the environment to slow down the rate at which resistance emerges. The control of antibiotics used in veterinary medicine, the strict application of hygienic measures in hospitals and the development of active immunization to reduce the risk of some infections are merely a few examples of such measures.

THE FUTURE OF EMERGING AND RE-EMERGING INFECTIONS

Infectious disease texts usually focus on microbes, pathogenicity and host defenses. In recent decades this narrow focus has been broadened to include a greater emphasis on human sexual behavior and a

NEOPLASTIC DISORDERS RELATED TO TRANSMISSIBLE AGENTS	
Disorder	Agent
Human T-cell leukemia	HTLV-1
Hairy cell leukemia	HTLV-2
Hepatocellular cancer	Hepatitis B and C viruses
Cervical cancer	Human papilloma viruses
Cutaneous cancer	Human papilloma viruses
Burkitt's lymphoma	Epstein–Barr virus
Nasopharyngeal lymphoma	Epstein–Barr virus
AIDS-related CNS lymphoma	Epstein–Barr virus
Gastric carcinoma	*Helicobacter pylori*
Maltoma	*Helicobacter pylori*
Kaposi's sarcoma	Herpesvirus type 8
AIDS-related body cavity lymphoma	Herpesvirus type 8
Castleman's disease	Herpesvirus type 8
Bladder cancer	Human papilloma virus

Fig. 5.10 Neoplastic disorders related to transmissible agents. Adapted from Lorber.[2]

PROBLEMS WITH ANTIMICROBIAL DRUGS FOR SOME BACTERIAL GROUPS	
Organism	Problem
Gram-positive cocci	Methicillin-resistant *Staphylococcus aureus* and coagulase-negative staphylococci, penicillin-resistant pneumococci, macrolide-resistant streptococci, vancomycin-resistant enterococci
Gram-negative cocci	Penicillin-resistant meningococci, quinolone-resistant gonococci
Gram-negative bacilli	*Enterobacter* spp. and other Enterobacteriaceae with chromosomal beta-lactamases; multidrug-resistant *Pseudomonas aeruginosa*, *Stenotrophomonas maltophilia*, *Acinetobacter* spp. with novel beta-lactamases, aminoglycoside-modifying enzymes and other resistance mechanisms; Enterobacteriaceae with extended-spectrum beta-lactamases; multidrug-resistant diarrheal pathogens (*Shigella* spp., *Salmonella* spp., *Escherichia coli*, *Campylobacter* spp.)
Acid-fast bacilli	Multidrug-resistant *Mycobacterium tuberculosis*; multidrug-resistant *Mycobacterium avium* complex

Fig. 5.11 Problems with antimicrobial drugs for some bacterial groups. Adapted from Kunin.[6]

1

5.5

recognition of the dangers of the hospital environment. A further expansion is warranted to include a focus on the broader socioeconomic issues that provide the milieu in which emerging and re-emerging infections arise and flourish.[19] Some of these issues are listed in Figure 5.12.

POPULATION GROWTH

Modern civilization dates from approximately 10,000 BC. It took until 1830 for the world population to reach 1 billion persons; however, from there the world population doubled in the next 100 years and reached 6 billion 70 years after that. Fertility rates are now falling; thus some of the developed countries have zero population growth, but the overall world population is growing at a rate of 1.5% per annum with a projected population doubling time of 46 years. It seems almost certain there will be 8 billion people on the earth by the year 2030.[20] Thereafter projections vary depending upon fertility assumptions (Fig. 5.13). By the end of the 21st century the world population could be between 10 and 14 billion persons and the final stable population could be between 11 and 18 billion. Whichever projection is used, it seems clear that the crowding that characterizes many areas today will increase – and crowding promotes the spread of infection. Some of the adverse effects that may result from a doubling or tripling of the world population are summarized in Figure 5.14.

POVERTY, MALNUTRITION AND EXPOSURE TO UNSAFE WATER

A reasonable estimate is that between one-quarter and one-third of the world's population live in poverty. Some 2 billion persons suffer from undernutrition or malnutrition; 1 billion experience hunger on a daily basis and at least 400 million suffer from dire poverty and major nutritional deprivation. Approximately 1.5 billion people lack access to basic health care. A similar number do not have access to safe water.[21] With a massive increase in population size expected in the 21st century, these disturbing figures could get substantially worse, even though a concerted effort may reduce the percentage of the world population suffering these deficiencies.[22]

The link between poverty and undernutrition or malnutrition is clear; so is the nexus between undernutrition and infectious diseases. Malnutrition influences incidence, prevalence, clinical appearance and clinical progression of a variety of infections. For example, lack of vitamin A in the diets of infants and small children results in a marked increase in the prevalence of respiratory tract infections and diarrheal disease. The adverse consequences of exposure to unsafe water are also fully established; diarrheal disease from water contaminated by bacteria, viruses and parasites accounts for billions of episodes each year and as a consequence billions of dollars in lost productivity, millions of deaths and an extraordinary toll in hardship and misery.

GLOBAL CLIMATE CHANGE

The climatologic event most likely to affect infectious diseases is global warming (Fig. 5.15).[23] The evidence for global warming gets progressively more convincing. It is likely that in the 21st century the earth will be 1.5–4.0°C warmer.[24] At least one-half the greenhouse gas

---

SOCIETAL ISSUES IN EMERGING AND RE-EMERGING INFECTIOUS DISEASES

- Population growth
- Poverty
- Malnutrition
- Unsafe water
- Global climate change
- Refugee populations
- Population aging
- Human activities
- Urbanization
- Travel
- Human behavior
- Warfare
- Public health infrastructure or policy breakdown
- Excessive antibiotic use

Fig. 5.12 Societal issues in emerging and re-emerging infectious diseases.

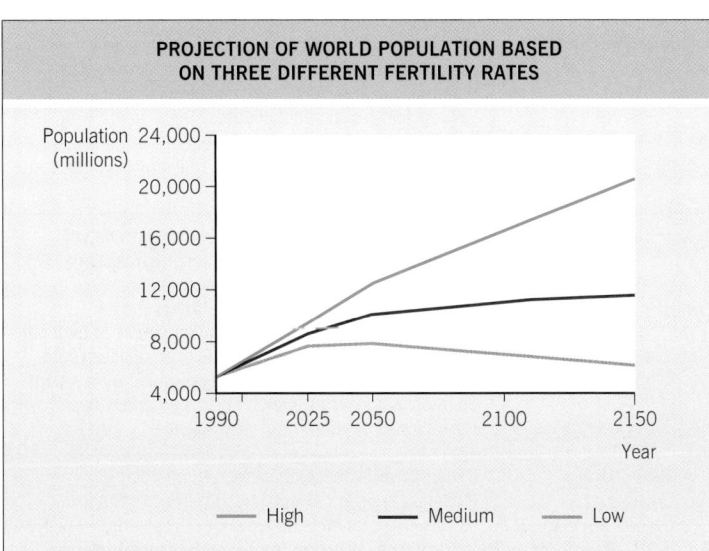

PROJECTION OF WORLD POPULATION BASED ON THREE DIFFERENT FERTILITY RATES

— High   — Medium   — Low

Fig. 5.13 Projection of world population growth based on three different fertility rates.

CONSEQUENCES OF WORLD POPULATION GROWTH			
	Eventual world population		
Areas of concern	10 billion	14 billion	20 billion
Increase in wars within or between nations	Certain	Certain	Certain
Major increases in internally displaced persons and refugees	Certain	Certain	Certain
Severe malnutrition and hunger (newer technologies could prevent or minimize)	Uncertain	Uncertain	Uncertain
Rainforest destruction	Certain: large percentage destroyed	Certain: virtually total destruction	Certain: virtually total destruction
Species loss	Very considerable	Massive	Catastrophic
Inadequate potable water supply (new technologies could prevent or minimize)	Likely	Very likely	Very likely
Increase in poverty (some insist this can be avoided by world economic growth)	Likely	Very likely	Almost certain
Wetland destruction	Certain: large percentage destroyed	Certain: very extensive destruction	Certain: massive destruction
Increased potential for disease spread	Likely	Very likely	Extremely likely
Perceptions that quality of life is diminished	Probable	Very likely	Extremely likely

Fig. 5.14 Consequences of world population growth. As the projection of the eventual world population rises, so the likelihood of adverse socioeconomic consequences increases.

burden is attributable to carbon dioxide. Methane (10–20%), chloro-fluorocarbons (10–20%) and nitrogen oxides (4–7%) are the other principal greenhouse gases. More than 25 billion tons of carbon dioxide are released yearly into the environment. Of that amount, about 60% results from industrial and home fossil fuel use and 10–20% from emissions from the more than 500 million cars and trucks used around the world. An additional 25% results from felling and burning trees in the world's ever diminishing forests. Atmospheric carbon dioxide concentrations have risen by 30% in the past 2 centuries; the current concentration of 360ppm could double by the end of the 21st century (Fig. 5.16).[25]

Greenhouse gas emissions, in the absence of vigorous actions, will inevitably rise in tandem with world population growth, with resultant increases in industrialization and irrigation required to provide the world with food, increase in the number of cars (to over 1 billion) and forest destruction. Global warming will increase productivity in some geographic areas, whereas others will suffer from severe floods or drought; both are guaranteed to raise the number and flow of refugees. Some 500 million people now live at or near sea level. Global warming and the resultant flooding that will likely follow will displace tens of millions, perhaps hundreds of millions, of these sea level inhabitants. Sea water incursions will destroy wetlands and contaminate fresh water supplies.

Although the current focus is on carbon dioxide, methane may be of equal concern in the 21st century. Methane now accounts for 10–20% of the greenhouse effect. It has an atmospheric half-life of about 12 years and is much more efficient in trapping heat than carbon dioxide. Atmospheric concentrations have been increasing sharply for the past 200 years; concentrations have more than doubled since the year 1800 (Fig. 5.16). Most of atmospheric methane results from anaerobic bacterial activity. Swamps, marshes, peat bogs and fens, other wetlands, rice paddies, landfills, the intestinal tracts of cattle and termites, oil and natural gas production and distribution, and coal extraction are the major planetary sources.[26] Most of the postindustrial revolution increase in methane concentrations is anthropogenic. As the world population increases, so will certain methane sources, including cattle and other ruminants needed to feed the growing population, rice paddies and the fossil fuels used to supply some of the increasing energy demands.

Changes in temperature will alter vector distribution and behavior. At higher temperatures some mosquitoes tend to be more active, eat more voraciously and bite more frequently. Additionally, they have shortened reproductive cycles and the extrinsic period for infectious agents (the time required for development in the mosquito) is lessened. Mosquitoes that have found higher elevations colder and less hospitable will be able to thrive in previously mosquito-free areas; this in turn will introduce certain diseases, such as malaria and dengue, to unexposed areas and therefore to nonimmune populations. For these populations, diseases will emerge that may have been endemic in their general geographic areas, but which they have escaped because their particular geographic subarea was free of the vectors. This introduction of infectious agents as a result of vector redistribution into nonimmune populations is likely to be one of the major worldwide consequences of global warming.[27–29]

Malaria, dengue and schistosomiasis lead the list of infections likely to increase in incidence and prevalence as a consequence of global warming (Fig. 5.17). The latter will probably also drive the tsetse fly southward, exposing new areas to sleeping sickness, a feared disease that results in populations leaving endemic areas. That exodus will be augmented by livestock trypanosomal infections that will increase poverty and malnutrition.

FORCED MIGRATION

There are currently about 50 million people who are refugees, either outside their own countries or within them but internally displaced (Fig. 5.18). That figure is likely to grow substantially in the 21st century, particularly if significant global warming occurs. Refugees are often crowded together in unhygienic circumstances, which encourages the emergence of a farrago of infectious diseases,[30] point-source epidemics and rapid person-to-person spread. During migration refugees are often exposed to, for them, new vectors carrying agents to which they have inadequate immunity. Additionally, some refugees carry micro-organisms (e.g. malaria, *Schistosoma haematobium*) with them that cause the spread of infection in the geographic areas to which the refugees migrate.

A historic paradigm of the potentially catastrophic role of migrants carrying organisms to nonimmune populations was the arrival of Europeans into the Americas. At the beginning of the 16th century there were an estimated 80 million Native Americans living on the American continent. One hundred years later their numbers had dwindled to less than 3 million, primarily because of newly introduced infections.

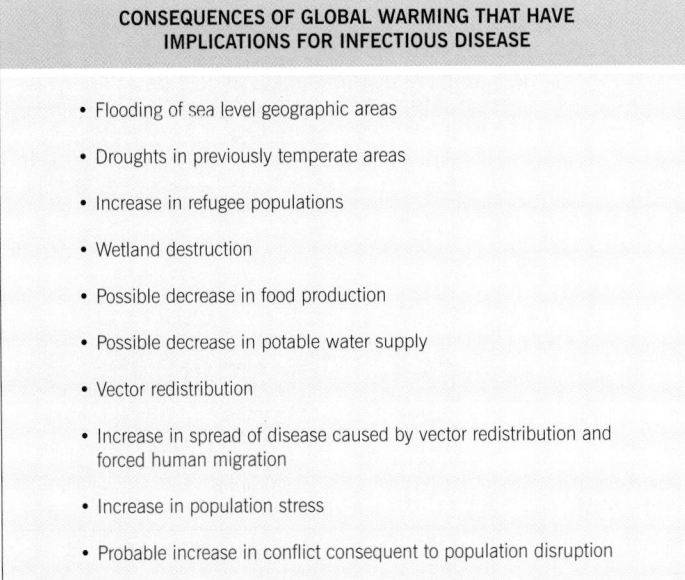

Fig. 5.15 Consequences of global warming that have implications for infectious disease.

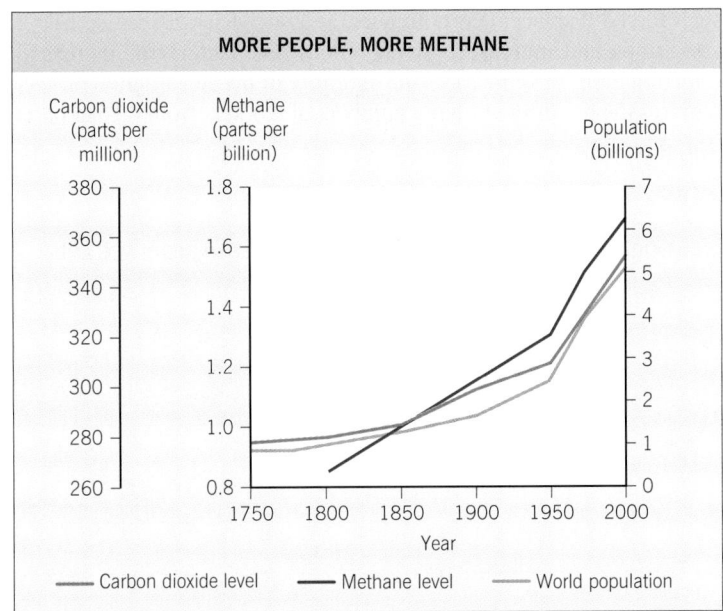

Fig. 5.16 The relationship between world population and methane levels, 1750–2000.

AN AGING POPULATION

By the year 2030, 25% of the US population will be 60 years of age or older; worldwide, the current 560 million persons over age 60 will have increased to 1.3 billion. The profound increase in the number of older persons will affect developed and developing areas of the world, but the latter will see the greatest percentage increases (Fig. 5.19). The change in the figures for the very old are even more dramatic and are illustrated by predictions for the USA: at present about 3 million people are aged 85 years or older; by the year 2040 that number will increase more than fivefold to an estimated 16–24 million persons. The percentage of the population over the age of 80 years will double in most areas of the world by the year 2030.[31]

Older persons as a group experience an array of deficits that may promote certain infections; the extent of the deficit varies greatly from individual to individual. The major defect is in delayed-type immunity and is manifested by an ever-increasing proportion of older people in each decade after the age of 60 years who are anergic to delayed-type cutaneous antigens.[32] Additionally, as a group, older persons show deficits in immunoglobulin production[33] and in polymorphonuclear leukocyte function.[34] These defects, together with their well established nutritional deficits, make older persons susceptible to a variety of emerging and re-emerging infections, particularly those handled by the lymphocyte–macrophage system; tuberculosis leads the list of re-emerging infections in older persons.[35,36]

HUMAN ACTIVITIES

Human activities have detrimental effects; nowhere is this more evident than in the infectious disease consequences of irrigation and dam construction.[37] During the 20th century, more than 38,000 large dams have been built and more than 1200 are under construction. In developing countries new infectious disease patterns have often been an untoward consequence of vector redistribution as a result of dam construction. Habitat advantages have been created, particularly for mosquitoes and snails (Fig. 5.20). The Aswan dam resulted in 200,000 new cases of Rift Valley fever and a marked increase in schistosomiasis and malaria among populations with a relatively low prevalence of both. In Ghana construction of a huge dam on the river Volta was followed by an increase in prevalence of *S. haematobium* in the Volta basin area, from approximately 10 to 90%. Similarly, in some areas filariasis and dracunculiasis have shown substantial increases in prevalence after dams have been constructed. Additionally, large dams such as the gargantuan one being constructed on the Yangtze River in China require relocation of tens of thousands, often millions of people; such forced displacement is frequently associated with worse living conditions and increased poverty, both risk factors for increased infection rates. In some cases the enormity of the construction project requires the recruiting of large numbers of workers from distant parts of the country or from other countries. These new 'temporary' immigrants bring their own infections with them, creating the potential for emerging or re-emerging infections in inadequately protected local populations. Furthermore, the newly created large bodies of water are subject to massive fecal contamination, increasing the likelihood of re-emerging pathogen epidemics (e.g. cholera).

Large irrigation projects and aquaculture (fish ponds) can have similar untoward consequences. Fish ponds in Kenya encouraged multiplication of malaria-transmitting mosquitoes. Irrigation in Cameroon was followed by a two- to three-fold increase in prevalence of urinary tract schistosomiasis.

Clearing forests can create aerosols of infected dusts; in Venezuela hundreds of cases of arenavirus hemorrhagic fever resulted from dust contaminated by urine and feces of the cotton rat.[38] Such deforestation can also change vector distribution. In South America, as forests were cleared, triatome vectors of Chagas' disease, deprived of both blood resources and natural shelters, invaded nearby human settlements.

As populations increase, especially in areas of the world affected by poverty, these disease-inducing activities of humans will inevitably proliferate. The increases in productivity and economic gain from dam construction and irrigation will have to be balanced in the final analyses against the economic loss caused by human and animal infections.

URBANIZATION

The latter half of the 20th century has been characterized by the creation of large cities with ever greater population densities that draw inhabitants from rural areas and often act as sink holes for hordes of newly landless people displaced by economic hardships or the ravages of war. Large

CAUSES OF FORCED MIGRATION
• Warfare
• Famine
• Poverty
• Loss of jobs
• Persecution
• Redrawing borders
• Construction (e.g. dams)

Fig. 5.18 Causes of forced migration.

MAJOR INFECTIOUS DISEASES LIKELY TO INCREASE IN INCIDENCE AND GEOGRAPHIC DISTRIBUTION THROUGH GLOBAL WARMING	
Almost certain substantial increase	Malaria
	Schistosomiasis
	Dengue
Probable increase	Leishmaniasis
	Arboviral diseases (other than dengue)
	Bancroftian and Brugian filariasis
	Trypanosomiasis
Possible increase	Onchercocerciasis

Fig. 5.17 Major infectious diseases likely to increase in incidence and geographic distribution as a result of global warming.

THE AGING POPULATION: PERCENTAGES OF TOTAL POPULATION, 1990 AND 2025				
Region	Year	65 years and over	75 years and over	80 years and over
Europe	1990	13.7	6.1	3.2
	2025	22.4	10.8	6.4
North America	1990	12.6	5.3	2.8
	2025	20.1	8.5	4.6
Asia	1990	4.8	1.5	0.6
	2025	10.0	3.6	1.8
Latin America/ Caribbean	1990	4.6	1.6	0.8
	2025	9.4	3.6	1.8
Near East/ North Africa	1990	3.8	1.2	0.5
	2025	6.4	2.2	1.1
Sub-Saharan Africa	1990	2.7	0.7	0.3
	2025	3.4	1.0	0.4

Fig. 5.19 The aging population: percentages of total population, 1990 and 2025. Data from US Bureau of the Census, International Population Reports, 1992.[31]

numbers of migrants often experience underemployment or no employment and become inhabitants of teeming slums. The crowded slums, often with inadequate sanitation and stagnant water, are not only ideal settings for point-source epidemics and rapid person-to-person transmission, but are also virtual breeding grounds for rodents, flies and mosquitoes. At the beginning of the 20th century about 15% of the world population of less than 2 billion people lived in cities; at the beginning of the 21st century approximately one-half of the world's 6 billion people will live in cities; that figure is expected to grow to 60–65% by the year 2030 (Fig. 5.21). Eighty per cent of this massive urbanization will take place in the so-called developing countries.[22] Individual cities have grown into massive population centers; at the beginning of the 21st century there will be at least be 26 mega-cities, each with more than 10 million inhabitants, and most of these will be in developing countries.

RAPID AND EXTENSIVE TRAVEL

In 1990 there were 280 million international airline travelers; by the year 2000 that figure will increase to between 400 and 600 million travelers. Some will already be carrying pathogens; others will be traveling to areas in which they will suffer unintended exposure to, for them, new pathogens that, potentially, they can introduce to their communities upon their return home.

The ease of travel between countries or continents also facilitates the spread of disease when frightened people flee an incipient epidemic in a given geographic area. Additionally, vector and micro-organisms often hitch rides on airplanes or boats; dengue virus-carrying mosquitoes and the bacilli of cholera are good examples.

EFFECTS OF DAM CONSTRUCTION AND IRRIGATION PROJECTS ON INCIDENCE AND PREVALENCE OF EMERGING AND RE-EMERGING PARASITIC INFECTIONS	
Change in prevalence	Infection
Major increase	Malaria
	Schistosomiasis
Some increase	Onchocerciasis
	Dracunculosis
	Bancroftian and Brugian filariasis

Fig. 5.20 Effects of dam construction and irrigation projects on incidence and prevalence of emerging and re-emerging parasitic infections.

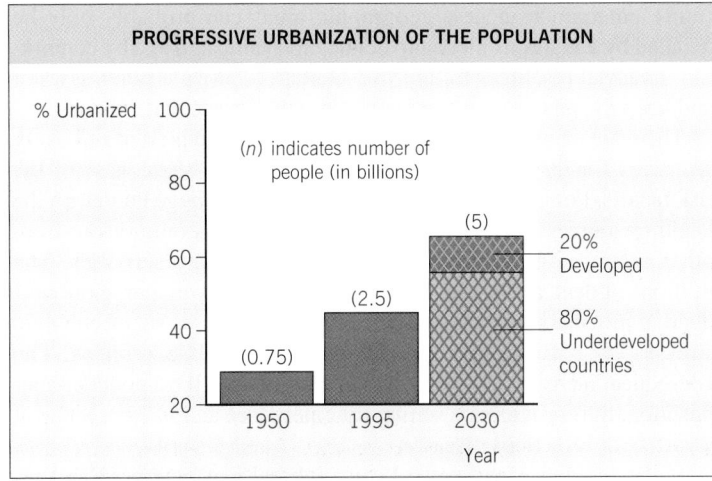

Fig. 5.21 Progressive urbanization of the population.

HUMAN BEHAVIOR

The quintessential example of human behavior affecting the spread of infection is the AIDS epidemic. In most of the world, where the virus is spread by heterosexual encounters, people's refusal to use condoms even when they knew the risks of unprotected sex and had condoms available contributed substantially to the spread of the epidemic and emergence of the disease in epidemic proportions in areas of previously very limited involvement. In other geographic areas, in particular the USA, and to a lesser extent, parts of Europe, the emergence of HIV and AIDS was related to male homosexual activity with multiple partners or to intravenous drug use.

There are many other examples. Much of the emergence (but probably not all) of the multidrug-resistant *M. tuberculosis* that appeared in the 1990s has been attributed to failure of compliance in regard to taking prescribed antituberculosis medications.

In hospitals, the single most important factor in the emergence of hospital epidemics caused by Gram-negative micro-organisms is neglect of the simple procedure of handwashing. In one reported mini-epidemic, no interventions stopped an epidemic of *Salmonella heidelberg*, resistant to all available antibiotics, until rigid handwashing requirements were implemented.[39]

Failure to follow basic hygienic principles by defecating into or close to water used for drinking or swimming promotes a variety of microbial epidemics.

WARFARE
The 20th century

Perhaps no human activity is so conducive to emergence or re-emergence of infectious diseases as warfare, a human behavior that, measured by the number of people involved, becomes more extensive every century (in part because of population growth). The 20th century has been the bloodiest in history. There have been 150 wars in the second half of the century, resulting in more than 23 million deaths, two-thirds of them civilians.[40]

Wars create the milieu for infection in many ways:
- massive injuries that invite microbial contamination;
- forced migration of nonimmunized persons into areas inhabited by disease-carrying vectors;
- crowding in refugee camps with inadequate sanitation facilities;
- migration of disease-carrying individuals into uninfected areas;
- exposure to disease-carrying rodents;
- malnutrition, even starvation; and
- destruction of public health infrastructures and safe water supplies.

Additionally, mass rape as an accepted or deliberately overlooked behavior of conquerors, or sometimes as an intentional military and governmental technique of intimidation and cruelty, can become a vehicle for spread of sexually transmitted diseases.

Future prospects

The prospects for less warfare are not good. Ethnic, religious, racial and tribal strife will be exacerbated by population growth, crowding and rivalries over increasingly depleted natural resources. In future decades competition for a decreasing supply of fresh water will be an ever more significant cause of war. Water shortages will result from a combination of population growth, increased irrigation requirements to feed the growing population and the effects of urbanization and industrialization. The depletion of water supplies by urbanization and industrialization can be mitigated by water treatment and recycling, but the resources required for such conservation are likely to be either insufficient or inadequately used in less affluent countries affected simultaneously by poverty, population explosion and uncontrolled urbanization.

Another type of warfare that by its very nature would create an emerging or re-emerging infection epidemic is germ warfare. There is reason to believe some rogue nations and extremist cults have been interested in the potential use of bacterial or viral agents as biologic weapons. A naturally occurring organism or one that is genetically engineered could create havoc.

PUBLIC HEALTH INFRASTRUCTURE OR POLICY BREAKDOWN

In April 1993, a breakdown at a water treatment plant handling water from Lake Michigan resulted in an estimated 400,000 cases of cryptosporidiosis in a small geographic area of the USA.[41] The attack rate was extraordinary; approximately one-half the people receiving water from one treatment facility became clinically sick with an illness characterized by watery diarrhea, abdominal cramps, fever and vomiting that lasted for a median of 3 days (range 1–38 days).

Cryptosporidiosis was first recognized as a human pathogen in 1976 among immunosuppressed individuals. A decade later small epidemics were recognized among immunocompetent hosts. The huge epidemic in Milwaukee, Wisconsin represents the completion of the disease spectrum of this ubiquitous parasite – first only immunocompromised hosts, then small numbers of immunocompetent persons and finally an enormous acute epidemic. In future cryptosporidiosis will re-emerge in small or large epidemics in areas in which it has not been observed for substantial time. Breakdown in public health infrastructures will be an important factor in the re-emergence of *Cryptosporidium* spp. in epidemic form and the emergence and re-emergence of other intestinal protozoans, including species of *Cyclospora* and *Microsporidia*.

THE INTER-RELATEDNESS OF SOCIAL, ECONOMIC AND ENVIRONMENTAL VARIABLES

Population growth, poverty, global warming, resource depletion and forced migration are all inextricably inter-related (Fig. 5.22). A world with 12 billion people that is simultaneously significantly warmer is likely to create a flow of refugees and internally displaced persons that would dwarf the current figure of 50 million. Hundreds of millions of displaced persons, some exposed to organisms to which they have no immunity and many living in poverty and suffering malnutrition and exposed to unsafe water, would create daunting challenges in the prevention and control of infectious diseases. The epidemiologic future of dengue, which now affects 100 million people worldwide each year, illustrates the concatenation of many of these variables: population growth, global warming, poverty, urbanization, flawed public health policy and the consequences of travel.[27,42]

The vector *Aedes aegypti* inhabits tropical areas between latitudes 30° north and 20° south. It does not thrive in colder areas above altitudes of 2000 feet and is urbanized, breeding particularly well in crowded ghettos where sanitation is inadequate and where water is stored or allowed to accumulate in a variety of containers. The disease spreads to new areas primarily through viremic travelers. Dengue virtually disappeared in the western hemisphere for the 30 years preceding 1977 as a result of an intensive mosquito eradication campaign. However, eradication was not complete in several islands in the Caribbean, in several countries in the northern regions of South America and in the southern USA. This failure to achieve full eradication, partly because of deficiencies in public health infrastructure and partly because of misguided policy decisions, permitted recolonization by the vector of previously vector-free areas and the re-introduction of all four dengue viruses, providing the setting for epidemic dengue and dengue hemorrhagic fever. As a result, dengue re-emerged with a vengeance in the 1970s and 1980s, causing millions of cases of illness in susceptible populations. The disease is spreading southward to Brazil, Bolivia, Paraguay, Ecuador and Peru, where the mosquito finds suitable breeding sites in increasingly crowded urban slums.

In the coming century the continuing population explosion will be accompanied by increasing urbanization. Because this population growth will occur predominantly in developing countries, an inevitable consequence will be creation of ever larger and more numerous overcrowded urban slums. These countries will often not have the financial resources (or sometimes the political will) to provide adequate sanitation and running water, thus encouraging *A. aegypti* to proliferate. Travel of dengue-infected persons to these mosquito breeding grounds will allow dengue to emerge in previously unaffected areas. In addition, the habitat of the mosquito will be further expanded by global warming that will permit it to breed in higher, previously inhospitable areas.

Much of this scenario could have been avoided if mosquito eradication had been complete in the 1940s and 1950s. The current spread of dengue into previously uninvolved areas and the predicted future emergence in new geographic areas can probably only be avoided by a vigorous mosquito eradication campaign and by committing financial resources to improve sanitation, provide running water and keep the pipes and water supply systems in adequate repair.

There are many other examples from the past and present and likely scenarios for the future that emphasize the inter-relatedness of the risk factors. For example, the HIV epidemic puts a huge burden on the health resources of developing countries, taking monies away from other infection-preventing or infection-controlling activities. The millions of dead and incapacitated are mainly the younger, more productive members of society. Their removal increases socioeconomic stresses, as will the presence of millions of AIDS orphans. The consequent increase in poverty will in turn increase the amount of malnutrition, thus providing a setting for emergence and re-emergence of a variety of infectious diseases.

If the incidence and severity of outbreaks of emerging and re-emerging infections is largely based on these social, economic and

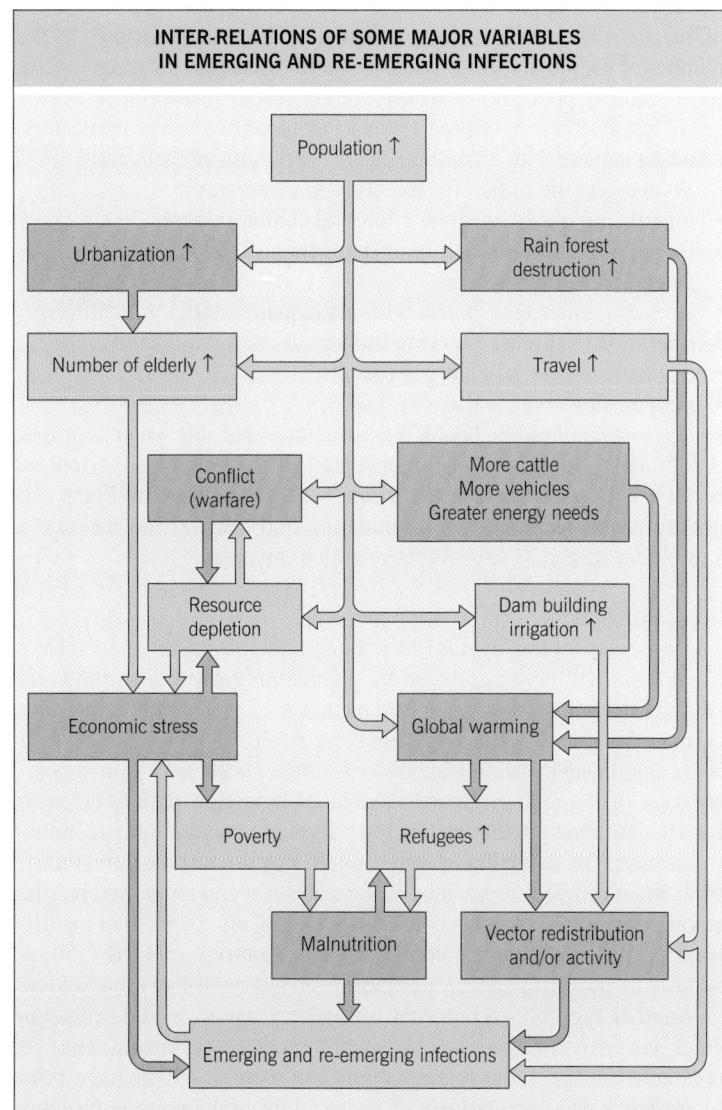

INTER-RELATIONS OF SOME MAJOR VARIABLES IN EMERGING AND RE-EMERGING INFECTIONS

Population ↑
Urbanization ↑
Rain forest destruction ↑
Number of elderly ↑
Travel ↑
Conflict (warfare)
More cattle More vehicles Greater energy needs
Resource depletion
Dam building irrigation ↑
Economic stress
Global warming
Poverty
Refugees ↑
Malnutrition
Vector redistribution and/or activity
Emerging and re-emerging infections

Fig. 5.22 Inter-relatedness of some major variables in emerging and re-emerging infections.

SOCIAL, ECONOMIC AND ENVIRONMENTAL VARIABLES THAT CAN BE MODIFIED TO REDUCE IMPACT OF INFECTIOUS DISEASE

Variables	Potential remedial or preventive actions
Population growth	Make population control a top priority
	Increase expenditures on family planning
Greenhouse effect	Decrease use of fossil fuels
	Increase use of renewable energy sources
	Decrease industrial and automobile emissions
	Control deforestation
Effects of urbanization	Better sanitation
	Adequate running water
	Better housing
Inadequate protection against disease	Commit the modest resources needed to immunize the world's children
Unsafe water	Commit modest resources to provide potable water; improve public health infrastructures
Inadequate water supply	Recycling, desalination
Swelling refugee populations	Control population growth and greenhouse effect
	Improve economic status
	Create international controls to stop wars
Construction of large dams, irrigation	Better planning
	Require infectious diseases impact statement before construction permitted
Overprescription of antibiotics	Institute better controls
	Consider developing more narrow-spectrum agents
Sexual behavior	Better education, greater availability of condoms
	Develop better vaginal microbicides
	Greater assumption of personal responsibility

Fig. 5.23 Social, economic and environmental variables that can be modified to reduce impact of infectious disease.

CDC STRATEGY: COMPLEMENTARY APPROACHES TO MONITORING INFECTIOUS DISEASES

- Strengthening the National Notifiable Disease System(s)
- Establishing population-based centers focused on epidemiology and prevention of emerging and re-emerging infections
- Establishing sentinel surveillance networks
- Developing a system for enhanced surveillance

Fig. 5.24 CDC strategy: complementary approaches to monitoring infectious diseases. Adapted from Sivard.[40]

Even with such an optimistic scenario, it seems evident that in the next century we will experience a variety of emerging and re-emerging infection epidemics. The nature of our world is such that some of them will be devastating, involving millions of people and moving with stunning rapidity. They will challenge our scientific ingenuity and our ability to respond. The frequency and severity of such emerging and re-emerging infection epidemics will to some extent be determined by our ability to predict their occurrence and by the vigor of our prospective actions either to prevent them entirely or to mitigate their consequences.

CONSEQUENCES OF EMERGING AND RE-EMERGING INFECTIONS FOR HEALTH CARE SYSTEMS

As a matter of public policy, there is a compelling need for monitoring and surveillance of emerging and re-emerging infections among humans and animals. The economic impact of a 'new' disease may be difficult to measure at the beginning of its dissemination but may represent a real threat and a source of concern.

The reaction of the infectious disease community and of governments to the threats posed by 'new' diseases should include increased surveillance, adequate public health infrastructure, primary prevention and adequate communication. The strategy developed by the Centers for Disease Control and Prevention (CDC) is briefly described in Figure 5.24.

To reach these goals, national and international sentinel networks, together with microbiology laboratories connected with central organizations such as the CDC, are needed to detect changes in the frequency and presentation of infectious diseases[43] and to perform prompt epidemiologic investigations. 'Lessons learned from the emergence of new diseases and the resurgence of old ones may help us prepare for future epidemics.'[44]

Development of efficient collaboration among agencies, optimal use of resources, diffusion of knowledge among doctors, health care workers and the public and the responsible use of drugs and vaccines are among the main priorities. Effective public health communication among countries may limit the extent of outbreaks and promote effective prevention strategies across borders.[43] A multidisciplinary holistic approach is essential for managing diseases of living organisms affecting humans as well as animals and plants.[45]

In the meantime, effective communication of the risk of infectious diseases is essential to avoid or minimize excessive fear, to engage patients and the public in decisions and actions aimed at reducing risks and to provide a basis for dialog among health providers, the public, scientists and health authorities.[46,47] As laboratory science provides cumulative refinement of health knowledge, social science can enhance the efficiency of communications of the risks of infectious diseases.

environmental variables, then infectious disease experts and other health personnel should examine the determinants of these variables and consider infectious disease scenarios for coming decades so that they may influence policy decisions that could beneficially affect the nature and severity of these determinants.

Most of the variables that promote infectious diseases are not immutable. They can potentially be modified by prudent human actions (Fig. 5.23). The vexing question is whether we have the foresight and willpower to take the necessary steps to avoid conditions that will promote emerging and re-emerging infections.

The future of infectious disease will be unalterably and unpredictably changed by the deciphering of the genome and the applications of gene modification, and by development of novel vaccines and vaccine vehicles. Once the genomic basis for susceptibility to or progression of certain infections is understood, scientists will have the tools to anticipate infections and potentially prevent them by gene modification or stabilization, or by administration of gene products. Alternatively, gene products or their derivatives will be used in the earlier phases of infections to prevent progression or hasten recovery.

It may well be that general resistance to a variety of infections will be genetically defined, opening the possibility of conferring such resistance on virtually everybody, and thereby altering profoundly the effects of some of the variables discussed above.

REFERENCES

1. The World Health Report 1996. Fighting disease. Fostering development. Geneva, Switzerland: WHO; 1996.

2. Lorber B. Are all diseases infectious? Ann Intern Med 1996;125:844–51.

3. Pinner RW, Teutsch SM, Simonsen L, et al. Trends in infectious diseases mortality in the United States. JAMA 1996;275:189–93.

4. Gao SJ, Moore PS. Molecular approaches to the identification of unculturable infectious agents. Emerg Infect Dis 1996;2:159–67.

5. Cohen ML. Epidemiology of drug resistance: implications for a post-antimicrobial era. Science 1992;257:1050–5.

6. Kunin CM. Resistance to antimicrobial drugs: a worldwide calamity. Ann Intern Med 1993;118:557–61.

7. Hossain MM, Glass RI, Khan MR. Antibiotic use in a rural community in Bangladesh. Int J Epidemiol 1982;11:402–5.

8. Wolff MJ. Use and misuse of antibiotics in Latin America. Clin Infect Dis 1993;17(suppl 2):S346–51.

9. Gold HS, Moellering RC Jr. Antimicrobial-drug resistance. N Engl J Med 1996;335:1445–53.

10. Seppälä H, Klaukka T, Lehtonen R, Nenonen E, The Finnish Study Group for Antimicrobial Resistance, Huovinen P. Outpatient use of erythromycin: link to increased erythromycin resistance in group A streptococci. Clin Infect Dis 1995;21:1378–85.

11. Nissinen A, Grönroos P, Huovinen P, et al. Development of β-lactamase-mediated resistance to penicillin in middle-ear isolates of Moraxella catarrhalis in Finnish children, 1978–1993. Clin Infect Dis 1995;21:1193–6.

12. Guillemot D, Carbon C, Balkan B, et al. Low dosage and long treatment duration of β-lactam: risk factors for the carriage of penicillin-resistant Streptococcus pneumoniae. JAMA 1998; in press.

13. Shay DK, Maloney SA, Montecalvo M, et al. Epidemiology and mortality risk of vancomycin-resistant enterococcal bloodstream infections. J Infect Dis 1995;172:993–1000.

14 Anti-tuberculosis drug resistance in the world. The WHO/IUATLD Global Project in Anti-tuberculosis drug resistance surveillance. Geneva, Switzerland: WHO;1997.

15. Park MM, Davis AL, Schluger NW, Cohen H, Rom WN. Outcome of MDR-TB patients, 1983–1993. Prolonged survival with appropriate therapy. Am J Respir Crit Care Med 1996;153:317–24.

16. Denning DW. Can we prevent azole resistance in fungi? Lancet 1995;346:454–5.

17. Kimberlin DW, Whitley RJ. Antiviral resistance: mechanisms, clinical significance and future implications. J Antimicrob Chemother 1996;37:403–27.

18. Condra JH, Schleif WA, Blahy OM, et al. In vivo emergence of HIV-1 variants resistant to multiple protease inhibitors. Nature 1995;374:569–71.

19. Louria DB. Emerging and re-emerging infections: the societal variables. Int J Infect Dis 1996;1:59–62.

20. Lutz W. The future of World population. Population Bulletin No 49. Washington DC: Population Reference Bureau; June 1994.

21. Hunter JM, Rey L, Chu KY, et al. Parasitic diseases in water resources development. Geneva: WHO; 1993.

22. Crews KA. Human needs and nature's balance. Population, resources and the environment. Washington DC: Population Reference Bureau; 1987.

23. Patz JA, Epstein PR, Burke TA, Balbus JM. Global climate change and emerging infectious diseases. JAMA 1996;275:217–23.

24. Haines A. Global warming and health: the changes expected in the world's climate will worsen health in many ways. Br Med J 1991;302:669–70.

25. Houghton JT, Filho LGM, Callander BA, et al. Climate change 1995. The science of climate change. Contribution of WGI to the second assessment report of the intergovernmental panel on climate change. Cambridge, England: Cambridge University Press; 1996.

26. Khalil MAK, ed. Atmospheric methane: sources, sinks and role in global change. Berlin, Heidelberg: Springer-Verlag; 1993.

27. Kuno G. Review of factors modulating dengue transmission. Epidemiol Rev 1995;17:321–35.

28. Rogers DJ, Packer MJ. Vector borne diseases, models, and global change. Lancet 1993;342:1282–4.

29. Cook GC. Effect of global warming on the distribution of parasitic and other infectious diseases: a review. J R Soc Med 1992;85:688–92.

30. Toole MJ, Waldman RJ. Refugees and displaced persons. JAMA 1993;270:600–5.

31. Kinsella K, Taeuber CM. An aging World II. US Bureau of the Census, International Population Reports, 1992, P-25 92–3. Washington DC: US Government Printing Office, 1992.

32. Wayne SJ, Rhyne RL, Garry PJ, Goodwin JS. Cell-mediated immunity as a predictor of morbidity and mortality in subjects over 60. J Gerontol 1990;45:M45–8.

33. Richter M, Jodouin CA. Immunoglobulin synthesis by the B cells of healthy ambulatory elderly is markedly delayed in culture. Aging: Immunology and Infectious Diseases 1991;3:1–10.

34. Nagel JE, Pyle RS, Chrest FJ, Adler WH. Oxidative metabolism and bactericidal capacity of polymorphonuclear leukocytes from normal young and aged adults. J Gerontol 1982;37:529–34.

35. Sen P, Middleton JR, Perez G, Gombert ME, Lee JD, Louria DB. Host defense abnormalities and infections in older persons. Infect Med 1994;11:364–71.

36. Louria DB, Sen P, Sherer CB, Farrer WE. Infections in older patients: a systematic clinical approach. Geriatrics 1993;48:28–34.

37. Gardner G, Perry J. Dam starts up. Vital Signs 1995. Worldwatch Institute. New York: WW Norton and Co; 1995:124–5.

38. Le Guenno B. Emerging viruses. Sci Am 1995;273:56–64.

39. Lintz D, Kapila R, Pilgrim E, et al. Nosocomial salmonella epidemic. Arch Intern Med 1976;136:968–73.

40. Sivard RL. World military and social expenditures. 1993 World Priorities. Washington DC; 1993.

41. MacKenzie WR, Hoxie NJ, Proctor ME, et al. A massive outbreak in Milwaukee of cryptosporidium infection transmitted through the public water supply. N Engl J Med 1994;331:161–7.

42. Halstead SB. Selective primary health care: strategies for control of disease in the developing world. XI Dengue. Rev Infect Dis 1984;6:251–64.

43. Berkelman RL, Bryan RT, Osterholm MT, et al. Infectious disease surveillance: a crumbling foundation. Science 1994; 264:368–70.

44. Levins R, Awerbuch T, Brinkmann U, et al. The emergence of new diseases. Am Sci 1994;82:52–60.

45. Vidaver AK. Emerging and reemerging infectious diseases. Perspectives on plants, animals and humans. American Society for Microbiology News 1996;62:583–5.

46. Glanz K, Yang H. Communicating about risk of infectious diseases. JAMA 1996;275:253–6.

47. Centers for Disease Control and Prevention. Addressing emerging infectious disease threats: a prevention strategy for the United States: executive summary. MMWR 1994;43(RR-5):1–18.

Syndromes by Body System

David T Durack, Roger G Finch & Allan R Ronald

2

Viral Exanthems

Barbara A Bannister

This chapter discusses those infections characterized by the eruption of widespread skin lesions (an exanthem). Although their etiologies differ, they share a number of features:
- many are highly infectious by the airborne route;
- the viral agents are shed in oropharyngeal secretions;
- exposure and infection usually occur in childhood;
- epidemics and large outbreaks are common in susceptible groups;
- infections in adults tend to be more severe, with complications; and
- infections in pregnancy can be detrimental to the fetus.

In spite of these similarities, each disease is discussed individually because each has its own etiology and clinical behavior.

MEASLES (RUBEOLA)

EPIDEMIOLOGY

Measles is highly infectious. In most populations, 95% or more of adults are seropositive. Transmission is usually by airborne droplet spread, which is important in hospitals and other institutions. Viruses are shed from the respiratory mucosa during the prodrome and evolution of the rash; in adults excretion can persist for 6 days after the rash begins.

In nonimmune communities, large epidemics occur in the spring and early summer of alternate years. Maternally derived immunity is effective up to age 6–9 months. The peak age of infection is about 4 years. In small and isolated communities, epidemics occur at less frequent intervals; they affect a wider age range and result in a higher mortality.

Death occurs in approximately 1 in 4000 cases in developed countries, usually in debilitated or immunocomprised individuals. In malnourished populations fatality rates reach 10–15%, mainly bacterial complications.

PATHOGENESIS AND PATHOLOGY

Measles virus is a member of the *Paramyxoviridae*, a family of enveloped, negative single-stranded RNA viruses. CD46 acts as a receptor for measles virus, probably in association with moesin. The virus also binds to CD46 on macrophages, inhibiting their participation in T-lymphocyte and cytotoxic natural-killer-cell activation.[1] Viral ribonucleocapsids are assembled in the host cell nucleus and accumulate as inclusion bodies in the cytoplasm. Virions acquire matrix protein, and leave the host cell by budding, deriving their envelope from the host cell membrane. Infected host cells often coalesce to form multinucleate giant cells.

Once virus has replicated in respiratory mucosal cells, it invades the local lymph nodes. Within 4–6 days viruses are detectable in the plasma and in blood mononuclear cells, particularly lymphocytes. By about 8 days the virus is detectable in the liver, spleen, lung, respiratory epithelia and eye, and has recently been demonstrated in endothelium in the central nervous system. The rash reflects viral invasion of the skin, with, accumulation of immune complexes and mononuclear cell infiltration.

In subacute sclerosing panencephalitis (SSPE) virus ribonucleocapsids are seen in neurons, but have defective expression of matrix protein; no virus release occurs and giant cells do not develop. In the presence of interferon-α these defects are rectified and the neuronal infection regains the ability to produce virus.[2]

PREVENTION

PRE-EXPOSURE PROPHYLAXIS

Live-attenuated measles vaccines, introduced in the 1960s, rapidly controlled epidemic disease. However, immunization before the age of 9–12 months produces short-lasting immunity, whereas immunization at the age of 1 year or more leaves a window of susceptibility between the loss of maternally derived protection and vaccine-induced protection; furthermore, vaccine uptake rates of over 95% are needed to prevent the spread of measles, emphasizing the need for effective immunization policies.[3]

A two-dose immunization program is used: the first dose at the age of 13 months (or at 6–9 months in developing countries in which measles threatens young infants), followed by a booster at 3–5 years of age. Adverse effects include:
- a mild feverish illness, rarely with a transient rash ('mini-measles') after 7 days in approximately 10% of first immunizations; and
- mild allergic reactions such as urticaria or other rashes (anaphylaxis is exceptionally rare).

About 96% of recipients seroconvert satisfactorily. Outbreak investigations show that approximately 4% of exposed vaccinees suffer from clinical measles.

Inactivated vaccine, available in the 1950s, was less effective; some recipients developed measles and suffered modified disease, with severe lung involvement and/or exfoliation. Other highly immunogenic vaccines exist and are effective at the age of 2–3 months, but there are concerns that their immunomodulatory effects may predispose recipients to other severe childhood infections.

POSTEXPOSURE PROPHYLAXIS

Human normal immunoglobulin is effective in preventing measles. It should be given early, preferably within 3 days of exposure. The recommended dose for immunoglobulin to prevent an attack of measles is as follows:
- age under 1 year – 250mg immunoglobulin,
- age 1–2 years – 500mg immunoglobulin,
- age 3 years and over – 750mg immunoglobulin.

CLINICAL FEATURES

THE PRODROMAL ILLNESS

After an incubation period of 9–11 days illness begins abruptly with high, swinging fever, irritability, nasal and conjunctival discharge, repetitive 'croupy' cough and, often, loose stools. Febrile convulsions are common in young children. Chest auscultation reveals many moist sounds, but impaired respiratory function is rare.

Koplik's spots are pathognomonic of prodromal measles. They appear in the buccal mucosa, usually opposite the upper premolars but may affect the whole inner cheek. White and irregular, their size varies from 'salt grains' to 'small breadcrumbs' and they are superimposed on a highly inflamed mucosa. They disappear by the second day of the rash and may be absent in the vaccinated individual.

EVOLUTION OF THE RASH
The rash begins on the third to fifth day of fever. It is maculopapular, extending downward from the ears and hairline, reaching the hips by the next day and the lower legs by the following one (Fig. 1.1). After 4 days, it changes from pink to purplish and the fever abates quickly, marking the end of viremia. The rash fades without desquamation in 4–7 days.

In dark-skinned patients the rash may be invisible, but the papular element causes a 'gooseflesh' appearance. In severe measles (which is more common in adults than children) or in immunosuppressed patients there may be a hemorrhagic component, with desquamation on healing.

OTHER FEATURES
There is often mild neutropenia, with a white cell count of $3-4 \times 10^9/L$.[4] Significant thrombocytopenia is rare. Liver transaminases and pancreatic amylase may be elevated, particularly in adults, although frank jaundice and pancreatitis are rare.

Marked suppression of cell-mediated immunity occurs during the illness and for weeks afterward, with negative recall skin-test reactions.

COMPLICATIONS
Secondary bacterial infections
These are common and often severe. Acute suppurative otitis media and pyogenic bronchopneumonia are the most frequent. In addition to *Streptococcus pneumoniae* and *Haemophilus influenzae*, *Staphylococcus aureus* is an important secondary invader (Fig. 1.2).

When poor hygiene, crowding or malnourishment exist, severe infection of macerated perioral or perinasal skin (cancrum oris) may be caused by pyogenic organisms, often accompanied by herpes simplex and/or anaerobic mouth flora (Fig. 1.3). A cloudy or punctate keratopathy with secondary bacterial keratoconjunctivitis may threaten sight. Tuberculosis may be unmasked or contracted during the immunosuppressed phase.

Postinfectious encephalitis
Postinfectious encephalitis occurs in approximately 1 in 800–1600 cases, and has a mortality of 12–15%. Up to 50% of survivors have neurologic sequelae of varying severity (see Chapter 2.20).

Subacute sclerosing panencephalitis
Subacute sclerosing panencephalitis occurs in approximately 1 in 1 million cases, particularly if measles occurred before the age of 2 years. After 3–10 years clumsiness and poor school performance herald the onset of myoclonic spasms with typical electroencephalographic changes; decerebration and death occur within 2 years.

Other associations of measles virus
Measles virus RNA has been demonstrated in the ossicles of patients with otosclerosis, and in osteoclasts of patients with Paget's disease. Crohn's disease has been described after intrauterine or early childhood measles, but the virus has not been demonstrated conclusively in affected bowel tissue.

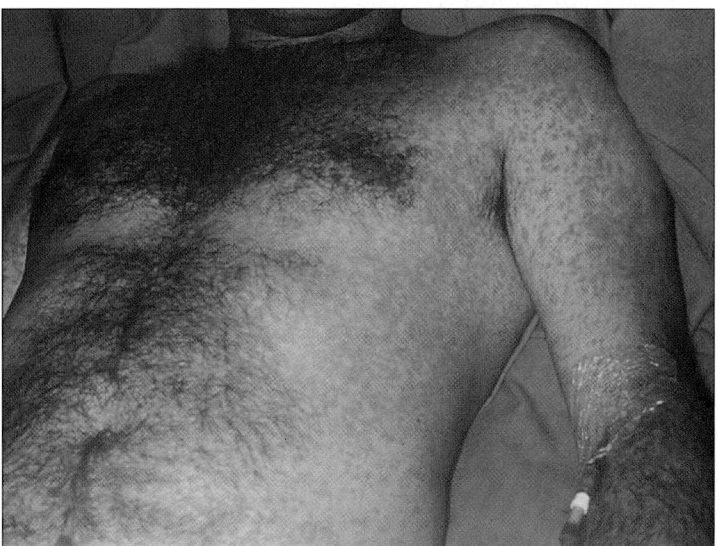

Fig. 1.1 The acute rash of measles. Marked conjunctivitis accompanied the maculopapular skin lesions in this unimmunized adult.

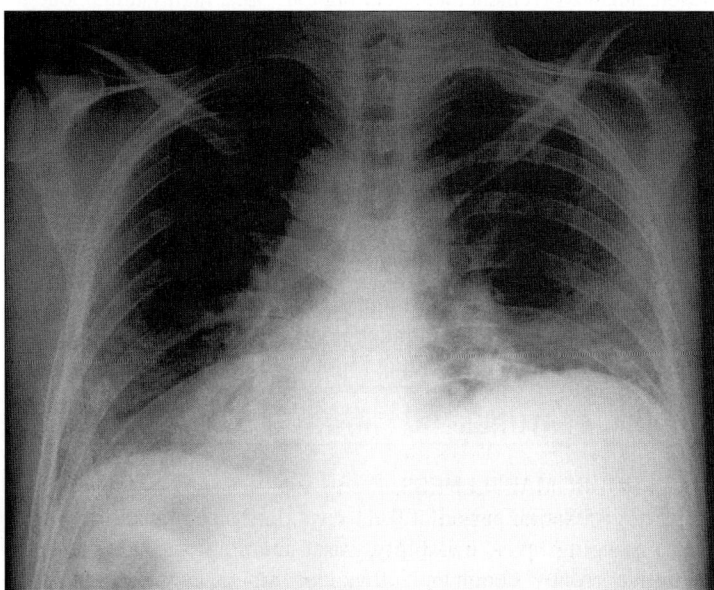

Fig. 1.2 Secondary invasion by S. *aureus* in measles. Ill defined basal opacities were seen in a patient who had moderate respiratory failure; S. *aureus* was isolated from sputum (same patient as Fig. 1.1).

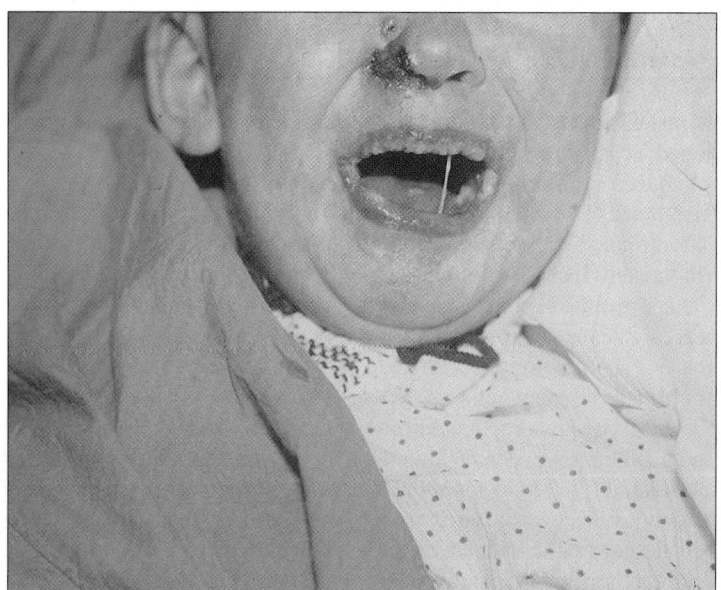

Fig. 1.3 Secondary infections complicating measles. Perioral infection and paranasal herpes simplex lesion in a 2-year-old girl.

DIAGNOSIS

Diagnosis is usually clinical but should be confirmed by laboratory tests, particularly during measles eradication programs.

Measles virus is difficult to recover from cell cultures, although it will grow in primary primate or human cell lines. Serodiagnosis is sensitive using IgM enzyme-linked immunosorbent assay (ELISA) detection in serum or saliva samples. In SSPE there are very high levels of IgG antibodies, with evidence of local production in the cerebrospinal fluid (CSF). High levels measles-specific of IgG are found in the perilymph in otosclerosis. Bronchial lavage may demonstrate multinucleate giant cells, intracytoplasmic inclusion bodies and measles capsid antigen using immunofluorescence, which is helpful in managing measles pneumonitis in adults and immunosuppressed patients.

MANAGEMENT

ANTIVIRAL DRUGS

Inhaled and intravenous (20–35mg/kg/day) ribavirin (tribavirin) has been used successfully in selected patients with severe viral pneumonitis.[5] Ribavirin does not readily enter the CSF and has not been evaluated in encephalitis, which is probably an immunolopathologic disorder.

Intrathecal interferon-α may delay deterioration in SSPE.

VITAMIN A

Measles mortality is inversely related to serum retinol concentrations. Children from developing countries or those from crowded urban areas of Western countries where health care and nutrition are suboptimal should receive oral vitamin A 10,000IU (age 1 year) or 20,000IU (age 1 year plus) at diagnosis.[6] Children with keratoconjunctivitis should have further doses 1 day and 1 month later.

High-dose vitamin A can be given with measles vaccine, although there is some evidence of reduced seroconversion, possibly because vitamin-induced immune enhancement reduces vaccine virus replication.

RUBELLA

EPIDEMIOLOGY

Rubella virus (rubivirus), a member of the *Togaviridae*, is transmitted from person to person by the airborne route and is only slightly less infectious than measles. An increase in cases occurs every 4–10 years, with larger epidemics every 10–20 years (Fig. 1.4). In susceptible populations the peak age of infection is between 5 and 9 years. In Western countries before the advent of immunization, 15–20% of individuals remained susceptible beyond the age of 20 years. In some tropical countries up to 40% of adults are susceptible.

Although rubella is mild in children and nonpregnant adults, in pregnant women the infection commonly causes severe disease and long-term damage to the developing fetus (see Chapter 2.55).

Recognition of rubella can be difficult, as it is often trivial, subclinical or atypical, mimicking other infections.[8]

PATHOGENESIS AND PATHOLOGY

Togaviridae are enveloped RNA viruses with cubical symmetry. Humans are the only known hosts of rubivirus, and only one serotype is recognized. Culture is possible in a variety of cell lines, but rarely produces a cytopathic effect. Positive cell cultures are identified by immunofluorescence, antigen-detecting ELISA or interference with infection by other viruses such as enteroviruses.

The virus attaches to and invades upper respiratory and pharyngeal mucosal cells. Viral construction and assembly occurs in the cytoplasm, and virions bud into intracytoplasmic vesicles, acquiring their envelope from the host cell membrane. Viral hemagglutinin molecules are

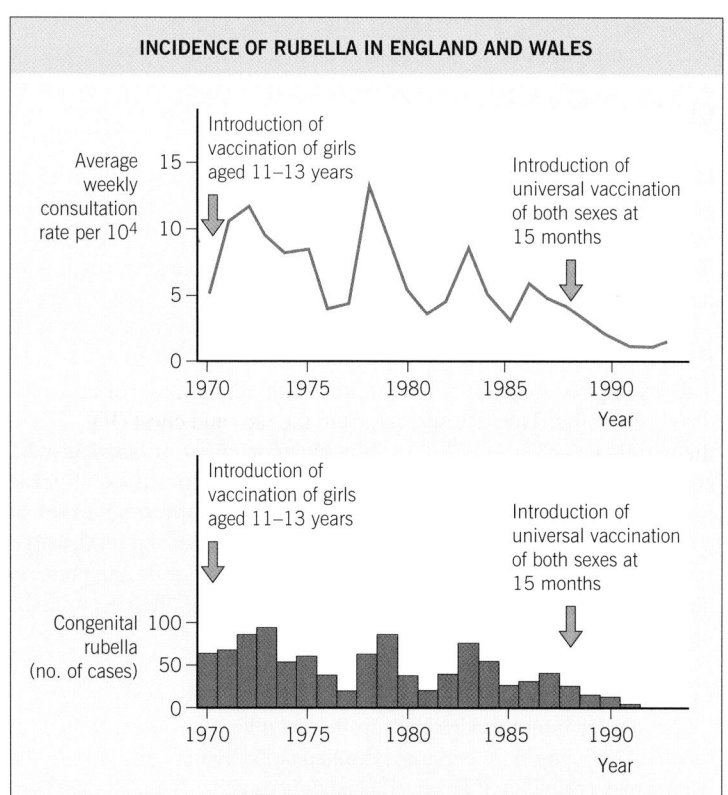

Fig. 1.4 Incidence of rubella in England and Wales. The effects of different immunization programs are shown. Data from Bannister *et al.*[7]

inserted into the envelope. Viremia and pharyngeal shedding are detectable 9 or 10 days after infection, and virus excretion continues for 14–21 days.

Most body tissues can be invaded, including lymphocytes, conjunctiva, synovium, uterine cervix and lymph nodes. Virus is excreted from the nasopharynx and in the stools and urine. The appearance of the rash marks the end of viremia and the production of neutralizing antibodies. Interestingly, men produce earlier and larger antibody responses than women to several rubella antigens, but only women seem to produce antibodies to the second envelope protein E2.[9] Capsid antigens are important in eliciting cytotoxic cell-mediated immunity.[10]

PREVENTION

Live-attenuated rubella vaccines became available in the late 1960s. About 95% of recipients seroconvert and develop hemagglutination-inhibiting antibodies (HI antibodies), which correlate with neutralizing antibody function. Vaccine virus is briefly excreted from the pharynx in the 4 weeks after immunization, but transmission to close contacts does not occur. Other members of a family may therefore be immunized even if a household member is pregnant.

Although HI antibodies decline over 10–16 years after immunization, resistance to re-infection by wild strains wanes little, indicating that vaccine-induced immunity is as durable as that which follows natural infection.[11] Between 1.5 and 4% of vaccinated individuals become re-infected (usually asymptomatically) and exhibit an IgM response after exposure to wild virus. Viremia is transient or absent during most re-infections. Congenital rubella rarely follows re-infection in naturally immune or vaccinated women. Effective immunization, vigilance and readily available screening and diagnostic testing are important in controlling outbreaks and protecting pregnant women.

Postexposure prophylaxis with human normal immunoglobulin has been attempted, but even high doses have not been reliably effective.

CLINICAL FEATURES

Postnatally acquired rubella is usually mild, and in most studies about one-half of seroconversions are asymptomatic. The incubation period is about 15 days (range 14–21 days). The clinical features may appear in any combination, usually developing simultaneously, although joint involvement often follows after 4–7 days.

RASH

This usually coincides with fever, although adults may suffer 1 or 2 days' prodrome. The rash spreads from the face and chest (Fig. 1.5) to the peripheries over 1 or 2 days. It is maculopapular or macular, with small elements, often fading to a 'peach-bloom' appearance after the first day. It rarely lasts more than 3 or 4 days. It mimics the rashes of parvovirus infection (see below), echovirus infections and mild scarlet fever or early Kawasaki disease, although it does not desquamate on healing. Conjunctival itching, soreness and reddening often occur at the onset of illness.

LYMPHADENOPATHY

Large, tender lymph nodes high in the occipital region are typical of rubella, although minor cervical lymphadenopathy may also occur. The patient may complain of localized head or neck pain. The nodes are hard and usually immobile, as they are tightly confined by the cervical fascia.

ARTHRALGIA AND ARTHRITIS

Many adults and some older children complain of marked joint pain late in the illness. The proximal finger joints and wrists are most often affected. Frank arthritis with effusions, soft tissue swelling and erythema can occur; larger joints may also be involved and women are affected more often than men.[12] In some individuals acute polyarthritis resembles rheumatoid arthritis, but subsides over weeks or months. Arthropathy also occurs in parvovirus infection.

COMPLICATIONS
Thrombocytopenia
A modest reduction in the platelet count is common and occasionally causes thrombocytopenic purpura, even if the original infection was subclinical. Severe bleeding is rare, but may occur late in the course of the rash. The platelet count recovers completely within a few weeks.

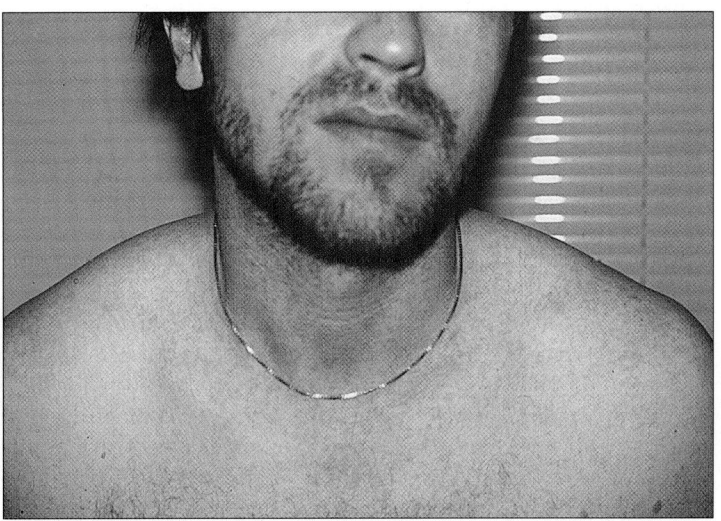

Fig. 1.5 Rubella. This patient had a typical early maculopapular rash, irritating conjunctivitis and painful occipital lymphadenopathy.

Encephalitis
Encephalitis is a rare complication, affecting approximately 1 in 5000 patients. It can occur up to 1 week after the appearance of the rash, but very rarely before it. The onset is abrupt, with irritability, headache and often stiff neck. Lumbar puncture reveals lymphocytes and mildly elevated CSF protein. The electroencephalogram shows widespread slow-wave abnormalities. Convulsions, altered consciousness or neurologic signs may follow, with varying severity. Polyradiculitis occurs rarely.[13] Almost all patients recover fully within 1 week or so, although fatalities and a chronic SSPE-like syndrome have occasionally been reported.

Individual reports exist of rubella-associated cases of hepatitis, pancreatitis and retinal vasculitis. Rubella antigens have been demonstrated in the chondrocytes of patients with Paget's disease.[14]

DIAGNOSIS

Rapid diagnosis depends on the detection of IgM antibodies, using antibody-capture or sandwich ELISA tests and particle agglutination techniques. Immunoglobulin M antibodies are detectable very early in infection and are also useful in diagnosing re-infection in those already immunized. Many polymerase chain reaction (PCR)-based tests are under investigation.

Screening tests for immunity are important, especially in antenatal care. Radial diffusion precipitin or radial hemolysis tests are the most frequently used techniques.

MANAGEMENT

Management is symptomatic. Nonsteroidal anti-inflammatory drugs are effective in treating arthralgia and arthritis, but should be substituted by simple analgesics if there is symptomatic thrombocytopenia.

Severe thrombocytopenia may be treated with prednisolone, or intravenous immunoglobulin followed by a brief reducing course of prednisolone.

Neither corticosteroids nor antiviral agents influence the course of rubella encephalitis.

PARVOVIRUS B19 INFECTION AND ERYTHEMA INFECTIOSUM

EPIDEMIOLOGY

Parvovirus B19, or human serum parvovirus, is the only member of the *Parvoviridae* pathogenic to humans. The *Parvoviridae* are very small, icosahedral, nonenveloped viruses whose genome is a single 5kb strand of DNA. The family includes the adeno-associated viruses, which replicate only in the presence of co-infection with a helper virus. Serologic evidence suggests that some can infect humans asymptomatically. Parvovirus-like structures (small round viruses or small round featureless viruses) can be seen in the stools of patients with acute gastroenteritis and have also been identified in some foods, but have not been speciated.

Parvovirus B19 is common worldwide and is highly transmissible from person to person via respiratory tract secretions; it has an incubation period of 6–10 days. Epidemics occur, peaking in the spring, every 3–5 years, with smaller outbreaks in intervening years. Infection is commonest between the ages of 4 and 10 years and usually manifests as erythema infectiosum (fifth disease or slapped cheek syndrome). In those with disorders causing short red blood cell survival, transient aplastic anemia occurs; in countries in which sickle-cell disease is common epidemics of aplasia occur. Infection probably confers lifelong immunity.

PATHOGENESIS AND PATHOLOGY

Viruses are adsorbed onto protein receptors of the host mucosa and are transported to the nucleus where they uncoat. DNA replication can only occur if the host cell is in the S phase of mitosis. In the mature host infection therefore affects rapidly replicating tissues, such as the bone marrow, reticuloendothelial system and, particularly, red-cell progenitors. The erythrocyte P-antigen acts as a virus receptor.[15] In the fetus, early infection may cause widespread damage and death of the conceptus, whereas later infections affect red-cell precursors (see Chapter 2.55).

Viral replication and assembly takes place in the host-cell nucleus; virions are released by lysis of the nuclear and cytoplasmic membranes. Virus is detectable in throat washings 1 week after infection, and an intense viremia (10^{10}–10^{12} virus particles/ml serum) occurs at the same time.

Viral excretion continues for about 5 days. Infection of erythrocyte precursors causes a profound reticulocytopenia during the second week, whereas the total leukocyte count falls to a lesser extent. Between days 10 and 14, IgM antibodies to capsid antigens appear, terminating the viremia. They remain detectable for 2–3 months. Between the third and fourth week IgG antibody levels rise; these decline slowly over a number of years.

PREVENTION

Parvovirus B19 is extremely difficult to cultivate in the laboratory, and this has delayed vaccine development. Attempts to engineer antigens, for instance in baculovirus systems, hold promise. Quarantine is not an effective means of interrupting transmission, as many infections are subclinical, and the infectious period is over by the time typical clinical features develop.

CLINICAL FEATURES

At least 50% of parvovirus infections are unrecognized. Most recognized infections present with a rash, but other features can occur alone.[16]

RASH (ERYTHEMA INFECTIOSUM)
After 2–4 days of malaise, fever and sweating, erythema of the cheeks appears, often with a slightly raised margin, as though the patient had been slapped (hence the name 'slapped cheek syndrome'). A macular rash appears 1 or 2 days later, spreading from the neck and shoulders to the peripheries in 2–3 days. Clear areas appear in the rash; these cause a reticulate pattern that can persist for 10–14 days, fading to violet and fluctuating with the skin temperature.

Other bizarre rashes may complicate the feverish, viremic phase of illness. Glove and sock purpura is well described, consisting of a mildly itchy, confluent erythema with a marked purpuric element that sometimes resembles a large bruise. I have seen similar rashes affecting the buttocks, perineum and thighs. Despite their intensity, these rashes resolve spontaneously in 4–6 days.

ARTHROPATHY AND ARTHRITIS
The incidence of arthritis is uncertain, as it can occur in the absence of rash or other features. In known cases it ranges from 10 to 33%, being highest in women and lowest in children. The commonest manifestation is polyarthralgia, with particular involvement of the wrists and proximal interphalangeal joints. Monoarthralgia and monoarthritis are also seen, and may cause concern when they manifest as pseudopalsy in a child. Young women may suffer acute polyarthralgia or polyarthritis, with or without rash but usually with noticeable preceding fever. Although most individuals recover in 1–2 weeks, pain and stiffness can persist for several months.

BLOOD AND BONE MARROW DISORDERS
Stem-cell and erythrocyte infection profoundly affect erythropoiesis during the viremic phase. The reticulocyte count is usually negligible or undetectable for 4–6 days, and bone marrow examination shows cessation of red-cell maturation and the presence of giant proerythroblasts. In normal patients this has little effect on the blood count, but in patients with sickle-cell disease, hereditary spherocytosis or severe nutritional anemias, there is transient, profound aplastic anemia. In tropical countries, epidemics of 'aplastic crises' can occur.

Other elements of the blood are less commonly affected; however, mild neutropenia and thrombocytopenia are common. Reticulocyte, platelet and neutrophil counts often rebound to levels well above normal in the 10 days after the fever.

OTHER CLINICAL FEATURES
Reports of hepatitis, meningitis, myocarditis, systemic vasculitis and nephritis have not been unequivocally attributed to parvovirus infection.

COMPLICATIONS
The most important complications are those affecting pregnancy, which include early fetal loss or second-trimester hydrops fetalis (see Chapter 2.55)

Hemophagocytic syndrome has been reported to complicate acute parvovirus infection.

Persistent aplastic anemia can occur when an immunocompromised patient fails to clear replicating virus from the bone marrow stem cells.

Polyarticular juvenile arthritis and refractory rheumatoid arthritis have been associated with an increased likelihood of seropositivity to parvovirus B19.

DIAGNOSIS

The presence of fever plus cytopenias or a very low reticulocyte count should arouse suspicion of parvovirus infection.

In the febrile phase, high titers of virus in the blood permit confirmation by ELISA or immunofluorescence methods of antigen detection or by PCR and identification of parvovirus DNA.

Immunoglobulin M antibodies become detectable at about the onset of the rash, allowing a reliable serologic diagnosis by the sixth to tenth day of illness.

MANAGEMENT

There is no specific antiviral treatment. Most individuals recover without sequelae in 1 or 2 weeks with symptomatic treatment alone. Non-steroidal anti-inflammatory drugs are helpful in persisting arthralgia and arthritis.

There may be enough neutralizing antibody in intravenous immunoglobulin to terminate or limit parvovirus replication in immunosuppressed patients with persisting aplastic anemia.

VARICELLA-ZOSTER VIRUS INFECTIONS (CHICKENPOX AND HERPES ZOSTER)

EPIDEMIOLOGY

Varicella-zoster virus (VZV) is an enveloped alpha-herpesvirus, with icosahedral symmetry and a linear, double-stranded DNA genome. Like other herpesviruses, it causes a primary infection (varicella or chickenpox) with seroconversion, and subsequent lifelong latency. Reactivation causes localized neurologic disease with an associated skin eruption (herpes zoster or shingles). Both primary and reactivation diseases are infectious, although there is less virus shedding from the rash of herpes zoster.

VARICELLA
In developed countries varicella causes winter and spring epidemics, mainly affecting schoolchildren, with a peak incidence at the age of

5–9 years. Maternally derived antibodies protect infants up to the age of 6–9 months. Likewise about 90% of adults are seropositive and immune. By contrast, in the tropics, varicella is less common in children, and seronegativity varies from 20 to 50% in adults.

Varicella-zoster virus is easily transmitted by respiratory secretions, on children's hands or by droplet spread. It also spreads along air currents in buildings such as hospitals.[17] In developed countries, exposure at home carries approximately an 80% risk of infection; in hospital or daycare centers this is about 40–60%. The incubation period varies from 10 to 25 days, averaging 15 days.

The incidence of adult varicella is increasing in several countries. In the UK reports of adult cases have doubled in the past 20 years. This is important, as the disease is more severe in adults; infection in pregnancy may cause fetal loss or damage (see Chapter 2.55). The fatality rate for varicella in the UK is about 1 per 6000 cases, but this rises to approximately 1 per 600 for those aged over 55 years.

HERPES ZOSTER

Herpes zoster reflects infection of a sensory nerve ganglion, its neurologic connections and associated dermatome. It complicates waning immunity, and therefore affects elderly, debilitated and immunocompromised individuals. It may be precipitated by such stresses as another illness, trauma or bereavement, or by immunodeficiency as a result of HIV infection, malignancy or immunosuppressive chemotherapy. There is usually an interval of years between the occurrence of varicella and the eruption of herpes zoster, although varicella in a fetus or infant may be followed by neonatal or childhood zoster.

Close contact with a patient with herpes zoster can lead to varicella in a seronegative person. It is possible that immunity is boosted throughout life by repeated exposure to varicella and zoster in the community.[17]

PATHOGENESIS AND PATHOLOGY

Varicella-zoster virus first infects the respiratory mucosa, where it replicates and invades the lymphatics, leading to asymptomatic primary viremia about 7 days after infection. Further viral replication occurs in most tissues; VZV DNA appears in the peripheral blood mononuclear cells and polymorphs at this stage. Virus replication and assembly takes place in the nucleus of affected cells, producing characteristic 'type A' intranuclear inclusions. Syncytium and giant cell formation occurs. In the skin large, balloon-shaped 'Tzanck' cells, with typical nuclear inclusions, are seen in scrapings from vesicular skin lesions. Varicella-zoster virus is strongly cell-associated, and is more readily demonstrated by antigen detection in respiratory or skin specimens than by culture of secretions or vesicle fluid.

Clinical disease begins with a secondary viremia about 15 days after infection. Focal lesions develop, containing giant cells with intranuclear inclusions. Organs infected include the skin, lungs, gut, reticuloendothelial system and occasionally the brain, retina or joint synovia. In the skin, cell damage and fluid collection separate the layers of the epidermis to produce blistering, at the base of which Tzanck cells are found. Giant-cell vasculitis may play a part in rare neurologic events that precede or follow the classic illness.

Humoral immunity was first demonstrable by fluorescence labeling of antibodies to membrane-associated antigens. These rise progressively throughout the illness, and no clear cut-off predicts susceptibility rather than immunity. Enzyme-linked immunosorbent assay tests are now used to detect IgM and IgG antibodies.[19] Varicella-zoster virus can be cultured, with cytopathic effects in human embryo cell lines.

In spite of cellular and humoral immunity, VZV persists in the body after primary infection. Unlike herpes simplex, it is not detectable by the presence of DNA 'latency sequences'.[20] Messenger ribonucleic acid has been demonstrated in trigeminal ganglion tissue. During reactivation, virus replication and assembly begins in sensory ganglion neurons, subsequently appears in glial cells and is accompanied by intense inflammation. Virus migrates along the dorsal root connections to the central nervous system, causing inflammation and nerve fiber degeneration, and along axons to the skin, where typical VZV skin lesions occur. Local meningeal inflammation surrounds the affected spinal segment and may proceed to a general, viral-type meningitis.

PREVENTION

PRE-EXPOSURE PROPHYLAXIS

Live-attenuated varicella vaccine contains the Oka strain of VZV. It is immunogenic in 94–99% of adolescents and adults when given in two doses 4–8 weeks apart. Breakthrough disease after exposure to wild varicella occurs in 12–20% of vaccinees 5–10 years after immunization, causing a similar secondary infection rate in immunized household contacts. However, the disease is mild, with a median of 20–40 vesicles.[21]

The vaccine can be given to selected immunocompromised individuals, for example children in remission from leukemia, or in the intervals between pulsed chemotherapy courses. A few recipients develop a sparse vesicular rash and may, rarely, infect close contacts with the vaccine strain. The vaccine virus exhibits latency, and can cause herpes zoster, earlier and more commonly in the immunosuppressed. Long-term follow-up will quantify the likelihood of later herpes zoster.

The vaccine is licensed for childhood use in some countries and is available for use on a 'named patient' basis in immunosuppressed individuals in other countries.

POSTEXPOSURE PROPHYLAXIS

Zoster immunoglobulin (ZIG) is a specific human immunoglobulin for intramuscular use, manufactured from the plasma of individuals with high VZV antibody levels (usually after recent varicella). It prevents or modifies varicella even when given 7–10 days after exposure.[22] Zoster immunoglobulin is recommended for:

- immunosuppressed individuals exposed to varicella or disseminated herpes zoster;
- nonimmune pregnant women who have been exposed to varicella or disseminated herpes zoster; and
- the neonate whose mother developed varicella between 7 days before and 28 days after delivery.

If ZIG cannot be given, particularly if intramuscular injection is contraindicated, there is evidence that intravenous immunoglobulin contains sufficient antibody to prevent infection.[23]

Varicella can occur after immunoglobulin prophylaxis. In neonates about 30% of these infections are severe, and in the immunosuppressed all infections are a threat. Antiviral chemotherapy should therefore be given to those with breakthrough infections.

Aciclovir alone has been given prophylactically, in household and institutional settings. A 10-day course prevented clinical disease in both, but larger studies are required to define the effective dose and duration of prophylaxis.[24]

CLINICAL FEATURES

VARICELLA

Childhood varicella is often first recognized when the rash appears. Adults more often have a 1–3 days' prodromal, influenza-like illness.

RASH

Lesions begin as papules, but progress within hours to clear vesicles surrounded by a variable halo of erythema. Vesicles are often oval, with the long axis parallel to skin creases, and are commonly pruritic. New lesions appear progressively over 5–7 days. The head and upper trunk are affected first and most densely, whereas the limbs have fewer lesions and these appear later. The rash is exaggerated and appears earlier in hot areas of skin, for instance under a diaper or occlusive dressing.

The vesicular fluid opacifies and in 2 or 3 days a central dimple appears. A crust then forms from this center outward, and falls away after about 5 days (Fig. 1.6). Unless secondary infection has occurred, scarring is limited to faint, pale outlines. The rash is accompanied by variable fever. Secondary cases in households are often more severely ill than the index case.

The density of the rash indicates the severity of varicella. Indicators of severe disease include confluence of the rash, multiple lesions in the mouth, pharynx and genital mucosae, and retrosternal or epigastric pain (presumably caused by tracheal and esophageal lesions).

Patients are infectious from the prodromal period until the skin lesions scab, although virus rapidly becomes undetectable after the sixth day of uncomplicated illness.

VARICELLA PNEUMONITIS
Varicella is always accompanied by a giant cell pneumonitis, but this is not usually clinically significant. Adolescents and adults (especially cigarette smokers) with severe rashes are at increased risk of respiratory disease. The first sign is a drop in arterial oxygen saturation (Fig. 1.7), followed within hours by respiratory symptoms, or abnormal sounds on auscultation. Pneumonitis varies widely in severity. In patients with severe pneumonitis there is cough with mucoid or blood-stained sputum and respiratory failure, which may prove fatal. Co-existing bacterial infection must always be suspected. The chest X-ray may show ground-glass changes, widespread nodular opacities (chickenpox lung) or segmental shadows.

HEPATITIS
Elevation of transaminase levels to three times the upper limit or more is most often seen in adults, particularly men, who suffer more severe disease. Clinical jaundice is rare.

THROMBOCYTOPENIA
Mild thrombocytopenia is common in adults, particularly men, and may cause a petechial rash and hematuria. The skin vesicles are then hemorrhagic. In severe varicella, platelet and vascular damage may lead to disseminated intravascular coagulation.

RARE FEATURES OF VARICELLA
Rare features of varicella include:
- transient cerebellar disturbance with ataxia and vertigo; this occurs in convalescence in about 1 in 4000 cases and mostly affects males;
- encephalitis, which may be of rapid onset with focal signs, seizures or coma; most patients recover, although a few, often those with imaging evidence of cerebral infarcts, suffer permanent sequelae;

- retinitis, which can occur immediately or after several weeks' delay, is often severe and may be associated with lasting visual impairment.

Occasionally, cerebral or retinal disease precedes the rash or occurs alone.

NEONATAL VARICELLA
Neonatal varicella affects neonates born to seronegative mothers and thus they lack maternally derived immunity. It is a severe, multisystem disease with lung, kidney, bone marrow and brain involvement, and a resulting case-fatality rate of 25–40%. The risk of severe disease rapidly decreases: after 4 weeks of age varicella is no longer dangerous. The source of varicella is often the perinatally infected mother. The infant will not acquire adequate antibody levels until the mother is 7 days into her clinical illness. Babies born before this, or exposed in the first 4 weeks of life, require varicella prophylaxis.

HERPES ZOSTER
Herpes zoster is heralded by pain in the dermatome served by the affected sensory root, which sometimes resembles pleurisy or abdominal pathology. Occasionally in children it manifests as a viral meningitis with increased lymphocytes in the CSF.

Groups of papules then appear at the sites where cutaneous nerves reach the skin. In a spinal nerve this is just lateral to the spine, in the midaxillary line and just lateral to the linea alba. This may not progress further; however, in adults it usually extends to fill the dermatome unilaterally. Some dermatomes are more often affected than others, possibly reflecting the denser areas of the preceding varicella rash.

The papules progress to vesicles, pustules and crusts but, unlike varicella, lesions may become confluent and form large, flaccid bullae that rupture to leave weeping bare areas. Uncomplicated lesions can heal in 4–6 days, but severe rashes may take 3–5 weeks. Nevertheless, skin depigmentation is often the only sequel. Scarring is rare.

OPHTHALMIC HERPES ZOSTER
The commonest cranial dermatome affected is the ophthalmic branch of the trigeminal nerve. The conjunctiva is usually inflamed and swollen, with associated edema of the eyelid; in severe cases, kerato-conjunctivitis can cause prolonged blurred vision and, rarely, corneal scarring. Nasociliary involvement (evidenced by vesicles on the tip of

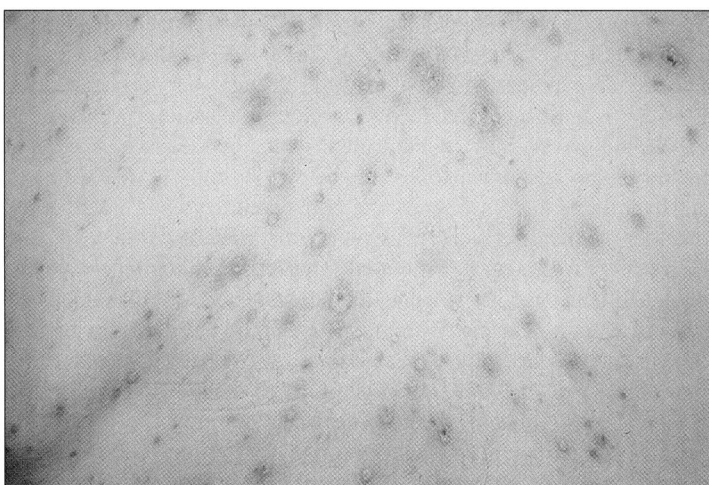

Fig. 1.6 The lesions of varicella. Papules, vesicles and pustules, some of which are beginning to crust from the center are seen.

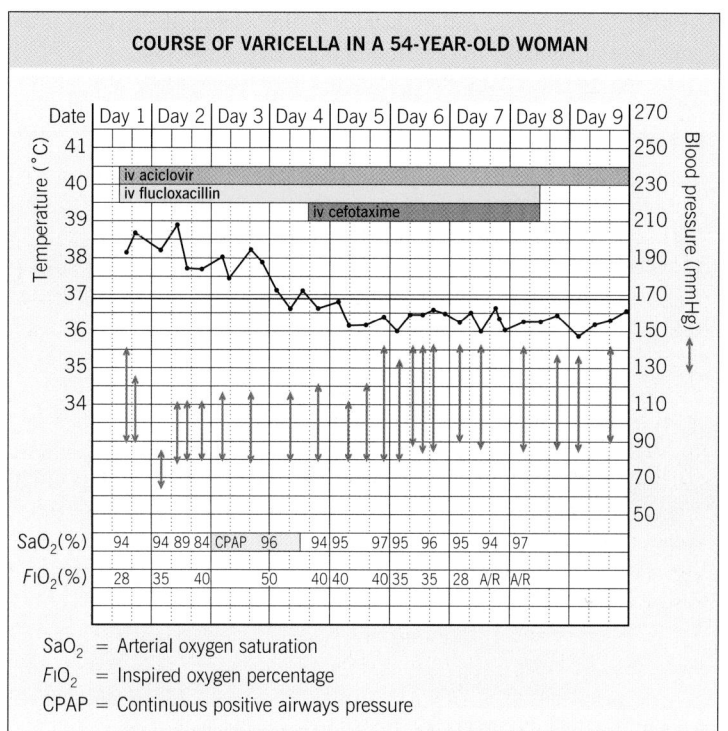

Fig. 1.7 Course of varicella in a 54-year-old woman. Low arterial oxygen saturation precedes respiratory and hemodynamic failure.

the nose) indicates inflammation of the uveal tract, with pain, blurred vision and the risk of synechiae of the iris.

GENICULATE HERPES ZOSTER (RAMSAY HUNT SYNDROME)

In this rare syndrome the geniculate nucleus of the facial nerve is involved, affecting sensory neurons that serve the skin in the external auditory meatus. Vesicles are often seen in the ear, but inflammation and swelling also compress the facial and auditory nerves. There is unilateral facial palsy, deafness and severe vertigo, often with prostration and vomiting. If the chorda tympani is involved, there is also loss of taste sensation on the anterior two-thirds of the tongue.

ZOSTER-ASSOCIATED PAIN AND POST-HERPETIC NEURALGIA

The tingling pain of herpes zoster recedes with healing, but older patients are at risk of persisting pain. This is often distressing, causalgic (not related in quality to the mild stimulus which causes it) and severe. Its average duration in those aged over 60 years is about 60 days, but it can last much longer and, rarely, persists permanently. This pain has been called post-herpetic neuralgia and has been given various definitions, for example pain after rash healing, or pain continuing more than 1 month after herpes zoster. It is now more correctly included in the whole continuum of pain caused by herpes zoster and is called zoster-associated pain (ZAP).

COMPLICATIONS

Secondary bacterial skin infection

Secondary bacterial skin infection is the commonest complication of varicella. Children are twice as likely as adults to have significant skin infection, particularly severe or toxin-mediated disease (Fig. 1.8). Eczema does not predispose individuals to more severe varicella or to worse secondary infection.

Bacterial infection of individual spots causes pain, induration and often abscess formation. The usual pathogens are *S. aureus* or *Streptococcus pyogenes*. Local extension can cause cellulitis or erysipelas. Bacteremia occasionally coexists. Children are particularly prone to staphylococcal or streptococcal toxic shock syndromes, perhaps because they lack antibodies to the exotoxins. Necrotizing fasciitis is rare and affects adults or children.

Secondary bacterial infection can also complicate herpes zoster, especially when severe and in the elderly. In ophthalmic herpes zoster, bacterial conjunctivitis or keratoconjunctivitis can occur.

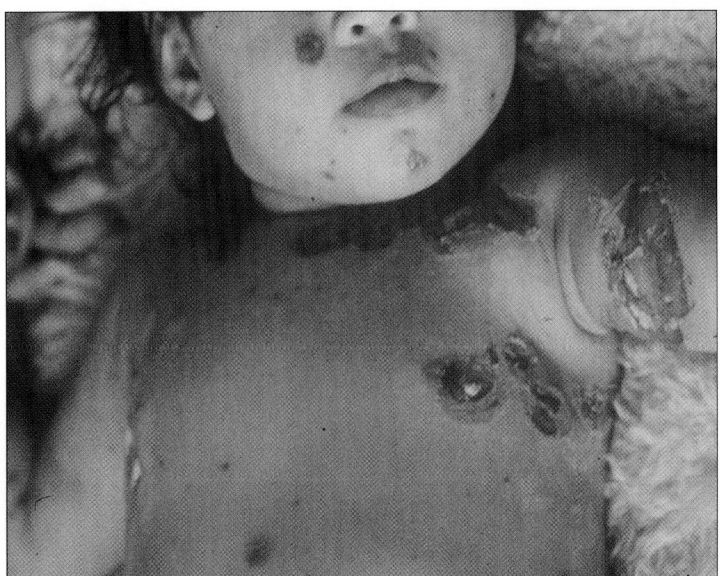

Fig. 1.8 Secondary staphylococcal infection of varicella lesions.
Staphylococcal pyrogenic exotoxin has caused a 'scalded skin' type of lesion surrounding the infected spots. Courtesy of Dr MG Brook.

Bacterial lung infections

These can exist alone or complicate varicella pneumonitis. They are less important than skin infections in children, even in those with a history of asthma, but are more common in adults.

Staphylococcus aureus is the commonest pathogen, but other chest pathogens occasionally occur. It is difficult to distinguish bacterial or mixed infection from viral pneumonia, especially as staphylococcal infection does not always cause an early neutrophilia. If doubt exists, bacterial infection should be assumed.

Motor paralysis in herpes zoster

Herpes zoster is occasionally associated with paralysis of muscle groups innervated from the affected dermatome. The quadriceps may be affected in lumbar zoster; diaphragmatic paralysis is sometimes seen in supraclavicular zoster. Transient paralytic ileus can occur in dorsal zoster. Electromyographic studies of affected muscles show evidence of axonal dysfunction. Gradual recovery is usual, but some residual weakness may persist.

Ascending myeloencephalitis

This is an exceptionally rare complication of herpes zoster, more common in immunosuppressed individuals. Successive involvement of higher spinal and cerebral levels first causes transverse myelitis, with pain, sensory and motor 'level's, and long-tract signs. These extend until cerebral irritability and coma supervene. There is a significant chance of recovery with vigorous antiviral treatment, depending on the severity of any underlying disease.

Varicella-zoster infection in the immunosuppressed

Cell-mediated immunosuppression predisposes individuals to severe VZV infections that result in progressive multisystem disease, often with a deceptively indolent onset. VZV is also recognized as one of the earlier opportunistic infections seen in patients who have AIDS (see Chapter 5.11). In severe immunosuppression, abnormal hemorrhagic lesions may develop without becoming vesicular, although the rash is distributed normally. Rarely, pneumonitis can exist without the rash, or retinitis occurs long after infection. Systemic corticosteroids during the incubation and prodrome are thought to predispose individuals to severe disease. A necrotizing cerebritis can appear in severely immuno-compromised hosts resulting in a syndrome resembling a brain abscess. A biopsy is necessary to establish the diagnosis.

Herpes zoster occurs earlier, more frequently and more severely in the immunosuppressed, often with deep, scarring lesions. Dissemination may occur, leading to varicella-like disease.

MANAGEMENT

VARICELLA-ZOSTER VIRUS INFECTIONS

The nucleoside analog aciclovir is licensed for the treatment of varicella. The oral dose is 800mg five times daily for 5–7 days, but, even with this maximal dose, predose troughs below the mean inhibitory concentration for VZV often occur. Valaciclovir, a prodrug of aciclovir, has much enhanced bioavailability, being well absorbed by the gut mucosa. It is hydrolyzed to release aciclovir. Famciclovir is similarly well absorbed and hydrolyzed to release penciclovir. Both prodrugs are licensed for the treatment of herpes zoster, but as yet not for varicella.

Antiviral treatment has minimal impact on mild childhood infections and is not recommended. In adolescents and in uncomplicated adult disease, oral aciclovir shortens the duration of illness by up to 1 day, and may reduce the risk of complications. Treatment commencing more than 1 or 2 days after the onset of rash is unlikely to influence the course of uncomplicated disease.

Intravenous aciclovir is the treatment of choice for severe or complicated VZV infections. A dose of 5–10mg/kg q8h is given by intravenous infusion over at least 1 hour. This avoids high peak blood levels and consequent renal impairment. Aciclovir is excreted by the kidney, and doses or dosing intervals must be altered if the creatinine clearance is below 60ml/min. Other side effects are mild and include nausea and occasional rashes. The dose may be increased to 15mg/kg in urgent cases, but renal function must be closely monitored.

In herpes zoster of the middle-aged and elderly, treatment started in the first 48 hours after the onset of the rash reduces the duration of the rash and the duration of ZAP. Ophthalmic and geniculate herpes zoster should always be treated in order to reduce the risk of severe eye inflammation or permanent facial or vestibular nerve damage.

SECONDARY BACTERIAL INFECTIONS

Secondary bacterial infection should be promptly treated. Skin lesions often respond to oral flucloxacillin (nafcillin) or cefaclor. Severely painful or necrotic skin lesions need inpatient treatment with intravenous flucloxacillin (nafcillin) 1.0g q6h for suspected staphylococcal infection. If streptococcal infection is suspected, benzylpenicillin 2.4g q4h or q6h is appropriate; for incipiently necrotic lesions, metronidazole 500mg q8h may be added, or clindamycin substituted.

Mild chest infections in children may respond to oral flucloxacillin, (nafcillin) but infection in adults usually requires parenteral treatment. If flucloxacillin alone is not effective, an early change to a broad-spectrum cephalosporin such as cefuroxime should be considered.

ZOSTER-ASSOCIATED PAIN

In acute herpes zoster simple analgesics are often effective. Opiates should not be withheld if pain is severe, although nausea and confusion may limit their use in the elderly. Late, causalgic pain responds poorly to any analgesic, but is often helped by amytryptyline (up to 25mg q8h). There is some evidence that this limits the duration of ZAP, if given early. Antiviral agents have no proven benefit on chronic post-herpetic neuralgia.

HUMAN HERPESVIRUS TYPE 6 AND ROSEOLA (EXANTHEM SUBITUM)

Human herpesvirus type 6 (HHV-6) was recovered from B lymphocytes by cocultivation. It exists as two variants, HHV-6A and HHV-6B;[25] both can infect humans, but only HHV-6B has been definitely associated with clinical disease. The virus is closely related to cytomegalovirus; a mononucleosis-like infection has occasionally been described. Infants are protected by maternally derived antibody detectable up to the age of 4–6 months. The virus can be found in the saliva of seropositive adults, suggesting that latent infection exists.

Almost all humans acquire infection and seroconvert in early childhood. Up to 60% of infected children develop roseola, in which 4 or 5 days of fever is followed by the sudden appearance of a macular

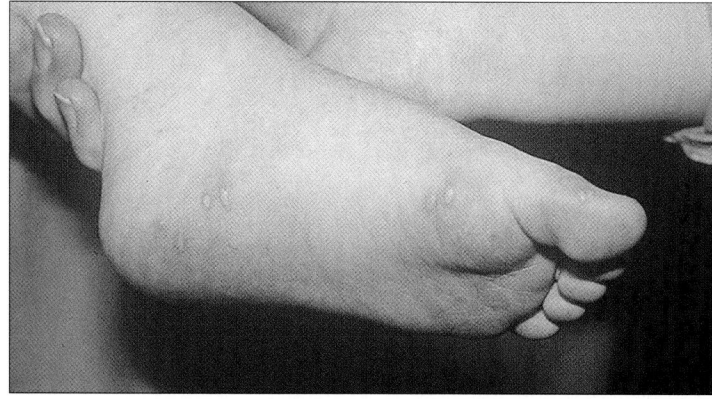

Fig. 1.9 Hand, foot and mouth disease. Typical vesicles are seen on the foot of a 3-year-old child.

or maculopapular rash, which quickly spreads across the neck, trunk and proximal limbs. The lesions fade in 1 or 2 days. Mild neutropenia is common in established infection. Occasional epidemics are recognized. The incubation period is about 10 days (range 5–15 days). Complications are few; febrile convulsions may accompany the high fever; occasional cases with encephalopathy or hepatic inflammation are described, rarely with lasting sequelae.[26] Some work suggests that the virus may be involved in the pathogenesis of multiple sclerosis.[27]

Treatment is symptomatic although the illness is usually trivial and self-limiting. Susceptibility to antiviral agents is similar to that of cytomegalovirus. Antipyretic medication is useful if the fever causes convulsions or other adverse effects.

HAND, FOOT AND MOUTH DISEASE

This is a systemic infection of young children that often occurs in local or household outbreaks and occasionally also affects adults. It is caused by coxsackie viruses, most commonly type A16.

After an incubation period of about 10 days, fever and mild generalized lymphadenopathy occur, followed after 2 or 3 days by the eruption of tense, clear vesicles on the palmar surfaces of the hands and feet (Fig. 1.9). Lesions also affect the mouth, tongue and pharynx. There is a papular or maculopapular rash on the buttocks and, rarely, on the back or thighs.

The illness is mild and self-limiting. Specific treatment is not available, but the lesions can be painful or tender and simple analgesics may help this.

REFERENCES

1. Starr SE. New mechanism of immunosuppression after measles. Lancet 1996;348:1257–8.
2. Segev Y, Ofir R, Salzberg S, et al. Tyrosine phosphorylation of measles virus nucleocapsid protein in persistently infected neuroblastoma cells. J Virol 1995;69:2480–5.
3. Calvert N, Cutts F, Irving R, Brown D, Marsh J, Miller E. Measles immunity and response to revaccination among secondary school children in Cumbria. Epidemiol Infect 1996;116:65–70.
4. Katz M. Clinical spectrum of measles. Curr Top Microbiol Immunol 1995;191:1–12.
5. Forni AL, Schluger NW, Roberts RB. Severe measles pneumonitis in adults: evaluation of clinical characteristics and therapy with intravenous ribavirin. Clin Infect Dis 1994;19:454–62.
6. Butler JC, Havens PL, Sowell AL, et al. Measles severity and serum retinol (vitamin A) concentration among children in the United States. Pediatrics 1993;91:1176–81.

7. Bannister B, Begg NT, Gillespie SH. Infectious disease. Blackwell Science: Oxford, 1996.

8. Shirly JA, Revill S, Cohen BJ, Buckley MM. Serological study of rubella-like illnesses. J Med Virol 1987;21:369–79.

9. Mitchell LA, Zhang T, Tingle AJ. Differential antibody reponses to rubella virus infection in males and females. J Infect Dis 1992;166:1258–65.

10. Lovett AE, Hahn CS, Rice CM, Frey TK, Wolinsky JS. Rubella virus-specific cytotoxic T-lymphocyte responses: identification of the capsid as a target of major histocompatibility complex class 1-restricted lysis and definition of two epitopes. J Virol 1993;67:5849–58.

11. Chu SY, Bernier RH, Stewart JA. Rubella antibody persistence after immunisation. JAMA 1988;259:3133–6.

12. Ueno Y. Rubella arthritis. An outbreak in Kyoto. J Rheumatol 1994;21:874–6.

13. Aguado JM, Posada I, Gonzalez M, et al. Meningoencephalitis and polyradiculitis in adults: don't forget rubella. Clin Infect Dis 1993;17:785–6.

14. Arnold W, Friedmann I. Detection of measles and rubella-specific antigens in the endochondral ossification zone in otosclerosis [in German] Laryngol Rhinol Otol 1987;66:167–71.

15. Brown KE, Anderson SM, Young NS. Erythrocyte P-antigen: cellular receptor for B-19 parvovoirus. Science 1993;262:114–7.

16. Cohen B. Parvovirus B19: an expanding spectrum of disease. Br Med J 1995;311:1549–52.

17. Leclair JM, Zaiz JA, Levin MJ, et al. Airborne transmission of chickenpox in a hospital. N Engl J Med 1980;302:450–3.

18. Garnett GP, Grenfell BT. The epidemiology of varicella-zoster infections: the influence of varicella on the prevalence of herpes zoster. Epidemiol Infect 1992;108:513–28.

19. Wiegle KA, Grose C. Molecular dissection of the humoral immune response to individual varicella-zoster viral proteins during chickenpox, quiescence, reinfection and reactivation. J Infect Dis 1984;149:741–9.

20. Meier JL, Straus SE. Comparative biology of latent varicella-zoster virus and herpes simplex virus infections. J Infect Dis 1992;166(suppl 1):S13–23.

21. Clements DA, Armstrong CB, Ursano AM, et al. Over five-year follow up of Oka/Merck varicella vaccine recipients in 465 infants and adolescents. Pediatr Infect Dis J 1996;14:874–9.

22. Salisbury DN, Begg NT. Varicella. Immunisation against infectious disease. London: HMSO; 1996:251–61.

23. Chen SH, Liang DC. Intravenous immunoglobulin prophylaxis in children with acute leukaemia following exposure to varicella. Pediatr Hematol Oncol 1992;9:347–51.

24. Asano Y Yoshikawa T, Suga S, et al. Postexposure prophylaxis of varicella in family contact by oral acyclovir. Pediatrics 1993;92:219–22.

25. Inoue N, Dambaugh TR, Pelett PE. Molecular biology of human herpesviruses 6A and 6B. Infect Agents Dis 1993;2:343–60.

26. Yamanishi K. Pathogenesis of human herpesvirus 6 HHV-6. Infect Agents Dis 1992;1:149–55.

27. Challoner PB, Smith KT, Pareker JD, et al. Plaque-associated expression of human herpesvirus 6 in multiple sclerosis. Proc Natl Acad Sci USA 1995;92:7440–4.

Cellulitis, Pyoderma, Abscesses and other Skin and Subcutaneous Infections

Dennis L Stevens

INTRODUCTION

Infections of the skin and/or subcutaneous tissues are highly diverse in respect to etiologic organisms, incidence, clinical manifestations, severity and complications. They may occur as single or recurrent episodes. Many cases are mild or self-limited, but some progress to cause scarring, loss of digits or limbs, or even death.

The terminology can be confusing because several different names, which are often not precisely defined, may be used to describe the same condition. Nomenclature for the most common infections is summarized in Figure 2.1.

When a patient presents with soft tissue infection, the clinician faces the challenge of establishing a specific diagnosis and prescribing definitive treatment. Important points in diagnosis are:
- the patient's symptoms;
- the general appearance of the infected site;
- historic clues such as contact with insects or animals, especially involving bites, travel to specific geographic areas, occupation or use of a hot tub (see Folliculitis, Furuncles and Carbuncles, below);
- the immune status of the host;
- chronicity; and
- anatomic distribution.

If the diagnosis cannot be established based upon the history, symptoms and signs, then needle aspiration, biopsy or surgical exploration may be necessary to obtain specimens for appropriate staining and culture.

As the antimicrobial susceptibility of these microbes varies greatly, treatment (particularly for severe infections) should be based upon the results of microscopy, Gram stain and culture whenever possible.

EPIDEMIOLOGY

Although the exact incidence of these infections in the general population is unknown, they are among the most common infections occurring in all age groups. Some are age-related, for example impetigo is more common in children, erysipelas is more common in older adults.

Infections of the skin and soft tissues can be caused by bacteria (including rickettsiae), fungi, viruses, parasites and spirochetes. Although there are hundreds of possible etiologic agents (Figs 2.1–2.4), two common species of Gram-positive cocci are the predominant causes of skin and soft tissue infections – *Staphylococcus aureus* and *Streptococcus pyogenes*. Skin and soft tissue infections caused by newly recognized or previously rarely encountered microbes are continually being described in immunocompromised patients, especially those who have AIDS.

Several noninfectious diseases can mimic infection of the soft tissues. For example, patients with contact dermatitis, pyoderma gangrenosum, gout, psoriatic arthritis with distal dactylitis, Reiter's syndrome, relapsing polychondritis or mixed cryoglobulinemia secondary to immune complex disease from chronic hepatitis C or B virus infection may present with erythematous rashes, with or without fever.

PATHOGENESIS

The integument is an organ that reacts to noxious, infectious, external and internal stimuli in a limited number of ways. It is therefore not surprising that infection can be mimicked by noninfectious inflammatory conditions. The rich plexus of capillaries beneath the dermal papillae provide nutrition to the stratum germinativum and the dermatocytes,

NOMENCLATURE, LOCATION AND ETIOLOGY OF COMMON SKIN AND SUBCUTANEOUS INFECTIONS			
Terminology	Subgroups	Location	Etiology
Pyoderma	Impetigo (impetigo contagiosa)	Skin	*Streptococcus pyogenes, Staphylococcus aureus*
	Bullous impetigo	Skin	*Staph. aureus* with group II phage
	Folliculitis (pustulosis)	Skin, hair follicles	*Staph. aureus*
	Folliculitis (sycosis) barbae	Skin, hair follicles of the beard	*Strep. pyogenes, Staph. aureus*
	Hot tub folliculitis	Skin	*Pseudomonas aeruginosa*
Abscesses	Furuncle (boil, subcutaneous abscess)	Subcutaneous tissue	*Staph. aureus*
	Hydradenitis suppurativa	Multiple furuncles in sweat glands: axilla, groins	*Staph. aureus* and other bacteria, including Gram-negative bacilli and anaerobes
	Carbuncle	Dense group of furuncles in areas of thick skin: back of neck, shoulders, buttocks	*Staph. aureus*
Cellulitis		Skin and subcutaneous tissue	*Staph. aureus, Strep. pyogenes*, Group C and G streptococci, *P. aeruginosa, Haemophilus influenzae*, or Gram-negative bacilli; fungi can cause cellulitis in immunocompromised hosts
	Erysipelas	Skin	*Strep. pyogenes*
Ecthyma		Skin and subcutaneous tissue	*Strep. pyogenes, Staph aureus*, or both; other bacteria
	Ecthyma gangrenosum	Skin and subcutaneous tissue in neutropenic patients	*P. aeruginosa*

Fig. 2.1 Nomenclature, location and etiology of some common skin and subcutaneous infections.

ETIOLOGY OF SOFT TISSUE INFECTIONS ASSOCIATED WITH SPECIFIC RISK FACTORS

Risk factor or setting	Likely etiologic agent
Cat bite	Pasteurella multocida
Dog bite	Pasteurella multocida, Capnocytophaga canimorsus (DF-2), Staphylococcus intermedius
Tick bite followed by erythema chronicum migrans rash	Borrelia burgdorferi
Hot tub exposure	Pseudomonas aeruginosa
Diabetes mellitus or peripheral vascular disease	Group B streptococci
Periorbital cellulitis (children)	Haemophilus influenzae
Saphenous vein donor site cellulitis	Groups C and G streptococci
Fresh water laceration	Aeromonas hydrophila
Sea water exposure, cirrhosis, raw oysters	Vibrio vulnificus
Cellulitis associated with stasis dermatitis	Groups A, C and G streptococci
Lymphedema	Groups A, C and G streptococci
Cat scratch	Bartonella henselae, Bartonella quintana
HIV-positive patient with bacillary angiomatosis	Bartonella henselae, Bartonella quintana
Fishmongering, bone rendering	Erysipelothrix rhusiopathiae
Fish tank exposure	Mycobacterium marinum
Compromised host with ecthyma gangrenosum	Pseudomonas aeuruginosa
Human bite	Eikenella corrodens, Fusobacterium spp., Prevotella spp., Porphorymonas spp., Streptococcus pyogenes

Fig. 2.2 Probable etiology of soft tissue infections associated with some specific risk factor or setting.

DIFFERENTIAL DIAGNOSIS OF BULLOUS SKIN LESIONS

Clinical condition	Etiology
Bullous impetigo	Staphylococcus aureus carrying group II phage
Erysipelas	Streptococcus pyogenes
Staphylococcal scalded skin syndrome	Staphylococcus aureus producing exfoliative toxin
Necrotizing fasciitis	Type I: mixed aerobic and anaerobic bacteria
	Type II: Strep. pyogenes
Gas gangrene	Clostridium perfringens, Clostridium septicum
Halophilic vibrio sepsis	Vibrio vulnificus
Pemphigoid	Immune mediated
Toxic epidermal necrolysis	Drug induced

Fig. 2.3 Differential diagnosis of bullous skin lesions.

DIFFERENTIAL DIAGNOSIS OF CRUSTED SKIN LESIONS

Clinical condition	Etiology
Impetigo	Staphylococcus aureus, Streptococcus pyogenes, or both
Ringworm	Dermatophytic fungi (e.g. Tinea rubrum)
Systemic fungal infections	Histoplasma capsulatum
	Coccidioides immitis
	Blastomyces dermatitidis
Cutaneous mycobacterial infection	Mycobacterium tuberculosis
	Mycobacterium marinum
Cutaneous leishmaniasis	Leishmania tropica
Nocardiosis	Nocardia asteroides

Fig. 2.4 Differential diagnosis of crusted skin lesions.

which are bound together by tight junctions and form the barrier to microbial invasion.

Once microbes have penetrated this barrier through a hair follicle, cut or bite, the dermal plexus of capillaries delivers the components of the host's defense – oxygen, complement, immunoglobulins, macrophages, lymphocytes and granulocytes – to the site of infection.

Perhaps the first clue available to the immune system of the presence of foreign material in the deep tissues is provided by the organisms themselves. Virtually all bacteria are comprised of proteins whose N-terminal amino acid sequence begins with an N-formyl-methionine group and these proteins are chemoattractive to phagocytes such as macrophages and granulocytes. Other microbial cell wall components such as zymosan of yeast, endotoxins of Gram-negative bacteria and peptidoglycans of Gram-positive bacteria activate the alternative complement pathway,[1] yielding serum-derived chemotactic factors. Chemotactic factors are therefore promptly produced at the site of infection by multiple mechanisms.

The efflux or diapedesis of phagocytes through endothelial cell junctions is dependent upon the orchestrated sequential expression of adherence molecules on the surface of the polymorphonuclear leukocyte (PMNL)[2,3] such as L-selectin and CD11b/CD18 in association with counter-receptors (adhesins) on the endothelial surface.[4] In vivo, surface expression of these molecules results first in 'rolling' of PMNLs along the endothelial surface, followed by tethering and finally firm adhesion of the PMNLs onto the surface of endothelial cells. Phagocytes actually leave the capillary through endothelial cell interstices bound by peripheral endothelial cell adherence molecules which are found only at these junctional sites.

Once diapedesis has occurred, the PMNL follows the gradient of chemotactic factors derived from the bacteria and serum to the site of active infection. Recent studies suggest that the activated endothelial cells also produce chemotactic cytokines such as interleukin (IL)-8.

Finally, activated granulocytes synthesize leukotriene B4 from arachidonic acid, and this too is a potent chemoattractant for leukocytes.

Production of proinflammatory cytokines such as IL-1, tumor necrosis factor-α, and IL-6 results in an augmentation of the immune functions described above. These cytokines induce fever, prime neutrophils, and increase antibody production and the synthesis of acute phase reactants such as C-reactive protein.[5,6] Cytokine-driven stimulation of endothelial cells also results in the generation of nitric oxide and prostaglandins, both of which cause vasodilation. The net physiologic effect is greater blood flow to the tissue. These processes results in the cardinal manifestations of inflammation:

- heat,
- swelling,
- erythema, and
- tenderness or pain.

At some locations, factors such as pressure, thrombosis or drugs may reduce or stop blood flow, resulting in inadequate oxygenation. Compounds such as corticosteroids, which inhibit phospholipase A_2 activity (necessary for releasing arachidonic acid from cell membranes), and nonsteroidal anti-inflammatory agents, which inhibit cyclooxygenase (the endogenous enzyme necessary for the synthesis of prostaglandins from arachidonic acid), reduce local blood flow to tissues. These drugs are therefore useful in the treatment of noninfectious inflammatory conditions because they reduce pain and swelling. However, if the inflammation is secondary to undiagnosed bacterial infection, these drugs may predispose the patient to more severe infection or mask the clinical signs, so delaying the correct diagnosis.

If tissue perfusion is moderately attenuated, tissues may remain viable, but the threshold for progression of infection may be lowered. Predisposing conditions in this category include:

- peripheral vascular disease affecting large arteries,
- diabetes mellitus causing microvascular disease; and
- chronic venous stasis causing postcapillary obstruction.

Necrosis of the skin and deeper tissue may occur if there is severe hypoxia. Two examples are pressure necrosis resulting in decubitus ulcers and compartment syndromes resulting in hypoxia then necrosis in muscles confined within tight fascial bundles.

When the host is physiologically, structurally and immunologically normal, only certain pathogens such as *Staph. aureus* and group A streptococci are able to cause disease by virtue of their potent virulence factors. This statement is supported by the observation that normal skin, although constantly exposed to many indigenous and exogenous microbes, rarely becomes infected. These bacteria, however, possess virulence factors such as toxins, capsules or dermonecrotic enzymes that confer ability to withstand the barrage of host defenses and to induce clinical disease.

In contrast, patients who have compromised skin integrity (e.g. burn patients), vascular defects (e.g. those with diabetes mellitus or pressure ulceration) or immunologic deficits may become infected with either virulent organisms (staphylococci or streptococci) or microbes that are usually saphrophytic, such as *Pseudomonas aeruginosa, Escherichia coli,* enterococci or *Fusarium* spp. Other defects such as complement deficiency, immunoglobulin deficiencies or neutropenia attenuate the host response to the invading pathogen and predispose to infection.

PREVENTION

Avoidance of cuts, scratches and other forms of trauma that disrupt the natural barrier function of the skin helps to prevent skin and soft tissue infections. For example, stopping shaving may prevent recurrent folliculitis in the beard area (sycosis barbae). Prompt cleansing, debridement and disinfection of such lesions are important for preventing infection, particularly in the case of bite wounds. Treatment of eczema reduces the risk of secondary bacterial superinfection.

Prevention of recurrent folliculitis or furunculosis is difficult to achieve, but there has been some success using intranasal applications of bacitracin or mupirocin ointment. pHisohex (hexachloraphene) baths may be tried to eliminate or reduce staphylococcal carriage in adults.[7] Prophylaxis with systemic antibiotics is of doubtful efficacy, and can result in the emergence of resistant strains; it should be tried only for severe cases.

Recurrent bacterial cellulitis of the lower extremities can often be prevented by topical antifungal treatment for dermatophyte infections such as tinea pedis because even minor or inapparent superficial fungal infection can serve as a portal of entry for Gram-positive cocci.

CLINICAL FEATURES, DIAGNOSIS AND MANAGEMENT OF SPECIFIC SOFT TISSUE INFECTIONS

FOLLICULITIS, FURUNCLES AND CARBUNCLES

Pustules or abscesses can develop when organisms permanently or transiently resident on the skin surfaces are introduced into deeper tissues (see Fig. 2.5). Pathogens can also seed the skin from hematogenous sources such as bacteremias, for example associated with staphylococcal endocarditis (see Fig. 2.6), or by contiguous spread from infectious foci in the lung or gastrointestinal tract. Most commonly, small focal abscesses develop in the superficial layers of the skin, where hair follicles serve as the portal of entry. Such lesions are called folliculitis.

Staphylococcus aureus accounts for most of these infections, but many different bacterial species can occasionally cause localized folliculitis.

Folliculitis can progress to form subcutaneous abscesses, called furuncles or boils, which usually drain and resolve spontaneously, but may progress to form a large, exquisitely painful group of contiguous furuncles, called a carbuncle (see Fig. 2.7). Carbuncles require surgical drainage as well as antibiotic treatment.[6]

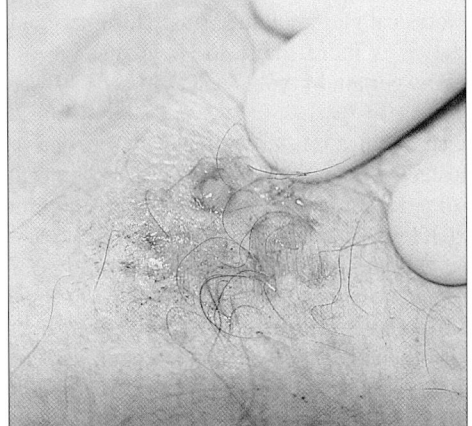

Fig. 2.5 Cutaneous infection at the previous insertion site of an intravenous catheter. Organisms from the skin were likely introduced into the dermis and subcutaneous tissue at the time of catheter insertion. Many of these infections remain superficial, but in this patient suppurative thrombophlebitis with bacteremia ensued.

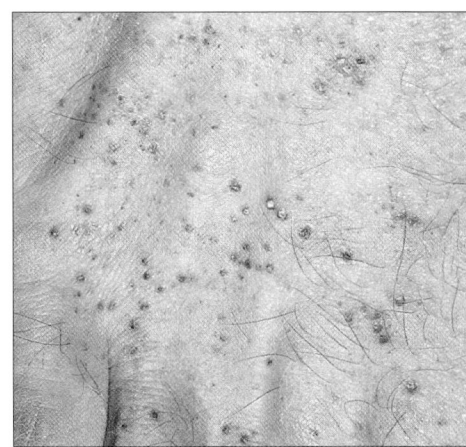

Fig. 2.6 Diffuse skin involvement with petechial lesions in a patient with *Staphylococcus aureus* bacteremia, endocarditis and acute aortic insufficiency.

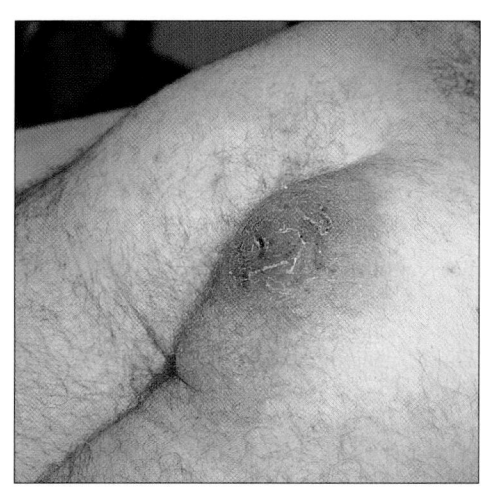

Fig. 2.7 Carbuncle of the buttock caused by *Staphylococcus aureus*. This large carbuncle developed over the course of 7–10 days and required surgical drainage plus treatment with antibiotics. The patient had previously experienced numerous episodes of *Staph. aureus* cutaneous abscesses. He carried the staphylococci in his anterior nares.

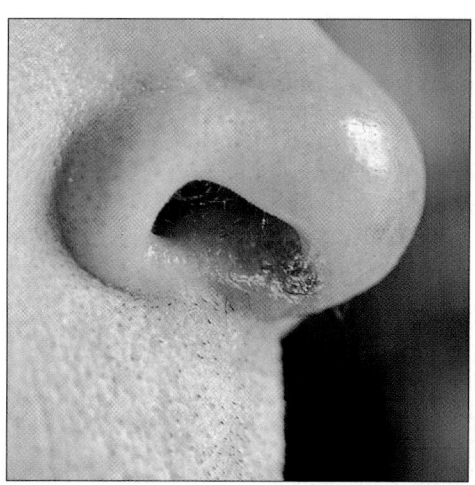

Fig. 2.8 Staphylococcal nasal carriage. This patient had a small staphylococcal abscess beneath the mucosa of the nose, illustrating how *Staphylococcus aureus*, which colonizes the nares, can infect skin and submucosa. Intact mucosa is highly resistant to infection; such infections usually occur as a result of defects in the mucosal membranes or via hair follicles inside the nose.

Recurrent furunculosis

Certain individuals seem to be predisposed to recurrent *Staph. aureus* skin infections (recurrent furunculosis). Most have one or more underlying factors such as poor hygiene, nasal carriage of staphylococci (see Fig. 2.8) or neurodermatitis. Although it has been suggested that diabetic patients are especially prone to boils and carbuncles, there are few data to support this concept. In contrast, it is well established that patients with Job's syndrome, who have eosinophilia and high levels of serum IgE antibody, are strongly predisposed to these focal *Staph. aureus* infections.

Treatment of recurrent furunculosis may require surgical incision and drainage as well as antistaphylococcal antibiotics such as oral dicloxacillin or parenteral nafcillin.

Predisposing factors

Superficial dermal trauma such as insect bites or abrasions can result in cutaneous abscesses.

Eczema may also serve as a portal of entry. Superinfected eczema may be difficult to distinguish from eczema itself because both result in crusted lesions, exudation and cutaneous erythema. The presence of lymphangitis, pustules or fever suggests infection. Because *Staph. aureus* is the most common cause of infected eczema, treatment with an oral antistaphylococcal antibiotic such as dicloxacillin is warranted.

Sebaceous glands empty into hair follicles; if the ducts become blocked they form sebaceous cysts, which may resemble staphylococcal abscess or become secondarily infected.

Chronic folliculitis is uncommon except in acne vulgaris where normal flora (e.g. *Propionibacterium acnes*) may play a role.

Recurrent folliculitis is most common in black males and associated with trauma from shaving (folliculitis barbae). Hidradenitis suppurativa occurs in either acute or chronic forms and can lead to recurrent axillary or pudendal abscesses.

Diffuse folliculitis

Diffuse folliculitis occurs in two distinct settings. The first, 'hot-tub folliculitis' is associated with water maintained at a temperature between 98.6 and 104°F that is insufficiently chlorinated and is caused by *P. aeruginosa*. The infection is usually self-limited, although serious complications of bacteremia and shock have occasionally been reported.

The second form of diffuse folliculitis, swimmer's itch (Fig. 2.9), occurs when the skin is exposed to water infected with avian freshwater schistosomes. Warm water temperatures and alkaline pH are suitable for mollusks that are the intermediate host between birds and humans. Free-swimming cercariae readily penetrate human hair follicles or pores, but quickly die. This triggers a brisk allergic reaction, causing intense itching and erythema. The infestation is self-limited, secondary infection is uncommon and antipruritics and topical corticosteroid cream promptly relieve the symptoms.

STAPHYLOCOCCAL SCALDED SKIN SYNDROME

This disorder has been described in all age groups, but it is usually seen in children under 5 years of age, including neonates.[8] The characteristics are a faint erythematous rash with the formation of flaccid bullae (Fig. 2.10). *Staphylococcus aureus* of phage group II is the causative organism. These organisms produce the toxin exfoliatin, which appears to affect the cell junctions of young dermal cells. Specifically, there is intraepidermal cleavage at the level of the stratum corneum. A classic clinical feature is Nikolsky's sign, in which lateral pressure on the skin results in shearing off of the top layer of skin (Fig. 2.11). The mortality of staphylococcal scalded skin syndrome is low, and fluid loss from the skin is minimal. Appropriate antibiotic therapy is the main component of treatment.

Staphylococcal scalded skin syndrome must be distinguished from toxic epidermal necrolysis, a condition that is more common in adults, usually secondary to a drug reaction and associated with high mortality (Fig. 2.11). Frozen section examination of a punch biopsy readily distinguishes these two entities:

- staphylococcal scalded skin syndrome shows a cleavage at the level of the stratum corneum; and
- toxic epidermal necrolysis shows deeper cleavage, at the stratum germinativum.

IMPETIGO

Impetigo contagiosa is a form of superficial pyoderma caused by streptococci and/or staphylococci. Currently, about half of impetigo cases are caused by *Staph. aureus*.[8] Staphylococci and group A streptococci can be co-isolated from impetiginous lesions in many cases. Group A streptococci alone currently cause less than half the cases. Staphylococcal impetigo tends to occur sporadically, whereas epidemics of impetigo caused by group A streptococci have been well described. Epidemics occur throughout the year in tropical areas or during the summer months in more temperate climates. Impetigo caused by group A streptococci is sometimes complicated by the development of poststreptococcal glomerulonephritis. This important nonsuppurative complication is more likely to occur during epidemics of impetigo caused by certain M types such as M type 49 (see Chapter 8.14).

Impetigo is characterized by thick crusted lesions with rounded or irregular margins, often located on the face (Fig. 2.12).[9] Streptococcal pyoderma frequently has a golden brown or honey color, resembling a plaque of dried serum. Children between 2 and 10 years of age are most commonly infected. Impetigo is often associated with poor socioeconomic conditions and poor hygiene.

Initially, colonization of unbroken skin occurs either exogenously from other infected persons (hence the term impetigo contagiosa) or endogenously by contamination of the skin with organisms carried in the anterior nares or oropharynx. Development of impetiginous lesions

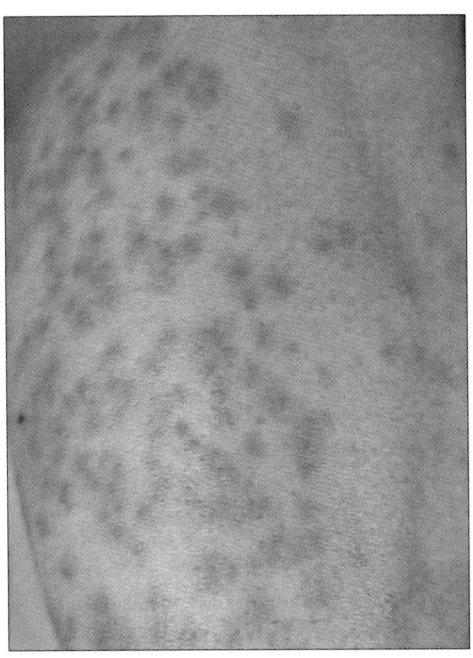

Fig. 2.9 Swimmer's itch. Diffuse folliculitis can be caused by *Pseudomonas aeruginosa* (hot tub folliculitis), schistosomes (swimmer's itch) or *Staphylococcus aureus* (folliculitis). This young man had been fishing in an alkaline lake in the western part of the USA. He had been fishing from a 'float tube' and had exposed only his hands and arms to the water. The rash was associated with severe itching. Although his white blood count was not elevated 35% of the white cells were eosinophils.

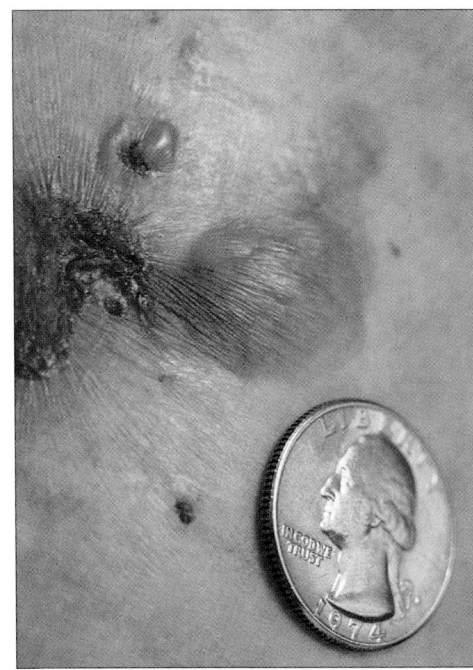

Fig. 2.10 Staphylococcal scalded skin syndrome. Flaccid bullae occur as single or multiple lesions. Examination of a frozen tissue section reveals that the cleavage plane is at the stratum corneum. This disease must be distinguished from toxic epidermal necrolysis (see Fig. 2.12).

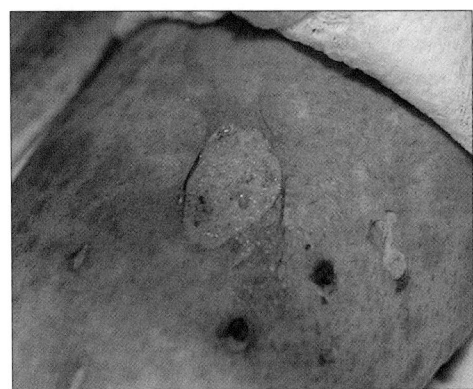

Fig. 2.11 Toxic epidermal necrolysis. This picture shows a skin slough (Nikolsky's sign), which resulted when lateral pressure was applied by the thumb in a plane parallel to the skin surface. This disorder is more common in adults, has a high mortality and is usually caused by medications.

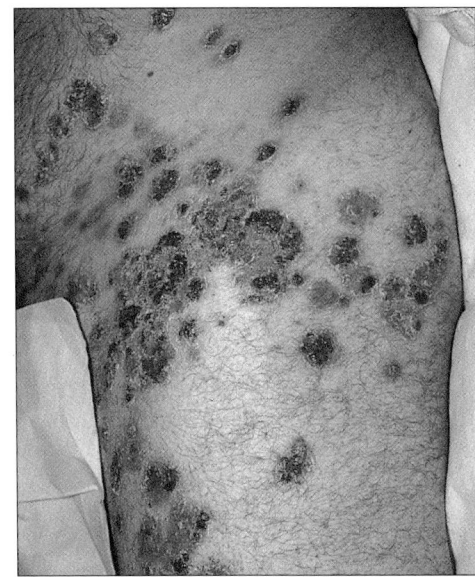

Fig. 2.12 Impetigo in a homeless man. Both *Staphylococcus aureus* and Group A streptococci were cultured from these lesions.

requires 10–14 days and likely is initiated through minor abrasions, insect bites and so on, all of which serve as a means of intradermal inoculation.

Patients should receive penicillin treatment, particularly when numerous sites of the skin are involved, although treatment may not prevent poststreptococcal glomerulonephritis. Topical treatment with an agent effective against Gram-positive bacteria such as bacitracin or mupirocin is also effective.

Bullous impetigo

Bullous impetigo is caused by strains of *Staph. aureus* harboring a group II bacteriophage that contains genetic elements coding for a toxin, which causes cleavage in the epidermis. This cleavage results in separation of the cellular planes at the level of the stratum corneum and this is responsible for the superficial flaccid bullae that characterize this condition. Several of these lesions may coalesce and spread to form large reddish plaques, usually involving the neck, face or chin. The superficial flaccid bullae are easily ruptured and may not be apparent at the time the patient is first seen. Because of the superficial nature of these infections, scarring does not occur. Appropriate treatment is with an antistaphylococcal antibiotic, which may be given orally.

ECTHYMA, PARONYCHIA AND BLISTERING DISTAL DACTYLITIS

Ecthyma, like impetigo, is characterized by dry crusted lesions of the skin and may be caused by *Staph. aureus*, group A streptococci or both. Unlike impetigo, this lesion extends into the dermis and may therefore lead to post-treatment scarring.[8]

Paronychia is an infection between the nail plate of a digit and the cuticle. It is associated with sucking of the fingers and occupations or hobbies involving prolonged immersion of the hands in water. Paronychia may occur in some immunocompromised patients. *Staphylococcus* is the most common etiologic agent, although oral anaerobes and streptococci may also be isolated. Fungi such as *Fusarium* spp. may be isolated from paronychias occurring in immunocompromised patients. Drainage is best accomplished between the nail plate and the cuticle. Antimicrobial agents are rarely needed in otherwise healthy individuals.

Blistering distal dactylitis is characterized by painful blisters on the finger pads of digits. It is most common in children. *Streptococcus pyogenes* is the most common organism isolated, although *Staph. aureus* can cause a similar lesion. Incision and drainage may be useful, in conjunction with an antibiotic appropriate for *Staph. aureus* or *Strep. pyogenes*.

ERYSIPELAS

Erysipelas is a specific variant of cellulitis caused by *Strep. pyogenes*, and occasionally by streptococci of groups B, C and D.[10,11] It is characterized by an abrupt onset of fiery red swelling of the face or extremities. Distinctive features are well-defined margins, particularly along the nasolabial fold, rapid progression and intense pain (see Fig. 2.13). Flaccid superficial bullae may develop during the second to third day of the illness, but extension to deeper soft tissues is rare.

Surgical debridement is rarely necessary, and treatment with penicillin is effective. Swelling may progress for a time despite appropriate treatment, even while fever, pain, and the intense red color are diminishing. Desquamation of the involved skin occurs after 5–10 days.

Erysipelas is most common in elderly adults, and the severity of systemic toxicity can vary from region to region. It seems to be less common and less severe today than in the past.

CELLULITIS

The term 'cellulitis' is commonly used by physicians, but is not well defined in the literature. It is a localized area of soft tissue inflammation characterized by:

- leukocytic infiltration of the dermis,
- capillary dilatation, and
- proliferation of bacteria.

Clinically cellulitis is recognized as an acute inflammatory condition of the skin characterized by localized pain, erythema, swelling and heat.[6] The area of erythema is a paler pink than the flaming red of erysipelas, and has indistinct margins (Fig. 2.14).

Cellulitis caused *Staphylococcus aureus* and *Streptococcus pyogenes*

Cellulitis is most commonly caused by indigenous flora such as *Staph. aureus* and *Strep. pyogenes,* which colonize the skin and appendages. Bacteria may gain access to the epidermis through cracks in the skin, abrasions, cuts, burns, insect bites, surgical incisions and intravenous catheters.

Cellulitis caused by *Staph aureus* spreads centripetally from a central localized infection such as an abscess (Figs 2.15 & 2.16), folliculitis or foreign body (e.g. a sliver, prosthetic device or intravascular catheter).

In contrast, cellulitis due to *Strep. pyogenes* is a more rapidly spreading diffuse process, frequently associated with lymphangitis (Fig. 2.17) and fever.[12] Recurrent streptococcal cellulitis of the lower extremities may be caused by group A, C or G streptococci in association with skin lesions such as chronic venous stasis (Fig. 2.18), saphenous venectomy for coronary artery bypass surgery,[13] or healed burns, especially if the skin is colonized by dermatophyte fungi. Streptococci also cause recurrent cellulitis among patients with chronic lymphedema resulting from irradiation, lymph node dissection, Milroy's disease or elephantiasis.

Recurrent staphylococcal cutaneous infections occur in individuals who have eosinophilia and elevated serum levels of immunoglobulin E (Job's syndrome) and among chronic nasal carriers of staphylococci.

Cellulitis associated with predisposing conditions

A number of other conditions predispose to infection by endogenous or exogenous pathogens (see Fig. 2.2). For example:

- *Streptococcus agalactiae* cellulitis occurs in people who have diabetes mellitus or peripheral vascular disease; and[14]
- *Haemophilus influenzae* causes periorbital cellulitis in children in association with sinusitis, otitis media or epiglottitis and will presumably become less common, as has *Haemophilus* meningitis, due to the impressive efficacy of the *H. influenzae* type b vaccine.

Cellulitis associated with bites

Many other species of bacteria can cause cellulitis. These often occur in special settings, and the history can provide useful clues to the diagnosis (see Fig. 2.2). Bites of various types may introduce specific organisms into the deeper tissues, resulting in soft tissue infections. For example, cellulitis associated with cat bites and, to a lesser degree, dog bites is commonly caused by *Pasteurella multocida*, although in the latter case *Staphylococcus intermedius* and *Capnocytophaga canimorsus* (DF-2) must also be considered. Cellulitis and abscesses associated with dog and human bites also contain a variety of anaerobic organisms.[15] *Pasteurella multocida* is resistant to dicloxacillin and nafcillin, but sensitive to all other beta-lactam antimicrobials as well as quinolones, tetracycline and erythromycin. Ampicillin–clavulanate, ampicillin–sulbactam or cefoxitin are good choices for treating animal or human bite infections.

Soft tissue infections may result from the bites of mosquitoes, horse flies and spiders; usually they cause only local allergic reactions with itching, swelling and erythema. Similarly, brown recluse spider bites may resemble acute infection at first, but later there is primary tissue destruction and central necrosis due to the action of dermonecrotic toxins. These infections may resemble pyoderma gangrenosum or may become secondarily infected with skin organisms. Mosquito bites may serve as a portals of entry for skin organisms such as *Staph. aureus* or *Strep. pyogenes*. Such infections are not uncommon in clinical practice, but given the number of individuals bitten by insects, infection is a relatively rare complication.

Cellulitis associated with water exposure

Aeromonas hydrophila causes a highly aggressive form of cellulitis in tissues surrounding lacerations that were sustained in fresh water lakes, rivers and streams. This organism is sensitive to aminoglycosides, fluoroquinolones, chloramphenicol, trimethoprim–sulfamethoxazole

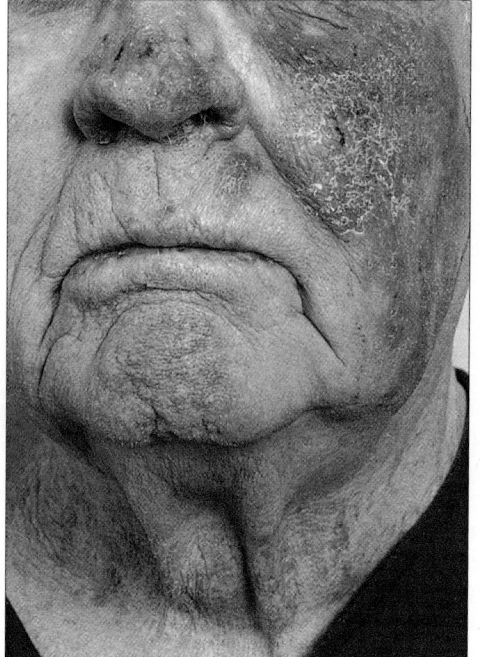

Fig. 2.13 Erysipelas. This form of cellulitis is caused by *Streptococcus pyogenes* and is most common in the elderly. Unique characteristics include a fiery red or salmon color, well-demarcated edges, desquamation after 5–7 days and location on the face or lower extemities. This picture was taken 48 hours after treatment with penicillin when the brilliant red salmon color had evolved to a reddish blue color. On the second day of treatment patients usually have less pain and fever subsides, but swelling may be more extensive.

Fig. 2.14 Cellulitis. In contrast to erysipelas, cellulitis is a pink color rather than brilliant red and has indistinct margins. *Staphylococcus aureus* and group A, C and G streptococci are the most common etiologies. Many other bacteria may cause cellulitis (see Fig. 2.1).

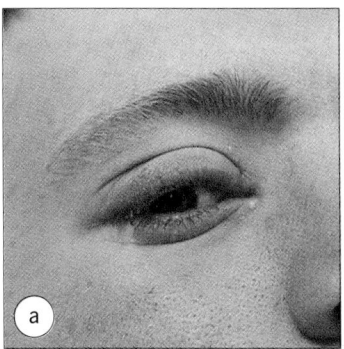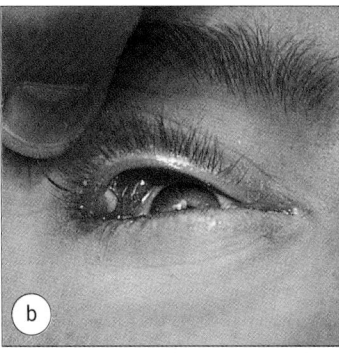

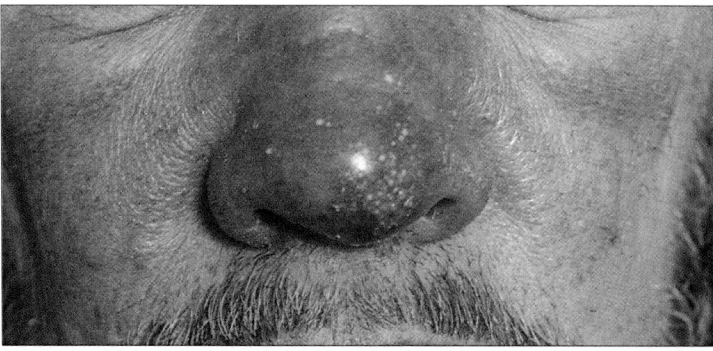

Fig. 2.15 Cellulitis. (a) This case was caused by *Staphylococcus aureus* and is spreading centripetally from a central localized focus of infection. The redness and swelling characteristic of cellulitis are apparent over the upper eyelid. (b) The cellulitis has actually developed from a localized staphylococcal abscess formed in a meibomian gland (chalazion).

Fig. 2.16 *Staphylococcus aureus* cellulitis of the nose. The focal lesion began in a hair follicle inside the nose, with redness, swelling and pain. Rarely, such lesions on the nose are complicated by extension into the cavernous sinus via veins draining the central part of the face.

(co-trimoxazole) and third-generation cephalosporins, but is resistant to ampicilllin.

Fish food containing the water fleas of the genus *Daphnia* can be contaminated with *Mycobacterium marinum,* which may cause cellulitis or granulomas on skin surfaces exposed to the water in aquariums or following injuries in swimming pools. Rifampin (rifampicin) plus ethambutol has been an effective treatment for some, although no comprehensive studies have been carried out. In addition, some strains of *M. marinum* are susceptible to tetracycline or trimethoprim–sulfamethoxazole .

Cellulitis caused by *Pseudomona* sp. and other Gram-negative bacteria

Pseudomonas aeruginosa causes four types of soft tissue infections:
*   ecthyma gangrenosum in neutropenic patients,
*   hot tub folliculitis,
*   burn wound sepsis, and
*   cellulitis following penetrating injury.

In the last of these *P. aeruginosa* is often introduced into the deep tissues by stepping on a nail, a scenario referred to as the 'sweaty tennis shoe syndrome'.

Treatment includes surgical inspection and drainage, particularly if the injury also involves bone or joint capsule. Choices for empiric treatment pending antimicrobial susceptibility data include aminoglycosides, third-generation cephalosporins such as ceftazidime, cefoperazone or cefotaxime, semisynthetic penicillins such as ticarcillin, mezlocillin or piperacillin, or fluoroquinolones. (The quinolones are not indicated in children under 13 years of age.)

Cellulitis caused by Gram-negative bacilli, including *P. aeruginosa* as described above, is most common in hospitalized immunocompromised hosts. Recently, *Stenotrophomonas maltophilia* has emerged as an important cause of nosocomial cellulitis in patients who have cancer.[16] The bacterium has been isolated from incubators, nebulizers, humidifiers and tap water in hospitals. The cellulitis may be related to intravenous catheters and in some circumstances may be metastatic via the bloodstream.

Trimethoprim–sulfamethoxazole , or ticarcillin–clavulanic acid, with or without ciprofloxacin are reasonable treatment choices, although cultures and sensitivities are important because of the high prevalence of antibiotic-resistant organisms in the health care environment.

Other causes of cellulitis

The Gram-positive aerobic rod, *Erysipelothrix rhusiopathiae,* which causes cellulitis in bone renderers and fishmongers, remains susceptible to erythromycin, clindamycin, tetracycline and cephalosporins, but is resistant to sulfonamides and chloramphenicol.

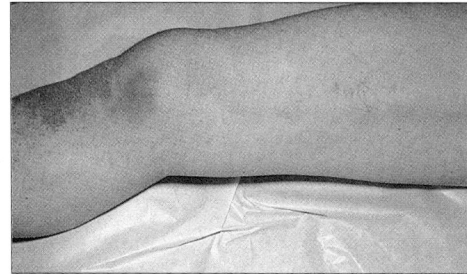

Fig. 2.17 Lymphangitis. Cellulitis caused by group A streptococci began below the knee and rapidly spread; about 4 hours later lymphangitis had spread up the inner aspect of the thigh.

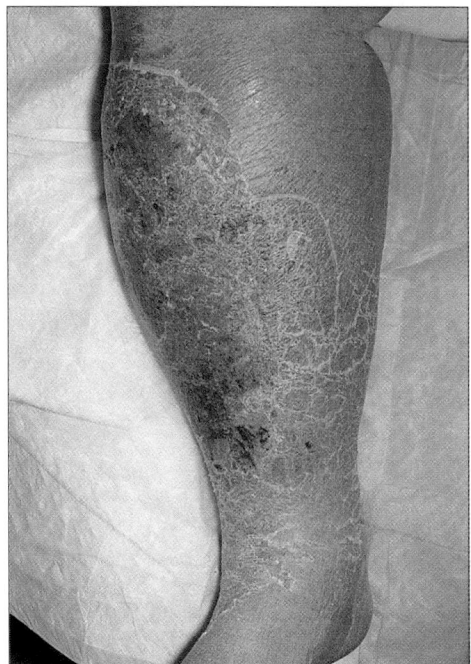

Fig. 2.18 Cellulitis of the lower leg associated with chronic venous insufficiency. Streptococci of groups A, B, C and G are the most common isolates. Group B streptococci seldom cause cellulitis in previously healthy hosts, but should be considered in people who have peripheral vascular disease or diabetes mellitus.

Differential diagnosis

The etiology of cellulitis can be suspected on the basis of the epidemiologic data supplied above. If there is drainage, an open wound or an obvious portal of entry, Gram stain and culture often can provide a definitive diagnosis (see Fig. 2.20). In the absence of these findings, the bacterial etiology of cellulitis may be difficult to establish. Even with needle aspiration from the leading edge or punch biopsy of the cellulitis itself, cultures are positive in only 20% of cases.[17] This suggests that relatively low numbers of bacteria may cause cellulitis and that the expanding area of erythema within the skin may be the direct result of extracellular toxins or the soluble mediators of inflammation elicited by the host.

Antibiotic treatment

Because many different microbes can cause cellulitis, the choice of initial empiric antibiotic therapy depends upon the clinical features described above. Once cultures and sensitivities are available, the choice is easier and more specific. The physician must first decide whether the patient's illness is severe enough to require parenteral treatment, either in hospital or on an outpatient basis.

Presumed streptococcal or staphylococcal cellulitis. For presumed streptococcal or staphylococcal cellulitis, nafcillin, cephalothin, cefuroxime, vancomycin, or erythromycin are good choices. Cefazolin and ceftriaxone have less activity against *Staph. aureus* than cephalothin, although clinical trials have shown a high degree of efficacy. Ceftriaxone is a useful choice for outpatient treatment because it can be given once daily. Similarly, teicoplanin, like vancomycin, has excellent activity against *Strep. pyogenes* and both *Staph. aureus* and *Staphylococcus epidermidis* and may be given once daily by intravenous or intramuscular injection.

For patients being treated orally dicloxacillin, cefuroxime axetil, cefpodoxime or erythromycin, clarithromycin or azithromycin are all effective treatments.

For known group A, B, C or G streptococcal infections, penicillin or erythromycin should be used orally or parenterally. For serious group A streptococcal infections such as necrotizing fasciculi or streptococcal toxic shock syndrome, clindamycin is more efficacious than penicillin.[18] This is probably because in this type of infection where there are large numbers of bacteria, streptococci are in a stationary growth phase and do not express a full complement of penicillin-binding proteins.[19] In contrast, the activity of clindamycin is not affected by inoculum size or growth phase. In addition, clindamycin suppresses the synthesis of many streptococcal exotoxins and surface proteins.[20]

Other types of cellulitis. For cellulitis associated with *Eikenella corrodens* useful antibiotics are penicillin, ceftriaxone, sulfamethoxazole–trimethoprim, tetracyclines and fluoroquinolones. Interestingly, this organism is resistant to oxacillin, cefazolin, clindamycin and erythromycin.

Cellulitis associated with cat bites may fail to respond to treatment with oral cephalosporins, erythromycins and dicloxacillin. Reasons for failure include resistance of *P. multocida* to oxacillin and dicloxacillin and the inadequate serum and tissue levels attained with older oral cephalosporins and erythromycins.

CUTANEOUS ULCERS

Infectious ulceration of the skin results from either:
- direct destruction of dermal cells by bacterial products, or
- an intense inflammatory reaction.

Cutaneous anthrax

This is an example of direct destruction of dermal cells by toxins produced by *Bacillus anthracis* (Fig. 2.20). This disease is contracted by direct inoculation of the skin of animal handlers, especially goat and sheep herders or hide processors.[21] The lesion begins as a papule that evolves into a bullus and then ulcerates. Sepsis may occur. The diagnosis is established by aspiration of the leading edge of the lesion, Gram stain and culture. Penicillin is appropriate therapy.

Cutaneous diphtheria

Since 1980 this has been recognized in homeless individuals who present with chronic nonhealing ulcers with an overlying dirty gray membrane. These lesions may mimic those of psoriasis, eczema or impetigo, but have a deeper base. Appropriate cultures of the ulcer are mandatory because organisms growing from routine cultures may be misidentified as diphtheroids.[22]

Cutaneous tularemia (ulceroglandular tularemia)

This occurs following a tick bite or handling of infected rodents or lagomorphs. It most commonly presents with regional lymphadenopathy associated with suppuration and fever, although pneumonic, oculoglandular, oropharyngeal and typhoidal forms have also been described. The characteristic lesion is a small ulceration with an eschar, which develops 2–10 days after exposure. Treatment with streptomycin has been successful, and doxycycline, chloramphenicol or a fluoroquinolone are alternatives.

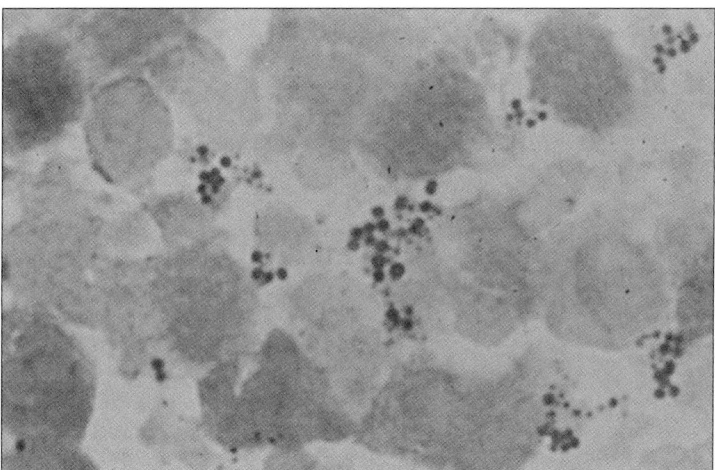

Fig. 2.19 Gram stain of purulent material demonstrating *Staphylococcus aureus*. The microbial etiology of cellulitis may be suspected based upon signs, symptoms and history; however, definitive diagnosis requires Gram stain and culture. If there is no portal of entry, aspiration or even punch biopsy of cellulitic skin yields a positive culture in only 20% of cases.

DIFFERENTIAL DIAGNOSIS OF ULCERATIVE SKIN LESIONS	
Clinical condition	Etiology
Anthrax	*Bacillus anthracis*
Cutaneous diphtheria	*Corynebacterium diphtheriae*
Ulceroglandular tularemia	*Francisella tularensis*
Bubonic plague	*Yersinia pestis*
Buruli ulcer	*Mycobacterium ulcerans*
Primary syphilis	*Treponema pallidum*
Chancroid	*Haemophilus ducreyi*
Lucio's phenomenon	*Mycobacterium leprae*
Decubitus (pressure) ulcer	Mixed aerobic and anaerobic bacteria
Leishmaniasis	*Leishmania tropica*
Ecthyma gangrenosum	*Pseudomonas aeruginosa*
Tropical ulcer	Idiopathic and nonspecific; mixed bacterial species

Fig. 2.20 Differential diagnosis of ulcerative skin lesions.

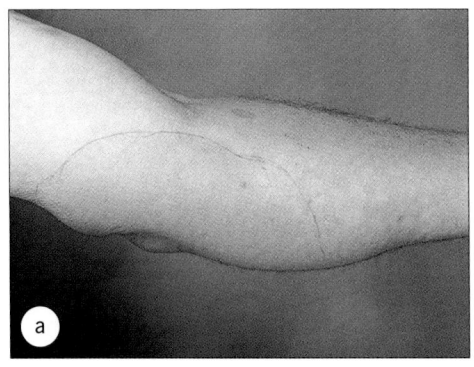

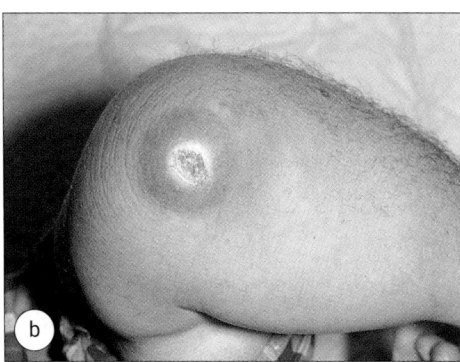

Fig. 2.21 Cellulitis at the elbow associated with olecranon bursitis. (a) Pale pink erythema on the inner aspect of the elbow. (b) Careful inspection demonstrates a focal infection over the point of the elbow. Fluid aspirated from the olecranon bursa yielded a pure culture of *Staphylococcus aureus*.

Buruli ulcer

This is caused by *Mycobacterium ulcerans*. It presents as a shallow ulcer, which slowly expands centripetally. It is uncommon in the USA and Europe, but is endemic in tropical climates, particularly Africa. Diagnosis is easily established by biopsy, acid-fast staining or culture. The organism is susceptible to isoniazid, rifampin and *para*-amino salicylic acid. Oral treatment with isoniazid and rifampin for 2–3 months is usually successful.

Leishmaniasis

Leishmaniasis also presents as a shallow ulcers with an expanding margin. Diagnosis should be suspected in patients residing in or returning from Central or South America. A biopsy from the raised edge stained with Giemsa or Wright's stain demonstrates the amastigote stage of *Leishmania tropica*. Treatment with antimony compounds is effective, but requires prolonged administration over 4–6 months.

Other causes of cutaneous ulcers

The differential diagnosis of cutaneous ulcers in genital areas should include:
- syphilis,
- chancroid,
- lymphogranuloma venereum, and
- herpes simplex virus infection.

Noninfectious causes of cutaneous ulceration include:
- Behçet's syndrome;
- cutaneous vasculitis, including lupus erythematosus;
- toxic epidermal necrolysis;
- pressure necrosis; and
- brown recluse spider bites.

Solitary shallow ulcers of skin and mucous membranes have also been described in disseminated histoplasmosis.

Herpes simplex can result in primary or recurrent cutaneous infections of the digits (herpetic whitlow) or head and neck. This viral infection is often misdiagnosed and mistreated as a bacterial condition, and occurs in those who are exposed to inoculation of the skin from oral secretions such as dentists, dental hygienists, nurses, anesthesiologists and wrestlers.

Orf is caused by a DNA virus similar to smallpox. It causes development of shallow ulcers (in general only one lesion) on the digits of animal handlers working with sheep or goats with mucous membrane lesions.[21]

BACILLARY ANGIOMATOSIS

This is a primary infection of endothelial cells that has important cutaneous manifestations.[23] The lesions may appear as purple nodules resembling Kaposi's sarcoma. They may also appear as scaly or ulcerated lesions and may have the appearance of superficial pink papules or plaques in blacks. This disease usually occurs in people who have HIV infection and is caused by *Bartonella henselae* or *Bartonella quintana*. The organisms can be acquired from cat bites and scratches

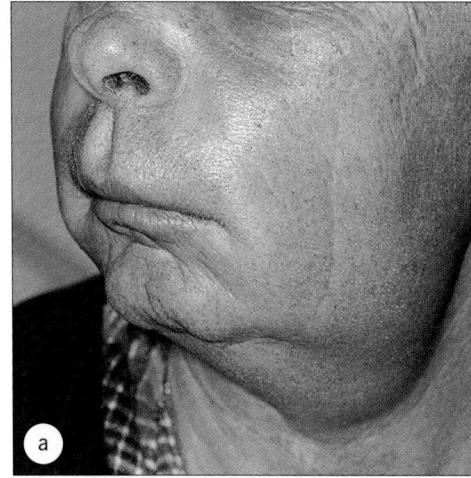

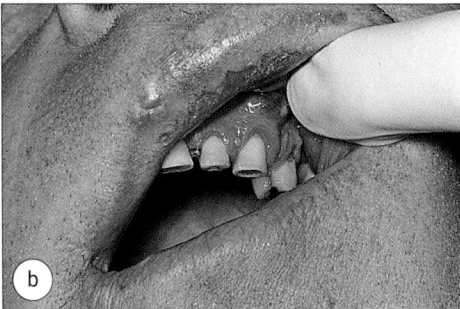

Fig. 2.22 Erythema and swelling of the face due to a tooth abscess. (a) Swelling of the face, on inspection resembling periorbital cellulitis. (b) Further inspection reveals a gingival abscess above the patient's left upper canine tooth.

or from cat fleas. The course and extent of infection is highly variable and depend upon the host's immune status.

Histopathology reveals capillary proliferation. The organisms can be visualized using Warthin–Starry silver stain or electron microscopy. Bacteriologic identification requires a special culture technique: lysed blood centrifugate or digested tissue is plated onto chocolate or Columbia agar and incubated for 10–14 days at 95°F in 5–7% carbon dioxide. Small dry adherent oxidase-negative colonies of Gram-negative curved rods with twitching motility can be identified as *Bartonella* spp. by fluorescent antibody, gas–liquid chromatography or biochemical tests.[24]

Resistance to penicillin, cephalosporins, sulfonamides and vancomycin has been described. The recommended therapy is erythromycin 500mg q6h.[23]

CUTANEOUS MANIFESTATIONS OF INFECTIONS OF DEEP SOFT TISSUES

Staphylococcal infections of deeper tissues may also cause superficial redness, warmth and swelling of the skin, even though the skin itself is not infected. Examples include olecranon bursitis (Fig. 2.21), septic arthritis, osteomyelitis, staphylococcal parotitis and other deep infections of the head and neck such as anaerobic infections, actinomycosis and tooth abscesses (Fig. 2.22).

REFERENCES

1. Greenblatt J, Boackle RJ, Schwab HJ. Activation of the alternate complement pathway by peptidoglycan from streptococcal cell wall. Infect Immun 1978;19:296–303.
2. Zimmerman GA, McIntyre TM. Neutrophil adherence to human endothelium *in vitro* occurs by CDw18 (Mo1, Mac-1/LFA-1, GP150,95) glycoprotein-dependent and independent mechanisms. J Clin Invest 1988;81:531–7.
3. Carlos TM, Harlan JM. Membrane proteins involved in phagocyte adherence to endothelium. Immunol Rev 1990;114:5–28.
4. Bevilacqua MP. Endothelial–leukocyte adhesion molecules. Ann Rev Immunol 1993;11:767–804.
5. Stevens DL. Cytokines; an updated compendium. Curr Opin Infect Dis 1995;8:175–80.
6. Stevens DL. Soft tissue infections. In: Isselbacher KJ, Braunwald E, Wilson JD, Martin JB, Fauci AS, Kasper DL, eds. Harrison's textbook of medicine, 13th ed. New York: McGraw–Hill; 1994:561–3.
7. Doebbeling BN, Reagan DR, Pfaller MA, Houston AK, Hollis RJ, Wenzel RP. Long-term efficacy of intransal mupirocin ointment: a prospective cohort study of *Staphylococcus aureus* carriage. Arch Intern Med 1994;154:1505–8.
8. Hirschmann J. Staphylococcal soft tissue infections. In: Stevens DL, ed. Atlas of infectious diseases. Philadelphia: Churchill Livingstone; 1995:2–10.
9. Dillon HC. Impetigo contagiosa: suppurative and nonsuppurative complications. Clinical, bacteriologic and epidemiologic characteristics of impetigo. Am J Dis Child 1968;115:530–41.
10. Bernard P, Bedane C, Mounier M, Denis F, Catanzano G, Bonnetblank JM. Streptocococcal cause of erysipelas and cellulitis in adults. Arch Dermatol 1989;125:779–82.
11. Norrby A, Eriksson B, Norgren M, *et al.* Virulence properties of erysipelas-associated group A streptococci. Eur J Clin Microbiol Infect Dis 1992;11:1136–43.
12. Bisno AL, Stevens DL. Streptococcal infections in skin and soft tissues. N Engl J Med 1996;334:240–5.
13. Baddour LM, Bisno AL. Non-group A beta-hemolytic streptococcal cellulitis: association with venous and lymphatic compromise. Am J Med 1985;79:155–9.
14. Stevens DL, Haburchak D, McNitt TR, Everett ED. Group B streptococcal osteomyelitis in adults. South Med J 1978;71:1450–1.
15. Goldstein EJC. Bite wounds and infection. Clin Infect Dis 1992;14:633–40.
16. Vartavarian SE, Papakadis KA, Palacios JA, Manning JT, Anaissie EJ. Mucocutaneous and soft tissue infections causes by *Xanthomonas maltophilia*. A new spectrum. Ann Intern Med 1994;121:969–73.
17. Duvanel T, Auckenthaler R, Rohner P, Harms M, Saurat HJ. Quantitative cultures of biopsy specimens from cutaneous cellulitis. Arch Intern Med 1989;149:293–6.
18. Stevens DL, Bryant AE, Yan S. Invasive group A streptococcal infection: new concepts in antibiotic treatment. Int J Antimicrob Agents 1994;4:297–301.
19. Stevens DL, Yan S, Bryant AE. Penicillin binding protein expression at different growth stages determines penicillin efficacy *in vitro* and *in vivo*: an explanation for the inoculum effect. J Infect Dis 1993;167:1401–5.
20. Gemmell CG, Peterson PK, Schmeling D, *et al.* Potentiation of opsonization and phagocytosis of *Streptococcus pyogenes* following growth in the presence of clindamycin. J Clin Invest 1981;67:1249–56.
21. Everett ED. Infections associated with animal contact. In: Stevens DL, ed. Atlas of infectious diseases. Philadelphia: Churchill Livingstone; 1995;5:2–8.
22. Megarbane B, Carbon C. Unusual presentations of bacterial skin and soft-tissue infections and their treatment. Curr Opin Infect Dis 1996;9:58–62.
23. Cockerell CJ, LeBoit PE. Bacillary angiomatosis: a newly characterized, pseudoneoplastic, infectious, cutaneous vascular disorder. J Am Acad Dermatol 1990;22:501–12.
24. Welch DF, Hensel DM, Pickett DA, San Joaquin VH, Robinson A, Slater LN. Bacteremia due to *Rochalimaea henselae* in a child: practical identification of isolates in the clinical laboratory. J Clin Microbiol 1993;31:2381–6.

Necrotizing Fasciitis, Gas Gangrene, Myositis and Myonecrosis

Dennis L Stevens

INTRODUCTION

The spectrum of infections of the deep soft tissues ranges from localized bacterial, viral and parasitic lesions to rapidly spreading, tissue-destructive infections such as necrotizing fasciitis and myonecrosis. For example, pyomyositis, which is common in the tropics but rare in temperate zones, is a focal infection of skeletal muscle that is usually caused by *Staphylococcus aureus*; it generally remains localized and rarely causes systemic complications. In contrast, necrotizing fasciitis and myonecrosis may be caused by single or multiple pathogens and often give rise to extensive tissue loss, bacteremia, organ failure, shock and death. Even the experienced clinician may have difficulty distinguishing between the different forms of deep soft-tissue infection during the early stages. Finally, despite early diagnosis and appropriate treatment, some patients will lose tissue, even limbs, whereas others will succumb to systemic complications. This chapter emphasizes the clinical clues that help to make early, specific diagnoses.

EPIDEMIOLOGY

Until the middle of the 20th century, wartime injuries were commonly complicated by gas gangrene caused by *Clostridium* spp. During the Civil War in the USA, nearly 50% of soldiers who sustained gunshot wounds developed infection, and many of these developed gas gangrene. Clostridial gangrene is typically a sporadic infection, but during the Civil War apparent epidemics of 'hospital gangrene' were described. Contributing factors included severe trauma, grossly contaminated wounds, crowded and dirty conditions, application of soiled dressings (often recycled from patients who had just died of infection) and primitive surgical techniques for debridement and fixation of open fractures. Group A streptococci undoubtedly caused some of these infections, but other major bacterial pathogens, including *Clostridium perfringens*, Gram-negative bacteria and mixed aerobic–anaerobic bacteria, also contributed.

Gas gangrene was also common during the First World War, particularly in the European theater, where the soil was rich and well fertilized with animal feces containing large numbers of vegetative spores of clostridia. In contrast, in North Africa, cases of gangrene following gunshot wounds were far less common, presumably because the desert sand contained few clostridial spores.[1] Gas gangrene has become uncommon in modern warfare because wounded soldiers are evacuated rapidly to well-equipped hospitals for surgical intervention, arterial reconstruction and antibiotic treatment, all of which have greatly reduced the prevalence of this feared disease.

In modern times, these serious deep soft tissue infections have become less common. Sporadic cases in the general population most often occur as occasional complications of penetrating trauma, compound fractures or septic abortions. For the first time in history, spontaneous gas gangrene caused by *Clostridium septicum* may be more common than trauma-associated gas gangrene caused by *C. perfringens*, *Clostridium histolyticum* or other *Clostridium* spp. (see Chapter 8.21).

Necrotizing fasciitis is a life-threatening form of soft tissue infection. It can occur in association with gas gangrene as a part of generalized tissue necrosis or as a separate clinical entity.[2] Two types of necrotizing fasciitis, types I and II, are recognized. Type I necrotizing fasciitis occurs in patients who have diabetes mellitus or severe peripheral vascular disease, or both;[3] it is usually caused by mixed aerobic and anaerobic bacteria. Although the risk for an individual diabetic patient is low, this type of deep soft tissue infection is the most common form of necrotizing fasciitis in the general population, because the total number of people who have diabetes is large.

Type II necrotizing fasciitis, formerly called streptococcal gangrene, is caused by group A streptococci. Since the mid-1980s, this disease been recognized with increasing frequency in many parts of the world, at a current annual incidence of 5–10 cases per 100,000.[4]

MORBIDITY AND MORTALITY

Before the availability of antibiotics, gas gangrene was usually fatal. Since then, mortality rates from gas gangrene caused by *C. perfringens* have improved, owing to aggressive antibiotic therapy, aggressive surgical therapy employing better surgical techniques, and hyperbaric oxygen therapy. The most important factors in determining outcome, reducing the need for amputations and preventing shock has been early recognition and aggressive treatment (see page 3.5).

The mortality and morbidity of group A streptococcal necrotizing fasciitis has evolved differently. In the pre-antibiotic era this infection carried a mortality rate of about 25% when treated with surgery (such as 'bear claw' fasciotomies) alone.[5] In modern times, mortality due to group A streptococcal necrotizing fasciitis has not decreased and continues to range from 30 to 70% despite antibiotics, appropriate surgical debridement and intensive supportive care. This suggests that more virulent strains must be responsible.

CLINICAL FEATURES

Pain, either generalized or localized, is the most common reason for patients who have deep-seated infection to seek medical care (Fig. 3.1). Although myalgia may occur with any febrile illness as part of the systemic immune response, in certain infectious diseases myalgia may provide an invaluable clinical clue. For example, diffuse myalgia is one of the cardinal manifestations of influenza. Severe, localized pain in a febrile patient is a common presentation for deep-seated bacterial infection. Early in the course of necrotizing fasciitis caused by group A streptococci, patients may have a viral-like prodrome with nausea, vomiting, diarrhea and fever; however, later in the course of the disease, patients seek medical assistance because of increasingly severe localized pain with continuing fever.

A portal of entry can be defined in the majority of cases of deep bacterial soft tissue infections such as type I necrotizing fasciitis and traumatic gas gangrene. In type I necrotizing fasciitis, infection begins at the site of a surgical incision, at a mucosal tear or at sites of skin breakdown in patients who have diabetes mellitus or peripheral vascular disease. Similarly, traumatic gas gangrene occurs at the site of major trauma such as a crush injuries or penetrating injuries severe enough to cause arterial damage. In these cases, the clinician has reason to suspect infection as a cause of fever or increasing pain. In

DIFFERENTIAL DIAGNOSIS OF INFECTIONS INVOLVING MUSCLE AND FASCIA					
Clinical feature	Necrotizing fasciitis type I	Necrotizing fasciitis type II	Gas gangrene	Pyomyositis	Myositis due to viruses or parasites
Fever					
Diffuse pain					Note 1
Localized pain		Note 2			
Systemic toxicity					
Gas in tissue					
Obvious portal of entry		Note 3	Note 4		
Diabetes mellitus					

Note 1: Pain with influenza is diffuse myalgia. Pleurodynia may be associated with severe localized pain (i.e. devil's grip). Pain with trichinosis may be severe and localized.

Note 2: Severe pain is present in necrotizing fasciitis associated with group A streptococcal necrotizing fasciitis. Necrotizing fasciitis type I is commonly seen in people who have diabetes mellitus who have peripheral neuropathy; hence the pain may not be severe.

Note 3: Fifty percent of patients who have necrotizing fasciitis caused by group A streptococci may not have an obvious portal of entry.

Note 4: Gas gangrene associated with trauma may be caused by *Clostridium perfringens*, *Clostridium septicum* and *Clostridium histolyticum* and there is always an obvious portal of entry. Spontaneous gas gangrene caused by *Clostridium septicum* is usually not associated with an obvious portal of entry. Organisms lodge in tissue as a result of bacteremia originating from a bowel portal of entry.

Fig. 3.1 Differential diagnosis of infections involving muscle and fascia. Red, severe; orange, moderate; yellow, mild-to-moderate; blue, mild; white, none.

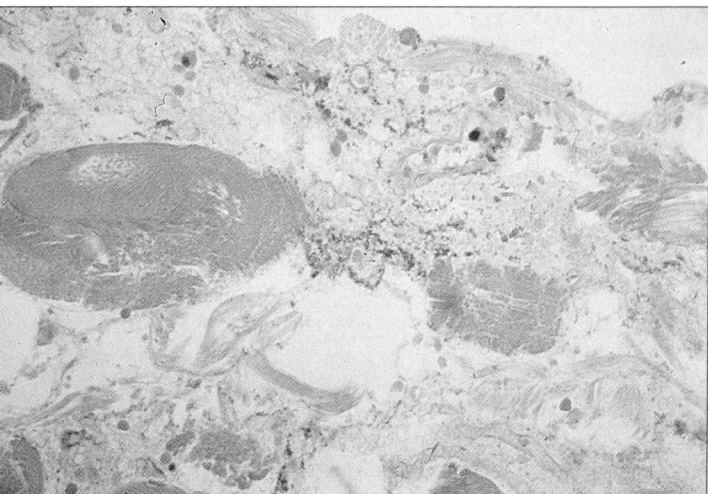

Fig. 3.2 Histopathologic examination of tissue from a patient who has necrotizing fasciitis with extension into the underlying musculature. Note the absence of acute inflammatory cells in the area of muscle necrosis. When present, infiltrating granulocytes can be seen at the interface between normal and necrotic tissue and are often massed within small postcapillary venules.

erythema is superseded by violaceous bullous lesions, massive local swelling becomes apparent and signs of systemic toxicity develop rapidly (see Chapter 8.19).

SPECIFIC TYPES OF DEEP SOFT TISSUE INFECTION

NECROTIZING INFECTIONS

Necrotizing infections of the skin and underlying soft tissues share the features of fulminant destruction of tissue and severe systemic signs of toxicity associated with high mortality (see Fig. 3.1). Few areas of infectious diseases have a more confusing nomenclature. This is partly because authors have named necrotizing infections on the basis of clinical features, whereas these diagnoses should be based on surgical or pathologic findings. Thus, many different names have been used to describe processes that share common pathologic features:

* extensive tissue destruction,
* thrombosis of blood vessels,
* abundant bacteria spreading along fascial planes, and
* relatively few acute inflammatory cells, although small collections of polymorphonuclear leukocytes or microabscesses have been described (Fig. 3.2).

For patients who have evidence of an aggressive localized soft tissue infection, prompt surgical exploration of that site is of extreme importance to determine whether a necrotizing process is present. The same is true for patients who have milder local features associated with severe systemic toxicity. In addition, although the clinical entity referred to as necrotizing fasciitis may occur alone, there is commonly also evidence of necrosis extending up to the dermis and down to underlying muscle (myonecrosis). Despite these common features, it is worth reviewing the many different types of necrotizing soft tissue infections that have been described in the literature because this may point to clinical clues leading to earlier surgical intervention and therefore an earlier diagnosis.

NECROTIZING FASCIITIS

Necrotizing fasciitis is a deep-seated infection of the subcutaneous tissue that results in progressive destruction of fascia and fat, although it may spare the skin itself.[8] Two clinical types exist.

Type I necrotizing fasciitis

Type I necrotizing fasciitis is a mixed infection caused by aerobic and anaerobic bacteria. It occurs most commonly after surgical procedures, in diabetic patients or in those who have peripheral vascular

contrast, patients who have either type II necrotizing fasciitis or spontaneous gas gangrene may have no apparent portal of entry.[6] Early in the course of infection in such patients, the only physical signs of infection may be fever and localized tenderness. Fever and localized pain are the cardinal clues to this diagnosis, but in some cases evidence of localized infection may not become apparent until after the development of systemic signs such as hypotension or organ failure.

Early in the course of deep infection associated with a defined portal of entry there is generally evidence of localized inflammation such as swelling, redness, warmth and tenderness. At that point the process may resemble simple cellulitis, which can be caused by any of a multitude of bacteria (see Chapter 2.2). In type I necrotizing fasciitis there is generally gas in the tissue, as there is in gas gangrene. Where there is no apparent portal of entry, the leading diagnoses to be considered are infection with group A streptococci (type II necrotizing fasciitis), *C. septicum* (spontaneous gangrene) or *Vibrio vulnificus*. The presence of gas in the tissue favors clostridial infection.

Gas may be detected by physical examination (crepitus) or by imaging (radiography, MRI or CT scan). Group A streptococci should be suspected if there is fever and severe pain and a history of blunt trauma or muscle strain. *Vibrio vulnificus* should be suspected in a patient who has cirrhosis of the liver, a history of ingestion of raw oysters or exposure to seawater in the south-east Atlantic Ocean or the Caribbean Sea.[7] Later, disease (see Fig. 3.1). Nonclostridial anaerobic cellulitis and synergistic necrotizing cellulitis are both variants of the same syndrome. It may not be important to distinguish these entities from one another, because all occur in diabetic patients and are caused by mixed anaerobic and aerobic bacteria.

Clinical features

These infections most commonly occur on or about the feet, with rapid extension along the fascia into the leg. Although cellulitis also occurs commonly in diabetic patients, necrotizing fasciitis should be considered in those who have cellulitis and systemic signs of infection such as tachycardia, leukocytosis, acidosis or marked hyperglycemia. In addition to its spontaneous occurrence in diabetic patients, type I necrotizing fasciitis may also develop as a result of a breach in the integrity of mucous membranes from surgery or instrumentation. In the head and neck region, bacterial penetration into the fascial compartments can result in a related syndrome known as Ludwig's angina (Fig. 3.3) or it may develop into necrotizing fasciitis. Group A streptococci may cause necrotizing fasciitis or a peritonsillar abscess, which can extend into the deep structures of the neck (Fig. 3.4).

Diagnostic tests

The first goal of management is to determine the depth and extent of the infection. Computed tomography or MRI scans are invaluable in this regard to determine whether the infection is localized or spreading along fascial planes. The second goal is to determine whether surgical intervention is necessary. Because of the proximity to vital structures of the neck, surgical consultation is of major importance because exploration, drainage and debridement may be necessary to prevent airway obstruction, to determine the level of soft tissue involvement and to establish which bacteria are involved.

Treatment

Both Ludwig's angina and necrotizing fasciitis of the head and neck are usually caused by mouth anaerobes such as *Fusobacterium* spp. anaerobic streptococci, *Bacteroides* spp. and spirochetes. Either penicillin or clindamycin is effective treatment largely because the Gram-positive aerobic cocci and anaerobes of the oropharynx are generally susceptible to both. In contrast, type I necrotizing fasciitis below the diaphragm requires ampicillin plus clindamycin and a fluoroquinalon to cover the *Bacteroides* spp. and enterobacteriacea.

Type II necrotizing fasciitis

Type II necrotizing fasciitis is caused by group A streptococci and was previously called streptococcal gangrene.[5] In recent years, there has been a dramatic increase in the number of invasive infections, including necrotizing fasciitis, caused by group A streptococci. In contrast to type I necrotizing fasciitis, type II may occur in any age group and among patients who do not have complicated medical illnesses. Predisposing factors include:

- a history of blunt trauma,
- muscle strain,
- childbirth,
- chickenpox,
- nonsteroidal anti-inflammatory agents,[9]
- intravenous drug abuse, or
- penetrating injury such as caused by a laceration or a surgical procedure.

In penetrating injuries, it is the skin rather than the mucous membranes that serve as the portal of entry for the streptococci. In contrast, among patients who do not have a defined portal of entry, hematogenous translocation of group A streptococci from the throat (asymptomatic or symptomatic pharyngitis) to the site of blunt trauma or muscle strain probably occurs.[10] The only other possibility, which is of course highly conjectural, is that group A streptococci reside in a dormant state in the deep tissue and trauma of various types reactivates their growth.

Group A streptococci are contagious microbes that in the past have caused epidemics of pharyngitis and scarlet fever in schools, rheumatic fever in military recruits and surgical wound infections in hospitalized patients. Thus, close contacts of a patient who have type II necrotizing fasciitis have a high likelihood of becoming colonized with a virulent strain. Clearly the risk of developing a secondary case of fulminant necrotizing fasciitis is very low, but it is probably higher than it is in the general population. In evaluating the risk to family members and hospital workers, the physician should consider the degree of exposure and the susceptibility of the host. Contacts who have conditions such as chickenpox or open wounds may benefit from prophylactic penicillin.

Pathogenesis

Pyrogenic exotoxins possess the unique ability to bind simultaneously to the MHC (major histocompatibility complex) class 11 portion of antigen-presenting cells, such as macrophage and specific Vβ (variable part of beta chain) segments of the T-lymphocyte receptor in the absence of classic antigen processing by the macrophage.[13] Thus, pyrogenic exotoxins are superantigens that can cause rapid proliferation of T lymphocytes bearing specific Vβ repertoires. Such stimulation of the host's immune cells is associated with production of both monokines [tumor necrosis factor (TNF)$_\alpha$], interleukin (IL)-1 and IL-6)] and the lymphokines (IL-2, interferon and TNF$_\beta$).[14] Expression of

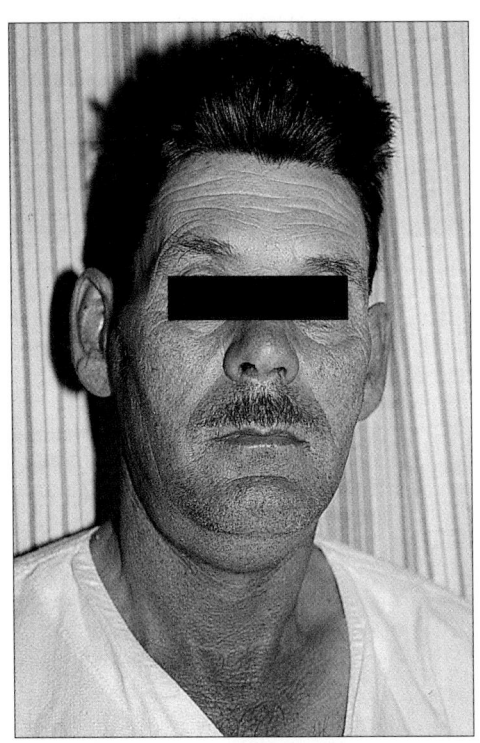

Fig. 3.3 Ludwig's angina. Infection begins with a break in the mucosal lining in the oropharynx; oral bacterial flora invade the soft tissues at the base of the tongue and penetrate through the floor of the mouth and into soft tissue of the neck. The floor of the mouth is elevated and patients talk as though they have a 'hot potato' in their mouth. Potential airway obstruction is a major concern. Although patients usually respond to penicillin, surgical consultation should be obtained, and CT or MRI scans are useful for determining whether a necrotizing process is present.

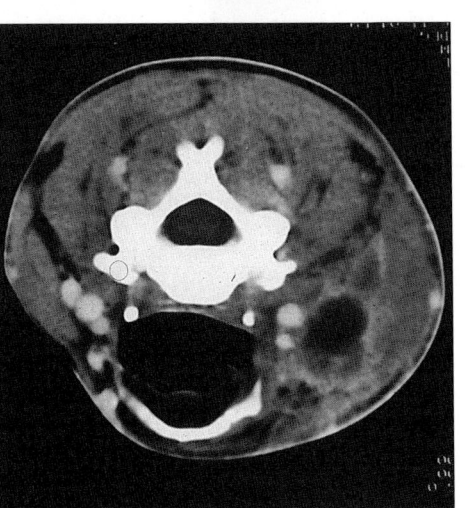

Fig. 3.4 Computed tomography of a soft tissue infection of the neck. This infection is caused by group A streptococci, which invaded as a rare complication of a previous 'strep throat'. Surgical drainage yielded a pure culture of group A streptococci and established a diagnosis. The patient was treated with intravenous penicillin for 10 days and made a good recovery.

these cytokines *in vivo* probably contributes to shock, organ failure and tissue destruction.[15]

Clinical features

Necrotizing fasciitis exhibits a remarkably rapid progression from an inapparent process to one associated with extensive destruction of tissue, systemic toxicity, loss of limb or death.[6,10,11] Unexplained pain that increases rapidly over time may be the first manifestation of infection.[6,10] The early signs and symptoms of infection may not be apparent, particularly in patients who have postsurgical infection, gunshot or knife wounds, or diabetes. In patients who have diabetes, the absence of pain may be related to neuropathy and anesthesia at the site of infection. In surgical patients, patients who have traumatic injuries and postpartum patients, the increasing pain may be assumed to be part of the normal convalescence rather than to be due acute infection. Such a delay in diagnosis may allow the disease to progress to later stages before appropriate antibiotics and surgical invention are initiated.

In addition to pain, there may also be fever, malaise, myalgias, diarrhea and anorexia during the first 24 hours; erythema, which may be diffuse or local, may also be present. However, in most patients excruciating pain in the absence of any cutaneous findings may be the only clue of infection. Within 24–48 hours, erythema may develop or darken to a reddish-purple color, frequently with associated blisters and bullae. Conversely, erythema may be absent and the characteristic bullae may develop in skin of normal appearance. The bullae are initially filled with clear fluid and rapidly take on a blue or maroon appearance (Fig. 3.5). When the bullous stage is observed, there is already extensive necrotizing fasciitis (Fig. 3.5) and patients usually exhibit fever and systemic toxicity.

Although many different M-types of group A streptococci have been associated with necrotizing fasciitis in the past, M type I and 3 have been the strains most commonly isolated from patients throughout the world.[10] These strains can produce one or more of the pyrogenic exotoxins A, B and C.[6,12] Necrotizing fasciitis caused by these strains is frequently associated with 'streptococcal toxic-shock syndrome'.[6] The hallmarks of this syndrome are the early onset of shock and multiple organ failure (see Chapter 8.14).

Diagnosis

Laboratory tests such as creatine phosphokinase, aspartate aminotransferase and serum creatinine usually show elevated levels and, together with leukocytosis with marked left shift, these findings should be sufficient to prompt surgical exploration.[6] Some experts have advocated punch biopsy and frozen section to establish the diagnosis; however, there may be false-negative findings if the deep tissue is not adequately sampled. Routine soft tissue radiographs, CT scans and MRI scans show soft tissue swelling.[16] Gas is not present and abscess formation is not apparent. These radiographic abnormalities are not unusual in uninfected patients who have trauma, or in postsurgical or postpartum patients (Fig. 3.6). In such cases, direct surgical exploration will determine whether necrotizing fasciitis is present, accomplish debridement of necrotic tissue and obtain material suitable for Gram stains and culture.

Management

The three main themes in treatment are surgical debridement, appropriate antibiotics and intensive supportive care. Some patients require mechanical ventilation and others need hemodialysis. Because of intractable hypotension and diffuse capillary leak, massive amounts of intravenous fluids (10–20 liters per day) are often necessary, although anasarca is a common complication. In some patients blood pressure improves with intravenous fluid alone. Pressors such as dopamine may be useful, but there is little controlled information from clinical or experimental studies in this specific infection. Although potent vasoconstrictors such as epinephrine (adrenaline) may improve blood pressure, symmetric gangrene may ensue, partly as a result of the

drug and partly as a result of poor perfusion caused by the bacteria, toxins and endogenous mediators.

Antibiotic selection is difficult in patients who have rapidly progressing infection. Recent studies suggest that clindamycin is superior to penicillin for treatment of experimental necrotizing fasciitis or myonecrosis caused by group A streptococci.[17] This corroborates studies done by Eagle more than 40 years ago, which demonstrated the failure of penicillin in this setting.[18] It seems likely that penicillin

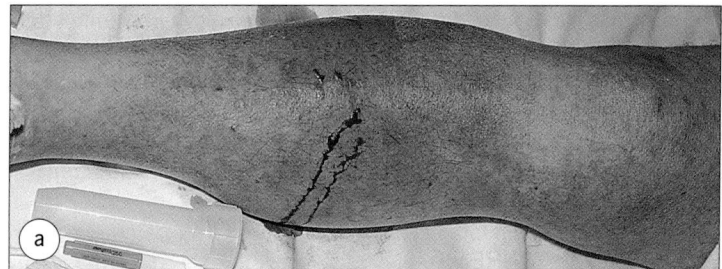
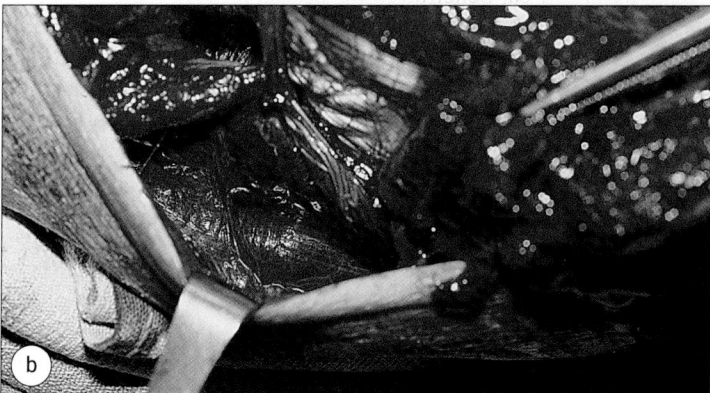

Fig. 3.5 Type II necrotizing fasciitis caused by group A streptococci. (a) This patient was a 60-year old man who had type II diabetes mellitus and who had a 3-day history of malaise, diffuse myalgia and low-grade fever. Over the course of 2–3 hours the pain became excruciating and was localized to the calf. During this time the calf swelled. Note that the skin over the anterior shin looks relatively normal, but that two small purple bullae are present. (b) Extensive necrotizing fasciitis was present on surgical exploration. In addition, myonecrosis was present beneath the fascia. The patient developed profound hypotension, acute respiratory distress syndrome and renal failure. He died despite aggressive surgical and medical management. There was no definable portal of entry, yet group A streptococci were grown from deep cultures and from blood.

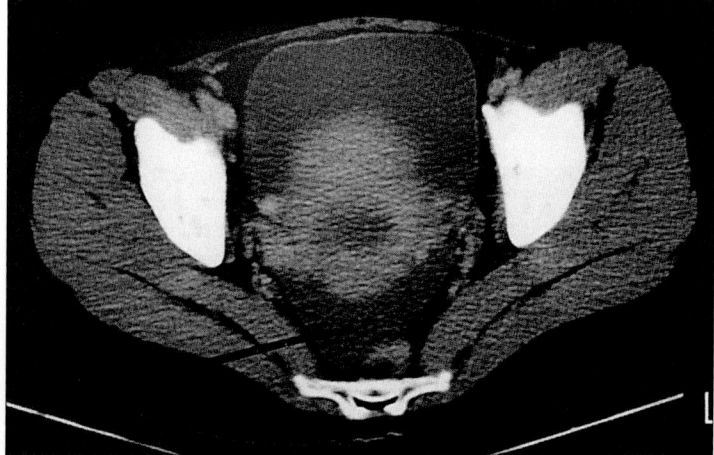

Fig. 3.6 Postpartum sepsis due to group A streptococci. The patient was a 24-year old woman who delivered a normal child. Thirty-six hours after delivery she developed fever, leukocytosis with marked left shift and increasing low abdominal pain. This MRI demonstrates swelling of the uterus, although not out of proportion for a recent delivery. There was no gas in the tissue. An emergency laparotomy revealed necrosis of the mucosa of the uterus, necrotizing fasciitis and myonecrosis of the uterus.

failure is due to the reduced expression of critical penicillin-binding proteins during the stationary phase of bacterial growth.[19] Clindamycin may be more efficacious because:

- it is not affected by inoculum size or stage of growth,
- it suppresses toxin production,
- it facilitates phagocytosis of *Streptococcus pyogenes* by inhibiting M-protein synthesis,
- it suppresses the production of regulatory elements that control cell wall synthesis, and
- it has a long postantibiotic effect.[20]

Neutralization of circulating streptococcal toxins is a desirable therapeutic goal and is advocated by some experts.[21-24] There seems little question that some batches of intravenous gammaglobulin contain neutralizing antibodies against some streptococcal toxins.[23] On the basis of two case reports[21,22] and a report of a nonrandomized clinical trial, there is a suggestion that this treatment may affect the mortality and morbidity of this fulminant infection.[24]

FOURNIER'S GANGRENE

In the perineal area, penetration of the gastrointestinal or urethral mucosa by bacteria may cause 'Fournier's gangrene', an aggressive infection caused by aerobic Gram-negative bacteria, enterococci and anaerobic bacteria such as *Bacteroides* spp. and peptostreptococci. These infections begin abruptly with severe pain and may spread rapidly to the anterior abdominal wall and the gluteal muscles; in males, infection frequently extends to the scrotum and penis (Fig. 3.7).

Surgical inspection, placement of drains and appropriate surgical debridement are necessary for both diagnosis and treatment. Antibiotic treatment should be based upon Gram-stain, culture and sensitivity information when available. An appropriate empiric regimen would be either ampicillin or ampicillin and sulbactam combined with either clindamycin or metronidazole. Alternatively, broader Gram-negative coverage might be advisable if the patient has had prior hospitalization or if antibiotics have been used recently. This could be accomplished by substituting ticarcillin–clavulanic acid or piperacillin–tazobactam for ampicillin, or by adding a fluorinated quinolone or an aminoglycoside.

MELENEY'S SYNERGISTIC GANGRENE

This rare variant occurs in postsurgical patients. The lesion is a slowly expanding, indolent ulceration that is confined to the superficial fascia. It results from a synergistic interaction between *S. aureus* and microaerophilic streptococci. As in other forms of necrotizing infection, antibiotic therapy together with surgical debridement are the mainstays of treatment.

NONCLOSTRIDIAL ANAEROBIC CELLULITIS

In nonclostridial anaerobic cellulitis, infection is associated with mixed anaerobic and aerobic organisms that produce gas in tissues. Unlike clostridial cellulitis, this type of infection is usually associated with diabetes mellitus, and it often produces a foul odor. Surgical exploration is required to distinguish this condition from necrotizing cellulitis, myonecrosis and necrotizing fasciitis by *Clostridium* spp.

CLOSTRIDIAL CELLULITIS

In clostridial cellulitis, infection is usually preceded by local trauma or recent surgery. *Clostridium perfringens* is the most common species causing this entity. Gas is invariably found in the skin; the fascia and deep muscle are spared. Although clostridial cellulitis differs from clostridial myonecrosis in that there is less systemic toxicity, it is mandatory that thorough surgical exploration and debridement should be performed to distinguish these entities. Magnetic resonance imaging or CT scans as well as a serum creatinine phosphokinase assay may also be useful for determining whether muscle tissue is involved. Treatment is discussed below under gas gangrene.

CLOSTRIDIAL GAS GANGRENE

Three types of clostridial soft tissue infections have been defined:[1]

- simple wound contamination or colonization,
- anaerobic cellulitis, and
- clostridial gas gangrene.

The first type, simple wound contamination or colonization, does not progress to true infection for various reasons (e.g. there may insufficient devitalized tissue to promote infection, or there may be effective host responses or effective medical and surgical management). Contamination is a very common occurrence; 30–80% of open traumatic wounds contain clostridial species.[25]

The second type, anaerobic cellulitis, occurs when there is devitalized tissue in a wound, sufficient for growth of *C. perfringens* or other strains. Although gas is produced locally and extends along fascial planes, bacteremia and invasion of healthy tissue does not occur. Appropriate medical and surgical management, including prompt removal of the devitalized tissue, is all that is necessary for cure, and mortality is generally nil.[1]

The third type is clostridial gas gangrene or myonecrosis. This is defined as an acute invasion of healthy living muscle that is undamaged by previous trauma or ischemia.[25] It is divided into three different subtypes:

- traumatic gas gangrene,
- spontaneous or nontraumatic gas gangrene, and
- recurrent gas gangrene caused by *C. perfringens*.

Traumatic gas gangrene is the most common subtype. It develops when a deep, penetrating injury that compromises the blood supply (e.g. knife or gunshot wounds, crush injury or car accident) creates an anaerobic environment that is ideal for clostridial proliferation. This type of trauma accounts for about 70% of cases of gas gangrene.

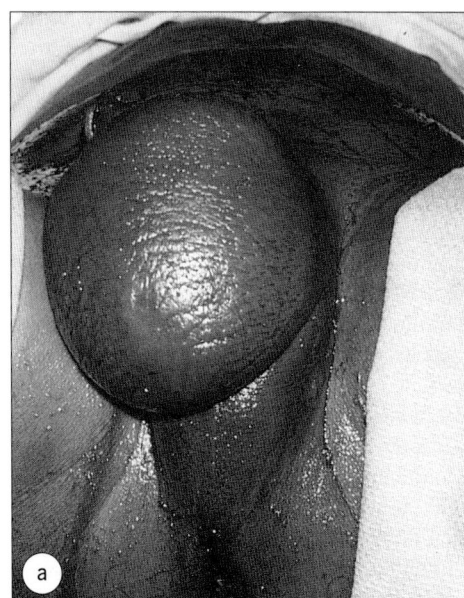

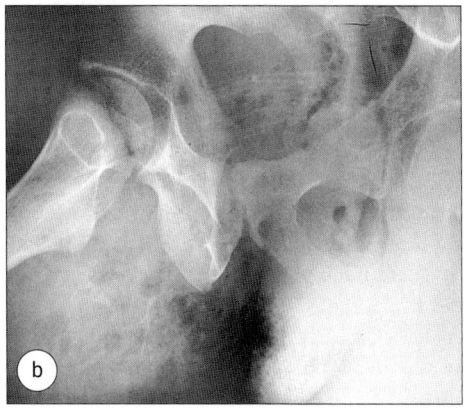

Fig. 3.7 Type I necrotizing fasciitis. A 24-year old man had been in good health but was awakened with severe perineal pain. (a) This photograph was taken 3 hours later. Note the massive swelling of the scrotum. (b) Soft tissue radiograph shows gas in the tissues of the thigh, buttocks, scrotum and anterior abdominal wall. Surgical inspection revealed brownish fluid in the scrotum, with gray, dull-colored, friable fascia but normal underlying musculature. Cultures grew *Enterococcus faecalis, Bacteroides fragilis, Escherichia coli* and anaerobic streptococci. The patient was treated with ampicillin, clindamycin and gentamicin for 3 weeks and surgical drains were placed in the scrotum, buttocks, thigh and anterior abdominal wall. There was an excellent clinical response. In some cases, surgery of a more radical nature may be necessary.

Clostridium perfringens is found in about 80% of such infections;[1] the remaining cases are caused by *C. septicum*, *Clostridium novyi*, *C. histolyticum*, *Clostridium bifermentans*, *Clostridium tertium* and *Clostridium fallax*. Other conditions associated with traumatic gas gangrene are bowel and biliary tract surgery, intramuscular injection of epinephrine, illegal abortion, retained placenta, prolonged rupture of the membranes and intrauterine fetal demise or missed abortion in postpartum patients.

Spontaneous or nontraumatic gas gangrene is less common. This is often caused by the more aerotolerant species *C. septicum*. As described later, most of these cases occur in patients who have a gastrointestinal portal of entry such as adenocarcinoma.

Third, and least common, is recurrent gas gangrene caused by *C. perfringens*. This has been described in people who have nonpenetrating injuries at sites of previous gas gangrene; residual spores of *C. perfringens* may remain quiescent in tissue for periods of up to 20 years, then germinate when minor trauma provides anaerobic conditions suitable for growth.[26]

TRAUMATIC GAS GANGRENE
Pathogenesis
The initiating trauma introduces organisms (either vegetative forms or spores) into the deep tissues, and produces an anaerobic niche with a sufficiently low redox potential and acid pH for optimal clostridial growth.[1,25] Necrosis progresses within hours. At the junction of necrotic and normal tissues few polymorphonuculear leukocytes are present, yet pavementing of these cells along the endothelium is apparent within capillaries and in small arterioles and postcapillary venules.[34,35] Later in the course of the illness there is leukostasis within larger vessels. Thus, the histopathology of clostridial gas gangrene is opposite to that seen in soft tissue infections caused by pyogenic organisms such as *S. aureus*, in which an early luxuriant influx of polymorphonuculear leukocytes localizes the infection without adjacent tissue or vascular destruction. Recent studies suggest that σ-toxin (Fig. 3.8), when elaborated in high concentrations at the site of infection, destroys host tissues and inflammatory cells.[36] As the toxin diffuses into surrounding tissues or enters the systemic circulation, σ-toxin promotes dysregulated adhesive interactions between polymorphonuculear leukocytes and endothelial cells and primes leukocytes for increased respiratory burst activity.[36] These actions lead to vascular leukostasis, endothelial cell injury and regional tissue hypoxia. Such perfusion deficits expand the anaerobic environment and contribute to the rapidly advancing margins of tissue destruction that are characteristic of clostridial gangrene.[1]

Shock associated with gas gangrene may be attributable, in part, to direct and indirect effects of toxins. α-Toxin (see Fig. 3.8) directly suppresses myocardial contractility *ex vivo*[37] and may contribute to profound hypotension via a sudden reduction in cardiac output.[38] In experimental models, σ-toxin causes 'warm shock', defined as a markedly reduced systemic vascular resistance combined with a markedly increased cardiac output.[37,38] It is clear that σ-toxin accomplishes this indirectly by inducing endogenous mediators that cause relaxation of blood vessel wall tension, such as the lipid autacoids prostacyclin or platelet-activating factor.[39] Reduced vascular tone develops rapidly and, in order to maintain adequate tissue perfusion, a compensatory host response is required; this either increases cardiac output or rapidly expands the intravascular blood volume. Patients who have Gram-negative sepsis compensate for hypotension by markedly increasing cardiac output; however, this adaptive mechanism may not be possible in shock induced by *C. perfringens* due to direct suppression of myocardial contractility by α-toxin.[37] The role of other endogenous mediators such as cytokines (e.g. TNF, IL-1, IL-6) as well as the potent endogenous vasodilator bradykinin have not been elucidated.

Prevention
Aggressive debridement of devitalized tissue and rapid repair of compromised vascular supply greatly reduce the frequency of gas gangrene

in contaminated deep wounds. Intramuscular epinephrine, prolonged application of tourniquets and surgical closure of traumatic wounds should be avoided. Patients who have compound fractures are at particular risk of gas gangrene if the wound is surgically closed. Patients who have contaminated wounds should receive prophylactic antibiotics.

Clinical findings
The first symptom is usually the sudden onset of severe pain at the site of recent surgery or trauma.[2,25] The mean incubation period is less than 24 hours, but it ranges from 6 to 8 hours to several days, probably depending on the degree of soil contamination or bowel contents spillage and the extent of vascular compromise.

The skin may initially appear pale, but it quickly changes to bronze then purplish red, becoming tense and exquisitely tender (Fig. 3.9). Bullae develop; they may be clear, red, blue or purple.

Gas in tissue may be obvious from physical examination, soft tissue radiographs, CT scan or MRI. Interestingly, none of these radiographic procedures have proved to be more specific or more sensitive than the

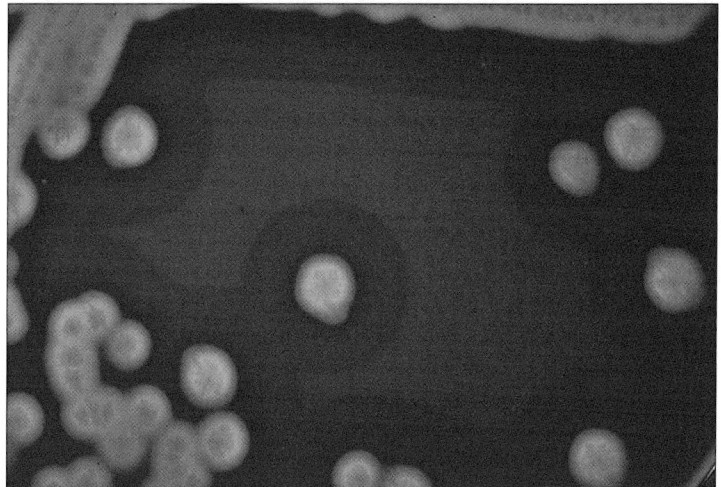

Fig. 3.8 Colonies of *Clostridium perfringens* growing on an anaerobic blood agar plate. σ-Toxin causes the clear zone of hemolysis closest to the colony. A second area of partial hemolysis is caused by α-toxin, an enzyme with phospholipase C activity.

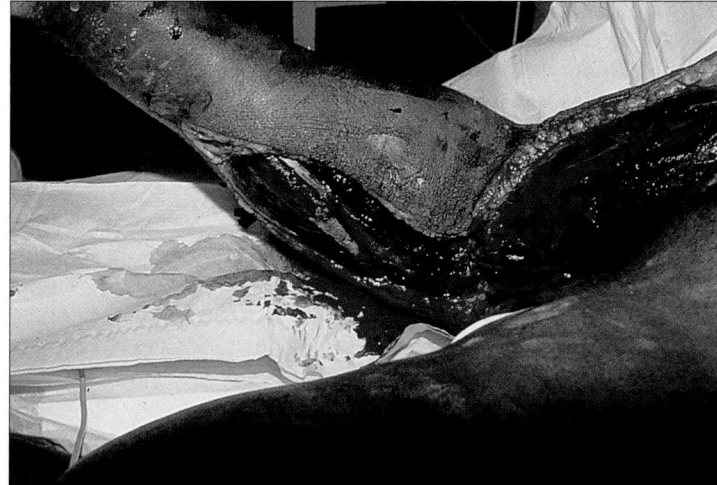

Fig. 3.9 Extensive gas gangrene of the arm due to *Clostridium perfringens*. A 35-year old man sustained a knife wound to the forearm. He did not seek medical care, but 36 hours later experienced severe pain in the upper arm and came to the emergency room. There was extreme tenderness of the arm, and crepitus was easily demonstrated. A radiograph also demonstrated gas in the deep soft tissues. Surgical debridement and antibiotics were instituted, but later amputation at the level of the shoulder was necessary. A pure culture of *Clostridium perfringens* was grown from the deep tissues.

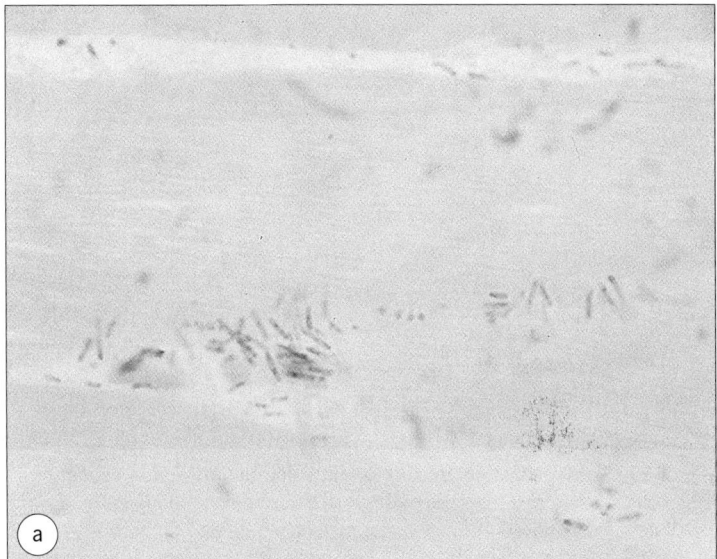
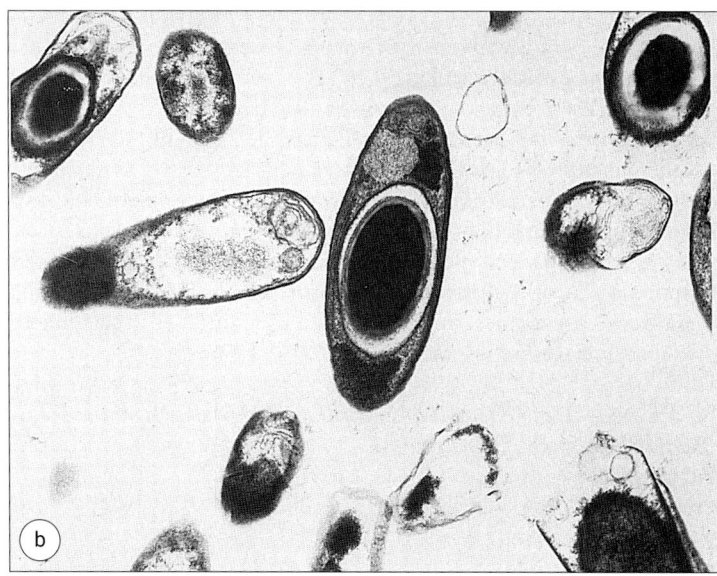

Fig. 3.10 *Clostridium perfringens* **in a patient who has extensive gas gangrene.** (a) Tissue Gram stain of tissue removed from the arm of the patient described in Figure 3.9. Note that the bacteria are rod shaped but Gram variable. Note also that there are few if any acute inflammatory cells at the site of infection. (b) Transmission electron micrograph of *Clostridium perfringens*. Note the endospores.

physical finding of crepitus in the soft tissue.[8] However, radiographic procedures are particularly helpful for demonstrating gas in deeper tissue such as the uterus.

Signs of systemic toxicity develop rapidly; these include tachycardia, fever and diaphoresis, followed by shock and multiple organ failure. Shock is present in 50% of patients at the time they presented to the hospital.[27] Bacteremia occurs in 15% of patients and may be associated with brisk hemolysis. In one patient, the hematocrit fell from 37 to 0% over a 24-hour period.[28] Subsequently, despite transfusion with 10 units of packed red blood cells over 4 hours, the hematocrit never exceeded 7.2%.[28] Based on my studies using recombinant α- and σ-toxins, it is clear that both toxins contribute to this marked intravascular hemolysis (unpublished). Not all cases of *C. perfringens* bacteremia have been associated with gas gangrene,[29] but 90% of *C. perfringens* and 100% of *C. septicum* isolates from blood were associated with clinically significant infection.[30]

Additional complications of clostridial myonecrosis include jaundice, renal failure, hypotension and liver necrosis. Renal failure is largely due to hemoglobinuria and myoglobinuria, but may it be a result of acute tubular necrosis caused by hypotension. Renal tubular cells are probably directly affected by toxins, but this has not been proved.

Diagnosis

Increasing pain at a site of previous injury or surgery, together with signs of systemic toxicity and gas in the tissues, support the diagnosis. Definitive diagnosis rests on demonstrating large, Gram-variable rods at the affected site (Fig. 3.10). Note that although clostridia stain Gram-positive when obtained from bacteriologic media, when visualized from infected tissues they often appear both Gram-positive and Gram-negative. In fresh specimens *C. perfringens* may appear to be encapsulated,[31] although this was not corroborated in gas gangrene associated with war-time trauma.[32] Surgical exploration is essential. The exposed muscle appears edematous, may be an abnormal reddish-blue to black color and does not bleed or contract when stimulated. Usually, some degree of necrotizing fasciitis and cutaneous necrosis are also present. Microscopic evaluation of biopsy material (see Fig. 3.10) demonstrates organisms among degenerating muscle bundles and characteristically an absence of acute inflammatory cells.[25,33]

Management

Penicillin, clindamycin, tetracycline, chloramphenicol, metronidazole and a number of cephalosporins have excellent in-vitro activity against *C. perfringens* and other clostridia. No controlled clinical trials have ever been conducted to compare the efficacy of these agents in humans. Based strictly on in-vitro susceptibility data, most textbooks state that penicillin is the drug of choice.[40,41] However, experimental studies in mice suggest that clindamycin has the greatest efficacy and penicillin the least.[42,43] Other agents with greater efficacy than penicillin include erythromycin, rifampin (rifampicin), tetracycline, chloramphenicol and metronidazole.[42,43] Slightly greater survival was observed in animals receiving both clindamycin and penicillin; in contrast, antagonism was observed with penicillin plus metronidazole.[43] Because between 2 and 5% of strains are resistant to clindamycin, a combination of penicillin and clindamycin is warranted. Based on his experimental studies and his vast clinical experience with gas gangrene, the late Dr William Altemeier recommended tetracycline and penicillin.[44] Thus, given an absence of efficacy data from a clinical trial in humans, the best treatment would appear to be clindamycin or tetracycline combined with penicillin. The failure of penicillin in experimental clostridial myonecrosis may be related to continued toxin production and filament formation rather than lysis.[45] In contrast, the efficacy of clindamycin and tetracycline may be related to their ability to inhibit toxin synthesis rapidly.[45]

Aggressive and thorough surgical debridement is mandatory to improve survival, preserve limbs and prevent complications.[40,41] The use of hyperbaric oxygen (HBO) is controversial, although some non-randomized studies have reported good results with HBO therapy when combined with antibiotics and surgical debridement.[27,46,47] Experimental studies in animals have demonstrated that HBO alone can be effective treatment if the inoculum is small and treatment is begun immediately.[48] In contrast, other studies have demonstrated that HBO was only of slight benefit when combined with penicillin.[49] However, survival was better with clindamycin alone than with either HBO alone, penicillin alone or HBO plus penicillin together.[49] The benefit of HBO, at least theoretically, is to inhibit bacterial growth,[50] to preserve marginally perfused tissue and to inhibit toxin production.[51] Interestingly, Altemeier did not use HBO and was able to realize a mortality rate of less than 15% using surgical debridement and antibiotics (tetracycline plus penicillin) alone.[44]

Therapeutic strategies directed against toxin expression *in vivo*, such as neutralization with specific antitoxin antibody or inhibition of toxin synthesis, may be valuable adjuncts to traditional antimicrobial regimens. Currently, antitoxin is no longer available. Future strategies may target endogenous proadhesive molecules such that toxin-induced vascular leukostasis and resultant tissue injury are attenuated.

Prognosis

Patients presenting with gas gangrene of an extremity have a better prognosis than those who have truncal or intra-abdominal gas gangrene, largely because it is difficult to debride such lesions adequately.[40,41,52] Hyperbaric oxygen could be useful in such patients, yet there is little data on this subject. In addition to truncal gangrene, patients who have associated bacteremia and intravascular hemolysis have the greatest likelihood of progressing to shock and death. In one study, of those patients who developed shock at some point in their hospitalization, 40% died, compared with 20% mortality in the group as a whole.[27] In another study, those who were in shock at the time of diagnosis had the highest mortality.[52]

SPONTANEOUS, NONTRAUMATIC GAS GANGRENE DUE TO *CLOSTRIDIUM SEPTICUM*

Pathogenesis

Predisposing factors include:[52–54]

- colonic carcinoma,
- diverticulitis,
- gastrointestinal surgery,
- leukemia,
- lymphoproliferative disorders,
- cancer chemotherapy,
- radiation therapy, and
- AIDS.

Cyclic or other forms of neutropenia are also associated with spontaneous gas gangrene due to *C. septicum,* and in such cases necrotizing enterocolitis, cecitis or distal ileitis are commonly found. These gastrointestinal pathologies permit bacterial access to the bloodstream; consequently, the aerotolerant *C. septicum* can become established in normal tissues.[1]

Clostridium septicum produces four toxins:

- α-toxin (lethal, hemolytic, necrotizing activity),
- β-toxin (deoxyribonuclease),
- γ-toxin (hyaluronidase), and
- δ-toxin (septicolysin, an oxygen labile hemolysin).

Clostridium septicum also produces a protease and a neuraminidase.[1]

The *C. septicum* α-toxin does not possess phospholipase activity and is thus distinct from the α-toxin of *C. perfringens.* Active immunization against α-toxin significantly protects against challenge with viable *C. septicum.*[55] The mechanism by which α-toxin contributes to *C. septicum* pathogenesis is unknown; however, the recent cloning and sequencing of this toxin should facilitate studies in this area (see Chapter 8.21).

Clinical features

The onset of disease is abrupt, often with excruciating pain, although the patient may sense only heaviness or numbness.[1,25,52–54] The first symptom may be confusion or malaise. Extremely rapid progression of gangrene follows. Swelling advances and bullae appear; these are filled with clear, cloudy, hemorrhagic or purplish fluid. The skin around such bullae also has a purple hue (Fig. 3.11), perhaps reflecting vascular compromise resulting from bacterial toxins diffusing into surrounding tissues.[52] Histopathology of muscle and connective tissues includes cell lysis and gas formation; inflammatory cells are notably absent.[52]

Diagnosis

Unlike the situation in traumatic gas gangrene, bacteremia precedes cutaneous manifestations by several hours. In the absence of the usual cutaneous manifestations of gas gangrene, other causes of fever and extremity pain such as deep vein thrombophlebitis or cellulitis are naturally considered first, delaying appropriate diagnosis and treatment, and as a consequence, increasing mortality.

Management

No comparative human trials have evaluated the efficacy of antibiotics or HBO for treating clinical cases of spontaneous gas gangrene. In-vitro

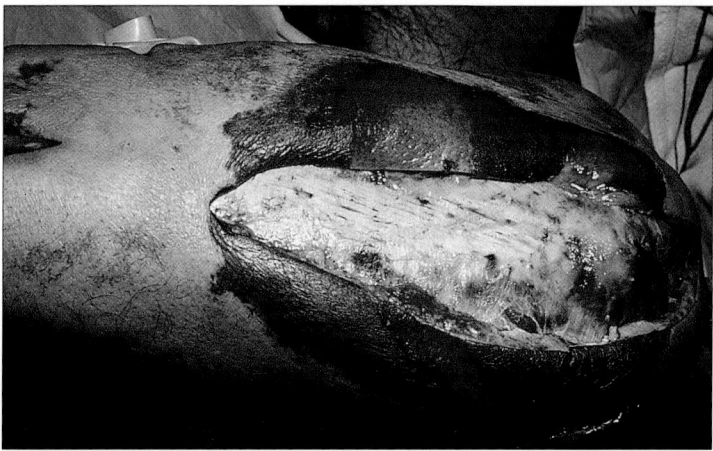

Fig. 3.11 Spontaneous necrotizing fasciitis due to *Clostridium septicum*. This patient developed the sudden onset of severe pain in the forearm. Swelling rapidly ensued and he sought medical treatment. Crepitus was present on physical examination and gas in the soft tissue was verified with routine radiographs. Immediate surgical debridement revealed necrotizing fasciitis but sparing of the muscle. Note the purple–violaceous appearance of the skin. See also Figure 3.12.

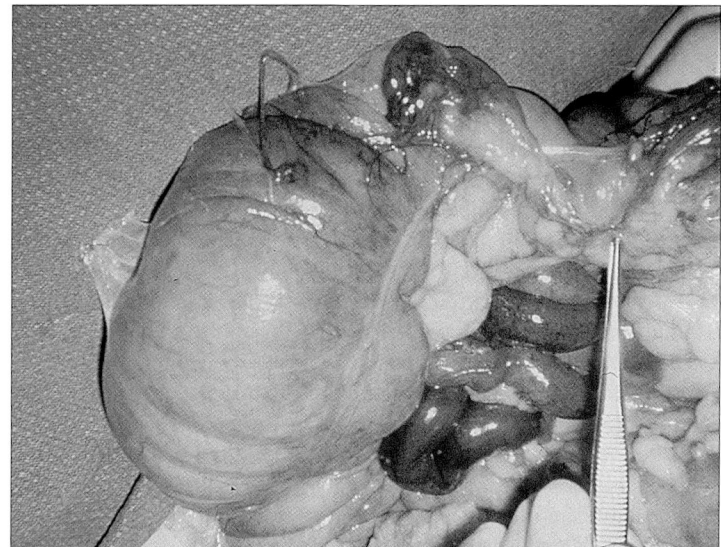

Fig. 3.12 Colonic carcinoma in a patient who has spontaneous gas gangrene caused by *Clostridium septicum*. The patient described in Figure 3.11 was found to have a mass in the colon. Surgical resection revealed an adenocarcinoma, which probably served as a portal of entry for the *Clostridium septicum* bacillus. Hematogenous seeding of the forearm resulted in spontaneous gas gangrene.

data indicate that *C. septicum* is uniformly susceptible to penicillin, tetracycline, erythromycin, clindamycin, chloramphenicol and metronidazole. The aerotolerance of *C. septicum* may reduce the likelihood that HBO therapy would be effective.[50]

Prognosis

The mortality of spontaneous clinical gangrene ranges from 67 to 100%, with the majority of deaths occurring within 24 hours of onset. Unfavorable factors include underlying malignancy and compromised immune status. All patients who survive bacteremia or spontaneous gangrene caused by *C. septicum* should have appropriate diagnostic studies of the gastrointestinal tract (Fig. 3.12). Occasionally, this has led to detection and cure of an unsuspected malignancy that might otherwise have been fatal.[52]

CLOSTRIDIUM SORDELLII INFECTIONS

Patients who have *C. sordellii* infection present with unique clinical features including edema, absence of fever, leukemoid reaction, hemoconcentration and later shock and multiple organ failure.[41] Often *C. sordellii* infections develop after childbirth or after gynecologic procedures,[56] and most represent endometrial infection. Rarely, other cases have occurred at sites of minor trauma such as lacerations of the soft tissues of an extremity. Unlike *C. perfringens* and *C. septicum* infections, pain may not be a prominent feature. The absence of fever and the paucity of signs and symptoms of local infection make early diagnosis difficult.[41] The mechanisms of diffuse capillary leak, massive edema and hemoconcentration are not well established but clearly are related to elaboration of a potent toxin or toxins. Hematocrits of 75–80% have been described and leukocytosis of 50,000–100,000 cells/mm³ with a left shift is common.[33,56]

CLOSTRIDIUM TERTIUM INFECTIONS

Clostridium tertium has been associated with spontaneous myonecrosis; however, it more commonly causes bacteremia in compromised hosts who have received long courses of antibiotics. Bacteremia probably arises from bowel sources and the presence of the organism in the bowel may be partly related to its relative resistance to penicillin, cephalosporins and clindamycin. *Clostridium*

tertium is, however, usually quite sensitive to chloramphenicol, vancomycin and metronidazole. Because this organism can grow aerobically, it may be mistakenly disregarded as a contaminant such as a diphtheroid or a *Bacillus* sp.[40,41]

PYOMYOSITIS

Most cases of pyomyositis occur in tropical areas. Local trauma is a common predisposing factor. Infection occurs within a single muscle group in most cases, with symptoms of localized pain, tenderness and fever (see Fig. 3.1). Diagnosis is confirmed by needle aspiration of pus, which usually yields *S. aureus* on culture. Most patients respond promptly to surgical drainage and appropriate antibiotics; severe systemic complications such as bacteremia and cardiovascular collapse are unusual.

Pyomyositis has been recognized with increasing frequency in North America among HIV-positive patients. *Staphylococcus aureus* remains the most common organism isolated in HIV-positive patients, although unusual organisms have been recovered in 20% of cases. Hospitalized immunocompromised patents who are HIV-negative occasionally develop pyomyositis caused by Gram-negative bacteria.

REFERENCES

1. Smith LDS. Clostridial wound infections. In: Smith LDS, ed. The pathogenic anaerobic bacteria. Springfield, Illinois: Charles C Thomas; 1975:321–4.
2. Weinstein L, Barza M. Gas gangrene. N Engl J Med 1972;289:1129.
3. Stevens DL. Clostridial myonecrosis and other clostridial diseases. In: Bennett JC, Plum F, eds. Cecil textbook of medicine, 20th ed. Philadelphia: WB Saunders; 1996:2090–3.
4. Schwartz B, Facklam RR, Brieman RF. Changing epidemiology of group A streptococcal infection in the USA. Lancet 1990;336:1167–71.
5. Meleney FL. Hemolytic streptococcus gangrene. Arch Surg 1924;9:317–64.
6. Stevens DL, Tanner MH, Winship J, et al. Reappearance of scarlet fever toxin A among streptococci in the Rocky Mountain West: severe group A streptococcal infections associated with a toxic shock-like syndrome. N Eng J Med 1989;321:1–7.
7. *Vibrio vulnificus* infections associated with eating raw oysters – Los Angeles, 1996. MMWR Morb Mortal Wkly Rep 1996;45:621–4.
8. Gozal D, Ziser A, Shupak A, Ariel A, Melamed Y. Necrotizing fasciitis. Arch Surg 1986; 121:233–5.
9. Stevens DL. Could nonsteroidal anti-inflammatory drugs (NSAIDs) enhance the progression of bacterial infections to toxic shock syndrome? Clin Infect Dis 1995;21:977–80.
10. Stevens D. Streptococcal toxic shock syndrome: spectrum of disease, pathogenesis and new concepts in treatment. Emerg Infect Dis 1995;1:69–78.
11. Chelson J, Halstensen A, Haga T, Hoiby EA. Necrotising fasciitis due to group A streptococci in western Norway: incidence and clinical features. Lancet 1994;344:1111–5.
12. Hauser AR, Stevens DL, Kaplan EL, Schlievert PM. Molecular analysis of pyrogenic exotoxins from *Streptococcus pyogenes* isolates associated with toxic shock-like syndrome. J Clin Microbiol 1991;29:1562–7.
13. Marrack P, Kappler JW. The staphylococcal enterotoxins and their relatives. Science 1990;248:705–11.

14. Hackett SP, Stevens DL. Superantigens associated with staphylococcal and streptococcal toxic shock syndromes are potent inducers of tumor necrosis factor beta synthesis. J Infect Dis 1993;168:232–5.
15. Stevens DL, Bryant AE, Hackett SP, et al. Group A streptococcal bacteremia: the role of tumor necrosis factor in shock and organ failure. J Infect Dis 1996;173:619–26.
16. Bisno AL, Stevens DL. Streptococcal infections in skin and soft tissues. N Engl J Med 1996;334:240–5.
17. Stevens DL, Gibbons AE, Bergstrom R, Winn V. The Eagle effect revisited: efficacy of clindamycin, erythromycin, and penicillin in the treatment of streptococcal myositis. J Infect Dis 1988;158:23–8.
18. Eagle H. Experimental approach to the problem of treatment failure with penicillin. I. Group A streptococcal infection in mice. Am J Med 1952;13:389–99.
19. Stevens DL, Yan S, Bryant AE. Penicillin binding protein expression at different growth stages determines penicillin efficacy in vitro and in vivo: an explanation for the inoculum effect. J Infect Dis 1993;167:1401–5.
20. Stevens DL, Bryant AE, Yan S. Invasive group A streptococcal infection: new concepts in antibiotic treatment. Int J Antimicrobial Agents 1994;4:297–301.
21. Barry W, Hudgins L, Donta S, Pesanti E. Intravenous immunoglobulin therapy for toxic shock syndrome. JAMA 1992;267:3315–6.
22. Yong JM. Letter. Lancet 1994;343:1427.
23. Norby-Teglund A, Kaul R, Low DE, McGeer A, Kotb M. Intravenous immunoglobulin and superantigen-neutralizing activity in streptococcal toxic shock syndrome patients [abstract]. 35th Annual Interscience Conference on Antimicrobial Agents and Chemotherapy, San Francisco, 1995.
24. Kaul R, McGeer A, Norby-Teglund A, Kotb M, Low D. Intravenous immunoglobulin therapy in streptococcal toxic shock syndrome: results of a matched case-controlled study [abstract LM68:339]. 35th Annual Interscience Conference on Antimicrobial Agents and Chemotherapy, San Francisco, 1995.

25. MacLennan JD. The histotoxic clostridial infections of man. Bacteriol Rev 1962;26:177–276.
26. Stevens DL, Laposky LL, Montgomery P, Harris I. Recurrent gas gangrene at a site of remote injury: localization due to circulating antitoxin. West J Med 1988;148:204–5.
27. Hart GB, Lamb RC, Strauss MB. Gas gangrene: I. A collective review. J Trauma 1983;23:991–1000.
28. Terebelo HR, McCue RL, Lenneville MS. Implication of plasma free hemoglobin in massive clostridial hemolysis. JAMA 1982;248:2028–9.
29. Gorbach SL, Thadepalli H. Isolation of *Clostridium* in human infections: evaluation of 114 cases. J Infect Dis 1975;131:S8–S85.
30. Brook I. Anaerobic bacterial bacteremia: 12–year experience in two military hospitals. J Infect Dis 1989;160:1071–5.
31. Butler HM. Pathogenicity of washed *Cl. welchii* and mode of development *Cl. welchii* infections in man. Med J Aust 1943;2:224–6.
32. Keppie J, Robertson M. The in vitro toxigenicity and other characters of strains of *Cl. welchii* type A from various sources. J Pathol Bacteriol 1944;56:123–6.
33. Stevens DL. Clostridial infections. In: Stevens DL, Mandell GL, eds. Atlas of infectious diseases. Philadelphia: Churchill Livingstone; 1995:13.1–13.9.
34. McNee JW, Dunn JS. The method of spread of gas gangrene into living muscle. Br Med J 1917;1:727–9.
35. Robb-Smith AHT. Tissues changes induced by *C. welchii* type a filtrates. Lancet 1945;2:362–8.
36. Bryant AE, Bergstrom R, Zimmerman GA, et al. *Clostridium perfringens* invasiveness is enhanced by effects of theta toxin upon PMNL structure and function: the roles of leukocytotoxicity and expression of CD11/CD18 adherence-glycoprotein. FEMS Immunol Med Microbiol 1993;7:321–6.
37. Stevens DL, Troyer BE, Merrick DT, Mitten JE, Olson RD. Lethal effects and cardiovascular effects of purified alpha- and theta-toxins from *Clostridium perfringens*. J Infect Dis 1988;157:272–9.
38. Asmuth DA, Olson RD, Hackett SP, et al. Effects of *Clostridium perfringens* recombinant and crude phospholipase C and theta toxins on rabbit hemodynamic parameters. J Infect Dis 1995;172:1317–23.

39. Whatley RE, Zimmerman GA, Stevens DL, Parker CJ, McIntyre TM, Prescott SM. The regulation of platelet activating factor synthesis in endothelial cells – the role of calcium and protein kinase C. J Biol Chem 1989;11:6325–33.

40. Gorbach SL. *Clostridium perfringens* and other clostridia. In: Gorbach SL, Bartlett JG, Blacklow NR, eds. Infectious diseases. Philadelphia: WB Saunders; 1992:1587–96.

41. Bartlett JG. Gas gangrene (other clostridium-associated diseases). In: Mandell GL, Douglas RG, Bennett JE, eds. Principles and practice of infectious diseases. New York: Churchill Livingstone; 1990:1851–60.

42. Stevens DL, Maier KA, Laine BM, Mitten JE. Comparison of clindamycin, rifampin, tetracycline, metronidazole and penicillin for efficacy in prevention of experimental gas gangrene due to *Clostridium perfringens*. J Infect Dis 1987;155:220–8.

43. Stevens DL, Laine BM, Mitten JE. Comparison of single and combination antimicrobial agents for prevention of experimental gas gangrene caused by *Clostridium perfringens*. Antimicrob Agents Chemother 1987;31:312–6.

44. Altemeier WA, Fullen WD. Prevention and treatment of gas gangrene. JAMA 1971;217:806–13.

45. Stevens DL, Maier KA, Mitten JE. Effect of antibiotics on toxin production and viability of *Clostridium perfringens*. Antimicrob Agents Chemother 1987;31:213–8.

46. Heimbach RD, Boerema I, Brummelkamp WH, Wolfe WG. Current therapy of gas gangrene. In: Davis JC, Hunt TK, eds. Hyperbaric oxygen therapy. Bethesda, Maryland: Undersea Medical Society; 1977:153–76.

47. Bakker DJ. Clostridial myonecrosis. In: Davis JC, Hunt TK, eds. Problem wounds: the role of oxygen. New York: Elsevir; 1988:153–72.

48. Hill GB, Osterhout S. Experimental effects of hyperbaric oxygen on selected clostridial species: II. In vivo studies on mice. J Infect Dis 1972;125:26–35.

49. Stevens DL, Bryant AE, Adams K, Mader JT. Evaluation of hyperbaric oxygen therapy for treatment of experimental *Clostridium perfrigens* infection. Clin Infect Dis 1993;17:231–7.

50. Hill GB, Osterhout S. Experimental effects of hyperbaric oxygen on selected clostridial species: I. In vitro studies. J Infect Dis 1972;125:17–25.

51. van Unnik AJM. Inhibition of toxin production in *Clostridium perfringens in vitro* by hyperbaric oxygen. Antonie Van Leeuwenhoek 1965;31:181–6.

52. Stevens DL, Musher DM, Watson DA, *et al*. Spontaneous, nontraumatic gangrene due to *Clostridium septicum*. Rev Infect Dis 1990;12:286–96.

53. Johnson S, Driks MR, Tweten RK, *et al*. Clinical courses of seven survivors of *Clostridium septicum* infection and their immunologic responses to a toxin. Clin Infect Dis 1994;19:761–4.

54. Alpern RJ, Dowell VR Jr. *Clostridium septicum* infections and malignancy. JAMA 1969;209:385–8.

55. Ballard J, Bryant A, Stevens D, Tweten RK. Purification and characterization of the lethal toxin (alpha-toxin) of *Clostridium septicum*. Infect Immun 1992;60:784–90.

56. McGregor JA, Soper DE, Lovell G, Todd JK. Maternal deaths associated with *Clostridium sordellii* infection. Am J Obstet Gynecol 1989;161:987–95.

Ectoparasites

Peter J Moss & Nicholas J Beeching

INTRODUCTION

Parasites depend on their hosts for sustenance; an ectoparasite is a parasite that lives or feeds on the surface of that host. Most ectoparasites of vertebrates are hematophagous, but a few feed on skin and tissue debris. Some spend their entire life on the host, others move from host to host as they develop, and many simply alight on the host to feed. The definition of 'ectoparasite' is usually extended to include those parasites that burrow into the epidermis as well as those that remain on the surface.

Humans are the preferred or only host of some ectoparasites, but the majority are catholic in their choice or turn to humans only when their primary host is unavailable. Ectoparasites can cause local skin disease as a direct result of their bites, as a result of secondary infection or as a result of hypersensitivity reaction. They can cause systemic disease by inducing an allergic response or by toxin release, and they can act as vectors for a large number of viral, bacterial and parasitic infections. This chapter reviews the clinical syndromes caused by ectoparasites, outlining the key features associated with each family.

SKIN PROBLEMS

TRANSIENT ECTOPARASITES
Clinical and pathologic features

The most common feature of ectoparasite infection is local reaction to the bite of a blood-feeding arthropod. Numerous species of insects and arachnids rely on blood meals from vertebrate hosts. Although the behavior and feeding methods differ by species, most uncomplicated arthropod bites produce a similar local reaction.

Initial contact in an unsensitized person may produce little or no response. After repeated bites typical raised pruritic lesions (papular urticaria) appear within 24–48 hours (Fig. 4.1), although delays of more than 1 week have been reported. Occasionally these lesions are bullous. With further exposure and increased sensitization, an immediate weal skin response may be seen, followed after some hours by papular urticaria. Some hypersensitive people may develop a pronounced immediate reaction with large areas of superficial edema. After prolonged and frequent biting, the delayed reaction often diminishes, and eventually there is no response to further bites. The term papular urticaria is also used to describe a condition (usually seen in children) in which widespread papular lesions occur distant from but temporally related to insect bites; this may represent reactivation of previously sensitized bite sites.

The lesions of papular urticaria consist of pruritic papules, often with a central puncture marking the site of the bite. Superficial erosion and ulceration resulting from scratching is common. Unlike most other types of urticaria, papular lesions may persist for several days, although this period tends to decrease with regular exposure. Histologically there is intense inflammatory infiltrate with a predominance of T lymphocytes; the response is thought to be a type 1 IgE-mediated reaction.[1] In some species of parasite a specific arthropod salivary allergen has been identified, but in other cases the stimulus remains obscure.

Treatment of uncomplicated bites is usually unnecessary, although severe pruritis may be relieved by systemic antihistamines. (Caution is needed with terfenadine and astemizole, which can cause prolongation of the cardiographic QT interval and have a synergistic cardiotoxic effect with certain antimalarial drugs.) Secondary bacterial infection is common in hot moist climates (see Fig. 4.2), and this may require antibiotic therapy. Such infection is usually due to Gram-positive cocci, but anaerobes are also found. Local lesions caused by various blood-feeding arthropods are usually indistinguishable, and diagnosis of the precise cause relies either on epidemiologic knowledge or on detection and identification of the parasite. This is often necessary in order to eradicate the source of infection.

The major species of transient-feeding ectoparasites responsible for this type of bite are discussed below.

Flies

The most common cause of local reactions are biting flies of the order Diptera. Mosquitoes, blackflies, horseflies, sandflies and midges are ubiquitous, whereas tsetse flies are essentially tropical. Only certain species of each family tend to attack humans, and in all except the tsetse fly only the females are blood-feeders. Culicid mosquitoes usually feed by inserting their proboscis directly into the capillary, whereas other species feed by inflicting local tissue damage and sucking the resultant blood (pool feeding). This may explain the relatively more severe irritation that complicates bites by some species, although host factors also play a significant part.

Fleas

Fleas occur worldwide and are a common cause of pruritic bites in humans. They are free living, only approaching their host in order to feed. The human flea, *Pulex irritans*, is found mainly in crowded and unhygienic living conditions and is relatively uncommon in the developed world. However, many species of animal and bird fleas will also feed on humans, and household infestations with cat and dog fleas (*Ctenocephalides felis* and *C. canis*) are increasing in frequency.

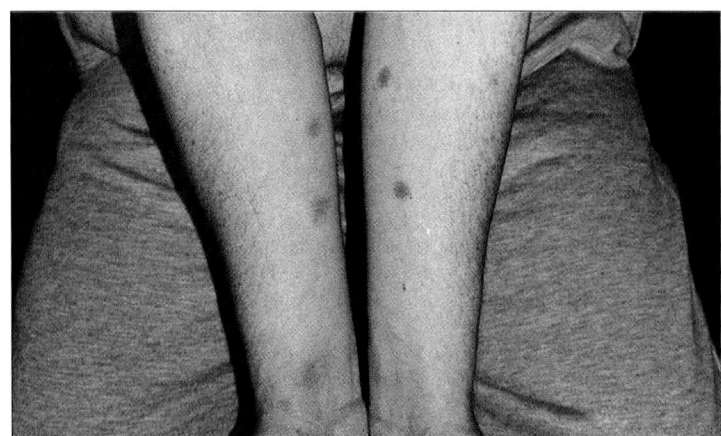

Fig. 4.1 Typical lesions of papular urticaria, caused in this case by bedbug bites.

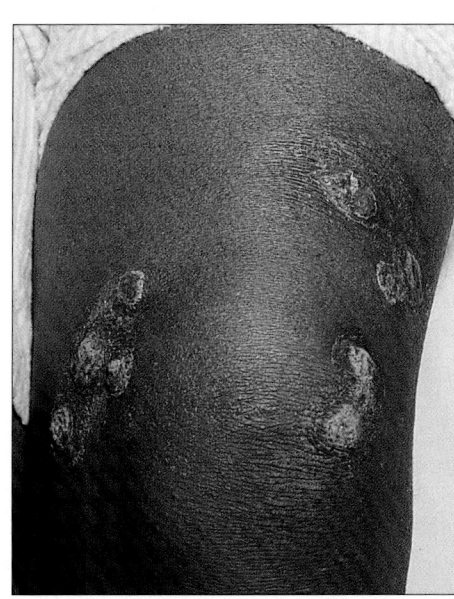

Fig. 4.2 Mosquito bites with secondary staphylococcal and streptococcal infection.

Flea bites provoke typical papular urticaria, although there may be a more severe reaction with bulla formation. The distribution of the lesions reflects the source of the infestation; for example, bites on the lower leg are usually due to cat and dog fleas, at least in adults. Diagnosis can be difficult; fleas are rarely seen on the human victim, and excoriation may mask the original nature of the lesions. If flea bites are suspected, careful inspection of the home environment is needed, although other sources of exposure (e.g. school, the workplace) should be considered. Household pets and their bedding should be checked thoroughly for fleas and droppings. Flea bites need no specific treatment unless there is secondary infection. Prevention depends on identifying the source of the infestation; in the case of pets, insecticides must be applied to both the animal and its environment.

Tungiasis, caused by the flea *Tunga penetrans*, is described in Chapters 6.6 and 6.14.

Bugs

Many members of the order Hemiptera (bugs) are blood feeders, but only two families include significant ectoparasites of humans. The Reduviidae cause relatively little local irritation, although hypersensitivity can develop with prolonged exposure; they are important principally as vectors of South American trypanosomiasis (see Chapter 6.33). Cimicidae (bedbugs) are voracious feeders and cause intense reactions. Bedbugs live and reproduce in crevices in walls and furniture, only approaching the host to feed (usually at night). They are found worldwide, the tropical bedbug (*Cimex hemipterus*) parasitizing humans in hot climates and the common bedbug (*C. lectularius*) in other areas. Bites cause papular lesions similar to those of other arthropods, but in unhygienic conditions infestations can be very heavy, and secondary iron-deficiency anemia has been reported.[2] Personal insect repellants and permethrin-impregnated bed nets provide some protection, but decontamination of the environment with residual insecticides may be necessary.

Ticks

Ticks are cosmopolitan ectoparasites of mammals, birds and reptiles. All stages of tick (larva, one or more nymphal instars and adults) attach to vertebrate hosts to feed; some species spend their entire life-cycle on a single animal (one-host ticks) while others drop off before moulting and then seek out a new host (multihost ticks). Although ticks are relatively host-specific, most will attack humans in the appropriate circumstances. Worldwide, hard ticks (family Ixodidae) are the more important parasites of humans, but soft ticks (family Argasidae) can cause a similar range of problems.

Most adult and immature ixodid ticks remain attached to the host for several days unless removed; argasid ticks feed more rapidly and may detach themselves after a few hours. The bite is often not irritating and passes unnoticed, especially in the early stages of attachment, an important factor in the role of the tick as a vector. Larval ticks are very small (<1mm in length) and are easily missed. In some cases, however (presumably when the host has been presensitized), tick-bites can cause itchy papular lesions with evidence of a type 1 hypersensitivity reaction. Elevated levels of specific IgE against tick saliva can be demonstrated in such people.[3] Local skin reactions may occur when tick attachment is prolonged (Fig. 4.3). Hypersensitive people may experience more generalized urticarial skin reactions and even systemic features of anaphylaxis (see below).

A characteristic necrotic lesion may be seen when the tick bite is associated with the transmission of certain rickettsial infections: the so-called eschar or *tâche noire* (Fig. 4.4; see Chapter 8.24).

Avoidance and management of tick bites. Ticks usually prefer certain types of vegetation, and most species are more commonly found during the spring and summer. A knowledge of the epidemiology of local tick species, as well as the wearing of long trousers and the use of permethrin-impregnated clothing, can decrease the incidence of tick bites and their complications.

Most ectoparasite vectors of infection feed rapidly, and length of time on the host probably does not influence likelihood of infection. Ixodid ticks, by contrast, can spend many days feeding, and the risk of transmission of some infections appears to be directly related to the duration of the bite. Tick paralysis is also dependent on prolonged feeding, and both infectious agents and toxins may be inoculated into the host by careless removal, which can also leave the barbed mouthparts embedded in the skin. As well as predisposing to bacterial infection this can also generate a chronic granulomatous response; in some cases local surgical excision is needed to relieve the symptoms. Early detection and appropriate detachment of ticks is therefore essential, especially in regions where tick-borne diseases are endemic. The ideal method of removal is to grasp the tick mouthparts as close to the skin as possible with fine forceps or tweezers, and gently lever the creature off. The body should not be squeezed, in order to prevent further inoculation. Any retained fragments should not be dug out, but the site cleaned and antiseptic applied. This method of removal is associated with a significantly lower incidence of rickettsial and borrelial infection following tick bites.[4]

In the particular case of Lyme disease, early antibiotic therapy after infection with *Borrelia burgdorferi* may provide some protection against the development of disease. Tick bites are very common and even in areas where the majority of vector species are infected, the rate of human infection is very low. Routine antibiotic prophylaxis following tick bites is not justified even in these areas. However, risk of infection rises dramatically once the tick has been feeding for more than 72 hours (from about 3% at <72 hours to 18–25% at >72 hours).[5] The approximate duration of attachment of the tick can be estimated

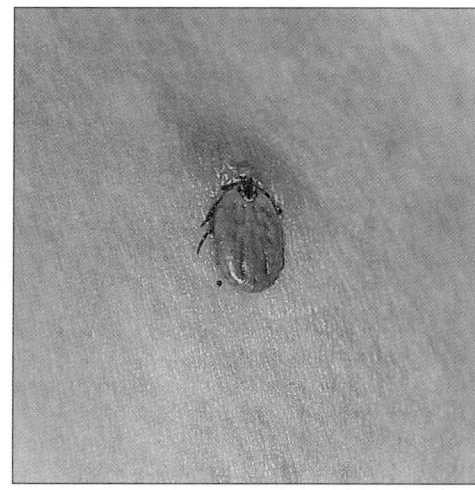

Fig. 4.3 Ixodid tick after feeding on the host for several days.

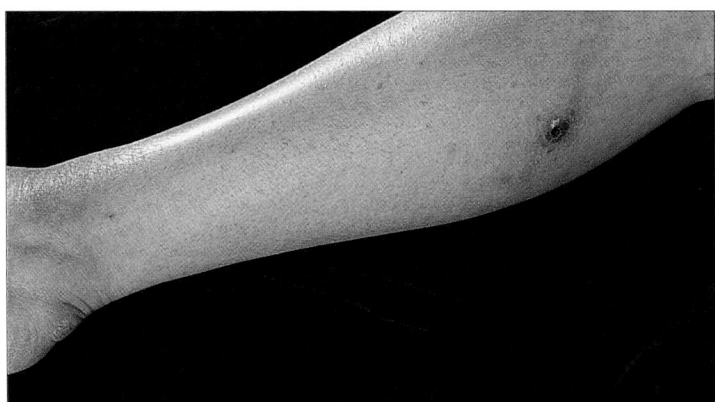

Fig. 4.4 Tick-bite eschar associated with African tick typhus.

from an index of tick engorgment (the scutal index), and antibiotics may be justified in cases where the tick had been feeding for more than 72 hours. Other attempts at predicting high-risk groups following tick bites (for example by testing the tick for *B. burgdorferi* infection) have not proved succesful.[5] There is no evidence that empiric antibiotic prophylaxis following tick bites has a role in the prevention of rickettsial infections such as Rocky Mountain spotted fever.[6]

Mites

The majority of mites that parasitize humans are not blood feeders, but feed on tissue fluids and cell debris. However, the effect of their bites is similar to those of other transient feeders. The human scabies mite (which is a resident parasite), follicle mites and the so-called food mites (which are not true human parasites) are discussed in Chapter 6.14.

Trombiculid mites ('chiggers') are found worldwide. The adult and nymphal stages are free-living predators, but the larvae parasitize many animals including humans. The mites inhabit areas of transitional vegetation (hence the alternative name of 'scrub mite'), often forming localized 'mite islands' in areas inhabited by a host species. Larval mites climb on to a human host who is passing through the vegetation, and crawl over the host's body to find a suitable area of skin to bite, such as the axillae or groins or areas of skin that are constricted by clothing. They feed for several days if undisturbed and then drop to the ground. The resulting lesions are similar to those caused by tick bites; the methods of prevention are similar.

Pyemotid mites are primarily predators of insects and their larvae, but they bite humans that come into contact with the grain or straw in which the mites live. The resulting papular urticarial rash, usually found on exposed surfaces or areas of thinner skin, goes under a number of occupational names, including 'straw itch', 'barley itch' and 'grain-shoveler's itch'.[7]

Cheyletiellid mites are ubiquitous tissue-feeding parasites of domestic dogs and cats. Bites follow close contact with infected animals, and lesions are usually seen on the thighs and abdomen after a pet has sat on someone's lap. Itchy papules similar to other arthropod bites result, and the diagnosis is made by finding mites on the animal. Some hematophagous animal mites also attack humans, causing typical lesions in areas that depend on the form of contact with the animal. Poultry, cage birds, wild and domestic rodents and snakes have all been incriminated.[7] In all these cases management is by removal or treatment of the principal animal host, with environmental acaricide if necessary.

INFESTATIONS OF RESIDENT HEMATOPHAGOUS PARASITES
Head and body lice

Epidemiology. Head lice (*Pediculus humanus capitis*) and body lice (*Pediculus humanus corporis*) are morphologically almost indistinguishable from each other, but they each tend to keep within their own territory on the host. The latter species clings to and deposits eggs on clothing fibers rather than hair shafts. It parasitizes those who do not change or wash clothing, unlike the head louse, which is not associated with poor hygiene alone. However, in both adults and children there is a correlation between lower socioeconomic groups and frequency of head louse infestation.[8] Children are more commonly infected with head lice than adults, and women are more frequently infected than men (at least in Western cultures). This is because the vast majority of infections are acquired by direct head-to-head contact, which is more likely in these groups. Overcrowding is also an important risk factor, but hair length is not. Head lice are more common in late summer, which probably reflects the need for high ambient temperature to hatch eggs. The role of fomites in transmission is controversial; there is little evidence that hats and brushes are important.

Clinical features. The main feature of head louse infestation is scalp itching, although secondary bacterial infection is not uncommon, and louse infection should be looked for in cases of scalp impetigo. Chronic infection can produce cervical lymphadenopathy. The diagnosis is made by finding empty egg-cases ('nits') stuck to the base of hair follicles; the highest concentration is usually in the occipital and parietal regions. In heavy infestations, developing eggs, nymphs and adult lice may be seen.

Management. Several insecticides are available for the treatment of head lice (see Fig. 4.5).[9] The acetylcholinesterase inhibitors malathion and carbaryl both have reasonable ovicidal and pediculicidal activity, although some resistance has been seen. Malathion, unlike carbaryl, has a residual action of several weeks, but two applications 10 days apart are necessary whichever agent is used. The synthetic pyrethroids, such as permethrin, also have good activity, although there are concerns about the rapid development of resistance to these compounds. Topical ivermectin has also been used with good effect, although there is little evidence to suggest that it is preferable to other agents.

Malathion and carbaryl need to remain on the scalp for 8–12 hours before they are washed off, and they are degraded by high temperatures (e.g. as occurs during the use of a hair dryer). Pyrethroids need only a short application. Lotion or mousse preparations are generally preferable to shampoos. Although there are numerous trials comparing different drugs and preparations, it is very difficult to draw general conclusions.[10] Resistance patterns vary from region to region, and there are many different formulations and preparations of drugs available. If possible, the choice of therapy should be based on a local policy designed to take into account existing resistance patterns and to prevent the development of resistance.

Systemic therapy has occasionally been used to treat head lice. Trimethoprim–sulfamethoxazole (co-trimoxazole) and ivermectin[11] have been reported to be effective, although repeated doses are necessary because they affect only the feeding stages of the parasite. In most cases topical treatment should be adequate. Older drugs, such as organochlorines and mercury-based preparations, are less effective and more toxic.

Body lice are associated with poor hygiene and unwashed clothing, and are principally parasites of vagrants and refugees. They can be found worldwide, but they are particularly found in cooler climates where clothing is rarely removed. Transmission is by direct body-to-body spread or by sharing infected clothing. Initially the bites are similar to those of other hematophagous ectoparasites, but the prolonged and persistent nature of the infestation leads to widespread excoriation and secondary infection and eventually to the hyperpigmented chronic skin condition known as 'vagabond's disease' or *morbus errorum*.

The diagnosis is made by finding lice and eggs in the clothing (particularly along seams), and treatment should be directed at the clothing rather than the patient. High-temperature washing, tumble-drying and malathion dusting powder are all effective at clearing garments of lice; permethrin-treated clothing may be protective for those at risk of infestation.[12]

Pubic lice

Pthirus pubis (often written as *Phthirus pubis*) is morphologically different from *Pediculus humanus* and is unique to humans. Infection is usually confined to the pubic region, although lice and eggs are sometimes found in axillary and facial hair, eyelashes, eyebrows and (especially in children) the scalp. Infection is transmitted by close, usually sexual, contact and is associated with other sexually transmitted diseases.

The main symptom is itching of the affected area, especially at night, although there may be few visible skin lesions. Close inspection may reveal eggs that are attached to the hair shafts, with adult lice clinging on close to the skin. Treatment is with the same insecticides as for head lice, with the proviso that alcohol-based preparations may irritate sensitive skin and mucous membranes. This is particularly true for the eyes, and eyelash infestations should always be treated with an aqueous formulation. It is usually advisable to treat the whole trunk and limbs in view of the possible spread to other hairy areas; where appropriate, sexual contacts should also be treated.

OTHER ECTOPARASITE INFESTATIONS
Scabies
Some infesting arthropod ectoparasites do not feed on blood at all, but cause disease in other ways. The most important of these is *Sarcoptes scabei*, the human scabies mite, which is found worldwide in conditions of poor hygiene. This skin-burrowing mite is not a blood-feeder, but ingests predigested dermal cells as it tunnels through the epithelium. Female mites live in small burrows in the skin, which they extend by 2–3mm daily, leaving a trail of eggs and feces behind them. The burrows are intensely itchy and are responsible for the features of scabies. They are usually found around the wrists, web spaces, toes and genitalia, although they may be more widespread; small papules are sometimes seen at the distal end adjacent to the female mite. Infestations are relatively light, with an average of 12 adult females found on an infected patient. Much heavier infestations are found in immunocompromised patients, causing 'crusted' or 'Norwegian' scabies.

Pseudoscabies
Sarcoptid mites are relatively host-specific, and mites acquired from animals do not usually cause prolonged infestations of humans. However, people in close contact with infected livestock (notably pigs, cows and dogs) may acquire temporary infestation, causing pruritic lesions but lacking the typical burrows of human scabies. No treatment is required except for avoidance of the source of infection.

Demodicidosis
Demodex folliculorum, the follicle mite, is a human ectoparasite that lives in the pilosebaceous follicles, where it feeds on cell contents. The mites are found in areas of high sebum production: the forehead, cheeks, nose and nasolabial folds. The role of follicle mites in skin disease is controversial; they are very common, and unless they are present in large numbers do not appear to cause problems. However, they have been described as a cause of papulopustular eruptions in children and immunocompromised subjects, and they have been implicated in the pathogenesis of other skin conditions such as pityriasis folliculorum and rosacea.[13]

Storage mites
The so-called storage mites include a number of mite species that live in stored products (e.g. flour, grain, straw, dried meat, dried fruit and cheese). When a person handles infested stock, mites crawl on to exposed areas and migrate under the horny layer of the skin. Here they can cause an acute dermatitis, with erythema and small papulovesicles, which is known by a number of occupational names, for example 'grocer's itch', 'baker's itch' and 'copra itch'.[7] It is uncertain whether the mites actually feed on skin cells, so they may not be true ectoparasites of humans.

Fig. 4.5 Commonly used topical preparations for the treatment of ectoparasite infestations. CSM, Committee on Safety of Medicines.

COMMONLY USED TOPICAL PREPARATIONS FOR THE TREATMENT OF ECTOPARASITE INFESTATIONS

Class	Agent	Uses	Toxicity	Comments
Acetyl-cholinesterase inhibitors	Malathion	Scabies Head lice Pubic lice		Good residual protection Recommended for pubic lice infestation of eyelashes
	Carbaryl	Head lice Pubic lice	Carcinogenic in animals; minimal risk to humans in therapeutic doses	Recent UK CSM warning regarding animal carcinogenicity: now prescription only in the UK
Organochlorines	Lindane	Head lice Pubic lice	Neurotoxic (potential for systemic absorption)	Increasing resistance; no longer available in the UK
Natural pyrethroids	Pyrethrin	Head lice Pubic lice		Less evidence of efficacy than synthetic pyrethroids
	Phenothrin	Head lice Pubic lice		Less evidence of efficacy than synthetic pyrethroids
Synthetic pyrethroids	Permethrin	Scabies Head lice Pubic lice	Rarely rash and local edema	Avoid in pregnancy and breast-feeding
Others	Benzyl benzoate	Scabies	Skin irritation	Avoid in pregnancy and breast-feeding
	Ivermectin	Head lice Scabies		Little evidence for efficacy Topical use possible
	Mercury preparations	Head lice	Contact dermatitis Systemic toxicity	Available over the counter in some European countries
	Monosulfiram	Scabies	'Antabuse' effect (alcohol should be avoided)	No longer available in the UK
	Sulfur ointment	Scabies	Skin irritation	Cheap, safe, reasonably effective

IMPORTANT ECTOPARASITE VECTORS OF HUMAN DISEASE				
Ectoparasite	Vector	Infective organism	Disease	Distribution
Flies (Diptera) Mosquitoes	*Anopheles* spp.	*Plasmodium* spp.	Malaria	Tropics and subtropics
	Anopheles spp. *Culex* spp. *Aedes* spp.	*Wuchereria bancrofti*	Lymphatic filariasis	Tropics
	Anopheles spp. *Mansonia* spp. *Aedes* spp.	*Brugia* spp.	Lymphatic filariasis	Southern Asia
	Aedes spp. *Culex* spp. *Anopheles* spp.	Arboviruses	Dengue, yellow fever Japanese encephalitis St Louis encephalitis	Specific to each disease
Black-flies (Simuliidae)		*Onchocerca volvulus*	Onchocerciasis	Sub-Saharan Africa, Central and South America
		Mansonella ozzardi	Mansonelliasis	Amazon basin
Sandflies	*Phlebotomus* spp.	*Leishmania* spp.	Visceral and cutaneous leishmaniasis	Sub-Saharan Africa, Asia and Mediterranean Europe
		Bunyaviridae	Sandfly fever	Central Asia, Mediterranean and North Africa
	Lutzomyia spp.	*Leishmania* spp.	Visceral and cutaneous leishmaniasis	Central and South America
		Bartonella bacilliformis	Bartonellosis (Oroya fever, Carrion's disease, verruga peruana)	South America
Midges	*Culicoides* spp.	*Mansonella perstans*	Mansonelliasis	Sub-Saharan Africa
		Mansonella ozzardi	Mansonelliasis	Amazon basin
Tsetse flies (Glossinidae)		*Trypanosoma* spp.	African trypanosomiasis	Sub-Saharan Africa
Deer flies (*Chrysops* spp.)		*Loa loa*	Loiasis	West Africa
		Francisella tularensis	Tularemia	Western USA
Fleas (Siphonaptera)	Various species	*Yersinia pestis*	Plague	Worldwide (patchy)
	Various species	*Rickettsia mooseri*	Murine typhus	Worldwide (patchy)
Bugs (Hemiptera)	Reduviidae	*Trypanosoma cruzi*	South American trypanosomiasis	Central and South America
Lice	Body louse (*Pediculus humanus corporis*)	*Rickettsia prowazeki*	Epidemic typhus	Worldwide (patchy)
		Bartonella quintana	Trench fever	Worldwide
	Body louse (*Pediculus humanus corporis*) and head louse (*Pediculus humanus capitis*)	*Borrelia recurrentis*	Louse-borne relapsing fever	Worldwide (patchy)
Ticks Ixodidae	Numerous hard tick (ixodid) species	*Rickettsia* spp.	Tick typhus and various rickettsial spotted fevers	Worldwide
		Borrelia burgdorferi	Lyme disease	USA, Europe, Eastern Asia, Australia
		Francisella tularensis	Tularemia	USA, Europe, Japan
		Babesia spp.	Babesiosis	USA, Europe
		Arboviruses	Tick-borne encephalitis, Congo–Crimea hemorrhagic fever and other arbovirus infections	
		Ehrlichia spp.	Ehrlichiosis	USA, Europe, North Africa, Eastern Asia
Argasidae	*Ornithodoros* spp.	*Borrellia* spp.	Tick-borne relapsing fever	Africa, Central Asia, North and South America
Mites	*Leptotrombidium* spp.	*Rickettsia tsutsugamushi*	Scrub typhus	South East Asia, Pacific and (rarely) West Africa
	Liponyssoides sanguineus	*Rickettsia akari*	Rickettsial pox	USA, South Africa, Eastern Asia

Fig. 4.6 Important ectoparasite vectors of human disease.

SKIN LESIONS DUE TO MYIATIC LARVAE

These parasites are covered in Chapter 6.14.

NONINFECTIVE SYSTEMIC PROBLEMS

TICK PARALYSIS/TOXICOSIS
Epidemiology
Paralysis and death of domestic animals and occasionally humans following tick bites has been documented in Australia and South Africa since the end of the 19th century, and more recently it has been observed in North America and Europe. This syndrome is not, as once thought, an infective process, but is caused by a toxin in the saliva of the pregnant females of certain ixodid species. Children are more often affected than adults, and the condition is most commonly seen in spring and early summer.

Clinical features
Tick paralysis almost always results from bites on the head, typically behind the ear where the tick may not be noticed. Symptoms appear only after the tick has been feeding for at least 48 hours. The usual presentation is an ascending flaccid paralysis, frequently with cranial nerve involvement, although atypical features such as isolated nerve lesions and cerebellar signs are occasionally seen. There is no sensory loss or decrease in consciousness, but if the condition is untreated death from respiratory failure can supervene. In the North American form the paralysis starts to improve within a few hours of removing the tick, but in the Australian form of the disease deterioration may continue for a further 24–48 hours.[14]

Management
The neurotoxin involved probably varies between different tick species. It has not been fully characterized, but there are many clinical and neurophysiologic similarities to the effects of botulinum toxin.[14] The essential treatment is to remove the tick carefully to prevent further transfer of toxin, followed by supportive care until the neurologic signs resolve. Although rare, the diagnosis should be considered in any progressive flaccid paralysis in an endemic area.

TICK ANAPHYLAXIS
The local allergic urticarial reactions to tick bites have already been discussed. Rarely, in hypersensitive people anaphylaxis can follow a bite, with bronchospasm, edema and hypotension. This is an IgE-mediated response to tick salivary antigens, which can occur soon after the tick first bites, or following careless removal.[15] Treatment is as for any form of anaphylactic reaction, and sensitive people in tick-infested areas may benefit from carrying adrenaline for inhalation or self-injection.

MITE ALLERGY
House dust mites (*Dermatophagoides* spp.) are cosmopolitan, free-living mites that feed principally on animal and human skin detritus. Although they are sometimes found on the skin surface they usually consume skin that has already been shed and are thus not true parasites. Their main medical importance is as a cause of allergic rhinitis and bronchial constriction.

ECTOPARASITES AS VECTORS FOR INFECTION

The principal importance of many human ectoparasites is their potential for transmitting a wide variety of viral, bacterial and protozoal infections. Figure 4.6 lists the major vector-borne human infections.

Bedbugs do not appear in the table; their role as potential vectors of infection remains controversial. Viable infective hepatitis B virus and other pathogens have been found in the gut of bedbugs weeks after their last blood meal, and a significant association has been shown between the presence of bedbugs and hepatitis B virus e antigenemia in Gambian children.[16] However, other community-based studies have failed to confirm that bedbugs have a significant role in hepatitis B transmission,[17] and attempts at transmitting infection among a group of chimpanzees using bedbugs were unsuccesful when the bugs fed normally.[18] Although HIV has been isolated from bedbugs up to 8 days after feeding on heavily infected blood under experimental conditions, there is no evidence to suggest transmission to humans by this route.[19]

REFERENCES

1. Jordaan HF, Schneider JW. Papular urticaria: a histopathologic study of 30 patients. Am J Dermatopathol 1997;19:119–26.
2. Venkatalachalam PS, Belavadi B. Loss of haemoglobin iron due to excessive biting by bedbugs. Trans R Soc Trop Med Hyg 1962;56:218–21.
3. Beaudouin E, Kanny G, Guerin B, Guerin L, Plenat F, Moneret-Vaytrin DA. Unusual manifestations of hypersensitivity after a tick-bite. Ann Allergy Asthma Immunol 1997;79:43–6.
4. Oteo JA, Martinez de Artola V, Gomez Cadinanos R, Casas JM, Blanco JR, Rosel L. Evaluation of methods of tick removal in human ixodidiasis. Rev Clin Esp 1996;196:584–7.
5. Sood SK, Salzman MB, Johnson BJ, et al. Duration of tick attachment as a predictor of Lyme disease in an area in which Lyme disease is endemic. J Infect Dis 1997;175:996–9.
6. Walker DH. Rocky Mountain spotted fever: a seasonal alert. Clin Infect Dis 1995;20:1111–7.

7. Blankenship ML. Mite dermatitis other than scabies. Dermatol Clin 1990;8:265–75.
8. Gillis D, Slepon R, Karsenty E, Green MS. Sociodemographic factors associated with *Pediculosis capitis* and *pubis* among young adults in the Israel Defence Forces. Public Health Rev 1990–91;18:345–50.
9. Burns DA. The treatment of human ectoparasite infection. Br J Dermatol 1991;125:89–93.
10. Vander Stichele RH, Dezure EM, Bogaert MG. Systematic review of clinical efficacy of topical treatments for head lice. Br Med J 1995;311:604–8.
11. Mumcuoglu KY, Miller J, Rosen LJ, Galun R. Systemic activity of ivermectin on the human body louse. J Med Entomol 1990;27:72–5.
12. Sholdt LL, Rogers EJ, Gerberg EJ, Schreck CE. Effectiveness of permethrin-treated military uniform fabric against human body lice. Milit Med 1989;154:90–3.
13. Burns DA. Follicle mites and their role in disease. Clin Exp Dermatol 1992;17:152–5.

14. Grattan-Smith PJ, Morris JG, Johnstone HM, et al. Clinical and neurophysiological features of tick paralysis. Brain 1997;120:1975–87.
15. Brown AFT, Hamilton DL. Tick bite anaphylaxis in Australia. J Accid Emerg Med 1998;15:111–3.
16. Vall Mayans M, Hall AJ, Inskip HM, et al. Risk factors for transmission of hepatitis B virus to Gambian children. Lancet 1990;336:1107–9.
17. Vall Mayans M, Hall AJ, Inskip HM, et al. Do bedbugs transmit hepatitis B? Lancet 1994;343:761–3.
18. Jupp PG, Purcell RH, Phillips JM, Shapiro M, Gerin JL. Attempts to transmit hepatitis B virus to chimpanzees by arthropods. South Afr Med J 1991;79:320–2.
19. Webb PA, Happ CM, Maupin GO, Johnson BJ, Ou CY, Monath TP. Potential for insect transmission of HIV: experimental exposure of *Cimex hemipterus* and *Toxorhynchites amboinensis* to human immunodeficiency virus. J Infect Dis 198;160:970–7.

Dermatologic Manifestations of Systemic Infections

Anthony C Chu

INTRODUCTION

The skin is the largest and most visible organ of the body. In addition to its role as a barrier separating the body from the external environment and its role in temperature regulation, the skin has a complex immune system that recognizes and attacks foreign antigens and microbes, but that also reacts to systemic disease to give characteristic clinical changes.

The skin may be affected by systemic infections in three ways:
- by direct involvement by the infectious agent,
- by specific reaction to an infection, and
- by nonspecific reaction to an infection.

DIRECT INVOLVEMENT OF THE SKIN BY AN INFECTIOUS AGENT DURING A SYSTEMIC INFECTION

VIRAL INFECTIONS
Chickenpox
Viral infection of the skin as part of a systemic infection is well demonstrated by chickenpox (see Chapter 2.1). After an incubation period of 14–21 days the patient develops 1–2 days of fever and malaise. This is followed by crops of unilocular vesicles, which quickly become pustular, appearing over 2–4 days (see Chapter 2.1). After the acute infection the virus persists in dorsal root nerve ganglion cells and on reactivation of the residual latent virus, herpes zoster or shingles develops.

Hand, foot and mouth disease
Hand, foot and mouth disease is caused by Coxsackie viruses A16, A5 and A10 (see Chapter 2.1). It occurs predominantly in children. After an incubation period of 5–7 days the patient develops painful stomatitis with oral vesicles that ulcerate. A more variable feature is that of small, thin-walled vesicles on the fingers and toes (see Chapter 2.1, Fig. 1.9). Viral particles can be identified in the vesicles on electron microscopy.

BACTERIAL INFECTIONS
Gonococcal infection
In disseminated gonococcal infection caused by *Neisseria gonorrhoeae*, characteristic skin lesions (called septic gonococcal dermatitis) may be observed. One or more crops of three or four macules or papules develop; these then become pustular or bullous. Gonococci can occasionally be cultured from the skin lesions.

Tuberculosis
In tuberculosis, skin involvement may occur as the result of contiguous involvement of the skin from underlying lymph nodes, joints or bones, a condition called scrofuloderma.[1] A bluish-red nodule develops over the affected bone, joint (Fig. 5.1) or lymph node and multiple fistulae develop. Diagnosis must be confirmed by biopsy, which shows tuberculous granulation tissue. *Mycobacterium tuberculosis* can often be isolated from involved tissue.

Skin involvement in tuberculosis may also occur secondary to hematogenous dissemination. In miliary tuberculosis, hematogenous dissemination can produce severe systemic symptoms and profuse crops of bluish papules, which become vesicular and then pustular. These often become necrotic, leading to ulceration of the skin.

Chronic hematogenous dissemination of tubercle bacilli in patients who have moderate or high degrees of immunity may present as one of the tuberculides:
- papulonecrotic tuberculid, in which there are symmetric crops of necrotic papules predominantly affecting the extremities;
- lichen scrofulosum, in which minute lichenoid papules appear predominantly on the limbs rather than on the trunk; and
- erythema induratum (or Bazin's disease), in which persistent or recurrent nodular lesions appear in the calves of the legs and may lead to ulceration (see Fig. 5.2); these nodular areas are very well defined and are generally asymptomatic.[2]

The tuberculides respond rapidly to antituberculous therapy.

Spirochetal infections
Disease caused by spirochetes tend to affect the skin as part of the their primary manifestation, but they may also involve the skin during subsequent, disseminated disease.

Syphilis. In syphilis, the primary lesion or primary chancre is often cutaneous or mucosal. Secondary syphilis starts approximately 3 months after the primary infection and gives rise to nonirritating, coppery red symmetric lesions, which start as macules and become papular (see Chapter 2.64, Fig. 64.3). Secondary syphilis is the 'great pretender'[3] and lesions of secondary syphilis can mimic acne, psoriasis and a number of other nonspecific dermatoses. Characteristically the palms and soles are affected. When mucosal surfaces are involved, 'snail tract' ulcers may develop. Later, chondylomata may occur perianally and on the vulva or penis. Patchy hair loss is a characteristic sign of secondary syphilis, giving rise to a moth-eaten appearance of the scalp.

Late or tertiary syphilis occurs after a latent period of up to 20 years. Both skin and mucous membranes may be affected. Nodular syphilides

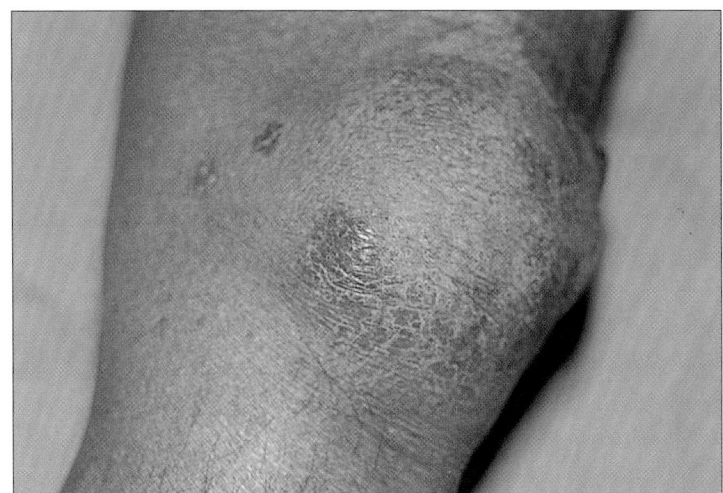

Fig. 5.1 Scrofuloderma in a 60-year old patient. A biopsy confirmed tuberculoid granulation tissue and the patient responded very well to antituberculous therapy.

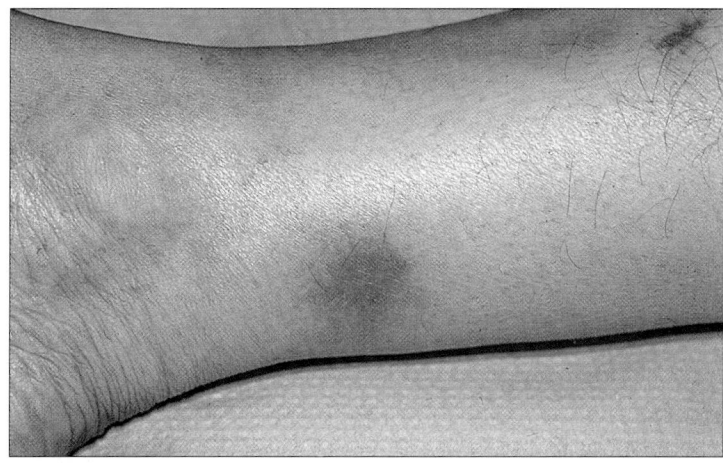

Fig. 5.2 Erythema induratum on the back of the leg of a 45-year old woman.

present as nodular subcutaneous lesions appearing in groups and tending to develop a circinate arrangement. These are more common on the extensor surfaces of the arms, the back and the face (Fig. 5.3), but they may occur in the oral cavity. Gummas are masses of syphilitic granulomatous tissue; they may originate in the subcutis, underlying bone or muscle. These masses ulcerate to produce punched-out ulcers.

Yaws. Yaws is a disease caused by the spirochete *Treponema pertenue*. The primary lesion of yaws produces a cutaneous erythematous papule, which becomes papillomatous and resembles a raspberry, giving rise to its name, 'fambesia'. After 2–4 months the secondary eruption of yaws develops, with multiple small papules developing into exudative papillomas (Fig. 5.4). Mucosal involvement does not occur in yaws. After 6 months to 3 years tertiary yaws occurs; this is characterized by ulcerated nodular and tuberous cutaneous lesions and keratoderma of the palms and soles.

Pinta. Pinta is caused by the spirochete *Treponema carateum*. The initial eruption starts in the skin as multiple erythematous papules and plaques. This is followed after months or years by generalized cutaneous lesions, where the skin becomes pale, pigmented or erythematosquamous. The late phase occurs 2–5 years after primary infection with irregular pigmentation, which can be grayish, steely or bluish in color. Areas of leukoderma, particularly around the elbows, knees, ankles and wrists, may develop. Hyperkeratosis occurs, particularly on the legs and arms, and is associated with areas of atrophy, particularly around the large joints (see Chapter 8.19).

Lyme disease
In infections with *Borrelia burgdorferi*, the primary lesion occurs at the site of the *Ixodes* tick bite, with a characteristic eruption: erythema

migrans.[4] The macular erythema starts up to 36 days after the bite and slowly increases in size by several centimeters each week. Subsequent dissemination leads to Lyme disease with involvement of the nervous system, heart and joints. One year or longer after the original infection, a late cutaneous manifestation may occur: acrodermatitis chronica atrophicans (see Chapter 2.45).[5] As this name suggests, this typically affects the hands and feet, but the elbows and knees may also be affected. Erythematous plaques develop and these slowly enlarge and become atrophic. *Borrelia burgdorferi* can be cultured from skin biopsies in this condition.

FUNGAL INFECTIONS
A number of deep fungal infections may have cutaneous involvement in the course of systemic disease. These fungal infections include blastomycosis, coccidiodioimycosis, cryptococcosis, histoplasmosis and paracoccidioidomycosis.

Cutaneous lesions in these deep fungal infections tend to be nonspecific, with papules, nodules and ulcers developing on different parts of the skin. In disseminated blastomycosis cutaneous lesions start as papules or nodules, which then ulcerate and evolve into serpiginous lesions with raised warty borders.

Disseminated coccidioidomycosis may result in cutaneous abscesses and granulomas and discharging sinuses. Disseminated cutaneous cryptococcosis is observed in patients on long-term immunosuppression. It presents as erythematous papules and nodules, which become exudative and eventually ulcerate (Fig. 5.5). Disseminated cutaneous cryptococcosis is seen most often in patients who have AIDS. The cutaneous lesions tend to be nonspecific, but molluscum contagiosum-like lesions are a recognized feature of this disease. These typically occur around the nose and mouth and eventually ulcerate to leave punched out, rolled edged ulcers.

SPECIFIC SKIN REACTIONS RESULTING FROM SYSTEMIC INFECTIONS

Systemic infections with viruses and bacteria can occasionally cause specific cutaneous reactions. These skin reactions can establish the diagnosis of the specific systemic infections and it is thus very important to recognize them.

VIRUSES
Roseola infantum and pityriasis rosea
Infection with human herpes virus 6 in the first 3 years of life gives rise to a specific dermatitis: roseola infantum (exanthem subitum) (see Chapter 2.1). After an incubation period of 10–15 days, fever starts abruptly and lasts for 3–5 days.[6] As the fever subsides a macular papular eruption, which is characteristically rose pink in color, develops on the neck and trunk. This later spreads to the arms, face and legs.

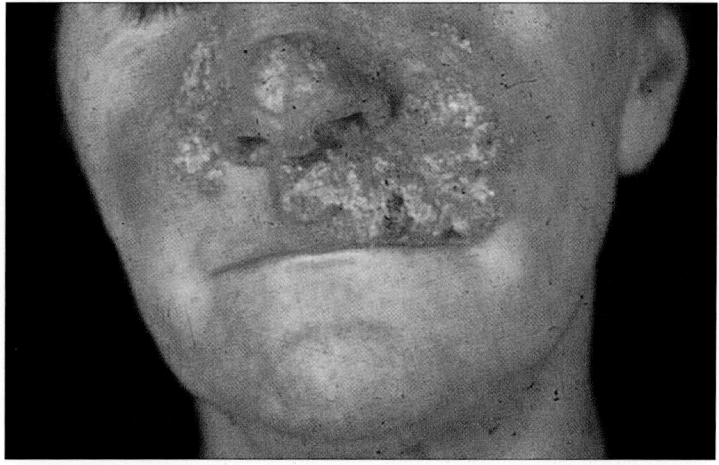

Fig. 5.3 Tertiary syphilis on the face of a 56-year old woman.

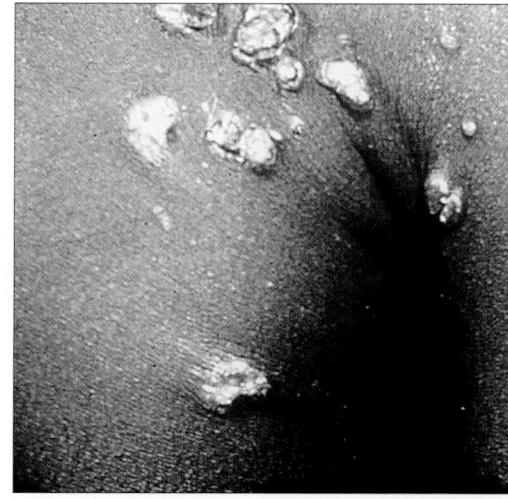

Fig. 5.4 Secondary yaws showing papular and rather vegetative lesions on the anterior chest wall.

The eruption subsides after 1–2 days, leaving no pigmentation or scaling of the skin.

A similar eruption is observed in adults; this is called pityriasis rosea. There is generally no prodromal syndrome but patients develop a single erythematous macular lesion, which may reach several centimeters in diameter, most commonly on the trunk, thigh or upper arm. The macule has a characteristic collarette of fine scales. This herald patch is followed after 5–15 days by a widespread eruption of small erythematous, scaly macules, which typically form a Christmas-tree pattern on the trunk and eventually spread down the limbs to subside after 6 weeks. Recent studies have implicated human herpes virus 7 in pityriasis rosea.[7]

Cutaneous changes associated with HIV infection

Infection with HIV is associated with a number of cutaneous changes. Some of these are characteristic enough to alert the physician to the possibility of infection with HIV. Kaposi's sarcoma is seen in about 34% of patients who have AIDS. The great majority of these patients are homosexual or bisexual men in developed countries (see Chapter 5.17).

Kaposi's sarcoma is a multicentric and endothelial cell neoplasm that often starts in the skin but may become disseminated to affect multiple organs.[8] It is associated with human herpes virus 8 infection. Skin lesions range in color from red to purple–brown and may be macules, papules, nodules or plaques. Cutaneous Kaposi's sarcoma in those who have AIDS is often multiple and very disfiguring (Fig. 5.6).

Oral hairy leukoplakia presents as asymptomatic white plaques on the lateral boarders of the tongue.[9] These may spread to involve the oral mucosa. Oral hairy leukoplakia is now considered to be due to a proliferation of Epstein–Barr virus within the epithelium of the tongue.

A common dermatosis in HIV-positive patients is a papulopruritic eruption or itchy folliculitis.[10] Small erythematous or skin-colored papules develop on the head, neck and trunk, and these are extremely pruritic. No infectious cause has been found for this, and histologic examination shows only a nonspecific perifollicular mixed cell infiltrate. This eruption does not respond well to topical corticosteroids, antihistamines or antimicrobials, but it may respond to ultraviolet light therapy.[11]

Another itchy papular eruption observed in HIV-positive patients is eosinophilic pustular folliculitis.[12] This condition starts as itchy erythematous papules on the head, neck, trunk and limbs, and may develop into plaques with a papular or vesicular boarder. Histology shows an eosinophil-rich perifollicular infiltrate. No infectious cause has been found for this condition. As with the itchy folliculitis, topical therapies and antihistamines tend to be ineffective but the condition often responds well to ultraviolet light.

Bacillary angiomatosis presents as small angioma-like lesions affecting both the skin and the internal organs.[13] In the skin, lesions start as pin-point red papules, which then enlarge to become nodular. Although seen mainly in HIV-positive patients, bacillary angiomatosis has also been described in other immunodeficient patients and is now known to be caused by *Bartonella* spp.

BACTERIAL INFECTIONS

Specific bacterial infections may cause a variety of cutaneous syndromes as a result of toxin production.

Scarlet fever

Scarlet fever complicates acute infection by *Streptococcus pyogenes* strains that produce a pyrogenic exotoxin. Production of the exotoxin appears to be depended on the presence of a temperate bacteriophage and is exclusive to the group A streptococci. Three antigenically distinct exotoxins can be produced: types A, B and C. Specific strains of *S. pyogenes* may produce one or more of these toxins.[14] After an incubation period of 2–5 days, fever develops with localized signs at the portal of entry (e.g. tonsillitis and lymphadenopathy or tenderness at a wound site).

The eruption of scarlet fever occurs on the second day of infection. It begins on the upper trunk with a punctate erythema that becomes generalized over a few hours to 3–4 days. A characteristic sign is the development of transverse red streaks at the sites of skin folds, owing to capillary damage; these are known as Pastia's lines. The face is erythematous but with a characteristic perioral pallor. After 7–10 days the eruption subsides with desquamation of the palms and soles.

Lyell's syndrome

Staphylococcal scalded skin syndrome, otherwise known as Lyell's syndrome, is caused by strains of *Staphylococcus aureus* that produce a specific epidermolytic toxin. Phage group 2 staphylococci predominate, but other phage groups have been implicated.

The epidermolytic toxin cleaves the epidermis just below the granular cell layer, resulting in the typical scalded skin appearance. The eruption usually starts suddenly with erythema and tenderness of the skin. Flaccid blistering occurs, which often rubs off leaving raw exudative areas. Staphylococci can usually be isolated from involved skin. This syndrome usually carries an excellent prognosis with resolution in 7–14 days.

The disease is one of infants and children. In the few reports of adults who have staphylococcal scaled skin syndrome there is generally an underlying medical problem, such as renal failure or immunosuppression and it is thought that reduced clearance of the toxin by the kidneys in these patients may be important in the development of the disease.[15]

Rheumatic fever

Group A β-hemolytic streptococci are implicated in the pathogenesis of rheumatic fever. A specific (although now rare) cutaneous manifestation of rheumatic fever is erythema marginatum rheumaticum.[16] This consists of rings or arcs of pale or dull red erythema, which are either macular or

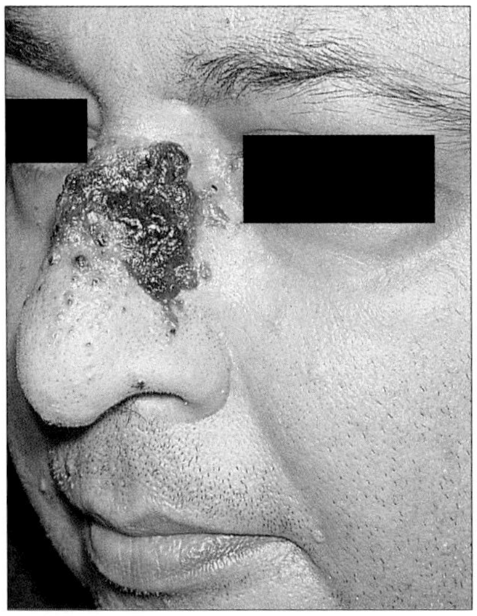

Fig. 5.5 Cutaneous cryptococcosis in a renal transplant patient. These lesions started as nodules that then rapidly ulcerated. Computed tomography of the patient's brain showed no abnormality but *Cryptococcus neoformans* was grown from the cerebrospinal fluid.

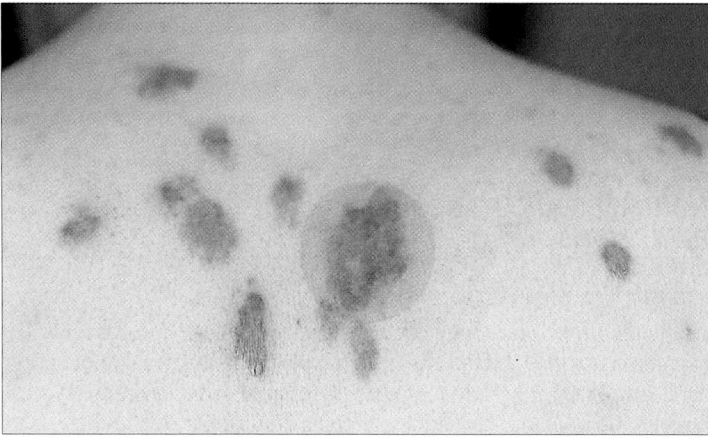

Fig. 5.6 Kaposi's sarcoma in a 20-year old man who had AIDS. One lesion on the patients back had been treated with radiotherapy resulting in disfiguring pigmentation at the site of treatment.

slightly thickened. The rings make a discrete or enlarged polycyclic pattern. These rings characteristically fade over a few hours or days and appear in recurrent crops, usually at different sites, over many weeks.

Sepsis

Sepsis caused by a variety of different bacteria can cause disseminated intravascular coagulation. This results in hemorrhagic skin lesions, particularly of dependant areas, followed by purpura and possibly ulceration of the skin. In acute meningococcal sepsis, 40–90% of patients develop these characteristic purpuric lesions, which are important diagnostic signs of this rapidly progressing infection.[17]

Henoch–Schönlein purpura

Henoch–Schönlein purpura has in the past been strongly associated with streptococcal infections but the link has become less impressive in recent years; other infectious agents, such as upper respiratory viruses, have been suggested. Henoch–Schönlein purpura has a characteristic appearance, with palpable purpuric papules developing on the lower legs and buttocks. This may be associated with arthritis, gastrointestinal syndromes and renal disease. Histologically there is a leukocytoclastic vasculitis and characteristic deposition of IgA within the walls of affected blood vessels.[18]

Leprosy

Mycobacterium leprae affects the skin in all forms of leprosy. In tuberculoid leprosy the skin lesions tend to be few or solitary (see Chapter 6.16, Fig. 16.2). They are often hypopigmented but they may have a rather indurated coppery color or a purple border. These patches tend to be hypoesthetic and dry with loss of hairs, and they show a negative histamine provocation test.

In lepromatous leprosy, multiple small macules, papules and nodules develop in a symmetric manner in all sites apart from the hairy scalp, the axillae and the groins, where the temperature tends to be higher. Patients often develop leonine facies because of diffuse involvement of the facial skin (Fig. 5.7). Borderline types of leprosy have clinical features between these extremes of immunologic reaction to the causative agent.

Three types of inflammatory reactions can occur during the course of leprosy. Type I leprae reaction occurs in borderline disease and is associated with upgrading of the condition. Existing skin lesions become more inflamed and painful or may ulcerate and new lesions may appear. This is associated with acute or insidious pain and tenderness of affected nerves.

Type II leprae reactions occur in patients who have lepromatous leprosy and borderline leprosy. These reactions may occur spontaneously or in response to treatment. The most common cutaneous manifestation is that of erythema nodosum leprosum, in which painful red nodules occur in the skin, most commonly on the face and extensor surfaces of the limbs.[19] Individual lesions are painful, red nodules, but they may ultimately ulcerate. Erythema nodosum leprosum may be accompanied by uveitis, myositis, lymphadenitis, neuritis, dactylitis, arthritis and orchitis.

The third type of reaction seen in leprosy is the so-called Lucio phenomenon.[20] This is due to deep cutaneous vasculitis leading to infarction of the overlying skin. Irregular erythematous patches develop, and these may necrose to leave deep painful ulcers.

NONSPECIFIC CUTANEOUS SIGNS OF SYSTEMIC INFECTIONS

ERYTHEMA MULTIFORME

Erythema multiforme may occur at any age. The lesions are usually asymptomatic and start as dull red macules and papules that occur on acral sites (particular the hands) and then spread more centrally. Typical target lesions occur; these have a central purpuric area and a raised rather edematous boarder (Fig. 5.8). Less commonly, the feet, elbows, knees, face, neck and trunk are affected.

In severe eruptions, bullae may develop over the individual lesions.

In the most severe form of the disease the oral mucosa shows extensive bullous formation with erosions affecting the lips and buccal mucosa. Genital lesions may also occur. This form is called the Stevens–Johnson syndrome. A variety of infectious agents have been implicated in causing erythema multiforme (Fig. 5.9).[21] The most common infectious cause of erythema multiforme is herpes simplex infection.

ERYTHEMA NODOSUM

Erythema nodosum is an acute type IV reaction to a number of different stimuli. The skin and subcutaneous fat are affected with a septal panniculitis. Clinically, there is a short prodrome of mild fever, myalgia and malaise. Erythematous nodules develop on the shins and more rarely on the arms, face and neck; these vary in diameter from 1cm to several centimeters (Fig. 5.10). The hallmark of erythema nodosum is pain and exquisite tenderness of the lesions. Initially, the lesions are bright red but as they subside over the next 3 weeks or so they undergo a bruise-like change from dusky purple–yellow and green before leaving mild scaling of the skin.

A number of infectious agents have been implicated in the etiology of erythema nodosum (Fig. 5.11).[22] These vary with the age of the patient and the country of residence. The most common infectious cause is an upper respiratory viral infection. Streptococcal sore throats are also a common cause in children, and tuberculosis is still a common cause in children where the disease is prevalent. Infections with *Chlamydia psittaci* have been responsible for small outbreaks of erythema nodosum in adults in the UK, where contact with birds and poultry may be an important clue in identifying the cause of the reaction. Infections with *Yersinia* spp. are a common cause of erythema nodosum in France and Finland but are rare in other countries.

Erythema nodosum may be related to inflammatory tinea capitis in children, particularly in association with kerion formation. Deep fungal infection, particularly coccidioidomycosis, blastomycosis and histoplasmosis have all been associated with erythema nodosum. More rarely, erythema nodosum has been reported in association with tularemia, salmonellosis, *Campylobacter* spp. infection and leptospirosis.

CUTANEOUS VASCULITIS

The clinical features of cutaneous vasculitis depend on the size of the blood vessels affected and on whether the vasculitis is acute or chronic. Acute leukocytoclastic vasculitis is caused by immune complex deposition in cutaneous blood vessels with complement fixation and damage caused by polymorphonuclear leukocyte infiltration and activation.

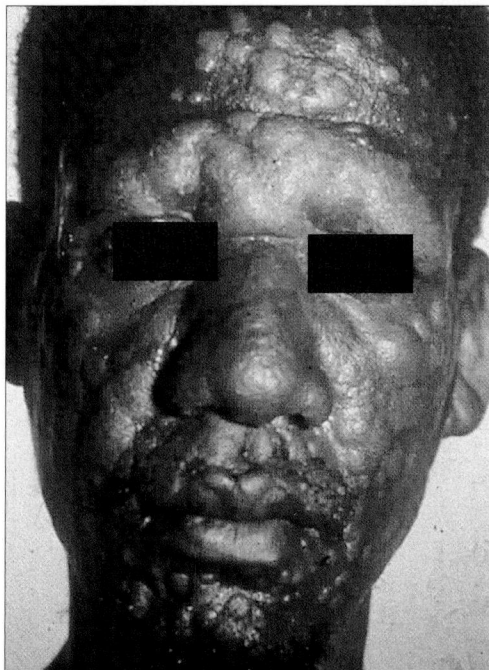

Fig. 5.7 Lepromatous leprosy, with multiple symmetric lesions on the face giving a leonine facies.

The targeted blood vessels tend to be small, superficial vessels and the clinical signs are of a purpuric macular or papular eruption on the lower legs and dependent areas; these eruptions may become bullous and ulcerate (Fig. 5.12). The most common bacterial infection associated with cutaneous vasculitis is a streptococcal sore throat,[23,24] which precedes the vasculitis by 1–3 weeks.

Subacute and chronic cutaneous vasculitis is associated with chronic foci of infection such as dental abscesses or asymptomatic chronic pyelonephritis.[23] In nodular vasculitis, tuberculosis has been blamed for the reaction; leprosy and syphilis should also be considered. *Neisseria gonorrhoeae*, *Mycoplasma pneumoniae* and *Rickettsia* spp. may also cause an acute vasculitis (Fig. 5.13).

Viruses can cause endothelial cell damage, platelet agglutination and immune complex formation. The best studied causes of viral vasculitis are influenza vaccines, hepatitis B virus[25] and the Bunyaviridae-induced hemorrhagic fever. Hepatitis C virus should also be considered in any vasculitis work up. Herpes simplex infection[26] and enterovirus infections[27] have also been implicated in cutaneous vasculitis.

Less commonly, fungal infections (including those with *Candida albicans*) have been reported in association with vascular damage and cutaneous vasculitis. Cryptococcosis may present with a widespread nodular vasculitis when complicating HIV infection.

GIANOTTI–CROSTI SYNDROME

Gianotti–Crosti syndrome is a cutaneous reaction to virus infection, characteristically seen in children aged between 6 months and 12 years. The majority of cases are associated with hepatitis B virus infection, usually with subtype ayw.[28] More recently, a number of other viruses have been causally linked with this syndrome, including Epstein–Barr virus, Coxsackie viruses A16, B4 and B5, echoviruses 7 and 9, poliovirus, cytomegalovirus, respiratory syncytial virus, hepatitis A virus and parainfluenza virus.[29,30]

The eruption presents acutely with dull red papules of 5–10mm diameter. These develop over 3–4 days, starting on the buttocks and thighs and spreading to the arms and face. The papules may become purpuric. In cases that are related to hepatitis B virus, the papules are not itchy, unlike those linked to other viruses. Lymphadenopathy of the axillae and groins is often present and may persist for several months after the eruption has settled, which generally occurs within 2–8 weeks to leave mild scaling but no scarring.

KAWASAKI DISEASE

Kawasaki disease is a diffuse vasculitic disease of unknown cause. A

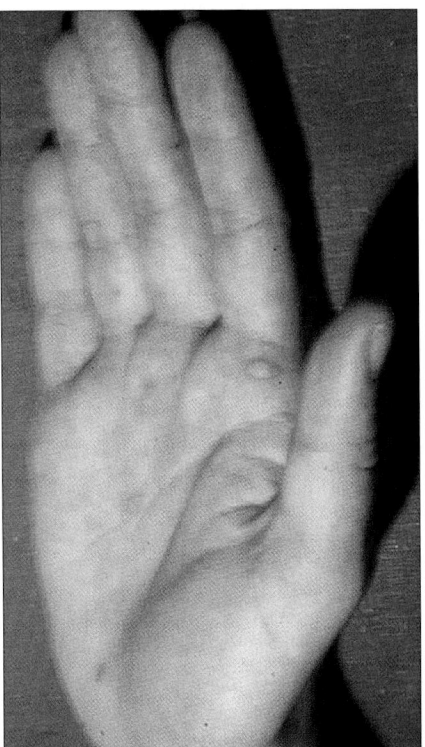

Fig. 5.8 Erythema multiforme showing target lesions and bullous lesions on the palms of the hands.

INFECTIVE CAUSES OF ERYTHEMA MULTIFORME
Herpes simplex virus
Mycoplasma pneumoniae
Lymphogranuloma inguinale
Psittacosis
Rickettsia spp.
Vaccinia
HIV infection
Hepatitis B virus
Enterovirus
Adenovirus
Orf
Infectious mononucleosis
Mumps
Poliomyelitis
Streptococcus pyogenes
Typhoid
Pseudomonas aeruginosa
Tularemia
Yersinia spp.
Tuberculosis
Syphilis
Legionnaires' disease
Histoplasmosis
Coccidioidomycosis

Fig. 5.9 Infective causes of erythema multiforme.

INFECTIONS ASSOCIATED WITH ERYTHEMA NODOSUM
Upper respiratory tract viruses
Streptococcal infections
Yersiniosis
Salmonellosis
Campylobacter spp.
Tuberculosis
Lymphogranuloma venereum
Cat-scratch disease
Psittacosis
Tularemia
Leptospirosis
Inflammatory dermatophyte infections
Coccidioidomycosis
Blastomycosis
Histoplasmosis

Fig. 5.11 Infections associated with erythema nodosum.

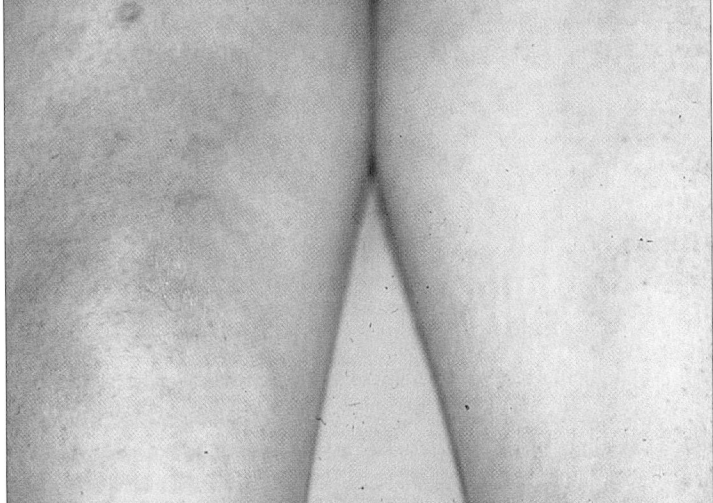

Fig. 5.10 Erythema nodosum on the lower legs. On investigation this patient was found to have a negative Mantoux even at 1 in 100, but the erythema nodosum subsided when the patient was started on antituberculous therapy.

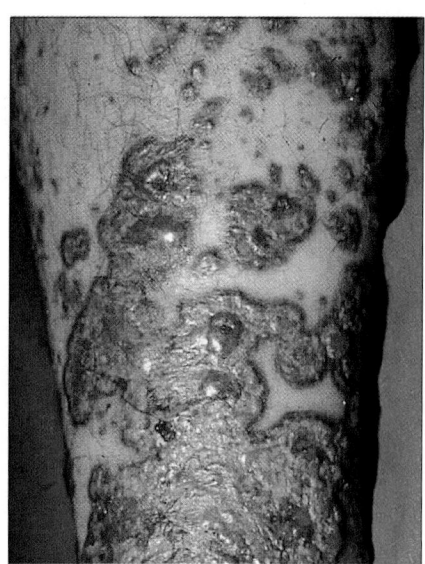

Fig. 5.12 Acute leucocytoclastic vasculitis showing bullous lesions on the lower leg. This patient was found to have a high antistreptolysin titer.

INFECTIONS ASSOCIATED WITH CUTANEOUS VASCULITIS
Streptococci
Dental abscesses
Chronic *Escherichia coli* infections
Tuberculosis
Leprosy
Syphilis
Gonorrhea
Hepatitis B virus
Hepatitis C virus
Enteroviruses
Hemorrhagic fever
Herpes simplex
Mycoplasma pneumoniae
Rickettsia spp.
Candidiasis
Cryptococcosis

Fig. 5.13 Infections associated with cutaneous vasculitis.

number of infectious agents have been implicated in its pathogenesis, including streptococci,[31] staphylococci,[32] *Leptospira* spp.,[33] *Pseudomonas* spp., *Rickettsia* spp., Epstein–Barr virus and other viruses. In most cases no agent is identified. The disease generally affects children under the age of 4 years and although it most commonly occurs in Japan it has been reported throughout the world.

The disease is acute in onset with a remittent fever. The conjunctivae become injected and the lips and tongue are red. At the onset of fever, a generalized polymorphic eruption develops on the trunk and proximal limbs; this is associated with redness and induration of the palms and soles. Cervical lymphadenopathy develops in 50–80% of patients. The fever lasts for more than 5 days and as this subsides the skin scales and the patient may develop arthralgias and arthropathy. Cardiac involvement develops at this stage of the illness in 20% of patients, with myocarditis, aneurysm, stenosis and obstruction of the coronary arteries, which is usually responsible for the 1% mortality seen in this disease.

REFERENCES

1. Ramesh V, Misra RS, Jain RK. Secondary tuberculosis of the skin: clinical features and problems in laboratory diagnosis. Int J Dermatol 1987;26:578–81.
2. Lebel M, Lassonde M. Eythema induratum of Bazin. J Am Acad Dermatol 1986;14:738–42.
3. Dunlop EMC. Some aspects of infectious syphilis today. Public Health 1964;78:259–67.
4. Berger BW. Erythema chronicum migrans of Lyme disease. Arch Dermatol 1984;120:1017–21.
5. Coulson IH, Smith NP, Holden CA. Acrodermatitis chronica atrophicans with co-existing morphoea. Br J Dermatol 1989;121:263–9.
6. Yamanishi K, Okuno T, Shiraki K, et al. Identification of human herpes virus 6 as a causal agent for exanthum subitum. Lancet 1988;i:1065–7.
7. Drago F, Ranieri E, Malaguti F, et al. Human herpesvirus 7 in patients with pityriasis rosea. Electron microscopy investigations and polymerase chain reaction in mononuclear cells, plasma and skin. Dermatology 1997;195:374–8.
8. Lemlich G, Schwam L, Lebwohl M. Kaposi's sarcoma and acquired immunodeficiency syndrome. J Am Acad Dermatol 1987;16:319–25.
9. Alessi E, Berti E, Cusini M, et al. Oral hairy leukoplakia. J Am Acad Dermatol 1990;22:79–86.
10. James WD, Redfield RR, Lupton GP, et al. A papular eruption associated with human T cell lymphotrophic virus type III disease. J Am Acad Dermatol 1985;13:563–6.
11. Gorin I, Lessana-Leibovitch M, Fortier P, et al. Successful treatment of the pruritus of human immunodeficiency virus infection and acquired immunodeficiency syndrome with psoralens and ultraviolet A therapy. J Am Acad Dermatol 1989;20:511–13.
12. Buchness MR, Lim HW, Hatcher VA, et al. Eosinophilic pustular folliculitis in the acquired immunodeficiency syndrome. N Engl J Med 1988;318:1183–6.
13. Cockerell CJ, LeBoit PE. Bacillary angiomoatosis: a newly characterised, pseudo-neoplastic, infectious, cutaneous vascular disorder. J Am Acad Dermatol 1990;22:501–12.
14. Schlievert PM, Bettin KM, Watson DW. Production of pyrogenic exotoxin by groups of streptococci: association with Group A. J Infect Dis 1979;140:676–81.
15. Melish ME, Chen FS, Murata MS. Epidermolytic toxin (ET) production in human and experimental staphylococcal infections. Clin Res 1979;27:114A.
16. Keil H. The rheumatic erythemas: a critical survey. Ann Intern Med 1937–38;11:2223–72.
17. Bannister B. Clinical aspects of meningococcal disease. J Med Microbiol 1988;26:161–87.
18. Wohlfarth B, Asamer H. Symptoms and immunology of Henoch–Schönlein syndrome. Arch Dermatol Res 1976;255:251–8.
19. Battacharya SK, Girgla HS, Singh G. Necrotising reaction in lepromatous leprosy. Lepr Rev 1973;44:29–32.
20. Rea TH, Ridley DS. Lucio's phenomenon: a comparative histological study. Int J Lepr 1979;47:161–6.
21. Huff JC, Weston WL, Tonnesen MG. Erythema multiforme: a critical review of characteristics, diagnostic criteria and causes. J Am Acad Dermatol 1983;8:763–75.
22. Doxiadis SA. Aetiology of erythema nodosum. Br Med J 1949;ii:844–5.
23. Parish WE. Microbial antigens in vasculitis. In: Wolff K, Winkelmann R, eds. Vasculitis. London: LLoyd Luke; 1980:129–50.
24. Ruiter M. Allergic cutaneous vasculitis. Acta Dermatol Venereol 1952;32:274–81.
25. Gower RG, Saysker WF, Komler P, et al. Small vessel vasculitis caused by hepatitis B virus immune complexes. J Allergy Clin Immunol 1978;62:222–8.
26. Cohen C, Trapukol S. Leucocytoclastic vasculitis associated with cutaneous infection by herpes virus. Am J Dermatol 1984;6:561–5.
27. Kirkpatrick CJ, Gruler H. Interaction between enterovirus and human endothelial cells in vitro. Am J Pathol 1985;118:15–25.
28. Crosti A, Gianotti F. Ulteriore contributo alla conoscenza dell' acrodermatite papulosa infantile. G Ital Dermatol 1964;105:477–81.
29. Draelos ZK, Hansen RC, James WD. Gianotti–Crosti syndrome associated with infections other than hepetitis B. JAMA 1986;256:2386–8.
30. Speak KH, Winkelman R. Gianotti–Crosti syndrome: review of ten cases not associated with hepatitis B. Arch Dermatol 1984;120:891–6.
31. Krensky AM, Teele R, Watkins J, et al. Streptococcal antigenicity in mucocutaneous lymph node syndrome and hydropic gallbladders [letter]. Pediatrics 1979;64:979–80.
32. Todd J, Fishaut M. Toxic shock syndrome associated with phage group I staphylococci. Lancet 1978;ii:1116–8.
33. Morens DM. Editorial: thoughts on Kawazaki disease etiology. JAMA 1979;241:399.

Superficial Fungal Infections

David W Warnock

INTRODUCTION

This chapter reviews the different fungal diseases of the skin, nails and hair. The most common of these diseases are dermatophytosis, candidiasis and pityriasis versicolor. Other, less frequent infections of the skin and hair include tinea nigra and piedra. In addition, there are a number of nondermatophytic molds that can cause nail disease (onychomycosis).

EPIDEMIOLOGY

The organisms that cause dermatophytosis are molds belonging to the genera *Trichophyton*, *Microsporum* and *Epidermophyton*.[1] Many of the 40 or so species that are recognized at present are worldwide in distribution, but others are confined to particular regions.[2] About 10 species are common human pathogens. The dermatophytes can be split into three ecologic groups depending on whether their usual natural habitat is the soil (geophilic species), animals (zoophilic species), or humans (anthropophilic species). Members of all three groups can cause human infections, but their different natural reservoirs have important implications in relation to the acquisition, site and spread of the disease. Infections originating from the soil are the least common. Infections having animal origins are more frequent, and particular species are often associated with particular animal hosts. Anthropophilic dermatophytes account for most human infections: these species are contagious and are readily transmitted from person to person.

Cutaneous candidiasis is a less common disease than dermatophytosis. *Candida albicans*, the predominant etiologic agent, is a commensal organism found in the mouth and gastrointestinal tract of a significant proportion of the normal population. It is seldom recovered from normal skin, being much less prevalent than *Candida parapsilosis*, but it is a frequent colonizer of moist or damaged skin and nails.

Malassezia furfur is a common commensal organism that colonizes the normal skin of the head and trunk during late childhood. In certain circumstances, such as hot humid climatic conditions, this lipophilic organism produces the disease pityriasis versicolor. In the tropics, up to 50% of the population may be affected. In patients with AIDS, *Malassezia furfur* can cause a widespread and severe folliculitis. *Malassezia furfur* can be transmitted from person to person, either through direct contact or through contaminated clothing or bedding. In practice, however, infection is endogenous in most cases, and spread between individuals is uncommon.

Tinea nigra is a chronic infection of the palms and soles. The disease is rare but has a worldwide distribution, although it is more common in the tropics and subtropics. The etiologic agent, *Phaeoannellomyces werneckii*, is a saprobic mold that is found in the soil and in decomposing vegetation. Human infection is thought to follow traumatic inoculation.

Black piedra is an uncommon hair infection that occurs in humid tropical regions. The natural habitat of the etiologic agent, *Piedraia hortae*, has not been identified. There are some reports of familial infection. White piedra is less common than black piedra. It is found worldwide, but it is more prevalent in the tropics and subtropics. The

etiologic agent, *Trichophyton beigelii*, has a widespread natural distribution, and is sometimes found on normal skin.

Onychomycosis is a nonspecific term used to describe fungal disease of the nails; tinea unguium is a more specific term used to describe dermatophyte nail infection. At least 80% of fungal nail infections and 90% of toenail infections are due to dermatophytes, in particular *T. rubrum*.[3] Between 5 and 10% of nail infections are due to *Candida* spp., and the remainder are attributable to nondermatophytic molds. Most prominent among these are *Scopulariopsis brevicaulis*, *Scytalidium dimidiatum* (*Hendersonula toruloidea*), *Aspergillus* spp. and *Fusarium* spp.[3] Unlike the dermatophytes these molds are not contagious. Onychomycosis is more prevalent in older people, and men are more commonly affected than women. Toenails are more frequently involved than fingernails.

PATHOGENESIS AND PATHOLOGY

The dermatophytes are keratinophilic fungi that are normally found growing only in the dead keratinized tissue of the stratum corneum, within and around hair shafts, and in the nail plate and keratinized nail bed. The clinical appearances of dermatophyte infections are the result of a combination of direct damage to the tissue by the fungus (mainly in the case of hair and nail infections) and of the immune response of the host. The damage to tissue is due to a combination of mechanical forces and enzymatic activities. Dermatophytes produce a number of keratinolytic proteinases that function best at an acidic pH, and these have been recognized as important virulence factors.[4]

The immune response to dermatophytes has been studied in human infections as well as in animal models.[5] The humoral response does not appear to help in the elimination of infection; the highest levels of antibodies are often found in patients with chronic dermatophytosis. Rather, it is the cell-mediated response that is important in ridding the stratum corneum of the infection.[6] Dermatophytes vary in their host interactions. Zoophilic species, such as *T. verrucosum*, often elicit intense inflammation in humans. This leads to enhanced epidermal proliferation and can result in spontaneous cure.[7] In contrast, anthropophilic species such as *T. rubrum* often produce chronic or recurrent lesions. Chronic dermatophytosis in otherwise healthy people may be mediated by fungal cell wall components, such as mannan, that diminish the local immune response.[7]

Except for neonatal infections, most cases of superficial candidiasis result from infection of the host from his own commensal flora. This shift in the host–fungus relationship results from a number of influences, of which host factors appear to be the most important. Local tissue damage is a critical factor in the pathogenesis of cutaneous candidiasis: most infections occur in moist, occluded sites and follow maceration of the tissue. Chronic mucocutaneous candidiasis is a rare condition that results from inherited defects in the cell-mediated immune response.[8]

Malassezia furfur is present on the normal skin from late childhood. Hot, humid environmental conditions are among the factors that predispose to the development of the cutaneous lesions of pityriasis versicolor.

PREVENTION

Prevention of dermatophytosis must take into account the site of the infection, the etiologic agent, and the source of the infection.

Tinea capitis is a common fungal infection in children. The predominant etiologic agents differ from continent to continent, but the anthropophilic species *T. tonsurans* has replaced *Microsporum audouinii* as the dominant cause of this infection in North, Central and South America.[2] Infections with this organism have also become much more common in the UK.[9] Anthropophilic tinea capitis is easily spread from child to child, both in the home and at school. Among the factors that favor its spread, *T. tonsurans* can exist in an asymptomatic carrier state in children.[9] Other less common causes of tinea capitis include the animal species, *Microsporum canis* and *T. verrucosum*.

To prevent the spread of anthropophilic tinea capitis in schools due to *M. audouinii*, contacts of infected children can be examined for infected fluorescent hairs with Wood's light (a source of ultraviolet light filtered through nickel oxide glass). In the more common non-fluorescent infection with *T. tonsurans*, detection is more difficult, but the scalp brush sampling method is often helpful in detecting subclinical disease.[10] All those found to be infected must be treated, and the importance of good personal hygiene should be stressed. It is seldom practical to exclude infected children from school.

In the case of tinea capitis and tinea corporis caused by zoophilic species, such as *M. canis* and *T. verrucosum*, it is important to locate the animal source. *Microsporum canis* infection of cats and dogs can often be detected with Wood's light examination. The subsequent course of action will depend upon the value placed on the infected animal. It is more difficult to detect and eliminate *T. verrucosum* infection in cattle, because infected hairs are not fluorescent and because the fungus can survive for long periods on hairs and scales that have been deposited on the walls of buildings and gates. Fungicidal washes have sometimes been effective in controlling this infection.

Tinea pedis is a contagious condition and is easily spread from person to person. Transfer within households has been reported, but the main spread occurs in communal baths and showers.[11] Educating infected people not to expose others to their infection by not walking barefoot on the floors of communal changing rooms and by avoiding public baths and showers can help to reduce the spread of this disease. Frequent hosing of the floors of public baths and the discouraging of antifungal foot dips near communal baths are helpful preventative measures. Prompt treatment of tinea pedis and the use of separate towels are sensible measures that can help to prevent tinea cruris, tinea manuum and tinea unguium.

Intertriginous candidiasis of the fingernails is often seen in people whose occupation necessitates frequent wetting of the hands. Wearing protective gloves can help to prevent this infection.

Good personal hygiene is important in preventing the spread of piedra. Infected people should not share hair brushes or combs with others.

CLINICAL FEATURES

The dermatophytes are the predominant causal organisms of fungal disease of the scalp, toe clefts, soles, palms and nails. In the temperate, developed countries, tinea pedis is the most common form of dermatophytosis. By contrast, in the tropics, tinea capitis and tinea corporis are the most prevalent.

TINEA CAPITIS

The clinical manifestations of tinea capitis are varied and depend on the species of dermatophyte involved and the degree of host response (Fig. 6.1). The appearance of the lesions can range from mild scaling and hair loss with minimal inflammation to severe inflammation with kerion formation.

In *M. audouinii* infection the lesions consist of well-demarcated patches of partial alopecia. Inflammation is minimal, but fine scaling is characteristic. Most of the hairs in these lesions are broken off near the surface of the scalp. In *M. canis* infection the picture is similar, but there is usually more inflammation. In both these infections the hair surface is coated with small arthrospores (ectothrix infection). The affected hairs show green fluorescence under Wood's light.

In *T. tonsurans* and *T. violaceum* infections the lesions are often inconspicuous, and inflammation may be minimal. The typical lesions are irregular patches of scaling. The affected hairs often break off at the surface of the scalp giving a 'black-dot' appearance. The hairs are filled with arthrospores (endothrix infection) and do not fluoresce under Wood's light.

The most florid form of tinea capitis is a kerion. A kerion is a painful inflammatory mass in which the hairs that remain are loose. Thick crusting with matting of adjacent hairs is common. Pus may be discharged from one or more points. A kerion may be limited in extent, but a large confluent lesion may develop (a severe form of kerion) that involves most of the scalp. In most cases this violent reaction results from infection with an animal dermatophyte such as *T. verrucosum* or *T. mentagrophytes* var. *mentagrophytes*. However, geophilic or anthropophilic organisms are sometimes involved. In *T. verrucosum* infections the hairs are covered with chains of large arthrospores but they do not fluoresce under Wood's light.

Favus is now rare, but it is still a distinctive form of fungal scalp infection. The causal organism is *T. schoenleinii*, an anthropophilic dermatophyte noted for its persistence. Favus presents with hair loss and the formation of cup-shaped crusts known as scutula. These give off a fetid odor and can amalgamate to form dense mats on part or all of the scalp. Long-standing favus can lead to permanent patches of cicatricial alopecia. Infected hairs give off a dull green fluorescence under Wood's light.

Tinea capitis must be distinguished from seborrheic dermatitis, psoriasis, bacterial folliculitis and cicatricial alopecia.

TINEA BARBAE

The animal species *T. verrucosum* and *T. mentagrophytes* var. *mentagrophytes* are the principal causes of dermatophyte infection of the beard and moustache areas of the face. *Microsporum canis* is a less common cause. The characteristic appearance is of a highly inflammatory pustular folliculitis (Fig. 6.2). Some infections are less severe and consist of circular, erythematous, scaling lesions.

TINEA FACIEI

The more common causes of dermatophyte infection of the face are *T. rubrum* and *T. mentagrophytes* var. *mentagrophytes*, but many other species may be involved, including *T. tonsurans* and *M. canis*. The typical annular lesions are erythematous, but scaling is often

SOME CHARACTERISTICS OF COMMON DERMATOPHYTES CAUSING SCALP INFECTION			
Organism	Arthrospore size	Arthrospore arrangement	Fluorescence under Wood's light
Microsporum audouinii	Small (2–3µm)	Ectothrix	Yes
Microsporum canis	Small (2–3µm)	Ectothrix	Yes
Trichophyton mentagrophytes	Small (3–5µm)	Ectothrix	No
Trichophyton soudanense	Large (4–8µm)	Endothrix	No
Trichophyton tonsurans	Large (4–8µm)	Endothrix	No
Trichophyton verrucosum	Large (5–10µm)	Ectothrix	No
Trichophyton violaceum	Large (4–8µm)	Endothrix	No

Fig. 6.1 Some characteristics of common dermatophytes causing scalp infection.

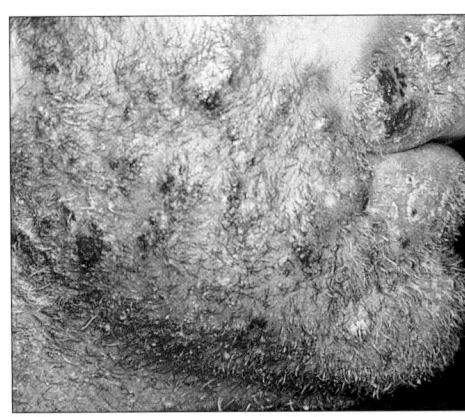

Fig. 6.2 Tinea barbae due to *Trichophyton verrucosum*.

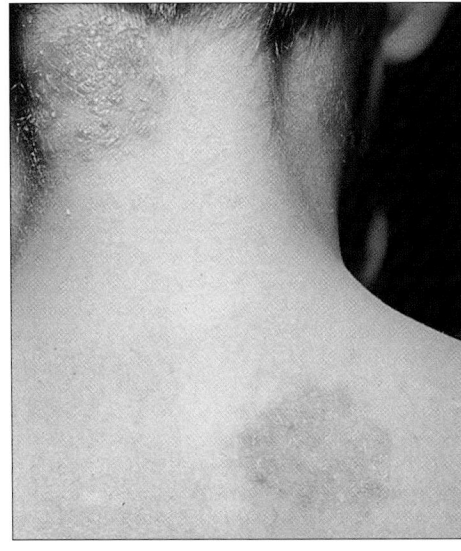

Fig. 6.3 Tinea corporis due to *Trichophyton. mentagrophytes* var. *mentagrophytes*.

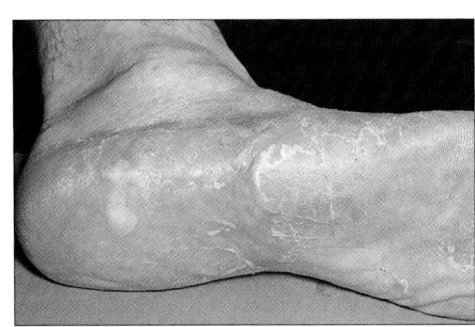

Fig. 6.4 Moccasin tinea pedis due to *Trichophyton rubrum*.

absent. The lesions are often pruritic and exacerbation after exposure to the sun is common.

TINEA CORPORIS

The clinical manifestations of tinea corporis are varied and often depend on the species of the infective organism. The disease often follows contact with infected animals, but occasional cases result from contact with contaminated soil. *Microsporum canis* is a frequent cause of human infection, and *T. verrucosum* infection is common in rural districts. Infections with anthropophilic species, such as *T. rubrum*, often follow spread from another site, such as the feet. Infections with *T. tonsurans* are sometimes seen in children with tinea capitis.

The characteristic lesion is an annular scaling plaque with a raised erythematous border and central clearing. In their most florid form the lesions can become indurated and pustular (Fig. 6.3). This is more common in infections with zoophilic organisms. The differential diagnosis includes discoid eczema, impetigo, psoriasis and discoid lupus erythematosus.

TINEA CRURIS

Infection of the groin and the perianal and perineal regions is more common in men. The predominant causes are the anthropophilic species, *T. rubrum* and *Epidermophyton floccosum*. The infection often follows spread from another site in the same person, but person-to-person spread (e.g. through contaminated clothing) is not uncommon.

In color, the lesions are erythematous to brown. They have raised scaling margins and radiate from the groin down the inner border of the thigh. Patients often complain of intense pruritus. The differential diagnosis includes intertriginous *Candida* spp. infection, bacterial intertrigo, psoriasis and seborrheic dermatitis.

TINEA IMBRICATA

This is a chronic infection that is characterized by the development of homogeneous sheets or concentric rings of scaling that can spread to cover large parts of the affected person. Most reports of tinea imbricata have come from the Pacific Islands and Melanesia but there have been occasional reports from South East Asia and Central and South America. The etiologic agent is the anthropophilic species, *T. concentricum*.

TINEA PEDIS

Infection of the feet is the most common form of dermatophytosis in the UK and North America. The main organisms involved are the anthropophilic species *T. rubrum* and, less commonly, *T. mentagrophytes* var. *interdigitale*.

The most common clinical presentation is interdigital maceration, peeling and fissuring, mostly in the spaces between the fourth and fifth toes. Itching is a common symptom.

Another common presentation associated with *T. rubrum* is hyperkeratosis of the soles, heels and sides of the feet. The affected sites are pink and covered with fine, white scales. This form of the disease is often chronic and resistant to treatment. If there is extensive involvement of the foot, then the term 'moccasin tinea pedis' is often applied (Fig. 6.4).

A third form of tinea pedis, associated with *T. mentagrophytes* var. *interdigitale*, is an acute vesicular infection of the soles. This severe form of the disease may resolve without treatment, but exacerbations tend to occur under hot humid conditions. There is often associated hyperhidrosis.

Tinea pedis can be difficult to distinguish from other infectious causes of toe web infection, such as *Candida* intertrigo and erythrasma. Noninfectious conditions that mimic tinea pedis of the soles include psoriasis and contact dermatitis.

TINEA MANUUM

Tinea manuum is usually unilateral, the right hand being more commonly affected than the left. Lesions on the dorsum of the hand appear similar to those of tinea corporis, with a distinct border and central clearing. Infection of the palms is more common. This presents as a diffuse scaling hyperkeratosis, with accentuation of the fissuring in the palmar creases. *Trichophyton rubrum* is the most common cause of tinea manuum. The differential diagnosis includes contact dermatitis, eczema and psoriasis.

TINEA UNGUIUM

The most common causes of dermatophyte infection of the nails are *T. rubrum* and *T. mentagrophytes* var. *interdigitale*, but many other species may be involved. Three clinical forms of tinea unguium are recognized. Distal or lateral subungual disease is the most common presentation (Fig. 6.5). This usually begins as a discoloration and thickening of the nail, and it can result in destruction of the entire nail plate and separation of the nail from the nail bed (Fig. 6.6). In superficial white onychomycosis, crumbling white lesions are evident on the nail surface, particularly in patients with AIDS. This condition is most commonly caused by *T. mentagrophytes* var. *interdigitale*. Proximal subungual disease is the least common presentation of dermatophyte nail infection.

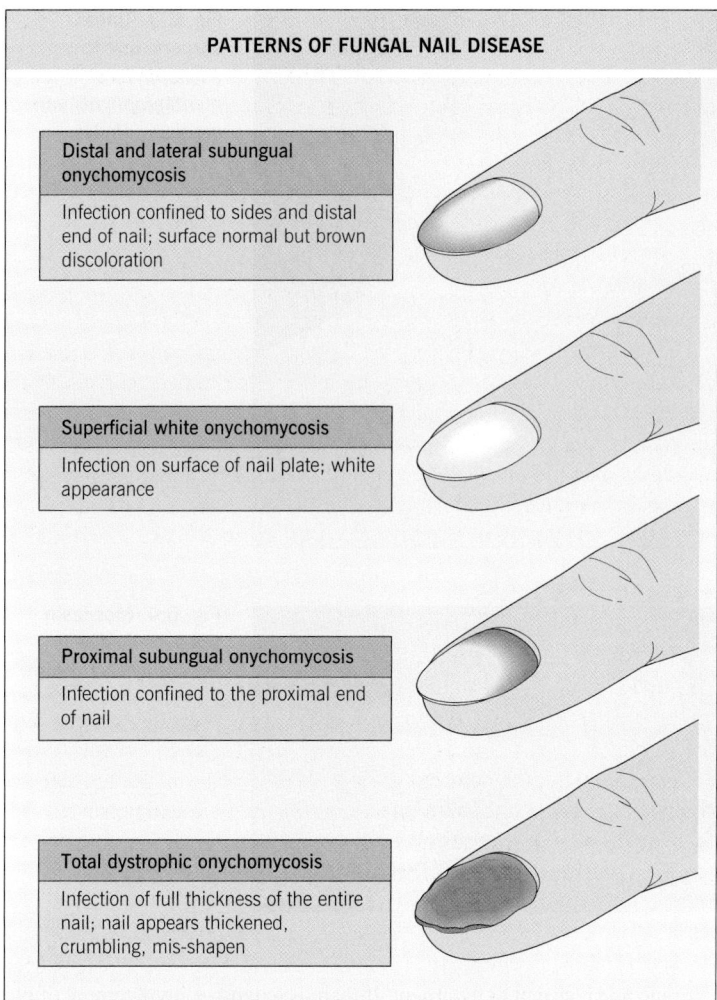

PATTERNS OF FUNGAL NAIL DISEASE

Distal and lateral subungual onychomycosis

Infection confined to sides and distal end of nail; surface normal but brown discoloration

Superficial white onychomycosis

Infection on surface of nail plate; white appearance

Proximal subungual onychomycosis

Infection confined to the proximal end of nail

Total dystrophic onychomycosis

Infection of full thickness of the entire nail; nail appears thickened, crumbling, mis-shapen

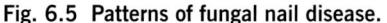

Fig. 6.5 Patterns of fungal nail disease.

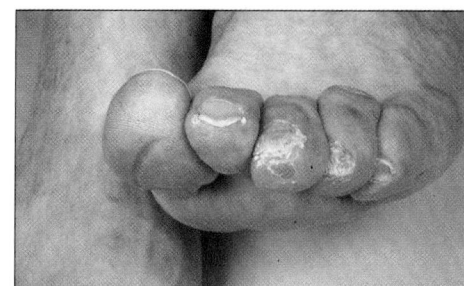

Fig. 6.6 Total dystrophic onychomycosis due to *Trichophyton rubrum*.

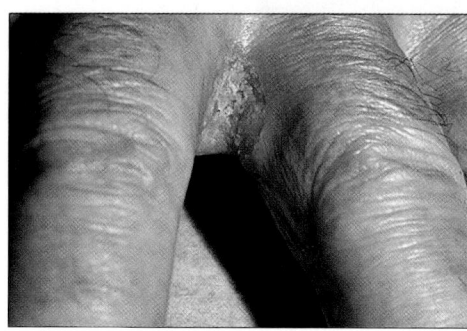

Fig. 6.7 Interdigital candidiasis.

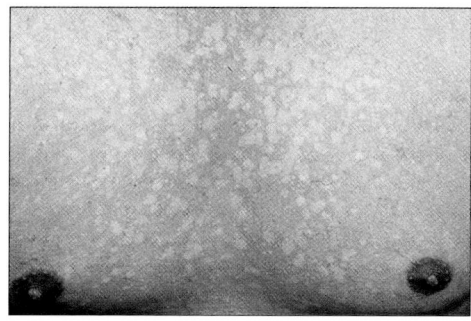

Fig. 6.8 Pityriasis versicolor showing depigmented lesions.

The differential diagnosis includes eczema, lichen planus, onychogryphosis and lichen planus. Unlike dermatophytosis, *Candida* infections of the nails often begin in the proximal nail plate and are associated with nail fold infection.

CANDIDIASIS

The lesions of cutaneous candidiasis (intertrigo) tend to develop in warm, moist sites such as the folds of the skin under the breasts and the groin. The infection is more common in overweight or diabetic people. The initial lesions are papules or vesicopustules that later enlarge and become confluent. The larger lesions are erythematous and have an irregular margin. Smaller, satellite lesions are often present. Soreness and itching is usual. The differential diagnosis includes dermatophytosis, seborrheic dermatitis, bacterial intertrigo and psoriasis.

Infection of the skin between the fingers or toes can also occur. Infection of the webs of the fingers presents as a macerated, erythematous lesion (Fig. 6.7). It is often uncomfortable and may be painful. This condition is usually seen in people whose occupations necessitate frequent immersion of the hands in water. Infection of the webs of the toes mimics tinea pedis, and many cases do occur in conjunction with this form of dermatophytosis.

Chronic mucocutaneous candidiasis (see Chapter 2.7) is a rare condition that affects people with underlying endocrinologic or immunologic disorders. The disease often develops during the first 3 years of life. The mouth is usually the first site to be affected, but lesions then appear on the scalp, hands, feet and nails. In some patients, disfiguring hyperkeratotic lesions develop on the scalp and face.

Three forms of *Candida* nail infection are recognized: infection of the nail folds (paronychia), distal nail infection, and total dystrophic onychomycosis. The last is a manifestation of chronic mucocutaneous candidiasis. Infection of the nail folds is more common in women than in men. The periungual skin is raised and painful, and a prominent gap develops between the fold and the nail plate. White pus may be discharged. The infection usually starts in the proximal nail fold, but the lateral margins are sometimes the first site to be affected. The nail plate may be invaded.

Distal *Candida* nail infection presents as onycholysis and subungual hyperkeratosis. It is often difficult to distinguish from dermatophytosis, but candidiasis tends to affect the fingernails rather than the toenails. In patients with chronic mucocutaneous candidiasis, the nail plate is invaded from the outset causing gross thickening and hyperkeratosis.

PITYRIASIS VERSICOLOR

Pityriasis versicolor is a disfiguring but otherwise harmless condition. The characteristic lesions consist of patches of fine brown scaling that are found particularly on the upper trunk, neck, upper arms and abdomen. In light-skinned people the affected skin may appear darker than normal. The lesions are light pink in color but grow darker, turning a pale brown shade. In dark-skinned or tanned people, the affected skin becomes depigmented (Fig. 6.8).

Hyperpigmented lesions must be distinguished from erythrasma, seborrheic dermatitis, pityriasis rosea, and tinea corporis. Hypopigmented lesions can be confused with pityriasis alba and vitiligo.

TINEA NIGRA

The lesions of tinea nigra, which are found on the palm or sole, consist of one or more, flat, dark brown or black, nonscaling patches with a well-defined edge. Inflammation is absent. The lesions, which are small at first, expand and become confluent. The disease is asymptomatic and may remain undiagnosed for long periods. Tinea nigra must be distinguished from malignant melanoma and chemical stains.

PIEDRA

Black piedra is most often seen on the scalp hair. Small, brown or black, hard nodules, which are difficult to remove, are formed on the distal hair shafts. The appearance of white piedra is similar, but the nodules are softer and pale in color. This condition affects the hairs of the beard and moustache. Less commonly it involves the scalp or pubic hair.

ONYCHOMYCOSIS

Up to 5% of cases of onychomycosis are due to nondermatophyte molds. With the exception of *Scytalidium dimidiatum*, these molds usually affect nails that have previously been diseased or damaged. This may account for the fact that these infections often affect only one nail. There is nothing specific about the clinical appearance of the lesions (Fig 6.9). Distal subungual hyperkeratosis with onycholysis of the distal nail plate is common (see Fig. 6.5). Superficial white lesions are another presentation.

DIAGNOSIS

Superficial fungal infections often present with characteristic lesions, but where this is not the case mycologic investigation can assist in diagnosis. Material should be collected from cutaneous lesions by scraping outwards from the margin. Cleansing the site with 70% alcohol before sampling will increase the likelihood of detecting fungus on direct microscopic examination. Nail specimens should be taken from discolored or dystrophic parts of the nail and should include the full thickness of the nail. If distal subungual lesions are present, debris should be collected from underneath the nail. If there is superficial nail plate involvement, the scrapings should be taken from the nail surface. Specimens from the scalp should include hair roots and skin scales. Wood's light can sometimes be useful for the selection of sites of active infection, especially if the lesions are inconspicuous or atypical.

Direct microscopic examination of skin and nail material is often sufficient for the diagnosis of a dermatophyte infection, but it gives no indication as to which species is involved. With hair specimens, the size and disposition of the arthrospores can give some indication as to the etiologic agent (see Fig 6.1; Chapter 8.29).

Culture is a more reliable method of diagnosis than microscopic examination. It permits the species of dermatophyte to be determined and this can aid the selection of the most appropriate form of treatment. If possible, both microscopic examination and culture should be performed on all specimens. If, however, there is insufficient material for both, microscopic examination should be performed.

Cutaneous candidiasis is often difficult to diagnose if the lesions are other than typical in appearance. Isolation of *C. albicans* from

scrapings is of doubtful significance because the organism is a common colonizer of cutaneous lesions in moist sites. Microscopic demonstration of the organism in scrapings is much more significant. Isolation of *C. albicans* from nails is seldom significant unless the organism is seen on direct microscopic examination.

Microscopic examination of scrapings from lesions will permit the diagnosis of pityriasis versicolor if there are clusters of round or oval cells together with short broad filaments (which are seldom branched). Because this appearance is pathognomonic for pityriasis versicolor, and because *Mal. furfur* is part of the normal skin flora, its isolation in culture is not helpful. Direct microscopic examination and culture of scrapings or epilated hairs will permit the diagnosis of tinea nigra and piedra.

It is not unusual to isolate molds other than dermatophytes from abnormal nails cultured on media from which cycloheximide has been omitted. In many cases, these molds are casual, transient contaminants, and direct microscopic examination of the material is negative. However, if filaments are seen on microscopic examination, but no dermatophyte is isolated, it is possible that the mold is the cause of the infection.

MANAGEMENT

There is now a good selection of topical and systemic agents for the treatment of superficial fungal infections. The choice of treatment and its duration depends on the causative organism, the site of infection and the extent of the disease, as well as on other factors for each individual patient, such as concurrent disease and medication. Topical agents can be used for localized skin infections, but they are seldom successful for sites with a thick keratin layer. The palms and soles, and certainly the nails and hair often require systemic antifungal treatment.

TINEA CAPITIS

Topical treatment is ineffective on its own in tinea capitis. Terbinafine 250mg/day and itraconazole 100mg/day are both effective oral treatments for scalp infection. In adults, either agent should be given for 2–4 weeks. Terbinafine is licensed in some countries for use in children and it appears to be a safe and effective agent in this group.[12] In other countries, the older drug griseofulvin must still be used in children. The recommended dose is 10mg/kg/day for at least 6–8 weeks.

TINEA CORPORIS AND TINEA CRURIS

The choice of topical or systemic treatment in these conditions depends on the extent of the disease. Localized lesions can be treated with topical antifungal preparations. Numerous imidazoles and allylamines are available in different formulations. These agents should be applied morning and evening for 2–4 weeks. To prevent relapse, treatment should be continued for at least 1 week after the lesions have cleared.

If the disease is widespread, or the patient fails to respond to topical preparations, oral treatment is usually indicated. Terbinafine 250mg/day for 2–4 weeks and itraconazole 100mg/day for 2 weeks are more effective than griseofulvin 10mg/kg/day for 4–6 weeks.

TINEA PEDIS

Tinea pedis is a chronic infection that seldom clears if left untreated. Infection of the webs of the toes will often respond to topical terbinafine, applied morning and evening for 1–2 weeks. Topical imidazoles can also be used, but they are less effective and must be applied for at least 4 weeks.[13] The recurrence rate following topical treatment is quite high and it is not uncommon for chronic infection to persist despite treatment.

If the disease involves the soles or if there is acute inflammation, oral treatment should be given. Terbinafine 250mg/day for 2 weeks has been shown to be effective in tinea pedis. Itraconazole 100mg/day is an alternative, but it must be given for 4 weeks.[14] Chronic tinea pedis is often associated with nail infection. Inadequate treatment of onychomycosis may result in re-infection of the feet.

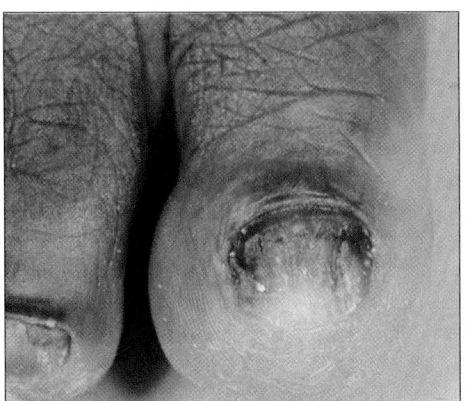

**Fig. 6.9
Onychomycosis due to *Scytalidium dimidiatum* (*Hendersonula toruloidea*).**

TINEA MANUUM

Local treatment with an imidazole or an allylamine will often suffice to clear tinea manuum. In cases that fail to respond to topical preparations, oral treatment is usually indicated. Infections of the palms are difficult to clear with griseofulvin, but oral terbinafine 250mg/day for 2–6 weeks has been shown to be highly effective.[15] Itraconazole 100mg/day for 4 weeks is an alternative.

CANDIDIASIS

Most patients with cutaneous candidiasis will respond to topical treatment with terbinafine or an imidazole such as clotrimazole or miconazole, applied for 2–4 weeks. However, relapse is common if any underlying problem is not controlled. If the infection is associated with an underlying skin disease, such as flexural eczema or diaper dermatitis, treatment with a combination preparation containing an azole agent together with hydrocortisone is often helpful.

Long term treatment with itraconazole or fluconazole has helped many patients with chronic mucocutaneous candidiasis. However, protracted treatment has led to the development of azole-resistant stains of *C. albicans* in some cases.[16]

PITYRIASIS VERSICOLOR

If left untreated, pityriasis versicolor will persist for long periods. Most patients with this disease respond to topical treatment with terbinafine, azole agents, or selenium sulfide shampoo, but more than half relapse within 12 months. Oral treatment with itraconazole 200mg/day for 1 week is indicated for extensive or recalcitrant lesions. Oral terbinafine and griseofulvin are ineffective.

TINEA NIGRA

Benzoic acid compound ointment or 10% thiabendazole solution can be applied morning and evening for 3–4 weeks. Topical imidazoles are also effective.

PIEDRA

Black piedra can be treated with a topical salicylic acid preparation or an imidazole cream. However, relapse is common. Shaving or clipping the affected hairs is often sufficient to clear white piedra. To help prevent recurrence, an imidazole lotion can be applied to the scalp after shampooing.

ONYCHOMYCOSIS

Topical agents should only be used where the infection is confined to the distal ends of the nails. Topical applications of tioconazole or amorolfine should be continued for at least 6 months for fingernails and 12 months or longer for toenails.

Oral terbinafine 250mg/day is the treatment of choice for proven dermatophyte infections of the nail (tinea unguium).[17] However, it is not appropriate for *Candida* infections, nondermatophytic mold infections, or mixed infections.[18] The optimum treatment period is 6–12 weeks for fingernails and 3–6 months for toenails. Treatment with terbinafine will also clear any associated skin infection without the need for additional topical treatment.

Itraconazole is also licensed for the oral treatment of nail infections at a dose of 200mg/day for 3–6 months. Pulsed treatment with itraconazole (in which 1 week of treatment is alternated with 3 weeks without treatment for 3–4 months) has also been advocated. It is at least as effective as continuous treatment while offering potential improvements in patient compliance and cost-effectiveness. Itraconazole has a broader spectrum than terbinafine and is more appropriate for patients who present with nondermatophyte or mixed nail infections.[18] Itraconazole interacts with a number of other drugs, and this can limit its usefulness in certain situations. Fluconazole is not licensed for use in fungal nail disease, but it is sometimes useful in severe *Candida* nail infections.

Oral griseofulvin is only effective in dermatophytosis. It is no longer regarded as a first-line choice for toenail infections, but it works quite well in fingernail infections if given over a 6–9-month period. It must be taken until the affected nail has fully grown out. It should be borne in mind that it has a number of side-effects and can interact with other medications.

Other interventions include chemical dissolution of the nail using 40% urea paste, and, in rare cases, surgical removal of the nail.

REFERENCES

1. Weitzman I, Summerbell RC. The dermatophytes. Clin Microbiol Rev 1995;8:240–59.
2. Rippon JW. The changing epidemiology and emerging patterns of dermatophyte species. Curr Top Med Mycol 1985;1:208–34.
3. Midgley G, Moore MK, Cook JC, Phan QG. Mycology of nail disorders. J Am Acad Dermatol 1994;31(Suppl):68–74.
4. Tsuboi R, Ko I, Takamori K, Ogawa H. Isolation of a keratinolytic proteinase from *Trichophyton mentagrophytes* with enzymatic activity at acidic pH. Infect Immun 1989;57:3479–83.
5. Calderon RA. Immunoregulation of dermatophytosis. Crit Rev Microbiol 1989;16:338–68.
6. Jones HE. Immune response and host resistance to human dermatophyte infection. J Am Acad Dermatol 1993;28(Suppl):12–8.
7. Dahl MV. Suppression of immunity and inflammation by products produced by dermatophytes. J Am Acad Dermatol 1993;28(Suppl):19–23.

8. Kirkpatrick CH. Host factors in defense against fungal infections. Am J Med 1984;77(Suppl 1):1–12.
9. Hay RJ, Clayton YM, De Silva N, Midgley G, Rossor E. Tinea capitis in south-east London: a new pattern of infection with public health implications. Br J Dermatol 1996;135:955–8.
10. Clayton YM, Midgley G. Scalp ringworm: simplified practical diagnostic method to study spread in children. Mod Med 1971;10:758–61.
11. Gentles JC, Evans EGV. Foot infections in swimming baths. Br Med J 1973;3:260–2.
12. Haroon TS, Hussain I, Aman S, *et al.* A randomized double-blind comparative study of terbinafine for 1, 2 and 4 weeks in tinea capitis. Br J Dermatol 1996;135:86–8.
13. Evans EGV, Dodman B, Williamson DM, Brown GJ, Bowen RG. Comparison of terbinafine and clotrimazole in treating tinea pedis. Br Med J 1993;307:645–7.

14. Hay RJ, McGregor JM, Wutte J, Ryatt JS, Ziegler C, Clayton YM. A comparison of two weeks terbinafine 250 mg/day with four weeks of itraconazole 100 mg/day in plantar tinea pedis. Br J Dermatol 1995;132:604–8.
15. White JE, Evans EGV, Perkins P. Successful two-week treatment with terbinafine for moccasin tinea pedis and tinea manuum. Br J Dermatol 1992;125:260–2.
16. Smith KJ, Warnock DW, Kennedy CTC, *et al.* Azole resistance in *Candida albicans*. J Med Vet Mycol 1986;24:133–44.
17. Brautigam M, Nolting S, Schopf RE, *et al.* Randomised double-blind comparison of terbinafine and itraconazole for treatment of toenail tinea infection. Br Med J 1995;311:919–22.
18. Denning DW, Evans EGV, Kibbler CC *et al.* Fungal nail disease: a guide to good practice (report of a Working Group of the British Society for Medical Mycology). Br Med J 1995;311:1277–81.

Deep Fungal Infections

Gerald P Bodey & Kenneth VI Rolston

FUNGAL INFECTIONS

Fungi are ubiquitous in the environment, but only a few genera are capable of causing human infection (Fig. 7.1). With the increasing number of immunocompromised and debilitated patients, genera previously considered to be nonpathogenic are being recognized as the cause of sporadic infections.[1] Historically, fungi causing human disease have been divided into two categories:
- the 'pathogenic' fungi, which can cause systemic infection in human hosts; and
- the 'opportunistic' fungi, which generally cause infection only in immunocompromised hosts.

These characterizations are not entirely satisfactory because:
- pathogenic fungi can cause serious infection in immunocompromised hosts; and
- opportunistic fungi can cause superficial, and occassionally, systemic infection in individuals with no discernible defects in host defenses.

Most of the pathogenic fungi are confined to specific geographic areas and can cause epidemics of infection under appropriate circumstances, while most opportunistic fungi cause infection worldwide and occasionally cause microepidemics that are nosocomial in origin.

HISTOPLASMOSIS

EPIDEMIOLOGY AND HOST FACTORS

Histoplasmosis is caused by *Histoplasma capsulatum*, a dimorphic fungus that is endemic in certain parts of North, Central and South America. It is the most common systemic mycosis in the USA, with most cases of infection occurring within the Ohio and Mississippi River valleys. Approximately 250,000–500,000 individuals are infected annually in the USA, the majority of whom remain asymptomatic.[2] Infection is acquired through inhalation of the organisms. There is a rough correlation between the number of organisms inhaled and the severity of illness.

The natural habitat of the mycelial form of the organism is the fertile soil of river valleys, where histoplasmosis is endemic. Heavily contaminated soils, which may harbor up to 10^5 viable particles per gram, are more common in environments populated by birds or bats, such as bird roosts, chicken coops, chimneys with plentiful bird droppings, old uninhabited buildings and caves with large numbers of bats. Disturbances of such environments by activities such as remodeling, demolition, earth removal, construction, cleaning chimneys, clearing shrubbery and recreational activities such as spelunking have resulted in epidemics of histoplasmosis.

Cell-mediated immunity plays a key role in protecting against spread of infection, and histoplasmosis has been recognized as an important opportunistic infection in individuals with impaired cell-mediated immunity, including patients who have AIDS.[3,4]

CLINICAL FEATURES

ACUTE INFECTION
The majority of patients remain asymptomatic or develop self-limited disease following exposure. Low inoculum exposure leads to symptoms in approximately 1% of individuals, but 99% have a clinically undetectable infection. Following a high inoculum exposure the frequency of symptomatic infection is much higher (approximately 50–100%).

FUNGI CAUSING INFECTION IN NORMAL AND COMPROMISED HOSTS					
Fungus		Incidence	Geographic distribution	Epidemics	Form
Pathogenic	*Histoplasma capsulatum*	Common*	River valleys between latitude 45°N and 30°S	Occasional	Dimorphic
	Coccidioides immitis	Common*	Southwestern USA, Central America, Argentina	Occasional	Dimorphic
	Blastomyces dermatitidis	Uncommon	Ohio and Mississippi River valleys	Uncommon	Dimorphic
	Sporothrix schenckii	Uncommon	Worldwide	Uncommon	Mold
	Paracoccidioides brasiliensis	Common*	Mexico – 23°N to Argentina – 34°S	Uncommon	Dimorphic
Opportunistic	*Candida* spp.	Common	Worldwide	Nosocomial contamination	Yeast
	Aspergillus spp.	Uncommon	Worldwide	Nosocomial; secondary to construction	Mold
	Cryptococcus neoformans	Uncommon	Worldwide associated with avian habitats	No	Yeast
	Mucorales	Rare	Worldwide	No	Mold
	Pseudallescheria boydii	Rare	Worldwide	No	Mold
	Malassezia furfur	Rare	Worldwide on human skin	No	Yeast
	Penicillium marneffei	Uncommon	South East Asia, Southern China	No	Mold
	Trichosporon beigelii	Rare	Worldwide	No	Yeast
	Fusarium spp.	Rare	Worldwide	No	Mold

Fig. 7.1 Fungi causing infection in normal and compromised hosts. *In endemic areas.

Most symptomatic patients develop pulmonary symptoms including a nonproductive cough and retrosternal or pleuritic chest pain, and a flu-like illness characterized by fever, myalgias, fatigue, chills, headache and anorexia.

Physical examination is usually normal, but may reveal the presence of rashes, cervical or supraclavicular lymphadenopathy, and pulmonary rales. Chest radiographs may reveal various findings including hilar or mediastinal adenopathy, patchy pulmonary infiltrates and, on rare occasions, pleural effusions. Miliary or diffuse pulmonary infiltrates may follow high inoculum exposure, but are distinctly uncommon, and are suggestive of disseminated disease.[5]

Most symptomatic patients recover without treatment within 2–3 weeks. Some, however, remain symptomatic and experience fatigue for several months, and may benefit from oral antifungal therapy.

Less than 10% of symptomatic patients with acute pulmonary histoplasmosis develop a more aggressive illness with chest pain, diffuse pulmonary infiltrates, respiratory insufficiency and/or obstructive symptoms due to enlarged lymph nodes, resulting in dysphagia or airway obstruction.

Some patients develop extrapulmonary manifestations including rheumatologic syndromes (arthritis, tenosynovitis) and pericarditis.[6] Synovial and pericardial cultures in such patients are negative. These symptoms generally respond to anti-inflammatory agents and do not require antifungal therapy.

CHRONIC PULMONARY HISTOPLASMOSIS

Chronic pulmonary histoplasmosis is more common in individuals with structural defects in the lung, such as emphysema. It is characterized by chronic pulmonary symptoms, which include cough and dyspnea, accompanied by progressive fibrotic and cavitary lesions, which are often found in the apical regions of the lungs.[7] Generalized symptoms, including fatigue, anorexia, weight loss, fever and sweats, are common.

All patients who have chronic pulmonary histoplasmosis require antifungal therapy. Without such treatment, the infection will progress to uninvolved areas of the same or opposite lung and lead to bronchopleural fistula formation and eventual dissemination.

DISSEMINATED HISTOPLASMOSIS

Disseminated histoplasmosis is defined as progressive disease with evidence of extrapulmonary involvement. Most of the manifestations are the result of involvement of the reticuloendothelial system. Exogenous primary infection or reinfection and endogenous reactivation of dormant infection in immunosuppressed individuals can both produce disseminated disease. Progressive disseminated histoplasmosis seldom develops in the absence of impaired cellular immunity and the most common predisposing conditions are AIDS, lymphoma, lymphocytic leukemia and immunosuppressive therapy. Old age may also predispose to dissemination.

The clinical manifestations include fever, anorexia, weight loss and sweats. Bone marrow involvement is common, resulting in anemia, thrombocytopenia and leukopenia.[8] Cutaneous and mucosal lesions, lymphadenopathy, hepatosplenomegaly, meningitis or cerebritis, endocarditis and adrenal insufficiency may also occur. Vaginal and penile ulcers, breast masses, bone and joint involvement, and epididymitis have also been reported, but are rare. Diffuse gastrointestinal involvement may result in protein and fat malabsorption.

Disseminated histoplasmosis occurs more frequently in AIDS patients, in whom it can be a rapidly progressive fatal illness, than in any other patient groups.[4] Central nervous system (CNS) involvement is also more common in people who have AIDS. All patients require therapy, without which the infection is uniformly fatal.[9]

MEDIASTINAL GRANULOMA AND FIBROSING MEDIASTINITIS

Important structures within the mediastinum may be obstructed, either due to the mass effect of large granulomas or secondary to fibrosis. Enlarged mediastinal nodes may compress the superior vena cava or pulmonary vessels, the esophagus and occasionally the large airways. Necrotic nodes may also rupture into a bronchus, the esophagus or the mediastinum, resulting in fistula formation. These events are rare and only 25% of patients with large mediastinal lymph nodes are symptomatic. Fibrosing mediastinitis is a rare and late complication of histoplasmosis, probably representing a late inflammatory reaction rather than active infection.

Superior vena cava obstruction and tracheobronchial obstruction are the most common manifestations. Obstruction of the pulmonary vessels, esophagus, inferior vena cava and thoracic duct are less common. Chest radiography may reveal a widened mediastinum or calcified hilar adenopathy.

DIAGNOSIS

Epidemiologic or historic evidence of exposure is usually elicited in cases of acute pulmonary histoplasmosis. Chronic pulmonary and disseminated histoplasmosis are best diagnosed by isolating *H. capsulatum* from clinical specimens. Most cultures become positive within 2–3 weeks. Cultures of bone marrow, blood, urine and sputum should be obtained from all patients suspected of having disseminated histoplasmosis. Among these the highest yield is from cultures of bone marrow, which are positive in up to 75% of cases. Blood cultures using the lysis centrifugation technique may be positive in up to 70% of cases, and sputum and urine cultures in 40–70% of cases of disseminated histoplasmosis. Sputum cultures yield the organisms in approximately 60% of cases of chronic pulmonary histoplasmosis, the yield being even higher if multiple samples are obtained (Fig. 7.2). Cultures are generally not useful in acute self-limited histoplasmosis.

A diagnosis of histoplasmosis can also be established by demonstrating the organisms in tissues using special stains:
- Wright's stain for peripheral blood or bone marrow; and
- Grocott–Gomori methenamine silver nitrate for other tissue samples.

Liver, lung, cutaneous lesions, brain, lymph nodes, mediastinal structures, bone or other potentially involved sites should be biopsied, especially if a rapid diagnosis is essential.

Another method for rapid diagnosis is detection of a polysaccharide antigen produced by *H. capsulatum*. This antigen can be detected in the urine of approximately 90% of patients with disseminated histoplasmosis and in the blood of approximately 50%. This test is also useful for monitoring therapeutic response because it disappears following successful treatment and reappears with relapse.

Histoplasmin skin testing is a useful epidemiologic tool, but has limited if any diagnostic use in individual patients. Skin testing may, in fact, lead to a false impression of recent infection because there is a rise in serum antibody titers in 15–25% of patients following histoplasmin injection.

Several methods for serologic testing are available, including immunodiffusion and complement fixation. These are also of limited diagnostic use since they are associated with relatively high rates of

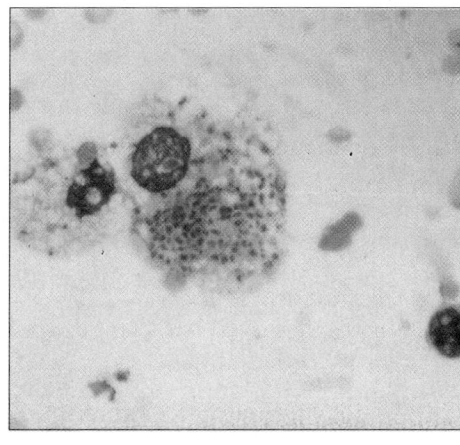

Fig. 7.2 Cytologic specimen from bronchoalveolar lavage fluid showing intracellular *Histoplasma capsulatum*.

false-positives and negatives. However, a positive serologic test in the appropriate clinical setting should prompt a thorough diagnostic evaluation and can serve as the basis for empiric antifungal therapy for patients with strongly suspected disseminated disease.

MANAGEMENT

Mild cases of acute histoplasmosis do not require any antifungal therapy. Severe acute pulmonary histoplasmosis warrants therapy with amphotericin B or itraconazole in addition to supportive care. The duration of antifungal therapy needed is, however, shorter than that for chronic pulmonary or disseminated infection.

Amphotericin B (50mg intravenously daily) is the recommended therapy for patients with severe pulmonary or disseminated disease and as initial therapy in immunosuppressed patients, including those who have AIDS.

Itraconazole and, to a lesser extent, ketoconazole are useful in the treatment of mild-to-moderate pulmonary or disseminated infection, and for maintenance therapy in patients who have AIDS or are immunosuppressed.[10,11] Itraconazole is usually administered at a loading dose of 200mg orally q8h for three days, followed by 200mg orally q12h. The value of fluconazole for treatment of histoplasmosis is still under investigation.[2,9,11]

The optimal duration of treatment for histoplasmosis remains to be established. Recommendations depend upon:
- the agent used;
- the nature and severity of infection; and
- host factors.

Patients being treated with oral azoles (ketoconazole, itraconazole, fluconazole) require more prolonged therapy than those treated exclusively with amphotericin B.[12] A 2 to 3-month course of oral azole therapy is sufficient for most patients with acute pulmonary histoplasmosis who require treatment. The high relapse rate among patients who have chronic pulmonary histoplasmosis necessitates treatment for at least 1 year. For immunocompetent patients with disseminated histoplasmosis, treatment should be given for at least 6 months.

All those with chronic pulmonary/disseminated disease (not just those with AIDS), should be monitored periodically for relapse following cessation of antifungal treatment.[11] Individuals with immunosuppressive disorders including AIDS require lifelong maintenance therapy: oral azole therapy is most convenient, although weekly intravenous amphotericin B is also effective.

Antifungal prophylaxis may be considered for immunosuppressed patients living in areas with high prevalence rates for histoplasmosis, but at present a firm recommendation for this cannot be made.

COCCIDIOIDOMYCOSIS

EPIDEMIOLOGY AND HOST FACTORS

Coccidioidomycosis is a fungal infection caused by *Coccidioides immitis*. It is endemic in certain regions of the Western Hemisphere including the Southwestern USA, Central America and Argentina.[13] In the USA, areas of highest endemicity include the southern San Joaquin Valley in California and southern Arizona.

Coccidioides immitis is found in the sandy soil of the lower Sonora Desert life zone. Infection occurs as a result of inhaling arthroconidia that have broken off from the parent mycelium. People of all ages can become infected, but the disease tends to be more aggressive in the very young and very old.

The spectrum of infection includes primary pulmonary infection, progressive pulmonary disease and extrapulmonary or disseminated disease. The incidence of primary pulmonary disease has no racial predilection, but disseminated disease is more common in certain racial groups, including people of Filipino, African-American, Hispanic,

native American and Oriental extraction. Extrapulmonary disease is also more common in women who acquire the infection in the latter part of pregnancy or early in the postpartum period and in diabetics.

Cell-mediated immunity is thought to be the primary host defense mechanism for containing the infection. Immunosuppressed patients, including those who have HIV infection, have an increased incidence and increased severity of infection with *C. immitis*.[14] Several major epidemics of coccidioidomycosis have been described in endemic areas of the southwestern USA, probably related to changes in climatic conditions.[15,16]

CLINICAL FEATURES

PRIMARY INFECTION
Inhalation of even one spore of *C. immitis* can result in infection. Approximately 60% of patients with primary pulmonary infection remain asymptomatic. Others develop an influenza-like respiratory illness characterized by fever, cough, headache and myalgias, which is generally self-limited and short-lived. In approximately 25% of symptomatic patients the initial manifestations are more severe and generalized. They include pulmonary symptoms such as pleuritic chest pain, arthralgias which can be symmetric and involve multiple joints, and skin manifestations, including erythema nodosum or erythema multiforme. This syndrome is also self-limited, representing an immune complex reaction and not disseminated disease.

CHRONIC PULMONARY DISEASE
Several types of pulmonary sequelae can develop after the initial infection. These include the formation of:
- pulmonary nodules (coccidioidomas);
- cavitary pulmonary lesions; and
- progressive pneumonia.

The nodules are typically solitary and 2–3cm in diameter, and represent granulomatous organization of coccidioidal pneumonia. They are often discovered on routine radiographic examination and are a source of diagnostic concern because they closely resemble lesions caused by primary lung cancer.[17]

Thin-walled cavities, which like nodules are generally peripheral in location, are seen in approximately 0.1% of all patients. Most of those with cavitary lesions are asymptomatic and the cavities are typically seen when radiographs are obtained for other purposes. Approximately 35–50% of these cavities close spontaneously within 2 years. Symptomatic patients with cavitary lesions usually develop hemoptysis, chest pain, fever, cough and sputum production. Occasionally a cavity ruptures and causes a pyopneumothorax. Some patients develop chronic fibrocavitary disease, which like pulmonary tuberculosis is frequently apical in location, is often bilateral and is slowly progressive.[18]

DISSEMINATED DISEASE
Dissemination occurs when infection spreads beyond the pulmonary parenchyma or hilar lymph nodes and is seen in approximately 1% of infected individuals. It occurs more frequently in:
- the very young or very old;
- certain racial groups;
- those who have HIV infection or are otherwise immunosuppressed; and
- those who acquire the infection in the second half of pregnancy or in the postpartum period.

Dissemination can involve virtually every organ and is seen most commonly in the skin, bones, joints and meninges. The classic skin lesions are verrucous in nature, although various other forms are seen, including subcutaneous abscesses and granulomas. Skeletal lesions show some predilection for the large joints of the extremities (knees, ankles, elbows and wrists). Tenosynovitis and sinus tract formation have been reported. Meningitis is the most serious manifestation. It may occur soon after the onset of pulmonary disease or may follow asymptomatic pulmonary infection. It may be rapidly progressive, but more often is indolent, progressing slowly over several months to 1–2 years. Hydrocephalus and neurologic deficits due to cranial nerve damage are not uncommon.[19] The entire spectrum of disseminated infection is seen in people who have HIV infection.[20]

DIAGNOSIS

The definitive means for establishing a diagnosis of coccidioidomycosis is isolation of the organism from a clinical specimen. The fungus grows readily on most culture media, usually within 7–10 days. Suspicion of the presence of coccidioidal infection is heightened if the patient has a history of exposure through travel or residence in an area of endemicity. In the absence of culture confirmation, a diagnosis of coccidioidomycosis may be established by visualization of the characteristic spherules (Fig. 7.3) on histopathologic examination of biopsy material or sputum. Stains such as hematoxylin–eosin and Grocott–Gomori methenamine silver nitrate are useful for such visualization. Newer techniques involving identification by DNA probes are being developed.

Serologic tests for the detection of coccidioidomycosis are quite sensitive and some are quite specific. These may be used to establish the diagnosis in the absence of positive cultures or histopathologic findings. Several tests are available, some that detect IgM antibodies and others that detect IgG antibodies. These include latex agglutination, immunodiffusion, enzyme immunoassay and complement fixation tests. The complement fixation test may be the most useful because it provides diagnostic as well as prognostic information, with high titers representing an increased risk of disseminated infection.

MANAGEMENT

Most patients with primary infection have self-limited disease and do not require therapy.

For nonmeningeal disease in patients who do not have a life-threatening infection, the new azoles itraconazole and fluconazole are effective in doses of 400mg/day. Prolonged therapy might be necessary to prevent relapses.

Although effective, amphotericin B therapy is now reserved for patients with life-threatening infection or for those who do not respond to the azoles as it is less convenient and more toxic.

Meninigitis remains the most difficult manifestation of coccidioidomycosis to treat. For many years the treatment of choice was intrathecal or intraventricular administration of amphotericin B. Recent data, however, indicate that fluconazole at a minimum daily dose of 400mg has become the treatment of choice for coccidioidal meningitis, and may be even more effective at higher doses. The role of itraconazole for the treatment of coccidioidal meningitis remains to be fully established.[10,21]

The newer liposomal or lipid formulations of amphotericin B may be useful in patients who require prolonged treatment with amphotericin B because of their diminished toxicity, which enables administration of higher dosages. These formulations are more expensive than other therapies.

BLASTOMYCOSIS

EPIDEMIOLOGY AND HOST FACTORS

Blastomycosis (sometimes called North American blastomycosis) is caused by the dimorphic fungus *Blastomyces dermatitidis*. Most cases occur in the states that surround the Ohio and Mississippi river valleys including Arkansas, Kentucky, North Carolina, Mississippi, Tennessee, Illinois, Louisiana, Minnesota and Wisconsin.[22]

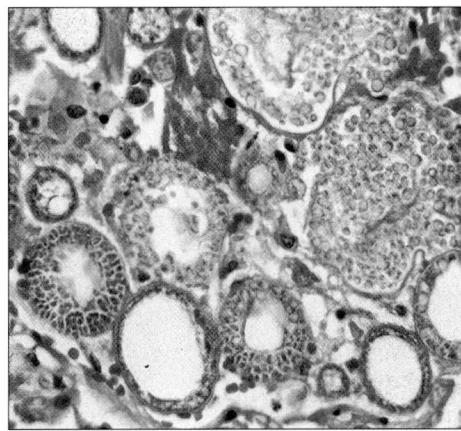

Fig. 7.3 Pulmonary coccidioidomycosis. Granuloma showing typical spherules.

The organism is found in soil, and epidemics have been reported following environmental exposure outdoors.[23,24] Infection begins with inhalation of spores into the lung, although cases have been reported following environmental or laboratory cutaneous inoculation. Most cases remain asymptomatic and the inhaled organisms are cleared by bronchopulmonary phagocytes. The organism spreads from the lung to various metastatic foci through lymphohematogenous channels. The development of immunity leads to granuloma formation in the lungs and various end-organs. Spontaneous resolution or endogenous reactivation may occur at pulmonary and extrapulmonary sites. Intact cellular immunity appears to be critical for preventing progressive infection.[25]

Although blastomycosis occurs in immunocompromised individuals, including those who have AIDS, it is much less frequent than other fungal infections such as histoplasmosis or cryptococcosis.

CLINICAL FEATURES

PULMONARY INFECTION

The spectrum of infection varies from subclinical disease to widely disseminated or miliary disease. Pulmonary blastomycosis can present as acute or chronic pneumonia:
- the acute pneumonia causes fever, chills, a productive cough and occasionally hemoptysis, so these patients are often thought to have acute bacterial pneumonia; and
- the chronic pneumonia causes fever, weight loss, malaise, fatigue, night sweats and a productive cough, and so these patients are often thought to have tuberculosis or a pulmonary neoplasm.

Radiographically, the pulmonary lesions appear most often as an alveolar or mass-like infiltrate; miliary or reticulonodular patterns are less common. Cavitary disease is uncommon.[26]

EXTRAPULMONARY INFECTION

The most common manifestations of extrapulmonary blastomycosis are cutaneous lesions (Fig. 7.4). These may be either ulcerative or verrucous (fungating) in nature. They can be mistaken for cancer in appearance and on histopathology due to the presence of hyperplasia and acanthosis.

Osteomyelitis due to *B. dermatitidis* occurs in about 25% of cases with extrapulmonary disease. Any bone may be involved, but the vertebrae, bones of the skull, pelvis, sacrum and ribs are most often affected.[27]

Extrapulmonary disease can also involve the genitourinary system. Extrapulmonary disease is more common in men; prostatitis and epididymo-orchitis are reported most often. In women, endometriosis and tubo-ovarian abscesses have been described, but are rare.

Central nervous system involvement results in meningitis or epidural or cranial abscesses.

In disseminated blastomycosis, lesions can be found in virtually every organ of the body. Subcutaneous lesions are most common, but abscesses may be found in the brain, bones, liver, spleen, prostate,

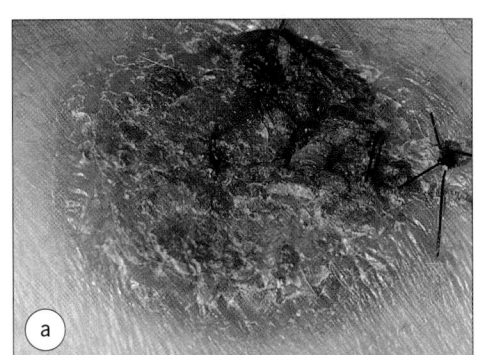

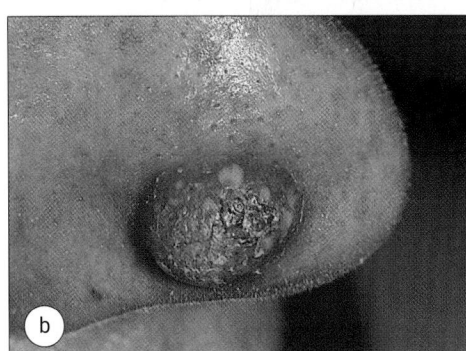

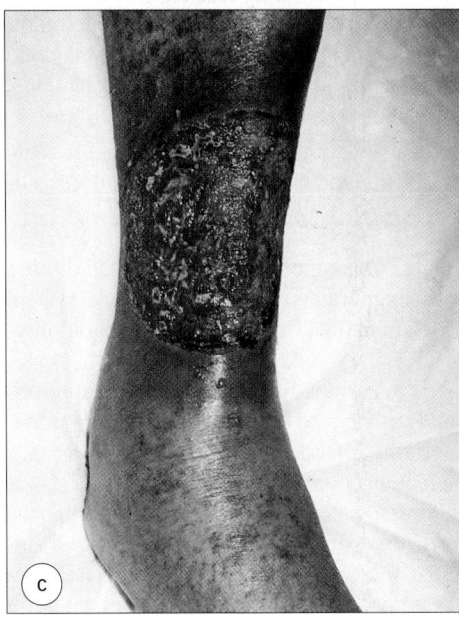

Fig. 7.4 Cutaneous blastomycosis. (a,b) Skin lesions caused by *Blastomyces dermatitidis* in a normal host. (c) A large cutaneous ulcer in a patient with multiple myeloma.

Symptomatic patients with pulmonary disease, and all patients with extrapulmonary disease, including cutaneous lesions, should receive antifungal therapy. For patients who do not have overwhelming or life-threatening blastomycosis, itraconazole 200mg/day orally for 6–12 months is regarded as the agent of choice.[21,29] Some patients fail to respond and need higher doses of itraconazole (200mg q12h).

Patients with meningitis, adult respiratory distress syndrome or other life-threatening forms of blastomycosis should receive therapy with amphotericin B initially. This may be switched to oral itraconazole after an initial response has been achieved and cultures are negative for *B. dermatitidis*.[21]

SPOROTRICHOSIS

EPIDEMIOLOGY AND HOST FACTORS

Sporotrichosis is an endemic fungal infection caused by the dimorphic fungus *Sporothrix schenckii*. It has been reported worldwide, but is most often seen in tropical and subtropical regions.[30]

The organism is often isolated from soil, sphagnum moss and plant debris such as timber, hay and straw.[31] Infection usually occurs following cutaneous inoculation of the organism during outdoor activities such as gardening and farming. Typically there is a history of scratches from rose thorns, conifer needles or timber. Natural infection also occurs in wild and domesticated animals. Zoonotic infections have been traced to bites and scratches from cats, birds, rodents and armadillos.

Cutaneous or lymphocutaneous disease follows local inoculation. Hematogenous dissemination can occur, leading to multifocal disease. Rarely, inhalation of organisms results in a granulomatous pneumonitis.

CLINICAL FEATURES

LYMPHOCUTANEOUS INFECTION
As a rule there is a localized infection with fixed cutaneous or lymphocutaneous manifestations at the site of inoculation without systemic complaints. The distal extremities are most often involved, although there may be lesions at any cutaneous site. These are raised, nodular, erythematous lesions that often ulcerate.[32] They vary in size from tiny punctate lesions to 2–4cm in diameter. Infection advances through local lymphatic channels, producing secondary lesions that are identical to the primary lesions.

Deep inoculation can lead to the development of tenosynovitis and nerve entrapment or carpal tunnel syndromes, and have even been reported in the absence of articular involvement.

Primary ocular sporotrichosis has been reported, presumably as a result of finger-to-eye transmission. Sites of involvement in the eye include the eyelids, conjunctiva, cornea, sclera, lacrimal sac, lacrimal canal and uveal tract.

EXTRACUTANEOUS INFECTION
Although uncommon, osteoarticular sporotrichosis is the most frequent form of extracutaneous infection. Single joint involvement is usual, with the major joints of the extremities being involved most often. The infection is usually indolent and progresses slowly. The involved joint is painful and swollen due to the presence of an effusion. The overlying skin may appear normal, although sinus tract formation has been reported. Other manifestations of osteoarticular infection include osteomyelitis, bursitis and tenosynovitis. Unifocal lesions are generally related to an extension of lymphocutaneous disease, whereas multifocal lesions are presumably related to hematogenous spread.[33]

Pulmonary sporotrichosis may result from inhalation of the organisms or as a result of dissemination from a cutaneous focus. Both upper and lower respiratory tract involvement may occur. The usual presentation is that of a pneumonitis with nonspecific respiratory

myocardium, pericardium and elsewhere. Recently, an overwhelming form of disseminated blastomycosis has been described in which the adult respiratory distress syndrome was the predominant feature.[28]

DIAGNOSIS

The presence of verrucous or ulcerated cutaneous lesions, alveolar or mass-like pulmonary infiltrates, or multiple osseous lesions in an appropriate environmental and geographic setting should heighten suspicion for a diagnosis of blastomycosis. A specific diagnosis is made by demonstrating the organisms in tissues, exudates or normally sterile fluids such as cerebrospinal fluid (CSF), or by growing the organism in culture. Various serologic tests have been developed, but are not sensitive or specific enough to be reliable diagnostic aids.

MANAGEMENT

A few patients with acute pulmonary blastomycosis will have become asymptomatic by the time a specific diagnosis is made. Observation without treatment is appropriate in such patients.

symptoms, including cough, dyspnea, chest pain and sputum production, and occasionally hemoptysis. Hilar or paratracheal adenopathy may occur, and chronic pulmonary infection may evolve into fibrocavitary disease. Pleural involvement is rare.[34]

DISSEMINATED SPOROTRICHOSIS

Systemic or disseminated sporotrichosis is uncommon and often occurs in a setting of impaired cellular immunity. Therapy with corticosteroids or other immunosuppressive agents, HIV infection and alcoholism appear to predispose to its development. Dissemination may result in cutaneous, osteoarticular, genitourinary, pulmonary or CNS involvement. The organism has also been recovered from blood and bone marrow. Meningitis is very rare and is usually an indolent process.

DIAGNOSIS

Cutaneous or lymphocutaneous lesions should heighten a clinical suspicion sporotrichosis. Similarly radiographs revealing pneumonitis or fibrocavitary disease with or without paratracheal or hilar adenopathy can suggest pulmonary sporotrichosis, but are nonspecific.

A specific diagnosis is generally made by isolating the organism from the affected site. A positive culture from any site strongly suggests the diagnosis because laboratory contamination with this organism is unusual, although rarely saprophytic involvement of the respiratory tract can occur. A positive blood culture is strongly indicative of disseminated disease and occurs most commonly in immunocompromised patients.

Histopathology reveals granulomatous lesions infiltrated with histocytes and polymorphonuclear leukocytes. Periodic acid–Schiff (PAS) staining may demonstrate cigar-shaped yeast forms, occasional hyphal forms and stellate eosinophilic material called asteroid bodies. Several serologic techniques have been developed and may be of use in establishing the diagnosis when the meninges or other obscure sites are involved.

MANAGEMENT

For localized infection, treatment with a saturated solution of potassium iodide (SSKI) is effective, but may be cumbersome and lead to poor compliance. Treatment is usually initiated as five drops in juice or water q8h, with weekly increments of five drops until a maximum 40–50 drops q8h (1g/ml) (25–40 drops for children) is reached. Therapy should be continued for 3–6 months. Although SSKI is inexpensive and most compliant patients respond to therapy, relapses do occur.[21,35]

Therapy of the various forms of sporotrichosis has changed considerably since the azole drugs became available. Itraconazole now appears to be the treatment of choice for lymphocutaneous sporotrichosis. A dose of 100–200mg/day for 3–6 months will produce excellent response rates, minimal side effects, and very few relapses.[35] Itraconazole, however, is relatively expensive compared with SSKI. Because the organism is sensitive to heat, cutaneous or lymphocutaneous lesions can be treated with local hyperthermia, particularly in pregnant patients and those who are intolerant of other drugs. Hyperthermia is not effective for systemic disease.

Osteoarticular sporotrichosis is best treated with itraconazole, 400mg/day orally, for as long as 1–2 years. Response rates are not as high as with cutaneous or lymphocutaneous disease, and relapses can occur. Amphotericin B is also effective, but is much more toxic. Intra-articular amphotericin B may be effective, but clinical experience with this form of therapy is limited.

Responses to all forms of therapy by patients with pulmonary sporotrichosis have been disappointing. Patients who are severely ill should receive initial therapy with amphotericin B, which can be changed to itraconazole once there is an improvement.[36] Patients who are less ill should receive itraconazole therapy initially. Prolonged therapy is indicated.

Patients with meningitis or disseminated sporotrichosis should be treated with amphotericin B initially. Disseminated infection in severely immunosuppressed patients such as those with AIDS probably requires lifelong therapy.[36] Itraconazole can be substituted for amphotericin B once there is an improvement. Surgery can play a useful adjunctive role for some localized sites of infection.

PARACOCCIDIOIDOMYCOSIS

EPIDEMIOLOGY AND HOST FACTORS

Paracoccidioidomycosis (South American blastomycosis) has a geographic distribution that is restricted to Latin America, from Mexico (23°N) to Argentina (34°S). Most cases have been reported from Brazil, Columbia, Venezuela, and Argentina.[13] Cases reported elsewhere have occurred in patients who previously resided in endemic countries.

The organism, *Paracoccidioides brasiliensis*, is a dimorphic fungus and is believed to lie dormant in the soil. It establishes a primary focus of infection in the lungs following inhalation.[30] Person-to-person transmission does not occur.

Clinical manifestations of the disease are rarely seen in people under 30 years of age. Men are more commonly affected than women in a ratio of approximately 15:1. Most primary infections are subclinical. Cell-mediated immunity appears to play a critical role in protection against infection, and reactivation may occur several years after primary infection, during periods of depressed cell-mediated immunity.[37] In recent years there have been descriptions of severe manifestations of paracoccidioidomycosis in immunosuppressed patients, especially those who have AIDS.[38] Alcoholism has also been shown to be an important predisposing factor.

CLINICAL FEATURES

Although primary infection occurs in the lungs, disseminated disease involving the skin, mucous membranes, reticuloendothelial system and adrenals is common.[39] Two distinct forms of paracoccidioidomycosis have been described:
- a subacute form, which is seen mostly in young adults (approximately 5% of cases) and is associated with relatively severe manifestations and a high mortality rate; and
- a more chronic form, which accounts for the majority of cases, is seen in older adults, and is associated with a much better prognosis.

Pulmonary involvement produces persistent cough, progressive dyspnea, purulent or blood-tinged sputum, chest pain, diffuse crackles on auscultation, and bilateral patchy nodular infiltrates, predominantly in the mid and lower portions of the lungs. Cavities and hilar adenopathy are less common. Longstanding cases often reveal fibrosis, and pulmonary hypertension may develop.

Mucosal lesions are common and involve the mouth, lips, gums, tongue, palate, larynx and pharynx. They are infiltrated or ulcerated, and generally painful. Cutaneous lesions are pleomorphic and tend to be located around body orifices. They may appear warty, crusted or ulcerated, and occasionally granulomatous. Adenopathy often involves cervical, axillary, mediastinal or mesenteric lymph nodes, and may be complicated by the formation of draining sinuses and fistulas.

Adrenal involvement can range from minimal dysfunction to overt insufficiency. Other organs (liver, CNS, spleen, vascular system, bones and male genitourinary tract) are involved less often. Disseminated disease often causes generalized symptoms including fever, malaise, weakness, weight loss and anorexia. The differential diagnosis includes tuberculosis (which co-exists in 10–25% of cases), other infections such as histoplasmosis, syphilis and leprosy, and neoplastic disorders.[40]

DIAGNOSIS

Laboratory diagnosis can occasionally be made by potassium hydroxide (KOH) examination of sputum or pus. Definitive diagnosis generally requires biopsy and demonstration of typical multiple budding yeasts, which often produce a characteristic 'pilot-wheel' appearance. Fungal cultures on Sabouraud–dextrose or yeast extract agar are also recommended. Several serologic tests are available including the agar gel immunodiffusion technique and the complement fixation test.[41] Other tests include immunoelectophoresis, counterimmunoelectrophoresis and enzyme-linked immunosorbent assay (ELISA). Some of these may be useful for diagnosis and for following response to therapy. Skin testing is also available, but is unreliable.

MANAGEMENT

Sulfonamides (4–6g/day), either alone or in combination with amphotericin B for prolonged periods, used to be the mainstay of therapy for paracoccidioidomycosis. Neither drug, either alone or in combination, produced satisfactory cure rates and the relapse rate was in the range of 20–30%. Ketoconazole, given in doses of 200–400mg/day for 6–18 months is associated with better response rates and fewer relapses. The newer triazole derivative, itraconazole, is now considered the drug of choice because it requires shorter duration of treatment (approximately 6 months), a lower daily dose (100mg), has fewer adverse effects, and is associated with response rates of around 85–95% and relapse rates of only 3–5%. Limited experience with fluconazole also indicates that this drug might be useful.

CRYPTOCOCCOSIS

EPIDEMIOLOGY AND HOST FACTORS

Cryptococcus neoformans is the only encapsulated pathogenic fungus. Although in the past it was considered to be an asexually reproducing yeast, mating types have been identified recently, and the fungus has been converted to its mycelial form known as *Filobasidiella neoformans*. However, when basidiospores are cultured in laboratory media or inoculated into mice they revert to the typical encapsulated yeast forms. It is uncertain whether the fungus exists in nature as the mycelial form. There are other *Cryptococcus* spp., but they are not human pathogens and do not usually grow at 98.6°F.

Cryptococcus neoformans is found worldwide. It can be recovered from avian droppings and other environmental sources. There are four serotypes based on capsular antigens, but serotype A, and to a lesser extent D, are responsible for most human infections. The variant *C. neoformans* var. *gattii* is found in tropical and subtropical environments, especially from Brazil. It is not associated with birds, but with species of eucalyptus trees. This variant belongs to serotypes B and C.

PATIENTS AT RISK

Although *C. neoformans* can cause illness in human hosts, including self-limited pneumonia and meningitis, most infections occur in immunocompromised hosts. The people who are most susceptible are those with defective cellular immunity, the leading causes being corticosteroid therapy, Hodgkin's disease, other lymphomas, chronic lymphocytic leukemia and AIDS, especially those with CD4+ T-lymphocyte counts of less than 200/mm³. In the USA at least 6% of AIDS patients develop cryptococcosis, accounting for 80–90% of all cryptococcal infections.[42] The frequency may be even higher in Africa. Other patients at risk include those receiving adrenal corticosteroid therapy, transplant recipients and pregnant women, and patients with other malignancies, diabetes mellitus, sarcoidosis, lupus erythematosus or Cushing's syndrome.

HOST DEFENSES

After initial inhalation, the organisms are ingested by neutrophils, monocytes and alveolar macrophages. Encapsulated organisms are more resistant to phagocytosis and killing. Phagocytosis by neutrophils may depend upon opsonization by complement and antibody directed at the capsule. Natural killer cells and T lymphocytes are important host defenses. The release of various cytokines enhances anticryptococcal activity. The organism produces no exotoxins, hence there is little organ dysfunction or necrosis until the infection is advanced. However, cryptococcal polysaccharide may be immunosuppressive and inhibit phagocytosis.

On histopathology, there are typically cystic clusters of cryptococci with a scant inflammatory response consisting of lymphocytes, plasma cells and macrophages, and giant cells containing ingested organisms.

CLINICAL FEATURES

Cryptococcal infection may be manifested as primary pneumonia, meningoencephalitis, skin lesions, osteomyelitis or disseminated infection.[43] Cryptococcal pyelonephritis has been reported as a cause of renal allograft rejection. Other uncommon forms of infection include endophthalmitis, sinusitis, endocarditis, esophagitis, hepatitis, peritonitis, myositis and prostatitis.

Infection is initiated by inhalation of aerosolized organisms into the lungs. Less than 15% of cases present with pneumonia. Pulmonary infection may be minimally symptomatic or may present with cough producing mucoid sputum, fever, chest pain and dyspnea.[44] A variety of abnormalities may be found on chest radiography including solitary lesions (often in the upper lobe), lobar pneumonia, bilateral infiltrates, miliary disease and pleural effusions. Cavitation is rare and calcification does not occur. Pulmonary infection often remains stable or resolves without specific therapy in human hosts. Occasional immunocompromised patients develop rapidly progressive bilateral pneumonia that may cause death from respiratory failure within a few weeks from the onset of first symptoms.

The most frequently encountered form of infection is meningoencephalitis.[45] Other forms of CNS infection include pure meningitis and cryptococcoma. Pulmonary infection is seldom detectable in patients with CNS infection even though the lung is the site of origin. Meningoencephalitis may be acute or insidiously chronic and early in the infection symptoms such as headache and confusion may wax and wane. Symptoms include progressive headache, fever, nausea, vomiting, dizziness, confusion, somnolence, personality changes and dementia. Some patients may be afebrile or have only mild fever. Some patients develop focal neurologic signs due to cranial nerve involvement and about 5% due to involvement of cranial blood vessels. Up to 30% of patients may develop visual loss due to papilledema. Seizures may occur late in the infection. Other neurologic signs include hyperreflexia, ankle clonus and extensor plantar responses. Only about 15% of patients have meningism.

Disseminated infection occurs in severely immunocompromised patients and involves the brain, heart, testis, prostate, eye, kidney and spleen. The skin and bone are frequently infected. Single or multiple, usually painless, skin lesions can be found on the face or scalp, but may appear anywhere. Lesions may be papules, pustules, plaques, ulcerations or acneiform or soft subcutaneous lesions. Those patients who have AIDS may develop umbilicated lesions resembling molluscum contagiosum. Cellulitis with necrotizing vasculitis may occur in transplant recipients. Osteolytic bone lesions often involve the cranium or vertebrae, are often multiple, cause swelling and pain, and can involve the bone marrow.

DIAGNOSIS

A diagnosis of CNS infection is usually indicated by abnormalities of the CSF, including elevated opening CSF pressure, decreased glucose and increased protein concentrations, and leukocyte counts of 20/mm³ or higher with a predominance of lymphocytes. Organisms may be detected in 20–50% of patients using an India ink preparation that

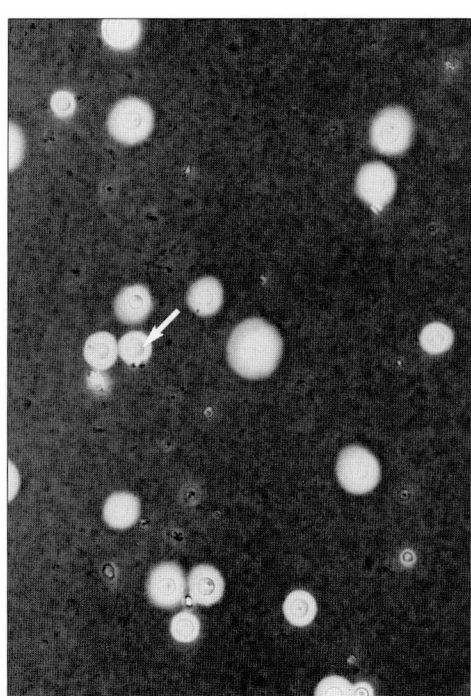

Fig. 7.5 India ink preparation of cerebrospinal fluid showing numerous *Cryptococcus neoformans* organisms. Note the easily identified capsule (arrow).

outlines the cell wall and capsule (Fig. 7.5). A positive culture is best obtained by centrifuging 5–10ml of CSF. The CSF may be normal in some patients with early disease.

A major advance in the diagnosis of cryptococcal meningitis is the latex agglutination test for detecting polysaccharide capsular antigen in CSF or serum. *Trichosporon beigelii* and *Capnocytophaga canimorsus* are rare causes of a false-positive antigen test. Commercially available kits usually include controls to detect non-specific rheumatoid factor in serum. The antigen is detected in the CSF of 90% and the serum of 70% of patients with meningitis. Patients who have AIDS usually have very high titers (and also many organisms on India ink preparations).

Cultures of sputum and bronchoalveolar fluid may be useful in making the diagnosis of cryptococcal pneumonia, but the organism may be a commensal in sputum. The organism can often be isolated from blood cultures of patients with disseminated disease and may be visualized in peripheral blood leukocytes or bone marrow macrophages in patients with extensive infection. It may also be cultured from urine specimens of some patients. The diagnosis can also be established from tissue biopsies using methenamine silver, PAS stain or Mayer's mucicarmine, which distinguishes cryptococci from other yeast-like fungi.

MANAGEMENT

A standard regimen for the treatment of cryptococcal meningitis is a 6-week course of amphotericin B (0.3–0.5mg/kg/day intravenously) plus flucytosine (150mg/kg/day, given in divided doses q6h).[46] Lower doses of flucytosine (75–100mg/kg/day), sufficient to maintain peak serum concentrations of 60μg/ml and trough concentrations of 25μg/ml can be used in the combination to minimize the toxicities of flucytosine. Flucytosine can cause diarrhea with dehydration, enhancing the likelihood of azotemia from amphotericin B, which then results in increased serum concentrations of flucytosine, enhancing the possibility of myelosuppression. Some physicians use daily doses of 0.5–0.7mg/kg of amphotericin B alone for 10 weeks. Rarely patients fail to respond to parenteral therapy and require intrathecal amphotericin B. Therapy should be continued until weekly India ink preparations are negative for 4 weeks. Abnormal protein concentrations should improve, but may remain abnormal for a prolonged period. Progressive pulmonary and disseminated infection requires similar aggressive therapy.

In a randomized trial among AIDS patients with cryptococcal meningitis, fluconazole (200–400mg/day) was as effective as amphotericin B 0.4–0.6mg/kg/day intravenously except for patients with positive blood cultures, antigen titers of at least 1:128 in the CSF, positive India ink preparations and impaired mental status. Among patients receiving amphotericin B, CSF cultures converted to negative in a median of 42 days compared to 64 days among patients receiving fluconazole. A currently recommended regimen for HIV positive patients is to administer amphotericin B (0.5–0.7mg/kg/day) plus flucytosine (75–100mg/kg/day) for several weeks and to follow this with fluconazole (200–400mg/day) once the disease has stabilized. Higher doses of fluconazole (800–1200mg/day) have been used successfully in a few patients who fail to respond to lower doses. Animal studies suggest that fluconazole plus flucytosine may interact synergistically.[47] Itraconazole is not a satisfactory substitute for fluconazole, at least not as currently formulated.

The overall mortality rate is about 25–30%. Some patients are left with residual neurologic defects such as hydrocephalus. The relapse rate in patients who do not have AIDS is less than 20%[48] so maintenance therapy is not necessary. However, more than 25% of AIDS patients experience recurrent disease, so these patients require maintenance therapy indefinitely. In a comparative trial of maintenance therapy, the relapse rate was 8% with fluconazole compared with 37% with amphotericin B.[49] The prostate may serve as a residual focus and site for relapse after apparently successful therapy in AIDS patients.

MUCORMYCOSIS

EPIDEMIOLOGY AND HOST FACTORS

The term mucormycosis applies to infections caused by a variety of fungi belonging to the order Mucorales. In the past these infections were referred to as zygomycosis or phycomycosis. The molds in this order are widely dispersed in the environment, especially in decaying materials, and can cause disease in many animals. The most common agents causing human disease are *Rhizopus* spp., followed by *Rhizomucor* spp.[50]

Infection is usually acquired by inhalation of spores, so sinus and pulmonary infections are most common. Occasional cases of primary cutaneous infection due to inoculation of spores in adhesive bandages have been described. Rare cases have originated from the gastrointestinal tract. Disseminated infection is uncommon.

As with *Aspergillus* spp., these molds have a propensity to invade blood vessels, causing thrombosis and tissue infarction. As for other molds, macrophages and neutrophils are primary host defenses against human infection. The host factors preventing infection are not fully delineated, but serum factors are involved. Patients susceptible to mucormycosis include those who have poorly controlled diabetes mellitus, acute leukemia, malnutrition or an organ transplant, and patients receiving adrenal corticosteroids or deferoxamine.[51] Patients with diabetic ketoacidosis are especially susceptible to the sino-orbital form of infection, whereas pulmonary infection is more common in patients who have leukemia. About 50 cases of mucormycosis have been described in patients with renal failure receiving deferoxamine for aluminum or iron overload.[52] The complex of iron deferoxamine abolishes the fungistatic effect of serum on *Rhizopus* spp.

CLINICAL FEATURES

SINO-ORBITAL INFECTION

The initial symptoms of sino-orbital infection are fever, retro-orbital pain or headache, often associated with circumorbital erythema. The infection usually progresses rapidly, with orbital cellulitis, conjunctivitis and loss of extraocular motor function resulting in proptosis and ultimately loss of vision. Destruction of the cheek, nasal and palatal structures may occur with erosion into the brain resulting in brain abscess or infarction and cavernous sinus or internal carotid thrombosis (Fig. 7.6). Radiographic procedures reveal mucosal thickening, air–fluid levels and bone destruction. Biopsy of infected tissue reveals large, broad, nonseptate hyphae with wide-angle branching.

PULMONARY INFECTION

Pulmonary infection may occur in immunocompromised hosts; it is the most common form of mucormycosis in leukemia patients. Some patients with pneumonia present with signs and symptoms suggesting acute pulmonary embolism because of the vascular thromboses and infarctions caused by these fungi. Most patients have only nonspecific signs suggesting pneumonia: fever, dyspnea, rales and pulmonary infiltrates on chest radiography. Lung infection is usually fulminant in neutropenic patients, but may be subacute in diabetics. Chest radiography may reveal a solitary or multiple nodules, wedge-shaped infarcts, cavitary lesions, lobar pneumonia or diffuse pneumonitis.

The organism is seldom recovered from sputum or bronchoalveolar lavage specimens and diagnosis usually requires pulmonary biopsy. This may be difficult to perform due to the presence of thrombocytopenia or compromised pulmonary function.

GASTROINTESTINAL INFECTION

Gastrointestinal infection has been described in patients with kwashiorkor, malnutrition, pellagra, amebic colitis, uremia and typhoid fever. About 35% of cases have been reported from South Africa. Presumably the organism is ingested and then invades the gastrointestinal tract. Organs most often infected are the stomach and large bowel. The blood vessels are invaded causing ischemia, ulceration, gangrene, necrosis and infarction of tissues. Symptoms include nausea, vomiting, abdominal pain, diarrhea, hematemesis and melena.

The diagnosis may be made by biopsy, but most cases are recognized only at autopsy examination. The infection is usually acute and rapidly fatal.

CUTANEOUS INFECTION

Cutaneous infection occurs primarily in patients with burn wounds or intravenous catheters. An epidemic in the 1970s resulted from contaminated bandage materials. Rarely, infection has followed superficial trauma in diabetics or intramuscular injections. Occasionally skin lesions are associated with disseminated infection.

Surgical excision is unlikely to be beneficial until the infection is under control. Major organ infections such as endocarditis, septic arthritis, osteomyelitis and brain abscesses have been described. Primary brain infections usually occur in intravenous drug addicts or after head trauma. Therapy for these infections is seldom effective.

MANAGEMENT

Mucorales are usually only marginally susceptible to amphotericin B. Successful therapy is infrequent and depends primarily upon recovery from the underlying disability. Whether the ability to administer much higher doses of amphotericin B in lipid formulations improves the efficacy of therapy needs to be determined. Other available antifungal agents are ineffective.

Successful therapy of sino-orbital infection requires extensive surgical debridement of infected and necrotic tissue. Some patients with pulmonary infection may also require surgical excision of necrotic tissue.

CANDIDIASIS

EPIDEMIOLOGY AND HOST FACTORS

There are approximately 200 species of *Candida,* although only about 10% of these have been recognized as causes of human disease. Most

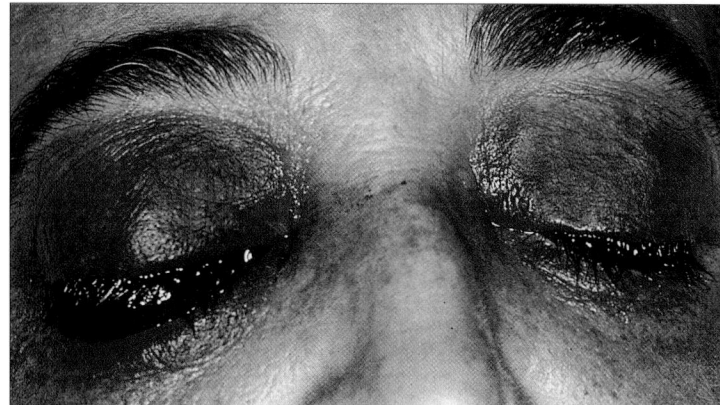

Fig. 7.6 Bilateral rhinocerebral mucormycosis in a patient who has acute leukemia.

infections are caused by *Candida albicans*, including over 50% of systemic infections.[53] *Candida tropicalis* is an increasing cause of systemic infections, now accounting for about 20%, and other species of medical importance include *Candida parapsilosis, Candida guilliermondii, Candida glabrata, Candida krusei* and *Candida lusitaniae*:[54]

- *C. tropicalis* appears to be more virulent than *C. albicans* as there is a much higher frequency of systemic infections among immunocompromised hosts who become colonized by *C. tropicalis*;
- *C. parapsilosis* is generally associated with vascular catheter-related infections and is a cause of nosocomial epidemics;
- *C. krusei* is inherently resistant to fluconazole, and increased colonization and infection by this organism has been reported in a few leukemia and bone marrow transplant units when fluconazole prophylaxis has been used; and
- *C. lusitaniae* is a rare cause of systemic infection, but is of concern because it may be inherently resistant to amphotericin B or may develop resistance during therapy.

The majority of *Candida* infections are derived from the patient's endogenous flora. There have been nosocomial epidemics resulting from contaminated equipment and fluids and probably human-to-human transmission. Infection in neonates may be acquired from the mother during delivery.

VIRULENCE FACTORS

The ability of some *Candida* spp. to adhere to mucosal surfaces is an important factor in the initiation of infection. Adherence to plastic polymers is a critical initial stage in the origin of catheter-associated infections. The virulence of different *Candida* spp. correlates with their capacity to adhere. *Candida albicans* produces proteinases and phospholipases that may contribute to pathogenesis. The formation of germ tubes or hyphae that can penetrate epithelial cell membranes also plays a role in the pathogenesis of infection.

HOST DEFENSES

Candida spp. are common colonizers of mucocutaneous surfaces, so infection is often a consequence of the loss of integrity of this barrier. Disruptions that follow trauma, chemotherapy-induced ulceration or insertion of intravascular catheters facilitate initiation of infection.[55] Alterations in the normal microbial flora may permit overgrowth of *Candida* spp. Excessive concentrations of *Candida* spp. in the gastrointestinal tract allow organisms to cross the intact epithelial surface by a process known as persorption, and enter the portal circulation.

CD4+ T lymphocytes probably play a significant role in protecting against superficial candidal infection because thrush and esophagitis are common in people who have AIDS who have deficient numbers of circulating CD4+ T lymphocytes.

The neutrophil is the primary cellular defense against systemic invasion by *Candida* spp. Neutrophils are able to ingest and kill candidal organisms and disseminated candidiasis is especially frequent among neutropenic patients. Aerosolized adrenal corticosteroid therapy is associated with superficial infection of the respiratory tract and systemic corticosteroid therapy is a predisposing factor for disseminated infection. Corticosteroids have many adverse effects on host defenses, including lympholysis and interference with macrophage function. Serum factors, including immunoglobulins, complement and cytokines also serve as host defenses against candidal infection.

CLINICAL FEATURES

DISSEMINATED CANDIDIASIS

Candidemia and disseminated candidiasis used to occur only in tertiary care centers, but recently these infections have emerged in primary community hospitals. The frequency of candidemia among hospitalized patients has doubled during the 1980s and *Candida* spp. have now become as common as enteric Gram-negative bacilli as a cause of sepsis. There are several reasons for this increase including:

- widespread use of intravascular catheters;
- increased number of immunocompromised hosts;
- extensive use of broad-spectrum antibacterial agents;
- the use of mechanical devices such as respirators and dialysis machines; and
- the ability to extend the lives of seriously ill patients.

There are two major dilemmas in the management of these infections: some patients have catheter-associated candidemia without deep tissue invasion, whereas other patients have disseminated candidiasis yet the organism cannot be isolated from blood culture specimens. It is therefore difficult to determine the true frequency of disseminated candidiasis.

Patients at risk

Disseminated candidiasis is predominantly a disease of immunocompromised and debilitated patients. Among those at risk are:

- neutropenic patients (especially those with acute leukemia);
- organ transplant (especially liver transplant) recipients;
- patients who have diabetes mellitus, cancer, hepatitis, hepatic cirrhosis, pancreatitis, lupus erythematosus, uremia, burn wounds or severe trauma;
- heroin addicts; and
- patients undergoing extensive or repeated gastrointestinal surgery.

Important predisposing factors include broad-spectrum antibacterial or adrenal corticosteroid therapy, intravascular catheters, tissue damage, parenteral alimentation, urinary catheters, hemodialysis, mechanical ventilation, major surgery and prolonged stay in an intensive care unit.

The excess mortality attributable to an episode of candidemia is estimated to be 38%. Factors that impact on prognosis include the number of positive blood cultures, duration of candidemia, age of patient, presence of major organ involvement and ability to correct underlying predisposing conditions such as neutropenia.

Intravascular catheters have been recognized as a source of candidemia for many years, especially if used for the administration of parenteral nutrition. Estimated rates of catheter-associated candidemia vary from less than 1 to 10%, depending upon duration of use. Although it is recognized that some patients with catheter-associated candidemia do not have invasive disease, it is now the general consensus that all patients with candidemia should receive antifungal therapy. In some instances when this has not been given patients have returned at a later date with serious candida infections such as ophthalmitis or vertebral osteomyelitis (Fig. 7.7). Among immunocompromised patients with candidemia, 70–80% have evidence of deep tissue invasion at autopsy examination. Most studies indicate that catheter removal reduces the duration of fungemia and facilitates recovery from infection. Some catheter-associated infections result in septic thrombophlebitis and metastatic foci of infection or candidal endocarditis.

There is no characteristic constellation of signs and symptoms to indicate a diagnosis of disseminated candidiasis. The usual presentation

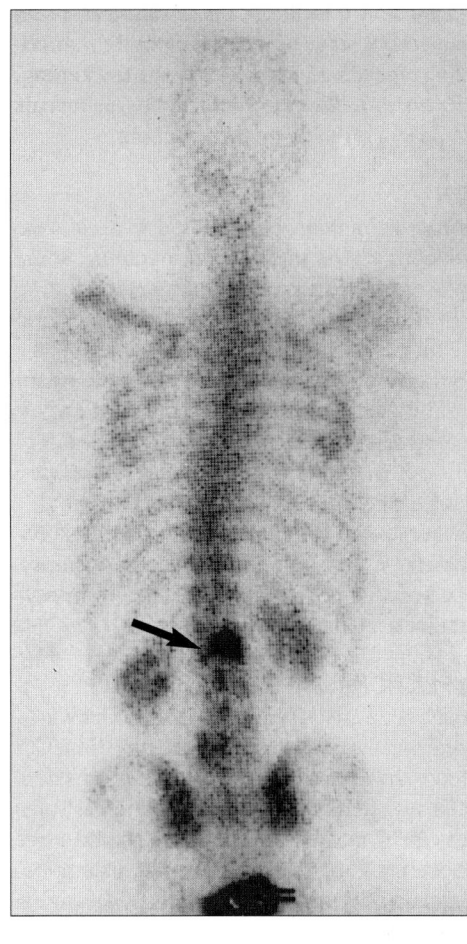

Fig. 7.7 Bone scan showing vertebral osteomyelitis (arrow) due to *Candida* spp. in a patient who has small cell carcinoma of the lung (posterior view).

is a seriously ill patient with persistent fever despite antibacterial antibiotics. Often the patient has deteriorating liver or renal function and a pulmonary infiltrate. Occasional patients may be hypothermic or normothermic, but usually these patients are receiving adrenal corticosteriods, which may mask fever. Because some of these patients have a preceding bacterial infection, the only clue to superinfection may be a change in the fever pattern. Occasional patients present with fever, hypotension, tachycardia and tachypnea suggestive of endotoxic shock.

The patient should be carefully examined for any signs suggestive of candidal infection. Eye involvement has been reported in 5–50% of patients, although these lesions are usually absent in neutropenic patients. The most common eye lesions are single or multiple fluffy white 'cotton ball' exudates on the retina, which progress to cause vitreous haze.[56] Some patients complain of ocular pain, blurred vision, scotomas, photophobia or 'floaters', whereas others notice no visual disturbances. Other manifestations include hemorrhagic exudates, Roth's spots, chronic uveitis, iritis and hypopyon. Most eye lesions occur in patients infected with *C. albicans*.

Characteristic skin lesions have been recognized in about 10% of patients, primarily those who are immunocompromised.[57] The lesions may be generalized or localized to the extremities and may be numerous or few. They are non-tender, firm nodules that are pink-to-red in color. The borders are usually discrete, but may coalesce as the infection progresses (Fig. 7.8). *Candida* spp. can be visualized in the dermis of tissue biopsies, but are isolated from only 50% of cultures. Some patients with skin lesions also have an associated myositis, which is exquisitely tender on palpation. It is most pronounced in the legs and most likely to be due to *C. tropicalis* infection.

Two distinct forms of disseminated candidiasis have been described:

- one in patients with acute leukemia; and
- the other in heroin addicts.

Chronic disseminated (hepatosplenic) candidiasis occurs predominantly in patients with acute leukemia. Fever develops during prolonged periods of neutropenia and fails to respond to antibacterial drugs.[58] After the

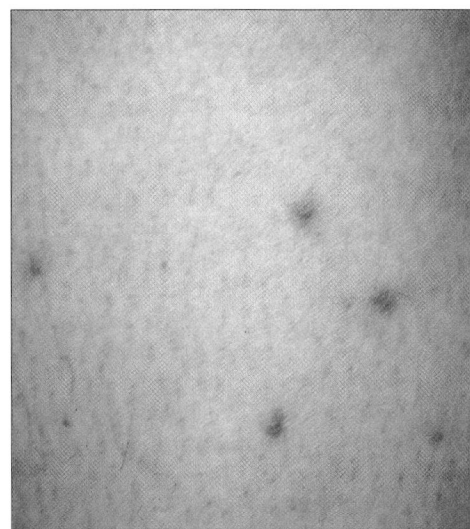

Fig. 7.8 Nodular skin lesion due to disseminated candidiasis.

patient achieves a remission of the leukemia and the neutrophil count recovers, the fever persists. The patient develops anorexia, weight loss and debilitation, and may acquire right upper quadrant or right pleuritic chest pain. About 50% of the patients develop hepatomegaly or splenomegaly or both. Characteristically, at this time the patient has a highly elevated serum alkaline phosphatase concentration and other liver function tests may be abnormal. Multiple lesions can be visualized in the liver and spleen, and occasionally in other organs by abdominal ultrasonography, CT scanning or MRI. A biopsy should be obtained, which will usually reveal hyphal elements, but the organism is cultured from only 50% of biopsy specimens. This is a chronic infection that may persist for several months despite therapy.

Since 1981 an unusual form of candidiasis has been reported in heroin addicts from Europe and Australia. The syndrome is characterized by skin lesions, ophthalmitis and osteoarthritis, occasionally with pulmonary or pleural infection. The initial symptoms begin a few hours to several days after an injection and consist of high fever, profuse sweating, severe headache and occasionally cholestasis. A few days later, cutaneous lesions appear, involving the scalp with multiple nodular painful abscesses. Other lesions include folliculitis or pustules, which may spontaneously drain thick pus. The lesions may spread to the beard area and involve regional lymph nodes. The lesions gradually resolve within 2–4 weeks if untreated, leaving areas of alopecia. Within a few days to 3 weeks of the septic phase more than 50% of patients develop eye lesions, which may be unilateral or bilateral. These lesions include chorioretinitis, episcleritis, hyalitis, anterior uveitis and endophthalmitis, and may be associated with photophobia and decreased visual acuity. Osteoarthritis, manifested as costochondritis or vertebral lesions, occurs 2 weeks to 5 months later. It is believed that this form of infection is due to the use of contaminated lemon juice to dissolve the heroin. The prevalence of this type of infection depends upon the products and practices in use by drug addicts at different times.

Diagnosis

A diagnosis of disseminated candidiasis may be difficult to establish, so therapy must often be initiated on the presumption of this infection.[59] In several autopsy series of disseminated candidiasis, candida were isolated from antemortem blood cultures in only 25–50% of the cases. In one series the yeast was cultured from the blood specimens of only 8% of patients during the first 48 hours after the onset of infection. The lysis–centrifugation technique may be superior with positive cultures antemortem in up to 70% of cases of autopsy-proven disseminated infection. To optimize the value of blood cultures:

- adequate volumes of blood should be collected;
- multiple specimens should be obtained; and
- the cultures should be maintained in aerobic conditions.

Candiduria in a susceptible patient without a urinary catheter is suggestive, but not diagnostic, of disseminated candidiasis.

Detection of circulating candidal antibodies has not proved useful for diagnosis. Considerable effort has focused on detection of circulating antigens such as cell mannan or glucans, enolase or metabolites such as D-arabinitol. None of these approaches has become widely accepted.

Management

Despite the availability of amphotericin B for many years, the optimum dosage schedule and duration of therapy for various types of candidal infection have not been definitively determined.[60] Furthermore, response to therapy often depends as much upon recovery from deficiencies in the patient's host defenses as on therapy. Because it is often difficult to establish a diagnosis of disseminated candidiasis, therapy may not be initiated until the disease is far advanced. The increasing use of empiric therapy further complicates the interpretation of results because patients may improve or worsen and not have candidal infection. There were no controlled trials of amphotericin B therapy until recent comparisons with fluconazole. Most data reported in the literature are derived from retrospective reviews of candidemia and disseminated candidiasis in which the outcomes of patients who received therapy are compared with outcomes of those who received no therapy.[61] Such studies have inherent biases because the sickest patients with the poorest prognosis are most likely to receive therapy and the less ill patients with a single positive blood culture are most likely to receive no therapy.

Mortality rates differ depending upon the patient's underlying diseases, age and other factors. Mortality rates at tertiary care centers have been reported to be about 60%. In these retrospective reviews, the mortality rates were about 65% among patients who received no therapy and 55% among those treated with amphotericin B.[61]

The results of therapy in cancer patients have generally been discouraging, especially in neutropenic patients. In several studies the mortality rates have been 90–100% unless the neutrophil count recovered, irrespective of whether the patients were treated with amphotericin B.[53] Among patients with neutrophil recovery, survival rates with amphotericin B therapy have been about 40%. Similarly poor results have been observed among bone marrow transplant recipients.[62] Results of amphotericin B therapy in surgical patients have been more encouraging, with survival rates of about 70% among treated patients.

The toxicities of amphotericin B (especially nephrotoxicity) can be ameliorated by administering the drug in a lipid formulation. This permits the administration of higher daily doses. Several of these formulations are available, each having different pharmacokinetic properties. They have been reported to be successful against serious candidal infections that have failed to respond to amphotericin B, although the higher doses were not more effective than the normal dose of amphotericin B in one randomized trial.

The antimetabolite, flucytosine, interacts synergistically with amphotericin B *in vitro* and in animal models. Although there are some clinical data suggesting that the combination may be superior to amphotericin B alone, especially against infections caused by *C. tropicalis*, an adequate comparative trial has never been performed. Flucytosine should not be used alone because some *Candida* strains are inherently resistant and others develop resistance during therapy. Care must be taken in using the combination because amphotericin B can cause renal impairment and flucytosine is excreted in the urine. Excessive serum concentrations of flucytosine can be associated with myelosuppressive toxicity, so serum concentrations should be monitored.

Fluconazole has been evaluated as an alternative to amphotericin B for the treatment of serious candidal infections in open and prospective randomized trials. In a randomized trial of non-neutropenic patients with candidemia, fluconazole and amphotericin B were similarly effective (70 versus 79%).[63] In this study, intravascular catheter removal was associated with a more rapid response. In a matched-cohort study of cancer patients and a prospective randomized trial that included neutropenic patients, both drugs were equivalent.[64] In all these studies there were significantly more side effects with amphotericin B. Although the dose of fluconazole was 400mg/day, there is some evidence that higher doses may be more effective. Other azoles have not been extensively evaluated for serious candidal infections.

Amphotericin B alone has been effective in about 55% of leukemia patients with chronic disseminated candidiasis and in 65% when combined with flucytosine. Lipid formulations are effective in about 75% of patients. Fluconazole 400mg/day orally appears to be the drug of choice, being effective in over 80% of cases, including those who have failed to respond to other therapies. The duration of therapy required is uncertain, but it should probably be continued for at least 1 month after symptoms abate.

MAJOR ORGAN INFECTION
Lung infection
The lung is involved in approximately 60–80% of patients with disseminated candidiasis and is more likely to be involved in patients without fungemia. Hematogenous pulmonary candidiasis is usually characterized on chest radiography by bilateral symmetrically distributed nodular lesions associated with small subpleural nodules. Primary candidal pneumonia is an uncommon infection, although it appears to be increasing in frequency. In one autopsy study of cancer patients only 8% of cases of pulmonary candidiasis represented primary infection. Most cases of primary pneumonia resulted from aspiration of infected oropharyngeal secretions.

The major clinical manifestations are fever and tachypnea, occasional chest pain, cough and sputum production. Radiographic examination of endobronchial infection is characterized by asymmetric lesions, primarily in the lower lobes.

The diagnosis is difficult to establish because culture of Candida spp. from sputum or bronchoalveolar lavage specimens usually reflect colonization. The diagnosis is made with certainty only by tissue biopsy, which is often not obtainable. The mortality rate from primary pneumonia may exceed 80%.

Joint infection
The frequency of septic arthritis is low. Predisposing factors include localized trauma, chronic articular disease and compromised host defenses. Most cases result from hematogenous dissemination and 70% involve a single joint. About 35% of the cases are indolent. The knee is most often infected.

The symptoms include fever, soft tissue swelling and effusion, joint pain, tenderness and restricted movement.

Synovial fluid examination reveals leukocytosis, but a normal glucose concentration.

In addition to systemic therapy, frequent aspirations of synovial fluid are helpful.

Candida spp. may also infect prosthetic joints. Infection usually occurs within 6 months of surgery. Therapy requires removal of the prosthesis in addition to systemic antifungal therapy with amphotericin B.

Bone infection
Bone disease, like joint involvement, is uncommon. Predisposing factors include diabetes mellitus, surgery, leukemia and intravenous heroin use. About 85% of cases are due to hematogenous dissemination, although less than 50% of patients have Candida spp. isolated from blood cultures. The most common bones involved are the vertebrae (especially lumbar), sternum and femur. Involvement of the ribs and long bones occurs mainly in individuals under 20 years of age, whereas vertebral osteomyelitis occurs almost exclusively in adults.

The most frequent symptom is local pain.

There are no unique radiologic features and the diagnosis is made by histopathologic examination and culture of biopsy tissue.

Most therapeutic experience has been obtained with amphotericin

B, but azoles may be useful alternatives, especially for long-term therapy. Surgical debridement is probably necessary for sternal, but not vertebral infection.

Abdominal organ infection
Candidal abscesses of the spleen are due to disseminated infection and are usually associated with hepatic infection. Splenic infection has occasionally resulted in hypersplenism. A few patients have large splenic abscesses and may benefit from splenectomy.

Candida spp. are occasionally cultured from bile or gallbladder tissue at surgery, often when there is infection in the liver and other organs. Infected patients present with the typical signs and symptoms of cholecystitis. Antifungal therapy is only required for neutropenic patients and patients with liver involvement or candidemia.

Candida spp. rarely cause pancreatic abscesses, usually as a polymicrobial infection with Gram-negative bacilli.

Candida pyelonephritis presents with fever, flank pain and systemic toxicity. Patients at risk include those with urinary obstruction, renal stones, diabetes mellitus, ureteral stents and nephrostomy tubes. Many of these patients have received prolonged antibacterial therapy. In diabetics the organism can migrate from the bladder to the renal pelvis forming bezoars, which may cause obstruction or necrotizing papillitis. The diagnosis cannot be made solely on urine culture. Visualization of candidal casts (fungal elements with cast-like impressions of the renal tubule) on microscopic examination is diagnostic, but requires special stains. Intravenous pyelography may fail to reveal bezoars in 30% of cases. The largest therapeutic experience has been with amphotericin B but fluconazole also has been successful.

Peritoneal infection
Peritoneal infections may result from perforation of the gastrointestinal tract, abdominal surgery or peritoneal dialysis. Recovery of Candida spp. from peritoneal fluid during or following surgery may be significant, although there has been considerable disagreement on this subject. In one autopsy series of 27 surgical patients from whom Candida spp. were cultured from peritoneal fluid, 33% had disseminated candidiasis and 30% had candidal peritonitis.[65]

The frequency of candidal peritonitis associated with dialysis is 7–18% over 2–7 years. Nearly 50% of these patients die or require hemodialysis. Dissemination to other organs is uncommon. Patients have been treated with intraperitoneal flucytosine or miconazole plus oral ketoconazole. Low-dose amphotericin B to produce a final concentration of 2–4µg/ml in the dialysate has been used, but it may cause abdominal pain, peritoneal adhesions and fibrosis mandating subsequent hemodialysis. Fluconazole penetrates well into peritoneal fluid and may prove to be more useful than other therapeutic agents. Successful therapy usually requires removal of the dialysis catheter. The overall cure rate is about 80%, but this falls to less than 30% without removal of the catheter. Some patients have been cured by catheter removal alone.

Central nervous system infection
Candidal meningitis may occur as a primary infection, but 50% of cases result from hematogenous dissemination. The incidence of cerebral infection associated with disseminated candidiasis is about 20% in most series, but occurs in 40% of patients who have endocarditis. Predisposing factors include prematurity, neurosurgery, neurosurgical shunts, trauma, intravenous drug use, alcohol abuse, malignant disease and immunosuppressive therapy. Lesions of CNS candidiasis include meningitis, abscesses, thrombosis and infarction, mycotic aneurysms, granulomas, transverse myelitis and hemorrhagic necrosis.

Patients with CNS candidiasis may present with headache, photophobia, nuchal rigidity, delirium, somnolence, disorientation, cranial nerve lesions or focal neurologic defects.

Examination of the CSF usually reveals pleocytosis with neutrophil or mononuclear predominance, normal or low glucose concentration, and elevated protein concentration. Yeasts may be visualized in up to 40% of cases, but the organism may be difficult to culture from CSF.

The usual therapy is amphotericin B 0.6–1.0mg/kg/day intravenously plus flucytosine for 4–8 weeks (150mg/kg/day, given in divided doses q6h). Foreign bodies such as shunts must be removed.

The cure rate for meningitis is about 65%, but patients with brain involvement have a very poor prognosis. As fluconazole crosses the blood–brain barrier, it may prove to be useful in this infection. A substantial proportion of patients with CNS infection develop long-term complications despite successful therapy.

Cardiac infection

Candida endocarditis occurs in four settings:
- primary infection associated with intravascular catheters or intravenous drug abuse;
- hematogenous dissemination;
- post-cardiac surgery of native or prosthetic valves; and
- superinfection of bacterial endocarditis.

Disseminated infection is also associated with myocardial abscesses or pericarditis.

Catheter-associated endocarditis usually occurs on native valves, most often the aortic or mitral valve. Up to 5% of cases of endocarditis in intravenous drug abusers are caused by *Candida* spp., and usually involve the left heart valves. *C. parapsilosis* is the most common species causing endocarditis in drug abusers. Surgical-associated infection of both native and prosthetic valves results from implantation of the organism at surgery. Prosthetic valve endocarditis usually occurs within 2 months of surgery, but may appear years later.

Cardiac vegetations tend to be bulky, friable and verrucous, and can become large enough to obstruct flow across the valve.

Usually these infections are asymptomatic, but they may cause cardiac arrhythmias and other complications. Symptoms of endocarditis include fever, malaise, fatigue, weight loss and repeated pulmonary emboli with cough, pleuritic pain and dyspnea. Usual signs such as splinter hemorrhages and Roth's spots are absent. Because the vegetations are large, emboli may obstruct large arteries, especially in the legs. Embolic lesions may also be found in the brain, kidney, spleen, liver, eye and coronary arteries.

Candida spp. can be isolated from blood cultures in 80% of cases. Echocardiography, especially transesophageal, may reveal bulky, highly echogenic lesions.

The optimal management is amphotericin B 0.6–0.8mg/kg/day to a total dose of 500mg, followed by valve replacement surgery and then an additional total dose of 1.0–1.5g amphotericin B. Before 1973, survival was less than 20%; now about 50% of patients survive.

ASPERGILLOSIS

EPIDEMIOLOGY AND HOST FACTORS

Only about 20 of the approximately 200 species of *Aspergillus* are pathogenic in man. Most infections have been caused by *Aspergillus fumigatus*, although *Aspergillus flavus* has emerged as an important pathogen at some institutions. Other pathogenic species include *Aspergillus glaucus*, *Aspergillus niger*, *Aspergillus terreus* and *Aspergillus nidulans*. These molds are ubiquitous in air, soil, water, organic debris, spices, potted plants and compost. In worldwide surveys of airborne molds *Aspergillus* spp. have accounted for 0.1–22% of total spores collected. Aspergillus spores remain suspended in the air for prolonged periods and remain viable for months in dry locations. The mold has been isolated from the oropharynx and gastrointestinal tract of healthy humans.

Microepidemics of aspergillosis have been reported in acute leukemia and bone marrow transplant units.[66] These epidemics have been associated with construction within or adjacent to the hospital.

Susceptible patients are at special risk when there is a disturbance of dust above false ceilings. A common source for a nosocomial epidemic may not always be discovered, but is usually related to the ventilation system. The risk of aspergillosis can be greatly reduced, but not eliminated, by the use of rooms with high-efficiency air filtration units for susceptible patients.

Aspergillus spp. can cause a wide variety of diseases in humans ranging from allergic disorders secondary to colonization to serious invasive infections in immunocompromised hosts (Fig. 7.9). Because *Aspergillus* spp. produce spores and are primarily inhaled respiratory pathogens, most infections involve the sinuses and lower respiratory tract. A few infections have arisen from cutaneous and gastrointestinal sources. Human hosts may also develop superficial infections such as otitis externa and keratitis and noninvasive fungus balls in the paranasal sinuses or pre-existent pulmonary cavities.[67] The severity of invasive infection often depends upon the extent of the deficiencies in host defenses. Basically aspergillosis can be divided into three disease categories:
- allergic manifestations;
- superficial and locally invasive infections; and
- major organ or disseminated infections.

HOST DEFENSES

A variety of factors predispose to the different forms of *Aspergillus* disease. Some infections have been attributed to exposure to an unusually heavy concentration of the organisms. Damage to the normal mucocutaneous barrier following trauma or ulceration due to antitumor agents

CLASSIFICATION OF ASPERGILLUS INFECTIONS
I. Disease in the normal host
A. Allergic manifestations
1. Asthma
2. Saprophytic bronchopulmonary aspergillosis
3. Extrinsic allergic alveolitis
4. Allergic bronchopulmonary aspergillosis
B. Superficial infection
1. Cutaneous infection
2. Otomycosis
3. Sinusitis
4. Tracheobronchitis
C. Invasive infection
1. Single organ
2. Disseminated
II. Infection associated with tissue damage or foreign body
A. Keratitis and endophthalmitis
B. Burn wound infection
C. Osteomyelitis
D. Prosthetic valve endocarditis
E. Vascular graft infection
F. Aspergilloma
G. Empyema and pleural aspergillosis
H. Peritonitis
III. Infection in the immunocompromised host
A. Primary cutaneous aspergillosis
B. Sino-orbital infection
C. Pulmonary aspergillosis
1. Invasive tracheobronchitis
2. Chronic necrotizing pulmonary aspergillosis
3. Acute invasive pulmonary aspergillosis
D. Central nervous system aspergillosis
E. Disseminated aspergillosis

Fig. 7.9 Classification of aspergillus infections.

may provide a focus for infection. Tissue damage due to previous bacterial infection is common in bone marrow transplant recipients and patients with acute leukemia. Most major organ and disseminated infections occur in patients who are severely immunocompromised.

In an animal model, the macrophage was found to be the primary defense against aspergillus spores. Adrenal corticosteroid administration permitted phagocytosis, but interfered with the fungicidal activity of macrophages. The neutrophil was found to be the primary defense against invasion by aspergillus mycelia.

VIRULENCE FACTORS

Invasive aspergillosis presumably follows the inhalation of conidia into the sinuses or lungs where they germinate. The hyphae invade blood vessels causing thrombosis and infarction, the necrotic tissue providing nutrients for subsequent fungal growth. Virulence of some aspergillus strains has been associated with their production of elastase, inhibitors of phagocytosis such as gliotoxin, and an inhibitor of complement activation. Among the toxic metabolites of *Aspergillus* spp. are aflatoxins, which do not appear to be involved in the infectious process, but may have long-term carcinogenic effects. *Aspergillus* spp. are allergenic and elicit antibody responses, which are involved in some disease processes. Aspergillus spores invade the lung through the alveoli or tracheobronchial tree. *Aspergillus* spp. invade small or large arteries and veins causing thrombosis and infarction. The organisms are capable of crossing fascial planes, cartilage and bone.

PATIENTS AT RISK

Human hosts rarely develop invasive aspergillosis (Fig. 7.10).[68] Those at risk include:
- patients who have prolonged neutropenia, such as those with acute leukemia, who have the highest risk of developing aspergillosis, especially pulmonary infection;
- those who have defects in neutrophil function, such as children with chronic granulomatous disease;
- people who have rheumatoid arthritis, sarcoidosis, lupus erythematosus or malignancy;
- recipients of chronic adrenal corticosteroid therapy or organ transplants;
- intravenous drug addicts;
- alcoholics;
- neonates; and
- people who have diabetes mellitus, chronic hepatitis and extensive burn wounds.

Bone marrow transplant recipients who develop chronic graft-versus-host disease are at special risk. Recently, patients who have advanced AIDS have developed tracheobronchial or pulmonary aspergillosis.[69]

CLINICAL FEATURES

INVASIVE PULMONARY INFECTION

Aspergillus infection of the respiratory tract may cause tracheobronchitis, chronic necrotizing pulmonary aspergillosis or acute invasive infection.

Tracheobronchitis and chronic necrotizing pulmonary aspergillosis
Tracheobronchitis and chronic necrotizing pulmonary aspergillosis occur in patients with mildly compromised host defenses (e.g. those who have diabetes mellitus, sarcoidosis or malnutrition, or who take aerosolized low-dose adrenal corticosteroid therapy). Pulmonary infection also occurs in patients with chronic pulmonary disease such as pneumoconiosis, radiation fibrosis or inactive tuberculosis.

Invasive tracheobronchitis causes dyspnea, wheezing, cough and mild hemoptysis. Chronic necrotizing pulmonary aspergillosis is slowly progressive, resulting in cavitation and aspergilloma formation. Patients are chronically ill with fever, weight loss, cough and sputum production.

Therapy of chronic nectrotizing pulmonary aspergillosis requires surgical resection or drainage plus intravenous amphotericin B. The

INVASIVE ASPERGILLUS INFECTIONS			
	System involved		Pathology
In normal hosts	Central nervous system		Pituitary abscess, cerebral granuloma, chronic meningitis, epidural abscess, cavernous sinus thrombosis
	Ophthalmic		Peri-orbital cellulitis, keratitis, endophthalmitis
	Cardiovascular		Endocarditis, pericarditis, mycotic aneurysm
	Respiratory		Sinusitis, bronchitis, pneumonia, empyema, laryngitis
	Thoracic		Esophagitis, mediastinitis
	Bone		Osteomyelitis
	Disseminated		Multiple organs
	System	Pathology	Surgical procedure/trauma
Following surgical procedures	Cardiovascular	Endocarditis	Valvuloplast, prosthetic valve placement
		Pseudo-aneurysm	Aortic bypass, coronary artery bypass
	Skin and skeletal	Infected prosthesis	Mammary implant
		Wound infection	Abdominal surgery
		Osteomyelitis, osteochondritis	Trauma, surgery
		Lumbar disc infection	Laminectomy
	Central nervous system	Chronic meningitis	Yttrium-90 pituitary implants
		Basilar artery aneurysm	Trans-sphenoidal hypophysectomy
		Cerebral granuloma	Trauma, craniotomy
	Pulmonary	Pneumonia	Carotid endarterectomy
		Empyema	Thoracotomy tube, pneumonectomy
	Ophthalmic	Keratitis, endophthalmitis	Trauma
	Disseminated		Prosthetic valve

Fig. 7.10 Invasive aspergillus infections.

value of intraconazole has not been determined in these cases. Many patients experience residual pulmonary damage and some develop recurrent infection.

Acute invasive pulmonary aspergillosis

Acute invasive pulmonary aspergillosis is the most common form of aspergillus infection in the immunocompromised host.[70] The majority of cases occur in patients who have acute leukemia, but it may also occur in transplant recipients and those who have hematologic malignancy.

A variety of types of pulmonary infection occur, including necrotizing bronchopneumonia, single wedge-shaped pulmonary infarctions, single or multiple nodular infarcts, single or multiple abscesses, lobar pneumonia, solitary granuloma and diffuse bilateral infiltrates.

About 30% of patients present with fever, the sudden onset of pleuritic chest pain, hemoptysis and a pleural friction rub suggestive of pulmonary embolization and infarction. Often the only evidence of infection is fever and the presence of pulmonary infiltrates that fail to respond to antibacterial agents. Occasional patients have a normal physical examination (other than fever) and a normal chest radiograph initially. A few patients develop exsanguinating pulmonary hemorrhage early in the course of the infection. Uncontrolled infection may cause pneumothorax or empyema, or extend into the ribs, vertebrae, mediastinum, esophagus or pericardium.

The earliest abnormality on chest radiograph is the appearance of single or multiple nodular lesions. These lesions may be visualized by CT in patients with normal chest radiographs. In some patients a nodular lesion can progress to a wedge-shaped infiltrate suggestive of pulmonary infarction. In others the lesions may evolve into lobar pneumonia or diffuse unilateral or bilateral infiltrates. Pulmonary lesions in patients whose infection is controlled often, develop cavities with thick walls that contain a fungus ball.

Although the clinical presentation and chest radiograph may suggest a diagnosis of pulmonary aspergillosis, confirmation can be difficult. The organism is cultured from sputum specimens in only 10–30% of cases, but bronchoscopy with culture of bronchoalveolar fluid can improved the yield only slightly, to about 40%.

Although the organism may be visualized on histopathologic examination of biopsy tissue, it is cultured from only about 40% of cases. However, when *Aspergillus* spp. are cultured from respiratory secretions of a susceptible patient, it is highly likely that the patient is either already infected or will develop infection in the near future.[71]

Despite considerable efforts to develop serologic tests for the diagnosis of aspergillosis, immunoprecipitation, immunodiffusion and counterimmunoelectrophoresis techniques have been unsatisfactory. Studies using ELISA for detecting circulating antigens have been more promising, but are not universally available.

PLEURITIS AND EMPYEMA
Pleural empyema usually occurs in previously damaged lung. The infection is often chronic, causing weight loss, malaise, cough and anemia.

Many of these infections are polymicrobial and the infection can be locally destructive producing intense fibrosis or cavitation. Early decortication and intravenous amphotericin B therapy may be helpful, but some patients require pneumonectomy.

INVASIVE CUTANEOUS ASPERGILLOSIS
Primary cutaneous aspergillosis has been recognized in recent years and is associated with intravascular catheters or armboards used to stabilize intravenous catheter sites. The organism may be implanted at the time of insertion or impregnated in adhesive dressings. *Aspergillus flavus* is the predominant species causing these infections.

The lesions occur mainly in neutropenic patients. They start as an erythematous indurated plaque that progresses to become a necrotic ulcer covered by a black eschar. If the lesion is located on an extremity, disseminated infection may result. If the catheter is placed in the subclavian vein, the organism may erode through the chest wall and cause pulmonary infection. Surgical excision should not be attempted until there is evidence of a response to antifungal therapy.[72] Occasional patients develop subcutaneous abscesses, granulomas or pustular lesions.

OPHTHALMIC AND PERIORBITAL INFECTION
Aspergillus spp. can cause eye infections by inoculation during trauma, secondary to extension from sino-orbital infection, or as a complication of hematogenous dissemination. Fungal keratitis has become more common in recent years due to the use of topical antibacterial agents and adrenal corticosteroids. These infections present as a slowly progressive epithelial erosion or infiltrate, and hypopyon is common.
Topical natamycin is effective if administered early, but about 20% of patients require surgical treatment. In some cases the infection progresses to endophthalmitis and requires enucleation.

Sino-orbital aspergillosis may extend from infected sinuses causing protopsis, orbital pain and loss of vision.

Endophthalmitis rarely occurs in human hosts, but is usually a complication of acute leukemia, endocarditis, organ transplantation or trauma.

Invasive sino-orbital infection is being observed with increasing frequency among patients with acute leukemia and bone marrow transplant recipients, and accounts for about 25% of invasive infections in these populations.[73] The maxillary sinus is most often involved, but pansinusitis is not uncommon (Fig. 7.11). The earliest symptoms are fever, headache, retro-orbital pain or periorbital erythema. Careful examination often reveals a black eschar on the nose, nasal septum or palate (Fig. 7.12). *Aspergillus* spp. are capable of invading across cartilage and bone causing extensive disfigurement of the face, necrosis of the palate, or invasion through the skull into the brain. About 50% of these infections progress to disseminated infection.

A diagnosis of aspergillus sino-orbital infection is usually not difficult to establish because the mycelia can be identified in tissue biopsies, although the organism may not be grown from culture specimens. Surviving patients often require surgical debridement.

CENTRAL NERVOUS SYSTEM ASPERGILLOSIS
Aspergillosis of the CNS can result from head trauma or surgery, extension of infection from the sinuses, or hematogenous dissemination. The latter two forms occur almost entirely in immunocompromised hosts. Five types of infection have been described:
- meningitis;
- meningoencephalitis;
- single brain abscess;
- multiple brain abscesses; and
- single granuloma.

Granulomatous infection may occur in human hosts and persist for many years. Examination of the CSF in cases of meningitis is not diagnostic, revealing only pleocytosis and elevated protein concentration. *Aspergillus* spp. are rarely cultured. Central nervous system infection is

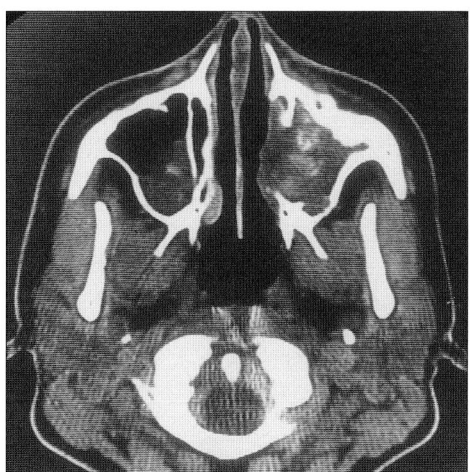

Fig. 7.11 Computerized tomography scan showing aspergillus infection of the maxillary sinuses.

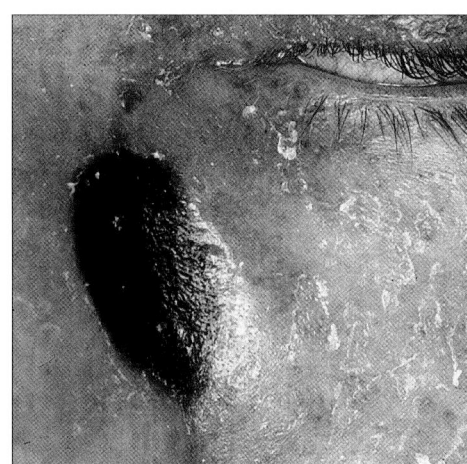

Fig. 7.12 Skin lesion on the nose of a patient who has aspergillus sinusitis.

manifested by seizures, neurologic defects or coma. Infection may cause cavernous sinus thrombosis or internal carotid artery occlusion. Computerized tomography reveals infarction or abscess formation.

CARDIOVASCULAR INFECTION

Most cardiovascular infections occur as a surgical complication or as an infection of prosthetic valves. Most involve the mitral or aortic valves where masses of infected thrombotic tissue may obstruct the orifice. Aspergillus valvular infections are usually associated with multiple embolic events, usually involving large arteries, the aortic bifurcation or major cerebral vessels.

Aggressive medical and surgical therapy is required to cure the endocarditis since medical therapy alone is ineffective. Therapy is effective only if all infected tissue is surgically removed. The prognosis remains poor.

OSTEOMYELITIS

Aspergillus osteomyelitis is rare, but may follow trauma, a surgical procedure, extension from other infected tissues or hematogenous dissemination. About 50% of the cases have occurred in children, most of whom have had chronic granulomatous disease. Infection usually involves the vertebrae or ribs and is due to contiguous spread from the lung.

About 50% of the patients have survived their infection with surgical debridement and intravenous amphotericin B.

GASTROINTESTINAL INFECTION

The esophagus is the most frequently involved gastrointestinal organ. Infection presents as ulcerative esophagitis, sometimes with pseudomembrane formation or as an abscess, and usually deeply invading the muscle. The large bowel may also be infected, with most lesions in the cecum. Gastrointestinal lesions can lead to perforation or massive hemorrhage. Rare cases of Budd–Chiari syndrome have resulted from thrombosis of the hepatic blood vessels.

DISSEMINATED ASPERGILLOSIS

Dissemination follows major organ infection in about 30–40% of patients who have acute leukemia and bone marrow transplant recipients. Any organ can be involved: the brain is involved in about 60% of cases and the gastrointestinal tract in 40%. Other organs that are frequently involved include kidneys, liver, spleen, heart and thyroid. Cutaneous lesions occur in about 5% of patients with disseminated infection. Usually there are only a few lesions, which begin as papular–pustular lesions and evolve into punched-out rounded lesions with sharply demarcated borders covered by a black eschar and surrounded by a thin erythematous halo. Adjoining lesions may gradually coalesce as the infection progresses.

MANAGEMENT

Treatment of invasive aspergillosis is often unsuccessful due to severe deficiencies in the host defense mechanisms or delays in initiating therapy. Amphotericin B has been the mainstay of therapy, although its activity against some *Aspergillus* spp. is marginal and success rates have not been impressive. The overall mortality rates for major organ or disseminated aspergillosis in immunocompromised hosts have been as low as 20% and as high as 100%. Therapeutic results are difficult to interpret because a critical factor in response to antifungal therapy is recovery of the patient's host defenses. Also the definition of response is complicated because these patients suffer extensive tissue destruction due to thrombosis and infarction and consequently residual organ damage may persist after the infection has been treated successfully. Patients with CNS, disseminated and valvular infections have particularly poor response rates. The appropriate dose of amphotericin B has not been determined, but should be at least 1.0mg/kg/day, and some physicians give doses as high as 1.5mg/kg/day until the creatinine exceeds 2.5–3.0mg/dl (220–266 μmol/L). Patients have developed aspergillosis while receiving doses of 0.6mg/kg/day amphotericin B.

The availability of lipid formulations of amphotericin B allows the administration of higher doses (5–6mg/kg/day) with less nephrotoxicity, but it is uncertain whether such a regimen is more effective.

The appropriate duration of therapy has not been defined. This becomes a major therapeutic dilemma because many patients have persistent tissue damage after the infection appears to have been controlled. Therapy should be continued for at least 1 month after improvement and stabilization. Patients with residual fungus balls are at risk of developing exsanguinating pulmonary hemorrhage, whereas patients with residual infection may experience a reactivation of infection during subsequent myelosuppressive or immunosuppressive therapy. For these reasons, judicial surgical debridement and excision should be considered when feasible. Small studies have shown that reactivation can be prevented during subsequent myelosuppressive therapy by administering amphotericin B during periods of neutropenia.

In-vitro data suggest that rifampin (rifampicin) and flucytosine may interact synergistically with amphotericin B against *Aspergillus* spp. Sporadic reports have suggested that combination therapy is more effective than amphotericin B alone, but no large comparative trials have been conducted.

Itraconazole is a promising agent for the treatment of aspergillosis, producing complete and partial response rates of 39–80%.[74] Response and mortality rates vary, depending upon the underlying disease process and the site of infection. For example, the response rate is about 45% for pulmonary infection, but less than 20% for sinus or CNS infection. Itraconazole can be used for long-term maintenance therapy in patients initially responding to amphotericin B, but is erratically absorbed from the gastrointestinal tract.

PSEUDALLESCHERIASIS

EPIDEMIOLOGY AND HOST FACTORS

This infection has had a confusing history because it has undergone several name changes in recent years (e.g. allescheriasis, petriellidiosis) and is caused by either the sexual form, *Pseudallescheria boydii,* or the asexual form, *Scedosporium apiospermium.* The fungus is worldwide in distribution and can be found in soil, manure, decaying vegetation and polluted streams. It is especially prevalent in areas of heavy rainfall.

The sexual form, *Pseudallescheria boydii* accounts for the majority of infections and has been identified as a cause of mycetoma. Infection occurs predominantly in younger men, aged 20–40 years who live in rural areas. It can cause infection in human hosts, in whom it is usually associated with trauma, and in immunocompromised hosts.

Subacute progressive pyogenic infections follow penetrating trauma of the bone, joint, eye, brain or subcutaneous tissue. Rare infections have been associated with surgery or intra-articular injections. The organism can chronically colonize the paranasal sinuses, external auditory canals, ectatic bronchi or pre-existing pulmonary cavities.

Most cases of pseudoallescheriasis have occurred in immunocompromised hosts, especially those who have acute leukemia, diabetes mellitus, an organ transplant, chronic granulomatous disease or AIDS, or are treated with high-dose adrenal corticosteroid therapy.

CLINICAL FEATURES

Pseudoallescheriasis has many features in common with aspergillosis. Vascular invasion is usual in the neutropenic patient, whereas tissue necrosis and pus formation predominate in other hosts. The organism can usually be cultured from infected tissues.

After mycetomas, pulmonary infection is the most common form and can be manifested as bronchial colonization, pulmonary colonization, pneumonia or fungus ball formation. Bronchial colonization is associated with wheezing and pulmonary congestion. Transient colonization is probably a common event. Pulmonary colonization usually

SOME EMERGING FUNGAL PATHOGENS					
Organism*		Natural sites	Major predisposing factors	Type of infection	Fatalities[†]
Yeasts	Rhodotorula rubra	Foods, air, soil, water	Catheters, leukemia	Fungemia	Uncommon
	Trichosporon beigelii	Soil, air, fruit	Leukemia	Pneumonia, disseminated	Common
	Blastoschizomyces capitatus	Soil, air, fruit	Leukemia	Disseminated	Common
	Hansenula anomala	Plants, soil, fruit	Catheters, neonates	Fungemia	Uncommon
	Malassezia furfur	Oily areas of skin	Catheters, lipid infusions, neonates	Pneumonitis, fungemia	Uncommon
Hyalohyphomyces	Fusarium spp.	Soil, plants, air, animals	Leukemia, burns	Sino-orbital, pneumonia, disseminated	Frequent
	Paecilomyces lilacinus	Air, soil, solutions	Eye surgery, prosthetics	Skin, eye, endocarditis	Rare, except endocarditis
	Penicillium marneffei	Bamboo rat	AIDS	Disseminated	Uncommon
	Scedosporium prolificans	Soil, water, animals	Trauma	Osteomyelitis, osteoarthritis	None
Phaeohyphomycetes	Alternaria alternata	Soil, vegetation	Trauma, allergic sinusitis	Skin, sinusitis	None
	Bipolaris spicifera	Soil, plants, animals	Allergic sinusitis	Sinusitis	None
	Curvularia lunata	Soil	Trauma, allergic sinusitis	Skin, sinusitis	None
	Wangiella dermatitidis	Soil, plants, animals	Trauma	Skin, disseminated	None, except disseminated
	Cladophialophora bantiana	Soil, wood, animals	Unknown	Brain	Common

*Predominant species causing human infection.
[†]Fatalities from most common types of infection when treated appropriately.

Fig. 7.13 Some emerging fungal pathogens.

occurs in preformed cavities or cysts. The most common predisposing factors are sarcoidosis, tuberculosis and previous bacterial infection. Surgical excision usually leads to recovery. Pneumonia occurs most often in immunocompromised hosts and often disseminates hematogenously. Rarely pneumonia or solitary pulmonary nodules occur in human hosts and infections have been reported following near-drowning in fresh or brackish water. Severe necrotizing pneumonia with fatal dissemination to the brain has occurred. Sputum cultures are often positive in patients with pulmonary infection, but diagnosis requires visualization of hyphae on smears or biopsies.

About 50% of the cases of invasive sinusitis have occurred in human hosts. Sinusitis also occurs in patients who have diabetes mellitus or acute leukemia and can invade into the brain.

Infection of the CNS presents as meningitis or brain abscess.[75] Meningitis usually occurs following trauma and a few patients have recovered after surgery. Brain abscesses can result from trauma, extension from sinusitis or hematogenous dissemination. The organism can be cultured from aspirated material. A combination of surgery plus intravenous therapy has been successful in some cases.

Osteoarthritis and osteomyelitis usually involve the knee following trauma.[76] These infections usually respond to surgery plus intravenous miconazole therapy.

Endocarditis usually occurs on prosthetic valves and the cure rate is about 65% with surgery plus miconazole therapy.

Hematogenous dissemination most often results in infections in the brain or thyroid, but can also cause endophthalmitis, and pulmonary, renal or myocardial infection.[77] The organism can usually be cultured from infected tissues, but is rarely isolated from blood during hematogenous dissemination.

MANAGEMENT

Surgical drainage and debridement is an important component of therapy in the normal host. Azoles are considered to be the therapy of choice. Itraconazole 200mg q12h is generally recommended, but patients have also responded to fluconazole and ketoconazole. The prognosis is usually good except in the severely immunocompromised host.

EMERGING FUNGI

EPIDEMIOLOGY AND HOST FACTORS

A wide variety of yeasts and molds have been described as causing occasional infections in humans (Fig. 7.13).[1,78] The mold infections are divided into two types:
- phaeohyphomycoses, which are caused by dematiaceous fungi producing light brown–black pigment (usually melanin) in the cell walls of hyphae or conidia; and
- hyalohyphomycoses, which are caused by non-pigmented fungi.

Infections range in severity from slowly progressive skin lesions following trauma such as those caused by *Alternaria alternata* to progressive fatal cerebral abscesses such as caused by *Cladophialophora*.

Paecilomyces spp. may contaminate 'sterile' solutions and cause infections of prosthetic devices, endophthalmitis after lens implantation, and skin lesions in bone marrow transplant recipients. All patients with prosthetic valve endocarditis have died of their infection.

Fusarium spp. cause sino-orbital, pulmonary and disseminated infection, predominantly in patients who have acute leukemia (Fig. 7.14). These patients usually die despite antifungal therapy unless their neutropenia resolves.

A few organisms cause localized cutaneous infections after minor trauma, including *Alternaria alternata* and *Wangiella dermatitidis*.

Several fungi, including *Hansenula anomala*, *Malassezia furfur* and *Rhodotorula rubra*, cause catheter-related fungemias.

Organisms that cause simple self-limited infections in human hosts such as *Fusarium* spp., *Scedosporium* spp. and *Wangiella dermatitidis* can cause serious and even fatal infection in people who are immunocompromised. Disseminated *Penicillium marneffei* infection is increasing in frequency among AIDS patients in South East Asia, but most survive if treated properly. *Trichosporon beigelii* and *Blastoschizomyces capitatus* usually cause disseminated infection that terminates fatally in patients who have acute leukemia.

Many molds cause sinusitis, varying from allergic disease caused by *Bipolaris spicifera*, *Curvuluria lunata* and *Exserohilum rostratum*, to chronic noninvasive sinusitis or acute or chronic invasive sinusitis.[79]

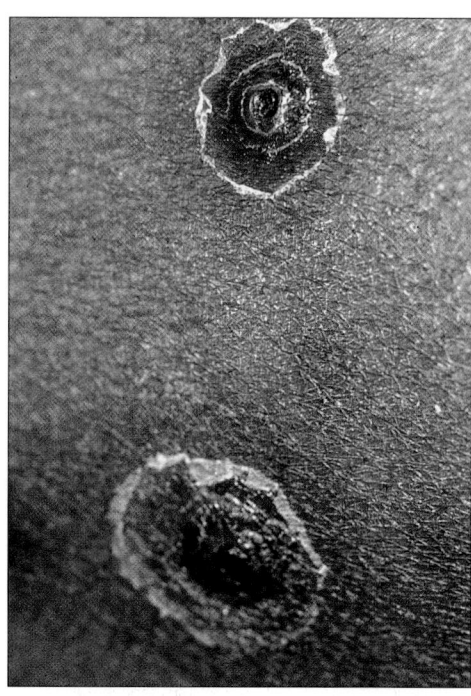

Fig. 7.14 Skin lesions due to disseminated fusarium infection.

Patients may therefore present with fever and renal, cardiac or pulmonary dysfunction. Some patients with severe hypoxemia have minimal abnormalities on chest radiography. Cardiac involvement may result in arrhythmias or congestive heart failure, whereas renal involvement may be manifested as hematuria, proteinuria and azotemia. Multiple maculopapular or nodular skin lesions are found in 30% of patients.

Azole agents appear to be more effective than amphotericin B, but recovery depends upon a resolution of neutropenia.

FUSARIUM SPP.

Several *Fusarium* spp. are capable of causing human disease. They are common soil and plant pathogens found worldwide. *Fusarium sporotrichioides* produces potent mycotoxins, which if ingested for long periods can cause aplastic anemia, neurologic symptoms and death. These fungi can cause superficial infections, endophthalmitis and osteomyelitis. Patients susceptible to serious infection include bone marrow transplant recipients and patients who have acute leukemia or burns.

The organism has a propensity for invading blood vessels causing thrombosis and tissue infarction and can be confused with *Aspergillus* spp. in the tissues. The majority of infections in immunocompromised hosts are sino-orbital, pulmonary or disseminated.[82] Sinus infection may extend to the orbit, eye and brain. Patients with pulmonary infection may present with a sudden onset of hemoptysis, pleuritic chest pain and a pleural friction rub. About 75% of infections are disseminated and involve the lungs, liver, spleen and brain. The organisms can be isolated from blood culture specimens in about 70% of cases. Many patients with disseminated infection develop multiple skin lesions, including grayish nodules or erythematous indurated lesions that progress to sharply demarcated rounded black eschars surrounded by a grayish halo. In-vitro susceptibility to antifungal agents is variable, but infection in neutropenic patients is usually rapidly fatal unless the neutrophil count recovers.

PENICILLIUM MARNEFFI

Penicillium marneffi is a thermally dimorphic fungus that is endemic to southern China, Vietnam and Thailand, where the natural reservoir is the bamboo rat. *Penicillium marneffi* infects cells of the mononuclear phagocytic system causing:
* granulomas in human hosts;
* focal necrosis in compromised hosts; and
* multiple abscesses in some patients.

The most common type of infection is disseminated and, although it may occur in human hosts, it has emerged as an important infection in AIDS patients, especially in Thailand.[83] The common signs and symptoms of infection include fever, weight loss, anemia, skin lesions, cough, diarrhea, generalized lymphadenopathy and hepatosplenomegaly. Patients may develop primary or hematogenous pneumonia, osteoarthritis, osteomyelitis and fungemia. Skin lesions usually involve the forehead, trunk, arms and abdomen. Most patients have a generalized papular rash, with some lesions resembling those of molluscum contagiosum.

The organisms can be isolated from 75% of blood specimens and 50% of bone marrow specimens collected from patients with disseminated infection. Treatment with itraconazole yields a 75% response rate after 8 weeks of treatment, but the relapse rate in AIDS patients exceeds 50%, indicating the need for long-term maintenance therapy.

It is critically important to identify the organism because they have differing susceptibilities to antifungal agents and it cannot be assumed that amphotericin B is the most appropriate therapy. Four of these occasional pathogens are discussed in more detail below.

MALASSEZIA FURFUR

Malassezia furfur is a saprophytic yeast that colonizes oily areas of the skin and causes tinea versicolor in human hosts. It causes folliculitis in patients who have AIDS, diabetes mellitus, trauma or cancer, organ recipients and patients receiving antibacterial or adrenal corticosteroid therapy. The folliculitis usually occurs over the shoulders, back and upper chest, and may spread rapidly. It is intensely pruritic and may persist for years. It usually responds to topical or oral azole agents, but infection in AIDS patients is highly resistant to therapy.

Neonates are susceptible to malassezia fungemia associated with the infusion of lipid emulsions through intravascular catheters.[80] Most of these patients have had severe gastrointestinal disorders. More than 50% of the children develop interstitial pneumonitis. Clinical symptoms and signs include fever, respiratory distress, hepatosplenomegaly and occasionally seizures. The organisms may not be isolated from routine blood cultures because they require fatty acids for growth. Catheter removal is an important component of successful management, along with discontinuation of lipid emulsions and probably a short course of amphotericin B therapy.

TRICHOSPORON BEIGELII

Trichosporon beigelii is widely distributed in soil, air and decaying fruit, but rarely on human skin or in the hospital environment. Most infections occur in males who have acute leukemia. *Trichosporon beigelii* can cause a variety of infections including pneumonia, but over 80% of cases are disseminated infection.[81] The organism is isolated from the blood cultures of most of these patients.

Clinical symptoms depend upon the organs predominantly infected.

REFERENCES

1. Rippon JW. Medical mycology, 3rd ed. Philadelphia: WB Saunders Company; 1988.
2. Bradsher RW. Histoplasmosis and blastomycosis. Clin Infect Dis 1996;22(Suppl 2):102–11.
3. Wheat J. Histoplasmosis and coccidioidomycosis in individuals with AIDS. A clinical review. Infect Dis North Am 1994;8:467–82.
4. Wheat J. Histoplasmosis: recognition and treatment. Clin Infect Dis 1994;19(Suppl 1):19–27.
5. Goodwin RA Jr, Des Prez RM. Pathogenesis and clinical spectrum of histoplasmosis. South Med J 1973;66:13–25.
6. Goodwin RA Jr, Des Prez RM. Histoplasmosis. Am Rev Respir Dis 1978;117:929–56.
7. Goodwin RA Jr, Owens FT, Snell JD, et al. Chronic pulmonary histoplasmosis. Medicine (Baltimore) 1976;55:413–52.
8. Goodwin RA Jr, Shapiro JL, Thurman GH, Thurman SS, Des Prez RM. Disseminated histoplasmosis: clinical and pathologic correlations. Medicine (Baltimore) 1980;59:1–33.
9. Wheat LJ, Connolly-Stringfield PA, Baker RL, et al. Disseminated histoplasmosis in the acquired immune deficiency syndrome: clinical findings, diagnosis and treatment, and review of the literature. Medicine (Baltimore) 1990;69:361–74.
10. Sharkey PK, Rinaldi MG, Dunn JR, Hardin TC, Fetchick RJ, Graybill JR. High-dose itraconazole in the treatment of severe mycoses. Antimicrob Agents Chemother 1991;35:707–13.
11. Wheat J, Hafner R, Korzun AH, et al. Itraconazole treatment of disseminated histoplasmosis in patients with the acquired immunodeficiency syndrome. Am J Med 1995;98:336–42.
12. Como JA, Dismukes WE. Oral azole drugs as systemic antifungal therapy. N Engl J Med 1994;330:263–72.
13. Rios-Fabra A, Morena AR, Isturiz RE. Fungal infection in Latin American countries. Infect Dis Clin North Am 1994;8:129–54.
14. Kirkland TH, Fierer J. Coccidioidomycosis: a reemerging infectious disease. Emerg Infect Dis 1996;2:192–9.
15. Einstein HE, Johnson RH. Coccidioidomycosis: new aspects of epidemiology and therapy. Clin Infect Dis 1993;16:349–56.
16. Galgiani JN. Coccidioidomycosis. Curr Clin Topics Infect Dis 1997;17:188–204.
17. Stevens DA. Coccidioidomycosis. N Engl J Med 1995;332:1077–82.
18. Stevens DA. Coccidioides immitis. In: Mandell GL, Bennett JE, Dolin R, eds. Mandell, Douglas and Bennett's principles and practice of infectious diseases, vol. 2, 4th ed. New York: Churchill Livingstone; 1995:2365–74.
19. Banuelos AF, Williams PL, Johnson RH, Bibi S, et al. Central nervous system abscesses due to Coccidioides species. Clin Infect Dis 1996;22:240–50.
20. McNeil MM, Ampel NM. Opportunistic coccidioidomycosis in patients infected with human immunodeficiency virus: prevention issue and priorities. Clin Infect Dis 1995;21(Suppl):111–13.
21. Kauffman CA. Newer developments in therapy for endemic mycoses. Rev Infect Dis 1994;19(Suppl 1):528–32.
22. Cockerill FR III, Roberts GD, Rosenblatt JE, Utz JP, Utz DC. Epidemic of pulmonary blastomycosis (Namekagon fever) in Wisconsin canoeists. Chest 1984;86:688–92.
23. Armstrong CS, Jenkins SR, Kaufman L, Kerking TM, Rouse BS, Miller GB Jr. Common-source outbreak of blastomycosis in hunters and their dogs. J Infect Dis 1987;155:568–70.
24. Klein BS, Vergeront JR, Weeks RJ, et al. Isolation of Blastomyces dermatitidis in soil associated with a large outbreak of blastomycosis in Wisconsin. N Engl J Med 1986;314:529–34.
25. Sarosi GA, Davies SF. Blastomycosis. Am Rev Respir Dis 1979;120:911–38.
26. Halvorsen RA, Duncan JD, Merten DF, Gallis HA, Putman CE. Pulmonary blastomycosis: radiologic manifestations. Radiology 1984;2:877–98.
27. Steele RW, Abernathy RS. Systemic blastomycosis in children. Pediatr Infect Dis 1983;2:304–7.
28. Meyer KC, McManus EJ, Maki DG. Overwhelming pulmonary blastomycosis associated with the adult respiratory distress syndrome. N Engl J Med 1993;329:1231–6.
29. Dismukes WE, Bradsher RW Jr, Cloud GC, et al. Itraconazole therapy of blastomycosis and histoplasmosis. Am J Med 1992;93:489–97.
30. Kwon-Chung KJ, Bennett JE. Medical mycology. Philadelphia: Lea & Febiger; 1992.
31. Dooley DP, Bostic PS, Beckius ML. Spook house sporotrichosis. A point-source outbreak of sporotrichosis associated with hay bale props in a Halloween haunted-house. Arch Intern Med 1997;157:1885–7.
32. Davis BA. Sporotrichosis. Derm Clin 1996;14:69–76.
33. Winn RE. A contemporary view of sporotrichosis. Curr Top Med Mycol 1995;6:73–94.
34. Winn RE. Sporotrichosis. Infect Dis Clin North Am 1988;2:899–911.
35. Kauffman CA. Old and new therapies for sporotrichosis. Clin Infect Dis 1995;21:981–5.
36. Bolao F, Podzamczer D, Ventin M, Gudiol F. Efficacy of acute phase and maintenance therapy with itraconazole in an AIDS patient with sporotrichosis. Eur J Clin Microbiol Infect Dis 1994;13:609–12.
37. Brummer E, Castaneda E, Restrepo A. Paracoccidioidomycosis: an update. Clin Microbiol Rev 1993;6:89–117.
38. Goldanii LZ, Sugar AM. Paracoccidioidomycosis and AIDS: an overview. Clin Infect Dis 1995;21:1275–81.
39. Manns BJ, Baylis BW, Urbanski SJ, Gibb AP, Rabin HE. Paracoccidioidomycosis: case report and review. Clin Infect Dis 1996;23:1026–32.
40. Restrepo A, Robledo M, Firaldo R, et al. The gamut of paracoccidioidomycosis. Am J Med 1976;61:33–42.
41. Restrepo AM. Paracoccidioides brasiliensis. In: Mandell GL, Bennett JE, Dolin R, eds. Mandell, Douglas and Bennett's principles and practice of infectious diseases, vol. 2, 4th ed. New York: Churchill Livingstone; 1995:2386–9.
42. Chuck SL, Sande MA. Infections with Cryptococcus neoformans in the acquired immunodeficiency syndrome. N Engl J Med 1989;327:794–9.
43. Hammerman KG, Powell KE, Christianson CS, et al. Cryptococcosis: clinical forms and treatment. Am Rev Respir Dis 1973;108:1116–25.
44. Woodring JH, Ciporkin G, Lee C, Worm B, Woolley S. Pulmonary cryptococcosis. Semin Roentgenol 1996;31:67–75.
45. Aberg JA, Powderly WG. Cryptococcosis. Adv Pharmacol 1997;37:215–51.
46. Bennett JE, Dismukes WE, Duma RJ, et al. A comparison of amphotericin B alone and combined with flucytosine in the treatment of cryptococcal meningitis. N Engl J Med 1979;301:126–31.
47. Aberg JA, Powderly WG. Cryptococcal disease: implications of recent clinical trials on treatment and management. AIDS Clin Rev 1998;229–48.
48. White M, Cirrincione C, Blevins A, Armstrong D. Cryptococcal meningitis: outcome in patients with AIDS and patients with neoplastic disease. Clin Infect Dis 1992;165:960–3.
49. Powderly WG, Saag MS, Cloud GA, et al. A controlled trial of fluconazole or amphotericin B to prevent relapse of cryptococcal meningitis in patients with the acquired immunodeficiency syndrome. N Engl J Med 1992;326:793–8.
50. Rinaldi MG. Zygomycosis. Infect Dis Clin North Am 1989;3:19–37.
51. Parfrey NA. Improved diagnosis and prognosis of mucormycosis. A clinopathiologic study of 33 cases. Medicine 1986;65:113–23.
52. Boelaret JR, Fenves AZ, Coburn JW. Mucormycosis among patients on dialysis. N Engl J Med 1989;321:190–4.
53. Bodey GP, ed. Candidiasis: pathogenesis, diagnosis, and treatment. New York: Raven Press; 1992.
54. Wingard JR. Importance of Candida species other than C. albicans as pathogens in oncology patients. Clin Infect Dis 1995;20:115–25.
55. Wey SB, Mori M, Pfaller MA, Wollson RF, Wenzel RP. Risk factors for hospital-acquired candidemia. Arch Intern Med 1989;149:2349–53.
56. Edwards JE, Foos RY, Mongomerie JZ, Guze JB. Ocular manifestations of candida septicemia. Review of 76 cases of hematogenous candida endophthalmitis. Medicine 1974;53:47–75.
57. Bodey GP, Luna MA. Skin lesions associated with disseminated candidiasis. JAMA 1974;229:1466–8.
58. Haron E, Feld R, Tuffnell P, Patterson B, Hasselback R, Matlow A. Hepatic candidiasis: an increasing problem in immunocompromised patients. Am J Med 1987;83:17–76.
59. Walsh TA, Chanock SJ. Laboratory diagnosis of invasive candidiasis: a rationale for complementary use of culture- and nonculture-based detection systems. J Infect Dis 1977;1(Suppl):11–9.
60. Gallas HA, Drew RH, Pickard WW. Amphotericin B: 30 years of clinical experience. Rev Infect Dis 1990;12:308–29.
61. Komshian SV, Uwaydah AK, Sobel JD, Crane LR. Fungemia caused by Candida species and Torulopsis glabrata in the hospitalized patient: frequency, characteristics and evaluation of factors influencing outcome. Rev Infect Dis 1989;11:379–90.
62. Goodrich JM, Reed E, Mori M, et al. Clinical features and analysis of risk factors for invasive candidal infection after marrow transplantation. J Infect Dis 1991;164:731–40.
63. Rex JH, Bennett JE, Sugar AM, et al. A randomized trial comparing flucaonazole with amphotericin B for the treatment of candidemia in patients without neutropenia. N Engl J Med 1994;331:1325–30.
64. Anaissie EJ, Darouiche RO, Abi-Said D, et al. Management of invasive candidal infections: results of a prospective, randomized, multicenter study of fluconazole versus amphotericin B and review of the literature. Clin Infect Dis 1996;23:964–972.
65. Solomkin J, Flohr A, Quie PG, Simmons RL. The role of Candida in intraperitoneal infections. Surgery 1980;88:524–30.
66. Bodey GP, Vartivarian S. Aspergillosis. Eur J Clin Microbiol Infect Dis 1989;8:413–37.
67. Riley EA, Tennenbaum J. Pulmonary aspergilloma or intracavitary fungus ball. Ann Intern Med 1962;56:896–909.
68. Karam GH, Griffin FM. Invasive pulmonary aspergillosis in nonimmunocompromised nonneutropenic hosts. Rev Infect Dis 1986;8:357–63.

69. Khoo SH, Denning DW. Invasive aspergillosis in patients with AIDS. Clin Infect Dis 1994;19(Suppl 1):41–8.

70. Young RC, Bennett JE, Vogel CL, Carbone PP, DeVita VT Jr. Aspergillosis. The spectrum of the disease in 98 patients. Medicine 1970;49:147–73.

71. Yu VL, Muder RR, Poorsattar A. Significance of isolation of aspergillus from the respiratory tract in diagnosis of invasive pulmonary aspergillosis: results from a three-year prospective study. Am J Med 1986;81:249–54.

72. Glorioso L, Webster GF. The role of surgery in the management of uncommon skin infections. Derm Surg 1995;21:136–44.

73. Viollier A, Peterson DE, De Jongh CA, et al. Aspergillus sinusitis in cancer patients. Cancer 1986;58:366–71.

74. Stevens DA, Lee JY. Analysis of compassionate use itraconazole therapy for invasive aspergillosis by the NIAID mycoses study group criteria. Arch Intern Med 1997;157:1857–62.

75. Berenger J, Diaz-Mediavilla J, Urra D, Munoz P. Central nervous system infection caused by *Pseudallescheria boydii*: case report and review. Rev Infect Dis 1989;11:890–6.

76. Hung LH, Norwood LA. Osteomyelitis due to *Pseudallescheria boydii*. South Med J 1993;86:231–4.

77. Lutwick LI, Galgiani JN, Johnson RH, Stevens DA. Visceral fungal infections due to *Petriellidium boydii* (*Allescheria boydii*). Am J Med 1976;61:632–40.

78. Bodey GP. New fungal pathogens. In: Remington JS, Swartz MN, eds. Current clinical topics in infectious diseases. Malden, MA: Blackwell Science; 1997:205–35.

79. Washburn RG, Kennedy DW, Begley MG, et al. Chronic fungal sinusitis in apparently normal hosts. Medicine (Baltimore) 1988;67:231–47.

80. Marcon MJ, Powell DA. Human infections due to *Malassezia* spp. Clin Microbiol Rev 1992;5:101–119.

81. Walsh TJ. Trichosporon. Infect Dis Clin North Am 1989;3:43–52.

82. Rabodonerina M, Piens MA, Monier MF, et al. Fusarium infections in immunocompromised patients: case reports and literature review. Eur J Clin Microbiol Infect Dis 1994;13:152–61.

83. Supparatpinyo K, Khamwan C, Baosoung V, et al. Disseminated *Penicillium marneffei* infection in Southeast Asia. Lancet 1994;334:110–3.

Practice Points

chapter
8

Approach to the acutely febrile patient who has a generalized rash

Edmund L Ong

INTRODUCTION

In assessing patients who have fever and rash, the following four points are essential.

- Is the patient well enough to give a further history?
- Is immediate cardiorespiratory support required?

- From the nature of the rash, does the patient require isolation precautions?
- Is immediate empiric antimicrobial therapy required?

The history obtained should give the following information:

- drugs taken within the past month,

MICROBIOLOGY OF CUTANEOUS MANIFESTATIONS ASSOCIATED WITH SYSTEMIC INFECTIONS			
Macular or papular rash		**Vesiculobullous eruptions**	
Viruses	Adenovirus Atypical measles Colorado tick fever Coxsackie viruses Cytomegalovirus Dengue virus Echoviruses Epstein–Barr virus Hepatitis B virus HIV-1 Human herpes virus 6 Lymphocytic choriomeningitis virus Parvovirus B19 (erythema infectiosum) Rubella (German measles) Rubeola (measles)	Viruses	Coxsackie viruses Echoviruses Herpes simplex virus (disseminated) Vaccinia Varicella (chickenpox) Varicella-zoster virus (disseminated)
Bacteria	*Bartonella bacilliformis* *Bartonella henselae* *Bartonella quintana* *Borrelia burgdorferi* (Lyme disease) *Borrelia* spp. (relapsing fever) *Chlamydia psittaci* *Francisella tularensis* *Leptospira* spp. *Mycobacterium haemophilium* *Mycoplasma pneumoniae* *Pseudomonas aeruginosa* *Rickettsia akari* (rickettsial pox) *Rickettsia prowazekii* (epidemic/louse-borne typhus) *Rickettsia rickettsii* (Rocky Mountain spotted fever) *Rickettsia tsutsugamushi* (scrub typhus) *Rickettsia typhi* (endemic/murine typhus) *Salmonella typhi* *Spirillum minus* (rat-bite fever) *Staphylococcus aureus* *Streptobacillus moniliformis* (rat-bite fever) Streptococci group A (scarlet fever) *Treponema pallidum* (secondary)	Bacteria	*Listeria monocytogenes* *Mycoplasma pneumoniae* *Rickettsia akari* (rickettsial pox) *Vibrio vulnificus*
		Petechial purpuric eruptions	
		Viruses	Adenovirus Atypical measles Congenital cytomegalovirus Coxsackie viruses Dengue virus Echoviruses Epstein–Barr virus Rubella (German measles) Viral haemorrhagic fevers Yellow fever
		Bacteria	*Borrelia* spp. (relapsing fever) *Capnocytophaga canimorsus* *Neisseria gonorrhoeae* *Neisseria meningitidis* *Rickettsia prowazekii* *Rickettsia rickettsii* *Staphylococcus aureus* *Streptobacillus moniliformis*
Fungi (disseminated)	*Blastomyces dermatitidis* *Candida* spp. *Coccidioides immitis* *Cryptococcus neoformans* *Fusarium* spp. *Histoplasma capsulatum*	Protozoa	*Plasmodium falciparum* (malaria)

Fig. 8.1 Microbiology of cutaneous manifestations associated with systemic infections.

SKIN LESIONS AND SYSTEMIC INFECTIONS

Lesion	Common pathogens	Time of appearance after onset of illness
Toxic erythema	Staphylococcus aureus, Streptococcus pyogenes	At presentation
Rose spots	Salmonella spp.	5–10 days
Purpuric lesions (in critically ill patients)	Neisseria meninigitidis, Rickettsia spp., Capnocytophaga canimorsus, Gram-negative bacteria	12–36 hours
Macronodular lesions	Candida spp., Cryptococcus neoformans, Histoplasma capsulatum, Fusarium spp.	Days
Erythema multiforme, bullous lesions, ecthyma gangrenosum	Pseudomonas spp., Vibrio vulnificus, Gram-negative bacteria	Days

Fig. 8.2 Skin lesions and systemic infections.

INFECTIOUS CAUSES OF ERYTHEMA MULTIFORME

Adenovirus
Chlamydia spp.
Coccidioides immitis
Coxsackie virus
Epstein–Barr virus
Herpes simplex infections
Histoplasma capsulatum
Mycobacterium tuberculosis
Mycoplasma pneumoniae
Salmonella typhi
Vaccinia
Yersinia spp.

Fig. 8.3 Infectious causes of erythema multiforme.

INFECTIOUS CAUSES OF ERYTHEMA NODOSUM

Chlamydia spp.
Coccidioides spp.
Hepatitis C virus
Histoplasma capsulatum
Mycobacterium leprae
Mycobacterium spp.
Streptococcal infections
Yersinia spp.

Fig. 8.4 Infectious causes of erythema nodosum.

- geographic itinerary of travel,
- immunizations,
- occupational exposure,
- sexually transmitted disease exposure,
- the immunologic status of the patient,
- any history of valvular heart disease,
- recent exposure to other ill febrile patients,
- exposure to wild or rural habitats and wild animals,
- exposure to domestic animals,
- prior medical history including allergies, and
- sun exposure.

PATHOGENESIS
Virtually any class of microbe can induce a local skin rash with fever if the microbes are allowed to penetrate the stratum corneum. The systemic effects of micro-organisms on the skin, however, can also produce cutaneous eruptions by:
- multiplying in the skin,
- toxin-mediated effects,
- inflammatory responses, and
- altering the vasculature of skin.

MICROBIOLOGY
The range of organisms causing systemic infections with prominent cutaneous manifestations are described in Figure 8.1 (see Chapters 2.1, 2.2, 2.5 & 2.7). There are other noninfectious causes of fever with a generalized rash, and these need to be borne in mind.

CLINICAL FEATURES
Physical examination should include the following:
- vital signs,
- general appearance,
- signs of toxicity,
- evidence of adenopathy,
- presence of mucosal, genital or conjunctival lesions,
- presence of hepatosplenomegaly,
- evidence of arthropathy, and
- signs of meningismus or neurologic dysfunction.

The rash should be assessed with regard to:
- its distribution,
- its pattern of progression,
- the timing of its development relative to the onset of illness and fever (Fig. 8.2), and
- its characteristics.

The morphology of skin lesions includes macules, papules, plaques, nodules, vesicles, bullae and pustules. Skin lesions are also characterized by their color and particularly by the presence or absence of hemorrhage. Lesions may also be hyperpigmented or hypopigmented. Blanching erythematous lesions are due to vasodilatation, whereas nonblanching erythemas may be due to extravasation of blood. Purpuric lesions are hemorrhages into the skin, and they may be small, petechial, or large and ecchymotic. Lesions of erythema multiforme usually begin as round or oval macules and papules that vary in size and have central erythema surrounded by a narrow ring of normal skin, which is also surrounded by another thin ring of erythema to form target lesions. Most cases are idiopathic, but the common infective causes are shown in Figure 8.3. The lesions of erythema nodosum are characterized by tender, erythematous nodules that vary in diameter from 1cm to several centimeters. Infectious agents are a major cause of this lesion (Fig. 8.4).

INVESTIGATIONS
Establishing the microbiologic diagnosis is of great importance in managing the patient. Blood cultures should form part of the essential investigations, along with full blood count and differential white cell count, liver function tests and renal function tests. Skin lesion aspirates or biopsy should be considered, particularly for the identification of meningococcal, staphylococcal and gonococcal infections. A punch biopsy of the maculopapular skin lesion of disseminated candidemia is sometimes diagnostic. Occasionally, a Gram stain of a routine buffy coat may reveal the responsible organisms (e.g. staphylococci, meningococci or Candida spp.) in a septic patient. Isolation of the causative organisms may be difficult, particularly with viruses and some bacteria. Serologic methods (e.g. serologic test for syphilis, paired viral complement fixation tests), molecular techniques (e.g. polymerase chain reaction for dengue fever virus) and immunofluoresence microscopy are useful methods for establishing the difficult culturable organisms.

FURTHER READING

Fitzpatrick TB, Johnson RA. Differential diagnosis of rashes in the acutely ill febrile patient and in life-threatening diseases. In: Jeffers JD, Scott E, White J, eds. Dermatology in general medicine. Textbook and atlas. 3rd ed. New York: McGraw–Hill;1987:21–2.

Weber JW, Cohen MS. The acutely ill patient with fever and rash. In: Mandell GL, Bennett JE, Dolin R, eds. Principles and practice of infectious diseases. 4th ed. Churchill Livingston;1955:549–61.

Management of the foot ulcer   *Sajeev Handa*

INTRODUCTION

Foot ulceration is a relatively common problem in clinical practice and one that sometimes poses difficult diagnostic and therapeutic dilemmas. Major complications are infection and, in more severe cases, the development of dry and wet gangrene. In certain cases making a determination of superinfection versus colonization can try even the most astute clinician.

PATHOGENESIS

This depends on the type and etiology.

Differential diagnosis of foot ulceration

The differential diagnosis includes:
- ischemic arterial ulceration;
- venous ulceration, due to increased venous hydrostatic pressure causing local edema, with its low exchange of oxygen and metabolites; edematous tissue, particularly skin, is more vulnerable to trauma than healthy tissue and is far less able to combat infection;
- neuropathic ulcers caused by diabetes, tabes dorsalis, leprosy, syringomyelia, or hereditary sensory (radicular) neuropathy; the protective pain sensation is ablated, resulting in loss of awareness of trauma, which can cause further deterioration of the ulcer;
- vasculitis; and
- infection, including acute pyogenic infections, tuberculous infections, tropical ulcer (chronic phagedenic ulcer secondary to Vincent's organisms), syphilis and yaws.

CLINICAL FEATURES

The ischemic arterial ulcer is typically located on the toes, heel, dorsum of the foot or lower third of the leg. The pain is severe and persistent and worsens at night. The ulcer is generally 'punched out' with a pale or necrotic base.

Venous ulcers are located in the 'gaiter' distribution around the ankle, especially around the medial malleoli. They are less painful, more diffuse and shallow and usually have some evidence of granulation tissue at the base.

Diabetic ulcers are usually located in the plantar or lateral aspect of the foot. They resemble arterial ulcers morphologically but are characteristically painless. Diabetic neuropathy (sensory, motor and autonomic), microvascular and macrovascular lesions, and diminished neutrophil function all conspire to generate diabetic foot ulcers.

All ulcers may become secondarily infected. Features of infection range from minimal cellulitis with lack of systemic toxicity to extensive cellulitis with associated lymphangitis, purulent drainage, sinus tract formation, osteomyelitis, septic arthritis, abscess formation and sometimes the development of gangrene. Systemic signs and symptoms often occur late and suggest severe infection.

INFECTED ULCER – DIAGNOSIS

A peripheral blood count may demonstrate a leukocytosis (this may be absent in severe cases, especially in diabetes); the erythrocyte sedimentation rate is usually raised. Blood cultures may be positive, especially if the patient is febrile and has not received prior antibiotic treatment.

Obtaining a swab culture of the ulcer itself is an unreliable means of establishing the causative organism(s) in superinfected ulcerations. Ulcers are typically colonized by a multitude of organisms that may or may not be pathogenic. Deep tissue cultures that avoid contact with the ulcer surface or other draining lesions are preferable. In osteomyelitis, bone cultures obtained by percutaneous biopsy or surgical excision are the best specimens for determining the etiology provided the incision site is away from the ulceration itself.

SELECTED EMPIRIC ANTIMICROBIAL REGIMENS FOR INFECTED FOOT ULCERS	
Nonlimb-threatening infection	
Oral regimen	Cephalexin Clindamycin Dicloxacillin/flucloxacillin Amoxicillin–clavulanate Quinolones Metronidazole
Parenteral regimens	Cefazolin Oxacillin or nafcillin
Limb-threatening infection	
Oral regimen	Clindamycin or metronidazole with a quinolone (consider trovafloxacin)
Parenteral regimens	Ampicillin–sulbactam with or without an oral quinolone or aminoglycoside Ticarcillin–clavulanate with an oral or parenteral quinolone or aminoglycoside Piperacillin–tazobactam with an oral or parenteral quinolone or aminoglycoside
Life-threatening infection	
Parenteral regimens	Imipenem–cilastatin Meropenem Vancomycin, metronidazole with either aztreonam or quinolone Piperacillin–tazobactam with an oral or parenteral quinolone or aminoglycoside

Fig. 8.5 **Selected empiric antimicrobial regimens for infected foot ulcers.** Note that if methicillin-resistant *Staphylococcus aureus* is a concern, vancomycin should be included in the regimen.

Plain radiographs of the affected area are useful in determining the presence of foreign bodies or air in the soft tissues, which may suggest the presence of gas-forming bacteria. Computed tomography scanning and MRI are useful for looking for abscesses as well as early osteomyelitis. The performance of technetium bone scanning for the diagnosis of osteomyelitis in the impaired foot is poor and use of a 24-hour indium-111 leukocyte scan is more sensitive than a bone scan in diagnosing osteomyelitis associated with a diabetic foot. However, this test is expensive and it may be difficult to interpret in the presence of local soft-tissue inflammation (Chapter 2.43).

MICROBIOLOGY

Mild ulcers may be infected by single organisms. Organisms frequently involved include:
- *Staphylococcus aureus,*
- *Streptococcus pyogenes,* and
- facultative Gram-negative bacilli and anaerobic organisms (which are isolated infrequently),

Severe ulcers, especially the diabetic foot, are usually polymicrobial with aerobic and anaerobic bacterial isolates, including:
- *S. aureus,*
- coagulase-negative staphylococci,
- aerobic streptococci and enterococci,
- Enterobacteriaceae (e.g. *Escherichia coli, Klebsiella* spp. and *Proteus* spp.),
- *Pseudomonas* spp.,
- *Corynebacterium* spp.,
- *Bacteroides* spp., and
- *Clostridium* spp.

THERAPY

Antibiotics are the mainstay of treatment (Chapter 2.2) and are recommended in the presence of a surrounding cellulitis, a foul-smelling lesion, fever or deep tissue infection. Empiric antibiotics are necessary until culture results are available (see Fig. 8.5).

The optimal duration of therapy is unclear; however, for infections that are limited to soft tissue, intravenous therapy may be administered for 7–10 days followed by oral therapy for an additional 14 days. For those in whom osteomyelitis is identified, a minimum of 6–8 weeks' parenteral therapy is recommended if the offending tissue is not removed in its entirety (Chapter 2.43). Limb-threatening infections require immediate hospitalization, bed rest and a strict nonweight-bearing regimen, even if signs and symptoms of systemic infection are absent. Although medical stabilization, metabolic and glycemic control (in diabetic patients) and antimicrobial therapy are important, debridement should not be delayed. Failure to debride necrotic, infected tissue and to drain purulent collections increases the risk of amputation. The initial debridement must be performed independently of the status of the arterial circulation and revascularization should be postponed until sepsis is controlled (Chapter 2.3).

It should be noted that definitive management of the ulcer will require treatment of the underlying cause. For example, up to 60% of diabetic patients with nonhealing ulcers have associated arterial insufficiency. Therefore the arterial circulation must be critically evaluated in all diabetics presenting with a foot ulcer. Once the ulcer has healed, a life-long program of proper footwear, education, and close follow-up for routine callus and nail care must be maintained. In addition, the tetanus vaccination status must be ascertained in all patients presenting with ulceration or infection.

FURTHER READING

Caputo GM, Cavanagh PR, Ulbrecht JS, *et al.* Assessment and management of foot disease in patients with diabetes. N Engl J Med 1994;331:854–60.

Lipsy BA, Pecoraro RE, Wheat LJ. The diabetic foot. Soft tissue and bone infection. Infect Dis Clin North Am 1990;4:409–32.

Grayson ML, Gibbons GW, Habershaw GH, *et al.* Use of ampicillin/sulbactam versus imipenem/cilastatin in the treatment of limb threatening foot infections in diabetic patients. Clin Infect Dis 1994;18:683–93.

Role of hyperbaric oxygen in the management of gas gangrene

Athena Stoupis

INTRODUCTION

Gas gangrene (clostridial myonecrosis) is one of the most serious, limb-threatening and possibly life-threatening infectious diseases (Chapter 2.3). It may occur as a complication of surgery or trauma or it may occur spontaneously. Rapid surgical decompression and excision of necrotic tissue along with antibiotic therapy have been the mainstay of treatment. Over the past 30 years, the use of hyperbaric oxygen (HBO; 100% oxygen at two to three times the atmospheric pressure at sea level) as an adjunct therapy has demonstrated diminished mortality rates and diminished tissue loss. However, its use remains controversial given the paucity of controlled clinical trials that have examined the specific efficacy of this modality.

PATHOGENESIS

Clostridial myonecrosis occurs when the oxygen tension (PO_2) of a necrotic wound is low, allowing the germination of clostridial spores and subsequent release of lethal toxins, which initiate the fulminant phase of hemolysis, loss of local host defenses and tissue necrosis.

Over 20 exotoxins are produced by *Clostridium perfringens*. The most virulent toxin appears to be the α-toxin. A tissue PO_2 of 250mmHg inhibits the production of α–toxin *in vitro*. Tissue oxygen levels of 300–400mmHg have been measured in patients during HBO therapy at 2 atmospheres. Once toxin production is halted, the disease cycle is broken and clinical improvement follows. Some investigators have shown direct inhibition of *Clostridium perfringens in vitro* by HBO therapy.

CLINICAL FINDINGS OF ACUTE GAS GANGRENE
Severe soft tissue pain Disproportionate tachycardia Skin changes (bullae, bronze discoloration) Gram-positive rods found on tissue smears Demonstrable myonecrosis and gas formation in imaging studies

Fig. 8.6 Clinical findings of acute gas gangrene.

COMPLICATIONS OF HBO THERAPY
Air embolism Combustion Confinement anxiety Ear or sinus pain Generalized tonic–clonic seizures Pneumothorax Transient myopia Tympanic membrane rupture

Fig. 8.7 Complications of hyperbaric oxygen therapy.

In addition, HBO increases the oxygen supply to the surrounding tissues of the wound, allowing normal phagocytosis and free radical formation by granulocytes, further assisting in the tissue repair process.

Low tissue oxygen tension levels reduce collagen synthesis. An increased oxygen supply enhances the rate of collagen synthesis and wound healing. Finally, although hyperoxia initially reduces the rate of capillary growth, a sharp increase of angiogenesis follows within the first 24 hours of oxygen therapy, allowing migration of cells into the previously hypoxic areas and further tissue proliferation.

MICROBIOLOGY

Clostridium spp. are Gram-positive, obligate anaerobic organisms. They are widespread in the environment, and they can be cultured from soil, clothing and the intestinal flora of humans.

Clostridium perfringens is the most commonly isolated organism in gas gangrene (80–95%). Other organisms less commonly implicated as the cause of gas gangrene include *Clostridium novyi* (10–40%) and *Clostridium septicum* (5–20%) (Chapter 8.21).

CLINICAL FEATURES

The incubation period of gas gangrene is usually less than 24 hours. The most significant clinical sign is intense pain that is out of proportion to the pain usually associated with the preceding injury or surgical procedure (Fig. 8.6). The patient rapidly becomes ill with fever, tachycardia, hemodynamic compromise and change in mental status.

Tense 'woody hard' edema in the vicinity of the wound develops. Bullae and vesicles may appear. Putrid serosanguinous drainage may develop in the overlying skin blebs and often drains from open wounds. Crepitus may develop, but it is a late sign of true gas gangrene.

INVESTIGATIONS

Early diagnosis is critical and is usually based on the clinical appearance of the patient. Demonstration of Gram-positive rods in the wound exudate gives rapid microbiologic identification that can be confirmed on subsequent anaerobic wound cultures. Blood cultures are usually negative and may not be helpful in establishing the diagnosis. Computized tomography scanning may show involvement of muscle and fascial planes.

MANAGEMENT

Early initiation of antibiotic therapy and rapid surgical decompression and removal of necrotic tissue are essential for a favorable outcome.

There is no consensus over the timing of adjuvant HBO therapy in relation to surgical intervention. The paucity of controlled randomized clinical trials for the use of HBO in gas gangrene has created controversy amongst investigators. Several studies have indicated that the combination of surgery, antibiotics and antecedent HBO therapy have reduced morbidity and mortality from 80–90% to 20–30% in both human and animal models.

In one study, a dog model of clinical gas gangrene infection was used. All of the infected controls and dogs randomized to surgery alone or HBO therapy alone died. Survival was 50% with antibiotics alone, 70% with antibiotics and surgery, and 95% with the combination of antibiotics, HBO therapy and surgery.

However, in human studies, the efficacy of HBO therapy was often determined retrospectively and the inclusion criteria of some of the cases was variable. Some investigators also argue that the large medical centers that have HBO chambers readily available also provide aggressive surgical and intensive care support, which may have an impact on morbidity and mortality outcomes.

However, most investigators advocate that HBO therapy before surgery has the following potential benefits:
- clearer demarcation of the borders between viable tissue and devitalized tissue, permitting more conservative tissue debridement; and
- substantial improvement and stabilization of the severely ill patient before surgery, with inhibition of toxin production.

Others advocate that surgery is indicated before HBO therapy, given the fulminant, life-threatening course of gas gangrene and the need for rapid debridement of necrotic tissue. Most clinical experience is weighted towards antecedent HBO therapy.

Surgical debridement should not be delayed when a HBO chamber is not readily available. Arrangements should be made for transfer to the appropriate institution that can provide HBO therapy after initial surgical debridement. If fasciotomy is indicated for relief of compartment syndrome, then it should be performed before HBO therapy.

To be effective, HBO must be inhaled directly through the atmosphere, through an endotracheal tube in a monochamber, or through tight-fitting masks or hoods or endotracheal tubes in a multiple occupancy chamber. For HBO, pressure is expressed in multiples of the atmospheric pressure at sea level, which is 1 atmosphere (760mmHg).

The standard HBO therapy protocol consists of multiple early treatment sessions administered at 3 atmospheres for 90 minutes or 2.5 atmospheres for 120 minutes. Three treatments are given during the first 24 hours, then 2 treatments per day for an average of 7 chamber treatments.

COMPLICATIONS OF HYPERBARIC OXYGEN THERAPY

The most common complaint during HBO treatment is the experience of ear or sinus pain (Fig. 8.7). Persistent pain may require myringotomy. Patients who have sinus infection also require nasal decongestants to avoid barotrauma.

Generalized seizures have also occurred with oxygen toxicity and are usually controlled with anticonvulsants. During the immediate seizure episode removal of the oxygen mask may promptly terminate seizures. Patients may also develop transient myopia, the cause of which is unknown. It is usually reversible within 2 months of completing therapy.

Another significant side effect is the development of tension pneumothorax secondary to barotrauma. Immediate recompression with the placement of a chest tube is required.

Claustrophobia is also a common side effect. Many patients require tranquilizers for relief of their confinement anxiety.

Complications of HBO therapy used for gas gangrene treatment fortunately are rare with the use of relatively low oxygen pressures (2–3 atmospheres) and with the short duration of HBO treatments.

FURTHER READING

De Mello FJ, Haglin JJ, Hitchcock CR. Comparative study of experimental *Clostridium perfringens* infection in dogs treated with antibiotic, surgery, and hyperbaric oxygen. Surgery 1973;73:936–41.

Grim PS, Gottlieb LJ, Boddie A, Batson E. Hyperbaric oxygen therapy. JAMA 1990;263:2216–20.

Hirn M. Hyperbaric oxygen in the treatment of gas gangrene and perineal necrotizing fasciitis. A clinical and experimental study. Eur J Surg 1993;Suppl 570:1–36.

La Van FB, Hunt TK. Oxygen and wound healing. Clin Plast Surg 1990;17:463–72.

Maapaniemi T, Nylander G, Sirsjo A, Larsson J. Hyperbaric oxygen reduces ischemia-induced skeletal muscle injury. Plast Reconstr Surg 1996;97:602–7.

Park MK, Myers RA, Marzella L. Oxygen tensions and infections: modulation of microbial growth, activity of antimicrobial agents, and immunologic responses. Clin Infect Dis 1992;14:720–40.

Tibbles PM, Edelsberg JS. Hyperbaric-oxygen therapy. N Engl J Med 1996;334:1642–8.

chapter

9

Generalized and Regional Lymphadenopathy

Ethan Rubinstein, Itzchak Levi & Bina Rubinovitch

The lymph nodes are major components of the body's surveillance system against foreign invaders; they function as a filter to trap microorganisms, cancerous cells and immune complexes. The lymphoid system grows rapidly during childhood and achieves twice the adult size by early adolescence. Although lymphoid tissue begins to regress during mid-adolescence, it does not reach adult maturity until the age of 20–25 years. Peripheral lymphadenopathy, therefore, is a common finding throughout late childhood, adolescence and young adulthood.[1] Lymphadenopathy (i.e. disease of lymph nodes) may be due to primary lymphoproliferative diseases as well as to secondary reactive (infectious and noninfectious) or infiltrative diseases. Figure 9.1 summarizes the differential diagnosis of lymphadenopathy.

EPIDEMIOLOGY

In children, the cause of lymphadenopathy is clinically apparent in most cases. In approximately 80% of cases it is benign, reactive, and most commonly due to an infectious cause. In contrast, lymphadenopathy in adults more often reflects serious disease. The probability of neoplasm affecting enlarged peripheral lymph nodes increases steadily with age; in those older than 50 years, more than 60% of the cases of lymphadenopathy are due to malignancy.[2,3] In tropical and subtropical parts of the world, lymphadenopathy requires other considerations.

PATHOGENESIS AND PATHOLOGY

Lymph nodes are widely distributed throughout the body, especially at potential portals of entry into the body (Fig. 9.2). The normal lymph

DIFFERENTIAL DIAGNOSIS OF LYMPHADENOPATHY	
Reactive	**Infectious diseases**
	Viral (e.g. infectious mononucleosis syndrome, rubella)
	Bacterial (e.g. pyogenic, cat-scratch disease)
	Mycobacterial (*Mycobacterium tuberculosis*, atypical mycobacteria)
	Spirochetal (e.g. syphilis, leptospirosis)
	Chlamydial (e.g. lymphogranuloma venereum)
	Fungal (e.g. coccidioidomycosis)
	Parasitic (e.g. toxoplasmosis)
	Noninfectious diseases
	Sarcoidosis
	Connective tissue diseases (e.g. systemic lupus erythematosus)
	Kawasaki's disease
	Rosai–Dorfman disease
	Kikuchi's disease
	Castleman's disease
	Drug hypersensitivity (e.g. to phenytoin)
	Silicone breast implantation
Infiltrative	**Malignant diseases**
	Metastatic carcinoma
	Metastatic melanoma, germ cell tumor
	Leukemia
	Nonmalignant diseases
	Lipid storage diseases (e.g. Gaucher's disease, Niemann–Pick disease)
	Amyloidosis
Primary lymphoproliferative diseases	Lymphoma (e.g. Hodgkin's, non-Hodgkin's)
	Angioimmunoblastic lymphadenopathy
	Lymphomatoid granulomatosis
	Malignant histiocytosis

Fig. 9.1 Differential diagnosis of lymphadenopathy.

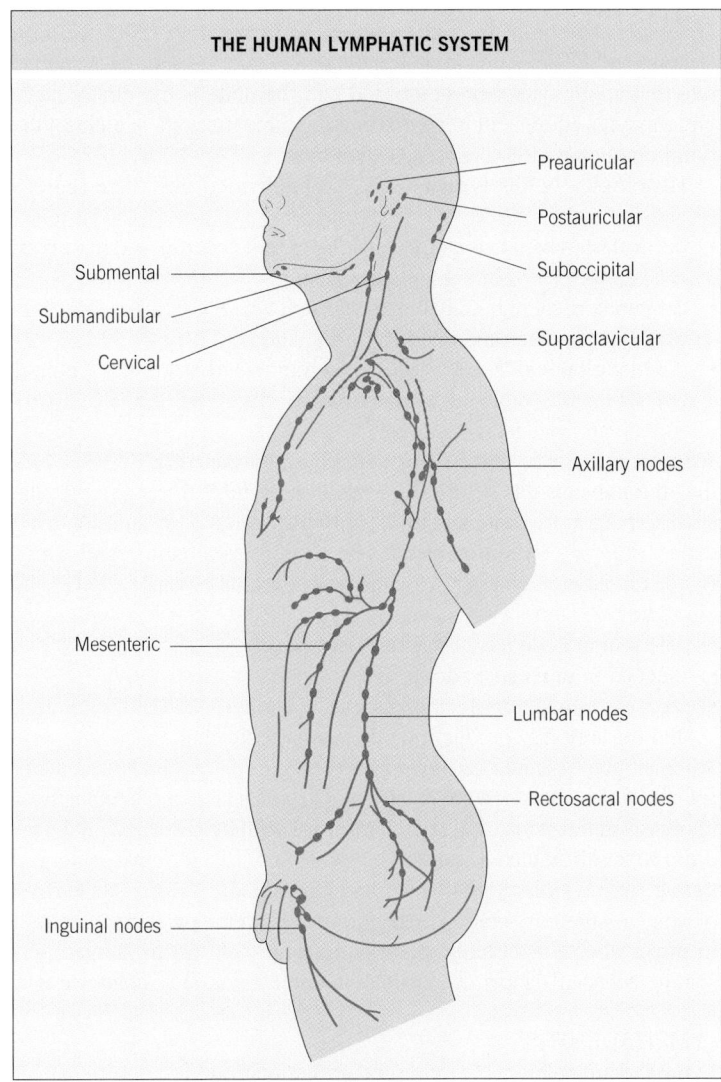

Fig. 9.2 The human lymphatic system.

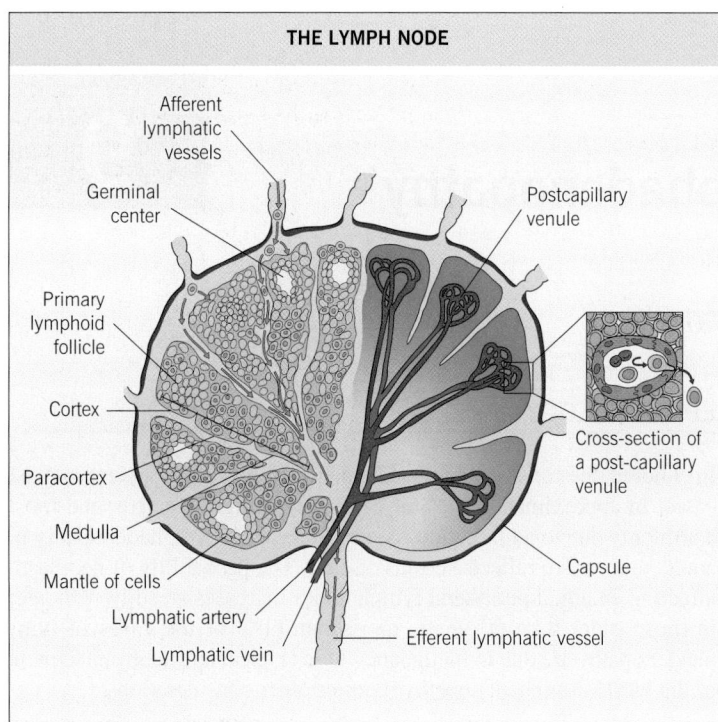

THE LYMPH NODE

Fig. 9.3 The lymph node.

GENERAL HISTOLOGIC CORRELATES OF SOME DISEASES THAT CAUSE LYMPHADENITIS	
Histologic feature	Type of disease and examples of causative organism
Acute suppurative lymphadenitis	Pyogenic infections (*Streptococcus pyogenes*, *Staphylococcus aureus*, *Yersinia pestis*)
Lymphadenitis with caseating necrosis	Tuberculosis (*Mycobacterium tuberculosis*)
	Atypical mycobacteria
Necrotizing granulomatous lymphadenitis	Cat-scratch disease (*Bartonella henselae*)
	Tularemia (*Francisella tularensis*)
	Leishmaniasis (*Leishmania braziliensis*, *L. major*)
	Lymphogranuloma venereum (*Chlamydia trachomatis*)
Non-necrotizing granulomatous lymphadenitis	Histoplasmosis (*Histoplasma capsulatum*)
	Coccidioidomycosis (*Coccidioides immitis*)
	Sarcoidosis
Necrotizing nongranulomatous lymphadenitis	Kikuchi's syndrome
	Systemic lupus erythematosus

Fig. 9.4 General histologic correlates of some diseases that cause lymphadenitis.

node is an oval, encapsulated, soft structure; the size ranges from 1cm to 2cm in diameter. The node contains a reticular network packed with lymphocytes, macrophages and dendritic cells. A single lymph node weighs about 1g and contains approximately 2000 million lymphocytes. The lymph node is a dynamic structure and the exchange rate of lymphocytes between blood and the node is extremely high: lymphocytes equivalent to approximately three times the weight of the lymph node pass into the lymph each hour.[4]

Histologically, the lymph node can be divided into three regions (Fig. 9.3):[5]

- the cortex, which is the outermost layer and is composed mainly of B lymphocytes and macrophages arranged in primary follicles;
- the paracortical region, below the cortex, which is composed mainly of T lymphocytes and dendritic cells; and
- the medulla, which is the innermost region and has fewer lymphocytes than the other regions but more plasma cells that actively secrete antibodies.

Afferent lymphatic vessels empty the lymph drained from the tissues into the subcapsular sinus; from there the lymph flows through the cortex, paracortex and medulla, allowing phagocytic and dendritic cells to trap any foreign material. The efferent lymphatic vessels carry lymph enriched in lymphocytes and antibodies; this lymph re-enters the circulatory system.

The lymph node has two main functions:

- it acts as a defensive barrier and
- it serves as a factory for lymphocyte maturation and differentiation and for antibody production during antigenic challenge.

After antigenic stimulation, the primary follicle enlarges into a secondary follicle, which contains a germinal center in which large proliferating lymphoblasts and plasma cells are interspersed with macrophages and dendritic cells surrounded by packed lymphocytes. The germinal center is a site where B lymphocytes are intensively activated and differentiated into plasma and memory cells. The dendritic cells in the paracortex are rich in major histocompatibility class II molecules and act as antigen presenting cells to T-helper cells, which in turn activate B lymphocytes.

LYMPHADENITIS

Lymphadenitis (Fig. 9.4) represents inflammation of the lymph node. The initial response to acute inflammation consists of swelling and hyperplasia of the sinusoidal lining cells and infiltration by leukocytes. The process may progress to abscess formation depending on the micro-organism involved and the host response.

Acutely inflamed nodes are most commonly caused by local trapping of microbes; acute inflammation commonly affects the cervical nodes in association with infections of the teeth or tonsils or the axillary or inguinal nodes in association with infections in the limbs. Generalized acute lymphadenopathy is characteristic of viral infections, bacteremias or diseases caused by exotoxins, as well as a variety of other noninfectious diseases. In acute lymphadenitis the lymph node becomes enlarged owing to cellular infiltration and edema. As a consequence of distension of the capsule, the node becomes tender. Abscess formation causes the node to become fluctuant. Penetration of the infection through the overlying subcutis and skin surface may produce draining sinuses, particularly when nodes have undergone suppurative necrosis. Control of the infection with resolution of the inflammatory changes leads to shrinkage of the node. Nodes resume their former macroscopic and microscopic appearance if the infection has not caused extensive tissue destruction. If severe scarring and fibrosis ensue, nodes may remain firm and palpable.

Chronic lymphadenitis is typically a proliferative response, with either follicular hyperplasia or paracortical lymphoid hyperplasia, depending on the cause of inflammation. Characteristically, the nodes are not tender.[6]

CLINICAL FEATURES

REGIONAL LYMPHADENOPATHY
Acute suppurative lymphadenitis

Acute suppurative lymphadenitis is commonly caused by a pyogenic infection. The inflammatory neutrophilic reaction arises due to drainage of bacteria – *Staphylococcus aureus* or group A streptococci – from an infected site. The most common sites of involvement are the submandibular, cervical, inguinal and axillary lymph nodes. The affected lymph node is extremely tender and firm, although it may be fluctuant, and the overlying skin may be red and warm. There are usually systemic manifestations. Acute cervical lymphadenitis due to a pyogenic infection is more common in children than adults. Nowadays it is commonly due to staphylococcal infections of the face or neck and, uncommonly, it may be a complication of streptococcal pharyngitis.[7] Acute pyogenic cervical lymphadenitis is unilateral. In contrast, acute bilateral cervical lymphadenitis is commonly due to viral upper respiratory infection, infectious mononucleosis, streptococcal pharyngitis or localized periodontal infections. Acute suppurative axillary lymphadenitis is a severe infection with prominent systemic manifestations and axillary pain that radiates to the shoulder and down to the arm. The axilla, arm, shoulder and supraclavicular and pectoral areas are markedly edematous, but there are no signs of skin infection or lymphangitis. The portal of entry of the infecting bacteria (group A streptococci or *S. aureus*) is often a traumatic lesion of the arm.[8] Acute suppurative inguinal lymphadenitis due to group A streptococci has been reported in patients infected with HIV with or without chronic lymphadenopathy. Rapidly enlarging lymph nodes may be accompanied by systemic manifestations, including toxic shock syndrome, without obvious genital or skin lesions.[9,10]

Patients with chronic granulomatous disease experience recurrent pyogenic infections, of which the most common manifestations are lower respiratory tract infections, suppurative lymphadenitis, subcutaneous abscesses and hepatic abscesses.[11] The infecting pathogens are catalase-positive organisms such as *S. aureus*, *Serratia marcescens*, *Burkholderia (Pseudomonas) cepacia* and *Aspergillus* spp. The histologic appearance of the lymph node is one of inflammation with granuloma formation and necrosis.[11,12]

Cat-scratch disease

Cat-scratch disease typically manifests after a cat scratch or bite as regional lymphadenopathy distal to the involved lymph node. The mode of transmission is presumably direct contact with the causative agent, *Bartonella henselae*. The disease occurs worldwide, with healthy children and adolescents being most frequently affected.[13] A history of a trivial cat scratch or a bite by a kitten can be elicited in most cases.[14] Rarely, a dog or monkey is implicated.

Tender lymphadenopathy develops within 1–3 weeks after inoculation. Commonly, an erythematous papule at the site of inoculation precedes the development of lymphadenopathy and may last for several weeks. Regional lymph node enlargement is the sole manifestation in one-half of the patients. Most commonly the cervical, axillary or epitrochlear lymph nodes are involved, but any peripheral nodes at multiple sites may be enlarged. In one-third of the patients, low grade fever is present, and about 15% have systemic manifestations such as malaise, headache, splenomegaly and sore throat. Unusual clinical manifestations occur in fewer than 10% of patients; the most frequent of these is the oculoglandular syndrome of Parinaud,[14,15] which is conjunctivitis with ipsilateral preauricular lymphadenitis (Fig. 9.5). The adenopathy subsides spontaneously within several months. Occasionally, aspiration of a suppurative lymph node is needed to relieve pain.

The diagnosis is based on epidemiologic exposure and can be confirmed by detection of serum antibody to *B. henselae*.[14] In atypical presentations or whenever a neoplastic or mycobacterial process is suspected, a lymph node biopsy or aspirate may be needed. Early in the course of the infection the involved lymph node shows lymphoid hyperplasia; later, granuloma formation with central areas of necrosis give the distinctive histopathologic appearance of necrotizing granulomatous lymphadenitis. The histologic reaction cannot differentiate cat-scratch disease from diseases such as tularemia, lymphogranuloma venereum and fungal and mycobacterial infections. Sometimes, small pleomorphic bacteria can be visualized with the Warthin–Starry silver stain in necrotic foci of early-stage microabscesses. A polymerase chain reaction (PCR) assay for detecting *B. henselae* DNA in clinical specimens has been found to be a sensitive and specific tool,[16] but it is not widely available.

Toxoplasmosis

Acute acquired infection with *Toxoplasma gondii* is common worldwide. The prevalence of seropositivity by the fourth decade of life in the USA is 30–50%, and higher than 90% in certain areas of western Europe.[17,18] Acute infection occurs primarily in patients in the second to fourth decade of life. In the immunocompetent host the infection is most often asymptomatic. In 10–20% of patients the infection is self-limiting, with lymphadenopathy being the most frequent clinical manifestation. In 90% of patients with clinically apparent infection, regional lymphadenopathy, usually of the head and neck, is the sole manifestation. A single node is usually involved, most commonly a posterior cervical, anterior cervical, axillary or suboccipital node; occasionally an inguinal node is involved. Retroperitoneal or mesenteric lymphadenopathy may occur and can cause abdominal pain. Cases of toxoplasmic hilar lymphadenopathy have also been reported.

On palpation, the lymph nodes are discrete, of varying firmness and may or may not be tender; they rarely suppurate and they do not ulcerate. The histologic appearance is distinctive but may sometimes be confused with lymphoma, cat-scratch disease or Kikuchi's lymphadenitis. Lymphadenopathy is associated with fever, headache, sore throat and myalgia in approximately 15% of patients. Toxoplasmosis may rarely cause a syndrome resembling mononucleosis. In uncommon situations lymphadenopathy may persist or recur for months and pose a diagnostic challenge.[17]

Toxoplasmosis has been estimated to cause between 3 and 7% of clinically significant lymphadenopathy. Of major importance is the diagnosis of infection in pregnant women and the subsequent management of the fetus, and the need to differentiate toxoplasmosis from neoplasia (Hodgkin's and non-Hodgkin's lymphoma and carcinoma). Failure to consider toxoplasmosis in the differential diagnosis frequently results in unnecessary surgical biopsies.[17]

In the immunocompetent host, serologic testing is sufficient for the diagnosis of toxoplasmic lymphadenitis because it occurs almost exclusively as a manifestation of the acute acquired infection. A negative result in the Sabin–Feldman dye test or a comparable test for detecting *Toxoplasma* IgG in the first 3 months practically excludes the diagnosis. Acute infection is likely if elevated IgM antibody titer on enzyme-linked immunosorbent assay is present. In patients with equivocal IgM antibody results (after 3 months), detection of IgA or IgE antibodies or an acute pattern in the differential agglutination titers may be helpful.[18]

Mycobacterial lymphadenitis

Tuberculous lymphadenitis is the most frequent form of extrapulmonary tuberculosis, and in Western countries it accounts for 5% of cases of tuberculosis.[19] In areas where both AIDS and tuberculosis are endemic (e.g. in central Africa), tuberculous lymphadenitis is the presenting sign of tuberculosis in 50% of young children and is often associated with intrathoracic disease; a contact with an index case is often apparent.[20] In the past, *Mycobacterium bovis* was a common cause of cervical lymphadenitis in countries with a high incidence of bovine tuberculosis.[9] Currently, most cases of mycobacterial cervical lymphadenitis are caused by *M. tuberculosis* or by atypical mycobacteria, especially *M. scrofulaceum* and *M. avium* complex (MAC). In the USA an abrupt change in the predominant etiologic agents from *M. scrofulaceum* to MAC was

OCULOGLANDULAR SYNDROMES		
Disease	Infecting organism	Features
Cat-scratch disease	*Bartonella henselae*	Parinaud's sign in 3% Conjunctivitis in 6%
Tularemia	*Francisella tularensis*	Parinaud's sign in 5%
Lymphogranuloma venereum	*Chlamydia trachomatis*	Parinaud's sign in <1%
Pharyngoconjunctival fever	Adenovirus 3, 7	Common in children
Epidemic keratoconjunctivitis	Adenovirus 8, 19, 37	Occasionally seen in adults
Chagas' disease	*Trypanosoma cruzi*	Romaña's sign

Fig. 9.5 Oculoglandular syndromes.

noted in the 1970s.[21] *Mycobacterium avium* complex is also seen in children in areas where *M. bovis* has been eradicated and *M. tuberculosis* is rare. Recent reports have documented rare cases of childhood lymphadenitis caused by other mycobacteria (*M. interjectum* or *M. malmoense*).[22–24]

Tuberculous cervical lymphadenitis (scrofula) is caused by spread of the infection from the lung, usually by the hematogenous or lymphatic route. When the source of infection is milk contaminated with *M. bovis*, the primary focus is in the tonsils or the pharynx.

Scrofula most often presents as a unilateral firm, red, painless mass located along the upper border of the sternocleidomastoid muscle or in the supraclavicular area.[23] Occasionally, tuberculous lymphadenitis may be found in the axilla (Fig. 9.6). The process progresses indolently and is usually not accompanied by systemic symptoms. Miliary tuberculosis should be suspected when the lymphadenopathy is generalized, localized outside the cervical chain, or accompanied by systemic symptoms.

In HIV-infected or otherwise immunocompromised patients, the course of the disease is severe with bilateral lymphadenopathy and systemic symptoms such as fever, night sweats and weight loss. Patients infected with HIV are more likely to develop extrapulmonary disease, often in conjunction with pulmonary tuberculosis.[25]

The diagnosis of mycobacterial lymphadenitis is confirmed by lymph node histology and bacteriology examinations. Fine-needle aspiration reveals the presence of granuloma but only rarely yields positive smears or cultures.[22] Bacteriology and histopathology examinations are complementary diagnostic tools, for *M. tuberculosis* has been cultured from lymph nodes without caseating granuloma and atypical mycobacteria have been cultured from lymph nodes with classic histopathologic appearance for tuberculosis. Acid-fast bacilli are only rarely seen in smears except in HIV-positive patients, in whom positive smear results are much more frequent because of the high density of organisms. Therefore, a specific culture of aspirated lymph node should be performed routinely. New diagnostic tools such as PCR and hybridization and blotting techniques hold promise for rapid and precise diagnosis.

INGUINAL LYMPHADENOPATHY

Sexually transmitted diseases (STDs) and metastatic genital neoplastic disease are the most common causes of inguinal lymphadenopathy. The differential diagnosis of infectious inguinal lymphadenopathy is shown in Figure 9.7.

Chancroid

Chancroid is caused by *Haemophilus ducreyi* and in some parts of the world (e.g. Thailand) it is one of the most common causes of genital ulcer with inguinal lymphadenopathy. The chancroid ulcer is a painful, nonindurated lesion that appears 1 day to several weeks after inoculation. Inguinal lymphadenitis occurs in between one-third and one-half of untreated cases. The lymph nodes are enlarged, painful and tender. The process is most commonly unilateral and, without treatment, it can progress to suppuration with periadenitis and involvement of the overlying skin (bubo). Coinfection with other organisms [e.g. herpes simplex virus (HSV) or *Chlamydia trachomatis*] is not uncommon. The differential diagnosis includes other STDs, especially syphilis, herpes simplex and lymphogranuloma venereum, secondary pyogenic infections of traumatic lesions and neoplasia.

Culture provides the definitive diagnosis; however, *H. ducreyi* is a fastidious organism and immediate direct inoculation into specific culture media is required for bacterial growth and isolation. Chemotherapy is sufficient in most uncomplicated cases but abscesses that are more than 5cm in diameter may need surgical drainage.[26]

Lymphogranuloma venereum

Lymphogranuloma venereum is a rare STD caused by *C. trachomatis* serovars L1, L2 and L3. The typical vesicular lesions appear 1–2 weeks after inoculation but the incubation period varies between 5 and 20 days. The lesions often go unnoticed by the patient. Inguinal lymphadenopathy appears 1–6 weeks after the vesicles disappear. The lymphadenopathy is most commonly unilateral but it is bilateral in 30–40% of the patients. The nodes are painful and the groove sign (cleavage of the enlarged nodes by the inguinal ligament) is seen in 25% of patients (Fig. 9.8). The involved lymph nodes frequently coalesce to form a bubo. If untreated, the nodes, which are filled with bacteria, rupture and a nonhealing fistula is formed. The anorectal syndrome, which occurs mainly in women and homosexual men, results from involvement of the pelvic lymph nodes. In the male, abscess formation may occur in the dorsal lymphatic of the penis and cause tissue destruction and elephantiasis of the penis. *Chlamydia trachomatis* can be isolated from both blood and aspirates of lymph nodes in approximately 30% of cases. Incision of the bubo is not warranted for diagnosis and positive serologic tests (complement fixation antibody test or microimmunofluorescence test) in the appropriate clinical setting are highly sensitive and specific for the diagnosis.[27]

Syphilis

The lymphadenopathy of primary syphilis is easily differentiated from chancroid and lymphogranuloma venereum because nodes involved in syphilis are firm, only moderately enlarged, nonsuppurative and painless. The classic primary chancre appears 14–30 days after inoculation and is a nonexudative, painless ulcer. In the immunocompetent patient only one chancre appears but in the immunocompromised patient, especially in patients with AIDS, multiple chancres may be seen. In women and homosexual men, the chancre may be located in the perianal region or in the anal canal. Regional painless lymphadenopathy is characteristic at this stage of disease. The chancre usually heals and disappears after 3–6 weeks, but the lymphadenopathy may persist for longer. The symptoms of secondary syphilis appear 2–8 weeks after the chancre has healed, with generalized lymphadenopathy and various skin lesions in the majority of patients. Epitrochlear lymphadenopathy suggests the diagnosis.[28]

Genital herpes

The typical vesicles associated with inguinal lymphadenopathy usually suggest the correct diagnosis. Rarely, lymph node enlargement may appear before the rash develops.[29] Herpes simplex virus is the most common cause of genital ulcers in the Western world. The incidence of genital herpes rose in the pre-AIDS era but it has been stable in the

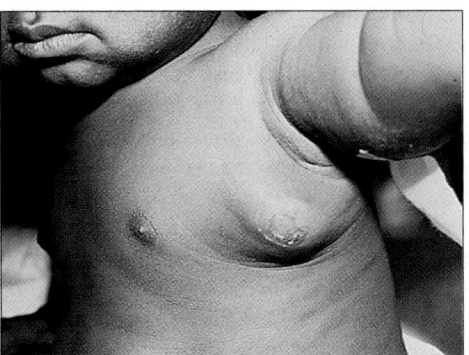

Fig. 9.6 Tuberculous lymphadenitis of the axilla.

DIFFERENTIAL DIAGNOSIS OF INFECTIOUS INGUINAL LYMPHADENOPATHY	
Sexually transmitted diseases	**Other diseases**
Syphilis	Pyogenic infections
Lymphogranuloma venereum	Cellulitis
Chancroid	Plague
Genital herpes	Filariasis
Granuloma inguinale	Onchocerciasis

Fig. 9.7 Differential diagnosis of infectious inguinal lymphadenopathy.

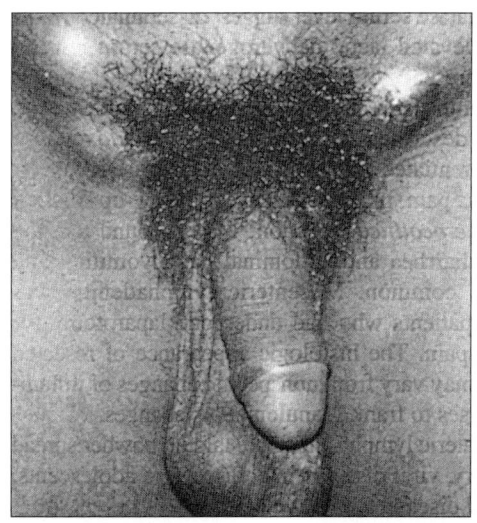

Fig. 9.8 Groove sign of lymphogranuloma venereum. There is cleavage of extensive lymphadenopathy by the inguinal ligament.

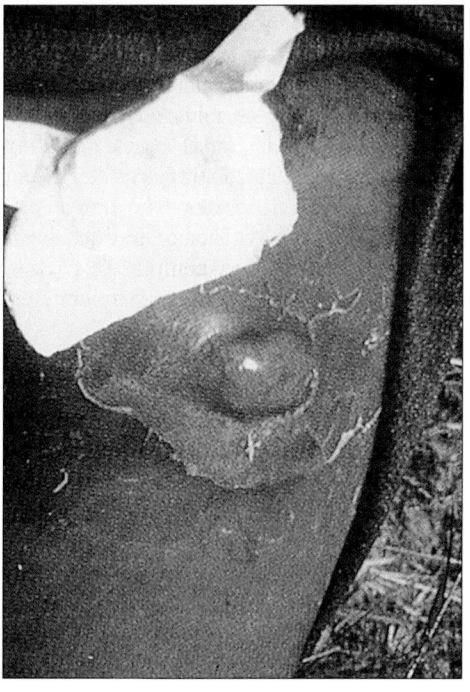

Fig. 9.9 Bubonic plague. Femoral lymph nodes matted together to form the classic bubo.

Granuloma inguinale

Granuloma inguinale (donovanosis) is caused by *Calymmatobacterium granulomatis*. The disease is rare in the Western world but it is a major cause of genital ulcer in southeast India, Brazil and some parts of Africa. The penile papules of granuloma inguinale appear within days of inoculation and rapidly ulcerate to form a red granulomatous painless ulcer with a characteristic surface that bleeds easily on contact. Subcutaneous spread into the inguinal region results in swellings (pseudobubos) that are not a true adenitis. Lymphedema and elephantiasis occasionally result from scarring and blockage of the lymphatics. Granuloma inguinale should be differentiated from other genital ulcerative lesions with inguinal lymphadenopathy. The diagnosis is established through the demonstration of the typical intracellular Donovan bodies in stained smears obtained from the lesions.[31]

Plague and tularemia

Plague and tularemia are both zoonotic infections that produce similar diseases, with fever and regional lymphadenitis.[32]

Plague is caused by *Yersinia pestis*. It is distributed worldwide (with the exception of Europe and Australia). Most human plague is of the bubonic form and is transmitted by bites of infected fleas. After an incubation period of 2–8 days, patients are affected by the sudden onset of fever, chills, malaise and headache. Usually at the same time or after a few hours, a painfully swollen regional lymph node appears in the draining area of the inoculation site, commonly in the axilla, neck or groin. The primary lesion is occasionally found at the bite site and may later develop into extensive cellulitis or abscess. Over the next few days, the discrete nodes become matted together to form the characteristic bubo (Fig. 9.9). If untreated, infection spreads hematogenously and results in a 'septic' phase with organ involvement, including secondary pneumonic plague.

Diagnosis of plague should be suspected in an acutely ill patient with an extremely tender cluster of lymph nodes when there has been the appropriate epidemiologic exposure. Isolation of *Y. pestis* from bubo aspirate, blood and any other involved organ is possible, but growth is slow and rapid identification of the bacteria is possible by Gram stain or Wayson stain. A patient suspected of having plague should be isolated, and treatment should begin immediately. The prognosis is favorable in patients who are treated early.

Tularemia is restricted to the northern hemisphere. Over 80% of infections are acquired by handling infected animals or by tick or deer fly bites. Infection commonly manifests as ulceroglandular syndrome. The most common portal of entry is the skin, with an ulcer or pustule developing 1–10 days after exposure; regional lymphadenopathy, usually axillary or epitrochlear, follows. The lymph nodes may suppurate. Systemic manifestations are common, but severe endotoxemia as seen in plague is uncommon. The oculoglandular syndrome is seen when the portal of entry is the conjunctiva (as happens when the eyes are contaminated with infected fluids). Conjunctivitis, conjunctival ulcerations and papules on the eyelids appear, and lymph nodes of the head and neck become inflamed. Diagnosis of typical ulceroglandular tularemia in a patient with the appropriate epidemiologic exposure is made on clinical grounds. In other less obvious settings diagnosis relies on serologic studies.

Filariasis and onchoceriasis should also be considered in the differential diagnosis of inguinal bubo formation; these are discussed below (See 'Lymphadenopathy of tropical origin').

MEDIASTINAL AND HILAR LYMPHADENOPATHY

Mediastinal or hilar lymph node enlargement may be detected because it causes symptoms (e.g. cough, dyspnea, hoarseness caused by recurrent laryngeal nerve compression, superior vena cava syndrome caused compression of the superior vena cava); on other occasions it is detected during routine chest radiographic screening. The presence of mediastinal lymphadenopathy is usually indicative of a significant disease and is frequently seen in lymphoma. In contrast, bilateral hilar

past decade. Women are reported to have higher rates of infection than men. Both HSV-1 and HSV-2 can cause genital herpes, but from epidemiologic studies it is estimated that HSV-2 causes more than 90% of genital herpes. The distinction between the two types of the virus is significant because HSV-1 infection is less severe and is less prone to recur than HSV-2.

Primary herpes genitalis infection is usually more severe than recurrent attacks. Genital lesions begin as macules and papules, followed by vesicles and ulcers that may appear and last for 2–3 weeks. Occasionally, primary infection is accompanied by systemic manifestations such as fever, malaise, aseptic meningitis (in 10% of patients) and extragenital lesions as well as dysuria and painful lymphadenopathy. In women, primary lesions appear on the vulva with involvement of the cervix. Lesions can also appear in the perineum, vagina, buttocks and perianal region. Urinary retention has been described in 15% of women. In males, the lesions are vesicular and are superimposed on an erythematous base. In homosexual men the lesions may appear on the buttocks and in the anal and perianal areas. The lymphadenopathy associated with primary herpes is either unilateral or bilateral and in severe cases generalized lymphadenopathy may also occur. Genital lesions and lymphadenopathy are common in genital herpes in the immunocompetent host; however, massive lymphadenitis is frequently seen in the immunocompromised patient. The diagnosis is based on isolation of HSV from a skin lesion, preferably from a vesicle.[30]

lymphadenopathy is more often benign and is seen in tuberculosis, sarcoidosis and endemic mycoses.[33]

Tuberculosis

Isolated mediastinal or hilar lymphadenopathy is an uncommon manifestation of tuberculosis, although tuberculosis should be considered, especially in high risk patients such as HIV-infected people or in people from Asia or Africa. Mediastinal and hilar lymphadenopathy can be a manifestation of primary disease or of reactivation of tuberculosis (Fig. 9.10). Isolated lymphadenopathy is relatively rare in postprimary tuberculosis.[34] Associated ipsilateral hilar or mediastinal adenopathy is almost universal in children with primary tuberculosis but it is less common in adults. In HIV-infected patients, mediastinal or hilar lymphadenopathy are usually present in tuberculosis even in the advanced stages of immunosuppression.

Endemic mycoses

Histoplasmosis. Histoplasmosis is a fungal infection acquired through inhalation. Histoplasmosis is endemic in the USA in the great river valleys of the Mississippi and Ohio. More than 90% of the primary infections are asymptomatic or only mildly symptomatic, although sudden enlargement of the hilar lymph nodes may cause substernal pain. Nonspecific systemic symptoms such as fever, headache, malaise and anorexia are common. Most patients recover within 2–6 weeks. Typical findings on chest radiography in symptomatic patients include patchy pneumonic infiltrates. Mediastinal and hilar lymphadenopathy is common in patients with or without parenchymal involvement. At times, extension of the infection from the pulmonary parenchyma to the adjacent mediastinal lymph nodes causes central caseating necrosis and granuloma formation with multinucleated giant cells. Resolution causes fibrosis of the affected nodes, which usually causes no symptoms. Rarely, the fibrotic lymph nodes invade mediastinal structures, resulting in esophageal stricture or compromise to the mediastinal blood or lymph vessels (fibrasing mediastinitis).[35]

Coccidioidomycosis. Coccidioidomycosis is endemic in the southwest USA, Mexico and Central and South America. The lymph nodes most commonly involved are the mediastinal and hilar lymph nodes. When there is involvement of the scalene or supraclavicular nodes, the organism can be isolated from these sites.[36]

Paracoccidioidomycosis. Paracoccidioidomycosis is endemic in Mexico and Central and South America. Most primary infections are asymptomatic. In 10% of patients there is lymphadenopathy, especially of the cervical, axillary and mediastinal nodes, with or without fistula formation. Characteristic budding yeasts may be demonstrated in aspirated material from lymph nodes.[37]

Sarcoidosis

Sarcoidosis is a multisystem granulomatous disease of unknown etiology. Bilateral symmetric hilar lymphadenopathy, usually with paratracheal adenopathy, is characteristic. Peripheral lymphadenopathy is rare. In the mild form of the disease (radiologic grading stage 1) mediastinal or hilar lymphadenopathy is usually discovered inadvertently in asymptomatic men undergoing a chest radiography for an unrelated cause. Computed tomography scanning can detect anterior mediastinal and subcarinal lymph nodes that are undetected by chest radiography. Biopsy of lung tissue, even without radiologic findings, is superior for histopathologic diagnosis than lymph node biopsy because it has a higher specificity. The lymph node often shows only nonspecific granuloma and therefore has a low diagnostic yield.[38]

ABDOMINAL AND RETROPERITONEAL LYMPHADENOPATHY

Abdominal and retroperitoneal lymphadenopathy are not usually inflammatory in origin but are frequently due to neoplasia. In the HIV-infected patient abdominal or retroperitoneal lymphadenopathy is commonly due to persistent generalized lymphadenopathy (PGL), disseminated MAC infection or lymphoma. Fever, night sweats and an elevated alkaline phosphatase serum level suggest disseminated MAC infection, whereas an elevated lactic dehydrogenase serum level is more suggestive of the presence of lymphoma.

Mesenteric lymphadenitis is frequently caused by *Y. enterocolitica*; some cases have been described with *Y. pseudotuberculosis*. The disease needs to be differentiated from appendicitis because it is manifested by right iliac fossa pain. In a recent 10-year follow-up study of 458 patients with *Y. enterocolitica* infection[39] it was found that the majority of cases had diarrhea and abdominal pain; vomiting and weight loss were also common. Mesenteric lymphadenitis was diagnosed in 43 of 56 patients who had undergone laparotomy for severe right iliac fossa pain. The histologic appearance of resected mesenteric lymph node may vary from nonspecific changes of inflammation and microabscesses to frank granulomatous changes.

Other causes of mesenteric lymphadenitis are talcum powder spread during abdominal surgery, viral diseases in children and adolescents, and inflammatory bowel disease.

GENERALIZED LYMPHADENOPATHY

Generalized lymphadenopathy is identified whenever three or more anatomically discrete groups of nodes are involved. Numerous infectious and noninfectious diseases cause generalized lymphadenopathy. Viral diseases predominate but systemic bacterial diseases, including tuberculosis, typhoid fever, brucellosis and leptospirosis, are not uncommon causes of generalized lymphadenopathy. The clinical setting is important in the differential diagnosis. The age of the patient, epidemiologic factors, accompanying physical findings (e.g. rash, organomegaly) or laboratory findings (e.g. atypical lymphocytes, eosinophilia) usually guide further diagnostic investigations.

INFECTIOUS MONONUCLEOSIS

Infectious mononucleosis is a syndrome that appears most commonly in children and young adolescents. It is classically characterized by acute onset of fever, tonsillopharyngitis, lymphadenopathy, splenomegaly and the appearance of atypical lymphocytes in peripheral blood.[40] In children and adolescents, Epstein–Barr virus (EBV) is the most frequent cause (80–90%) followed by cytomegalovirus (CMV; 8–16%).[41] It is usually a benign and self-limiting process. Patients may exhibit generalized lymphadenopathy, localized lymph node enlargement in unusual sites (e.g. the inguinal nodes), and lymphadenopathy without systemic manifestations. Rarely, a progressive, fatal disease develops in patients with X-linked lymphoproliferative disorder and in other immunocompromised patients.[40]

Complete recovery generally occurs within 1–26 weeks after onset of disease, although postinfectious asthenia is not an uncommon complication. Serious complications, sequelae and death are exceedingly

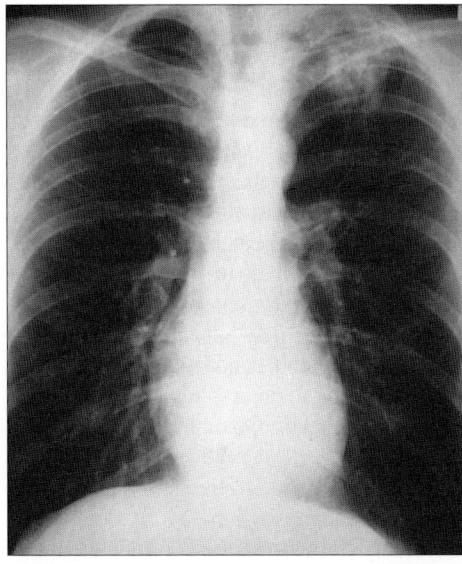

Fig. 9.10 Pulmonary tuberculosis.

rare, occurring in fewer than 1 case in 3000. Other complications are meningoencephalitis with seizures, splenic rupture, upper airway obstruction, interstitial pneumonitis with hypoxemia and severe hepatitis with liver failure.

Lymphadenopathy is present in the vast majority of children and young adults but in only 45% of patients older than 40 years old.[40] Lymph nodes are usually moderately enlarged throughout the body, principally in the posterior cervical, axillary and groin region. They are usually nontender or only minimally tender (Fig. 9.11). Lymph node histology demonstrates paracortical immunoblastic proliferation, as seen in most viral infections.[42]

Mononucleosis-like syndrome may occasionally be caused by *T. gondii* (1% of infectious mononucleosis cases)[17] and by other viruses, such as hepatitis A virus, HSV, rubella, adenovirus and human herpes virus type 6; it may also be caused by allergic reactions to various drugs.[40] Acute retroviral syndrome caused by HIV infection may manifest as mononucleosis-like syndrome and is discussed below.

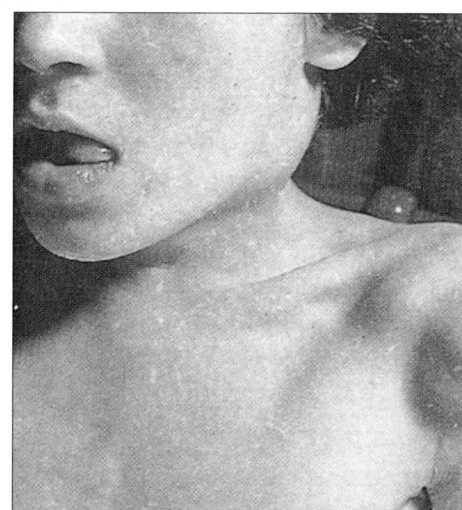

Fig. 9.11 Posterior cervical lymphadenopathy in infectious mononucleosis.

LYMPHADENOPATHY RELATED TO HUMAN IMMUNODEFICIENCY VIRUS

Clinically, the acute retroviral syndrome presents as a mononucleosis-like syndrome in 50–70% of patients.[43] Common manifestations are fever, lymphadenopathy, pharyngitis, arthralgia and rash. A variety of laboratory abnormalities such as thrombocytopenia, leukopenia and elevated liver enzyme levels are common. At this initial stage of the infection, lymph nodes enlarge owing to widespread dissemination of the virus throughout the lymphatic system, causing reactive nonspecific hyperplasia, which reflects the profound immunologic reactions induced by the virus.[43,44] Initially, the virus is entrapped in the lymph nodes and actively replicates, infecting hitherto uninfected T-helper cells traveling through the node. During the advanced stages of the disease the lymph nodes are destroyed, the follicles disappear and the virus enters the blood stream.[45]

Two-thirds of patients develop PGL during the course of HIV infection.[46] The most frequently involved nodes are the posterior cervical, anterior cervical, occipital, submandibular and axillary groups. Enlarged nodes are symmetric and painless, with a diameter of 2cm or less. Persistent generalized lymphadenopathy may persist for as long as the virus is contained in the infected lymph nodes.

At times, a patient with AIDS develops lymphadenopathy caused by a neoplastic disease (e.g. lymphoma or Kaposi's sarcoma) or an opportunistic infection. Sudden enlargement, pain or tenderness of a lymph node warrants aspiration or biopsy. Enlarged mesenteric or retroperitoneal lymph nodes can be part of the PGL syndrome, but if nodes are large or if there are symptoms such as fever, abdominal pain or diarrhea, a mycobacterial disease or lymphoma should be suspected. Mediastinal or hilar lymphadenopathy is not a part of the PGL syndrome and, whenever isolated intrathoracic lymphadenopathy is detected, a thorough investigation for mycobacterial disease is recommended. In such cases tuberculosis is found in more than half of the patients.[47]

HUMAN T-LYMPHOCYTE LEUKEMIA VIRUS 1

Lymphadenopathy is the most common finding in patients with adult T-lymphocyte leukemia or lymphoma caused by human T-lymphocyte leukemia virus 1(HTLV-1). Other characteristic findings include skin lesions, hepatomegaly, splenomegaly, hypercalcemia, lymphocytosis with abnormal circulating lymphocytes, hyperimmunoglobulinemia and rapid clinical deterioration. Histologic diagnosis of the disease requires immunophenotypic analysis, and these high-grade tumors often show loss of pan-T antigens.[48] Peripheral lymphadenopathy may also be observed in association with tropical spastic paraparesis and myelopathy caused by HTLV-1 which is endemic in some tropical areas.[49]

LYMPHADENOPATHY OF A PRESUMED TROPICAL ORIGIN
Leishmaniasis

Enlarged lymph nodes (mean diameter 3.6cm and up to 10.5cm) occur in 77% of patients with parasitologically confirmed cutaneous leishmaniasis in South America, and in patients with *Leishmania major* in equatorial Africa.[50,51] Lymphadenopathy precedes the skin lesion in two-thirds of cases by some 2 weeks. Cultures of the enlarged lymph nodes for *Leishmania* spp. are more frequently positive (86%) than cultures of the skin. Lymph node histology frequently shows necrotizing or suppurative granulomas, sometimes with discharging sinuses. Patients with leishmanial lymphadenopathy often have fever, hepatomegaly, splenomegaly and more intense leishmanin skin reactions and lymphocyte proliferation in response to antigenic stimulation, but fewer previous infections. Therefore, in endemic areas unexplained lymphadenopathy should prompt a search for leishmaniasis.

Leptospirosis

Lymphadenopathy may appear in up to one-third of the patients with leptospirosis. Other common signs of this infection include fever, headache, myalgia and the classic clinical findings of conjunctival irritation, jaundice and impairment of renal function.[52]

Filariasis

The most common symptomatic manifestations of filarial infection are recurrent episodes of high fever, occasionally with shaking chills, accompanied by lymphadenitis and a distinctive lymphangitis extending retrogradely from the lymph node where the filaria resides to the periphery. The attacks may last for 3–7 days and occur between six and 12 times a year. The attacks subside spontaneously without any specific therapy. The affected lymph nodes are characteristically enlarged and painful and the lymphatic vessels around them appear inflamed and indurated. Sometime local lymphedema appears as well. Occasionally local thrombophlebitis may also occur. With infection by *Brugia malayi*, an abscess of the entire local lymphatic apparatus may develop with characteristic scars. The involved area is most commonly in the inguinal region. With the continuation of lymphangitis and lymphadenitis, pitting edema of the skin develops; this is transformed into brawny edema of the involved area, resulting in thickening of the subcutaneous tissue and hyperkeratosis. There is coarsening of the skin, with deep fissuring and nodular and papillomatous hyperplastic changes. The damage to the lymphatic vessels leads to the development of elephantiasis, particularly in the legs but also in the lower arms and breasts.[53]

Onchocerciasis

The major manifestations of onchocerciasis are dermatitis, onchocercomas, lymphadenitis and visual impairment or blindness. The frequency and distribution of these symptoms vary according to the duration of exposure and the age and geographic location of the patient. Mild-to-moderate lymphadenopathy is common, particularly in the inguinal and femoral areas. Involved nodes are firm and nontender; at times they may reach gigantic proportions and be associated with local lymphatic obstruction and elephantiasis ('hanging groin'). In a recent survey of 770 patients in Uganda,[53] the most common manifestations of onchocerciasis were troublesome skin itching, chronic papular onchodermatitis and depigmentation; lymphadenopathy appeared only in conjunction with bacterially infected skin lesions associated with the itch.

Wuchereria bancrofti infection
In contrast to the situation in onchocerciasis, lymphadenopathy may be a striking feature of infection with *Wuchereria bancrofti*. Filaria are frequently present in the lymph nodes. The histology of the lymph node may not show the intense eosinophilia present in the peripheral blood smear or in other invaded organs. At times the genitalia may also be involved, with funiculitis, epidydimitis, scrotal pain and anatomic disfiguration of the penis and scrotum. Scrotal lymphedema, hydrocele and elephantiasis may ensue. In addition, characteristic swelling of the leg below the knee and of the arm below the elbow develop as a result of lymphatic involvement and subsequent elephantiasis. Occasionally, obstruction of the retroperitoneal lymphatics occurs, leading to rupture of lymphatic vessels into the kidneys and the appearance of chyluria.

African trypanosomiasis
Lymphadenopathy is observed in up to 80% of patients with African trypanosomiasis. The supraclavicular or posterior cervical lymph nodes are the most frequently involved. The nodes are usually soft, rubbery, discrete, painless and nontender. They appear at the second stage of the disease. The skin chancre, the hallmark of the first stage of the disease, appears 1 week after the bite and lasts for 2–3 weeks; the skin chancre disappears without leaving a scar. During the second stage, when enlarged lymph nodes are present, pyrexial episodes lasting 1–6 days occur and alternate with afebrile intervals lasting several weeks. Anemia, monocytosis, elevated serum IgM and involvement of the central nervous system with elevated protein and immunoglobulins in the cerebrospinal fluid are characteristic of African trypanosomiasis in endemic areas. In light-skinned travelers to endemic areas, a characteristic extensive erythematous skin rash with circinate patches on the chest or back may appear and disappear several times and therefore suggest the correct diagnosis.[54]

American trypanosomiasis (Chagas' disease)
Lymphadenopathy is an integral part of the first two stages of American trypanosomiasis, which is caused by *Trypanosoma cruzi*. The initial cutaneous lesion (the so-called 'inoculation chagoma'), which consists of a small raised reddish tender nodule with an indurated base, is accompanied by swelling of the regional lymph nodes.

Symptomatic acute Chagas' disease, which usually affects children and adolescents, is manifested by a lesion at the portal of entry in 50% of vector-infected patients. Regional lymphadenitis (iliac, axillary or cervical) may occur. Romaña's sign (Fig. 9.12) is a painless, unilateral indurated erythematous edema of the eyelids, accompanied by conjunctivitis and auricular lymphadenopathy. Local symptoms may be accompanied by rash, mild fever, hepatomegaly and acute myocarditis.

Occasionally fatal meningoencephalitis occurs in young infants. Generalized enlargement of the lymph nodes, liver and spleen begins to develop during the second week of the infection, with accompanying subcutaneous edema of the face, legs and feet. The lymph nodes are usually isolated and discrete, nontender, nonadherent and painless. During this stage, myocarditis ensues; this is the hallmark of the disease and manifests itself with sinus tachycardia and a variety of conduction defects.[55]

NONINFECTIOUS CAUSES OF LYMPHADENOPATHY
Postvaccination lymphadenopathy
Postvaccination lymphadenopathy is rare nowadays. In the past, smallpox (vaccinia) vaccination was the most common cause of postvaccination lymphadenopathy. Regional lymphadenopathy may occur from several days up to 2 weeks after measles vaccination; it is not usually accompanied by systemic manifestations. The histopathologic findings of an excised node are similar to primary viral lymphadenitis,[56] and characteristic Warthin–Finkeldey multinucleated giant cells can be seen. An outbreak of axillary lymphadenitis has been documented in children receiving BCG vaccination. *Mycobacterium bovis* was isolated from a minority of these patients.[57]

Drug-induced lymphadenopathy
Certain drugs are known to cause hypersensitivity reactions associated with lymphadenopathy associated with fever, rash, arthralgia and eosinophilia. Liver enzyme abnormalities and pancytopenia are occasionally seen as well.[58] Phenytoin is the most common drug responsible for such cases.[58,59] Moreover, some anticonvulsants (e.g. phenytoin and carbamazepine) can cause a pseudolymphoma syndrome, which is characterized by fever, erythematous rash, marked lymphadenopathy and organomegaly.[60] Most patients have taken the implicated drug for only a short time, usually less than 3–4 months, but in some patients many months elapse between initiation of the drug and the appearance of the clinical syndrome. In most patients lymphadenopathy spontaneously regresses 1–2 weeks after stopping the drug.

Lymphadenopathy and autoimmune disease
Generalized lymphadenopathy is common in some autoimmune disease. Studies have shown that lymphadenopathy occurs in up to 75% of patients with rheumatoid arthritis, 43% of patients with juvenile rheumatoid arthritis and up to 65% of patients with active systemic lupus erythematosus.[42]

Kawasaki disease (mucocutaneous lymph node syndrome)
Kawasaki disease is an acute inflammation of small and medium-sized arteries that affects young children. The clinical manifestations include fever, conjunctivitis, oral mucositis, skin rash and cardiac involvement. Lymphadenopathy occurs in 75% of the patients, most frequently in the cervical area.[61] The most devastating complications of this disease include coronary artery aneurysm, coronary thrombosis and myocarditis. The histopathologic features of the lymph nodes are not characteristic; there are scattered necrotic foci associated with thrombi of the adjacent microvasculature.[42] The diagnosis is made on clinical grounds and at least five features should be present. The differential diagnosis of Kawasaki disease includes staphylococcal scalded skin syndrome, scarlet fever and hypersensitivity reactions. The presence of lymphadenopathy, however, suggests Kawasaki disease.

Rosai–Dorfman disease (sinus histiocytosis with massive lymphadenopathy)
Rosai–Dorfman disease (sinus histiocytosis with massive lymphadenopathy) is a rare, idiopathic and generally benign, self-limiting disease that affects children and adolescents. Massive lymphadenopathy, most commonly involving the cervical nodes, is the hallmark of the disease. Nearly 50% of the patients have some extranodal

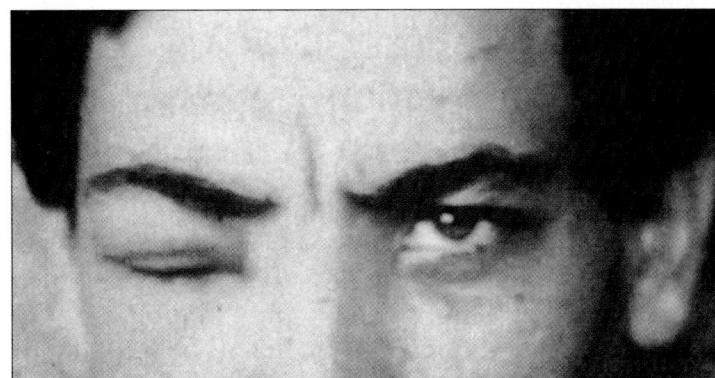

Fig. 9.12 Romaña's sign in acute Chagas' disease. There is unilateral edema of the eyelid accompanied by conjunctivitis and auricular lymphadenopathy.

involvement, most of them occurring in the head and neck where they involve the nose, paranasal sinuses and parotid gland. About 10% of the patients have an associated immunologic disorder.

The involved lymph nodes show a marked sinus expansion by numerous histiocytes with abundant clear cytoplasm containing engulfed small lymphocytes and a small bland nucleus. The clinical setting is usually a child or adolescent presenting with marked cervical adenopathy associated with fever, neutrophilic leukocytosis, elevated erythrocyte sedimentation rate and polyclonal hypergammaglobulinemia. Although the disease is usually self-limiting, the prognosis is unfavorable in patients with immunologic disorders.[42,62]

Kikuchi's disease

Kikuchi's disease is a histiocytic necrotizing lymphadenitis that was first described in 1972 in Japan as a benign lymphadenopathy of the neck.[63] Kikuchi's disease affects women more often than men and, owing to its association with systemic lupus erythematosus and Still's disease, it is suspected of being an autoimmune disorder. The clinical features of Kikuchi's disease include fever and lymphadenopathy, which is usually cervical.[64] The differential diagnosis includes infectious disease and malignant disease. Biopsy is important for diagnosis and exclusion of lymphoma.

Castleman's disease

This condition, originally called angiofollicular lymph node hyperplasia, was first described as a rare cause of a mediastinal mass seen on chest X-ray. It sometimes caused mild systemic symptoms of fever and night sweats, and was associated with an elevated erythrocyte sedimentation rate. More recently a variant has been described in which there is generalised lymphadenopathy and more systemic signs. There may be an association with the so-called POEMS syndrome: peripheral neuropathy, organomegaly, endocrinopathy a monoclonal paraprotein and skin lesions. The etiology of Castleman's disease is unknown. Severe cases may require corticosteroid therapy.

Infiltrative lymphadenopathy

Inborn errors of metabolism (Gaucher's disease, Niemann–Pick disease), amyloidosis, histiocytosis X and metastatic malignancy cause infiltration of various organs, including the lymph nodes. The nodes in these cases are characteristically firm and nontender; they may constitute the first clue to a systemic infiltrative process.

Lymphadenopathy and silicone breast implant

In recent years there has been a growing body of evidence concerning the immune response to silicone and its breakdown products. In women with silicone breast implants, leakage of silicone causes axillary lymph node enlargement. The histopathology is characteristic for foreign body reaction.

MANAGEMENT

Lymphadenopathy may be the presenting sign in many diseases. Techniques for palpation and assessment of lymph nodes are essential for providing the physician with useful information on which diagnostic and therapeutic decisions can be based. In adults, small lymph nodes can normally be palpated in the inguinal area, and in children in the suboccipital area. Enlarged supraclavicular, scalenal, axillary and epitrochlear lymph nodes are usually pathologic and require appropriate investigation with possible aspiration or biopsy of the node. The investigation of lymphadenopathy can be organized according to the following categorizations:

- the mode of presentation (an acutely ill, chronically ill or asymptomatic patient, and any pertinent associated clinical manifestation;
- the patient's age, epidemiologic exposure and immune status;
- the physical characteristic of the enlarged node or nodes; and
- the location of the lymphadenopathy.

MODE OF PRESENTATION

In acutely ill patients with a tender, enlarged lymph node a pyogenic bacterial infection is most commonly found. A search for skin and soft tissue infection in the region drained by the involved lymph node is indicated. A thorough ear, nose and throat examination is mandatory if the adenitis is in the head and neck area. Fluctuant abscesses should be aspirated, Gram stained and cultured, and appropriate antibiotic treatment be instituted. Group A streptococcal and *S. aureus* infections cannot be differentiated on the basis of clinical presentation. In endemic regions plague should be suspected and treated promptly. The acutely ill patient who is found to have generalized lymphadenopathy should be evaluated for systemic infections such as streptococcal and staphylococcal bacteremia, infectious mononucleosis, typhoid fever, rickettsiosis, leptospirosis, miliary tuberculosis and reactive noninfectious diseases, depending on any associated clinical features. In the asymptomatic or mildly symptomatic young patient with generalized lymphadenopathy and without localizing clinical features, the most plausible etiology is a viral disease, usually caused by EBV, CMV or HIV; appropriate serologic or culture studies are called for.

In the elderly, acute EBV or CMV infections cause lymphadenopathy less frequently than they do in younger patients. The differential diagnosis includes primary lymphoproliferative and metastatic disease as well as reactive processes.

Figure 9.13 summarizes the clinical presentation of infectious lymphadenitis.

DISEASE PROGRESSION

Lymphadenopathy of long duration mandates further evaluation. Although lymphadenopathy due to cat-scratch disease or toxoplasmosis may persist for months, a presumptive diagnosis of toxoplasmic lymphadenitis should be questioned if adenopathy persists longer than 6 months, and lymph node biopsy or aspiration should be performed. Fine-needle aspiration is suitable for diagnosing infection or metastatic disease but a lymph node biopsy is required for the diagnosis of lymphoma. Analysis of biopsied lymph node yields a diagnosis in 50–60% of patients. Among patients in whom a diagnosis is not established by biopsy, 25% will develop a definable disease, mostly lymphoma, within a year. Therefore, close follow up and repeated biopsies should be performed in patients with a nondiagnostic initial biopsy.

AGE

Lymphadenopathy is common in the pediatric age group and represents a benign process in approximately 80% of cases. Therefore, in a child with lymphadenopathy and other features suggesting a possible bacterial infection, a trial of antibiotic may be appropriate. In adults, especially in patients older than 50 years, any finding of lymphadenopathy requires a thorough evaluation and consideration of a lymph node biopsy.

PHYSICAL CHARACTERISTICS OF THE ENLARGED LYMPH NODE

The size, consistency and relation to underlying tissue are important clues to the etiology of the enlarged nodes. Lymph nodes involved by an infective process tend to be large, soft and tender. Signs of local inflammation may be present, and draining sinuses are commonly seen in mycobacterial lymphadenitis. This presentation may be mistaken for orocervicofacial actinomycosis, which seldom spreads to the lymphatic vessels to cause lymphadenopathy. Nodes involved in lymphomas are rubbery, matted together and nontender. Metastatic lymph nodes due to carcinomas are usually firm, nontender and fixed to the underlying tissues.

LOCATION

Specific locations of enlarged lymph nodes are associated with specific etiologies (Fig. 6.14). Intra-abdominal or intrathoracic lymphadenopathy

CLINICAL PRESENTATION OF INFECTIOUS LYMPHADENITIS

Disease		Infecting organism	Lymphadenopathy		Systemic manifestations
			Regional	Generalized	
Bacterial	Pyogenic	Group A streptococci Staphylococcus aureus	Yes	No	Prominent
	Cat-scratch disease	Bartonella henselae	Yes	No	Occasional, mild
	Scrofula	Mycobacterium tuberculosis, nontuberculous mycobacteria	Yes	No	No, unless AIDS is present
	Miliary tuberculosis	Mycobacterium tuberculosis	No	Yes	Prominent
	Syphilis	Treponema pallidum	Yes	Yes	Variable
	Plague	Yersinia pestis	Yes	No	Prominent
	Tularemia	Francisella tularensis	Yes	No	Common, mild to moderate
	Chancroid	Haemophilus ducreyi	Yes	No	No
	Leptospirosis	Leptospira	No	Yes	Prominent
Viral	Infectious mononucleosis	Epstein–Barr virus, cytomegalovirus, HIV	Yes	Yes	Common, mild to moderate
	Rubella	Rubella virus	Yes	Yes	Common, mild
	Genital herpes (primary infection)	Herpes simplex virus 2	Yes	No	Common, mild to moderate
	Persistent generalized lymphadenopathy	HIV	Yes	Yes	Variable
	Pharyngoconjunctival fever	Adenovirus 3, 7	Yes	No	Common, mild
	Epidemic keratoconjunctivitis	Adenovirus 8, 19, 37	Yes	No	Occasional, mild
Chlamydial	Lymphogranuloma venereum	Chlamydia trachomatis	Yes	No	Common, moderate
Rickettsial	Spotted fever	Rickettsia rickettsii, R. conori	No	Yes	Prominent
Fungal	Histoplasmosis	Histoplasma capsulatum	Yes	Yes	Uncommon
	Coccidioidomycosis	Coccidioides immitis	Yes	No	Uncommon
Protozoan	Toxoplasmosis	Toxoplasma gondii	Yes	No	Uncommon
	Chagas' disease	Trypanosoma cruzi	Yes	Yes	Common, mild to moderate
	African trypanosomiasis	Trypanosoma brucei	Yes	No	Common, mild to moderate
	Leishmaniasis	Leishmania spp.	Yes	No	Variable
Helminthic	Filariasis	Brugia malayi	Yes	No	Common
		Wuchereria bancrofti	Yes	No	No
	Onchocerciasis	Onchocerca vulvulus	Yes	No	No

Fig. 9.13 Clinical presentation of infectious lymphadenitis.

are not accessible to palpation, and imaging should be undertaken whenever they are suspected. Suggested investigations for regional lymphadenopathy are discussed below according to its site.

Head and neck lymphadenopathy
Any lymph node enlargement in the head and neck region should stimulate a thorough search for an infection in the oropharyngeal and nasal cavities. Symmetric lymph node enlargement usually suggests self-limiting viral disease, and unilateral node enlargement may be viral in origin but evokes a broader differential diagnosis, including cat-scratch disease, toxoplasmosis and neoplasia. Unilateral enlarged tender lymph nodes usually indicate an acute infection, but may be due to a rapidly proliferating process. If asymptomatic cervical node enlargement persists and serologic testing for toxoplasmosis is negative, a lymph node biopsy or aspiration should be performed. An abnormal chest radiograph in children and young adults with cervical lymphadenopathy has been found to be strongly associated with malignant neoplasm, mostly lymphoma. Furthermore, 80% of patients with cervical lymphadenopathy, abnormal chest radiograph and nondiagnostic lymph node biopsies are

subsequently found to have malignant or granulomatous disease. We recommend a lymph node biopsy, and not aspiration, as the diagnostic procedure of choice when asymptomatic cervical lymphadenopathy persists in the presence of an abnormal chest radiograph. Supraclavicular lymphadenopathy without any other enlarged nodes, particularly in adults, is often of neoplastic origin and should therefore be biopsied.

In children and adolescents other causes of lumps in the neck, such as epidermoid thyroglossal or branchial cysts and parotid gland enlargement, should be differentiated from cervical lymphadenopathy.

Axillary lymphadenopathy
Infectious causes of unilateral axillary lymphadenopathy include local infectious processes of the arm and hand, hydradenitis suppurativa, streptococcal and staphylococcal lymphadenitis, cat-scratch disease, toxoplasmosis and tularemia. Conventional bacteria are easily differentiated from cat-scratch disease and toxoplasmosis on clinical grounds and should be treated accordingly. Asymptomatic unilateral axillary lymphadenopathy should be evaluated for neoplasia in both adults and adolescents. In the younger age group, however, a serologic test for the

CORRELATION BETWEEN THE SITE OF LYMPHADENOPATHY AND DISEASE	
Enlarged lymph node	Associated disease or condition
Occipital	Scalp infections, insect bites, head lice
Posterior auricular	Rubella, ear piercing, HIV
Anterior auricular	Eye or conjunctival infections
Posterior cervical	Toxoplasmosis
Submental	Dental infections
Anterior cervical or submandibular	Oral cavity infections, Epstein–Barr virus, HIV, tuberculosis
Supraclavicular	Neoplasia
Mediastinal	Sarcoidosis, tuberculosis, histoplasmosis, neoplasia (Hodgkin's or non-Hodgkin's lymphoma, metastases)
Axillary	Cat-scratch disease, pyogenic infection of the upper arm, neoplasia (breast, lymphoma)
Epitrochlear	Viral diseases, cat-scratch disease, tularemia, hand infection, secondary syphilis
Abdominal/retroperitoneal	Tuberculosis, neoplasia, yersiniosis
Inguinal	Genital herpes, syphilis, lymphogranuloma venereum, filariasis, neoplasia

Fig. 9.14 Correlation between the site of lymphadenopathy and disease.

presence of *Toxoplasma* antibodies should precede the biopsy. Bilateral axillary lymphadenopathy can by caused by a variety of viral and bacterial infections as well as by neoplasms and immunologic disorders.

Thoracic lymphadenopathy

The principal differential diagnosis of intrathoracic lymphadenopathy includes neoplasia, tuberculosis, sarcoidosis and endemic mycoses. Unilateral or bilateral mediastinal lymphadenopathy in children without additional findings is the characteristic feature of primary tuberculosis. However, malignant lymphoma in the pediatric age group may also manifest in this way. Therefore, if a tuberculin skin test is found to be strongly reactive in such circumstances, antituberculous therapy should be started. However, if the tuberculin skin test is nondiagnostic or nonreactive and remains so on retesting 10–14 days later, an invasive diagnostic procedure is indicated.

Mediastinal lymphadenopathy in adults without any accompanying complaints or findings is usually indicative of a neoplasm requiring an invasive diagnostic procedure. An exception to this is the HIV-infected patient or one who arrives from an endemic area in whom tuberculosis may be as frequent as a neoplasia. In the appropriate epidemiologic settings, endemic mycosis is also a diagnostic possibility requiring specific tests.

These considerations also apply to patients with unilateral hilar lymphadenopathy. Bilateral hilar lymphadenopathy in the asymptomatic young patient is commonly caused by sarcoidosis. In patients who have parenchymal infiltration on radiography in addition to intrathoracic lymphadenopathy, bronchoscopy should be performed if sputum smear for *M. tuberculosis* is negative, regardless of age.

In the future, it is possible that new laboratory procedures such as PCR may reduce the need for invasive procedures. In patients without lung parenchymal involvement the diagnostic yield of sputum examination is low. Bronchoscopy increases the diagnostic yield of tuberculosis to 50–75%, especially if mucosal biopsy specimens are taken from ulcerating granuloma seen during the procedure.[46] Video-assisted thoracic surgery and mediastinotomy increase the diagnosis to 100% of patients, whereas mediastinoscopy supports the diagnosis of tuberculosis in 85–90%.[47]

Abdominal lymphadenopathy

Abdominal lymphadenopathy may be detected as an isolated finding during the investigation of abdominal complaints. In such cases, the etiology of the lymph node enlargement lies in the abdominal organs that drain into the enlarged nodes. The appropriate diagnostic approach should be directed at investigating and, if appropriate, biopsying a particular organ. Exceptions to this may be intra-abdominal lymphoma and abdominal tuberculosis (mesenteric lymphadenitis), in which the abdominal lymph nodes may be the primary site involved. In cases with abdominal lymphadenopathy, a careful search for peripheral lymph node enlargement is mandatory.

Inguinal lymphadenopathy

The main causes of inguinal lymphadenopathy include infectious diseases (STDs and others) and neoplasm (lymphoma or metastatic carcinoma). If an STD is suspected or a genital ulcer is detected, serologic tests (e.g. Venereal Disease Research Laboratory, complement fixation test, microimmunofluorescence test for *Chlamydia spp.*), bacteriologic investigations (dark field, immediate culture), virologic investigations (herpesvirus culture) should be performed. According to epidemiologic considerations, the presence of one STD could indicate the possibility of another STD. Therefore, it is recommended that multiple infectious etiologies such as HIV and HBV are ruled out.

PRACTICAL SUMMARY

- The size of an enlarged peripheral lymph node often is not helpful in determining the cause of lymphadenopathy or the need for biopsy.
- Empiric antibiotic treatment for suspected suppurative lymphadenitis is indicated and should be primarily directed toward *Strep. pyogenes* and *Staph. aureus*.
- In immunosuppressed patients (e.g. patients who have acute leukemia), or in diabetic patients with foot ulcers and inguinal lymphadenitis, aspiration of pus from the involved node should be performed and therapy modified accordingly.
- Do not attempt drainage of a scrofula: it may cause fistula formation. Total excision is the treatment of choice in such cases. If in doubt, excision is the preferred approach.
- Consult a hematologist before processing an excised lymph node. It is essential that the biopsy material should be handled properly to allow possible ancillary tests, such as immunoperoxidase staining, cytogenetic analysis and molecular clonality studies.
- Aspirated or excised material should be of sufficient amount to ensure recovery of suspected organisms.
- Specimens for bacterial and fungal diagnosis should be processed for Gram stain, acid-fast stain, Giemsa or Wright stain and methenamine silver stain.
- Specimens for parasitic diseases should be fixed in 100% alcohol and not in formalin.
- Specimens for viral cultures should be transported in appropriate transport media.
- For PCR assays, consult the local laboratory.
- The patient who has acute HIV infection manifesting as mononucleosis-like syndrome is typically HIV-antibody negative. In order to rule out the possibility of acute retroviral syndrome, a negative serum p24 antigen or HIV PCR are required.
- In suspected tropical lymphadenitis or lymphadenopathy, appropriate serologic tests are mandatory and tissue specimens should be processed accordingly.
- Lymphadenopathy caused by dual infections or by an infectious process and a noninfectious one has been described; if, for example, lymphadenopathy attributed to toxoplasmosis on the basis of serologic investigations persists for more than 6–8 months, lymph node biopsy should be performed to exclude other diagnoses.

REFERENCES

1. Slap BG, Brooks SJ, Schwartz S. When to perform biopsies of enlarged peripheral lymph nodes in young patients. JAMA 1984;252:1321–6.
2. Buchino JJ, Jones VF. Fine needle aspiration in the evaluation of children with lymphadenopathy. Arch Pediatr Adolesc 1994;148:1327–30.
3. Sinclair S, Beckman E, Ellman L. Biopsy of enlarged superficial lymph nodes. JAMA 1974;228:602–3.
4. Hay JB, Cahill RNP. In: Hay JB, ed. Animal models of immunological processes. London: Academic Press; 1982:97–134.
5. Kuby J. In: Kuby J, ed. Immunology. New York: WH Freeman and Company; 1992:64–5.
6. Cotran RS, Kumar V, Robbins SL, eds. Pathologic basis of disease. 5th ed. WB Saunders, Philadelphia; 1994:632–3.
7. Yamauchi T, Ferrieri P, Anthony BF. The etiology of acute cervical adenitis in children. serological and bacteriologic studies. J Med Microbiol 1980;13:37–43.
8. Boyce JM. Severe streptococcal axillary lymphadenitis. N Engl J Med 1990; 323:655–8.
9. Janssen F, Zelinky-Gurung A, Caumes E, et al. Group A streptococcal cellulitis–adenitis in apatient with AIDS. J Am Acad Dermatol 1991;24:363–5.
10. Ho DD, Murata GH. Streptococcal lymphadenitis in homosexual men with chronic lymphadenopathy. Am J Med 1984;77:151–3.
11. Liese JG, Jendrossek V, Jansson A, et al. Chronic granulomatous disease in adults. Lancet 1996;347:220–3.
12. Mouy R, Fischer A, Vilmer E, et al. Incidence, severity and prevention of infections in chronic granulomatous disease. J Pediatr 1989;114:550–60.
13. Jackson LA, Perkins BA, Wenger JD. Cat-scratch disease in the United States. Am J Public Health 1993;83:1707–11.
14. Zangwill KM, Hamilton DH, Perkins BA, et al. Cat-scratch disease in Connecticut. Epidemiology, risk factors, and evaluation of a new diagnostic test. N Engl J Med 1993;329:8–13.
15. Wear DJ, Malatry RH, Zimmerman LE, et al. Cat-scratch bacilli in the conjunctiva of patients with Parinaud's oculoglandular syndrome. Ophthalmology 1985;92;1282–7.
16. Anderson B, Sims K, Regnery R, et al. Detection of B. henselae DNA in specimen from cat scratch disease patients by PCR. J Clin Microbiol 1994;32:942–8.
17. McCabe RE, Brooks RG, Dorfman RF, et al. Clinical spectrum in 107 cases of toxoplasmic lymphadenopathy. Rev Infect Dis 1987;9:754–74.
18. Momtoya JG, Remington JS. Studies on the serodiagnosis of toxoplasmic lymphadenitis. Clin Infect Dis 1995;20:781–9.
19. Summers GD, McNicol MW. Tuberculosis of superficial lymph nodes. Br J Dis Chest 1980;74:369–373.
20. Bem C, Patil PS, Bharucha H, et al. Importance of human immunodeficiency virus associated lymphadenopathy and tuberculous lymphadenitis in patients undergoing lymph node biopsy in Zambia. Br J Surg 1996;83:75–8.
21. Grzybowski S, Allen EA. History and importance of scrofula. Lancet 1995;346:1472–4.
22. Wolinsky E. Mycobacterial lymphadenitis in children. A prospective study of 105 nontuberculous cases with long term follow-up. Clin Infec Dis 1995; 20:954–63.

23. Haas WH, Kirschner P, Ziesing S, et al. Cervical lymphadenitis in a child caused by a previously unknown mycobacterium. J Infec Dis 1993;167:237–40.
24. Hoffner SE, Henriques B, Petrini B, et al. Mycobacterium malmoense, an easily missed pathogen. J Clin Microbiol 1991;29:2673–4.
25. Shriner KA, Mathisen GE, Goetz MB, et al. Comparison of mycobacterial lymphadenitis among persons infected with human immunodeficiency virus and seronegative controls. Clin Infect Dis 1992;15:601–5.
26. Hammond GW, Slutchuk M, Scatiff J, et al. Epidemiologic, clinical, laboratory and therapeutic features of an urban outbreak of chancroid in North America. Rev Infect Dis 1980;2:867–79.
27. Perine PL, Osoba AO. Lymphogranuloma venereum. In: Holmes KK, Mardth PA, Sparling PF, et al., eds. Sexually transmitted diseases, 2nd ed. New York: McGraw-Hill; 1990:195–204.
28. Chapel TA. The signs and symptoms of secondary syphilis. Sex Transm Dis 1980;7:161.
29. Miliauskas JR, Leong AS. Localized herpes simplex lymphadenitis. Report of three cases and review of the literature. Histopathology 1991;19:355–60.
30. Mertz GJ. Genital herpes simplex virus infection. Med Clin North Am 1990:74:1433–54.
31. Sehgal VN, Shyam Prasad AL. Donovanosis. Current concepts. Int J Dermatol 1986:25:8–16.
32. Craven RB, Barnes AM. Plague and tularemia. Infect Dis Clin North Am 1991;5:165–75.
33. Winterbauer RH, Belic N, Moores KD. A clinical interpretation of bilateral hilar adenopathy. Ann Intern Med 1973;78:65–71.
34. Woodring HJ, Vandiviere M, Lee C. Intrathoracic lymphadenopathy in postprimary tuberculosis. South Med J 1988;81:992–7.
35. Goodwin RA, Jr, Shapiro JL, Thurman GH, et al. Disseminated histoplasmosis. clinical and pathologic correlations. Medicine (Baltimore) 1980;59:1–33.
36. Sagel SS. Common fungal diseases of the lung. I. Coccidioidomycosis. Radiol Clin North Am 1973;11:153–161.
37. Manns BJ, Baylis BW, Urbanski SJ, et al. Paracoccidioidomycosis. Case report and review. Clin Infect Dis 1996;23:1026–32.
38. Kirks RD, Greenspan HR. Sarcoidosis. Radiol Clin North Am 1973;11:279–94.
39. Saeb A, Lassen J. Acute and chronic gastrointestinal manifestations associated with Yersinia enterocolitica infection. A Norwegian 10-year follow-up study on 458 hospitalized patients. Ann Surg 1992;215:250–5.
40. Al-Hajjar S, Hussain Quadri SM. Epstein–Barr virus. Infect Dis Pract 1996;20:41–4.
41. Lajo A, Borque C, DelCastilo F, et al. Mononucleosis caused by EBV and CMV in children. A comperative study of 124 cases. Pediatr Infect Dis J 1994;13:56–60.
42. Segal GH, Perkins SL, Kjeldsberg CR. Benign lymphadenopathies in children and adolescents. Semin Diagn Pathol 1995;12:288–302.
43. Kinloch-de Loes S, deSaussure P, Saurat JH, et al. Symptomatic primary infection due to human immunodeficiency virus type 1: review of 31 cases. Clin Infect Dis 1993;17:59–65.
44. Pantaleo G, Graziosi C, Fauci AS. The role of lymphoid organs in the pathogenesis of HIV infection. Semin Immunol 1993;5:157–63.
45. Pantaleo G, Graziosi C, Fauci AS. New concepts in the immunopathogenesis of human immunodeficiency virus infection. N Eng J Med 1993;328:327–35.

46. Chadburn A, Metroka C, Mouradian J. Progressive lymph node histology and its prognostic value in patients with acquired immunodeficiency syndrome and AIDS related complex. Hum Pathol 1989;20:579–87.
47. Said JW. AIDS-related lymphadenopathies. Semin Diagn Pathol 1988;5:365–75.
48. Nakamura S, Suchi T, Koshikawa T, et al. Clinicopathological study of 212 cases of peripheral T-cell lymphoma among the Japanese. Cancer 1993;72:1762–72.
49. Plumelle Y, Pascaline N, Nguyen D, et al. Adult T cell leukemia–lymphoma. a clinicopathological study of 26 cases in Martinique. Hematol Pathol 1993;7:251–62.
50. Sousa A, De Qi Paarise ME, et al. Bubonic leishmaniasis. a common manifestation of Leishmania (Viannia) braziliensis infection in Ceara (Brazil). Am J Trop Med Hyg 1995;53:380–5.
51. Gaafar A, Ismail A, El-Kadaro AY, et al. Necrotizing suppurative lymphadenitis in Leishmania major infections. Trop Med Int Health 1996;1:243–50.
52. Van Crevel R, Speelman P, Gravekamp C, et al. Leptospirosis in travelers. Clin Infect Dis 1994;19:132–4.
53. Okello DO, Ovuga EB, Ogwal-Okeny JW. Dermatological problems of onchocerciasis in Nebbi district, Uganda. East Afr Med J 1995;72:295–8.
54. Foulkes JR. Human trypanosomiasis in Africa. Br Med J 1981;283:1172–4.
55. Coura JR. Evolutive pattern in Chagas' disease and the life span of Trypanosoma cruzi in human infection. New approaches in American trypanosomiasis research. Scientific Publication 318. Pan American Health Organisation; 1976:378–82.
56. Dorfman RF, Herweg JC. Live, attenuated measles virus vaccine. Inguinal lymphadenopathy complicating administration. JAMA 1966;198:230–1.
57. Praveen KN, Smikle MF, Prabhakar P, et al. Outbreak of bacillus Calmette–Guérin associated lymphadenitis and abscesses in Jamaican children. Pediatr Infect Dis J 1990;9:890–3.
58. Wolkenstein P, Revuz J. Drug induced severe skin reactions. Incidence, management and prevention. Drug Saf 1995;13:56–68.
59. Abratt RP, Sealy R, Uys CJ, et al. Lymphadenopathy associated with diphenylhydantoin therapy. Clin Oncol 1982;8:351–6.
60. Saltzstein SI, Ackerman LV. Lymphadenopathy induced by anticonvulsant drugs and mimicking clinically and pathologically malignant lymphomas. Cancer 1959;12:164–82.
61. Nadel S, Levin M. Kawasaki disease. Curr Opin Pediatr 1993;5:34–9.
62. Foucar E, Rosai J, Dorfman RF. Sinus histiocytosis with massive lymphadenopathy (Rosai–Dorfman disease). Review of the entity. Semin Diagn Pathol 1990;7:19–73.
63. Pilevi S, Kikuchi M, Helborn D, et al. Histiocytic necrotizing lymphadenitis without granulocytic infiltration. Virchows Arch [A] 1982;395:257.
64. Turner RR, Martin J, Dorfman RF. Necrotizing lymphadenitis. A study of 30 cases. Am J Surg Pathol 1983;7:115–23.
65. Roux SP, Bertucci GM, Ibarra JA, et al. Unilateral axillary adenopathy secondary to a silicone wrist implant. Report of a case detected at screening mamography. Radiology 1996;198:345–6.

Practice Point

Management of the solitary enlarged lymph node

Martin Dedicoat &
Martin J Wood

PATHOGENESIS

Enlargement of a lymph node may result from:
- infiltration by metastatic malignancy;
- acute inflammation secondary to infectious agents being filtered from afferent lymphatics or blood; or
- proliferation of lymphocytes and other mononuclear cells in response to antigenic stimuli or due to a primary lymphoproliferative disorder.

In certain infections there is nonspecific abscess formation and suppuration, whereas in others there is a more distinctive histologic appearance. Caseation necrosis suggests mycobacterial (or occasionally fungal) infection; a granulomatous reaction with or without stellate necrosis is typical of sarcoidosis, cat-scratch disease, tularemia, lymphogranuloma venereum and Kikuchi's disease; and follicular hyperplasia with epithelioid histiocytes is seen in toxoplasmosis. In other cases it is usually not possible to determine the infecting organism from the histologic appearances.

MICROBIOLOGY

Many infections can result in a solitary enlarged lymph node, but most (particularly viral and protozoal infections) are much more likely to cause a generalized lymphadenitis. The organisms listed in Figure 10.1 are those that need particular consideration. Causes of lymphadenopathy other than infection are listed in Figure 10.2.

CLINICAL FEATURES

A patient may present with an enlarged lymph node or it may be a chance finding. Palpable lymph nodes do not always have a pathologic cause; a submandibular or cervical node less than 1cm in diameter or an inguinal node less than 2cm in diameter in an adult may be considered to be normal. Solitary nodes in other areas are more likely to have a pathologic cause. Evaluation requires an assessment of the duration and progression of the enlargement and any associated systemic or local (related to the area drained by the enlarged lymph node) symptoms or signs. The patient's occupation, exposure to animals, sexual behavior and travel history will indicate whether diseases listed in Figures 10.1 and 10.2 can be excluded or should be considered more seriously.

Examination of the mass should first focus on ensuring that it is a lymph node (Fig. 10.3) and an enlarged node should be assessed for its size, texture, tenderness and any discharge. An acutely enlarged, very tender (perhaps fluctuant), cervical, submandibular, axillary or epitrochlear node with overlying skin erythema and fever, particularly in a child, suggests a streptococcal or staphylococcal etiology. Suppurative iliac lymphadenitis in a child is also usually caused by *Staphylococcus aureus*, but in an adult several sexually transmitted diseases, particularly lymphogranuloma venereum, also need to be considered. In an appropriate geographic location and with animal exposure, plague and tularemia should be considered in an acutely ill person who has inguinal buboes.

In the absence of fever and tenderness, an indolent suppurative painless lymphadenitis, particularly in the cervical or submandibular region, suggests mycobacterial infection. In children this is is often caused by atypical mycobacteria such as *Mycobacterium scrofulaceum* or *Mycobacterium avium-intracellulare.* Peripheral tuberculous lymphadenitis occurs particularly in young adult women immigrants from areas where tuberculosis is endemic. Similar slowly progressive regional lymphadenitis is a feature of cat-scratch disease, which is caused by *Bartonella henselae,* and most patients who have this infection have been scratched or bitten by a cat. Hard immobile nodes are suggestive of malignancy and rubbery painless nodes may indicate a lymphoproliferative process. The area drained by any enlarged node should be examined for signs of skin inflammation or malignancy.

INVESTIGATIONS

Investigations should be tailored to the clinical findings. Basic tests include a full blood count and blood film and antibody test for mononucleosis. Swabs should be taken from the throat (for cervical nodes), and any ulcerative lesions or sinus tracts. A fluctuant node can be aspirated and the pus stained with Gram and Ziehl–Neelsen stains and cultured for bacteria, including mycobacteria, and fungi. Any material from a submandibular swelling can also be sent for cytology because this may be helpful in differentiating a submandibular node from a branchial cyst containing cholesterol crystals. If the patient is febrile blood cultures should be obtained. A chest radiograph is useful if the node is supraclavicular because it may show a pulmonary infiltrate, mediastinal or other masses, or hilar adenopathy due to sarcoidosis. Patients who have an enlarged cervical node without a visible cause should have a thorough ear, nose and throat examination and any suspicious mucosal lesions should be biopsied.

Serologic tests can be helpful in supporting a diagnosis of streptococcal, viral or rickettsial infection, toxoplasmosis and cat-scratch disease. Immunologic tests such as antinuclear antibody, dsDNA and rheumatoid factor may be indicated if systemic lupus erythematosus or rheumatoid arthritis are thought likely. A tuberculin test (Mantoux or Heaf) can suggest tuberculosis as a cause, but needs to be interpreted carefully, particularly for patients who have lived in Asia and other countries where the disease is endemic and previous infection is likely, and in those who have had previous BCG immunization. It is often falsely negative in patients who have HIV infection.

Other investigations such as CT imaging should be guided by clinical suspicion. A single stony-hard supraclavicular node suggests an intra-abdominal malignancy.

MANAGEMENT

If there is a cause for the enlarged node found on examination or after initial investigations, including microscopy of any purulent material obtained after aspiration, the management is usually straightforward and directed at the underlying disease. An acutely ill patient who has suppurative lymphadenitis or an enlarged node accompanied by lymphangitis can be treated with a penicillinase-resistant penicillin such as flucloxacillin. Cervical nodes secondary to presumed pharyngotonsillar infection can be treated with penicillin, which may need to be given intravenously at first until the patient is able to swallow. More chronic suppurative lymphadenitis might be treated empirically as tuberculosis, an atypical mycobacterial infection or cat-scratch disease, depending upon the epidemiologic features. A single lymph node infected by atypical mycobacteria is usually treated by surgical excision alone.

If no specific diagnosis is suggested by the history and initial investigation a decision has to be made about performing an excision biopsy. If a node is less than 1cm in diameter and there are no suspicious features (hard, fixed, painless node or supraclavicular location) in an otherwise well patient under 40 years of age it can usually be observed on a regular basis every few weeks and in many cases will regress or the disease process will manifest itself. Biopsy is indicated for:
- nodes that fail to regress or have enlarged despite empiric antibiotic therapy directed at the disease thought to be the most likely cause;
- a node over 2cm in diameter; and
- a progressively enlarging hard node or one with associated local symptoms or signs (e.g. hoarseness, nasal obstruction or mucocutaneous ulceration and induration).

It needs to be stressed, however, that if an enlarged node is thought to due to metastasis from a primary malignancy elsewhere the patient needs referral for a surgical assessment and an exhaustive search for the primary before any lymph node biopsy.

FURTHER READING

Artenstein AW, Kim JH, Williams WJ, Chung RC. Isolated peripheral tuberculous lymphadenitis in adults: current clinical and diagnostic issues. Clin Infect Dis 1995;20:876–82.

Bass JW, Vincent JM, Person DA. The expanding spectrum of bartonella infections: 2. Cat scratch disease. Pediatr Infect Dis J 1997;16:163–79.

Kelly CS, Kelly RE. Lymphadenopathy in children. Pediatr Clin North Am 1998;45:875–88.

Norris A, Krasinskas A, Salhany K, Gluckman S. Kikuchi-Fujimoto disease: a benign cause of fever and lymphadenopathy. Am J Med 1996;171:401–5.

Shahidi H, Myers JL, Kvale P. Castleman's disease. Mayo Clin Proc 1995;70:969–77.

Zumla A, James DG. Granulomatous infections: etiology and classification. Clin Infect Dis 1996;23:146–58.

INFECTIOUS CAUSES OF A SOLITARY LYMPH NODE

Infecting agent		Site	Comments
Viruses	Herpes simplex virus, type 2	Inguinal	Not always associated with mucocutaneous lesions
	Adenoviruses	Cervical or preauricular	Associated with pharyngitis or conjunctivitis
Bacteria	Group A streptococci	Cervical	Tender, may suppurate
	Staphylococcus aureus	Regional	Search for skin focus
	Mycobacterium tuberculosis	Regional (particularly cervical)	Particularly in certain ethnic groups and in people who have HIV infection
	Atypical mycobacteria	Cervical	Scrofula; particularly in children
	Treponema pallidum (syphilis)	Inguinal	In primary disease; painless lymphadenitis; search for chancre
	Haemophilus ducreyi (chancroid)	Inguinal	Painful papules and suppurative nodes
	Yersinia pestis (plague)	Inguinal or femoral	Extremely tender node and acute systemic illness; exposure to rodents or fleas
	Francisella tularensis (tularemia)	Regional	Painful ulcer at site of inoculation; tender node; exposure to rodents
	Bartonella henselae (cat-scratch disease)	Regional (usually axillary, epitrochlear or cervical)	History of cat scratch or bite; skin lesion may have healed; not usually systemically ill; node moderately tender
Rickettsia/ chlamydia	Rickettsia tsutsugamushi (scrub typhus)	Regional	Travel to Asia or Australasia; history of mite bite with eschar at site
	Rickettsia akari (rickettsialpox)	Regional	Travel to South Africa, Korea or North America; papule at site of mite bite and generalized vesicular rash
	Chlamydia trachomatis (lymphogranuloma venereum)	Inguinal	Fixed, tender, matted nodes above and below inguinal ligament (groove sign); foci of suppuration and fistulas
Fungi	Histoplasma capsulatum var. duboisii	Regional	West Africa; cutaneous lesion
	Paracoccidioides brasiliensis (paracoccidioido-mycosis)	Cervical	Central and South America; usually chronic mucocutaneous lesions present
Protozoa	Toxoplasma gondii	Cervical	Mononucleosis-like illness; often generalized lymphadenopathy
	Trypanosoma brucei (African trypanosomiasis)	Cervical	African travel or residence; often generalized lymphadenopathy

Fig. 10.1 Infectious causes of a solitary enlarged lymph node.

NONINFECTIOUS CAUSES OF A SOLITARY ENLARGED LYMPH NODE

Immunologic	Rheumatoid arthritis (Felty's syndrome)
	Systemic lupus erythematosus
Malignant	Leukemia
	Lymphoma
	Metastatic malignancy
Miscellaneous	Sarcoidosis
	Drugs (carbamazepine, phenytoin)
	Castleman's disease (possibly related to human herpesvirus-8)
	Kikuchi's disease (histiocytic necrotizing lymphadenitis; possibly an infectious etiology)
	Histiocytosis X

Fig. 10.2 Noninfectious causes of a solitary enlarged lymph node.

MASSES OFTEN CONFUSED WITH ENLARGED LYMPH NODES

Name of mass	Usual site	Comment
Branchial cyst	Over the midpoint of the sternomastoid muscle	Contains sterile pus and many cholesterol crystals
Dermoid cyst	In the midline at any line of embryologic fusion	Fluctuant mass containing cheesy epithelial debris
Thyroid nodule	In region of the thyroid gland	Moves on swallowing
Thyroglossal cyst	In midline of throat	Moves on protruding the tongue
Onchocercal nodule	Associated with bony prominence such as the iliac crest or occiput	Travel or residence in Africa or Latin America; may be associated skin changes or visual problems
Femoral hernia	Below inguinal ligament	Cough impulse; reducible

Fig. 10.3 Masses often confused with enlarged lymph nodes.

Conjunctivitis, Keratitis and Infections of Periorbital Structures

chapter
11

Luke Herbert

CONJUNCTIVITIS

Conjunctivitis is inflammation of the conjunctiva. It is not a diagnosis, but a description of a clinical syndrome. There may be redness, dilated blood vessels, follicles, papillae and a watery-to-purulent discharge. Follicles are germinal centers of conjunctival lymphoid tissue and are predominant in viral conjunctivitis. They are small (typically <1mm) pale bumps under the tarsal, and sometimes limbal, conjunctiva. Small papillae are nonspecific and give the tarsal conjunctiva a velvety appearance. Giant papillae are a sign of chronic inflammation,give the upper tarsal conjunctiva a cobblestone appearance and may lead to reticular scarring on resolution.

Decreased vision or photophobia are associated with keratitis or uveitis, which can accompany conjunctivitis.

NONINFECTIVE CONJUNCTIVITIS

Endogenous causes of noninfectious conjunctivitis include dry eye and acute and chronic inflammatory conditions of the conjunctiva such as Stevens–Johnson syndrome or mucous membrane pemphigoid. Exogenous causes include pollution and medication (conjunctivitis medicamentosa). Rarely conjunctival or eyelid tumors can cause conjunctivitis (masquerade syndrome).

The distinction between noninfective and infectious causes is usually clear from the history. Except for chlamydial conjunctivitis, infectious conjunctivitis rarely lasts longer than 3 weeks, beginning to resolve after 10 days. Conjunctivitis medicamentosa can be a difficult condition to diagnose and may follow an infectious conjunctivitis. Clues include a history of initial improvement on starting a new type of eye drops followed by worsening and complaints that the eye-drops sting. Thorough history taking is necessary as patients may not recall all the different eye drops they have been using during an episode of conjunctivitis. Withdrawal of all topical medication and reassessment 2 or 3 days later is helpful.

In allergic conjunctivitis there is often a history of atopy and chronic mucus discharge and there are giant papillae.

INFECTIOUS CONJUNCTIVITIS

BACTERIAL CONJUNCTIVITIS
Epidemiology
Bacterial conjunctivitis is ubiquitous and is commoner in warmer months and regions. It is transmitted by contact with ocular or upper respiratory tract discharges of people who have the infection, fomites, medical equipment or shared cosmetics. In some areas insect vectors are involved.

Clinical features
Tearing, irritation and sticky discharge without preauricular lymphadenopathy are early clinical features. The conjunctiva is pink (not red). The lids may be stuck together by a mucopurulent exudate on awakening.

Diagnosis
Microbiologic investigation is necessary only in neonatal, hyperacute, severe, unusual or chronic cases. Microscopy of conjunctival smears can be useful and conjunctival swabs on blood agar and, especially in children, chocolate agar are used. *Haemophilus influenzae* biogroup *aegyptius* and *Streptococcus pneumoniae* are common causes. *Haemophilus influenzae* type b and *Moraxella* and *Branhamella* spp., *Neisseria meningitidis* and *Corynebacterium diphtheriae* are also involved. In infants the main organisms are *H. influenzae* biogroup *aegyptius,* gonococci, *S. pneumoniae,* viridans streptococci, entero-cocci and rarely *Pseudomonas aeruginosa.*[1,2]

Management
Topical broad-spectrum antibiotic drops are used two hourly until the symptoms subside, which should occur rapidly. In Europe, chloramphenicol, and in the USA, neomycin, polymyxin and bacitracin are used. Gentamicin and tobramycin are useful against Gram-negative organisms, but cause a higher rate of local toxic reactions. Erythromycin or the quinolones may also be used.

HYPERACUTE CONJUNCTIVITIS
Hyperacute conjunctivitis is characterized by copious discharge, chemosis and lid swelling. Membranes may form on the tarsal conjunctiva and there may be a tender preauricular lymphadenopathy. Corneal involvement is common and severe, and corneal perforation can occur within 24 hours. It is caused by *Neisseria gonorrhoeae* and *N. meningitidis*.

Management
The drug of choice is an extended-spectrum cephalosporin such as ceftriaxone 1g (25–40mg/kg) every 12 hours for 3 days. Repeated irrigation of the conjunctival sac is recommended to reduce inflammatory microbial mediators to the cornea.

BRAZILIAN PURPURIC FEVER
This is caused by a rare invasive clone of *H. influenzae* biogroup *aegyptius*. Systemic disease occurs in children 1–3 weeks after an episode of conjunctivitis. It is seen over a widespread area in Brazil and there is a case mortality of 70%. The clinical picture is similar to that of meningococcal sepsis.

Management
The Brazilian purpuric fever clone of *H. influenzae* biogroup *aegyptius* is resistant to trimethoprim, but is sensitive to chloramphenicol and ampicillin. During epidemics systemic rifampin (rifampicin) (20mg/kg/day for 2 days) may be used as prophylaxis against Brazilian purpuric fever for children who have conjunctivitis.

OPHTHALMIA NEONATORUM
Ophthalmia neonatorum is any conjunctivitis in the first 3 weeks of life. The most serious cause is gonococcal conjunctivitis, which can be life threatening. Commoner causes are *Chlamydia trachomatis*, chemical irritation and herpes simplex virus.

Epidemiology

Ophthalmia neonatorum occurs worldwide, but is uncommon where there is adequate infant eye prophylaxis. Globally gonococcal ophthalmia neonatorum is an important cause of blindness. The risk of ophthalmia neonatorum for a child born to an infected mother is 30–50% for gonorrhea[3] and 15–35% for chlamydial infection.[4] Transmission usually occurs in the birth canal.

Prevention

Topical prophylaxis was described in 1881 by Credé. His silver nitrate eye drops substantially reduced the incidence of gonococcal conjunctivitis, but are inactive against chlamydia and toxicity is common. Recently, 2.5% aqueous povidone–iodine has been shown to be safer, cheaper and more effective.[5,6] Maternal treatment before birth is the best prevention.

Clinical features

Gonococcal conjunctivitis presents 24–48 hours after birth and earlier after premature rupture of membranes. Lid edema, chemosis and a discharge, which is serosanguineous and rapidly becomes purulent, progress to corneal ulceration. Perforation can occur soon afterwards.

Chlamydial conjunctivitis presents 5–12 days after birth with a watery discharge, which becomes purulent more slowly. Follicles are absent because the conjunctival lymphoid tissue in infants is immature. Untreated the condition usually resolves in 3–4 weeks, but can take 1 year. Rarely membranes and micropannus form, resulting in significant stromal scarring in later life. Pneumonitis, rhinitis, vaginitis and otitis can follow the conjunctivitis.

Diagnosis

Cultures on blood and chocolate agar for gonococci, and viral culture and immunofluorescent testing, enzyme immunoassay or DNA probing for chlamydia antigen should be performed.

Management

Neonates who have a purulent discharge are presumed to have gonococcal infection and are treated with ceftriaxone 25–50mg/kg intramuscularly or intravenously to a maximum of 125mg. Frequent irrigation removes bacteria and microbial products. A single intramuscular dose of 125mg of ceftriaxone is effective therapy for gonococcal ophthalmia neonatorum.[7] Parents should be screened for sexually transmitted diseases.

Treatment of chlamydial ophthalmia neonatorum comprises 2 weeks of erythromycin 10mg/kg q12h for the first week and q8h for the second week of life.

CHLAMYDIAL CONJUNCTIVITIS: TRACHOMA

Chlamydial infection results in three distinct clinical pictures. Trachoma is a scarring condition of the conjunctiva and cornea in adults caused by recurrent childhood infection with *C. trachomatis*. Adult inclusion conjunctivitis is an acute condition associated with sexually transmitted chlamydial infection. Neonatal chlamydial conjunctivitis is described above.

Epidemiology

Trachoma occurs worldwide and is endemic in poorer rural areas of developing countries. Blindness due to trachoma is still common in parts of the Middle East, northern and sub-Saharan Africa, parts of the Indian subcontinent, South East Asia and China. There are pockets of infection in South America, among Australian Aborigines, in the Pacific islands and in native American reservations in southwest USA.

Prevention

The infection is transmitted by contact with ocular or nasopharyngeal secretions, either directly through fomites or insect vectors (the flies *Musca sorbens* in Africa and the Middle East and *Hippelates* spp. in the Americas). Untreated active lesions can be infectious for years.

Prevention of transmission is the most important public health measure.[8] Education about personal hygiene and regular washing of the face is very important and these hygiene measures require only a tiny amount of water. There has been mass treatment of the population with topical tetracycline or erythromycin in hyperendemic areas.

Clinical features

The acute conjunctivitis is characterized by a diffuse follicular reaction in the conjunctiva of the superior tarsal plate and at the limbus with soft follicles. Papillary hypertrophy is a nonspecific sign. With resolution of the follicles there is subconjunctival scarring and a loss of conjunctival mucin-producing goblet cells. Blinding complications result from chronic re-infection,[9] severe dry eyes and entropion leading to corneal scarring, bacterial superinfection and ulceration.

Diagnosis

The diagnosis is made on clinical grounds in endemic areas.

Expressed follicles have a characteristic microscopic appearance involving macrophages (Leber's cells), plasma cells and lymphoblasts.

Chlamydia trachomatis types A–C are involved. Secondary bacterial superinfection is common and causes severe disease. Antibodies to *C. trachomatis* can be demonstrated in the tears and serum.

Management

Prevention of the chronic sequelae by treatment in childhood is a public health priority. Once scarring has occurred management is with lubricants and surgery.

CHLAMYDIAL CONJUNCTIVITIS: ADULT INCLUSION CONJUNCTIVITIS

Clinical features

The conjunctivitis presents with a mucopurulent discharge after a 4- to 12-day incubation period. It is often monocular and develops into a chronic follicular conjunctivitis, often with epithelial keratitis and limbal follicles. Tender preauricular lymphadenopathy is common. Untreated the disease has a chronic course and may progress to keratitis and possibly iritis.

Diagnosis

Enzyme-linked immunoassay or immunofluorescent monoclonal antibody stains of conjunctival scrapings are rapid and convenient ways to make the diagnosis.[10]

Management

Treatment is with 3 weeks of systemic doxycycline 100mg q12h or erythromycin stearate 500mg q6h. Topical treatment is relatively ineffective.

VIRAL CONJUNCTIVITIS

EPIDEMIOLOGY

Viral conjunctivitis is common and occurs worldwide. Epidemics frequently occur and may be propagated by eye clinics. Transmission is by direct or indirect contact with ocular or upper respiratory tract secretions. Viral particles can remain infectious on surfaces for more than 1 month.

The incubation period is from 2 days to 2 weeks and infected people remain contagious for up to 2 weeks after the symptoms begin.

CLINICAL FEATURES

The main patterns of viral conjunctivitis are:
- epidemic keratoconjunctivitis (EKC),
- pharyngoconjunctival fever (PCF), and
- acute hemorrhagic conjunctivitis (AHC).

The symptoms and signs of these patterns of infection are similar, but vary in degree. All present as an acute follicular conjunctivitis, with watering, grittiness, redness, ecchymosis and lid edema, often with flu-like symptoms. Preauricular lymphadenopathy and bilateral involvement are common.

In EKC most patients have some focal epitheliopathy and photophobia by 2 weeks. Subepithelial opacities appear after 2 weeks in 50% of patients and occasionally impair vision. These lesions cause occasional recurrences of grittiness. The natural history is of slow resolution, which can take more than 1 year.

In PCF there is a similar ophthalmic picture, but the systemic features are more pronounced.

In AHC ecchymosis is more prominent and the onset of symptoms more rapid. Rarely a polio-like radiculopathy follows AHC.

DIAGNOSIS

Several methods are available for typing the viruses that cause acute conjunctivitis, most of which are time-consuming and expensive. More recently, polymerase chain reaction (PCR) and restriction fragment length polymorphism analysis have allowed faster diagnosis. Immunochromatography promises almost instant results.[11] These tests will be useful for epidemiology.

Most epidemics of viral conjunctivitis are caused by adenoviruses, commonly serotypes 8, 19, 37 for EKC, and types 3 and 8 for PCF. Picornaviruses such as enterovirus type 70 and Coxsackie virus type A24 cause AHC. Conjunctivitis can be a feature of many other viral diseas es including influenza, rubella, rubeola, chickenpox and glandular fever.

MANAGEMENT

The management of viral conjunctivitis is supportive with warm or cold compresses reducing symptoms of itch, and lubrication and cycloplegics if there is an element of keratitis (see below). Antibacterial prophylaxis is probably unnecessary and can cause an allergic or toxic conjunctivitis.

KERATITIS

Keratitis is an inflammation of the cornea. Microbial keratitis is suppurative inflammation of the cornea produced by a replicating micro-organism. It carries a high risk of visual loss and can be caused by bacteria, fungi, viruses or parasites. A large variety of bacteria and fungi can infect the cornea.[12]

Typical acute microbial keratitis is the major syndrome. Patients present with a corneal epithelial defect and a stromal infiltrate (Fig. 11.1). The other main clinical problems are herpesvirus infections, with recurrent inflammation leading to scarring, and infection in a 'compromised' cornea (i.e. after local or systemic immunosuppression, injury or chronic disease). Acanthamoeba keratitis, which used to be rare, is a problem in contact lens wearers. Noninfectious keratitis is important in that it can be confused with infectious keratitis.

Algorithms for the initial division of keratitis into the main clinical situations are shown in Figure 11.2.

INFECTIOUS KERATITIS

TYPICAL ACUTE MICROBIAL KERATITIS
Epidemiology
Microbial keratitis is responsible for 30% of cases of blindness in some developing countries. In hot climates fungal infection is more frequent, although bacterial keratitis still accounts for 60% of cases.[13]

Contact lens wear increases the risk of developing bacterial keratitis.[14] The annual incidence is 5/10,000 for daily wear of soft lenses and 20/10,000 for overnight wear of soft lenses, although estimates tenfold higher than this have been made. It has been estimated that over 65% of all new cases of keratitis in London, UK are due to contact lens wear.[15] The largest risk factor is overnight soft lens wear. This increases the risk by a factor of 5 compared to daily lens wear, and by a factor of 20 compared to rigid lens wear.[16]

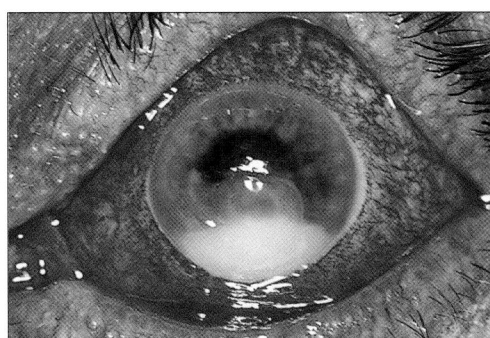

Fig. 11.1
Typical microbial keratitis. Note accumulation of inflammatory cells at the dependent part of the anterior chamber of the eye (hypopyon) and mid-corneal defect. Courtesy of Myron Yanoff.

Surgery, particularly corneal grafts and corneal sutures, and concomitant use of topical corticosteroids increase the risk of infection. Other than vitamin A deficiency systemic predisposing conditions are relatively unimportant clinically. Vitamin A deficiency is particularly important in children who are malnourished and who have a concomitant infection, especially measles, where keratomalacia (corneal melting) can occur suddenly.

Pathogenesis and pathology
Four principal groups of bacterial pathogens are responsible for most cases of infective keratitis. Micrococci (*Staphylococcus* and *Micrococcus* spp.), *Streptococcus* and *Pseudomonas* spp. and the Enterobacteriaceae (*Citrobacter, Klebsiella, Enterobacter, Serratia* and *Proteus* spp.) accounted for 87% of cases of bacterial keratitis in one series.[17]

Pseudomonas infection is recognized for its swift suppurative course to perforation secondary to proteolytic enzyme release. It is particularly common in contact lens wearers (hard and soft). *Serratia marcescens* corneal ulcers have been associated with contact lens wear and contaminated eye drops. *Neisseria gonorrhoeae, C. diphtheriae* and *Haemophilus* and *Listeria* spp. are capable of penetrating an intact corneal epithelium. Other bacteria and fungi produce disease only after a loss of corneal epithelial integrity.

Following invasion by micro-organisms several chemotactic substances are released leading to an inflammatory cell infiltrate and consequent phagocytosis, cell death, release of proteolytic enzymes and corneal stromal damage.

Clinical features
The clinical appearance is not pathognomonic for any particular infecting organism, although some patterns are characteristic. Stromal ring infiltrates imply a massive immune response characteristic of infection by *Bacillus* and *Pseudomonas* spp. They are also seen in infections by *Streptococcus, Listeria, Proteus* and *Acanthamoeba* spp.

Staphylococcal infection can present early without an infiltrate, but with pain, localized edema and a ring of keratic precipitates (inflammatory cells adherent to the endothelium). Developing ulcers due to *Staphylococcus aureus* infection are round or oval and tend to progress in depth rather than area.

Diagnosis
Diagnosis is by microscopy and culture of a corneal scrape. In contact lens wearers the lenses and lens case should be cultured.

In some parts of the world broad-spectrum therapy is used without initial investigation and it has been suggested that this practice could be extended.[18] If microbiologic services are not available there is little choice. However, the current high success rates of this treatment may not continue and in some areas antibiotic resistance is developing. Corneal scraping also debrides the ulcer, allows antibiotics to enter the base of the ulcer and provides microbiologic data (provided that antimicrobial therapy has not been given within the previous 24 hours).

The cornea is anesthetized with nonpreserved amethocaine 1%, five or six drops at 2-minute intervals. Using a slit-lamp, necrotic material

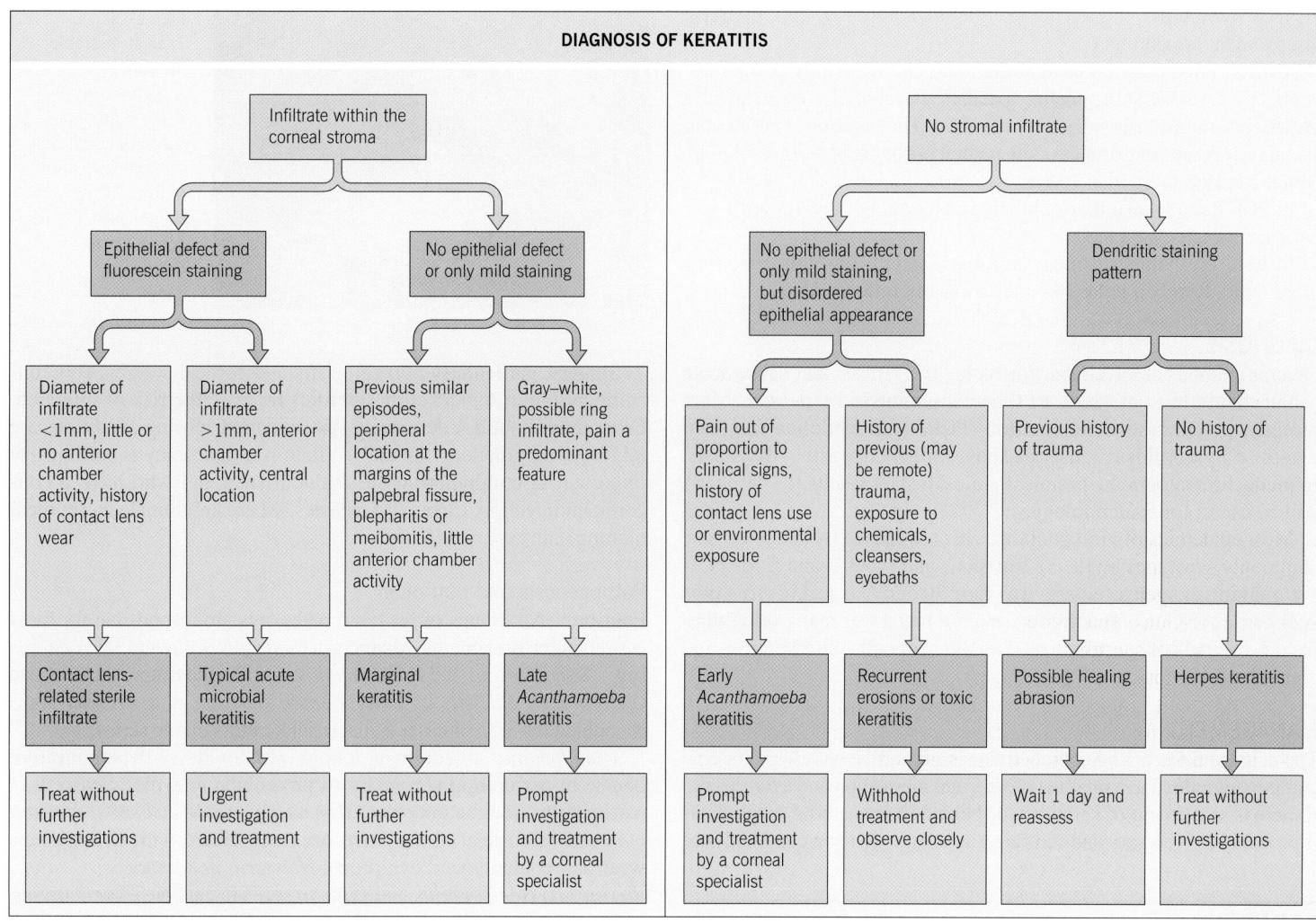

Fig. 11.2 Diagnosis of keratitis.

is removed from the center of the ulcer. A 23 gauge needle tip is scraped parallel to the cornea to remove infected tissue. A fresh needle is used for each specimen. If a slit-lamp is not available scraping with a scalpel blade is safer than using a needle. The diagnostic yield is greater from the sides of the ulcer than from necrotic areas.

Slides should be made for Gram stain and Giesma stain, and appropriate bacterial cultures (and fungal cultures if suspected) should be prepared directly from the needle. Bending the tip of the needle before use facilitates this. The sharp side is used to scrape the cornea and the smooth surface used to plate out the specimen without penetrating the surface of the agar.

Management
Either gentamicin 1.5% with cefuroxime 5% or the fluoroquinolones ofloxacin 0.3% or ciprofloxacin 0.3% are effective against 90% of expected isolates in most clinical settings.[19,20]

Aminoglycosides are toxic to the epithelium in moderate doses and quinolones are preferred as monotherapy. In cases where streptococci are likely (e.g. chronic ocular surface disease, children) there may be quinolone resistance and combination with cefuroxime 5% is recommended.

Initial treatment is with drops every hour day and night for 2 days, followed by review.[21] If the clinical picture has improved or not worsened treatment is reduced to drops every hour by day for 3 days. After this time the ulcer should be sterile. Treatment is reduced to prophylactic levels q6h until the epithelium has healed.

If the clinical picture progresses after 2 days of treatment the patient should be admitted to hospital for supervised treatment. If after the first week there is no response to therapy, consider stopping

therapy and re-culturing or switching to a different antibiotic guided by antibiotic sensitivity testing.

FUNGAL KERATITIS
Fungal infections are seen in two distinct clinical settings. In hotter climates the cornea is inoculated with infected vegetable matter as a result of agricultural or other trauma. Infection can then occur in otherwise healthy eyes. In temperate climates infection most often occurs in association with chronic ocular surface disease or prolonged corticosteroid use.

The septate filamentous fungal species, especially *Fusarium* and *Aspergillus* spp., are the most common cause of fungal keratitis. With increasing distance from the equator the relative incidence of candidal infection increases. Dematiaceous filamentous fungi such as *Curvularia* spp. are of low virulence and cause indolent infections.

Prevention
The main cause of fungal keratitis worldwide is trauma. In the developed world risk factors include protracted epithelial ulceration, therapeutic soft contact lens wear, corneal transplant and topical corticosteroid therapy. Patients who have exposure keratitis and a history of previous herpes simplex or herpes zoster keratitis are at risk.

Clinical features
Fungal keratitis usually presents as a typical microbial keratitis. It is not possible to diagnose the type of infection on clinical grounds. Clinical context is the most important guide to appropriate investigation and therapy. In filamentary fungus keratitis the corneal surface is gray or dull. Satellite lesions are common in the surrounding stroma and may

be seen with an intact epithelium (Fig. 11.3). Candidal lesions appear in corneas that are already abnormal. They are often quite localized at first with a collar button configuration.

Diagnosis

Diagnosis is by culture of corneal scrapes. In indolent cases corneal biopsy is indicated.

Management

Historic data are the best guide to selecting antifungal therapy.[22] The greatest experience in the use of antifungals for keratitis comes from India. However, this experience may not apply to situations where there is a local or systemic disorder of immunity.

No currently available antifungal agent has a favorable profile of activity and toxicity. Response to antifungal treatment is poor compared with that to antibacterial treatment. Surgical management (corneal transplant) may be necessary.

Combined topical and systemic therapy is often used and is usually prolonged. Corneal drug penetration is helped by daily scraping of the epithelium and necrotic stroma.

The choice of antifungal is often dictated by availability. Most topical antifungal agents have to be made locally from tablets or intravenous preparations. The following preparations have been used with various degrees of success.

Polyenes. Amphotericin B is fungicidal, but is toxic to the eye in high concentrations. It is used diluted in sterile water at 0.1–0.15% 2–4 times every hour for the first 1–2 days.

Natamycin 5% has poor corneal penetration, but is useful for superficial filamentary fungal infections.

Pyrimidines. Flucytosine 1% can be prepared from a commercially available intravenous or tablet form and is used in combination only (early resistance occurs) with amphotericin B for candidal keratitis. Concomitant systemic use may be helpful.

Imidazoles. Miconazole 10mg/ml in polyethoxylated castor oil (intravenous preparation) was effective in more than 60% of cases in a prospective trial in India[23] when used topically every 2 hours.

Ketoconazole 2% prepared as an aqueous solution from tablets is probably effective against *Aspergillus flavus*, but not *Aspergillus fumigatus* or *Fusarium* spp. Systemic and topical administration is often combined.

Econazole 1% is used topically in combination with systemic itraconazole, and clotrimazole 1% vaginal cream has also been used.

Fluconazole is given systemically or as a 0.2–0.5% topical aqueous solution.

Itraconazole used orally has an improved spectrum against filamentous fungi. It has poorer tissue penetration, but a good clinical response when used against candidal infections. *Fusarium* spp. respond less well.

Other agents. Silver sulfadiazine 1% is used for antibiotic prophylaxis in patients who have burns. It has moderate antifungal activity *in vitro*, but has been widely used in developing countries as a topical antifungal with good rates of success, particularly against *Fusarium* spp.

Chlorhexidine gluconate 0.2% solution is at least as effective as natamycin in treating fungal infections and is suggested as an inexpensive agent for use in the developing world.[24]

Initial treatment for fungal keratitis depends upon local experience. In London, UK we use topical econazole 1% (or amphotericin B 0.15 or 0.3%) hourly for 48 hours, then 2 hourly for 72 hours and then reduce the dosage depending upon the initial response. Long-term treatment is required. Systemic treatment is used as an adjunct: itraconazole 200mg daily initially, reduced to 100mg for longer term use. If surgical debridement is performed a 2mm clear margin is advised. The inflammatory reaction results from live organisms and fungal debris. As most antifungals are fungistatic, reduction of inflammation also depresses local immunity so that the organisms are not killed. Concomitant corticosteroid use is therefore not recommended for fungal keratitis.

ACANTHAMOEBA KERATITIS

Epidemiology

Acanthamoeba histolytica was not recognized as a cause of keratitis until the 1970s, and the incidence has increased since. *Acanthamoeba histolytica* live in soil and water, including swimming pools, water storage tanks and contact lens cases (see Chapter 8.33).[25] Approximately 10–15% of cases are associated with agricultural and other trauma, but most are associated with contact lens use. The annual incidence during 1985 through 1987 was estimated at 1.65–2.01/million contact lens wearers.[26] Poor lens hygiene by soft contact lens wearers and using homemade saline- or chlorine-based disinfection systems are risk factors. Disposable lens wearers have a particularly high risk, although this may be related to care systems used with the lenses.[27]

In the UK the use of tank-stored water by contact lens wearers to rinse lenses or lens cases may have introduced *Acanthamoeba histolytica* into their lens care systems.[28] The free-living protozoa have been seen grazing on bacterial slime on the bottom of contact lens cases.

Acanthamoeba histolytica can also cause scleritis and chorioretinitis.

Prevention

Good lens hygiene, the use of hydrogen peroxide 3% for at least 3 hours[29] and avoidance of tap water in contact lens care are important preventive measures.

Clinical features

In early epithelial disease there may be punctate keratopathy, pseudodendrites, epithelial wrinkling, diffuse or focal subepithelial infiltrates and radial perineural infiltrates. Ring infiltrates and corneal ulceration may present later.[30,31] Pain out of proportion to the clinical signs is common, but not constant. The clinical picture may resemble herpetic or fungal keratitis, and a high index of suspicion is warranted in contact lens wearers who have apparent herpetic disease. Bacterial coinfection or superinfection in late disease occurs in around 10% of cases and causes an atypical presentation.

The clinical course of *Acanthamoeba histolytica* keratitis is prolonged. Early diagnosis is important, but treatment started before proper diagnostic tests are carried out only confuses the clinical picture. Unlike bacterial keratitis there is no justification for starting therapy without investigation. A delay of a 1–2 days while a patient is referred for expert opinion and investigation is less harmful than early inappropriate therapy. The grave prognosis of *Acanthamoeba histolytica* keratitis in the past was due to the slow inexorable progression of disease rather than fulminant corneal destruction.

Diagnosis

Diagnosis is made by microbiologic and histopathologic examination of tissue specimens. The epithelium is removed for examination by epithelial biopsy. In cases where only the stroma appears to be involved corneal biopsy (described above) is necessary. If culture is negative, tear fluid PCR has been suggested as an adjunctive investigation.[32]

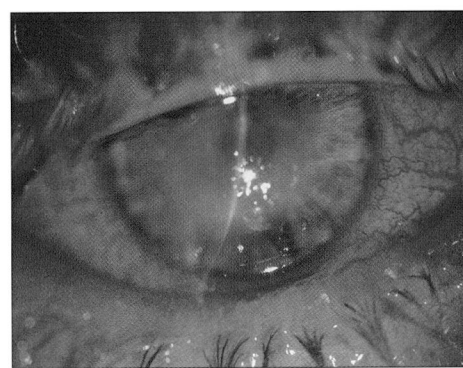

Fig. 11.3 Fungal keratitis. The corneal surface looks rough, and there are several satellite lesions best seen here at the periphery on the left side of the cornea. Courtesy of Myron Yanoff.

Microbiology. Specimens[33] can be plated on non-nutrient agar, which is later overlain with *Escherichia coli* in the laboratory. Tracks of bacterial clearing show where the amebae have been grazing.

Bacterial and fungal cultures should also be obtained.

Microscopy techniques vary. Fluorescent microscopy can be carried out using calcofluor white, which stains the walls of cysts, or with acridine orange or an immunofluorescent antibody. An immunoperoxidase test is used in some laboratories. Confocal microscopy of a wet preparation can be used to identify motile trophozoites, which have a large karyosome and a contractile vacuole.

Biopsy specimens should also be stained with hematoxylin and eosin, periodic acid–Schiff and methenamine silver to demonstrate *Acanthamoeba histolytica* cysts.

Sensitivity testing, although useful in screening for amebicides, is less useful in the management of individual cases,[34,35] perhaps because *Acanthamoeba histolytica* encysts in infected tissues.

Management

The diamidines, propamidine isethionate 0.1% and hexamidine 0.1% and the cationic antiseptics, polyhexamethyl biguanide (PHMB) 0.02% and chlorhexidine 0.02% are probably the most effective medications,[31,36] although availability can be a problem. Local manufacture of chlorhexidine or PHMB may be possible from 20% disinfectant preparations. The azoles (clotrimazole, fluconazole, ketoconazole and miconazole) have also been suggested for use as a third agent.

Initial treatment starts immediately after the epithelium is debrided using a cationic antiseptic and a diamidine, each hour day and night for 48 hours, then hourly by day for 3 days. Dosage is then reduced to 3-hourly to reduce local toxicity. If toxicity is suspected the frequency of the diamidine should be reduced.

It may take 2 weeks to achieve a response to treatment. Pain relief with systemic nonsteroidal anti-inflammatory agents and cycloplegia are very important.

The use of corticosteroids in controlling inflammation is controversial. Some authorities say that they are contraindicated at any stage. Others advocate the use of weak topical corticosteroid to control inflammation after at least 2 weeks of antiamebic therapy, emphasizing the importance of continued antiamebic therapy until several weeks after the corticosteroid is stopped.

VIRAL KERATITIS – HERPES SIMPLEX VIRUS TYPE 1 OR 2
Epidemiology

Herpes simplex keratitis has an annual incidence of new cases of 8/10,000. The incidence peaks in individuals aged 5–10 and 35–40 years. Males are affected twice as often as females. Approximately 50% of patients have a history of herpes labialis. Primary ocular infection occurs in 5%.[37]

Corneal infection is usually (98% of cases) with herpes simplex virus type 1, except in neonatal herpes infection when 80% of cases are due to herpes simplex virus type 2.

Pathogenesis and pathology

The pattern of dendritic ulcers is caused by direct infection of corneal epithelium. It is thought that delayed type hypersensitivity to viral antigens causes the inflammation that leads to disciform keratitis.[38]

Clinical features

Primary ocular infection is usually asymptomatic, although a vesicular reaction may be seen. Occasionally there is a follicular conjunctivitis. Corneal damage is caused by recurrent disease.

Recurrence occurs in around 10% of cases at 1 year and 50% by 20 years. Triggers include fever, trauma and ultraviolet light. Recurrence is a consequence of latency.[39] Latency develops as virus spreads to a sensory ganglion and remains dormant there. It is thought that infection can spread across a ganglion, for instance

from the mandibular to the ophthalmic division of the trigeminal nerve, and hence from lip to eye. Spread from eye to eye is uncommon except if there is atopy where delayed-type hypersensitivity is impaired. These patients are at risk from bilateral disease, larger geographic ulcers and disseminated infection.

With each recurrence corneal scarring increases, and it is thought that viral particles remaining within the cornea cause the continuing inflammation and edema seen in disciform keratitis.

Diagnosis

Viral culture or immunofluorescence[40] can be used to confirm infection, but in practice the diagnosis is clinical. In epithelial disease there is a characteristic dendritic ulcer (Fig. 11.4). Corneal sensation is often impaired, and there is usually a history of similar attacks in the past.

Management

Untreated herpes simplex keratitis usually resolves within 1–2 weeks, but it can progress, resulting in the development of geographic ulcers. Resolution is more rapid if the dendritic ulcer is debrided. Antiviral treatment also speeds up resolution, and no benefit has been shown for a combination of debridement and antivirals when compared with the use of antivirals alone. The choice of antiviral depends upon availability. In Europe aciclovir 3% ophthalmic ointment 5 times a day is almost universally preferred because it is effective and has a low incidence of toxicity.[41] In the USA, trifluridine 1% 2-hourly is used.

Oral aciclovir or famciclovir is effective, but comparatively expensive. It may be useful when there is a desire to reduce corneal exposure to topical agents. Systemic antiviral treatment is recommended as prophylaxis against encephalitis for infants who have primary infection.

Prophylactic treatment with oral aciclovir 400mg q12h reduces the recurrence rate of stromal (severe) disease from 28 to 14%.[42]

The management of the chronic sequelae of herpes simplex keratitis may require topical corticosteroid therapy under close ophthalmic supervision. Topical antiviral treatment reduces recurrence rates in these patients.[43]

VIRAL KERATITIS – HERPES ZOSTER OPHTHALMICUS
Epidemiology

The varicella-zoster virus is a herpesvirus that causes chickenpox as a primary infection and shingles on recurrence. Around 90% of adults are seropositive for varicella-zoster virus. The rate of recurrence increases with age, and second recurrences can occur in those who have impaired immunity.

Pathogenesis and pathology

Reactivated virus replicates in the ganglion, producing local inflammation and premonitory pain before traveling down peripheral nerves to the skin or eye. A perineuritis and vasculitis occurs, and in the eye a disciform keratitis, iritis and cyclitis are common manifestations.

Clinical features

The clinical appearance is typical. Symptoms of eye involvement include photophobia and decreased vision. Hutchinson's sign, a rash on the side of the nose, is associated with ocular inflammation (Fig. 11.5).

Management

Oral aciclovir 800mg five times a day for 7 days accelerates skin healing and reduces the incidence of episcleritis, keratitis and iritis and probably acute pain.[44] The newer antivirals famciclovir and valaciclovir have improved bioavailability and are increasingly used instead of aciclovir. There is little role for topical antivirals.

Disciform keratitis, iritis and cyclitis respond to conventional corticosteroid treatment, but require prolonged therapy, sometimes for years.

INFECTIONS OF PERIORBITAL STRUCTURES

PERIORBITAL CELLULITIS

The orbit is the bony structure surrounding the eye. Infection of the contents of the bony orbit is called orbital cellulitis. Orbital infection commonly occurs as a result of contiguous spread from adjacent structures. Periorbital cellulitis is divided into preseptal or postseptal (orbital) depending upon the site of infection. Orbital cellulitis is sight and occasionally life threatening.

Preseptal cellulitis is 5–10 times more common than orbital cellulitis in infants and toddlers and is not sight or life threatening, but can rarely spread to become orbital cellulitis. It is commonly caused by *Haemophilus influenzae* or *Streptococcus* spp. and follows an upper respiratory tract infection. In adults it is most often seen after minor trauma such as an infected bite or scratch.

The source and agents of infection causing orbital cellulitis vary with age. The paranasal (ethmoid, maxillary and frontal) sinuses are the main sources. Orbital cellulitis is uncommon in neonates, but when it occurs it is usually secondary to conjunctivitis or a developmental abnormality such as a ruptured dacryocele. In infants respiratory tract infections may cause preseptal cellulitis. In older children and adults dental abscesses and trauma become important causes. Endogenous orbital cellulitis is rare.

Clinical features
In adults there is frequently a history of sinusitis, headache or recent tooth extraction or abscess. Children often have an antecedent upper respiratory tract infection.

Preseptal cellulitis is characterized by usually unilateral mainly upper eyelid swelling and edema. Lower lid swelling occurs when the cellulitis is secondary to dacryocystitis. Edematous conjunctiva can prolapse between the lids.

In orbital cellulitis features of preseptal cellulitis are variably present, but there is also proptosis, decreased ocular mobility and even decreased vision or a relative afferent pupil defect. These signs are caused by increased intraorbital pressure due to edema or abscess. If a subperiosteal abscess forms there may be nonaxial displacement of the globe and a palpable fluctuant mass in the orbit. Headache, fever and leukocytosis are common.

Diagnosis
Blood and local cultures are mandatory.

A CT scan can distinguish between preseptal and orbital cellulitis and show the site of an orbital or subperiosteal abscess:[45]
- preseptal cellulitis produces edema of the lids and tissues anterior to the orbital septum; and
- orbital cellulitis produces edema of the orbital tissues and proptosis.
Orbital cellulitis is often associated with signs of primary or secondary sinus disease.

Staphylococcus and *Streptococcus* spp. and, in those under 4 years of age, *H. influenzae* are the main pathogens that cause preseptal and orbital cellulitis in children. In subperiosteal abscesses in children over 9 years of age and adults there is often a mixed infection of aerobes and anaerobes[46] from extending sinus or dental infections.

Management
Preseptal cellulitis responds well to systemic antibiotics. Broadspectrum agent(s) that cover *Staphylococcus* and *Streptococcus* spp. and *H. influenzae* should be used. A response is usual within 24 hours.

Orbital cellulitis requires prompt diagnosis and treatment with intravenous antibiotics as an inpatient. Monitoring of vision, pupillary reaction, extraocular movements and central nervous system function should be carried out during the first 1–2 days until the infection begins to resolve. If a subperiosteal abscess or sinusitis is identified and the clinical picture is not improving after 24 hours surgical manage-

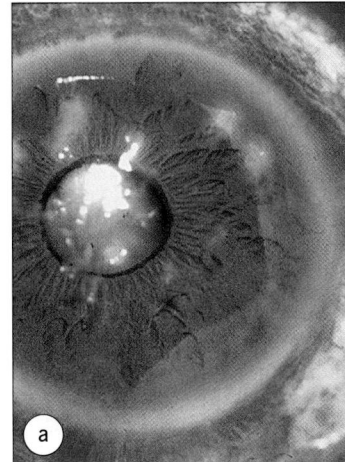 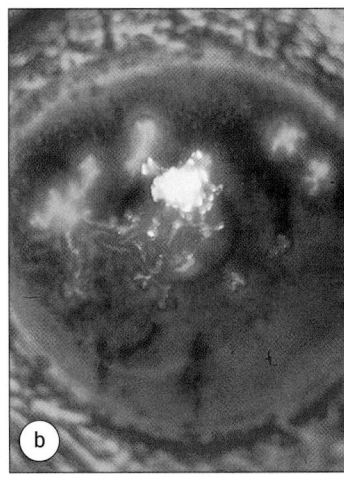

Fig. 11.4 Herpes simplex virus dendritic keratitis, showing branching epithelial lesions seen (a) without staining and (b) with rose bengal staining. Rose bengal stains the devitalized cells at the edges of the dendritic lesions. Courtesy of Myron Yanoff.

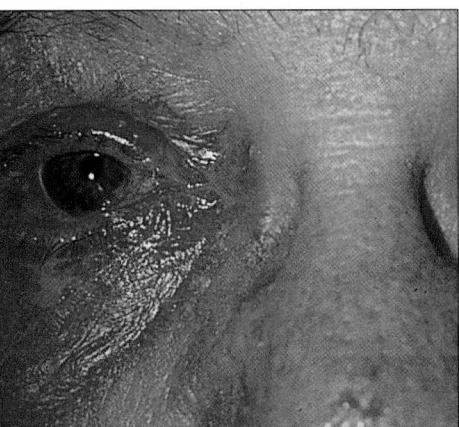

Fig. 11.5 Herpes zoster ophthalmicus. Inflamed right periorbital skin, with conjunctivitis and a lesion on the nose. Courtesy of Myron Yanoff.

ment is required. Orbital or brain abscesses are less common, and should be drained immediately.

LACRIMAL SYSTEM INFECTIONS

DACRYOADENITIS
Dacryoadenitis is usually due to a viral infection of the lacrimal gland. Patients present with adenopathy, fever, malaise and leukocytosis. The causes include infectious mononucleosis, herpes zoster, mumps, trachoma, syphilis, tuberculosis and sarcoidosis. It occasionally occurs in dehydrated patients as an ascending staphylococcal infection associated with a purulent discharge. On CT scanning there is diffuse lacrimal gland swelling without bony defects.

Diagnosis
The condition is usually self-limiting. Investigation other than CT scanning is reserved for chronic cases, who should be referred for specialist investigation to exclude neoplasia.

Management
Treatment is generally symptomatic. Corticosteroids can help speed up resolution. It can be difficult to distinguish dacryoadenitis from idiopathic lacrimal gland inflammation (pseudotumor), although the presence of enlarged preauricular lymph nodes makes a viral diagnosis more likely.

CANALICULITIS
There are chronic and acute forms. Acute dacryoadenitis may be caused by herpes simplex or herpes zoster and is often unrecognized except as a conjunctivitis and by its sequelae: scarred closed canaliculi and punctum.

Chronic canaliculitis is usually unilateral and characterized by pain or tenderness at the inner canthus. A chronic conjunctivitis may mask the more specific signs. The lacrimal punctum may pout and 'sulfur granules' may be expressed. These sulfur granules are pathognomonic of infection with *Actinomyces israelii*, an anaerobic Gram-positive branching filamentous bacterium. Less common causes are *Aspergillus* and *Candida* spp.

Treatment is by incision of the infected canaliculus and washout of all 'sulfur' material, usually with a penicillin-containing irrigation fluid.

DACRYOCYSTITIS
Pathogenesis and pathology
This condition occurs in chronic and acute forms. In infants it is usually an indolent condition resulting from incomplete development of the lacrimal drainage system. There is a mucopurulent discharge and recurrent conjunctivitis. Colonization is usual with *H. influenzae, Streptococcus pneumoniae,* staphylococci and *Klebsiella* and *Pseudomonas* spp.

In adults an acquired block of the lacrimal drainage system can cause an acute or chronic infection. An acute infection can be precipitated by instrumentation for investigation of a suspected blocked lacrimal duct. For this reason, mucoceles or chronic dacryocystitis should not be probed or syringed.

Acute dacrocystitis presents with a painful swelling over the lacrimal sac.

Treatment is with warm compresses and systemic antibiotics. A large abscess should be drained by a stab through the skin or inferior fornix conjunctiva. A dacryocystorhinostomy will prevent recurrence.

REFERENCES

1. Liesegang TJ. Bacterial keratitis. Infect Dis Clin N Am 1992;6:815–29.
2. Limberg MB. A review of bacterial keratitis and bacterial conjunctivitis. Am J Ophthalmol 1991;112:2–9.
3. Laga M, Meheus A, Piot P. Epidemiology and control of gonococcal ophthalmia neonatorum. Bull World Health Organ 1989;67:471–7.
4. Talley AR, Garcia-Ferrer F, Laycock KA, *et al.* Comparative diagnosis of neonatal chlamydial conjunctivitis by polymerase chain reaction and McCoy cell culture. Am J Ophthalmol 1994;117:50–7.
5. Isenberg SJ, Apt L, Yoshimori R, Leake RD, Rich R. Povidone–iodine for ophthalmia neonatorum prophylaxis. Am J Ophthalmol 1994;118:701–6.
6. Isenberg SJ, Apt L, Wood M. A controlled trial of povidone–iodine as prophylaxis against ophthalmia neonatorum. N Engl J Med 1995;332:562–6.
7. Laga M, Naamara W, Brunham RC, *et al.* Single-dose therapy of gonococcal ophthalmia neonatorum with ceftriaxone. N Engl J Med 1986;315:1382–5.
8. Munoz B, West S. Trachoma: the forgotten cause of blindness. Epidemiol Rev 1997;19:205–17.
9. Beatty WL, Byrne GI, Morrison RP. Repeated and persistent infection with chlamydia and the development of chronic inflammation and disease. Trends Microbiol 1994;2:94–8.
10. Haller EM, Auer-Grumbach P, Stuenzner D, *et al.* Detection of antichlamydial antibodies in tears: a diagnostic aid? Ophthalmology 1997;104:125–30.
11. Uchio E, Aoki K, Saitoh W, Itoh N, Ohno S. Rapid diagnosis of adenoviral conjunctivitis on conjunctival swabs by 10-minute immunochromatography. Ophthalmology 1997;104:1294–9.
12. Armstrong M. The laboratory investigation of infective keratitis. Br J Biomed Sci 1994;51:65–72.
13. Liesegang TJ, Forster RK. Spectrum of microbial keratitis in South Florida. Am J Ophthalmol 1980;90:38–47.
14. Liesegang TJ. Contact lens-related microbial keratitis: part I: epidemiology. Cornea 1997;16:125–31.
15. Dart JK, Stapleton F, Minassian D. Contact lenses and other risk factors in microbial keratitis. Lancet 1991;338:650–3.
16. Dart JK. The epidemiology of contact lens related diseases in the United Kingdom. CLAOJ 1993;19:241–6.
17. Jones DB. Polymicrobial keratitis. Trans Am Ophthalmol Soc 1981;79:153–67.
18. McLeod SD, Kolahdouz-Isfahani A, Rostamian K, Flowers CW, Lee PP, McDonnell PJ. The role of smears, cultures, and antibiotic sensitivity testing in the management of suspected infectious keratitis. Ophthalmology 1996;103:23–8.
19. Parks DJ, Abrams DA, Sarfarazi FA, Katz HR. Comparison of topical ciprofloxacin to conventional antibiotic therapy in the treatment of ulcerative keratitis. Am J Ophthalmol 1993;115:471–7.
20. Hyndiuk RA, Eiferman RA, Caldwell DR, *et al.* Comparison of ciprofloxacin ophthalmic solution 0.3% to fortified tobramycin–cefazolin in treating bacterial corneal ulcers. Ciprofloxacin Bacterial Keratitis Study Group. Ophthalmology 1996;103:1854–62.
21. Allan BD, Dart JK. Strategies for the management of microbial keratitis. Br J Ophthalmol 1995;79:777–86.
22. O'Day DM. Selection of appropriate antifungal therapy. Cornea 1987;6:238–45.
23. Mohan M, Panda A, Gupta SK. Management of human keratomycosis with miconazole. Aust NZ J Ophthalmol 1989;17:295–7.
24. Rahman MR, Johnson GJ, Husain R, Howlader SA, Minassian DC. Randomised trial of 0.2% chlorhexidine gluconate and 2.5% natamycin for fungal keratitis in Bangladesh. Br J Ophthalmol 1998;82:919–25.
25. Martinez AJ, Visvesvara GS. Free-living, amphizoic and opportunistic amebas. Brain Pathol 1997;7:583–98.
26. Schaumberg DA, Snow KK, Dana MR. The epidemic of acanthamoeba keratitis: where do we stand?. Cornea 1998;17:3–10.
27. Radford CF, Bacon AS, Dart JK, Minassian DC. Risk factors for acanthamoeba keratitis in contact lens users: a case–control study. Br Med J 1995;310:1567–70.
28. Seal D, Stapleton F, Dart J. Possible environmental sources of *Acanthamoeba* spp. in contact lens wearers. Br J Ophthalmol 1992;76:424–7.
29. Moore MB. Acanthamoeba keratitis and contact lens wear: the patient is at fault. Cornea 1990;9(Suppl 1):33–5.
30. Bacon AS, Frazer DG, Dart JK, Matheson M, Ficker LA, Wright P. A review of 72 consecutive cases of acanthamoeba keratitis, 1984–1992. Eye 1993;7:719–25.
31. Illingworth CD, Cook SD. Acanthamoeba keratitis. Surv Ophthalmol 1998;42:493–508.
32. Lehmann OJ, Green SM, Morlet N, *et al.* Polymerase chain reaction analysis of corneal epithelial and tear samples in the diagnosis of acanthamoeba keratitis. Invest Ophthalmol Vis Sci 1998;39:1261–5.
33. Walker CW. Acanthamoeba: ecology, pathogenicity and laboratory detection. Br J Biomed Sci 1996;53:146–51.
34. Osato MS, Robinson NM, Wilhelmus KR, Jones DB. In vitro evaluation of antimicrobial compounds for cysticidal activity against acanthamoeba. Rev Infect Dis 1991;13(Suppl 5):431–5.
35. Elder MJ, Kilvington S, Dart JK. A clinicopathologic study of in vitro sensitivity testing and acanthamoeba keratitis. Invest Ophthalmol Vis Sci 1994;35:1059–64.
36. Duguid IG, Dart JK, Morlet N, *et al.* Outcome of acanthamoeba keratitis treated with polyhexamethyl biguanide and propamidine. Ophthalmology 1997;104:1587–92.
37. Norn MS. Dendritic (herpetic) keratitis. I. Incidence – seasonal variations – recurrence rate – visual impairment – therapy. Acta Ophthalmol (Copenh) 1970;48:91–107.
38. Pepose JS. Herpes simplex keratitis: role of viral infection versus immune response. Surv Ophthalmol 1991;35:345–52.
39. Fraser NW, Spivack JG, Wroblewska Z, *et al.* A review of the molecular mechanism of HSV-1 latency. Curr Eye Res 1991;10(Suppl):1–13.
40. Baker DA, Pavan-Langston D, Gonik B, *et al.* Multicenter clinical evaluation of the Du Pont Herpchek HSV ELISA, a new rapid diagnostic test for the direct detection of herpes simplex virus. Adv Exp Med Biol 1990;263:71–6.
41. Grant DM. Acyclovir (Zovirax) ophthalmic ointment: a review of clinical tolerance. Curr Eye Res 1987;6:231–5.
42. Acyclovir for the prevention of recurrent herpes simplex virus eye disease. Herpetic Eye Disease Study Group. N Engl J Med 1998;339:300–6.
43. Wilhelmus KR, Dawson CR, Barron BA, *et al.* Risk factors for herpes simplex virus epithelial keratitis recurring during treatment of stromal keratitis or iridocyclitis. Herpetic Eye Disease Study Group. Br J Ophthalmol 1996;80:969–72.
44. Cobo M. Reduction of the ocular complications of herpes zoster ophthalmicus by oral acyclovir. Am J Med 1988;85:90–3.
45. Gutowski WM, Mulbury PE, Hengerer AS, Kido DK. The role of C.T. scans in managing the orbital complications of ethmoiditis. Int J Pediatr Otorhinolaryngol 1988;15:117–28.
46. Harris GJ. Subperiosteal abscess of the orbit. Age as a factor in the bacteriology and response to treatment. Ophthalmology 1994;101:585–95.

Endophthalmitis

Michael Whitby & Lawrence Hirst

Endophthalmitis is fortunately an uncommon condition; however, it may result in severe visual impairment or loss of an eye.

EPIDEMIOLOGY

DEFINITION AND NOMENCLATURE
Endophthalmitis is an infection within the vitreous and may involve the cornea and, in severe cases, the sclera (panophthalmitis). A number of classifications of this condition have been published, but from a practical point of view, categorization by the clinical setting, taking into account such factors as the events preceding infection and the time to diagnosis, is most appropriate. Categories include postoperative endophthalmitis [acute (within 2 weeks of operation), delayed onset (more than 2 weeks after operation), conjunctival filtering bleb-associated], post-traumatic endophthalmitis and endogenous endophthalmitis. Each of these subtypes may have characteristic clinical features and a spectrum of common causative pathogens (Fig. 12.1).

INCIDENCE AND PREVALENCE OF ENDOPHTHALMITIS
Although recent eye surgery is the most common cause of endophthalmitis, accounting for more than 70% of cases, the incidence of infection after cataract extraction, the most commonly performed eye surgery, continues to decline. Reported infection rates after extra-capsular cataract extraction, with or without intraocular lens implantation, is approximately 0.1–0.2%.[1] Endophthalmitis may occur after any other form of ocular surgery, but appears to be more common after glaucoma filtering procedures.

Endophthalmitis after penetrating ocular trauma is common, representing 7–30% of all endophthalmitis cases; 3–26% of penetrating eye injuries develop infection. It is more common when trauma is associated with a retained intraocular foreign body or when the injury is contaminated with vegetable matter.[2] The leading organisms are staphylococci, especially *Staphylococcus aureus* and *Bacillus* spp.

Endogenous bacterial and fungal endophthalmitis are the least common forms, accounting for less than 2–8% of cases – they usually follow bloodstream spread of organisms and are commonly associated with a number of chronic medical conditions, such as diabetes mellitus, chronic renal failure, immunocompromised patients, invasive medical procedures, including urinary catheterization and intravascular central lines, and intravenous drug abuse.

PATHOGENESIS AND PATHOLOGY

Although a broad range of organisms can cause endophthalmitis, the most common causative infectious agents are bacteria. Virtually any bacterium, including those usually accepted as saprophytes, can cause infection, although members of the normal ocular microflora are the most commonly implicated.

ACUTE POSTOPERATIVE ENDOPHTHALMITIS
In over 70% of cases, the pathogenic organism is a Gram-positive bacterium. *Staphylococcus epidermidis* and other coagulase-negative staphylococci are now the most frequently isolated bacteria both from postsurgical and from post-traumatic endophthalmitis, representing 50–55% of all culture-positive cases.[3] *Staphylococcus aureus* and *Streptococcus* spp. are cultured from 10–30% of postoperative infections, whereas Gram-negative organisms, including *Pseudomonas* spp., *Proteus* spp. and *Citrobacter* spp., are implicated in only 7–20%. The change in prevalence of *S. epidermidis* probably represents, at least in part, a past failure to recognize coagulase-negative staphylococci as potential ocular pathogens.

Infecting organisms are usually introduced into the eye via incisions at the time of surgery. Nosocomial outbreaks of endophthalmitis caused by contaminated irrigation fluids, intraocular lenses and donor corneas have been recognized. Infiltration of pathogens in the immediate postoperative period may be associated with inadequately buried sutures, suture removal or the presence of vitreous wicks.

DELAYED POSTOPERATIVE ONSET ENDOPHTHALMITIS
Delayed onset endophthalmitis is often caused by less aggressive organisms, including *S. epidermidis*, *Corynebacterium* spp. and *Candida* spp. A specific syndrome of chronic localized infection may occur with *Propionibacterium acnes*.

MICROBIAL ETIOLOGY OF ENDOPHTHALMITIS		
Category of endophthalmitis		Common causative organisms
Postoperative	Acute	Coagulase-negative staphylococcus
		Staphylococcus aureus
		Streptococcus spp.
		Gram-negative bacilli
		Pseudomonas spp.
	Delayed	*Staphylococcus epidermidis*
		Propionobacterium acnes
		Candida spp.
	Filtering bleb	*Streptococcus* spp.
		Haemophilus influenzae
		Staphylococcus aureus
Post-traumatic	Bacterial	*Staphylococcus aureus*; other staph spp.
		Bacillus spp.
		Pseudomonas spp.
		Other Gram-negative bacilli; anaerobes; corynebacteria; streptococci
	Fungal	*Penicillium* spp; *Fusarium* spp; *Acremonium* spp; other filamentous fungi
Endogenous	Bacterial	Enteric Gram-negative bacilli
		Fungi (including *Candida albicans*, *Aspergillus* spp.)
		Streptococcus spp.
	Fungal	Yeasts (*Candida albicans*, *Cryptococcus* spp.)
		Filamentous fungi (*Aspergillus* spp., *Acremonium* spp., *Fusarium* spp., *Paecilomyces* spp.)

Fig. 12.1 Microbial etiology of endophthalmitis.

FILTERING BLEB ENDOPHTHALMITIS

Filtering bleb endophthalmitis is frequently caused by streptococci (60%) and *Haemophilus influenzae* (20%), although *S. aureus* remains a prominent pathogen.[4]

POST-TRAUMATIC ENDOPHTHALMITIS

Post-traumatic infection may be polymicrobial (10%) and rarely, although more commonly than seen in postoperative infection, can be caused by anaerobic organisms, especially *Clostridium* spp. *S. aureus* remains a common agent, although saprophytes such as *Bacillus* spp. may induce fulminating endophthalmitis.[5] Spread of organisms through corneal abrasions and penetrating corneal ulcers, particularly those involving *S. aureus* or *Pseudomonas aeruginosa*, may lead to endophthalmitis.

ENDOGENOUS ENDOPHTHALMITIS

Endogenous infection may be associated with a recognizable infective focus elsewhere in the body and this may provide an indication as to the likely causative organism. Ocular involvement, however, may also be the first and only manifestation of systemic infection. Two to three decades ago, the most commonly associated bacteria were meningococci and pneumococci related to meningitis and infective endocarditis, respectively; more recently, *Streptococcus* spp. other than *Streptococcus pneumoniae*, *S. aureus* and Enterobacteriaceae from gastrointestinal sources have become more prominent.[6] Intravenous drug use may be associated with infection with *Candida* spp., *Aspergillus* spp. and *Bacillus cereus*, although more common pathogens, including *S. aureus*, may be involved.

FUNGAL ENDOPHTHALMITIS

Fungal endophthalmitis may occur as exogenous or endogenous infection. Postoperative fungal infection is fortunately exceedingly rare; however, after trauma, fungal endophthalmitis may represent up to 10% of cases, particularly if penetration with vegetable matter has occurred.[7] Extension of a fungal corneal ulcer may also lead to endophthalmitis. Fungi most commonly identified in this situation are usually saprophytic and may include *Aspergillus* spp., *Fusarium* spp., *Acremonium* spp. and *Paecilomyces* spp. Endogenous fungal endophthalmitis has been seen with increasing frequency over the past two decades, concurrent with an increased recognition of systemic fungal infections. *Candida albicans* is the most frequently reported causative agent after hematogenous dissemination from other infected body sites, particularly infected central venous catheters, and often in immunocompromised patients.[8] Direct intravenous inoculation as a result of narcotic abuse or contaminated infusion solutions has also been reported. Other fungi less commonly implicated in endogenous fungal endophthalmitis include *Cryptococcus neoformans*, *Aspergillus* spp. and *Paecilomyces* spp.

PREVENTION

The prevention of endophthalmitis is based on identification and pretreatment of high-risk patients, and reduction in the conjunctival commensal flora.

PREOPERATIVE PRECAUTIONS
High-risk patients

Host factors that lower resistance to infection, such as chronic immunosuppression or diabetes mellitus, have been reported as significant risk factors for postoperative endophthalmitis. Reduction in immunosuppressive medications when possible, and optimal control of blood glucose is essential in such groups. Pre-existing infection of external ocular tissue, for example chronic blepharitis, conjunctivitis and lacrimal outflow obstruction, should be identified and treated with appropriate topical antibiotics.

Antimicrobial prophylaxis

The aim of preventative treatment is to reduce eyelid and ocular surface microflora; this may be achieved by using topical antibiotics, topical antiseptic agents or subconjunctival antibiotics at the time of surgery.

Topical antibiotics. Although there is no consensus as to the optimal use of preoperative topical antibiotics in intraocular surgery, several studies have demonstrated significant falls in bacterial colonization of the conjunctiva with the application of topical antibiotics and have thus suggested a reduction in the incidence of postoperative endophthalmitis with the use of such antibiotics preoperatively. Topical antibiotics have been reported to be most effective in decreasing conjunctival bacterial colony counts when administered 2 hours before surgery.[9] Until the early 1980s, gentamicin (3mg/ml) was consistently found to be the most effective antibiotic in this situation compared with other agents such as chloramphenicol (5mg/ml), bacitracin (10mg/ml), neomycin (5mg/ml) and polymixin (2.5mg/ml).[10] However, the increase in gentamicin resistance among *S. epidermidis*, now the most common cause of postoperative endophthalmitis, suggests that it may no longer be the optimal agent for prophylaxis.[11] Vancomycin, when used prophylactically, has been shown to be active against staphylococci, but the risk of emerging resistance in enterococci and to a lesser extent in methicillin-resistant *S. aureus* has led the US Department of Health and Human Services Centers for Disease Control and Prevention to publish recommendations discouraging the prophylactic use of vancomycin.[12] Although no specific recommendations have been developed for ophthalmology, it seems appropriate to restrict the use of vancomycin to the treatment of, for example serious keratitis, endophthalmitis or orbital cellulitis caused by beta-lactam resistant Gram-positive organisms, or alternatively to the treatment of enterococci and *S. aureus* in patients unable to tolerate beta-lactam antibiotics. More recently, fluoroquinolones (all compounded at a concentration of 3mg/ml), for example ciprofloxacin, norfloxacin and ofloxacin, have been shown to be very effective in reducing conjunctival and eyelid bacterial flora when used preoperatively.[13]

Subconjunctival antimicrobials. Subconjunctival antibiotics can be administered after intraocular surgery based on the rationale that, at the completion of the ocular procedure, it is appropriate to inhibit growth of any bacteria that may have gained entry into the eye during surgery. During routine cataract surgery, aqueous fluid samples have been demonstrated to be culture positive in up to 43% of cases.[14] Conflicting results as to the value of this modality have been reported, and penetration into the vitreous is relatively poor.

Topical antiseptics. Application of 5% aqueous povidone–iodine solution alone has been shown to be nontoxic and to decrease perioperative conjunctival bacterial colony counts and reduce the incidence of postoperative endophthalmitis significantly.[15] In combination with topical antibiotics, povidone–iodine has been found to sterilize the conjunctiva in more than 80% of treated patients.[16]

INTRAOPERATIVE PRECAUTIONS

Although the judicious use of preoperative antibiotics can reduce infection rates considerably, they do not replace meticulous aseptic technique in intraocular procedures. An appropriate operating room environment, with efficient ventilation to reduce bacterial contamination, is essential; surgical techniques should be modified to minimize entry of ocular surface microbes into the eye during the surgical procedure, and adhesive-backed plastic drapes to isolate the eyelids and lashes from the operative field are essential.

Implantation of intraocular lenses with prolene haptics appears to increase the risk of endophthalmitis, probably because coagulase-negative staphylococci bind well to this particular plastic. Binding to polymethylmethacrylate material is less, therefore its use may reduce risk.[17] Care must be taken to minimize contact with the external eye during insertion of an intraocular lens to prevent contamination with conjunctival flora. There is always the threat of infection from personnel and equipment in the operating room, and from contaminated irrigation solutions.

CLINICAL FEATURES

Clinical signs of endophthalmitis vary greatly depending on the preceding events, the nature of the infecting organism, the degree of tissue inflammation and the duration of disease. Early diagnosis requires the maintenance of a high index of suspicion.

ACUTE POSTOPERATIVE ENDOPHTHALMITIS

Acute postoperative endophthalmitis usually occurs within 2 weeks of surgery, whereas the presentation of infection after penetrating trauma will often be more rapid. As a general principle, the more rapid the onset of symptoms, the more virulent the organism, with *S. aureus*, *Streptococcus pyogenes*, *Bacillus* spp. and Gram-negative bacilli being implicated in very rapid onset of infection within 24–72 hours of surgery. This presentation is characterized by marked anterior chamber inflammation and by the rapid development of a fibrinous anterior chamber exudate with hypopyon, which produces severe pain, more prominent than general postoperative discomfort, and by a progressive decrease in visual acuity. A marked vitreous inflammatory reaction, often obscuring visualization of the retina, frequently follows (Figs 12.2, 12.3 & 12.4). Associated features may include marked conjunctival, lid and corneal edema, but systemic features are virtually never seen.

DELAYED ONSET POSTOPERATIVE ENDOPHTHALMITIS

Delayed onset endophthalmitis has a more insidious course and frequently overlaps with acute postoperative endophthalmitis if less virulent organisms are implicated. Symptoms may not manifest until weeks or even months after surgery, although early mild clinical features with progressive worsening over time are not uncommon (Fig. 12.5). When delayed onset endophthalmitis is caused by *P. acnes*, it usually develops months after cataract extraction; patients will often have a history of steroid-responsive postoperative inflammation with a fluctuating course over many months. The most common clinical signs are posterior capsular deposits and chronic iridocyclitis.[18]

Fungal infection may also have a delayed clinical onset. Anterior chamber reaction with progressive white infiltrates often adherent to the iris and posterior corneal surface is seen (Figs 12.6 & 12.7). Fluffy white fungal ball infiltrates ('string of pearls') occurring in the vitreous are characteristic (Fig. 12.8). Patients who have chronic postoperative endophthalmitis caused by coagulase-negative staphylococci may present with a hypopyon and diffuse vitritis, which occasionally obscures the view of the fundus. Visual loss is usually more severe than that in endophthalmitis caused by *P. acnes* or fungi.

FILTERING BLEB ENDOPHTHALMITIS

A conjunctival filtering bleb is a collection of fluid under the conjunctiva resulting from the formation of a fistula at operation through the sclera from the anterior chamber in an endeavor to reduce pressure in the anterior chamber. Endophthalmitis associated with a conjunctival filtering bleb is actually an acute presentation of endophthalmitis, but may occur months to years after the operation with rapid development of symptoms. Intraocular spread occurs from an initial bacterial penetration through the mucosa of the bleb, often in association with bacterial conjunctivitis. A purulent discharge and an injected bleb are commonly seen, ultimately in association with typical signs of endophthalmitis.

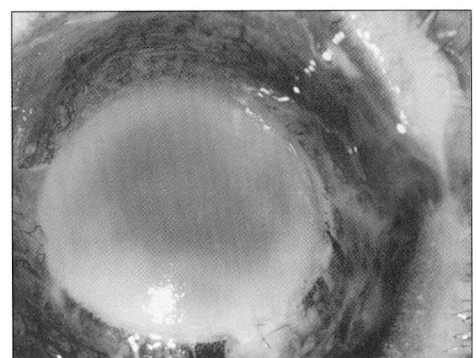

Fig. 12.2 Corneal edema and fibrinous anterior chamber exudate in a traumatic foreign body induced endophthalmitis. Any posterior vitreal or retinal view is obscured by the anterior corneal and aqueous haze.

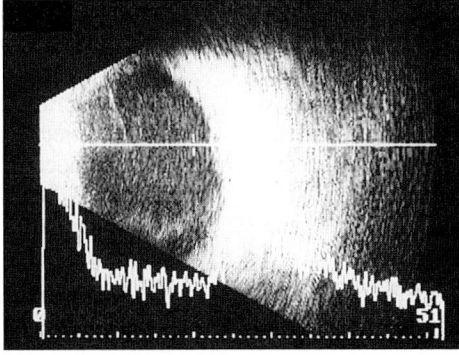

Fig. 12.3 B-scan ultrasound of the eye showing total vitreous opacity of a severe endophthalmitis in patient seen in Figure 12.2. This horizontal 'cut' through the eye shows the normally 'transparent' vitreous cavity to be filled with inflammatory debris, but there is no obvious retinal detachment.

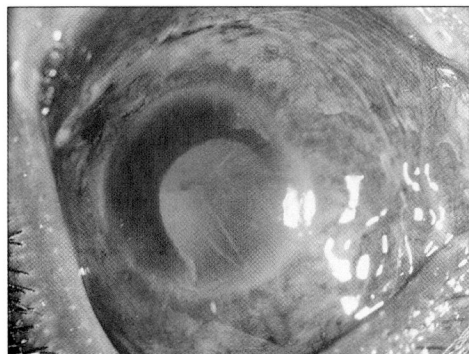

Fig. 12.4 A dense vitreous abscess in advanced endophthalmitis. This partially treated postoperative endophthalmitis has vitreous cellular and protein deposits obscuring the retinal view.

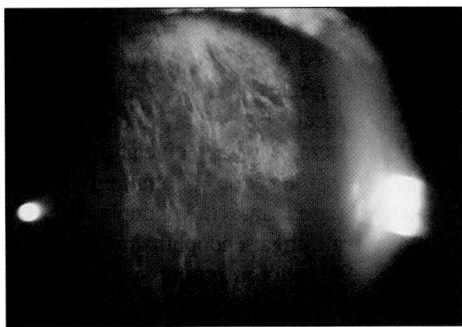

Fig. 12.5 The typical posterior capsular opacities seen in a late-onset S. epidermidis endophthalmitis. These deposits are actual coccal colonies, which are frequently removed at subsequent vitrectomy surgery to open up the capsular bag to intraocular antibiotics.

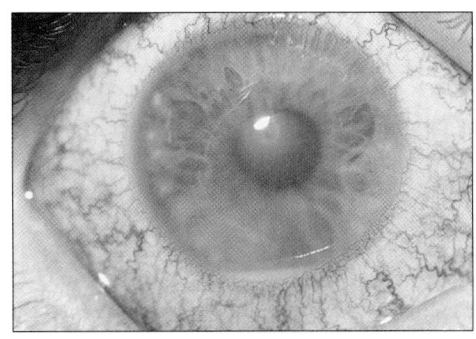

Fig. 12.6 A 'quiet' endogenous fungal endophthalmitis with small hypopyon. This eye is relatively quiet with little chemosis, injection and pain, but has a small hypopyon and some small fungal 'balls' on the temporal iris.

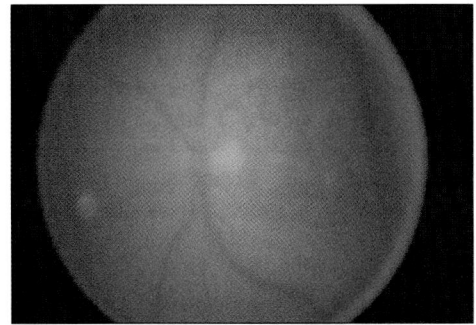

Fig. 12.7 The degraded ophthalmoscopic retinal view obtained in patient seen in Figure 12.6. The corneal edema and anterior chamber activity makes vitreous and retinal observation difficult.

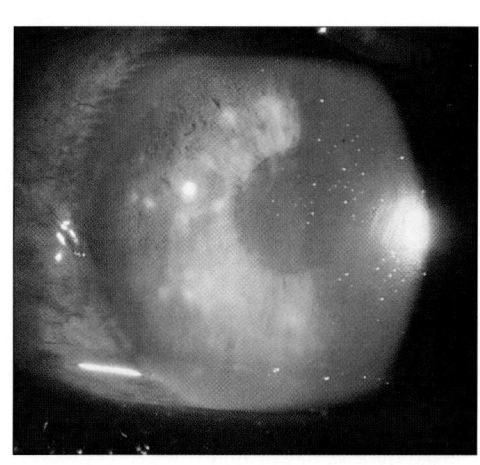

Fig. 12.8 Fungal 'fluff balls' on the iris seen in a fungal endophthalmitis. Although these are not pathognomonic, their appearance raises the real possibility that the infection is of fungal origin.

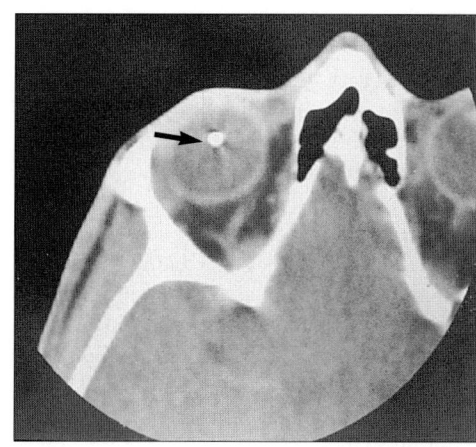

Fig. 12.9 Horizontal CT scan section of eye seen in Figures 12.2 and 12.3 revealing metallic intraocular foreign body in vitreous cavity (arrow). This CT scan demonstrates that the vitreous opacity seen by ultrasound is 'invisible' to this investigation.

POST-TRAUMATIC ENDOPHTHALMITIS

Presentation will vary depending on the nature and severity of the ocular trauma, or the type of retained foreign body, for example steel or vegetable matter, and the virulence and concentration of the organism initially deposited into the intraocular tissues (Fig. 12.9). The more virulent this organism, including *S. aureus* and *B. cereus*, the more rapid the onset of pain and associated ophthalmic features of infection. *Bacillus cereus*, fungi, and to a lesser extent nocardia and atypical mycobacteria should be considered when injury to the eye is related to plant or vegetable matter.[19]

ENDOGENOUS ENDOPHTHALMITIS

Endogenous endophthalmitis usually has an insidious onset with a slow decrease in visual acuity caused by vitritis and localized areas of chorioretinitis. It may be suspected when other systemic symptoms of infection are present, or in certain groups of patients, including those in whom bacteremia or fungemia is common, such as those with infective endocarditis and those with intravascular or urinary catheters, or patients who abuse intravenous drugs. Rarely, a fungal endophthalmitis, with a predilection for *Paecilomyces* infection, may occur in otherwise healthy individuals with no antecedent trauma.[20]

DIFFERENTIAL DIAGNOSIS

The differential diagnosis of postoperative inflammation includes sterile uveitis related to retained lens cortex, operative complications such as vitreous loss, hemorrhage and iris trauma, pre-existing uveitis and toxicity of foreign material such as irrigation solutions introduced during surgery. These presentations are often difficult to distinguish from similar symptoms caused by infective endophthalmitis, and careful sequential monitoring of such eyes or intraocular sampling for culture is appropriate to facilitate early diagnosis and treatment.

DIAGNOSIS

MICROBIOLOGIC INVESTIGATIONS IN ENDOPHTHALMITIS

Confirmation of the diagnosis of infective endophthalmitis is essential to rational management. Because most postoperative infections are caused by normal ocular flora, there is some correlation between the results of external swabs of the eyelid margins and conjunctivae with intraocular isolates.[21] These should not be used to determine causative pathogens; routine preoperative cultures have a low predictive value and are not recommended. The optimal specimen for laboratory processing in endophthalmitis is an intraocular aspirate; aqueous and vitreous specimens should be obtained, although the latter is the most reliable, as some 30–55% of concomitant aqueous specimens are negative in the presence of positive vitreous isolates.[22] In the case of late endophthalmitis, any available capsule and lens material should also be cultured. Foreign bodies should be processed in traumatic endophthalmitis, whereas a swab of the bleb may assist in bleb-associated infections.

Because specimen volumes are often very limited, the traditional approach of direct inoculation onto culture media for aerobic and anaerobic bacteria, and fungi, remains important. Direct inoculation of specimens into blood culture bottles is of more limited value, but is useful in circumstances in which appropriate media are not readily available. Rapid results by microscopy of Gram stains are useful, with positive results occurring in some 50–70% of well collected vitreous aspirates.[23] An appropriate clinical history should accompany specimens to the laboratory so that culture can be prolonged for fastidious organisms, and so that skin commensals such as *P. acnes* are not routinely discarded as contaminants.

MANAGEMENT

ANTIBIOTIC CHEMOTHERAPY

Early institution of antimicrobial therapy is essential to optimal outcome in the management of infective endophthalmitis – controversy continues as to the best therapeutic approach.

Intravitreal antibiotics

Intravitreal injection of antibiotics is the most effective way of achieving high intraocular antibiotic levels. Direct intravitreal injections of nonpreserved (i.e. intravenous) formulations of antibiotics are now the recommended route of administration in endophthalmitis treatment. The rationale of such therapy is that, although antibiotics when administered topically, subconjunctivally or systemically may attain therapeutic concentrations in the anterior chamber, concentrations in the vitreous are much lower. Intravitreal injections may produce significant retinal toxicity, although single injections have been shown to be safe and effective.

The optimal combination of antibiotics in empiric therapy normally covers Gram-positive and Gram-negative organisms. Over recent years, vancomycin has replaced first generation cephalosporins for Gram-positive activity because of the increasing incidence of *S. epidermidis* infection resistant to methicillin and other beta-lactam drugs. Reports of retinal toxicity caused by gentamicin led to the use of amikacin to cover Gram-negative organisms, as this later antibiotic was believed to be less toxic. Amikacin has now been used widely in controlled and uncontrolled clinical situations. However, more recently, gentamicin and amikacin have been associated with macular infarction,[24] and this has led to increased use of other broad-spectrum Gram-negative antimicrobial agents, particularly ceftazidime. Repeat injections of aminoglycosides should be avoided, except in severe cases. Intravitreal amphotericin B injections (1–5mg) can be utilized in fungal endophthalmitis, with a single repeat inoculation after 72–96 hours in progressive infection; again, however, toxicity limits longer duration of therapy.

Subconjunctival antibiotics

The data regarding subconjunctival antibiotic penetration is conflicting, possibly because of varying degrees of inflammation in the eye or poor and variable sampling techniques. Penetration is affected by the transscleral and transcorneal permeability of the agent, but high aqueous levels can be achieved with vancomycin, gentamicin and beta-lactam antibiotics for up to 4 hours; however, vitreous concentrations are generally poor. Subconjunctival injections are an irritant and are painful, thus limiting duration of this form of therapy to a few days.

Topical antibiotic therapy
The efficacy of topical antibacterial applications in endophthalmitis is not well studied, although significant concentrations of antibiotics in the anterior segment can be obtained with frequent administration of highly concentrated (fortified) solutions. A combination of vancomycin and gentamicin provides a broad-spectrum cover, but solutions must be prepared by a qualified pharmacist if they are not commercially available. Third-generation cephalosporins, such as cefotaxime and ceftazidime, and fluoroquinolones, such as ciprofloxacin, may be used to replace gentamicin to provide appropriate Gram-negative cover. The use of collagen shields to produce frequent topical application of antibiotic solutions has been explored, but is limited by potential corneal toxicity. Ionotophoresis also increases anterior chamber concentrations, but its efficacy remains unproved.

Systemic antibiotics
In humans, intraocular penetration of systemically administered antibiotics is generally poor. However, intravenous antibiotics are a common adjunctive therapy in endophthalmitis, justified in that they may enhance concentrations of antibiotics achieved with intravitreal agents and extend the duration of therapeutic activity. Intraocular inflammation and/or performance of a vitrectomy may alter the blood–retina barrier to allow improved intraocular penetration.

Posterior chamber concentrations of newer and broad-spectrum agents, including ceftazidime, imipenem and ciprofloxacin, appear improved, particularly in terms of efficacy against Gram-negative bacilli such as *Pseudomonas* spp. However, none is reliably active against *S. epidermidis*, the most common cause of postoperative endophthalmitis, and resistance may develop rapidly.

A recent multicenter randomized trial, the Endophthalmitis Vitrectomy Study (EVS), sponsored by the National Eye Institute of the National Institutes of Health, followed a cohort of 420 patients who had clinical evidence of endophthalmitis within 6 weeks after cataract surgery or secondary intraocular lens implantation.[25] Patients were randomly assigned to therapy, with or without pars plana vitrectomy and with or without systemic antibiotics of ceftazidime and amikacin, but each with an intravitreal injection of vancomycin and amikacin. When outcome was assessed 9–12 months after the operation, no difference in final visual acuity or media clouding between groups with and without systemic antibiotics could be determined. Well conducted as this study was, a number of questions remain unanswered, particularly in relation to generalization of the results – do the results, for example, extrapolate to Gram-negative infection or to other categories of ocular surgery? Moreover, a significant percentage of coagulase-negative staphylococci and *Streptococcus* spp., the most common Gram-positive pathogens, are resistant to ceftazidime and amikacin.

Duration of therapy is very variable – in spite of the presence of an ocular foreign body such as an intraocular lens, endophthalmitis caused by *S. epidermidis* will settle rapidly with appropriate management. Length of therapy can be assessed by a reduction in cellular activity both in the anterior and in the posterior chambers and by improvement in visual acuity.

Fungal endophthalmitis poses a particular problem – itraconazole, a lipophilic antifungal imidazole, has been shown to be efficacious in *Aspergillus* endophthalmitis.[26] Fluconazole, a hydrophilic imidazole, achieves useful concentrations in intraocular tissue and has also proved successful in *Candida* endophthalmitis.[27] Amphotericin B, often the only available therapy in filamentous fungal infections other than those caused by *Aspergillus* spp., does not achieve significant concentrations in intraocular tissue – nevertheless, it is widely used in fungal endophthalmitis with some evidence of success.

Specific recommendations
Endophthalmitis may cause irreparable visual loss within 24–48 hours. Initial therapy must frequently be empiric, both because of the low sensitivity of Gram stain film and the 24–48 hour delay until culture results become available. Antibiotic therapy should be chosen to cover the spectrum of pathogens likely to be implicated. In this situation classification of endophthalmitis by clinical setting provides useful information. Suggested initial antibiotic therapy for acute postoperative, filtering bleb and post-traumatic endophthalmitis is illustrated in Figure 12.10.

Localized bleb infection without endophthalmitis can usually initially be managed with topical therapy. Because of the increased prevalence of *H. influenzae* in this infection, a combination of antibiotics that covers this pathogen and provides broad-spectrum activity against Gram-positive and Gram-negative organisms should be chosen.

ADJUNCTIVE THERAPY
Vitrectomy
The place of pars planum vitrectomy remains a controversial issue in the management of endophthalmitis. The theoretic rationale for such a procedure is that it offers a reduction in organism load, a reduction in traction effect on the retina with less potential for detachment, collection of adequate culture material and possibly improved distribution of intravitreal antibiotics. Evidence for its efficacy has been conflicting, often as a result of poorly controlled studies. The EVS was designed to determine definitively the value of vitrectomy in the presence of intravitreal antibiotics. The final conclusions of this study were that visual acuity was improved significantly in patients treated with vitrectomy only if the initial vision was light perception, but not if initial vision was hand movements or better, that is, the most severe cases on presentation benefited most from vitrectomy.[25]

Corticosteroids
The use of corticosteroids to reduce the inflammatory response to infection and thus preserve ocular tissue is widely practiced with administration by several routes, including intraocular, periocular, topical and systemic, but its place in therapy remains contentious. Experimental animal studies demonstrate superior outcomes utilizing corticosteroids with antibiotics even in endophthalmitis caused by pseudomonads and fungi. In general, clinical studies do not report deterioration in outcomes if corticosteroids are used in combination with antibiotics, at least at the ocular level.[28]

Management of intraocular lens
In most cases of acute postoperative pseudophakic endophthalmitis, removal of the intraocular lens is not necessary and does not influence outcome. In fact, it may be hazardous and predispose to anterior segment hemorrhage and retinal detachment. Exceptions may occur when the pathogen is a fungus, and in cases of late onset endophthalmitis caused by *P. acnes* when conservative treatment with intravitreal vancomycin and corticosteroids is unsuccessful. In such cases, complete capsulectomy and lensectomy may be necessary to provide cure.

OUTCOME
Up to 50% of patients who have endophthalmitis suffer major visual loss within 24–48 hours of onset, emphasizing the essential need for early diagnosis and prompt treatment.[29] Approximately 30% of patients in recent studies of endophthalmitis achieved a final visual acuity of 20/60 or better after treatment.[1,30] Certain factors are highly correlated with poor visual outcome; these include severity of infection, delay in time to diagnosis and institution of treatment, virulence of infecting organisms and intraocular complications such as vitreous hemorrhage and retinal detachment. Poor visual perception at the time of diagnosis correlates with either a virulent organism, such as *Bacillus* spp., *Streptococcus* spp., or Gram-negative bacilli or fungi, or a delay in diagnosis even with a low virulence organism. Normally, however, *S. epidermidis* endophthalmitis has an excellent outcome, although even in this situation some 10% of patients develop

ANTIMICROBIAL THERAPY OF ENDOPHTHALMITIS				
Category of endophthalmitis	Antimicrobial therapy			
		Topical	Intravitreal	Systemic

Postoperative	Acute	Cefazolin (5mg/ml)
		  + gentamicin (8–15mg/ml)
		  or amikacin (25–50mg/ml)
			Cefazolin (2.25mg)
			  + amikacin (400mg)
				Cefazolin (2gm q8h) + gentamicin (4–5mg/kg q24h)*
				  or amikacin (15mg/kg q24h)*

		Vancomycin (50mg/ml)
		  + gentamicin
		  or amikacin
		  or ceftazidime (5mg/ml)
		  or ciprofloxacin (3mg/ml)
			Vancomycin (1mg)
			  + amikacin
			  or ceftazidime (2.25mg)
				Vancomycin + gentamicin
				  or amikacin
				  or ceftazidime (2g 8h)
				  or ciprofloxacin (400mg q12h)

	Delayed	Vancomycin + gentamicin
		  or amikacin
		  or ceftazidime
		  or ciprofloxacin
			Vancomycin + amikacin
			  or ceftazidime
				Vancomycin + gentamicin
				  or amikacin
				  or cefotaxime (2g q6h)
				  or ceftazidime
				  or ciprofloxacin

	Filtering bleb	Vancomycin + ceftazidime
		  or ciprofloxacin
			Vancomycin + ceftazidime	Vancomycin +/or cefotaxime,
				  ceftazidime,
				  ciprofloxacin

Post-traumatic		Vancomycin + gentamicin
		  or amikacin
		  or ceftazidime
		  or ciprofloxacin
			Vancomycin + amikacin
			  or ceftazidime
				Vancomycin + gentamicin
				  or amikacin
				  or ceftazidime
				  or ciprofloxacin

Fig. 12.10 Initial empiric recommendations for antimicrobial therapy of endophthalmitis. Dosages given in brackets apply to all citations of each specific drug within the relevant column. (*Dosages must be adjusted to reflect the patient's age, body weight and renal function.)

blindness.[31] Culture-negative cases of endophthalmitis generally have a better visual outcome than do culture-positive groups, which may relate to the lower virulence of more fastidious organisms or to the veracity of diagnosis.

The outcome of post-traumatic endophthalmitis and endophthalmitis related to a conjunctival filtering bleb is poor, probably because of the intrinsic virulence of organisms implicated in this form; however, for converse reasons, prognosis in delayed ophthalmitis, including that caused by *P. acnes*, is usually more favorable.

The primary complication of endophthalmitis is retinal detachment that may occur at any time before, during or after treatment. Prognosis in this situation is extremely poor.

REFERENCES

1. Kattan HM, Flynn HW, Pflugfelder SC, Robertson C, Foster RK. Nosocomial endophthalmitis surgery: current incidence of infection after intraocular surgery. Ophthalmology 1991;98:227–38.
2. Thompson JT, Parver LM, Enger CL, Mieler WF, Liggett PE. Endophthalmitis after penetrating ocular injuries with retained intraocular foreign bodies. National Eye Trauma System. Ophthalmology 1993;100:1468–74.
3. Shrader SK, Band JD, Lauter CB, Murphy P. The clinical spectrum of endophthalmitis: incidence, predisposing factors and features influencing outcome. J Infect Dis 1990;162:115–20.
4. Mandelbaum S, Forster RK, Gelender H, Culbertson W. Late onset endophthalmitis associated with the filtering blebs. Ophthalmology 1985;92:964–72.
5. Schemmer GB, Driebe WT Jr. Post-traumatic *Bacillus cereus* endophthalmitis. Arch Ophthalmol 1987;105:342–4.
6. Okada AA, Johnson RP, Liles WC, D'Amico DJ, Baker AS. Endogenous bacterial endophthalmitis: report of a ten year retrospective study. Ophthalmology 1994;101:832–8.
7. Pflugfelder SC, Flynn HW, Zwickey TA, et al. Exogenous fungal endophthalmitis. Ophthalmology 1988;95:19–30.
8. Donahue SP, Greven CM, Zurauleff JJ, et al. Intraocular candidiasis in patients with candidemia: clinical implications derived from a prospective multicenter study. Ophthalmology 1994;101:1302–9.
9. Whitney CR, Anderson RP, Allansmith MR. Preoperatively administered antibiotics: their effect on bacterial counts of the eyelids. Arch Ophthalmol 1972;87:155–60.
10. Fahmy JA. Bacterial flora in relation to cataract extraction. V: effects of topical antibiotics on the preoperative conjunctival flora. Acta Ophthalmol (Copenh) 1980;58:567–75.
11. Davis JL, Kaidou-Tsiligianni A, Pflugfelder SC, et al. Coagulase negative staphylococci endophthalmitis: increase in antimicrobial resistance. Ophthalmology 1988;95:1404–10.
12. Hospital Infection Control Practitioners Advisory Committee (HICPAC). Recommendations for preventing the spread of vancomycin resistance. Infect Control Hosp Epidemiol 1995;16:105–13.
13. Leeming JP, Diamond JP, Trigg R, et al. Ocular penetration of topical ciprofloxacin and norfloxacin drops and their effect upon eyelid flora. Br J Ophthalmol 1994;78:546–8.
14. Dickey JB, Thompson KD, Jay WM. Anterior chamber aspirate cultures after uncomplicated cataract surgery. Am J Ophthalmol 1991;112:278–82
15. Apt L, Isenberg S, Yoshimori R, Paez JH. Chemical preparation of the eye in ophthalmic surgery. III. Effect of povidone iodine on the conjunctiva. Arch Ophthalmol 1984;102:728–9.
16. Apt L, Isenberg S, Yoshimori R, Spierer A. Outpatient topical use of povidone–iodine in preparing the eye for surgery. Ophthalmology 1989;96:289–92.
17. Dilly PN, Sellors PJ. Bacterial adhesion to intraocular lenses. J Cataract Refract Surg 1989;15:317–20.
18. Winward KE, Pflugfelder SC, Flynn HW Jr, Roussel TJ, Davis JL. Postoperative *Proprionobacterium* endophthalmitis. Treatment strategies and long term results. Ophthalmology 1993;100:447–51.
19. Thompson JT, Parver LM, Enger CL, Mieler WF, Liggett PE. Infectious endophthalmitis after penetrating injuries with retained intraocular foreign bodies. National Eye Trauma System. Ophthalmology 1993;100:1468–74.
20. Hirst LW, Sebban A, Whitby M, Nimmo GR, Stallard K. Non-traumatic mycotic keratitis. Eye 1992;6:391–5.
21. Speaker MG, Milch FA, Shah MK, Eisner W, Kreiswirth BN. Role of external bacterial flora in the pathogenesis of acute postoperative endophthalmitis. Ophthalmology 1991;98:639–49.
22. Weber DJ, Hoffman KL, Thoft RA, Baker AS. Endophthalmitis following intraocular lens implantation: report of 30 cases in a review of the literature. Rev Infect Dis 1986;8:12–20.
23. Bode DD, Gelender H, Forster RK. A retrospective review of endophthalmitis due to coagulase negative staphylococci. Br J Ophthalmol 1985;69:915–9.
24. Campochiaro PA, Conway BP. Aminoglycoside toxicity – a survey of retinal specialists: implications for ocular use. Arch Ophthalmol 1991;109:946–50.
25. Endophthalmitis Vitrectomy Study Group. Results of the Endophthalmitis Vitrectomy Study: a randomised trial of immediate vitrectomy and of intravenous antibiotics for the treatment of postoperative bacterial endophthalmitis. Arch Ophthalmol 1995;113:1479–96.
26. Oxford KW, Abbot RL, Fung WE. *Aspergillus* endophthalmitis after sutreless cataract surgery. Am J Ophthalmol 1995;120:534–5.
27. Akler ME, Vellend H, McNeely DM, Walmsley SL, Gold WL. Use of fluconazole in the treatment of candidal endophthalmitis. Clin Infect Dis 1995;20:657–64.
28. Mao LK, Flynn HW Jr, Miller D, Pflugfelder SC. Endophthalmitis caused by *Staphylococcus aureus*. Am J Ophthalmol 1993;116:584–9.
29. Bohigian GM, Olk RJ. Factors associated with a poor visual result in endophthalmitis. Am J Ophthalmol 1986;101:332–41.
30. Speaker MG, Menikoff JA. Prophylaxis of endophthalmitis with topical povidone iodine.Ophthalmology 1991;98:1769–75.
31. Ormerod LD, Ho DD, Becker LE, et al. Endophthalmitis caused by coagulase negative staphylococci. I: disease spectrum and outcome. Ophthalmology 1993;100:715–23.

chapter

13

Infectious Retinitis and Uveitis

Jay S Duker & Michael Barza

The classic definition of uveitis is inflammation of one or more parts of the uveal tract of the eye, namely, the choroid, the iris and the ciliary body. In practice, uveitis has come to mean any inflammation of the intraocular structures, regardless of the precise anatomic sites involved. Inflammation localized to certain structures can be denoted by more specific terms. For example, inflammation of the iris (iritis) or ciliary body (cyclitis) is called 'anterior uveitis'. Inflammation of the vitreous (vitritis), retina (retinitis) or choroid (choroiditis) is called 'posterior uveitis'. Inflammation of the entire globe is called 'pan-uveitis'. Inflammation localized to the outer coats of the eye or optic nerve without adjacent or accompanying intraocular inflammation (e.g. scleritis, keratitis, optic neuritis) does not usually fall under the heading of uveitis.

The 'anterior segment' of the eye consists of the cornea, anterior chamber, lens, iris, posterior chamber and ciliary body; the 'posterior segment' refers to the vitreous cavity and posterior structures including the retina and optic nerve (Fig. 13.1).

The location, distribution and ophthalmoscopic appearance of inflammatory lesions are useful to the ophthalmologist in suggesting likely causes of uveitis (Fig. 13.2).[1] Intermediate uveitis centers about the equator of the eye between the anterior and posterior parts of the uveal tract, whereas anterior uveitis involves the anterior chamber and posterior uveitis involves the posterior segment of the eye. Chronic intermediate uveitis with certain morphologic characteristics may be termed the 'pars planitis' syndrome. The diagnosis of retinal vasculitis is made by the finding of inflammatory sheathing of the retinal vessels on ophthalmoscopic examination and by the evidence of leakage of dye from the involved vessels on fluorescein angiography (Fig. 13.3).[1] Retinal vasculitis is sometimes isolated but more commonly it occurs in conjunction with posterior uveitis. It is a nonspecific finding and can occur in ischemic conditions as well as in infection. Endophthalmitis, although it overlaps to some degree with uveitis and retinitis, is considered separately (see Chapter 2.12).

There are many known causes of uveitis, including infections, autoimmune disorders, various other systemic diseases and trauma, including surgical trauma. In some instances, the ocular lesions are only one manifestation of an underlying multisystem disorder, whereas in others the eye represents the only site of overt disease. Many cases of uveitis remain of uncertain origin despite extensive investigation. In trying to determine the cause of any particular case of uveitis, the ophthalmologist considers a number of features, including the distribution and morphologic characteristics of the lesions, the chronicity of the disorder and the presence of underlying systemic diseases.

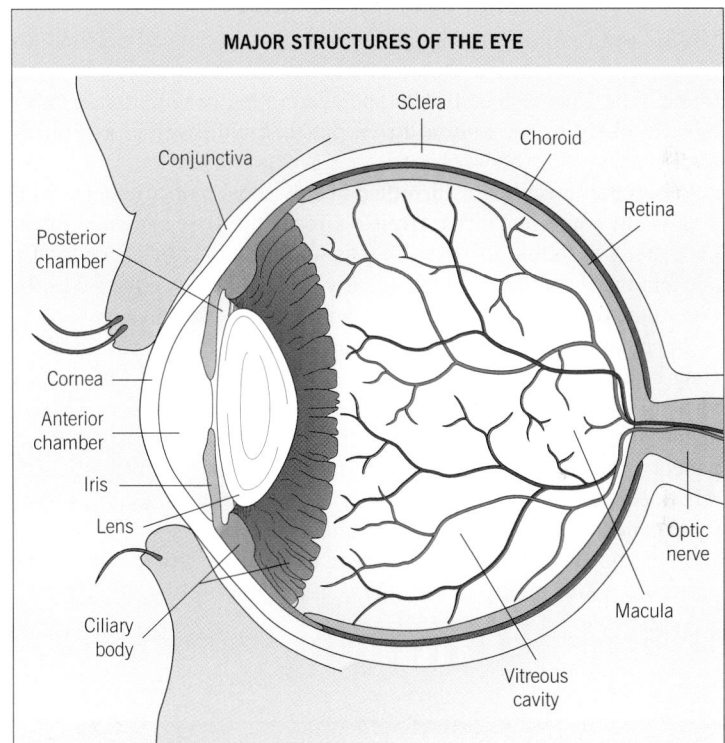

MAJOR STRUCTURES OF THE EYE

Fig. 13.1 Major structures of the eye.

Fig. 13.2 Anterior, posterior and intermediate uveitis. Definitions and common symptoms.

ANTERIOR, POSTERIOR AND INTERMEDIATE UVEITIS			
	Anterior uveitis	Intermediate uveitis	Posterior uveitis
Ophthalmoscopic signs that define the type of uveitis	Inflammatory cells in the anterior chamber with or without keratic precipitates or iris lesions	Inflammatory cells more highly concentrated in anterior vitreous than in anterior chamber	Inflammation of retina, choroid, retinal vessels, posterior vitreous humor, or a combination of these
Additional clinical signs	Ciliary flush (perilimbal injection of the sclera) Posterior synechiae	Macular edema Inflammatory exudate on pars plana	Retinal vasculitis Optic disc edema Macular edema
Symptoms	Pain Redness Photophobia	Floaters	Floaters Blurred vision

Among the diagnostic tests commonly done to determine the cause of uveitis are:

- chest X-ray to detect sarcoidosis and tuberculosis,
- full blood count,
- erythrocyte sedimentation rate,
- serologic tests for syphilis,
- HLA-B27 antigen, and
- angiotensin converting enzyme.

Within the broad categories of retinitis and uveitis, there are certain distinctive syndromes, such as acute retinal necrosis (ARN), progressive outer retinal necrosis (PORN) and pars planitis, which allow the ophthalmologist to make a syndrome diagnosis on clinical grounds.

This chapter describes the major manifestations of uveitis and retinitis, with an emphasis on the infectious causes of these syndromes. Uveitis and retinitis in immunosuppressed patients and neonates are considered separately because the causative agents differ from those in immunocompetent and adult patients. Only the infectious aspects pertinent to the eye will be discussed. Because significant uveitis and retinitis must be managed by an experienced ophthalmologist, detailed regimens of locally applied anti-infective and anti-inflammatory agents have not been given.

EPIDEMIOLOGY

Uveitis and retinitis are uncommon problems in clinical practice. In Minnesota, USA, the annual incidence of new cases of uveitis has been found to be 17 cases per 100,000 population.[2] A general ophthalmologist is likely to see only a dozen patients with uveitis or retinitis each year.

A specific cause can be identified in only about half of patients with uveitis. In some instances, uveitis affords the first evidence of an underlying systemic disease. Uveitis and retinitis can occur at any age and the incidence is about equally divided between the sexes. In one study, the mean age of patients with uveitis was 45 years.[1]

Infectious uveitis or retinitis in neonates is almost always the result of congenital infection [toxoplasmosis, rubella, cytomegalovirus, herpes virus (TORCH) syndrome; see Chapter 2.55]. Each of the TORCH agents can involve the uvea or retina. Among immunosuppressed patients, uveitis or retinitis is found most commonly in patients with AIDS. However, hematogenous fungal endophthalmitis occurs primarily in patients with other forms of immunosuppression.

Although uveitis does not appear to be more prevalent in any particular parts of the world, there is geographic variation in the underlying causes. For example, acquired ocular toxoplasmosis is quite common in Brazil and rare in the rest of the world. Behçet's disease is prevalent in Turkey and the Middle East but unusual elsewhere. Leprosy has been eradicated in most developed countries but can still be found in less developed regions. Onchocerciasis (river blindness) primarily affects the cornea but it can produce retinitis and choroiditis. It is seen only in equatorial Africa and Central America.

CLINICAL FEATURES

Common symptoms of intraocular inflammation, irrespective of the cause, are ocular pain, photophobia, 'floaters' (specks that appear to float in the visual field) and impaired vision (Fig. 13.2). Both eyes may be affected simultaneously but unilateral involvement does not rule out a systemic cause. Anyone with these symptoms should have an ophthalmologic evaluation employing pharmacologic dilatation of the pupil with examination by slit lamp and indirect ophthalmoscopy. Because most of the uveal tract can be readily visualized in this fashion, precise definition of the morphology of the lesions is possible. The findings allow the process to be characterized as anterior, intermediate, or posterior uveitis, or panuveitis (Fig. 13.2).

Additional clinical signs include conjunctival injection, anterior segment cells and 'flare' (protein floating in aqueous fluid, seen on slit lamp examination), iris nodules (granulomas), posterior synechiae, posterior segment cells, optic disc edema, retinal vasculitis, retinitis and choroiditis. A hypopyon refers to layered inflammatory cells that settle gravitationally in the inferior aspect of the anterior chamber (Fig. 13.4). In cases of severe acute uveitis, there may be so much intraocular inflammation that a cloudy media results. This may preclude visualization of the inner aspects of the eye. In such cases ocular ultrasonography should be performed.

Chronic uveitis can lead to cataract formation, epiretinal membrane formation, iris, retinal, or choroidal neovascularization, and retinal detachment. A rare sequel of healed diffuse retinitis or choroiditis is known as 'salt-and-pepper fundus' because of the stippled appearance of the retinal pigment epithelium. The lesions are nonspecific and may be seen following a variety of infectious and inherited disorders (Fig. 13.5).

The characteristic causes and clinical presentations of uveitis seen in a general community-based ophthalmologic practice and in a tertiary referral center have been found to differ (Fig. 13.6).[1] In the community ophthalmic practice, about 90% of uveitis was anterior and most cases of anterior uveitis were acute. By contrast, in patients seen in the tertiary referral center, intermediate and posterior uveitis and panuveitis

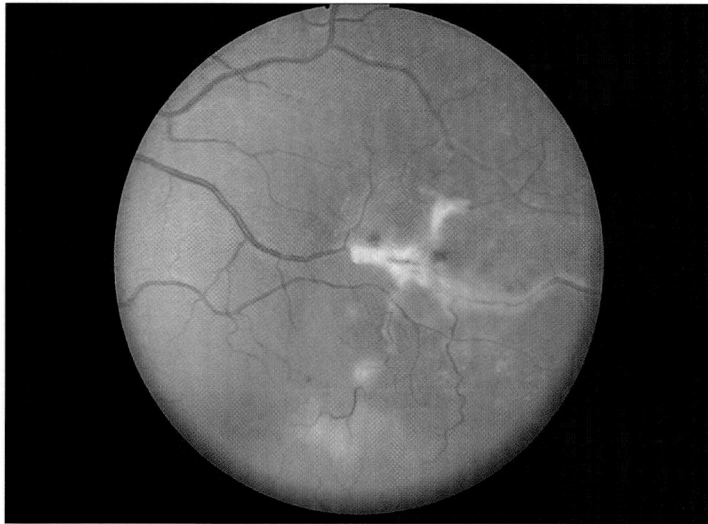

Fig. 13.3 Retinal inflammatory vascular sheathing (vasculitis).

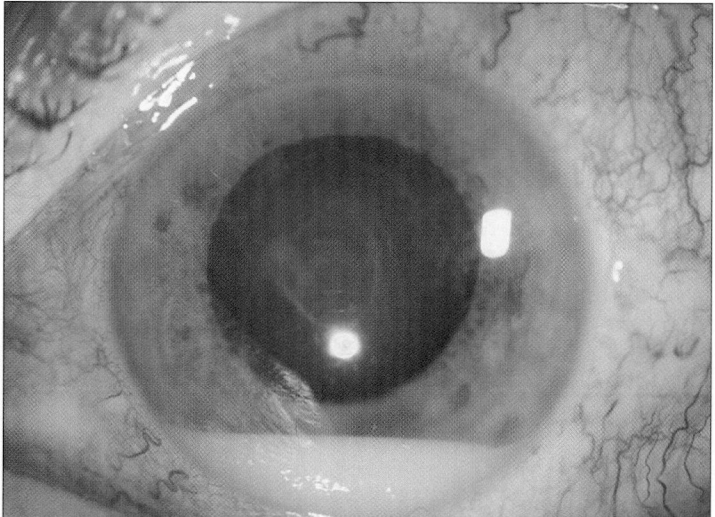

Fig. 13.4 Hypopyon. The finding of a hypopyon (layered inflammatory cells in the anterior chamber of the eye) usually denotes a severe anterior uveitis.

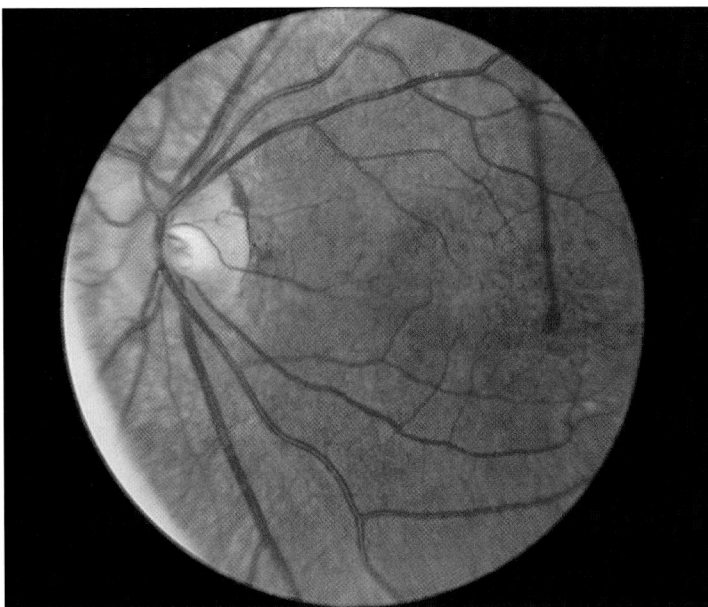

Fig. 13.5 'Salt-and-pepper' fundus. The pigment alterations in the macula give a 'dirty' appearance to the retina. The lesion occurred following congenital rubella infection. The vertical black line across the fovea is a focusing stick.

UVEITIS IN COMMUNITY-BASED AND TERTIARY OPHTHALMOLOGY CENTERS

	Patients in community-based ophthalmology practice	Patients in tertiary referral center
Mean age of patients	46 years	45 years
Males	49%	52%
Percentage with: Anterior uveitis Intermediate uveitis Posterior uveitis Panuveitis and other	91% 1% 5% 3%	60% 12% 15% 13%
Percentage of cases of anterior uveitis that are chronic	9%	63%
Percentage in which specific diagnosis was made	47%	58%
Percentage attributable to infection	14%	21%
Percentage associated with systemic disease (including infections)	13%	9%
Most common causes of uveitis	HLA-B27-associated anterior uveitis (15%) CMV retinitis (7%) Traumatic uveitis (5%) VZV uveitis (4%) *Toxoplasma* retinochoroiditis (4%)	CMV retinitis (33%) HLA-B27-associated anterior uveitis (8%) Pars planitis syndrome (6%) HSV-associated uveitis (5%) *Toxoplasma* retinochoroiditis (4%)
Most common causes of posterior uveitis	CMV retinitis *Toxoplasma* retinochoroiditis	CMV retinitis *Toxoplasma* retinochoroiditis

Fig. 13.6 Uveitis in community-based and tertiary ophthalmology centers. The characteristics of uveitis seen in a community-based ophthalmology practice and in a tertiary referral center. The figures for the proportion of cases in which a specific diagnosis was made are based on data gathered at, or requested at, the first visit; cases of CMV retinitis and 'masquerade' syndrome are omitted. The figures for the proportion of cases associated with systemic disease include cases due to varicella, candidiasis, coccidioidomycosis and syphilis. Data from McCannel *et al.*, 1996.[1]

were more prevalent and much of the anterior uveitis was chronic. In both settings, a specific diagnosis could be made in only about half of patients from data gathered at the initial visit. An infectious cause was documented in 21% of the referred patients and 14% of the community-based patients. The uveitis was attributed to a systemic disease, usually rheumatologic, in a smaller number of patients. The most common causes of uveitis in both settings were HLA-B27-associated anterior uveitis; cytomegalovirus (CMV) retinitis; herpesvirus-associated uveitis, caused either by herpes simplex virus (HSV) or varicella-zoster virus (VZV); and *Toxoplasma* retinochoroiditis (Fig. 13.6). Thus, three of the four most common causes of uveitis were infectious, but infectious causes accounted for well under half of all cases of uveitis in either setting.

Anterior uveitis is much more common than posterior uveitis, and the specific cause is more likely to be identifiable. When infectious, anterior uveitis commonly arises from systemic disease that is clinically obvious, whereas posterior uveitis may arise from an infection that has no extraocular manifestations. This is the case in uveitis caused by *Toxoplasma gondii*, *Toxocara canis* and *Histoplasma capsulatum*. The lesions of anterior uveitis not uncommonly remit without treatment, whereas those of posterior uveitis tend to persist or progress.

PATHOGENESIS AND PATHOLOGY

Most of the infections discussed in this chapter gain access to the ocular structures via hematogenous spread of micro-organisms from other sites. The uveal tract is highly vascular, offering a ready target for seeding by blood-borne microbes. Some organisms (e.g. herpesviruses, *T. gondii*) seem to have a propensity for the retina itself. Furthermore, circulating inflammatory cells and mediators of inflammation have a potent impact on the uveal tract and adjacent structures. These inflammatory cells include T and B lymphocytes, macrophages and monocytes, mast cells and eosinophils. Inflammatory mediators include cytokines, complement and antibodies. In some types of infectious uveitis (e.g. tuberculous and possibly spirochetal uveitis), the inflammation may be produced by a combination of microbial invasion and immunologic mechanisms. Occasionally, uveitis occurs as a 'sympathetic' reaction to an adjacent infection (e.g. anterior uveitis in patients with HSV keratitis). Other infections are hypothesized to gain access to the eye by spreading along nerves (e.g. the ARN syndrome associated with VZV).

The eye is unique among organs in showing a neovascular response to certain stimuli, especially prolonged inflammation. New vessels may form in the cornea, iris, retina, optic nerve and choroid, presumably as a result of the production of various protein growth factors such as vascular endothelial growth factor. These neovascular vessels themselves can cause severe loss of vision. Together with specific treatment of the underlying cause, laser photocoagulation may be needed to treat ocular neovascularization.

Many of the pathogens in uveitis are organisms associated with an intracellular location (viruses, spirochetes, mycobacteria, fungi, parasites). Some tend to persist indefinitely and to produce episodic exacerbations. The eye may be the only site of clinically evident inflammation.

PREVENTION

Patients with systemic infections associated with an appreciable risk of intraocular infection should be screened by an ophthalmologist for early detection and treatment. An example is the periodic examination of patients with HIV infection and a low CD4+ lymphocyte count to detect CMV retinitis. Likewise, patients with HIV infection who develop ophthalmic zoster are at risk of developing ARN and are candidates for ophthalmologic screening examination. Patients with *Candida* fungemia merit ocular examination to detect metastatic retinitis. Neonates with congenital HSV infection must be screened

VIRAL CAUSES OF RETINITIS AND UVEITIS			
Viral infection	Systemic infection	Features of retinitis or uveitis	Other ocular disease
Measles	Uveitis occurs 1–2 weeks after onset of rash	Common: anterior uveitis Rare: chorioretinitis or neuroretinitis	Common: conjunctivitis, keratitis Rare: optic neuritis
SSPE (see Fig. 13.8)	Uveitis occurs some years after infection	Chorioretinitis involves macula	Papillitis; motility disturbances
Herpes simplex virus	Primary infection; lids and conjunctiva	Common: anterior uveitis Rare: uveitis, retinitis, ARN	Dendritic corneal ulcer common
Varicella-zoster virus	Convalescence from varicella or trigeminal zoster (often with nasociliary branch involved)	Common: mild, anterior uveitis, self-limited; rarely, chorioretinitis or ARN	Granulomatous keratic precipitates; synechiae; glaucoma, cataract
Epstein–Barr virus	Infectious mononucleosis	Rare: mild anterior uveitis or chorioretinitis	Common: follicular conjunctivitis
Influenza, adenovirus, mumps	Systemic infection usually evident	Rare: bilateral, mild, self-limited, anterior uveitis Rare: neuroretinitis or optic neuritis	None

Fig. 13.7 Viral causes of retinitis and uveitis. These ocular problems are seen in immunocompetent adults and children.

carefully for ocular lesions, which may first appear up to several months after birth.

MANAGEMENT

There are two major principles of therapy for intraocular infections. The first principle is to treat the infection. Drugs for the treatment of ocular diseases may be given by topical administration, periocular injection, systemic administration (orally or intravenously, or both) and intravitreal injection.

The second principle is to suppress intraocular inflammation, lest there be persisting damage to the retina and other crucial structures. This is usually accomplished by the use of corticosteroids, which may be given by various routes.

UVEITIS IN IMMUNOCOMPETENT ADULTS AND CHILDREN
Viral causes of uveitis

Uveitis, especially anterior uveitis, may occur in the course of many viral infections, most commonly rubeola and infections caused by the herpesvirus family (Fig. 13.7). The uveitis is generally self-limiting and does not require treatment.

Measles often causes conjunctivitis and keratitis; the keratitis rarely leads to bacterial ulceration and perforation of the cornea. There may be anterior uveitis. Other rare complications are chorioretinitis or neuroretinitis; these may occur, together with measles encephalitis, 1–2 weeks after the onset of rash.[3]

The ocular lesions are generally self-limiting and there is no specific treatment available. Involvement of the optic disc (optic neuritis) may cause severe visual loss but this may improve spontaneously over subsequent months. There may be residual pigmentary retinopathy with a 'salt-and-pepper' appearance (Fig. 13.5).

Subacute sclerosing panencephalitis (SSPE), which results from measles infection in very early life, commonly causes chorioretinitis, usually about the time that the neurologic signs of the disease become evident. The chorioretinitis is often focal, involving the macula, and there is mild vitritis (Fig. 13.8). Cortical blindness may occur. The prognosis of the ocular lesions is poor. There is no specific treatment.[4]

Herpes simplex virus infection of the eye in children and adults usually presents as recurrent keratitis with characteristic dendrites (see Chapter 8.5). There may be an associated anterior uveitis (iridocyclitis). Rarely, HSV keratitis may spread along the axons to produce

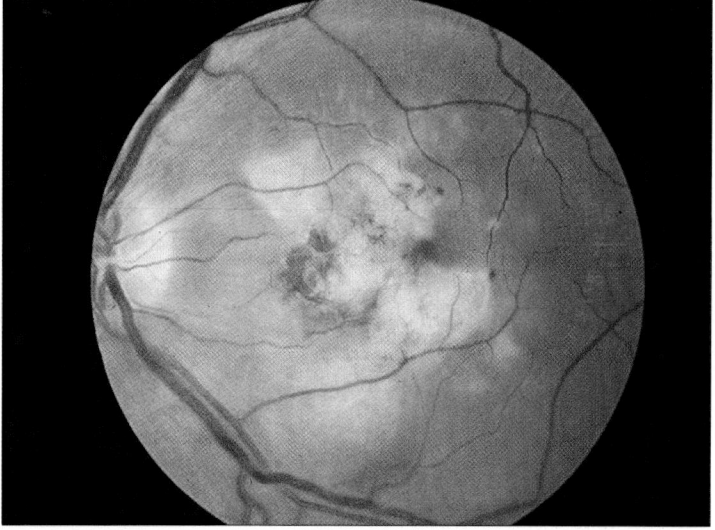

Fig. 13.8 Macular retinitis from a patient with subacute sclerosing panencephalitis.

retinitis and posterior uveitis.[5] Another rare manifestation of HSV ocular infection is ARN, which is discussed below. Retinitis and posterior uveitis are usually treated by antiviral agents such as acyclovir given intravenously in high dosage. Anterior uveitis alone may be treated topically except, perhaps, in immunosuppressed patients.

Varicella, especially in the convalescent stage, may cause a mild, self-limiting anterior uveitis. Treatment is not usually necessary, but corticosteroid drops may be applied. A more serious lesion, keratitis, may develop in patients with trigeminal zoster, especially during convalescence from zoster that has involved the nasociliary branch of the trigeminal nerve. The keratitis may be dendritiform or geographic. It may be accompanied by anterior uveitis with granulomatous keratic precipitates (clumps of inflammatory cells on the corneal endothelium) and posterior synechiae (adhesions between the iris and the anterior surface of the lens).[6]

The uveitis may be treated with 1% trifluridine ophthalmic drops. Rarely, trigeminal zoster may lead to chorioretinitis and the ARN syndrome (see below). In such cases, intravenous aciclovir and

BACTERIAL CAUSES OF RETINITIS AND UVEITIS			
Bacterial infection	Systemic infection	Features of retinitis or uveitis	Other ocular disease
Yersinia spp.	Infection occult, not proven	Suggested important cause of anterior uveitis in patients with HLA-B27 antigen	None
Borrelia burgdorferi	Features of extraocular Lyme disease	Nonspecific anterior or posterior uveitis	Conjunctivitis
Treponema pallidum	Uveitis usually during secondary syphilis; interstitial keratitis is delayed manifestation of congenital syphilis	Common: bilateral anterior uveitis Rare: choroiditis (large white lesions), retinal vasculitis, papillitis	Acute bilateral interstitial keratitis (age 5–10 years, after congenital infection)
Bartonella spp. (see Fig. 13.10)	Nonspecific systemic symptoms antedate ocular symptoms	Bilateral papillitis; optic disc edema; white retinal lesions; vitritis	None
Metastatic endophthalmitis	Often extraocular source is evident	Often bilateral; focal or diffuse uveitis or retinitis	None

Fig. 13.9 Bacterial causes of retinitis and uveitis. These ocular problems are seen in immunocompetent adults and children.

corticosteroids may be administered. There are reported cases with primary varicella infection of childhood (chickenpox).[7]

During infectious mononucleosis caused by Epstein–Barr virus (EBV) infection, a bilateral, mild, follicular conjunctivitis may be seen. Rarely, a mild anterior uveitis can occur, as well. Recently, a chorioretinitis resembling that seen with histoplasmosis, but with vitritis, has been ascribed to EBV infection.[8,9]

Other viral infections may produce uveitis on occasion. Influenza virus infection may cause a mild, transient, bilateral anterior uveitis during the acute infection or neuroretinitis during convalescence.[10] No treatment is needed.

One of the characteristic manifestations of adenovirus infection is epidemic keratoconjunctivitis. There may be concomitant anterior uveitis, for which either no treatment or topical corticosteroid treatment may be given.

Mumps virus infection may cause a mild, evanescent, bilateral anterior uveitis, which may appear up to 4 weeks after the onset of clinical infection. Optic neuritis, sometimes with neuroretinitis, may occur after mumps infection, but it nearly always resolves spontaneously and no treatment is needed.[11]

HLA-B27-associated uveitis

An autoimmune form of recurrent, bilateral anterior uveitis is quite common in patients who harbor the HLA-B27 antigen. HLA-B27-associated uveitis is the most common type of nonidiopathic anterior uveitis. Although usually considered immune-mediated rather than infectious, it may be triggered by systemic infection with Gram-negative bacteria, *Mycoplasma* spp., or *Chlamydia trachomatis*, as seen in Reiter's syndrome. Reiter's syndrome consists of the triad of conjunctivitis, urethritis, and uveitis.[12] Several serologic studies from Scandinavian countries and Australia suggest that *Yersinia* infections may be important contributors.[13]

Bacterial causes of uveitis

Many bacterial species are associated with ocular infections (Fig. 13.9). *Borrelia burgdorferi* infection may cause a wide variety of ocular problems. Conjunctivitis and keratitis occur commonly in the early stages of infection, probably on an immunologic basis. In later stages of Lyme disease there may be iridocyclitis, retinal vasculitis, exudative retinal detachment, vitritis and optic disc edema. Orbital pseudotumor and orbital myositis have also been described.[14–16] The

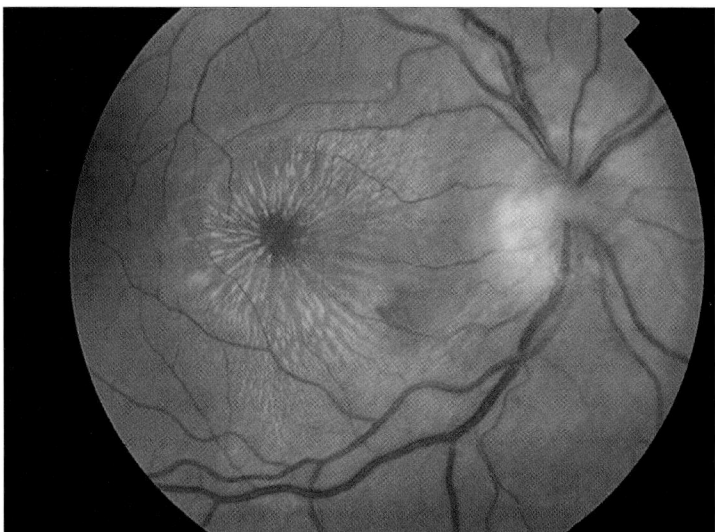

Fig. 13.10 Neuroretinitis with a macular star associated with *Bartonella* infection. Note the swelling of the optic disc with stellate hard exudate in the macula.

treatment is with systemic antibiotics, using regimens appropriate for the stage of the disease (see Chapter 8.19).

Ocular lesions are common in the course of secondary syphilis (*Treponema pallidum* infection). The most common manifestation is a bilateral anterior uveitis, sometimes with iris nodules (granulomas). Less common is a choroiditis with large, white, 'geographic' lesions. There may also be retinal vasculitis, vitritis and papillitis.[17–19] Syphilis should be considered in the differential diagnosis of any posterior segment inflammation or any bilateral anterior segment inflammation. The diagnosis is made serologically and treatment is according to the stage of the syphilis (see Chapter 2.64).

Bartonella henselae in immunocompetent patients has recently been reported as a cause of 'stellate neuroretinitis', also known as 'macular star' (Fig. 13.10), and of Parinaud's oculoglandular fever with retinitis. Macular star can also seen in *Toxocara canis* infection in children and as a benign postviral illness. Cats are thought to be an important reservoir of *B. henselae*, and most infections have occurred in patients with a clear-cut history of exposure to cats.[20] *Bartonella* infection should be suspected in any patient with optic disc edema and intraocular inflammation, especially if retinal lesions are seen.[21]

The infectious agent of Whipple's disease, *Tropheryma whippelii*, is associated with a multisystem disorder, which can include pan-uveitis, retinitis and choroiditis. The diagnosis can be made by biopsy of affected tissue.[22]

Rarely, other bacterial infections have been associated with uveitis distinct from endogenous endophthalmitis. The list includes lepto-spirosis,[23] brucellosis,[24] and tularemia.[25]

Mycobacterium tuberculosis infection can cause anterior uveitis, posterior uveitis or isolated choroiditis. This infection should be a consideration in every case of nonspecific uveitis of unknown cause. There is nearly always active extraocular disease. The anterior uveitis may be acute or chronic, unilateral or bilateral, and there may be gran-ulomatous keratic precipitates. A periphlebitis resembling that seen in sarcoidosis may occur along with choroidal infiltrates; these infiltrates represent miliary tubercles. The uveitis usually improves within 2 weeks of the start of specific antituberculous treatment.

Infection with *Mycobacterium leprae* also may result in ocular inflammation. Corneal complications caused by peripheral nerve damage is the most common ocular complication, and uveitis is seen in only 2% of cases.[26]

Bacterial endophthalmitis is considered in detail in Chapter 2.12. Whereas most instances of bacterial endophthalmitis are exogenous, following surgery or trauma, between 2 and 8% of cases arise from metastatic (endogenous) infection of the eye in the course of bacteremic illness.[27] The possibility of metastatic endophthalmitis should be con-sidered in all patients with unexplained ocular inflammation, especially in those with significant underlying medical diseases. The ophthalmic findings are variable, but generally falls within the following patterns:

- one or more focal areas of inflammation within the uveal tract or retina;
- diffuse involvement of the anterior segment but sparing of the retina, choroid, and vitreous;
- diffuse involvement of the retina, choroid and vitreous, but sparing of the anterior segment; and
- panophthalmitis.

The diagnosis can usually be made by blood cultures, identification of a primary source of infection, and, if necessary, aspiration and culture of the vitreous. Treatment typically does not salvage vision.

Fungal causes of uveitis

The most common fungal species that cause metastatic endophthalmitis are *Candida* spp. (Fig. 13.11), especially *C. albicans* (see Chapter 2.7). The hallmark lesion is a yellow–white, fluffy patch of retinitis with indistinct borders (Fig. 13.12), almost always associated with vitritis. The lesions may mimic those of toxoplasmosis but inactive reti-nal scars are not seen in *Candida* infection. However, some cases of *Candida* endophthalmitis have an indolent course and some even improve spontaneously. The diagnosis is suspected from the appear-ance of the lesions in a typical clinical setting. Blood cultures may assist in the diagnosis, and vitreous culture may prove it. Patients with *Candida* fungemia should be considered candidates for routine ophthalmoscopic screening. Treatment of *Candida* endophthalmitis is discussed in Chapter 7.16.

Whereas metastatic *Candida* infection usually occurs in a setting of active fungemia, *Histoplasma* ocular infection usually occurs without evident extraocular infection (Fig. 13.11). The lesions arise from pre-vious hematogenous spread to the choroid, producing a granuloma that usually becomes an inactive scar.[28] Vitritis is rare but disc edema with optic neuritis can occur acutely. As a late complication, choroidal neovascular membranes can penetrate the old choroidal scars leading

FUNGAL CAUSES OF RETINITIS AND UVEITIS			
Fungal infection	Systemic infection	Features of retinitis or uveitis	Other ocular disease
Candida spp. (see Fig. 13.12)	Risk factors for candidemia	Whitish fluffy patch of retinitis and some vitritis	Anterior segment cells with hypopyon; corneal abscess
Histoplasma capsulatum (see Fig. 13.13)	History of residence in an endemic area; no extraocular infection evident	Choroidal granulomas, scars; optic neuritis; no vitritis	No anterior segment inflammation

Fig. 13.11 Fungal causes of retinitis and uveitis. These ocular problems are seen in immunocompetent adults and children.

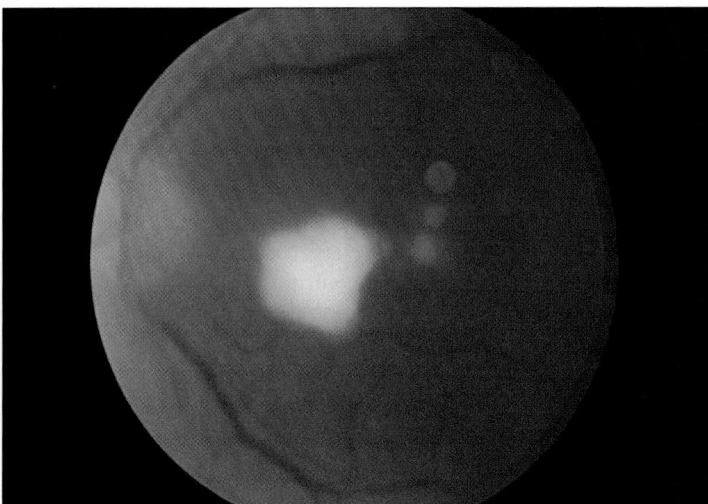

Fig. 13.12 A focal area of superficial retinitis and vitritis secondary to *Candida albicans*.

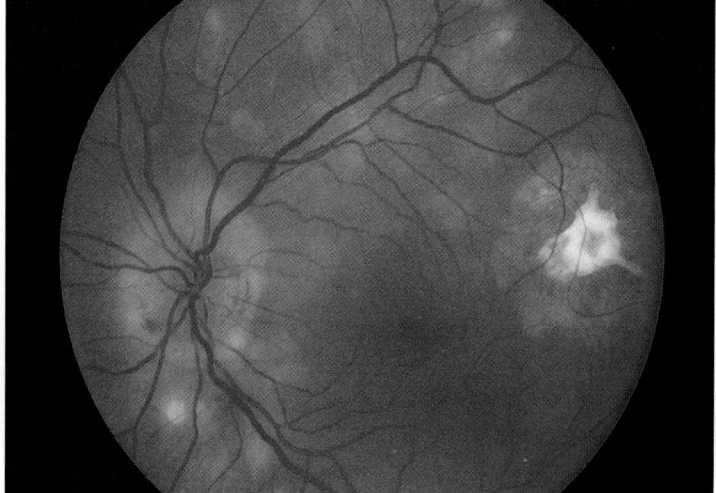

Fig. 13.13 The classic ocular findings of previous histoplasmosis. Note the peripapillary atrophy and punched-out yellowish chorioretinal scars. An old choroidal neovascular membrane is present in the center of the histoplasmosis scar temporal to the macula.

to retinal edema, hemorrhage and decreased vision. The diagnosis of ocular histoplasmosis is suspected by the finding of characteristic choroidal lesions (Fig. 13.13) in a patient who has resided in an area endemic for the fungal infection. Serologic or skin tests for histoplasmosis are usually positive but do not prove the diagnosis. The organisms have never been cultured from an intraocular source so the relation to *Histoplasma* infection is inferential.

The treatment of ocular histoplasmosis depends on the stage of infection. Corticosteroids may be used to treat the acute choroidal granulomas but have little role in the chronic, neovascular stage when there is no active inflammation. Laser photocoagulation is usually employed if there is a choroidal neovascular membrane that is not subfoveal; surgery may be done for subfoveal lesions because the laser would cause a blind spot. There is no indication for antifungal treatment.

Rarely, other fungi such as *Coccidioides*, *Blastomyces* and *Aspergillus* spp. and *Cryptococcus neoformans* may cause chorioretinitis by hematogenous spread. *Nocardia* species (Fig. 13.14) also occasionally cause chorioretinitis. Although rare overall, these infections are more common in the immunosuppressed. The diagnosis should be suspected based on confirmation of the associated systemic infection. Systemic antifungal treatment is required.

Parasitic causes of uveitis

Ocular infection by *Toxocara canis*, the dog roundworm, is found in young children, especially boys, aged from 6 months to 4 years (Fig. 13.15). *Toxocara cati*, the cat roundworm, also has been implicated but the organisms have never been positively identified in the human eye. The typical presenting complaint is decreased vision, strabismus, or leukocoria (a whitish lesion seen in the pupil). *Toxocara* infection is acquired by the ingestion of soil contaminated with embryonated eggs (see Chapter 8.35). There may be a history of pica. The larvae are believed to reach the eye by hematogenous spread. However, most affected children do not have a history or current evidence of visceral larva migrans. The ocular findings are generally unilateral.

There are several ophthalmoscopic presentations of ocular toxocariasis (Fig. 13.16). The features they have in common are a whitish or yellowish retinal mass, representing a granuloma surrounding the larva, and the eventual formation of traction bands between the vitreous and the granuloma, which may result in retinal folds and exudative retinal detachment.[29] There may be diffuse posterior uveitis, sometimes called 'nematode endophthalmitis'. There is usually dense vitreous inflammation. Unlike bacterial endophthalmitis, there is little or no pain or anterior segment inflammation. Other presentations include

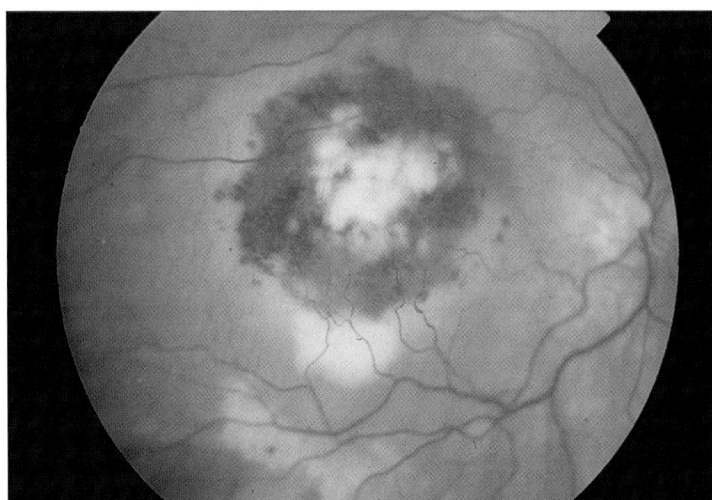

Fig. 13.14 A *Nocardia* chorioretinal abscess in the macula of a patient following heart transplant.

PARASITIC CAUSES OF RETINITIS AND UVEITIS			
Parasitic infection	Systemic infection	Features of retinitis or uveitis	Other ocular disease
Toxocara canis (see Fig. 13.16)	Children 6 months to 4 years of age; no extraocular infection	Usually unilateral; pale granulomatous mass or focal retinitis; traction bands; vitritis	No anterior segment inflammation
Toxoplasma gondii (see Figs 13.17 & 13.18)	Usually acquired *in utero* but not evident systemically	Recurrent self-limiting attacks of chorioretinitis and vitritis ('headlight in the fog')	May be keratic precipitates (granulomatous reaction) in anterior chamber

Fig. 13.15 Parasitic causes of retinitis and uveitis. These ocular problems are seen in immunocompetent adults and children.

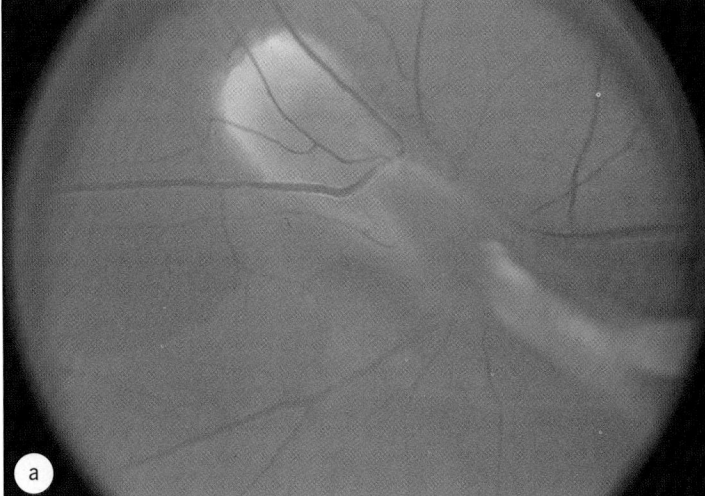

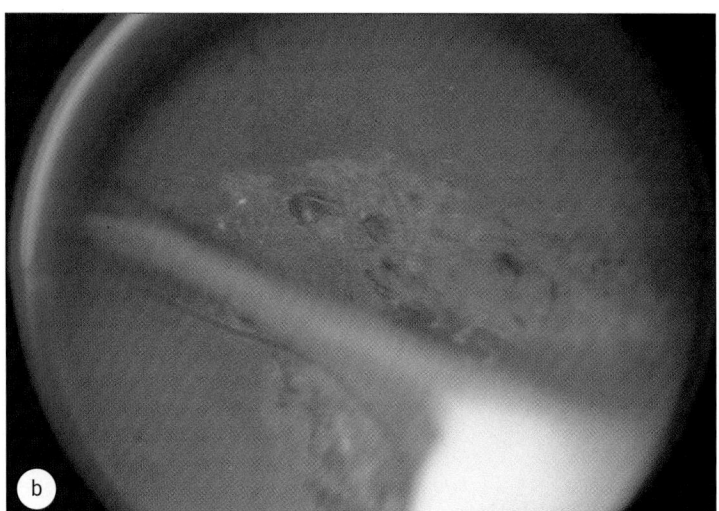

Fig. 13.16 Ocular toxocariasis. (a) The posterior pole of a left eye affected by toxocariasis. There is severe macular distortion and dragging of the retina toward a granuloma in the inferotemporal retinal periphery. (b) The periphery of the inferotemporal retina in the same eye showing the granuloma.

localized retinitis affecting the macula or the peripheral retina, and acute optic neuritis in which the granuloma overlies the optic disc. A 'macular star' (neuroretinitis), which is characteristic of toxocariasis, certain viral infections and bartonellosis, may be seen as a result of leakage from vessels in the optic disc.

The major differential diagnoses of ocular toxocariasis are non-infectious diseases such as retinoblastoma and Coats' disease, a congenital vascular disorder. Peripheral blood eosinophilia is rare in ocular toxocariasis. A serum enzyme-linked immunosorbent assay (ELISA) antibody titer to the parasite of 1:8 or more supports the diagnosis. A positive ELISA titer of the intraocular fluid, which may be found even if the serum titer is negative, is highly indicative of the infection. Treatment is directed toward stemming the intraocular inflammation, clearing any media opacity and preventing permanent distortion in the retinal architecture. Corticosteroids, usually applied locally in the eye, and cataract or vitrectomy surgery are the mainstays of treatment.

Toxoplasma gondii infection is a common cause of posterior segment inflammations in children and adults (Fig. 13.15). In the immunocompetent, it represents the most common cause of posterior uveitis. In many countries, including the USA, almost all cases of ocular toxoplasmosis are thought to follow intrauterine infection (see Chapter 2.55) with hematogenous spread to the eye. Postnatally acquired infection is followed by ocular toxoplasmosis in fewer than 5% of cases. Nevertheless, in some countries, such as Brazil, postnatally acquired infection is the more common antecedent of ocular toxoplasmosis. The infection as it presents in immunosuppressed patients is discussed later in this chapter.

The lesions of ocular toxoplasmosis are found preferentially in the nerve fiber layer of the retina but can affect any layer including the choroid.[30] Healed lesions of congenital toxoplasmosis are flat, atrophic, chorioretinal scars that have a propensity for the macular area of the fundus (Fig. 13.17). There may be recurrent bouts of uveitis, caused by the rupture of cysts to release trophozoites. Most patients have their first reactivation before 30 years of age. Ophthalmoscopic examination shows vitritis and one or more white retinal lesions that are usually round or oval and not more than 5mm in diameter. There may be many such lesions surrounding an old scar (Fig. 13.18). Aggregates of vitreous cells over the active lesions are the rule. The appearance of the vitreous haze and the white granuloma has been likened to a 'headlight in the fog'. There may be retinal hemorrhages, sheathing of arterioles and venules, and papillitis. There may be a granulomatous reaction in the anterior chamber with keratic precipitates and conjunctival injection.

The diagnosis of ocular toxoplasmosis is made by the characteristic appearance of the lesions together with a positive serum antibody test for *T. gondii* (see Chapter 8.34). Other possible causes of localized necrotizing retinitis with vitritis, such as syphilis or tuberculosis, should be considered (Fig. 13.19). Further support for the diagnosis can be obtained by determining the ratio of *Toxoplasma* antibody between serum and a sample of ocular fluid.[31]

In otherwise healthy persons, flare-ups of ocular toxoplasmosis tend to be self-limiting over a period of weeks to months. Not all active lesions need to be treated. The highest priority for treatment is for lesions that threaten the fovea or the optic nerve or large areas of the nerve fiber layer, as well as those that produce enough vitritis to impair vision. Once the fovea is directly involved, visual acuity is usually permanently compromised.

Treatment is the same as for other systemic forms of toxoplasmosis – pyrimethamine, sulfadiazine and clindamycin (see Chapter 7.17). Many ophthalmologists avoid pyrimethamine initially because of its marrow-suppressive effects, preferring to rely on the other two agents. Corticosteroids are often used concomitantly, but not without the anti-infective drugs. Laser photocoagulation may be used for active lesions that are unresponsive to medication and pars plana vitrectomy may be used to clear vitreous opacities.

Rarely, uveitis may occur in other parasitic infections such as cysticercosis, myiasis and onchocerciasis.

UVEITIS IN NEONATES

There are several causes of uveitis in neonates (Fig. 13.20).

Herpes simplex virus

Congenital infection by HSV is usually acquired directly from the infected birth canal, but it sometimes occurs transplacentally or through the amniotic fluid. The congenital infection may mainly affect the skin, eyes and oral cavity; the internal organs ('disseminated disease'); or the central nervous system. However, the eyes may be involved in any of these presentations. Ocular findings may first appear from 1 week to several months after birth, and must be carefully sought by periodic ophthalmoscopic examination of infants at risk. About 80% of isolates are HSV-2; this strain is associated with more severe ocular infections than HSV-1.

Congenital HSV infection may cause a wide variety of ocular lesions. In the anterior segment, conjunctivitis and keratitis (punctate, dendritic, or geographic) are most common, and are usually seen in the acute phase of the infection. There is often an associated anterior uveitis. Peripheral anterior and posterior synechiae and secondary cataracts may be seen.

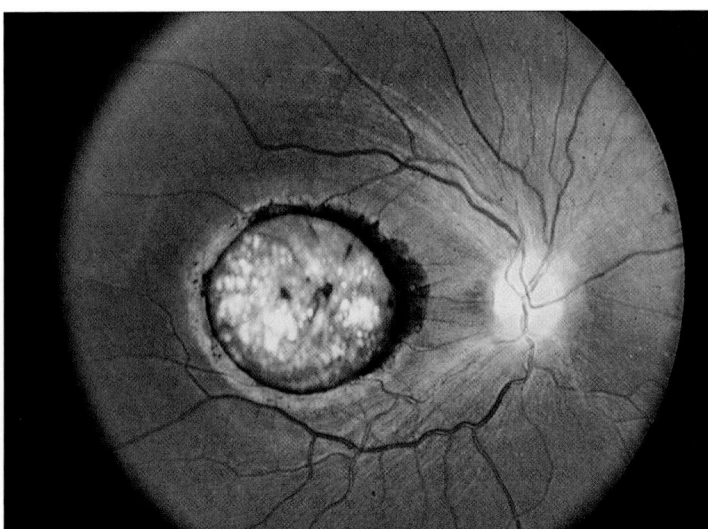

Fig. 13.17 An old, inactive congenital macular toxoplasmosis scar. The patient's vision was 20/400.

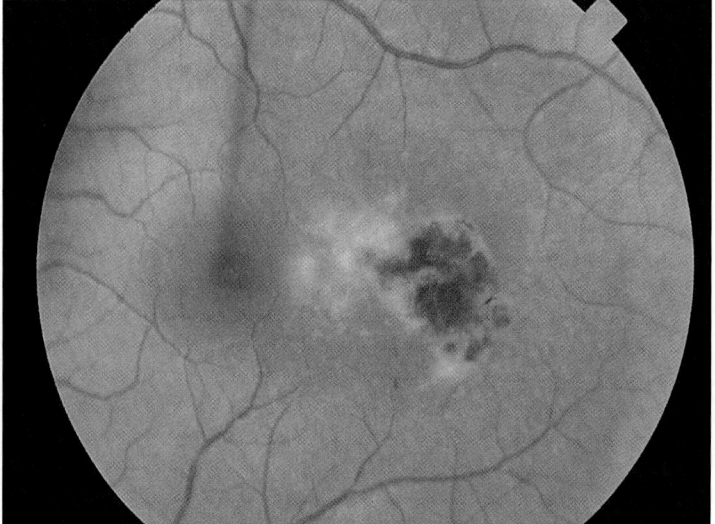

Fig. 13.18 A reactivated area of retinal toxoplasmosis. The lesion is the area of whitening and is adjacent to an old scar, just temporal to the macula of the left eye.

CHARACTERISTICS OF SOME INFECTIONS CAUSING POSTERIOR UVEITIS/RETINITIS WITHOUT EXTRAOCULAR MANIFESTATIONS

	Usual number of lesions	Appearance of lesions	Distribution of lesions	Accompanying vitritis
Toxoplasma gondii (see Figs 13.17 & 13.18)	One to a few	'Headlight in fog'	Random, but heavier in macular area	Almost always
Toxocara canis (see Fig. 13.16)	One	Granuloma	Macular, optic disc or periphery	Always
Histoplasma capsulatum (see Fig. 13.13)	Multiple	Choroidal granulomas	Various	Almost never
Treponema pallidum	Diffuse retinochoroiditis	Bilateral anterior uveitis; large white geographic choroidal lesions	Random	Always
Borrelia burgdorferi	Focal or diffuse	Anterior uveitis, retinal vasculitis, exudative retinal detachment	Random	Usually
Mycobacterium tuberculosis	One or a few	Retinitis or chorioretinitis	Random	Usually

Fig. 13.19 Characteristics of some infections causing posterior uveitis/retinitis without extraocular manifestations.

INFECTIOUS RETINITIS AND UVEITIS IN NEONATES

	Systemic infection	Features of uveitis/retinitis	Other ocular disease
Viral infections			
Herpes simplex virus	Disseminated infection usually evident	Anterior uveitis early; optic neuritis, retinal hemorrhages and necrosis later; sparing of choroid	Conjunctivitis, keratitis common
Varicella-zoster virus	Features of congenital varicella-zoster (rare)	Chorioretinitis	Microphthalmia; cataracts
Cytomegalovirus	Features of congenital cytomegalovirus infection	Retinitis in 20–25% of infants with symptomatic cytomegalovirus infection; resembles that seen in adults with AIDS	None
Rubella	Congenital rubella syndrome	Mild, self-limiting chorioretinitis + vitritis in 25–50% with congenital rubella syndrome; unilateral or bilateral; eventual 'salt-and-pepper' fundus	None
Bacterial infections			
Treponema pallidum	Stigmata of congenital lues	'Salt-and-pepper' fundus; occasionally optic atrophy, retinal vascular sheathing	Delayed manifestation: acute interstitial keratitis (age 5–10 years)
Fungal infections			
Candida spp. (see Fig. 13.12)	*Candida* fungemia; risk factors	Whitish fluffy patch of retinitis, some vitritis	None
Parasitic infections			
Toxoplasma gondii (see Figs 13.17 & 13.18)	Rarely, encephalitis, hydrocephalus at birth	Rarely, chorioretinitis at birth	None

Fig. 13.20 Infectious retinitis and uveitis in neonates.

Posterior segment changes tend to occur later in the infection.[32] There may be disc edema with optic neuritis. Retinal involvement ranges from scattered hemorrhages to widespread retinal necrosis similar to that seen in the ARN syndrome. There may be retinal vasculitis and vitritis, and retinal detachments in severe cases. Residual changes include pigment migration and clumping ('salt-and-pepper' appearance), macular chorioretinal scars, optic atrophy and preretinal neovascularization.

The diagnosis and treatment of neonatal HSV infection are reviewed in Chapter 7.15. Because the ocular lesions are part of a generalized infection, systemic treatment is required. In the exceptional instances in which the anterior segment of the eye is the only evident site of the suspected infection, viral cultures of the conjunctiva should be performed and topical treatment alone may be given.

Varicella-zoster virus

Congenital infection by VZV is very rare (see Chapters 2.55 & 8.5). The ocular findings in the neonate are microphthalmia, chorioretinitis, and cataract formation. If there is active chorioretinitis, an antiviral agent such as acyclovir should be given intravenously.

Cytomegalovirus

Congenital infections by CMV are usually asymptomatic (see Chapters 2.55 & 8.5). With symptomatic infections, retinitis occurs in 20–25% of cases. If retinitis is not evident at birth, it is unlikely to occur later. The retinitis resembles that seen in adult patients with HIV infection (see below).

Rubella

In the congenital rubella syndrome, ocular manifestations occur in 25–50% of affected children.[33] The classic finding is a mild, self-limiting chorioretinitis that may be unilateral or bilateral. There may be vitritis. Vision is usually not impaired. A common sequel is a 'salt-and-pepper' fundus, caused by changes in the retinal pigment epithelium (Fig. 13.5). A similar appearance is produced by congenital syphilis and influenza. Other ocular manifestations of congenital rubella include cataracts and a mild anterior uveitis that may cause posterior synechiae. There is no specific treatment.

Syphilis

The most common ocular manifestation of congenital syphilis (see Chapter 2.64) is 'salt-and-pepper fundus'. The lesions are almost always bilateral but may be sectoral or exclusively peripheral. They are the result of chorioretinitis, which may be evident at birth or appear in the first few years of life. Visual acuity is rarely affected. In more severe cases, there may be diffuse sheathing of the retinal vessels, optic atrophy and migration of the retinal pigment epithelium in a manner resembling retinitis pigmentosa.[34] Acute interstitial keratitis is a delayed manifestation of congenital syphilis. It may be accompanied by anterior uveitis and secondary glaucoma may develop. The lesions of keratitis are self-limited but treatment of the syphilitic infection is indicated.

Candida spp. may cause retinitis and vitritis in neonates. The infection is acquired after birth and the ocular infection is usually hematogenous. Risk factors are prematurity, low birth weight, sepsis, malnutrition and treatment with broad-spectrum antibiotics. The clinical presentation and treatment are as for adults (see Chapter 7.16).

Toxoplasma chorioretinitis is usually acquired *in utero*. Although the ocular complications usually present long after the neonatal period, they are sometimes evident at birth in the TORCH syndrome (see Chapter 2.55). Manifestations include encephalitis, hydrocephalus and bilateral chorioretinitis. Treatment is described in Chapter 7.17.

THE ACUTE RETINAL NECROSIS SYNDROME

The ARN syndrome is a recently described, rare syndrome of a vaso-obliterative retinal and choroidal vasculitis, diffuse retinal necrosis and vitritis. It is bilateral in one-third of patients, although the two eyes need not be affected simultaneously. It has been reported in children as young as 8 years of age but it occurs most often in adults. Conclusive evidence now exists that VZV is the primary cause; HSV is a less common cause.[35] Patients infected with HIV who develop zoster of the first division of the trigeminal nerve appear to have a high risk of subsequent ARN, often bilateral, over the next few weeks to months.[36]

Acute retinal necrosis causes diffuse arteritis and phlebitis with sheathing of the retinal vessels and striking white areas of retinal necrosis (Fig. 13.21). Broad areas of the peripheral retina are involved early on, but the macula is usually spared initially. There is often mild inflammation of the anterior segment. As the disease progresses, there is increasing vitritis. Optic neuropathy with edema of the disc may appear.

Retinal detachment follows in 75% of patients. The detachments are notoriously difficult to repair. Prior prophylactic laser treatment of healthy retina, posterior to the areas of necrosis, reduces the incidence of retinal detachment.

The mainstay of treatment for ARN is aciclovir, given in high dosage intravenously (e.g. 12–15 mg/kg q8h for 7–14 days). Oral aciclovir should be continued for 2–3 months to lessen the risk of fellow eye involvement. Systemic corticosteroids are given as well, to decrease inflammation. Retinal detachments require complex vitreoretinal surgery for successful repair. It has been suggested that patients with AIDS who develop ophthalmic zoster be given long-term oral prophylaxis with aciclovir, but there is no proof of benefit from this approach.[36]

UVEITIS AND RETINITIS IN IMMUNOSUPPRESSED PATIENTS

Because of the AIDS pandemic, ophthalmologists are now encountering a variety of intraocular infections that previously were either unknown or extraordinarily rare.

Cytomegalovirus retinitis

The most common ocular infection in HIV-positive adult patients is CMV retinitis. Although CMV retinitis occurs at some time in the course in about 35% of adult patients with AIDS, it represents the AIDS-defining diagnosis in fewer than 5%. Cytomegalovirus retinitis rarely occurs in patients who have CD4+ lymphocyte counts over 50 cells/mm^3.[37] Pediatric patients who have AIDS have a much lower incidence of CMV retinitis than adults, presumably because most children have not been exposed to CMV. In one study of African patients with AIDS, there were no cases of CMV retinitis.[38]

Symptoms of CMV retinitis tend to be absent or minimal at the start. Floaters, decreased peripheral vision, or metamorphopsia are occasionally seen. Often, an active infection is noted on a routine

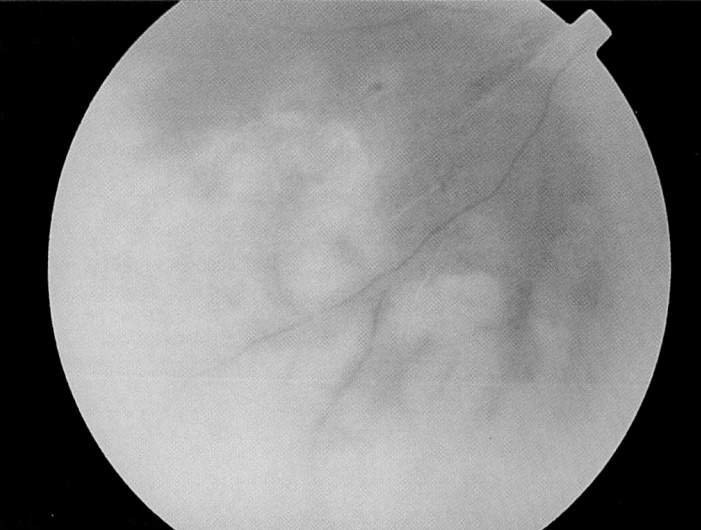

Fig. 13.21 Typical appearance of the retina in the acute retinal necrosis syndrome. There is dense peripheral retinal whitening with a geographic border. Satellite lesions are common. The view is hazy owing to vitritis.

ophthalmologic screening examination. In 40% of patients with CMV retinitis, the lesions are bilateral at presentation. Nearly 75% of patients will present to the ophthalmologist with disease that is considered immediately sight-threatening. Pain, redness, or more than a mild anterior uveitis are highly unusual with CMV retinitis.

The hallmark lesion of CMV retinitis is a necrotizing, full-thickness retinitis resulting in retinal cell death (Fig. 13.22). Consistent with the theory that CMV is hematogenously spread, retinal tissue adjacent to major retinal blood vessels or the optic disc is often affected initially. The areas of active retinitis have a granular appearance and are dirty-white in color. Hemorrhage is common, owing to damage to vascular endothelial cells. The appearance has been likened to a 'brush fire' and to 'ketchup and cottage cheese'. The retinitis spreads contiguously as well as by producing satellite lesions. It is common to see areas of healed retinitis alongside areas of active necrosis. Areas of burned out necrosis show an absence of retinal tissue while the underlying retinal pigment epithelium assumes a 'salt-and-pepper' appearance.

Loss of vision occurs both because of the death of retinal cells and because of retinal detachment. About 10–20% of eyes with CMV retinitis can be expected to suffer detached retina. The risk is time dependent; after 1 year the risk approaches 50%. Although vitreous surgery to repair the detached retinas is successful in more than 90% of instances, visual results are often limited by the underlying disease process.[39]

There are three agents available for systemic administration for the treatment of CMV retinitis: ganciclovir, foscarnet, and cidofovir.[40] Although all three are typically effective initially, they all have potential side effects and disadvantages that limit their long-term utility. The mean time to progression of the retinitis is only 2 months for all three medications, making long-term efficacy the major problem with intravenous therapy. Orally administered ganciclovir is even less effective than intravenous therapy. Thus, systemically administered agents are most useful for preventing progression of the extraocular infection that often accompanies or follows CMV retinitis.

Direct intraocular treatment in the form of intravitreal injections of ganciclovir or foscarnet or intravitreal insertion of a sustained release ganciclovir implant can achieve much higher intraocular concentrations of drugs than intravenous therapy. The long-term efficacy of such local forms of therapy is superior to that of intravenous therapies. The mean time to progression of newly diagnosed CMV retinitis treated with a ganciclovir implant is 220 days (7 months), which is approximately the designed life span of the device. If the devices are replaced before the end of their estimated life span, however, at least 75% of eyes can be expected to suffer no progression until death.[41] High-dose

(2mg per dose) weekly intravitreal injections of ganciclovir appear to have similar long term efficacy.[42]

Implants and intravitreal injections carry the risks of invasive ocular procedures. Intravitreal injections must be given at least once a week, whereas ganciclovir implants only need to be placed at intervals of 6–8 months. If no concurrent systemic anti-CMV medication is given to patients treated with local therapy, there is a risk of systemic CMV. The incidence of systemic CMV infection in the year following initiation of exclusively local treatment for CMV retinitis is reportedly 11–30%.[41]

Other causes of uveitis and retinitis

About 75% of patients with HIV-1 infection have a nonsight threatening retinopathy that may be caused by the HIV-1 itself.[43] The lesions are multiple, bilateral, cotton-wool spots and scattered retinal hemorrhages (Fig. 13.23). If there is concern that such lesions may be due to CMV, close observation over a period of days to weeks with documentation by photographs is recommended. Cytomegalovirus retinitis will invariably progress, whereas cotton-wool spots caused by HIV will resolve.

Opportunistic infections with *Pneumocystis carinii*, *Histoplasma capsulatum*, *Cryptococcus neoformans* and atypical mycobacteria, may produce multifocal choroiditis in patients with AIDS. These infections are rarely sight-threatening but they should alert the clinician to the presence of a systemic infection. Unfortunately, it is generally not possible for the ophthalmologist to distinguish among these possible opportunistic infections on the basis of the eye examination alone.[43]

Other important posterior segment infections that can occur in HIV-positive patients include toxoplasmosis, syphilis, and infection with HSV and VZV. Whereas toxoplasmosis in immunocompetent patients produces a slowly progressive, focal, relapsing chorioretinitis, in immunocompromised patients it can produce a severe, diffuse retinitis.[44] Serologic testing may be helpful. Nearly one-third of patients with AIDS and *Toxoplasma* retinitis will have concurrent toxoplasmosis of the central nervous system. Ocular syphilis can also mimic CMV retinitis but the lesions of secondary syphilis are usually a choroiditis, rather than a retinitis.[45] Syphilis is diagnosed serologically. Neuroretinitis caused by *Bartonella* infection has been reported in a patient with AIDS.[20]

Acute retinal necrosis syndrome

The ARN syndrome (see above) occurs in both healthy and immunosuppressed people, including those with AIDS. Acute retinal necrosis differs from CMV retinitis in that the lesions of ARN are typically

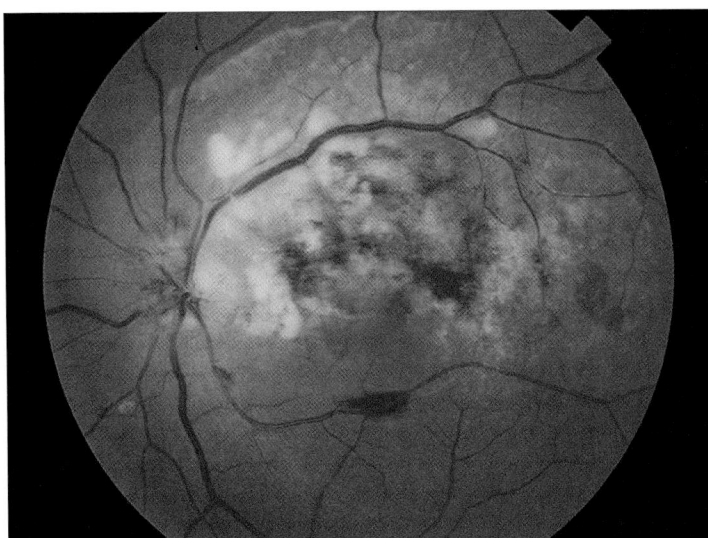

Fig. 13.22 Cytomegalovirus infection with granular retinal whitening along the major blood vessels with mild hemorrhage. The view is clear because there is only mild vitritis.

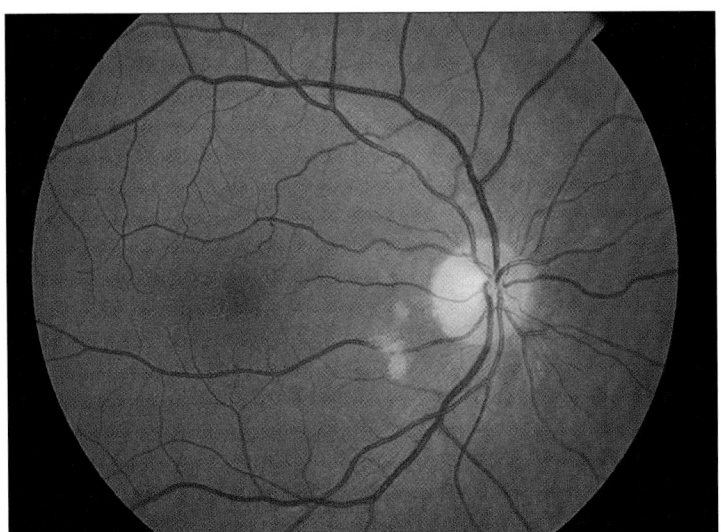

Fig. 13.23 HIV retinopathy. There are multiple superficial white patches in the retina (cotton-wool spots). These do not affect vision and typically wax and wane over time.

peripheral and the course is much more rapid. In addition, significant vitreous cells are a prominent feature of ARN but not of CMV retinitis. Patients infected with HIV who develop zoster of the first division of the trigeminal nerve appear to have a high risk of subsequent ARN, often bilateral, over the next few weeks to months.[36] Thus, when the rash of ophthalmic zoster appears, AIDS patients should be followed carefully for signs of ARN.

A specific type of rapidly progressive ARN has been described in AIDS patients. It has been called progressive outer retinal necrosis (PORN) and is due to VZV infection.[46] Without aggressive therapy, PORN results in total loss of vision within days to weeks. The recommended treatment is a combination of foscarnet, together with either ganciclovir or aciclovir, given intravenously or intravitreously.

Perhaps the most common cause of noninfectious anterior uveitis in HIV-positive patients is a dose-related reaction to rifabutin. Patients receiving rifabutin for prophylaxis against *Mycobacterium avium intracellulare* in conjunction with another agent that interferes with the metabolism of rifabutin (such as clarithromycin, fluconazole, or ritonavir) are at particular risk.[47] The incidence of rifabutin-induced uveitis is 20% among AIDS patients taking the medication but it has been reported in the HIV-negative patients as well. Treatment with corticosteroids and discontinuation of the medication usually results in prompt reversal of the inflammation.[48] Systemic cidofovir has also been reported to cause uveitis in AIDS patients.

REFERENCES

1. McCannel CA, Holland GN, Helm CJ, *et al.* Causes of uveitis in the general practice of ophthalmology. Am J Ophthalmol 1996;121:35–46.
2. Darrell RW, Wagner HP, Kurland LT. Epidemiology of uveitis: incidence and prevalence in a small urban community. Arch Ophthalmol 1962; 68:502–14.
3. Bell WE, Blodi CF. Measles. In: Gold DH, Weingeist TA, eds. The eye in systemic disease. Philadelphia: Lippincott; 1990:258–9.
4. Robb RM, Watters GW. Ophthalmic manifestations of subacute sclerosing pancencephalitis. Arch Ophthalmol 1970;83:426–9.
5. Pavan-Langston D, Brockhurst RJ. Herpes simplex panuveitis. Arch Ophthalmol 1969;81:783–7.
6. Karbassi M, Raizman MB, Schuman JS. Herpes zoster ophthalmicus. Surv Ophthalmol 1992;39:395–410.
7. Capone A, Meredith TA. Central visual loss caused by chickenpox retinitis in a 2-year-old. Am J Ophthalmol 1992;113:592–3.
8. Raymond LA, Wilson CA, Lenneman CC, *et al.* Punctate outer retinitis in acute Epstein–Barr virus infection. Am J Ophthalmol 1988;104:424–5.
9. Tiedeman JS. Epstein-Barr viral antibodies in multifocal choroiditis and retinitis. Am J Ophthalmol 1987;103:659–63.
10. Rabon RJ, Louis GJ, Zegarra H, Gutman FA. Acute bilateral posterior angiopathy with influenza A viral infection. Am J Ophthalmol 1987;103:289–93.
11. Wilhelmus KR. Mumps. In: Gold DH, Weingeist TA, eds. The eye in systemic disease. Philadelphia: Lippincott; 1990:262–4.
12. Lee DA, Barker SM, Su WP, Allen GL, Liesegang TJ, Ilstrup DM. The clinical diagnosis of Reiter's syndrome. Ophthalmology 1986;93:350–6.
13. Wakefield D, Stahlberg TH, Toivanen A, Granfors K, Tennant C. Serologic evidence of *Yersinia* infection in patients with anterior uveitis. Arch Ophthalmol 1990;108:219–21.
14. Fedorowski JJ, Hyman C. Optic disk edema as the presenting sign of Lyme disease. Clin Infect Dis 1996;23:639–40.
15. Lesser RL, Kornmehl EW, Pachner AR, *et al.* Neuro-ophthalmologic manifestations of Lyme disease. Ophthalmology 1990;97:699–706.
16. Karma A, Seppala I, Mikkila H, Kaakkola S, Viljanen M, Tarkkanen A. Diagnosis and clinical characteristics of ocular Lyme borreliosis. Am J Ophthalmol 1995;119:127–35.
17. Gass JDM, Braunstein RA, Chenoweth RG. Acute syphilitic posterior placoid chorioretinitis. Ophthalmol 1990;97:1288–97.
18. Margo CE, Hamed LM. Ocular syphilis. Surv Ophthalmology 1992;37:203–20.
19. Tamesis RR, Foster CS. Ocular syphilis. Ophthalmology 1990;97:1281–7.
20. Wong MT, Dolan MJ, Lattuada CP Jr, *et al.* Neuroretinitis, aseptic meningitis, and lymphadenitis associated with *Bartonella* (Rochalimaea) infection in immunocompetent patients and patients infected with human immunodeficiency virus type 1. Clin Infect Dis 1995;21:352–60.
21. Bafna S, Lee AG. Bilateral optic disc edema and multifocal retinal lesions without loss of vision in cat scratch disease. Arch Ophthalmol 1996;114:1016–7.
22. Rickman LS, Freeman WR, Green WR, *et al.* Uveitis caused by *Tropheryma whippelii* (Whipple's bacillus). N Eng J Med 1995;332:363–6.
23. Levin N, Nguyen-Khoa JL, Charpentier D, Strobel M, Fournie-Amazourz E, Denis P. Panuveitis with papillitis in leptospirosis. Am J Ophthalmol 1994;117:118–9.
24. Walker J, Sharma OP, Rao NA. Brucellosis and uveitis. Am J Ophthalmol 1992;114:374–5.
25. Marcus DM, Frederick AR Jr, Hodges T, Allan JD, Albert DM. Typhoidal tularemia. Ophthalmology 1990;108:118–9.
26. Shields JA, Waring GO, Monte LG. Ocular findings in leprosy. Am J Ophthalmol 1974;77:880–90.
27. Okada AA, Johnson RP, Liles WC, D'Amico DJ, Baker AS. Endogenous bacterial endophthalmitis. Report of a ten-year retrospective study. Ophthalmology 1994;101:832–8.
28. Nussenblatt RB, Palestine AG. Ocular histoplasmosis. In: NEED EDS. Uveitis. Fundamentals and clinical practice. Chicago: Year Book Publishing: 1989:379–85.
29. Shields JA. Ocular toxocariasis: a review. Surv Ophthalmol 1984;28:361–81.
30. Mets MB, Holfels E, Boyer KM, *et al.* Eye manifestations of congenital toxoplasmosis. Am J Ophthalmol 1996;122:309–24.
31. Baarsma GS, Luyendijk L, Kijlstra A, *et al.* Analysis of local antibody production in the vitreous humor of patients with severe uveitis. Am J Ophthalmol 1991;112:147–50.
32. Reynolds JD, Griebel M, Mallory S, Steele R. Congenital herpes simplex retinitis. Am J Ophthalmol 1986;102:33–6.
33. Hara J, Fujimoto F, Ishibashi T, Seguchi T, Nishimura K. Ocular manifestations of the 1976 rubella epidemic in Japan. Am J Ophthalmol 1979;87:642–653.
34. Pulido JS, Corbett JJ, McLeish WM. Syphilis. In: Gold DH, Weingeist TA, eds. The eye in systemic disease. Philadelphia: Lippincott; 1990:233–9.
35. Duker JS, Blumenkranz MS. Diagnosis and management of the acute retinal necrosis (ARN) syndrome. Surv Ophthalmol 1991;35:327–43.
36. Sellitti TP, Huang AJW, Schiffman J, Davis JL. Association of herpes zoster ophthalmicus with acquired immunodeficiency syndrome and acute retinal necrosis. Am J Ophthalmol 1993;116:297–301.
37. Gross JS, Bozzette SA, Matthews WC, *et al.* Longitudinal study of cytomegalovirus retinitis in acquired immune deficiency syndrome. Ophthalmology 1990;97:681–6.
38. Kestelyn P, Van de Perre P, Rouvoy D, *et al.* A prospective study of the ophthalmologic findings in the acquired immune deficiency syndrome in Africa. Am J Ophthalmol 1985;100:230–8.
39. Regillo CD, Vander JF, Duker JS, Fischer DH, Belmont JB, Kleiner R. Repair of retinitis-related retinal detachments with silicone oil in patients with acquired immune deficiency syndrome. Am J Ophthalmol 1992;113:21–7.
40. Studies of ocular complications of AIDS research group (SOCA). Mortality in patients with the acquired immune deficiency syndrome treated with either foscarnet or ganciclovir for cytomegalovirus retinitis. N Engl J Med 1992;326:213–20.
41. Martin DF, Parks DJ, Mellow SD, *et al.* Treatment of cytomegalovirus retinitis with an intraocular sustained-release ganciclovir implant. Arch Ophthalmol 1994;112:1531–9.
42. Young SH, Morlet N, Heery S, Hollows FC, Coroneo MT. High dose intravitreal ganciclovir in the treatment of cytomegalovirus retinitis. Med J Aust 1992;157:370–3.
43. Jabs DA, Green WR, Fox R, Polk BF, Bartlett JG. Ocular manifestations of acquired immune deficiency syndrome. Ophthalmology 1989;96:1092–9.
44. Cochereau-Massin I, LeHoang P, Lautier-Frau M, *et al.* Ocular toxoplasmosis in human immunodeficiency virus-infected patients. Am J Ophthalmol 1992;114:130–5.
45. McLeish WM, Pulido J, Holland S, Culbertson WW, Winward K. The ocular manifestations of syphilis in the human immunodeficiency virus type 1-infected host. Ophthalmol 1990;97:196–203.
46. Forster DJ, Dugel PU, Frangieh GT, Liggett PE, Rao NA. Rapidly progressive outer retinal necrosis in the acquired immune deficiency syndrome. Arch Ophthalmol 1990;110:341–8.
47. Havlir D, Torriani F, Dube M. Uveitis associated with rifabutin prophylaxis. Ann Intern Med 1994;121:510–2.
48. Saran BR, Maguire AM, Nichols C, *et al.* Hypopyon uveitis in patients with acquired immunodeficiency syndrome treated for systemic Mycobacterium avium complex infection with rifabutin. Arch Ophthalmol 1994;112:1159–65.

Practice Points

Management of red eye

Renée Ridzon

INTRODUCTION
There are many causes of red eye, both infectious and noninfectious. When evaluating this problem, the clinician must make an accurate and rapid diagnosis. Some causes are treated with supportive therapy; others are sight-threatening and must be referred to an ophthalmologist for immediate attention. There are elements of the patient history and physical examination that will aid the clinician in proper diagnosis of the disorder so that appropriate therapy can be administered (see Chapters 2.11 & 2.13).

PATHOGENESIS
Less serious causes of the red eye include conjunctivitis, which may be a result of trauma or a foreign body, burns, chemical irritation, allergic reaction or infection, subconjunctival hemorrhage or disorders of the adnexal structures of the eye. Acute angle-closure glaucoma, keratitis, acute iridocyclitis, and corneal ulcers are more serious causes that can lead to vision loss. Abnormal lid function with inability to close the eye completely (e.g. in Bell's palsy) can result in a red eye. Red eye may also be a manifestation of a systemic disorder such as Kawasaki's disease, hemorrhagic viral infections, Stevens–Johnson syndrome or connective tissue disorders.

MICROBIOLOGY
The common pathogens causing acute conjunctivitis in adults are *Streptococcus pneumoniae* and *Staphylococcus aureus*. In children, common bacterial causes include *Strep. pneumoniae, Staph. aureus* and *Haemophilus influenzae*. Chronic bacterial conjunctivitis is most commonly caused by *Staph. aureus* or *Moraxella lacunata*. *Neisseria gonorrhoeae* and *Chlamydia trachomatis* cause conjunctivitis both in the newborn and in adults.

The most common cause of viral conjunctivitis is adenovirus, which can cause an epidemic form. Another causative virologic agent is herpes simplex virus, which usually produces an accompanying keratitis.

As in the case of conjunctivitis, keratitis is most often caused by bacteria and viruses. The common causative agents include *Staph. aureus, Strep. pneumoniae,* and *Pseudomonas aeruginosa*. Keratitis due to *N. gonorrhoeae* may result from untreated conjunctivitis. Herpes simplex virus types 1 and 2 as primary infection and reactivation disease are the most common viral etiologies. Varicella-zoster virus may involve the cornea when, on reactivation, there is involvement of the ophthalmic division of the trigeminal nerve. Fungus may be a rare cause of keratitis, and fungal keratitis may occur after corneal trauma. In people who use soft contact lenses, *Acanthamoeba* spp. can cause keratitis.

CLINICAL FEATURES
A focused history and physical examination are essential to the prompt diagnosis of red eye. The history should include past diagnoses of systemic illness; recent exposure to potential irritants, allergens or other ill people; trauma; and recent symptoms of illness and ocular-related symptoms such as blurred vision, ocular pain, photophobia, itching and

exudation. The physical examination of the eye should include measurement of visual acuity, measurement of intraocular pressure if needed, characterization of exudate, if present, and examination of the pupil, conjunctiva and cornea. Fluorescein may be needed to look for defects in the cornea or the conjunctiva.

Conjunctivitis is characterized by hyperemia of the conjunctiva. The congestion of blood vessels tends to be less intense near the limbus than at the peripheral part of the sclera. The etiology may be noninfectious or infectious. The patient may have complaints of itching or burning, and papillae may be found on the palpebral conjunctiva. Infectious conjunctivitis begins unilaterally and then subsequently involves both eyes. Secretions are usually present, and may vary from watery in viral infections to purulent in bacterial infection. Chlamydial and *N. gonorrhoeae* conjunctivitis in the newborn are both marked by a hyperpurulent discharge and are acquired during birth. Chronic bacterial conjunctivitis may be accompanied by blepharitis. Adenoviral conjunctivitis may present with pharyngoconjunctival fever, characterized by fever, sore throat and conjunctivitis; preauricular adenopathy may be present. Corneal involvement may produce eye pain and photophobia. Certain enterovirus strains cause acute hemorrhagic conjunctivitis with hemorrhages in the bulbar conjunctiva.

Infectious keratitis usually presents unilaterally with complaints of pain, photophobia, tearing and blurred vision. Corneal clouding, ulceration and hypopyon may be present, but discharge is generally absent. Herpes simplex virus keratitis may be accompanied by vesicles on the eyelid, follicular conjunctivitis, and dendritic ulcers within the cornea. Bacterial keratitis is the most likely microbial infection to cause corneal opacification, scarring and rapid progression to perforation. A ciliary flush of hyperemia may be seen surrounding the limbus in bacterial keratitis. Immunosuppression and use of corticosteroids are risk factors for bacterial keratitis. Use of soft contact lenses, especially extended-wear lenses, increases the risk of *P. aeruginosa* keratitis.

A red eye with a dilated pupil and absent light response suggests acute angle-closure glaucoma and necessitates immediate attention by an ophthalmologist. Iridocyclitis presents with a small pupil with poor light response and is associated with connective tissue disease.

INVESTIGATIONS
Most initial therapy for infectious conjunctivitis is empiric, and cultures or scrapings usually are not obtained. Chlamydial infection of the newborn can be diagnosed clinically or through Giemsa staining or an immunofluorescence assay of material from a palpebral–conjunctival scraping. Herpes simplex keratitis is usually diagnosed clinically, although scrapings can be obtained for culture or immunoassay. Corneal scrapings for culture may be obtained to ensure appropriate antibiotic coverage.

MANAGEMENT
Any patient who presents with a vision-threatening form of red eye should be referred to an ophthalmologist for immediate attention (Fig. 14.1; see Chapter 2.13).

Because of the difficulty in distinguishing viral conjunctivitis from bacterial conjunctivitis, some physicians recommended that all conjunctivitis should be treated with topical antibiotics. Drops are usually best for adults because there is less interference with vision; however, infants and children should receive ointment because it stays in the eyes better with crying than do drops. There are a number of different antibiotics available as topical ophthalmologic preparations, including cephalosporins, penicillins, aminoglycosides, fluoroquinolones and amphotericin B. Inadequate response to topical antibiotics should prompt reassessment of the patient, culture and possible referral. Mothers of infants who have *C. trachomatis* or *N. gonorrhoeae* conjunctivitis and their sexual partners and sexual partners of adults who have *C. trachomatis* conjunctivitis should receive therapy. Chronic conjunctivitis may be accompanied by blepharitis, and treatment needs to be directed at the lid as well as the conjunctiva. Adenoviral conjunctivitis is highly contagious during the first 2

weeks and it is recommended that children should be kept out of school during this time.

Keratitis can be sight-threatening condition and needs to be treated promptly; this is especially true for the bacterial form because it may be rapidly progressive.

FURTHER READING

Baum J. Infections of the eye. Clin Infect Dis 1995;21:479–88.
Durand M. Infections of the eyelid, lacrimal system, conjunctiva and cornea. Curr Clin Top Infect Dis 1996;16:125–50.
Ghezzi K, Renner GS. Ophthalmologic disorders. In: Rosen P, Barkin RM, Braen CR, *et al*, eds. Emergency medicine: Concepts and Clinical Practices, 3rd ed, Vol III. St Louis: Mosby-Year Book; 1992:2427–59.
Papastamelos AG, Tunkel AR. Antibacterial agents in infections of the central nervous system and eye. Infect Dis Clin North Am 1995;9:615–37.
Syed NA, Hyndiuk AA. Infectious conjunctivitis. Infect Dis Clin North Am 1992;6:789–805.

SUGGESTED TREATMENT OF INFECTIOUS CAUSES OF RED EYE			
Disorder	Causes	Clinical features	Treatment
Conjunctivitis		Conjunctival injection, exudate	
Viral conjunctivitis		Starts unilaterally, progresses to both eyes in 2–10 days	
Epidemic keratoconjunctivitis	Adenovirus	Preauricular lymph nodes preceded by upper respiratory infection and fever	None
Acute hemorrhagic conjunctivitis	Enterovirus, Coxsackie virus, adenovirus 11	Unilateral pain, seromucous discharge, photophobia	None
Acute bacterial conjunctivitis	*Staphylococcus aureus* *Streptococcus pneumoniae* *Haemophilus influenzae*	Purulent exudate	Topical antibiotic ointment q4–q6h for 5–7 days
	Neisseria gonorrhoeae	Unilateral, mucopurulent exudate	Infants: penicillin 50,000–100,000U/kg/day iv in 4 doses for 7 days; if resistance is suspected or confirmed ceftriaxone 25–50mg/kg/day iv or im Adults: penicillin 2,400,000U im q12h for 3–5 days
	Chlamydia trachomatis	Bilateral in infants appears 3–10 days after birth accompanied by large follicles in adults	Infants: erythromycin syrup, 50mg/kg/day po in 4 doses for 14 days Adults: doxycycline 100mg q12h po for 7 days (some ophthalmologists treat for 21 days)
Chronic bacterial conjunctivitis	*Staphylococcus aureus*, *Moraxella lacunata*		Lid hygiene; erythromycin ointment q4–q6h for 5–7 days
Allergic conjunctivitis		Itching, tearing	Topical antihistamines or corticosteroids
Keratitis		Conjunctival injection, ciliary flush, corneal opacification, visual changes, pain, photophobia, corneal ulceration, corneal perforation	
Viral keratitis	Herpes simplex virus 1 and 2	Usually unilateral; dendritic forms on cornea	Trifluridine 1% eyedrops (1 drop per hour 9 times a day for 3–5 days, then 1 drop 5 times a day); avoid topical corticosteroids
	Varicella-zoster virus	Vesicular eruption in ophthalmic division of trigeminal nerve	Aciclovir 800mg 5 times a day po for 10 days; role of corticosteroids is disputed
Bacterial keratitis		Corneal opacity	
	Staphylococcus aureus, *Streptococcus pneumoniae*		Cefazolin 5% eyedrops and gentamicin 1.5% eyedrops every 15–60min for 24–72 hours, with slow dose reduction over several weeks
	Pseudomonas aeruginosa	Associated with soft contact lenses	Piperacillin or ticarcillin 0.6–2% eyedrops and tobramycin 1.5% eyedrops loading dose followed by 1 drop every 15–30min with slow reduction over weeks
Fungal keratitis	*Aspergillus* spp. *Fusarium* spp. *Candida* spp.	Associated with preceding corneal trauma; slowly progressive; treat only after confirmation	Amphotericin B 0.15% eyedrops or natamycin 5% every 2–3 hours with slow reduction over weeks
Parasitic keratitis	*Acanthamoeba* spp.	Associated with soft contact lenses; treat only after confirmation	Propamidine 0.1% eyedrops and neomycin 5% eyedrops for several months to 1 year

Fig. 14.1 Suggested treatment of infectious causes of red eye. Cases of conjunctivitis do not normally need to be referred to an ophthalmologist; cases of keratitis do.

Eye problems and the patient in the intensive care unit

Harminder Singh Dua

INTRODUCTION

The critically ill patient in an intensive care unit (ICU) is particularly vulnerable to bacterial corneal infections, which are by far the most serious ocular problems encountered in these patients. Exposure keratitis and associated corneal abrasions are other, relatively minor problems, although they are significant because they are often the precursors of serious corneal infection (see Chapter 2.11). Despite considerable awareness of the problem and various protocols followed by ICUs the world over, bacterial keratitis with sequelae of corneal scarring and visual impairment continues to occur in ICU patients.

OCULAR SURFACE DEFENSE

The exposed position of the eyes ensures constant encounters with environmental pathogens. However, the ocular surface is equipped with a wide range of protective mechanisms. The lids provide physical and mechanical protection. The blink reflex aids flow of tears across the eye surface and helps in flushing contaminating organisms down the nasolacrimal passages into the nasopharynx, where they are effectively dealt with by the lymphoid tissue. The conjunctiva is also provided with lymphoid tissue, which can mount a competent humoral and cell-mediated immune response against invading organisms. Constant evaporation of tears keeps the ocular surface temperature down and so makes it less favorable to bacterial growth. Furthermore, tears have several important antimicrobial constituents such as immunoglobulins, lysozyme, lactoferrin, complement components, ceruloplasmins, defensins and betalysins. The integrity of the corneal surface epithelium is the single most important defense against bacterial invasion. In critically ill ICU patients, several of the above factors are breached or compromised, predisposing to infection.

RISK FACTORS FOR EYE INFECTION IN INTENSIVE CARE UNIT PATIENTS

Important risk factors for bacterial keratitis in the setting of an ICU are listed in Figure 14.2. Exposure, inadequate blinking and drying (leading to epithelial erosions and abrasions) are important factors that make a critically ill patient susceptible to ocular surface infection. When intermittent positive-pressure ventilation is employed, it leads to venous stasis, body fluid retention and conjunctival edema. Edematous and chemosed conjunctiva prolapses through the lids with consequent drying and bacterial contamination. Infected respiratory tract secretions are a common source of bacterial contamination of the eyes. Suction of copious tracheobronchial secretions when carried out over the patient's head, across the eyes, is known to cause bacterial dispersion and ocular contamination. *Pseudomonas aeruginosa* is the most common pathogen isolated from corneal ulcers in ICU patients.

MANAGEMENT

Prevention, by eliminating or addressing the risk factors, is the key to management of ocular surface infections in critically ill patients. The eyes should be frequently inspected, every 4–6 hours at least (Fig. 14.3). Sterile artificial tear drops should be instilled at each inspection and proper lid closure should be maintained at all times. This prevents drying of the corneal surface.

RISK FACTORS FOR CORNEAL AND CONJUNCTIVAL INFECTION IN PATIENTS IN ICU's

Dry eye
Inadequate tear production
Poor or absent blink reflex (e.g. because of coma or the use of paralyzing and sedating drugs)
Exposure as a result of proptosis or poor closure of lids (lagophthalmos), leading to excessive evaporation

Microtrauma
Tips of eye medication dispensers
Cotton wool or gauze wipes or patches applied over open lids

Conjunctival contamination
Nosocomial pathogens, commensals
Infected body fluids (droplets) related to suction from respiratory tract
Conjunctivitis, conjunctival edema (chemosis as a result of ventilation support), with protrusion of conjunctiva through lids
Retained contact lens

Poor host resistance
Malnutrition, chronic alcoholism, immunodeficiency, prolonged corticosteroid medication, diabetes mellitus, overwhelming systemic infection

Fig. 14.2 Risk factors for corneal and conjunctival infection in patients in intensive care units.

SUGGESTED PROTOCOL FOR EYE CARE IN PATIENTS IN ICUs

At the outset
Assess condition of eyes (A to C)
Ensure patient is not wearing contact lenses (soft or rigid)
In road traffic accident patients, exclude conjunctival sac foreign bodies (seek ophthalmic opinion if necessary)

A Eyes are clean and moist, and lids close adequately
If blink reflex preserved:
 Inspect eyes at regular intervals (4–6 hours)
 Ensure that eyelids remain closed at all times
 Keep eyes moist by instillation of simple eye ointment or artificial tear drops at each inspection
If blink reflex is absent:
 The lids can be lightly taped shut

B There is conjunctival edema, drying of ocular surface or eyes tend to remain open
Nurse patient with head up (if possible) to encourage dispersion of conjunctival fluid
Remove any obstruction to jugular venous drainage (e.g. with endotracheal tube harness)
Instil drops or ointment as above
Close eyes fully with adhesive tape or polyacrylamide gel patches
Ensure polyacrymide gel patches are kept hydrated with sterile normal saline
Inspect at 4–6 hours intervals for first 24 hours
If eyes remain moist and satisfactory, continue as above
If dryness increases or epithelial abrasions develop, increase frequency of simple paraffin eye ointment and consider topical antibiotic prophylaxis (gentamicin or ciprofloxacin), particularly if patient has infection at any other site

C The eyes are/become red, inflamed and sticky
Suspect conjunctivitis or keratitis
If there is conjunctival discharge, the eyes should not be patched or taped shut
Allow free drainage of discharge, irrigate with sterile normal saline, culture swabs from conjunctival sac and commence (prophylactic) antibiotics
Because eyes are open, risk of drying becomes greater
Increase frequency of inspections and instillation of ocular lubricants
Refer to an ophthalmologist

Avoid
Touching tips of drop or ointment applicators to ocular surface
Using the same drop or ointment units for right and left eyes
Placing patch or tape over partially open eyes
Patching of eyes with discharge
Suction of secretions across the head of the patient and suction without covering the eyes
Routine eye swabs for culture in all patients in intensive care units
Embarrassment of leaving contact lens *in situ*

Fig. 14.3 Suggested protocol for eye care in patients in intensive care units. Modified from protocol used in the intensive care unit of the University Hospital, Queen's Medical Centre, Nottingham, UK (Dr Bernard Riley, personal communication).

Lid closure can be achieved by placing a strip of micropore adhesive tape horizontally across the closed lid margins. Constant removal and reapplication of adhesive tape can lead to excoriation of the lid skin. The Donaldson eye patch, which is shaped like a 'T' with an adhesive horizontal arm applied to the upper lid and the long arm provided with a Velcro mechanism, allows repeated opening and closure of the lids without any abrasive effect. Alternatively a temporary 'Frost suture' can be passed through the upper or lower lid. A 4 0' or 5 0' silk suture mounted on a cutting needle is passed horizontally through the skin of the lid, close to the lid margin (upper or lower). At this site, the skin is fairly firmly adherent to the underlying tissues and provides good anchorage to the suture (Fig. 14.4). The two ends are left 2–3 inches (4.5–7.5cm) long and taped to the cheek (or brow). The suture is used as a handle to open or close the lids. Eye patches or sutures can be discontinued when the blink reflex returns to normal. When the lids cannot be apposed owing to rigidity or loss of tissue, as occurs after injury or burns, or when chemosed conjunctiva protrudes through the palpebral aperture, polyacrylamide gel patches of high water content or cling wrap can be used. These provide adequate cover and protection and conserve moisture. Gel patches need to be kept constantly hydrated with sterile normal saline. Instruments used to cut gel patches or cling wrap to appropriate size must be sterile.

Suction of secretions should be carried out from the side of the head rather than over the top of the head. At all times, the eyes should be adequately covered and shielded during suction manuvers. In the presence of respiratory or other infections, eye swabs should be taken every 1–2 days to detect early colonization of the conjunctival sac. In the presence of a positive swab, prophylactic antibiotic drops should be commenced. Chloramphenicol or ciprofloxacin drops provide a broad range of cover. Gram staining helps to tailor the choice of antibiotic. Antibiotic ointments smeared on the surface of the lid skin will make it difficult to retain adhesive tape.

Early detection of infection is the next best step in management. Appearance of lid swelling and conjunctival swelling and redness are important signs. Any discharge or crusting of the lid margins should be viewed with suspicion. Early signs of corneal involvement include loss of the normal shine or luster, corneal haziness and localized white infiltrates. Corneal staining with 2% fluorescein is a useful bedside test and if positive indicates corneal abrasion or ulcer. Instil a drop or two of 2% fluorescein, close and open the eyelid to ensure even spread, irrigate with a few drops of sterile saline 20–30 seconds later and view the cornea with a blue light (pen lights with cobalt blue filter attachments are widely available). Any area of the cornea denuded of epithelium will fluoresce green.

Treatment of established corneal infection constitutes an ocular emergency and an ophthalmologist must be involved at the outset. Corneal ulcer, particularly those caused by *Pseudomonas* spp., can progress rapidly with perforation of the cornea and loss of the eye. The usual protocol is to take corneal scrapes for Gram stain and culture (aerobes and anaerobes and fungi) and sensitivity. Eye drops of gentamicin (15mg/ml) and cefuroxime (5 or 10%) (or vancomycin 25mg/ml if hypersensitive

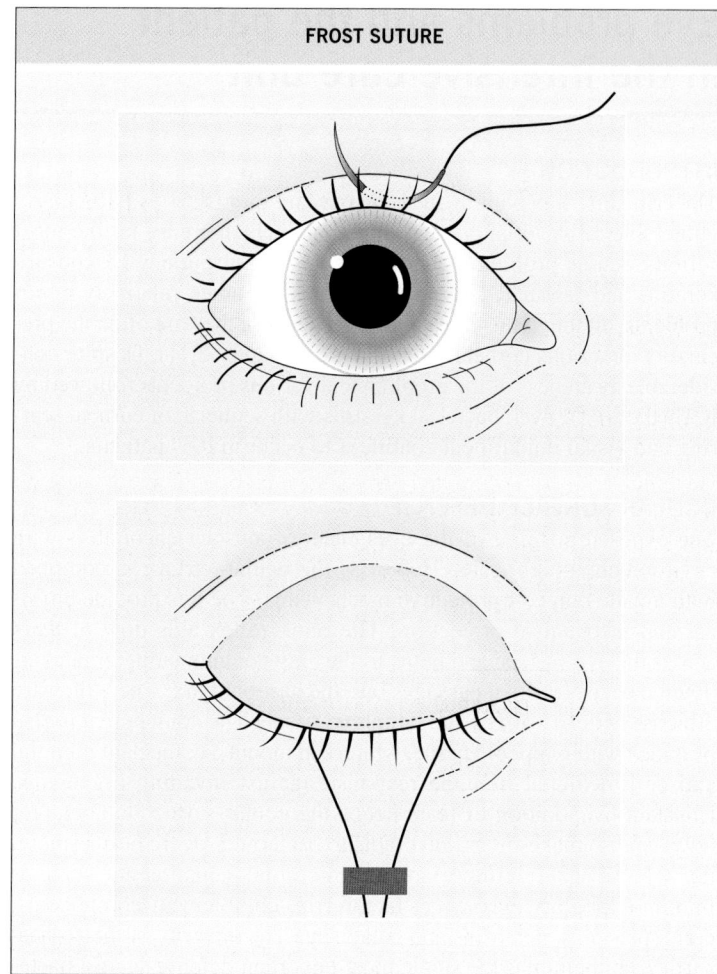

FROST SUTURE

Fig. 14.4 Frost suture. A 5 0' silk suture is placed at the upper lid margin through half the tissue thickness (above), and used to tape the lid shut (below).

to beta-lactams) are commenced at 1-hourly intervals, each drop alternating every half hour, round the clock, for 24–48 hours. Treatment is tapered or modified according to clinical response and sensitivity results. Ciprofloxacin 0.3% is a useful option, especially if *Pseudomonas* spp. are suspected. For all drops, an initial intensive loading regimen of 1–2 drops every 15 minutes for 4–6 hours is beneficial.

FURTHER READING

Hilton E, Uliss A, Samuels S, Adams AA, Lesser ML, Lowy FD. Nosocomial bacterial eye infections in intensive-care units. Lancet 1983;1:1318–20.
Parkin B, Turner A, Moore E, Cook S. Bacterial keratitis in the critically ill. Br J Ophthalmol 1997;81:1060–3.

Acute and Chronic Meningitis

Stephen L Leib & Martin G Täuber

INTRODUCTION

Meningitis is the most common serious manifestation of infection of the central nervous system (CNS). Inflammatory involvement of the subarachnoid space with meningeal irritation leads to the classic triad of headache, fever and meningism, and to a pleocytosis in the cerebrospinal fluid (CSF). Meningitis is divided clinically into acute and chronic disease; acute meningitis develops over hours or days, whereas the symptoms of chronic meningitis evolve over weeks or even months.

Acute meningitis is caused by a variety of infectious agents (Fig 15.1). The most serious form of acute meningitis is caused by pyogenic bacteria, such as *Streptococcus pneumoniae*, *Neisseria meningitidis*, *Haemophilus influenzae*.[1–3] Group B streptococci (*Streptococcus agalactiae*), Enterobacteriaceae and *Listeria monocytogenes* are the major pathogens in the neonatal period (Fig. 15.2).[3]

Aseptic meningitis, in which no bacterial pathogen can be isolated by routine cultures, can mimic bacterial meningitis, but the disease has a much more favorable prognosis. Many cases of aseptic meningitis are caused by viruses, primarily enteroviruses, but bacteria such as *Mycobacterium tuberculosis*, *Leptospira* spp., *Brucella* spp., *Borrelia burgdorferi* and noninfectious etiologies also cause meningitis with negative cultures.[2]

Patients with aseptic meningitis show signs of meningeal inflammation and lymphocytic pleocytosis in the CSF, in which no etiologic bacterial pathogen can be identified. Because the term 'aseptic meningitis' existed before routine tests to detect viruses were available, it is imprecise and is often used synonymously with viral meningitis. Although viruses are the most common cause of aseptic meningitis (Fig. 15.3), there are numerous nonviral etiologies (including spirochetes and rickettsiae) and noninfectious etiologies (see Fig. 15.1).[2] The most common group of viruses causing viral aseptic meningitis are the enteroviruses, including Coxsackie viruses.[4]

Chronic meningitis is defined by symptoms of meningeal inflammation with CSF pleocytosis that persist for more than 4 weeks.[5] The diagnosis is based on the history, clinical evidence of meningitis, CSF examination, and often on imaging studies. The differential diagnosis is broad (see Fig. 15.1). The predominant CSF cell type can provide clues to the underlying disease (Fig. 15.4).

EPIDEMIOLOGY

INCIDENCE
Acute bacterial meningitis
The incidence of acute bacterial meningitis in the USA is approximately 5–10 cases per 100,000 persons per year.[1] Up to 15,000 and 25,000 cases of bacterial meningitis are estimated to occur annually in the USA. The very old and the very young are more commonly affected. The organisms that cause bacterial meningitis vary with the age of the patient (see Fig. 15.2). Neonatal meningitis has been reported in 1 child per 200–500 live births; at present approximately 75% of these cases are caused by *Streptococcus agalactiae*. Until recently, young children aged 1 month to 2 years have had the highest incidence of meningitis, with *H. influenzae* type b as the predominant pathogen. The use of new conjugate *H. influenzae* type b vaccines has reduced the incidence of invasive *H. influenzae* infection, including meningitis, by more than 90% in developed countries, where the vaccine is widely used.

The incidence of bacterial meningitis shows a peak in winter and early spring and varies greatly in different areas of the world. This variability is accounted for primarily by the epidemiology of *N. meningitidis*, which can cause either sporadic cases or epidemics of meningitis. Small

MICROBIAL CAUSES OF MENINGITIS		
Acute bacterial meningitis		
Common etiologic species	*Haemophilus influenzae* *Neisseria meningitidis* *Streptococcus pneumoniae*	*Listeria monocytogenes* *Streptococcus agalactiae*
Other etiologic species	*Staphylococcus aureus* *Staphylococcus epidermidis* *Escherichia coli* *Klebsiella pneumoniae* *Pseudomonas aeruginosa* *Nocardia* spp. Viridans streptococci *Enterobacter* spp. *Proteus* spp. *Citrobacter* spp.	*Flavobacterium* spp. *Moraxella* spp. *Propionibacterium acnes* *Enterococcus faecalis* *Salmonella* spp. Group A streptococci *Serratia* spp. *Acinetobacter* spp. *Pasteurella multocida* *Aeromonas* spp.
Other organisms	Spirochetes Mycobacteria *Borrelia* spp. Rickettsiae	*Leptospira* spp. *Brucella* spp. *Naegleria* spp. *Acanthamoeba* spp.
Chronic meningitis		
Viruses	Lymphocytic Choriomeningitis virus Mumps virus Herpes simplex virus	Varicella-zoster Arbovirus Flavivirus Echovirus
Bacteria	*Mycobacterium tuberculosis* *Brucella* spp. *Treponema pallidum* *Borrelia* spp.	*Leptospira* spp. *Nocardia* spp. *Actinomyces* spp. *Listeria monocytogenes*
Fungi	*Cryptococcus neoformans* *Coccidioides immitis* *Histoplasma capsulatum* *Candida* spp.	*Blastomyces dermatitidis* *Sporothrix schenckii* *Aspergillus* spp.
Parasites	*Cysticercus* spp. *Angiostrongylus cantonensis* *Paragonimus westermani* *Gnathostoma spinigerum*	*Schistosoma* spp. *Echinococcus* spp. *Strongyloides* spp.
Aseptic meningitis		
Viruses	Enteroviruses Mumps Herpes viruses Lymphocytic choriomeningitis Adenoviruses	HIV Morbillivirus Rubivirus Epstein–Barr virus Arboviruses

Fig. 15.1 Microbial causes of meningitis.

BACTERIAL CAUSES OF ACUTE MENINGITIS RELATED TO AGE AND PREDISPOSING FACTORS

Age	Pathogen	Predisposing factors
0–4 weeks	Streptococcus agalactiae	Birth complications
	Escherichia coli	Birth complications
	Listeria monocytogenes	Maternal infection
	Streptococcus pneumoniae	CSF leak, asplenia
1–3 months	Escherichia coli	Nosocomial colonization
	Haemophilus influenzae	CSF leak, sinusitis, otitis
	Listeria monocytogenes	Immunodeficiency
	Neisseria meningitidis	Complement deficiencies, immunodeficiency
	Streptococcus agalactiae	Nosocomial colonization
	Streptococcus pneumoniae	CSF leak, immunodeficiency
3 months–18 years	Haemophilus influenzae	Age 3 months–6 years, CSF leak, otitis media, sinusitis
	Neisseria meningitidis	Epidemics, terminal complement deficiencies
	Streptococcus pneumoniae	CSF leak, otitis media, sinusitis, asplenia
18–50 years	Neisseria meningitidis	Epidemics, immunodeficiency
	Streptococcus pneumoniae	CSF leak, otitis media, sinusitis, asplenia, alcoholism
>50 years	Listeria monocytogenes	Immunodeficiency, diabetes mellitus
	Streptococcus pneumoniae	CSF leak, otitis media, sinusitis, asplenia, alcoholism
Not age-related	Enterobacteriaceae	Neurosurgery, nosocomial acquisition
	Staphylococcus aureus	Neurosurgery, CSF leak, endocarditis, abscesses
	Propionibacterium acnes	Neurosurgery, CSF leak, dermal sinus

Fig. 15.2 Bacterial causes of acute meningitis related to age and predisposing factors.

CHARACTERISTIC FEATURES OF ASEPTIC MENINGITIS BY ETIOLOGY

Agent	Season	Clinical signs	Special features
Enteroviruses	Summer–autumn	Nonspecific	Children and young adults; culture throat and stool
Coxsackie virus	Summer–autumn	Petechial rash, pleurodynia, herpangina, myopericarditis, conjunctivitis	Children and young adults; culture throat and stool
Echovirus	Summer–autumn	Dermatomyositis	Children and young adults; culture throat and stool
Arboviruses	Spring, autumn (vector dependent)	Encephalitis prominent	Serology and local epidemiology important for diagnosis
Herpes simplex virus	No seasonal pattern	May accompany primary genital herpes	CSF glucose may be low; CSF PCR positive
Cytomegalovirus	No seasonal pattern	Very rare complication of CMV infection	
Epstein–Barr virus	No seasonal pattern	Complication of mononucleosis	
Mumps	Spring	Orchitis, oophoritis, pancreatitis	Children and young adults; CSF glucose may be low
Lymphocytic choriomeningitis	Autumn–winter	Exposure to rodents; alopecia, orchitis, arthritis, myopericarditis	CSF glucose may be low; CSF pleocytosis may be >1000/mm^3
HIV	No seasonal pattern	Mononucleosis-like syndrome	Check serology; if negative, recheck in 3 months
Syphilis	No seasonal pattern	During acute infection and in neurosyphillis	CSF serology
Lyme disease	Summer–autumn	History of tick bite or erythema migrans	Check blood serology
Leptospirosis	Summer–autumn	Biphasic illness after rodent or water exposure	First phase – check blood and CSF cultures; second phase – check urine cultures and serology

Fig. 15.3 Characteristic features of aseptic meningitis by etiology.

outbreaks typically occur in populations of young adults living in close quarters, such as dormitories of military camps or schools. Major epidemics, which dramatically increase the incidence of the disease, have occurred periodically in certain parts of the world, including sub-Saharan Africa (the so-called 'meningitis belt'), Europe (particularly Scandinavia), Asia and South America. During these epidemics, attack rates can reach several hundred per 100,000 people, with devastating consequences, particularly in areas with limited medical resources.[6]

Special clinical circumstances affect the spectrum of bacterial pathogens likely to cause meningitis in a particular patient. Age is the single most important determinant in this regard (see Fig. 15.2). Other important factors include various forms of immunosuppression, surgery, trauma and focal suppurative infections of the head (see Fig. 15.2).[7–9]

Aseptic meningitis

In the USA, aseptic meningitis has an incidence similar to that of bacterial meningitis, up to 10 cases per 100,000 people per year. A recent report noted 8,000–13,000 cases of aseptic meningitis over a 7-year period in the USA.[2] The true incidence rate is likely to be higher because aseptic meningitis often is not reported. The disease preferentially affects children and young adults. Children are exposed to enteroviruses in day-care centers and at school, where many of the people looking after them are young adults, the population most frequently infected with enteroviruses. Other populations at risk are those prone to acquire sexually transmitted diseases, including HIV, herpes simplex and syphilis, and those exposed to mosquitoes (which transmit arboviruses), ticks (Lyme disease, Colorado tick fever), or animals or animal products (lymphocytic choriomeningitis, *Brucella*). There is marked seasonal variation in the incidence of the disease, with rates in the summer to autumn months that are often four to seven times the rates observed in winter (see Fig. 15.3). This is a direct reflection of the seasonal variation in the acquisition of the systemic enteroviral infections that can lead to aseptic meningitis – enteroviruses are most common in the summer and early autumn, and arboviruses infections typically occur in the summer when the insect vectors are most prevalent.

PATHOGENS AND CLINICAL FEATURES OF CHRONIC MENINGITIS

Pathogen		Predominant type of CSF pleocytosis	Predisposition and risk factors	Associated clinical manifestations
Bacteria	*Actinomyces* spp.	Neutrophils	Mouth and ear lesions	CNS lesions, endophthalmitis
	Borrelia burgdorferi (Lyme disease)	Lymphocytes	Tick bite	Cranial nerve palsy (VII nerve)
	Brucella spp.	Lymphocytes, neutrophils	Unpasteurized dairy products	Undulant fever, hepatomegaly
	Leptospira spp.	Neutrophils	Exposure to urine of infected animals	Hepatomegaly, hepatitis, thrombocytopenia
	Mycobacterium tuberculosis	Neutrophils, monocytes, lymphocytes	Immunodeficiency, high endemic prevalence	Cranial nerve palsy (VI nerve)
	Nocardia spp.	Neutrophils	Immunodeficiency	Abscesses
	Treponema pallidum	Eosinophils, lymphocytes	Sexually transmitted diseases	Cranial nerve palsy (VII and VIII nerves)
Viruses	Cytomegalovirus	Lymphocytes; neutrophils (in HIV)	Immunodeficiency	Fever, retinitis
	Echovirus	Lymphocytes	Agammaglobulinemia	Dermatomyositis
	Lymphocytic choriomeningitis virus	Lymphocytes	Exposure to rodents	Orchitis, leukocytopenia, thrombocytopenia
	Mumps virus	Neutrophils	No vaccination	Parotitis, orchitis, oophoritis
	HIV	Lymphocytes	HIV risk factors	Mononucleosis-like illness
Fungi	*Aspergillus* spp.	Lymphocytes or neutrophils	Immunodeficiency, surgery	Lung involvement
	Candida spp.	Neutrophils	Antibiotics, surgery, immunodeficiency	Disseminated disease
	Coccidioides spp.	Lymphocytes	Endemic areas	Lung involvement
	Cryptococcus spp.	Lymphocytes	Immunodeficiency	Encephalitis, headache
	Histoplasma spp.	Lymphocytes	Endemic areas, immunodeficiency	Fever, oral lesions, hepatosplenomegaly
	Pseudallerescheria spp.	Neutrophils	Immunodeficiency	Skin lesions, endophthalmitis
	Sporothrix spp.	Neutrophils	Immunodeficiency	Skin lesions, endophthalmitis
Parasites	*Taenia solium*	Eosinophils	Endemic areas	Elevated intracranial pressure, calcified lesions on head imaging
	Angiostrongylus spp.	Eosinophils	Raw sea food	Fever

Fig. 15.4 Pathogens and clinical features of chronic meningitis.

Chronic meningitis

The epidemiology of chronic meningitis is quite varied, being determined by the specific etiologic agent (see Fig. 15.4).[5] Meningitis caused by *M. tuberculosis* predominantly affects young children and the elderly, with an increased incidence in developing countries and in patients with low socioeconomic status or HIV infection.[10,11] Some causes of chronic meningitis have defined geographic distributions, such as coccidioidomycosis, histoplasmosis, blastomycosis, paracoccidioidomycosis, Lyme disease, cysticercosis, angiostrongyloidiasis and sarcoidosis. Those exposed to animals and animal products are at risk of brucellosis and other zoonoses. Areas with high rates of HIV infection also have higher incidences of chronic meningitis associated with AIDS; the specific etiologies may also be influenced by the geographic location (for example, cryptococcosis, coccidioidomycosis, histoplasmosis and tuberculosis).

AGENTS OF MENINGITIS
Acute bacterial meningitis

Gram-positive pathogens. *Streptococcus pneumoniae*, an encapsulated Gram-positive diplococcus, causes a severe form of bacterial meningitis that often leaves neurologic sequelae in survivors and is fatal in up to 30% of patients. The organism can affect all age groups and causes the most severe disease in the very young and the very old. There are at least 84 serotypes identified among pneumococcal isolates, but a few serotypes predominate as the causes of meningitis. Different serotypes cause invasive disease in children (14, 6, 18, 19, 23, 4, 9) than in adults (1, 3, 4, 7, 8, 9, 12, 14).[12,13] Group B streptococci (*Streptococcus agalactiae*) is a pathogen of the neonatal period, and it often causes a devastating sepsis and meningitis. It colonizes the birth canal of women, from where it is

transmitted to the child. The colonized newborn can develop group B streptococcal disease of early onset (developing at less than 7 days of age; median 1 day) or late onset (developing later than 7 days of age). Early onset disease presents as a sepsis-like disease with a very high mortality; late onset disease presents primarily as meningitis.[14,15]

Listeria monocytogenes is a Gram-positive rod that causes meningitis in neonates, in adults with underlying conditions such as alcoholism and long-term treatment with corticosteroids, and in pregnant women. There is often an encephalitic component to presentation, with early mental status alterations, neurologic deficits and seizures.[16]

Staphylococci rarely cause meningitis except in the setting of intraventricular shunts, or as a consequence of staphylococcal bacteremia in patients with endocarditis, intravascular devices, or suppurative foci.[17] Streptococci (other than *S. pneumoniae*), enterococci and Gram-positive anaerobes are rare causes of bacterial meningitis.

Gram-negative pathogens. *Haemophilus influenzae* is a Gram-negative coccobacillus that is serotyped based on its capsule. Of the six encapsulated serotypes (a–f), type b causes almost all cases of invasive disease, including meningitis. *Haemophilus influenzae* meningitis is a disease of young children.[18] *Neisseria meningitidis*, a Gram-negative diplococcus, is mainly responsible for bacterial meningitis in young adults; it causes both sporadic cases and epidemics. The organism is transmitted from person to person by droplets, a form of transmission that is favored by crowded conditions.[19,20] Enterobacteriaceae (e.g. *Escherichia coli*, *Klebsiella* spp. and *Serratia* spp.) cause meningitis in neonates and in patients undergoing neurosurgical procedures. *Pseudomonas aeruginosa* can cause meningitis in neutropenic patients and in patients after neurosurgery.[21]

Acute aseptic meningitis

Viruses. Viruses are the most common cause of aseptic meningitis (see Fig. 15.3).[22,23] Enteroviruses account for more than 80% of cases of aseptic meningitis in which the cause is identified. Enteroviruses that cause meningitis include Coxsackie viruses A and B, echovirus and poliovirus. Enteroviruses are transmitted by the fecal–oral route and are spread through close contact in households and day-care centers. Affected groups include infants, young children and those looking after them. Infections are more frequent in the late summer and early autumn, but they can occur at any time of year, especially in tropical climates.

Mumps, a paramyxovirus, is spread by respiratory droplets and is usually seen in the late winter and early spring. Neurologic complications range from encephalitis to meningitis. Young children are most commonly affected, and boys are more often affected than girls by a ratio of between 2:1 and 5:1. Mumps meningitis follows mumps parotitis, and there is often no salivary gland involvement at the time of presentation of aseptic meningitis.[24]

Lymphochoriomeningitis virus is an arenavirus that is spread by contact with rodent urine or feces. The disease was most prevalent in young adults and in impoverished populations, but lymphochoriomeningitis virus has become a rare cause of meningitis. Patients present with the typical symptoms of acute meningitis. After an initial improvement, some patients relapse into a second phase of meningitis, which is believed to be immune-mediated.[25]

Patients infected with arboviruses (St Louis encephalitis virus, Western equine encephalitis virus, California encephalitis virus and Eastern equine encephalitis virus) usually present with symptoms of encephalitis rather than meningitis. However, a minority of patients have meningitis, with a paucity of symptoms suggestive of encephalitis.

Many of the herpesviruses cause neurologic complications, including aseptic meningitis. Primary genital herpes caused by herpes simplex virus type 2 is the most common cause. By recent estimates, one-third of women and one-eighth of men have aseptic meningitis associated with their primary herpetic infection. Aseptic meningitis is much less likely to complicate recurrent outbreaks of herpes. Herpes aseptic meningitis is a benign and self-limited illness that must be distinguished from herpes encephalitis, which is a serious illness that often has devastating neurologic consequences and often causes death.[26]

Varicella-zoster virus, cytomegalovirus, and Epstein–Barr virus can also cause aseptic meningitis. More recently, HIV-1 has been identified as a cause of aseptic meningitis. Seroconversion of HIV-1 often causes a mononucleosis-like illness with fever, malaise, rash, myalgias and arthralgias, and this is sometimes associated with aseptic meningitis.[27] Other less important viral etiologies of aseptic meningitis include adenovirus, measles, and rubella.

Bacteria. Some bacterial infections can cause an aseptic meningitis syndrome.[28] Patients with bacterial meningitis who have been partially treated with antibiotics may have symptoms of meningitis with a CSF profile very similar to that of aseptic viral meningitis. Parameningeal bacterial foci following infections can be associated with culture-negative meningitis, usually with a predominantly granulocytic CSF pleocytosis. Symptoms of meningitis are generally mild or absent. Bacterial endocarditis can cause a cerebritis, which is characterized by vasculitis of the small cerebral vessels; it can also be associated with aseptic meningitis. Spirochetes commonly cause brain infections with meningeal inflammation and a CSF profile similar to that of viral meningitis. Secondary syphilis rarely (in about 1% of all cases) causes acute, aseptic meningitis that can be associated with hydrocephalus, cranial nerve palsies and encephalitic changes. Aseptic meningitis is also a manifestation of early Lyme disease and is frequently associated with cranial and peripheral neuropathies.[29] Both the early and second phase of leptospirosis can cause an aseptic meningitis.[30] The CSF shows a moderate lymphocytic pleocytosis and is sterile. The meningitis resolves without specific therapy over the course of a few weeks. Rickettsiae, including *Coxiella burnetii* and *Ehrlichia* spp., can cause an aseptic meningitis with lymphocytic pleocytosis and elevated protein concentrations as part of the meningoencephalitis that characterizes infections by these intracellular pathogens.

Amebae. Naegleria fowleri, and rarely *Acanthamoeba* spp., can cause an acute meningoencephalitis that occurs most commonly in children and young adults and resembles bacterial meningitis with signs indicating severe brain involvement. The organism is acquired by swimming in fresh water. The CSF shows a polymorphonuclear pleocytosis with increased protein and decreased glucose concentrations, many erythrocytes and a negative Gram stain. A fresh, warm sample of CSF should be examined microscopically for evidence of motile amebae. The disease is fatal in more than 95% of cases.[31]

Noninfectious causes. Neurosurgery involving the posterior fossa can result in aseptic meningitis ('posterior fossa syndrome'). Signs of meningitis appear rapidly, but patients often do not look very ill. The CSF has a polymorphonuclear pleocytosis with elevated protein and low glucose mimicking bacterial meningitis, but cultures remain negative. The syndrome is diagnosed after excluding infectious causes (particularly bacteria) and is treated by high doses of glucocorticoids for several days.

Other noninfectious diseases causing aseptic meningitis include carcinomatous meningitis, sarcoidosis, systemic lupus erythematosus and Behçet's disease. Many drugs have been linked to aseptic meningitis, most importantly trimethoprim–sulfamethoxazole (co-trimoxazole), nonsteroidal anti-inflammatory drugs and OKT3, an antibody directed against T lymphocytes.[32] Mollaret's meningitis is a recurrent lymphocytic meningitis, usually seen in young women. The cause is unknown but is thought by some to be related to herpes simplex virus. The episodes are benign and self-limiting, the prognosis is good.

Chronic meningitis

Bacterial. Worldwide, tuberculous meningitis, which results from the rupture of a tubercle into the adjacent subarachnoid space, is the most important cause of chronic meningitis. The presentation is typical for chronic meningitis – slowly progressive headache and signs of meningeal irritation, followed by cranial nerve involvement, other neurologic deficits and progressive mental status changes over a period of weeks. Tuberculous meningitis may be a consequence either of primary infection or of reactivation of disease. The diagnosis can be confirmed by a positive CSF culture; however, *M. tuberculosis* is recovered from the CSF in only 38–88% of cases. A moderate lymphocytic pleocytosis is most common. The glucose can be very low; the protein is often very high. Cerebrospinal fluid smears for acid-fast bacilli are positive only in a minority of cases (10–20%). Skin tests for delayed hypersensitivity to tuberculin are frequently negative in tuberculous meningitis, whether resulting from primary infection or reactivated disease.[11]

Chronic meningitis is an unusual complication of brucellosis. Symptoms of *Brucella* meningitis tend to progress over an extended period of months to years. The diagnosis should be entertained when there is a history of exposure to farm animals, consumption of undercooked meats or unpasteurized dairy products from endemic areas.[33]

Secondary syphilis may cause chronic meningitis. The disease is slowly progressive, and generally symptoms have been present for more than 1 month before presentation. Cranial nerve palsies are common; the facial and acoustic nerves are the most frequently affected. Diagnosis is based on a positive Venereal Disease Research Laboratory test in CSF.[34]

The diagnosis of meningitis associated with Lyme disease, caused by *Borrelia burgdorferi*, should be considered in patients who live or have traveled through endemic regions, particularly those with a history of a tick bite or erythema chronicum migrans. Meningitis may persist for weeks and may be associated with cranial nerve palsies and peripheral neuropathies.[29] Syphilis, other spirochetal diseases and collagen vascular diseases may result in a false positive Lyme serology.

Fungi. Chronic meningitis caused by *Cryptococcus neoformans*, an encapsulated, ubiquitous fungus, has presentations ranging from a subacute meningoencephalitis to fever of unknown origin. Patients at highest risk are those with defects in cellular immunity such as occurs in AIDS, hematologic malignancies and prolonged use of high dose corticosteroids, even though a significant number of patients with cryptococcal meningitis in the pre-AIDS era had no identifiable immune defect. The CSF shows a moderate lymphocytic pleocytosis, but in patients with AIDS, inflammation may be virtually absent. Cryptococcal antigen latex agglutination is positive in more than 90% of cases, whereas microscopy of India ink preparations to visualize the yeast in CSF is less sensitive.[35]

Coccidioides immitis grows in the dry sandy soils of the southwest USA, and Central and South America. Acute infection is acquired by inhalation of the spores, and meningitis develops within a few months later. There are few distinguishing features of the disease; some patients with generalized disease have erythema nodosum; hydrocephalus is a common complication. Cerebrospinal fluid eosinophilia in patients who have lived or traveled though endemic regions should alert the clinician to the possibility of *Coccidioides* meningitis. Complement-fixing antibodies are present in the CSF in 75–95% of cases, and CSF cultures are positive in more than 50%.

Histoplasma meningitis is a rare complication of histoplasmosis. The diagnosis should be entertained in patients who live or have traveled through endemic regions – the Ohio River Valley of the USA, the Caribbean, and South America. Cerebrospinal fluid cultures are positive in 27–65% of cases. Blood cultures should be done and a buffy coat of the blood should be examined for the presence of the fungus.[36] *Histoplasma* polysaccharide antigen is found in the urine, blood, or CSF in 61% of patients and in an even higher proportion of patients with AIDS.

Candida meningitis is rare and is most commonly a result of disseminated infection or placement of a ventricular shunt. Risk factors for candidemia are the prolonged use of antibiotics or corticosteroids, hyperalimentation, abdominal surgery, intravenous drug use and intravenous catheterization. Neonates are particularly prone to disseminated infection. Cerebrospinal fluid cultures are diagnostic.

Parasites. Neurocysticercosis is endemic in Mexico, South America and Asia. Infection is acquired by eating food contaminated with eggs of *Taenia solium*. Seizures are the most common manifestation. Intraventricular and basilar cysts (racemose cysticercosis) may present with signs of obstructive hydrocephalus. The CSF has a lymphocytic pleocytosis with eosinophils. Computed tomography scans of the head show multiple calcified lesions. Serology of blood and CSF may provide support for the diagnosis.[37]

Angiostrongylus cantonensis, the rat lung worm, is most prevalent in Asia and the Pacific Islands and is acquired by the ingestion of raw or inadequately cooked shellfish or snails. Symptoms are typical of chronic meningitis, and rash with pruritus is also common. Infection results in peripheral eosinophilia and chronic eosinophilic meningitis, which resolves spontaneously within 2 months. There is no effective therapy.[38]

Other less common causes of infectious chronic meningitis are organisms that usually cause abscesses but that may leak into the subarachnoid space to cause chronic meningitis. These conditions include blastomycosis, paracoccidioidomycosis, phaeohyphomycoses, mucor, actinomycosis, nocardiosis and toxoplasmosis. Less common fungi causing this syndrome include *Sporothrix schenckii*, chromoblastomycoses and *Aspergillus* spp.

Noninfectious causes. Meningeal carcinomatosis may cause a chronic meningitis that is difficult to distinguish from infectious causes. Neurosarcoidosis is an uncommon complication of sarcoidosis. Basilar inflammation is a prominent feature, resulting in cranial nerve palsies. The CSF shows a lymphocytic pleocytosis and usually a normal glucose. Less common noninfectious causes include granulomatous angiitis, Behçet's disease and Vogt–Koyanagi–Harada syndrome.

PATHOGENESIS AND PATHOLOGY

PATHOGENESIS

The pathogenesis of meningitis is best known from studies on bacterial meningitis, where the role of mucosal colonization, bloodstream invasion, CNS colonization and multiplication within the CSF have been elucidated in experimental systems (Fig. 15.5).

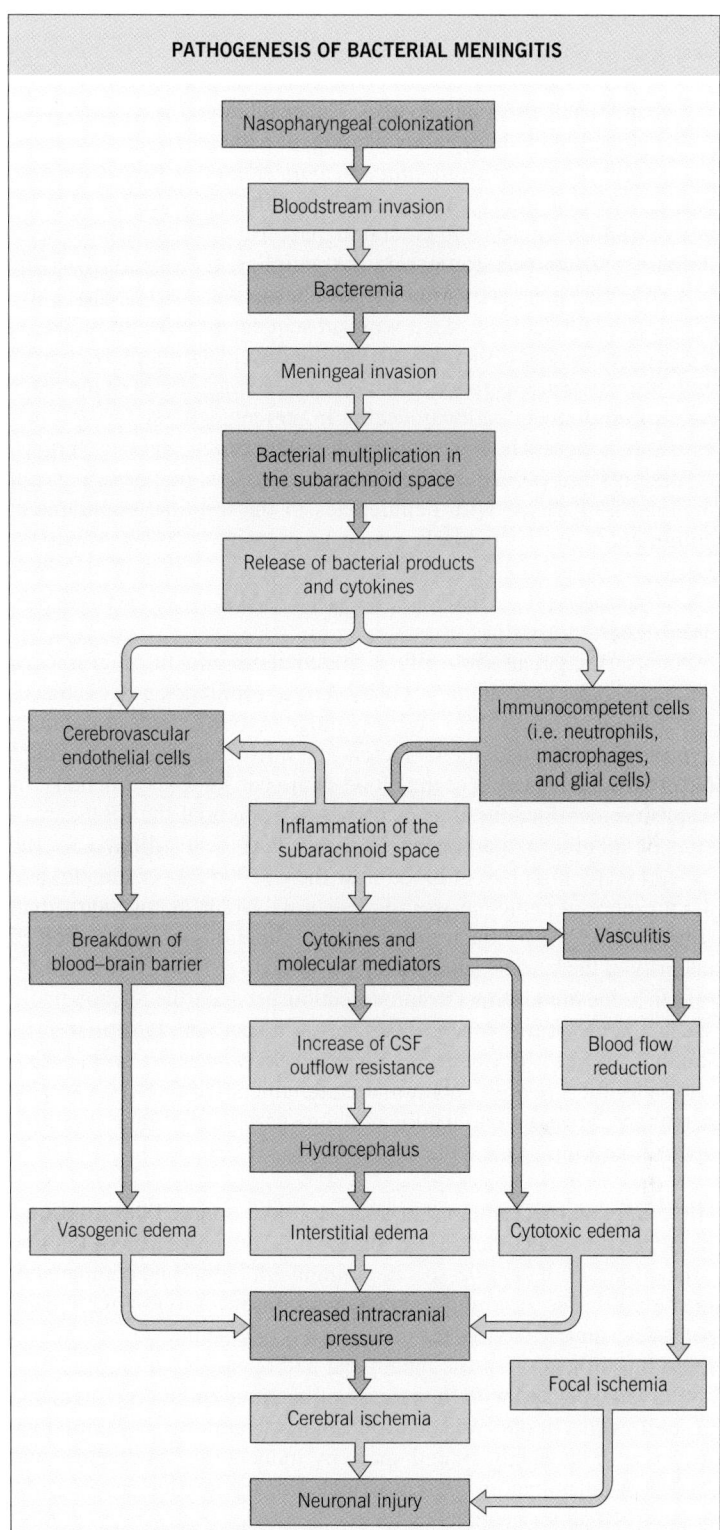

PATHOGENESIS OF BACTERIAL MENINGITIS

Nasopharyngeal colonization → Bloodstream invasion → Bacteremia → Meningeal invasion → Bacterial multiplication in the subarachnoid space → Release of bacterial products and cytokines → Cerebrovascular endothelial cells; Immunocompetent cells (i.e. neutrophils, macrophages, and glial cells) → Inflammation of the subarachnoid space → Breakdown of blood–brain barrier; Cytokines and molecular mediators; Vasculitis → Increase of CSF outflow resistance; Blood flow reduction → Hydrocephalus → Vasogenic edema; Interstitial edema; Cytotoxic edema → Increased intracranial pressure; Focal ischemia → Cerebral ischemia → Neuronal injury

Fig. 15.5 Pathogenesis of bacterial meningitis. These events lead to CSF infection, subsequent subarachnoid space inflammation, pathophysiologic changes and ultimately neuronal injury.

Nasopharyngeal colonization and invasion

Specific bacterial virulence factors for meningeal pathogens include specialized surface components (e.g. the polysaccharide capsule with specific epitopes and fimbriae or pili). These factors are crucial for adherence to the nasopharyngeal epithelium, the evasion of local host defense mechanisms and subsequent invasion of the bloodstream. Lack of specific antibodies correlates with an increased risk of invasive disease. Viral infection of the respiratory tract may also promote invasive disease. From the nasopharyngeal surface, encapsulated organisms cross the epithelial cell layer and invade the small subepithelial blood vessels.[39]

Intravascular survival

In the bloodstream, bacteria must survive host defenses, including circulating antibodies, complement-mediated bactericidal mechanisms and neutrophil phagocytosis. Encapsulation is a shared feature of the principal hematogenous meningeal pathogens (*H. influenzae*, *N. meningitidis*, *S. pneumoniae*, *E. coli* K1 and group B streptococci). The capsule is instrumental in inhibiting neutrophil phagocytosis and complement-mediated bactericidal activity. Several defense mechanisms counteract the antiphagocytic activity of the bacterial capsule. Activation of the alternative complement pathway results in cleavage of C3 with subsequent deposition of C3b on the bacterial surface, thereby facilitating opsonization, phagocytosis and intravascular clearance of the organism. Impairment of the alternative complement pathway occurs in patients with sickle-cell disease and in those who have undergone splenectomy, and these groups of patients are predisposed to the development of pneumococcal meningitis. Patients with deficiencies in the terminal complement components are particularly prone to invasive infections with *N. meningitidis*.[20,40]

Meningeal invasion

Studies on the pathogenesis of experimental bacterial meningitis show that cells in the choroid plexus and cerebral capillaries possess receptors for adherence of meningeal pathogens. For *E. coli*, a complex interplay between endothelial factors and microbial genes orchestrates the crossing by bacteria of the blood–brain barrier. Experimental evidence has identified the choroid plexus as a potential site for the invasion of meningeal pathogens, and this may be facilitated by the exceptionally high rate of blood flow there (200ml/g per minute) and the presence of pathogen-specific receptors. Nonhematogenous invasion of the CSF by bacteria occurs in situations of compromised integrity of the barriers surrounding the brain (e.g. in otitis media, mastoiditis, sinusitis). Direct communication between the subarachnoid space and the skin or mucosal surfaces as a result of malformation or trauma give rise to meningeal infection with bacterial species that vary with the site of the abnormal communication. Bacteria can also reach the CSF as a complication of neurosurgery, spinal anesthesia, or ventriculostomy placement.[20,40]

Host defense mechanisms in subarachnoid space inflammation

Pathogens reaching the CSF are likely to survive because of the low concentrations of capsule-specific immunoglobulins and complement in the CSF. The resulting deficiency in opsonization of meningeal pathogens greatly reduces the effectiveness of granulocytes and allows rapid multiplication of the meningeal pathogens. Bacterial multiplication is associated with the release of bacterial products (fragments of cell wall, lipopolysaccharide) that trigger the inflammatory response in the subarachnoid space by inducing the production and release of inflammatory cytokines (including the interleukins IL-1, IL-6 and IL-8, tumor necrosis factor-α, chemokines and others), upregulate adhesion molecules on brain vascular endothelial cells and promote the recruitment of granulocytes into the CSF. It is this granulocytic inflammation that appears to be primarily responsible for the complex pathophysiologic CNS alterations associated with bacterial meningitis.[41–43]

Blood–brain barrier

The blood–brain barrier separates the brain from the intravascular compartment and maintains homeostasis within the CNS. The permeability of the blood–brain barrier increases in meningitis; this increase occurs at the level of the choroid plexus epithelium and the cerebral microvascular endothelium. The increase in permeability results from separation of intercellular tight junctions and from increased pinocytosis. As a result, molecules in blood, including antibiotics, penetrate at increased rates into the CSF during meningitis, with an approximately five-fold increase for most antibiotics.[44,45]

Increased intracranial pressure

The major element leading to increased intracranial pressure in bacterial meningitis is the development of cerebral edema, which may be vasogenic, cytotoxic, or interstitial in origin. Vasogenic cerebral edema is primarily a consequence of increased blood–brain barrier permeability.

Cytotoxic edema results from an increase in intracellular water following alterations of the cell membrane and loss of cellular homeostasis. Cytotoxic mechanisms include ischemia and the effect of excitatory amino acids. Secretion of antidiuretic hormone also contributes to cytotoxic edema by making the extracellular fluid hypotonic and increasing the permeability of the brain to water.

Interstitial edema occurs by an increase in CSF volume, either through increased CSF production via increased blood flow in the choroid plexus, or decreased resorption secondary to increased CSF outflow resistance.[46,47]

Cerebral vasculitis and alterations in cerebral blood flow

Bacterial meningitis is associated with marked changes in cerebral blood flow. In the early phase of the disease, an increase in blood flow is observed, and this appears to be mediated by nitric oxide and oxidative radicals. In advanced meningitis, cerebral blood flow is reduced. Several clinical studies have found an association between severe cerebral blood flow reduction and adverse outcomes both in children and adults with meningitis, suggesting that ischemia is an important mediator of brain damage in meningitis. Cerebral blood flow reduction during meningitis can be global, as a result of reduced cerebral perfusion pressure (resulting from increased intracranial pressure or systemic hypotension, or both), or focal, as a result of vascular involvement of cerebral arteries and veins by the subarachnoid space inflammation (Figs 15.6 & 15.7).[48–50]

Neuronal injury

The mechanisms of neuronal injury during meningitis have not been conclusively identified. Studies in experimental models of bacterial meningitis and inference from clinical studies point to ischemia as a critical factor leading to brain damage. Whether additional mechanisms of injury, for example direct neurotoxic effects of inflammatory mediators or products from granulocytes, also play a role has not been conclusively shown. Experimental evidence points to a role of excitatory

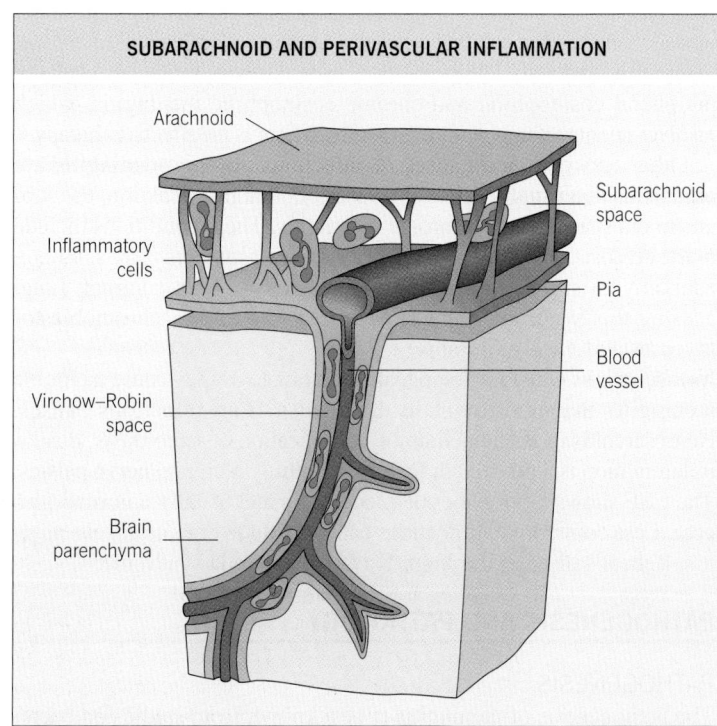

Fig. 15.6 Subarachnoid and perivascular inflammation in meningitis. The inflammation in the subarachnoid space extends into the Virchow–Robin spaces along the vasculature.

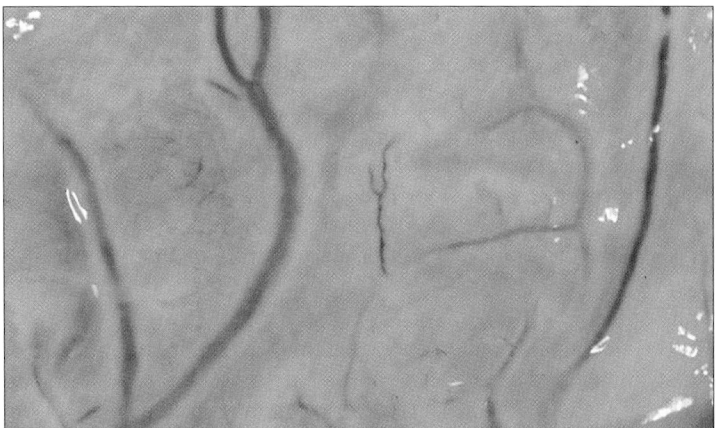

Fig. 15.7 Arachnoid membrane in purulent meningitis. Close-up view of the arachnoid membrane covering the purulent subarachnoid space, with penetrating blood vessels exhibiting inflammatory vasculitis and thrombosis. Courtesy of Dr M Tolnay, University of Basel, Switzerland.

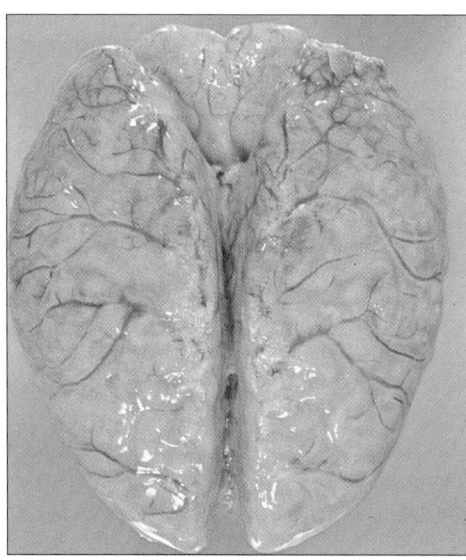

Fig. 15.8 Brain with inflammatory exudate covering the cortical hemispheres in purulent meningitis. Courtesy of Dr M Tolnay, University of Basel, Switzerland.

amino acids in causing neuronal damage. Reactive oxygen intermediates and nitric oxide also appear important in experimental models, both as agents of neuronal injury and as regulators of cerebral blood flow. The role of these molecules in humans has not been evaluated.[42,49,51]

PATHOLOGY

Important pathologic findings in patients with meningitis include:
- subarachnoid space inflammation;
- inflammatory involvement of the cerebral vasculature; and
- parenchymal brain damage.

The subarachnoid space inflammation appears as a grayish yellow-to-green exudate covering the base and convexities of the brain (Figs 15.7 & 15.8). The exudate consists predominantly of granulocytes in acute bacterial meningitis, and of a mixture of lymphocytes, macrophages and granulocytes in subacute and chronic forms of meningitis. On the surface of the brain, the involvement of the vasculature is often macroscopically obvious (see Fig. 15.7). Histologic examination shows infiltration of vessel walls by inflammatory cells with consecutive thrombosis of the vessel lumen (Fig. 15.9). Vascular involvement is most prominent in acute bacterial meningitis, but it is also seen in chronic meningitis, especially tuberculous.

Inflammation also involves the inner ear, to which it gains access via the cochlear aqueduct connecting the subarachnoid space with the endolymphatic space. Toxic effects of the inflammation on hair cells of the inner ear appear to be responsible for the hearing impairment associated with bacterial meningitis (Fig. 15.10).

Damage to the brain parenchyma is evidenced by the presence of brain edema (including signs of cerebral herniation), by areas of cerebral infarction resulting from ischemia and by histologic changes. The histologic changes include loss of neurons, most prominently in patients who survive acute bacterial meningitis for several days before succumbing to the disease. This loss of neurons is associated with a marked reaction of astrocytes and microglia. The extent and localization of neuronal loss probably determines the type of neurologic sequelae resulting from meningitis (see Fig. 15.10).[40,52]

PREVENTION

The most effective prevention for bacterial meningitis is provided by vaccination. This has been most impressively documented with *H. influenzae* type b, where the new conjugated vaccines have led to a reduction of more than 90% in the number of cases in vaccinated populations.[18,53] Current recommendations are to vaccinate all children against *H. influenzae* type b with one of several available vaccines, beginning at 3 months of age. Unfortunately, this is not possible in many countries, for economic reasons.

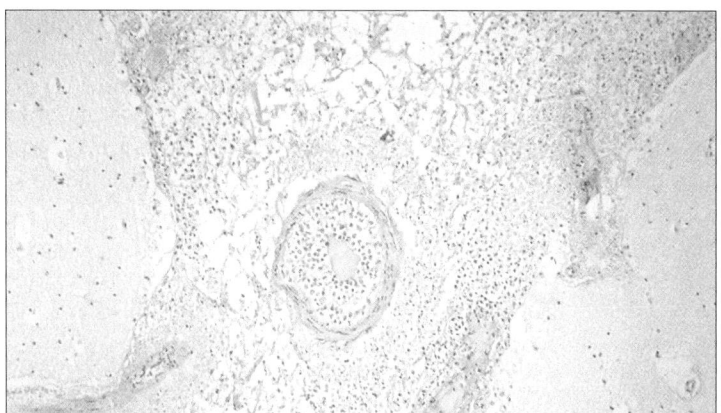

Fig. 15.9 Histopathology of the subarachnoid space in meningitis. Note the inflammatory involvement of the blood vessels and the small vessel leading into the brain parenchyma sourrounded by inflammation in the Virchow–Robin space. Courtesy of Dr M Tolnay, University of Basel, Switzerland.

The efficacy of currently available pneumococcal vaccines in reducing pneumococcal meningitis has not been conclusively proven. Nevertheless, the vaccine should be offered to people at increased risk of invasive pneumococcal disease, such as the elderly, those with underlying diseases and immunocompromising conditions, asplenic patients, patients with sickle cell disease and those with anatomic defects that predispose to meningitis.[54,55]

In the case of meningococcal meningitis, vaccines are available for all major serotypes except type B, which has a poorly immunogenic polysaccharide capsule. For the other types, vaccination is effective in the setting of ongoing epidemics, but is not routinely performed except in epidemic conditions.[56]

Prevention of neonatal meningitis is a focus of intense efforts. Prophylactic antibiotic treatment of women known to be colonized with group B streptococci, of their newborn children after birth, or of both have been attempted. Most promising appears to be an approach in which women who are colonized with group B streptococci and who have risk factors for neonatal infection (prematurity, prolonged rupture of the membranes, signs of infection during labor) are treated with a short course of ampicillin prior to delivery.[14] Vaccine development against group B streptococci has not reached the clinical stage, but conjugated vaccines similar to those developed for *H. influenzae* type b are promising.

Antibiotics are widely used for the prevention of meningitis associated with neurosurgery and the placement of intraventricular shunts. In patients undergoing craniotomy, perioperative antibiotic prophylaxis appears to reduce the number of postoperative infections. Whether antibiotic prophylaxis during implantation of a ventricular shunt is effective in preventing subsequent shunt infections is not well established, but a recent meta-analysis suggested some benefit. The use of antibiotics for prophylaxis should be limited to 24 hours.[57]

CLINICAL FEATURES

BACTERIAL MENINGITIS

Meningitis is the most likely diagnosis in patients who present with the classical triad of fever, headache and a stiff neck, which is present in at least 80% of patients. Other signs and symptoms occur less frequently (Fig. 15.11), and patients complaining of headache or presenting with altered mental status must be carefully examined for evidence of meningeal irritation (i.e. meningism, with Kernig's sign, Brudzinski's sign, or both). Bacterial meningitis can be present in patients in whom the clinical diagnosis is not obvious. This is particularly true in small children and in the elderly. In children under 2 years of age, signs of meningeal inflammation are frequently absent, and the most common clinical presentations include fever and altered mental status (irritability, lethargy), which are present in over 90% of patients. Similarly, in elderly patients, fever may be minimal, and mental status changes may be the most obvious symptom. In patients with suspected meningitis, a careful skin examination for the characteristic purpuric or petechial skin rash of *N. meningitidis* should be performed (Fig. 15.12). Other clues derived from the history and physical examination may help in the differential diagnosis of meningitis (Fig. 15.13).

COMMON NEUROLOGIC SEQUELAE OF BACTERIAL MENINGITIS	
Deficit	Approximate frequency (%)
Hearing loss	15–30
Parenchymal damage	5–30
Cerebral palsy	5–10
Learning disabilities	5–20
Seizure disorder	<5
Cortical blindness	<5
Cerebral herniation	3–20
Hydrocephalus	2–3

Fig. 15.10 Common neurologic sequelae of bacterial meningitis.

Untreated bacterial meningitis is characterized by progressive loss of consciousness, commonly associated with other neurologic signs including seizures and focal deficits, leading to coma and death. The extent of mental status changes, with profound coma as the most extreme, provides a clinical indication of the severity of the disease. Patients presenting in coma have a very high mortality (up to 50%). Systemic complications of the infectious process include septic shock, disseminated intravascular coagulation (particularly with meningococcal infections), and acute respiratory distress syndrome.

ASEPTIC MENINGITIS

The clinical manifestations of aseptic meningitis are often indistinguishable from those of bacterial meningitis. Acute onset of fever, headache, photophobia, nausea with vomiting and meningism are most common. On the other hand, severe neurologic findings, including seizures, are very uncommon in most forms of aseptic meningitis. Overall, symptoms are generally milder than those of pyogenic meningitis. Most cases of aseptic meningitis are self-limiting and do not lead to sequelae even though constitutional symptoms can persist for several weeks. Depending on the causative pathogen, signs of meningeal inflammation may be associated with other clinical findings (see Fig. 15.3).

CHRONIC MENINGITIS

Symptoms and signs of chronic meningitis evolve over several days to weeks. Most prominently, patients complain of headaches, often associated with constitutional signs of infection (fever, anorexia). Nuchal rigidity may be subtle or absent in cases of chronic meningitis. Many forms of chronic meningitis involve the base of the brain and lead to cranial nerve palsies, often affecting eye movements and facial musculature. As the syndrome progresses, signs of brain involvement with seizures, mental status changes, confusion or hallucinations, and focal neurologic deficits develop. Hydrocephalus and increased intracranial pressure may also accompany the syndrome.

DIAGNOSIS

CEREBROSPINAL FLUID EXAMINATION

Examination of CSF is of paramount importance for the diagnosis of all forms of meningitis (Fig. 15.14). Accordingly, a lumbar puncture should be performed in patients with suspected meningitis once a mass lesion that may lead to cerebral herniation has been ruled out on clinical grounds or by CT scan of the head. Evidence for mass lesions consists of the combination of focal neurologic signs (focal seizures,

COMMON SIGNS AND SYMPTOMS IN ACUTE MENINGITIS AND ENCEPHALITIS			
Meningitis	Adult	Headache	Kernig's sign
		Fever	Brudzinski's sign
		Neck and back pain	Photophobia
		Meningism	Lethargy or coma
		Nausea and vomiting	Seizures
	Infant	Fever	Bulging fontanelles
		Irritability	Convulsions
		Lethargy	Ophisthotonus
		Refusal to feed	Seizures
		Strange cry	
Encephalitis		Fever	Stupor or coma
		Vomiting	Seizures
		Psychiatric alteration	Electroencephalographic changes
		Focal neurologic deficits	

Fig. 15.11 Common signs and symptoms in acute meningitis and encephalitis.

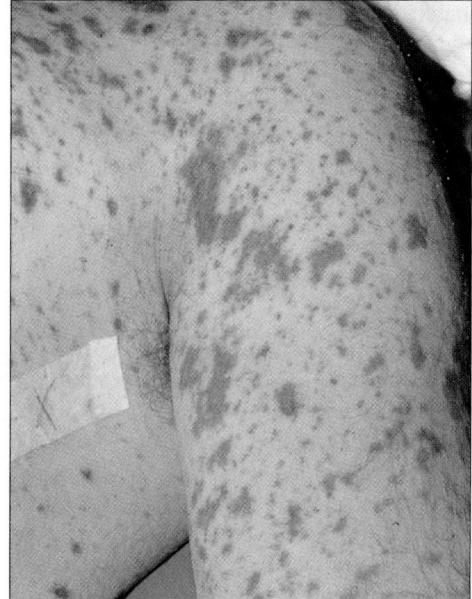

Fig. 15.12 Skin lesions in acute meningococcemia. Characteristic purpura with petechiae and ecchymoses in a patient with fulminant sepsis and meningitis due to *Neisseria meningitidis*. Courtesy of Professor W Zimmerli, University of Basel, Switzerland.

sensorimotor and visual defects) and clinical evidence of increased intracranial pressure (headache, vomiting, impaired mental status, papilledema). In patients without such a combination of signs indicating possible mass lesion, imaging studies prior to lumbar puncture are not necessary. While performing the lumbar puncture, CSF pressure should be recorded.

Immediate examination of the CSF provides valuable information. A Gram stain of uncentrifuged CSF (if the CSF is turbid) or centrifuged CSF (if it is not) indicates the presence of white blood cells, their approximate differential count (mononuclear versus polymorphonuclear) and whether bacteria are present.

Cultures for bacteria and fungi should always be performed, even in patients already treated with antibiotics. Tests for the detection of bacterial antigens by immunologic methods, such as latex particle agglutination, have sensitivities in the range of the Gram stain or culture and are of doubtful utility when used routinely, but they can sometimes identify organisms in patients with partially treated bacterial meningitis and negative Gram stain and culture.

Cerebrospinal fluid concentrations of protein, glucose and lactate, in addition to number and type of white blood cells, are helpful in the differential diagnosis of various forms of meningitis (see Fig. 15.14).[58]

In addition to the routine tests performed on all CSF samples, specific tests may be indicated under special circumstances. Viral cultures are mostly negative in CSF from patients with aseptic meningitis, and they should not be performed routinely. However, nucleic acid detection by polymerase chain reaction and related tests is highly sensitive for detection of selected pathogens, particularly herpes viruses such as herpes simplex virus and cytomegalovirus. Serologic tests in CSF can establish the etiology of cases of chronic meningitis (syphilis, coccidioidomycosis). Isolation of enteroviruses should be attempted from throat washes or stool, because after the first 3 days of symptoms enteroviruses are recovered only from these sites.

SYSTEMIC PARAMETERS

Signs of inflammation are most pronounced in acute bacterial meningitis, and in some cases of chronic meningitis (e.g. tuberculosis, fungal meningitis). In bacterial meningitis, differential blood count will frequently show a leukocytosis with a left shift. Erythrocyte sedimentation rate and other acute phase reactants are typically elevated.

Blood cultures should be performed in all patients with suspected meningitis prior to initiation of antibiotic therapy. They yield the infecting organism in more than 60% of cases of acute bacterial meningitis, should be sterile in aseptic meningitis, and rarely can reveal the organism in chronic meningitis (*Brucellosis* spp., *Nocardia* spp., fungi).

Patients with acute meningitis should be examined for evidence of electrolyte imbalance. Hyponatremia is common and may indicate dehydration (in which case the urine sodium concentration is low) or the syndrome of inappropriate antidiuretic hormone (SIADH); in which case the urine sodium concentration is high, an assessment that is important for correct choice of fluid substitution, particularly in children with acute meningitis.

Evidence for disseminated intravascular coagulation is most commonly seen in patients with meningococcal meningitis. Platelet count, prothrombin time, partial thromboplastin time, fibrinogen levels, and fibrin d-dimers should be measured in patients with suspected disseminated intravascular coagulation.

IMAGING STUDIES

In patients with bacterial meningitis, the possibility of focal infections of the head (sinusitis, otitis media) must be considered, and in selected cases, an appropriate radiologic test (e.g. a CT scan of the head) may be necessary. A CT scan of the head is also indicated in patients with suspected intracerebral mass lesions or parameningeal foci. Chest X-rays in patients with acute bacterial meningitis may reveal pneumonia, and in patients with chronic meningitis it may show evidence of pulmonary involvement by tubercle bacilli or fungi.

CLUES FROM THE HISTORY AND PHYSICAL EXAMINATION IN THE DIFFERENTIAL DIAGNOSIS OF MENINGITIS	
Clinical feature	Likely organism
Purpura, petechiae	*Neisseria meningitidis*
Cellulitis of the face	*Staphylococcus aureus, Haemophilus influenzae*
Otitis media, sinusitis, mastoiditis	*Streptococcus pneumoniae, Haemophilus influenzae*
Cerebrospinal fluid fistula	*Streptococcus pneumoniae*
Parotitis	Mumps
Endocarditis (peripheral stigmata, murmur)	*Staphylococcus aureus*
Pericarditis	*Neisseria meningitidis, Streptococcus pneumoniae*
Pneumonia	*Streptococcus pneumoniae, Haemophilus influenzae*
Spondylodiscitis	*Staphylococcus aureus, Mycobacterium tuberculosis*
Septic arthritis	*Staphylococcus aureus, Streptococcus pneumoniae*
Focal signs	*Listeria monocytogenes,* brain abscess, encephalitis
Alcoholism, liver cirrhosis	*Listeria monocytogenes, Streptococcus pneumoniae*
Pregnancy	*Listeria monocytogenes*
Neurosurgery	Staphylococci, Enterobacteriaceae, *Pseudomonas aeruginosa*
Kidney, heart transplantation	*Listeria monocytogenes, Cryptococcus neoformans*
Neutropenia	Gram-negative rods, fungi
HIV infection	*Cryptococcus neoformans, Nocardia* spp., *Listeria monocytogenes, Mycobacterium tuberculosis*

Fig. 15.13 Clues from the history and physical examination in the differential diagnosis of meningtis.

Fig. 15.14 Differential diagnosis of meningitis based on CSF findings.

DIFFERENTIAL DIAGNOSIS OF MENINGITIS BASED ON CSF FINDINGS						
Diagnosis	Pressure (cmH$_2$O)	White blood cells (x10^6/l)	Polymorpho-nucleocytes (%)	Glucose (ratio)	Protein (g/l)	Lactate (mmol/l)
Normal	<20	1–2	<1	>0.5	<0.45	<2
Acute bacterial meningitis	>20	>1000	>50	<0.4	>1	>4
Chronic meningitis	Variable	>1000	Variable	<0.4	>0.45	>2
Aseptic (viral) meningitis	<20	<1000	<50	>0.4	Variable	<2

MANAGEMENT

Treatment of meningitis includes two main goals:
- eradication of the infecting organism; and
- management of CNS and systemic complications.

Bacterial meningitis represents a medical emergency, particularly in patients with rapidly progressive disease and severely impaired CNS function. In these patients, we recommend initiation of empiric therapy without delay. One or two blood cultures should be obtained before administering the first antibiotic dose. We also administer adjunctive therapy with dexamethasone in these severely ill patients concomitantly with the first antibiotic dose (for more detail, see below). Once empiric therapy has been initiated, further diagnostic work-up is performed. Further therapy will depend on the CSF findings. In patients who are clinically stable and are unlikely to be adversely affected if antibiotics are not administered immediately, including those with suspected viral or chronic meningitis, a lumbar puncture represents the first step, unless there is clinical suspicion of a mass lesion. Findings in the CSF and on CT scan, if performed, will guide the further diagnostic work-up and therapy in all patients.

ANTIBIOTIC CHEMOTHERAPY
Empiric antibiotic therapy

Figure 15.15 summarizes empiric antibiotic regimens designed to cover the likely pathogens in different patient populations with suspected bacterial meningitis. Antibiotics should be administered intravenously by bolus infusion at the highest clinically validated doses, corrected for age and renal function. High doses are needed because only a small fraction of the serum concentration (between 3 and 15% for most beta-lactam antibiotics) penetrates into the CSF and because only antibiotic concentrations that exceed the MBC by a factor of 10–30 are rapidly bactericidal in the CSF.

Empiric therapy is primarily based on the age of the patient, with modifications if there are positive findings on CSF Gram stain or if the patient presents with special risk factors (see Fig. 15.2). It is safer to choose regimens with broad coverage, as they can usually be modified within 24–48 hours when antibiotic sensitivities of the infecting organism become available. An important factor in the choice of empiric antibiotic therapy is the emergence of organisms with increasing resistance to antibiotics. Most importantly, pneumococci that are relatively resistant to penicillin (MIC 0.1–1.0μg/ml) or highly resistant to penicillin (MIC >1.0μg/ml) are increasingly important in many parts of the world. Many of the penicillin-resistant organisms have reduced sensitivity to cephalosporins, and failure of these drugs in the treatment of pneumococcal meningitis caused by resistant organisms has occurred. Empiric therapy with dual antibiotic coverage effective against betalactam-resistant pneumococci may therefore be prudent, unless a patient is highly unlikely to have pneumococcal meningitis (e.g. a Gram stain indicates other etiology) or the local incidence of highly resistant pneumococci is very low. Patients at risk of infection with *L. monocytogenes* must be covered with ampicillin. In patients at risk of infections caused by difficult-to-treat Gram-negative bacilli with a high likelihood of resistance to many beta-lactam drugs, inclusion of an aminoglycoside in the empiric therapy regimen is recommended (Fig. 15.15).[8]

In patients with chronic meningitis, empiric antibiotic therapy should be directed at the suspected pathogen (Fig. 15.16). Often, a definite diagnosis is not available for several days, in which case empiric therapy may have to be initiated. It is important to cover the treatable causes of chronic meningitis, for which the outcome is poor if treatment is delayed. For example, empiric antituberculous therapy should be instituted promptly in cases of suspected tuberculous meningitis.

Definitive antibiotic therapy

Identification and sensitivity testing of the causative organism is followed by adjustment of antibiotic therapy to provide optimal but narrow coverage (Figs 15.16 & 15.17). Information on antibiotic

Patients and special modifying circumstances	Antibiotic	Dosage (intravenous)	
		Children	Adults
Neonate or infant under 3 months	Ampicillin plus cefotaxime or gentamicin	50–100mg/kg q6h 50mg q6–8h 2.5mg/kg q8h	
Neonate (pre-term, low birth weight)	Vancomycin plus ceftazidime	10mg/kg q12h 50mg/kg q12h	
3 months to 50 years	Ceftriaxone or cefotaxime	50mg/kg q12h 50mg/kg q6h	2–4g q24h 2g q4h
Over 50 years or impared cellular immunity	Ceftriaxone or cefotaxime plus ampicillin or penicillin G		2–4g q24h 2g q4h 2g q4h 3–4 million units q4h
Drug resistant *Streptococcus pneumoniae*	Ceftriaxone plus rifampin (rifampicin) or vancomycin	50mg/kg q12h 10–20mg/kg q24h 10–15 mg/kg q6h	2–4g q24h 600mg q24h 0.5g q6h
Neurosurgery, CSF shunt, or head trauma	Ceftazidime plus nafcillin (or vancomycin plus aminoglycoside)	50mg/kg q8h 50mg/kg q6h 10–15mg/kg q6h 2.5mg/kg q8h	2g q8h 2g q4h 0.5g q6h 1.5–2mg/kg q8h

Fig. 15.15 Recommendations for empiric antibiotic therapy of bacterial meningitis.

sensitivities is crucial in the case of the pneumococci (see above), *H. influenzae* and Gram-negative rods or staphylococci commonly causing bacterial meningitis in neurosurgical patients. Optimal duration of treatment of bacterial meningitis has not been carefully studied, but a total of 7 days appears adequate if the disease is caused by *H. influenzae* type b or *N. meningitidis*, although treatment should be extended to 10–14 days for the other common organisms, including pneumococci, and to 21 days for neonatal meningitis. Duration of treatment of chronic meningitis depends on the pathogen and can vary from days (syphilis) to months (tuberculosis, cryptococcosis) to indefinitely (coccidioidomycosis).

ADJUNCTIVE THERAPY

Several recent clinical trials have indicated that adjunctive therapy with dexamethasone improves the neurologic and audiologic outcome in bacterial meningitis. This has been shown primarily in children with *H. influenzae* meningitis; the data are more limited for children with pneumococcal and meningococcal meningitis, and only scant for adults with bacterial meningitis.[59–61] Experimental and clinical data suggest that the maximum benefit of dexamethasone is achieved when the drug is given either shortly before or at the same time as the first antibiotic dose. This is probably related to the fact that corticosteroids reduce the release of proinflammatory cytokines that are stimulated by bacterial products liberated from the pathogen by the bactericidal action of antibiotics.

Based on the available data, dexamethasone is recommended in all children over 6 weeks of age with bacterial meningitis, beginning if possible 10–15 minutes before the first antibiotic dose. The recommended dose is 0.15 mg/kg intravenously q6h, for a duration of 2–4 days. The role of dexamethasone for the newborn is presently unclear. Dexamethasone therapy should not be restricted to children with severe disease, because prevention of hearing loss has also been achieved in children with relatively mild disease.

In the absence of controlled data for adult patients, a conservative approach could consist of giving dexamethasone (in the same dose as in children) to patients who have clinical evidence of impaired CNS physiology with altered mental status, high CSF pressure, signs of brain edema on CT scan, hearing impairment, or rapidly progressive

TREATMENT RECOMMENDATIONS FOR COMMON TREATABLE CAUSES OF NONPYOGENIC MENINGITIS

Agent	Therapy	Dose	Route
Herpesviruses	Aciclovir	10mg/kg q8h	iv
Mycobacterium tuberculosis	Isoniazid	10mg/kg/day (up to 300mg/day)	po or iv
	Rifampin (rifampicin)	10mg/kg/day (up to 600mg/day)	po or iv
	Ethambutol	25mg/kg/day	po or iv
	Pyrazinamide	25mg/kg/day (up to 2.5g/day)	po or iv
Brucella spp. (>8 years)	Doxycycline plus	100mg q12h	po
	gentamicin	1.7–2mg/kg q8h	iv
Brucella spp. (<8 years)	Trimethoprim–sulfamethoxazole	5mg/kg trimethoprim q12h 25mg/kg sulfamethoxazole q12h	po po
	plus gentamicin	2mg/kg q8h	iv
Treponema pallidum	Penicillin G	2g q4h	iv
Borrelia spp.	Ceftriaxone	2–3g q24h	iv
Cryptococcus spp.	Amphotericin B plus	0.5–0.8mg/kg/day	iv
	flucytosine	37.5mg/kg q6h	po
Coccidioides spp.	Fluconazole	400–600mg/day	po

Fig. 15.16 Treatment recommendations for common treatable causes of nonpyogenic meningitis. Note that the dose of flucytosine must be reduced or the drug omitted in patients with AIDS, owing to increased bone marrow toxicity.

RECOMMENDATIONS FOR ANTIBIOTIC THERAPY IN PATIENTS WITH A POSITIVE CSF GRAM STAIN OR CULTURE

Bacteria		Antibiotic	Alternative antibiotic (in the case of allergy)
Gram stain	Culture		
Gram-positive diplococci	*Streptococcus pneumoniae*, penicillin-resistant or sensitivity unknown	Ceftriaxone plus vancomycin or rifampin (rifampicin)	Vancomycin plus rifampin
	Streptococcus pneumoniae, penicillin-sensitive	Penicillin G	Ceftriaxone or chloramphenicol
Gram-positive cocci	β-hemolytic streptococci	Penicillin or ampicillin	Cefotaxime, chloramphenicol, or vancomycin
Gram-negative coccobacilli	*Haemophilus influenzae*	Ceftriaxone or cefotaxime	Chloramphenicol
Gram-negative diplococci	*Neisseria meningitidis*	Penicillin G	Ceftriaxone or chloramphenicol
Gram-positive bacilli	*Listeria monocytogenes*	Ampicillin plus gentamicin	Trimethoprim–sulfamethoxazole
Gram-negative bacilli	Enterobacteriaceae	Ceftriaxone plus gentamicin	Quinolones
Gram-negative bacilli	*Pseudomonas aeruginosa*	Ceftazidime plus tobramycin	Quinolones

Fig. 15.17 Recommendations for antibiotic therapy in patients with a positive CSF gram stain or culture.

MEASURES TO REDUCE INCREASED INTRACRANIAL PRESSURE IN ACUTE MENINGITIS

Intracranial pressure monitoring

Normalization of systemic blood pressure

Dexamethasone, 0.15mg/kg q6h

Head elevation of more than 30° to the horizontal

Mannitol, 1–1.5 g/kg iv over 15 min; repeat once

Hyperventilation [arterial partial pressure CO_2 between 28 to 32mmHg (3.7–4.2kPa)]

Intraventricular shunt with CSF drainage in cases where there is evidence of hydrocephalus

Fig. 15.18 Measures to reduce intracranial pressure in acute meningitis.

disease. When instituting dexamethasone therapy, it is mandatory to confirm the bacterial etiology of meningitis. If this cannot be achieved within 24–48 hours, it is safer to stop the anti-inflammatory drug and to reassess the appropriateness of the chosen antimicrobial therapy. At present, there is no evidence that treatment with dexamethasone for 1–2 days has any adverse effects on outcome of viral meningitis. It is important that patients who are given dexamethasone should be closely monitored for evidence of gastrointestinal blood loss.

There is no recognized benefit from either prophylactic or full anti-coagulation in the management of patients with bacterial meningitis, and the involvement of the cerebral vasculature by the inflammation is likely to increase the risk of cerebral hemorrhages in anticoagulated patients with bacterial meningitis.

SUPPORTIVE CARE

In critically ill patients with bacterial meningitis, intensive supportive care may be needed, indicating admission to a critical care unit. Patients with severe meningitis are often neurologically depressed and prone to seizures; they may need intubation for airway protection or assisted ventilation.

Children may have complex requirements for fluid supplementation, with the need for a careful clinical assessment of fluid status, repletion of fluid deficits and monitoring for SIADH. If SIADH is present (indicated by falling serum sodium and reduced urine output with urine sodium concentration of more than 50mmol/l), fluids should be reduced to two-thirds of the maintenance level until the SIADH has resolved. Resolution within 1–2 days is usual.

In addition, active attempts to reduce intracranial hypertension should be undertaken in patients with increased intracranial pressure and severely impaired CNS function. Although there is only a small amount of controlled experience in the reduction of intracranial pressure in meningitis, several measures can be attempted (Fig. 15.18).

MONITORING DURING THERAPY

Repeat CSF examination should be performed in patients in whom there is doubt about the success of therapy or the accuracy of the initial diagnosis, but not in patients who respond promptly to therapy. Recurrent fever after an initial response to therapy is a common problem in patients with meningitis, particularly in children, and is most commonly due to infected intravenous lines, secondary infectious foci (e.g. septic arthritis, purulent pericarditis, pleural or intracranial empyema), or drug fever. Sterile subdural effusions, which occur in approximately one-third of children with meningitis, do not require drainage, unless symptoms or signs of intracranial hypertension are present. Obstructive hydrocephalus, which occurs in less than 5% of patients, usually manifests within the first few weeks of infection and should be treated with ventriculoperitoneal shunting. Neurologic sequelae, including hearing impairment, cranial nerve palsies and motor deficits, can improve for several months after the acute illness, and appropriate, individually tailored supportive therapies should be arranged for patients who are left with sequelae from the disease.

REFERENCES

1. Schuchat A, Robinson K, Wenger JD, et al. Bacterial meningitis in the United States in 1995. N Engl J Med 1997;337:970–6.
2. Connolly KJ, Hammer SM. The acute aseptic meningitis syndrome. Infect Dis Clin North Am 1990;4:599–622.
3. Segreti J, Harris AA. Acute bacterial meningitis. Infect Dis Clin North Am 1996;10:797–809.
4. Rotbart HA. Enteroviral infections of the central nervous system. Clin Infect Dis 1995;20:971–81.
5. Swartz M. Chronic meningitis–– many causes to consider. N Engl J Med 1987;317:957–9.
6. Haelterman E, Boelaert M, Suetens C, Blok L, Henkens M, Toole MJ. Impact of a mass vaccination campaign against a meningitis epidemic in a refugee camp. Trop Med Intern Health 1996;1:385–92.
7. Riordan FA, Thomson AP, Sills JA, Hart CA. Bacterial meningitis in the first three months of life. Postgrad Med J 1995;71:36–8.
8. Quagliarello VJ, Scheld WM. Treatment of bacterial meningitis. N Engl J Med 1997;336:708–16.
9. Smith AL, Haas J. Neonatal bacterial meningitis. In: Scheld WM, Whitley RJ, Durack DT, eds. Infections of the central nervous system. New York: Raven Press; 1991:313–33.
10. Porkert MT, Sotir M, Parrott-Moore P, Blumberg HM. Tuberculous meningitis at a large inner-city medical center. Am J Med Sci 1997;313:325–31.
11. Verdon R, Chevret S, Laissy JP, Wolff M. Tuberculous meningitis in adults: review of 48 cases. Clin Infect Dis 1996;22:982–8.
12. Dagan R. Epidemiology of pediatric meningitis caused by Haemophilus influenzae B, Streptococcus pneumoniae and Neisseria meningitidis in Israel. Isr J Med Sci 1994;30:351–5.
13. Engelhard D, Pomeranz S, Gallily R, Strauss N, Tuomanen E. Serotype-related differences in inflammatory response to Streptococcus pneumoniae in experimental meningitis. J Infect Dis 1997;175:979–82.
14. Poulain P, Betremieux P, Donnio PY, Proudhon JF, Karege G, Giraud JR. Selective intrapartum anti-bioprophylaxy of group B streptococci infection of neonates: a prospective study in 2454 subsequent deliveries. Eur J Obstet Gynecol Reprod Biol 1997;72:137–40.
15. Wald ER, Bergman I, Taylor HG, Chiponis D, Porter C, Kubek K. Long-term outcome of group B streptococcal meningitis. Pediatrics 1986;77:217–21.
16. Schwarzkopf A. Listeria monocytogenes – aspects of pathogenicity. Pathol Biol 1996;44:769–74.
17. Lerche A, Rasmussen N, Wandall JH, Bohr VA. Staphylococcus aureus meningitis: a review of 28 consecutive community-acquired cases. Scand J Infect Dis 1995;27:569–73.
18. Liptak GS, McConnochie KM, Roghmann KJ, Panzer JA. Decline of pediatric admissions with Haemophilus influenzae type b in New York State, 1982 through 1993: relation to immunizations. J Pediatr 1997;130:923–30.
19. Arango CA, Rathore MH. Neonatal meningococcal meningitis: case reports and review of literature. Pediatr Infect Dis J 1996;15:1134–6.
20. Virji M. Meningococcal disease: epidemiology and pathogenesis. Trends Microbiol 1996;4:466–9; discussion 469–70.
21. Haile-Mariam T, Laws E, Tuazon CU. Gram-negative meningitis associated with transsphenoidal surgery: case reports and review. Clin Infect Dis 1994;18:553–6.
22. Ratzan KR. Viral meningitis. Med Clin North Am 1985;69:399–413.
23. Hammer SM, Connolly KJ. Viral aseptic meningitis in the United States: clinical features, viral etiologies, and differential diagnosis. Curr Clin Top Infect Dis 1992;12:1–25.
24. Saito H, Takahashi Y, Harata S, et al. Isolation and characterization of mumps virus strains in a mumps outbreak with a high incidence of aseptic meningitis. Microbiol Immunol 1996;40:271–5.
25. Roebroek RM, Postma BH, Dijkstra UJ. Aseptic meningitis caused by the lymphocytic choriomeningitis virus. Clin Neurol Neurosurg 1994;96:178–80.
26. Bergstrom T, Vahlne A, Alestig K, Jeansson S, Forsgren M, Lycke E. Primary and recurrent herpes simplex virus type 2-induced meningitis. J Infect Dis 1990;162:322–30.
27. Price RW. Neurological complications of HIV infection. Lancet 1996;348:445–52.
28. Elmore JG, Horwitz RI, Quagliarello VJ. Acute meningitis with a negative Gram's stain: clinical and management outcomes in 171 episodes. Am J Med 1996;100:78–84.
29. Pachner AR. Early disseminated Lyme disease: Lyme meningitis. Am J Med 1995;98(suppl):37–43.
30. Torre D, Giola M, Martegani R, Zeroli C, Fiori GP, Ferrario G, Bonetta G. Aseptic meningitis caused by Leptospira australis. Eur J Clin Microbiol Infect Dis 1994;13:496–7.
31. Barnett ND, Kaplan AM, Hopkin RJ, Saubolle MA, Rudinsky MF. Primary amoebic meningoencephalitis with Naegleria fowleri: clinical review. Pediatr Neurol 1996;15:230–4.
32. River Y, Averbuch-Heller L, Weinberger M, Meiner Z, Mevorach D, Schlesinger I, Argov Z. Antibiotic induced meningitis. J Neurol Neurosurg Psychiatry 1994;57:705–8.
33. Bouza E, Garcia de la Torre M, Parras F. Brucellar meningitis. Rev Infect Dis 1987;9:810–22.
34. Chapel TA. The signs and symptoms of secondary syphilis. Sex Transm Dis 1980;7:161–63.
35. Jones GA, Nathwani D. Cryptococcal meningitis. Br J Hosp Med 1995;54:439–45.
36. Wilhelm C, Ellner JJ. Chronic meningitis. Neurol Clin 1986;4:115–41.
37. Oka Y, Fukui K, Shoda D, et al. Cerebral cysticercosis manifesting as hydrocephalus – case report. Neurol Med Chir 1996;36:654–8.
38. Clouston PD, Corbett AJ, Pryor DS, Garrick R. Eosinophilic meningitis: cause of a chronic pain syndrome. J Neurol Neurosurg Psychiatry 1990;53:778–81.
39. Rubin LG, Moxon ER. Pathogenesis of bloodstream invasion with Haemophilus influenzae type b. Infect Immun 1983;41:280–4.
40. Quagliarello V, Scheld WM. Bacterial meningitis: Pathogenesis, pathophysiology, and progress. N Engl J Med 1992;327:864–72.
41. Low PS, Lee BW, Yap HK, Tay JS, Lee WL, Seah CC, Ramzan MM. Inflammatory response in bacterial meningitis: cytokine levels in the cerebrospinal fluid. Ann Trop Paediatr 1995;15:55–9.
42. Pfister HW, Fontana A, Täuber MG, Tomasz A, Scheld WM. Mechanisms of brain injury in bacterial meningitis: workshop summary. Clin Infect Dis 1994;19:463–79.
43. Tunkel AR, Scheld WM. Pathogenesis and pathophysiology of bacterial meningitis. Annu Rev Med 1993;44:103–20.
44. Kim KS, Wass CA, Cross AS. Blood–brain barrier permeability during the development of experimental bacterial meningitis in the rat. Exp Neurol 1997;145:253–7.
45. Tunkel AR, Wispelwey B, Quagliarello VJ, et al. Pathophysiology of blood–brain barrier alterations during experimental Haemophilus influenzae meningitis. J Infect Dis 1992;165:S119–20.
46. Täuber MG, Sande E, Fournier MA, Tureen JH, Sande MA. Fluid administration, brain edema, and cerebrospinal fluid lactate and glucose concentrations in experimental Escherichia coli meningitis. J Infect Dis 1993;168:473–6.
47. Koedel U, Bernatowicz A, Paul R, Frei K, Fontana A, Pfister HW. Experimental pneumococcal meningitis: cerebrovascular alterations, brain edema, and meningeal inflammation are linked to the production of nitric oxide. Ann Neurol 1995;37:313–23.
48. Pfister HW, Borasio GD, Dirnagl U, Bauer M, Einhäupl KM. Cerebrovascular complications of bacterial meningitis in adults. Neurology 1992;42:1497–504.
49. Leib SL, Kim YS, Chow LL, Sheldon RA, Täuber MG. Reactive oxygen intermediates contribute to necrotic and apoptotic neuronal injury in an infant rat model of bacterial meningitis due to group B streptococci. J Clin Invest 1996;98:2632–9.
50. Tureen J. Effect of recombinant human tumor necrosis factor-alpha on cerebral oxygen uptake, cerebrospinal fluid lactate, and cerebral blood flow in the rabbit: role of nitric oxide. J Clin Invest 1995;95:1086–91.
51. Leib SL, Kim YS, Ferriero DM, Täuber MG. Neuroprotective effect of excitatory amino acid antagonist kynurenic acid in experimental bacterial meningitis. J Infect Dis 1996;173:166–71.
52. Waggener JD. The pathophysiology of bacterial meningitis and cerebral abscesses: an anatomical interpretation. Adv Neurol 1974;6:1–17.
53. Progress toward elimination of Haemophilus influenzae type b disease among infants and children-United States, 1987–1995. MMWR Morb Mortal Wkly Rep 1996;45:901–6.
54. Hattotuwa KL, Hind CR. Pneumococcal vaccine. Postgrad Med J 1997;73:222–4.
55. Zangwill KM, Vadheim CM, Vannier AM, Hemenway LS, Greenberg DP, Ward JI. Epidemiology of invasive pneumococcal disease in southern California: implications for the design and conduct of a pneumococcal conjugate vaccine efficacy trial. J Infect Dis 1996;174:752–9.
56. Bushra HE, Mawlawi MY, Fontaine RE, Afif H. Meningococcal meningitis group A: a successful control of an outbreak by mass vaccination. East Afr Med J 1995;72:715–8.
57. Brodie HA. Prophylactic antibiotics for posttraumatic cerebrospinal fluid fistulae. A meta-analysis. Arch Otolaryngol Head Neck Surg 1997;123:749–52.
58. Tunkel AR, Scheld WM. Acute bacterial meningitis. Lancet 1995;346:1675–80.
59. Schaad UB, Kaplan SL, McCracken G Jr. Steroid therapy for bacterial meningitis. Clin Infect Dis 1995;20:685–90.
60. Townsend GC, Scheld WM. The use of corticosteroids in the management of bacterial meningitis in adults. J Antimicrob Chemother 1996;37:1051–61.
61. Bonadio WA. Adjunctive dexamethasone therapy for pediatric bacterial meningitis. J Emerg Med 1996;14:165–72.

Acute and Chronic Encephalitis

Kevin A Cassady & Richard J Whitley

Viral infections of the central nervous system (CNS) occur infrequently and most often result in relatively benign, self-limiting disease. Nevertheless, these infections have great importance because of the potential for significant neurologic impairment, if not death. Brain tissue is exquisitely sensitive to metabolic derangements and, if injured, recovers slowly and often incompletely.[1] Numerous factors in addition to viral serotype, receptor preference, viral load and cell tropism influence the clinical manifestations of viral CNS infections, including an individual's age, immune history, cultural practices and genetic make-up. Changes in behavior, cultural beliefs and modification of the environment result in changes in disease patterns and exposure to new infectious agents. Therefore, CNS infections must be examined in a geographic, cultural and environmental context, as well as at the cellular, molecular and genetic levels. Indeed, tumors, infections and autoimmune diseases of the CNS often produce similar signs and symptoms.[2] Improvements in our ability to diagnose CNS infections will produce a better understanding of the pathogenesis and true extent of CNS viral disease. The history and clinical presentation, although frequently suggestive of a diagnosis, remain unreliable methods for determining the specific etiology of CNS disease. Different diseases may share a common pathogenic mechanism and therefore result in a similar clinical presentation. The subject of viral infections of the CNS has been reviewed in detail.[3]

The definition of viral infection of the CNS is often based on virus tropism and disease duration. Encephalitis refers to inflammation of parenchymal brain tissue. Acute encephalitis begins abruptly (hours to days) whereas a chronic encephalitis is insidious in onset, occurring over weeks to months. The temporal course of slow viral infections of the CNS (e.g. kuru, visna) overlaps with the chronic encephalitides. Slow viral diseases are distinguished by their long incubation period and eventually result in death or extreme neurologic disability over months to years.[4]

Viral disease in the CNS can also be classified by pathogenesis. Neurologic disease is frequently categorized as either primary or postinfectious. Primary encephalitis results from direct viral entry into the CNS that produces clinically evident cortical or brainstem dysfunction.[5] Subsequent damage is caused by the host immune response but invasion by the pathogen initiates CNS damage. The parenchyma exhibits neuronophagia and the presence of viral antigens or nucleic acids. A postinfectious or parainfectious encephalitis produces signs and symptoms of encephalitis that are temporally associated with a systemic viral infection, but there is no evidence of direct viral invasion of the CNS. Pathologic specimens demonstrate demyelination and perivascular aggregation of immune cells, but no evidence of virus or viral antigen; this leads some to hypothesize an autoimmune etiology.[5,6] The presence of immune cells distinguishes primary and postinfectious encephalitis from an encephalopathy.

Inflammation occurs at multiple sites in the brain and accounts for the myriad of clinical descriptors of viral neurologic disease. Inflammation of the spinal cord, leptomeninges, dorsal nerve roots or nerves results in myelitis, meningitis, radiculitis and neuritis, respectively. Aseptic meningitis is a misnomer frequently used to refer to a benign, self-limiting, viral infection that causes inflammation of the leptomeninges.[7] The term hinders epidemiologic studies, as the definition fails to differentiate between infectious (bacterial, fungal, tuberculous, viral or other infectious etiologies) and noninfectious causes. Meningitis and encephalitis can represent separate clinical entities; however, a continuum exists between these distinct forms of CNS disease. A change in a patient's clinical condition can reflect disease progression with involvement of different regions in the CNS. Epidemiologic data in many cases provide clues to the etiology of the illness. An overview is difficult, as each pathogen fills a different ecologic niche with unique seasonal, host and/or vector properties (Figs. 16.1 & 16.2).[1] Instead it is useful to analyze the prototypes of viral CNS infection, meningitis and encephalitis, and the approach to patients with presumed viral infections of the CNS. This chapter addresses the issues of acute and chronic encephalitis. Acute and chronic meningitis, including those caused by viruses, are discussed in Chapter 2.15.

VIRAL ENCEPHALITIS

EPIDEMIOLOGY

Passive reporting systems underestimate the incidence of viral encephalitis, as they do for viral meningitis. The CDC received 740–1340 annual reports of persons who have encephalitis between 1990 and 1993. A review of the cases in Olmsted county, Minnesota from 1950 to 1980 found the incidence of viral encephalitis was at least twice that reported by the CDC. Studies performed in Finland, a country with few arboviral infections, estimate the incidence of encephalitis at anywhere between 8.8 and 12.6 cases per 100,000 population.[14] Herpes simplex virus infections of the CNS occur without seasonal variation, affect all ages and constitute the majority of fatal cases of endemic encephalitis in the USA.[10] Arboviruses, a group of over 500 arthropod-transmitted RNA viruses, are the leading cause of encephalitis worldwide and in the USA. Arboviral infections occur in epidemics and show a seasonal predilection, reflecting the prevalence of the transmitting vector. Asymptomatic infections vastly outnumber those that are symptomatic. Patients with symptomatic infections may develop a mild systemic febrile illness or a viral meningitis.[11] Encephalitis occurs in a minority of persons with arboviral infections, but the case fatality rate varies from 5 to 70%, depending upon viral etiology and age of the patient.

Japanese B encephalitis and rabies constitute the majority of cases of encephalitis outside of North America. Japanese B encephalitis virus, a member of the *Flavivirus* genus, occurs throughout Asia and causes epidemics in China despite routine immunization.[1] In warmer locations, the virus occurs endemically.[15] The disease typically affects children, although adults with no history of exposure to the virus are also susceptible.[5] As with the other arboviral infections, asymptomatic infections occur more frequently than symptomatic infections. However, the disease has a high case fatality rate and leaves one-half of the survivors with a significant degree of neurologic morbidity.[15] Rabies virus remains endemic around the world. Human infections in

DNA VIRUSES AND CNS INFECTIONS

Virus	Viral agent	CNS disease	Temporal course	Transmission	Pathway to CNS	Frequency	Laboratory confirmation
Herpetoviridae	Herpes simplex virus (HSV) type 1 and type 2	Encephalitis, meningitis meningo-encephalitis	Acute Latent reactivation	Human	Blood and neuronal	+++	Gold standard is CSF PCR or cell culture of brain biopsy sample if PCR is unavailable
	Cytomegalovirus (CMV)	Encephalitis (immunosuppressed and neonate)	Acute	Human	Blood	++	Gold standard is PCR Brain biopsy or CSF culture can also detect CMV
	Epstein–Barr virus (EBV)	Encephalitis, meningitis, myelitis, Guillain–Barré	Acute	Human	Blood	+	Serologic evidence
	Varicella-zoster virus (VZV)	Cerebellitis, encephalitis, meningitis, myelitis, zoster ophthalmicus	Postinfectious Acute and latent reactivation (zoster)	Human	Blood and neuronal	++	Clinical findings, cell culture from a lesion, brain biopsy, or autopsy rarely
	Human herpesvirus 6 (HHV-6)	Encephalitis, febrile seizures, latent form?	Acute Latent infection	Human	?	?	Culture, PCR (high frequency of detection; significance unknown)
	B Virus	Encephalitis	Acute	Animal bite and human	Neuronal	+	Culture
Adenoviridae	Adenovirus	Meningitis, encephalitis	Acute	Human	Blood	+	Cell culture of CSF or brain
Poxviridae	Vaccinia	Encephalomyelitis	Postinfectious	Vaccine	Blood	Extinct	Recent vaccination

Frequency: +++ = frequent, ++ = infrequent, + = rare, ? = unknown

Fig. 16.1 DNA viruses and CNS infections: type of disease, epidemiology and pathogenesis.

the USA have decreased over the past decades to 1–3 cases per year because of the immunization of domestic animals. Recently, a resurgence of cases linked to infected coyotes has occurred in Texas. In areas outside the USA, annual cases of rabies encephalitis number in the thousands.[16]

Postinfectious encephalitis, an acute demyelinating process, accounts for approximately 100 additional cases of encephalitis reported to the CDC annually. The disease historically produced approximately one-third of the encephalitis cases in the USA and was associated with measles, mumps and other exanthematous viral infections.[5] Postinfectious encephalitis is now associated with antecedent upper respiratory virus (notably influenza virus) and varicella infections in the USA. Measles continues to be a leading cause of postinfectious encephalitis worldwide and complicates 1 out of every 1000 measles infections.

Most viruses can cause infection of the CNS, resulting in either encephalitis or meningitis; however, rabies and B virus only cause encephalitis. Fortunately, encephalitis is a rare complication of viral infection.

HERPESVIRUS INFECTIONS

Herpes simplex virus causes encephalitis (HSE) in individuals of all ages and remains the most common cause of sporadic fatal encephalitis in the USA, accounting for approximately 1250 cases yearly.[17] Two distinct antigenic types exist: HSV-1 and HSV-2. Both cause CNS disease.[18] Herpes simplex virus is a large, dsDNA virus with an icosadeltahedral capsid, a surrounding tegument and an envelope with glycoprotein spikes. The virus establishes latency after primary infection. The molecular biology of HSV is reviewed elsewhere (see Chapter 8.5).[19]

Varicella-zoster virus causes chickenpox (varicella) and shingles (herpes zoster). Overall, 1 in 1000 patients develop CNS disease.[17,20] Cerebellar ataxia is the most common manifestation of CNS viral infection. Although encephalitis can follow varicella, usually 5–20 days after the onset of the rash, it is uncommon. The mortality from encephalitis is low. The occurrence of CNS involvement after herpes

zoster is more common, as 40% of patients develop CSF pleocytosis, which is usually asymptomatic. Mortality from herpes zoster is as high as 20% in immunosuppressed patients with CNS complications.[21] Contralateral granulomatous arteritis is a complication of zoster ophthalmicus in elderly individuals.[17,20]

Cytomegalovirus is associated with distinctive cytopathic enlargement of infected cells. Although CMV is a rare cause of encephalitis in healthy adults, congenital infection with CNS involvement occurs in at least 1 in 1000 live births; furthermore, CNS disease in the immunocompromised host, particularly those with HIV infection, is increasingly recognized.

Epstein–Barr virus was isolated from the cells of a patient with Burkitt's lymphoma.[22] This virus, the principal cause of infectious mononucleosis, occasionally results in acute encephalitis.[17] Mortality associated with EBV encephalitis is low.

Human herpesvirus 6 (HHV-6) is associated with roseola; however, cases of CNS disease have been reported. Brain disease is rarely fatal.

B virus appears to be the only nonhuman primate herpesvirus that is pathogenic for humans.[23] The resulting encephalitis is severe, and mortality associated with infection exceeds 75% in the absence of therapy.

ARBOVIRUS INFECTIONS

Arthropod-borne viruses include the alphaviruses, flaviviruses, bunyaviruses and, in at least one case, a reovirus. Mosquitoes and ticks transmit the viral infection from animal hosts to humans, leading to encephalitis. The annual incidence is variable for most of the arboviral encephalitides and reflects the dynamic relationship between mosquito and animal vector populations. Inapparent infection is generally more common than encephalitis for most arboviral infections but this ratio differs according to the infecting virus.

Alphaviruses are small, positive, ssRNA enveloped viruses. The CDC reports approximately five cases of Eastern equine encephalitis (EEE) annually. Mortality ranges from 50 to 75% and the rate of symptomatic infection is high.[11] Western equine encephalitis (WEE) causes about 13 cases annually. Western equine encephalitis has a lower mortality (3–9%). Venezuelan equine encephalitis (VEE) virus

RNA VIRUSES AND CNS INFECTIONS

Virus	Viral taxonomy	Vector	CNS disease	Disease pattern	Geographic distribution	Frequency	Case fatal	Laboratory confirmation
Togaviridae – Alphavirus (Arbovirus)	Western equine encephalitis virus	Mosquito, birds	Encephalitis, meningitis	Epidemic	USA – west of Mississippi River	++	3–10%	Serologic titers (HI, CF, NA, IFA), viral antigen detection in brain. Rarely culture
	Eastern equine encephalitis virus	Mosquito, birds	Encephalitis, meningitis	Sporadic	USA – Atlantic and Gulf Coast states	+	>30%	Viral culture or antigen detection in brain, serologic titers (HI, CF, NA, IFA), CSF IgM ELISA
	Venezuelan equine encephalitis virus	Mosquito, horses	Encephalitis, meningitis	Sporadic, epidemic	C and S America, SW USA, Florida	+	<1%	Serologic titers (HI, CF, NA, IFA), CSF IgM ELISA
Flaviviridae – Flavivirus (Arbovirus)	Japanese B encephalitis virus	Mosquito, swine, bird	Encephalitis, meningitis	Epidemic, endemic	Japan, China, Korea, Taiwan, SE Asia, India, Nepal	+++	25%	Peripheral blood ELISA, serologic titers (HI, CF, NA, IFA), CSF antigen tests
	St Louis encephalitis virus	Mosquito, swine, bird	Encephalitis, meningitis	Epidemic, endemic	USA	+++	7%	CSF IgM ELISA, serologic titers (HI, CF, NA, IFA). Rarely culture
	West Nile fever virus	Mosquito, swine, bird	Encephalitis, meningitis	Epidemic, endemic	Uganda, Egypt, Israel	+	Rarely	Culture (rare), serology (HI, IFA)
	Murray Valley virus	Mosquito, swine, bird	Encephalitis	Epidemic, endemic	Australia	++	20–60%	Viral culture, serologic titer (HI, CF, NA)
	Tick-borne encephalitis virus (TBE complex)	Tick, unpasteurized milk	Encephalitis	Epidemic, sporadic	Eastern Russia and Central Europe	++	20%	Serologic titer (HI, CF, N), IgM ELISA
Bunyaviridae (Arbovirus)	California (La Crosse) encephalitis virus	Mosquito, rodents	Encephalitis, meningitis	Endemic	Northern Midwest and NE USA	+++ (LCV) + (CEV)	<1%	Viral culture, CSF IgM ELISA, serologic titers (HI, CF, NA, IFA), CIE
Reoviridae – Orbivirus (Arbovirus)	Colorado tick fever virus	Tick, rodents	Encephalitis, meningitis	Endemic	Rocky Mountains, Pacific Coast states USA	+	<1%	Antigen detection on RBC membrane, viral culture, serologic titers (HI, CF, NA, IFA)
Picornaviridae (Enterovirus)	Poliovirus	Fecal–oral	Meningitis, myelitis	Endemic	Worldwide	++	4.5–50%*	Viral culture CSF or brain, viral culture from other site. Serologic testing for some serotypes. PCR becoming gold standard
	Coxsackievirus	Fecal–oral	Meningo-encephalitis, meningitis, myelitis	Endemic	Worldwide	+++	Rarely†	
	Echovirus	Fecal–oral	Meningo-encephalitis, meningitis, myelitis	Endemic	Worldwide	+++	Rarely†	
Paramyxoviridae (Exanthematous virus)	Measles virus	Postinfectious, blood	Encephalitis, SSPE	Sporadic	Worldwide	++	20–30%	Serology, ELISA, clinically
	Mumps virus	Blood	Encephalitis, meningitis, myelitis	Sporadic	Worldwide	+++	<1%	CSF viral culture
Orthomyxoviridae (Upper respiratory virus)	Influenza viruses	Postinfectious	Encephalitis	Sporadic	Worldwide	+	<1%	Viral culture from another site
Rhabdoviridae	Rabies	Mammal	Encephalitis, encephalomyelitis	Sporadic	Worldwide	+++	~100%	Antigen detection in brain, serologic tests (IFA, CF, HA, CIE), viral culture
Retroviridae	Ultimately 100% HIV 1	Human	Encephalopathy, encephalitis, leukoencephalopathy	?	Worldwide	++	~100%	PCR autopsy samples/MRI findings
Arenaviridae	Lymphocytic choriomenigitis virus	Rodent	Encephalitis, meningitis	Sporadic	Worldwide	+	<2.5%	CSF, blood culture. Urine culture, serology

Fig. 16.2 RNA viruses and CNS infections: type of disease, epidemiology and pathogenesis. *Case fatality from poliomyelitis is increased in sporadic cases. Vaccination has decreased the epidemic forms of polio and consequently morbidity. In turn, the calculated case fatality rate in the USA has increased as sporadic and vaccine-associated disease has increased relative to the number of cases of disease. †Rarely fatal except in the neonate and agammaglobulinemic patient, in whom fatality rates can approach 50% even with treatment. SSPE, subacute sclerosing panencephalitis.

causes 20 nonfatal cases per year on average, occurring concomitantly with equine fatalities. Mortality associated with VEE is reported to be 1% but is higher in children less than 5 years of age. Everglades virus has also been associated with encephalitis.

Flaviviruses are positive ssRNA viruses that have similar morphology to alphaviruses but a distinctive genomic structure and replication cycle.[24,25] St Louis encephalitis virus causes epidemics throughout the USA but outside of the New England region.[26,27] The mortality from the disease is 2–20%, depending upon the patient's age. In the elderly, St Louis encephalitis virus produces more severe disease, resulting in higher mortality and morbidity.

Japanese B encephalitis has caused several epidemics. Mortality associated with Japanese B encephalitis is between 20 and 50%. Murray Valley (Australian X) encephalitis epidemics have occurred with a mortality rate of 70%. Other encephalitic flaviviruses include Rocio, West Nile, Kysanur Forest disease, Powassan, Ilheus, Negishi, Russian spring–summer, louping-ill and Central European.

Bunyaviruses are negative ssRNA viruses.[6] Encephalitis from bunyaviruses is associated with La Crosse encephalitis virus, the most common cause of arbovirus infection in the USA. Mortality is less than 1%; however, neurologic sequelae, including seizure disorder and personality problems, have been reported in up to 15% of infected children. Other causes of encephalitis in this group include Jamestown Canyon, snowshoe hare and Tahyna viruses. These viruses collectively comprise the California serogroup of bunyaviruses.

Reoviruses are dsRNA viruses without an envelope. Colorado tick virus is the most common member of this family and causes encephalitis in humans.

RHABDOVIRUSES
Rabies is a ssRNA virus with a bullet-shaped envelope (see Chapter 8.8).[28] Rabies is uniformly fatal in unimmunized individuals. Prevention is the mainstay of treatment and consists of immunization of domestic animals and potentially exposed individuals. Postexposure treatment consists of thorough cleaning of the bite wound, administration of rabies immunoglobulin at the site of the animal bite and postexposure vaccination using rabies human diploid cell vaccine. Treatment after the onset of clinical illness invariably fails and may exacerbate symptoms.[16]

The Semple rabies vaccine causes an encephalitis that appears to be an autoimmune response to myelin in the vaccine. Because of its low cost, this vaccine is still widely used worldwide. The associated mortality is low.

ARENAVIRUSES
Arenaviruses are bisegmented single-stranded ambisense (contains a negative single-stranded and a pseudo-positive single-stranded) RNA enveloped viruses that include lymphocytic choriomeningitis virus and Lassa virus. Lymphocytic choriomeningitis virus usually produces meningitis, although cases of encephalitis, myelitis and bulbar paralysis have been reported.

PARAMYXOVIRUSES
Paramyxoviruses are negative single-stranded enveloped RNA viruses (see Chapter 8.2). Two members of the genus cause CNS disease: mumps and measles. Approximately 0.5–2.3% of cases of mumps encephalitis are fatal. The pathologic findings of post-measles encephalitis suggests a postinfectious encephalomyelitis.[29] Measles remains a major public health problem in many areas of the world where infection continues unabated, and it has an associated mortality of 1.5 million people annually.[30,31] Most deaths attributed to measles are not the consequence of encephalitis, but rather to opportunistic infections occurring as a consequence of the immune deficiency associated with infection. Measles encephalitis has a mortality of about 20%.

ENTEROVIRUSES
Enteroviruses are members of the picornavirus family (see Chapter 8.3). They are small ssRNA viruses without an envelope and include polioviruses, echoviruses and coxsackie viruses. In the USA, poliomyelitis (see Chapter 2.22) occasionally follows the administration of the attenuated oral polio vaccine to individuals who are not recognized as immunocompromised. Worldwide wild strain poliomyelitis remains common in areas where vaccination is not routine (see Chapter 2.22). Poliovirus is targeted for worldwide eradication by the World Health Organization. Echoviruses and coxsackieviruses usually cause aseptic meningitis but can also result in encephalitis.[32,33] These viruses are usually associated with a low mortality except in patients with X-linked agammaglobulinemia.

ORTHOMYXOVIRUSES
The prototype member of this family is influenza, causing a post-influenza encephalitis syndrome.[8] Encephalitis usually occurs in children and has a low mortality.

MISCELLANEOUS AGENTS
Acute hemorrhagic leukoencephalitis usually follows an upper respiratory tract infection. Although it is presumed to be of viral etiology, no agent has been identified. Focal neurologic signs develop. Surviving patients usually have significant neurologic impairment. The CT scan has a characteristic appearance with widespread, bilateral white matter involvement.

PATHOGENESIS AND PATHOLOGY

The pathogenesis of encephalitis requires that viruses reach the CNS by hematogenous or neuronal spread. Similar to meningitis, viruses most frequently access the CNS after secondary viremia and cell-free or cell-associated CNS entry. Other than direct entry via cerebral vessels, viruses can initially infect the meninges and enter the parenchyma across either ependymal cells or the pial linings. Viruses exhibit differences in neurotropism and neurovirulence. For example, reovirus types 1 and 3 produce different CNS diseases in mice on the basis of differences in receptor affinities. Viral hemagglutinin receptors on reovirus type 3 binds to neuronal receptors enabling a fatal encephalitis. Reovirus type 1 has a distinct hemagglutinin antigen and binds to ependymal cells and produces hydrocephalus and ependymitis.[12,15] Receptor difference is only one determinant of viral neurotropism; other viral factors may exert influence. For example, enteroviruses with similar receptors produce very different diseases. Five coxsackie B viruses (B1–B5) readily produce CNS infections, whereas type B6 rarely produces neurologic infection.[7,34] Viral genes have been discovered that influence neurovirulence of HSV-1. Mutant HSV-1 viruses with either $\gamma_1$34.5 gene deletions or stop codons inserted into the gene have a decreased ability to cause encephalitis and death after intracerebral inoculation in mice compared with wild-type virus.

In addition to viral factors, host physiology is also important in determining the extent and location of viral CNS disease, including age, sex and genetic differences.[9] Host age influences the clinical manifestations and sequelae of a viral infection. For example, Sindbis virus infection produces a lethal encephalitis in newborn mice, whereas weanling mice experience a persistent but nonfatal encephalitis. The reason for the difference in outcome is two-fold. Mature neurons resist viral-induced apoptosis and older mice have an improved antibody response that limits viral replication. Macrophage function and processing capacity change with age in humans.[8] In addition to age, physical activity may be an important host factor that determines the severity of infection. Exercise has been associated with increased risk of paralytic poliomyelitis and may result in an increased incidence of enteroviral myocarditis and aseptic meningitis.[7]

Herpes simplex virus and rabies are pathogens that infect the CNS by neuronal spread as illustrated in Figure 16.3. Sensory and motor

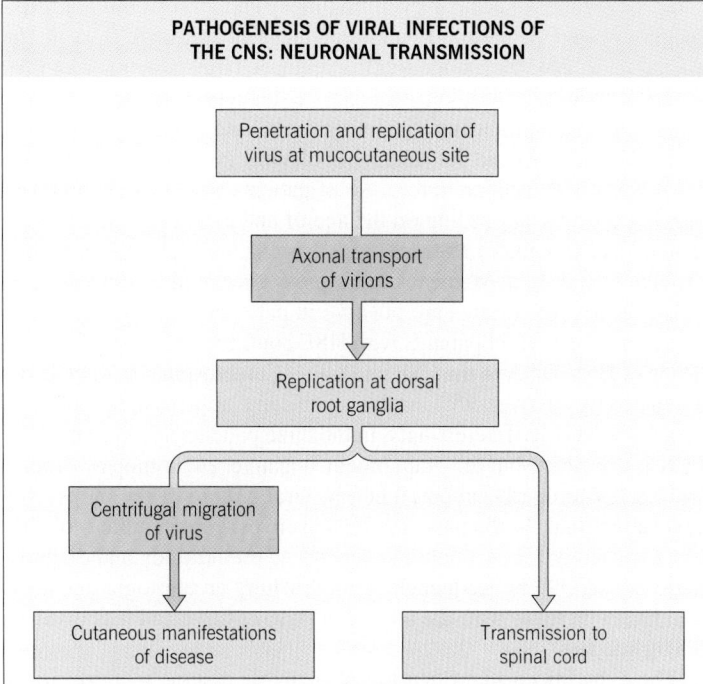

Fig. 16.3 Pathogenesis of viral infections of the CNS: neuronal transmission.

PATHOGENESIS OF VIRAL INFECTIONS OF
THE CNS: NEURONAL TRANSMISSION

Penetration and replication of
virus at mucocutaneous site

Axonal transport
of virions

Replication at dorsal
root ganglia

Centrifugal migration
of virus

Cutaneous manifestations
of disease

Transmission to
spinal cord

neurons contain transport systems that carry materials along the axon to (retrograde) and from (anterograde) the nucleus. Historically, the peripheral neural pathway was considered the only route for viral neurologic infection.[8] Recent data, however, show that the bloodstream is the principal pathway for CNS infections in humans. Peripheral or cranial nerves provide access to the CNS and shield the virus from immune regulation.

Rabies classically infects by the myoneural route and provides a prototype for peripheral neuronal spread.[16] Rabies virus replicates locally in the soft tissue after a bite from a rabid animal. After primary replication, the virus enters the peripheral nerve by binding to the acetylcholine receptor. Once in the muscle, the virus buds from the plasma membrane and may cross myoneural spindles or enters the nerve by the motor endplate.[8,16] Investigators have also demonstrated rabies entry via sensory nerves before soft tissue replication; however, this occurs less frequently.[11] The virus travels by anterograde and retrograde axonal transport to infect neurons in the brainstem and limbic system. Eventually the virus spreads from the diencephalic and hippocampal structure to the remainder of the brain, killing the animal.[16]

Viruses also infect the CNS through cranial nerves. Animal studies have shown that HSV can infect the brain through the olfactory system as well as the trigeminal nerve. The pathogenesis of human HSV infections, however, is less clear. Despite data supporting olfactory and trigeminal spread of virus to the CNS, definitive proof is lacking. The association of viral latency in the trigeminal ganglia, the relative infrequency of HSE and the confusing data regarding encephalitis from HSV reactivation suggest that the pathogenesis is very complex.[1]

The parenchyma in patients with acute encephalitis exhibits neuronophagia and cells containing viral DNA or antigens.[5] The pathologic findings are unique for different viruses and reflect differences in pathogenesis and virulence. In the case of HSV, a hemorrhagic necrosis occurs in the inferomedial temporal lobe with evidence of perivascular cuffing, lymphocytic infiltration and/or neuronophagia.[35] Pathologic specimens in animals with rabies encephalitis demonstrate microglial proliferation, perivascular infiltrates and neuronal destruction. The location of the pathologic findings can be limited to the brainstem areas (dumb rabies) or the diencephalic, hippocampal and hypothalamic areas (furious rabies), depending on the immune

response mounted against the infection.[16] Pathologic findings differ based on the viral etiology and are discussed in subsequent sections.

PREVENTION OF INFECTIONS OF THE CNS

Mumps, historically the most frequent cause of viral CNS disease, has largely been eliminated through vaccination. Live attenuated vaccines against measles, mumps and rubella have resulted in a dramatic decrease in the incidence of encephalitis in industrialized countries. Measles continues to be a leading cause of postinfectious encephalitis in developing countries, however, and complicates 1 out of every 1000 measles infections.[36,37] Vaccination has also changed the character of previously common viral CNS disease. In 1952, poliomyelitis affected 57,879 US inhabitants.[38] Widespread vaccination has eradicated the disease in developed countries. Vaccines exist for some arboviral infections. Vaccination against Japanese B encephalitis virus has reduced the incidence of encephalitis in Asia; however, in China, where 70 million children are immunized for Japanese B encephalitis virus, 10,000 cases still occur annually.[39]

Vaccination is not cost effective for preventing all viral infections. For example, vector avoidance, the use of mosquito deterrents and mosquito abatement programs are less costly strategies for preventing arboviral encephalitides. Ideally, chemoprophylaxis taken during outbreaks would provide the least costly and most effective prevention; however, no drug currently exists.[11] Pre- and immediate postexposure prophylaxis are the only ways known to prevent death in individuals exposed to rabies. Case reports exist of patients surviving symptomatic rabies; however, all of these patients had some prior immunity or received postexposure prophylaxis before symptoms developed. Individuals with frequent contact with potentially rabid animals (veterinarians, animal control staff, workers in rabies laboratories and travelers to rabies-endemic areas) should receive preexposure vaccination.

CLINICAL FEATURES

Although patients with encephalitis have clinical and laboratory evidence of parenchymal disease, infection rarely involves only the brain parenchyma. Some viruses (rabies, B virus) produce a true encephalitis picture; however, most patients with encephalitis have a concomitant meningitis. Most patients also have a prodromal illness with myalgias, fever and anorexia, reflecting the systemic viremia. Neurologic symptoms can range from fever, headache and subtle neurologic deficits or change in level of consciousness to severe disease with seizures, behavioral changes, focal neurologic deficits and coma.[10] Clinical manifestations reflect the location and degree of parenchymal involvement, and differ according to the viral etiology. For example, HSE infects the inferomedial frontal area of the cortex, resulting in focal seizures, personality changes and aphasia. These symptoms reflect the neuroanatomic location of infection, with inflammation near the internal capsule, and limbic and Broca's regions.[1] Paraesthesias near the location of the animal bite and change in behavior correlate temporally with the axoplasmic transport of rabies and viral infection of the brainstem and hippocampal region.[1,16] Rabies has a predilection for the basal ganglia and limbic system, producing personality changes. The damage spares cortical regions during this phase, allowing animals to vacillate between periods of calm normal activity and short episodes of rage and disorientation.[16] In contrast, Japanese B encephalitis virus initially produces a systemic illness with fever, malaise and anorexia, followed by photophobia, vomiting, headache and changes in brainstem function. Most children die from respiratory failure and frequently have evidence of cardiac and respiratory instability, reflecting viremic spread via the vertebral vessels and infection of brainstem nuclei.[5] Other patients have evidence of multifocal CNS disease that involves the basal ganglia, thalamus and lower cortex, and develop tremors, dystonia and parkinsonian symptoms. Encephalitis, unlike meningitis, has a higher mortality and complication rate. Case fatality rates differ according to the viral etiology and unique host factors.[1] For example, St Louis encephalitis virus has an overall case mortality rate of 10%; however, in children the mortality rate is only 2%. The virus produces more severe disease in the elderly, with a mortality rate of 20%.[10] Other viruses like WEE and EEE produce higher mortality and morbidity in children than in adults.

Some viruses do not directly infect the CNS but produce immune system changes that result in parenchymal damage. In patients with postinfectious encephalitis, focal neurologic changes and altered consciousness correlate temporally with a recent (1–2 week) viral infection or immunization. Pathologic specimens, although they show evidence of demyelination, do not demonstrate evidence of viral infection in the CNS by culture or antigen tests. Patients with postinfectious encephalitis have subtle differences in their immune system and some authors have proposed an autoimmune reaction as the pathogenic mechanism of disease.[5,6] Viruses most frequently associated with postinfectious encephalitis are measles, VZV, mumps, influenza and parainfluenza. With immunization, the incidence of postinfectious encephalitis has decreased in the USA; however, measles continues to be a leading cause of postinfectious encephalitis worldwide.[5]

DIAGNOSIS

Establishing a diagnosis requires a meticulous history, knowledge of epidemiologic factors and a systematic evaluation of possible treatable diseases.[10] Encephalitis can occur as a separate clinical entity; however, meningitis frequently co-exists. Laboratory findings such as a CSF pleocytosis usually occur in encephalitis although they are by no means necessary for the diagnosis. Most patients undergo a lumbar puncture in order to assess the CSF indices. Supratentorial and cerebellar tumors can produce increased intracranial pressure and can mimic encephalitis. A careful fundoscopic examination should be performed to rule out any evidence of papilledema and increased intracranial pressure before CSF is obtained. A CSF pleocytosis typically exists. The cell counts number in the 10s to 100s in viral encephalitis, although higher counts occur.[10] Cerebrospinal glucose levels are usually normal, although some infections (e.g. EEE) produce CSF findings consistent with an acute bacterial meningitis. Some viruses (HSV) produce a hemorrhagic necrosis and the CSF exhibits this with moderately high protein levels and evidence of red blood cells.

Unlike meningitis, encephalitis often requires additional laboratory and radiologic tests to establish the diagnosis. The clinical circumstances of the patient and the likely etiologies dictate specific laboratory and radiologic evaluations. Historically, the gold standard for diagnosis has been brain biopsy and viral culture. Recently, some authors have advocated the use of PCR of the CSF in patients with symptoms and radiologic findings consistent with encephalitis.[40] Radiographic studies that are useful in the diagnosis of encephalitis are CT scan and MRI. Magnetic resonance imaging detects parenchymal changes earlier than CT scan and better defines the extent of a lesion. Furthermore, MRI can distinguish acute viral encephalitis from postinfectious encephalitis on the basis of location of the lesions and evidence of mass effect. The increased sensitivity of MRI to alterations in brain water content and the lack of bone artifacts make this the neuroradiologic modality of choice for CNS infections.[41] Electroencephalograms (EEGs) provide another sensitive method to detect CNS dysfunction. Patients with viral encephalitis frequently have diffuse or focal epileptiform discharges with background slowing. These EEG changes precede CT scan evidence of encephalitis and provide a more sensitive, although nonspecific, diagnostic test than CT. Electroencephalogram changes in the temporal lobe area strongly support the diagnosis of HSE, but the absence of these changes does not rule it out.

Historically, patients with viral encephalitis required a battery of different diagnostic tests. Herpes simplex encephalitis, for example,

could be diagnosed acutely by brain biopsy and viral culture, or retrospectively by CSF antibody and convalescent serologic tests.[35] The diagnosis of enterovirus meningitis requires virus isolation from the throat or rectum acutely or serologic studies retrospectively. The use of PCR has revolutionized viral diagnostics and is rapidly becoming the new gold standard for diagnosis of viral infections of the CNS. Viral DNA is detectable in the CSF of patients with encephalitis with varying success, depending on the age of and extent of disease in the patient. The laboratory test is relatively rapid, has high sensitivity and provides a less invasive means to diagnose encephalitis. For example, only 4% of CSF cultures are positive in patients with sporadic HSE; however, 53 out of 54 patients with HSE confirmed by biopsy had evidence of HSV DNA in the CSF by PCR.[40] Cerebrospinal fluid PCR has a sensitivity of over 95% and a specificity approaching 100% in patients with HSE. Interestingly, in the three patients in whom the CSF PCR was positive but the brain biopsy negative, either biopsy samples had been improperly prepared before viral culture or the biopsy site was suboptimal. In the past, 50–75% of investigations failed to identify an etiology for encephalitis, depending on the study and diagnostic tests used.[10] The frequency of establishing an etiologic diagnosis will likely increase with the advent of this sensitive and less invasive diagnostic test.

The expeditious identification of treatable disease is a priority in patients presenting with neurologic changes. During the National Institute of Allergy and Infectious Disease Collaborative Antiviral Study Group clinical trials of vidarabine or aciclovir treatment of HSE, patients underwent brain biopsy for confirmation of disease before study enrolment. Of the 432 patients in the study only 195 (45%) had biopsy-confirmed HSE. A second group of 95 patients (22%) had another etiology established by brain biopsy. Of these 95 patients 38 had a treatable disease (9% of the entire study group) such as bacterial abscess, tuberculosis, fungal infection, tumor, subdural hematoma or autoimmune disease. The majority of the 57 identifiable but untreatable causes for encephalitis were of viral etiology. A third group of 142 patients (33%) went undiagnosed even after brain biopsy, CT scan, technetium brain scan, EEG and additional bacterial, fungal and virologic studies (culture from multiple sites and serologic studies).[2]

Pathologic processes in the CNS have limited clinical expressions and thus often produce similar signs and symptoms.[2] Mass lesions in the CNS (tumor, abscess or blood) can cause focal neurologic changes, fever and seizures similar to those of encephalitis. Metabolic (hypoglycemia, uremia, inborn errors of metabolism) and toxin-mediated disorders (ingestions, tick-paralysis or Reye's syndrome) can cause decreased consciousness, seizures and evidence of background slowing on EEG. Limbic encephalitis can produce a protracted encephalitis and is caused by paraneoplastic phenomena. Furthermore, nonviral infectious causes of encephalitis need to be vigorously investigated as these are frequently treatable. Mycoplasma produces a demyelinating brainstem encephalitis in 0.1% of infections. Diseases that mimic viral encephalitis are listed in Figure 16.4.

MANAGEMENT

Patients with encephalitis, depending on the etiology and extent of CNS involvement, require management to be tailored to their clinical situation.

Currently, few antiviral medications are available to treat CNS infections. Antiviral therapy exists for HSV-1, HSV-2, VZV and CMV. The introduction of aciclovir and vidarabine has resulted in a sharp decline in mortality and morbidity from herpes infections. Neonatal mortality from disseminated HSV disease and HSE has declined from 70 to 40% since the development of aciclovir and vidarabine. Antiviral treatment of disseminated HSE decreases the morbidity from 90 to 50% of survivors and reduces the severity of their neurologic impairment. Varicella immunoglobulin and aciclovir have reduced the complications from primary VZV infection and zoster in the neonate

DIFFERENTIAL DIAGNOSIS IN ENCEPHALITIS AND MENINGITIS

Infectious	Bacterial	*Mycoplasma*, *Ureaplasma*, *Legionella* and *Chlamydia* spp.
		Mycobacteria
		Spirochetes (*Treponema*, *Borrelia* and *Leptospira* spp.)
		Rickettsia, *Ehrlichia* and *Bartonella* spp.
		Nocardia and *Actinomyces* spp.
		Brucella and *Listeria* spp.
		Partially treated bacterial infection, CNS abscess, parameningeal infection, endocarditis
		Toxin-mediated
	Fungal	*Blastomyces*, *Candida*, *Histoplasma*, *Coccidioides*, *Aspergillus* and *Sporothrix* spp. and Zygomycetes
	Protozoa and parasites	Toxoplasmosis, *Taenia solium*, *Echinococcus* spp., *Strongyloides* spp., *Schistosoma* spp., *Acanthamoeba* spp., *Naegleria fowleri*, *Entamoeba histolytica*, *Trypanosoma* spp., *Plasmodium* spp.
Postinfectious	Guillain–Barré	
	Brainstem encephalitis	
	Miller–Fischer syndrome?	
	Viral postinfectious (VZV, measles, parainfluenza, influenza, RSV)	
Noninfectious	Drug-induced	Sulfa antibiotics, non-steroidal anti-inflammatory drugs, immunoglobulin, intrathecal injections, INH, penicillin, carbamazepine, ARA-C, azathioprine
	Rheumatologic disease	Systemic lupus erythematosus, sarcoidosis, Beçhet's and vasculitic diseases
	Tumors and masses	Brain tumors (gliomas, meningioma, medulloblastoma, etc.), CNS lymphomas, carcinomatous processes
		Arteriovenous malformation
	Poisonings and toxins	Lead, mercury, arsenic
		Reye's syndrome
		Drug ingestion
	Demyelinating disease	Multiple sclerosis
		Adrenal leukodystophy
	Vascular insult or trauma	Cerebrovascular accident or subarachnoid hemorrhage

Fig. 16.4 Differential diagnosis in encephalitis and meningitis. RSV, respiratory syncytial virus; ARA-C, cytarabine; INH, isoniazid.

and immunocompromised patient. Although controlled trials have not evaluated the efficacy of aciclovir in VZV encephalitis, it is routinely used to treat this complication. Antiviral medications have influenced the mortality and morbidity of VZV and HSV infections; however, with the emergence of aciclovir-resistant herpesviruses in immunocompromised patients, novel antiviral agents are needed for continued effective treatment of alphaherpesvirus infections.[13] With the increase of HIV infection, diseases previously limited to the neonatal and postnatal period now occur with increasing frequency in the adult population. Ganciclovir and foscarnet are used for the treatment of CMV encephalitis although clinical trials have not confirmed the efficacy of treatment. This is discussed in Chapter 4.4.

APPROACH TO THE PATIENT WITH VIRAL CNS DISEASE

The approach to a patient with a presumed CNS viral infection must be tailored to the severity of neurologic involvement Legient. Distinctions between meningitis and encephalitis are of little consequence as there

is significant overlap of syndromes. Disease severity is of greatest relevance. One approach is summarized in Figure 16.5. A single method for managing a patient with presumed viral CNS disease is not possible as the degree of diagnostic and therapeutic intervention differs according to the type of CNS disease. For example, a patient with photophobia and nuchal rigidity, but a nonfocal neurologic examination does not require invasive intracranial pressure monitoring like a patient with encephalitis and evidence of increased intracranial pressure. The first step of any intervention hinges on establishing the correct diagnosis. A history and physical examination are logical first steps in establishing a diagnosis. The thoroughness of the initial history and physical examination is tailored to the stability of the patient. A

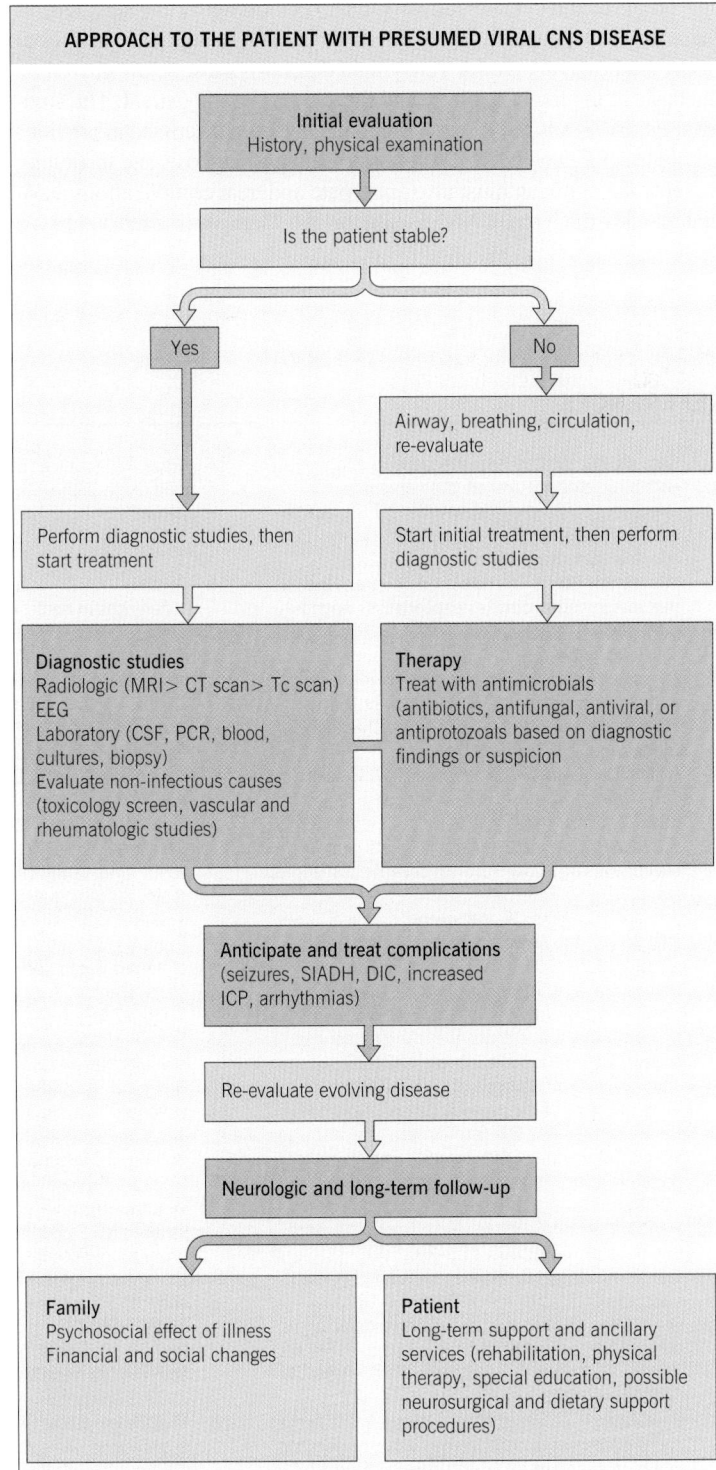

Fig. 16.5 Approach to the patient with presumed CNS viral infection. SIADH, syndrome of inappropriate antidiuretic hormone secretion; DIC, disseminated intravascular coagulation; ICP, intracranial pressure.

comatose individual with apneustic respirations requires immediate intervention, whereas in an individual with nuchal rigidity and photophobia there is time for a more detailed investigation for the etiology of the symptoms before any therapy is instituted. After establishing the degree of CNS disease by history and physical examination, and stabilizing the patient (airway, breathing, circulation), the clinician must ascertain a diagnosis.

Treatable causes of CNS dysfunction require rapid evaluation and intervention before further or permanent CNS damage ensues. Potentially treatable diseases (fungal CNS infections, partially treated bacterial meningitis, tuberculous meningitis, parameningeal infection, mycoplasma and fastidious bacterial infections) can mimic viral CNS disease and should be thoroughly and promptly investigated before the illness is attributed to an untreatable viral etiology. Treatable viral infections and noninfectious etiologies also must be thoroughly investigated, as these frequently require timely intervention. The radiographic and laboratory studies available for verifying a diagnosis must be prioritized on the basis of the likely etiology and the stability of the patient. The studies used to diagnose CNS viral infection have been discussed in previous sections (see Chapter 2.15). After establishing a diagnosis and instituting therapy, the clinician must also anticipate and treat complications associated with the viral CNS disease or the therapeutic interventions.

Seizures secondary to direct viral CNS damage, inflammatory vasculitis and electrolyte changes require anticonvulsant therapy with benzodiazepines, phenytoin and barbiturates. Patients with cerebral edema may require intracranial pressure monitoring and hyperventilation, osmotic therapy and CSF removal in an attempt to maintain cerebral pressures less than 15 torrs.[10] The risks of increased intracranial pressure from aggressive fluid resuscitation and/or the syndrome of inappropriate antidiuretic hormone secretion necessitate meticulous fluid management and frequent electrolyte monitoring. Cardiac arrhythmias can also develop in patients with encephalitis secondary to electrolyte changes or brainstem damage. Cardiac and respiratory arrest can occur early in disease; therefore, equipment for intubation and cardioversion should be readily available for a patient with encephalitis. In addition to the direct damage the virus can cause in the CNS, it can also produce systemic damage that complicates the management of the CNS disease. Patients can develop overwhelming hepatitis, pneumonitis, disseminated intravascular coagulation and shock. Intracranial pressures can rise to dangerous levels as capillary leak complicates the patient's course. Patients in coma from encephalitis can recover after long periods of unconsciousness. The physician should limit the amount of iatrogenic damage and vigorously support the patient during the acute phase of the illness.

REFERENCES

1. Cassady KA, Whitley KJ. Pathogenesis and pathophysiology of viral central nervous system infections. In: Scheld WM, Whitley RJ, Durack DT eds. Infections of the central nervous system. 2nd ed. New York: Raven Press; 1997:7–22.
2. Whitley RJ, Cobbs CG, Alford CA Jr, et al. Diseases that mimic herpes simplex encephalitis: diagnosis, presentation and outcome. JAMA 1989;262:234–9.
3. Cassady KA, Whitley RJ. Central nervous system infections. In: Richman DD, Whitley RJ, Hayden FG, eds. Clinical virology. New York: Churchill Livingstone; 1997:35–53.
4. Adams DH, Bell TM. Definition of slow viruses. In: Slow viruses. Reading: Addison–Wesley; 1976:7–15.
5. Johnson RT. The pathogenesis of acute viral encephalitis and postinfectious encephalitis. J Infect Dis 1987;155:359–64.
6. Johnson RT, Mims CA. Pathogenesis of viral infections of the nervous system. N Engl J Med 1968;278:23–30.
7. Rotbart HA. Viral meningitis and the aseptic meningitis syndrome. In: Scheld WM, Whitley RJ, Durack DT, eds. Infections of the central nervous system. New York: Raven Press; 1991:19–40.
8. Johnson RT. Pathogenesis of CNS infections. In: Viral Infections of the nervous system. New York: Raven Press; 1982:37–60.
9. Wilfert CM, Lehrman SN, Katz SL. Enteroviruses and meningitis. Pediatr Infect Dis J 1983;2:333–41.
10. Ho DD, Hirsch MS. Acute viral encephalitis. Med Clin North Am 1985;69:415–29.
11. Tsai TF. Arboviral infections in the United States. Infect Dis Clin North Am 1991;5:73–102.
12. Rotbart HA. Nucleic acid detection systems for enteroviruses. Clin Microbiol Rev 1991;4:156–68.
13. Whitley RJ, Gnann J. Acyclovir: a decade later. N Engl J Med 1992;327:782–9.
14. Rantakallio P, Leskinen M, von Wendt L. Incidence and prognosis of central nervous system infections in a birth cohort of 12,000 children. Scand J Infect Dis 1986;18:287–94.
15. Vaughn DW, Hoke CH Jr. The epidemiology of Japanese encephalitis: prospects for prevention. Epidemiol Rev 1992;14:197–221.
16. Mrak RE, Young L. Rabies encephalitis in humans: pathology, pathogenesis and pathophysiology. J Neuropathol Exp Neurol 1994;53:1–10.
17. Whitley RJ. Viral encephalitis. N Engl J Med 1990;323:242–50.
18. Nahmias AJ, Dowdle WR. Antigenic and biologic differences in herpesvirus hominis. Prog Med Virol 1968;10:110–59.
19. Roizman B, Sears AE. Herpes simplex viruses and their replication. In: Roizman B, Whitley RJ, Lopez C, eds. The human herpesviruses. New York: Raven Press; 1993:11–68.
20. Griffin DE. Viral infections of the central nervous system. In: Galasso GJ, Whitley RJ, Merigan TC, eds. Antiviral agents and viral diseases of man. New York: Raven Press; 1990:461–95.
21. Chretien F, Gray F, Lescs MC, et al. Acute varicella-zoster virus ventriculitis and meningo-myelo-radiculitis in acquired immunodeficiency syndrome. Acta Neuropathol 1993;86:659–65.
22. Burnett FM, Lush D, Jackson AV. The propagation of herpes B and pseudorabies viruses on the chorioallantois. Aust J Exp Biol Med Sci 1939;17:35.
23. Gay FP, Holden M. Isolation of herpes virus from several cases of epidemic encephalitis. Proc Soc Exp Biol Med 1933;30:1051–3.
24. Umenai T, Krzysko R, Bektimirov TA, et al. Japanese encephalitis: current worldwide status. Bull WHO 1985;63:625–31.
25. Monath TP. Alphavirus (Eastern, Western, and Venezuelan equine encephalitis). In: Mandell GL, Douglas RG Jr, Bennett JE, eds. Principles and practice of infectious diseases. New York: Churchill Livingstone; 1990:1241–2.
26. Luby JP. St Louis encephalitis. Epidemiol Rev 1979;1:55–73.
27. Monath TP, Tsai TF. St Louis encephalitis: lessons from the last decade. Am J Trop Med Hyg 1987;37(Suppl 3):40–59.
28. Murphy FA, Bauer SP, Harrison AK, et al. Comparative pathogenesis of rabies and rabies-like viruses: viral infection and transit from inoculation site to the central nervous system. Lab Invest 1973;28:361–76.
29. Adams RD, Kubik CS. The morbid anatomy of the demyelinative diseases. Am J Med 1952;12:510–46.
30. Johnson RT, Griffin DE, Hirsch RL, et al. Measles encephalomyelitis-clinical and immunological studies. N Engl J Med 1984;310:137–41.
31. Johnson RT. The virology of demyelinating diseases. Ann Neurol 1994;36(Suppl):54–60.
32. Kaplan MH, Klein SW, McPhee J, et al. Group B coxsackie virus infections in infants younger than three months of age. Rev Infect Dis 1983;5:1019–32.
33. Modlin JF. Perinatal echovirus infection: insights from a literature review of 61 cases of serious infection and 16 outbreaks in nurseries. Rev Infect Dis 1986;8:918–26.
34. Cherry JD. Enteroviruses: polioviruses (poliomyelitis), coxsackieviruses, echoviruses, and enteroviruses. In: Feigin RD, Cherry JD, eds. Textbook of pediatric infectious diseases. Philadelphia: WB Saunders; 1987:1729–841.
35. Nahmias AJ, Whitley RJ, Visintine AN, et al. Herpes simplex encephalitis: laboratory evaluations and their diagnostic significance. J Infect Dis 1982;145:829–36.
36. Assaad F. Measles: summary of worldwide impact. Rev Infect Dis 1983;5:452–9.
37. Johnson RT, Griffin DE, Gendelman HE. Postinfectious encephalomyelitis. Semin Neurol 1985;5:180–90.
38. Strebel PM, Sutter RW, Cochi SL, et al. Epidemiology of poliomyelitis in the United States one decade after the last reported case of indigenous wild virus-associated disease. Clin Infect Dis 1992;14:568–79.
39. Rosen L. The natural history of Japanese encephalitis virus. Ann Rev Microbiol 1986;40:395–414.
40. Lakeman FD, Whitley RJ, National Institute of Allergy and Infectious Disease CASG. Diagnosis of herpes simplex encephalitis: application of polymerase chain reaction to cerebrospinal fluid from brain biopsied patients and correlation with disease. J Infect Dis 1995;171:857–63.
41. Smith RR. Neuroradiology of intracranial infection. Pediatr Neurosurg 1992;18:92–104.

Brain Abscess and Other Focal Pyogenic Infections

Gregory C Townsend

A number of entities can be considered focal pyogenic infections of the central nervous system (CNS). These include brain abscess, spinal cord abscess, subdural empyema, epidural abscess and suppurative intracranial phlebitis. The year 1993 marked the 100th anniversary of the publication of *Pyogenic infective diseases of the brain and spinal cord* and *Atlas of head sections*, by Sir William MacEwen, which were landmarks in the descriptions of the anatomy and natural history of focal suppurative brain processes and of their management.[1]

As noted by MacEwen, these conditions are characterized by the presence of one or more localized and well defined collections of purulent material within the confines of the CNS (i.e. within the cranial vault or the paraspinal space). They exert their effects largely by direct involvement and destruction of the parenchyma of the brain or spinal cord, by encroachment on parenchyma, by elevation of intracranial pressure or by interference with flow of blood or of cerebrospinal fluid (CSF).

Infections in contiguous structures tend to lead to infections in certain areas of the cranial vault because of their anatomic relationships (Fig. 17.1). The frontal and ethmoidal paranasal sinuses underlie the anterior cranial fossa, so that infections in these sinuses often lead to infections in or near the frontal lobe. The sphenoid sinus neighbors the sella turcica, temporal lobes and cavernous sinuses; sphenoid sinusitis may lead to infections in the frontal or temporal lobes or the pituitary gland or to cavernous sinus thrombosis. Infections in the middle ear and mastoids may spread to the temporal lobe, cerebellum or brainstem. Because of the focal nature of these infections in the CNS, they often become manifest by focal neurologic deficits, rather than by more global CNS dysfunction such as may be seen with bacterial meningitis or with encephalitis. This chapter addresses the more common of these diseases (brain abscess, subdural empyema and epidural abscess) and touches only briefly on the others.

BRAIN ABSCESS

Brain abscess is a focal suppurative process of the parenchyma of the brain. The diagnosis and management of brain abscess have undergone considerable changes during the past few years as a result of a number of advances, including the introduction and widespread availability of noninvasive radiographic diagnostic techniques, the development and use of antimicrobial agents that demonstrate adequate penetration across the blood–brain barrier and into abscesses, and the refinement of minimally invasive surgical procedures.

EPIDEMIOLOGY

Although one of the more common of the focal pyogenic CNS infections, brain abscess is still an uncommon condition. Autopsy series report a cumulative lifetime incidence of approximately 1%.[2] Recent reports have indicated that brain abscesses account for approximately 1 in 10,000 hospital admissions in the USA.[3]

The predominant age of patients with brain abscesses depends on the predisposing factors; brain abscesses as a complication of otitis media are most common among young children and older adults, whereas those

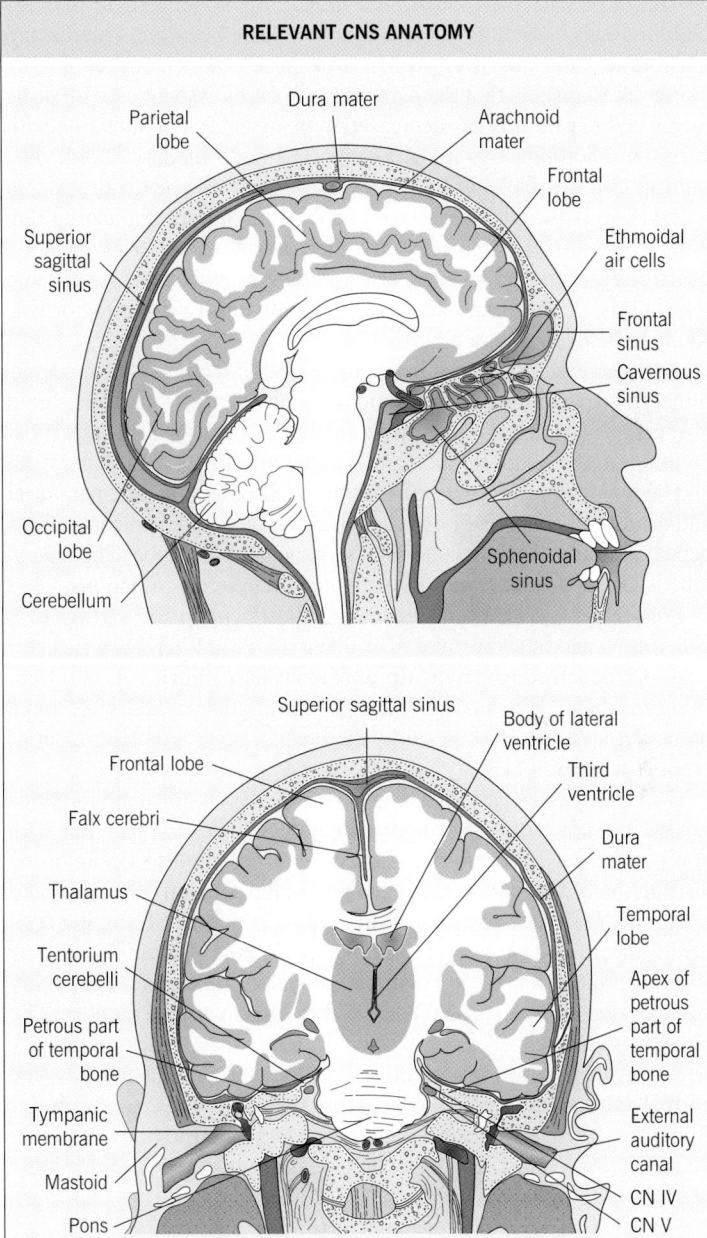

RELEVANT CNS ANATOMY

Fig. 17.1 Anatomic relationships between potential contiguous sources of infection and sites at which focal pyogenic central nervous system infections may occur.

caused by paranasal sinusitis are most common among older children and young adults.[3–6] Although there have been conflicting reports on the possibility of a male predominance, three series published within the past 10 years indicated that brain abscesses are approximately two to three times as common among males as among females.[3,5,7]

Several major clinical settings that predispose to brain abscess have been identified:

- association with a contiguous focus of infection (e.g. sinusitis, otitis media),
- after trauma (e.g. penetrating head injury, neurosurgery),
- hematogenous spread from a distant focus (e.g. in association with lung abscess), and
- cryptogenic (no recognized focus).

Brain abscesses associated with a contiguous focus account for approximately 40–50% of the total; the percentage of cases without an identified predisposing factor has been reduced to approximately 15% with the use of new sensitive imaging procedures.[6–8] In addition to these settings, brain abscesses have been reported after cerebrovascular accidents.

The most commonly identified underlying conditions in patients with brain abscess in developed countries have been otitis media and mastoiditis, and this may still be true in less developed countries. However, it appears that the percentage of cases associated with otitis media and mastoiditis has decreased in many areas in association with early antimicrobial therapy for suspected otitis media. Recent data indicate that the risk of brain abscess in patients who have otitis media is less than 0.5%.[9,10] There have been several reports indicating that brain abscess is associated with other conditions such as cyanotic heart disease and trauma at least as often as with otitis media and mastoiditis.[7,11] In Turkey, the most common predisposing factor was found to be bacterial meningitis.[12]

As noted earlier, the location of focal CNS infections is often determined by proximity to a contiguous focus of infection. Thus, brain abscesses associated with otitis media and mastoiditis are most common in the temporal lobe and cerebellum (Fig. 17.2). Other head and neck infections associated with brain abscesses include paranasal and dental infections. Brain abscesses associated with sinus infections occur primarily in the frontal lobe or in the temporal lobe. The frontal lobe is also the most commonly affected after dental infections.

Post-traumatic brain abscesses usually occur in the setting of a penetrating wound, but may also occur in closed-head injuries, for example penetrating pencil tip and lawn dart injuries in children. Presentation of the abscess may occur months or years after the precipitating event. In one study, the median time to development of brain abscess was 113 days.[13]

Brain abscesses that occur at a distant site with hematogenous spread are often multiple; approximately 10–15% of patients with brain abscesses have multiple abscesses. They tend to occur in the distribution of the middle cerebral artery at the junction of the gray and white matter, where microcirculatory flow is poorest. Cyanotic congenital heart disease and chronic pyogenic lung diseases (e.g. lung abscess, bronchiectasis) are common predisposing factors. Hereditary hemorrhagic telangiectasia (Osler–Weber–Rendu disease) is also associated with brain abscess; it is thought that in these cases pulmonary arteriovenous malformations allow septic microemboli to bypass the normal pulmonary filter and gain access to the cerebral circulation.[14,15] Brain abscesses have been reported after dental extractions and other manipulations, dilatation of esophageal strictures and endoscopic sclerosis of esophageal varices.

PATHOGENESIS AND PATHOLOGY

The main pathogenetic factors responsible for the development of brain abscesses are a source of virulent micro-organisms and the presence of ischemic or devitalized brain tissue. The vulnerability of compromised tissue to brain abscess is illustrated by the occurrence of brain abscesses after trauma or after cerebrovascular accident, their association with cyanotic heart or lung disease and their predilection for areas of poor local perfusion such as the junction of gray and white matter.

Experimental models have demonstrated differences in the abilities of various micro-organisms to induce brain abscesses. Not only are certain species (i.e. *Escherichia coli* and *Staphylococcus aureus)* more likely to

SITE OF BRAIN ABSCESS BASED ON PREDISPOSING CONDITION	
Predisposing condition	Site
Otitis media or mastoiditis	Temporal lobe Cerebellum
Paranasal sinusitis	Frontal lobe Temporal lobe
Dental infection/manipulation	Frontal lobe
Trauma/neurosurgery	Related to wound
Meningitis	Cerebellum Frontal lobe
Cyanotic heart disease	Middle cerebral artery distribution
Pyogenic lung disease	
Bacterial endocarditis	
Gastrointestinal source	
T-lymphocyte deficiency	
Neutropenia	

Fig. 17.2 Site of brain abscess based on predisposing condition.

cause abscesses than others (e.g. *Streptococcus pyogenes*) but there are also differences between strains, such as possession of a capsule.[16,17]

Two mechanisms have been postulated by which brain abscess may occur in association with a contiguous focus of infection: direct extension through infected bone; or hematogenous spread through emissary veins or diploic veins or spread through local lymphatics. Infections associated with otogenic infections may also spread through the internal auditory canal, between suture lines or through cochlear aqueducts. Brain abscesses developing after trauma or after neurosurgical procedures may follow deep wound injury with direct inoculation into the brain parenchyma, or may be a result of extension of a superficial infection through compromised tissue.

The areas of the brain most commonly involved by solitary brain abscess are the frontal and temporal lobes, followed by the frontoparietal region, and parietal, cerebellar and occipital lobes.[18] These areas are the most likely to be associated with a contiguous focus of infection or hematogenous seeding. Although rare, abscesses in other areas, such as the pituitary gland, thalamus, basal ganglia and brainstem, may occur and may be associated with specific predisposing conditions. For example, abscesses of the pituitary are often associated with pre-existing pituitary adenomas and with sphenoidal sinusitis.

Experimental animal data, surgery and autopsy findings and radiographic examinations indicate that brain abscesses develop in a four-stage process.[19] These stages are early and late cerebritis (days 1–3 and 4–9, respectively) and early and late capsule formation (days 10–13 and day 14 and later, respectively), and represent a continuum rather than discrete steps. The evolution of this process is dependent upon the causative organism, local factors, host immunologic status and antimicrobial therapy.

The microbiology of brain abscess is dependent upon the site of the initiating infection, the patient's underlying condition and geographic location (Fig. 17.3). The organisms most commonly isolated are streptococci, the Enterobacteriaceae, anaerobes, *S. aureus* and fungi; approximately 30–60% are polymicrobial. Fungi were the organisms most commonly isolated in a report from Saudi Arabia.[20] Fungi are particularly common causes of brain abscesses in immunocompromised patients; *Aspergillus* spp. are especially common in patients with bone marrow and solid organ transplants.[21] Patients with defects in T-lymphocyte immunity (including patients who have AIDS) are predisposed to infections with organisms such as *Toxoplasma gondii*, *Nocardia* spp., *Cryptococcus neoformans*, *Mycobacterium* spp. and fungi.

Infections acquired in the tropics have a broader differential diagnosis, including several parasites (e.g. amebiasis) (see Chapters 6.5 & 6.20).

PREVENTION

The primary means of prevention of brain abscesses and of other focal CNS infections is the appropriate use of antibiotics in patients with predisposing infections such as otitis media and mastoiditis. Other preventive measures include those taken to correct or to prevent other predisposing conditions. These include surgical correction of cyanotic congenital heart disease, maintenance of dental hygiene, management of pyogenic lung infections and attention to proper sterile techniques during neurosurgical procedures. In patients with underlying T-lymphocyte defects, measures to prevent exposure to *T. gondii* are recommended.

LIKELY PATHOGENS AND SUGGESTED EMPIRIC THERAPY FOR BRAIN ABSCESS

Predisposing condition	Likely pathogens	Empiric therapy
Otitis media or mastoiditis	Streptococci (anaerobic and aerobic)	Third-generation cephalosporin + metronidazole
	Bacteroides spp.	A penicillin
	Enterobacteriaceae	
Paranasal sinusitis	Streptococci	Third-generation cephalosporin ± metronidazole
	Bacteroides spp.	
	Enterobacteriaceae	
	Staphylococcus aureus	
Dental infection or manipulation	Streptococci	Penicillin ± metronidazole
	Fusobacterium spp.	
	Bacteroides spp.	
Trauma or neurosurgery	*Staphylococcus aureus*	Antistaphylococcal penicillin + third-generation cephalosporin
	Coagulase–negative staphylococci	
	Enterobacteriaceae	
	Streptococci	Vancomycin
	Pseudomonas aeruginosa	
Cyanotic heart disease	Streptococci	Third-generation cephalosporin
	Haemophilus spp.	
Pyogenic lung disease	Streptococci	Penicillin or third-generation cephalosporin + metronidazole
	Nocardia asteroides	
	Actinomyces spp.	
	Fusobacterium spp.	
	Bacteroides spp.	
Bacterial endocarditis	Viridans streptococci	Ampicillin and gentamicin ± antistaphylococcal penicillin
	Staphylococcus aureus	
	Enterococci	
	Haemophilus spp.	
Gastrointestinal source	Enterobacteriaceae	Third-generation cephalosporin
T-lymphocyte deficiency	*Toxoplasma gondii*	Variable
	Nocardia spp.	
Neutropenia	Enterobacteriaceae	Third- or fourth-generation cephalosporin, meropenem
	Pseudomonas aeruginosa	
	Fungi, especially *Aspergillus* and *Mucor*	Amphotericin B

Fig. 17.3 Likely pathogens and suggested empiric therapy for brain abscess based on predisposing condition.

CLINICAL FEATURES

As noted earlier, the clinical manifestations of brain abscess and other focal suppurative CNS processes are largely caused by the presence of a space-occupying lesion.[18,22,23] The most common symptom is headache, which is usually hemicranial. Other common symptoms include fever, focal neurologic findings (especially hemiparesis), nausea and vomiting and seizures (usually generalized). Nuchal rigidity may occur if the abscess is contiguous with or near the meninges.

Other signs and symptoms vary depending on the stage, size and anatomic location of the abscess. Those of the frontal lobe are characterized by global mental status changes, hemiparesis and expressive speech disturbances. Temporal lobe abscesses may manifest with headache and aphasia (if the abscess involves the dominant hemisphere). Cerebellar abscesses are associated with vomiting, ataxia, nystagmus and dysmetria. Vomiting, hemiparesis, dysphagia and facial weakness may be seen with brainstem abscesses. Rapid deterioration with new onset of nuchal rigidity suggests the possibility of rupture of an abscess into the intraventricular or subarachnoid space.

Routine laboratory findings may include a peripheral leukocytosis and a left shift, but approximately 40% of patients with brain abscess have normal leukocyte concentrations. The erythrocyte sedimentation rate is often elevated. An elevated C-reactive protein has been found to be sensitive (77–90%) and specific (77–100%) when used to distinguish brain abscess from cerebral neoplasms.

The differential diagnosis of brain abscess includes subdural empyema, epidural abscess, bacterial meningitis, cerebral neoplasm, cerebrovascular accident and encephalitis.

DIAGNOSIS

Radiographic imaging with contrast-enhanced CT or MRI have contributed greatly to the diagnosis and management of brain abscess. They have obviated the need for more invasive techniques such as pneumoencephalography and myelography. Plain skull radiographs are insensitive but the presence of air indicates the need for further evaluation. Technetium-99 (^{99m}Tc) brain scanning is very sensitive and is the procedure of choice when CT or MRI is unavailable; there is some evidence that ^{99m}Tc scanning may be more sensitive than CT in the early cerebritis stage. ^{99m}Tc-hexamethylpropyleneamine oxime-labeled leukocyte single-photon emission CT has been examined as a potential means of distinguishing brain abscess from other focal cerebral parenchymal lesions, such as neoplasms. Ultrasonography may also be used if other techniques are unavailable.

The characteristic appearance of brain abscess on CT scan varies with the stage of the disease.[24] During the cerebritis stage, cerebral edema is prominent; no abnormalities may be seen in the early cerebritis stage. As capsule formation progresses, the abscess appears as a lesion with a hypodense center composed of necrotic debris surrounded by ring enhancement, which may in turn be surrounded by hypodense cerebral edema (Fig. 17.4). Although highly sensitive, CT scanning is not specific. These findings may also be seen in patients with cerebral neoplasms, cerebrovascular accidents or granulomas.

Magnetic resonance imaging is more sensitive than CT in the early cerebritis stage of brain abscess; the latter appears as slightly low intensity on MRI T1-weighted images and very low intensity on MRI T2-weighted images. Magnetic resonance imaging may be more sensitive in diagnosing possible lesions in the posterior fossa because of the absence of bone artifact (Fig. 17.5).[25] Also, MRI may allow distinction of abscess fluid from CSF, which may be important if intraventricular rupture is suspected. Enhancement with gadolinium–DTPA allows evaluation of disruption of the blood–brain barrier, and permits greater distinction of the radiographic appearance of the central abscess, capsule and surrounding edema. Examination by means of ^{1}H magnetic resonance spectroscopic imaging has been proposed as a means of distinguishing brain abscess from other focal cerebral parenchymal lesions.

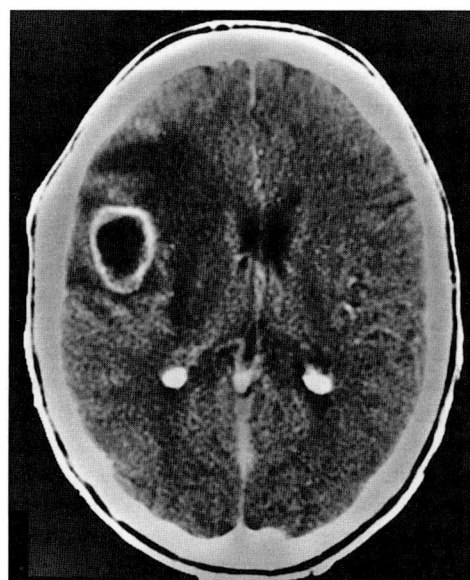
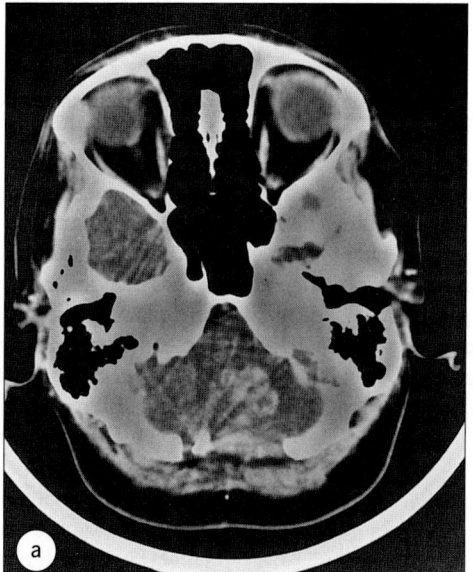
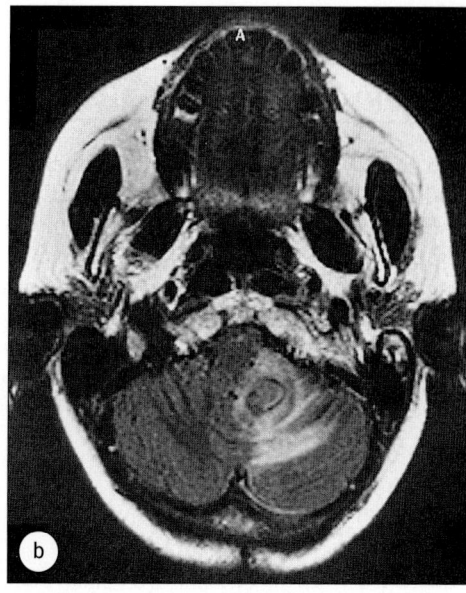

Fig. 17.4 Contrast-enhanced CT scan of the head in the coronal projection of a 43-year-old man with an atrial septal defect that persisted after attempts at surgical repair. The patient presented with seizures after undergoing dental work for which he did not receive antimicrobial prophylaxis. Note the ring-enhancing lesion in the right frontoparietal region with edema and mass effect.

Fig. 17.5 Contrast-enhanced CT and MRI scans of the head in the coronal projection of a 43-year-old woman with headaches after a recent fall on her head. (a) CT scan image reveals a cystic ring-enhancing lesion in the left cerebellum. Note the prominent bone artifact. (b) T1-weighted MRI scan image reveals an enhancing cystic lesion in the left cerebellum with significant surrounding edema. Bone artifact is absent. Both CT and MRI scans were felt to be most consistent with a primary or metastatic neoplasm, but culture of material obtained at stereotactically guided aspiration grew *Staphylococcus aureus*.

It must be noted that the appearance of edema and contrast enhancement on CT and MRI may be diminished or absent in immunocompromised patients, possibly because of the poor host inflammatory response.

Lumbar puncture should be avoided in patients with known or suspected brain abscess. The yield from CSF culture is low (less than 10% positive) and the risk of herniation is considerable (approximately 15–30%). In patients who may have meningitis, blood cultures should be obtained and appropriate empiric therapy should be initiated, then an imaging procedure should be performed. Lumbar puncture may be performed if there is no evidence of a mass lesion.

MANAGEMENT

Most patients with brain abscess require surgical drainage. In addition to its role as a therapeutic measure, drainage also allows for collection and microbiologic evaluation of abscess material, which may be important in guiding antimicrobial therapy. It is now clear that aspiration is as effective as excision in most patients, and is less invasive, and thus has become the procedure of choice. Stereotaxic CT-guided aspiration permits accurate access even to areas that had been difficult to reach by aspiration, such as the brainstem, cerebellum and thalamus.[26] Multiple abscesses may thus be drained. Neuroendoscopic aspiration has also been used with success in a small number of patients.

Abscess material should be examined by Gram stain and by aerobic and anaerobic cultures at a minimum. The clinical setting may also dictate the use of special stains and cultures for fungi, mycobacteria and protozoa. Polymerase chain reaction examination of CSF may be useful in diagnosing tuberculous brain abscesses.

Antibiotics used in the management of brain abscess should be parenteral, have activity against the pathogens that are likely in a given clinical situation, penetrate abscess fluid (and the site of any underlying infection) in adequate concentrations and be bactericidal. The combination of penicillin or a third-generation cephalosporin (cefotaxime or ceftriaxone) plus metronidazole is effective as empiric therapy for most patients (see Fig. 17.3). An antistaphylococcal

penicillin (such as nafcillin, oxacillin or flucloxacillin) should be used if staphylococci are suspected. Vancomycin should be used instead if methicillin resistance is suspected or identified. In patients with intraventricular rupture of brain abscess, it has been recommended that optimal management should include open craniotomy with debridement, intraventricular lavage and intraventricular as well as intravenous antibiotics. Changes in therapy in all cases should be guided by results of microbiologic examination and by clinical and radiographic progress. Fungal brain abscess has a very poor prognosis; it's management is discussed in more detail in Chapters 4.5 & 8.26.

There is a great deal of evidence that there are certain circumstances under which brain abscess may be treated without surgical drainage. Small abscesses (less than 3cm in diameter) and abscesses in the cerebritis stage may respond to antimicrobial therapy alone. Medical therapy alone may also be indicated if the patient is a poor surgical candidate. In these cases, prolonged courses of antibiotics (at least 8 weeks of parenteral therapy) and close monitoring with sequential CT or MRI scans are necessary; MRI may be especially useful here because of its lack of ionizing radiation.

Although the optimal duration of antimicrobial therapy for brain abscess after surgical drainage has not been established, many authorities recommend 4–6 weeks of parenteral antibiotics. Radiographic imaging procedures should be used for monitoring of therapy. Radiographic abnormalities may persist for months after successful therapy of brain abscesses (Fig. 17.6).

Adjunctive therapy with corticosteroids, mannitol and hyperventilation may be indicated in patients with evidence of increased intracranial pressure. The routine use of corticosteroids in the absence of increased intracranial pressure cannot be recommended.

The prognosis for patients with brain abscess has improved considerably, particularly since the introduction of CT scanning. Mortality is now less than 30% in most series. Long-term sequelae may occur in about one-third of patients and include mental retardation, seizures and focal neurologic deficits. Poor prognostic factors include delayed or missed diagnosis, multiple lesions, deep-seated lesions, intraventricular rupture, coma, fungal etiology and extremes of age.

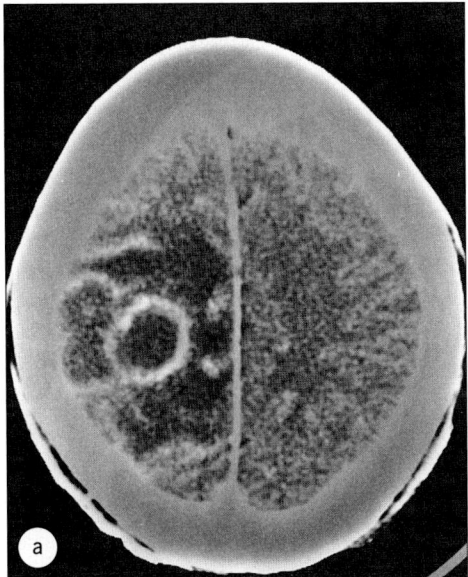

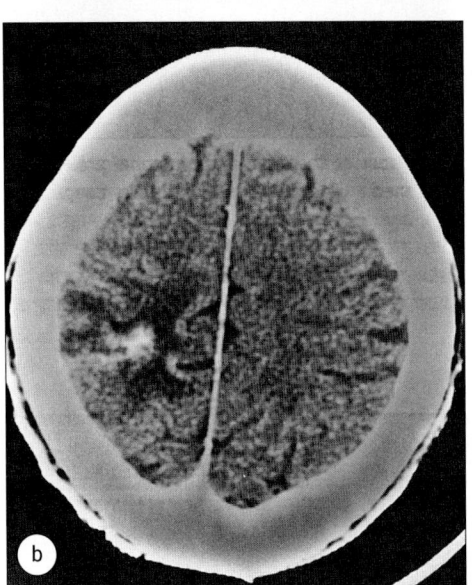

Fig. 17.6 Contrast-enhanced CT scans of the head in the coronal projection of a 66-year-old woman with a group B streptococcal brain abscess demonstrating evolution of the abscess during and after surgical and antimicrobial therapy. (a) The original scan demonstrates a hypodense necrotic center surrounded by an enhancing capsule and hypodense edema. (b) Seven weeks later, after stereotactically guided aspiration and a full course of antimicrobial therapy, the central cavity can no longer be seen, although the enhancement and surrounding edema persists to a small degree.

Considerable advances have been made in the diagnosis and management of brain abscess, and these have been associated with improved patient outcomes. Further advances in imaging, surgical techniques and antimicrobial therapy may lead to further reductions in morbidity and mortality.

SUBDURAL EMPYEMA AND INTRACRANIAL EPIDURAL ABSCESS

Subdural empyema and epidural abscess are focal collections of purulent material between the dura mater and arachnoid mater, and outside of the dura mater, respectively. Subdural empyema accounts for approximately 15–20% of all focal intracranial infections.

EPIDEMIOLOGY

Subdural empyema in adults is most often a complication of acute or chronic bacterial paranasal sinusitis, otitis media or mastoiditis.[27,28] It is the most common intracranial complication of sinusitis, accounting for approximately 60% of such cases.[29] The frontal and ethmoidal sinuses are the foci in well over one-half of the cases. Hematogenous spread from a distant source may also occur. In children the most common predisposing condition is bacterial meningitis. Other predisposing conditions include trauma (such as neurosurgical procedures) and infection of

a pre-existing subdural hematoma. As with brain abscess, there is a male predominance among patients with subdural empyema.

Intracranial epidural abscess usually follows paranasal sinusitis (particularly frontal), otitis media, mastoiditis or cranial trauma.

PATHOGENESIS AND PATHOLOGY

As with brain abscesses, extension of infection into the epidural or subdural space from a contiguous focus may occur by extension through infected bone or by hematogenous seeding through emissary veins. Intracranial epidural abscess is almost always associated with subdural empyema and with overlying osteomyelitis. In patients with subdural empyema, infection can spread rapidly through the subdural space until limited by its natural boundaries. These include the falx cerebri, tentorium cerebelli, base of the brain, foramen magnum posteriorly and the anterior spinal canal. Within the compartments defined by these boundaries, as the infection progresses it behaves as an expanding mass lesion.

As the lesion expands, intracranial pressure increases and the cerebral parenchyma is compromised. Interference with flow of blood or of CSF may cause cerebral edema and hydrocephalus. Septic thrombosis of veins within the affected subdural or epidural space may lead to thrombosis of cavernous sinuses or cortical veins, leading to infarction of brain tissue.

Organisms commonly isolated from adult patients with subdural empyema and intracranial epidural abscess include anaerobes, aerobic streptococci, staphylococci, *Streptococcus pneumoniae*, *Haemophilus influenzae* and other Gram-negative bacilli. Polymicrobial infections are common. In children, the most common causative agents are those that are responsible for the underlying meningitis. In the past, this has been *H. influenzae* in children over 3 months of age, but as the relative frequency of *H. influenzae* meningitis declines it is likely that its role in subdural empyema will also diminish.

CLINICAL FEATURES

The most prominent early symptoms associated with subdural empyema and intracranial epidural abscess are fever and headache. The headache is often focal at onset but may become generalized. These symptoms are usually followed by focal neurologic defects. Abscesses near the petrous portion of the temporal bone may be associated with V and VI cranial nerve palsies, causing unilateral facial pain and lateral rectus muscle weakness. Signs of increased intracranial pressure (such as vomiting, gait disturbances and mental status changes) and of meningeal irritation may follow, and may be accompanied by seizures, hemiparesis and hemisensory defects.

DIAGNOSIS

The procedures of choice in the diagnosis of subdural empyema and epidural abscess are CT or MRI scanning. Imaging reveals a hypodense lesion with displacement of the arachnoid mater in both entities, with accompanying displacement of the dura mater noted in patients with subdural empyema. Mass effect is more common with subdural empyema than with epidural abscess (Fig. 17.7). Capsule formation with contrast enhancement may be seen in either condition, but is more common with epidural abscess (Fig. 17.8). Cranial osteomyelitis may also be noted in patients with underlying contiguous foci of infection. Gadolinium-enhanced MRI may detect lesions not noted on CT (because the lesions may be isodense with the cerebral tissue on CT). As with brain abscess, lumbar puncture is contraindicated in patients with known or suspected subdural empyema or epidural abscess (see Chapters 4.5 & 8.26).

MANAGEMENT

Surgical evacuation is necessary for management of most patients with subdural empyema and intracranial epidural abscess. This should

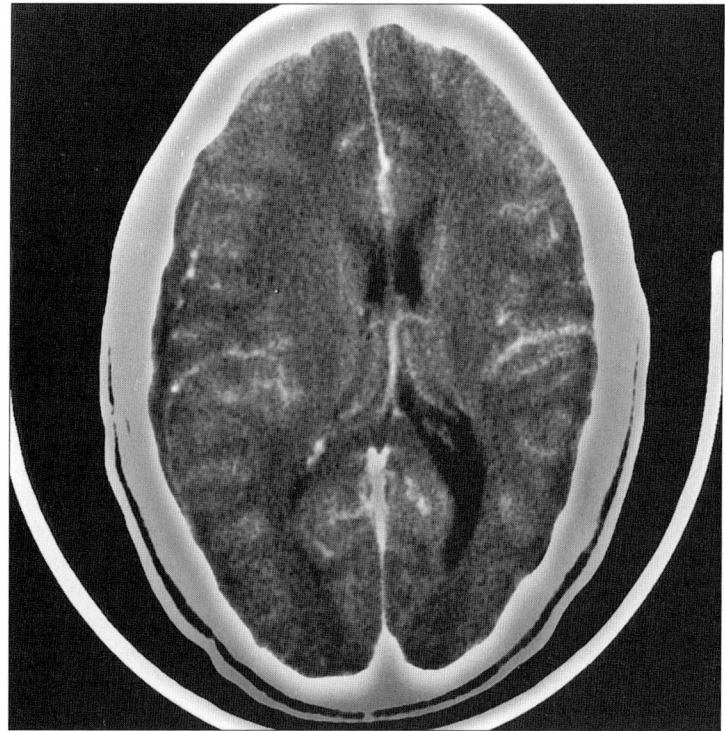

Fig. 17.7 Contrast-enhanced CT scan of the head in the coronal projection of a 23-year-old man with fever and headache. There is a small isodense extra-axial fluid collection in the subdural space on the right, with significant mass effect shown by right-to-left midline shift and effacement of the right lateral ventricle. There was also opacification of the frontal and ethmoid sinuses, suggesting sinusitis as the source of this subdural empyema.

Fig. 17.8 Contrast-enhanced CT scan of the head in the coronal projection of a 19-year-old man with otitis media who presented with sinus congestion 1 week earlier. Plain films of the sinuses revealed opacification of the right maxillary and ethmoidal sinuses, and an intracranial air–fluid level. Note the intracranial gas in the right frontal region abutting a hypodense region in the epidural space with ring enhancement and surrounding edema, representing an intracranial epidural abscess.

be accomplished by craniotomy or by the use of burr holes. It may also be necessary to debride the primary source of infection. Samples should be submitted for Gram stain and aerobic and anaerobic cultures. Antimicrobial therapy alone may be used for a limited number of patients with very small collections of fluid.

The choice of empiric antimicrobial therapy is dependent upon the age of the patient and the site of the primary infection (Fig. 17.9). In adults, the wide variety of possible pathogens and the potential for polymicrobial infection dictates the use of broad-spectrum therapy. In children, therapy should be directed against the likely causes of meningitis. Parenteral antimicrobial therapy should be continued for 3–6 weeks, with close monitoring of clinical status and radiographic appearance.

SUPPURATIVE INTRACRANIAL PHLEBITIS

Suppurative intracranial phlebitis is inflammation of the blood vessels within the cranium as a result of infection.[30]

PATHOGENESIS AND PATHOLOGY

These infections usually follow infections of the paranasal sinuses, middle ear, mastoids, face and oropharynx. They may also occur in association with subdural empyema, epidural abscess or bacterial meningitis. Conditions associated with increased blood viscosity or hypercoagulability increase the risk of suppurative intracranial phlebitis.

Spread generally occurs along emissary veins. The venous sinuses most commonly involved are the cavernous sinus, lateral sinus and superior sagittal sinus. If there is sufficient involvement of the vasculature, cerebral edema and hemorrhagic infarction may result. The infarcts tend to occur in venous watershed regions. Involvement of the superior sagittal sinus or of the lateral sinuses may block reabsorption of CSF and lead to hydrocephalus and increased intracranial pressure.

PATHOGENS AND SUGGESTED EMPIRIC ANTIBIOTIC REGIMENS FOR SUBDURAL EMPYEMA AND INTRACRANIAL EPIDURAL ABSCESS

Predisposing condition	Likely pathogens	Empiric therapy
Paranasal sinusitis	Streptococci *Bacteroides* spp. *Staphylococcus aureus* Enterobacteriaceae *Haemophilus influenzae*	Third-generation cephalosporin + metronidazole ± antistaphylococcal penicillin or A penicillin
Otitis media or mastoiditis	Streptococci *Bacteroides* spp. *Staphylococcus aureus* Enterobacteriaceae *Pseudomonas aeruginosa*	Third-generation cephalosporin + metronidazole ± antistaphylococcal penicillin or A penicillin
Trauma	*Staphylococcus aureus* Coagulase-negative staphylococci Enterobacteriaceae	Vancomycin + third-generation cephalosporin
Dental infection	*Bacteroides* spp. Streptococci *Fusobacterium* spp.	Penicillin or third-generation cephalosporin + metronidazole
Neonate	Enterobacteriaceae Group B streptococci *Listeria monocytogenes*	Third-generation cephalosporin + ampicillin
Infant or child	*Streptococcus pneumoniae* *Haemophilus influenzae* *Neisseria meningitidis*	Third-generation cephalosporin ± Vancomycin

Fig. 17.9 Pathogens and suggested empiric antibiotic regimens for subdural empyema and intracranial epidural abscess based on underlying condition.

There may also be subsequent involvement of contiguous structures leading to brain abscess, subdural empyema, epidural abscess, meningitis or distant seeding and infection of the lungs and other organs.

The microbiology of suppurative intracranial phlebitis is similar to that of subdural empyema and intracranial epidural abscess, with *S. aureus*, streptococci and anaerobes being most commonly identified.

CLINICAL FEATURES

The clinical manifestations of suppurative intracranial phlebitis vary with the location of the involved venous sinuses or cortical veins.

Cavernous sinus thrombosis is associated with palsies of cranial nerves III, IV, V and VI, producing loss of corneal reflexes, ophthalmoplegia and hypesthesia over the upper part of the face. Papilledema and visual loss may result from obstruction of retinal venous return.

Lateral sinus thrombosis involves cranial nerves V and VI, resulting in altered facial sensation and lateral rectus muscle weakness. Obstruction of venous CSF resorption may cause communicating hydrocephalus and increased intracranial pressure. Cranial nerves IX, X and XI may also be affected.

Involvement of the superior sagittal sinus may also diminish CSF resorption. In addition, obstruction of venous drainage from the motor cortex region of the cerebral hemispheres may lead to weakness of the legs.

Cortical vein thrombosis may be neurologically silent or produce only transient defects if collateral venous drainage can compensate for thrombosis. If collateral flow is inadequate, the lesion will manifest as progressive neurologic defects. The precise nature of the defects depends on the location of the veins involved. Unilateral or bilateral extremity weakness, hemiparesis, aphasia, seizures and changes in mental status may be seen.

DIAGNOSIS

The diagnostic procedure of choice is MRI as it is more sensitive than CT. The appearance of suppurative intracranial phlebitis on MRI is that of increased signal within the involved vessel (Fig. 17.10). Sensitivity of MRI can be enhanced by the use of magnetic resonance angiography. Computed tomography may be used when MRI is unavailable. If CT or MRI are unremarkable and suppurative intracranial phlebitis is still suspected, angiography should be performed.

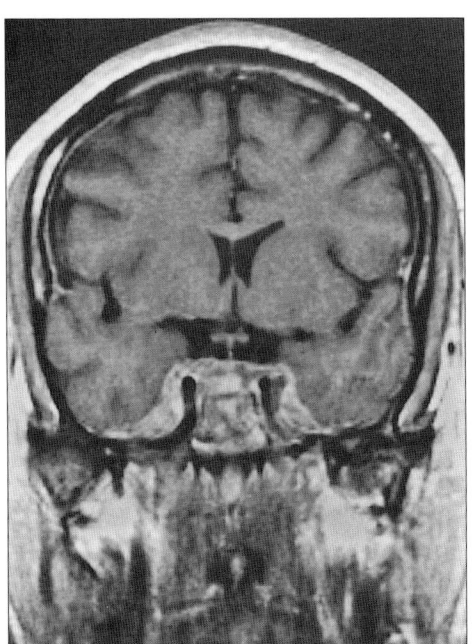

Fig. 17.10 Contrast-enhanced MRI scan of the head in the sagittal projection of a 29-year-old man with sinus congestion and headache. There is nonuniform signal intensity of the cavernous venous sinuses, indicating cavernous sinus thrombosis. The sphenoid, ethmoidal and maxillary paranasal sinuses also demonstrated abnormal signal intensity.

MANAGEMENT

Empiric antimicrobial therapy is similar to that employed for subdural empyema and intracranial epidural abscess (see Fig. 17.3). It may be necessary to control increased intracranial pressure with adjunctive measures such as corticosteroids, hyperosmolar agents and hyperventilation. Anticoagulant therapy has been used with some success, but carries with it the risk of hemorrhagic infarction. Surgery may be required for drainage of associated abscesses.

SPINAL EPIDURAL ABSCESS

Spinal epidural abscess is focal infection of the paraspinal epidural space.

PATHOGENESIS AND PATHOLOGY

Spinal epidural abscess may be secondary to a contiguous source of infection, such as vertebral osteomyelitis, penetrating trauma or decubitus ulcers, or may arise by hematogenous spread from a distant source.[27,31,32] A history of back trauma is common. In addition to pulmonary infections and infective endocarditis, as seen in patients with brain abscess and subdural empyema, possible sources for hematogenous seeding of the spinal epidural space include intra-abdominal, pelvic and genitourinary infections. Spread from these sources occurs via the paravertebral venous plexus.

In most cases in adults, the thoracic spine is involved, whereas cervical and lumbar involvement are more common in children. There is a male predominance.

The organism responsible for the majority of cases of spinal epidural abscess is *S. aureus*. Aerobic and anaerobic streptococci, *E. coli* and *Pseudomonas aeruginosa* are also common. Polymicrobial infections may occur, but are uncommon.

CLINICAL FEATURES

Four clinical stages have been described for spinal epidural abscess:
* fever and focal back pain;
* nerve root compression with nerve root pain;
* spinal cord compression with accompanying deficits in motor and sensory nerves and bowel and bladder sphincter function; and
* paralysis (respiratory compromise may also be present if the cervical cord is involved).[33]

Progression tends to be rapid with infection caused by direct hematogenous spread, and may be accompanied by severe pain. Progression to the second stage tends to occur slowly in patients with abscesses secondary to vertebral osteomyelitis, but may accelerate after that.

Headache, meningismus and focal tenderness are common signs and symptoms. Laboratory evaluation often reveals leukocytosis and elevated erythrocyte sedimentation rate in acute cases.

DIAGNOSIS

Gadolinium-enhanced MRI has supplanted CT and myelography as the diagnostic procedure of choice for spinal epidural abscess (Fig. 17.11).[34] Magnetic resonance imaging is highly sensitive and can identify osteomyelitis and intramedullary spinal cord lesions. If MRI is not available, myelography should be performed.

MANAGEMENT

Surgical drainage is indicated for the management of most patients with spinal epidural abscess. This should ordinarily be achieved by laminectomy, but CT-guided aspiration may be performed in selected patients. Antimicrobial therapy alone may be considered in patients who have not progressed to the third stage of the illness (i.e. those

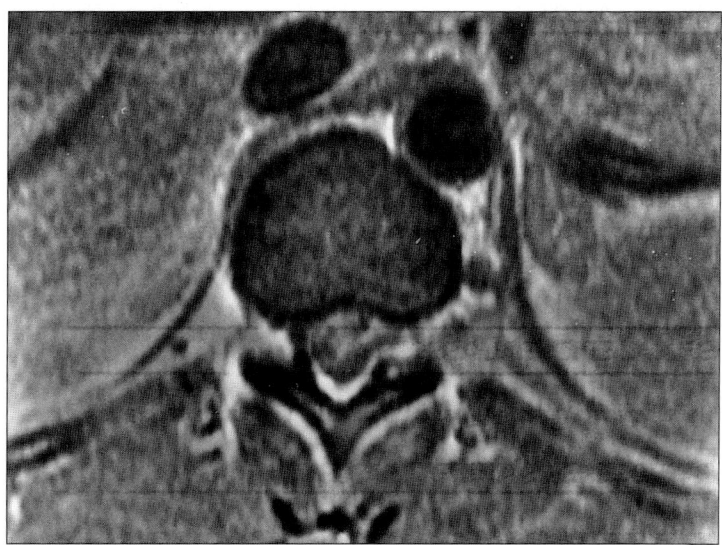

Fig. 17.11 Contrast-enhanced MRI scan of the spine in the coronal projection of a 28-year-old man with a 1-week history of headache, fever and sweats. Physical examination demonstrated meningismus but no focal neurologic deficits. Scans in the sagittal section demonstrated a substance nearly isointense with the spinal cord and running nearly the length of the cord. This scan clearly demonstrates impingement and anterior displacement of the cord by the spinal epidural abscess.

without neurologic deficits). Such patients should be monitored closely for worsening pain, fever or the appearance of neurologic deficits.

An antistaphylococcal penicillin should be instituted as empiric therapy in all patients; vancomycin may be used in patients with penicillin allergies. Antibiotics active against Gram-negative organisms (such as a third-generation cephalosporin) and anaerobes (such as metronidazole)

should be added in patients whose underlying source may have been an intra-abdominal, pelvic or genitourinary infection. The duration of parenteral therapy should be at least 3–4 weeks; if osteomyelitis is present, therapy should be continued for a total of 8 weeks (see Chapter 2.43).

SPINAL CORD ABSCESS

Intramedullary spinal cord abscess is a rare condition that can be defined as a focal suppurative process of the parenchyma of the spinal cord. It usually involves the thoracic segment of the spinal cord, and is generally hematogenous in origin. The lungs are usually the source of infection, and there have been reports of such abscesses in drug users who inject. Spinal cord abscesses may also arise secondary to congenital dermal sinuses. The organisms that have been isolated in patients with spinal cord abscesses have included *S. aureus*, streptococci, *Listeria monocytogenes* and *Burkholderia* (formerly *Pseudomonas*) *cepacia*.[35] The symptoms of spinal cord abscess mimic those of spinal epidural abscess. Diagnosis may be made by CT, MRI or myelography and aspiration if not contraindicated. Treatment consists of surgical debridement and prolonged antimicrobial therapy. Antibiotics should be directed against *S. aureus* and possibly Gram-negative bacilli, or as directed by cultures.

The diagnosis of focal pyogenic infections of the CNS has been revolutionized in the past 2 decades with the introduction and widespread use of CT and MRI scanning. Because of its high sensitivity, ability to delineate infections in surrounding tissues and absence of ionizing radiation, MRI is generally preferable to CT for diagnosis. Management has also been altered by the refinement of minimally invasive surgical techniques, such as CT-guided aspiration, and by studies demonstrating the efficacy of medical management alone in defined situations. It is to be hoped that further advances in management will lead to greater improvements in patient outcomes.

REFERENCES

1. Canale DJ. William Macewen and the treatment of brain abscesses: revisited after one hundred years. J Neurosurg 1996;84:133–42.
2. Nicolosi A, Hauser WA, Musicco M, et al. Incidence and prognosis of brain abscess in a defined population: Olmstead County, Minnesota, 1935–1981. Neuroepidemiology 1991;10:122–31.
3. O'Donoghue M, Green H, Shaw D. Cerebral abscess on Merseyside, 1980–1988. J Infect 1992;25:163–72.
4. Rosenfeld EA, Rowley AH. Infectious intracranial complications of sinusitis, other than meningitis, in children: 12-year review. Clin Infect Dis 1994;18:750–4.
5. Seydoux C, Franciloi P. Bacterial brain abscesses: factors influencing mortality and sequelae. Clin Infect Dis 1992;15:394–401.
6. Yang SY. Brain abscess: a review of 400 cases. J Neurosurg 1981;55:794–9.
7. Yen PT, Chan ST, Huang TS. Brain abscess: with special reference to otolaryngologic sources of infection. Otolaryngol Head Neck Surg 1995;113:15–22.
8. Yang SY, Zhao CS. Review of 140 patients with brain abscess. Surg Neurol 1993;39:290–6.
9. Browning G. The unsafeness of safe ears. J Laryngol Otol 1984;98:23–6.
10. Kangsanarak J, Navacharoen N, Fooanant S, Ruckphaopunt K. Intracranial complications of suppurative otitis media: 13 years' experience. Am J Otol 1995;16:104–9.
11. Hlavin ML, Kaminski HJ, Fenstermaker RA, White RJ. Intracranial suppuration: a modern decade of postoperative subdural empyema and epidural abscess. Neurosurgery 1994;34:974–80.
12. Ersahin Y, Mutluer S, Guzelbag E. Brain abscess in infants and children. Childs Nerv Syst 1994;10:185–9.

13. Patir R, Sood S, Bhatia R. Post-traumatic brain abscess: experience of 36 patients. Br J Neurosurg 1995;9:29–35.
14. Finkelstein R, Engel A, Simri W, Hemil J. Brain abscesses: the lung connection. J Intern Med 1996;240:33–6.
15. Press O, Ramsey P. Central nervous system infections associated with hereditary hemorrhagic telangiectasia. Am J Med 1984;77:86–92.
16. Costello G, Heppe R, Winn H, et al. Susceptibility of brain to aerobic, anaerobic, and fungal organisms. Infect Immun 1983;41:535–9.
17. Kline M, Kaplan S, Hawkins E, et al. Pathogenesis of brain abscess formation in an infant rat model of *Citrobacter diversus* bacteremia and meningitis. J Infect Dis 1988;157:106–12.
18. Nielsen H, Glydensted C, Harmsen A. Cerebral abscess: aetiology and pathogenesis, symptoms, diagnosis, and treatment. Acta Neurol Scand 1982;65:609–22.
19. Britt R, Enzmann D, Yeager A. Neuropathological and computed tomographic findings in experimental brain abscess. J Neurosurg 1981;55:590–603.
20. Jamjoom AB, al-Hedaithy SA, Jamjoom ZA, et al. Intracranial mycotic infections in neurosurgical practice. Acta Neurochirurg 1995;137:78–84.
21. Hagensee ME, Bauwens JE, Kjos B, Bowden RA. Brain abscess following marrow transplantation: experience at the Fred Hutchinson Cancer Research Center, 1984–1992. Clin Infect Dis 1994;19:402–8.
22. Brewer N, Maccarty C, Wellman W. Brain abscess: a review of current experience. Ann Intern Med 1975;82:571–6.
23. Samson D, Clark K. A current review of brain abscess. Am J Med 1973;54:201–10.

24. Whelan M, Hilal S. Computed tomography as a guide in the diagnosis and follow-up of brain abscess. Radiology 1980;135:663–71.
25. Wispelwey B, Scheld W. Brain abscess. Semin Neurol 1992;12:273–8.
26. Shahzadi S, Lozano AM, Bernstein M, Guha A, Tasker RR. Stereotactic management of bacterial brain abscesses. Can J Neurol Sci 1996;23:34–9.
27. Silverberg A, DiNubile M. Subdural empyema and cranial epidural abscess. Med Clin North Am 1985;69:361–74.
28. Harris L, Haws F, Triplett JJ. Subdural empyema and epidural abscess: recent experience in a community hospital. South Med J 1987;80:1254–8.
29. Singh B, Van Dellen J, Ramjettan S, Maharaj TJ. Sinogenic intracranial complications. J Laryngol Otol 1995;109:945–50.
30. Southwick F, Richardson E, Swartz M. Septic thrombosis of the dural venous sinuses. Medicine 1986;65:82–106.
31. Nussbaum E, Rigamonti D, Standiford H, et al. Spinal epidural abscess: a report of 40 cases and review. Surg Neurol 1992;38:225–31.
32. Darouich R, Hamill R, Greenberg S, Weathers S, Musher D. Bacterial spinal epidural abscess: review of 43 cases and literature survey. Medicine 1992;71:369–85.
33. Heusner A. Nontuberculous spinal epidural infections. N Engl J Med 1948;239:845–54.
34. Numaguchi Y, Rigamonti D, Rothman M, et al. Spinal epidural abscess: evaluation with gadolinium-enhanced MR imaging. Radiographics 1993;13:545–59.
35. Bartels R, Gonera E, van der Spek J, et al. Intramedullary spinal cord abscess: a case report. Spine 1995;20:1199–204.

Toxin-Mediated Disorders: Tetanus, Botulism and Diphtheria

Martin J Wood

The three diseases described in this chapter are caused by exotoxins that conform to the general A–B model, each being composed of an enzymatic (A) portion and a binding (B) portion. The biological activity resides in the A portion whereas the B subunits may bind to target cells but are biologically inactive. Common to all the three toxins described, A and B are domains of a single protein that is cleaved by proteolytic activity of the bacterium.

TETANUS

Tetanus is caused by tetanospasmin, a neural toxin that interferes with inhibition of spinal cord reflexes and is produced by the obligate anaerobic bacterium *Clostridium tetani*.

EPIDEMIOLOGY

Tetanus is still common in developing tropical countries, where it is an important cause of death, particularly in neonates. The World Health Organization estimated in 1990 that there were about 715,000 deaths worldwide from neonatal tetanus. In the developed world, however, active immunization and better hygiene, wound care and management of childbirth have meant that the disease is now rare. The annual incidence of tetanus has fallen from nearly 4 to 0.2 per million population in the USA since 1947 (Fig. 18.1); mortality has dropped even more, with the death:case ratio falling from about 50% to below 30%.[1] In England and Wales there were only 9 cases of tetanus (and 3 deaths, all in elderly women) in the period 1993–1994.

Neonatal tetanus usually occurs within 3–14 days of birth in infants delivered under nonsterile conditions to nonimmunized women. The umbilical cord stump is the usual portal of entry, particularly if cultural practices dictate the application of animal dung to the stump. At other ages acute wounds are the portal of entry for *C. tetani* in about 80% of cases, with the remainder associated with chronic decubitus ulcers, gangrene, abscesses, or parenteral drug abuse. Tetanus is more likely to occur in the summer when gardening and other pastimes bring people into contact with soil.

PATHOGENESIS AND PATHOLOGY

Spores of *C. tetani* contaminate a wound and germinate under anaerobic conditions. The proliferating organisms elaborate tetanospasmin (tetanus toxin), one of the most potent of the known poisons, with an estimated lethal dose of 2.5ng/kg bodyweight. It is produced by a plasmid-encoded gene and is synthesized as a 151kDa polypeptide. As with botulinum and diphtheria toxins, tetanospasmin consists of a binding (B) domain and an enzymatic (A) domain which are separated by clostridial proteolytic cleavage into the light (L) chain (approximately 50kDa and containing the A domain) and heavy (H) chain, containing the B domain (approximately 100kDa).

Most of the toxin gets into the bloodstream, but it must then gain entry into CNS via neurons to exert its toxicity. The effect of tetanus toxin is via a three-stage process: binding, internalization and induction

of paralysis. The H chain interacts with the ganglioside GT_1 of neurons at neuromuscular junctions, both locally and distally (via the bloodstream), and enables the L chain to enter the cytoplasm of the neuron. The tetanospasmin is then transported intra-axonally at 75–250mm/day in a retrograde manner to the cell body in the ventral horns of the spinal cord and the motor nuclei of cranial nerves and then, via transsynaptic spread, to other neurons within the CNS (Fig. 18.2). Within the neurons tetanospasmin acts as a zinc-dependent protease that cleaves synaptobrevin, a protein component of synaptic vesicles,[2] and prevents release of neurotransmitters at the presynaptic membrane.

The predominant adverse effect is disinhibition of spinal cord reflex arcs as a result of interference with the release of the neurotransmitters glycine and γ-aminobutyric acid from presynaptic inhibitory Renshaw cells and 1a fibres of α motor neurons. Excitatory reflexes, freed from inhibition, thus lead to multiple, intense muscle spasms. Tetanospasmin also interferes with presynaptic acetylcholine release at the neuromuscular junction (similar to the effect of the botulinum toxin; see below) and disinhibits sympathetic reflexes at the spinal level, producing autonomic dysfunction.

There are no specific gross or histologic abnormalities in tetanus. Any changes described in fatal cases reflect terminal hypoxia and autonomic dysfunction.

PREVENTION

Tetanus is a preventable disease. Generally, concentrations of antibody to tetanospasmin as low as 0.01IU/ml are regarded as protective against clinical tetanus, although cases have occurred in patients with antibody concentrations at least ten-fold higher than this. Active immunization with tetanus toxoid is extremely effective. A primary series of three doses of tetanus toxoid given in infancy, either with diphtheria toxoid and pertussis (DTP) or with diphtheria toxoid alone (DT), with a

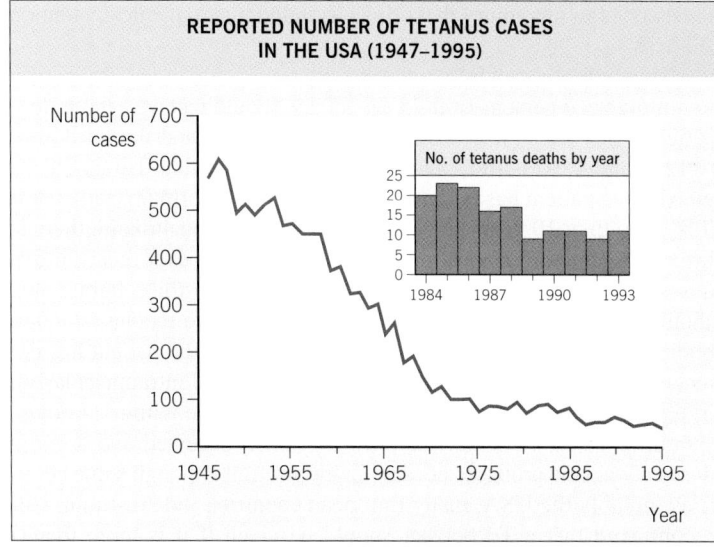

Fig. 18.1 Reported number of tetanus cases in the USA (1947–1995).

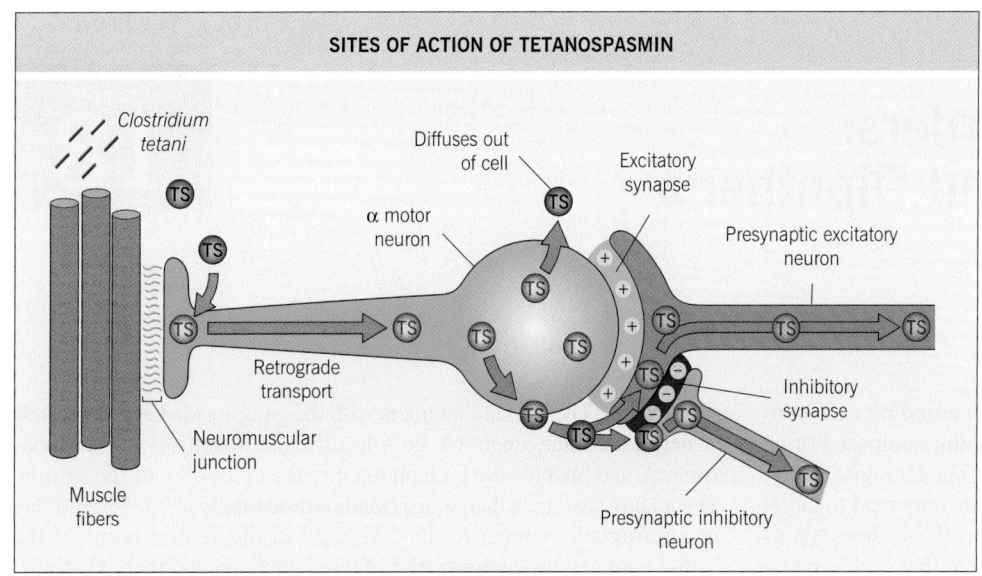

Fig. 18.2 Sites of action of tetanospasmin.
Tetanospasmin (TS) is produced by *Clostridium tetani* at the site of the wound and binds and internalizes at the neuromuscular junction into the α motor neuron. It then travels by retrograde axonal flow to the cell body and diffuses out into the synapses and extracellular space of the CNS. It enters other neurons and travels further into the CNS. Its major effect is to inhibit transmitter release from the glycinergic presynaptic inhibitory neuron but it can also inhibit release of transmitters at the the excitatory synapses and of acetylcholine at the neuromuscular junction.

RECOMMENDATIONS FOR USE OF TETANUS PROPHYLAXIS IN WOUND MANAGEMENT

History of tetanus toxoid administration	Clean, minor wounds		All other wounds	
	Tetanus toxoid vaccine*	Immunoglobulin	Tetanus toxoid vaccine*	Immunoglobulin
Unknown or less than three doses	Yes and proceed with basic immunization	No	Yes and proceed with basic immunization	Yes (250U human tetanus immunoglobulin or 3,000U equine tetanus antitoxin)
More than three doses	No, unless >10 years since last dose	No	No, unless >5 years since last dose	No

Fig. 18.3 Recommendations for use of tetanus prophylaxis in wound management.
*Administered as Td (i.e. low adult dose of diphtheria toxoid).

booster at school entry is virtually 100% effective for 5–10 years. After this, routine boosters, usually given with the adult low-dose form of diphtheria toxoid (as Td vaccine) should be given every 10 years for life. Neonatal tetanus can be prevented by ensuring that all pregnant women are immune. Failure to boost immunity means that many elderly individuals no longer have protective levels of tetanus antibodies.[3]

The need for both active and passive immunization against tetanus with specific human tetanus immunoglobulin (HTIG) should be reviewed after any injury that brings an individual to medical attention (Fig. 18.3).

Clean, minor wounds do not need any special treatment. Previously nonimmunized persons over 7 years of age should receive a three-dose series of Td, the first two doses 4–8 weeks apart and the third after 6–12 months. Although many protocols suggest that Td should be given if the patient has not previously completed a primary series or if it is more than 10 years since the last dose of tetanus toxoid, there is little justification for boosting if the individual has ever received five doses of toxoid.[4] All other wounds, including frostbite, burns, etc., should be considered to render the patient prone to tetanus. Foreign bodies and ischemic tissue should be removed. If the patient has not received a primary series then Td and HTIG (250U intramuscularly), or equine tetanus antitoxin if HTIG is not available within 24 hours, should be given. Patients who have previously received five or more doses of vaccine probably need no immunization although some countries (notably the USA, many European countries and Australia) still recommend that a Td booster should be given if it is more than 5 years since the last dose of tetanus toxoid.

CLINICAL FEATURES

Although tetanus can occur at any age, those over 60 years of age are at most risk in the developed world because they have lowest immunization levels: elderly women are at greatest risk because they are less likely to have been immunized in childhood.

The incubation period to the first symptom ranges from 1 day to several months, but most cases start between 3 and 21 days after an acute injury. There is a correlation between the distance of the injury from the CNS and the duration of the incubation period. The time between the first symptom and the first reflex spasm is termed 'the period of onset'.

There are four clinical forms of tetanus, neonatal disease and localized, cephalic and generalized tetanus, depending on the predominant site of toxin action.

Localized tetanus consists of fixed muscle rigidity and painful spasms, sometimes lasting weeks or months, confined to an area close to the site of the injury. It is rare and generally mild but may herald generalized tetanus. Cephalic tetanus is a particular form of localized tetanus associated with wounds to the head or face or with chronic otitis media, and is manifested by atonic palsies involving the motor cranial nerves. The incubation period is often only 1–2 days and generalized tetanus may follow

Generalized tetanus (which is by far the most common form) typically starts with rigidity and spasm of the masseter muscles, causing trismus or lockjaw and the characteristic risus sardonicus – a grimace through clenched teeth and closed mouth with wrinkled forehead and raised eyebrows (Fig. 18.4). Other muscles, first the neck, then the thorax, back and extremities, become rigid and go into spasms

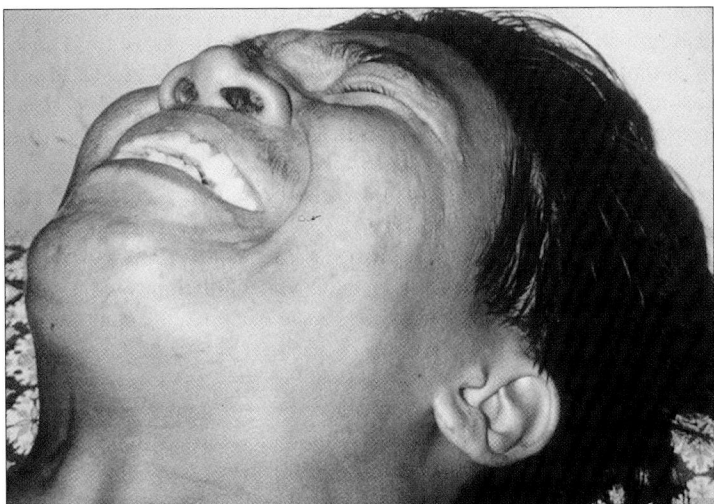

Fig. 18.4 Facial spasm and risus sardonicus in a Filipino patient who has tetanus.

RATING SCALE FOR SEVERITY AND PROGNOSIS OF TETANUS		
Score 1 point for each of the following		
• Incubation period <7 days		
• Period of onset <48 hours		
• Acquired from burns, surgical wound, compound fracture, septic abortion		
• Narcotic addiction		
• Generalized tetanus		
• Fever >104°F (40°C)		
• Tachycardia >120 beats/min (>150 beats/min in neonates)		
Total score indicates severity and prognosis		
Score	Severity	Mortality (%)
0–1	Mild	<10
2–3	Moderate	10–20
4	Severe	20–40
5–6	Very severe	>50

Fig. 18.5 Rating scale for severity and prognosis of tetanus.

producing opisthotonos, abdominal rigidity and apnea. Tetanospasms are intermittent, irregular and unpredictable, although they are often triggered by external stimuli, sometimes very trivial such as a sudden noise or puff of cold air, or even the internal stimulus of a distended bladder or bowel. Each spasm is sudden, painful and generalized, resulting in opisthotonos, leg extension and arm flexion; pharyngeal spasm causes dysphagia, and spasm of the glottis may cause immediate asphyxiation and death. Cognitive functions are not affected. Severe tetanus is accompanied by abnormalities of the autonomic nervous system, including hypo- or hypertension, arrhythmias and flushing.

Neonatal tetanus typically starts with poor sucking and irritability, followed by trismus and tetanospasms. It has a higher death:case ratio than tetanus at other ages.

With intensive care the death rate from tetanus (which is due to respiratory dysfunction or autonomic cardiovascular instability) may be as low as 10–20%, with higher rates in infants and in the elderly. A rating scale for the severity and prognosis of tetanus (Fig. 18.5) may be used. In general, the more rapid the evolution of symptoms and signs the worse the prognosis, but the belief that a short incubation period leads to a worse prognosis has been challenged by recent data from US cases.[5]

Complications related to spasms include vertebral and long bone fractures, glottic obstruction and asphyxia, and intramuscular haematomas. Rhabdomyolysis is common in generalized tetanus. Other complications are those related to general debility and prolonged intensive care.

Strychnine poisoning is the only true mimic of tetanus, although there are several other diseases that may overlap to some extent. Strychnine poisoning develops more rapidly than tetanus and there is usually no muscle rigidity between spasms; serum analysis for strychnine should be performed in suspect cases. Other causes of trismus include dystonic reactions to phenothiazines, which may be ruled out by administration of benztropine 1–2mg intravenously or diphenhydramine 50mg intravenously, and dental abscesses. Tetany from hypocalcemia or alkalosis tends to affect the extremities rather than the axial muscles and there is no trismus.

DIAGNOSIS

The diagnosis of tetanus depends upon clinical features and epidemiologic history, and laboratory tests are usually unhelpful. There is often a moderate leukocytosis but the CSF is normal, except for increased pressure. Neither electroencephalography nor electromyography is helpful. Occasionally, characteristic Gram-positive bacilli with terminal or subterminal spores may be visualized in aspirates from a wound, but anaerobic cultures are rarely positive and the organism may be grown from wounds in the absence of disease.

MANAGEMENT

A guide to the general management of the patient with tetanus has been published.[6] Human tetanus immunoglobulin 500IU as a single intramuscular injection,[7] should be given at the time of diagnosis in order to prevent further circulating toxin from reaching the CNS. The use of intrathecal HTIG to neutralize toxin that has entered but is not yet fixed to nervous tissue has not been consistently beneficial and is not routinely recommended; intrathecal injections are potent stimuli for tetanospasms.

The source of toxin should be removed by wound debridement and removal of foreign bodies. Therapy with metronidazole (15mg/kg intravenously followed by 20–30mg/kg/day intravenously for 7–14 days) should be used to eradicate *C. tetani*, even though antibiotics are not likely to penetrate into the anaerobic conditions that support growth of the organism.[8] Penicillin is theoretically less suitable (it acts as a central γ-aminobutyric acid antagonist), although it is still used in much of the world. Only vegetative forms of *C. tetani* will be susceptible to antibiotics.

A benzodiazepine (midazolam administered intravenously at 5–15 mg/h is suitable) should be used to produce sedation, decrease rigidity and control spasms. Airway protection during spasms is paramount. If the patient's ventilation is compromised they should be sedated, intubated, provided with a soft nasal feeding tube and moved to a quiet and darkened area. A tracheostomy may be needed. If benzodiazepines do not adequately control the spasms then the patient will need long-term neuromuscular blockade.

The management over the next few weeks is that of any ventilated patient, plus specific therapy for autonomic nervous system complications and control of spasms.[9] Sympathetic hyperactivity is treated with combined α- and β-blockade or morphine. Epidural blockade with local anesthetics may be needed. Hypotension requires fluid replacement and dopamine or norepinephrine (noradrenaline) administration. Parasympathetic overactivity is rare but if bradycardia is sustained then a pacemaker may be needed.

Clinical tetanus does not induce immunity against further attacks of the disease and all patients should be fully immunized with tetanus toxoid (in the form appropriate for their age) during convalescence.

BOTULISM

Botulism is caused by ingestion of neurotoxins (antigenic types A, B, E and F cause human disease) produced by groups I or II of *Clostridium botulinum*, an anaerobic, spore-forming bacillus (Fig. 18.6). There are three forms of the illness: food-borne botulism from ingestion of preformed toxin; wound botulism; and botulism from intestinal colonization, usually, but not universally, in infants.[10,11]

EPIDEMIOLOGY

All three forms of botulism occur throughout the world, but for food-borne botulism the causative strains, the responsible foods and the resulting illness vary in different geographic areas.

Accurate data about the incidence of botulism are difficult to obtain but it is estimated that, in France, there were about 300 food-borne outbreaks between 1979 and 1988; in the USA there were 474 outbreaks involving nearly 1050 persons between 1950 and 1990. Outbreaks were most frequent in the summer or autumn. In the UK the incidence is much lower than in Europe or the USA, with only nine outbreaks between 1922 and 1988. In 1989 the largest ever outbreak of food-borne botulism in the UK affected 27 people who had eaten hazelnut yoghurt. The illness was caused by type B toxin formed by bacteria growing in canned hazelnut conserve used to flavor the yoghurt that had been inadequately heat treated.[12]

Nearly 1000 cases of infant botulism (roughly equally divided between type A and type B *C. botulinum*) were reported in the USA between 1976 and 1990. Almost half the cases were reported from California, with an incidence of 7 per 100,000 live births. Cases occur most frequently in the second month of life and 95% of cases are in infants less than 6 months old.[10]

Most cases of food-borne botulism are associated with home preserved meats, fish and vegetables, but the common vehicles are often idiosyncratic to a country or culture.[13] In the USA (apart from Alaska), Spain, Italy and China most cases follow consumption of home preserved vegetables (home-canned asparagus, beans and peppers in the USA, home-fermented bean curd in China) contaminated with type A *C. botulinum*; in Alaska, Japan, Canada and Scandinavia cases are usually caused by type E toxin and follow eating preserved fish products; in central continental Europe cases typically arise from home-cured meats and are caused by nonproteolytic strains of type B *C. botulinum*. Commercially prepared foods are only rarely implicated. There is a significant association between infant botulism and ingestion of honey.

Occasionally botulism can follow wound infections with *C. botulinum*. The wounds are often compound fractures or penetrating wounds: cases have also been reported in intravenous drug users and to complicate sinusitis in chronic cocaine sniffers.[14]

PATHOGENESIS AND PATHOLOGY

In food-borne botulism there is ingestion of preformed toxin, but in other forms of the syndrome the toxin is produced *in vivo* and released when vegetative cells lyse. The toxin is not released from spores. Botulinum toxins are the most poisonous substances known to man and are synthesized as a polypeptide of molecular weight 150–165kDa, which is then broken into an H chain of about 100kDa and an L chain joined by a disulfide bond (Fig. 18.7). The mechanism of action is similar or identical to that of tetanospasmin, resulting in cleavage of synaptobrevin and inhibition of release of acetylcholine at peripheral cholinergic synapses.[2] The H chain of the toxin binds rapidly to the membrane of the presynaptic α motor neuron and then some or all of the toxin molecule translocates through the membrane. Finally, there is a slow paralytic step that may partially depend upon temperature and activity of the neuron. The process is irreversible and the synapse is

permanently damaged; recovery of function depends upon the budding and growth of new presynaptic end plates.

Infant botulism[15] results from colonization of the infant's gastrointestinal tract with as many as 10^8 proteolytic *C. botulinum* organisms per gram of feces. The mechanisms that relate to colonization and toxin absorption from the infant gut are unclear and both the organism and toxin may sometimes continue to be excreted in the feces for several months after the illness has resolved. Wound botulism typically results from soil contamination of severe head wounds, as occurs in warfare.

Death results from respiratory paralysis and there are no specific pathologic findings on gross or histologic examination in any of the forms of botulism.

PREVENTION

The key to the prevention of botulism is adequate processing and storage of food to destroy spores, and prevent their germination and toxin production. Spores are not killed by boiling at 212°F (100°C) but are destroyed by heating at 250°F (109°C) for 2.5 minutes (the type of temperature achieved under pressure processing of low-acid foods). Once toxin is formed, it can be inactivated by boiling or heating at 176°F (72°C) for 30 minutes.

Toxin production by strains of *C. botulinum* is inhibited at a pH below 4.6, in NaCl and at low temperatures [below 38°F (3°C)]; the respective values differ somewhat for different strains. Commercial canneries pay particular attention to less acidic (pH >4.6) fruit and vegetables; the canning and curing of meats rely on reduced heat treatment to kill vegetative bacteria and sodium chloride and nitrite to inhibit spore growth. Vacuum packaging of food may encourage the growth of anaerobes and there are concerns that botulinum toxin may be produced before spoilage is obvious. Toxin has been detected in mushrooms and coleslaw kept in modified atmosphere packaging. This should be preventable by piercing the packaging of fresh vegetables with air holes to allow sufficient oxygen to be present.

Honey has been associated with infant botulism and is not recommended for infants less than 1-years-old.

CHARACTERISTICS OF GROUPS OF *C. BOTULINUM* AND THE TOXINS THAT PRODUCE HUMAN DISEASE				
Group	Toxins produced	Proteolysis	Heat resistance of spores	Disease severity
Group I	A, B, F	Yes	High	Severe
Group II	B, E, F	No	Low	Less severe

Fig. 18.6 **Characteristics of groups of *Clostridium botulinum* and the toxins that produce human disease.**

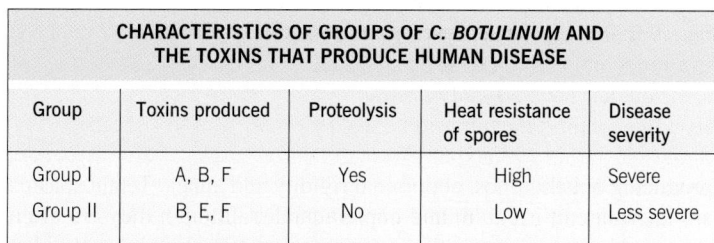
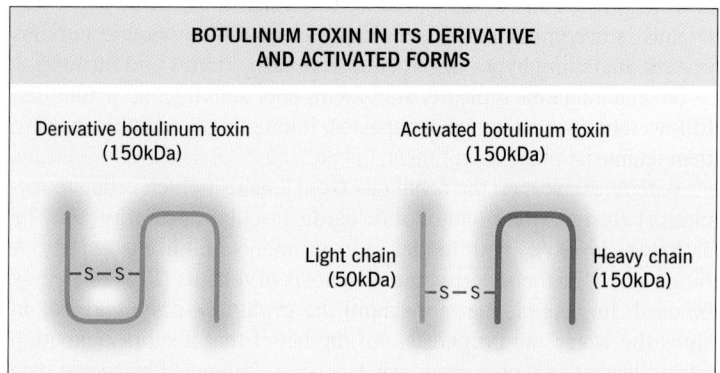

BOTULINUM TOXIN IN ITS DERIVATIVE AND ACTIVATED FORMS

Derivative botulinum toxin (150kDa)

Activated botulinum toxin (150kDa)

Light chain (50kDa)

Heavy chain (150kDa)

—S—S—   —S—S—

Fig. 18.7 **Botulinum toxin in its derivative and activated forms.**

CLINICAL FEATURES

Food-borne botulism usually develops 12–36 hours after ingestion of the toxin, although the interval may be as short as 6 hours or as long as 10 days. Patients who have type E toxin-mediated disease tend to have shorter, and those who have type B tend to have longer, incubation periods. Wound botulism occurs at a mean of 7.5 days (range 4–18 days) after the injury.[16]

Typically, botulism first affects the muscles supplied by the cranial nerves with disturbances of vision and difficulties in swallowing and speech followed by descending weakness of muscles of the trunk and extremities that is bilateral but not necessarily symmetric. Cardiovascular, gastrointestinal and urinary autonomic dysfunction may follow. The presentation may be related to the type of toxin; autonomic symptoms occur earlier and are more prominent in intoxication with type B and E toxins.

Common presenting symptoms are diplopia, dysphagia, dysarthria, dry mouth and fatigue (Fig. 18.8).[17] Ptosis and ophthalmoplegia are common physical signs, together with facial weakness and a decreased gag reflex. The pupils are dilated or fixed in less than 50% of cases. Frequently there is weakness of the extremities, although deep tendon reflexes are usually normal. Patients are usually afebrile and have no sensory deficits. Patients who have wound botulism have a similar presentation but acute gastrointestinal symptoms are lacking.

Constipation is the first sign of infant botulism, with neurologic signs developing either concurrently or up to several weeks later. The neurologic signs progress in a similar manner to those in other forms of botulism but they may be overlooked by the parents, who merely note the infant is irritable, lethargic or unable to suck. There is a wide range of clinical illness associated with infant botulism; 50% of cases develop ventilatory failure. Although some studies suggested that infant botulism was responsible for 5% of cases of the sudden infant death syndrome (SIDS) in California, no evidence of botulism has been found in any SIDS cases elsewhere in the USA.

COMPLICATIONS

The severity and duration of food-borne botulism is related to the amount of toxin ingested. Respiratory failure occurs in 20–35% of patients; the mean duration of respiratory support is 7 weeks for those requiring mechanical ventilation. Recovery from botulism is usually complete but persistent dysphagia, diplopia and prolonged weakness is a rare complication of severe cases.[18,19]

There has been a steady decline in mortality associated with botulism this century: the rate was about 70% in the period 1910–1919 and about 9% during 1980–1989. The mortality is higher in type A disease than in type B.[20]

The prognosis for infants hospitalized with botulism and given meticulous supportive care is very good, with less than 1.3% case fatality, and full recovery.

DIFFERENTIAL DIAGNOSIS

The diseases most often confused with botulism are Guillain–Barré syndrome (particularly the Miller–Fisher variant confined to the cranial nerves), myasthenia gravis and the Eaton–Lambert myasthenic syndrome, other forms of food-poisoning and tick paralysis. Guillain–Barré syndrome frequently has sensory complaints and the Miller–Fisher syndrome includes prominent ataxia. The myasthenias lack autonomic dysfunction and are less fulminant than botulism. In tick paralysis a careful search will reveal the *Dermacentor* tick still attached.

DIAGNOSIS

Routine laboratory tests are not helpful in the diagnosis of botulism. The diagnosis is best confirmed by assay of botulinum toxin in the patient's blood, gastric washings or feces by means of toxin neutralization tests in mice. Toxin may also be demonstrated in the incriminated food. This

FREQUENCY OF SYMPTOMS IN TYPES A, B AND E FOOD-BORNE BOTULISM			
Symptoms	Type A disease (% of cases)	Type B disease (% of cases)	Type E disease (% of cases)
Dry mouth	26–83	96–100	55–88
Dysphagia	25–96	77–100	63–90
Vomiting	70	50–100	88–100
Diarrhea	35	8–14	10
Constipation	73	17–100	25–38
Fatigue	8–92	69–100	Not known
Dizziness	8–86	30–100	63
Diplopia	50–90	57–100	85
Dysarthria	25–100	69–100	50
Paresthesia	20	12–14	Not known
Weakness of arm	16–86	64–86	Not known
Weakness of leg	16–76	64–86	Not known
Dyspnea	35–91	34	88

Fig. 18.8 Frequency of symptoms in types A, B and E food-borne botulism.[17]

test takes anything from 6 to 96 hours to perform and the initial diagnosis must, therefore, be based on clinical findings.

Clostridium botulinum may be cultured or the toxin detected by an enzyme-linked immunosorbent assay in the patient's feces, particularly in infant botulism and other cases resulting from intestinal colonization.

Electrophysiologic studies show normal nerve conduction velocities but the electromyogram is often abnormal with facilitation (an incremental increase) of the compound muscle action potential when high frequency (20–50 per second) repetitive stimuli are applied. These abnormalities may persist for several months after the onset of illness.

MANAGEMENT

Elimination of any unabsorbed toxin from the gastrointestinal tract should be encouraged in patients with suspected botulism, administration of an emetic or gastric lavage is recommended if ingestion of the suspect food has occurred within the last few hours and (unless there is a paralytic ileus) purgation or high enemas should be administered even several days after food ingestion.

The mainstay of therapy for botulism is meticulous supportive care. Patients should be admitted to an intensive care unit and their respiratory function monitored by repeat vital capacity measurements. Intubation should be performed if vital capacity falls below 12ml/kg.

Equine antitoxin, containing antibodies to types A, B and E toxin, is available from public health laboratories in the UK. Its availability in other countries should be sought through public health services. There are few data concerning its use in humans but it is clearly effective in experimental animals. It has to be given as early as possible in the course of the illness but its use needs careful consideration in view of the risk of serious anaphylaxis or serum sickness. A test dose is administered into the skin or the conjunctiva. If there is no hypersensitivity, one vial is given intravenously and one vial intramuscularly for an average adult: there is no need for repeated doses. In view of the good prognosis in infant botulism, the risks of equine antitoxin probably preclude its use. The potential role of human or monoclonal botulism immunoglobulin is under investigation in infant botulism.

Although guanidine hydrochloride (which increases release of acetylcholine from nerve terminals in response to nerve stimulation) has theoretical advantages, there was no improvement in recovery in a controlled study of patients with type A disease. Guanoxan and 3,4-diaminopyridone are investigational. Antibiotics do not help.

The relevant public health authorities should be notified promptly of a suspected case of botulism so that the necessary investigation may be conducted.

DIPHTHERIA

EPIDEMIOLOGY

The incidence of diphtheria has fallen dramatically in the technically developed world over the past 50 years but the disease remains endemic in many parts of the Third World, including India, Nigeria, Brazil, Indonesia and the Philippines. Since 1990 there has been a considerable epidemic of diphtheria in Russia and other parts of the former Soviet Union, and by 1995 nearly 50,000 cases had occurred, including some in tourists and other visitors.[21]

Spread of *Corynebacterium diphtheriae* takes place via respiratory droplets or by direct contact with infected respiratory secretions and 3–5% of healthy persons may harbor the organism in their throats. Epidemics have also resulted from contaminated milk. Skin infections are important reservoirs of infection and sources of dissemination of diphtheria in tropical countries, and, among alcoholic persons in urban areas of the West, person-to-person spread by exudate from infected skin lesions is relatively easy.[22] Occasional cases of diphtheria are caused by toxigenic strains of *Corynebacterium ulcerans*, which is usually transmitted by unpasteurized cows' or goats' milk. [23]

Although immunization with toxoid does have a dramatic effect upon the incidence of diphtheria, the disease incidence started to decline well before the widespread use of immunization and other factors are also important. Toxoid after all only attenuates the effects of toxin and does not prevent colonization with the organism; carriage rates should, therefore, remain high and there should be frequent epidemics among the relatively large proportion of individuals with subprotective antitoxin levels. The evidence, however, points to an extremely low carrier rate and disease is very rare in most developed countries. It is still unclear why this should be so.

PATHOGENESIS AND PATHOLOGY

Corynebacterium diphtheriae is not very invasive and organisms remain in the superficial layers of the respiratory mucosa or skin. Its major virulence is the result of the exotoxin, which inhibits protein synthesis in mammalian cells. Exotoxin production by *C. diphtheriae* is the result of a lysogenic β-phage which carries the *tox+* gene into the bacterium. Toxin production in a phage-bearing strain depends upon genetic and nutritional factors, especially a deficiency of iron in the environment. The toxin is secreted as a 62kDa polypeptide comprising two segments; the B segment binds to specific receptors on the cell surface and after endocytosis, and the toxic segment A is released by proteolytic cleavage. Segment A catalyses the cleavage of nicotinamide adenine dinucleotide leading to ribosylation and inactivation of elongation factor-2 (EF-2), which is necessary for the interaction of mRNA and tRNA. Its inactivation prevents the addition of further amino acids to the developing polypeptide chain (Fig. 18.9).[24] The toxin is very potent; a single molecule can inactivate all the EF-2 in a cell and stop protein synthesis within a few hours.

All cells are affected by the toxin but the major effects are local in the vicinity of bacterial growth, and distant, on the heart, nerves and kidneys.

Within a few days of respiratory infection the toxin produces a local necrotic coagulum of fibrin, dead epithelial cells and cellular infiltrate, which represent the adherent pseudomembrane. This gray–green or black membrane can be local or extend widely to cover the entire pharyngeal or tracheobronchial mucosa. There is a marked underlying soft tissue edema and regional lymphadenitis, producing the bull neck appearance.

Myocarditis, renal tubular necrosis and demyelination, and axon degeneration within cranial or peripheral nerves are prominent features of the more severe infections with *C. diphtheriae*.

PREVENTION

Diphtheria can be prevented by active immunization with formalin-detoxified diphtheria toxin (toxoid). Mass immunization with three or four injections of diphtheria–pertussis–tetanus is given to infants in most developed countries, but immunity declines over time and 20–80% of adults have antibody titers below the level of 0.01IU/ml that is considered protective. Indeed, epidemic diphtheria may occur when more than 70% of a population have antitoxin titers below 0.01IU/ml. In order to maintain population immunity to diphtheria a booster is recommended every 10 years in adults. Persons over age 7 years have a higher incidence of constitutional symptoms in response to the concentration of diphtheria toxoid in diphtheria–pertussis– tetanus and hence an adult vaccine with low dose purified toxoid and without the pertussis component (Td) is used. The resurgence of diphtheria in the former Soviet Union emphasizes the need to ensure that population immunity is maintained by booster immunization of adults.[21]

CLINICAL FEATURES

Symptoms of diphtheria may be divided into two groups: those that occur locally as a result of noninvasive infection of the respiratory tract or skin, and those that occur at distant site secondary to dissemination of diphtheria toxin.

After an incubation period of 2–4 days the onset of diphtheria is usually insidious with a mild sore throat and fever; local symptoms and signs of inflammation may then develop at various sites within the respiratory tract. Infection limited to the anterior nares is generally a mild disease, with a thin blood-stained or purulent nasal discharge and a delicate membrane on the nasal mucosa. Toxin absorption from the nasal mucosa is poor and there are usually few systemic symptoms or toxin-mediated problems. The most common site for clinical diph-

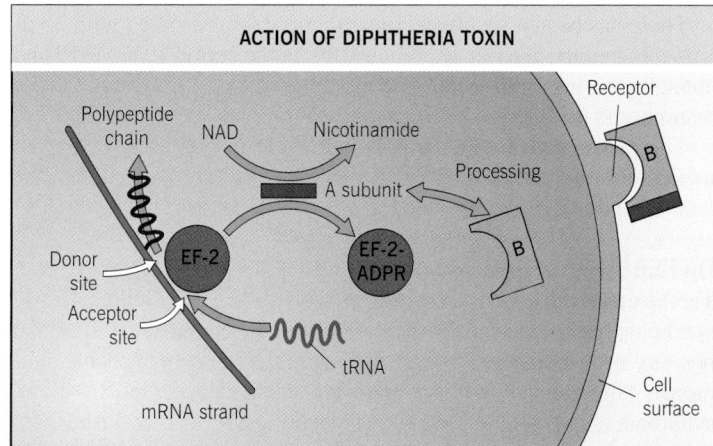

Fig. 18.9 Action of diphtheria toxin. The binding subunit attaches to the cell surface and the toxin enters the cell. After endocytosis the toxin is cleaved and the active A subunit is released. This then catalyses the cleavage of nicotinamide adenine dinucleotide (NAD) and the transfer of adenine diphosphate ribose (ADPR) to elongation factor-2 (EF-2). EF-2 is essential for ribosomal reactions at the acceptor and donor site, whereby the mRNA code is transferred via tRNA to an amino acid sequence and the building of a polypeptide chain. EF-2–ADPR is incapable of adding amino acids to a polypeptide chain and protein synthesis is stopped.

theria is the posterior structures of the mouth and pharynx. The membrane develops typically on the tonsil(s) and spreads locally. The membrane is initially translucent and thin but rapidly becomes thicker and develops a gray–green color with patches of necrosis. It is adherent to the underlying tissues and its removal produces bleeding. The patient is feverish and there are enlarged lymph glands in the neck. In severe cases the membrane spreads rapidly over the uvula, palate, oropharynx and nasopharynx; the extent of the membrane correlates with the severity of the local and systemic symptoms. In the most severe cases there is a weak thready pulse, profound exhaustion and muscle weakness. Severe cervical lymphadenopathy and edema of the anterior cervical tissues creates the bull neck appearance and may cause respiratory embarrassment.

Spread of the membrane downward leads to laryngeal diphtheria; the voice becomes hoarse and there is a bovine cough and stridor. The child becomes cyanosed and anxious, and requires urgent intubation and removal of the membrane if death is to be prevented.

In tropical areas C. diphtheriae is a cause of skin infections, which may be impetiginous or appear as chronic ulcers with a grayish slough or membrane. Outbreaks of cutaneous diphtheria have been recorded among vagrants and other impoverished, homeless groups.[25] Cutaneous infection rarely causes clinical disease but is an important reservoir for the organism.

It is the later effects of diphtheria toxin on the heart and the nervous system that produce the most severe complications. Some degree of cardiac toxicity is detectable in most cases of diphtheria with a widespread membrane and in about 50% of those with a moderate local exudate. Myocarditis characteristically begins during the first 1–2 weeks of the illness, often as the local respiratory disease is settling. First degree heart block or ST-T wave changes on the electrocardiogram and raised serum aspartate aminotransferase concentrations develop early and warn of more severe forms of heart block or life-threatening arrhythmia. Myocarditis is a poor prognostic sign, increasing the mortality three- or four-fold. Bundle-branch block or complete heart block has a mortality rate of up to 90% and the survivors are often left with conduction defects.

Some form of neuritis occurs in 10–20% of patients with diphtheria and in up to 75% of those with severe primary disease. Bilateral paralysis of the palate and posterior pharyngeal wall often appears in the first week of the illness and produces rhinolalia, dysphagia and nasal regurgitation of swallowed liquids. Other manifestations of neuritis are oculomotor and accommodation defects, facial paralysis and a peripheral motor neuropathy. The latter is usually a delayed effect, developing 6 weeks or more after the onset of diphtheria. The degree of dysfunction is variable but foot-drop is particularly common. Sensory neuropathies are rare complications of diphtheria. Although it may be slow, recovery from diphtheritic neuropathy is usually complete.

The differential diagnosis includes infectious mononucleosis, streptococcal tonsillitis and acute epiglottitis. The tonsillar exudate of infectious mononucleosis is creamy in color, does not extend beyond the tonsil and does not produce bleeding if removed. Streptococcal pharyngotonsillitis is associated with moresevere local symptoms and a higher fever. Epiglottitis is more acute in onset and is not associated with membrane formation.

DIAGNOSIS

The need to initiate antitoxin therapy as soon as possible means that the diagnosis of diphtheria needs to be presumptive and made on clinical grounds. It must be suspected whenever there is a membrane in the throat or nares. Many individuals have diphtheroids in their throats and hence microscopy for C. diphtheriae is unreliable; confirmation of the diagnosis of diphtheria depends upon isolation of a toxin-producing strain of C. diphtheriae. The organism can be cultured on selective media and isolates tested for toxin production by inoculation of guinea pigs or by the Elek's plate method (immunoprecipitation of toxin in agar cultures by overlaid diphtheria antitoxin-containing filter paper strips) (see Chapter 8.15).

MANAGEMENT

Administration of diphtheria antitoxin (DAT) is the crucial therapeutic measure in diphtheria. It will only neutralize extracellular toxin and hence needs to be administered as early as possible, often before the disease can be microbiologically confirmed. It is an equine antiserum, however, and all patients must be tested for hypersensitivity to horse protein; this is done by instilling diluted DAT into the conjunctival sac or injecting 0.1ml of a 1:100 dilution subcutaneously, while taking appropriate precautions for anaphylaxis. Even if hypersensitivity is shown, DAT will need to be administered, but only after desensitization procedures. The therapeutic dose and route of administration of DAT depends upon the extent of the disease. The recommended doses (the minimum therapeutic dose has never been determined) are as follows: for mild disease of less than 48 hours' duration, 20,000–40,000IU (or 500IU/kg body weight) given half intramuscular and half by intravenous infusion over 30 minutes; for more severe disease or illness more than 3 days old, 80,000–120,000IU (up to 2500IU/kg) by intravenous infusion.

Erythromycin [2g/day for 6 days, then 1g/day for 8 days (50% of these dosages for children <6 years)] or procaine penicillin [1.2 million IU/day for 6 days, then 600,000 IU/day for 8 days (50% of these dosages for children <6 years)] should be administered for 14 days to eradicate C. diphtheriae and terminate toxin production, and the patient should be kept in strict isolation during this period until three throat swabs taken after therapy are culture negative. Patients with diphtheria caused by C. ulcerans do not need isolation because person-to-person spread has never been documented. Supportive measures are also important. Patients should be confined to bed and their electrocardiogram monitored daily until the danger of myocarditis has passed: those who develop cardiac toxicity will need full support and effective therapy for any conduction abnormalities. Corticosteroid therapy does not prevent myocarditis or neuritis in diphtheria.[26] Respiratory monitoring needs to be vigilant and early tracheostomy and intubation is sensible for those with laryngeal diphtheria.

Because clinical infection does not always induce immunity, a course of toxoid should be commenced at the end of the first week of illness and completed during convalescence.

Those exposed to a case of diphtheria who have been fully immunized need to be observed for 7 days. Those with incomplete or unclear immunity should have their throats swabbed and be started on erythromycin (7 days of oral therapy) or benzathine penicillin (a single intramuscular dose of 1.2 million IU) and a course of toxoid. The antibiotic can be stopped if the cultures are negative; those initially carrying the organism need to have eradication confirmed 2 weeks after completing therapy.

REFERENCES

1. Izurietta HS, Sutter RW, Strebel PM, *et al.* Tetanus surveillance – United States, 1991–1994. MMWR Morb Mort Wkly Rep 1997;46:15–25.

2. Schiavo G, Benfenati F, Poulain B, *et al.* Tetanus and botulinum-B neurotoxins block neurotransmitter release by proteolytic cleavage of synaptobrevin. Nature 1992;359:832–5.

3. Gergen PJ, McQuillan GM, Kiely M, Ezzati-Rice TM, Sutter RW, Virella G. A population-based serologic survey of immunity to tetanus in the United States. N Engl J Med 1995;332:761–6.

4. Bowie C. Tetanus toxoid for adults – too much of a good thing. Lancet 1996;348:1185–6.

5. Sutter RW, Orenstein WA, Wassilak SG. Tetanus. In: Hoeprich PD, Jordan MC, Ronald AR, eds. Infectious diseases: a treatise of infectious processes, 5th ed. Philadelphia: JB Lippincott Company; 1994:1175–85.

6. Bleck TP. Tetanus. In: Scheld WM, Whitley RJ, Durack DT, eds. Infections of the central nervous system. New York: Raven Press; 1991:603–24.

7. Blake PA, Feldman RA, Buchanan TM, *et al.* Serologic therapy of tetanus in the United States. JAMA 1976;236:42–4.

8. Ahmadsyah I, Salim A. Treatment of tetanus: an open study to compare the efficacy of procaine penicillin and metronidazole. Br Med J 1985;291:648–50.

9. Wright DK, Lalloo UG, Nayiager S, Govender P. Autonomic nervous system dysfunction in severe tetanus: current perspectives. Crit Care Med 1989;17:371–5.

10. Arnon SS. Infant botulism: anticipating the second decade. J Infect Dis 1986;154:201–6.

11. Bartlett JC. Infant botulism in adults. N Engl J Med 1986;315:254–5.

12. O'Mahoney MO, Mitchell E, Gilbert RJ, *et al.* An outbreak of foodborne botulism associated with contaminated hazelnut yoghurt. Epidemiol Infect 1990;104:389–95.

13. Hauschild AHW. *Clostridium botulinum*. In: Doyle MP, ed. Foodborne bacterial pathogens. New York: Marcel Decker; 1989:111–89.

14. MacDonald KL, Rutherford GW, Friedman SM, *et al.* Botulism and botulism-like illness in chronic drug abusers. Ann Intern Med 1985;102:616–18.

15. Schreiner MS, Field E, Ruddy R. Infant botulism: a review of 12 years' experience at the Children's Hospital of Philadelphia. Pediatrics 1991;87:159–65.

16. Merson MH, Dowell VR. Epidemiologic, clinical, and laboratory aspects of wound botulism. N Engl J Med 1973;289:1105–10.

17. Woodruff BA, Griffin PM, McCroskey LM, *et al.* Clinical and laboratory comparison of botulism from toxin types A, B, and E in the United States 1975–1988. J Infect Dis 1992;166:1281–6.

18. Mann J. Prolonged recovery from type A botulism. N Engl J Med 1983;309:1522–3.

19. Wilcox P, Andolfatto G, Fairbarn MS, *et al.* Long-term follow-up of symptoms, pulmonary function, respiratory muscle strength, and exercise performance after botulism. Am Rev Resp Dis 1989;139:157–63.

20. Hughes JM. Botulism. In: Scheld WM, Whitley RJ, Durack DT, eds. Infections of the Central Nervous System. New York: Raven Press Ltd; 1991:589–602.

21. Hardy IRB, Dittman S, Sutter RW. Current situation and control strategies for resurgence of diphtheria in newly independent states of the former Soviet Union. Lancet 1996;347:1739–44.

22. Bowler ICJ, Mandal BK, Schlecht B, Riorden T. Diphtheria – the continuing hazard. Arch Dis Child 1988;63:194–210.

23. De Carpentier JP, Flanagan PM, Singh IP, Timms MS, Nassar WY. Nasopharyngeal *Corynebacterium ulcerans;* a different diphtheria. J Laryngol Otol 1992;106:824–6.

24. Pappenheimer AM. The diphtheria bacillus and its toxin: a model system. J Hyg (Camb) 1984;93:397–440.

25. Harnish JP, Tronca E, Nolan CM, Turck M, Holmes KK. Diphtheria among alcoholic urban adults. A decade of experience in Seattle. Ann Intern Med 1989;111:71–82.

26. Thisyakorn U, Wongvanich J, Kumpeng V. Failure of corticosteroid therapy to prevent diphtheritic myocarditis or neuritis. Pediatr Infect Dis 1984;3:126–8.

Transmissible Spongiform Encephalopathies of Humans and Animals

Glenn C Telling & John Collinge

The transmissible spongiform encephalopathies, or prion diseases, are a group of closely related neurologic conditions of humans and animals with the unique property of being both inherited and infectious diseases. The recent era of scientific interest in these diseases is notable for the award of two Nobel Prizes for Physiology or Medicine: in 1976 to D Carleton Gajdusek at the US National Institutes of Health for 'discoveries concerning new mechanisms for the origin and dissemination of infectious diseases', which he shared with Baruch S Blumberg; and in 1997 to Stanley B Prusiner at the University of California San Francisco 'for his discovery of prions – a new biological principle of infection'. In recent years prion diseases have captured the public attention with the emergence of the bovine spongiform encephalopathy (BSE) epidemic in Europe, and more recently with the appearance of a new variant of Creutzfeldt–Jakob disease (nvCJD) in humans, which appears to be caused by exposure to BSE.

The unifying hallmark of the prion diseases is the aberrant metabolism of the prion protein (PrP), which exists in at least two conformational states with different physicochemical properties. The normal form of the protein, referred to as PrP^C, is expressed on the surface of neurons via a glycophosphatidyl inositol anchor in both infected and uninfected brains. The normal form of PrP is a sialoglycoprotein of molecular weight 33–35kDa with a high content of α-helical secondary structure that is sensitive to protease treatment and soluble in detergents. The disease-associated isoform, referred to as PrP^{Sc}, is found only in infected brains and is partially resistant to protease treatment and insoluble in detergents, has a high content of β-pleated sheet and forms aggregates.

Although the precise molecular structure of the prion still eludes definitive identification, considerable evidence argues that prions are devoid of nucleic acid and composed largely, if not entirely, of an abnormal isoform of PrP. During the disease process, PrP^{Sc} coerces PrP^C to adopt to the infectivity-associated conformation, an event that is central to prion propagation (see Chapter 8.12).[1]

EPIDEMIOLOGY

ANIMAL PRION DISEASES

Scrapie is the prototypic prion disease (Fig. 19.1). It has been recognized as an enzootic disease of sheep and goats for more than 250 years. In the UK, 0.5–1% of the sheep population is affected annually, although other areas of the world with large sheep populations claim to have eradicated the disease. The etiology of natural scrapie has been the subject of intense debate for many years, but it is now clear that it is an infectious disease for which susceptibility is genetically modulated by the host.

Since its discovery in 1985, BSE has reached epidemic proportions, affecting over 170,000 cattle in the UK and lesser numbers in certain other European countries. It has been estimated that up to 1 million cattle were infected with BSE in the UK.[2] Epidemiologic studies point to contaminated offal used in the manufacture of meat and bone meal and fed to cattle as the source of prions responsible for BSE.[3] Because the UK has a relatively large sheep population in

which scrapie is endemic, it was hypothesized that scrapie-contaminated sheep offal was the initial source of BSE. An alternative view is that BSE prions originated spontaneously in cattle and that infection was subsequently amplified by recycling of infected cattle that had subclinical disease. As sheep were also fed meat and bone meal, it is not unreasonable to expect that a BSE-like disease with characteristics different from conventional scrapie strains might also appear in the sheep population, although there is currently no evidence that this has occurred.

The host range of BSE appears to be unusually wide, affecting many other animal species (Fig. 19.1). Foodstuffs contaminated with BSE have caused disease in several other animal species in the UK, including feline spongiform encephalopathy (FSE) in domestic cats, exotic ungulates and captive cats in zoos. In addition to these 'natural' infections, BSE has been experimentally transmitted to a wide variety of species. Outbreaks of transmissible mink encephalopathy and chronic wasting disease in captive populations of mink, mule deer and elk in certain regions of the USA have also been attributed to prion-infected foodstuffs, although the origin of infection is less certain in this diseases. Epidemiologic studies suggest intraspecific lateral transmission as the most plausible explanation for the spread of chronic wasting disease in captive populations of Rocky Mountain elk. Chronic wasting disease has also been diagnosed in free-ranging mule deer, Rocky Mountain elk and white-tailed deer from north–central Colorado.[4]

ANIMAL PRION DISEASES		
Disease	Host	Etiology
Scrapie	Sheep and goats	Thought to involve both horizontal and vertical transmission
Transmissible mink encephalopathy	Captive mink	Probably food-borne, although the origin of infectious prions is uncertain
Chronic wasting disease	Captive and free-ranging mule deer and Rocky Mountain elk	Origin unknown There is evidence for horizontal transmission
Bovine spongiform encephalopathy (BSE)	Cattle	Food-borne in the form of contaminated meat and bone meal
Feline spongiform encephalopathy	Domestic and zoo cats	Feed contaminated with bovine spongiform encephalopathy
Exotic ungulate encephalopathy	Captive bovidae	Feed contaminated with bovine spongiform encephalopathy

Fig. 19.1 Animal prion diseases.

HUMAN PRION DISEASES			
Disease	Incidence	Etiology	Age of onset or incubation period and duration of illness
Sporadic Creutzfeldt–Jakob disease	1 case per 1 million population	Unknown but hypotheses include somatic mutation or spontaneous conversion of PrPC into PrPSc	Age of onset is usually age 45–75 years; age of peak onset is 60–65 years; 70% of cases die in under 6 months
Familial Creutzfeldt–Jakob disease, Gerstmann–Straussler–Scheinker syndrome, fatal familial insomnia	10–20% of cases of human prion disease	Autosomal dominant PRNP mutation	Average age of onset for Gerstmann–Straussler–Scheinker syndrome is 45 years with a mean duration of illness of 5 years
Kuru (1957–1982)	>2500 cases among the Fore people in Papua New Guinea	Infection through ritualistic cannibalism	Incubation period 60–360 months; duration of illness 3–12 months
Iatrogenic Creutzfeldt–Jakob disease	About 80 cases to date	Infection from contaminated human growth hormone, human gonadotropin, depth electrodes, corneal transplants, dura mater grafts, neurosurgical procedures	Incubation periods of cases from human growth hormone 4–30 years; duration of illness 6–18 months
New variant Creutzfeldt–Jakob disease	30 young adults in the UK and France	Infection by bovine spongiform encephalopathy prions	Mean age of onset 26 years; mean duration of illness 14 months

Fig. 19.2 Human prion diseases. Onset tends to be earlier in familial CJD compared to sporadic CJD. Mean onset of FFI is about 50 years; the mean duration is about 1 year. PrPC, normal form of prion protein; PrPSc, disease-associated isoform of prion protein; PRNP, prion protein gene.

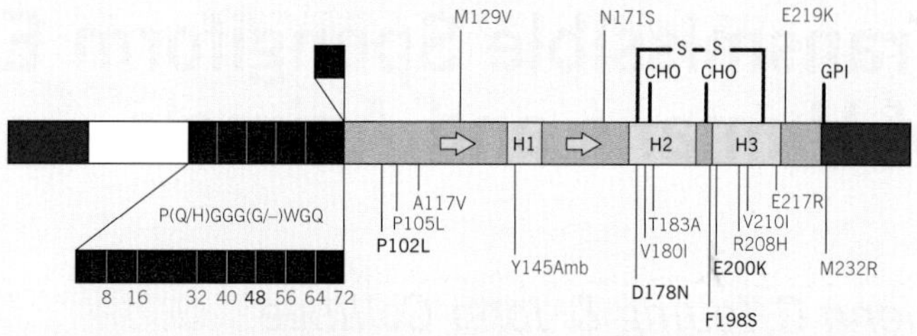

Fig. 19.3 Pathogenic mutations, polymorphisms and structural features of the human prion protein. The human PrP gene, PRNP, encodes a 253-amino-acid residue translation product, which is processed by removal of an amino-terminal signal peptide of 22 amino acids and a carboxyl-terminal hydrophobic peptide of 23 amino acids (both shown in blue). After cleavage of the carboxyl-terminal peptide a glycosyl phosphatidylinositol (GPI) anchor is added. The three α-helices (designated H1, H2 and H3) and two short sections forming a β-pleated sheet (shown by arrows) that have been identified by nuclear magnetic resonance spectroscopy of recombinant mouse PrP expressed in Escherichia coli are shown in yellow. The α-helix H1 extends from amino acid residue 144 to amino acid residue 154; H2 extends from amino acid residue 175 to amino acid residue 193; and H3 extends from amino acid residue 200 to amino acid residue 219. The two regions making up the β-pleated sheet extend from amino-acid residues 128 to 131 and amino acid residues 161 to 164 (mouse PrP numbering). The amino-terminal portion of the molecule is unstructured and contains a tandem array of five octapeptide repeats between codons 51 and 90. The octarepeat amino acid sequence is shown below, represented by single letter amino acid code. Aspargine-linked oligosaccharides are attached at residues 181 and 197, and H2 and H3 are connected by a disulfide bond that joins codons 179 and 213. The amino-terminal 66 or so amino acids of PrPSc are cleaved by proteinase K. This protease-resistant core is shown in gray. The pathogenic mutations associated with human prion disease are shown below the PrP coding sequence. These consist of 8, 16, 32 40, 48, 56, 64 and 72 amino acids insertions within the octarepeat region between codons 51 and 91, and various point mutations causing nonconservative missense amino acid substitutions. Point mutations are designated by the wild-type amino acid preceding the codon number, followed by the mutant residue, using single letter amino acid conventions. The mutations for which genetic linkage with familial Creutzfeldt–Jakob disease, Gerstmann–Straussler–Scheinker syndrome and fatal familial insomnia has been established are shown in bold type. Deletion of a single octapeptide repeat is not associated with disease. Other polymorphisms found at codons 129, 171 and 219 are also shown above the coding sequence.

HUMAN PRION DISEASES

The human prion diseases are unique in biology in that they are manifest as sporadic, genetic and infectious diseases (Fig. 19.2). The majority of cases of human prion disease occur sporadically as Creutzfeldt–Jakob disease (CJD) at a rate of roughly 1 per 10[6] population across the world, with an equal incidence of disease in men and women. The aetiology of sporadic CJD is unknown, although hypotheses include somatic mutation of the PrP gene (referred to as PRNP), and the spontaneous conversion of PrPC into PrPSc as a rare stochastic event. There is a common benign polymorphism at codon 129 of PRNP encoding either methionine or valine (Fig. 19.3). Homozygosity at this position predisposes people to the development of sporadic and iatrogenic CJD.[5,6]

Approximately 10–20% of human prion diseases are inherited with an autosomal dominant mode of inheritance. Inherited human prion diseases have been shown to segregate with more than 20 different missense and insertion mutations in the coding sequence of PRNP (see Fig. 19.3), and five PRNP mutations have been genetically linked to loci controlling familial Creutzfeldt–Jakob disease, Gerstmann–Straussler–Scheinker syndrome

and fatal familial insomnia, which are inherited human prion diseases that can be transmitted to experimental animals.[7]

In order to provide a model of how a mutation in the PrP gene could result in a disease that was both inherited and infectious, transgenic mice were engineered to express a PrP gene mutation associated with Gerstmann–Straussler–Scheinker syndrome. These mice spontaneously developed clinical and neuropathologic symptoms similar to mouse scrapie between 150 and 300 days of age.[8,9] Importantly, the serial propagation of infectivity from the brains of these spontaneously sick mice to indicator mice that express low levels of mutant protein but that do not otherwise get sick demonstrated that infectious prions had been produced de novo in the brains of these spontaneously sick mice.[9,10]

Although the human prion diseases are experimentally transmissible, the acquired forms have, until recently, been confined to rare and unusual situations. For example, kuru is thought to have been spread by cannibalism among the Fore linguistic group of the Okapa district of the Eastern Highlands in Papua New Guinea.[11] The disease had its origins at the beginning of the 20th century and was the leading cause of death in this population by the middle of the century, killing over 3000 people in the total population of 30,000. Mainly adult women as well as children of both sexes were affected, to give an annual disease-specific mortality of approximately 3%. It is thought that the roughly seven-fold higher incidence of disease in adult women than adult men was the result of higher exposure of women to infectious brain material. Since the cessation of cannibalistic practices around 1956, the disease has all but died out, with only a handful of cases currently occurring in older people who were presumably exposed to kuru as young children.

Other examples of acquired human prion diseases have resulted from iatrogenic transmission of CJD during corneal transplantation, contaminated electroencephalographic electrode implantation and surgical operations using contaminated instruments or apparatus. In addition, iatrogenic CJD has occurred as a result of implantation of dura mater grafts and treatment with growth hormone or gonadotropin derived from the pituitary glands of human cadavers.[12]

The appearance of CJD cases in teenagers and young adults in the UK during the mid-1990s prompted considerable concern that they might have acquired the illness as a result of exposure to BSE. By March 1996, it became clear that the unusual clinical presentation and neuropathology was remarkably consistent in these new cases.[13] In the past three years, more than 30 cases of nvCJD have been reported in teenagers and young adults in the UK and a single case of nvCJD has been reported in France. All reported cases of nvCJD have been homozygous for methionine at the polymorphic codon 129.[14] Molecular strain typing, which focuses on the biochemical properties of PrP^{Sc} from the brains of BSE-infected cattle and patients who have CJD, has demonstrated that nvCJD is different from sporadic CJD but similar to BSE.[15,16] Moreover, the incubation times and profile of neuropathologic lesions of nvCJD and BSE prions are indistinguishable in inbred lines of mice.[17] These data argue that BSE and nvCJD are the same strain.

PATHOGENESIS AND PATHOLOGY

The animal and human prion diseases share a number of characteristic features, the most consistent being the neuropathologic changes that accompany disease in the central nervous system. Indeed, it was the neuropathologic similarities between scrapie and kuru that strongly suggested that the two diseases might be closely related, and that kuru, like scrapie, might also be transmissible by inoculation.[18] Subsequently, brain extracts from patients who have kuru produced a progressive neurodegenerative condition in inoculated chimpanzees after a prolonged incubation period of 18–21 months.[19] The neuropathologic similarities between kuru and CJD prompted similar transmission experiments from CJD patients.[20]

Although the brains of patients or animals who have prion disease frequently show no recognizable abnormalities on gross examination, microscopic examination of the central nevous system typically reveals characteristic histopathologic changes, consisting of neuronal vacuolation and degeneration, which gives the cerebral gray matter a microvacuolated or 'spongiform' appearance (Fig. 19.4), and a reactive proliferation of astroglial cells, which is often out of all proportion to the degree of nerve cell loss. Although spongiform degeneration is frequently detected, it is not an obligatory neuropathologic feature of prion disease; astrocytic gliosis, although not specific to the prion diseases, is more constantly seen. The lack of an inflammatory response is also an important characteristic. Although it is by no means a constant feature, some examples of prion disease are characterized by deposition of amyloid plaques composed of insoluble aggregates of PrP (see Fig. 19.4). Amyloid plaques are a notable feature of kuru and Gerstmann–Straussler–Scheinker syndrome but they are infrequently found in the brains of patients who have sporadic CJD.

Although there is wide variation in the neuropathologic profiles of different forms of human prion disease, the histopathologic features of nvCJD are remarkably constant and distinguish it from other human prion diseases. Large numbers of PrP-positive amyloid plaques are a constant feature of nvCJD but they differ in morphology from the plaques seen in kuru and Gerstmann–Straussler–Scheinker syndrome in that the surrounding tissue takes on a microvacuolated appearance, giving the plaques a florid appearance.[13] It is noteworthy that transmission of BSE to three macaques produced disease with neuropathologic features similar to those reported in cases of nvCJD in humans.[21]

Detection of PrP^{Sc} in brain material by immunohistochemical or immunoblotting techniques is considered to be diagnostic of prion

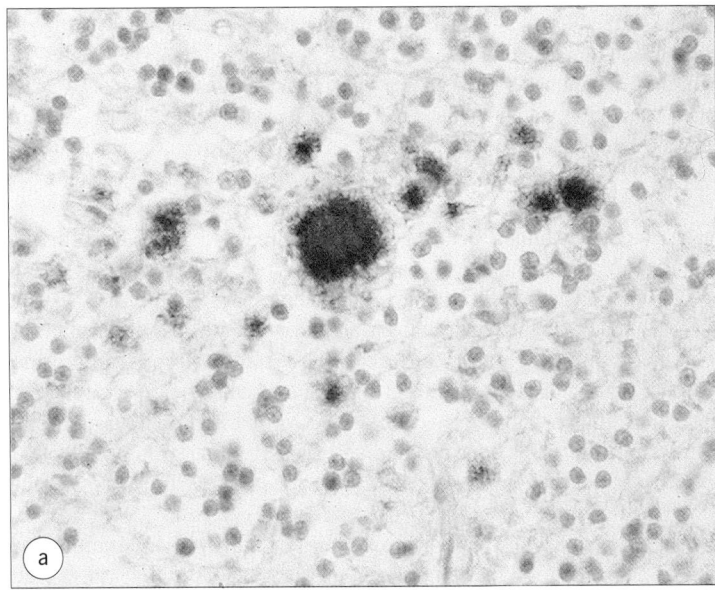

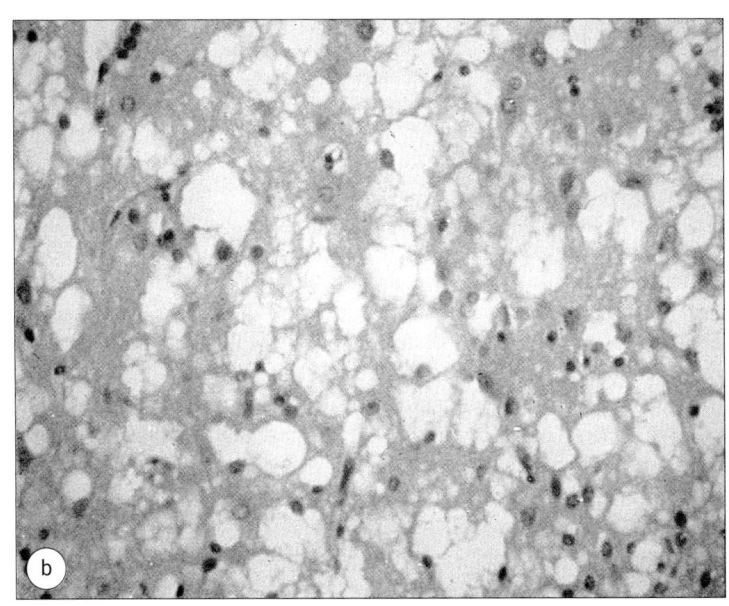

Fig. 19.4 Neuropathology of prion disease. (a) Amyloid deposition in prion disease. The insoluble aggregates of prion protein are demonstrated by hydrolytic autoclaving and immunoreactivity with antiprion protein antibody.

(b) Spongiform degeneration in prion disease. There is severe neuronal loss and vacuolation in this patient who has Creutzfeldt–Jakob disease (hematoxylin and eosin stain). Courtesy of Dr Stephen DeArmond.

disease. However, certain examples of natural and experimental prion disease occur without accumulation of detectable protease-resistant PrP^{Sc},[9,22,23] and the time course of neurodegeneration is not equivalent to the time course of PrP^{Sc} accumulation in mice expressing lower than normal levels of PrP^C.[24] Moreover, PrP^{Sc} is not toxic to cells that do not express PrP^C.[25] Thus, it appears that accumulation of PrP^{Sc} may not be the sole cause of pathology in prion diseases. An alternative mechanism of PrP-induced neuronal degeneration has been suggested from recent studies of mutant forms of PrP that disrupt the regulation of PrP biogenesis in the endoplasmic reticulum.[26]

Mice in which the PrP gene has been disrupted (referred to as $Prnp^{0/0}$) and that express no PrP^C fail to propagate infectivity and do not develop the neuropathologic hallmarks of scrapie when inoculated with prions.[27–29] Gene-targeted $Prnp^{0/0}$ mice have also been studied to probe the normal function of PrP^C. Two independently generated lines of gene-targeted $Prnp^{0/0}$ mice developed normally and appeared to suffer no gross phenotypic abnormalities.[28,30] The relative normality of these PrP null mice could result from effective adaptive changes during development. However, cerebellar Purkinje cell degeneration has been reported in a third line of $Prnp^{0/0}$ mice[31] and several other phenotypic defects are being investigated in $Prnp^{0/0}$ mice, including altered circadian rhythms and sleep patterns,[32] alterations in superoxide dismutase activity[33] and defects in copper metabolism.[34] Electrophysiologic studies have demonstrated that fast inhibition and long-term potentiation mediated by γ-aminobutyric acid receptors were impaired in hippocampal slices from $Prnp^{0/0}$ mice[35,36] and that calcium-activated potassium currents were disrupted.[37] These abnormalities of synaptic inhibition are reminiscent of the neurophysiologic defects seen in patients who have CJD and in scrapie-infected mice.[35]

Although the pathologic consequences of prion infection occur in the central nevous system and experimental transmission of these diseases is most efficiently accomplished by intracerebral inoculation, most natural infections do not occur by these means. Indeed, administration to sites other than the central nevous system is known to be associated with much longer incubation periods, which may extend to 20 years or more. Experimental evidence suggests that this latent period is associated with clinically silent prion replication in the lymphoreticular tissue, whereas neuroinvasion may take place later.[38] Mice with severe combined immune deficiency are largely resistant to disease after extracerebral inoculation with prions,[21,39] and corticosteroid treatment substantially delays disease in mice that are intraperitoneally challenged with scrapie prions.[40] Recent studies have indicated that differentiated B lymphocytes may be crucial for prion neuroinvasion.[41]

PREVENTION

Because there are currently no treatments for these invariably fatal diseases, prevention is particularly important. Perhaps the most effective example of prevention was the cessation of cannibalistic practices among the Fore people of Papua New Guinea in the 1950s, which resulted in the disappearance of kuru. The replacement of growth hormone derived from the pituitary glands of human cadavers with recombinant growth hormone was implemented to avoid the continued iatrogenic transmission of CJD to young children who have growth hormone deficiency. Similarly, because CJD has resulted from the use of prion-contaminated surgical instruments or apparatus after neurosurgical or ophthalmic procedures, it is advised that surgical instruments be incinerated in cases where CJD is suspected so as to avoid future iatrogenic transmission of prion disease. Because of the involvement of the lymphoreticular system in prion disease, treatments that inhibit prion replication in lymphoid organs may represent a viable strategy for rational secondary prophylaxis after accidental exposure.[42] Future studies on the peripheral pathogenesis of prion disease should identify the crucial steps in the spread

of prions from the periphery that may be amenable to pharmacologic intervention.

When it was realized that BSE was caused by feeding prion contaminated foodstuffs to cattle, a number of preventive measures were introduced in the UK. In July 1988 a ban on feeding ruminant-derived protein to other ruminants was introduced to break the cycle of infection via feed. Because the available evidence indicates that nvCJD has resulted from human exposure to bovine prions via the food chain, the BSE epidemic prompted concerns over the safety of prion-contaminated foodstuffs. A ban on specified bovine offals was introduced in the UK in 1989 to prevent inclusion in the human food chain of bovine tissues thought to contain the highest titer of prions; these included tissues from the lymphoreticular system and the central nevous system. The European Union imposed a worldwide ban on the export of British cattle, products derived from them (with the exception of products for technical uses) and mammalian meat and bonemeal in March 1996 after the announcement that BSE and nvCJD may be linked. Since then, more than 1.35 million cattle over 30 months old have been culled in the UK in a further attempt to limit human exposure to BSE. The cost of tackling BSE to the British and European taxpayer has been estimated at £3500 million (approximately $US5600 million). Because BSE infectivity has also been detected in dorsal root ganglia, which may on occasion be included in meat for human consumption, the UK government also introduced a controversial ban on the sale of 'beef on the bone' in 1997. Although there is no evidence that disease can be transmitted via blood or blood products, the long incubation period of prion diseases and the possibility of increased numbers of future cases of CJD as a result of exposure to BSE has raised the issue of blood as a possible vehicle for iatrogenic disease. As a protective measure against this theoretic risk, the UK government decided in 1998 that all blood donations should be leukodepleted.

CLINICAL FEATURES

The incubation times of the prion diseases are long and range from months to decades (see Fig. 19.2). For example, since the cessation of cannibalistic practices among the Fore people, kuru has all but died out, but a handful of cases still occur in older people who were presumably exposed to kuru as young children over 40 years ago. Although incubation times are long, once clinical symptoms have appeared the progression to death is relatively rapid with a duration of illness usually lasting no more than 6–12 months.

In scrapie, affected animals exhibit behavioral changes that are characterized by anxiousness and hypersensitivity, followed by intense pruritus. (Indeed, the term 'scrapie' derives from the tendency of affected animals to rub or scrape themselves against walls and fences, thus removing much of their fleece.) Later stages of the disease are characterized by unsteady gait, eventually resulting in severe ataxia; animals become recumbent in the terminal phase of the disease.

The clinical features of BSE are also well described and include temperament changes, postural abnormalities, co-ordination problems and terminal recumbence.

Classic CJD is a rapidly progressive dementia accompanied by myoclonus. Decline to akinetic mutism and death is rapid and often occurs within 3–4 months. Cerebellar ataxia, extrapyramidal and pyramidal features and cortical blindness are also frequently seen. These clinical symptoms are usually accompanied by characteristic periodic sharp wave complexes on electroencephalography. Atypical cases of CJD are, however, well recognized and can present diagnostic difficulties.

The clinical features of kuru consist of a progressive cerebellar ataxia accompanied by dementia in the later stages and death, which usually occurs within 9 months.

The clinical presentation of nvCJD resembles kuru more than classic CJD and consists of behavioral and psychiatric disturbances, peripheral sensory disturbance and early cerebellar ataxia. The duration of disease is longer in nvCJD with mean patient survival times of about 14 months, compared with about 4 months for sporadic CJD. Moreover, whereas classical CJD is predominantly a late onset disease with a peak onset between 60 and 65 years, the median age of onset of nvCJD is 26 years.

The diagnosis of CJD is confirmed by the appearance of characteristic neuropathologic features by brain biopsy or at necropsy. Analysis of mutations in the coding sequence of the prion protein gene (see Fig. 19.3) may also be diagnostic and used for presymptomatic testing in affected families.[42] PrPSc from specific CJD cases with different codon 129 genotypes can be typed according to the size and extent of glycosylation of the protease-resistant fragments by immunoblotting after proteinase K treatment and Western blotting of brain material.[15,43] A characteristic banding pattern of PrPSc found in nvCJD patients and BSE-infected animals distinguishes nvCJD PrPSc from the patterns observed in other types of CJD.[15,16] Because it is possible to detect PrPSc in biopsies of tonsillar tissue from nvCJD patients, this method can be used to diagnose nvCJD before death while avoiding brain biopsy.[44]

REFERENCES

1. Cohen FE, Pan KM, Huang Z, Baldwin M, Fletterick RJ, Prusiner SB. Structural clues to prion replication. Science 1994;64:530–1.
2. Anderson RM, Donnelly CA, Ferguson NM, et al. Transmission dynamics and epidemiology of BSE in British cattle. Nature 1996;382:779–88.
3. Wilesmith JW, Wells GA, Cranwell MP, Ryan JB. Bovine spongiform encephalopathy: epidemiological studies. Vet Rec 1988;123:638–44.
4. Spraker TR, Miller MW, Williams ES, et al. Spongiform encephalopathy in free-ranging mule deer (Odocoileus hemionus), white-tailed deer (Odocoileus virginianus) and Rocky Mountain elk (Cervus elaphus nelsoni) in north–central Colorado. J Wildl Dis 33:1–6.
5. Palmer MS, Dryden AJ, Hughes JT, Collinge J. Homozygous prion protein genotype predisposes to sporadic Creutzfeldt–Jakob disease. Nature 1991;352:340–2.
6. Collinge J, Palmer MS, Dryden AJ. Genetic predisposition to iatrogenic Creutzfeldt–Jakob disease. Lancet 1991;337:1441–2.
7. Collinge J. Human prion diseases and bovine spongiform encephalopathy (BSE). Hum Mol Genet 1997;6:1699–705.

8. Hsiao KK, Scott M, Foster D, Groth DF, DeArmond SJ, Prusiner SB. Spontaneous neurodegeneration in transgenic mice with mutant prion protein. Science 1990;250:1587–90.
9. Telling GC, Haga T, Torchia M, Tremblay P, DeArmond SJ, Prusiner SB. Interactions between wild-type and mutant prion proteins modulate neurodegeneration transgenic mice. Genes Dev 1996;10:1736–50.
10. Hsiao KK, Groth D, Scott M, et al. Serial transmission in rodents of neurodegeneration from transgenic mice expressing mutant prion protein. Proc Natl Acad Sci USA 1994;91:9126–30.
11. Gajdusek DC. Unconventional viruses and the origin and disappearance of kuru. Science 1977;197:943–60.
12. Brown P, Preece MA, Will RG. 'Friendly fire' in medicine: hormones, homografts, and Creutzfeldt–Jakob disease. Lancet 1992;340:24–7.
13. Will RG, Ironside JW, Zeidler M, et al. A new variant of Creutzfeldt–Jakob disease in the UK. Lancet 1996;347:921–5.
14. Collinge J, Beck J, Campbell T, Estibeiro K, Will RG. Prion protein gene analysis in new variant cases of Creutzfeldt–Jakob disease. Lancet 1996;348:56.

15. Collinge J, Sidle KCL, Meads J, Ironside J, Hill AF. Molecular analysis of prion strain variation and the aetiology of 'new variant' CJD. Nature 1996;383:685–90.
16. Hill AF, Desbruslais M, Joiner S, Sidle KCL, Gowland I, Collinge J. The same prion strain causes vCJD and BSE. Nature 1997;389:448–50.
17. Bruce ME, Will RG, Ironside JW, et al. Transmissions to mice indicate that 'new variant' CJD is caused by the BSE agent. Nature 1997;389:498–501.
18. Hadlow WJ. Scrapie and kuru. Lancet 1959;ii:289–90.
19. Gajdusek DC, Gibbs CJJ, Alpers MP. Experimental transmission of a kuru-like syndrome to chimpanzees. Nature 1966;209:794–6.
20. Gibbs CJJ, Gajdusek DC, Asher DM, et al. Creutzfeldt–Jakob disease (spongiform encephalopathy): Transmission to the chimpanzee. Science 1968;161:388–9.
21. Lasmézas CI, Deslys JP, Demaimay R, et al. BSE transmission to macaques. Nature 1996;381:743–4.
22. Collinge J, Palmer MS, Sidle KCL, et al. Transmission of fatal familial insomnia to laboratory animals. Lancet 1995;346:569–70.

23. Medori R, Montagna P, Tritschler HJ, *et al*. Fatal familial insomnia: a second kindred with mutation of prion protein gene at codon 178. Neurology 1992;42:669–70.

24. Bueler H, Raeber A, Sailer A, Fischer M, Aguzzi A, Weissmann C. High prion and PrP^Sc levels but delayed onset of disease in scrapie-inoculated mice heterozygous for a disrupted PrP gene. Mol Med 1995;1:19–30.

25. Brandner S, Isenmann S, Raebe, A, *et al*. Normal host prion protein necessary for scrapie-induced neurotoxicity. Nature 1996;379:339–43.

26. Hegde RS, Mastrianni JA, Scott MR, *et al*. A transmembrane from of the prion protein in neurodegenerative disease. Science 1998;279:827–34.

27. Bueler H, Aguzzi A, Sailer A, *et al*. Mice devoid of PrP are resistant to scrapie. Cell 1993;73:1339–47.

28. Manson JC, Clarke AR, Hooper ML, Aitchison L, McConnell I, Hope J. 129/Ola mice carrying a null mutation in PrP that abolishes mRNA production are developmentally normal. Mol Neurobiol 1994;8:121–7.

29. Sakaguchi S, Katamine S, Shigematsu K, *et al*. Accumulation of proteinase K-resistant prion protein (PrP) is restricted by the expression level of normal PrP in mice inoculated with a mouse-adapted strain of the Creutzfeldt–Jakob disease agent. J Virol 1995;69:7586–92.

30. Bueler H, Fischer M, Lang Y, *et al*. Normal development and behaviour of mice lacking the neuronal cell-surface PrP protein. Nature 1992;356:577–82.

31. Sakaguchi S, Katamine S, Nishida N, *et al*. Loss of cerebellar Purkinje cells in aged mice homozygous for a disrupted PrP gene. Nature 1996;380:528–31.

32. Tobler I, Gaus SE, Deboer T, *et al*. Altered circadian activity rhythms and sleep in mice devoid of prion protein. Nature 1996;380:639–42.

33. Brown DR, Schulz-Schaeffer WJ, Schmidt B, Kretzschmar HA. Prion protein-deficient cells show altered response to oxidative stress due to decreased SOD-1 activity. Exp Neurol 1997;146:104–12.

34. Brown DR, Qin K, Herms JW, *et al*. The cellular prion protein binds copper *in vivo*. Nature 1997;390:684–7.

35. Collinge J, Whittington MA, Sidle KCL, *et al*. Prion protein is necessary for normal synaptic function. Nature 1994;370:295–7.

36. Whittington MA, Sidle KCL, Gowland I, *et al*. Rescue of neurophysiological phenotype seen in PrP null mice by transgene encoding human prion protein. Nature Genet 1995;9:197–201.

37. Colling SB, Collinge J, Jefferys JGR. Hippocampal slices from prion protein null mice: disrupted Ca^{2+}-activated K^+ currents. Neurosci Lett 1996;209:49–52.

38. Blattler T, Brandner S, Raeber AJ, *et al*. PrP-expressing tissue required for transfer of scrapie infectivity from spleen to brain. Nature 1997;389:69–73.

39. Kitamoto T, Muramoto T, Mohri S, Doh-ura K, Tateishi J. Abnormal isoform of prion protein accumulates in follicular dendritic cells in mice with Creutzfeldt–Jakob disease. J Virol 1991;65:6292–5.

40. Outram GW, Dickinson AG, Fraser H. Reduced susceptibility to scrapie in mice after steroid administration. Nature 1974;249:855–6.

41. Klein MA, Frigg R, Flechsig E, *et al*. A crucial role for B cells in neuroinvasive scrapie. Nature 1997;390:687–90.

42. Aguzzi A, Collinge J. Post-exposure prophylaxis after accidental prion inoculation. Lancet 1997;350:1519–20.

43. Collinge J, Poulter M, Davis MB, *et al*. Presymptomatic detection or exclusion of prion protein gene defects in families with inherited prion diseases. Am J Hum Genet 1991;49:1351–4.

44. Parchi P, Castellani R, Capellari S, *et al*. Molecular basis of phenotypic variability in sporadic Creutzfeldt–Jakob disease. Ann Neurol 1996;39:669–80.

chapter 20

Postinfectious and Vaccine-Related Encephalitis

Rodney E Willoughby Jr. & Edwin J Asturias

INTRODUCTION

Infections or immunizations can cause disease by aberrant host responses directed against brain, spinal cord or peripheral nerves. Pathogenesis is divided by anatomic differences in myelin into diseases of the central nervous system (CNS) and peripheral nervous system (PNS). The CNS syndromes discussed below are encephalomyelitis, transverse myelitis, cerebellar ataxia, optic neuritis (ON), Sydenham's chorea (SC), encephalopathy and Reye's syndrome. The PNS syndromes are Guillain-Barré syndrome (GBS), brachial neuritis and cranial neuropathies.

ENCEPHALOMYELITIS, TRANSVERSE MYELITIS, AND RELATED CONDITIONS

EPIDEMIOLOGY

The most important of the various postinfectious CNS syndromes are:
- acute disseminated encephalomyelitis (ADEM): an inflammatory demyelinating disease, probably autoimmune in nature, that characteristically follows a monophasic course.[1] Acute hemorrhagic leukoencephalitis is a hyperacute necrotizing form of ADEM;
- postinfectious encephalomyelitis (PIE): a subset of ADEM affecting brain and spinal cord after an infection;
- postvaccinal encephalitis (PVE): follows various immunizations;
- acute cerebellar ataxia (ACA): characterized by predominant cerebellar dysfunction;
- acute transverse myelitis (ATM): a distinctive syndrome affecting the spinal cord; and
- optic neuritis (ON): inflammation of the ophthalmic nerve, which can occur in isolation or with multifocal CNS involvement.

Although postinfectious CNS syndromes are differentiated by their predominant anatomic involvement, they probably represent similar pathologic mechanisms: overlapping syndromes and variants may occur. Encephalitis associated with antecedent bacterial infections displays a predilection for basal ganglia, producing SC or stereotypic behaviors.

The incidence of ADEM varies by country as a function of endemic diseases, intercurrent epidemics and use of international or locally developed vaccines. Seasonality, reported in some case series, might reflect underlying epidemics that trigger these rare diseases. With the introduction of vaccines against common childhood diseases, the proportion of PIE decreased from 33 to 15% of acute encephalitis cases in the USA and Europe.[2] The incidence of PIE in the USA is approximately 1/100,000 population. The incidence after immunization is generally much lower than after natural infection (Fig. 20.1). Annual incidence of ATM is 0.8/100,000 USA population.[3] The incidence of SC in the USA and Europe is approximately 0.1/100,000 population. There are no population-based estimates for ON or ACA.

The association of ON with subsequent development of multiple sclerosis (MS) is well established. The autoimmune, demyelinating, but multiphasic phenotype of MS is an invariable contrast to these monophasic postinfectious syndromes. The prevalence of MS is 60/100,000 population. For comparison with ADEM, adrenoleukodystrophy, a rare genetic demyelinating syndrome, occurs with a prevalence of 2/50,000 males.

PATHOGENESIS AND PATHOLOGY

The pathogenesis of postinfectious syndromes of the CNS has been best delineated following measles infection and immunization against rabies.[4,5] The pathology of encephalomyelitis following measles infection is perivenular mononuclear inflammation, edema and demyelination, with relative sparing of axons. Lipid-laden macrophages are present in areas of demyelination. Almost identical pathology is seen in PVE and experimental models of allergic encephalomyelitis (EAE). The pathology of ACA, which is benign and self-limited, is rarely described; the pathology of ON and ATM is similar to that of PIE. The pattern of demyelination observed in postinfectious syndromes is distinct from the demyelination seen in progressive multifocal leukoencephalopathy due to papovavirus infection, human T-cell leukemia/lymphoma virus (HTLV)-1 infection or MS.[6] Repeated attempts to recover infectious agents from brain tissue (culture, viral antigen or nucleic acid) have been mostly unsuccessful. Intrathecal production of interferons or antibodies, which are indicators of CNS infection, are frequently absent.[1,4]

Patients with major neurologic complications after rabies vaccine or measles infection have elevated levels of antibody reactive to brain white matter or myelin basic protein (MBP), as well as increased lymphoproliferative responses to MBP.[4,5] The animal model of EAE, using repeated immunization with brain tissue, induces inflammatory demyelinating lesions in the CNS similar to those in PIE or PVE. The pathogenesis is by cell-mediated attack on CNS myelin. The incidence of PIE is low relative to the prevalence of associated infectious agents (Fig. 20.2). Genetic factors predisposing to autoimmunity or enhanced CNS inflammation are important in EAE and may determine which individuals develop ADEM.[7]

INCIDENCE OF PIE AND PVE		
Disease	Disease-associated	Vaccine-associated
Smallpox	1/2000	1/20,000
Rabies	Fatal disease	Semple vaccine 1/400
		Suckling mouse vaccine 1/7500
		Duck embryo vaccine 1/50,000
		Human diploid vaccine: none
Measles	1/1000	1.2/million
Rubella	1/6000	<1/million
Mumps	1/6000	<1/million
Pertussis	1/125	1/140,000
Varicella	1/4000	<1/100,000

Fig. 20.1 Incidence of postinfectious encephalomyelitis (PIE) and postvaccinal encephalomyelitis (PVE).

INFECTIONS ASSOCIATED WITH POSTINFECTIOUS CNS SYNDROMES
Nonspecific upper respiratory infections
Nonspecific gastrointestinal infections
Measles
Mumps
Rubella
Varicella-zoster virus
Epstein–Barr virus
Herpes simplex virus
Influenza
Smallpox (variola)
Mycoplasma pneumoniae
Streptococcus pyogenes
Campylobacter jejuni
Vaccines
Smallpox (vaccinia)
Rabies
Measles
Oral poliovirus
Diphtheria-tetanus (DT and Td) and tetanus toxoid vaccines
Haemophilus influenzae type b
Plasma-derived hepatitis B
Inactivated *Vibrio cholerae*
Japanese B encephalitis

Fig. 20.2 Infections associated with postinfectious CNS syndromes.

The pathogenesis of CNS autoimmunity following bacterial infections is less clear. Mycoplasma are associated with PIE; mycoplasma antigens cross-react with brain tissue.[8] Limited pathologic descriptions in SC indicate neuronopathy rather than demyelination. Antibodies of IgG subclass reactive against subthalamic and caudate nuclei are detected more frequently in patients with acute rheumatic fever or SC than in controls. Children with tics or obsessive–compulsive disorder with attention deficit-hyperactivity disorder can have antibodies to caudate and putamen.[9] The role of cell-mediated immunity has not been defined.

Common infections are frequently associated with postinfectious ADEM (Fig. 20.2). Acute cerebellar ataxia is especially common after chickenpox, occurring in 35% of cases of ADEM associated with varicella-zoster virus (VZV).[10]

PREVENTION

The incidence of PIE has decreased over the past 30 years, probably related to successful immunization against many viral diseases as well as to development of more purified vaccines (see Fig. 20.1).[2] Although vaccines can trigger ADEM, the probability of this event is much higher after wild-type virus infection. Although vaccinia virus vaccines are no longer in use, Semple rabies vaccines are still produced in some countries. A change to human diploid cell rabies vaccines virtually eliminates the risk of PVE. New vaccine technology, including recombinant proteins and DNA vaccines, should further reduce incidence of PVE.

CLINICAL FEATURES

The age-specific incidences of infectious encephalitis versus PIE are distinct. The incidence of encephalitis is highest in infancy (22.5/100,000), although PIE is rare under in children under 1 year of age.[11] The age distribution of PIE and PVE generally coincides with the epidemiology of associated pathogens or vaccines. Most patients with ACA are 1–6 years of age; a viral prodrome is present in 64%.[10] The incidence of ATM has distinct peaks in adolescence, middle age and the elderly; a viral prodrome is present in 30%.[12] The incidence of ON is highest in young-to-middle-aged adults; a viral prodrome is present in 50%.[13] Unlike most postinfectious CNS syndromes, the sex-specific incidence of ON is unequal, favoring females with a ratio of 2:1. Sydenham's chorea affects school-aged children; a similar age distribution is reported for the onset of childhood tics and obsessive–compulsive disorders.[9]

The onset of PIE is usually abrupt, occurring 5–14 days after infection. The illness begins with a recurrence of fever and a depressed level of consciousness. Neurologic manifestations are classically multifocal. Signs range from lethargy and irritability, to convulsions (50%), involuntary movements (18%), ataxia (10%), hemiplegia (12%), visual disturbances and cranial nerve deficits. Recovery can begin within days, but complete resolution occurs over weeks or months. The mortality ranges from 5 to 20%, with highly variable morbidity. A poor prognosis is associated with coma, focal neurological deficits and extreme or persistent fever.

POSTVACCINAL ENCEPHALITIS

This is best characterized for Semple rabies vaccines.[5] Prodromal fever, headache and myalgia develop 6–14 days after the first immunization. Within 1–4 weeks, patients develop neurologic signs of lethargy (50%), meningisms (33%), focal neurologic deficits (50%) and sphincter disturbances (33%). The duration of illness is less than 2 weeks and 80% of patients recover completely; the associated mortality is 15%.

Distinguishing between infectious encephalomyelitis and PIE can be challenging, especially when caused by the same infectious agent.[8,14] The differential diagnosis of PIE and PVE includes infectious encephalitis, progressive multifocal leukoencephalitis (papovavirus), MS, vasculitis, cerebral emboli, cerebral vein thrombosis, chronic meningitis, sarcoidosis, intracranial hemorrhage, malignancy, mitochondrial disorders (mitochondrial encephalomyopathy–lactic acidosis–stroke-like episodes syndrome) and metabolic disorders (adrenoleukodystrophy).

ACUTE CEREBELLAR ATAXIA

This develops suddenly with vomiting, inco-ordination, truncal ataxia and dysarthria. Refusal to walk and mutism are common presenting signs in children.[10] Cerebellitis is a frequent component of general encephalomyelitis and can be complicated by acute hydrocephalus. Acute cerebellar ataxia must be distinguished from drug ingestion, GBS, benign paroxysmal vertigo associated with migraine, peroxisomal disorders, metabolic diseases, inherited ataxias, Wernicke encephalopathy, paraneoplastic syndromes (myoclonus–opsoclonus syndrome) and posterior fossa tumors.

ACUTE TRANSVERSE MYELITIS

This is an acute syndrome mimicking transection of the spinal cord. Prodromal symptoms include fever, rash and pain in the legs, interscapular region or back. Peak neurologic dysfunction is reached within 2 hours in 15% of the patients, and within 24 hours in 50%, but progression up to 14 days has been reported. Neurologic deficit is commonly localized to the thoracic region, but 20% of patients are affected in the cervical or lumbar area. Muscular weakness is accompanied by decreased or absent deep tendon reflexes. Some degree of asymmetry can be observed during early evolution of the disease; significant asymmetry suggests other diagnoses. Loss of sensation to pain and temperature below a clear demarcated level is universal; loss of perception of touch and proprioception are common. Sphincter disturbances and dysautonomia are usually described. Recovery to independent ambulation occurs in 50% of pediatric and 35% of adult cases. Improvement may continue beyond 6 months. Pulmonary emboli, urinary tract infections and decubitus ulcers are common complications.

Transverse myelitis must be differentiated from MS, acute epidural abscesses, hematomas or arteriovenous malformations, tumors, anterior spinal artery syndrome associated with lupus, syphilis or schistosomiasis, dissecting aneurysm, tropical paraparesis (HTLV-1), as well as infections by VZV, cytomegalovirus (CMV) and toxoplasmosis in immunocompromised hosts.

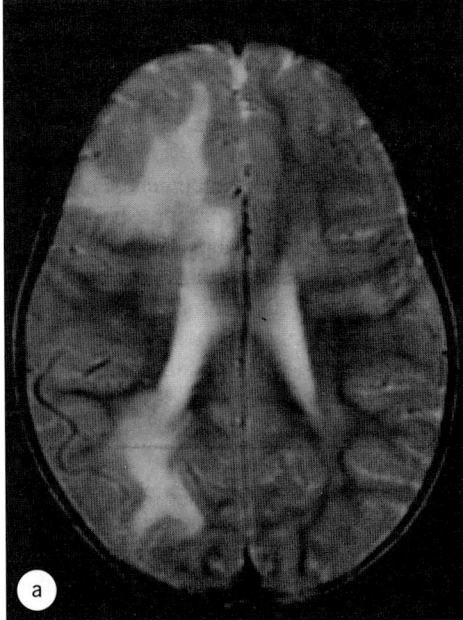 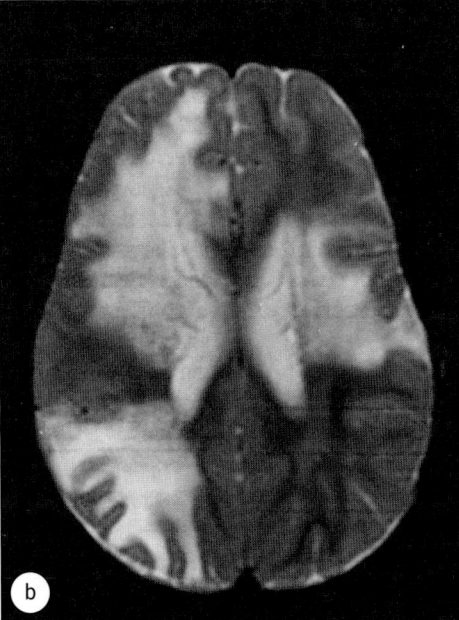 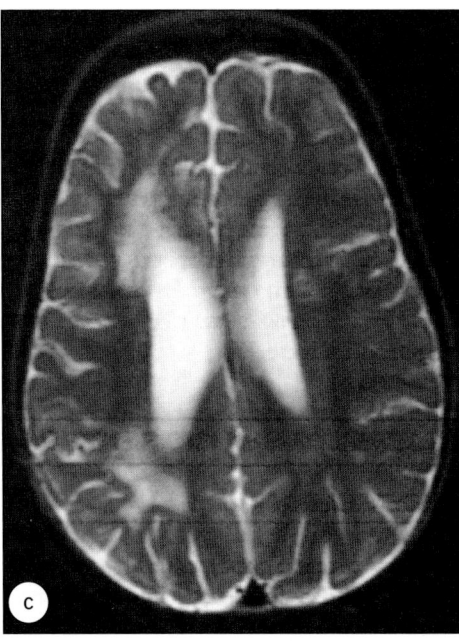

Fig. 20.3 Postinfectious encephalomyelitis. (a, b) Magnetic resonance imaging of brain at presentation showing asymmetric demyelination of cortical white matter. Basal ganglia were also involved bilaterally (not shown). (b) At 7 weeks, the distribution is more symmetric. (c) Residual lesions at 4 months, with full clinical recovery.

OPTIC NEURITIS

This is heralded by pain above or behind the eye aggravated by movement, loss of color discrimination and progressive central visual impairment. Total blindness of the eye may follow within a few hours to days. Single eye involvement is present in 90% of adult cases; bilateral neuritis occurs in up to 40% of pediatric cases. Most patients recover within 4 weeks. The reported incidence of MS following ON varies widely (5–57%), but is less in children.[13]

The differential diagnosis of ON includes MS, hereditary retinal diseases, vasculitis (giant cell arteritis, lupus), intoxications, parasellar tumors, granulomatous meningitis, neuroborreliosis, syphilis and infection with *Bartonella henselae*.

SYDENHAM'S CHOREA

Chorea is a smooth rapid movement that flows from joint to joint. Sydenham's chorea, which is associated with 15% of cases of rheumatic fever, can include dyskinesias such as tics, athetosis (worm-like movements) and ballismus (violent flinging movement). The prodrome includes emotional lability, obsessive–compulsive symptomatology and hyperactivity. The onset is insidious, with a latency of from 2 weeks to several months after streptococcal pharyngitis. Recovery varies, taking from several weeks to more than 6 months. Rheumatic carditis recurs in 20% of patients with chorea.

The differential diagnosis of basal ganglia lesions includes metabolic disease (Wilson's disease, organic acidemias), cerebral palsy, post-pump cardiac surgery, adverse drug reactions, cerebral vein thrombosis and lupus erythematosus (lupoid sclerosis).

DIAGNOSIS

It is challenging to differentiate postinfectious syndromes from infectious encephalitis (see Chapter 2.16). Magnetic resonance imaging is more sensitive than CT; CT scans are frequently normal;[15] MRI findings are large white matter lesions with initially asymmetric distribution and variable enhancement with contrast (Fig. 20.3). There is limited correlation between clinical signs and neuroradiologic imaging. White matter lesions may take up to 18 months to resolve, and new lesions may appear despite clinical improvement.[16]

Cerebrospinal fluid (CSF) findings are not specific. Elevated intracranial pressure is uncommon and the CSF profile is often normal. Pleocytosis, if present, is mononuclear and rarely exceeds 200 cells/μl.

With extreme inflammation (hemorrhagic leukoencephalitis), neutrophils and erythrocytes are seen. A mild elevation of CSF protein is common. Presence of MBP in the CSF is indicative of oligodendroglial damage and demyelination; the sensitivity is 60%.

Magnetic resonance imaging is recommended for ACA or ON to delineate multifocal CNS disease and to exclude vascular and space-occupying lesions. For ATM, exclusion of treatable causes of cord compression is essential. Computerized tomography scan or MRI of the spine has replaced myelography in the diagnostic approach; myelograms are usually normal in ATM. Despite clinical 'transection', MRI shows cord inflammation extending along many segments. Cerebrospinal fluid analyses are similar to those in PIE. Testing for syphilis, schistosomiasis, HIV and HTLV-I (often coincident) is important in patients from endemic areas with unexplained myelopathy. Polymerase chain reaction (PCR) best detects CMV, VZV and toxoplasmosis in CSF of immunocompromised hosts.

Culture of CSF is indicated, but rarely informative in cases of ADEM. Results of genetic amplification assays such as PCR can be useful when interpreted properly. DNA or RNA derived from infectious agents can persist for weeks, and should not necessarily be construed as evidence of active infection; it can identify antecedent infection.[17,18] Genetic material can mislead when detected as false positives or 'innocent bystanders' in areas of inflammation.[19] Cerebrospinal fluid antibody titers are of limited use. An absence of CSF antibodies is consistent with PIE, but CSF antibodies may be longlived and unrelated to the acute process.[4,20] Simultaneous seroconversions to several pathogens are common, and antibodies to *Mycoplasma pneumoniae* are cross-reactive with brain tissue.[8]

MANAGEMENT

There is no proven treatment for PIE. It is difficult to distinguish postinfectious myelitis from neurosurgical emergencies; early use of CT or MRI is indicated. Lumbar puncture should include pressure measurement. Antiviral therapy is not indicated, but initial exclusion of treatable infectious encephalitis can be difficult and empiric therapy is often given. Immunoglobulin and corticosteroid therapies have no demonstrated benefit in ADEM, although corticosteroids have been used to treat swelling of the cord.[21]

Management of seizures with anticonvulsants and administration of antipyretics is recommended; autonomic instability should be treated with short-acting drugs. Protection of the airway and control of intracranial pressure are often necessary. Management of ATM requires meticulous care to avoid complications during a prolonged recovery. Pneumonia, sepsis, renal failure and autonomic disturbances, including arrhythmias, are acute life-threatening complications. Urinary tract infection is very common; intermittent catheterization is preferable to use of an indwelling catheter to minimize this risk. Good nursing and, in some cases, anticoagulation should minimize the risk of pulmonary embolism. Psychologic support is necessary for both the patient and his or her family. Corticosteroids are sometimes given in high doses for ON to obtain a rapid improvement but have no significant effect on long-term outcome.[22]

ENCEPHALOPATHY AND REYE'S SYNDROME

EPIDEMIOLOGY

The term encephalopathy is used when CNS dysfunction is not associated with histologic or indirect evidence (CSF pleocytosis, MRI findings) of inflammation. Encephalopathy following infection or immunization does not appear to be a single syndrome. The Vaccine Safety Committee, Institute of Medicine, Washington DC, has modified case definitions used in the National Childhood Encephalopathy Study (NCES); (Fig. 20.4). Reye's syndrome is an encephalopathy associated with liver dysfunction.

The incidence of postinfectious and postvaccinal encephalopathy varies by country, reflecting national immunization practices and sanitation. The incidence of postvaccine encephalopathy is less than 10.5/million immunizations.[23] Age-specific incidences of vaccines and postvaccinal encephalopathy overlap the ages of onset of many childhood neurologic conditions.[24,25] The incidence of encephalopathies associated with typhoid and other enteric pathogens is highest during the summer or the rainy season. The seasonality of Reye's syndrome corresponds to antecedent varicella or influenza infections. The incidence of Reye's syndrome was 0.31/100,000 individuals under 18 years of age in 1980; milder forms of the encephalopathy occur in 5.6/100,000 children.[26] Reye's syndrome associated with salicylate use has become less common since the educational campaigns discouraging aspirin use in children.[27]

Whole-cell pertussis (wP) is the vaccine most frequently associated with encephalopathy. Controversy over the neurologic complications of the diphtheria, tetanus and wP (DTwP) vaccine reduced the immunization rate in the UK to 31% in 1977; this, in turn, gave rise to the largest epidemic of pertussis observed in 20 years. The NCES, a case–control study of the association of DTwP immunization with serious neurologic diseases, was undertaken from 1976 to 1979. Estimated attributable risk for acute encephalopathy, atypical seizures, infantile spasms and Reye's syndrome was 1/110,000 doses.[24] A 10-year follow-up study confirmed that all serious acute neurologic events, irrespective of association with DTwP, might be associated with important neurologic sequelae.[25] Evidence is consistent with, but does not establish, a causal relationship of DTwP vaccine with encephalopathy; there were no associations of DTwP with infantile spasms or Reye's syndrome. Declining reactogenicity of DTwP vaccines and recent licensing of acellular pertussis vaccines may change the incidence of this syndrome.

PATHOGENESIS AND PATHOLOGY

The pathogenesis of postinfectious or postvaccinal encephalopathy is not known. Latency between infection or vaccination and encephalopathy is highly variable, ranging from hours up to 6 weeks. Autopsy series of postinfectious encephalitis include cases of encephalopathy; findings demonstrate cerebral edema without inflammation. Hypoxic insult, electrolyte disorders and endogenous toxins are often invoked to explain this pathology.[28,29] Some cases of postvaccinal encephalopathy

may result from unmasking or precipitation of an underlying neurologic condition by the vaccine.[23] Postinfectious encephalopathy is associated with nonspecific respiratory and gastrointestinal tract infections, measles, pertussis and typhoid infections.[30,31] Whole-cell pertussis, DT/Td/tetanus toxoid, measles, mumps and vaccinia vaccines have been associated with encephalopathy.[23]

Liver pathology in Reye's syndrome is pathognomonic. Panlobular accumulation of small lipid droplets occurs without evidence of cholestasis or inflammation. By electron microscopy, the mitochondria are large and irregular, with diminished matrix granules. There may be a proliferation of peroxisomes and smooth endoplasmic reticulum, and depletion of glycogen. The pathogenesis is not known. Underlying metabolic disorders cause some cases of Reye's syndrome.[32]

PREVENTION

Repeat immunization with the specific vaccine is contraindicated in instances of postvaccinal encephalopathy not due to another identifiable cause. Licensing of acellular pertussis vaccines will reduce the incidence of this syndrome. Avoidance of aspirin use for common fevers and for analgesia in children effectively minimizes the risk of Reye's syndrome. Reye's syndrome following the administration of live varicella vaccine to patients on chronic salicylate therapy has not been described. The decision whether to give this vaccine to such patients must be individualized.

CLINICAL FEATURES

Postinfectious encephalopathy is a disease of early childhood, occurring at a mean age of 18 months. In contrast, PIE is rare in children under 2 years of age.[29] Encephalopathy after pertussis infection occurs mostly during the first 6 months of life.[30] In contrast to postinfectious and postvaccinal encephalopathy, Reye's syndrome affects school-aged children and adolescents.

Encephalopathy is indistinguishable clinically from encephalitis.[28,29] Fever and seizures are common, but the presence of focal neurologic

DEFINITION OF ENCEPHALOPATHY
Acute encephalopathy
Children <24 months:
Significantly decreased level of consciousness (stupor or coma) lasting for at least 24 hours, not attributable to postictal state or medication
Children ≥24 months:
Condition lasting for at least 24 hours, characterized by two of following:
Confusional state or a delirium, or a psychosis, not medication related
Significantly decreased level of consciousness (stupor or coma), independent of seizure and not attributed to medication
Seizure associated with loss of consciousness
Increased intracranial pressure is consistent with the diagnosis at any age
Excluded conditions: Sleepiness Persistent inconsolable crying Bulging fontanelle Seizures
Chronic encephalopathy
Persistence of acute findings over several months to years beyond the acute episode
Excluded conditions: Return to normalcy, followed by chronic encephalopathy Chronic encephalopathy secondary to genetic, prenatal or perinatal factors

Fig. 20.4 Definition of encephalopathy. Modified from Vaccine Safety Committee, Institute of Medicine.[3]

deficits is unusual. No specific neurologic syndrome has been described after DTwP vaccination. The onset of encephalopathy after wP vaccination typically occurs in the first 3 days, and is rare after 7 days, although encephalopathy after pertussis infection occurs in the second or third week. Reye's syndrome is heralded by severe repetitive vomiting refractory to common interventions, followed by altered consciousness.

The differential diagnosis of encephalopathy is similar to that for PIE. In infants, shaken baby syndrome, cerebral vein thrombosis and hyperpyrexic shock with encephalopathy must be considered. In many countries, shigellosis, acute typhoid fever and malaria cause diagnostic confusion.

Encephalopathy is frequently complicated by aspiration pneumonia. Intracranial hypertension, inappropriate antidiuretic hormone secretion, electrolyte disorders and hypoxic–ischemic injury may exacerbate it and produce secondary brain damage. Cerebral edema can be severe and lead to cerebral herniation. Children suffering severe neurologic syndromes temporally associated with wP vaccine administration carry a five-fold relative risk for chronic neurologic disease over asymptomatic vaccine recipients.[25]

DIAGNOSIS

There is no diagnostic test for postinfectious encephalopathy. The CSF is frequently under increased pressure, but is otherwise normal by routine analysis. In Reye's syndrome there must be evidence of liver disease consisting of elevated liver transaminases or elevated plasma ammonia. The blood glucose concentration is frequently low; bilirubin is normal.

A diagnosis of postvaccinal encephalopathy is by temporal association; proof of causation is impossible in individual cases.

MANAGEMENT

Therapy is supportive. Electrolyte or metabolic disorders and intoxications are excluded by history and laboratory analysis. Magnetic resonance imaging may reveal encephalomyelitis, cerebral edema or other pathology. Plasma and urine samples for metabolic analysis should be obtained early. Intravenous glucose is important for brain metabolism and reversal of gluconeogenesis and hyperammonemia. Complications of encephalopathy include aspiration and cerebral herniation. Intubation and mechanical ventilation are commonly indicated.

GUILLAIN–BARRÉ SYNDROME

EPIDEMIOLOGY

Guillain–Barré syndrome is an acute, ascending, symmetric paralytic disorder diagnosed by consensus clinical criteria. Acute inflammatory demyelinating polyneuropathy (AIDP) is the classic form of GBS. Variants include:
- acute motor axonal neuropathy (AMAN, Chinese paralysis syndrome);
- acute motor sensory axonal neuropathy (AMSAN);
- hyperacute GBS; and
- Miller Fisher syndrome (MFS).
Other forms may exist.

Guillain–Barré syndrome has replaced poliomyelitis as the most common cause of acute flaccid paralysis worldwide. In the temperate Americas, Europe and Australia, GBS occurs without seasonality.[33,34] In China, middle latitudes of the Americas, and possibly the Indian subcontinent, the number of cases increases during summer months.[35] Geographic or familial clustering is rare with either form. Guillain–Barré syndrome and axonal variants are coincident and the incidence of GBS is estimated to be 0.4–1.5/100,000 population in temperate climates.

Guillain–Barré syndrome is associated with most antigenic triggers

of PIE, including minor respiratory infections in 50% of cases. *Campylobacter jejuni* infections are associated with 26–40% of GBS cases in industrialized nations and in up to 90% of cases in China.[34] Fewer than 5% of cases are vaccine-associated.[36]

PATHOGENESIS AND PATHOLOGY

The pathogenesis of GBS is heterogeneous.[37,38] Peripheral nerve myelin is distinct from CNS myelin and mechanisms of demyelination in the CNS and PNS may differ. Major proteins in peripheral myelin include P_0, MBP and P_2. The G_{M1} ganglioside is enriched in paranodal regions of both nerve and myelin, although the G_{Q1b} ganglioside is similarly enriched in oculomotor nerves.

Classic GBS (AIDP) is an acute monophasic demyelinating syndrome of peripheral nerves.[33] It is multifocal, with a predilection for nerve roots and internodes. Demyelination is associated with deposits of antibody and complement as well as macrophage 'stripping' of outer myelin lamellae. Inflammation at the nerve roots is believed to lead to disruption of the CNS blood–brain barrier, with leakage of serum proteins into the CSF. In AIDP, axonal loss is correlated with severe inflammation.

Experimental allergic neuritis (EAN), caused by repeated immunization with peripheral nervous tissue, is clinically, electrophysiologically and pathologically similar to GBS. Immunologic mechanisms may differ between EAN and GBS. Passive transfer of lymphocytes sensitized to P_0 or P_2 myelin proteins reproduces EAN; transfer of serum does not. In contrast, human T lymphocyte activation against myelin proteins is variable, although sera from GBS patients causes nerve demyelination in tissue culture. Antibodies against G_{M1} and related sialylated gangliosides are detected in up to 60% of patients with *C. jejuni*-associated GBS. Strains of *C. jejuni* contain membrane glycolipids with identical glycoconjugate structures to those of peripheral nerve gangliosides. This is antigenic identity rather than oft-quoted mimicry. Antibodies against ganglioside G_{Q1b} are described in 90% of cases of MFS, a GBS variant with ophthalmoplegia.

Acute motor sensory axonal neuropathy and AMAN variants, although clinically similar to demyelinating GBS (AIDP), are characterized by axonal degeneration with or without sensory nerve involvement, respectively.[37,38] Both syndromes are frequently associated with *C. jejuni*. Axonal degeneration correlates with macrophage infiltration of internodal and periaxonal spaces.[37] A chicken model of *C. jejuni*-associated AMAN has been reported.

CONDITIONS ASSOCIATED WITH GBS

Nonspecific respiratory tract symptoms
Campylobacter jejuni
Mycoplasma pneumoniae
Cytomegalovirus
Epstein–Barr virus
Human immunodeficiency virus-1
Japanese encephalitis virus
Hodgkin's disease
Lymphoma
Systemic lupus erythematosus
Surgery
Parturition

Vaccines
  Vaccinia
  Rabies
  Influenza A/New Jersey/76
  Oral poliovirus in Finland

Fig. 20.5 Conditions associated with Guillain–Barré syndrome (GBS).

Infectious and other antigenic triggers associated with GBS are common (Fig. 20.5). Campylobacter can induce several autoimmune conditions; reactive arthritis and GBS do not cosegregate. Specific matches of bacterial serotype and host genotype may be required; these may differ in Asia and North America or Europe.[39,40]

PREVENTION

Guillain–Barré syndrome associated with *C. jejuni* infections is prevented by improvements in local sanitation, water and food supplies. Control of common diseases such as CMV, HIV, mycoplasma infection and Japanese encephalitis should reduce the incidence of GBS and other postinfectious syndromes. Replacement of whole-cell or tissue-derived vaccines with purified component vaccines may also diminish the incidence of GBS.

CLINICAL FEATURES

The annual incidence of GBS in the USA increases with age, from 0.8/100,000 individuals under 18 years of age to 3.25/100,000 in those over 60.[36] There is an overall male to female preponderance of 1.5 to 1 for GBS occurring in later life.[34] Acute motor axonal neuropathy in China affects children and young adults, with a mean age of 19 years.[35]

Guillain–Barré syndrome is an acute afebrile paresis that progresses over a few days to weeks. Diagnosis is by consensus criteria; there is no specific laboratory diagnosis (Fig. 20.6).[41] Paresthesias in toes or fingertips variably precede motor findings. Weakness is generally more profound in the legs, but may predominantly affect the arms or cranial nerves in up to 10% of cases each. Weakness begins distally and progresses centrally; progression may be quite rapid. As GBS evolves, general symmetry of paresis is the rule. Dysautonomia may be prominent, but bowel or bladder incontinence is rare. Pain is common, involving the large muscles of the legs and back.

Examination shows relatively symmetric motor weakness, absent or greatly diminished tendon reflexes, and minimal loss of sensation despite sensory complaints. In severe cases, respiration, airway control and autonomic function are affected.

Miller Fisher syndrome comprises ophthalmoplegia, ataxia and areflexia, with little weakness. Axonal neuropathy (AMAN or AMSAN) is clinically indistinguishable from demyelinating disease (AIDP). Curiously, axonal involvement is important for the prognosis of the adult but not the pediatric form of AMAN.[35,42]

Phases of GBS include:
- progression (2–4 weeks),
- plateau (2–4 weeks), and
- recovery (weeks to months).

Respiratory failure develops in 20% of children and 40% of adults; pneumonia occurs in 25% of patients and urinary tract infections in 40%. Mean duration of intubation is 15–30 days with current therapy. Guillain–Barré syndrome is complicated by lability of blood pressure, cardiac arrhythmias or thrombosis in 20, 25 and 3% of adults, respectively. Mortality with optimal supportive care and treatment is under 5%.

A rapid onset of severe paresis, need for mechanical ventilation, increasing age, antibodies to *C. jejuni* and G_{M1}, and axonal neuropathy are associated with slow or incomplete recovery.[43] Mean time to ambulation with current therapy is 40–50 days; 15% of cases do not walk at 48 weeks. Most (80%) eventually pursue normal activities, but show mild residual effects under careful examination. The outcomes for children and adults are probably similar.

Guillain–Barré syndrome must be distinguished from a variety of diseases of the CNS and PNS. Chronic inflammatory demyelinating polyneuropathy, a relapsing demyelinative disease, and chronic progressive demyelinating polyneuropathy are clinically indistinguishable at onset from GBS.

CRITERIA FOR DIAGNOSIS OF GBS	
Required	Muscle weakness
	Progressive motor weakness of more than one limb, and/or bulbar and facial paralysis (30%), and/or external ophthalmoplegia (6%)
	Areflexia
Supportive	Clinical
	Progression over 2–4 weeks
	Relative symmetry
	Mild sensory signs
	Cranial nerve involvement (without sphincter involvement; 50%)
	Recovery after interval of 2–4 weeks after nadir
	Autonomic dysfunction (20%)
	Absence of fever at onset
	Cerebrospinal fluid
	Cerebrospinal fluid protein rising after first week
	Cerebrospinal fluid leukocytosis less than 10/µl, (mononuclear cells)
	Nerve conduction studies, in two or more motor nerves
	Partial conduction block or decreased M responses, or both (75%)
	Nerve conduction velocity <70% of normal, several weeks into illness (60%)
	Abnormalities in late responses (F-waves, H-reflexes; 46%)
	Features discordant for GBS
	Marked persistent asymmetry of weakness
	Sphincter dysautonomia at onset or persistent
	Cerebrospinal fluid leukocytosis >50/µl, or neutrophils in CSF
	Sharp sensory level
	Systemic illness or constitutional symptoms
Exclusionary	–

Fig. 20.6 Criteria for diagnosis of Guillain–Barré syndrome (GBS). Required criteria must be present for diagnosis. Supportive criteria strongly support the diagnosis, but may not be present initially and in all cases. Exclusionary criteria suggest an alternate diagnosis is likely. Modified from Asbury and Cornblath.[41]

DIAGNOSIS

Diagnosis requires examination of the CSF and nerve conduction studies (Fig. 20.6). Cerebrospinal fluid pressure should be normal and contain fewer than 10 leukocytes/µl. Cerebrospinal fluid protein may be normal during the first 48 hours of illness and is not reliably elevated until the second week of illness. Nerve conduction studies must include several nerves because demyelination is patchy. Conduction studies may not become abnormal until several weeks into the illness; up to 20% of patients never have abnormal studies. Conduction velocity is usually less than 60% of normal. F-wave responses, which measure nerve root disease, are a useful indicator of the disease.[41]

Stool cultures for *C. jejuni* are often positive in patients with GBS, especially those with axonal neuropathy. Diarrhea is an insensitive (70%) predictor of carriage of *C. jejuni*. Enrichment methods may improve yield from culture.[34] Serology for recent *C. jejuni* infection is of limited use. Cases may be culture positive for *C. jejuni*, but not mount an antibody response; IgM antibodies are cross-reactive with Salmonella and *Yersinia* spp. Approximately 50% of cases colonized with *C. jejuni* have serum antibodies against G_{M1} ganglioside. Anti-G_{M1}

antibodies of IgM class are present in acute and chronic motor neuropathies, including axonal GBS; IgG class antibodies are more specific for classic GBS (AIDP).[44] Serologic evidence of infections with Epstein–Barr virus (EBV), CMV and mycoplasma are reported in 15, 8 and 5%, respectively, of GBS cases occurring in childhood and young adulthood.[45,46] Cold agglutinins are often positive and result from EBV, CMV or mycoplasma infection. Rheumatoid factor may cause false IgM seropositivity.

MANAGEMENT

The management of GBS is a challenge to the clinician because laboratory features are often absent until the second week of illness. It is essential to exclude competing diagnoses requiring emergent management, especially epidural abscess of the spine. Initial evaluation should include CT or MRI of the spine. Lumbar puncture is performed and repeated a week or two later. Nerve conduction studies are necessary for diagnosis, and have prognostic significance for the course of recovery. Stool cultures with enrichment for *C. jejuni* provide corroborative data. Analysis for antiganglioside and anticampylobacter antibodies remains a research tool. Serology for syphilis and HIV are frequently ordered; some experts test for antibodies against EBV, CMV and mycoplasma.

During evolution of the illness, it is imperative to monitor evolving respiratory paralysis by objective measures of vital capacity. In children unable to comply with standard testing, range of serial counting, alphabets or song in a single breath is useful at the bedside. Intensive care is indicated for rapidly declining vital capacities or those below 18ml/kg. Disease is intermittently progressive up to 4 weeks after onset.

Several large controlled studies have demonstrated use for plasma exchange (PE) or immunotherapy with intravenous immunoglobulin (IVIG).[42,43,47] Use of corticosteroids is not effective.[33] The natural history of GBS, with spontaneous full recovery in 80% of cases, limits statistical power for detecting differences in therapy. Therapy for MFS has not been well studied; pediatric representation in studies is low. Complications limit therapy in 14% of PE and 3% of IVIG therapies. Combination therapy with PE and IVIG results in comparable efficacy but additive toxicities.[42] Anecdotal reports suggest better outcome after treatment with IVIG over PE in cases with both G_{M1} and *C. jejuni* antibodies.[48] Relapses occur after either therapy in 10% of cases.[33] Although therapy with IVIG can be performed at many clinics, most experts agree that GBS requires expert diagnosis and management available at tertiary referral centers. An international support group, GBS Foundation International, is accessible on the internet at http://www.webmast.com/gbs/.

BRACHIAL NEURITIS

EPIDEMIOLOGY AND PATHOGENESIS

Brachial neuritis (brachial plexus neuropathy, neuralgic amyotrophy) is a well-described but poorly understood axonopathy. Annual incidence is approximately 1.6/100,000 individuals.[3] About 15% of cases are associated with immunizations or administration of antiserum; outbreaks have been reported. Administration of tetanus toxoid carries an excess risk of 0.5–1.0/100,000 doses. Latency from immunization to disease is 6–21 days, consistent with an immunologic mechanism.[3]

CLINICAL FEATURES

Brachial neuritis begins with severe aching pain of the shoulder and upper arm. Weakness develops as pain subsides. Motor and sensory deficits are consistent with lesions in the brachial plexus. There is no correlation of laterality of brachial neuritis and antecedent immunization; the syndrome is bilateral in up to one-third of cases. Recovery, requiring regeneration and collateral innervation of axons, begins within 1 month of onset and requires 2–3 years. Brachial neuritis can be complicated by paresis of the diaphragm.

Brachial neuritis must be distinguished from injection damage to the nerve, poliomyelitis at the site of an antecedent injection, cervical ribs, cord compression and Lyme disease. In the infant, perinatal traction injury, syphilitic pseudoparalysis and occult trauma or osteomyelitis must also be considered.

DIAGNOSIS AND MANAGEMENT

Nerve conduction studies are consistent with axonal neuropathy without a conduction block. Radiologic study of the affected arm and shoulder is often performed to exclude alternate diagnoses. Serologic testing for syphilis and Lyme disease may be indicated. There are no controlled studies on the therapy of this uncommon disorder. Psychologic support is essential during prolonged rehabilitation.

CRANIAL NEUROPATHIES

EPIDEMIOLOGY AND PATHOGENESIS

Peripheral cranial nerves can be affected singly or as a multifocal process following infections or immunizations. Facial palsy is the most common cranial neuropathy, with incidence of 35/100,000 population. Bell's palsy or isolated acute peripheral facial paralysis of unknown etiology accounts for 73% of facial palsies. Similar etiologies for GBS and Bell's palsy were suggested in one study.[36] Although a postinfectious etiology is presumed, recent molecular data implicate reactivation by HSV-1.[49] Bulbar nerve palsies and ophthalmoplegia occur most commonly in association with GBS (30 and 6% of GBS cases, respectively).

CLINICAL FEATURES

Mean age of onset of facial palsy is 46 years with equal sex distribution. The onset frequently follows a respiratory tract infection. The paresis is sudden, without systemic illness. Simultaneous, bilateral disease occurs in less than 1% of cases in adults, and may be associated with subclinical neuropathy of other cranial or peripheral nerves. Bilateral disease is more frequent in children. Resolution occurs within 6 weeks in 80% of cases. Bulbar nerve palsies present with a weak voice or cry, nasal intonation, nasal reflux and difficulty handling oral secretions. Ophthalmoplegia can present as torticollis or diplopia, and be associated with retro-orbital pain.

In areas of endemicity, *Borrelia burgdorferi* causes 30% of facial, and most bilateral, palsies.[50] Herpes simplex and VZV cause facial palsy by primary infection or reactivation. Although HIV-1 is associated with facial palsy, paresis during severe immunodeficiency usually indicates another etiology. Causes of facial paresis include GBS, MS, skull fractures, suppurative otitis, acoustic neuroma, carcinomatous or granulomatous meningitis, sarcoidosis, leprosy, diphtheria and Kawasaki disease.[51] Causes of ophthalmoplegia include chronic meningitis, intracranial hypertension and botulism. Bulbar paresis occurs in GBS, diphtheria, botulism, poliomyelitis and paraneoplastic syndromes.

DIAGNOSIS

Polymerase chain reaction detected HSV-1 genome in 79% of endoneural fluids from a surgical series with Bell's palsy.[49] Extrapolation to PCR testing of other sterile fluids, such as CSF, is uncertain. Serologic diagnosis of Lyme borreliosis or antecedent herpes simplex virus or VZV infection in facial palsy is complicated by limitations of test sensitivities and specificities.[50] Simultaneous seroconversions to several viruses are common.[51] In areas endemic for Lyme disease, physicians frequently evaluate facial palsy after empiric oral therapy against *B. burgdorferi*. Given the self-limited nature of Bell's palsy, it is poor logic to make a causal diagnosis based on reponse to therapy for Lyme disease.

MANAGEMENT

Management of isolated Bell's palsy varies. Evaluation of bilateral facial palsies or other cranial neuropathies includes investigation for GBS and CNS demyelinating disease. There are few controlled therapeutic trials to address therapeutic strategies; corticosteroid therapy is no more effective than placebo.

REFERENCES

1. Griffin DE. Monophasic autoimmune inflammatory diseases of the CNS and PNS. In: Waksman BH, ed. Immunologic mechanisms in neurologic and psychiatric disease. New York: Raven Press; 1990:91–104.
2. Koskiniemi M, Vaheri A. Effect of measles, mumps, rubella vaccination on pattern of encephalitis in children. Lancet 1989;1:31–4.
3. Vaccine Safety Committee Institute of Medicine. Adverse events associated with childhood vaccines. Evidence based on causality. Washington, DC: National Academy Press; 1994:241.
4. Johnson RT, Griffin DE, Hirsch RL, et al. Measles encephalomyelitis – clinical and immunologic studies. N Engl J Med 1984;310:137–41.
5. Hemachudha T, Phanuphak P, Johnson RT, Griffin DE, Ratanavongsiri J, Siriprosomsup W. Neurological complications of Semple type rabies vaccine: clinical and immunological studies. Neurol 1987;37:550–6.
6. Itoyama Y, Webster HdeF, Sternberger NH, et al. Distribution of papovavirus, myelin-associated glycoprotein, and myelin basic protein in progressive multifocal leukoencephalopathy lesions. Ann Neurol 1982;11:396–407.
7. Woody RC, Steele RW, Charlton RK, Smith V. Histocompatibility determinants in childhood postinfectious encephalomyelitis. J Child Neurol 1989;4:204–6.
8. Lehtokoski-Lehtiniemi E, Koskiniemi M-L. *Mycoplasma pneumoniae* encephalitis: a severe entity in children. Pediatr Infect Dis J 1989;8:651–3.
9. Kiessling LS, Marcotte AC, Culpepper L. Antineuronal antibodies: tics and obsessive–compulsive symptoms. J Dev Behav Pediatr 1994;15:421–5.
10. Gieron-Korthals MA, Westberry KR, Emmanuel PJ. Acute childhood ataxia: 10-year experience. J Child Neurol 1994;9:381–4.
11. Miller HG, Stanton JB, Gibbons JL. Para-infectious encephalomyelitis and related syndromes. A critical review of the neurological complications of certain specific fevers. Q J Med 1956;25:427–504.
12. Altrocchi PH. Acute transverse myelopathy. Arch Neurol 1963;9:21–9.
13. Francis DA. Demyelinating optic neuritis: clinical features and differential diagnosis. Br J Hosp Med 1991;45:376–9.
14. Koenig H, Rabinowitz S, Day E, Miller V. Post-infectious encephalomyelitis after successful treatment of herpes simplex encephalitis with adenine arabinoside. N Engl J Med 1979;300:1089–93.
15. Caldemeyer KS, Smith RR, Harris TM, Edwards MK. MRI in acute disseminated encephalomyelitis. Neuroradiology 1994;36:216–20.
16. Kesselring J, Miller DH, Robb SA, et al. Acute disseminated encephalomyelitis. MRI findings and the distinction from multiple sclerosis. Brain 1990;113:291–302.
17. Kimberlin DW, Lakeman FD, Arvin AM, et al. Application of the polymerase chain reaction to the diagnosis and management of neonatal herpes simplex virus disease. J Infect Dis 1996;174:1162–7.

18. Puchhammer-Stockl E, Popow-Kraupp T, Heinz FX, Mandl CW, Kunz C. Detection of varicella–zoster virus DNA by polymerase chain reaction in the cerebrospinal fluid of patients suffering from neurological complications associated with chicken pox or herpes zoster. J Clin Microbiol 1991;29:1513–6.
19. Jay V, Becker LE, Otsubo H, et al. Chronic encephalitis and epilepsy (Rasmussen's encephalitis): detection of cytomegalovirus and herpes simplex virus 1 by the polymerase chain reaction and *in situ* hybridization. Neurol 1995;45:108–17.
20. Vandvik B, Sköldenberg B, Forsgren M, Stiernstedt G, Jeansson S, Norrby E. Long-term persistence of intrathecal virus-specific antibody responses after herpes simplex virus encephalitis. J Neurol 1985;231:307–12.
21. Boe J, Solberg CO, Saeter T. Corticosteroid treatment for acute meningoencephalitis: a retrospective of 346 cases. Br Med J 1965;Apr (vol 1):1094–5.
22. Beck RW, Trobe JD, Optic Neuritis Study Group. The optic neuritis treatment trial. J Neuro-Ophthalmol 1995;15:131–5.
23. Advisory Committee on Immunization Practices. Update: vaccine side effects, adverse reactions, contraindications, and precautions. MMWR Morb Mortal Wkly Rep 1996;45:1–35.
24. Miller DL, Ross EM, Alderslade R, Bellman MH, Rawson NSB. Pertussis immunisation and serious acute neurological illness in children. Br Med J 1981;282:1595–9.
25. Miller D, Madge N, Diamond J, Wadsworth J, Ross E. Pertussis immunisation and serious acute neurological illnesses in children. Br Med J 1993;307:1171–6.
26. Lichtenstein PK, Heubi JE, Daugherty CC, et al. Grade I Reye's syndrome. A frequent cause of vomiting and liver dysfunction after varicella and upper respiratory tract infection. N Engl J Med 1983;309:133–9.
27. Committee on Infectious Diseases. Aspirin and Reye syndrome. Pediatrics 1982;69:810–2.
28. Spillane JD, Wells CC. The neurology of Jennerian Vaccination. Brain 1964;87:1–44.
29. Lyon G, Dodge PR, Adams RD. The acute encephalopathies of obscure origin in infants and children. Brain 1961;84:680–708.
30. Litvak AM, Gibel H, Rosenthal SE, Bosenblatt P. Cerebral complications in pertussis. J Pediatr 1948;32:357–79.
31. Osuntokun BO, Bademosi O, Ogunremi K, Wright SG. Neuropsychiatric manifestations of typhoid fever in 959 patients. Arch Neurol 1972;27:7–12.
32. Rowe PC, Newman SL, Brusilow SW. Natural history of symptomatic partial ornithine transcarbamylase deficiency. N Engl J Med 1986;314:541–7.
33. Ropper AH. The Guillain–Barré syndrome [Review]. N Engl J Med 1992;326:1130–6.
34. Rees JH, Soudain SE, Gregson NA, Hughes RA. *Campylobacter jejuni* infection and Guillain–Barré syndrome. N Engl J Med 1995;333:1374–9.
35. McKhann GM, Cornblath DR, Griffin JW, et al. Acute motor axonal neuropathy: a frequent cause of acute flaccid paralysis in China. Ann Neurol 1993;33:333–42.

36. Schonberger LB, Jurqitz ES, Katona P, Holman RC, Bregman DJ. Guillain–Barré syndrome: its epidemiology and associations with influenza vaccination. Ann Neurol 1981;9 (Suppl):31–8.
37. Griffin JW, Li CY, Ho TW, et al. Pathology of the motor–sensory axonal Guillain–Barré syndrome. Ann Neurol 1996;39:17–28.
38. Griffin JW, Li CY, Ho TW, et al. Guillain–Barré syndrome in northern China. The spectrum of neuropathological changes in clinically defined cases. Brain 1995;118:577–95.
39. Rees JH, Vaughan RW, Kondeatis E, Hughes RA. HLA-class II alleles in Guillain–Barré syndrome and Miller Fisher syndrome and their association with preceding *Campylobacter jejuni* infection. J Neuroimmunol 1995;62:53–7.
40. Yuki N, Ichikawa H, Doi A. Fisher syndrome after *Campylobacter jejuni* enteritis: human leukocyte antigen and the bacterial serotype. J Pediatr 1995;126:55–7.
41. Asbury AK, Cornblath DR. Assessment of current diagnostic criteria for Guillain–Barré syndrome. Ann Neurol 1990;27(Suppl):21–4.
42. Plasma exchange/Sandoglobulin Guillain–Barré syndrome trial group. Randomised trial of plasma exchange, intravenous immunoglobulin, and combined treatments in Guillain–Barré syndrome. Lancet 1997;349:225–30.
43. van der Meche FG, Schmitz PIM, Dutch Guillain–Barré Study Group. A randomized trial comparing intravenous immune globulin and plasma exchange in Guillain–Barré syndrome. N Engl J Med 1992;326:1123–9.
44. Kornberg AJ, Pestronk A, Bieser K, et al. The clinical correlates of high-titer IgG anti-GM1 antibodies. Ann Neurol 1994;35:234–7.
45. Goldschmidt B, Menonna J, Fortunato J, Dowling P, Cook S. Mycoplasma antibody in Guillain–Barré syndrome and other neurological disorders. Ann Neurol 1980;7:108–12.
46. Dowling PC, Cook SD. Role of infection in Guillain–Barré syndrome: laboratory confirmation of herpesviruses in 41 cases. Ann Neurol 1981;9(Suppl):44–55.
47. The Guillain–Barré Syndrome Study Group. Plasmapheresis and acute Guillain–Barré syndrome. Neurol 1985;35:1096–1104.
48. Jacobs BC, Schmitz PI, van der Meche FG. *Campylobacter jejuni* infection and treatment for Guillain–Barré syndrome. N Engl J Med 1996;335:208–9.
49. Murakami S, Mizobuchi M, Nakashiro Y, Doi T, Hato N, Yanagihara N. Bell palsy and herpes simplex virus: identification of viral DNA in endoneurial fluid and muscle. Ann Intern Med 1996;124:27–30.
50. Hansen K, Lebech AM. The clinical and epidemiological profile of Lyme neuroborreliosis in Denmark 1985–1990. A prospective study of 187 patients with *Borrelia burgdorferi* specific intrathecal antibody production. Brain 1992;115:399–423.
51. Morgan M, Nathwani D. Facial palsy and infection: the unfolding story. Clin Infect Dis 1992;14:263–71.

Infections in Hydrocephalus Shunts

Roger Bayston

Hydrocephalus shunts drain excess cerebrospinal fluid (CSF) from the cerebral ventricles to the peritoneal cavity [ventriculoperitoneal (VP)], to the right cardiac atrium [ventriculoatrial (VA)], or less commonly to other sites (Fig. 21.1). Cerebrospinal fluid is also sometimes drained from the lumbar spinal theca to the peritoneal cavity [lumboperitoneal (LP)].

EPIDEMIOLOGY

The incidence of infection varies according to the age at which the shunt is inserted. Up to 25% of operations in premature infants with hydrocephalus after periventricular hemorrhage result in infection, whereas in older children the incidence is 3–8%.[1-3] There is no difference in infection rates between VA and VP routes.[4] Although the incidence of shunt infections has generally fallen, it is still unacceptably high. Some centres have reported rates of infection near to zero.[5]

PATHOGENESIS AND PATHOLOGY

The source of the organisms is almost invariably the patient's skin, from which they gain access to the device during its insertion.[6,7] Where there is a serious breakdown in surgical asepsis, or where the operating theater environment or air is grossly contaminated, these may be alternative sources. Although the bacterial population on the surface of the patient's skin can be reduced to almost zero by agents such as alcoholic chlorhexidine, recolonization by resident bacteria occurs rapidly. It is therefore usual to find coagulase-negative staphylococci in the incision during the procedure. In nonimplant surgery these are irrelevant, but where a biomaterial or device is inserted they are highly likely to adhere to and colonize the device. Coagulase-negative staphylococci, and particularly *Staphylococcus epidermidis*, predominate in shunt infections. After adhering to the shunt material, they multiply and produce copious amounts of exopolysaccharide ('slime'), enabling the formation of a biofilm. Because of nutrient depletion, growth is very slow and this accounts for the often long periods between surgery and clinical presentation of infection. *Staphylococcus aureus* causes a different clinical picture, and is more frequently involved in external shunt infections (Fig. 21.2).[4] Unlike *S. epidermidis*, it produces α-toxin, which protects it from phagocytosis. A very active inflammatory response is also evoked, leading to erythema and suppuration.

The clinical presentation of infection in VA shunts differs from that in VP shunts (Fig. 21.3). In the former, bacteria enter the bloodstream directly to cause intermittent fever, which, in infections caused by *S. epidermidis*, propionibacteria or coryneforms, may continue for months or years with little other evidence of infection. However, antibody to bacterial components is produced in large quantities, and immune complex disease may ensue, with deposits of C3, C4, IgG and IgM on the synovial and glomerular basement membranes. Hypertension, renal failure (shunt nephritis) and arthropathy may result.[8] In VP and LP shunt infections, the bacteria are discharged into the peritoneal cavity, provoking the greater omentum to seal off the distal catheter. This and associated adhesions give rise to shunt obstruction and raised CSF pressure (Fig. 21.4). Occasionally, peritoneal

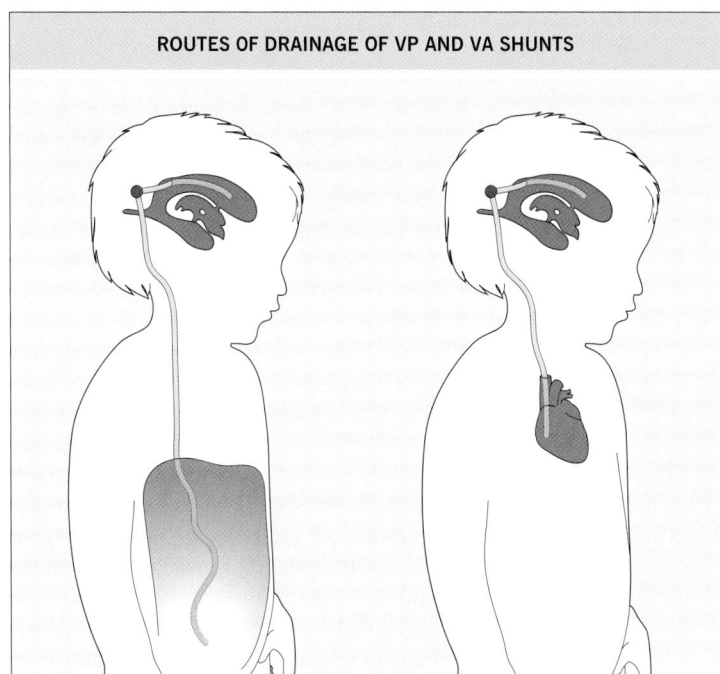

Fig. 21.1 Routes of drainage of VP and VA shunts. Ventriculoperitoneal shunts drain CSF from the cerebral ventricles to the peritoneal cavity via catheter tubing implanted superficially over the rib cage. The lower end of the peritoneal catheter lies free in the abdomen. Ventriculoatrial shunts drain CSF via a convenient neck vein such as the jugular and the superior vena cava to the right atrium.

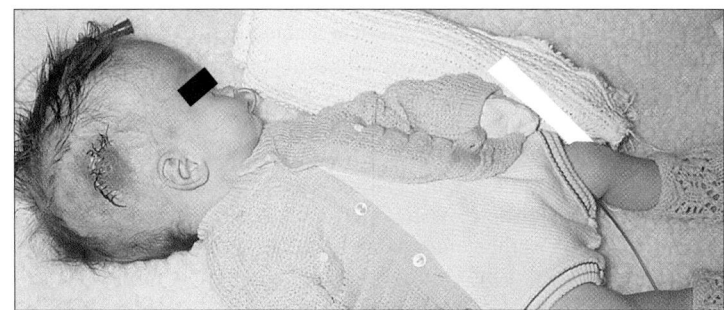

Fig. 21.2 External shunt infection in a premature infant with poor nutritional status. The infection can be caused by organisms introduced at surgery, or they may gain access through minor skin abrasions and pressure necrosis. Differing from the more common internal shunt infections, they are usually caused by *Staphylococcus aureus* and constitute a wound infection enhanced by a foreign material.

abscesses are seen. In all types of shunts ventriculitis is seen in most cases, although the inflammatory response is usually feeble. Only a few shunt infections are due to causes other than surgery. In babies or adults whose nutritional status is poor, erosion of the skin over the shunt can take place, leading to secondary infection with *S. aureus* or

CLINICAL FEATURES OF VA AND VP SHUNT INFECTIONS OF SURGICAL ORIGIN		
	VA shunts	VP shunts
Time from surgery to presentation	Weeks, months, several years	<9 months
Intermittent fever	75%	<50%
Anorexia, lassitude, poor sleep pattern	>80%	>50%
Shunt obstruction	<1%	>75%
Other features	Chills, rigors: 20% Arthralgia: 50% [late onset cases (1–15 years)] Rash: 70% [late onset cases (1–15 years)] Nephritis: 30% [late onset cases (1–15 years)]	Abdominal pain, bloating: >75% Swelling, erythema over shunt tubing: >60% Headache, vomiting etc. (i.e. recurrence of hydrocephalus): 75%

Fig. 21.3 Clinical features of VA and VP shunt infections of surgical origin. Percentages indicate the approximate proportion of cases in which features are present. It is important to realise that each case is different, and that many of these features may be absent or modified.

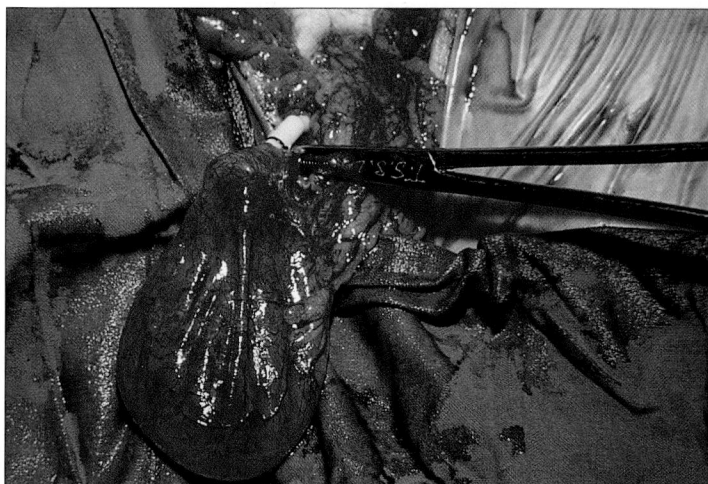

Fig. 21.4 Cystic obstruction of a VP shunt caused by shunt infection with *Staphylococcus epidermidis*. Bacteria and bacterial products entering the peritoneal cavity via the shunt catheter evoke an inflammatory response involving the greater omentum, which seals off the catheter outlet. The resulting cyst fills with CSF, giving rise to recurrence of the hydrocephalus. Cystic obstruction can occur from noninfective causes, but unlike those cases caused by infection, which present within 6–9 months of surgery, they can arise at any time.

Gram-negative bacteria. An unusual but well-documented cause of VP shunt infection is visceral perforation by the distal catheter, which results in polymicrobial infection of the cerebral ventricles.[9] However, peritonitis from this cause is rare.

No cases of hematogenous spread, including to VA shunts, have been documented. Cerebrospinal fluid shunts appear to be unusually free of risk from this source. However, VP shunts can become infected during abdominal surgery or continuous ambulatory peritoneal dialysis.

PREVENTION

In view of the source of infection, most attempts at prevention have been targeted at the surgical procedure. Alcohol-based povidone–iodine and chlorhexidine should be used for skin preparation, the latter having the greater activity. Assiduous surgical technique is extremely important, but infection rates are rarely reduced below 3–5% for adults and 10% for infants. The use of prophylactic antibiotics would appear to be reasonable, but they have not been found to have a statistically significant beneficial effect in properly designed trials.[10] Those who feel obliged to use them despite this are advised to administer 10mg vancomycin hydrochloride in 1–2ml sterile water for injection intraventricularly as soon as the ventricular catheter is inserted (this should be inserted first), and 1.5g cefuroxime (25mg/kg for children) intravenously at induction of anesthesia.

External shunt infections (involving the tissues around the outside of the shunt) are not sufficiently common to merit the routine use of prophylaxis, but where a special problem exists a first or second generation cephalosporin should be administered intravenously at induction. Because of the general lack of success in further reducing the infection rate beyond acceptable minima, several innovative processes have been developed for treatment of biomaterials and devices in order to reduce bacterial adherence. To date these have not proved effective outside the laboratory, and very few are suitable for central nervous system (CNS) implantation. Often, only the outside surface of the shunt is modified, so no significant effect on the majority of shunt infections can be expected. One process (Bactiseal) consists of introducing rifampin (rifampicin) and clindamycin into the molecular

matrix of the silicone in such a way that high-level protection of all surfaces can be conferred for over 2 months in long-term in-vitro tests. Antibacterial activity is undiminished in the presence of protein conditioning film, such as that found in infants with high CSF protein levels after hemorrhage or meningitis, who are at greatest risk of shunt infection.[11] The results of clinical trials are awaited.

CLINICAL FEATURES

The clinical features of VA shunt infection differ considerably from those of VP and LP shunts (Fig. 21.3). Although the shunt lumen becomes colonised at implantation, in VA shunts symptoms considered serious enough to warrant specialist medical attention may not appear for months or years.[8] Many patients have intermittent low-grade fever, but some do not. Some report chills and occasionally rigors. Transient rashes are common. Sore throat and muscular and joint pains are common complaints. Anemia is almost universally found and there is increasing lassitude, anorexia, irritability and poor sleep. Dyspepsia may also be a problem. In later stages, arthralgia becomes more common. Unfortunately these features are nonspecific and are often mistaken for those of other conditions. As the disease progresses, nephritis and vasculitis may appear. The vasculitic rash is usually confined to the lower extremities, and can be frankly hemorrhagic and ulcerate. Nephritis is indicated by hypertension, hematuria and proteinuria, edema and often loin pain.

In contrast, infections in VP and LP shunts almost always present within 6 months of surgery.[12,13] Fever is present in fewer than 50% of cases and is usually intermittent and mild. Chills and rigors are rare. There may be abdominal discomfort, bloating, pain or tenderness, and occasionally persistent flatulence. In cases presenting within 1 or 2 weeks of surgery, there may be failure of the abdominal wound to heal, with CSF leak and sometimes catheter protrusion. In LP shunts there is often spinal pain. However, the most constant symptoms are those of hydrocephalus caused by obstruction at the distal end, and the differential diagnosis is between infective and noninfective shunt obstruction. In the former there is often erythema and tenderness over the lower shunt track, whereas these features are absent in noninfective obstruction. In addition, distal VP shunt obstruction occurring more than 9 months after shunt surgery is very unlikely to have an infective cause.[13,14] A very small number of cases present as acute abdomen, with fever, abdominal pain and tenderness suggesting appendicitis or peritonitis.[15] These may present at any time, and may lead to unnecessary laparotomy. The tenderness is not necessarily associated with the location of the shunt tip.

Ventriculoperitoneal shunt infections can also present at any time after perforation of the bowel or vagina. The distal catheter often protrudes from the anus or vagina and CSF leaks from these sites. They usually present as meningitis rather than shunt obstruction or peritonitis, with few abdominal features. Considering the often large numbers of bacteria seen in the CSF in these cases, the patients are not usually severely ill and recovery is often uneventful after shunt removal, without need for laparotomy.

DIAGNOSIS

Blood should be drawn for culture in all cases of suspected shunt infection. However, in infected VP and LP shunts the positive culture rate is less than 5%, except where *S. aureus* or Gram-negative bacilli are involved. In VA infections the positivity rate is much higher and blood should be drawn for culture on several occasions. In longstanding infections blood cultures may remain negative, possibly because of high antibody and opsonin titres. All isolates, however doubtful, should be saved until a definitive diagnosis is made. Attempts should be made to compare consecutive isolates, by antibiograms and by proprietory kits such as API Staph, or by molecular typing techniques if available. Differentiation between contaminants and pathogens, however, remains a problem. In addition, despite claims that a positive test for adherence or 'slime' production indicates a likely pathogen rather than a contaminant,[16,17] critical evaluation shows that these tests, as currently formulated, are of no value in the diagnostic laboratory.[18]

Aspiration of CSF from the shunt reservoir carries little risk of introducing infection. The CSF sample should be examined promptly and a portion should be centrifuged for Gram film and culture, whatever the cell count, because bacteria are not infrequently found in the absence of a significant cellular response. As with blood cultures, isolates should be kept and identified, although the isolation of an organism from a shunt aspirate, particularly if it is also seen on Gram film, is diagnostic of shunt infection. It is important to realise that no isolate should be disregarded, whatever its identity.

It should be noted that the shunt can be infected distal to the reservoir. In such cases reservoir aspiration may yield normal CSF that is culture-negative.

In the presence of symptoms and a suggestive history, negative blood and CSF cultures cannot rule out shunt infection completely, and a high index of suspicion should be retained. If symptoms persist consideration should be given to removing the shunt empirically, and it is then imperative that it is sent immediately to the laboratory in a sterile container for Gram stain and culture. Cultures should be incubated for at least 5 days. The Gram stain is very important; where organisms are isolated on culture without being seen on microscopy they are almost invariably contaminants, except where antimicrobials have been given immediately before shunt removal.

In view of the difficulties both of laboratory and of clinical diagnosis, serologic tests have been developed. For example, a whole-cell agglutination test using *S. epidermidis* has proved useful in diagnosing VA shunt infections.[8] The agglutinin titer in individuals without shunts rises with age. In patients who have VA shunt infection caused by coagulase-negative staphylococci, the titer rises before symptoms appear and, over several months, it can rise to 15–30 times the normal level for age. It can therefore be used as a screening test. When used in this way, shunt nephritis is not seen because a diagnosis is invariably made sufficiently early for it to be avoided.[8] Ventriculoperitoneal and LP shunts do not discharge directly into the bloodstream, which may

explain why the agglutination test is not useful in these cases. The plasma C-reactive protein can also be helpful in distinguishing between infective and noninfective distal VP shunt obstruction.[19]

MANAGEMENT

Three factors are important in the antimicrobial chemotherapy of shunt infections. The first is the inherent multiresistance of many strains of coagulase-negative staphylococci. Almost all are resistant to penicillin and at least 50% are resistant to methicillin, and therefore to cephalosporins. Resistance to aminoglycosides is also common. However, all clinical isolates of *S. epidermidis* are currently susceptible to vancomycin, although some strains of *Staphylococcus haemolyticus* and a few of *S. epidermidis* are resistant to teicoplanin. Similarly the incidence of resistance to rifampin and lincosamines is low in most centers.

The second factor is the lack of a vigorous inflammatory response in the CNS to most shunt infections, and most systemically administered antimicrobials fail to penetrate the CSF, this being particularly true of aminoglycosides, beta-lactams, glycopeptides and streptogramins. Of the few drugs that give acceptable CSF concentrations in such circumstances, chloramphenicol is bacteriostatic and ineffective in treating shunt infections; rifampin is highly active against most organisms causing shunt infections but cannot be given alone because of rapid development of resistance; and trimethoprim is active against fewer Gram-positive bacteria than rifampin.

The third factor is the mode of growth of the organisms in the shunt lumen. Bacteria that grow as a biofilm have much lower growth rates and produce exopolymers. The concentration of antimicrobials required to kill biofilm organisms is often several logs higher than the conventional MIC.[20]

These factors explain the generally disappointing results achieved whenever attempts are made to treat shunt infections without shunt removal. The shunt should therefore be removed early and an external ventricular drain (EVD) inserted to control CSF pressure (Fig. 21.5). This course of action is supported by many reports, clearly indicating that shunt retention is associated with a greater chance of relapse, a longer hospital stay and a greater risk of death.

Antimicrobials should be begun as soon as the diagnosis is confirmed. Vancomycin is recommended for coagulase-negative staphylococci, *S. aureus*, coryneforms and for those enterococci that are susceptible. As the drug does not give adequate CSF concentrations when given intravenously,[4] it should be given intraventricularly via a reservoir or through the clamped EVD tube. A Rickham reservoir should be incorporated in the system if the chosen EVD does not have a reservoir or injection port. Alternatively an Ommaya reservoir can be inserted contralaterally. The standard dose of intraventricular vancomycin is 20mg daily, although this should be reduced to 10mg daily for those with small ventricles. It should be noted that the dose depends

---

TREATMENT OF SHUNT INFECTIONS CAUSED BY *S. EPIDERMIDIS*, OTHER COAGULASE-NEGATIVE STAPHYLOCOCCI, AND OTHER SUSCEPTIBLE GRAM-POSITIVE BACTERIA

Shunt removal, insertion of external drain

Intraventricular vancomycin 20mg daily plus intravenous/oral rifampin 15mg/kg per day (pediatric) or 600mg/day (adults), both in two divided doses

After 7–10 days of treatment, reshunt if necessary. Stop both antibiotics on this day

Fig. 21.5 Treatment of shunt infections caused by *Staphylococcus epidermidis*, other coagulase-negative staphylococci and other susceptible Gram-positive bacteria.

on ventricular volume rather than on age or body weight. The vancomycin should be diluted in 1–2ml sterile water for injection. In addition to vancomycin, rifampin should be given intravenously in a total dose of 15mg/kg per day (two divided doses) for children or 300mg q12h for adults. The drug can be given orally in most cases after a few days. Alternatively, trimethoprim can be given intravenously, 3mg/kg q8h for children and 250mg q12h for adults. Teicoplanin offers no obvious advantage over vancomycin. Intraventricular vancomycin given in the doses recommended above leads to CSF concentrations that commonly reach 5–10 times the expected plasma concentrations, but no toxicity has been encountered. Attempts should not be made to titrate the dose to keep the CSF concentrations below the toxic plasma levels. There is no indication for the use of intravenous vancomycin in addition to that given by the intraventricular route except in the case of methicillin-resistant *S. aureus* shunt infections, for which vancomycin might be the only available agent. The drug may be given by the intravenous route alone if the CSF cell count and protein concentration are sufficiently raised to indicate a vigorous inflammatory response.

Using this regimen, coagulase-negative staphylococci should no longer be detectable in the CSF on microscopy or culture by day 4, and any fever should have resolved. A new shunt, if needed, can be inserted by day 7–10 of the regimen, the last dose of vancomycin and rifampin being given on that day. It is unwise to wait for a few days after stopping treatment, as this is the period of greatest risk for secondary infection from the EVD. Using this regimen for coagulase-negative staphylococci, *S. aureus*, coryneforms and propionibacteria, successful eradication and reshunting within 10 days without relapse can be expected in almost all cases.[21]

For shunt infections caused by Gram-negative bacilli, the shunt should again be removed and the treatment for Gram-negative meningitis (Chapter 2.15) instituted.

A notable exception to the rule of shunt removal is community-acquired bacterial meningitis in shunted persons. Such patients should be treated in the same way as those without shunts, and can be expected to respond at least as well. On no account should these patients be subjected to shunt removal.[4]

REFERENCES

1. Pople IK, Bayston R, Hayward RD. Infection of cerebrospinal fluid shunts in infants: a study of etiological factors. J Neurosurg 1992;77:29–36.
2. Renier D, Lacombe J, Pierre-Khan A, Sainte-Rose C, Hirsch JF. Factors causing acute shunt infection. J Neurosurg 1984;61:1072–8.
3. Key CB, Rothrock SG, Falk JL. Cerebrospinal fluid shunt complications: an emergency medicine perspective. Pediatr Emerg Care 1995;11:265–73.
4. Bayston R. Hydrocephalus shunt infections. London: Chapman and Hall Medical; 1989.
5. Choux M, Gentori L, Lang D, Lena G. Shunt implantation: reducing the incidence of shunt infection. J Neurosurg 1992;77:875–80.
6. Bayston R, Lari J. A study of the sources of infection in colonised shunts. Dev Med Child Neurol 1974;16(suppl 32):16–22.
7. Shapiro S, Boaz J, Kleiman M, Kalsbeck J, Mealey J. Origins of organisms infecting ventricular shunts. Neurosurg 1988;22:868–72.
8. Bayston R, Swinden J. The aetiology and prevention of shunt nephritis. Zeit Kinderchir 1979;28:377–84.
9. Brook I, Johnson N, Overturf G, Wilkins J. Mixed bacterial meningitis: a complication of ventriculo- and lumbo-peritoneal shunts. J Neurosurg 1977;47:961–4.
10. Brown EM, de Louvois J, Bayston R, et al. Antimicrobial prophylaxis in neurosurgery and after head injury: British Society for Antimicrobial Chemotherapy Working Party Report on the Use of Antibiotics in Neurosurgery. Lancet 1994;344:1547–51.
11. Bayston R, Lambert E. Duration of activity of cerebrospinal fluid shunt catheters impregnated with antimicrobials to prevent bacterial catheter-related infection. J Neurosurg 1997;87:247–51.
12. Piatt JH. Cerebrospinal fluid shunt failure: late is different from early. Pediatr Neurosurg 1995;23:133–9.
13. Ronan A, Hogg GG, Klug GL. Cerebrospinal fluid shunt infections in children. Pediatr Infect Dis J 1995;14:782–6.
14. Bayston R, Spitz L. Infective and cystic causes of malfunction of ventriculoperitoneal shunts for hydrocephalus. Zeit Kinderchir 1977;22:419–24.
15. Reynolds M, Sherman J, McLone DG. Ventriculoperitoneal shunt Infection masquerading as an acute surgical abdomen. J Pediatr Surg 1983;18:951–4.
16. Davenport DS, Massanari RM, Pfaller MA, et al. Usefulness of a test for slime production as a marker for clinically significant infections with coagulase-negative staphylococci. J Infect Dis 1986;153:332–9.
17. Diaz-Mitoma F, Harding GKM, Hoban DJ, et al. Clinical significance of a test for slime production in ventriculoperitoneal shunt infections caused by coagulase-negative staphylococci. J Infect Dis 1987;156:555–60.
18. Bayston R, Rogers J. Production of extracellular slime by staphylococcus epidermidis during stationary phase of growth: its association with adherence to implantable devices. J Clin Pathol 1990;43:866–70.
19. Castro-Gago M, Sanguinedo P, Garcia C, et al. Valor de la proteina C-reativa (PCR) en le diagnostico de las complicaciones infecciosas de los 'shunts' en nos niños hidrocefalos. Ann Esp Pediatr 1982;16:47–52.
20. Brown MR, Collier PJ, Gilbert P. Influence of growth rate on susceptibility to antimicrobial agents; modification of cell envelope and batch and continuous culture studies. Antimicrob Agents Chemother 1990;34:1623–8.
21. Bayston R, de Louvois J, Brown EM, et al. Treatment of infections associated with shunting for hydrocephalus: British Society for Antimicrobial Chemotherapy Working Party Report on Use of Antibiotics in Neurosurgery. Br J Hosp Med 1995;53:368–73.

Neurotropic Virus Disorders

Martin J Wood

The diseases described in this chapter are all the result of infections of or infection-mediated damage to cells within the spinal cord, the dorsal root ganglia adjacent to the cord, or the brainstem.

POLIOMYELITIS

EPIDEMIOLOGY

The incidence of acute paralytic poliomyelitis has fallen dramatically over the past 4 decades as a result of mass vaccination campaigns and the target set by the World Health Organization in 1988 to eradicate the disease worldwide by the year 2000. From 1988 to 1995 reported cases of paralytic polio declined by 80% – from more than 35,000 to just over 6200 (Fig. 22.1)[1] – and the Western hemisphere was declared free of transmission of indigenous wild poliovirus in 1994. Within the European region wild polio remains endemic in Turkey and the Central Asian Republics of the former Soviet Union. In 1996 a large outbreak occurred in Albania, which had been free of polio since 1985, confirming the high risk of importation and transmission of polio in unvaccinated and incompletely vaccinated populations that had been seen elsewhere.[2]

In countries where poliovirus is endemic, most paralytic disease is caused by serotype 1 or, to a lesser extent, serotype 3. Vaccine-associated cases, of which two-thirds occur in nonimmunized contacts of vaccine recipients and the remainder in the vaccine recipients themselves, now account for many reported cases.[3] In the USA, of the 133 confirmed cases of paralytic poliomyelitis reported during the period 1980–1994, 94% were associated with oral poliovirus vaccine (OPV; Fig. 22.2).[4]

Poliovirus is usually transmitted by direct fecal–oral contact, indirect contact with saliva or feces, or from contaminated water. Disease occurs all year round in the tropics, and occurs during the summer and autumn in temperate countries. Children are more susceptible to infection but the risk of paralytic disease after infection is higher in adults.

PATHOGENESIS AND PATHOLOGY

After exposure poliovirus multiplies in the lymphoid tissue of the tonsils and, particularly, in the Peyer's patches of the ileum. The virus passes to the regional lymph nodes, a primary viremia subsequently distributing the virus to the entire reticuloendothelial system. In most instances the immune system then controls the infection and viral replication ceases at this point. In a minority of persons, however, further replication in the reticuloendothelial system occurs and there is a major disseminating viremia. It is believed that virus enters the CNS as a result of this hematogenous dissemination, but this may be only part of the story. The cell-surface receptor for poliovirus is a member of the immunoglobulin-like superfamily of proteins.[5] Experiments in transgenic mice containing the human gene for this receptor suggest that poliovirus spreads from muscle to the anterior horn cells via nerve pathways.[6]

Within the CNS poliovirus primarily targets motor neurons in the brainstem and the anterior horn of the spinal cord. Neurons at these sites and, to a lesser extent, those in the mesencephalon, cerebellum and precentral gyrus of the cerebral cortex are destroyed and surrounded by an inflammatory infiltrate of polymorphonuclear leukocytes and mononuclear cells (Fig. 22.3).

PREVENTION

Poliovirus causes an acute nonpersistent illness; humans are the only reservoir and virus survival in the environment is finite. These facts, combined with the ability of polio immunization to interrupt virus

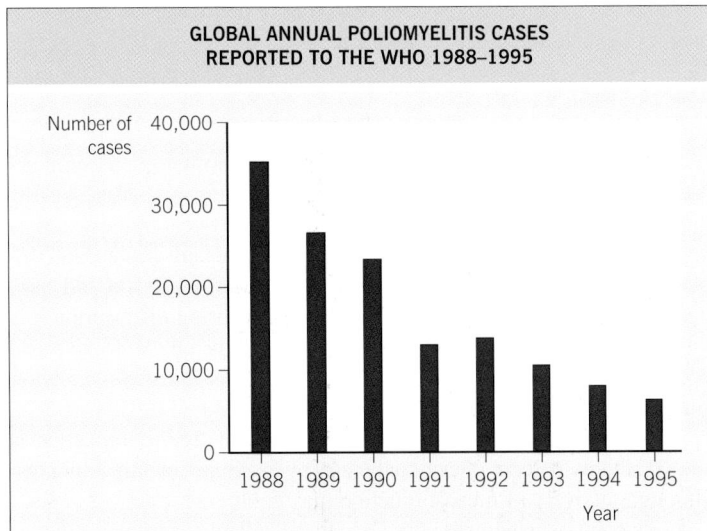

Fig. 22.1 Global annual poliomyelitis cases reported to the World Health Organization in 1988–1995.[1]

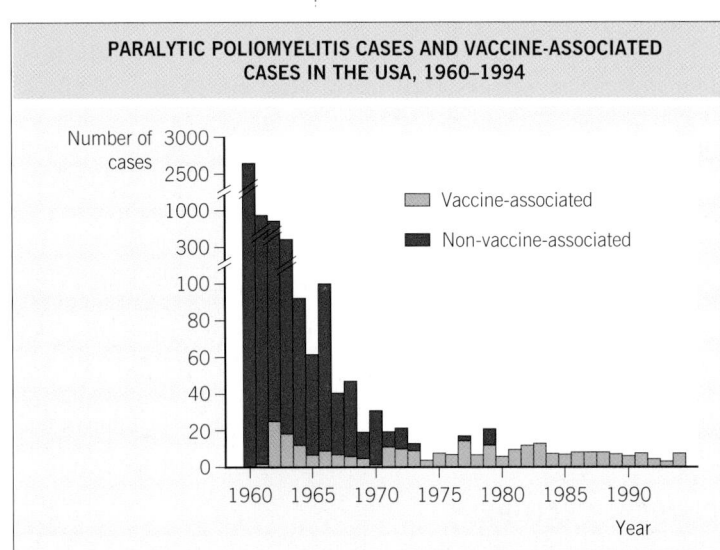

Fig. 22.2 Total number of cases of paralytic poliomyelitis and number of vaccine-associated cases in the USA in 1960–1994.[4]

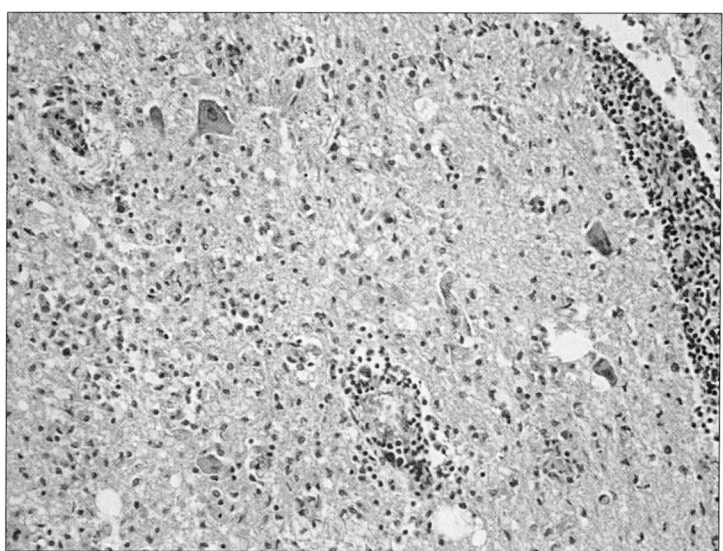

Fig. 22.3 Appearance of anterior horn in poliomyelitis. Damaged and destroyed anterior horn neuron cell bodies are surrounded by an inflammatory infiltrate.

transmission, make poliovirus a candidate for eradication by the World Health Organization.[7]

Two types of poliovirus vaccine are available: the orally administered Sabin vaccine (OPV), consisting of live attenuated strains of all three serotypes of poliovirus, and the Salk inactivated poliovirus (IPV) vaccine. After one dose and three doses of OPV, 50% and more than 95% of recipients, respectively, develop long-lasting immunity. Administration of OPV interferes with subsequent infection with wild poliovirus. Of children, 90–100% develop protective antibody to all three serotypes of poliovirus after two doses of IPV. Persons vaccinated with IPV may still be infected with and excrete wild-type strains of poliovirus, although epidemiologic studies have confirmed that IPV reduces circulation of wild-type virus considerably.

The strategies for global eradication of poliomyelitis by the year 2000 include the following measures aimed at interrupting transmission of wild poliovirus in endemic countries: high vaccination coverage of children younger than 1-year-old with three doses of OPV; effective surveillance systems; and supplemental vaccination on national immunization days, when two doses of OPV are given to all children younger than 5-years-old, irrespective of previous immunization. The scale of this undertaking can be judged from the fact that, in India alone, more than 125 million children were immunized on January 18 1997.

Orally administered Sabin vaccine can be complicated by paralytic poliomyelitis; the risk is one in 2.4 million doses, although for children receiving their first dose of OPV it is one in 750,000 doses. Immunodeficient persons, particularly those with hypogammaglobulinemia, are at greatest risk (a 3000–7000-fold higher risk than in the immunocompetent recipient). Where routine immunization has been widespread and wild poliovirus has been almost eradicated (e.g. the USA), most cases of paralytic poliomyelitis are caused by OPV. In these circumstances a sequential IPV–OPV vaccination schedule has been recommended. The USA guidelines for vaccination, for example, suggest that IPV is given at 2 months and 4 months, and that OPV should be given at 12–18 months and at age 4–6 years. The use of IPV is designed to induce high levels of protection by the time of the first dose of OPV, which should theoretically reduce the incidence of vaccine-associated paralytic disease while maintaining population immunity at high levels.

CLINICAL FEATURES

The incubation period of poliomyelitis is probably about 10–14 days, but most (at least 95%) poliovirus infections are asymptomatic. Indeed,

in most symptomatic cases there is merely a nonspecific febrile illness corresponding to the enteric and primary viremic phase of viral replication. This illness lasts a few days and is followed in a small percentage of cases by the major illness of aseptic meningitis and paralytic disease. The onset of this phase is abrupt, with meningitic symptoms and muscle pains, often in the neck or back, followed a few days later by the gradual onset, in less than 1% of poliovirus infections, of paralytic disease. Risk factors for paralytic disease are a large inoculum of virus, increasing age, pregnancy, recent tonsillectomy, strenuous exercise and intramuscular injections during the incubation period.[8]

The typical clinical features of paralytic poliomyelitis are due to viral lysis of motor neurons of the anterior horn of the spinal cord and/or the brain stem. There is fever and muscle pain, and rapid progression over 2–4 days to maximal paralysis. Spinal paralysis is typically asymmetric and is more severe proximally. Bulbar paralysis may affect swallowing and respiration. Fasciculation is often evident and the deep tendon reflexes are absent or diminished. Autonomic disturbance is often evident. Although sensory symptoms are common, the presence of sensory signs should alert the clinician to another diagnosis.

The mortality from paralytic poliomyelitis is between 2 and 10% and is generally caused by bulbar involvement and/or respiratory failure. After the acute illness there is often a degree of recovery of muscle function over the subsequent 6 months or more.

After many years of stable neurologic impairment, in 25–40% of patients new neuromuscular symptoms (weakness, pain and fatigue) develop, a disorder termed the post-polio syndrome.[9] It has been suggested that post-polio syndrome is the result of progressive deterioration in the function of surviving motor neurons caused by immunologic mechanisms, normal aging or overburden of neurons from re-innervation.[8] In many patients, however, late functional deterioration after polio is caused by orthopedic factors or radiculopathies.[10]

The most important disease likely to be confused with paralytic poliomyelitis is the Guillain–Barré syndrome (GBS). The illnesses can usually be distinguished by the symmetric paralysis and sensory signs of GBS and the elevated protein but relatively normal cell count in the CSF of GBS patients.

DIAGNOSIS

In the preparalytic phase there is nothing to distinguish poliomyelitis from other causes of viral meningitis. There is an increased number of mononuclear leukocytes in the CSF but poliovirus is rarely isolated from the CSF. The diagnosis may be confirmed by serologic testing of paired acute and convalescent sera, or by isolation of poliovirus from throat swabs taken during the first week of the disease, or from feces cultured up to several weeks after the onset. Polymerase chain reaction methods have been developed for detection of poliovirus but are not yet used in routine diagnostic laboratories.[11]

MANAGEMENT

Management of the acute phase of paralytic poliomyelitis is supportive and symptomatic. Patients need hospitalization and bedrest during the first week or so. Light splints and passive physical therapy to prevent contractures, moist hot packs for muscle pain and spasms, and frequent turning to prevent bedsores are important. Nutrition and fluid balance need to be maintained and close monitoring of respiration is vital. If the vital capacity falls below 50% of predicted values, hypoxia occurs; if there is pooling of pharyngeal secretions, assisted ventilation should be started.

When the fever subsides active physiotherapy and mobilization is started. Eighty percent of eventual recovery is attained within 6 months, although recovery of muscle function may continue for up to 2 years.

Long-term management of the paralysed patient is complex and outside the scope of this account.

HERPES ZOSTER IN THE NORMAL HOST

EPIDEMIOLOGY

Studies of the incidence of herpes zoster in the USA and UK suggest there are about 3 cases per 1000 persons per year.[12,13] These figures suggest that in the USA there may be 900,000 cases of herpes zoster and that in the UK there may be 200,000 cases of herpes zoster annually. There are no reliable data for other areas of the world. The incidence increases dramatically after middle age (Fig. 22.4). There is no sex difference, but owing to population demographics in developed countries most cases are seen in females in the sixth and seventh decades of life. Children or adolescents who acquired their varicella-zoster virus (VZV) infection *in utero* or in the first year of life have an up to 20-fold greater risk of developing herpes zoster before the age of 20 years. Almost 20% of individuals in the UK will develop herpes zoster at some stage; about 5% of immunocompetent patients can expect to suffer a second episode, and less than 1% a third episode.[12,13]

Typically, herpes zoster occurs unexpectedly with no seasonality. There is no evidence that it is more common during chickenpox outbreaks.

PATHOGENESIS AND PATHOLOGY

Identification of VZV nucleic acids within sensory ganglia and demonstration that VZV isolates from varicella and herpes zoster in the same patient are identical have proved that the disease is caused by reactivation of VZV from within the sensory ganglia, where it has been resident since the primary attack of chickenpox usually many years earlier. During this latent period it is believed that host immunity to VZV is repeatedly boosted by re-exposure to VZV antigens, either from exogenous sources or from episodes of endogenous replication that did not lead to herpes zoster. The molecular mechanisms that establish and maintain VZV latency are not fully understood, but reactivation of the virus is clearly related to declining VZV-specific cell-mediated immunity (CMI). In the elderly the risk of herpes zoster is proportional to the marked decline in VZV-specific CMI associated with advancing age.[14]

After reactivation of VZV from latency, the virus replicates within the neuron and travels down the nerve to the skin that nerve innervates. As this occurs the neurons are destroyed and there is a marked inflammatory neuritis with cellular infiltrate and hemorrhage. Once it reaches the skin the virus replicates within the epidermis and produces the characteristic vesicular rash. Histologically, the lesion is indistinguishable from that of varicella or herpes simplex, consisting of an intra-epidermal blister with multinucleate giant cells in its floor.

The pathogenesis of postherpetic neuralgia (PHN) is poorly understood, but recent research has suggested that the increased transmission of nociceptive impulses during the period of acute neuritis induces central sensitization and hyperexcitability of spinal neurons. This is then maintained by a changed peripheral imput and by excitotoxic damage in the dorsal horn of the spinal cord.[15]

PREVENTION

The development of herpes zoster in an individual previously infected with VZV might be prevented by measures designed to boost their declining CMI to the virus. This can be accomplished by administering the live attenuated Oka strain vaccine; when this vaccine is given to seropositive elderly adults (mean age 67 years), most have a long-lasting boost in their VZV-specific CMI to a level similar to that of normal 40-year-olds, a group with a relatively low-risk of herpes zoster.[16,17] Whether this will reduce the frequency and severity of herpes zoster in vaccinees is still to be tested in a controlled trial.

CLINICAL FEATURES

Herpes zoster infection is almost always unilateral. The dermatome most frequently affected (10–15% of cases) is the ophthalmic division of the trigeminal nerve. Otherwise, each dermatome is affected at a similar rate. Hence, more than 50% of herpes zoster involves one or more of the thoracic dermatomes and the cervical and lumbosacral dermatomes are each affected in 10–15% of cases.

The chief clinical features of acute herpes zoster are pain and rash.[18] Systemic symptoms and signs may also occur, including headache, malaise, nausea and vomiting, fever and regional lymphadenopathy. Pain and paresthesia within the affected dermatome often precede the rash by several days; prolonged periods of prodromal pain have been reported. The pain is extremely variable in its character, periodicity and severity, and because it is similar to that found in a wide range of other conditions, the true nature of the cause is not usually recognized until the rash appears. The pain usually increases for a few days and then declines in severity somewhat slowly, often in parallel with skin healing.

The rash of herpes zoster (Fig. 22.5) usually appears proximally in the involved dermatome and spreads distally over the following few days.[18] It begins as erythematous maculopapules that vesiculate within 12 hours or so. After 3–4 days the vesicles become cloudy pustules and these then gradually dry and crust during the subsequent 7–10 days, thereafter persisting for a further 1–2 weeks. New lesions continue to appear for a mean of 2–3 days and only 10–15% of immunocompetent individuals have new lesions beyond 4 days. Virus can be cultured

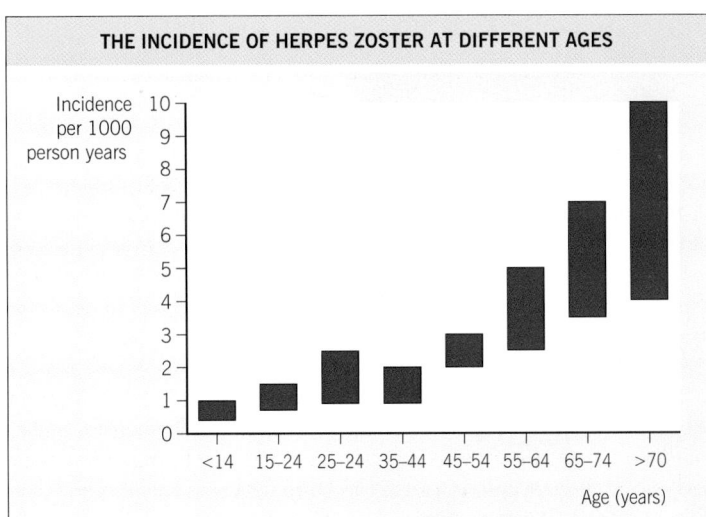

Fig. 22.4 **The incidence of herpes zoster at different ages.**[12, 13]

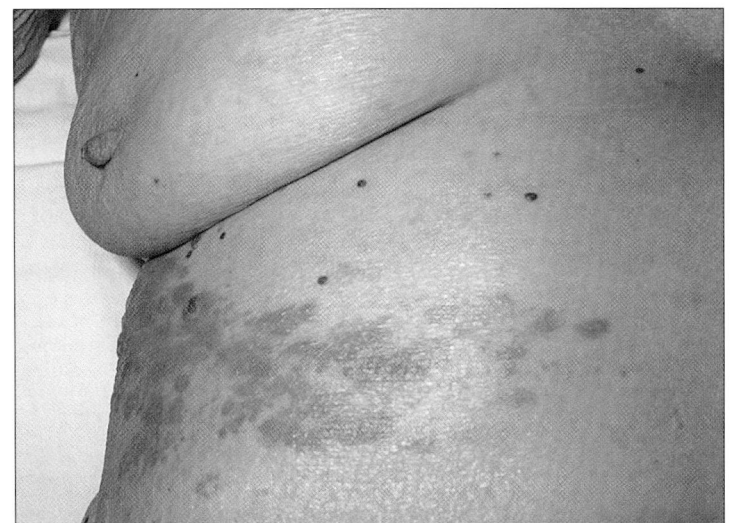

Fig. 22.5 **Typical dermatomal rash of herpes zoster.**

from the vesicles for only a few days, although in 15% of cases it is recoverable from lesions for 1 week. Occasionally, especially in the very elderly or those with poor nutrition, the rash may become necrotic, ulcerative and gangrenous. The appearance of a score or so of lesions outside the primary dermatome within a few days of rash onset is not unusual in otherwise healthy adults, but widely disseminated cutaneous disease is rare.

Although most cases of herpes zoster in the immunocompetent host are self-limiting, in 15–20% one or more complications occur (Fig. 22.6). The major complication and cause of morbidity after herpes zoster in the immunocompetent host is chronic pain or PHN. Postherpetic neuralgia is an arbitrarily defined term; some definitions include any pain after rash healing, whereas others limit PHN to pain persisting for 30 days or longer.[19] Pain persists for more than 4 weeks after the resolution of the rash in 10–15% of adult patients with herpes zoster; only 5–10% are still in pain after 3 months and 2–5% after 12 months.[18,19] In the elderly, prolonged pain is more common. At 1, 3 and 6 months after the illness only 50–60%, 25% and 9–13%, respectively, of patients over 60-years-old are still suffering pain. The other factors that influence the likelihood of prolonged pain after herpes zoster infection are the severity of the acute pain, prolonged prodromal pain, distress and psychologic conviction.

Some ocular involvement is common in patients with ophthalmic zoster. Up to 85% of patients with involvement of the nasociliary branch of the trigeminal nerve [clinically suggested by Hutchinson's sign, the rash involving the lateral tip of the nose; (Fig. 22.7)] will develop ocular complications, but ocular involvement can occur even if this sign is absent. Every ocular tissue can be affected by VZV.[20] Although conjunctivitis is the most frequent complication, anterior uveitis and keratitis are of greater significance. Keratitis may manifest as epithelial or subepithelial punctate changes, dendritic or disciform ulceration, or corneal vascularization. Eyes with stromal disease may be rendered blind.

Localized motor paralysis is observed in less than 5% of patients with herpes zoster, predominantly in cases involving the trigeminal nerve or the cervical or lumbosacral dermatomes. The true incidence of motor weakness is much greater, but there is great difficulty in assessing weakness of intercostal or abdominal musculature, the most common sites of a herpes zoster rash. Motor signs usually develop abruptly with or shortly after the rash and reach a peak within a few days; in most cases there is complete functional recovery, although this may be prolonged. A particularly common motor complication is the Ramsay Hunt syndrome (vesicles in or around the external auditory meatus and a lower motor neuron facial palsy). Encephalitis and myelitis are uncommon complications of herpes zoster in otherwise healthy patients and are probably caused by direct extension of virus from the dorsal root ganglion to the meninges and the brain. A variety of other neurologic complications, such as aseptic meningitis,

transverse myelitis, necrotizing myelopathy, cerebral angiitis and GBS have been described in association with clinical herpes zoster.

There is no evidence of any risk to fetal development if a pregnant woman suffers from herpes zoster infection.[21]

Aspects of herpes zoster infection in the immunocompromised host are discussed in Chapter 4.5.

DIAGNOSIS

The diagnosis of herpes zoster is essentially clinical, based on the characteristic appearance and distribution of the rash. The only condition that is likely to be confused with herpes zoster with any regularity is herpes simplex virus (HSV) infection. Zosteriform rashes may be caused by HSV but the latter usually causes a much less extensive rash than does herpes zoster; the individual lesions of HSV are smaller and tend to recur. Patients with recurrent herpes zoster of the buttocks or thighs almost always have HSV type II infection. Confirmation of VZV infection can be obtained by polymerase chain reaction examination or culture of the vesicular fluid.

MANAGEMENT

Although steps should be instituted to ease the inflammation and irritation caused by the skin lesions, the management of herpes zoster is primarily aimed at reducing the pain and complications of the illness.[22] Adequate analgesia is very important while antiviral therapy limits the degree of neuronal damage by VZV. Placebo-controlled studies have shown that oral aciclovir (800mg five times daily for 7 days), if started within 72 hours of rash onset, reduces the severity and duration of the acute illness in the normal host with herpes zoster. A meta-analysis of the placebo-controlled data has confirmed that aciclovir also reduces the duration of the pain.[23] In patients with ophthalmic zoster, aciclovir reduces the incidence of ocular complications. All patients with ophthalmic zoster should also be examined by an ophthalmologist. The L-valine ester prodrug of aciclovir (valaciclovir) is rapidly converted to aciclovir after oral administration, and overcomes the poor bioavailability of the latter. Valaciclovir, 1000mg q8h for 7 days, significantly shortens the duration of pain compared with a standard course of oral aciclovir in immunocompetent individuals with herpes zoster. The time to rash resolution was similar for the two drugs.[22] The oral prodrug of penciclovir, famciclovir, is also effective for lesion healing and resolution of pain in uncomplicated herpes zoster when given either as 500mg q8h (the dosage licensed in the USA) or as 250mg q8h (the dosage licensed in Europe) for 7 days. The clinical efficacy of the three drugs seems very similar and a choice between them may depend on fiscal constraints and personal experience.[22] As yet, famciclovir therapy has not been studied in ophthalmic zoster.

COMPLICATIONS OF HERPES ZOSTER IN THE IMMUNOCOMPETENT INDIVIDUAL	
Complication	Examples
Postherpetic neuralgia	
Ocular complications	Conjunctivitis
	Uveitis
	Keratitis
	Glaucoma
	Retinal necrosis
Motor weakness	Ramsay Hunt syndrome
Encephalitis, transverse myelitis, etc.	
Cerebral angiitis	

Fig. 22.6 Complications of herpes zoster in the immunocompetent individual.

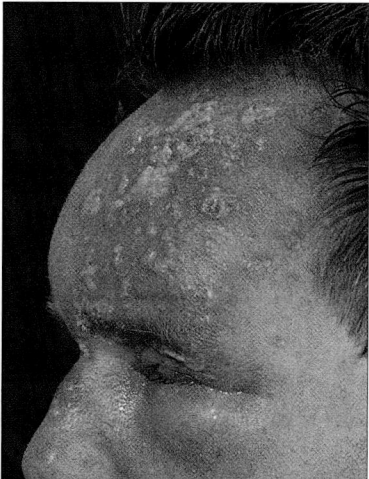

Fig. 22.7 Hutchinson's sign. When the rash of herpes zoster involves the skin at the tip and side of the nose it indicates that the nasociliary branch of the trigeminal nerve is involved. There is an increased risk of uveal tract inflammation and ocular damage.

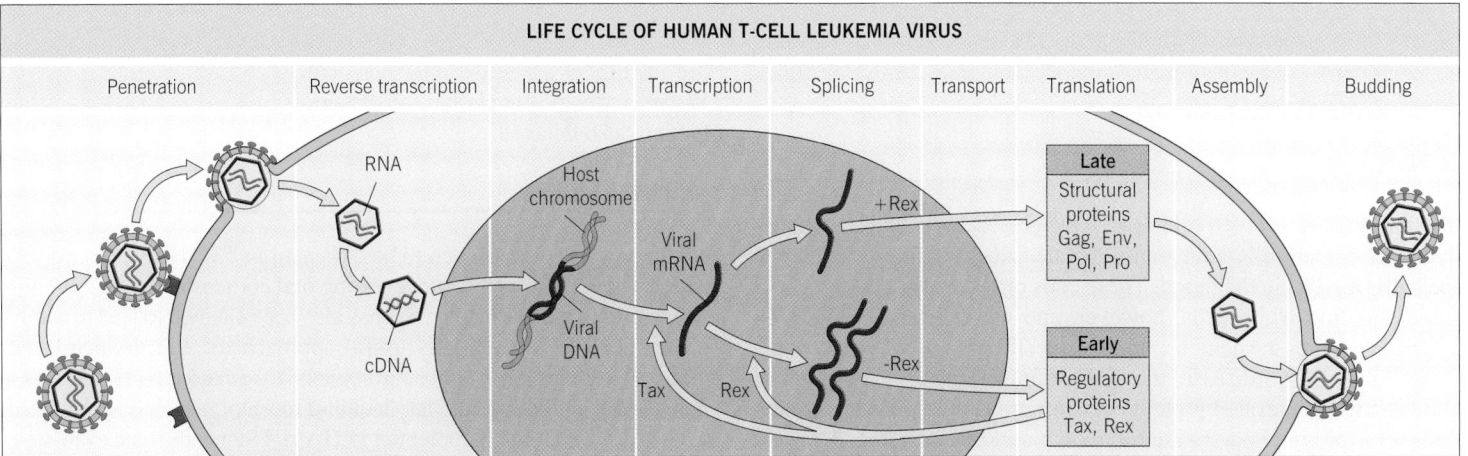

Fig. 22.8 The life cycle of human T-cell leukemia virus. HTLV-I infection is initiated by cell-free virions or, more commonly, by cell-to-cell virus transmission. The two RNA genome copies are converted into double-stranded DNA provirus by the viral enzyme reverse transcriptase and the proviral DNA is integrated into the host chromosome. Transcription is activated by the viral Tax protein. In the early stages of infection, both Tax and Rex proteins are produced. The Rex protein directs the preferential transport of unspliced or singly spliced viral messages to the cytoplasm for translation into structural proteins for virion assembly.

Whichever drug is used the benefits have only been demonstrated if treatment is started within 72 hours of the appearance of the herpes zoster rash (except in ophthalmic zoster, where the ocular complications are reduced even if aciclovir is started 7 days after rash onset).

HUMAN T-CELL LEUKEMIA VIRUS 1 (HTLV-I)

Human T-cell leukemia virus type I (HTLV-I), was the first human retrovirus to be discovered. In addition to its role in adult T-cell leukemia (ATL), it causes a progressive myelopathy termed tropical spastic paraparesis (TSP) in the West Indies and several other countries, or HTLV-I-associated myelopathy (HAM) in Japan.

EPIDEMIOLOGY

Human T-cell leukemia virus-I infection is found endemically in southwestern Japan, where 20% of the population is seropositive, and in the Caribbean basin (including northern South America and the southeastern USA) where the seropositivity approaches 5%. Studies have also shown high seroprevalence rates of HTLV-I in west Africa, the islands of Melanesia in the Pacific and the Middle East. Infection is also found in immigrant populations from these areas, including West Indians in the UK.

Human T-cell leukemia virus-I can be transmitted by sexual intercourse, inoculation of infected blood or blood products and perinatal exposure. Sexual transmission is primarily via semen from which it can be isolated. Epidemiologic data from Japan suggest a very low rate of transmission from females to males in serologically discordant couples.[24] Breast-milk is an important vehicle of transmission since seroconversion is rare in infants who are not breast-fed, even if their mother is infected. The risk of seroconversion after receiving blood infected with HTLV-I is high (up to 80% after receipt of fresh blood products).[25] In endemic populations the prevalence of infection increases with age and clusters in families. Infection is lifelong. Not unexpectedly, HTLV-I is more prevalent in intravenous drug users and homosexual males than in the general population.

PATHOGENESIS AND PATHOLOGY

Human T-cell leukemia virus-I can infect a variety of human cells but only CD4+ T lymphocytes are transformed by the virus; the specific receptor has not been identified but the HTLV-I envelope glycoprotein (gp46) is the probable attachment molecule. Within the cell, reverse transcription, integration of proviral DNA and transcription and virus replication are typical of retrovirus replication (Fig. 22.8).

There are two hypotheses for the pathogenesis of HAM/TSP.[26] In one, HTLV-I infects glial cells and the cytotoxic immune response against infected cells causes demyelination. In the second the HTLV-I infection induces an autoimmune process. Although indirect evidence favors the first hypothesis, direct demonstration of HTLV-I infection of CNS cells is lacking.

Gross pathology shows spinal cord atrophy but a normal brain. The histology shows a diffuse inflammatory encephalomyelitis, with predominantly mid-thoracic cord involvement. The inflammatory infiltrate of mononuclear cells is mostly perivascular and there is hyaloid thickening of the vascular adventitia and media.[27] Demyelination and significant axonal loss is the final result of the inflammatory process.

PREVENTION

Prevention of HTLV-I infection depends upon screening blood to minimize the risk of transfusion-related disease. This is policy in France, the USA, Canada and Japan. Health educational programs should also promote condom use and warn seropositive mothers of the risks of transmission by breast-feeding. No effective vaccine has been developed.

CLINICAL FEATURES

Only a small proportion of those infected with HTLV-I develop ATL or HAM/TSP: the lifetime risk of these diseases in HTLV-I-infected Japanese is estimated at 2–4% and 0.25%, respectively.[26] The usual age at onset of HAM/TSP is the fifth decade of life and more women than men are affected.

The myeloradiculopathy produced by HTLV-I mainly affects the pyramidal tracts and, to a lesser extent, the sensory system. HAM and TSP have identical features; they are clinically characterized by a chronic syndrome with a combination of upper- and lower-motor neuron signs. Patients often complain of difficulty walking, dragging pains and stiffness of the legs, together with numbness and paresthesia, urinary retention and/or incontinence and impotence. About one-third of patients have weakness in the upper limbs, but the cranial nerves are only very rarely involved. Examination reveals a symmetric spastic paraparesis with mild sensory abnormalities indicative of posterior column involvement (diminished vibration and proprioception). Most patients progress gradually over months or years.

There may be confusion of HAM/TSP with multiple sclerosis.

There is, however, a lack of optic neuritis or ocular movement problems in the former and the latter tends to run a relapsing–remitting course. The World Health Organization has published diagnostic guidelines for HTLV-I myelopathy.[28]

DIAGNOSIS

The hallmark of HTLV-I infection is the presence of 'flower lymphocytes' (T-helper cells with multilobulated nuclei that are similar to the cells of ATL) in the blood. These cells only comprise about 1% of the circulating white cells, however, and the diagnosis of HTLV-I infection requires the demonstration of specific antibodies in the serum.

In HTLV-I CNS disease, the CSF examination may be normal or show a slightly elevated protein concentration and a mild lymphocytosis. Flower lymphocytes are found in a minority of cases. A definitive diagnosis of HAM/TSP requires detection of HTLV-I DNA in the CSF by polymerase chain reaction or evidence of intrathecal synthesis of HTLV-I antibody.

Myelography and CT scanning is usually normal apart from spinal cord atrophy. The imaging of choice is MRI, which shows diffuse high-intensity signals in the thoracic cord on T2-weighted images. Similar lesions are sometimes seen in the periventricular white matter. Visual evoked potentials and somatosensory evoked potentials from the legs are also delayed.

MANAGEMENT

No therapy has been proven to be of benefit in TSP/HAM. Occasional patients have improved while receiving oral corticosteroids or systemic α-interferon, and plasmapheresis has also been claimed to lead to a temporary benefit. A potentially useful approach for ATL (which has a much poorer prognosis than neurologic disease caused by HTLV-I) is a monoclonal antibody to the interleukin-2 receptor, which is upregulated by HTLV-I infection. Its potential in HAM/TSP needs to be evaluated.

At present the management of HAM/TSP is similar to that of myelopathies of any cause, with supportive therapy of spasticity and urinary sphincter disturbance.

REFERENCES

1. de Quadros CA. Global eradication of poliomyelitis. Int J Infect Dis 1997;1:125–9.
2. Oostvogel PM, van Wijngaarden JK, van der Avoort H, et al. Poliomyelitis outbreak in an unvaccinated community in the Netherlands 1992–1993. Lancet 1994;344:665–70.
3. Querfurth H, Swanson PD. Vaccine-associated paralytic poliomyelitis: regional case series and review. Arch Neurol 1990;47:541–4.
4. Centers for Disease Control and Prevention. Paralytic poliomyelitis – United States, 1980–1994. MMWR Morb Mortal Wkly Rep 1997;46:79–83.
5. Mendelsohn CL, Wimmer E, Racaniello VR. Cellular receptor for poliovirus: molecular cloning, nucleotide sequence, and expression of a new member of the immunoglobulin superfamily. Cell 1989;56:855–65.
6. Ren R, Racaniello VR. Polio spreads from muscle to the central nervous system by neural pathways. J Infect Dis 1992;166:747–52.
7. Cochi SL, Hull HF, Sutter RW, Wilfert CM, Katz SL. Global poliomyelitis eradication initiative: status report. J Infect Dis 1997;175 (Suppl 1):1–3.
8. Kidd D, Williams AJ, Howard RS. Classic diseases revisited: poliomyelitis. Postgrad Med J 1996;72:641–7.
9. Dalakas MC, Hallett M. The post polio syndrome. In: Plum F, ed. Advances in contemporary neurology. Philadelphia: FA Davis; 1988:51–94.
10. Kidd D, Howard RS, Williams AJ, et al. Late functional deterioration following paralytic poliomyelitis. Q J Med 1997;90:189–96.
11. WHO Memorandum. New approaches to poliovirus diagnosis using laboratory techniques. Bull WHO 1992;70:27–33.

12. Hope-Simpson RE. The nature of herpes zoster: a long-term study and a new hypothesis. Proc Roy Soc Med 1965;58:9–20.
13. Ragozzino MW, Melton LJ III, Kurland LT, Chu CP, Perry HO. Population-based study of herpes zoster and its sequelae. Medicine 1982;61:310–6.
14. Miller AE. Selective decline in cellular immune response to varicella zoster in the elderly. Neurology 1980;30:582–7.
15. Woolf CJ, Thompson SWN. The induction and maintainance of central sensitization is dependent on n-methyl-D-aspartic acid receptor activation: implications for the treatment of post-injury pain hypersensitivity states. Pain 1991;44:293–9.
16. Levin MJ, Murray M, Zerbe GO, White CJ, Hayward A. Immune responses of elderly persons 4 years after receiving a live attenuated varicella vaccine. J Infect Dis 1994;170:522–6.
17. White CJ. Varicella-zoster virus vaccine. Clin Infect Dis 1997;24:753–63.
18. Wood MJ, Easterbrook P. Shingles, scourge of the elderly: the acute illness. In: Sacks SL, Straus SE, Whitley RJ, Griffiths PD, eds. Clinical management of herpes viruses. Amsterdam: IOS Press; 1995:193–209.
19. Easterbrook P, Wood MJ. Post-herpetic neuralgia: what do drugs really do? In: Sacks SL, Straus SE, Whitley RJ, Griffiths PD, eds. Clinical management of herpes viruses. Amsterdam: IOS Press; 1995:211–35.
20. deLuise VP. Ocular involvement in herpes zoster. In: Watson CPN, ed. Herpes zoster and postherpetic neuralgia. Amsterdam: Elsevier; 1993:87–96.

21. Enders G, Miller E, Cradock-Watson J, Bolley I, Ridehalgh M. Consequences of varicella and herpes zoster in pregnancy: prospective study of 1739 cases. Lancet 1994;343:1548–51.
22. Wood MJ. Herpes zoster in the normal and immunocompromised host. In: Arvin AM, ed. Herpes virus infections. London: Ballière Tindall; 1996:439–55.
23. Wood MJ, Kay R, Dworkin RH, Soong S, Whitley RJ. Oral acyclovir therapy accelerates pain resolution in patients with herpes zoster: a meta-analysis of placebo-controlled trials. Clin Infect Dis 1996;22:341–7.
24. Kajiyama W, Kashiwaga S, Ikematsu H, et al. Intrafamilial transmission of adult T cell leukemia virus. J Infect Dis 1986;154:851–7.
25. Sullivan MT, Williams AE, Fang CT, et al. Transmission of human T-lymphotropic virus types I and II by blood transfusion. A retrospective study of recipients of blood components (1983 through 1988). The American Red Cross HTLV-I/II Collaborative Study Group. Arch Intern Med 1991;151:2043–8.
26. Höllsberg P, Hafler DA. Pathogenesis of diseases induced by human lymphotropic virus type I infection. N Engl J Med 1993;328:1173–82.
27. Montgomery RD, Cruikshank EK, Robertson WB, McMenemey WH. Clinical and pathological observations in Jamaican neuropathy. A report on 206 cases. Brain 1964;87:425–62.
28. World Health Organization. Virus diseases: human T lymphotropic virus type I, HTLV-I. Wkly Epidemiol Rec 1989;64:382–3.

Practice Points

chapter
23

Neuroradiology – what and when?

Verka Beric

Infections of the central nervous system remain life threatening despite the reduction in mortality observed since the introduction of antibiotics. This reduction has been attributed as much to the advent of CT, with its facilitation of earlier and more accurate diagnoses, as to improvements in chemotherapy and surgical technique. Magnetic resonance imaging, which appeared a decade after CT, has had a less marked effect because modern CT effectively remains the first choice for excluding intracranial emergencies. Computed tomography is generally more readily available and, unlike MRI, it is not subject to specific contraindications or to limitations imposed by requiring compatible life support systems. However, MRI is far superior to CT in detecting lesions in the spinal cord and brain stem and often demonstrates lesions in the brain at an earlier stage in the disease process. With the benefits of cross-sectional imaging, other modalities such as plain radiography, angiography and nuclear medicine now have little to offer. In neonates, transcranial sonography has a role to play, but CT or MRI are still often required to clarify the nature and extent of the abnormalities shown.

Suitable imaging for suspected diagnoses are considered below in the broad categories of brain abscess, intracranial empyema, meningitis and encephalitis.

BRAIN ABSCESS
Brain abscesses are most commonly bacterial in origin but they may be tuberculous, parasitic or fungal. They arise in the cerebral

parenchyma 10–14 days after diffuse infection (cerebritis), which is usually limited to the white matter. Early cerebritis is rarely seen on CT, but MRI can demonstrate increased signal on T2-weighted images. Unfortunately, this finding is of limited clinical value as patients rarely present at this early stage. A developing abscess is well demonstrated on both CT and MRI. Necrosis develops in the region of cerebritis and becomes walled off by a fibrovascular capsule that is in turn surrounded by edema. The capsule enhances intensely with CT and MRI contrast agents and tends to be thinner on its medial side, so that it appears to 'point' towards the ventricles (Fig. 23.1). Complications such as ependymitis and ventriculitis or daughter abscesses may occur if the abscess ruptures. If the diagnosis is in doubt, a radiolabeled leukocyte scan may confirm the presence of focal parenchymal infection. However, because percutaneous CT- or MRI-guided stereotactic needle aspiration is usually required for microbial analysis, especially if there is a poor response to empiric treatment, such isotope studies are rarely necessary. Response to treatment is best assessed by serial cross-sectional imaging, for which CT is usually adequate, and is seen as a gradual reduction in the size of the abscess and surrounding edema.

A tuberculous abscess (tuberculoma) is known to follow an episode of tuberculous meningitis; it may also arise through hematogenous spread from an extracranial source, usually of pulmonary origin. It may be solid or cavitating with a thick capsule, is often small and multiple, and is demonstrated on both contrast-enhanced CT and MRI.

Worldwide, cysticercosis (caused by *Taenia solium*) is the most common parasitic infection to affect the central nervous system. Patients may have hundreds of larvae-containing cysts scattered throughout the brain, ventricles and subarachnoid spaces. Acute illness occurs many months after initial infection when the larvae die and incite an intense local inflammatory reaction. At this stage, CT and MRI reveal contrast-enhancing nodular or ring lesions surrounded by extensive localized edema. The edema is most clearly seen on T2-weighted MRI. Later in the disease process, the dead larvae appear as punctate calcifications without a surrounding mass effect and are most readily visible on CT.

Hydatid disease (caused by *Echinococcus* spp.) results in a large cyst that contains fluid of the same desnsity as cerebrospinal fluid (CSF); the cyst does not display contrast enhancement or surrounding edema. Magnetic resonance imaging confers no particular advantage over CT.

Toxoplasma gondii is a common opportunistic infection in patients who have AIDS. Multiple ring-enhancing and nodular lesions are the hallmark of toxoplasmosis but the appearances are nonspecific and are similar to that of multiple brain abscesses, lymphoma or metastatic disease. Because toxoplasmosis is the most common cause of a mass lesion in the central nervous system in HIV-positive patients, empiric

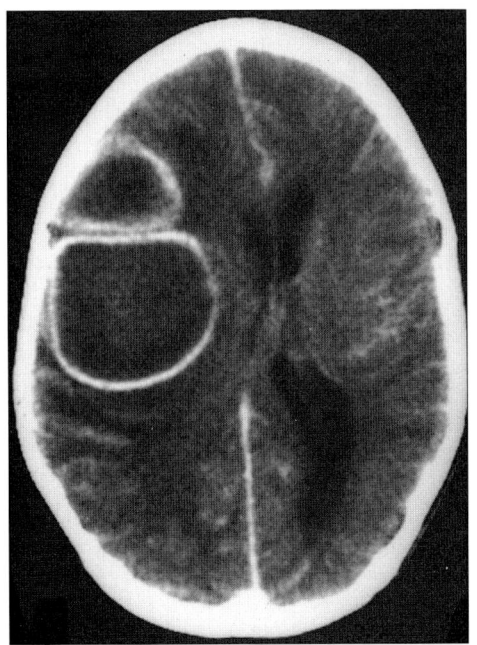

Fig. 23.1 Cerebral abscess. Contrast enhanced axial CT demonstrating two cerebral abscesses with surrounding edema and mass effect. Thin, smooth enhancing capsules surround cavities of nonenhancing necrotic tissue. Courtesy of Dr I Colquhoun.

treatment is usually commenced if CT or MRI suggest an abnormality. Biopsy may be required for definitive diagnosis if clinical or radiologic improvements are not demonstrated. Alternatively, a thallium-201 single photon emission CT (SPECT) scan may be helpful. This shows increased uptake in lymphoma and thus aids in differentiation from brain damage that is due to an infectious agent, such as toxoplasmosis.

INTRACRANIAL EMPYEMA

An intracranial empyema is an abscess that has developed in the subdural or epidural space. Subdural empyemas are more common, rapidly progressive and result in significant mortality if a delay in diagnosis occurs. Extradural empyemas cause less neurologic deficit because the dura mater minimizes the pressure exerted on the brain. Computed tomography scans and MRI demonstrate similar features. A subdural empyema is cresent-shaped, following the contour of the skull, and often extends into the interhemispheric space, where it appears linear. An extradural empyema has a lentiform shape and does not expand into the interhemispheric fissure (Fig. 23.2). Subdural empyemas may be easily overlooked on initial CT studies but then become clearly apparent a few days later. Small lesions may be obscured by the overlying bone on CT scans but should be readily detected on coronal MRI scans.

MENINGITIS

Meningitis may present as an acute life-threatening situation. In this case it is most commonly of bacterial origin and is diagnosed from both clinical and laboratory findings, as CT and MRI scans are very often normal at the time of presentation. Viral meningitis also presents acutely but is benign and self-limiting. Imaging findings are also normal unless coexisting encephalitis ensues. Granulomatous meningitis, due for example to tuberculosis, and fungal meningitis often present in a chronic indolent fashion. Their hallmark of exudative thickened basal meninges are usually visible on contrast-enhanced CT and MRI scans.

In general, in all cases of suspected infection of the central nervous system, CSF sampling for microbial and biochemical analysis is indicated as a matter of urgency, but this is particularly so when meningitis is suspected. Computed tomography or MRI scans should be performed before CSF sampling if the patient's conscious state is depressed or if focal neurologic signs or papilledema are present, because these clinical features may indicate the presence of an intracranial mass or raised intracranial pressure. If there is raised intracranial pressure, withdrawal of CSF may result in the potentially catastrophic clinical event known as coning (or cerebral herniation). This is attributed to impaction of the cerebellar tonsils in the foramen magnum with consequent compression of the medulla. However, coning may occur in the context of a normal CT or MRI scan. Therefore, if uncomplicated meningitis is suspected, CSF sampling and treatment should not be delayed in order to obtain brain imaging because this delay is likely to result in a greater risk of clinical deterioration than would have occurred with the possibility of coning.

Computed tomography and MRI scans are useful for demonstrating the development of complications of meningitis, such as ventriculitis, infarctions, subdural effusions and hydrocephalus, in the patient who has responded poorly to initial treatment.

ENCEPHALITIS

Encephalitis refers to diffuse inflammation and edema of the brain. It is usually viral in origin. Many cases are due to herpes simplex virus, which is associated with high mortality and, in surviving patients, considerable morbidity. The most sensitive imaging modality is T2-weighted MRI, which demonstrates the characteristic edema of the medial temporal lobes, inferior frontal lobes and the insula as areas of increased signal (Fig. 23.3). Computed tomography mirrors these findings but changes may be minimal in the first few days despite severe neurologic impairment. Morbidity associated with biopsy of herpes-involved tissue is considered significant enough to allow empiric treatment based on MRI findings and the clinical history alone.

Human immunodeficiency virus encephalopathy is a form of subacute encephalitis caused by HIV itself. It presents as a progressive subcortical dementia and is usually a manifestation of end-stage AIDS. Computed tomography shows global atrophy and diffuse hypodense areas in the deep white matter, particularly in the frontal lobes. The lesions are usually bilateral, essentially symmetric and do not enhance with intravenous contrast. Again, T2-weighted MRI is the most sensitive imaging modality.

Progressive multifocal leukoencephalopathy is an indolent infection caused by the JC papovavirus. It is acquired in childhood but

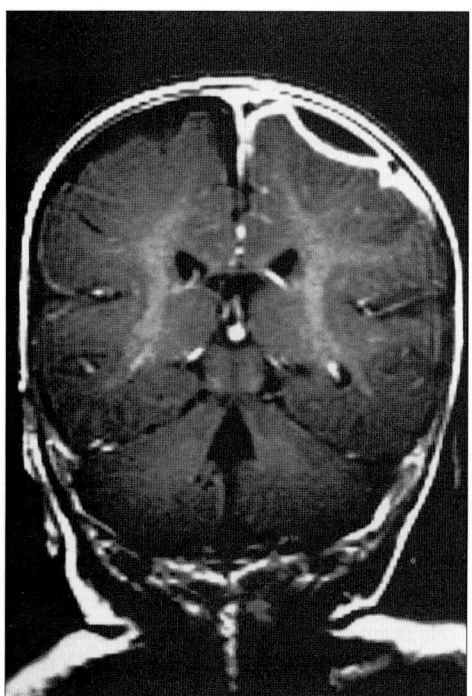

Fig. 23.2 Extradural empyema. Contrast-enhanced T1-weighted coronal MRI demonstrating lentiform extradural collection surrounded by enhancing dura mater. Courtesy of Dr K Chong.

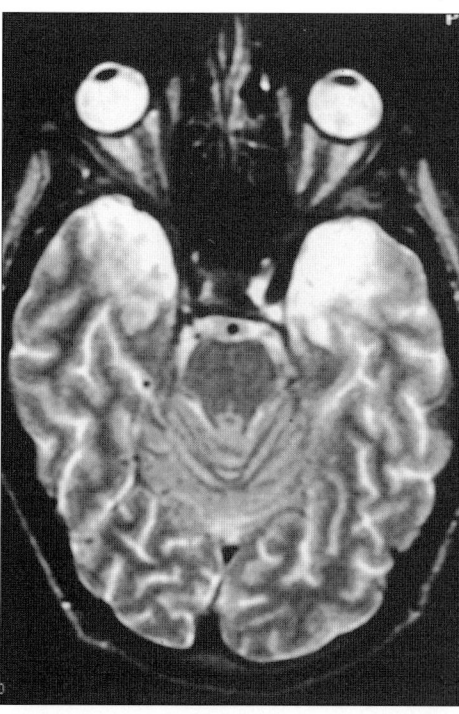

Fig. 23.3 Herpes simplex encephalitis. T2-weighted axial MRI demonstrating characteristic involvement of medial temporal lobes with high signal edema. Courtesy of Dr K Chong.

reactivates during periods of immunosuppression, such as occurs in AIDS. It results in asymmetric demyelination, usually of the posterior parietal white matter. Computed tomography shows non-enhancing, hypodense, ill-defined lesions. However, T2-weighted MRI is more reliable and may be positive early in the disease process when CT scans still appear normal. The relatively defined scalloped margins, multiple involved areas and asymmetry distinguish it from HIV encephalopathy.

FURTHER READING

Archer BD. Computed tomography before lumbar puncture in acute meningitis: a review of the risks and benefits. Can Med Assoc J 1993;148(6):961–5.
Osborn AG, Tong KA. Intracranial infections and inflammation. In: Handbook of neuroradiology: brain and skull. St Louis: Mosby; 1996:413–93.
Stevens JM. Infections of the central nervous system. In: Butler P, ed. Imaging of the nervous system. London: Springer; 1990:107–30.
Thurnher MM, Thurnher SA, Schindler E. CNS involvement in AIDS: spectrum of CT and MRI findings. Eur Radiol 1997;7:1091–7.

Lumbar puncture – when to do and what tests to order   *Linsey Philip*

INTRODUCTION
The analysis of cerebrospinal fluid (CSF) is essential in the evaluation of the patient who has suspected infection of the central nervous system. Lumbar puncture (LP) must be performed whenever meningitis or encephalitis is suspected.

COLLECTION OF CEREBROSPINAL FLUID
Before performing an LP, always exclude raised intracranial pressure by examining the ocular fundi. Computed tomography scanning of the head, preferably with contrast, is indicated before an LP in the patient who has focal neurologic deficit, recent head trauma, diminished level of consciousness or AIDS. Antibiotic therapy should not be withheld for these procedures to be performed. Measure the opening pressure whenever possible. Draw a minimum of 10ml of CSF in adults for baseline analysis in three or four tubes. In doubtful situations collect an extra fluid, label it and have it stored. Measurement of CSF closing pressure may be helpful. Normal CSF pressure is 60–150mmH$_2$0. The CSF pressure has prognostic value in a patient who has cryptococcal meningitis. Figure 23.4 lists the quantities of CSF suggested for analysis.

TRANSPORTATION AND STORAGE OF CEREBROSPINAL FLUID
As with other body fluids, universal precautions apply to CSF. Cerebrospinal fluid should be transported to the laboratory without delay. It is hypotonic and therefore neutrophils may lyse; neutrophil counts may decrease by 32% after 1 hour and 50% after 2 hours in CSF specimens held at room temperature. *Neisseria meningitidis, Haemophilus influenzae* and *Streptococcus pneumoniae* are fastidious organisms that may not survive long transit times or variations in temperature. Cerebrospinal fluid should be stored at −94°F for future viral cultures. Store CSF at 39°F for antigen detection tests.

INDICATIONS FOR LUMBAR PUNCTURE
The indications for lumbar puncture are:
- acute bacterial meningitis, which presents with headache, fever, stiff neck, lethargy, vomiting and confusion, although the signs and symptoms may be subtle or absent at extremes of age;
- chronic meningitis, which presents with fever, lethargy, headache, nausea, vomiting and cranial nerve palsies or focal neurologic deficits lasting 1–4 weeks before presentation; fungal and mycobacterial cultures should be done and it is important to store enough CSF for further testing;
- acute nonbacterial meningitis (aseptic meningitis): viral meningitis is the usual cause and it is usually seasonal in nature; if the initial CSF shows a predominance of polymorophonucleocytes then a repeat LP done 18–24 hours later will show a shift towards lymphocytes. Bacterial causes of aseptic meningitis-like syndromes include syphilis, *Borrelia burgdorferi* and *Bartonella henselae*. Noninfectious causes are medications (e.g. nonsteroidal anti-inflammatory drugs), malignant diseases, tumors, systemic lupus erythematosus, sarcoidosis, Behçet's syndrome and Mollaret's meningitis. Parameningeal infections such as brain abscess, epidural abscess, sinusitis and retropharyngeal abscess can also present as aseptic meningitis;

OPTIMAL QUANTITIES OF CEREBROSPINAL FLUID FOR LABORATORY ANALYSIS	
Test	Amount of cerebrospinal fluid
Protein	1ml
Glucose	0.5ml
Gram stain and culture (bacterial)	2–5ml
Venereal disease research laboratory	0.5ml
India ink preparation	0.3ml
Cryptococcal antigen	1ml
Mycobacterial culture	5–10ml
Fungal culture	5–10ml
Viral culture	3–5ml
Cytology	10ml
Coccidioidomycosis antibody	1ml
Serology (others)	1ml
PCR for herpesvirus, enterovirus	1ml

Fig. 23.4 Optimal quantities of cerebrospinal fluid for laboratory analysis.

- acute encephalitis, which presents with fever, headache, behavioral changes, speech disturbances, seizures and focal neurologic signs; herpes encephalitis may present with symptoms of temporal lobe seizures and fever;
- infection with HIV plus a positive serologic test for syphilis, dementia, progressive lumbosacral polyradiculopathy (in which cytomegalovirus is probably an important pathogen), focal neurologic deficits (including cranial nerve palsies), unexplained change in mental status, or unexplained changes in MRI or CT scan of head;
- relief of intracranial pressure in cryptococcal meningitis; about 30ml should be removed daily while the pressure is elevated or the headache is worsening;
- unexplained or worsening headache in an immunocompromised patient; and
- the administration of medications such as intrathecal gentamicin or vancomycin.

TESTS TO ORDER
The findings in normal CSF are:
- cell count 0–5 lymphocytes or mononuclear cells per ml,
- glucose 45–80mg/dl or two-thirds of the serum value, and
- total protein 15–50mg/dl.

Gram stain
The Gram stain is a simple, rapid, reliable and inexpensive method of detecting bacteria and inflammatory cells. It is most reliable at detecting >10^5 bacteria per ml of body fluid. Bacteria have been observed in:
- 90% of cases of meningitis caused by *S. pneumoniae* and *Staphylococcus* spp.;
- 86% of cases caused by *H. influenzae*;
- 75% of cases caused by *N. meningitidis*;
- 50% of cases caused by Gram-negative bacilli; and
- <50% of cases caused by *L. monocytogenes* and anaerobic bacteria.

The chances of observing bacteria in CSF can be increased up to 100-fold by cytospin centrifugation. Morphologic and Gram stain properties may be altered in partially treated bacterial meningitis.

Culture

Routine bacterial cultures should be performed in all cases where a diagnostic LP is performed. Mycobacterial and fungal cultures should be done in immunocompromised patients and when mycobacterial and fungal infection is clinically suspected. The yield is higher with larger volumes of CSF. Viral culture is indicated for suspected viral meningitis and acute encephalitis and in HIV-positive patients.

Leukocyte count with differential

A total CSF leukocyte count of $2000 \times 10^6/l$ or a polymorphonucleocyte count $>1180 \times 10^6/l$ have a high predictive value in acute bacterial meningitis. Neutrophilic pleocytosis is usually seen in bacterial meningitis but it may also be present in early viral meningitis. Eosinophils in the CSF is an uncommon finding (Fig. 23.5). Helminthic infection of the CSF is the most common cause of eosinophilia.

Protein

Protein levels in the CSF are commonly elevated in bacterial meningitis, and very high protein levels are seen in tuberculous meningitis.

Glucose

A ratio of CSF glucose to blood glucose below 0.23 is a strong predictor of acute bacterial meningitis. Hypoglycorrhachia <45mg/dl is seen in a variety of conditions, including:

• viral infections (herpes simplex virus, mumps, lymphocytic choriomeningitis),
• bacterial infections (bacterial meningitis, tuberculosis, syphilis, leptospirosis, brucellosis), and
• fungal infections (cryptococcosis, histoplasmosis, blastomycosis).

Miscellaneous causes include sinusitis, brain abscess, endocarditis, meningeal carcinomatosis and amebic meningoencephalitis.

Acid-fast stains

Acid-fast stains are positive in only 10–20% of patients who have tuberculous meningitis whereas cultures are positive in 60–80% of cases. Yield is increased if 20–40ml of CSF is submitted for staining. Assays to detect mycobacterial antigens have a sensitivity of 50–80% and a specificity >90% for *Mycobacterium tuberculosis*. Polymerase chain reaction may be the most useful technique in tuberculous meningitis.

Cryptococcal antigen

Cryptococcal antigen is more sensitive (>90%) than India ink (75%) in cryptococcal meningitis.

Rapid bacterial antigen detection tests

Latex agglutination is the most frequently performed rapid bacterial antigen detection test. Its use is controversial and most hospital laboratories have stopped performing these tests because of false-positives and false-negative results and a lack of cost effectiveness. These tests may have some value in partially treated meningitis because the cultures are frequently negative.

CAUSES OF EOSINOPHILIA OF THE CEREBROSPINAL FLUID	
Parasitic infestations of the central nervous system	**Bacterial infections**
Taenia solium	*Treponema pallidum*
Angiostrongylus cantonensis	*Mycobacterium tuberculosis*
Toxocara cati	**Others**
Toxocara canis	Lymphoma
Gnathostoma spinigerum	Multiple sclerosis
	Foreign material in the CNS
Fungal infections	Viral meningitis
Coccidioides immitis	

Fig. 23.5 Causes of eosinophilia of the cerebrospinal fluid.

Serologic tests

Serologic test for syphilis should be performed in all cases of suspected neurosyphilis. Sensitivity varies from 48 to 84%. A variety of antibody tests is available (e.g. for Lyme disease, arboviruses, coccidioidomycosis and histoplasmosis) and these should be performed on the basis of clinical suspicion.

Polymerase chain reaction

Polymerase chain reaction assays are increasingly being used. They are 98% sensitive, 94% specific in herpes simplex virus infections and 80% sensitive in progressive multifocal leukoencephalopathy. They are quicker and more sensitive than viral cultures in enteroviral meningitis and superior to brain biopsy in herpes encephalitis. Polymerase chain reaction is being tested in a variety of other bacterial and viral infections.

Direct examination

Direct examination of the CSF is useful in amebic meningoencephalitis.

FURTHER READING

Durand ML, Calderwood SB, Weber DJ, *et al*. Acute bacterial meningitis in adults – a review of 493 episodes. N Engl J Med 1993;328:21–8.

Gray L, Fedorko D. Laboratory diagnosis of bacterial meningitis. Clin Microbiol Rev 1992;5:130–45.

Jeffery K, Read SJ, Peto T, Mayon–White, Bangham CR. Diagnosis of viral infections of the central nervous system: clinical interpretation of PCR results. Lancet 1997;349:313–7.

Kuberski T. Eosinophils in the cerebrospinal fluid. Ann Intern Med 1979;91:70–5.

Lakeman F, Whitley R. Diagnosis of herpes simplex encephalitis: application of polymerase chain reaction to cerebrospinal fluid from brain-biopsied patients and correlation with disease. J Infect Dis 1995;171:857–63.

Perkins M, Mirrett S, Reller LB. Rapid bacterial antigen detection is not clinically useful. J Clin Microbiol 1995;33:1486–91.

Powderly W. Recent advances in the management of cryptococcal meningitis in patients with AIDS. Clin Infect Dis 1996;22(Suppl 2):119–23.

Shanholtzer C, Schaper P, Peterson L. Concentrated gram stain smears prepared with a cytospin centrifuge. J Clin Microbiol 1982;16:1052–6.

Spanos A, Harrell F, Durack D. Differential diagnosis of acute meningitis. JAMA 1989;262:2700–7.

Varki A, Puthuran P. Value of second lumbar puncture in confirming a diagnosis of aseptic meningitis. Arch Neurol 1979;36:581–2.

Verdon R, Chevret S, Laissy J-P, Wolff M. Tuberculous meningitis in adults: review of 48 cases. Clin Infect Dis 1996;22:982–8.

Approach to the patient who has fever and headache

Iain Stephenson & Martin Wiselka

INTRODUCTION

Fever and headache are common presenting signs with a wide differential diagnosis. The physician needs to be able to recognize the early features of bacterial meningitis and initiate appropriate treatment without delay as the consequences of a missed diagnosis or inadequate treatment can be fatal. Investigations for other causes of fever and headache can be initiated once meningitis has been excluded.

PATHOGENESIS

Inflammation of the meninges may result from a number of pathologic processes including infection, acute vasculitis, malignant infiltration and subarachnoid hemorrhage. Organisms enter the meninges via the nasopharyngeal mucosa or after blood-borne spread. Direct invasion can follow skull fracture or neurosurgery. Relatively poor host defenses and low complement levels in the cerebrospinal fluid (CSF) may facilitate the spread of infection.

Bacterial meningitis is associated with acute inflammation stimulated by bacterial antigens and cytokines. This results in a fibrinous neutrophilic exudate across the leptomeninges and may be associated with the systemic features of sepsis syndrome and circulatory collapse. The increased permeability of the blood–brain barrier, raised intracranial pressure and vasculitic changes around the vessels traversing the subarachnoid space may result in brain ischemia. Tuberculous and fungal infections tend to have a more insidious onset but they may begin fairly abruptly. A CSF pleocytosis with negative Gram stain and culture is termed an aseptic meningitis (Fig. 23.6). Viral infections cause disease either by direct invasion of the leptomeninges and brain, or indirectly by postinfective immune-mediated phenomena.

MICROBIOLOGY

Fever and headache may be nonspecific features of many infections but they may result from infection of the meninges (meningitis) or brain tissue (encephalitis). The organisms causing bacterial meningitis vary with age and geographic region (Fig. 23.7). *Neisseria meningitidis, Streptococcus pneumoniae* and *Haemophilus influenzae* type b cause about 80% of cases of adult meningitis.

The incidence of *H. influenzae* meningitis in children has declined dramatically following the introduction of *H. influenzae* type b vaccine. Pneumococcal meningitis may follow an initial otitis media, sinus infection or pneumonia and most cases occur in infants and the middle-aged or elderly. Meningococcal meningitis is most common in infants, children and young adults. Outbreaks of infection occur in nurseries, schools, universities and residential accommodation. Cases of meningococcal infection occur more frequently during the winter months and may be associated with influenza infection. In Europe and North America meningococci belonging to groups B and C most commonly cause disease, whereas group A strains have been responsible for serious outbreaks of infection in sub-Saharan Africa. Typing of infection is relevant because the current meningococcal vaccine gives protection against groups A and C strains but has no effect on group B disease.

Rare causes of bacterial meningitis include *Listeria monocytogenes*, which is associated with pregnancy and underlying immunosuppression or malignancy. Following trauma or neurosurgery, meningitis caused by Gram-negative organisms such as *Escherichia coli, Pseudomonas* spp., *Klebsiella pneumoniae* and *Enterobacter* spp. can occur.

SOME CAUSES OF LYMPHOCYTIC CEREBROSPINAL FLUID	
Viruses	Enteroviruses
	Mumps virus
	Herpes simplex virus
Bacteria	Partially treated bacterial meningitis
	Early bacterial meningitis
	Cerebral abscess
	Tuberculosis
	Brucellosis
	Spirochetes (treponemes, leptospirosis, *Borrelia* spp.)
Fungi	Cryptococcosis
	Histoplasmosis
Protozoa	Toxoplasmosis
	Amebiasis
Inflammatory conditions	Seropositive conditions (e.g. lupus)
	Seronegative conditions (e.g. Behçet's syndrome, Kawasaki's disease)
	Sarcoidosis
Chemicals	Irritants
Carcinomatous conditions	Usually secondary deposits

Fig. 23.6 Some causes of lymphocytic cerebrospinal fluid.

LIKELY ORGANISMS AND POSSIBLE EMPIRIC TREATMENT REGIMENS FOR BACTERIAL MENINGITIS		
Group of patients	Likely organisms	Treatment
Neonates	Group B streptococci *Escherichia coli* *Listeria monocytogenes*	Ampicillin and gentamicin Cefotaxime
Children	*Neisseria meningitidis* *Streptococcus pneumoniae* *Haemophilus influenzae*	Ceftriaxone Cefotaxime (vancomycin if resistant pneumococcus)
Adults	*Neisseria meningitidis* *Streptococcus pneumoniae* *Haemophilus influenzae* *Listeria monocytogenes*	Ceftriaxone (vancomycin if resistant pneumococcus) Ampicillin
Elderly people/ underlying malignancy	*Neisseria meningitidis* *Streptococcus pneumoniae* *Haemophilus influenzae* *Listeria monocytogenes* Gram-negative organisms	Ceftriaxone (vancomycin if resistant pneumococcus) Ampicillin
Post-traumatic surgery	*Streptococcus pneumoniae* *Haemophilus influenzae* *Escherichia coli* *Klebsiella pneumoniae* *Enterobacter* spp. *Pseudomonas* spp. *Staphylococcus aureus*	Ceftriaxone Ceftazidime Carpabenem

Fig. 23.7 Likely organisms and possible empiric treatment regimens for bacterial meningitis.

Viral meningitis is predominantly caused by the enteroviruses (70%), including Coxsackie viruses A and B and the echoviruses. The mumps virus causes about 10% of the diagnosed cases of viral meningitis in the UK with the remainder being caused by herpes simplex virus, varicella-zoster virus, measles virus, adenoviruses or Epstein–Barr virus. Herpes simplex encephalitis can cause necrotic edematous changes that may be asymmetric and localized in the temporal lobes.

CLINICAL FEATURES
The cardinal features of meningeal inflammation are:
- headache,
- neck stiffness, and
- photophobia.

Meningococcal meningitis and sepsis are associated with a petechial or purpuric rash. An exantham may be present in viral infections. The history can often localize the source of infection or may suggest a generalized febrile illness. The presence of intracranial shunts, previous head trauma, recent travel history and underlying immunosuppression will influence the range of potential pathogens. Symptoms and signs of meningitis may be nonspecific in very young or elderly patients. Wakening or early morning headache, with or without vomiting, that is worse on coughing and bending forward or that is associated with visual disturbance are symptoms of raised intracranial pressure.

On examination, vital signs must be documented and the skin should be fully exposed to look for a rash and for the presence of cervical or other lymphadenopathy. Signs of meningism should be sought, including evidence of neck stiffness, photophobia and the presence of Kernig's sign. To elicit Kernig's sign, the patient is placed supine and the lower limb is flexed at the hip and the knee is extended. Patients who have meningism resist by contracting the hamstrings. Assessment of focal neurologic signs, including cranial nerve assessment and funduscopy for papilledema, is important. Examination of the tympanic membrane may reveal an underlying otitis media. Urinary dipstick examination should be performed. Acute meningococcal meningitis associated with a florid purpuric rash is usually unmistakable, but patients may be relatively well with equivocal signs or have a more insidious illness.

INVESTIGATIONS
The aim of investigation is to establish the cause of fever and headache and to identify any infecting organisms. A blood count is helpful because bacterial infections are usually accompanied by a neutrophilia. Biochemical and clotting profiles can indicate the development of systemic complications. Cultures of body fluids (blood, sputum, urine, CSF, throat swab and skin scrapings) may reveal the causative pathogen. Antigen-detection kits are also available and give rapid results. Meningococcal, tuberculosis, herpes simplex and enterovirus genome detection by the polymerase chain reaction (PCR) is now available from reference laboratories. Comparison of meningococcal antibody titers in acute and convalescent serum samples can yield a retrospective diagnosis.

Chest and sinus radiographs may be helpful in revealing underlying infection. Computed tomography or MRI scans of the head can identify the presence of cerebral edema, hydrocephalus or a mass effect and exclude alternative diagnoses of intracranial hemorrhage, subdural collection or abscess formation. Examination of the CSF remains important in many cases; routine analysis includes cell count, protein and glucose estimation, culture and Gram stain.

Acute bacterial meningitis is usually associated with polymorphonuclear leukocytosis in the CSF with raised protein and low glucose levels. Viral meningitis characteristically gives a lymphocytosis with normal protein and glucose levels. However, there is a wide differential diagnosis of a lymphocytic CSF, which can be investigated by Ziehl–Neelsen and Indian ink staining, cytology, direct immunofluorescence and viral PCR (see Fig. 23.6). A low CSF glucose ($<^2/_3$

serum glucose) usually indicates a bacterial, fungal, tuberculous or carcinomatous cause.

MANAGEMENT
Immediate management
The possibility of meningitis should be considered in all patients who have fever and headache. Patients who appear reasonably well with no obvious source of infection need to be observed closely because the signs of meningitis may evolve very rapidly.

If bacterial meningitis is suspected, immediate hospital admission should be arranged and blood cultures and intravenous antibiotic therapy should be instituted without delay. Resuscitation may be required and all patients who have suspected or confirmed bacterial meningitis should be closely monitored, preferably in a high-dependency or intensive care unit.

There is compelling evidence that immediate empiric antibiotic therapy can improve the outcome of meningococcal sepsis and meningitis. In the UK, general practitioners are advised to give intravenous or intramuscular benzylpenicillin to any patient who has suspected bacterial meningitis. The only contraindication is a previous anaphylactic reaction to penicillin.

Following admission and any immediate resuscitation the two major questions for the clinician managing the patient are whether to do a head scan (CT or MRI) or a lumbar puncture.

Role of head scanning
Computed tomography and MRI scanning is unhelpful in uncomplicated viral meningitis, when it is safe to perform a lumbar puncture. The indications for performing an urgent scan before lumbar puncture include focal neurologic signs, altered level of consciousness, papilledema or symptoms suggestive of raised intracranial pressure, convulsions and suspected subarachnoid hemorrhage.

Role and safety of lumbar puncture
The safety of lumbar puncture in patients who have bacterial meningitis has recently been questioned because occasional patients who have unsuspected cerebral edema have developed brain stem coning and death after the procedure. This occurs most commonly in patients who have fulminant meningococcal disease and early lumbar puncture should therefore be avoided in patients who have purpuric rash. Lumbar puncture may be considered at a later stage in these patients if there has been no improvement on empiric treatment.

The value of lumbar puncture is also declining with increasing use of antibiotics before the procedure and the availability of newer diagnostic techniques. Nevertheless, the lumbar puncture remains a very important investigation in patients who have suspected viral meningitis, in whom it allows the diagnosis to be established, and in the atypical causes of meningitis. If the CSF is clear, further investigations should be performed to establish the cause of fever and headache. In these circumstances a chest radiograph is helpful to exclude pneumonia and urinalysis is useful to exclude a urinary tract infection, because these conditions may present with signs of meningism.

Choice of antibiotic therapy
Empiric therapy should cover all likely pathogens; treatment can then be modified if any organisms are identified. When considering antibiotic choice, the agent used must penetrate the CSF to achieve an adequate inhibitory concentration. Antibiotic penetration is initially good because the blood–brain barrier is impaired owing to the inflamed meninges, but as the disease resolves penetration becomes less. Ceftriaxone and cefotaxime are third-generation cephalosporins that will cover the meningococcus, the pneumococcus, *H. influenzae* and most other organisms (see Fig. 23.7) and they are frequently used as empiric therapy. Cephalosporins have little activity against *Listeria* spp. and ampicillin should be added if listeriosis is suspected. Penicillin-resistant pneumococci are occurring with increasing

frequency in many areas and benzylpenicillin is therefore inadequate as empiric therapy for bacterial meningitis.

The treatment of lymphocytic meningitis is difficult because the diagnosis is often uncertain and there is a wide range of potential pathogens. It is occasionally necessary to treat patients with empiric antibiotics, antiviral therapy (aciclovir), antituberculous therapy and antifungal therapy, with the possible addition of corticosteroids. Patients who have lymphocytic meningitis can present a major diagnostic and therapeutic challenge.

Role of corticosteroids

Early dexamethasone treatment has been shown to be associated with an improved outcome in meningitis caused by *H. influenzae*, but the effect of corticosteroids is less clear in other forms of bacterial meningitis because there have been few large, well-controlled studies. In view of the lack of evidence regarding the use of corticosteroids, clinicians differ widely in their practice; however, it seems sensible to give corticosteroids as early as possible to have a maximal effect.

Management of the complications of meningitis

Bacterial meningitis may be accompanied by all the features of sepsis syndrome, with multiple-organ failure requiring intensive care support. It has been suggested that hemofiltration may have a therapeutic role by removing bacterial toxins and unwanted cytokines, although there are no controlled studies. A sensible approach is to consider early hemofiltration in seriously ill patients who have hypotension and oliguria. The role of extracorporeal membrane oxygenation is also uncertain, but this should be considered if the patient is failing to respond to conventional ventilation and circulatory support.

Seizures are managed with anticonvulsants or sedation and ventilation. Metastatic seeding of infection can form cerebral or epidural abscesses and progress to a subdural empyema. The blockage or interruption of CSF circulation at the foramina, aqueduct or subarachnoid granulations can produce hydrocephalus. Raised intracranial pressure can result in sinus thrombosis, cerebral edema with herniation, cranial nerve palsies or brain ischemia. Sensorineural deafness occurs in about 10% of patients who have pneumococcal meningitis and a smaller proportion of patients who have meningococcal meningitis, and audiologic assessment is recommended for all patients who have recovered from bacterial meningitis.

PUBLIC HEALTH ISSUES

Public health physicians should be notified immediately of any patients who have known or suspected meningitis so that appropriate action can be taken. Cases of meningitis are often associated with considerable local publicity and anxiety in the community. The role of the public health physician is to provide appropriate information and to organize antibiotic prophylaxis for close contacts of patients who have meningococcal or *Haemophilus* meningitis and more extensive prophylaxis and vaccination campaigns if these are indicated. There are published national guidelines for the management of clusters or epidemics of meningococcal disease.

Empiric antimicrobial therapy for suspected infection of the central nervous system

Marc A Tack

INTRODUCTION

Acute bacterial infections of the central nervous system (CNS) are almost uniformly life threatening, and the initial antimicrobial therapy is usually empiric. The key clinical determinants of antimicrobial selection are the age and immune status of the patient and the clinical presentation. Careful attention must be taken to assess the patient's risk of immune dysfunction because this may result in an expanded list of potential etiologic agents and thus alter the selection of empiric therapy. A previously healthy adult who has acute bacterial meningitis poses different etiologic considerations from those of a patient with AIDS who has acute bacterial meningitis. Similarly, if the blood–brain barrier has been compromised, such as in the case of placement of an intrathecal catheter or other surgical manipulation, empiric antimicrobial therapy must be targeted toward pathogens that gain entry by these routes.

PATHOGENESIS

Infection of the CNS may occur as a result of several mechanisms. Bacterial penetration of the CNS is frequently associated with bacteremia and the pathogenesis in these cases is hematogenous spread. Extension of local infections, such as sinusitis and otitis, have been implicated as frequent causes of brain abscesses. Implanted foreign bodies, such as a ventriculoperitoneal shunt, pose a risk for infection and direct seeding of the CNS. Lastly, trauma may provide a portal of entry for direct inoculation of pathogens.

MICROBIOLOGY

The most frequent pathogens associated with bacterial meningitis in a previously healthy host are *Streptococcus pneumoniae* and *Neisseria meningitidis*. *Haemophilus influenzae*, formerly a frequently isolated organism, is now rarely implicated owing to routine pediatric immunization. In neonates, *Streptococcus agalactiae* is frequently isolated. In elderly or immunocompromised patients, *Listeria monocytogenes* must be included in the differential diagnosis of acute bacterial meningitis (Fig. 23.8).

In patients who have foreign bodies or who have undergone recent neurosurgical procedures, *S. aureus* and coagulase-negative staphylococci are the most common pathogens, although a host of other organisms including fungi have been reported. Aerobic Gram-negative bacilli have also been encountered in post-trauma and postoperative patients. A detailed review of bacterial meningitis is found in Chapter 2.15.

CLINICAL FEATURES

The most common presenting clinical features of acute bacterial meningitis are fever, headache and meningismus. This triad of symptoms is seen in over 85% of cases and should be easily recognizable to the experienced clinician. Confusion and altered sensorium are also frequently noted.

Presumptive evidence of meningococcal meningitis may be apparent on physical examination. Of patients who have meningococcemia, with or without meningitis, 50% manifest a macular erythematous papular rash early in the course of the disease. This rash rapidly appears petechial and then becomes purpuric.

In neonates, the presentation of acute bacterial meningitis may be subtle. In this group, meningismus is infrequently noted, and irritability and temperature instability may be the only indication of meningitis. Refusal to feed, lethargy, a high-pitched cry, vomiting, diarrhea and respiratory distress should alert the clinician to this diagnosis.

Elderly patients, especially those who have comorbid disease, often present with subtle manifestations. Fever is frequently absent and confusion or altered level of consciousness may be the only clinical finding.

Other less common causes of meningitis may frequently present with varying clinical syndromes. Cryptococcal meningitis in a patient who has AIDS typically presents as an insidious illness; persistent fever and headache over several days or even weeks is often the only

COMMON BACTERIAL PATHOGENS ASSOCIATED WITH PREDISPOSING FACTORS FOR MENINGITIS	
Predisposing factor	Common bacterial pathogens
CFS shunt	Coagulase-negative staphylococci, *Staphylococcus aureus*, Gram-negative bacilli
Postneurosurgery or post-trauma	*Staphylococcus aureus*, coagulase-negative staphylococci, Gram-negative bacilli
Immunocompromise	*Streptococcus pneumoniae*, *Neisseria meningitidis*, *Listeria monocytogenes*, Gram-negative bacilli
Skull fracture	*Streptococcus pneumoniae*, group A streptococci, *Staphylococcus aureus*

Fig. 23.8 Common bacterial pathogens associated with predisposing factors for meningitis.

COMMON BACTERIAL PATHOGENS CAUSING MENINGITIS ACCORDING TO THE AGE OF PATIENT	
Age of patient	Most common bacterial pathogens
0–4 weeks	*Streptococcus agalactiae*, *Escherichia coli*, *Listeria monocytogenes*, *Klebsiella pneumoniae*
4 weeks to 2 years	*Streptococcus agalactiae*, *Streptococcus pneumoniae*, *Haemophilus influenzae*
2–18 years	*Haemophilus influenzae* (decreasing), *Neisseria meningitidis*, *Streptococcus pneumoniae*
18–60 years	*Streptococcus pneumoniae*, *Neisseria meningitidis*
Over 60 years	*Streptococcus pneumoniae*, *Listeria monocytogenes*, others

Fig. 23.9 Common bacterial pathogens causing meningitis according to the age of patient.

clinical complaint. Lyme meningitis, more common in highly endemic areas, often presents as a subacute basilar meningitis with cranial nerve palsies and radiculopathy as common findings. Tuberculous meningitis may also present in an insidious manner, necessitating a high index of suspicion for early recognition and successful treatment.

The clinical manifestations of a brain abscess are usually more attributable to the space-occupying effect of the lesion than to the actual infection. The classic triad (fever, headache and a focal neurologic deficit) is seen in only 50% of patients. Headache, which is usually moderate or severe, is the most common manifestation; the next most common is fever. Eventually, altered mentation, ranging from confusion to coma, ensues. Neurologic findings may be focal, but this depends on the size and location of the abscess. Seizures as well as papilledema are more common in brain abscess than in meningitis.

INVESTIGATIONS

Early diagnosis and rapid initiation of appropriate antimicrobial therapy is essential in patients who present with manifestations of acute infection of the CNS. A lumbar puncture should be performed in all patients unless there are specific contraindications to this procedure. Patients who present with papilledema or focal neurologic findings should undergo a CT scan before lumbar puncture to determine whether there is a space-occupying lesion under increased intracranial pressure; it will determine the presence of a brain abscess in most cases as well. In patients who have a shunt or reservoir, cerebrospinal fluid (CSF) samples may be obtained from these sites.

Samples of CSF should be examined, preferably using a cytospin technique, for the presence of bacterial and fungal pathogens using appropriate stains. Glucose and protein levels in the CSF should be obtained together with a simultaneous serum glucose level for comparison. Cultures of CSF for bacterial, fungal and mycobacterial organisms should be obtained. If cryptococcal meningitis is suspected, a cryptococcal antigen assay should be performed on CSF as well. Bacterial latex agglutination tests are frequently used but are of limited benefit in clinical practice owing to their high false-negative rate.

In addition to studies of the CSF, blood cultures should be sent in all cases because of the high rate of concomitant bacteremia. Other specimens, such as sputum, urine and sinus aspirates, should be obtained and evaluated when clinically appropriate.

MANAGEMENT

The rapid initiation of appropriate antimicrobial therapy in acute bacterial meningitis is imperative. The initiation of antibiotics should not be delayed while awaiting an imaging study before lumbar puncture.

In general, the patient should receive the first dose of antibiotics within 30 minutes of arrival at the hospital if bacterial meningitis is suspected. Appropriate therapy should be based on the age, clinical presentation and predisposing factors, and therapy should be modified if indicated when the etiologic agent is identified (Fig. 23.9).

The empiric antibiotic of choice is a third-generation cephalosporin (ceftriaxone or cefotaxime). In patients aged under 3 months or over 60 years, ampicillin should be included to the empiric regimen for the treatment of potential listeriosis.

One area of controversy is the inclusion of vancomycin in the empiric regimen to treat high-level, beta-lactam resistant *S. pneumoniae*. In my opinion, vancomycin should be used in conjunction with a third-generation cephalosporin in areas where 10% or more of the community isolates of *S. pneumoniae* demonstrate resistance to penicillin. In order to help decrease the emergence of vancomycin-resistant bacteria, vancomycin should be discontinued if the isolate is sensitive to penicillin or third-generation cephalosporins.

Patients who develop a CNS infection after trauma or postoperatively are at higher risk of Gram-negative bacillary infections. An antipseudomonal cephalosporin (ceftazidime or cefepime) in combination with vancomycin is an appropriate empiric regimen. Vancomycin is used because of the frequent beta-lactam resistance seen with coagulase-negative staphylococci, which are often identified as the pathogen in this setting. This is also the empiric regimen I suggest for patients who have foreign bodies in place.

In patients who have a brain abscess, streptococci, Gram-negative bacilli and anaerobes are frequent pathogens, and empiric antimicrobial therapy must target these pathogens and penetrate purulent collections. A third-generation cephalosporin (ceftriaxone or cefotaxime) in combination with metronidazole is useful in this clinical setting. The diagnosis and treatment of brain abscess is presented in detail in Chapter 2.17.

Although there are no controlled clinical trials, most clinicians treat acute bacterial meningitis for 7–14 days. The duration of therapy for brain abscesses is prolonged and determined by clinical and radiographic response. Patients who have AIDS who are infected with cryptococcal meningitis require prolonged therapy followed by chronic suppression (see Chapters 5.12 & 8.26 for further discussion).

FURTHER READING

Durand ML, Calderwood SB, Weber DJ, *et al*. Acute bacterial meningitis in adults: a review of 493 cases. N Engl J Med 1993;328:21–8.

Schuchat A, Robinson K, Wenger JD, *et al*. Bacterial meningitis in the United States in 1995. N Engl J Med 1997;337:970–6.

Spanos A, Harrell EE, Durack DT. Differential diagnosis of acute meningitis, an analysis of the predictive value of initial observations. JAMA 1989;262:2700–7.

Pharyngitis, Laryngitis and Epiglottitis

Dennis A Clements

This chapter describes some of the most common infections of mankind, the upper respiratory infections, which include pharyngitis, laryngitis and epiglottitis. Although viruses play a significant role in the pathogenesis of many of these infections, bacteria and other organisms are responsible for many others. This chapter details the importance of these infections and provides a practical guide to diagnosis and management.

EPIDEMIOLOGY

DEFINITION AND NOMENCLATURE

Pharyngitis, commonly called 'sore throat', is an inflammatory process of the pharynx, hypopharynx, uvula and tonsils that can be caused by viral or bacterial pathogens, and occasionally both (Fig. 24.1). Pharyngitis can be separated into one group of illnesses with

COMMON CAUSES OF PHARYNGITIS, LARYNGITIS AND EPIGLOTTITIS						
	Organism/entity	Disease/syndrome	Pharyngitis	Nasopharyngitis	Laryngitis	Epiglottitis	Complications
Bacteria	*Arcanobacterium haemolyticum*	Pharyngitis +/– scarlatiniform rash	++				
	Corynebacterium diphtheriae	Diphtheria with pseudomembrane	+++				
	Corynebacterium spp. (other)	Pharyngitis	++	+++			
	Haemophilus influenzae	Pharyngitis	+++				
	Legionella pneumophila	Pharyngitis	++	++	·	+++ (type b)	Epiglottitis, meningitis
	Neisseria gonorrhoeae	Pharyngitis	++				Pneumonia
	Neisseria meningitidis	Pharyngitis	++				Septic arthritis
	Streptococcus pyogenes (group A β-hemolytic)	Pharyngitis (scarlet fever)	+++++				Meningitis, sepsis
	Streptococcus spp. (groups B, C and G)	Pharyngitis	+++		+		Rheumatic fever, acute glomerulonephritis
	Treponema pallidum	Secondary syphilis	+		+		
	Yersinia entercolitica	Pharyngitis and enterocolitis	++		+		
Viruses	Adenoviruses	Nasopharyngitis		+++			Pneumonia
	Coronavirus	Nasopharyngitis		++			
	Coxsackie A virus	Herpangina	++	++			
	Cytomegalovirus	Mononucleosis syndrome		+++			Prenatally: birth defects
	EBV	Mononucleosis syndrome	++	+++			
	HSV	Pharyngitis with ulcerations	+++		++		Systemic disease
	HIV-1	Pharyngitis and lymphadenopathy	++				AIDS
	Influenza A and B	Nasopharyngitis, myalgia, headache		++	+++		Pneumonia
	Measles	Measles disease	+++	+++			Conjunctivitis, pneumonia, meningitis
	Parainfluenza viruses	Cold and croup		++	+++		Pneumonia
	Reoviruses (1–3)	Nasopharyngitis (uncommon)	+	+			
	RSV	Pharyngitis		+++			Bronchiolitis
	Rhinovirus	Nasopharyngitis		+++			
Other organisms	*Candida* spp.	Pharyngitis	++				
	Chlamydia pneumoniae	Pharyngitis	++		+		Pneumonia
	Coxiella burnetii	Nasopharyngitis		+			
	Mycoplasma pneumoniae	Pharyngitis	++	+			Pneumonia
Unknown etiology	Aphthous stomatitis	Ulcerative gingivitis	+				
	Behçet's syndrome	Pharyngitis with ulcerations	+++				
	Kawasaki's disease	Pharyngitis, conjunctivitis	+++				Coronary artery aneurysms
	Stevens–Johnson syndrome	Pharyngitis, stomatitis, ulcerations	+++				Shock

Fig. 24.1 Common causes of pharyngitis, laryngitis and epiglottitis.

associated nasal symptoms (which are most commonly viral in origin) and another that cause only pharyngitis. It is important to distinguish between these infections because rheumatic fever and acute glomerulonephritis may complicate untreated group A β-hemolytic streptococcal infections, but they can usually can be prevented by appropriate antibiotic treatment.

Laryngitis, or inflammation of the larynx (subglottic area), is almost always secondary to a viral infection. Lower voice pitch, hoarseness and aphonia frequently occur. It is important to differentiate laryngitis from other infectious forms of obstructive airway disease, such as epiglottitis, which may be life-threatening. Laryngitis in small children often gives a 'croup' syndrome. Children with laryngitis are often noted to 'bark' like seals. These illnesses are generally self-limited and require only supportive care.

Epiglottitis (bacterial cellulitis of the epiglottis), or supraglottitis, is an inflammatory process of the epiglottis and/or supraglottic structures that is almost always caused by *Haemophilus influenzae* type b (HIB). It is usually rapidly progressive, particularly in young children, and needs immediate antibiotic treatment and often intubation to avoid possible respiratory obstruction.

INCIDENCE, PREVALENCE AND SEASONALITY

Infections of the upper respiratory system are more common than any other acute infectious malady. The self-limited viral infections are most frequently caused by adenoviruses, rhinoviruses, coronaviruses, enteroviruses and parainfluenza viruses (see Fig. 24.1). Other viral infections, such as respiratory syncytial virus (RSV) and Epstein–Barr virus (EBV), are less common, but still frequently occur. Bacterial causes of upper respiratory infections are led by group A β-hemolytic streptococci (GAS), but can also be caused by *Haemophilus influenzae*, *Bordetella pertussis*, *Chlamydia pneumoniae*, *Corynebacterium haemolyticum*, *Mycoplasma pneumoniae* and *Yersinia enterocolitica* among others.

These upper respiratory infections are often difficult to differentiate, and hence difficult to diagnose, frequently leading to futile overtreatment in many cases. Further complicating the issue is the fact that primary viral infections are often succeeded by secondary 'opportunistic' bacterial infections, making under-treatment a problem in a significant minority of infections. Additionally, individuals with allergies or structural defects are sometimes more prone to secondary bacterial infections. The clinician is therefore challenged to weigh multiple factors involved in deciding whether an infection is viral or bacterial in origin, and whether antibiotic treatment is warranted.

It is estimated that children in day care in the USA have an upper respiratory infection approximately every 3 weeks from the age of 6 months to 2 years.[1] The incidence then decreases with the upshot that by the time of school entry a child has about 3–6 episodes of upper respiratory infection per year. Most of these infections include pharyngitis and/or laryngitis. Young children often have pharyngitis on inspection but do not complain of sore throat; this symptom is more common in adolescents and adults. Often the only sign of pharyngitis in young children is refusal to eat and/or drink.

Viral upper respiratory infections frequently occur in mini-epidemics (RSV, parainfluenza, influenza, varicella, measles). They are more common in the winter except for those caused by enteroviruses, which are more common in the summer.[2] Some viral infections occur year round, with no seasonal pattern (adenoviruses). Group A β-hemolytic streptococcal infections are more common in the winter, but many other nonviral respiratory infections do not appear to be seasonally linked (*Chlamydia* and *Mycoplasma* spp.). Some bacterial infections appear to be linked to preceding viral infections and hence occur more commonly in the winter. Pharyngeal colonization may occur throughout the year. Fortunately, epiglottitis is rare now that HIB immunization is routine for infants in many countries.

MORBIDITY, MORTALITY, HISTORIC CHANGE AND RISK FACTORS

Influenza infections vary significantly from year to year. In the USA one subtype was predominant each year until about 10 years ago, after which time both H3N2 and H1N1 strains have been circulating simultaneously. When there is a major shift in antigen type, significant excess morbidity occurs as the new strain infects the community. Increasing air travel has accelerated the rate at which the influenza viruses travel around the world and has perhaps been responsible for the increasing frequency with which the viruses are detected. The shifted strain outbreaks have most affected the elderly and children with congenital heart and lung disease. Minor influenza drifts have occurred also, but cause less disease. There has also been a recent decrease in the average age that children acquire upper respiratory diseases because of the increasing use of day care for children. The long-term effect of this is unknown. In the short term it appears that it has been responsible for a significant increase in the number of ear infections in children less than 2 years old.[3]

Rheumatic fever, a complication of group A β-hemolytic streptococcal pharyngitis, has waxed and waned in importance.[4] After a century of prominence, the disease was in considerable decline in developed countries for 40 years. Recently, clusters of cases of rheumatic fever have occurred, for example in Salt Lake City, Utah, USA, where it is hypothesized that the re-emergence of certain M-types have been responsible.

Before HIB vaccination was instituted there were approximately 20,000 cases of HIB disease each year in the USA. Since the advent of HIB immunization the incidence of this disease has decreased by 95%.

PATHOGENESIS AND PATHOLOGY

The pathogenesis of the sore throat due to pharyngitis is poorly understood. Volunteers given rhinoviral infections produce bradykinin and lysylbradykinin, which are known inflammatory mediators that can excite nerve endings in the pharynx to cause pain.[5] There is also suggestive evidence from laboratory animals that adenovirus, RSV and other viral infections directly invade the pharyngeal cells and produce an inflammatory response. This leads to the well described 'red, sore throat'. Additionally, adenovirus and EBV often produce lymphoid hyperplasia and tonsillar exudation. Herpes simplex virus (HSV) and coxsackievirus infections frequently lead to ulcerations of the oral mucosa. Herpes simplex virus ulcers are more common in the anterior part of the mouth and coxsackievirus ulcers occur more frequently in the posterior part of the pharynx, but this is only a guide and both viruses can cause ulcers in any part of the oropharynx.

Streptococcal pharyngitis often inflames the posterior pharynx, with petechiae on the uvula and soft palate.[6] When one sees this clinical sign, GAS are often isolated by throat culture. A confusing factor is that up to 10% of patients who have EBV infections will have a secondary group A β-hemolytic streptococcal pharyngitis during their illness. *Corynebacterium diphtheriae* can also cause pharyngitis, producing a characteristic gray membrane across the structures of the posterior pharynx. This is seldom seen today except in a few geographic areas where diphtheria outbreaks are currently occurring, such as Russia. There are also noninfectious causes of pharyngitis, such as Behçet's syndrome, Kawasaki's disease and Stevens–Johnson syndrome.

Laryngitis may be an isolated event, but more commonly is part of a more extensive upper respiratory infection. Young children with croup cannot inform us of the extent of their symptoms, and refusal to swallow and/or eat may be their only sign of difficulty. Adults with laryngitis often had croup as children and these two entities may be one and the same illness, the only difference being that the adult subglottic airway is larger and thus adults are less likely to develop stridor. Parainfluenza viruses are the most common cause of croup,[7] but adenoviruses, influenza and RSV also cause laryngitis/croup. Normally there is a mild coryza and sore throat followed by an inflammatory process of the larynx, trachea and subglottic area. There can be significant pain during

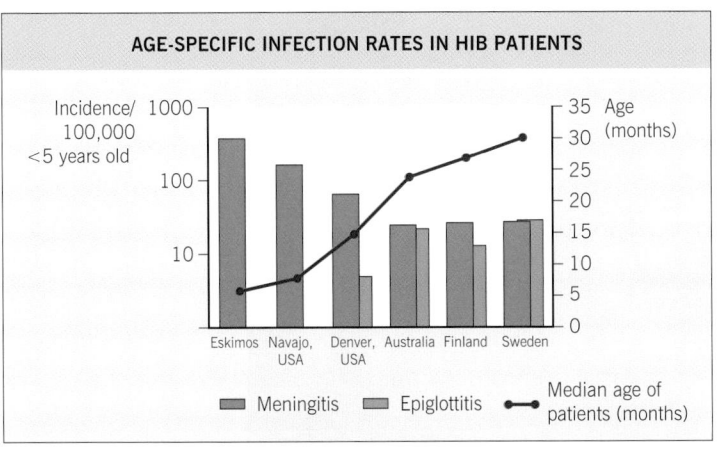

AGE-SPECIFIC INFECTION RATES IN HIB PATIENTS

Fig. 24.2 Incidence and median age of HIB disease. Disease type and geographic location per 100,000 children less than 5 years of age is shown.

coughing. The subglottic area swells, and because it is located in an area of the nondistensible cricoid cartilage, it can only swell into the airway. This gives the characteristic croupy cough and stridor in a child and laryngitis in an adult. It is of interest that croup is more pronounced after sunset and at night, when the child is lying down. During the daytime the symptoms are often markedly improved. Occasionally the distention into the airway progresses enough to cause airway compromise, and intubation is necessary. Fortunately, this is a rare event.

Epiglottitis is an acute cellulitis of the epiglottis and/or surrounding tissue that has the potential to cause complete obstruction of the airway. It is almost always caused by HIB. In Melbourne, Australia, HIB was isolated from 114 (93%) out of 123 blood cultures collected from epiglottitis patients, and no other pathogens were isolated.[8] The usual patient is 1–5 years old (Fig. 24.2) and onset is sudden, with sore throat and fever, with head forwardly extended, often with drooling. Respirations appear delicate, with little movement of the head. There may be a raspy sound when breathing. Fever may cause tachycardia. The mood of some affected children may seem dull or anxious. Visualization of the pharynx reveals a 'cherry red' epiglottis, but sometimes the epiglottis is less red than the surrounding peri-epiglottic structures or base of the tongue. Visualization of the epiglottis must be performed with care because respiratory arrest may occur if there is laryngeal spasm while probing the mouth.

PREVENTION

Preventing pharyngitis is desirable, but difficult to achieve. Viral pharyngitis is spread mostly by aerosolized oral secretions, hand-to-mouth contact with multiple individuals and the use of common utensils, glassware, etc. Certain viruses are known to be particularly resilient; RSV has been cultured from table tops hours after being

inoculated there.[9] Measles has been known to be contracted from the air in a physician's waiting room, as long as 1 hour after the child with measles had left the room. Other viruses may be less durable and less contagious, but close contact is obviously not necessary to transmit many of these agents. Prevention of disease depends mainly on good handwashing and preventing the spread of oral secretions. Masks and handkerchiefs inoculated with antiviral drugs have been used in experimental trials, but after several minutes of breathing, when the mask becomes wet, the benefit seems to diminish. There are vaccines available to prevent some of these diseases. Effective measles vaccines have been used for approximately 30 years, so the disease has decreased dramatically in most countries. Certain adenoviral vaccines have been used with some degree of success, mostly in military personnel. Vaccines for RSV and parainfluenza viruses are currently under development. These vaccines could have a significant effect on the population's health, particularly on that of the youngest children.

Transmission of streptococcal pharyngitis seems to require closer contact than for most viruses. Studies performed in the military during World War II showed that soldiers in barracks sleeping on either side of the index case were more likely to have disease than those further away.[10] To date there are no immunizations available to prevent streptococcal disease, although trials evaluating group B and group A vaccines are underway. For patients who have had prior group A disease and subsequent rheumatic fever, penicillin prophylaxis is recommended. Most patients receive intramuscular benzathine penicillin, 1.2 million units, once per month, although oral regimens are acceptable but have poorer compliance rates.

Vaccines against parainfluenza viruses would have the most impact on preventing laryngitis and croup. These are still experimental. The ability of influenza vaccine to prevent laryngitis has not been studied. To date, no other preventive measures against laryngitis are available.

In the only study to date seeking specific risk factors for epiglottitis, day care attendance was the strongest predictor for disease but the association was modified by whether the subject had had an upper respiratory illness in the previous 4 weeks.[11] There was also the suggestion that northern European ancestry was a risk factor as well. Fortunately, the incidence of epiglottitis (and meningitis) has decreased markedly since the advent of HIB vaccination. Whether the incidence of HIB disease in adults may change in the future is unknown, because long-term immunity from vaccination may prove to be either more or less effective than that due to natural infection.

CLINICAL FEATURES

PHARYNGITIS

Pharyngitis is a ubiquitous infection. A 'sore throat' affects most people at least once every year. Most cases of viral pharyngitis are associated with an upper respiratory infection (nasopharyngitis), as

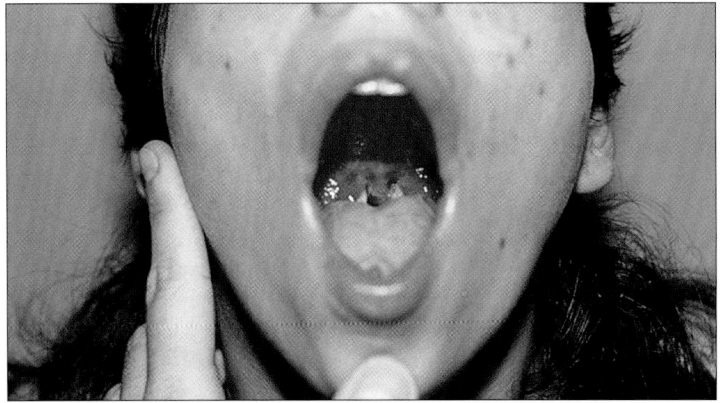

Fig. 24.3 Epstein–Barr virus (mononucleosis or glandular fever) pharyngitis.

Fig. 24.4 Adenoviral pharyngitis.

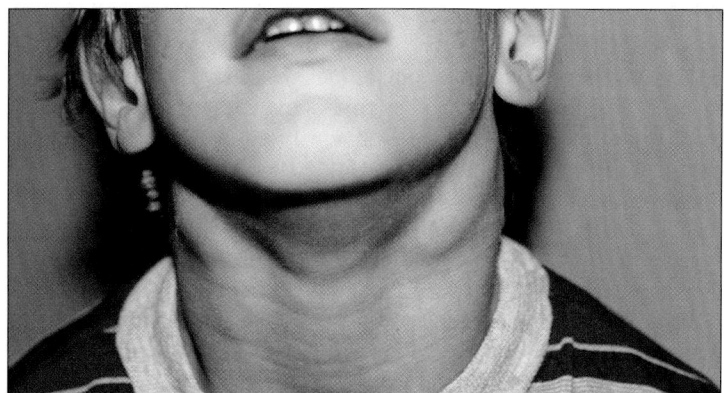

Fig. 24.5 Adenopathy associated with EBV.

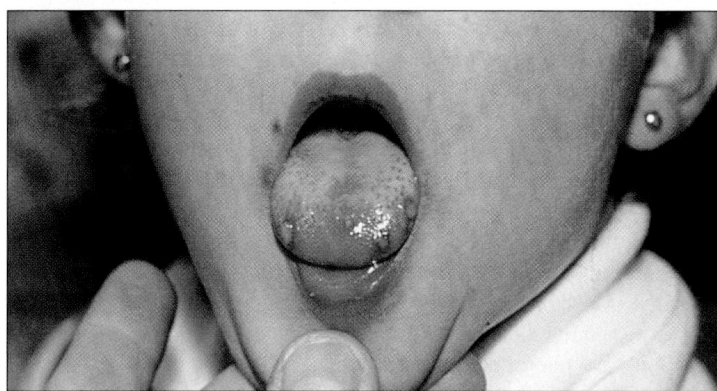

Fig. 24.6 Herpes simplex virus stomatitis.

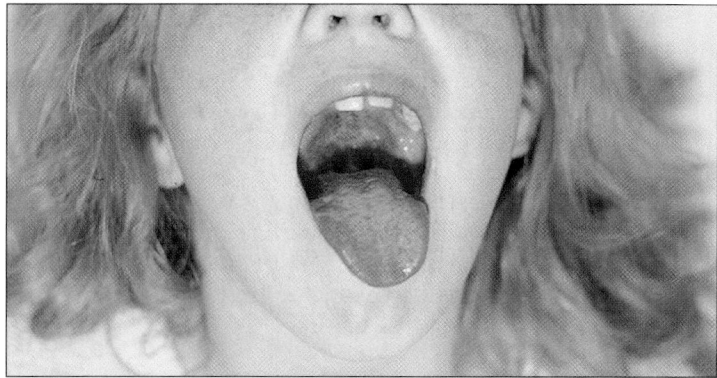

Fig. 24.7 Pharyngitis associated with GAS infection. Exudates are not always present.

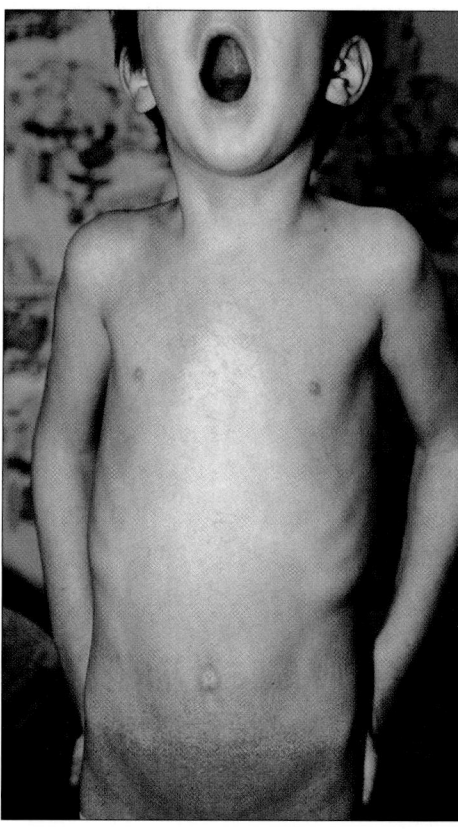

Fig. 24.8 Scarlet fever. Skin rash and pharyngitis associated with GAS infection.

shown in Figure 24.1. Generally nasopharyngitis has a prodrome that may include malaise, diaphoresis, fever, headache and general aches and/or pains. Coryza and sore throat then begin. Many infections will progess to produce a cough and/or laryngitis. Some viral infections produce predominantly coryza, others more pharyngitis, and others more cough or laryngitis. Coxsackieviruses often cause ulcers in the posterior pharynx along with a sore throat. Measles can cause a severe pharyngitis, but the associated symptoms of conjunctivitis, rash and Koplik spots make the disease easily diagnosable. Parainfluenza and influenza viruses can give a particularly painful pharyngitis, with frequently associated symptoms of cough and laryngitis.

The DNA viruses [EBV (Fig. 24.3), adenovirus (Fig. 24.4), cytomegalovirus and HSV] can produce significant pharyngitis. They also tend to last longer than the other viral causes of pharyngitis. These viruses produce other upper respiratory symptoms such as nontender cervical adenopathy (Fig. 24.5) or, in the case of HSV, tongue and mouth ulcers (Fig. 24.6). Herpes simplex virus pharyngitis has been described as a disease in which 'the gums swell-up and swallow the

teeth'. Rhinoviruses and RSV infections give upper respiratory symptoms as well as pharyngitis in infants. Respiratory syncytial virus also causes.

The syndrome of acute HIV infection ('seroconversion illness') is well described, and may cause symptoms in up to 50% of patients (see Chapter 5.8). It is a mononucleosis-like illness with pharyngitis being a prominent feature. Patients will also have fever, lymphandenopathy, rash and myalgias. The symptoms are nonspecific.

It is important to diagnose bacterial causes of pharyngitis because, unlike viral causes, many can be treated specifically with antibiotics. Proper treatment can avoid significant morbidity and/or mortality. Pharyngitis caused by GAS is the most common infection causing significant pharyngeal edema, frequently with petechiae on the soft palate and uvula (Fig. 24.7). Tender, cervical nodes are common. Small children may complain of abdominal pain, which may be due to mesenteric adenitis. Headache and raised temperature are also common. Some patients who have a streptococcal sore throat have a characteristic red 'scarlet fever' rash that begins in the groin and axillary areas and spreads over the body (Fig. 24.8). The rash is sandpaper-like, and may itch. A strawberry tongue is also often present. Other patients have a characteristic rash on the face (Fig. 24.9). Without treatment the illness usually resolves over 3 or 4 days, but rheumatic fever may ensue. The recommended treatment is penicillin, or erythromycin for those allergic to penicillin. Other β-hemolytic streptococcal infections (groups C, G and B) can cause pharyngitis but not rheumatic fever. For these, antibiotic treatment may provide symptomatic relief. Occasionally, pharyngitis can be secondary to an abscess in the peritonsillar area. This is usually easily diagnosed by an asymmetry of the tonsillar pillars. The affected side is asymetrically enlarged and protrudes anteriorly into the mouth.

Haemophilus influenzae (nontypable and types a–f) can cause pharyngitis, and type b can also cause epiglottitis or meningitis. The appearance of pharyngitis is nondiagnostic. Many individuals are carriers but are not ill. *Corynebacterium diphtheriae* causes diphtheria, which is easily diagnosed because of the gray pseudomembrane in the posterior pharynx along with pharyngitis. The disease has recently become endemic in parts of the former Soviet Union. *Arcanobacterium*

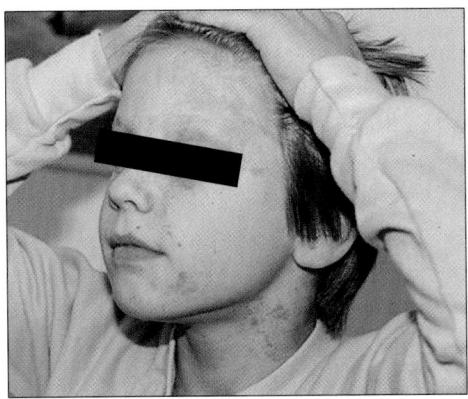

Fig. 24.9 Facial rash associated with GAS infection.

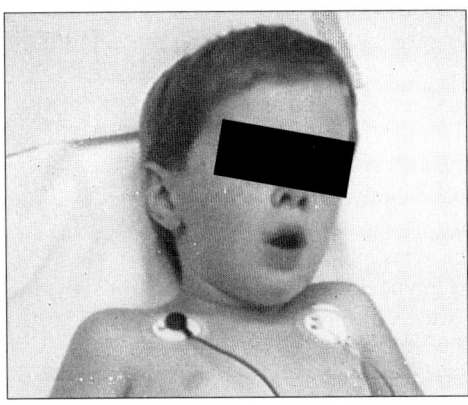

Fig. 24.10 Child with epiglottitis. Courtesy of Intensive Care Unit, Royal Children's Hospital.

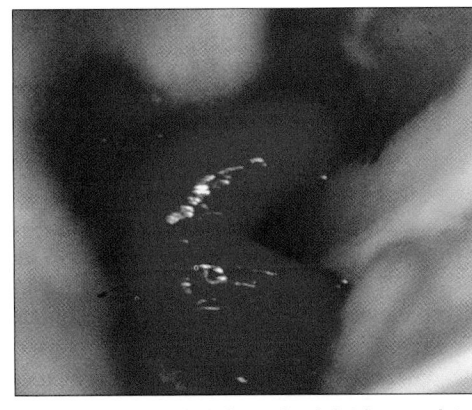

Fig. 24.11 Acutely inflamed epiglottis associated with HIB. The epiglottis protrudes upwards and is cherry red from the bottom of the figure. Courtesy of Intensive Care Unit, Royal Children's Hospital.

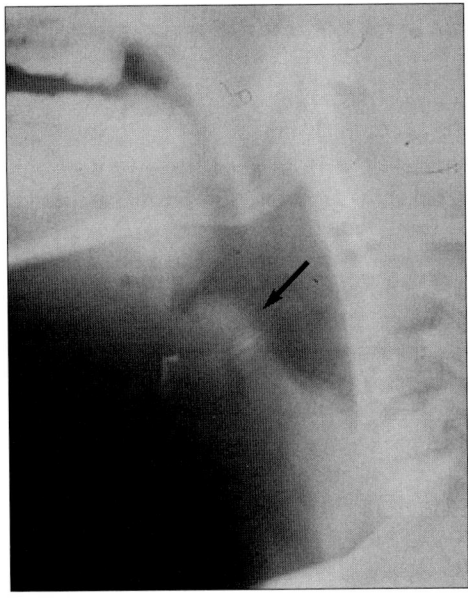

Fig. 24.12 Lateral neck radiograph of a child with acute epiglottitis demonstrating an enlarged hypopharynx due to forward neck extension and an enlarged 'thumb-shaped' epiglottis (arrow). Courtesy of Dr Donald Frush.

(previously *Corynebacterium*) *haemolyticum* is a common cause of pharyngitis and can also cause a scarlatiniform rash. It is the cause of many non-GAS throat infections.[12] *Neisseria gonorrhoeae* can also cause pharyngitis. The appearance of the pharyngitis is nondiagnostic, so a heightened awareness is required to make this diagnosis.[13]

Chlamydia pneumoniae and *Mycoplasma pneumoniae* can cause pharyngitis, but generally will go on to cause cough also, often with wheezing and pneumonia.[14,15] *Candida albicans* can cause pharyngitis but normally only in the immunocompromised host. The pharyngitis is hyperemic, with white plaques on the buccal mucosa.

Aphthous stomatitis is a common cause of mouth ulcers. The etiology is unclear. Small painful ulcers appear on the buccal mucosa, but can also appear in the posterior pharynx. The ulcers are usually stress related and last approximately 1 week. Very extensive aphthous ulceration can also be seen as a complication of HIV infection. Behçet's syndrome may cause pharyngitis. Kawasaki's disease, most common in children, can cause significant pharyngitis. Most children with Kawasaki's disease also have fever, a strawberry tongue and, importantly, conjunctivitis. This condition is frequently confused with streptococcal disease. Stevens–Johnson syndrome can result in pharyngitis, stomatitis and perioral swelling and ulcerations.

LARYNGITIS

Laryngitis is inflammation of the subglottic area and is generally of viral etiology although there is evidence that some individuals with *M. pneumoniae* infection can also develop hoarseness.[16] The most common cause of laryngitis and croup in infants is parainfluenza virus. The order of frequency is type 3>type 1>type 2. Because the infant airway is relatively narrower, croup with a 'barky' cough is much more common in infants. Older children, adolescents and adults tend to have laryngitis only. The hoarseness lasts from 2–5 days. A sore throat is common. Other common causes of laryngitis are influenza, RSV and adenovirus infections.

The feared complications of laryngitis are respiratory arrest, particularly in children with croup, and bacterial tracheitis in anyone with croup/laryngitis, particularly those that might have had recent trauma to the subglottic area.[17] Croup is worse at night and when lying down. Cool air and an upright posture are the treatments of choice. Temperature may be slightly elevated, but fever is not a characteristic of the disease. Bacterial tracheitis, when it occurs, is usually heralded by the sudden onset of fever and dyspnea.[18] The syndrome may be clinically indistinguishable from epiglottitis, except that the epiglottis is normal. The most common causes of the infection are *Staphylococcus aureus*, GAS and HIB. Immediate antibiotic treatment is indicated. Sometimes intubation is necessary.

EPIGLOTTITIS

Patients with epiglottitis often have an underlying illness, presumed to be viral. They then have sudden onset of fever, with the neck extended forward, drooling and air hunger. Affected children are anxious and lean forward to open their airway (Fig. 24.10). The diagnosis is easily made by viewing the epiglottitis, which is swollen and red (Fig. 24.11). Intubation is often required. *Haemophilus influenzae* type b is almost always obtained by culturing swabs from the epiglottis in children. In adults other pathogens may be obtained.[19] Some children have been discharged without intubation after receiving only one dose of ceftriaxone when the epiglottis did not appear reddened, but subsequent epiglottic and blood cultures have been positive for HIB. They were cured completely. The duration of hospital treatment averages 3 days. Intubation is needed for less than 24 hours in most cases.[20]

DIAGNOSIS

The most common treatable cause of pharyngitis is GAS infection. This can be diagnosed with a simple latex antigen test directly from a throat swab, but this procedure is not widely used outside North America. The latex test has a high specificity and an adequate sensitivity,[21] but bacterial culture is the gold standard. Group B, C and G streptococci can also cause significant morbidity, but only group A leads to rheumatic fever, so the reason for treatment is not only to eliminate the pharyngitis but also to prevent the subsequent rheumatic disease. Viral causes of pharyngitis do not normally require specific diagnosis, but serologic tests are available for mononucleosis (EBV) and cytomegalovirus. Adenoviruses, RSV and parainfluenza viruses can be diagnosed using rapid antigen tests, which are available but rarely used in uncomplicated community-acquired infections.

Laryngitis is not normally diagnosed by laboratory tests, and radiographs are of little use except to exclude foreign body aspiration or epiglottitis.

The white blood cell count in epiglottitis is often elevated, with an increase in the percentage of neutrophils and band forms. A culture of the epiglottis is usually positive for HIB but the result may not be available until the child is ready for discharge. Blood cultures are frequently positive for HIB in children, although there are usually fewer of these organisms per milliliter than in children with meningitis. Efforts to determine whether there are organism subtype differences that predispose to meningitis versus epiglottitis have been equivocal. In adults, the disease is reported to be caused principally by HIB, but pneumococci, *H. parainfluenzae* and streptococci are also reported. At the time of admission, if time permits, a radiogram of the lateral neck show may 'the thumb sign' (Fig. 24.12), demonstrating an enlarged epiglottis. Absence of such a finding does not eliminate epiglottitis as a diagnosis, but it provides reassurance that the pharynx can be visualized without threat of airway obstruction.

Visualization of the posterior pharynx is the best way to confirm the diagnosis of epiglottitis. Because airway obstruction is the most feared complication of this disease, this examination should be performed in a manner and place where immediate intubation can be performed if necessary.[20] At hospitals where the disease has been seen frequently it is common to give an inhaled anesthetic to allow a quick examination of the pharynx with an anesthesiologist, anesthetist or intensive care specialist standing by. Culture of the epiglottis should be performed by obtaining a swab during the examination.

MANAGEMENT

Antibiotic dosages are shown in Figure 24.13. For group A streptococcal pharyngitis the recommended therapy is 7–10 days of oral penicillin or amoxicillin. Erythromycin and clindamycin are acceptable alternatives. There have been studies showing that one dose of ceftriaxone intramuscularly or oral azithromycin for 5 days are equally effective at eliminating carriage of GAS, but recurrent pharyngeal colonization occurs with all treatment regimens. Viral causes of pharyngitis can be most suitably treated with supportive measures: gargles, lozenges, etc. *Mycoplasma* and *Chlamydia* spp. infections can be treated with erythromycin or tetracycline (depending on age). Diphtheria and *Arcanobacterium* spp. infection should be treated

ANTIBIOTIC DOSAGES FOR THE TREATMENT OF RESPIRATORY INFECTIONS			
Antibiotic	Dosage	Oral maximum dose	IV/IM maximum dose
Azithromycin	10mg/kg 1st day, 5mg/kg days 2–5	500mg	NA
Cefotaxime	100–200mg/kg/day im/iv, q6–8h	NA	12g/24h
Ceftriaxone	50–75mg/kg/day im/iv, q12–24h	NA	4g/24h
Clindamycin	20–40mg/kg/day, q6–8h	1.8g/24h	4.8g/24h
Doxycycline†	3–5mg/kg/day, q12h	300mg/24h	NA
Erythromycin	20–40mg/kg/day, q6–8h	2.4g/24h*	2.4g/24h*
Penicillin	penV-potassium 25–50mg/kg/day, q6h	500mg/dose	NA
Tetracycline†	25–50mg/kg/day, q6h	500mg/dose	NA

* Erythromycin base
† Preferable to use other antibiotics in children under age 8 because of tooth enamel staining

Fig. 24.13 Antibiotic dosages for the treatment of respiratory infections.

with erythromycin or penicillin. *Legionella* spp. infections should be treated with tetracycline. *Haemophilus influenzae* type b and *Yersinia enterocolitica* should be treated with a third-generation cephalosporin.

Causes of laryngitis are generally viral, therefore having no specific treatment. For supportive care, cool air and humidity often relieve some of the symptoms. Patients with bacterial superinfection (tracheitis) should be treated for presumed staphylococcal superinfections with nafcillin (flucloxacillin) or vancomycin, depending on whether the infection was acquired while in the hospital and therefore more likely to be methicillin-resistant.

Treatment of epiglottitis in children is with cefotaxime or ceftriaxone and immediate intubation if needed. Ampicillin should not be used due to the high frequency of ampicillin-resistant strains of HIB. Even if the airway is patent at the time of diagnosis, intubation is recommended because progression to airway obstruction is common until antibiotic therapy has begun. Most children can be successfully extubated after 24 hours of antibiotic therapy and some extubate themselves before that time has expired. Family members and day-care contacts should receive rifampin (rifampicin) prophylaxis (300mg q12h for 2 days) to avoid secondary infection.

REFERENCES

1. Loda FA, Glezen WP, Clyde WA Jr. Respiratory disease in group day care. Pediatrics 1972;49:428–37.
2. Denny FW. Acute respiratory infections in children: etiology and epidemiology. Pediatr Rev 1987;9:135–46.
3. Clements DA, Langdon ML, Bland CL, Walter EB. Influenza A vaccine decreases the incidence of otitis media in 6–30 month old day care children. Arch Pediatr Adolesc Med 1995;149:1113–7.
4. Denny FW, Wannamaker LW, Brink WR, Rammelkamp CH, Custer EA. Prevention of rheumatic fever. JAMA 1950;143:151–3.
5. Proud D, Reynolds CJ, Lacapra S, et al. Kinins are generated in nasal secretions during natural rhinovirus colds. J Infect Dis 1990;161:120–3.
6. Dyment PG, Klink LB, Jackson DW. Hoarseness and palatal petechiae as clue in indentifying streptococcal throat infections. Pediatrics 1968;41:822–3.
7. Downham MAPS, McQuillin J, Gardner PS. Diagnosis and clinical significance of parainfluenza virus infections in children. Arch Dis Child 1974;49:8–15.
8. Gilbert GL, Clements DA. *Haemophilus influenzae* type b infections in Victoria, Australia 1985–87. A population based study to determine the need for

9. immunization. Pediatr Infect Dis J 1990;9:252–7.
9. Hall CB, Douglas RG. Modes of transmission of respiratory syncytial virus. J Pediatr 1981;99:100–3.
10. Rammelkamp CH, Denny FW, Wannamaker LW. Studies on the epidemiology of rheumatic fever in the armed forces. In: Thomas L, ed. Rheumatic fever. Minneapolis: University of Minnesota Press; 1952:72–89.
11. Clements DA, Weigle, K, Guise I, Gilbert GL. A case–control study examining risk factors for invasive *Haemophilus influenzae* type b disease in Victoria, Australia 1988–90. J Paediatr Child Health 1995;31:513–8.
12. Miller RA, Brancato F, Holmes KK. *Corynebacterium hemolyticum* as a cause of pharyngitis and scarlatiniform rash in young adults. Ann Intern Med 1986;105:867–72.
13. Hutt DM, Judson FN. Epidemiology and treatment of oropharyngeal gonorrhea. Ann Intern Med 1986;104:655–8.
14. Grayston JT. Infections Caused by *Chlamydia pneumoniae* Strain TWAR. Clin Infect Dis 1992;15:757–63.

15. Denny FW, Clyde WA, Glezen WP. *Mycoplasma pneumoniae* disease: clinical spectrum, pathophysiology, epidemiology and control. J Infect Dis 1971;123:74–92.
16. Denny FW, Murphy TF, Clyde WA Jr, et al. Croup: an 11-year study in a pediatric practice. Pediatrics 1983;71:871–6.
17. Edwards KM, Dundon MC, Altemeier WA,. Bacterial tracheitis as a complication of viral croup. Pediatr Infect Dis 1983;2:390–1.
18. Dudin AA, Thalji A, Rambaud-Cousson A. Bacterial tracheitis among children hospitalized for severe obstructive dyspnea. Pediatr Infect Dis 1990;9:293–5.
19. MayoSmith MF, Hirsch PJ, Wodzinski SF, Schiffman FJ. Acute epiglottis in adults. N Engl J Med 1986;314:1133–9.
20. Butt W, Shann F, Walker C, et al. Acute epiglottitis: a different approach to management. Crit Care Med 1988;16:43–7.
21. Kellogg JA. Suitability of throat culture procedures for detection of group A streptococci and as reference standards for evaluation of streptococcal antigen detection kits. J Clin Microbiol 1990;28:165–9.

Otitis, Sinusitis and Related Conditions

Stephen I Pelton

OTITIS MEDIA

EPIDEMIOLOGY

Acute otitis media (AOM) is a common and frequently recurrent illness associated with upper respiratory tract infection. It has been diagnosed more frequently over the past decade. Although many risk factors such as male sex, bottle feeding, an 'immature' immune system and familial predisposition have been associated with an increased incidence,[1] the change in child rearing patterns resulting in early entry into the day care setting has been considered to be the critical factor in the increased incidence of acute otitis media.[2] This hypothesis has been supported by an observed two- to three-fold increase in AOM among children in day care compared with home care.

A pattern of AOM in a prospective study of children followed from birth through 7 years of age has been described.[3] The peak incidence of disease was in the second 6 months of life. Almost two-thirds of children had at least one episode by the age of 1 year, and age at first episode was highly predictive for recurrent otitis media. Three or more episodes was relatively common during the first 4 years of life but became unusual by year 6 or 7.

PATHOGENESIS

Evidence suggests that host factors as well as infectious agents contribute significantly to the occurrence of AOM (Fig. 25.1). Two well-established host factors are eustachian tube dysfunction and immunologic abnormalities.[4,5] Otitis media is nearly universal in children with cleft palate and the associated functional eustachian tube obstruction. In other children, reflux of nasopharyngeal secretions (and presumably bacterial pathogens) into the middle ear has been demonstrated. Children who have immunologic deficiencies (especially hypogammaglobulinemia) suffer recurrent mucosal surface infections including otitis media. More recently, recurrent otitis has been reported in children who have IgG subclass deficiency, IgA deficiency and HIV disease.[6,7] Finally, passive immunization with antibacterial polysaccharide immunoglobulins has been demonstrated to reduce the incidence of type specific pneumococcal otitis media.[8] These studies suggest that children who have humoral immune deficiencies are more susceptible to AOM. Respiratory viral pathogens also appear to be important in the pathogenesis of AOM, most often as a cofactor rather than as a direct invader. During seasonal respiratory syncytial virus outbreaks, the incidence of AOM increases significantly.[9]

PREVENTION

Strategies for the prevention of acute and recurrent otitis media have focused on reducing disease caused by specific bacterial pathogens or on immunoprophylaxis against respiratory viral infection. Studies of pneumococcal polysaccharide vaccine in the early 1980s demonstrated that immunization with an octavalent or 14-valent pneumococcal polysaccharide resulted in a reduction in disease caused by serotypes that

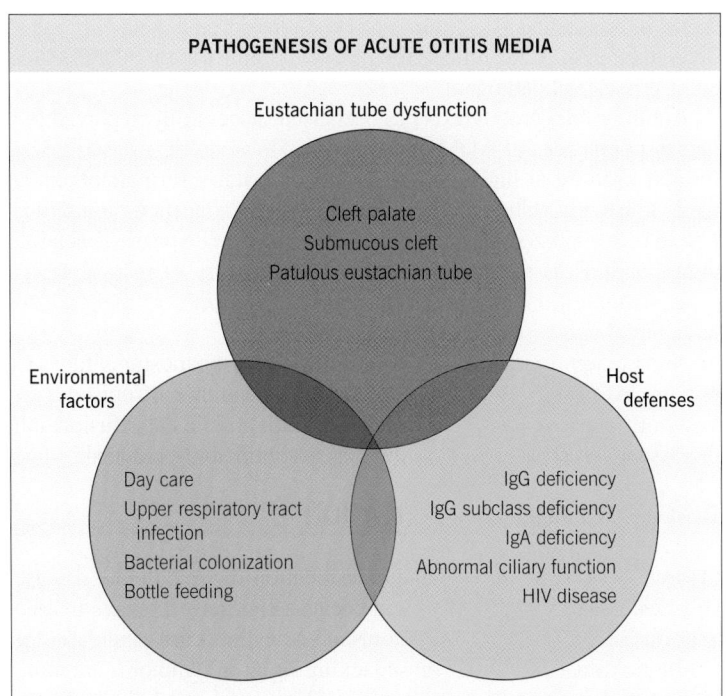

Fig. 25.1 Pathogenesis of acute otitis media.

were associated with a good serum antibody response.[10,11] Unfortunately, no reduction was observed in children less than 7 months of age, and in one of the studies the effect was limited to the first 6 months after immunization.

Recently, studies of passive immunoprophylaxis with bacterial polysaccharide immunoglobulin both in experimental animals and in infants has confirmed that high serum levels of antibodies to bacterial surface antigens are sufficient to provide protection against acute middle ear infection.[7,12,13] This has been demonstrated in experimental models for disease caused both by nontypable *Haemophilus influenzae* and *Strep. pneumoniae*, and in clinical trials for disease due to *Strep. pneumoniae*.

New formulations of pneumococcal polysaccharide conjugated to protein haptens (pneumococcal conjugate vaccine) have demonstrated enhanced immunogenicity in children immunized at 2, 4 and 6 months of age, protection against serotype-specific invasive disease and a modest effect on nasophayngeal carriage of *Strep. pneumoniae*.[14–16] These preliminary results hold promise that pneumococcal conjugate vaccine will be more effective than the polysaccharide vaccine for prevention of otitis media and sinusitis. Current recommendations for the use of pneumococcal vaccine for prevention of otitis media target high-risk children such as those undergoing myringotomy and tympanostomy tube placement who are older than 2 years of age.

Prevention of AOM through immunoprophylaxis against respiratory virus infection has been demonstrated using influenza vaccine.[17,18] A reduction in cases of influenza virus A infection as well as a 36% decline in otitis media was observed in a day care center during a community outbreak of influenza.

Respiratory syncytial virus is the viral pathogen most closely associated with AOM. Considerable progress has been made in the immunoprophylaxis of RSV disease, and two approaches have been shown to be effective.[19,20] First, the use of immunoglobulin with high titers of neutralizing antibody against RSV, has been shown to reduce a proprietary incidence and severity of lower respiratory tract disease due to RSV. It has also been shown to reduce the frequency of AOM from 0.78 episodes per child to 0.15 episodes. These studies did not permit discrimination between the anti-RSV effect and a nonspecific effect of passive administration of immunoglobulin with antibody directed against a spectrum of pathogens. Most recently, studies of an RSV monoclonal antibody demonstrated protection against lower respiratory disease caused by RSV but failed to diminish episodes of AOM in recipients. This finding has been interpreted as showing that the reduction in AOM reflects the passive administration of antibodies against bacterial pathogens.

Antimicrobial prophylaxis has been used successfully in preventing recurrent episodes of AOM and sinusitis. However, its use should be limited to those at high risk.[21,22] Selection criteria for patients most likely to benefit include multiple episodes within a recent 6-month time period or recognized immunologic defects that predispose to bacterial complications of respiratory infection and history of recurrent disease. Amoxicillin (20mg/kg/day) and sulfisoxazole (500mg q12h) have both been used successfully.

Another approach has been the insertion of tympanostomy tubes to prevent AOM.[23] Although the reduction in number of episodes of acute otitis has been limited, time spent with middle ear effusion and the associated conductive hearing loss is significantly reduced.

DIAGNOSIS AND CLASSIFICATION

Optimal diagnostic criteria and classification for middle ear disease (Fig. 25.2) are critically important because children who have middle ear effusion and signs and symptoms of acute illness are candidates for antibiotic therapy, whereas those lacking signs or symptoms are more likely to suffer from otitis media with effusion and are unlikely to benefit significantly from antimicrobial therapy.

The hallmark of middle ear disease is the presence of middle ear effusion or otorrhea. Therefore, pneumatic otoscopy has become the diagnostic method of choice. The pneumatic otoscope permits visualization of the tympanic membrane as well as assessment of its mobility. The healthy tympanic membrane moves briskly inward when pressure is applied to the attached rubber bulb and it returns with the release of the bulb pressure. When middle ear effusion is present, the tympanic membrane has reduced or absent mobility on both positive and negative pressure. When AOM is present, the tympanic membrane usually has signs of inflammation (erythema, diminished translucency, loss of light reflex) and the child has localized clinical manifestations (earache or tenderness) or systemic manifestations (e.g. fever, irritability, vomiting). It is important to distinguish AOM from otitis media with effusion because antimicrobial therapy is not considered effective against otitis media with effusion.

Acute otitis media with otorrhea must be distinguished from external otitis media. The history of relief from earache when drainage begins and the presence of a perforation of the tympanic membrane helps to distinguish these two diagnoses. The pain in external otitis usually continues to increase even after drainage begins, and the canal is frequently swollen so that its diameter is significantly reduced.

Chronic suppurative otitis media without cholesteatoma is a condition with persistent drainage and chronic perforation, with or without a myringotomy tube, lasting for longer than 6 weeks. The disease usually occurs in particular populations such as the Inuit, native Americans, Australian Aborigines, young infants and children who have immunodeficiency, or postmyringotomy and tube insertion. The pathogenesis and treatment for chronic suppurative otitis media is very different from that of AOM.

MICROBIOLOGY

The pathogens isolated in AOM as defined by aspiration and culture of middle ear fluid are most frequently *Strep. pneumoniae*, *H. influenzae*, *Moraxella catarrhalis* and group A streptococci. The relative frequency of each pathogen varies throughout the world (Fig. 25.3).[24] A higher frequency of infection with group A streptococci is observed in Europe than in the USA, specifically in children older than 2 years of age. An increased proportion of cases due to *M. catarrhalis* has recently been reported from Finland, mainly in infants less than 2 years of age.[25] *Haemophilus influenzae* has been demonstrated as an important pathogen in all age groups, including adults.[26]

Viruses, *Mycoplasma* spp., *Chlamydia* spp. and less common bacterial pathogens have on occasion been identified as etiologic agents in AOM. Recent studies have identified viral antigens or viruses in some children who have AOM, most frequently in combination with bacterial pathogens. Respiratory syncytial virus has been found most commonly,[27] but influenza virus, enteroviruses and rhinoviruses have also been reported. Polymerase chain reaction technologies have identified RNA from *Chlamydia pneumoniae* in middle ear fluid from children who have AOM and otitis media with effusion.[28] *Mycoplasma pneumoniae* has been cultured from one case and has been proposed as the etiology of AOM associated with bullous myringitis in patients who have concomitant pneumonia.[29]

Less common bacterial pathogens include *Staphylococcus aureus* and *Pseudomonas aeruginosa*. Both of these are frequently found in children who have chronic suppurative otitis media but they have only

	CLASSIFICATION OF OTITIS MEDIA		
Diagnosis	Middle ear effusion or otorrhea	Inflammation of tympanic membrane	Symptoms
Acute otitis media	Effusion	Erythema	Fever, irritability, vomiting, ear ache
Otitis media with effusion	Effusion	Usually absent, may be opaque	Asymptomatic, may have difficulty sleeping
Chronic suppurative otitis media	Otorrhea	Perforated	Frequently painless, diminished hearing

Fig. 25.2 Classification of otitis media.

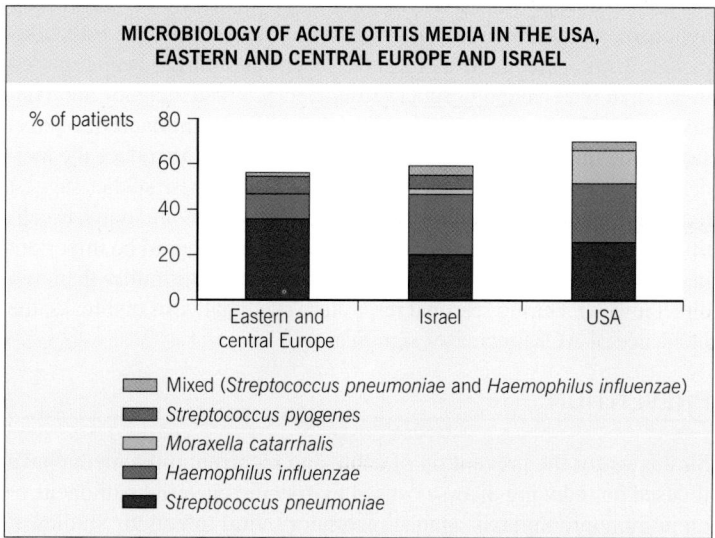

Fig. 25.3 Microbiology of acute otitis media in the USA, eastern and central Europe and Israel. Culture results of middle ear aspirates from children. Adapted from Jacobs *et al.*, 1995.[24]

occasionally have been isolated from children with intact tympanic membranes. *Mycobacterium tuberculosis* and *Pneumocystis carinii* have been isolated from the middle ear in unusual cases of otitis media.[30]

Otitis media in the first 6 weeks of life warrants special consideration. Although most children will have the usual respiratory pathogens (*Strep. pneumoniae, H. influenzae* and *M. catarrhalis*), enteric bacteria have been identified in 15% of cases and *Staph. aureus* in 10% of cases (Fig. 25.4).[31] Thus neonates, especially those less than 2–3 weeks of age, require a different management strategy with careful evaluation, parenteral administration of broad-spectrum antimicrobial agents and close observation.

EFFECT OF ANTIMICROBIAL THERAPY ON THE OUTCOME OF ACUTE OTITIS MEDIA

The rapid increase in isolates of *Strep. pneumoniae* with reduced susceptibility to penicillin and a recognition of the dramatic rise in antibiotic

MICROBIOLOGY OF OTITIS MEDIA IN THE FIRST 6 WEEKS OF LIFE	
Respiratory Pathogens	49.7%
Streptococcus pneumoniae	18.3%
Haemophilus influenzae	12.4%
Streptococcus pneumoniae and *Haemophilus influenzae*	3.0%
Staphylococcus aureus	7.7%
Streptococci group A or group B	3.0%
Moraxella catarrhalis	5.3%
Enteric Pathogens	18.3%
Escherichia coli	5.9%
Klebsiella spp. and *Enterobacter* spp.	5.3%
Pseudomonas aeruginosa	1.8%
Other	5.3%
No Pathogens Recovered	32.0%

Fig. 25.4 Microbiology of otitis media in the first 6 weeks of life.
Microbiology in 169 infants less than 6 weeks of age who have acute otitis media. Data from Shurin.[31]

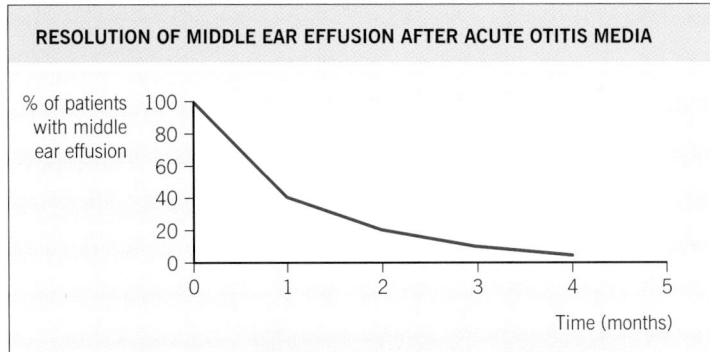

Fig. 25.5 Resolution of middle ear effusion after acute otitis media.
Adapted from Klein *et al.*, 1992.[1]

VARIABILITY IN REPORTED INCIDENCE OF SINUS DISEASE IN PEDIATRIC PRACTICE		
	Cases per month	
Clinical diagnosis	Mean	Range
Acute sinusitis	18	1–200
Recurrent sinusitis	13	4–100
Chronic sinusitis	7.5	1–40

Fig. 25.6 Variability in reported incidence of sinus disease in pediatric practice.

prescriptions written each year for otitis media has resulted in a renewed evaluation of the role of antibiotics in the treatment of AOM. Studies comparing antibiotic and control-treated children who have AOM, historic reflection on the frequency of suppurative complications of AOM, and limited data from isolated areas where antibiotic therapy is often initially deferred for the diagnosis of AOM have provided evidence that antimicrobial treatment is associated with a shorter duration of local and systemic signs and symptoms such as fever, irritability and earache.[32,33] The use of antibiotics for AOM has also been associated with a reduction in acute suppurative mastoiditis over the past three decades and is further supported by recent reports of a rising incidence of mastoiditis associated with the withholding of initial antimicrobial therapy in children who have AOM.[34] Outcome measures such as resolution of signs and symptoms at 2 weeks after diagnosis, presence of middle-ear fluid at 4–6 weeks and frequency of recurrent infection appear to be unrelated to initial antibiotic therapy. In most studies, middle ear effusion is found in up to 40% of children 1 month after an episode AOM; this gradually resolves over several months in most children (Fig. 25.5).

Studies comparing antibiotic-treated children with untreated controls demonstrate that age is a critical feature in identifying the patients that are most likely to benefit from antimicrobial therapy.[35] Children under 3 years of age are at highest risk of having persistence of signs and symptoms and suppurative complications if untreated, whereas children over 3 years of age are likely to have resolution of their signs and symptoms without complications even if not treated with antibiotics.

COMPLICATIONS

Mastoiditis is an uncommon complication of AOM that is seen predominantly in children under 2 years of age. The children are usually acutely ill with toxicity and localized pain and tenderness over the mastoid process. Bulging of the external ear secondary to subperiosteal abscess or inflammation or paralysis of the facial nerve are classic manifestations. Partially treated (subacute) mastoiditis may manifest itself as persistent fever, tenderness of the mastoid process and otorrhea. In contrast to uncomplicated AOM, the bacterial pathogens of mastoiditis are more virulent. Group A streptococci and *Strep. pneumoniae* are the two most common. *Haemophilus influenzae* type b was seen frequently before universal immunization, and it should be considered in children who have not been adequately vaccinated. *Staphylococcus aureus* and Gram-negative enteric bacteria have been identified in patients who have subacute mastoiditis.

Therapy for acute mastoiditis is parenteral antibiotics with close observation for the development of possible complications such as intracranial abscess, venous sinus thrombosis, osteomyelitis or hydrocephaly. Myringotomy is necessary if facial nerve palsy is present. Prolonged therapy for 2–4 weeks is generally required.

SINUSITIS

EPIDEMIOLOGY

SINUSITIS IN CHILDREN
The recognition and diagnosis of sinus disease in children remains difficult. The signs and symptoms frequently lack specificity and overlap with nasal allergy or airway obstruction. Physicians often have divergent views on what criteria are sufficient to warrant intervention. There is a wide variance in the monthly incidence of acute and chronic sinusitis reported by pediatric practitioners.[36] Figure 25.6 summarizes the mean number of episodes and range reported by different physicians. The wide disparity and incidence probably reflects differences in diagnostic criteria rather than true differences in incidence.

CLINICAL FEATURES

The presentation of acute sinusitis changes with increasing age. In young children persistent rhinorrhea (which is often purulent), daytime and night-time cough, foul breath and, less commonly, fever are the hallmarks of sinus disease. Less frequently, high fever, purulent rhinorrhea and facial tenderness or swelling signal the likely presence of acute sinusitis (Fig. 25.7). The overlap between uncomplicated upper respiratory tract infection and sinusitis is large. Most children who have signs and symptoms of less than 7 days duration have uncomplicated upper respiratory tract infection. Concern for sinusitis is appropriate when signs and symptoms persist beyond 7–10 days or when localized signs are present.

In older children and adults, symptoms and signs are more localized. Frontal headache, facial pain or pressure, and nasal congestion are frequent complaints. Facial tenderness or swelling over the maxillary or frontal sinus may be present. Nasal congestion, or even obstruction, is almost universally present except when sinus disease is of dental origin.

In chronic sinusitis, cough is especially prominent. The cough is usually present throughout the day, and it occasionally precipitates post-tussive emesis, especially soon after awakening. Chronic headache may also be part of the typical cluster of symptoms reported by patients. The pain is often dull; it often radiates to the top of the head or it may be bitemporal in nature. Nasal congestion and mucopurulent or purulent nasal discharge often complete the cluster of signs.

DIAGNOSIS

Defining the microbiology of paranasal sinus disease requires sampling sinus secretions without contamination from normal respiratory flora. Sampling involves a transnasal approach and attempted sterilization of the area through which the trocar will be passed. Because complete sterilization is usually impossible, investigators have frequently used a colony count of $\geq 10^4$ cfu/ml to define infection.

Wald et al. have contributed greatly to our understanding of the microbial pathogenesis.[37] Streptococcus pneumoniae is the most frequent pathogen isolated from children who have acute sinusitis (Fig. 25.8). Other pathogens are bacterial species commonly found as part of the normal respiratory flora; these include nontypable H. influenzae, M. catarrhalis and group A streptococci.

Two distinct clinical settings require special knowledge, because the bacterial pathogens are likely to differ from there in patients who have concomitant upper respiratory tract infection. The microbiology of sinusitis in the intensive care unit includes Staph. aureus, P. aeruginosa and other Gram-negative enteric bacteria. In addition, anaerobes and yeasts are frequently isolated in combination with aerobes. In this setting, sinusitis is recognized as a cause of cryptogenic fever or in association with fulminant sepsis. Disease in this setting requires sinus aspiration to identify the specific pathogen. Initial antimicrobial therapy should be directed against nosocomial pathogens and then modified once the specific bacterial etiology has been identified.

A foul-smelling discharge and a recent history of dental pain or a dental procedure should suggest an odontogenic etiology for sinus disease. Bacterial pathogens from the oropharynx invade devitalized tissue in the gingiva and spread to the sinus. Mixed anaerobic infection with Bacteroides spp. and anaerobic streptococci are commonly identified. Antimicrobial therapy, in combination with debridement or drainage of devitalized tissue or periapical abscess, is usually necessary.

IMAGING

Sinus radiographs must be interpreted with the knowledge that at birth and through early childhood only the maxillary and ethmoid sinuses are

aerated. The frontal sinuses do not appear routinely until the age of 5–7 years and may be further delayed in some patients. Sinus opacification without clinical signs or symptoms of sinus disease has been seen in some young infants undergoing radiologic studies for alternative diagnoses such as head trauma. One study reported 60% incidence of sinus opacification in normal children under 1 year of age.[38] These observations limit the usefulness of routine sinus radiographs in the first year of life and demand that radiographic interpretations should be performed with consideration of clinical parameters.

Opacification (especially when asymmetric), mucosal swelling or air–fluid levels are all potential abnormalities in patients who have sinus infection (Fig. 25.9).

Computed tomography and MRI provide anatomic detail of the sinuses. These techniques are especially revealing when complications or extension of disease are suspected. Specific examples and indications are discussed in the section on complications (page 25.5).

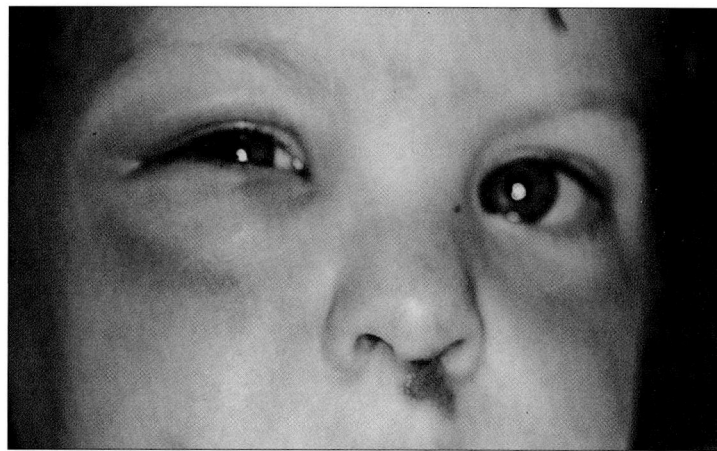

Fig. 25.7 Acute sinusitis with facial swelling and periorbital edema.

BACTERIAL SPECIES CULTURED FROM SINUS ASPIRATES PERFORMED IN CHILDREN			
Bacterial species	Single isolate	Mixed culture	Total (%)
Streptococcus pneumoniae	14	8	22 (37.9)
Moraxella catarrhalis	13	2	15 (25.9)
Haemophilus influenzae	10	5	15 (25.9)
Streptococcus spp.	2	3	5 (8.6)
Eikenella corrodens	1	0	1 (1.7)

Fig. 25.8 Bacterial species cultured from sinus aspirates performed in children. Data from Wald et al.[37]

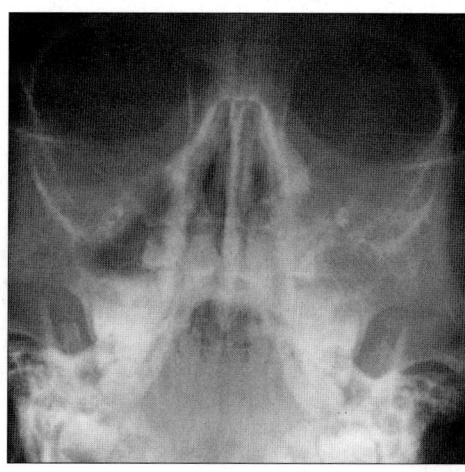

Fig. 25.9 Left maxillary sinusitis.

COMPLICATIONS

The course of untreated sinus disease and response to therapy in non-toxic children has been evaluated in placebo-controlled trials.[39] In these trials, half of the children have persistent or worsening signs or symptoms 3 days after diagnosis, and 40% are considered 'failures to improve' 10 days after diagnosis.

In comparison with children treated with antimicrobial agents such as amoxicillin or amoxicillin–clavulanate, the placebo-treated children are less likely to have a rapid resolution within 3 days of their signs and

NATURAL HISTORY OF ACUTE PARANASAL SINUSITIS IN 35 CHILDREN		
	Number (%)	
Outcome	Day 3	Day 10
Cure	4 (11)	15 (43)
Improvement	14 (40)	6 (17)
No change	11 (32)	0
Failure (worsening or persistence of symptoms)	6 (17)	14 (40)

Fig. 25.10 Outcome of placebo- versus antibiotic-treated children who had acute paranasal sinusitis. Data from Wald et al.[39]

CLASSIFICATION OF ORBITAL CELLULITIS		
Group	Classification	Descriptions
I	Preseptal	Erythema and edema of eyelids, normal vision and full range of motion
II	Orbital cellulitis without abscess	Diffuse edema (of orbit) but no abscess
III	Orbital cellulitis with subperiosteal abscess	Abscess adjacent to lamina papyracea; clinically there is proptosis, changes in vision and possibly pain on movement of the eye
IV	Orbital cellulitis with abscess in the orbital fat	Proptosis, limited motility of globe, loss of vision
V	Cavernous sinus thrombosis	Bilateral disease

Fig. 25.11 Classification of orbital cellulitis. Data from Chandler et al.[40]

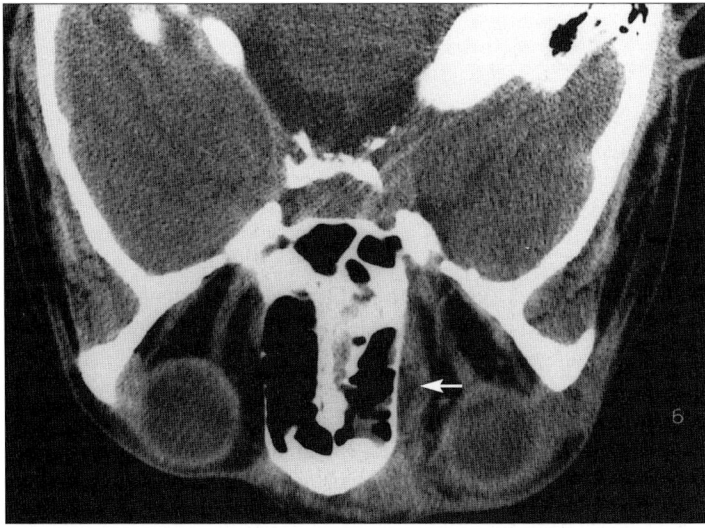

Fig. 25.12 Computed tomography scan of a patient who has right subperiosteal abscess (arrow) adjacent to the lamina papyracea. Note the partial opacification in the right ethmoid sinus.

symptoms and are also less likely to ultimately achieve complete cure by day 10 (Fig. 25.10).[39] However, if end points beyond 10 days are selected, many investigators have been unable to demonstrate any beneficial effect of antimicrobial agents on the outcome of sinus disease.

The complications of sinus disease frequently cause substantial morbidity and may require surgical intervention. The most common complications of sinusitis arise primarily from bacterial spread to the orbit, frontal bone or central nervous system. Extension of infection is usually direct through a complex network of venous channels and not the result of hematogenous spread. Occasionally, hematogenous dissemination will produce bacterial complications at distant sites.

Orbital cellulitis is the most common serious complication of sinusitis and is most frequently associated with ethmoiditis. The clinical manifestations represent a spectrum of severity and they often predict the response to antibiotic therapy or the need for surgical drainage. A widely accepted classification system is that proposed by Chandler (Fig. 25.11).[40] Proptosis, motility of the globe and visual acuity are the key features that differentiate the various spectra of diseases. A Marcus–Gunn pupil in the swinging flashlight test (pupillary dilatation when the light is moved from the normal eye to the affected eye) is diagnostic of optic nerve compression and a hallmark of advanced disease. Even with this classification scheme, it is often very difficult to distinguish cases that require surgical intervention from those that will respond to medical management. Computed tomography scans should be performed if the patient has ophthalmoplegia or visual loss or if the patient is not responding to treatment. Differentiating 'inflammatory phlegmon' from abscess may still be difficult (Fig. 25.12).

Medical management requires a team approach and involves the pediatric infectious disease specialist, the otolaryngologist and the ophthalmologist. Initial therapy is directed against likely pathogens. A history of trauma or facial cellulitis can be helpful in predicting whether *Staph. aureus* is likely, whereas previous or concomitant sinusitis suggests *Strep. pneumoniae*, *H. influenzae*, group A streptococci or *M. catarrhalis*. However, the severity of illness and potential for complications mandate broad-spectrum parental therapy such as ceftriaxone, cefotaxime, amoxicillin–clavulanate or clindamycin in combination with aztreonam or chloramphenicol. The need for surgical intervention varies, and the decision is based on the response to antimicrobial therapy, visual acuity and motility, and the results of CT scanning. Drainage of the involved sinus may also be necessary for rapid healing.

Intracranial complications from sinusitis are most common in adolescents and adults.[41] Brain abscess in the frontal lobe or subdural abscess are most frequent. These complications are often difficult to diagnose clinically and may present without signs or symptoms of increased intracranial pressure or toxicity. Fever, signs of meningeal irritation without toxicity, and focal neurologic abnormalities are the hallmarks. Less specific signs and symptoms include headache, behavioral changes and seizures. Currently, the diagnosis is best made by CT scan with contrast. Magnetic resonance imaging may be more sensitive for detection of small abscesses and cerebritis and for differentiation of epidural from subdural abscesses.

The mucosa of the frontal sinus and the marrow of the frontal bone have a common venous drainage. Thus, bacterial invasion of the marrow and subsequent osteomyelitis (Pott's puffy tumor) are recognized complications of frontal sinusitis. This entity was first described clinically by Sir Percival Pott in 1795, but it was not until 1879 that Lamel Oryne defined its pathology. Computed tomography scanning is useful for defining the extent of frontal bone involvement and whether intracranial extension has occurred.

THERAPY FOR ACUTE OTITIS MEDIA AND ACUTE SINUSITIS

The goal of antibiotic therapy is sterilization of the middle ear. Eradication of the bacterial pathogen in the middle ear is highly correlated with a successful clinical response.[42] Antibiotics should be

ANTIMICROBIAL AGENTS COMMONLY USED IN THE THERAPY OF ACUTE OTITIS MEDIA

Drug	Pediatric dosage	Penicillin-sensitive *Streptococcus pneumoniae*	Beta-lactamase-producing *Haemophilus influenzae*	Advantages and concerns
Amoxicillin	13.3mg/kg per dose q8h; maximum dose 500mg q8h	++++	–	1. Low cost, well tolerated 2. Emerging high-level (MIC≥2.0μg/ml) resistance among *Streptococcus pneumoniae* isolates
Amoxicillin–clavulanate	15mg/kg amoxicillin per dose with 2.4mg/kg clavulanic acid q8h; maximum dose 875mg q12h	++++	+++	1. Broad spectrum 2. Frequent diarrhea 3. Emerging high-level (MIC≥2.0μg/ml) resistance among *Streptococcus pneumoniae* isolates
Cefaclor	20mg/kg per dose q12h; maximum dose 1g/day	++	+	1. Infrequent occurrence of serum sickness 2. Limited activity against penicillin-intermediate (MIC 0.12–1.0mg/ml) and highly resistant isolates
Cefdinir	7mg/kg per dose q12h or 14mg/kg per dose q24h	+++	+++	1. Limited activity against resistant *Streptococcus pneumoniae* (MIC≥2.0mg/ml) 2. Diarrhea
Cefixime	4mg/kg per dose q12h or 8mg/kg per dose q24h; maximum dose 400mg q24h	++	++++	1. Limited activity against penicillin-intermediate (MIC 0.12–1.0mg/ml) and highly resistant isolates 2. Potent activity against beta-lactamase-producing *Haemophilus influenzae* 3. High cost
Cefprozil	15mg/kg per dose q12h; maximum dose 1g q24h	++++	+	1. High cost 2. Active against penicillin-intermediate *Streptococcus pneumoniae* 3. Less active against *Haemophilus influenzae*
Ceftibuten	9mg/kg per dose q24h; maximum dose 400mg q24h	+	+++	1. Not approved for acute otitis media caused by *Streptococcus pneumoniae* 2. High cost
Ceftriaxone	50mg/kg/dose im	+++	++++	1. Parenteral administration 2. Multiple doses required for resistant *Streptococcus pneumoniae*
Cefuroxime axetil	15mg/kg per dose q12h; maximum dose 1g/day	++++	++	1. Significant after taste 2. Active against penicillin-intermediate *Streptococcus pneumoniae* 3. High cost
Cefpodoxime	5mg/kg per dose q12h or 10mg/kg per dose q24h; maximum dose 400mg q24h	++++	++++	1. Significant after taste 2. Active against penicillin-intermediate *Streptococcus pneumoniae* 3. High cost
Erythromycin sulfisoxazole liquid	12.5–16.6mg/kg erythromycin with 42.5–50mg/kg sulfisoxizole per dose q6h or q8h; maximum dose 2g erythromycin per day	++++	+++	1. Low cost 2. Gastric distress frequent 3. Four times daily dosing 4. Emerging macrolide resistantance reported among *Streptococcus pneumoniae* with increasing use
Loracarbef	15mg/kg per dose q12h; maximum dose 800mg/day	+++	+	Limited activity against penicillin-intermediate *Streptococcus pneumoniae*
Trimethoprim–sulfamethoxazole (co-trimoxazole)	4mg/kg trimethoprim with 20mg/kg sulfamethoxazole per dose q12h	++++	++++	1. In-vitro resistance among *Streptococcus pneumoniae* reported at 20–50% 2. Rare occurrences of Stevens–Johnson syndrome
Clarithromycin	7.5mg/kg per dose q12h; maximum dose 1g/day	++++	+	1. Undesireable after taste 2. Emerging resistance among *Streptococcus pneumoniae*
Azithromycin	10mg/kg per day on day 1, 5mg/kg per day on days 2–5; maximum dose 500mg on day 1	++++	++	1. Undesireable after taste 2. Emerging resistance among *Streptococcus pneumoniae*

Fig. 25.13 Antimicrobial agents commonly used in the therapy of acute otitis media.

chosen for their ability to achieve drug concentrations in the middle ear that exceed the MIC for the likely pathogens. Successful sterilization of middle ear infection occurs when drug concentrations exceed the MIC for approximately 50% of the dosing interval.[43] Presumptive therapy should be directed against nontypable strains of *H. influenzae*, *Strep. pneumoniae* and *M. catarrhalis*. In AOM with perforation, activity against group A streptococci should be included.

Figure 25.15 lists the antimicrobial agents commonly used for therapy of AOM and acute sinusitis, the dose, the relative activity of each agent against penicillin-sensitive isolates of *Strep. pneumoniae* and beta-lactamase-producing nontypable *H. influenzae*, and characteristics

of special significance. Although studies of clinical outcome have rarely demonstrated significant differences, studies with microbiologic end points often suggest that sterilization of the middle ear may be more frequently achieved with antimicrobial agents that attain adequate levels in the serum and middle ear and are active *in vitro* against nontypable *H. influenzae* and *Strep. pneumoniae*. Amoxicillin remains the drug of first choice because of its ability to sterilize middle ear infection due to most isolates of *Strep. pneumoniae* and nontypable *H. influenzae*, its low cost and its excellent safety record. None of the antimicrobials listed in Figure 25.13 has been demonstrated, in appropriate trials, to be more effective than amoxicillin as initial therapy of AOM or acute sinusitis.

DURATION OF THERAPY

Decreasing the duration of therapy reduces cost, may diminish the emergence of resistance among respiratory pathogens and should be associated with fewer adverse events. Several studies have demonstrated that by day 5 the middle ear can be successfully sterilized by antimicrobial agents with appropriate in-vitro activity.[44] Therefore, 'short-course' therapy is likely to be successful in resolving signs and symptoms caused by highly susceptible isolates. Unfortunately, the duration of acute therapy appears not to affect either the resolution of effusion at long-term follow-up or the risk of recurrence.

Recent studies that compared short courses (5 days) with traditional courses have consistently demonstrated higher failure rates with the short course in children younger than 2 years of age, especially those attending group day care.[45,46] These studies suggest that recommendations for short-course therapy should be limited to children older than 2 years of age. Further studies in children who have diseases caused by multidrug-resistant *Strep. pneumoniae* suggest that short course therapy is inadequate and should not be recommended in this setting.

TREATMENT FAILURES

When a child's symptoms fail to respond within 3 days or the tympanic membrane remains bright red and angry in appearance, the likelihood of persistent middle ear infection is high. Increasingly, a pathogen resistant to the initial antimicrobial agent prescribed is the likely problem. A broader-spectrum antimicrobial agent that is active against beta-lactamase-producing nontypable *H. influenzae* and penicillin-intermediate *Strep. pneumoniae* should be considered next (see Fig. 25.13). Small studies suggest that amoxicillin–clavulanate and cefuroxime are effective against both of these pathogens.

EMERGENCE OF PENICILLIN-RESISTANT ISOLATES OF *STREPTOCOCCUS PNEUMONIAE*

In South Africa, France and Spain, and now in the USA, strains of *Strep. pneumoniae* with MIC greater than or equal to $2.0\mu g/ml$ to penicillin have been isolated from the middle ear or sinus of children who have AOM or sinusitis.[47,48] These children have often already failed treatment with an antibiotic. The risk features that characterize these children include:
- recent antimicrobial treatment, most often with expanded spectrum cephalosporins;
- age under 5 years; and
- attendance at a day care center.

Clusters of cases have occurred in well-defined geographic areas.[49]

Limited information is available about therapeutic regimens effective for children who have AOM caused by these isolates. Experience from Kentucky with a large cluster of cases and from Europe suggests high dose amoxicillin (80–150mg/kg/day), amoxicillin (40mg/kg/day)

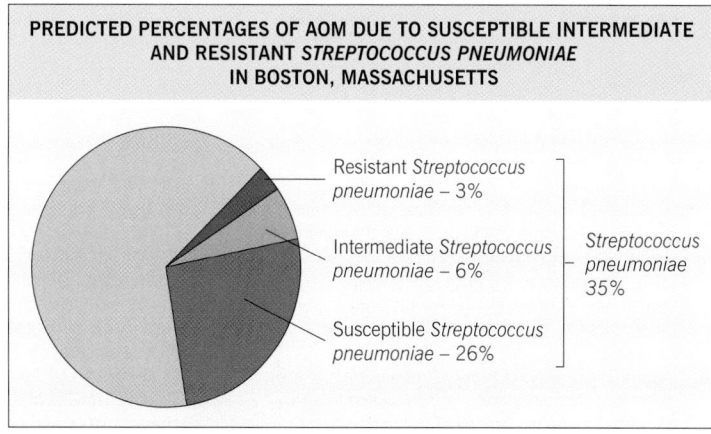

PREDICTED PERCENTAGES OF AOM DUE TO SUSCEPTIBLE INTERMEDIATE AND RESISTANT *STREPTOCOCCUS PNEUMONIAE* IN BOSTON, MASSACHUSETTS

Resistant *Streptococcus pneumoniae* – 3%

Intermediate *Streptococcus pneumoniae* – 6%

Susceptible *Streptococcus pneumoniae* – 26%

Streptococcus pneumoniae 35%

Fig. 25.14 Predicted percentages of acute otitis media due to susceptible, intermediate and resistant *Streptococcus pneumoniae* in Boston, Massachusetts.

plus amoxicillin–clavulanic acid (45mg/kg/day), ceftriaxone (50mg/kg/day) and clindamycin (50mg/kg/day) will successfully sterilize the middle ear and resolve symptoms.[49]

Disease caused by resistant isolates of *Strep. pneumoniae* remains infrequent among unselected cases of AOM and sinusitis. In Boston, we estimate that 3% of current unselected cases would be due to resistant *Strep. pneumoniae* (Fig. 25.14). Initial therapy targeted at this pathogen is not recommended. However, in cases where initial and second courses of treatment fail, as well as in cases with significant toxicity, antimicrobial agents effective against resistant isolates of *Strep. pneumoniae* should be selected.

PENICILLIN ALLERGY

For the child who has hives or anaphylaxis to penicillin, there is a limited selection of antimicrobial agents for therapy because aminopenicillins and cephalosporins have significant cross-reactivity. Trimethoprim–sulfamethoxazole (TMP-SMX; co-trimoxazole) has been effective, is low in cost and relatively safe. However, resistance rates of 20–50% among isolates of *Strep. pneumoniae* have raised questions about the potential for clinical failure.

Alternatives to TMP–SMX are macrolides, including clarithromycin and azithromycin, which may be less effective against nontypable *H. influenzae*, or combination therapy with a macrolide and sulfisoxazole. Erythromycin sulfisoxazole has a profile of efficacy, low cost and safety, but suggested dosing is three to four times per day. Another potential selection is clindamycin in combination with sulfisoxazole.

REFERENCES

1. Klein JO, Teele DW, Pelton SI. New concepts in otitis media: results of investigations of the greater Boston otitis media study group. In: Barness L, ed. Advances in pediatrics. Boston, Massachusetts: Mosby-Year Book; 1992:127–56.
2. Wald ER, Dashefsky B, Byers C, et al. Frequency and severity of infections in day care. J Pediatr 1988;112:540–6.
3. Teele DW, Klein JO, Rosner BA, et al. Epidemiology of otitis media during the first seven years of life in children in Greater Boston: a prospective, cohort study. J Infect Dis 1989;160:83–94.
4. Bluestone CD, Paradise JL, Beery QC. Physiology of the eustachian tube in the pathogenesis and management of middle ear effusions. Laryngoscope 1972;82:1654–70.

5. Berdal P, Brandtzag P, Froland S, et al. Immunodeficiency syndromes with otorhinolaryngological manifestations. Acta Otolaryngol (Stockh) 1976;82:185–92.
6. Umetsu DT, Ambrosino DM, Quinti I, et al. Recurrent sinopulmonary infection and impaired antibody response to bacterial capsular polysaccharide antigens in children with selective IgG-subclass deficiency. N Engl J Med 1985;313:1247–51.
7. Barnett ED, Klein JO, Pelton SI, Luginbuhl LM. Otitis media in children born to human immunodeficiency virus-infected mothers. Pediatr Infect Dis J 1992;11:360–4.
8. Shurin PA, Rehmis JM, Johnson CE, et al. Bacterial polysaccharide immune globulin for prophylaxis of acute otitis media in high-risk children. J Pediatr 1993;123:801–10.

9. Henderson FW, Collier DM, Sanyal MA, et al. A longitudinal study of respiratory viruses and bacteria in the etiology of acute otitis media with effusion. N Engl J Med 1982;306:1377–83.
10. Teele DW, Klein JO, The Greater Boston Collaborative Otitis Media Study Group, et al. Use of pneumococcal vaccine for prevention of recurrent otitis media in infants in Boston. Rev Infect Dis 1981;3(Suppl):113–8.
11. Makela PH, Leinonen M, Pukander J, Karma P. A study of the pneumoccal vaccine in prevention of clinically acute attacks of recurrent otitis media. Rev Infect Dis 1981;3(Suppl):124–30.
12. Shurin PA, Giebink GS, Wegman DL, et al. Prevention of pneumococcal otitis media in chinchillas with human bacterial polysaccharide immune globulin. J Clin Microbiol 1988;26:755–9.

13. Barenkamp SJ. Protection by serum antibodies in experimental nontypable *Haemophilus influenzae* otitis media. Infect Immun 1986;52:572–8.

14. Anderson EL, Kennedy DJ, Geldmacher KM, *et al*. Immunogenicity of heptavalent pneumococcal conjugate vaccine in infants. J Pediatr 1996;128:649–53.

15. Black S, Shinefield H, Ray P, *et al*. Efficacy of Heptavalent conjugate pneumococcal vaccine in 37,000 infants and children: results of the northern california kaiser permanente efficacy trial (abstract LB-9). Presented at the 38th Interscience Conference on Antimicrobial Agents and Chemotherapy, September 1998, San Diego, California.

16. Dagan R, Givon N, Yagupsky P, *et al*. Effect of a 9-valent pneumococcal vaccine conjugated to crm$_{197}$ on nasopharyngeal carriage of vaccine type and non-vaccine type *S. pneumoniae* strains among day care center attendees (abstract G 52). Presented at the 38th Interscience Conference on Antimicrobial Agents and Chemotherapy, September 1998, San Diego, California.

17. Heikkinen T, Ruuskanen O, Waris M, *et al*. Influenza vaccination in the prevention of acute otitis media in children. Am J Dis Child 1991;145:445–8.

18. Belshe RB, Mendelman PM, Treanor J, *et al*. The efficacy of live attenuated, cold-adapted, trivalent, intranasal influenza virus vaccine in children. N Eng J of Med 1998;338:1405–12.

19. Simoes EA, Groothuis JR, Tristram DA, *et al*. Respiratory syncytial virus-enriched globulin for the prevention of acute otitis media in children. J Pediatr 1996;129:214–9.

20. The IMpact-RSV Study Group. Palivizumab, a humanized respiratory syncytial virus monoclonal antibody, reduces hospitalization from respiratory syncytial virus infection in high-risk infants. Pediatrics 1998;102:531–7.

21. Mandel EM, Casselbrant ML, Rockette HE, *et al*. Efficacy of antimicrobial prophylaxis for recurrent middle ear effusion. Pediatr Infect Dis J 1996;15:1074–82.

22. Williams RL, Chalmers TC, Stange KC, *et al*. Use of antibiotics in preventing recurrent acute otitis media and in treating otitis media with effusion. A meta-analytic attempt to resolve the brouhaha. JAMA 1993;270:1344–51.

23. Casselbrant ML, Kaleida PH, Rockette HE, *et al*. Efficacy of antimicrobial prophylaxis and of tympanostomy tube insertion for prevention of recurrent acute otitis media: results of a randomized clinical trial. Pediatr Infect Dis J 1992;11:278–86.

24. Jacobs MR, Bajaksouzian S, Burch D, Poupard J, Appelbaum PC. Activity of amoxicillin ± clavulanate against *Streptococcus pneumoniae* strains from patients with acute otitis media in Eastern Europe, Israel and USA (abstract). 35th Interscience Conference on Antimicrobial Agents and Chemotherapy, September 1995, San Francisco, California.

25. Takala AK, Syrjänen R, Herva E, Eskola J. Bacteriological etiology of acute otitis media (AOM) among Finnish children less than two years of age; a cohort study of 329 children in a special study clinic designed for diagnosis and treatment of AOM (abstract). Copenhagen Otitis Media Conference (Third Extraordinary International Symposium on Recent Advances in Otitis Media), 1–5 June 1997, Copenhagen, Denmark.

26. Herberts G, Jeppson PH, Nylen O, Branefors-Helander P. Acute otitis media: etiological and therapeutic aspects of acute otitis media. Pract Otorhinolaryngol 1971;33:191–202.

27. Deka K, Howie VM, Owen MJ, *et al*. Patient characteristics and prevalence of respiratory syncytial virus (RSV) infection in acute otitis media (AOM). In: Lim DJ, Bluestone CD, *et al*., eds. Recent advances in otitis media (Proceedings of the sixth international symposium). Hamilton, Ontario: BC Decker; 1996:315–7.

28. Storgaard M, Ostergaard L, Jensen JS, *et al*. *Chlamydia pneumoniae* in otitis media (abstract 79). Copenhagen Otitis Media Conference (Third Extraordinary International Symposium on Recent Advances in Otitis Media), 1–5 June 1997, Copenhagen, Denmark.

29. Klein JO, Teele DW. Isolation of viruses and mycoplasma from middle ear effusions: a review. Am Otol Rhinol Laryngol 1976;85:140–4.

30. Kenna MA, Rosane BA, Bluestone CD. Medical management of chronic suppurative otitis media without cholesteatoma in children. Laryngoscope 1986;46:146–51.

31. Shurin PA. Otitis media and mastoiditis. In: Jensen HB, Baltimore RS, eds. Pediatric infectious diseases. Norwalk, Connecticut: Appleton and Lange; 1995:923–35.

32. Rudberg RD. Acute otitis media: comparative therapeutic results of sulfonamide and penicillin administered in various forms. Acta Otolaryngol (Stockh) 1954;113:1–79.

33. Kaleida PH, Casselbrant ML, Rockette HE, *et al*. Amoxicillin or myringotomy or both for acute otitis media: Results of a randomized clinical trial. Pediatrics 1991;87:466–74.

34. Hoppe JE, Köster S, Bootz F, Niethammer D. Acute mastoiditis – relevant once again. Infection 1994;22:178–82.

35. Van de Heyning PH, Cohen R, Pricippi N, Hende L, Behre U. Eurotitis study, a prospective bacteriological survey of pathogens cultured from middle ear fluid in children with clinical failure of first line antibacterial therapy for acute otitis media (abstract 143). Copenhagen Otitis Media Conference (Third Extraordinary International Symposium on Recent Advances in Otitis Media), 1–5 June 1997, Copenhagen, Denmark.

36. Muntz HR, Lusk RP. Signs and symptoms of chronic sinusitis. In: Lusk RP, ed. Pediatric sinusitis. New York: Raven Press; 1992:1–7.

37. Wald ER, Reilly JS, Casselbrant M, *et al*. Treatment of acute maxillary sinusitis in childhood: a comparative study of amoxicillin and cefaclor. J Pediatr 1984;104:297–302.

38. Maresh MM, Washburn AH. Paranasal sinuses from birth to late adolescence: size of paranasal sinuses as observed on routine posteroanterior roentgenogram. Am J Dis Child 1940;60:841–61.

39. Wald ER, Chiponis D, Ledesma-Medina J. Comparative effectiveness of amoxicillin and amoxicillin–clavulanate potassium in acute paranasal sinus infection in children: a double-blind, placebo-controlled trial. Pediatrics 1986;77:795–800.

40. Chandler JR, Langenbrunner DJ, Stevens ER. The pathogenesis of orbital complications in acute sinusitis. Laryngoscope 1970;80:1414–28.

41. Lusk RP, Tychsen L, Park TS. Complication of sinusitis. In: Lusk RP, ed. Pediatric sinusitis. New York: Raven Press; 1992:127–46.

42. Marchant CD, Carlin SA, Johnson CE, Shurin PA. Measuring the comparative efficacy of antibacterial agents for acute otitis media: the 'Pollyanna phenomenon'. J Pediatr 1992;120:72–7.

43. Craig W, Andes D. Pharmacokinetics and pharmacodynamics of antibiotics in otitis media. Pediatr Infect Dis J 1996;15:255–9.

44. Howie VM. Eradication of bacterial pathogens from middle ear infections. Clin Infect Dis 1992;14(Suppl 2):209–10.

45. Cohen R, Levy C, Boucherat M, *et al*. A multicenter, randomized, double blind trial of 5 versus 10 days of antibiotic therapy for acute otitis media in young children. J Pediatr 1998;133:634–9.

46. Hoberman A, Paradise J, Burch DJ, *et al*. Equivalent efficacy and reduced occurrence of diarrhea from a new formulation of amoxicillin/clavulanate potassium (Augmentin) for treatment of acute otitis media in children. Pediatr Infect Dis J 1997;16:463–70.

47. Appelbaum PC. Antimicrobial resistance in *Streptococcus pneumoniae*: an overview. Clin Infect Dis 1992;15:77–83.

48. Welby PL, Keller DS, Cromien JL, Tebas P, Storch GA. Resistance to penicillin and non-beta-lactam antibiotics of *Streptococcus pneumoniae* at a children's hospital. Pediatr Infect Dis J 1994;13:281–7.

49. Block SL, Harrison CJ, Hedrick JA, *et al*. Penicillin-resistant *Streptococcus pneumoniae* in acute otitis media: risk factors, susceptibility patterns and antimicrobial management. Pediatr Infect Dis J 1995;14:751–9.

Bronchitis, Bronchiectasis and Cystic Fibrosis

James R Yankaskas

Inflammatory airways diseases are highly prevalent, causing significant morbidity and mortality. Genetic, environmental, and infectious factors can contribute to acute and chronic inflammation of the airways of the lung. The nature, severity and duration of these insults may produce acute or chronic inflammation with associated cough, dyspnea, sputum production and obstructive lung disease. Clinically, these are classified as bronchitis (acute or chronic), the main symptoms of which are cough and sputum, or bronchiectasis, in which the airways are structurally damaged and become dilated. The ability to stop the progression of these diseases is often limited by chronic inflammation and by structural alterations in the airways. Nevertheless, antibiotics, anti-inflammatory drugs and other forms of therapy can modulate acute exacerbations and, potentially, the progression of these diseases. Cystic fibrosis (CF) is a common genetic disease that leads to progressive bronchitis and bronchiectasis. Knowledge about the molecular, cellular and organ-level pathogenesis of CF has increased greatly in the past decade and new treatments are being developed.

BRONCHITIS EPIDEMIOLOGY

Bronchitis is defined as inflammation of the bronchial mucous membranes. Acute bronchitis is manifested by the development of a cough, with or without sputum, that typically occurs during the course of an acute viral illness. Such cough commonly develops in the first week of upper respiratory infections (URIs) induced by rhinoviruses, in 30% of patients.[1] Acute bronchitis develops in 60% of patients during influenza A infections.[2] In the USA over 34 million annual office visits are for acute sinusitis, bronchitis or URIs. The majority of these patients are treated with antibiotics, and such prescriptions comprise 31% of the total antibiotic prescriptions written.[3]

Chronic bronchitis is defined by the clinical criteria of productive cough for more than 3 months per year for at least 2 years.[4] More than 12 million Americans, or about 5% of the population, have chronic bronchitis. The male:female distribution is about 2:1, but the prevalence is increasing in females. Chronic bronchitis is a major category of chronic obstructive pulmonary disease (COPD) and accounts for significant morbidity and mortality, especially in individuals aged over 55 years. In the USA COPD accounted for nearly 83,000 deaths in 1989 and was the fifth leading cause of death;[5] it was also a contributing factor in death in other illnesses, such as heart disease.

PATHOGENESIS AND PATHOLOGY

Acute bronchitis is most commonly due to infection of the respiratory epithelium with viruses, such as rhinoviruses, adenoviruses and influenza. Acute bronchitis may also be caused by infections with *Mycoplasma pneumoniae*, *Chlamydia pneumoniae* or *Bordetella pertussis*. The pathogenic effects of these organisms are incompletely understood, but they infect and directly damage airway epithelia, cause release of proinflammatory cytokines, increase production of secretions and decrease mucociliary clearance. Airways damaged by such infections may be more susceptible to irritation by inhaled toxins or bacteria. The role of secondary bacterial infections in the development of symptoms is not clear.

Chronic bronchitis develops as the result of a recurring or persistent injury and the resultant inflammatory responses. Cigarette smoking is the principal etiologic factor. Air pollutants, such as sulfur dioxide, or occupational exposures may also contribute. The pathologic effects are an increase in the proportion of goblet cells in the surface epithelium and an increase in the size of submucosal glands (Fig. 26.1). The distribution of these pathologic changes along the airway tree depends in part on the composition of the inhaled toxins, and may involve peripheral bronchioles as well as central bronchi. There is an influx of polymorphonuclear leukocytes, surface epithelial cell hyperplasia and metaplasia, and inflammatory mucosal edema. These effects may be amplified by genetic diseases that impair airway defenses. Primary ciliary dyskinesia[6] decreases mucociliary transport secondary to altered ciliary structure and function. Deficiency in α1-antitrypsin produces an imbalance in the defenses against neutrophil elastase and leads to pan-acinar emphysema and bronchitis, particularly in smokers.[7]

PREVENTION

Chronic bronchitis primarily develops in cigarette smokers. Avoidance of inhaled toxins, particularly cigarette smoke, is of paramount importance in reducing the incidence and progression of chronic bronchitis. The loss of lung function, as measured by spirometry, is more rapid in active cigarette smokers. Such individuals can gain significant benefits from stopping or significantly decreasing their cigarette consumption. Sputum production usually decreases within weeks. The accelerated decline of lung function seen in smokers slows to that of affected nonsmokers of the same age.[8] Thus, the importance of avoiding primary and secondary cigarette smoke cannot be overemphasized.

CLINICAL FEATURES

Acute bronchitis typically develops during the course of an acute URI. Pharyngitis, coryza, low-grade fever and malaise precede the development of a cough with scanty sputum. Dyspnea is rare. In the absence of other lung disease, most symptoms subside over several days, although the cough may persist for weeks to several months. The quantity of sputum and frequency of cough decrease with time, and no long-term sequelae occur.

The key symptoms of individuals with chronic bronchitis are chronic cough, production of sputum, wheezing and exertional dyspnea. These symptoms develop insidiously, often over many years. Presentation for medical care typically occurs during an acute exacerbation. Upon direct inquiry, patients often recall persistent dyspnea and sputum production following URIs for several years before presentation. The sputum is purulent, yellow or green, and may be blood-streaked. The daily volume ranges from scanty up to about 60ml. The cough and sputum are usually most severe soon after awakening. Exertional dyspnea and fatigue are first noticed during exacerbations, and later become persistent.

Acute or subacute exacerbations are characterized by increases in cough, sputum production, dyspnea and wheezing.[9] These symptoms

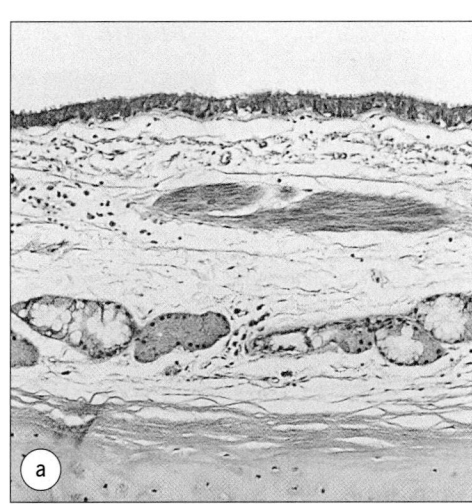

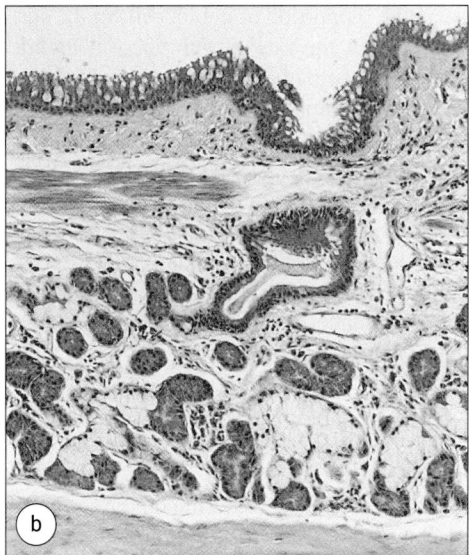

Fig. 26.1 Bronchial wall. (a) The bronchial wall from normal patient. Normal pseudostratified columnar epithelia with few goblet cells, overlie smooth muscle and a submucosal gland. Cartilage is at the bottom of the figure (H&E stain, ×100). (b) Bronchial wall from a patient who has chronic bronchitis. Hyperplastic epithelia with mucous cell metaplasia overlie a hypertrophied submucosal gland. (H&E stain, ×100).

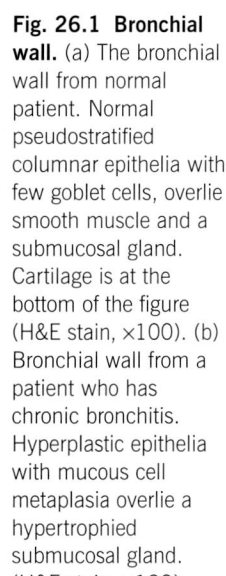

VIRAL AND BACTERIAL PATHOGENS IN BRONCHITIS	
Common	Viruses: (rhinoviruses, adenoviruses, influenza A and B, parainfluenza)
	Haemophilus influenzae
	Haemophilus parainfluenzae
	Moraxella catarrhalis
	Neisseria spp.
	Streptococcus pneumoniae
Uncommon	*Chlamydia pneumoniae*
	Klebsiella pneumoniae
	Mycoplasma pneumoniae
	Pseudomonas aeruginosa

Fig. 26.2 Viral and bacterial pathogens in bronchitis.

often follow URIs and tend to be more frequent during winter months. The sputum often changes in color to darker yellow or green. Sputum cultures may identify one of the bacterial pathogens listed in Figure 26.2, but the pathogenic role of these microbes is not certain.[10,11] Pulmonary function decreases during such exacerbations and may lead to further complications. The progressive disease often leads to increasingly frequent exacerbations, further loss of lung function and worse symptoms.

Patients who have severe obstructive airways disease may develop the serious complications of hypoxemic and/or hypercapnic respiratory failure. Hypoxemia develops initially during exercise or sleep, and may cause morning headaches. Prolonged hypoxemia may cause cyanosis, polycythemia, pulmonary hypertension and cor pulmonale. Secondary signs of right heart failure, such as jugular venous distention, hepatomegaly and peripheral edema, develop in late disease and may become chronic. The respiratory acidosis that signals hypercapnic respiratory failure may be of gradual onset and be compensated for by a metabolic alkalosis through renal retention of bicarbonate. Individuals with scanty sputum production and greater degrees of emphysema often achieve adequate oxygenation and ventilation until late in the course of the disease. Exacerbations in the setting of severe disease often produce superimposed acute respiratory failure that is life-threatening and requires intensive care.

DIAGNOSIS

The history of persistent cough and daily sputum is essential to the diagnosis of chronic bronchitis. The extent and duration of cigarette smoking quantifies the major risk factor. The presence of antecedent reactive airways disease, for example childhood asthma, may increase

the risk for developing chronic bronchitis and COPD. Physical examination reveals tachypnea and late expiratory wheezes on auscultation. Patients who have advanced disease develop hyperinflation of the lungs with increased anterior–posterior diameter of the thorax and a depressed diaphragm. In such patients, breath sounds and heart sounds are muted. Patients who have severe disease may use accessory muscles of respiration and/or pursed-lip breathing. Medium or coarse inspiratory crackles appear in patients who have bronchitis and excess airway secretions. Patients who have severe disease may develop central and peripheral cyanosis, or neck vein distention, hepatomegaly and peripheral edema as signs of hypoxemia and right heart failure.

Pulmonary function tests are essential to establish the diagnosis of obstructive lung disease, to measure the severity of airway obstruction and to follow the course of illness. Spirometry performed before and after inhaled β-adrenergic agonists often reveals decreased forced expiratory volume in 1 second (FEV_1) and decreased FEV_1:forced vital capacity ratio. Improved flows after inhaled β-adrenergic agonists indicate the presence of reversible bronchoconstriction. Forced vital capacity is also decreased in patients who have very severe obstruction. In such individuals, lung volumes should be measured to differentiate restrictive from obstructive respiratory impairments and to quantify lung hyperinflation and gas trapping. The diffusing capacity for carbon monoxide may be reduced in patients who have severe obstruction or emphysema. The chest X-ray shows increased lung volumes; in patients who have emphysema the heart may appear low and the bronchovascular markings may be decreased. Patients who have chronic bronchitis often have enlarged hearts, engorged apical vessels, bronchial cuffing and other signs of fluid overload. Arterial blood gases may reveal mild to severe hypoxemia. Patients who have severe disease may develop respiratory acidosis and a compensatory metabolic alkalosis. The complete blood count may reveal polycythemia and the serum electrolytes a metabolic alkalosis. Sputum Gram stain and culture are important to assess the abundance of polymorphonuclear leukocytes and to help identify bacterial pathogens that may be associated with acute exacerbations.

MANAGEMENT

Acute bronchitis is best managed with symptomatic treatment. Nonsteroidal anti-inflammatory drugs and decongestants are useful for pharyngitis, sinusitis and coryza. Antibiotics are indicated for clinically significant bacterial bronchitis, but such a complication is difficult to distinguish from viral bronchitis. Antibiotics are taken by 53–66% of patients who have acute sinusitis, bronchitis or URIs,[3] indicating overprescription. This practice promotes the development of antibiotic-resistant bacteria, which may lead to greater morbidity in the community. Therefore, antibiotics should be reserved for patients with acute bronchitis who have increased numbers of polymorphonuclear leukocytes and numerous bacteria in Gram-stained sputum samples, or who do not respond to symptomatic therapy.

The most important feature of managing chronic bronchitis is the avoidance of exposure to irritants, particularly cigarette smoke. Thus, smoking cessation is of primary importance for each individual. Support for smoking cessation can be provided by individual counseling, provision of smoking cessation literature or through smoking cessation groups. Nicotine gum or transdermal nicotine may be useful to reduce withdrawal symptoms.

No specific therapy is available to treat chronic bronchitis. Symptomatic therapy is directed at reducing mucosal edema, mucus hypersecretion, bronchial smooth muscle constriction and airway inflammation (Fig. 26.3). Inhaled β-adrenergic agonists and anticholinergic drugs may be of benefit to patients who have reactive airways disease, as demonstrated on pulmonary function tests.[12] Theophylline may be useful in patients who have nocturnal symptoms or severe hyperinflation and respiratory muscle fatigue. In addition to relaxing bronchial smooth muscle, β-adrenergic agonists enhance mucociliary clearance. Inhaled drugs with intermediate (4–6 hours) and long (8–12 hours) duration of action are available. These are generally preferred to systemic treatments. Metered dose inhalers (MDIs) appear to have an efficacy similar to that of nebulizers, but effective treatment requires co-ordination of MDI actuation and the breathing cycle. The beneficial effects can be enhanced by the use of a spacer to improve deposition of drugs in the lungs. Anticholinergic drugs relax bronchial smooth muscle, and have an intermediate duration of action (4–6 hours). Ipratropium bromide is available as an MDI. The effects of anticholinergics and β-agonists appear to be roughly equivalent.[13] The responses of individual patients to such drugs must be assessed to determine the optimum treatment.

Systemic and inhaled corticosteroids provide a beneficial effect by reducing severity of airway inflammation. This typically results in decreased airway obstruction and decreased mucus secretion. Long-term use of systemic corticosteroids may be complicated by osteoporosis, central obesity and/or glucose intolerance. Once a beneficial effect of corticosteroids has been demonstrated with systemic therapy, these side effects can be minimized by use of moderate-to-high doses of inhaled corticosteroids. Typical drugs include beclomethasone, 800–1600µg/day and fluticasone, 350–2640µg/day. Other forms of therapy, such as cromolyn sodium, expectorants and chest physiotherapy, have not been demonstrated to have significant effects in chronic bronchitis or COPD.

The role of bacterial infection in causing acute exacerbations of chronic bronchitis is controversial. It is likely that less than half the cases of acute exacerbation are due to bacterial infection. A number of controlled studies have failed to show significant benefit of antibiotic therapy.[14,15] Nevertheless, antibiotics may be effective in patients who have a significant increase in the number of polymorphonuclear leukocytes in expectorated sputum and dominant bacteria on Gram stain or in culture. Previous positive responses to antibiotic therapy may also support repeated use in individual patients. Antibiotics effective against the common bacterial species are listed in Figure 26.4. Patients who have exacerbations of sufficient severity to require hospitalization should be treated with parenteral antibiotics with comparable antibacterial spectra, and the treatment modified based on sputum culture results.

Hypoxemia may be diagnosed by ambulatory, exercise or nocturnal pulse oximetry, as well as by arterial blood gases. Patients who have significant hemoglobin desaturation (arterial oxygen saturation <90%) should receive supplemental oxygen. Nocturnal oxygen has been shown to improve survival[16] and continuous treatment has greater effects than nocturnal treatment alone.[17] Some patients who have COPD also have obstructive sleep apnea, and detailed sleep studies may be required to establish the effectiveness of oxygen and/or continuous positive airway pressure by nasal mask to prevent nocturnal hypoxemia.[18] Noninvasive assisted ventilation by nasal mask has been used for some patients who have severe hypercapnic respiratory failure.[19] Patients who have acute respiratory failure and significant respiratory acidosis or hypoxemia often require hospitalization, parenteral antibiotics, intensive care unit care and mechanical ventilation.[20]

BRONCHIECTASIS

EPIDEMIOLOGY

Bronchiectasis is defined as abnormal dilatation of bronchi.[21,22] It typically involves medium-sized bronchi and results from destruction of the muscular and elastic components of the airway walls. Bronchiectasis is classified as cystic, cylindrical or varicose, on the basis of the morphologic structure of the airways. Chronic airway inflammation is the essential pathologic feature, resulting from genetic abnormalities that impair airway defense mechanisms or from chronic respiratory infections. Such infections have become relatively rare in the USA; the current prevalence of bronchiectasis is less than 1 in 10,000.

THERAPEUTIC OPTIONS FOR ACUTE EXACERBATIONS OF CHRONIC BRONCHITIS

Option	Agent/measure	Examples	Notes
Bronchodilators	β-adrenergic agonists	Albuterol, salmeterol	Inhaled administration preferred
	Anticholinergics	Ipratropium bromide	Inhaled administration mandatory
	Theophylline		Second-line agent
Anti-inflammatory agents	Corticosteroids	Prednisone, fluticasone	Administration by inhalation may reduce side effects
Expectorants	Recombinant human DNase	Dornase α	Efficacy in COPD not established
	Iodinated compounds	Iodinated glycerol	Limited efficacy
	Reducing agents	N-acetyl cysteine	Limited efficacy
Airway clearance measures	Controlled coughing		Efficacy not established
	Physical		Efficacy not established
Supplemental oxygen			Correct significant hypoxemia
Antibiotics	See Figure 26.4	See Figure 26.4	Indications and efficacy controversial

Fig. 26.3 Therapeutic options for acute exacerbations of chronic bronchitis.

ORAL ANTIBIOTICS FOR ACUTE EXACERBATIONS OF CHRONIC BRONCHITIS

Agent	Dose
Amoxicillin	250–500mg q8h
Amoxicillin/clavulanic acid	875/125mg q8h
Ampicillin	500mg q6h
Azithromycin	500mg day 1, then 250mg q24h
Cefaclor	500mg q8h
Cephalexin	500mg q6h
Ciprofloxacin	500–750mg q12h
Clarithromycin	500mg q12h
Doxycycline	100mg q12h
Erythromycin	250–500mg q6h
Ofloxacin	400mg q12h
Tetracycline	250–500mg q6h
Trimethoprim–sulfamethoxazole	80/400mg q12h

Fig. 26.4 Oral antibiotics for acute exacerbations of chronic bronchitis.

PATHOGENESIS AND PATHOLOGY

The principal diseases that cause bronchiectasis are listed in Figure 26.5. The genetic diseases cause deficits in airway defense or in immunologic mechanisms that permit the development of chronic bacterial infections in the airways. Bacterial and inflammatory cell-derived proteolytic and oxidative molecules cause progressive airway wall damage that eventually produces bronchiectasis. Immune reactions to fungi can produce the central bronchiectasis that is associated with allergic bronchopulmonary aspergillosis. Chronic infections with *Mycobacterium tuberculosis*[23] or nontuberculous mycobacteria (particularly *Mycobacterium avium* complex),[24] and *Bordetella pertussis* are recognized infectious causes. Bacteria that secondarily infect damaged airways after other injuries probably propagate airway damage, but the time course and relative contributions of the different organisms have not been established.

CLINICAL FEATURES

Daily cough and production of purulent sputum are the most typical symptoms of bronchiectasis. Sputum production can range from less than 10ml to greater than 150ml daily, and tends to correlate with disease extent and severity. Bronchiectasis associated with CF, which becomes generalized and progresses relentlessly, is described in greater detail below. Occasional individuals have no discernible sputum production ('dry bronchiectasis'). The clinical course is usually of progressive symptoms and respiratory impairment. Airway obstruction progresses and leads to increasing exertional and resting dyspnea. Acute exacerbations may be precipitated by viral or newly acquired bacterial pathogens, as with chronic bronchitis. The main clinical feature differentiating bronchiectasis from chronic bronchitis is the quantity of sputum production. In addition to progressive respiratory failure, patients who have bronchiectasis are prone to hemoptysis due to hypertrophied bronchial arteries that are closely apposed to the inflamed airways.[25] Hemoptysis from this source can be massive, even fatal.

DIAGNOSIS

Diagnosis is suggested by clinical symptoms and a physical examination with hyperinflated chest and medium- to low-pitched inspiratory crackles and sometimes expiratory wheezes. Chest X-ray may demonstrate hyperinflation and bronchiectatic cysts or dilated bronchi with thickened walls forming tram track patterns radiating from the lung hila. High-resolution chest CT scans readily demonstrate mild and severe forms of bronchiectasis. Computed tomography scans have largely replaced bronchography as a diagnostic examination. Sputum culture may identify characteristic pathogens, including *Haemophilus influenzae*, *Streptococcus pneumoniae* and/or *Pseudomonas aeruginosa*. Sputum acid-fast bacillus smears and cultures should be performed to evaluate mycobacterial disease. Spirometry is essential to determine the severity of airway obstruction and to evaluate the course of disease.

MANAGEMENT

Specific causes, such as tuberculosis, should be identified and treated whenever possible. Standard therapy includes measures to clear excess secretions from the airways. Chest physiotherapy based on chest percussion and postural drainage is accepted as the most effective technique. Alternatives such as pneumatic vests, aerobic exercise or flow interrupter valves may be effective, but their use must be individualized. Bronchodilators have a role in patients who have objective spirometric or subjective clinical responses. Acute exacerbations are managed with intensification of airway clearance measures and the use of antibiotics directed at pathogens identified in recent sputum cultures. The use of prophylactic oral or inhaled antibiotics has been advocated

PRINCIPAL CAUSES OF BRONCHIECTASIS	
Genetic	Cystic fibrosis
	Immunoglobulin deficiency
	Primary ciliary dyskinesia
Infectious	*Bordetella pertussis*
	Tuberculosis
	Nontuberculous mycobacteria (especially *Mycobacterium avium* complex)
Inflammatory	Allergic bronchopulmonary aspergillosis
	α1-antitrypsin deficiency
	Bronchial obstruction
Other	Bronchopulmonary sequestration
	Congenital cartilage abnormalities
	Yellow nail syndrome

Fig. 26.5 Principal causes of bronchiectasis.

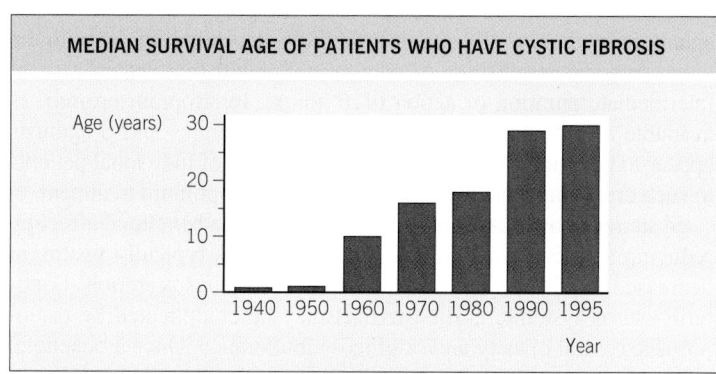

Fig. 26.6 The median survival of CF patients 1940–1995. The median survival of CF patients has increased dramatically. Data from Stacey FitzSimmons.

to control the major symptoms of bronchiectasis, and such treatment must be tailored to the individual responses. Surgical resection of localized bronchiectatic lung is occasionally useful.[26]

CYSTIC FIBROSIS

EPIDEMIOLOGY

Cystic fibrosis is the most common lethal genetic disease in Caucasians.[27] This autosomal recessive disease is caused by mutations in the cystic fibrosis transmembrane conductance regulator (CFTR) gene located on chromosome 7. The incidence is 1 in every 3300 live Caucasian births, with a gene carrier rate of 1 in 29. Other ethnic groups have lower carrier rates, with the Hispanic birth incidence 1 in 9500, Native American 1 in 11,200, African-American 1 in 15,300 and Asian 1 in 32,100 live births.

When CF was first described in 1938, survival past infancy was rare. Improved treatments for pancreatic insufficiency, lung infections and other complications have increased the median survival from less than 1 year to more than 31 years (Fig. 26.6). Over 21,000 CF patients have been identified in the USA.[28] The median survival in 1996 was 31.3 years. Adults (>18 years old) now account for 35.6% of CF patients, and survival can now extend to as long as 71 years.[28]

PATHOGENESIS

The CFTR gene encodes a 1480 amino acid protein, with 12 membrane-spanning regions, two nucleotide binding folds and a

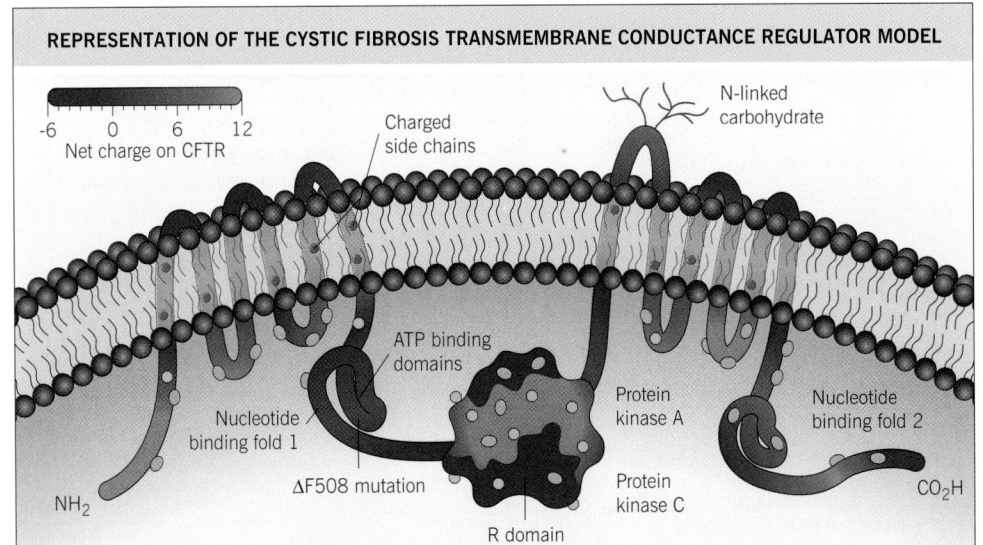

REPRESENTATION OF THE CYSTIC FIBROSIS TRANSMEMBRANE CONDUCTANCE REGULATOR MODEL

Fig. 26.7 Representation of the CFTR model, based on structural, hydropathy and expression studies. The membrane-spanning domains are arranged in groups of six, each associated with a nucleotide binding fold (NBF). These features are similar to those of the multidrug resistance 'P' glycoprotein. The 'R' domain is unique to CFTR. Adapted from Riordan J, *et al*. Science 1989;245:1071 and Hooper C, Journal of NIH Research, Nov–Dec 1989;1:79.

regulatory ('R') domain (Fig. 26.7). This protein is localized to the apical membranes of epithelia lining the organs affected by the disease, particularly the airways, pancreatic duct, sweat gland ducts, intestines and reproductive tract. The CFTR protein acts as a chloride-channel[29] and as a regulator of epithelial sodium channels[30] and other chloride channels.[31] Over 700 different mutations in the CF gene have been identified, encompassing several functional abnormalities (Fig. 26.8). Class I mutations prevent protein production. Class II mutations produce proteins that fail to traffic to the apical cell membrane. The most common CF mutation, ΔF508, is in this class; it accounts for 68% of US cases of CF. Class III mutations traffic properly, but have defective regulation. Class IV mutations traffic properly, but have defective chloride conductance. Some exon splice-site mutations have been labeled class V mutations and may permit transcription of some normal CFTR mRNA, conferring a less severe clinical phenotype.[32] All classes of mutations alter chloride permeability and regulation of ion transport in the affected epithelial cells.

The pathogenesis of airways disease in CF is not completely understood. Cystic fibrosis transmembrane conductance regulator mutations produce decreased chloride permeability and increased net sodium absorption by bronchial epithelial cells. The effects on bronchiolar epithelial cells and on submucosal gland secretion are not fully understood. It has been suggested that CF mutations lead to relative dehydration, abnormal mucus sulfation or abnormal function of peptide antimicrobial molecules (defensins) in the airway surface liquid.[33] These abnormalities cause impaired mucociliary clearance, secondary bacterial infection and airways inflammation. This chronic infection and inflammation form a vicious circle that produces progressive airway obstruction, bronchiectasis and, eventually, respiratory failure. This scheme of pathogenesis is illustrated in Figure 26.9. Some existing and potential treatments, directed at the specific pathogenic processes, are indicated.

CLINICAL FEATURES

Cystic fibrosis is classically recognized from the triad of bronchiectatic airways disease, exocrine pancreatic insufficiency and elevated sweat chloride. Most patients have onset of cough and chronic respiratory tract infections during infancy or childhood. Early respiratory tract pathogens include *Staphylococcus aureus* and *H. influenzae*. *Pseudomonas aeruginosa*, particularly mucoid variants, appears in greater prevalence with increasing age and becomes the dominant pathogen by the teenage years (Fig. 26.10). It is common to isolate several different bacteria from the sputum of adolescent and adult CF patients. Pathologically, there is inflammation and obstruction both of

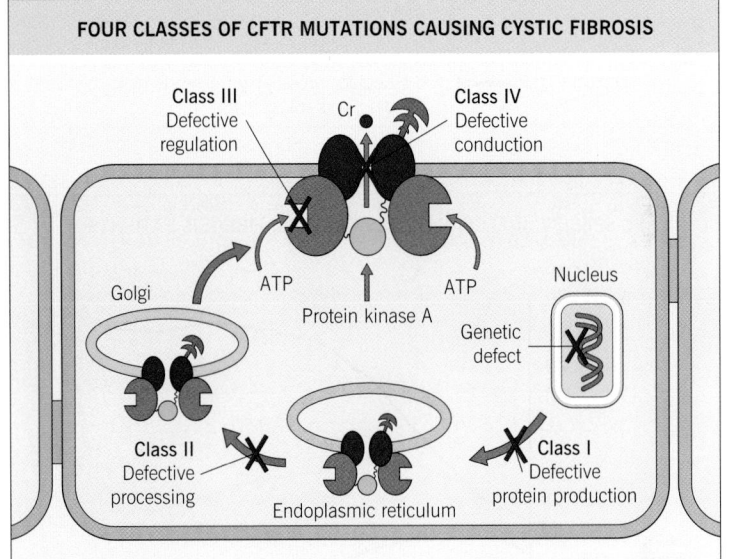

FOUR CLASSES OF CFTR MUTATIONS CAUSING CYSTIC FIBROSIS

Fig. 26.8 Mutations in the CFTR causing CF. Mutations in the CFTR are divided into classes on the basis of mechanisms of dysfunction. See text for detailed descriptions.

bronchioles (Fig. 26.11) and of bronchi, with submucosal gland hypertrophy (Fig. 26.12). Bronchiectasis tends to start in the upper lobes and becomes generalized. Chest X-ray shows hyperinflated lungs, cystic bronchiectasis and, occasionally, upper lobe atelectasis (Fig. 26.13).

The clinical course of chronic cough, mucus hypersecretion and airway obstruction is progressive and is punctuated by acute exacerbations. When such exacerbations are effectively treated, pulmonary function may return to baseline levels. With more severe disease, exacerbations become more frequent and less reversible, culminating in fatal respiratory failure (Fig. 26.14).

DIAGNOSIS

The standard diagnostic criteria for CF are the combination of characteristic lung disease with airway obstruction, bronchiectasis and infection with typical bacterial pathogens; exocrine pancreatic insufficiency, which occurs in more than 85% of CF patients; and elevated sweat chloride, which occurs in more than 98% of patients. The diagnosis initially may be suggested by a family history of CF or by the presence of meconium ileus at birth, noted in 17% of cases. Of patients reported to the CF Foundation Patient Registry, 51% presented with

TREATMENT APPROACHES TO CYSTIC FIBROSIS AIRWAYS DISEASE

Abnormality	Solution	Approach	
		Available	Investigational
Abnormal CF gene	Provide normal gene		Gene therapy
Abnormal CFTR protein	Provide normal protein Activate mutant form		Protein therapy ?Phosphodiesterase inhibitors ?Phosphatase inhibitors ?Others
Abnormal salt transport	Block Na⁺ uptake Increase Cl⁻ efflux		Amiloride UTP
?Abnormal mucus	Decrease viscosity	Dormase α (rhDNase) (in vitro)	Gelsolin
Impaired clearance	Augment ciliary action	Airway clearance techniques	
?Pseudomonas infection	Reduce bacterial count	Antibiotics	
Inflammatory response	Decrease host reaction	Anti-inflammatory drugs (corticosteroids, ibuprofen)	Antiproteases Pentoxifylline IVIG
Bronchiectasis	Replace irreversibly damaged areas	Lung transplantation	

Fig. 26.9 Treatment of CF airways disease. The pathogenesis of CF lung disease is based on a vicious circle of airway infection, inflammation and obstruction (first column). Treatment can be directed at different pathogenic mechanisms (second column). Currently available and proposed treatment options are shown in final columns. Data from Stacey FitzSimmons.

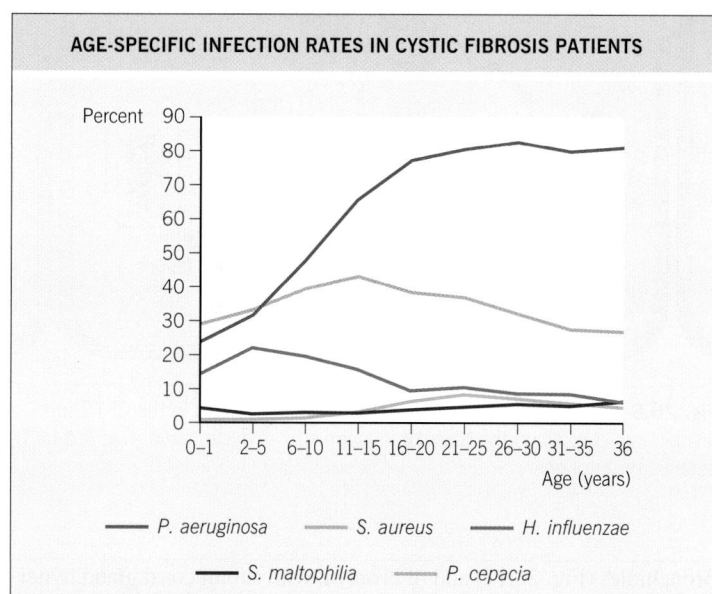

AGE-SPECIFIC INFECTION RATES IN CYSTIC FIBROSIS PATIENTS

Legend:
— P. aeruginosa — S. aureus — H. influenzae
— S. maltophilia — P. cepacia

Fig. 26.10 Age-specific infection rates in CF patients. Bacteria isolated from CF sputum samples vary with age and demonstrate the trend toward *Pseudomonas aeruginosa* as the dominant pathogen. Data from Stacey FitzSimmons.

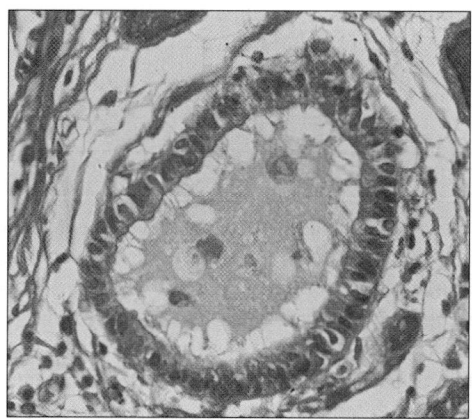

Fig. 26.11 A CF bronchiole is completely occluded by mucoid secretions and surrounded by fibrotic tissue. (H&E stain.)

acute or persistent respiratory symptoms, 42% with failure to thrive or malnutrition, 35% with steatorrhea and 19% with meconium ileus or intestinal obstruction.

Developments in the understanding of the molecular and physiologic pathogenesis of CF have led to additional diagnostic criteria. Cystic fibrosis transmembrane conductance regulator mutational analysis is offered by several companies that test for 6–70 common mutations and can detect mutations in about 95% of CF cases. Abnormal CFTR function in airway epithelia can be assessed by in-vivo measurements of nasal electric potential difference and its response to selected modulators of ion transport.[34] The clinical application of these tests has been summarized by a CF Foundation sponsored consensus committee.[35]

MANAGEMENT

Exocrine pancreatic insufficiency and malnutrition are managed with oral pancreatic enzyme supplementation and dietary supplements. Pulmonary disease causes the major morbidity in CF, and eventually death in 95% of patients. Daily clearance of airway secretions is essential.[36,37] This can be accomplished by chest physiotherapy, which enhances sputum production and increases pulmonary function.[38] Physical exercise augments airway clearance and improves cardiovascular function. Special breathing techniques, including forced expiratory technique, autogenic drainage and active cycle of breathing,[39] have been useful in some individuals. Mechanical devices, including the flutter valve[40] and external thoracic compression devices, may improve patient independence, but their efficacy is less well established.

Antibiotics are used extensively. Acute exacerbations are treated with intravenous antibiotics directed at the major pulmonary pathogens, especially *Pseudomonas* spp. and *Staphylococcus aureus*. Because of the high bacterial burden, two antibiotics with different mechanisms of action and with in-vitro efficacy against each major bacterium are selected. Pharmacokinetic studies of beta-lactams, aminoglycosides and sulfa drugs demonstrate increased clearance in CF patients, necessitating the use of higher doses. Typical antibiotic choices are listed in Figure 26.15. Home intravenous antibiotic therapy has cost and convenience advantages,[41] but its clinical efficacy in

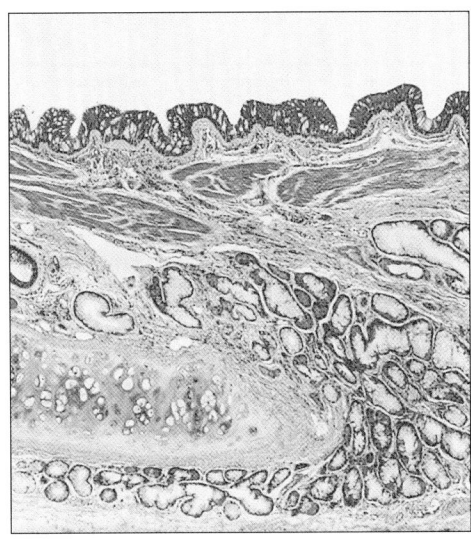

Fig. 26.12 A CF submucosal gland demonstrates marked hypertrophy and dilated gland ducts with mucoid secretions. The surface epithelium has marked goblet cell metaplasia. (H&E stain.)

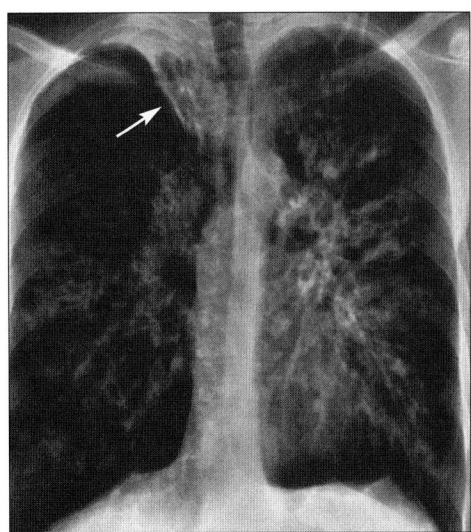

Fig. 26.13 A typical postero-anterior chest radiograph of a 24-year-old man with CF. The lungs are hyperinflated due to airway obstruction and bronchiectasis. The right upper lobe atelectasis (arrow) is chronic.

TYPICAL CLINICAL COURSE FOR CYSTIC FIBROSIS

Fig. 26.14 Typical clinical course of CF. Serial pulmonary function measurements of FEV_1 demonstrate a typical clinical course. Measurements are connected by solid lines during therapy for acute exacerbations, and by dotted lines between such therapy. The lower bars indicate periods of hospital treatment. Pulmonary function decreases and the exacerbations are more frequent and less responsive to treatment in advanced disease. H, Haemophilus; S, Staphylococcus aureus; P, Pseudomonas aeruginosa.

INHALED AND PARENTERAL ANTIBIOTICS COMMONLY USED FOR CF

Parenteral (normally two effective agents against each bacterial isolate)		
Class	Drug	Pertinent efficacy
Aminoglycosides	Gentamicin	Staphylococcus aureus, Haemophilus influenzae, Pseudomonas spp.
	Tobramycin	S. aureus, H. influenzae, Pseudomonas spp.
Beta-lactams	Ceftazidime	Pseudomonas spp.
	Piperacillin	H. influenzae, Pseudomonas spp.
	Ticarcillin/ clavulanate	S. aureus, H. influenzae, Pseudomonas spp.
Monobactam	Aztreonam	Pseudomonas spp.
Carbapenem	Imipenem– cilastatin	S. aureus, H. influenzae, Pseudomonas spp.
Fluoroquinolones	Ciprofloxacin	S. aureus, H. influenzae, Pseudomonas spp.
Sulfa drugs	Trimethoprim– sulfamethoxazole	S. aureus, Burkholderia cepacia
Glycopeptides	Vancomycin	Oxacillin-resistant S. aureus
Aerosolized		
Drug	Common doses	
Tobramycin	80–300mg q12h to q8h	
Colistimethate sodium	75–150mg q12h to q8h	

Fig. 26.15 Inhaled and parenteral antibiotics commonly used for CF. Higher doses of aminoglycosides, beta-lactams and sulfa drugs are required because of increased clearance in CF.

this setting has not been rigorously established. The benefits of chronic oral antibiotics are controversial, but some aerosolized antibiotics have demonstrated efficacy.[42]

Cystic fibrosis patients are particularly susceptible to the complications of massive hemoptysis and pneumothorax. Episodes of massive hemoptysis, defined as more than 240ml blood per 24 hours, are managed with antibiotics, transient cough suppression and reduction in chest physiotherapy, and bronchial artery embolization.[43] Such therapy is usually effective and does not compromise candidacy for eventual lung transplantation. Large pneumothoraces are managed by chest tube drainage. Recurrent pneumothoraces may require repeated chest tubes or abrasion pleurectomy.[44] Hypoxemia is best treated with supplemental oxygen plus standard pulmonary therapy. Ventilatory assistance can be effectively provided by mask ventilation.[45,46]

Lung transplantation has become an effective form of therapy.[47] From the first heart–lung transplant for CF in 1983 to mid-1996, more than 750 heart–lung or sequential double lung transplants (the preferred operation in the USA) for CF have been performed worldwide. Transplant evaluation is indicated when natural survival is expected to be slightly longer than the waiting time for donor organ availability, currently about 2 years. The highly variable progression of CF disease makes prediction difficult, but an FEV_1 of less than 30% predicted or increasing functional impairment with frequent hospitalizations is an accepted referral criterion. The 1 and 5-year survival rates after lung transplantation for CF are 70% and 48%, respectively. These are comparable to the survival rates of patients who receive lung transplants for other diseases. Deaths in the first year are primarily due to operative complications and infections. After one year most deaths are caused by obliterative bronchiolitis, the pathologic marker of chronic rejection. The scanty number of donor organs limits the availability of lung transplantation, and many patients wait more than 2 years after being accepted as a transplant candidate. Living donor transplantation (sequential transplantation of a lower lung lobe from each of two donors) has become an effective alternative in some centers.[48]

REFERENCES

1. Gwaltney JM, Hendley JO, Simon G, Jordan WS. Rhinovirus infections in an industrial population. JAMA 1967;202:494–500.

2. Gwaltney JM. Rhinoviruses. In: Evans AS, Kaslow RA, eds. Viral infections of humans, epidemiology and control, 4th ed. New York: Plenum Medical Book Co; 1997:815–38.

3. Gonzales R, Steiner JF, Sande MA. Antibiotic prescribing for adults with colds, upper respiratory tract infections, and bronchitis by ambulatory care physicians. JAMA 1997;278:901–4.

4. Dantzker DR, Pingleton SK, Pierce JA, et al. Standards for the diagnosis and care of patients with chronic obstructive pulmonary disease (COPD) and asthma. Am Rev Respir Dis 1987;136:225–44.

5. Adams PF, Benson V. Current estimates from the National Health Interview Survey, 1991. National Center for Health Statistics. Vital and Health Statistics 1992; Series 10, No. 184:1–30.

6. Eliasson R, Mossberg B, Camner P, Afzelius BA. The immotile-cilia syndrome. N Engl J Med 1977;297:1–6.

7. Jones DK, Godden D, Cavanagh P. Alpha-1-antitrypsin deficiency presenting as bronchiectasis. Br J Dis Chest 1985;79:301–4.

8. Higgins MW, Keller JB, Becker M, et al. An index of risk for obstructive airways disease. Am Rev Resp Dis 1982;125:144–51.

9. Chodosh S. Treatment of acute exacerbations of chronic bronchitis: state of the art. Am J Med 1991;91(Suppl 6A):87–92.

10. Murray PR, Washington JA. Microscopic and bacteriologic analysis of expectorated sputum. Mayo Clin Proc 1975;50:339–44.

11. Fagon J, Chastre J, Trouillet J, et al. Characterization of distal bronchial microflora during acute exacerbation of chronic bronchitis. Am Rev Resp Dis 1990;142:1004–8.

12. Ferguson GT, Cherniack RM. Management of chronic obstructive pulmonary disease. N Engl J Med 1993;328:1017–22.

13. Easton PA, Jadue C, Dhingra S, Anthonisen NR. A comparison of the bronchodilating effects of a beta2-adrenergic agent (albuterol) and an anticholinergic agent (ipratropium bromide), given by aerosol alone or in sequence. N Engl J Med 1986;315:735–9.

14. Anthonisen NR, Manfreda J, Warren CPW, et al. Antibiotic therapy in exacerbations of chronic obstructive pulmonary disease. Ann Intern Med 1987;106:196–204.

15. Murphy TF, Sethi S. Bacterial infection in chronic obstructive pulmonary disease. Am Rev Respir Dis 1992;146:1067–83.

16. Medical Research Council Working Party. Long-term domiciliary oxygen therapy in hypoxemic cor pulmonale complicating chronic bronchitis and emphysema. Lancet 1981;1:681–6.

17. Nocturnal Oxygen Therapy Trial Group. Continuous or nocturnal oxygen therapy in hypoxemic chronic obstructive pulmonary disease. Ann Intern Med 1980;93:391–8.

18. Petrof BJ, Kimoff RJ, Levy RD, Cosio MG, Gottfried SB. Nasal continuous positive airway pressure facilitates respiratory muscle function during sleep in severe chronic obstructive pulmonary disease. Am Rev Respir Dis 1991;143:928–35.

19. Strumpf DA, Millman RP, Carlisle CC, et al. Nocturnal positive-pressure ventilation via nasal mask in patients with severe chronic obstructive pulmonary disease. Am Rev Respir Dis 1991;144:1234–9.

20. Irwin RS, Pratter MR. A physiologic approach to managing respiratory failure. In: Rippe JM, Irwin RS, Fink MP, Cerra FB, eds. Intensive Care Medicine, 3rd ed. Boston: Little, Brown and Company; 1996:581–6.

21. Barker AF, Bardana EJ. Bronchiectasis: update of an orphan disease. Am Rev Respir Dis 1988;137:969–78.

22. Luce JM. Bronchiectasis. In: Murray JF, Nadel JA, eds. Textbook of respiratory medicine, 2nd ed. Philadelphia: WB Saunders Company; 1996:1398–417.

23. Rosenzweig DY, Stead WW. The role of tuberculosis and other forms of bronchopulmonary necrosis in the pathogenesis of bronchiectasis. Am Rev Respir Dis 1966;93:769–85.

24. Wallace RJ, Glassroth JG, Griffith DE, Olivier KO, Cook JL, Gordin F. Diagnosis and treatment of disease caused by nontuberculous mycobacteria. Am J Respir Crit Care Med 1997;156(Suppl 2):1–25.

25. Liebow AA, Hales MR, Lindskog GE. Enlargement of the bronchial arteries and their anastomoses with the pulmonary arteries in bronchiectasis. Am J Pathol 1949;25:211–31.

26. George SA, Leonardi HK, Overholt RH. Bilateral pulmonary resection for bronchiectasis: a 40 year experience. Ann Thorac Surg 1979;28:48–53.

27. Davis PB, Drumm M, Konstan MW. Cystic fibrosis. Am J Respir Crit Care Med 1997;154:1229–56.

28. Cystic Fibrosis Foundation, Patient Registry. 1996 Annual Data Report. Bethesda, Maryland: Cystic Fibrosis Foundation; August:1997.

29. Bear CE, Li C, Kartner N, et al. Purification and functional reconstitution of the cystic fibrosis transmembrane conductance regulator (CFTR). Cell 1992;68:809–18.

30. Stutts MJ, Canessa CM, Olsen JC, et al. CFTR as a cAMP-dependent regulator of sodium channels. Science 1995;269:847–50.

31. Gabriel SE, Clarke LL, Boucher RC, Stutts MJ. CFTR and outward rectifying chloride channels are distinct proteins with a regulatory relationship. Nature 1993;363:263–6.

32. Highsmith WE, Burch LH, Zhou Z, et al. A novel mutation in the cystic fibrosis gene in patients with pulmonary disease but normal sweat chloride concentrations. N Engl J Med 1994;331:974–80.

33. Smith JJ, Travis SM, Greenberg EP, Welsh MJ. Cystic fibrosis airway epithelia fail to kill bacteria because of abnormal airway surface fluid. Cell 1996;85:229–36.

34. Knowles MR, Paradiso AM, Boucher RC. In vivo nasal potential difference: techniques and protocols for assessing efficacy of gene transfer in cystic fibrosis. Hum Gene Ther 1995;6:445–55.

35. Rosenstein BJ, Cutting GR. The diagnosis of cystic fibrosis: a consensus statement. J Pediatr 1998;132:589–95.

36. Ramsey BW. Management of pulmonary diseases in patients with cystic fibrosis. N Engl J Med 1996;335:179–88.

37. Noone PG, Knowles MR. Standard therapy of cystic fibrosis lung disease. In: Yankaskas JR, Knowles MR, eds. Cystic fibrosis in adults. Philadelphia: Lippincott-Raven Inc.; 1998:145–73

38. Thomas J, Cook DJ, Brooks D. Chest physical therapy management of patients with cystic fibrosis. A meta-analysis. Am J Respir Crit Care Med 1995;151:846–50.

39. Hardy KA. A review of airway clearance: new techniques, indications and recommendations. Respir Care 1994;39:440–5.

40. Konstan MW, Stern RC, Doershuk CF. Efficacy of the Flutter device for airway mucus clearance in patients with cystic fibrosis. J Pediatr 1994;124:689–93.

41. Gilbert DN, Dworkin RJ, Raber SR, Leggett JE. Outpatient antimicrobial-drug therapy. N Engl J Med 1997;337:829–38.

42. Ramsey BW, Dorkin HL, Eisenberg JD, et al. Efficacy of aerosolized tobramycin in patients with cystic fibrosis. N Engl J Med 1993;328:1740–6.

43. Fellows KE, Khaw KT, Schuster S, Shwachman H. Bronchial artery embolization in cystic fibrosis; technique and long-term results. J Pediatr 1979;95:959–63.

44. Egan TM. Thoracic surgery for patients with cystic fibrosis. In: Orenstein DM, Stern RC, eds. Treatment of the hospitalized cystic fibrosis patient. New York: Marcel Dekker, Inc.; 1997:231–47.

45. Hodson ME, Madden BP, Steven MH, Tsang VT, Yacoub MH. Noninvasive mechanical ventilation for cystic fibrosis patients: a potential bridge to transplantation. Eur Respir J 1991;4:524–7.

46. Piper AJ, Parker S, Torzillo PJ, Sullivan CE, Bye PTP. Nocturnal nasal IPPV stabilizes patients with cystic fibrosis and hypercapnic respiratory failure. Chest 1992;102:846–50.

47. Yankaskas JR, Mallory GB. Lung transplantation in cystic fibrosis: consensus conference statement. Chest 1998;113:217–226.

48. Starnes VA, Barr ML, Cohen RG, et al. Living-donor lobar lung transplantation experience: Intermediate results. J Thorac Cardiovasc Surg 1996;112:1284–91.

Community-Acquired Pneumonia

David R Baldwin & John T Macfarlane

Pneumonia can be discussed in a number of different ways. We have chosen the scheme illustrated in Figure 27.1. This chapter concentrates largely on community-acquired pneumonia (CAP) and Chapter 2.28 on hospital-acquired pneumonia, including ventilator-associated pneumonia. Other subjects are covered elsewhere.

EPIDEMIOLOGY

DEFINITION AND CLASSIFICATION

Pneumonia acquired outside hospital is termed CAP. It may be a primary disease occurring at random in healthy individuals or may be secondary to a predisposing factor such as chronic lung disease or diabetes mellitus. It is important to understand that community-acquired lower respiratory tract infection (LRTI) is not synonymous with CAP and only 5–10% of patients who have LRTI actually have pneumonia characterized by radiologic evidence of lung parenchymal disease, which may include lobar or segmental opacification, patchy nonsegmental shadowing or diffuse disease. Figure 27.1 shows a clinically relevant classification of CAP; categories are based on severity and the presence of pre-existing disease. Management of patients in the different categories differs in terms of general supportive measures and specific antimicrobial therapy.

INCIDENCE

Several large studies have measured the incidence of CAP and have reported rates that vary more than 10-fold.[1] A large community study in Seattle, USA in the 1960s and 1970s showed an overall prevalence of 12 per 1000 population for all ages, which was similar to the rate in Finland in 1993 (11.6 per 1000).[2] In England in 1985, a lower rate of 1–3 per 1000 was found for adults, and in Spain in 1992 a similar rate of 2.6 per 1000 was found.[3,4] This difference may in part be explained by differences in the criteria used to define pneumonia. However, when the same criteria

are used, it can be shown that a variety of factors influence incidence: age, race, social deprivation indices,[5] recent admission for pneumonia and host defense factors.[6] In the North American study, prevalence was higher in 0–4 year olds (12–18 per 1000), and in the Finnish study it was higher in 2–5 year olds (36 per 1000) and in those aged over 70 years (34 per 1000). A more recent study from the Mayo Clinic has also shown a rate of pneumonia of 30 per 1000 for patients aged over 65 years.[7]

The attack rate is also influenced by the seasonal pattern of pathogens either causing or predisposing to pneumonia (such as viruses).[8] The seasonal pattern of common pathogens is shown in Figure 27.2. Most respiratory pathogens are more common in the winter months, but notably, legionellosis is more common in the summer and mycoplasma infection occurs in worldwide epidemics every 3–4 years, when it is responsible for approximately 20% of cases of pneumonia. At other times *Legionella* cases are sporadic and account for fewer than 10% of pneumonia cases. Bacterial pneumonia, including that caused by *Streptococcus pneumoniae*, *Haemophilus influenzae* and *Staphylococcus aureus*, are seen at times of peak activity of the influenza virus. Virus infections predispose bacteria normally contained in the nasopharynx to colonize the lower airway. Furthermore, viral infections may encourage more severe infection by impairing host defense mechanisms (see Pathogenesis and pathology). *Streptococcus pneumoniae*, *H. influenzae*, *S. aureus* and *Moraxella catarrhalis* are carried in the nasopharynx to varying degrees (50, 50, 30 and 5–50%, respectively). During epidemics of mycoplasmosis, pharyngeal carriage rates of 13.5% have been reported.[9] *Haemophilus influenzae* and *M. catarrhalis* can also colonize the lower respiratory tract in patients who have chronic obstructive pulmonary disease (COPD). This may reflect their ability to persist in a lower respiratory tract compromised by impaired defenses by producing only a low-grade inflammatory response and thereby not inducing a vigorous immune response.

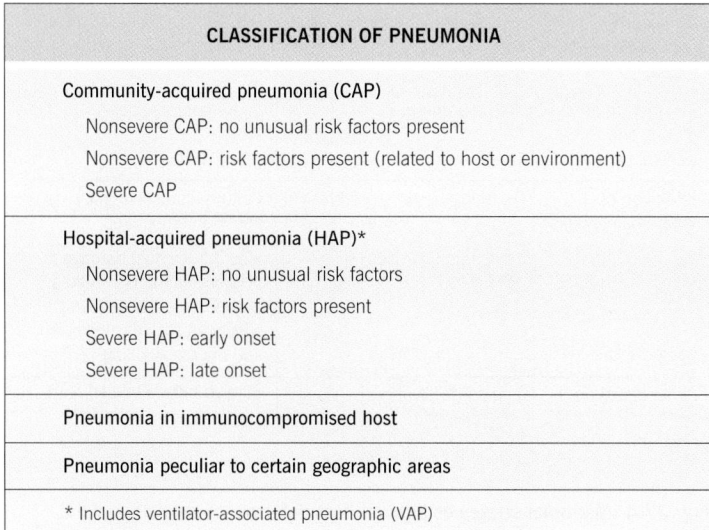

CLASSIFICATION OF PNEUMONIA

Community-acquired pneumonia (CAP)

  Nonsevere CAP: no unusual risk factors present
  Nonsevere CAP: risk factors present (related to host or environment)
  Severe CAP

Hospital-acquired pneumonia (HAP)*

  Nonsevere HAP: no unusual risk factors
  Nonsevere HAP: risk factors present
  Severe HAP: early onset
  Severe HAP: late onset

Pneumonia in immunocompromised host

Pneumonia peculiar to certain geographic areas

* Includes ventilator-associated pneumonia (VAP)

Fig. 27.1 Classification of pneumonia. This classification is designed to provide a practical approach to likely pathogens and their appropriate management.

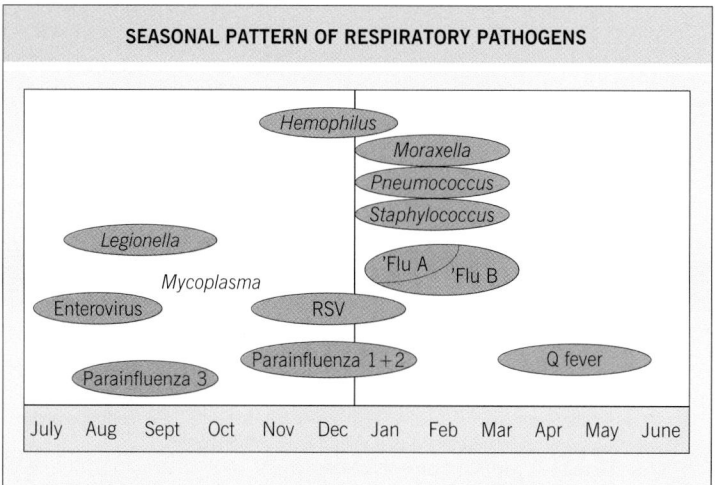

SEASONAL PATTERN OF RESPIRATORY PATHOGENS

Hemophilus
Moraxella
Pneumococcus
Staphylococcus
Legionella
'Flu A
'Flu B
Mycoplasma
Enterovirus
RSV
Parainfluenza 1 + 2
Q fever
Parainfluenza 3

July   Aug   Sept   Oct   Nov   Dec   Jan   Feb   Mar   Apr   May   June

Fig. 27.2 Seasonal pattern of respiratory pathogens in the northern hemisphere. Most respiratory pathogens are commoner in the winter months with the notable exceptions of *Legionella* spp. and *Coxiella burnetii* (Q fever). With permission from Macfarlane.[8]

When *Legionella*, psittacosis and Q fever infections occur in clusters, an environmental source should be sought. *Legionella* infections occur worldwide and are usually sporadic. Their occurence in the summer months may partly be explained by foreign travel and exposure to risk factors such as water systems in public buildings and hotels. Debilitated or immunocompromised patients are particularly vulnerable. *Legionella* organisms are found in native waters, including rivers, lakes, thermal springs and under ice, in industrial coolant water and in water circulating in large buildings and domestic systems. *Legionella* spp. have been cultured from many hot water systems in homes, hotels and hospitals. The organisms are killed by drying but may survive for more than a year in domestic tap water. There is no human or animal reservoir, although algae and amebae may act as environmental hosts. Legionellosis epidemics have occurred in hotels and hospitals; indeed the disease was first recognized in 1976 when an outbreak of severe pneumonia occurred among members of the Pennsylvanian branch of the American Legion who had stayed at a hotel. For an outbreak to occur, it is necessary to have a reservoir, such as an infected water system; bacterial amplification facilitated by stagnation, dirt or sludge; and a water temperature between 68 and 113°F. The bacteria then have to be disseminated via showers, fans, air conditioning, respiratory therapy equipment and possibly, spray taps. Finally the strain of *Legionella* must be pathogenic to humans and be inhaled in sufficient quantity to cause infection.[10]

MORBIDITY AND MORTALITY

Pneumonia is the sixth leading cause of death in the USA and the commonest fatal infectious disease. In the USA as many as 4 million cases occur annually of which one-fifth require hospitalization. Mortality rates vary but are estimated between 1 and 5% overall and up to 25% among patients admitted to hospital. In severe pneumonia mortality rates are higher and may be up to 50% in patients requiring ventilatory support.[11,12] Mortality, as well as attack rate, is influenced by comorbidity. The majority of adult patients who die from CAP have one or more comorbidities such as COPD, ischemic heart disease, diabetes mellitus, malignancy and neurologic disease. These are more often present in the elderly, which partly explains the rising mortality with age.

PATHOGENESIS AND PATHOLOGY

The mode of acquisition varies by pathogen. Most bacterial infections result from aspiration of endogenous organisms resident in the nasopharyngeal secretions, although inhalation of infected droplets may occur from other patients (viral infections), from animals (psittacosis) or from environmental sources (legionellosis).

HOST–PATHOGEN INTERACTIONS

The distal lung contains few commensal micro-organisms despite large numbers present in inspired air and upper airway secretions. A multifaceted defense system maintains this relatively sterile environment, which is overcome or subverted in pneumonia. Figures 27.3 and 27.4 summarize these host defenses and the tactics used by pathogens to overcome them. The majority of bacteria entering the lungs are rapidly removed by local mechanisms such as the mucociliary escalator and cough reflex in combination with local secretory IgA and phagocytosis by macrophages. With more invasive infections, there is a progressive host response with recruitment of circulatory inflammatory cells, augmented by a specific immune response. In normal lungs, over 85% of the cells recovered from the lower airways by bronchoalveolar lavage are alveolar macrophages, but with infection this changes dramatically as outside cells are recruited. Greatly increased numbers of neutrophils

HOST DEFENSE MECHANISMS		
Host defense mechanisms		Mechanism of lung defense
Physical defenses	Nose	Filtering of larger particulate matter
	Cough	Bulk clearance of microbes in secretions
	Mucociliary escalator	
Nonspecific cellular and humoral factors	Immunoglobulins (principally IgA)	Binding of microbes to facilitate removal by the mucociliary escalator or ingestion and destruction by alveolar macrophages or removal via pulmonary lymphatics
	Complement	
	Antiproteases	
	Opsonins	
	Lactoferrin	Depletion of essential nutrients for some bacteria
	Alveolar macrophage	Endocytosis of bacteria and release of toxic oxygen and nitrogen radicals and lysosomal enzymes
		Direct and antibody dependent cytotoxicity, secretion of IFN-γ, TNF and transferrin
	Neutrophil	Endocytosis and generation of oxygen and nitrogen radicals, lactoferrin and lysozyme
Specific immune response	Specific antibody production	Enhanced production of a variety of cytokines, including IFN-γ, IL-2, IL-12, TNF-β, IgA, IgG, IgM, perforins and granzymes
	Macrophage–T-lymphocyte interaction	
	Recruitment of neutrophils, lymphocytes, and natural killer cells	

Fig. 27.3 Host defense mechanisms. The lung has several levels of defense, from mechanical barriers to a specific immune response. These processes have overlapping cellular and humoral effects.

MICROBIAL STRATEGIES AGAINST HOST DEFENSE		
Microbial strategy	Organism	Mediators/mechanisms
Inhibition of ciliary function	*Pseudomonas aeruginosa*	Phenazine pigments
	Streptococcus pneumoniae	Pneumolysin
	Haemophilus influenzae	Unidentified low molecular weight compound
Damage to cilia	*Pseudomonas aeruginosa*	Pyocyanin (a phenazine pigment)
	S. pneumoniae	Pneumolysin
	H. influenzae	Lipopolysaccharide (endotoxin)
Adherence to components of mucus	*H. influenzae, P. aeruginosa*	Pili, fibrils
Penetration of mucus and adherence	Influenza viruses	Viral neuraminidases
Inhibition of inflammatory cells	*H. influenzae*	Culture filtrates inhibit neutrophil migration
	Respiratory viruses	May induce host damage to phagocytes through cellular expression of foreign antigen effects on mobility, ingestion and microbial killing
Avoid detection	*Legionella*, fungi, mycobacteria	Survive intracellularly
	Respiratory viruses	

Fig. 27.4 Microbial strategies against host defense. A knowledge of the mechanisms of microbial counter-defense can be useful in the clinical setting. For example, it is important to use antibacterial agents that are active in the intracellular environment when treating *Legionella* and mycobacterial infections.

are seen in conventional bacterial pneumonias such as those produced by the pneumococcus. In *Legionella* and viral infections, a lymphocyte infiltrate often predominates. Other inflammatory cells are found in lesser numbers, for example natural killer cells.[13,14]

INFLAMMATORY CELL RECRUITMENT

Recruitment of cells from the lung interstitium and blood to the site of infection occurs through nonspecific and specific immune reactions. Nonspecific reactions include the local production of a variety of chemotactic and proinflammatory cytokines by resident lung macrophages and epithelial cells. In addition, a specific immune response is generated. Macrophages and dendritic cells process antigens to smaller molecules that are displayed on the cell surface as part of the major histocompatibility complex (MHC) locus. Antigen presentation requires direct CD4+ T-lymphocyte–macrophage/dendritic cell contact via intercellular adhesion molecules. The T-lymphocyte receptor binds to MHC class II molecules on the antigen presenting cell and at the same time binds the intracellular adhesion molecule-1 to its ligand lymphocyte function associated antigen-1. The latter provides additional costimulation of lymphocytes. Antigen presentation may occur in the lung interstitium, the bronchus-associated lymphoid tissue and the intrapulmonary lymph nodes. As a result a variety of cytokines are produced; interleukin (IL)-1 is secreted by antigen presenting cells, and this in turn induces IL-2 production by memory T lymphocytes. Interleukin-2 in a potent inducer of T-lymphocyte activation and proliferation.[15]

CELL-MEDIATED ANTIMICROBIAL ACTIVITY

T-lymphocyte activation and cytokine production stimulate other cells to increase antimicrobial function. For example, interferon (IFN)-γ increases macrophage antimicrobial function by enhancing MHC expression and augmenting oxygen-dependent and -independent microbial killing. This mechanism acts on intracellular pathogens and inhibits growth of respiratory pathogens such as *Legionella* spp., mycobacteria, pathogenic fungi, *Pneumocystis carinii* and *Chlamydia* spp. There are many other host defense cytokines (see Fig. 27.3) that may interact and have common activities. They may act to stimulate or suppress host defense reactions. When viruses reach the lower airways they interact with macrophages that normally resist invasion and replication through the production of IFNs. Macrophages can also reduce virus replication in neighboring cells. If a specific antibody to the virus is present, this can neutralize virus via induction of natural killer cells, T lymphocytes, IFN-γ secretion and lysis by complement.

COUNTER-DEFENSE MECHANISMS EMPLOYED BY PATHOGENS

Pathogenic organisms have a variety of virulence factors that may contribute to the inhibition of normal defense mechanisms. For example, many bacteria inhibit ciliary function, thus decreasing the efficacy of clearance from the lung (see Fig. 27.4). Others may exist in the mucous layer without stimulating a significant host response, thus subverting detection and, when clearance is impaired as in COPD, may colonize the airway. Other bacteria may avoid host defenses by surviving and replicating intracellularly such as *Legionella* and *Mycobacterium* spp.; the former exist inside membrane-bound vacuoles, which resist lysosomal fusion and acidification. Respiratory viruses can interfere with the mucociliary escalator and also produce factors such as neuraminidases, which facilitate penetration of mucus and attachment to the epithelial cells. This predisposes to bacterial colonization and secondary infection. Viruses affect phagocytic mobility, ingestion and microbial killing. Specific antibodies directed against defense cells expressing viral antigens may further impair their function.[16]

GROSS PATHOLOGY AND HISTOLOGY

The interactions between host and pathogen result in the histopathologic features of pneumonia. Initially there is alveolar congestion and an exudate rich in fibrin and red blood cells. Macroscopically the consolidated lung appears rather like liver, hence the term 'red hepatization'. Later in the course of the illness the lung becomes more gray (gray hepatization) as a result of infiltration with neutrophils and other inflammatory cells. The consolidated lobe sometimes shows multiple abscess formation (Fig. 27.5) or, occasionally, frank necrosis. These features are more often present in *S. aureus*, *Klebsiella pneumoniae* and anaerobic infections.

ETIOLOGY

A key factor guiding therapy for CAP is knowledge of the spectrum of potential pathogens. Major factors that influence this spectrum are age (infection in children differs from that in adults and the elderly); severity (as defined by clinical criteria); and the presence of comorbidity, commonly chronic cardiorespiratory disease, diabetes mellitus, neurologic deficit or immunodeficiency as a result of drugs or disease. Geographic variation is also important, for example tuberculosis is a relatively common cause of CAP in Hong Kong[17] and Q fever in Nova Scotia, Canada and northern Spain. The causative pathogens and their approximate relative frequencies are summarized in Figure 27.6.[18–21]

In adults, 60–80% of CAP cases are caused by bacteria, 10–20% are 'atypical' and 10–15% are viral. *Streptococcus pneumoniae* is the commonest pathogen and is responsible for 30–50% of cases. In most series, no pathogen is identified in 30% of cases. The majority of these are also thought to be pneumococcal infections in which identification has not been made because of prior antibiotic therapy or lack of sputum for microbiologic investigations during the initial phase of the illness. The frequency of viral and atypical pneumonias may also be underestimated because the acute and convalescent serum samples required for diagnosis are often not obtained. During epidemics, *Mycoplasma pneumoniae* is the next most common pathogen, accounting for up to 23% of cases. Nontypeable (unencapsulated) *H. influenzae* is the next most common pathogen. It may cause pneumonia in previously healthy individuals but is more common in patients who have pre-existing lung disease. In some series, in which subgroups of patients who have COPD have been studied, *H. influenzae* is more common.[22]

Influenza virus is the most common cause of viral pneumonia and frequently precedes secondary bacterial pneumonia. Psittacosis, Q fever and *Legionella* spp. each account for 2% of cases. *Legionella* infection is more often found in hospital-based surveys of CAP and exhibits a geographic variation such that studies in Spain have shown up to 14% of cases caused by *Legionella* spp., slightly less than that for the pneumococcus (15%). Community-acquired pneumonia caused by *S. aureus* is uncommon but important because of its severity even in previously healthy individuals. A similar pattern of causative organisms is found in studies from Europe, Australia and New Zealand, but studies in North America more frequently report enteric Gram-negative bacilli (EGNB), aspiration and staphylococcal infections. This may be explained by the higher proportion of debilitated patients and drug and alcohol misusers in the study population. Two large studies from the USA and Canada found the pneumococcus to be a less frequent cause of CAP, but this may reflect different criteria for diagnosis of pneumonia.[23,24]

In children, the spectrum of pathogens and disease is different (Fig. 27.6). The major LRTIs are bronchiolitis in infants under 6 months of age, pneumonia in the first 2 years of life and laryngotracheobronchitis in the second and third years of life. Respiratory syncytial virus (RSV) is the main cause of bronchiolitis, although adenovirus, parainfluenza virus type 3, rhinovirus and influenza A have been implicated. There are two important subtypes of RSV, type A and B. Epidemics occur yearly and coincide with the coldest winter month. Respiratory syncytial virus type A is the most common and tends to be the most severe. Pneumonia in children under the age of 2 years is usually caused by RSV, parainfluenza, influenza or adenovirus, but less commonly by enterovirus, rhinovirus, measles virus, varicella-zoster virus and *Coxiella burnetii*. Respiratory syncytial virus is the most important cause in infants. Neonatal pneumonia usually follows premature rupture of the membranes, allowing the fetus to swallow amniotic fluid contaminated with vaginal organisms. Perinatal pneumonia is usually hospital acquired secondary to invasive procedures and therefore is usually caused by EGNB and *S. aureus*.

In a study of 121 children hospitalized for LRTI in Helsinki, a cause was found in 69%: bacterial infection in 25%, viral in 25% and multiple organisms in 20%. *Mycoplasma pneumoniae* was more common with increasing age, as were bacterial infections. In Finland, 195 children hospitalized with pneumonia were surveyed over 12 months.[25] A viral infection alone was indicated in 19%, a bacterial infection alone in 15% and a mixed viral and bacterial infection in 16% of patients; 46% of the 69 patients who had viral infection and 52% of the 62 patients who had bacterial infection had a mixed viral and bacterial etiology. Respiratory syncytial virus was identified in 52 patients and *S. pneumoniae* in 21%. The next most common agents were nontypeable *H. influenzae* (9%), adenoviruses (5%) and *Chlamydia* spp. (4%). In Uruguay etiology was determined in 47.7% of 541 cases; 38.6% were viruses and 12.6% bacteria. Viral and mixed etiologies were more frequent in children under 12 months of age. Bacteria predominated in infants aged between 6 and 23 months. Among the viruses, RSV predominated (66%). The bacterial pneumonias accounted for 12.2% of the recognized etiologies. The most important bacterial agents were *S. pneumoniae* (64%) and *H. influenzae* (19%).[26]

PREVENTION

Methods for the prevention of CAP include vaccination, prophylactic antibiotic therapy, elimination of environmental sources and maintenance of good hygiene. In practice the only vaccines used to prevent CAP are pneumococcal, influenza, measles and *H. influenzae* b vaccines. Measles vaccine helps to prevent pneumonia, which may follow this disease, especially in malnourished children. Similarly, influenza may predispose to secondary bacterial pneumonia in addition to causing primary CAP. Influenza viruses A and B (especially A) regularly alter their surface hemagglutinin and neuraminidase antigens. It is essential therefore that influenza vaccine contains the components of the prevalent strains, which are defined each year by the World Health Organization. Influenza vaccine is recommended for all ages and especially the elderly with the following conditions: chronic respiratory disease, including asthma; chronic heart disease; chronic renal failure; diabetes mellitus and other endocrine disorders; and immunosuppression

as a result of disease or treatment. Residents of nursing or residential homes for the elderly or other long-term care institutions should also be vaccinated. Currently, influenza vaccines give 70–80% protection against vaccine strains, although this is less in the elderly.[27]

A 23-valent capsular polysaccharide vaccine provides immunity against the most common serotypes causing pneumococcal pneumonia. It covers nearly 90% of those serotypes that cause severe disease in the UK. Overall efficacy in preventing bacteremic pneumococcal pneumonia is 60–70%, although the vaccine is not effective in children under 2 years of age or in the immunocompromised. It has been relatively ineffective in patients who have multiple myeloma, Hodgkin's and non-Hodgkin's lymphoma (especially during treatment) and in chronic alcoholism. It does not prevent otitis media in children or reduce the frequency of exacerbations of chronic bronchitis. It is also uncertain whether it prevents nonbacteremic CAP. In the UK, immunization is recommended to all those over the age of 2 years who are at special risk of pneumococcal infection or in whom infection might be unusually severe. This includes patients who have homozygous sickle-cell disease, asplenia or severe dysfunction of the spleen, chronic renal disease or nephrotic syndrome, immunodeficiency or immunosuppression as a result of disease or treatment (including HIV disease), chronic heart, lung or liver disease (including cirrhosis) and diabetes mellitus.[27]

Varicella-zoster immunoglobulin therapy is indicated to prevent infections in exposed, susceptible individuals, who may develop severe fulminating pneumonia. Such patients include the immunocompromised, neonates and pregnant women, and those who possess no antibodies to varicella-zoster virus and have had significant exposure to chicken pox or herpes zoster.[27] Oral aciclovir or famciclovir may also be used to prevent varicella-zoster infection in this population.

Prophylactic antibacterial drugs have only limited use in the prevention of CAP. Long-term oral penicillin is recommended in patients

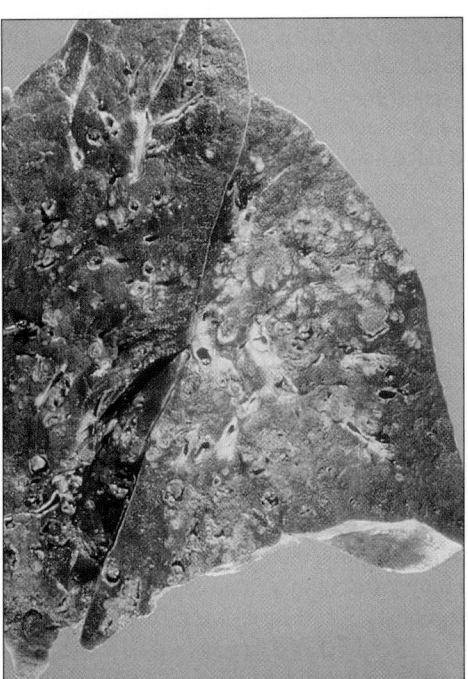

Fig. 27.5 Multiple discrete areas of consolidation with abscess formation is a classic feature of *S. aureus* pneumonia. With permission from Macfarlane JT, Finch RG, Colton RE. A colour atlas of respiratory infections. London: Chapman & Hall, 1993.

USUAL CAUSES OF COMMUNITY-ACQUIRED PNEUMONIA			
Age group	Pathogens		Percentage of total
Adults and the elderly	Core pathogens	*Streptococcus pneumoniae*	30–50
		Respiratory viruses	15
		Mycoplasma pneumoniae (during epidemics)	5–23
	Additional risk factors present	*Haemophilus influenzae*	15–35
		Staphylococcus aureus	4
		Moraxella catarrhalis	2–10
		Legionella pneumophila	0.5
		Influenza virus	5
Severe (adults and elderly)	Core pathogens	*S. pneumoniae*	30
		L. pneumophila	15
		S. aureus	4
	Unusual	*M. pneumoniae*	2
		H. influenzae	1
		Klebsiella pneumoniae	
		Varicella-zoster	
Children – less than 2 years	Core pathogens	Respiratory syncytial virus	25
		Other viruses	13
		Mixed viral and bacterial	25
		S. pneumoniae	8
		H. influenzae type b	2
2–15 years	Core pathogens	*S. pneumoniae*	25
		M. pneumoniae	10
		Mixed infections	15
		S. aureus	5
		H. influenzae type b	2

Fig. 27.6 Usual causes of community-acquired pneumonia. The most common pathogens in each category are shown with estimates of the overall percentage contributions. Core pathogens are those most commonly encountered and may be modified in severe adult CAP and by the presence of risk factors such as pre-existing lung disease and debility (see also Fig. 27.9).

under 16 years of age at particular risk of pneumococcal infection, for example after splenectomy.

Prevention may also require identification and elimination of an environmental source of infection. If two or more cases of *Legionella* pneumonia, psittacosis or Q fever occur, a search for a potential reservoir of infection should be made. The relevant public health officials should be informed. For legionellosis, contaminated water systems should be cleaned and sterilized by hyperchlorination and heat. *Legionella* colonization can be prevented by the use of correctly designed water systems, including sealed tanks, and regular heat or hyperchlorination treatment.

CLINICAL FEATURES

GENERAL SYMPTOMS AND SIGNS

Symptoms may be constitutional and nonspecific, such as malaise, anorexia, headache, myalgia, arthralgia, sweating and rigors. Specific symptoms to pneumonia or a specific pathogen also occur. In viral and mycoplasma infections, constitutional symptoms may be preceded by upper respiratory tract symptoms of sore throat, sneezing, nasal discharge and blockage. High pyrexia and rigors are common in the young who have pneumococcal and *Legionella* infections. In contrast, the elderly or seriously ill may have minimal or no fever. Cough is the most common respiratory symptom and is present in over 80% of cases, followed by dyspnea in 60–70%, pleural pain in 60%, new sputum production in over 50% and hemoptysis in 15%.[11,28] Sputum is initially mucoid or absent, particularly with atypical and *Legionella* infections. Purulent sputum develops later, although in patients who have pre-existing chronic bronchitis or bronchiectasis it is present at the outset.

Nonrespiratory symptoms may be more prominent and mask the diagnosis. Marked confusion may occur with any pneumonia, especially in the elderly who may have no physical signs other than an elevated respiratory rate and localizing chest signs. Confusion is also more common in *Legionella* and psittacosis pneumonias. A prominent headache in association with confusion or impaired consciousness raises the possibility of *Legionella* infection or co-existent meningitis, especially in pneumococcal pneumonia. Lower lobe pneumonia may present with abdominal pain mimicking acute abdominal or urinary tract pathology.

The duration of history is variable. Usually, symptoms have been present for several days before hospital admission; however, it is important to realize that patients who have pneumococcal or staphylococcal infection may become critically ill within hours, whereas in mycoplasma infection symptoms can be present for 2–3 weeks.

Classic signs of lobar consolidation are infrequent and it is more common to hear localized crackles. If pneumonia is complicated by parapneumonic pleural effusion or empyema, lower zone dullness to percussion and reduced breath sounds may be present. Abdominal tenderness is not unusual, especially in lower lobe pneumonia or if there is associated hepatitis. There are no specific symptoms and signs that permit a confident clinical diagnosis of a particular etiology, although some pathogens are more often associated with a particular pattern.[29] Commonly recognized patterns of pneumonic illness are described in Figure 27.7 and the pathogens that may be responsible are listed. Occasionally a specific clinical feature or characteristic pattern may suggest a specific pathogen. For example, herpes labialis is more common in pneumococcal pneumonia, and erythema nodosum and erythema multiforme in *Mycoplasma* infection. The rash of chickenpox is always present with varicella pneumonia. *Mycoplasma* pneumonia and Q fever have a variety of extrapulmonary manifestations that, if present, may point to the diagnosis. Classic and some specific features of the more common pathogens are shown in Figure 27.8. Figure 27.9 gives a more comprehensive list of clues in the history and examination that may suggest a specific pathogen.

DIFFERENTIAL DIAGNOSIS OF PNEUMONIA

Pneumonia is most commonly confused with pulmonary infarction and pulmonary edema, and indeed may co-exist with either of these conditions. Careful attention to the exact sequence of the events in the history, for example when establishing whether there was a prodrome of symptoms suggesting upper respiratory infection, may help point to pneumonia. Even with expert interpretation of examination findings and basic investigations the diagnosis may still be obscure and further investigations may be indicated. In practice, treatment is often given for more than one condition whilst further investigations are awaited. Pulmonary embolism may need to be excluded by ventilation perfusion scanning or pulmonary angiography. Less common differential diagnoses include primary or metastatic lung cancer, pulmonary eosinophilia and acute allergic or cryptogenic alveolitis. Hepatic or subphrenic abscess, pancreatitis or perforated peptic ulcer may mimic basal pneumonia.

DIAGNOSIS

The purpose of investigations in CAP are:
- to confirm the diagnosis of pneumonia,
- to determine etiology,
- to assess severity,
- to determine the impact of the illness on any underlying conditions, such as COPD or cardiac failure, and
- to provide data for epidemiologic purposes.

They can be broadly divided into general investigations, which help with the first three, and those that are mainly aimed at determining etiology.

CHEST RADIOGRAPHY, BIOCHEMISTRY AND HEMATOLOGY

A chest radiograph is required for diagnosis of CAP and usually shows lobar or segmental opacification in bacterial pneumonias and in the majority of atypical infections. Less commonly patchy peribronchial shadowing or more diffuse nodular or ground-glass opacification is seen, particularly in viral and atypical infections. The lower lobes are most commonly affected in all types of pneumonia, and small pleural effusions can be detected in about one-quarter of cases, especially if a lateral decubitus film is taken. Multilobar pneumonia is a feature of severe disease, and spread to other lobes despite appropriate antibiotics is seen in *Legionella* and *M. pneumoniae* infections. Hilar lymphadenopathy is unusual except in *Mycoplasma* pneumonia, particularly in children. Cavitation is uncommon but is a classic feature of *S. aureus* and *S. pneumoniae* serotype 3 infections.

Clearance of radiographic changes usually occurs after about 8 weeks but varies from 2 weeks to many months depending on the age of the patient, the severity of pneumonia, the presence of pre-existing lung disease and the pathogen. The rates of resolution of radiographic pulmonary shadows in different pneumonias are shown in Figure 27.10.[30] Bacteremic pneumococcal pneumonia and *Legionella* infections are particularly slow to clear. After resolution of the illness it is important to arrange a further chest radiograph, as unsuspected malignant disease is surprisingly common. One study revealed the presence of unsuspected malignant disease in 7% of pneumonia cases (17% if limited to smokers) in patients over the age of 60 years.[3]

A full blood count, renal, electrolyte and liver biochemical profiles, a blood glucose and an erythrocyte sedimentation rate or C reactive protein are useful general investigations. In most cases of pneumonia caused by *S. pneumoniae* or *H. influenzae*, the white blood cell count is above 15×10^9/l; it is usually marginally raised in *Legionella* infections ($11–15 \times 10^9$/l). Mildly raised hepatic enzymes and bilirubin are not uncommon in bacterial pneumonias, particularly if there is bacteremia. Raised blood urea, hyponatremia, hypokalemia, hypoalbuminemia, hyperglycemia, proteinuria and hematuria can be present in all severe pneumonias, but none indicates etiology. Hyponatremia is seen in 50% of patients who have *Legionella* pneumonia.

MICROBIOLOGIC INVESTIGATIONS

For identification of the pathogen, sputum and pleural fluid (if an effusion is present) should be Gram stained and cultured. Sputum Gram staining can provide a specific and rapid diagnosis in about one-fifth of cases of pneumococcal and staphylococcal pneumonia, when large numbers of a predominant organism are usually seen. Sputum culture is less specific because it is often contaminated with upper respiratory tract organisms, and it is not produced in one-quarter to one-third of patients in the early stages of pneumonia. In addition, even a single dose of antibiotic can prevent a positive culture of *S. pneumonia* and *H. influenzae*, and this occurs in over one-half of patients admitted to hospital in the UK. Even in the presence of untreated bacteremic pneumococcal pneumonia, sputum culture is negative in over one-half of the patients. Blood cultures are positive in less than one-quarter of patients who have bacterial pneumonia who present to hospital, but when they are positive they are usually specific.

Antigen detection, serology and other investigations

Antigen detection is useful for diagnosis of CAP caused by *S. pneumoniae*, encapsulated forms of *H. influenzae*, *Mycoplasma* and *Chlamydia* spp. (including specific identification of *Chlamydia pneumoniae*), and *Legionella pneumophila* serogroup 1. Detection of pneumococcal polysaccharide capsular antigen is particularly helpful as it may be detected in 80% of sputa, 36–45% of urine and 9–23% of serum.[31,32] Mycoplasma antigen detection is a new test that improves the rate of diagnosis; *Legionella* antigen is present in urine in the first

week of the illness before serum antibodies are detectable. The most useful diagnostic tests are shown in Figure 27.11.

Serologic methods are used to diagnose viral, atypical and *Legionella* infections. A four-fold or greater increase in specific antibody titer in blood taken early in the course of the illness and after 10–14 days is evidence of recent infection, and high unchanging titers are suggestive. The main limitation of serology is that the diagnosis is obtained too late to influence initial management. This forces the adoption of an empiric approach to the choice of antibiotic. Specific IgM antibody detection can be used to obtain a more rapid diagnosis in mycoplasma and *Legionella* infections, although their sensitivity and specificity varies. Direct fluorescent antibody tests are available for staining respiratory secretions to detect *Legionella* spp. and some viruses, although these are

---

PATHOGENS AND THEIR USUAL PATTERN OF CLINICAL PRESENTATION

Clinical presentation	Organism
Abrupt onset of severe pneumonia, with fever, rigors and signs of lobar consolidation	*Streptococcus pneumoniae*, *Staphylococcus aureus*, *H. influenzae*, *Legionella* spp., *Streptococcus pyogenes*, *Klebsiella pneumoniae*, *Neisseria meningitidis*, *Yersinia pestis* (plague), *Pseudomonas pseudomallei* (rare)
Indolent or low-grade infection associated with pre-existing lung disease	*Haemophilus influenzae*, *S. pneumoniae*, *Moraxella catarrhalis*, *Chlamydia pneumoniae*, *Pasteurella multocida*, *Pseudomonas aeruginosa* *Staphylococcus aureus*
Prodromal flu-like or predominantly upper respiratory tract symptoms, followed by pneumonia	*Mycoplasma* spp., *Chlamydia* spp., *Legionella* spp., *Coxiella burnetii*, Respiratory viruses
Extrapulmonary manifestations	*Mycoplasma* spp. (variety see Fig. 27.9), *Coxiella* spp. (variety see Fig. 27.9), Herpesviruses (skin and mucocutaneous), *Yersinia pestis* (lymphadenopathy), *Leptospirosis* (renal and hepatic), *Legionella* spp.
Tuberculosis-like illness	*Klebsiella pneumoniae* (chronic form), *Pseudomonas pseudomallei* (melioidosis), *Mycobacteria* spp., e.g. *kansasii*, *Cryptococcus neoformans*
Locally invasive disease with abscess and sinus formation	*Actinomycetes* spp., *Nocardia* (immunocompromised host), *Pseudomonas mallei* (Glanders), *Eikenella corrodens*
Diarrhea	*Legionella* spp., *S. pneumoniae* *Coxiella burnetii*, tularemia (*Francisella tularensis*)
Organisms that may cause pneumonia as a rare complication of main infection	*Salmonella typhi* or *paratyphi* (Enteric fever), *Brucella abortus* (Brucellosis), *Bacillus anthracis* (Anthrax), *Listeria monocytogenes*

Fig. 27.7 Pathogens and their usual pattern of clinical presentation. Although it is usually not possible to say which pathogen is responsible for CAP on clinical criteria alone, it is helpful to have some understanding of the usual pattern of illness for common pathogens.

CLASSIC FEATURES OF MORE COMMON PATHOGENS AND CLINICAL POINTERS TO DIAGNOSIS

Organism	Classic features
Streptococcus pneumoniae	Abrupt onset over hours with rigors, fever, malaise, tachycardia and tachypnea. Dry cough initially, then productive of 'rusty' sputum. Less acute presentation (possibly modified by antibiotics). Worsening of cardiac or respiratory failure, confusion or general physical deterioration in elderly or debilitated. Herpes labialis.
Staphylococcus aureus	Rapid onset of fever, confusion and respiratory distress, often after influenza. May be secondary to infected intravenous cannulae or right-sided endocarditis. Multiple pulmonary abscesses, empyema. Look for a potential source.
Haemophilus influenzae	Two forms: typable strains cause acute severe infection with lobar consolidation in children; vaccination has dramatically reduced this. Nontypeable strains cause patchy bronchopneumonia with persistent purulent sputum and malaise. Subacute bronchopneumonia in patients with pre-existing lung disease.
Legionella spp.	Two forms: Pontiac fever – acute self-limiting flu-like illness. Pneumonia – abrupt onset with high fever, rigors, malaise and myalgia. Slight cough, in half, severe headache, confusion and delirium, diarrhea and abdominal pain. Neurologic (cerebellar) signs. Renal failure.
Klebsiella spp.	Acute severe pneumonia with thick, tenacious bloodstained sputum, commonly affects the right upper lobe. Dense consolidation on chest radiograph with 'bulging fissures'.
Mycoplasma spp.	Upper respiratory tract symptoms such as sore throat and coryza followed after 4–7 days by fever, dry cough and dyspnea. In some cases erythema nodosum, erythema multiforme, Stevens–Johnson syndrome, myringitis, splenomegaly, generalized lymphadenopathy and salivary gland enlargement.
Chlamydia spp.	Psittacosis – mild flu-like illness to fulminating pneumonias with multiple organ failure. Macular rash (Horden's spots) rarely in psittacosis. Diarrhea occurs in 25%. *Chlamydia pneumoniae* commonly causes sore throat, prominent cough, prolonged bronchitis in young adults and mild pneumonia.
Coxiella spp.	Q Fever manifests with a flu-like illness and pneumonia of varying severity. Multisystem involvement – arthritis, thrombophlebitis, arteritis, pericarditis, myocarditis and chronic endocarditis, particularly of the aortic valve.
Influenza	Flu symptoms – fever, rigors, myalgias may be followed by severe pneumonia or by secondary bacterial pneumonia. Epidemics (occasionally pandemics) in winter months.
Viruses*	Coryzal infection, cough and rarely pneumonia.
Herpesvirus	Both varicella-zoster and herpes simplex may cause severe pneumonia, which follows 2–3 days after clinical evidence of infection (cutaneous lesions). Rash of chickenpox in varicella. Cold sore or primary oral lesions in herpes simplex.

* Parainfluenza, RSV, adenovirus, coronavirus, coxsackie virus

Fig. 27.8 Classic clinical features of pneumonia caused by specific pathogens. Although classic clinical features are described in most texts, in practice there may be considerable overlap.

not universally available. Cold agglutinins are present in about 50% of *Mycoplasma* infections but are a nonspecific finding.

Viral isolation, culture and identification is a lengthy process and is of little practical value in most cases. However, in difficult cases when no diagnosis has been reached and there is no resolution it may provide a diagnosis, particularly in the immunocompromised host. Amplification of DNA from a variety of pathogens using the polymerase chain reaction has been attempted but these techniques remain under investigation.

In patients in whom the diagnosis is obscure, who fail to respond to empiric treatment or who are particularly ill or immunocompromised, invasive techniques may be indicated to sample lower respiratory secretions or lung tissue. These include fiberoptic bronchoscopy with lavage, quantitative culture and protected bronchial brush (see Invasive

techniques Chapter 2.28), percutaneous needle aspiration and lung biopsy (transbronchial or open). Whenever invasive techniques are used and when an unusual diagnostic test is indicated, it is most important for clinicians and as microbiologists, to liaise. This allows a decision about the most appropriate tests and the correct samples and ensures the laboratory is ready to process the samples.

MANAGEMENT

The management of CAP depends on the severity of the illness, the presence of underlying disease and the age of the patient. At best, immediate diagnostic tests may identify the pathogen in fewer than 30% of cases and therefore an empiric antibiotic regimen is necessary. The spectrum of organisms in the elderly and younger adult is similar, but it differs in children. In severe pneumonia, *Legionella* infection is more frequently found and hence different empiric antibiotics are required. Similarly, *H. influenzae* is more often found in patients who have pre-existing lung disease.

ASSESSMENT OF SEVERITY
Studies of CAP have identified several prognostic factors on the basis of clinical and investigative features (see Fig. 27.12). The most consistent early predictors of death are:
- a respiratory rate >30/min,
- a diastolic blood pressure of ≤60mmHg, and
- a blood urea of >7mmol/l.

If two or more of these features are present, the chance of death is increased 9- to 20-fold.[11,33]

GENERAL MANAGEMENT
All patients who have CAP, whether managed at home or in hospital, should rest in bed, have adequate oral fluids and should not smoke. Simple analgesics or nonsteroidal anti-inflammatory drugs can be given for pleural pain and fever. Chest physiotherapy is only

HISTORY AND EXAMINATION FINDINGS THAT SUGGEST A SPECIFIC DIAGNOSIS	
History	Pathogen
Alcoholism	*Klebsiella pneumoniae, S. pneumoniae* *S. aureus,* anaerobes
Chronic obstructive pulmonary disease	*S. pneumoniae, H. influenzae* *M. catarrhalis*
Animal exposure	
Birds	*Chlamydia psittaci* (psittacosis)
Rats, squirrels, rabbits	*Yersinia pestis* (plague), tularemia
Rats, mice	*Leptospira* spp.
Horses	*Pseudomonas mallei* (glanders)
Cats	*Coxiella burnetii* (Q fever), *Pasteurella multocida*
Cattle, sheep, goats	*C. burnetii*
Corticosteroid therapy	*S. aureus, M. tuberculosis, Pneumocystis carinii, Legionella* spp.
AIDS/immunocompromised/iv drug abuse	*Mycobacterium* spp., *Pneumocystis carinii,* fungal diseases, cytomegalovirus
Travel	
Thailand, SE Asia	*Pseudomonas pseudomallei* (melioidosis)
Asia, Africa, Central and South America	*Paragonimus westermani* (paragonimiasis)
Exposure to contaminated water systems	*L. pneumophila*
Examination	Pathogen
Skin	
Erythema multiforme	*Mycoplasma pneumoniae*
Maculopapular rash	Measles
Erythema nodosum	*Chlamydia pneumoniae*
Erythema gangrenosum	*M. tuberculosis, Pseudomonas aeruginosa, Serratia marcescens*
Mouth	
Dental caries	Anaerobic pneumonia
Herpes simplex	*S. pneumoniae*
Ears	
Bullous myringitis	*M. pneumoniae*
Neurology	
Poor gag reflex; altered conscious level; recent seizure	Aspiration
Cerebellar ataxia	*M. pneumoniae, L pneumophila*
Encephalitis	*M. pneumoniae, C. burnetii*

Fig. 27.9 History and examination findings that suggest a specific diagnosis. Specific clinical features may occasionally point to a specific pathogen and may influence management.

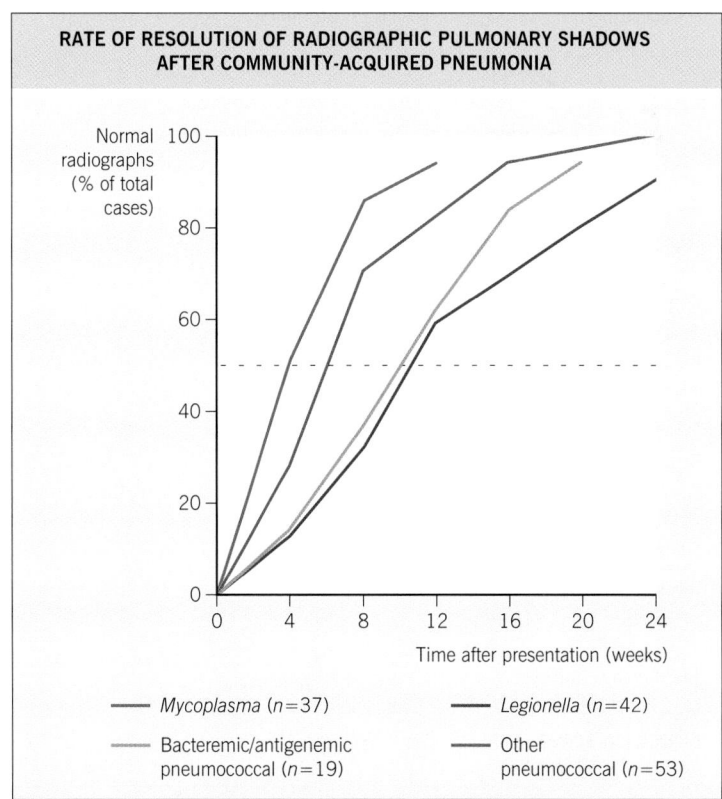

RATE OF RESOLUTION OF RADIOGRAPHIC PULMONARY SHADOWS AFTER COMMUNITY-ACQUIRED PNEUMONIA

Normal radiographs (% of total cases)

Time after presentation (weeks)

— *Mycoplasma* (*n*=37)   — *Legionella* (*n*=42)
— Bacteremic/antigenemic pneumococcal (*n*=19)   — Other pneumococcal (*n*=53)

Fig. 27.10 Rate of resolution of radiographic pulmonary shadows after community-acquired pneumonia. Pneumonia can take 4–8 weeks to clear radiographically even in less severe cases such as *Mycoplasma* pneumonia. More severe pneumonias such as *Legionella* and bacteremic pneumococcal pneumonia take longer to resolve, sometimes up to 6 months. Data from Macfarlane *et al.*[30]

INVESTIGATIONS AIMED AT DETERMINING ETIOLOGY OF CAP

Investigation		Comments
General microbiology	Sputum Gram stain	Rapid and widely available
		Low sensitivity (10%)
		High specificity if positive (70–80%)
	Sputum culture	Prior antibiotics and contamination with oropharyngeal bacteria is a problem
	Blood culture	Positive in 20–25% of bacterial pneumonias and relates to etiology and prognosis
	Pleural fluid stain and culture	Essential to exclude empyema
	Nasopharygeal swabs	Useful in children, used to diagnose viral infections
Serologic tests	Acute and convalescent sera	Retrospective diagnosis of viral, atypical and *Legionella* infections
	Cold agglutinins	Positive in about 50% of cases of *Mycoplasma* infection
	Antigen detection	Pneumococcal-sputum positive in 80%, urine in 36–45%, serum in 9–23% *Legionella* spp., encapsulated forms of *Haemophilus influenzae*, *Mycoplasma* spp., *Chlamydia* spp. and specifically *Chlamydia pneumoniae* and *Legionella pneumophila* serogroup 1
Invasive tests	Transtracheal aspiration, bronchoalveolar lavage (BAL), protected specimen bronchial brush (PSB), percutaneous needle biopsy, lung biopsy	Consider in patients who are immunocompromised, who fail to respond. Bronchoalveolar lavage and PSB are most often used

Fig. 27.11 Investigations aimed at determining etiology of community-acquired pneumonia. Immediate diagnosis is only possible in about 15% of cases of CAP. Even in research studies in which extensive investigations have been performed, no causative organism is identified in 30% of cases.

FEATURES DISTINGUISHING SEVERE PNEUMONIA (FROM DIFFERENT SOURCES)

Features associated with poor outcome	Factors associated with increased mortality (from a large meta-analysis[11])	OR/CI (95%)
Clinical	Clinical	
Age >60 years	Male sex	1.3 (1.2–1.4)
Pre-existing medical illness	Hypothermia	5.0 (2.4–10.4)
Confusion	Systolic hypotension	4.8 (2.8–8.3)
New atrial fibrillation	Tachypnea	2.9 (1.7–4.9)
Respiratory rate >30/min*	Diabetes mellitus	1.3 (1.1–1.5)
Diastolic blood pressure ≤60mmHg*	Neoplastic disease	2.8 (2.4–3.1)
Cyanosis	Neurologic disease	4.6 (2.3–8.9)
Investigations	Investigations	2.8 (2.3–3.6)
White blood cells < 4 x 10⁹/l or > 30 x 10⁹/l	Bacteremia	2.5 (1.6–3.7)
	Leukopenia	3.1 (1.9–5.1)
Blood urea >7mmol/l*	Multilobar radiographic shadows	
Hypoxia (PaO_2 <8kPa)		
Multilobar or spreading radiographic shadows		

*Two or more of these three features increase risk of death by 9- to 21-fold.[29]

Fig. 27.12 Features distinguishing severe pneumonia. Severity of pneumonia has been determined by identifying those factors that are associated with increased risk of death. Some (*) are consistently identified in different studies and are used as a basis for guiding management.

useful if patients have a pre-existing lung disease, such as chronic bronchitis or bronchiectasis, that may lead to sputum retention. patients who have moderate or severe CAP should be admitted to hospital and receive oxygen supplementation by face mask. Patients who have severe pneumonia should be monitored in a high dependency unit and if necessary transferred to intensive care. The danger period is in the first 3–4 days after admission. In severe CAP the onset of progressive cardiorespiratory failure can be very rapid and assisted ventilation with inotropic support can preserve life while a response to antibiotics is awaited. Generally, previously fit adults will require ventilation if they are unable to maintain a PaO_2 of 8kPa with maximum supplemental oxygen. Assisted ventilation may be required for many days or weeks before successful weaning. In one study of severe CAP some patients weaned after 4 weeks of ventilation have survived.[34] An algorithm for the management of CAP in adults is shown in Figure 27.13.

ANTIBIOTIC THERAPY

Appropriate empiric antibiotic therapy choices are based on guidelines from five different countries (Fig. 27.14).[12,35–37] The choices vary according to age, severity of illness, history of pre-existing

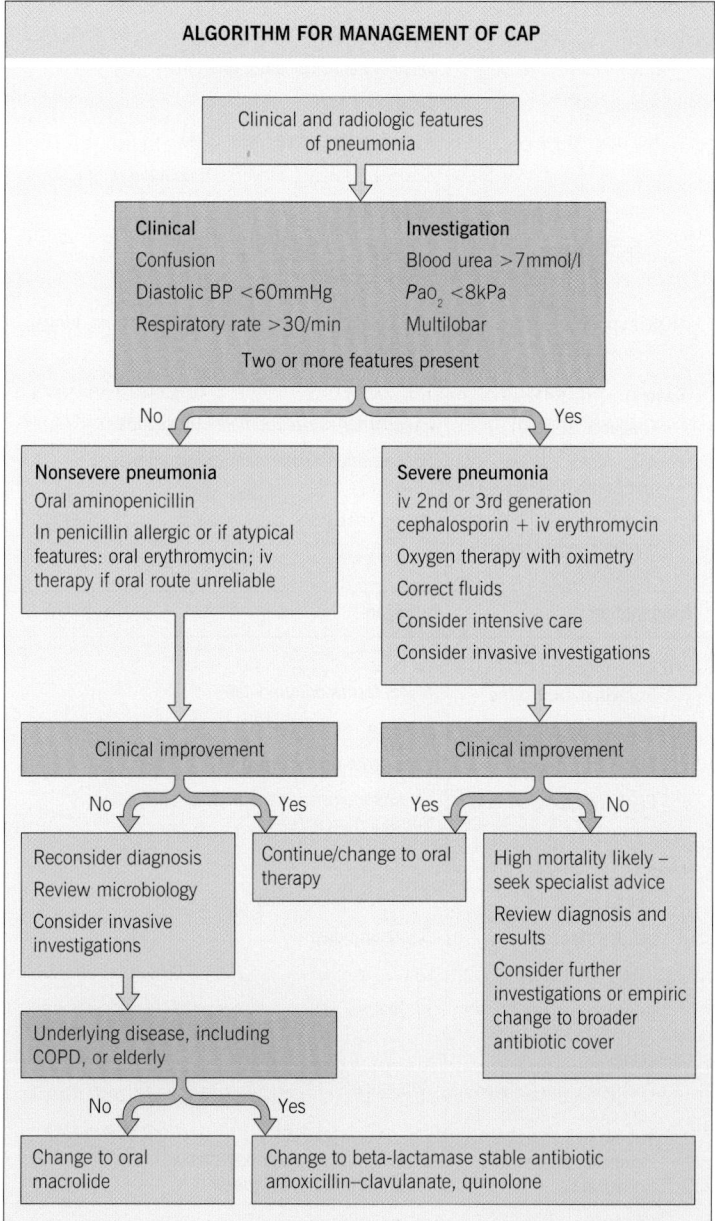

Fig. 27.13 Algorithm for the management of community-acquired pneumonia. Adapted from the Nottingham City Hospital CAP Guidelines, 1996.

	Guidelines from different countries	Age <60 years; no comorbidity	Age >60 years† and/or comorbidity	Patients requiring hospitalization but not intensive care	Patients with severe pneumonia requiring intensive care
1st choice	American/Canadian	Macrolide	2nd generation cephalosporin	2nd or 3rd generation cephalosporin	Macrolide + 3rd generation cephalosporin with antipseudomonal activity
	British	Aminopenicillin	Aminopenicillin	Aminopenicillin	Macrolide + 2nd or 3rd generation cephalosporin
	French	Amoxicillin	Oral cephalosporin		Macrolide + 3rd generation cephalosporin
	Spanish	Penicillin/ampicillin	2nd or 3rd generation cephalosporin		Macrolide + 3rd generation cephalosporin
2nd choice	American/Canadian	Tetracycline	Trimethoprim–sulfamethoxazole or beta-lactam + beta-lactamase inhibitor or macrolide	Macrolide or beta-lactam + beta-lactamase inhibitor	Macrolide + imipenem–cilastin ciprofloxacin or other broad-spectrum antipseudomonal
	British	Macrolide or 2nd or 3rd generation cephalosporin	Macrolide or 2nd or 3rd generation cephalosporin		Ampicillin + flucloxacillin + macrolide
	French	Macrolide	Amoxicillin–clavulanate (co-amoxyclav)		Macrolide + amoxicillin–clavulanate
	Spanish	Macrolide*	Amoxicillin–clavulanate		Quinolone + 3rd generation cephalosporin

EMPIRIC ANTIBIOTIC THERAPY FOR COMMUNITY-ACQUIRED PNEUMONIA

* Spanish guidelines state that macrolides should be used if an atypical syndrome is present.
† French >75 years.

Fig. 27.14 Empiric antibiotic therapy for community-acquired pneumonia. A summary of recommendations from five countries is shown. Not all countries give specific recommendations for all categories of pneumonia.

chest disease and presence of penicillin hypersensitivity. In practice, most patients who have mild or moderate pneumonia can be managed with oral antibiotics, although there are large differences between oral and intravenous blood and tissue concentrations for some agents. Penicillins and quinolones are well absorbed and generally have an oral bioavailability of over 60% of serum. The newer third-generation cephalosporins have approximately 30% oral bioavailability, which may fall if the patient is not eating. Newer macrolides also have approximately 30% oral bioavailability but the most commonly used, erythromycin, has only 5–11%, depending on the preparation; thus a 500mg dose will at best be equivalent to only 50mg given intravenously. Antibiotics vary in their gastrointestinal side effects. The penicillins, quinolones and tetracyclines are relatively well tolerated, cephalosporins (especially oral third-generation) and new macrolides less so, and erythromycin causes enough side effects to warrant discontinuation of treatment in 10–30% of patients (depending on the preparation).

Adult nonsevere community-acquired pneumonia

In this category, *S. pneumoniae* is the most common organism, although other organisms may be a reason for a poor response. In the presence of pre-existing lung disease *H. influenzae* must be considered. An aminopenicillin such as oral amoxicillin or intravenous ampicillin is an appropriate choice. In patients allergic to penicillin, erythromycin can be substituted. If there is no improvement after 48 hours then the diagnosis should be reviewed and therapy adjusted if the pathogen has been identified. If pre-existing chest disease is present amoxicillin–clavulanate, a quinolone (ofloxacin or ciprofloxacin) or a parenteral cephalosporin such as cefuroxime can be substituted to cover beta-lactamase producing *H. influenzae* or *M. catarrhalis*. If there is no underlying pulmonary disease then erythromycin may be substituted to cover *M. pneumoniae* infections. Erythromycin is a less satisfactory choice for elderly patients because of the infrequency of atypical pathogens in this group and its poor activity against *H. influenzae*.

Adult severe community-acquired pneumonia

In severe infection, *Legionella* spp. becomes more important and therefore erythromycin and a beta-lactamase stable beta-lactam (such as cefuroxime or amoxicillin–clavulanate) is recommended initially.

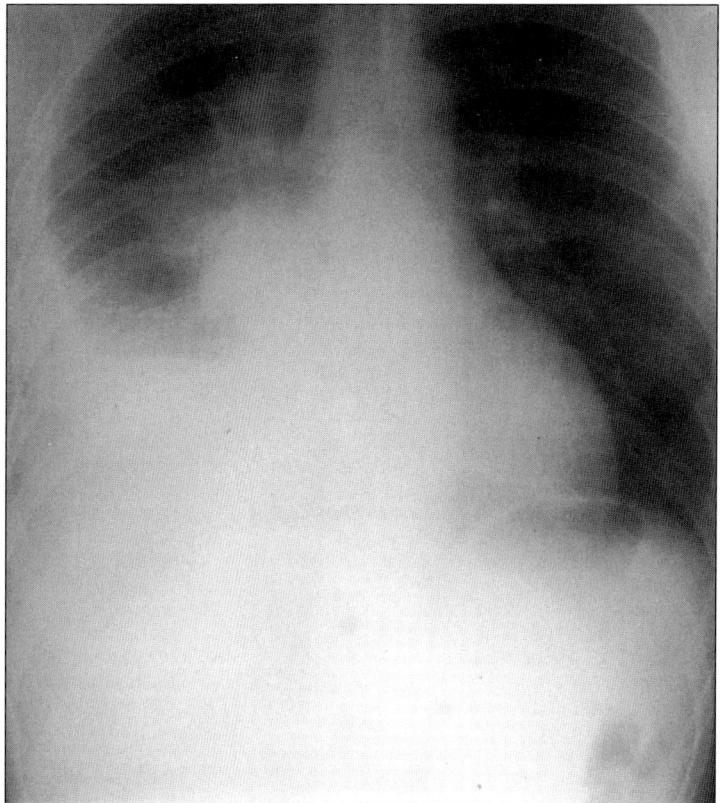

Fig. 27.15 Chest X-ray showing a right sided lobar pneumonia with right empyema in a 25-year old man who was training for the British Rowing Team. Prompt treatment with intercostal drainage ensured he recovered without loss of lung function.

This will cover all likely pathogens, including the commoner (pneumococcal, staphylococcal and *Legionella*) infections. It is important to start antibiotic therapy as soon as possible and to use the intravenous route, although once there is clear clinical improvement this can be changed to the oral route. If there is no response to treatment, specialist advice should be sought. The diagnosis should be reviewed with all available clinical and laboratory data and consideration given to invasive diagnostic techniques. If *Legionella* infection is thought to be a possible cause, then rifampin or ciprofloxacin may be added to erythromycin. Some studies have suggested that clarithromycin may be more effective than erythromycin, but there have been no randomized controlled trials. Consideration should also be given to the possibility of secondary hospital-acquired pneumonia and appropriate antibiotics administered.

The duration of antibiotic therapy is debatable and is best dictated by clinical improvement associated with some knowledge of the half-life of the drug in plasma and tissues. In uncomplicated mild or moderate pneumonia a 5- to 7-day course is usually adequate. Patients started on intravenous therapy may be transferred to oral therapy 24 hours after there has been a clear improvement with resolution of fever, and they should receive antibiotics for 5–10 days thereafter. Prolonged therapy may be required if lung cavitation occurs.

COMPLICATIONS

Most patients recover from CAP without complications. In about one-quarter of patients a small proteinaceous sympathetic effusion develops and resolves spontaneously. Such effusions may cause persistent fever after resolution of pneumonia even if all organisms have been eliminated. They should always be sampled to exclude empyema, which, if present, will require drainage (Fig. 27.15). Pulmonary abscess and pneumothorax are important complications which are discussed in Chapter 2.28.

REFERENCES

1. Macfarlane JT. An overview of community acquired pneumonia with lessons learned from the British Thoracic Society Study. Semin Respir Infect 1994; 9:153–65.
2. Jokinen C, Heiskanen L, Juvonen H, *et al.* Incidence of community-acquired pneumonia in the population of four municipalities in eastern Finland. Am J Epidemiol 1993;137:977–88.
3. Woodhead MA, Macfarlane JT, McCracken JS, Rose DH, Finch RG. Prospective study of the aetiology and outcome of pneumonia in the community. Lancet 1987;i:671–4.
4. Almirall J, Morato I, Riera F, *et al.* Incidence of community-acquired pneumonia and *Chlamydia pneumoniae* infection: a prospective multicentre study. Eur Respir J 1993;6:14–8.
5. Victora CG, Fuchs SC, Flores JA, Fonseca W, Kirkwood B. Risk factors for pneumonia among children in a Brazilian metropolitan area. Pediatrics 1994;93:977–85.
6. Hedlund JU, Ortqvist AB, Kalin M, Scalia-Tomba G, Giesecke J. Risk of pneumonia in patients previously treated in hospital for pneumonia. Lancet 1992;340:396–7.
7. Houston MS, Silverstein MD, Suman VJ. Community-acquired lower respiratory tract infection in the elderly: a community-based study of incidence and outcome. J Am Board Fam Pract 1995;8:347–56.
8. Macfarlane J. Community-acquired pneumonia. Br J Dis Chest 1987;81:116–27.
9. Gnarpe J, Lundback A, Sundelof B, Gnarpe H. Prevalence of *Mycoplasma pneumoniae* in subjectively healthy individuals. Scand J Infect Dis 1992;24:161–4.
10. Meyer RD. *Legionella* infections: a review of five years of research. Rev Infect Dis 1983;5:258–78.
11. Fine MJ, Smith MA, Carson CA, *et al.* Prognosis and outcomes of patients with community-acquired pneumonia. A meta-analysis. JAMA 1996;275:134–41.
12. Niederman MS, Bass JB Jr, Campbell GD, *et al.* Guidelines for the initial management of adults with community-acquired pneumonia: diagnosis, assessment of severity, and initial antimicrobial therapy. American Thoracic Society. Medical Section of the American Lung Association. Am Rev Respir Dis 1993;148:1418–26.
13. Rose RM. The host defense network of the lungs: an overview. In: Niederman MS, Sarosi GA, Glassroth J, eds. Respiratory infections. A scientific basis for management. Philadelphia: WB Saunders; 1994:3–16.

14. Stockley RA. Humoral and cellular mechanisms. In: Brewis RA, Corrin B, Geddes DM, Gibson GJ, eds. Respiratory medicine, 2nd ed. London: WB Saunders; 1995:192–218.
15. Flores I, Casaseca T, Martinez-A C, Kanoh H, Merida I. Phosphatidic acid generation through interleukin 2 (IL-2)-induced alpha-diacylglycerol kinase activation is an essential step in IL-2-mediated lymphocyte proliferation. J Biol Chem 1996;271:10334–40.
16. Jakab GJ, Warr GA. Immune enhanced phagocytic dysfunction in pulmonary macrophages infected with parainfluenza 1 (Sendai) virus. Am Rev Respir Dis 1981;124:575–81.
17. Hui KP, Chin NK, Chow K, *et al.* Prospective study of the aetiology of adult community acquired bacterial pneumonia needing hospitalisation in Singapore. Singapore Med J 1993;34:329–34.
18. Bohte R, van Furth R, van den Broek PJ. Aetiology of community-acquired pneumonia: a prospective study among adults requiring admission to hospital. Thorax 1995;50:543–7.
19. Ortqvist A, Hedlund J, Grillner L, *et al.* Aetiology, outcome and prognostic factors in community-acquired pneumonia requiring hospitalization. Eur Respir J 1990;3:1105–13.
20. Venkatesan P, Gladman J, Macfarlane JT, *et al.* A hospital study of community acquired pneumonia in the elderly. Thorax 1990;45:254–8.
21. Anonymous. Community-acquired pneumonia in adults in Br hospitals in 1982–1983: a survey of aetiology, mortality, prognostic factors and outcome. The British Thoracic Society and the Public Health Laboratory Service. Q J Med 1987;62:195–220.
22. Carr B, Walsh JB, Coakley D, Mulvihill E, Keane C. Prospective hospital study of community acquired lower respiratory tract infection in the elderly. Respir Med 1991;85:185–7.
23. Marrie TJ, Durant H, Yates L. Community-acquired pneumonia requiring hospitalization: 5-year prospective study. Rev Infect Dis 1989;11:586–99.
24. Fang GD, Fine M, Orloff J, *et al.* New and emerging etiologies for community-acquired pneumonia with implications for therapy. A prospective multicenter study of 359 cases. Medicine 1990;69:307–16.
25. Nohynek H, Eskola J, Laine E, *et al.* The causes of hospital treated acute lower respiratory tract infection in children. Am J Dis Child 1991;145:618.
26. Hortal M, Suarez A, Deleon C, *et al.* Etiology and severity of community acquired pneumonia in children from Uruguay: a 4-year study. Revista do Instituto de Medicina Tropical de Sao Paulo 1994;36:255–64.

27. Anonymous. Immunisation against infectious disease. London: HMSO; 1996.
28. Woodhead MA, Macfarlane JT. Comparative clinical and laboratory features of legionella with pneumococcal and mycoplasma pneumonias. Br J Dis Chest 1987;81:133–9.
29. Farr BM, Kaiser DL, Harrison BD, Connolly CK. Prediction of microbial aetiology at admission to hospital for pneumonia from the presenting clinical features. British Thoracic Society Pneumonia Research Subcommittee. Thorax 1989;44:1031–5.
30. Macfarlane JT, Miller AC, Roderick Smith WH, Morris AH, Rose DH. Comparative radiographic features of community acquired Legionnaires' disease, pneumococcal pneumonia, mycoplasma pneumonia, and psittacosis. Thorax 1984;39:28–33.
31. Miller J, Sande MA, Gwaltney JM Jr, Hendley JO. Diagnosis of pneumococcal pneumonia by antigen detection in sputum. J Clin Microbiol 1978;7:459–62.
32. Spencer RC, Savage MA. Use of counter and rocket immunoelectrophoresis in acute respiratory infections due to *Streptococcus pneumoniae*. J Clin Pathol 1976;29:187–90.
33. Farr BM, Sloman AJ, Fisch MJ. Predicting death in patients hospitalized for community-acquired pneumonia. Ann Intern Med 1991;115:428–36.
34. Woodhead MA, Macfarlane JT, Rodgers FG, Laverick A, Pilkington R, Macrae AD. Aetiology and outcome of severe community-acquired pneumonia. J Infect 1985;10:204–10.
35. Anonymous. Guidelines for the management of community-acquired pneumonia in adults admitted to hospital. The British Thoracic Society. Br J Hosp Med 1993;49:346–50.
36. Mandell LA, Marrie TJ, Niederman MS. Initial antimicrobial treatment of hospital acquired pneumonia in adults: a conference report. Can J Infect Dis 1993;4:317–21.
37. Woodhead M. Empirical antibiotic therapy and lower respiratory tract infections: European guidelines and current practices. Monaldi Arch Chest Dis 1995;50:472–6.
38. Chien SM, Pichotta P, Siepman N, Chan CK. Treatment of community-acquired pneumonia. A multicenter, double-blind, randomized study comparing clarithromycin with erythromycin. Canada-Sweden Clarithromycin-Pneumonia Study Group. Chest 1993;103:697–701.
39. Schonwald S, Barsic B, Klinar I, Gunjaca M. Three-day azithromycin compared with ten-day roxithromycin treatment of atypical pneumonia. Scand J Infect Dis 1994;26:706–10.

Hospital-Acquired Pneumonia

John T Macfarlane & David R Baldwin

EPIDEMIOLOGY

DEFINITION

Hospital-acquired pneumonia (HAP) is defined as pneumonia that occurs more than 48 hours after hospital admission, excluding any infection incubating at the time of admission.[1] Ventilator-associated pneumonia (VAP) can be regarded as a particular subgroup of HAP for which the incidence, etiology, investigation and outcome are somewhat different. It should be remembered that patients recently discharged from hospital who develop pneumonia may have an illness with features more in keeping with hospital-acquired rather than community-acquired infection.

INCIDENCE AND SIZE OF THE PROBLEM

Pneumonia is the third most common type of infection acquired in hospital after urinary tract and surgical wound infection and is associated with the highest mortality. Hospital-acquired pneumonia is estimated to occur in 300,000 hospitalized patients each year in the USA. It adds 5–9 days to the hospital stay of survivors[2,3] and billions of dollars to health care costs. Up to 1% of hospitalized patients may acquire nosocomial lung infection;[2,3] the incidence varies with type of hospital and ward. The incidence is lowest in district hospitals and on general medical and pediatric wards, and higher in teaching hospitals (presumably because of the increased complexity of medical cases). The highest incidence is found in the intensive care unit (ICU). The attack rate of pneumonia for patients receiving assisted ventilation rises progressively with length of stay in the ICU;[4,5] prevalences of up to 50% have been reported after 7 days of mechanical ventilation.[6,7]

MORTALITY

Crude mortality rates for HAP range up to 70%.[8] This is misleading as pneumonia may not be the true cause of death in patients who have multiple pathology. Pneumonia has been estimated to be the 'attributable cause' of death in one-third to one-half of patients who develop HAP.[1,2,8]

PATHOGENESIS AND ETIOLOGIC AGENTS

PATHOGENESIS

Factors associated with the pathogenesis of HAP are summarized in Figure 28.1.[9] Hospital-acquired pneumonia is usually caused by the aspiration of bacteria that colonize the upper respiratory tract into the lungs. Aspiration of upper respiratory tract secretions is usually the result of impaired mechanical host defense; subsequent colonization of the lower airway is facilitated by debility, defective host defense and changes in bacterial mucosal adherence factors. Less commonly other mechanisms may be involved, including hematogenous spread of infection to the lungs from a distant focus and inhalation of pathogens aerosolized either from contaminated respiratory equipment (e.g. ventilator or nebulizer equipment) or from the hospital environment (e.g. showers and water systems colonized with *Legionella* bacteria).

Microaspiration of pharyngeal secretions is usually clinically silent and occurs even in healthy subjects during sleep but becomes very frequent in patients who have reduced consciousness.[2] Aspiration is almost inevitable in intubated patients because the normal laryngeal barrier between the oropharynx and the lower respiratory tract is compromised. Secretions pool above the cuff of the endotracheal tube from where they leak into the lower airway. In the healthy individual, aspirated secretions can be dealt with effectively by lung defenses, including mucociliary clearance and alveolar macrophages. When host defenses are impaired, bacteria are able to proliferate and cause pneumonia.

The oropharynx of debilitated patients becomes colonized rapidly by enteric Gram-negative bacteria (EGNB). These bacteria are not normally present in the upper respiratory tract and the frequency of colonization increases with increasing severity of the underlying illness. Up to three-quarters of critically ill patients become colonized within a few days of hospital admission.[2,3] Oropharyngeal colonization is often a harbinger of subsequent pneumonia.[10]

Colonization of the lower respiratory tract is facilitated by changes in respiratory epithelial cells that favor bacterial adherence. Alteration of cell surface carbohydrates, loss of surface fibronectin and alteration of epithelial cell bacterial receptors all contribute to enhanced colonization by pathogenic bacteria.[2,10,11]

CAUSATIVE ORGANISMS

The pathogens associated with HAP have been studied extensively. However, variations in the patient populations studied, the methods used to obtain and analyze specimens and the definitions used for HAP have, until recently, made it difficult to obtain a sensible overview of the problem. Fortunately, guidelines from the American Thoracic Society,[1] the Canadian Consensus Conference[12] and other reviews[8] are now in existence; these propose a classification of the pathogens causing HAP that is both sensible and practical. The approach relies on assessing three factors, including disease severity, the presence of comorbid disease and other risk factors for specific pathogens, and the time of onset of the pneumonia, in considering likely pathogens and therefore guiding initial antibiotic selection.

The spectrum of potential pathogens associated with HAP is different from that of community-acquired pneumonia. The bacterial pathogens most frequently associated with HAP are EGNB and *Staphylococcus aureus*. Mixed infections are not unusual, particularly in VAP. The role of viruses has not been widely studied, but is likely to be important, especially at times of community outbreaks of viral infection, when staff and visitors may transmit viral infection to hospitalized patients.

A group of 'core' pathogens must be considered in all cases of HAP. These include EGNB (e.g. *Enterobacter* spp., *Escherichia coli*, *Klebsiella* spp., *Proteus* spp. and *Serratia marcescens*) *Haemophilus influenzae* and Gram-positive organisms such as *Streptococcus pneumoniae* and methicillin-sensitive *S. aureus*. Other pathogens, in addition to the 'core' pathogens, must be considered in certain circumstances. These include resistant Gram-negative organisms such as *Pseudomonas aeruginosa*, *Enterobacter* spp., *Klebsiella pneumoniae* and *Acinetobacter* spp., methicillin-resistant *S. aureus* (MRSA), *Legionella* spp. and anaerobic organisms. The potential pathogens can be categorized into three groups depending on the severity of the pneumonia, the presence of comorbid disease or prior antibiotic therapy, and the length of hospitalization.

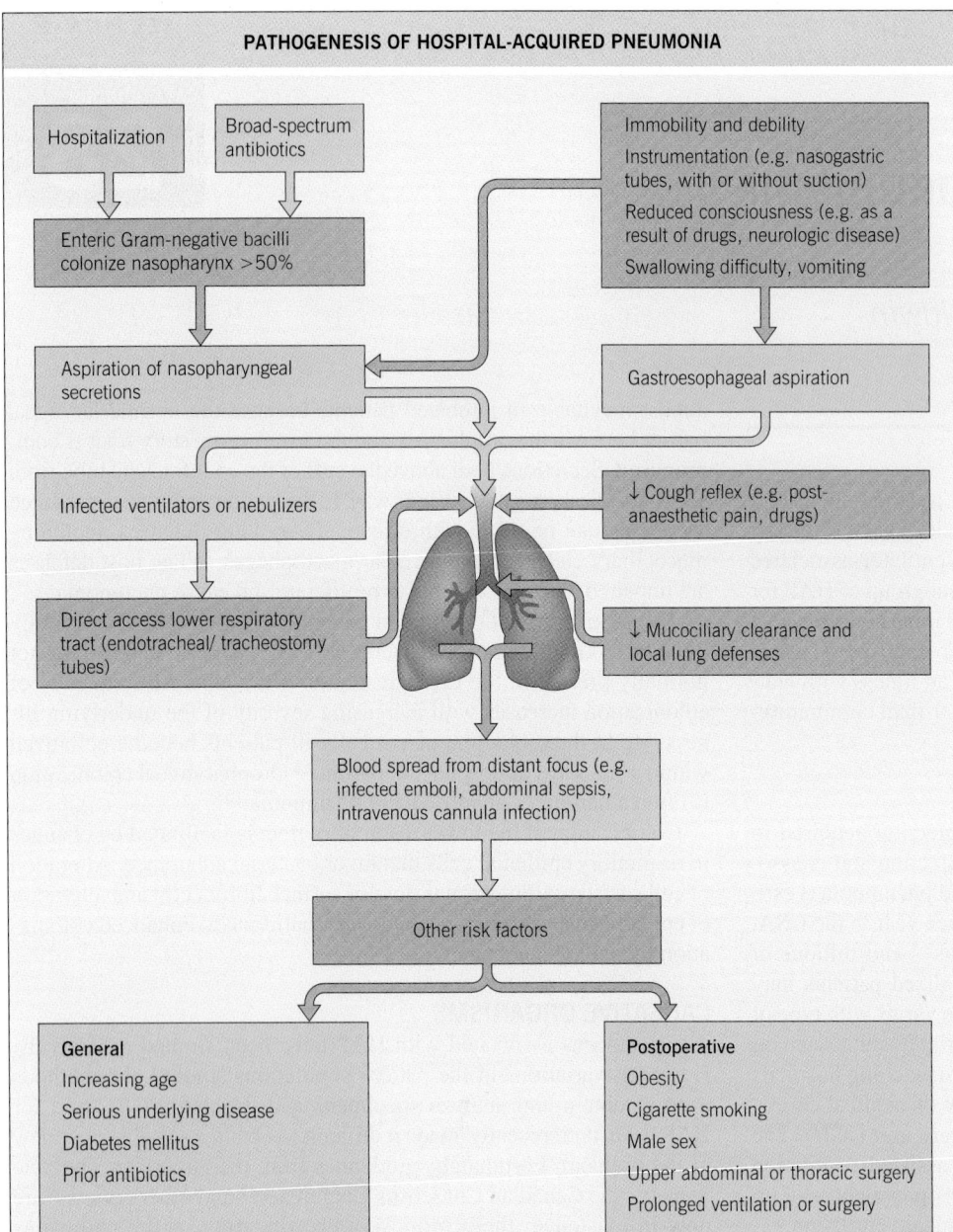

Fig. 28.1 **Factors involved in the pathogenesis of hospital-acquired pneumonia.** With permission from Macfarlane, 1986.[9]

PATHOGENESIS OF HOSPITAL-ACQUIRED PNEUMONIA

Hospitalization → Enteric Gram-negative bacilli colonize nasopharynx >50%

Broad-spectrum antibiotics → Enteric Gram-negative bacilli colonize nasopharynx >50%

Immobility and debility

Instrumentation (e.g. nasogastric tubes, with or without suction)

Reduced consciousness (e.g. as a result of drugs, neurologic disease)

Swallowing difficulty, vomiting

Enteric Gram-negative bacilli colonize nasopharynx >50% → Aspiration of nasopharyngeal secretions

Gastroesophageal aspiration

Infected ventilators or nebulizers

↓ Cough reflex (e.g. post-anaesthetic pain, drugs)

Direct access lower respiratory tract (endotracheal/ tracheostomy tubes)

↓ Mucociliary clearance and local lung defenses

Blood spread from distant focus (e.g. infected emboli, abdominal sepsis, intravenous cannula infection)

Other risk factors

General
Increasing age
Serious underlying disease
Diabetes mellitus
Prior antibiotics

Postoperative
Obesity
Cigarette smoking
Male sex
Upper abdominal or thoracic surgery
Prolonged ventilation or surgery

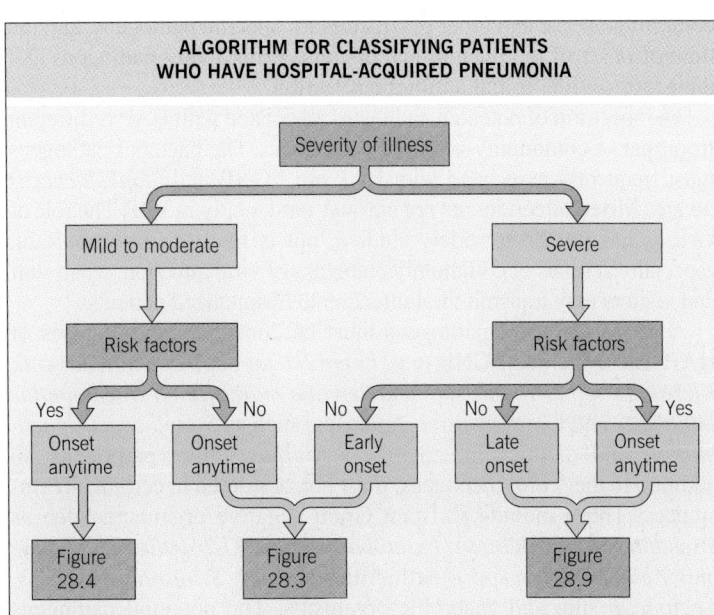

ALGORITHM FOR CLASSIFYING PATIENTS WHO HAVE HOSPITAL-ACQUIRED PNEUMONIA

Severity of illness

Mild to moderate → Risk factors → Yes: Onset anytime (Figure 28.4); No: Onset anytime (Figure 28.3)

Severe → Risk factors → No: Early onset (Figure 28.3); No: Late onset; Yes: Onset anytime (Figure 28.9)

Fig. 28.2 **Algorithm for classifying patients who have hospital-acquired pneumonia to provide a basis for empiric antibiotic management.** Adapted from Figure 1 in the American Thoracic Society consensus statement.[1]

For all grades of severity of HAP the length of hospital stay before the development of infection has the same broad influence. If HAP occurs within 5 days of hospitalization, *S. pneumoniae*, *H. influenzae* and *S. aureus* are the most frequently isolated pathogens.[13–15] Enteric Gram-negative bacteria become more common with increasing duration of hospital stay, presumably because the 'community' pathogens initially colonizing the oropharynx are replaced by 'hospital' pathogens. An algorithm for classifying patients who have HAP is shown in Figure 28.2. The three groups are considered below.

Patients who have mild to moderate HAP, no unusual risk factors and onset any time, or patients who have severe HAP with early onset

In this situation the 'core' pathogens are most likely and the antibiotic choice should reflect this possibility (Fig. 28.3).

Patients who have mild to moderate HAP, risk factors and onset at any time

In addition to the 'core' pathogens shown in Figure 28.3, other bacteria must be considered, depending on which risk factor is present (Fig. 28.4). Aspiration of anaerobic organisms is more likely in certain patients, for example those with swallowing problems, poor dental hygiene or impaired consciousness. Using invasive techniques and

ETIOLOGY AND MANAGEMENT OF NONSEVERE HAP WITH NO UNUSUAL RISK FACTORS, AND EARLY ONSET SEVERE HAP	
'Core' organisms	'Core' antibiotics
Escherichia coli	2nd or 3rd generation cephalosporins
Klebsiella spp.	or
Proteus spp.	
Serratia marcescens	Beta-lactam/beta-lactamase inhibitor combination
Enterobacter spp.	
Haemophilus influenzae	If penicillin-allergic, fluoroquinolone or clindamycin + aztreonam
Streptococcus pneumoniae	
Staphylococcus aureus (methicillin-sensitive)	

Fig. 28.3 A guide to likely 'core' pathogens and empiric antibiotic choice for patients who have early onset severe HAP or nonsevere HAP without any unusual risk factors, occurring at any time. Adapted from Table 1 in the American Thoracic Society consensus statement.[1]

ETIOLOGY AND MANAGEMENT OF NONSEVERE HAP; RISK FACTORS PRESENT; ONSET AT ANY TIME		
Core organisms plus:	Core antibiotics plus:	
Organism	Risk factor	Antibiotics
Anaerobes	Recent thoracoabdominal surgery	Clindamycin or beta-lactam
	Impaired swallowing	Beta-lactamase inhibitor (alone)
	Witnessed aspiration	
	Dental sepsis	
Staphylococcus aureus	Coma	Consider adding vancomycin if MRSA possible
	Head trauma	
	Neurosurgery	
	Diabetes mellitus	
	Renal failure	
Legionella spp.	High-dose corticosteroids	Erythromycin +/– rifampicin +/– fluroquinolone
	Organism endemic in hospital	
Pseudomonas aeruginosa	Prior antibiotics	Treat as severe HAP (see Fig. 28.10)
	High-dose corticosteroids	
	Prolonged ICU stay	
	Structured lung disease such as bronchiectasis	

Fig. 28.4 A guide to likely additional pathogens and antibiotic therapy required for patients who have mild to moderate HAP and additional risk factors present. Adapted from Table 2 in the American Thoracic Society consensus statement.[1]

DEFINITION OF SEVERE HAP	
Chest radiographs	Multilobar, cavitating or rapidly progressing lung shadowing
	Admission required to ICU
Respiratory failure	Need for mechanical ventilation or
	Need for >35% oxygen to maintain arterial oxygen saturation >90%
Evidence of severe sepsis	Shock (systolic BP <90mmHg or diastolic BP <60mmHg)
	Need for vasopressors for more than 4 hours
	Urine output <80ml in 4 hours
	Renal dialysis required

Fig. 28.5 Definition of severe HAP accepted by the American Thoracic Society. Adapted from Table 4 in the American Thoracic Society consensus statement.[1]

specific anaerobic cultures,[16] such organisms can be identified in up to one-third of all patients who have HAP, but the true significance of these findings is debated in the absence of clear risk factors for anaerobic infection.[1] Staphylococcus aureus infection is particularly associated with early infection in comatose patients, after multiple trauma or neurosurgical operations. The cause for this is not clear. However, MRSA is unlikely in this situation unless the patient has received multiple antibiotics before hospitalization.

Severe HAP

The definition of severe HAP is less developed than that for community-acquired pneumonia. Pointers to the presence of severe pneumonia are given in Figure 28.5.

When severe HAP occurs within 5 days of admission, the patient is likely to be infected by the core organisms, in particular H. influenzae and Gram-positive pathogens (see Fig. 28.3). With increasing length of hospital stay, factors such as critical illness, mechanical ventilation, respiratory tract instrumentation, exposure to antibiotics, corticosteroids and other drugs and the ubiquitous presence of pathogenic organisms within the hospital, especially in the ICU, become increasingly important. In such circumstances resistant organisms such as P. aeruginosa, Acinetobacter spp. and MRSA must also be covered by initial therapy. Infection with these organisms themselves denotes severe pneumonia, as the mortality attributable to these organisms is greater than with other types of infection.

PREVENTION

With the enormous impact that HAP has on the workings and economy of hospitals, it is perhaps surprising that few evidence-based guidelines on prevention are available.[1,2,17] The principles of prevention relate to minimizing the risk factors for nosocomial infection. Before elective surgery, increasing the level of fitness for an operation is likely to be of benefit. This should include cessation of smoking, weight reduction in the obese and improving control of coexisting disease such as chronic obstructive pulmonary disease, diabetes mellitus or cardiac failure. Short preoperative hospital stays and operation times may be beneficial. Strict airway management during and after surgery is essential and nasogastric and endotracheal tubes should be removed as early as possible. Each staff member can contribute by adherence to a strict handwashing regimen between patient contacts. Patient contact with staff harboring a viral respiratory infection should be avoided and influenza vaccination of staff during periods of high influenza activity should be ensured. Evaluation of swallowing should be a routine procedure for patients who have impaired consciousness or neuromuscular swallowing problems, with oral intake restricted as necessary.

It is now recognized that gastric acidity plays an important role in preventing EGNB from ascending the gastroesophageal tract and contaminating the respiratory tree. Routine therapy with H_2 antagonists and proton pump inhibitors to reduce gastric acidity and 'prevent' stress gastric ulceration is no longer recommended. Sucralfate therapy is being seen as a safer alternative. Enthusiasm for selective decontamination of the gastrointestinal tract with oral antibiotics has waxed and waned and has not become routine management in most ICUs (see Kollef MH[29]).

One of the most important factors for prevention is probably the circumspect use of antibiotics and the adoption of a sensible hospital antibiotic policy, together with regular surveillance for HAP outbreaks and the antibiotic-resistant patterns of likely pathogens.

CLINICAL FEATURES AND DIFFERENTIAL DIAGNOSIS

The diagnosis of pneumonia may be obvious in the hospitalized patient who develops the classic symptoms of fever, malaise, cough, purulent sputum, localizing chest signs and consolidation on the chest radiograph. All too often, however, the situation is less straightforward, with the list of differential diagnoses lengthening in proportion to the complexity of the underlying problem:

- pulmonary infarction,
- adult respiratory distress syndrome,
- pulmonary edema,
- pulmonary hemorrhage,
- pulmonary vasculitis,
- underlying disease (e.g. malignancy),
- iatrogenic lung shadowing (e.g. drug toxicity or radiation pneumonitis) and
- pre-existing lung disease (e.g. fibrosing alveolitis).

Hospital-acquired pneumonia should be considered in the context of an illness developing 48 hours after hospital admission and characterized by fever, leukocytosis, purulent sputum or tracheobronchial secretions and new or persisting infiltrates on the chest radiograph. However, the accuracy of a clinical diagnosis is poor compared with a microbiologic or pathologic diagnosis. In one study in an ICU less than one-half of the patients who have fever and probable pneumonia diagnosed on clinical grounds had the diagnosis confirmed microbiologically.[18]

The difficulties in making an accurate diagnosis from simple clinical features has led to more complicated diagnostic criteria being developed, particularly for VAP. For example, a 'clinical pulmonary infection score' has been suggested; this would take account of temperature, white blood cell count, presence of purulent secretions, oxygenation requirements and chest radiograph infiltrates, combined with a clinical course consistent with a diagnosis of pneumonia, the lack of any alternative source of sepsis, or histologic confirmation of pneumonia.[4,19]

An alternative approach is to consider ventilated patients 'at risk' of pneumonia if they develop new lung infiltrates and have purulent tracheal aspirates. A diagnosis of 'definite' VAP then requires microbiologic confirmation from quantitative culture from protected specimen brochial brush (PSB) samples or the presence of intracellular bacteria in cells from a bronchoalveolar lavage (BAL) cytospin.[6]

DIAGNOSIS

GENERAL INVESTIGATIONS (HEMATOLOGY, IMMUNOLOGY AND RADIOLOGY)

Patients who have suspected hospital-acquired pneumonia should have a full blood count measured; neutrophilia may point to infection as might a raised serum C reactive protein. Biochemical tests are often indicated to assess the impact of the pneumonia on the underlying condition and to assess renal and hepatic function. Oxygenation should be assessed by pulse oximetry or arterial blood gas estimation. The chest radiograph will show new or worsening lung shadowing, although it is not usually diagnostic of infection. Cavitation is suggestive of infection, particularly by enteric Gram-negative bacteria, anaerobes or fungi, but can be seen with pulmonary infarction.

GENERAL MICROBIOLOGIC INVESTIGATIONS

Blood cultures should always be obtained. A positive culture identifies the pathogen and is equated with a worse prognosis. However, only about 20% of blood cultures in hospital-acquired pneumonia patients are positive, indicating high specificity and low sensitivity.[1] The sources of the bacteremia, other than the lung, should always be considered. Pleural fluid should always be sampled to identify an impending empyema (see Fig. 28.6). Serologic tests for viral and atypical pathogens are rarely of value, unless nosocomial *Legionella* pneumonia is a possibility or specific IgM tests are available.

SPECIAL INVESTIGATIONS AND TECHNIQUES TO OBTAIN LOWER RESPIRATORY TRACT SAMPLES

Ideally, there would exist a widely available and accepted technique to obtain uncontaminated secretions from the site of a lung infection that was simple, safe and inexpensive to perform. Although the past 10 years has seen a rapid expansion in the use of different techniques for sampling in HAP, none fulfils the above criteria. The techniques can be broadly divided into three groups (Fig. 28.7). A major limitation of studies that have attempted to validate these techniques is the lack of a clear 'gold standard' for the diagnosis of pneumonia. In some studies, investigations have been performed just before death and the diagnosis of infection made postmortem. This is probably a better gold standard than lung biopsy, but does not reflect normal clinical practice, in which the diagnosis is attempted at an earlier stage of the illness. It is with these limitations in mind that the following techniques are described.

Noninvasive techniques

Expectorated sputum. The problems of sputum collection are well known and include contamination of the specimen by upper respiratory tract flora, making it unrepresentative of lower respiratory tract secretions. This is a particular problem in the nosocomial setting, when EGNB commonly colonize the upper respiratory tract and pathogens can be isolated with equal frequency in patients who have and without pneumonia.[3] The incidence of false-positive results for Gram-positive pathogens is relatively low but may rise to 50% for EGNB.[20] Only one-third to one-half of sputum cultures provide reliable information compared with blood cultures, transtracheal aspirates and PSB samples.[16,20–22] Contamination of sputum by oral secretions should be suspected if the sputum Gram stain contains <25 polymorphonuclear neutrophils and >10 squamous cell epithelial cells per low-power field. The presence of elastin fibers in potassium hydroxide preparations of sputum equates well with the presence of pneumonia, although the test is not widely available.[19]

Endotracheal aspirates. Aspiration via the endotracheal tube is the simplest method of obtaining secretions in patients on mechanical ventilation. Experience has indicated a high sensitivity but a very low

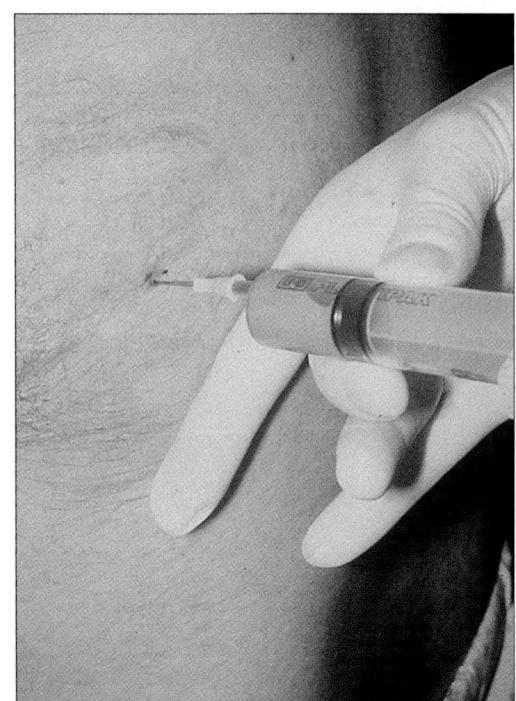

Fig. 28.6 Pleural fluid, if present, should always be sampled in a patient who has pneumonia to assess etiology. In this case, purulent fluid was detected suggestive of an empyema. Reproduced from Macfarlane JT, Finch RG, Cotton RE. A Colour Atlas of Respiratory Infections. London: Chapman & Hall; 1993.

TECHNIQUES USED TO OBTAIN RESPIRATORY SPECIMENS FROM PATIENTS WITH SUSPECTED HAP		Special equipment required (bedside + lab)	Skill required	Risk of technique	Sensitivity	Specificity
Noninvasive techniques	Expectorated sputum	0	0/+	0	+	+
	Endotracheal aspirate	+	+	0/+	++	+
	Blind distal airways sampling	+++	++	+	++	++
Perbronchoscopic invasive procedures	Protected specimen brush	+++	+++	++	+++	++++
	Bronchoalveolar lavage	+++	+++	++	++++	+++
	Protected bronchoalveolar lavage	++++	++++	++	++++	++++
Nonbronchoscopic invasive procedures	Percutaneous lung needle aspirate	+	+++	+++	++	++++
	Transtracheal aspiration	+++	++++	+++	+++	++
	Pleural fluid sampling	+	++	+	+	++++
Oral lung biopsy invasive procedures		++++	++++	+++	++++	++++

Fig. 28.7 Assessment of the advantages and disadvantages of the different techniques used to obtain respiratory secretions from patients who have suspected HAP. It is based on an arbitrary scale from 0 (very low/little) to ++++ (very high/much).

specificity, suggesting that a negative rather than a positive culture is of greater value to the clinician. Quantitative cultures with a high cut-off level improve specificity but adversely affect sensitivity. Daily quantitative bacterial cultures may identify a rapid rise in bacterial counts a few days before the development of new pulmonary infiltrates; regular surveillance with endotracheal aspirates may, therefore, be helpful.[20] The identification of elastin fibers and antibody-coated bacteria may increase the ability to differentiate between colonization and pneumonia.[19]

Nonbronchoscopic techniques for sampling the distal airways. Nonbronchoscopic techniques have the advantage of being less invasive and simple to perform; small endotracheal tubes (such as in children) can be used, although samples cannot be obtained reliably from the area of the lung where infection is suspected. The simplest technique involves distal, nondirected bronchial lavage through a standard aspiration catheter.[4] In one study mean bacterial colony counts increased significantly during the 2 days preceding the clinical onset of pneumonia, with counts falling significantly after appropriate antibiotic therapy. Blind techniques using plugged catheters or PSB samples and quantitative culture have reported sensitivities between 61 and 100% and specificity at a similar level.[20]

Bronchoscopic invasive procedures

Much has been published about the value of invasive techniques for managing HAP. However, questions as to who, when and how to perform these tests and the reliability of the results remain unresolved as does the applicability of published results to everyday clinical situations.[1,18,19]

Fiberoptic bronchoscopy provides direct visual access to the lower airways. Bronchoscopic techniques are relatively simple to perform in patients receiving mechanical ventilation, but such patients have often received prior antibiotics, reducing the value bronchoscopic studies. It is likely that invasive techniques would be most useful in patients who have moderate or severe HAP before antibiotic therapy is started. In practice immediate access to bronchoscopic techniques may be limited and the procedure itself may on occasions precipitate cardiorespiratory failure in a spontaneously breathing but hypoxic patient, necessitating ventilatory support earlier than anticipated.

Protected specimen brush. The double catheter PSB (Fig. 28.8) is effective in avoiding contamination during passage through the bronchoscopic suction channel. Attention to correct technique is

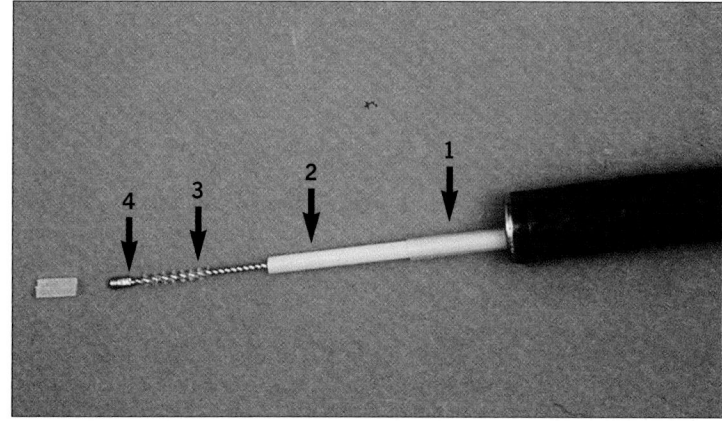

Fig. 28.8 An extended protected specimen brush protruding from the end of a fiberoptic bronchoscope. Note the outer plastic sheath (arrow 1) and the inner protective yellow plastic cover (arrow 2) with the microbiologic brush pushed out (arrow 3). The protective gelatin plug occludes the end of the outer cover (arrow 4) until ejected before obtaining the specimen. Reproduced from Macfarlane JT, Finch RG, Cotton RE. A Colour Atlas of Respiratory Infections. London: Chapman & Hall; 1993.

important for obtaining the specimen and transferring the brush to transport medium for quantitative culture.[19] Briefly, the brush catheter is passed bronchoscopically to the segment from which the sample is to be obtained; the inner sheath is then extended, thus expelling the wax plug. Next, the brush is extended and then withdrawn back into the inner sheath. The catheter is then removed from the bronchoscope and the brush cut aseptically, once it has been advanced from the inner sheath, into 1ml sterile normal saline. The sample is then immediately vortex mixed and plated out in dilutions for quantitative culture. Numerous studies have reported a sensitivity of 62–100% and a similar specificity, using a threshold concentration of $>10^3$cfu/ml on quantitative bacterial culture.[20]

Bronchoalveolar lavage. For BAL, the bronchoscope is wedged into a subsegmental airway and the bronchoalveolar area is lavaged; volumes of over 100ml sterile normal saline are required to reach the distal alveoli (Fig. 28.9).

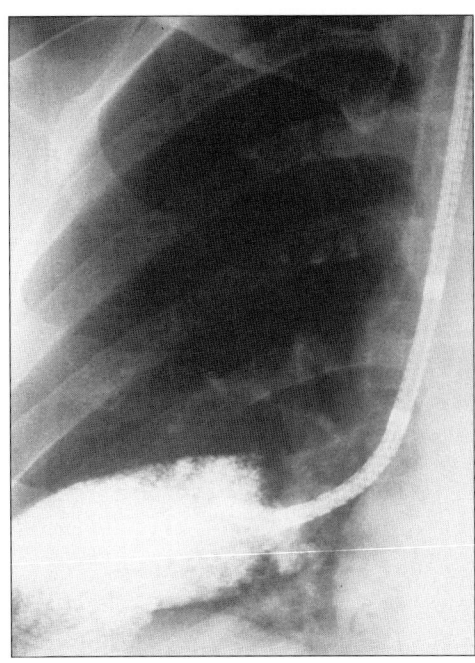

Fig. 28.9 Limited bronchoalveolar lavage of right middle lobe using radiopaque solution. Note alveolar filling pattern. Reproduced from Macfarlane JT, Finch RG, Cotton RE. A Colour Atlas of Respiratory Infections. London: Chapman & Hall; 1993.

The advantage is that a large part of the lung is sampled and the specimen allows microscopic analysis to assess the presence of intracellular bacteria, neutrophils and elastin fibers and cytologic evaluation if required. This can be particularly useful if the diagnosis of pneumonia is in doubt and malignancy is a diagnostic possibility. Contamination of the BAL fluid in the bronchoscopic channel is one disadvantage and a careful technique is required to avoid this. After wedging the tip of the bronchoscope in the relevant subsegment, 50ml normal saline at 37°C is instilled. This aspirate samples airways rather than the alveoli, is best referred to as a 'bronchial wash'[23] and is more likely to be contaminated with bacteria present in the suction channel. This sample should therefore be processed separately from the second, third and, if necessary, fourth aliquots of 50ml, which should be pooled. Sensitivity and specificity of BAL quantitative cultures have ranged from 72 to 100% and 69 to 100%, respectively, using threshold concentrations of $>10^4$cfu/ml.

When compared with PSB performed at the same time, BAL has greater sensitivity but a marginally reduced specificity. Combining both techniques overcomes this problem and appears to provide the best results in experienced centers.[20,24]

An alternative is to perform a protected BAL using a balloon tipped catheter (to allow effective wedging and isolation of a pulmonary subsegment) with a distal ejectable plug. This is reported to improve specificity compared with BAL and sensitivity compared with PSB.[20,25]

Percutaneous invasive techniques

Percutaneous lung needle aspirate. Percutaneous lung needle aspirate (PLNA) has been used successfully to investigate nonventilated patients who have lung shadowing. The technique can be performed at the bedside with minimal equipment. The use of a 25-gauge ultrathin needle reduces the chance of pneumothorax. In one study of 98 patients who had HAP outside the ICU, the sensitivity was 61%, the specificity 100% and the pneumothorax complication rate 3.5%. The latter reduces the usefulness of this technique in patients receiving mechanical ventilation. Animal models suggest a high sensitivity and specificity.[19] When compared with histologic diagnosis of pneumonia on lung biopsy immediately postmortem as a 'gold standard', PLNA had the lowest sensitivity (25%) but the highest specificity (79%) of the invasive techniques discussed. However, recent studies have questioned the value of immediate, postmortem lung biopsies as the 'gold standard' for the diagnosis of pneumonia.[18,26]

Transtracheal aspiration. Transtracheal aspiration is now rarely used due to the ready availability of fiberoptic bronchoscopy. However, its value was demonstrated for the investigation of patients who have suspected HAP on general medical and surgical wards.[16] More recent studies have reaffirmed its potential usefulness as a bedside technique to obtain uncontaminated lower respiratory secretions in patients not receiving mechanical ventilation.

The influence of invasive techniques on management of HAP. The literature supports the view that PSB and BAL specimens cultured quantitatively can provide useful and reliable information about the likely presence and cause of HAP, particularly in the ICU.[20] Their value is considerably diminished if the patient is already receiving antibiotics, which is unfortunately the usual situation. The effect of PSB results on management was shown in one study of 110 mechanically ventilated patients who had suspected HAP.[27] Antibiotics were stopped in the majority before PSB was performed. Quantitative PSB culture supported the clinical diagnosis of pneumonia in only 41% of patients. The PSB results suggested that the initial treatment was appropriate in one-third of all patients, inappropriate in a further one-third (patients were receiving antibiotics that were not considered necessary) and the situation was unclear in the remaining one-third. Of the patients who had pneumonia, over one-third had their antibiotics changed because of the PSB result.

Although this suggests that invasive techniques may influence immediate management, the literature does not show that using these techniques improves outcome. It is suggested that invasive techniques should only be performed if the clinical and laboratory expertise is available and if the results are consistently applied to management decisions as part of an agreed management protocol.[1,20] In practice, quantitative culture is time-consuming and demanding and is not performed routinely in all laboratories, which limits its usefulness in many hospitals.

MANAGEMENT

GENERAL FACTORS

The general management of the patient who has HAP is important. Such patients frequently have underlying disease, which may be worsened by the infection and require additional therapy. Careful attention to fluid balance and oxygenation is essential and chest physiotherapy may be helpful. Not infrequently the diagnosis of HAP may be uncertain and additional empiric therapy (e.g. anticoagulation for possible pulmonary embolus) may be started, pending results of appropriate investigations. Even with effective management, the prognosis may be poor because of the underlying disease or overwhelming infection. In only a proportion of patients dying with HAP is death directly attributable to the infection.

GUIDELINES FOR EMPIRIC ANTIBIOTIC THERAPY

Guidelines from the American Thoracic Society[1] and the Canadian Consensus Conference[3,12] have been published and provide a useful basis for the practical, empiric management of HAP. The decision tree is summarized in Figures 28.2, 28.3, 28.5 and 28.10 and depends on assessment of severity, the description of 'core' pathogens, the identification of risk factors for specific pathogens and time of onset to guide empiric antibiotic therapy. In a similar way to the empiric management of community-acquired pneumonia, patients who have severe infection are identified early and start by receiving combination antibiotic therapy to cover all likely pathogens. For nonsevere HAP, single antibiotic therapy is usually appropriate to cover the 'core' pathogens, unless additional risk factors are present.[8,28]

Mild to moderate HAP; no risk factors for other pathogens; 'core' pathogens likely

In this situation a single agent effective against the 'core' pathogens, including Gram-positive organisms, *H. influenzae* and EGNB is appropriate.[8,28] Options include a second- or third-generation cephalosporin, such as cefuroxime, ceftriaxone or cefotaxime, or a combination of a beta-lactam antibiotic with a beta-lactamase inhibitor (e.g. amoxycillin or ticarcillin, together with clavulanic acid) or a quinolone (see Fig. 28.3). Oral therapy can be used if appropriate.

ETIOLOGY AND MANAGEMENT OF PATIENTS WITH SEVERE HAP, APART FROM THOSE WITH EARLY ONSET INFECTION AND NO UNUSUAL RISK FACTORS	
Core organisms plus:	Antibiotics
Pseudomonas aeruginosa	Combination of: • Aminoglycoside or ciprofloxacin plus one of:
Acinetobacter spp.	• Antipseudomonal beta-lactamase stable beta-lactam antibiotic • Imipenem • Aztreonam†
MRSA in some hospitals	• +/– Vancomycin
†Does not give cover for Gram-positive or *Haemophilus influenzae* infections	

Fig. 28.10 A guide to likely pathogens and appropriate empiric antibiotic therapy for patients with severe HAP. Those with early onset severe HAP without unusual risk factors present are managed as shown in Figure 28.3. Adapted from Table 3 in the American Thoracic Society consensus statement.[1]

Mild or moderate HAP; risk factors present for specific pathogens in addition to 'core' pathogens

In this situation the specific risk factors will provide some guidance as to whether additional antibiotic therapy may be required to cover such pathogens as anaerobes, more resistant EGNB and *Legionella* infection as well as the 'core' pathogens. Combination therapy may be required, including the antibiotic appropriate to cover the 'core' organisms (see Fig. 28.4).

Severe HAP

'Early' severe HAP occurring soon after hospital admission is likely to be caused by the 'core' organisms, in particular *S. pneumoniae*, *S. aureus* and *H. influenzae* and is treated like nonsevere infection (see Fig. 28.3). For 'late' severe HAP occurring after 5 days of hospitalization, empiric therapy should cover *P. aeruginosa* and *Acinetobacter* spp. in addition to the 'core' organisms. Combination antibiotics providing antipseudomonal cover are required, including an antipseudomonal beta-lactam antibiotic together with either an aminoglycoside or a fluoroquinolone, or both. Methicillin-resistant *S. aureus* may be a problem in some institutions (Fig. 28.10).

FACTORS TO CONSIDER WHEN A PATIENT WITH HAP FAILS TO RESPOND TO THERAPY	
Factor	Action
Improvement expected too soon	Continue therapy – review again
Deterioration in underlying disease	Optimise general management
Diagnosis of hospital-acquired pneumonia incorrect	Review situation Consider differential diagnosis
Additional pathologic process present	Review situation Consider differential diagnosis
Additional or unexpected pathogen present Pathogen resistant to antibiotic	Review microbiologic data Consider alternative or invasive tests
Local intrathoracic complication (e.g. empyema, lung abscess)	Review chest radiographs Consider CT scan, bronchoscopy
Metastatic infective complication (e.g. endocarditis, arthritis, abscess)	Detailed clinical examination and appropriate tests
Reason for pneumonia persisting (e.g. aspiration, bacteremia from distant focus)	Review history Repeat blood cultures
Secondary complications (e.g. intravenous line infection, pulmonary emboli)	Detailed clinical examination and further studies (e.g. V/Q scan)
General factors (e.g. dehydration, nutrition, hypoxia)	Manage appropriately
Allergic reaction to antibiotics (often after several days of therapy)	Look for rash and recurrence of fever Consider stopping/changing antibiotic
Patient not actually receiving or taking the antibiotic	Check

Fig. 28.11 Factors to consider when a patient with hospital-acquired pneumonia is not improving with initial management.

Factors to consider when assessing response

Assessment of the response of the patient who has HAP is difficult because of the complex relationship between the infection and the underlying disease. Factors to consider if the patient is not responding to empiric therapy are shown in Figure 28.11, and have been reviewed elsewhere.[1]

REFERENCES

1. Anonymous. Hospital-acquired pneumonia in adults: diagnosis, assessment of severity, initial antimicrobial therapy, and preventive strategies. A consensus statement, American Thoracic Society, November 1995. Am J Respir Crit Care Med 1996;153:1711–25.
2. Dal Nogare AR. Nosocomial pneumonia in the medical and surgical patient. Risk factors and primary management. Med Clin North Am 1994;78:1081–90.
3. Giamarellou H. Nosocomial pneumonia: pathogenesis, diagnosis, current therapy and prophylactic approach. Int J Antimicrob Agents 1993;3:S87–S97.
4. A'Court CD, Garrard CS, Crook D, et al. Microbiological lung surveillance in mechanically ventilated patients, using non-directed bronchial lavage and quantitative culture. Q J Med 1993; 86:635–48.
5. Fagon JY, Chastre J, Domart Y, et al. Nosocomial pneumonia in patients receiving continuous mechanical ventilation. Am Rev Respir Dis 1988;139:877–84.

6. Fagon JY, Chastre J, Hance AJ, et al. Nosocomial pneumonia in ventilated patients: a cohort study evaluating attributable mortality and hospital stay. Am J Med 1993;94:281–8.
7. Rello J, Quintana E, Ausina V, et al. Incidence, etiology, and outcome of nosocomial pneumonia in mechanically ventilated patients. Chest 1991;100:439–44.
8. Niederman MS. An approach to empiric therapy of nosocomial pneumonia. Med Clin North Am 1994;78:1123–41.
9. Macfarlane JT. Pneumonia. Med Int 1986;36:1498–1506.
10. Niederman MS. The pathogenesis of airway colonisation: lessons learned from the study of bacterial adherence. Eur Respir J 1994;7:1737–40.
11. Pennington JE. Hospital-acquired pneumonia. In: Pennington JE ed. Respiratory infections diagnosis and management, 3rd ed. New York: Raven Press; 1994:207–27.

12. Mandell LA, Marrie TJ, Niederman MS. Initial antimicrobial treatment of hospital acquired pneumonia in adults: a conference report. Can J Infect Dis 1993;4:317–21.
13. Costabel U, Teschler H, Schoenfeld B, et al. BOOP in Europe. Chest 1992;102:14S–20S.
14. Schleupner CJ, Cobb DK. A study of the etiologies and treatment of nosocomial pneumonia in a community-based teaching hospital. Infect Control Hosp Epidemiol 1992;13:515–25.
15. Rello J, Ricart M, Ausina V, Net A, Prats G. Pneumonia due to *Haemophilus influenzae* among mechanically ventilated patients. Incidence, outcome, and risk factors. Chest 1992;102:1562–5.
16. Bartlett JG, O'keefe P, Tally FP, Louie TJ, Gorbach SL. Bacteriology of hospital acquired pneumonia. Arch Intern Med 1986;146:868–71.
17. Dal Nogare AR. Nosocomial pneumonia outside the intensive care unit. In: Niederman MS, Sarosi GA, Glassroth J eds. Respiratory infections A scientific basis for management. Philadelphia: WB Saunders; 1994:139–46.

18 . Brun-Buisson C. Diagnosis of ventilator acquired pneumonia. Thorax 1995;50:1128–30.

19. Torres A, Gonzalez J, Ferrer M. Evaluation of the available invasive and non-invasive techniques for diagnosing nosocomial pneumonias in mechanically ventilated patients. Intensive Care Med 1991;17:439–48.

20. Griffin JJ, Meduri GU. New approaches in the diagnosis of nosocomial pneumonia. Med Clin North Am 1994;78:1091–122.

21. Bryan CS, Reynolds KL. Bacteraemic nosocomial pneumonia. Analysis of 172 episodes from a single metropolitan area. Am Rev Respir Dis 1984;129:668–71.

22. Pollock HM, Hawkins EL, Bonner JR, et al. Diagnosis of bacterial pulmonary infections with quantitative protected catheter cultures obtained during bronchoscopy. J Clin Microbiol 1983;17:255–9.

23. Kelly CA, Kotre JC, Ward C, Hendrick DJ, Walters EH. Anatomical distribution of bronchoalveolar lavage fluid as assessed by digital radiography. Thorax 1987;42:626–9.

24. Violan JS, de Castro FR, Luna JC. Comparative efficacy of bronchoalveolar lavage and telescoping plugged catheter in the diagnosis of pneumonia in mechanically ventilated patients. Chest 1993;103:386–90.

25. Barreiro B, Dorca J, Manresa F, et al. Protected bronchoalveolar lavage in the diagnosis of ventilator-associated pneumonia. Eur Respir J 1996;9:1500–7.

26. Torres A, el-Ebiary M, Padro L, et al. Validation of different techniques for the diagnosis of ventilator-associated pneumonia. Comparison with immediate postmortem pulmonary biopsy. Am J Respir Crit Care Med 1994;149:324–31.

27. Rodriguez de Castro F, Sole Violan J, Leon E, et al. Do quantitative cultures of protected brush specimens modify the initial empirical therapy in ventilated patients with suspected pneumonia? Eur Respir J 1996;9:37–41.

28. La Force FM. Systemic antimicrobial therapy of nosocomial pneumonia: monotherapy versus combination therapy. Eur J Clin Microbiol Infect Dis 1989;8:61–8.

29. Kollef MH. The role of selective digestive tract decontamination on mortality and respiratory tract infections: a meta-analysis. Chest 1994;105:1101–8.

Lung Abscesses and Pleural Abscesses

Julie E Mangino & Robert J Fass

Lower respiratory tract infections (LRTIs) are a major indication for antimicrobial therapy in developed countries. Although many LRTIs are self-limiting, those caused by necrotizing organisms are invariably serious; they may lead to abscess formation in the lung and can spread to the pleural space.

EPIDEMIOLOGY

The etiologies of lung abscess and pleural abscess, or empyema, vary in different parts of the world. The common denominator is usually aspiration pneumonia, acquired either in the community or the hospital. Nosocomial pneumonia is a major cause of morbidity and lengthened hospital stay, with enormous economic impact. Aspiration pneumonia leading to necrotizing pneumonia or lung abscess, with or without empyema, is a continuum; any stage or all stages may be encountered. Underlying diseases, associated trauma or surgery, and the timeliness of appropriate therapy are the major factors in determining clinical presentation and prognosis.

LUNG ABSCESS

A lung abscess is arbitrarily defined as a localized area of pulmonary necrosis caused by infection, with a solitary or dominant cavity measuring at least 2cm in diameter. When cavities are multiple and smaller than 2cm, the infection is usually referred to as a necrotizing pneumonia.[1–3] Most abscesses are suppurative bacterial infections caused by aspiration.

Primary lung abscesses typically present in patients who have no predisposing disease other than a predilection to aspirate oral secretions; they are more common in males than in females. Secondary lung abscesses occur in patients with an underlying condition such as a partial bronchial obstruction or lung infarct, or in those who are otherwise immunocompromised because of chemotherapy, malignancy, organ transplantation, or HIV infection. Lung abscesses may be termed nonspecific or putrid, referring, respectively, to the often unclear etiology or the offensive odor of the sputum.[3,4]

Over the past 5 decades, the incidence of bacterial lung abscess in the USA has diminished considerably, and the mortality rate has decreased from 30–40% to 5–10%. Factors associated with a worse prognosis include advanced age, prolonged symptoms, concomitant disease, nosocomial infection and (according to some studies) larger cavity size. In the past, tuberculosis was responsible for a higher proportion of lung abscesses. In recent years, more lung abscesses have been associated with pulmonary malignancies or other underlying conditions.[3–7]

EMPYEMA

A pleural effusion associated with pneumonia, lung abscess, or bronchiectasis is referred to as a parapneumonic effusion. These occur in up to 40% of people with bacterial pneumonia; they are the most common cause of exudative pleural effusion in the USA.[8] Empyema, or pleural pus, is an infected parapneumonic effusion with characteristic changes in the composition of the pleural fluid. It has been declining in frequency and changing in etiology.[6] Mortality ranges from approximately 2 to 50%, with the lowest rates in young, healthy people

and the highest rates in the elderly and immunocompromised. The prognosis is poorer when pathogens are resistant to antimicrobial drugs or when appropriate treatment is delayed.[8–10]

PATHOGENESIS AND PATHOLOGY

Micro-organisms gain access to the lower respiratory tract by a variety of routes, including inhalation of aerosolized particles, aspiration of oropharyngeal secretions, and hematogenous spread from distant sites (Fig. 29.1). Less frequently, infection occurs by direct extension from a contiguous site. Lung abscess is caused only by organisms that cause necrosis, but empyema can result from infection by any pathogen that reaches the pleural space.

LUNG ABSCESS

Of the inhaled respiratory pathogens, only the mycobacteria (see Chapter 2.30) and the dimorphic fungi (see Chapter 2.7) commonly cause lung abscesses. Bacterial abscesses are usually caused by aspiration of oropharyngeal secretions or, occasionally, by hematogenous seeding.[1]

Aspiration of small quantities of oropharyngeal secretions probably occurs intermittently in everyone, particularly during sleep. Despite the frequency of aspiration, the airways below the level of the larynx are normally sterile owing to highly efficient clearing mechanisms, including cough, a mucociliary system that escalates particles cephalad to be swallowed, phagocytosis by alveolar macrophages and neutrophils aided by opsonizing antibodies and complement, and lymphatic trapping with sequestration in regional lymph nodes. Risk factors for pneumonia after aspiration include conditions that increase the inoculum of pathogenic organisms in aspirated secretions, conditions that increase the likelihood of aspiration and conditions that increase the volume of the aspirate (Fig. 29.2). Under these circumstances, aspirated oropharyngeal secretions are more likely to cause chemical irritation and infection. When an anaerobic pleuropulmonary infection occurs in an edentulous patient, the diagnosis of bronchogenic carcinoma should be considered.[1–3,11]

The composition of the oropharyngeal flora at the time of aspiration determines the potential etiologic agents for LRTIs. Those organisms that are most numerous or virulent proliferate and emerge as single or predominant pathogens. Although the classic non-necrotizing respiratory pathogens *Streptococcus pneumoniae* and *Haemophilus influenzae* can cause disease by this mechanism, normal oropharyngeal secretions contain many more streptococci of various species and more anaerobes (approximately 10^8 organisms/ml) than aerobes (approximately 10^7 organisms/ml). Some of the streptococcal species are microaerophilic (i.e. they require supplemental carbon dioxide to grow on artificial media).[12,13] The pneumonia that follows aspiration, with or without abscess formation, is typically polymicrobial with between two and four bacterial species present in large numbers. In general, 50% or more of these infections are caused by purely anaerobic bacteria, 25% are caused by mixed aerobes and anaerobes, and 25% or fewer are caused by aerobes only. Among hospitalized patients, progressive colonization with *Staphylococcus aureus*, Enterobacteriaceae and *Pseudomonas aeruginosa* occurs, and these aerobic

SYNDROMES BY BODY SYSTEM

CAUSES OF LOWER RESPIRATORY TRACT INFECTIONS IN ADULTS

Organisms	Inhalation	Aspiration — Community-acquired	Aspiration — Hospital-acquired	Hemato-genous
Haemophilus influenzae	■	■	□	
Streptococcus pneumoniae	■	■	□	
Oropharyngeal streptococci and anaerobes		■	■	
Staphylococcus aureus	■		■	■
Enterobacteriaceae			■	
Pseudomonas aeruginosa			■	
Legionellaceae	■			
Mycoplasma pneumoniae	■			
Chlamydia pneumoniae	■			
Viruses	■			
Histoplasma capsulatum	■			
Blastomyces dermatitidis	■			
Coccidioides immitis	■			
Mycobacteria	■			

■ Common cause of infection   □ Less common cause of infection

Fig. 29.1 Causes of lower respiratory tract infections in adults. Oropharyngeal streptococci and anaerobes, *Staphylococcus aureus*, Enterobacteriaceae, *Pseudomonas aeruginosa*, the dimorphic fungi (*Histoplasma capsulatum*, *Blastomyces dermatidis*, *Coccidioides immitis*), and mycobacteria frequently cause necrosis and subsequent abscess formation.

RISK FACTORS FOR ASPIRATION PNEUMONIA AND LUNG ABSCESS

Increased bacterial inoculum	Periodontal disease, gingivitis, tonsillar or dental abscess, drugs that decrease gastric acidity
Impairment of consciousness	Drugs, alcohol, general anesthesia, metabolic encephalopathy, coma, shock, cerebrovascular accident, cardiopulmonary arrest, seizures, surgery, trauma
Impaired cough and gag reflexes	Vocal cord paralysis, intratracheal anesthesia, endotracheal tube, tracheostomy, myopathy, myelopathy, other neurologic disorders
Impairment of esophageal function	Diverticula, achalasia, strictures, disorders of gastrointestinal motility, neoplasm, tracheoesophageal fistula, pseudobulbar palsy
Emesis	Nasogastric tube, gastric dilatation, ileus, intestinal obstruction

Fig. 29.2 Risk factors for aspiration pneumonia and lung abscess.

ANAEROBIC BACTERIA ASSOCIATED WITH PLEUROPULMONARY INFECTIONS

	Gram-negative bacteria	Gram-positive bacteria
Bacilli	*Bacteroides fragilis* group *Fusobacterium nucleatum* *Fusobacterium necrophorum* *Porphyromonas* spp. *Prevotella* spp.	*Actinomyces* spp. *Bifidobacterium* spp. *Clostridium* spp. *Eubacterium* spp. *Lactobacillus* spp. *Propionibacterium* spp.
Cocci	*Veillonella* spp.	*Gemella morbillorum* *Peptostreptococcus* spp. *Streptococcus* spp.

Fig. 29.3 Anaerobic bacteria associated with pleuropulmonary infections.
(Note: *Porphyromonas* spp. include organisms previously named *Bacteroides melaninogenicus* subsp. *asaccharolyticus*, *B. endodontalis* and *B. gingivalis*. *Prevotella* spp. include organisms previously named *B. melaninogenicus* subspp. *melaninogenicus* and *intermedius*, *B. oralis* and *B. denticola*. *Gemella morbillorum* was previously named *Streptococcus morbillorum*. *Peptostreptococcus* spp. include organisms previously named *Peptococcus* spp.)

organisms are frequent causes of nosocomial aspiration pneumonia and lung abscess.[6,12,14,15]

The anaerobic organisms that are associated with pleuropulmonary infection, using current nomenclature,[16,17] are shown in Figure 29.3. The primary pathogens are *Streptococcus* spp., *Peptostreptococcus* spp., *Fusobacterium nucleatum* and *Prevotella* spp. Additionally, *Porphyromonas* spp. are commonly associated with periodontal disease and may also be isolated. Although not consistently part of the normal oropharyngeal flora, the *Bacteroides fragilis* group of organisms are isolated from approximately 15% of patients.[2,11–14,16]

A variety of virulence factors associated with oropharyngeal streptococci and anaerobes have been identified. Properties that facilitate attachment include capsular polysaccharides, fimbriae, hemagglutinin and lectin. Tissue breakdown and the metabolic activity of organisms provide reducing substances and a low redox potential, and these factors facilitate bacterial proliferation. Volatile fatty acids, sulfur compounds, indoles, amines and hydrolytic enzymes (hyaluronidase, chondroitin sulfatase and heparinase) produced by damaged tissue lead to subsequent abscess formation.[18]

The pathology of aspiration pneumonia is characterized by alveolar edema and infiltration with inflammatory cells. Foci of aspiration pneumonia most commonly develop in the subpleural regions of the gravity-dependent segments of the lungs, particularly the superior segments of the lower lobes and the posterior segments of the upper lobes. The right lung is the more frequent location, presumably because of the less acute angle in the take-off of the right main stem bronchus. In general, the right upper and lower lobes are most commonly involved, followed by the left lower lobe and right middle lobe.[1,3,19,20]

The degree and rate of progression of aspiration pneumonia vary considerably. These infections may be acute, subacute, or chronic, depending on differences in etiology, size of inoculum and host factors. If the process is indolent, fibrosis limits the spread of infection. Abscesses typically communicate with a bronchus, producing the familiar air-filled cavity, often with an air–fluid level that can be seen on radiographs. These are usually not apparent until the infection has been present for 1–2 weeks, when multiple adjacent microscopic abscesses filled with necrotic material (pulmonary gangrene) slough to form a gross cavity (Fig. 29.4).[5]

29.2

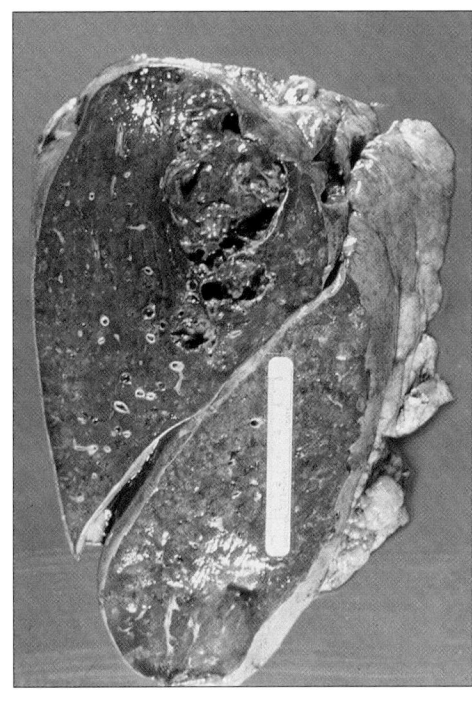

Fig. 29.4 Cross-section of a lung abscess.

Although less common than aspiration, hematogenous seeding of the lung, or septic emboli, may also result in lung abscesses or necrotizing pneumonia. There may be a solitary infiltrate or cavity or, more often, multiple bilateral lesions. The most common etiologic agents are the nosocomial pathogens, *Staph. aureus* and aerobic Gram-negative bacilli (Fig. 29.1). When the primary focus is in the abdomen, anaerobes, particularly *B. fragilis*, may be present.

Infective endocarditis (predominantly right-sided), intravenous drug injection and indwelling right atrial catheters placed for vascular access are commonly associated with septic pulmonary emboli. Any organism that is part of the skin flora or contaminants in injected material may be responsible. *Staphylococcus aureus* and streptococci are the most common pathogens, but *P. aeruginosa* and *Candida* spp. may also be responsible, causing serious infections.[21]

Some uncommon causes of lung abscess should be considered in appropriate circumstances. Inhaled micro-organisms such as *Legionella* spp., *Chlamydia* spp., *Mycoplasma pneumoniae* and viruses are rare causes of lung abscesses. *Cryptococcus*, *Aspergillus* and *Rhizopus* spp. occasionally cause disease in normal hosts, but are more commonly opportunistic pathogens. Patients with advanced HIV disease may have cavitary lesions caused by atypical *Mycobacteria* spp., particularly *Mycobacterium kansasii*, and other organisms such as *Rhodococcus equi* and *Nocardia asteroides*.[22] *Pseudomonas pseudomallei* is endemic to South East Asia, particularly Thailand, and typically causes upper lobe cavities. In endemic areas, the parasites *Paragonimus westermani* and *Entamoeba histolytica* may cause abscess by contiguous extension.

EMPYEMA

The pleural space is normally sterile. It is most commonly contaminated by direct extension from a contiguous focus of infection, usually pulmonary, or by direct inoculation at the time of trauma or surgery (Fig. 29.5).[8,23,24] The pleural space may also become involved owing to hematogenous seeding from a distant focus of infection, particularly in the presence of hemothorax or pleural malignancy.

The initial stage in the pathogenesis of empyema associated with pneumonia is the development of a sterile parapneumonic effusion, which has varying characteristics depending on its stage of evolution (Fig. 29.6).[8,24] The effusion is initially transudative but rapidly becomes exudative with an influx of leukocytes and increasing permeability of the visceral pleura. Neutrophils, lactate dehydrogenase (LDH) and protein increase, glucose and pH decrease. Fibrin is deposited on the pleural surfaces and loculations may occur. With time, a final organizing stage occurs in which pleural fibroblasts produce an inelastic membrane or pleural peel that encases the lung and restricts inflation. Invasion with bacteria accelerates the fibropurulent reaction. Empyema

Fig. 29.5 Causes of empyema.

CAUSES OF EMPYEMA	
Pulmonary infection	Pneumonia
	Lung abscess
	Bronchiectasis
Mediastinal disease	Tracheal fistula
	Esophageal perforation
Subdiaphragmatic infection	Subphrenic abscess
	Hepatic abscess
Skeletal infection	Paravertebral abscess
	Vertebral osteomyelitis
Direct inoculation	Trauma
	Thoracentesis
Postoperative	Hemothorax (infected)
	Pneumothorax (infected)
	Bronchopleural fistula

CHARACTERISTICS OF PLEURAL FLUID ASSOCIATED WITH BACTERIAL LOWER RESPIRATORY TRACT INFECTIONS				
		Exudate		
Pleural fluid characteristic	Transudate	Uncomplicated parapneumonic effusion	Complicated parapneumonic effusion	Empyema
Appearance	Clear	Variable	Variable	Pus
White blood cell count (cells/ml)	<1000	Variable	Variable	>15,000
Differential cell count	Variable	Neutrophils	Neutrophils	Neutrophils
Protein (g/dl)	<3.0	>3.0	>3.0	>3.0
Glucose (mg/dl)	Same as serum	>60	40–60	<40
pH	Greater than serum	>7.2	7.0–7.2	<7.0
Lactate dehydrogenase (units/ml)	<200	<1000	>1000	>1000
Bacteria	Absent	Absent	Absent	Present

Fig. 29.6 Characteristics of pleural fluid associated with bacterial lower respiratory tract infections. The values may overlap. Complicated pleural effusions are those with fluid characteristics that indicate the potential need for tube drainage. When the glucose is 40–60mg/dl or the pH is 7.0–7.2, repeat thoracentesis may be helpful. When the glucose is <40mg/dl or the pH is <7.0, a chest tube is indicated even if bacteria are not present by smear or culture. Data from Light[8] and Sokolowski, et al.[33]

fluid is relatively deficient in opsonins and complement, and it becomes progressively more acidic as the infection ensues. Occasionally, an empyema may spontaneously drain through necrotic lung tissue into a bronchus (bronchopleural fistula) or communicate through the chest wall (empyema necessitans).[8,10,24]

The various respiratory pathogens have different propensities to causing empyema. *Streptococcus pneumoniae*, the most common cause of pneumonia, is frequently associated with a parapneumonic pleural effusion, yet pneumococcal empyema is relatively uncommon. Aspiration pneumonia more frequently progresses to empyema.[8] Empyema is also more common with organisms such as *Staph. aureus* and *P. aeruginosa* that produce potent extracellular enzymes that breach the integrity of the pleura, allowing penetration to the pleural space.

Overall, the relative frequencies of various organisms causing empyema has changed over time. Prior to the antibiotic era, most empyemas were caused by *Strep. pneumoniae* and, to a lesser extent, by *Staph. aureus* and *Streptococcus pyogenes*. Between 1955 and 1965, penicillin-resistant *Staph. aureus* was the predominant pathogen.[8,25] In the early 1970s, coinciding with a surge of interest in anaerobic infections, anaerobic empyemas were recognized more frequently (Fig. 29.7).[26,27] At that time, about 50% of empyemas were caused by aerobes, with Gram-positive cocci being more common than Gram-negative bacilli. About 25% were caused by anaerobes; and about 25% were mixed aerobic–anaerobic infections. *Streptococcus pneumoniae* was most frequent in young ambulatory patients, anaerobes were most frequent after aspiration, and *Staph. aureus* and aerobic Gram-negative bacilli were most frequent after thoracotomy.[9,27–29] Because one-quarter of all empyemas are now associated with trauma or surgery, there has been a relative increase in the proportion of staphylococcal infections and a decrease in anaerobic infections.[8] With the widespread use of *H. influenzae* type b vaccination, empyema due to this organism, previously common in children, has become rare.

PREVENTION

Minimizing the risks of aspiration in people who are unconscious, undergoing anesthesia, or subject to seizures will reduce the incidence of pneumonia with subsequent abscess formation or empyema. If pneumonia does occur, the timely administration of appropriate antibiotics reduces the likelihood of progression. Pleural effusions should be aspirated for diagnosis and drained, if indicated, to abort progressive suppurative complications.

CLINICAL FEATURES

LUNG ABSCESS
Aspiration is usually subtle and unrecognized, but it may lead to pneumonia and lung abscess. If overt, it may be followed by symptoms and signs such as choking, cough, wheezing, cyanosis, or asphyxia, which are related to the particulate, liquid and chemical nature of the material aspirated. Within hours, there may be fever, tachypnea, diffuse rales and hypoxemia.[11,29] If pneumonia develops, patients usually present within 1 week with a productive cough, a temperature over 102°F (38.9°C) and a leukocyte count of more than 15,000 cells/mm³.[29] Aspiration pneumonia is not readily distinguishable from pneumococcal pneumonia, although true rigors are uncommon in aspiration pneumonia and symptoms have usually been present for longer before presentation for medical care; a condition predisposing to aspiration is also more likely to be present. Among community-acquired cases, common conditions that predispose to aspiration are alcoholism, seizures and drug overdose. Among hospital-acquired cases, patients tend to have neurologic disorders, such as cerebrovascular accidents and brain tumors, or metabolic disorders that result in stupor or coma. Only a minority of patients with aspiration pneumonia have putrid sputum, which, if present, tends to develop 1–2 weeks into the course when an abscess has formed.[6,12,14,29]

FREQUENCY OF ORGANISMS ISOLATED FROM BACTERIAL EMPYEMAS

Organism	% of isolates		
	1971–1973[27] (n = 214)	1969–1978[9] (n = 93)	1973–1985[28] (n = 343)
Haemophilus influenzae	<1	0	3
Streptococcus pneumoniae	2	7	20
Other streptococci (including microaerophiles)	13	22	8
Staphylococcus aureus	8	8	17
Enterobacteriaceae	9	10	11
Pseudomonas spp.	5	9	3
Other aerobes	5	2	2
Bacteroides spp.	11	14	8
Anaerobic cocci	15	9	10
Fusobacterium spp.	7	8	6
Prevotella spp.	6	4	6
Other anaerobes	19	7	6

Fig. 29.7 Frequency of organisms isolated from bacterial empyemas.

Lung abscesses may also present in a more indolent fashion with weeks to months of productive cough, malaise, weight loss, low-grade fever, night sweats, leukocytosis and anemia. The patient may become debilitated as if with tuberculosis. Findings that are suggestive of a suppurative lung abscess rather than tuberculosis include a shorter duration of symptoms, putrid sputum and leukocytosis. Lung abscess must also be distinguished from a necrotic neoplasm. Patients with neoplasms often lack risk factors for aspiration, symptoms of respiratory infection, fever and leukocytosis. The possibility of tuberculosis or a noninfectious cause of a lung cavity (neoplasm, infarct, or vasculitis) should be suspected in a patient treated for presumed lung abscess who does not respond to appropriate antimicrobial therapy.

In the pre-antibiotic era, lung abscess characteristically ran a chronic course with the potential for sudden, severe complications. These included brain abscess, massive hemoptysis, endobronchial spread to other portions of the lung, and rupture into the pleural space with the development of a bronchopleural fistula and pyopneumothorax. With modern antimicrobial therapy, these complications have become rare.

EMPYEMA
Symptoms of empyema include fever, chills, cough, dyspnea and chest pain associated with a recent pulmonary or contiguous infection in the oropharynx, mediastinum, or subdiaphragmatic area. The occurrence of persistent fever and leukocytosis with pleural effusion despite appropriate antibiotics should suggest the presence of empyema. There may also be severe constitutional manifestations such as shock, tachypnea, altered consciousness and respiratory failure. Typical findings on physical examination include diminished breath sounds, dullness to percussion and a pleural friction rub. Patients with an empyema that is secondary to an aerobic pneumonia tend to present with an acute illness, whereas those with an anaerobic pneumonia have subacute or indolent illness with findings such as putrid sputum to suggest the etiology.[1,5,29]

DIAGNOSIS

RADIOGRAPHY
Both lung abscess and empyema may be suspected from clinical symptoms, but the chest radiograph is the primary tool for diagnosing these infections. Radiographs obtained soon after aspiration usually demon-

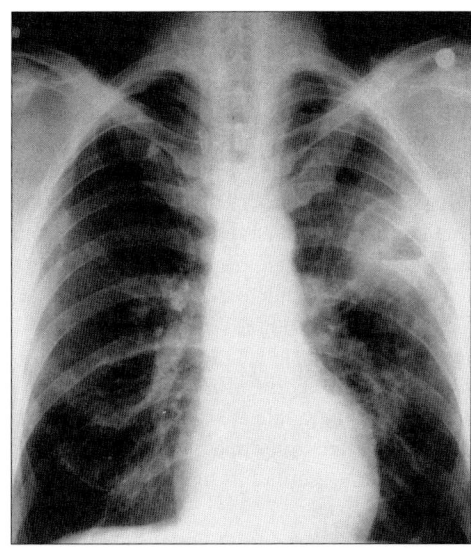

Fig. 29.8 A lung abscess showing an air–fluid level.

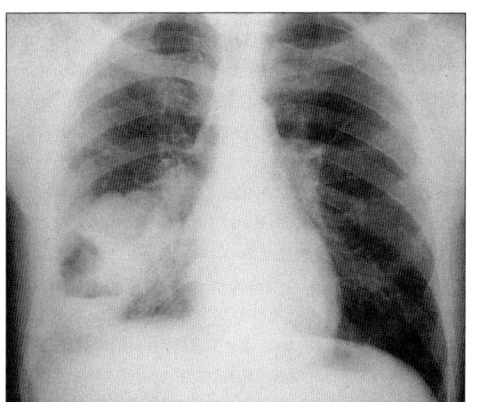

Fig. 29.9 A lung abscess associated with a multinodular bronchogenic carcinoma.

thinner walls with a smooth luminal margin and exterior.[30] Both ultrasound and CT may be used to guide aspiration of fluid from abscesses or the pleural space.

DIAGNOSIS

The first step in determining the specific etiology of any LRTI is the evaluation of lower respiratory tract secretions by Gram-stain. These are most likely to be useful if they are obtained before the administration of effective antimicrobial treatment. If stains of expectorated specimens show neutrophils and alveolar macrophages, without squamous epithelial cells (indicative of contamination with saliva), they are useful for defining the offending pathogen or pathogens. In aerobic pneumonia there is usually a single predominant organism; in aspiration pneumonia there is usually a mixed flora, representing the diverse morphotypes of the oropharyngeal flora. Typically, there are various sizes of Gram-positive cocci and pleomorphic Gram-negative coccobacilli and bacilli, which may be tapered and are generally smaller and poorer staining than the Enterobacteriaceae (Fig. 29.9).[1,2,11,13,31] Although some of the individual organisms may resemble pathogenic aerobes such as *Strep. pneumoniae*, there is no predominant pathogen.

Invasive procedures, such as endotracheal aspiration and bronchoscopy, may be useful to obtain lower respiratory secretions for evaluation. Tracheal aspiration through the nose or the mouth is of limited use because these specimens are often contaminated with oropharyngeal flora. Bronchoscopy with bronchoalveolar lavage is useful because large samples can be obtained with relatively little contamination. They can be concentrated by cytocentrifugation, permitting multiple microbiologic and cytologic evaluations. The bronchoscopic techniques of protected catheter aspiration and protected specimen brushing reduce contamination considerably, but they provide relatively scanty specimens and rely on quantitative cultures to help distinguish the significance of cultures. In general, counts that indicate more than 10^5 cfu/ml of respiratory secretions for an appropriate organism (Figs 29.1 & 29.3) are indicative of infection.[1,5,15,32]

Specimens of lower respiratory tract secretions that have passed through the mouth should be cultured for aerobes, but not for anaerobes. Growth of recognized aerobic pathogens is helpful for interpreting Gram stains and for providing isolates for susceptibility testing. The absence of aerobic pathogens in specimens from untreated patients should indicate the possibility of anaerobic infection. When specimens are contaminated by saliva, the streptococci and anaerobes that comprise the normal oropharyngeal flora will always grow in culture, whether or not infection is present, and they provide no insight into the pathogenicity of the organisms isolated.

The problem of contamination of respiratory tract secretions by saliva can be avoided if specimens of lower respiratory secretions are obtained by transtracheal aspiration. A catheter is passed through the cricothyroid membrane and specimens are collected by suction.[1,12,14] Although infrequently used today, this technique established the role of anaerobes in suppurative pleuropulmonary infections in the early 1970s. Another method for obtaining uncontaminated material for culture is percutaneous transthoracic needle aspiration (percutaneous abscess drainage). Today, this procedure is more frequently performed under fluoroscopic or CT guidance for the diagnosis of malignancy than to obtain material for culture. It can be used, however, to aspirate peripheral abscesses, particularly if bronchoscopy does not provide an adequate specimen for microbiologic diagnosis.

If appropriate specimens from the lower respiratory tract are obtained for culturing anaerobes, they should be expeditiously transported to the laboratory, with minimal exposure to air, for proper processing. If tuberculosis or fungal infection is in the differential diagnosis, appropriate smears and cultures should be requested. If a malignancy is suspected, cytologic stains should be performed.

In addition to lower respiratory tract secretions, blood and pleural fluid, if present, should also be sent to the laboratory for microbiologic

strate localized or diffuse alveolar infiltrates within 1–2 days. There is nothing distinctive about the appearance of aspiration pneumonia except that infiltrates are usually in dependent segments of the lung.

The characteristic appearance of a lung abscess is that of a density or mass with a cavity, frequently with an air–fluid level indicating communication with the tracheobronchial tree (Fig. 29.8). The time required for cavitation after a known episode of aspiration is about 1–2 weeks. With necrotizing pneumonia, multiple small lucencies in circumscribed areas of opacification may develop more rapidly.[2,5,6] Abscesses due to tuberculosis are less likely to have an air–fluid level and are more likely to have a dense fibronodular infiltrate that surrounds the cavities.[20] Those associated with a malignancy may be more sharply defined or have an eccentric-shaped cavity with a thick, irregular wall (Fig 29.9).

A pleural effusion that is visible on posterior–anterior and lateral upright chest radiographs suggests the possibility of empyema. On a decubitus film, with the suspect side down, free pleural fluid can be visualized between the chest wall and the dependent lung. If the layer of pleural fluid is greater than 1cm thick, it should be aspirated for diagnostic studies. A decubitus film with the suspect side up is also useful because it permits assessment of any underlying parenchymal infiltrate, less obscured by the effusion.[8,24]

Ultrasound and CT may be helpful in defining pleuropulmonary lesions. Ultrasound can define loculated collections of pleural fluid, and portable equipment is available for unstable or critically ill patients; CT can define abscesses that are not apparent on plain radiographs and can distinguish between parenchymal and pleural disease. Loculated empyema with a bronchopleural fistula may resemble a lung abscess. Features on CT that tend to favor lung abscess are the presence of thick walls and lesions that are round or oblong, whereas empyemas have evaluation. In anaerobic lung infections, blood cultures are rarely positive. Pleural fluid, if present, requires analysis of protein, lactate dehydrogenase, and glucose and determination of pH, as well as microbiologic evaluation. With empyema, the Gram stain usually indicates the pathogens.[8]

MANAGEMENT

LUNG ABSCESS

In the past, penicillin G was the preferred drug for treating aspiration pneumonia and lung abscesses, as well as for all anaerobic infections above the diaphragm caused by oropharyngeal flora. In a study of over 70 patients hospitalized with lung abscesses in the 1960s, nearly all responded to intravenous penicillin G. Oral penicillin V in a dose of 3g/day was also effective and those rare patients who failed to respond to penicillin could be satisfactorily treated with tetracycline.[6]

In the 1970s, when transtracheal aspiration was used to define the microbiology of pneumonia and lung abscesses, concern over the use of penicillin was raised because of occasional therapeutic failures and the isolation of penicillin-resistant *B. fragilis* from some patients.[1,14] However, in one study[34] that compared clindamycin, a drug that is active against *B. fragilis*, with penicillin G in the treatment of aspiration pneumonia and primary lung abscess, there was no difference in rates of defervescence, radiographic clearing or ultimate outcome. Notably, 7 patients from whom *B. fragilis* was isolated responded to penicillin. Subsequently, in a 1983 prospective study of 39 patients with lung abscess,[35] there were 0/19 failures with clindamycin and 4/20 failures with penicillin G. Resolution of fever and putrid sputum was more rapid with clindamycin (4.4 days) than penicillin G (7.6 days) and patients who did not respond to penicillin G ultimately responded to clindamycin. In a 1990 study of 37 patients with lung abscess or necrotizing pneumonia,[36] only 1 of 19 patients failed to respond to clindamycin, whereas 8 of 18 failed with penicillin G. In this study, patients underwent transtracheal aspiration or protected specimen brushing to culture for anaerobes; 9/10 of the penicillin G resistant strains were beta-lactamase producers. It is now recognized that there has been a change in the susceptibilities of the oropharyngeal Gram-negative anaerobes since the 1970s. Many, in addition to *B. fragilis*, are now beta-lactamase producers and resistant to penicillin. In a study of 449 isolates, which included *Bacteroides* spp. other than *B. fragilis*, *Fusobacterium* spp., *Prevotella* spp. and *Porphyromonas* spp. from 28 US medical centers, 57.9% of isolates were beta-lactamase producers.[37]

Today, transtracheal aspiration and other invasive procedures are rarely performed to determine the microbiologic etiology of aspiration pneumonia and lung abscesses in nonimmunocompromised patients. Treatment is usually empiric and largely effective.[6] Clinical outcome for most anaerobic infections seems to correlate with in-vitro data as broadly applied, and detailed study of individual cases does not seem to be necessary. Monitoring trends in susceptibility patterns and detailed study in problematic individual cases suffices.[29]

The in-vitro spectrum and clinical utility of antimicrobials for the treatment of lower respiratory tract bacterial infections is summarized in Figure 29.11. For community-acquired infections that result from aspiration, and where oropharyngeal streptococci and anaerobes are the likely pathogens, penicillin G (or ampicillin or amoxicillin) remains an excellent foundation for treatment, but the addition of a beta-lactamase inhibitor or metronidazole is advisable owing to the frequency of beta-lactamase production among Gram-negative anaerobes.[29,37,38] Clindamycin is also a primary therapeutic agent, despite in-vitro resistance among some *Bacteroides* and *Fusobacterium* spp. Resistance rates vary significantly in different geographic areas, so surveillance of resistance is important in assessing the utility in a given area.[4,6,31,38,39] Metronidazole alone is not effective because of its inactivity against the aerobic and microaerophilic streptococci.[6,38,40]

For hospital-acquired infections, where *Staph. aureus* and aerobic Gram-negative bacilli are common components of the oropharyngeal flora, piperacillin or ticarcillin (rather than penicillin or ampicillin) with a beta-lactamase inhibitor provide better coverage of likely pathogens. Appropriate alternatives are imipenem alone, clindamycin plus an aminoglycoside or ciprofloxacin, or an expanded spectrum cephalosporin such as cefotaxime, ceftizoxime, ceftriaxone, or cefoperazone plus metronidazole. Many cephalosporins, for example, ceftazidime, have little or no activity against anaerobes and should not be used unless the etiology has been defined and found to be due to aerobic Gram-negative bacilli.[6,10,40]

Tetracyclines, which were used for lung abscess and empyema in the 1960s, are no longer recommended for the treatment of aerobic–anaerobic pleuropulmonary infections because of high rates of resistance. Chloramphenicol has an excellent spectrum of activity, but it is rarely recommended because of potential hematotoxicity and the availability of alternative agents.[6,40] The macrolides and azalides have inconsistent in-vitro activity against oropharyngeal anaerobes and there is little clinical precedent for their use.[41] Aminoglycosides and quinolones should be used only for their activity against aerobic Gram-negative bacilli and need to be combined with a drug that is active against streptococci and anaerobes. Some new quinolones, such as trovafloxacin, have greater activity than ciprofloxacin or ofloxacin against oropharyngeal streptococci and anaerobes, and might prove to be more useful.[42] Other agents that have suboptimal or no activity against oropharyngeal streptococci and anaerobes include aztreonam and trimethoprim–sulfamethoxazole (co-trimoxazole). The antistaphylococcal penicillins and vancomycin should be reserved for staphylococcal infections.

The duration of antimicrobial therapy necessary to treat pleuropulmonary infections is variable: 1–2 weeks may suffice for simple aspiration pneumonia, but necrotizing pneumonia and lung abscesses may require 3–12 weeks of treatment. Parenteral therapy is generally employed until the patient is afebrile (most are afebrile in 7 days) and able to have a consistent enteral intake.[29] For most community-acquired infections, amoxicillin–clavulanate and clindamycin are excellent oral drugs that can be used for continued treatment after initial parenteral therapy. A less costly oral alternative is penicillin V plus metronidazole. If aerobic Gram-negative bacilli are present, oral treatment is more problematic and must be based on the results of susceptibility tests; ciprofloxacin or ofloxacin plus a penicillin or clindamycin may be appropriate. It is probably best to treat until the cavity is gone or until serial radiographs show considerable improvement or only a small stable residual scar. The time to cavity closure depends largely on the size of the cavity when treatment is initiated and the condition of the patient.

Surgical drainage of lung abscesses is rarely indicated because drainage occurs naturally via the tracheobronchial tree. If spontaneous drainage is not adequate, even with the aid of postural drainage and percussion, clinical improvement is impeded, and CT-guided

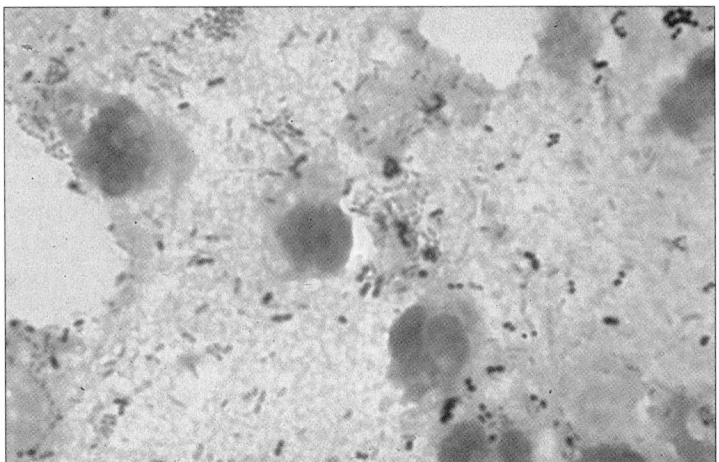

Fig. 29.10 Gram stain of lower respiratory tract secretions. The patient had a lung abscess caused by oropharyngeal streptococci and anaerobes.

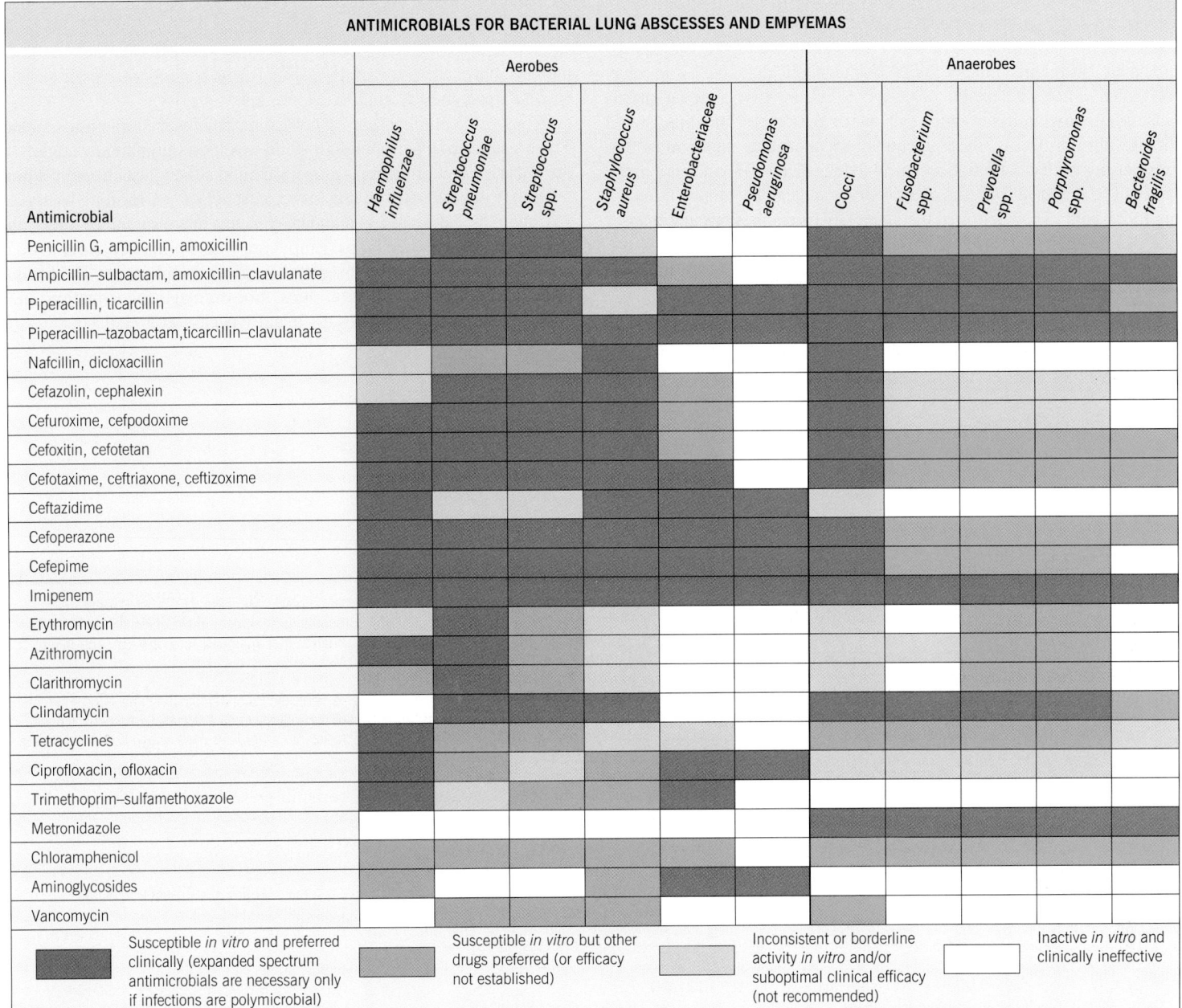

Fig. 29.11 Antimicrobials for bacterial lung abscesses and empyemas. Information for *Streptococcus pneumoniae* is for penicillin-susceptible strains – selected cephalosporins or vancomycin should be used for resistant strains. Information for *Staphylococcus aureus* is for methicillin-susceptible strains – vancomycin should be used for resistant strains. Vancomycin is the drug of choice for beta-lactam-resistant Gram-positive organisms.

percutaneous abscess drainage may then be beneficial. The drainage catheter can be left in place until there is clinical improvement and drainage has diminished, usually within several days to 1 week. This technique may also be used to reduce the risk of endobronchial spread of infection to other areas of the lungs as well as in patients who are too ill to undergo lung resection to remove necrotic tissue, persistent cavities, or nonfunctional lung.

EMPYEMA

The antimicrobial treatment of empyema is similar to that of aspiration pneumonia and lung abscess, but single organism infections with a defined etiology are more common, thus facilitating antibiotic choice. Antibiotics should be administered in full doses for 2–4 weeks. Therapy may need to be prolonged further, particularly if drainage is not optimal. Antibiotic levels in pleural fluid are comparable to those in serum, so standard systemic doses provide adequate pleural fluid levels.[24]

The proper assessment and management of parapneumonic effusions associated with LRTIs is critical for a successful outcome. Most small

effusions clear with antimicrobial treatment and need not be drained. However, if fluid persists more than a few days or layers to more than 1cm on a decubitus radiograph with the involved side dependent, it should be aspirated and analyzed. The characteristics of the fluid are used to determine the need for tube drainage (Fig. 29.6).

Effusions are termed 'complicated' when characteristics indicate a potential need for tube drainage. Complicated effusions are termed 'empyemas' if they are frankly purulent and bacteria are present; tube drainage is mandatory. Chest tubes are placed using negative pressure until the lung is expanded, and then to an underwater drainage system until the fluid is scanty and clear, and then gradually withdrawn over a period of several days. Lack of prompt clinical improvement may indicate the need for repositioning the tube to facilitate and continue drainage.

Chest tube drainage of complicated parapneumonic effusions is successful in most patients. It should not be delayed, because these effusions can progress from free-flowing to loculated fluid rapidly. When the fluid becomes loculated, drainage by repeated thoracentesis or tube insertion may not be adequate. The presence of loculated fluid should be suspected if the patient remains ill or febrile or has a persistent leukocytosis. After appropriate evaluation by ultrasound or CT, options for management include image-guided percutaneous drainage by an interventional radiologist[43] or the instillation of thrombolytic agents (urokinase or streptokinase) through a catheter or chest tube.[44] If administered before fibrosis occurs, these agents attack the fibrin membranes that are causing the loculations. Successful therapy leads to an increase in the amount of drainage from the pleural space and can be administered for up to 2 weeks. Thoroscopy to mechanically lyze adhesions and inspect the pleural cavity has also been used to assist in management.[8]

If patients do not respond to the above measures, contrast material can be injected into the chest tube to evaluate the empyema cavity. Open drainage, evacuation of all infected material and decortication of the pleura should be considered. This is a major surgical procedure that requires rib resection; it may not be tolerated by debilitated patients. Open drainage, without decortication, may be better tolerated in these patients but it is followed by a prolonged period of convalescence with an open chest wound.[8]

A serious complication of empyema is a bronchopleural fistula. The presence of a peripheral air–fluid level radiographically suggests the presence of a bronchopulmonary fistula, although such an air–fluid level may occasionally be due to the presence of gas-forming bacteria. Adequate tube drainage is mandatory to minimize spread of infection to other portions of the lungs. Empyema with a bronchopleural fistula after pneumonectomy is a disastrous surgical complication. The fistula often does not close with antibiotics, tube drainage and irrigation, and complex surgical procedures are usually necessary.[8]

REFERENCES

1. Bartlett JG, Finegold SM. Anaerobic infections of the lung and pleural space. Am Rev Respir Dis 1974;110:56–77.
2. Bartlett JG, Gorbach SL, Tally FP, et al. Bacteriology and treatment of primary lung abscess. Am Rev Respir Dis 1974;109:510–8.
3. Pohlson EC, McNamara JJ, Char C, et al. Lung abscess: a changing pattern of the disease. Am J Surg 1985;150:97–101.
4. Hammond JM, Potgieter PD, Hanslo D, et al. The etiology and antimicrobial susceptibility patterns of microorganisms in acute community-acquired lung abscess. Chest 1995;108:937–41.
5. Bartlett JG. Anaerobic bacterial infections of the lung. Chest 1987;91:901–9.
6. Bartlett JG. Antibiotics in lung abscess. Semin Respir Infect 1991;6:103–11.
7. Harber P, Terry PB. Fatal lung abscesses: review of 11 years' experience. South Med J 1981;74:281–3.
8. Light RW. Parapneumonic effusions and empyema. In: Retford DC, ed. Pleural diseases. Baltimore: Williams and Wilkins; 1995:129–53.
9. Varkey B, Rose HD, Kutty CPK, et al. Empyema thoracis during a ten-year period. Analysis of 72 cases and comparison to a previous study (1952–1967). Arch Intern Med 1981;141:1771–6.
10. Bartlett JG. Bacterial infections of the pleural space. Semin Respir Infect 1988;3:308–21.
11. Finegold SM. Aspiration pneumonia. Rev Infect Dis 1991;13(Suppl 9):737–42.
12. Bartlett JG, Gorbach SL, Finegold SM. The bacteriology of aspiration pneumonia. Am J Med 1974;56:202–7.
13. Gorbach SL, Bartlett JG. Anaerobic infections. N Engl J Med 1974;290:1237–45.
14. Lorber B, Swenson RM. Bacteriology of aspiration pneumonia. A prospective study of community- and hospital-acquired cases. Ann Intern Med 1974;81:329–31.
15. Wiblin RT. Nosocomial pneumonia. In: Wenzel RP, ed. Prevention and control of nosocomial infections, 3rd ed. Baltimore: Williams and Wilkins; 1997:807–19.
16. Finegold SM. Overview of clinically important anaerobes. Clin Infect Dis 1995;20(Suppl 2):205–7.
17. Summanen P. Microbiology terminology update: clinically significant anaerobic Gram-positive and Gram-negative bacteria (excluding spirochetes). Clin Infect Dis 1995;21:273–6.

18. Duerden BI. Virulence factors in anaerobes. Clin Infect Dis 1994;18(Suppl 4):253–9.
19. Cameron JL, Mitchell WH, Zuidema GD. Aspiration pneumonia. Clinical outcome following documented aspiration. Arch Surg 1973;106:49–52.
20. Israel RH, Poe RH, Greenblatt DW, et al. Differentiation of tuberculous from nontuberculous cavitary lung disease. Respiration 1985;47:151–7.
21. Chan P, Ogilby JD, Segal B. Tricuspid valve endocarditis. Am Heart J 1989;117:1140–6.
22. Furman AC, Jacobs J, Sepkowitz KA. Lung abscess in patients with AIDS. Clin Infect Dis 1996;22:81–5.
23. Schachter EN. Suppurative lung disease: old problems revisited. Clin Chest Med 1981;2:41–9.
24. Bryant RE, Salmon CJ. Pleural empyema. Clin Infect Dis 1996;22:747–64.
25. Weese WC, Shindler ER, Smith IM, et al. Empyema of the thorax then and now. A study of 122 cases over four decades. Arch Intern Med 1973;131:516–20.
26. Sullivan KM, O'Toole RD, Fisher RH, et al. Anaerobic empyema thoracis. Arch Intern Med 1973;131:521–7.
27. Bartlett JG, Thadepalli H, Gorbach SL, et al. Bacteriology of empyema. Lancet 1974;i:338–40.
28. Brook I, Frazier EH. Aerobic an anaerobic microbiology of empyema. A retrospective review in two military hospitals. Chest 1993;103:1502–7.
29. Bartlett JG. Anaerobic bacterial infections of the lung and pleural space. Clin Infect Dis 1993;16(Suppl 4):248–55.
30. Stark DD, Federle MP, Goodman PC. Differentiating lung abscess and empyema: radiography and computed tomography. Am J Roentgenol 1983;141:163–7.
31. Civen R, Jousimies-Somer H, Marina M, et al. A retrospective review of cases of anaerobic empyema and update of bacteriology. Clin Infect Dis 1995;20(Suppl 2):224–9.
32. Pollock HM, Hawkins EL, Bonner JR, et al. Diagnosis of bacterial pulmonary infections with quantitative protected catheter cultures obtained during bronchoscopy. J Clin Microbiol 1983;17:255–9.
33. Sokolowski JW, Burgher LW, Jones FL, et al. Guidelines for thoracentesis and needle biopsy of the pleura. Am Rev Respir Dis 1989;140:257–8.
34. Bartlett JG, Gorbach SL. Treatment of aspiration pneumonia and primary lung abscess. Penicillin G vs clindamycin. JAMA 1975;234:935–7.

35. Levison ME, Mangura CT, Lorber B, et al. Clindamycin compared with penicillin for the treatment of anaerobic lung abscess. Ann Intern Med 1983;98:466–71.
36. Gudiol F, Manresa F, Pallares R, et al. Clindamycin vs penicillin for anaerobic lung infections. High rate of penicillin failures associated with penicillin-resistant Bacteroides melaninogenicus. Arch Intern Med 1990;150:2525–9.
37. Appelbaum PC, Spangler SK, Jacobs MR. β-Lactamase production and susceptibilities to amoxicillin, amoxicillin-clavulanate, ticarcillin, ticarcillin-clavulanate, cefoxitin, imipenem and metronidazole of 320 non-Bacteroides fragilis Bacteroides isolates and 129 fusobacteria from 28 US centers. Antimicrob Agents Chemother 1990;34:1546–50.
38. Finegold SM, Wexler HM. Present status of therapy for anaerobic infections. Clin Infect Dis 1996;23(Suppl 1):9–14.
39. Rasmussen BA, Bush K, Tally FP. Antimicrobial resistance in anaerobes. Clin Infect Dis 1997;24(Suppl 1):110–20.
40. Perlino CA. Metronidazole vs clindamycin treatment of anaerobic pulmonary infection. Failure of metronidazole therapy. Arch Intern Med 1981;141:1424–7.
41. Fass RJ. Erythromycin, clarithromycin and azithromycin: use of frequency distribution curves, scattergrams and regression analysis to compare in vitro activities and describe cross-resistance. Antimicrob Agents Chemother 1993;37:2080–6.
42. Spangler SK, Jacobs MR, Appelbaum PC. Activity of CP 99,219 compared with those of ciprofloxacin, grepafloxacin, metronidazole, cefoxitin, piperacillin, and piperacillin-tazobactam against 489 anaerobes. Antimicrob Agents Chemother 1994;38:2471–6.
43. Klein JS, Schultz S, Heffner JE. Interventional radiology of the chest: image-guided percutaneous drainage of pleural effusions, lung abscess, and pneumothorax. Am J Roentgenol 1995;164:581–8.
44. Robinson LA, Moulton AL, Fleming WH, et al. Intrapleural fibrinolytic treatment of multiloculated thoracic empyemas. Ann Thorac Surg 1994;57:803–14.

Tuberculosis

Jon S Friedland

Mankind has been plagued throughout history by tuberculosis. It has been identified in skeletons over 6000 years old and remains the most prevalent infectious disease in the world. Among a long list of notable patients are Samuel Johnson, Jean-Jacques Rousseau, John Keats and Fyodor Dostoyevsky. This chapter focuses on current understanding of the pathophysiology, epidemiology and clinical aspects of tuberculosis.

EPIDEMIOLOGY

WORLDWIDE INCIDENCE AND PREVALENCE

Mycobacterium tuberculosis is estimated to infect 1.6 billion people worldwide or approximately one-third of the world's population.[1] Usually infection is contained by the immune system so that about 15 million people have clinical disease at any one time. Tuberculosis kills around 3 million people each year, which is more than any other single infectious disease. Recent data on tuberculosis notification rates are shown in Figure 30.1. However, such notification data are notoriously incomplete, with under-reporting of cases.[2] Confounding factors in the global collection of incidence and prevalence data include effects of treatment, difficulties in identifying extrapulmonary disease and those associated with tuberculin testing (see Testing for exposure). However, the size of the tuberculosis problem is such that it has been uniquely identified as a 'global emergency' by the World Health Organization (WHO).

Over 96% of tuberculosis-related deaths occur in the poorer nations of the world and the disease has huge social and economic costs. In wealthier nations, rates of tuberculosis have been falling over the past 80 years, partly as a result of the development of effective treatments, active case-finding and use of the BCG vaccine. Recently, this trend has been halted in some countries because of the increased incidence of tuberculosis in high-risk population groups, including poorer communities, immigrants and patients who have HIV infection. Levels of disease in homeless populations in developed countries can be as high as 2%.[3]

Impact of HIV

Approximately 8 million people are co-infected with HIV and tuberculosis, the majority of whom live in sub-Saharan Africa, the Indian subcontinent and Southeast Asia (Fig. 30.2). HIV-seropositive patients appear more susceptible to infection by *M. tuberculosis*. Subsequently, approximately 50% of patients who have dual infection will develop clinical tuberculosis, and reactivation rates may be over 20 times greater than in similarly aged controls.[4] Clinical tuberculosis is associated with shorter survival in AIDS patients.[5]

In many developed countries (for example USA, France, Germany and The Netherlands) HIV infection has led to well–documented increases in localized and disseminated tuberculosis. In the USA, tuberculosis patients are offered screening for HIV. Miliary tuberculosis accounted for less than 1.5% of cases of tuberculosis in the

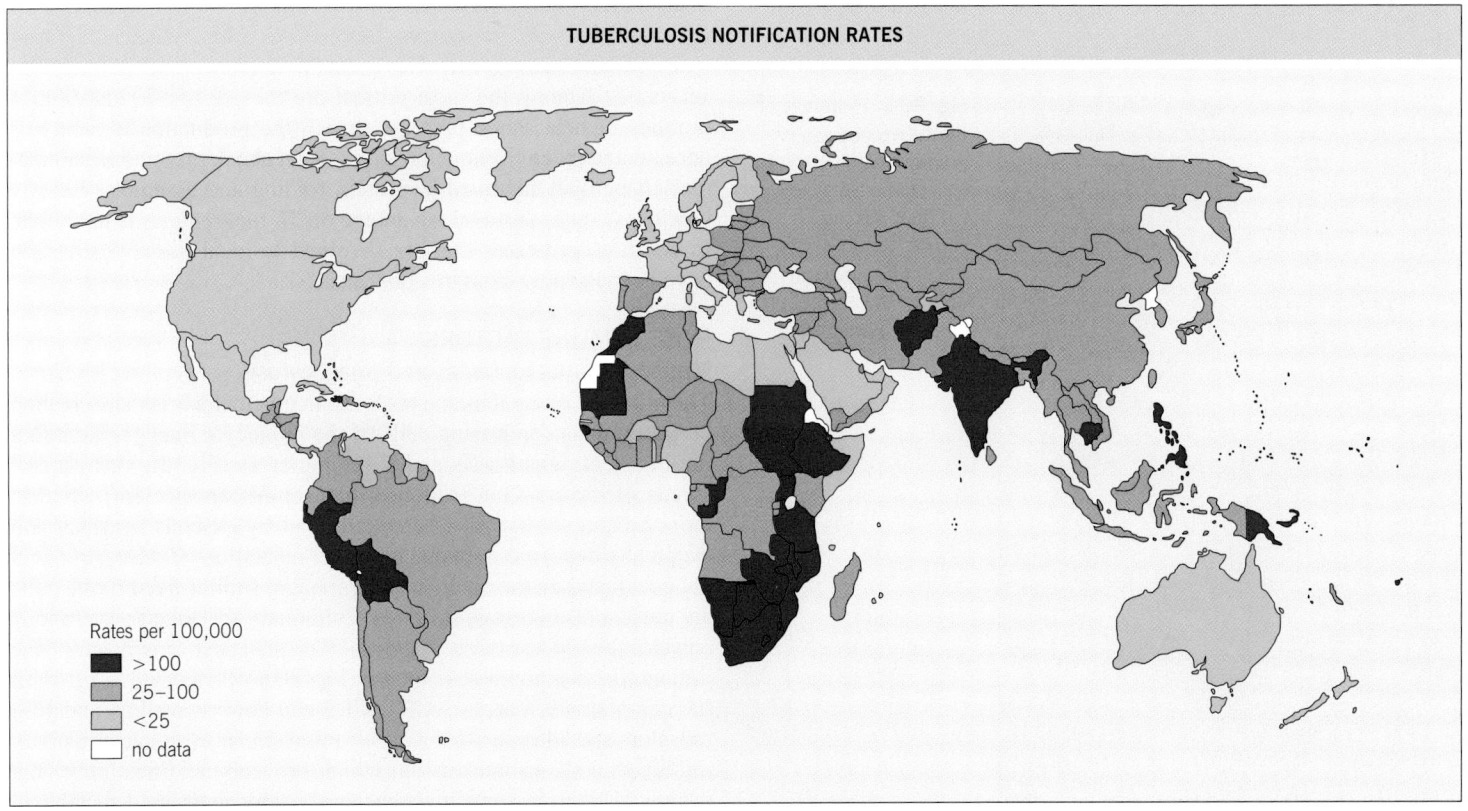

TUBERCULOSIS NOTIFICATION RATES

Rates per 100,000
- ■ >100
- ▓ 25–100
- ▒ <25
- □ no data

Fig. 30.1 Tuberculosis notification rates worldwide. Data from the Global Tuberculosis Program, WHO (1996).

USA for 20 years, but recently, in some areas, disseminated disease accounted for up to 10% of tuberculosis cases.[6] In contrast, in the UK and some Scandinavian countries, the increased incidence of tuberculosis has been associated with economic deprivation rather than with HIV infection.[7]

Diagnosis of dual infection may be difficult because HIV also predisposes to atypical, nodal and extrapulmonary tuberculosis. In addition to HIV increasing the incidence of clinical tuberculosis, infection with *M. tuberculosis* appears to increase viral replication and HIV disease progression.[8] This is in part because tuberculosis activates nuclear factor kappa B (NF-κB) dependent transcription of the HIV genome.[9,10] (See Chapter 5.6).

SPREAD OF INFECTION

Spread of infection is dependent on inhalation of aerosols from individuals with pulmonary infection. Proximity to and duration of association with an index case are critical factors. Up to one-quarter of household contacts of an index case may acquire infection, although the extent to which individual genetic predisposition or immunologic impairment contributes to this is uncertain. The role of factors such as

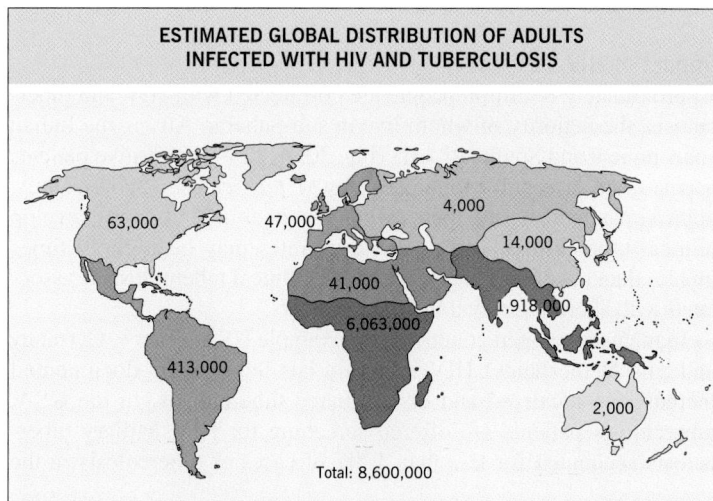

ESTIMATED GLOBAL DISTRIBUTION OF ADULTS INFECTED WITH HIV AND TUBERCULOSIS

63,000

47,000

4,000

14,000

41,000

1,918,000

6,063,000

413,000

2,000

Total: 8,600,000

Fig. 30.2 Estimated global distribution of adults co-infected with tuberculosis and HIV. Data from same source as Figure 30.1.

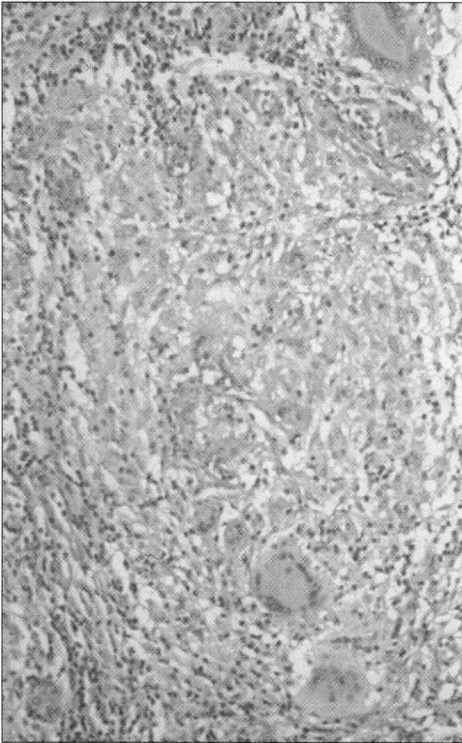

Fig. 30.3 Histology of the tuberculous granuloma. Monocytic cells and smaller T lymphocytes are shown, together with multinucleate giant cells on the edge of an area of caseation.

vitamin D deficiency and iron overload in the spread of tuberculosis are unknown. Spread of infection is quite separate to development of disease, which occurs in less than 10% of infected persons and is significantly increased by impaired cell mediated immunity (see Clinical risk factors). Congenital transmission of tuberculosis is not a significant factor in the natural spread of disease.

Transmission in closed institutions

Overcrowding contributes to the spread of tuberculosis among the poor. Close proximity to infected individuals is a significant issue in any closed institution and for health care workers. Many countries have specific guidelines for tuberculosis control in institutions (see Prevention). Genetic techniques using restriction fragment length polymorphism (RFLP) analysis – often of the insertion sequence IS6110 – to provide DNA fingerprints has proved useful in documenting local outbreaks of tuberculosis, including those involving multidrug resistant organisms.[11]

In prisons, the situation is complicated by the fact that often inmates have an increased prevalence of HIV, are regularly moved to other prisons or back into the community with little warning and are frequently poorly managed in terms of health services. Because release of prisoners is often into poor circumstances and crowded hostels, the consequence of undetected or inadequately treated tuberculosis may be rapid spread of disease. An effective public health program with an active community care component can overcome such problems.

PATHOGENESIS AND PATHOLOGY

THE PATHOGEN

Mycobacterium tuberculosis is a member of the order Actinomycetales, which is characterized by a complex cell wall rich in mycolic acids together with peptidoglycan and arabinogalactan, a complex polysaccharide molecule, that surrounds the cell membrane. Many cell wall components are of pathogenic significance. Lipoarabinomannan (LAM) stimulates monocyte proinflammatory activity principally by binding to the CD14 receptor, also the binding site for bacterial lipopolysaccharide. The mycobacterial genome has a high G + C content. Details of metabolic pathways within *M. tuberculosis* and of assimilation of nutrients such as iron, which is stored in association with mycobactins, are reviewed elsewhere.[12] Mycobacteria contain many proteins associated with growth, virulence and intracellular survival.[13] Among the most critical are the 10, 65, 70 and 90kDa families of heat shock proteins (hsps), the production of which is upregulated by environmental stress. Heat shock proteins are molecular chaperones involved in protein folding and assembly. Exactly how hsps confer survival advantage on *M. tuberculosis* is unknown. In addition, proteases that are involved in local tissue destruction have been isolated from mycobacteria.

HOST IMMUNE FACTORS

Monocytes, macrophages and phagocytosis

The principal tissue immune response in tuberculosis is the formation of granulomas comprising cells of the monocyte lineage, including multinucleate giant cells and T lymphocytes (Fig. 30.3). In initial stages of the immune response, neutrophils are present, whereas more advanced disease is characterized by caseous necrosis and eventually deposition of calcium. After inhalation, *M. tuberculosis* is phagocytosed by the alveolar macrophage; similar fixed tissue cells are present elsewhere in the body. Pulmonary surfactant protein may enhance the process of phagocytosis. The phagocytosing macrophage initiates the host immune response (Fig. 30.4). Phagocytosis involves the complement receptors CR1, CR3 and CR4 as well as mannose receptors and adhesion molecules.[14] Intracellular mycobacteria partly inhibit phagolysosome fusion, which prevents acidification of the vacuole. However, some mycobacterial components are detectable in the cytoplasm.

Phagocytosis is a potent stimulus to gene expression and secretion of proinflammatory cytokines such as tumor necrosis factor (TNF), interleukin (IL)-1 and IL-6. Phagocytosis of *M. tuberculosis* activates the transcription factors NF-IL-6 and NF-κB, both of which are important in proinflammatory cytokine gene activation.[15] The known consequences of TNF secretion include fever and cachexia, two prominent symptoms in tuberculosis. Tumor necrosis factor also has a pivotal role in granuloma formation and is found at sites of human infection. Injection of anti-TNF antibodies in a murine model decreased granuloma formation and increased replication of *Mycobacterium bovis*, BCG strain.[16] At early stages of infection, cellular recruitment to the granuloma is essential, and macrophage-derived chemokines are important in this process.[17] The granuloma in tuberculosis is well circumscribed and it is likely that down regulatory cytokines such as IL-10 are involved in limiting inflammatory responses. Interestingly, when monocytes die by apoptosis there may be associated killing of intracellular mycobacteria, although how crucial this is in humans is unknown.[18] Surprisingly little is known about what exactly kills *M. tuberculosis* in humans.

Infected macrophages are probably involved in the tissue damage characteristic of tuberculosis. Macrophages secrete proteases such as collagenase and gelatinase, the actions of which are opposed by tissue inhibitors of metalloproteinases (TIMPs). TIMP genes are closely regulated, with the transcription factor activator protein-1 having a central role, and their expression is increased by macrophage-derived cytokines TNF and IL-1β. Other monocyte-derived proteins involved in tissue destruction include lysosomal proteases such as cathepsins, which function best at acid pH, and the plasminogen activator urokinase. Activation of the plasminogen system is followed by activation of the clotting system and laying down of fibrous tissue, a process in which macrophage-derived transforming growth factor-β has a central role.[19]

T lymphocytes

In immunity to tuberculosis αβ and γδ CD4+ T lymphocytes are critical. Patients who have reduced T lymphocyte function or numbers are at higher risk of clinical tuberculosis. *Mycobacterium tuberculosis* may impair macrophage antigen presentation to T lymphocytes by downregulating the co-stimulatory molecule B7–1. Cells of the T-helper (T_H)1 subclass, which secrete interferon-γ and IL-2, are central to the control of infection in murine models. In human disease the situation is more complex with T_H1, T_H2 (which produce IL-4, -5, -6, -10 and -13) and intermediate cell types detectable,[20] although T_H1 cells appear to concentrate at sites of infection such as pleura.[21] The dual presence of T_H1 and T_H2 cells may account for the fact that, although tuberculosis is limited within the granuloma, the organism is not usually completely killed off by the immune response.

The involvement of γδ T lymphocytes in immunity to human tuberculosis remains controversial, although they appear critical in murine models of infection. The percentage of γδ cells at sites of tuberculosis in the few studies performed in patients have been conflicting but their presence has been correlated with effective immune responses. These cells have the potential to recognize important, conserved mycobacterial antigens such as the 65kDa hsp.[22] γδ T lymphocytes may be involved in macrophage aggregation and activation, in lysis of infected cells and in cytokine secretion.[20,23]

Other T-cell phenotypes involved in immunity to tuberculosis include CD8+ lymphocytes,[24] although their exact role in humans is still to be defined. In addition, there are double-negative T lymphocytes lacking CD4 and CD8, which recognize mycobacterial lipoglycan antigens presented via CD1, proteins that have distant homology to the major histocompatibility complex.[25]

Humoral response

Many proteins, carbohydrates and lipids of *M. tuberculosis* contain epitopes that stimulate antibody production. Such antibodies have been used to characterize important antigens of *M. tuberculosis*, such as the 12, 65 and 72kDa hsps. However, in terms of pathogenesis, it has proved difficult to identify specific antibody responses in sera of tuberculosis patients of importance in host defense. Interest in antibody responses in tuberculosis has centered upon the development of diagnostic tests.

Local tissue responses

Granuloma formation is the consequence of a complex interaction between the organism, the immune system and local release of tissue factors and proteases. Gross pathology reflects the relative influence of these factors in a particular patient. This process may be modulated by systemic or local production of hormones such as 1,25-dihydroxy-vitamin D_3.[26] Caseous necrosis, typical of mycobacterial granulomas, is probably caused by the delayed type hypersensitivity response, although it is not known why it is so very rare in nontuberculous granulomas.

HOST GENETIC FACTORS

There is a undoubtedly a genetic component to host resistance to *M. tuberculosis*. Identical twins have been shown to be concordant for tuberculosis and it has been suggested in the USA that black patients are more susceptible to infection.[27] Human leukocyte antigen (HLA) haplotypes associated with susceptibility to tuberculosis include A8, A10, B8, Bw15 and DR2. It is likely that many genetic polymorphisms influence susceptibility to tuberculosis to varying degrees. Much interest has focused on non-HLA linked genes such as the *bcg* gene, located on human chromosome 2. Its product, the protein *Nramp* (natural resistance associated membrane protein), is a major determinant of disease susceptibility in murine systems[28] but its importance in humans is less clear. Certain families that are susceptible to atypical mycobacterial infections have recently been shown to have deletions in the interferon-γ receptor gene (see Newport *et al.*[75]).

PREVENTION

PUBLIC HEALTH MEASURES

Strategies to prevent spread of tuberculosis aim first to identify and promptly treat infectious patients and second to prevent spread of infection. Many countries have a system, often legally enforced, of infectious patient notification to a central body that traces infected contacts of index cases. In addition, high-risk patients or communities,

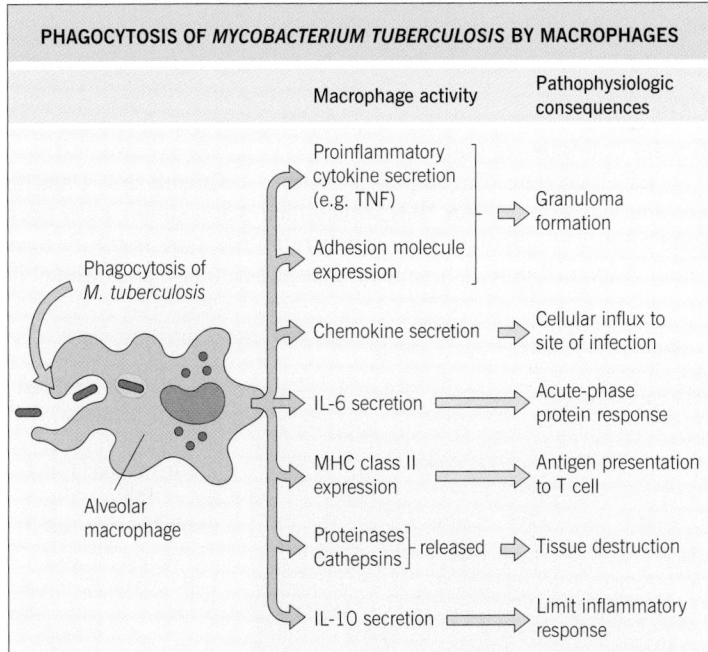

Fig. 30.4 Phagocytosis of *Mycobacterium tuberculosis* by macrophages. Phagocytosis initiates many critical pathways involved in host defense to infection.

such as intravenous drug users, may be screened so that definitive or prophylactic therapy may be instituted. In its simplest form, case-finding involves clinical assessment and examination of sputum smears, although radiologic examination may be a useful adjunct. Skin testing may be appropriate in countries with low rates of infection and no routine immunization of the population. It is important to distinguish between disease relapse and reinfection, and RFLP analysis has proved useful.[29] Prevention programs may require incentives for successful implementation; they should be linked to educational initiatives and involve social services.

Infectious patients should be isolated until effective treatment has been instituted. In the USA, laminar airflow and negative pressure ventilation rooms are provided for patients who have known or suspected tuberculosis, particularly those with multidrug resistant disease. Detailed guidelines have been produced in the USA from several sources which are useful[30] but are potentially extremely costly to implement.[31] For example, expensive respirator masks have been advocated but are likely to represent a poor use of funds, particularly in developing countries. Shortwave ultraviolet illuminators to kill organisms in clinics and shelters have been used, although their efficacy has yet to be tested in comparative trials with other control methods. In many parts of the globe, basic patient isolation and possibly specified, ventilated rooms for procedures that generate aerosols is all that is feasible. Appropriate control measures should be defined in advance in high-risk procedure rooms, during patient transport and in all at-risk institutions.

TESTING FOR EXPOSURE
Mantoux test
This is the commonest test used to screen for tuberculosis exposure and depends on the intradermal injection of a specified quantity of an internationally standardized purified protein derivative (PPD) of tuberculin. PPD solution should not be left in syringes because it may be variably adsorbed to their surface. Tuberculin positivity manifests as induration at the site of testing after 48 hours. Induration less than 5mm after a standard injection of 10 units PPD is regarded as negative and greater than 15mm as positive. However, PPD may have a booster effect on immunologic memory and a second Mantoux test should be performed a week after a negative test to confirm the finding.

Induration in the 5–15mm range may be indicative of exposure to mycobacteria, previous immunization or disease in the immuno-suppressed patient, which have unpredictable confounding effects on Mantoux testing. In the USA, induration greater than 5mm is taken as positive in patients who have HIV, a close contact with tuberculosis or a fibrotic chest radiograph, and induration above 10mm is positive in any other high-risk group. Patients who are immunosuppressed, such as those with HIV (particularly if CD4+ T-lymphocyte count is below 400/ml) or who have measles or sarcoidosis, have a strong tendency to anergy. Systemic illness, including miliary tuberculosis, is also associated with anergy. The Centers for Disease Control and Prevention, Atlanta, USA has recommended concurrent testing for generalized anergy, but the relationship between general anergy and tuberculin negativity is unclear. False-negative tests may also occur at the extremes of age in patients on high dose corticosteroids, after use of inadequately stored tuberculin or as a result of poor injection technique. Skin testing is not a useful exercise in low-risk children. PPD may re-stimulate previous hypersensitivity producing the booster Mantoux effect whereby a second Mantoux test 8 weeks after a negative test becomes positive. To avoid confusion negative Mantoux tests should be repeated within 2 weeks.

Heaf test
This test involves placing PPD on the skin of a subject and then using a multiple puncture gun to pierce the skin in six places; the response is then graded (Figs 30.5 & 30.6). Heaf guns must be resterilized between patients; a disposable head is preferred.

Tine test
The Tine test is similar to the Heaf test except that the puncture needles (usually four not six) are precoated with tuberculin. There has been considerable controversy as to the reliability of this technique and it is fading from general use.

CHEMOPROPHYLAXIS
Chemoprophylaxis may be primary in unexposed individuals or secondary in those exposed to *M. tuberculosis* who do not have clinical disease. Secondary prophylaxis is practiced most commonly and successfully in tuberculosis control programs in the USA. This approach, which is based on regular skin prick testing, is not possible when vaccination is common or resources inadequate. Isoniazid, 300mg daily for 6–12 months, is the usual preventative regimen and, as in treatment schedules, is associated with a significant incidence of (principally hepatic) toxicity, which is particularly important because the subjects are well. In addition, with the increase in drug resistance, it is likely that significant numbers of organisms will not respond to isoniazid. Chemoprophylaxis has been advocated in all HIV-seropositive patients because of the increased incidence of clinical disease in patients exposed to *M. tuberculosis*. However, if diagnostic facilities are poor, there must be a significant chance of inadvertently treating established tuberculosis, which would hasten the emergence of isoniazid resistance. The issues, which include economic factors, are complex and the validity of prophylaxis in HIV vigorously debated.[32] In contrast, the use of secondary chemoprophylaxis in potential transplant recipients is established. Chemoprophylaxis should be deferred in pregnant women, a group who may be more prone to isoniazid hepatitis.

VACCINES
Bacille Calmette–Guerin
The BCG vaccine, developed by Albert Calmette and Camille Guerin, was first used in 1921. Since then many strains have been used clinically, although the current reference type is the Pasteur strain. Vaccination leads to a local immune response and ultimately

HEAF TEST GRADES	
Heaf test grade	Response
0	No induration at puncture sites
1	Discrete induration at a minimum of four needle sites
2	Induration at needle sites merge to form ring but leave clear center
3	One large induration site seen (5–10mm diameter)
4	Induration over 10mm diameter

Fig. 30.5 The Heaf test grades.

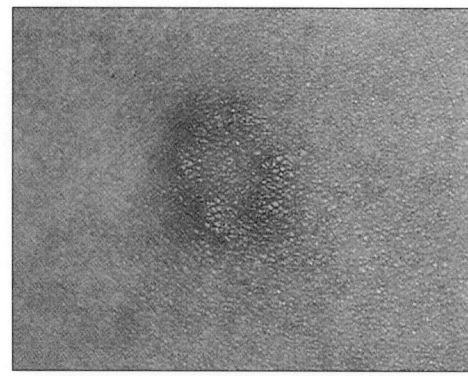

Fig. 30.6 A Heaf test grade 2 response. With permission from James DG and Studdy PR, Colour atlas of respiratory diseases, 2E, London: Mosby; 1992.

scar formation (Fig. 30.7). Keloid may form in susceptible individuals. Adverse reactions other than local irritation are uncommon and anaphylaxis extremely rare. Local abscesses or ulcers usually reflect poor technique. Adenitis, sometimes suppurative, occurs at a rate of 25 cases per 1,000,000 vaccinations. Lupoid reactions, infected osteitis and disseminated BCG disease are very rare, the latter two necessitating therapy with rifampin (rifampicin) and isoniazid (BCG is resistant to pyrazinamide).

Extent of immunity after BCG vaccination depends on the strain used, environmental factors, the genetics of the population being vaccinated and individual host factors such as age. There is a poor correlation between tuberculin reactivity after vaccination, which develops to maximal levels within 3 months, and protection against disease. Reviews indicate that BCG vaccine efficacy is about 60–80%,[33] although in certain parts of the world, such as Malawi, even repeated vaccination offered no protection against tuberculosis; it did, however, decrease *Mycobacterium leprae* infection rates.[34] Giving BCG to infants provides significant protection from tuberculosis in household contacts.

Novel vaccines
There are three novel vaccine approaches. The first of these involve using an environmental commensal *M. vaccae* to enhance protective immune responses but it proved unsuccessful.[35] The second approach involves naked DNA vaccines encoding for immunogenic mycobacterial antigens. This has been successfully used in an animal model in which injection of the DNA coding for the mycobacterial 65kDa hsp was protective against challenge with virulent *M. tuberculosis*.[36] Third, there is research interest in subunit, recombinant or genetically engineered vaccines in which either BCG serves as a vector for specific antigens of *M. tuberculosis*, or an attenuated *M. tuberculosis* is created by deletion of specific virulence factors, or antigens are administered, possibly with an adjuvant.

CLINICAL FEATURES

In this section, the diverse clinical presentations of primary, pulmonary and miliary tuberculosis are reviewed together with the characteristic changes found on radiologic examination. The principal extra-pulmonary manifestations of tuberculosis are also covered. Diagnostic approach and treatment strategies for tuberculosis are in later sections of this chapter.

PRIMARY AND CHILDHOOD INFECTION
Primary tuberculosis is acquired by inhalation of infected particles, usually in childhood, although in affluent countries the first encounter with tuberculosis may be as an adult. A single bacillus can cause disease but usually 50–200 organisms are required for development of active infection. Inhaled bacilli pass into the lung where damage is often but not always confined to one segment with concurrent involvement of draining, frequently hilar, lymph nodes. This gives rise to the primary Ghon complex. Clinical disease develops in less than 5% of people exposed to *M. tuberculosis*, although infection is established in about 30% of cases. After initial infection, the only sequelae may be scar tissue, which is often calcified and later may be identified on routine chest X-ray. After the first year of infection, there is a 3–5% lifetime chance of reactivation of disease in non-HIV infected individuals. In addition, a patient exposed to tuberculosis may be infected by a second strain of *M. tuberculosis* later in life and this may account for up to one-third of adult clinical presentations.

Symptomatic patients present with cough with variable amounts of sputum and hemoptysis, together with localized pleuritic chest pain and dyspnea. In addition, systemic features such as fever, night sweats, anorexia and weight loss occur. A minority of patients have retrosternal pain, sometimes exacerbated by swallowing and increased by sternal pressure that is thought to relate to lymphadenopathy. Primary tuberculosis is seen as asymmetric hilar adenopathy and associated consolidation on chest X-ray. In children, isolated lymphadenopathy is more common. Less typical chest X-rays of primary infection include those that appear normal or have widespread disease, lobar consolidation and pleural effusions. An unusual complication of primary tuberculosis is bronchial obstruction caused by pressure of a node on a main bronchus. This phenomenon, sometimes called epituberculosis, may lead to secondary bronchiectasis. Untreated primary disease will progress to involve the entire lung and will also disseminate. Symptoms are present at this stage and may be severe, with continuous cough and sputum production, severe dyspnea, high fevers, drenching sweats and cachexia. Chest X-ray reveals widespread patchy consolidation, with areas of collapse and cavitation.

Endobronchial tuberculosis is usually a complication of primary infection, although it may occur during reactivation. It may follow adhesion of inflamed lung parenchyma or lymph nodes to bronchi or may arise via lymphatic or hematogenous spread of infection and even from direct seeding of inhaled bacilli. Endobronchial tuberculosis probably frequently goes undiagnosed as it was found in over 400 of 1000 consecutive autopsies on patients who have tuberculosis.[37] The classic clinical presentation is with a barking cough and wheeze. Sputum production may be exacerbated when the mucosa is breached and caseous material extruded. Parasternal pain, dyspnea, symptoms caused by collapse and consolidation of distal lung tissue and systemic manifestations of tuberculosis may be found. The most important late complication of endobronchial infection is bronchiectasis.

PULMONARY INFECTION
Risk factors for reactivation
The majority of cases of tuberculosis are caused by reactivation of infection acquired years earlier. The stimulus to reactivation may be frank immunosuppression or may be more subtle when factors such as malnutrition and vitamin D deficiency are involved. The role of corticosteroids in reactivation of tuberculosis has not been fully defined. High doses may cause reactivation, which often presents atypically or is detected belatedly because the symptoms of infection may mimic symptoms of the disease for which corticosteroids were

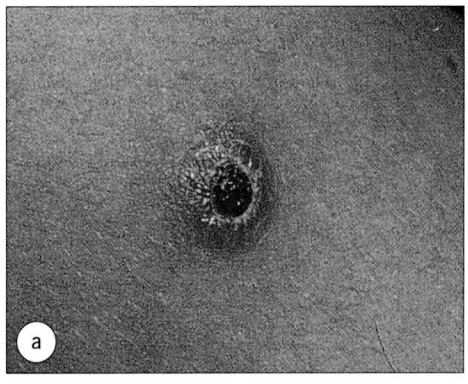
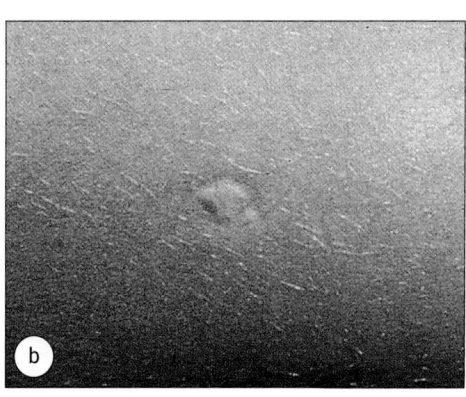

Fig. 30.7 BCG response at 6 weeks. (a) Clinical evidence of a cell-mediated immune response is clearly apparent at 6 weeks; (b) the healed BCG scar. With permission from James DG and Studdy PR.[73]

being prescribed. However, tuberculosis does not appear more common in asthmatics maintained on daily low-dose prednisolone. Other conditions associated with reactivation of tuberculosis are end-stage renal disease, diabetes mellitus, silicosis, gastrectomy and transplantation; in the latter, disease usually results from immuno-suppression, although occasionally infection is transmitted with the implanted organ. Although tuberculosis and lung malignancy may coexist and the symptoms of tuberculosis may mimic those of cancer, tuberculosis is not a risk factor for lung cancer. However, lung malignancy is a systemic risk factor for reactivation of tuberculosis and may invade and disrupt old tuberculous lesions leading to active infection. Tuberculosis has frequently been found to be associated with sarcoidosis. Some workers have detected mycobacterial DNA in patients who have sarcoid but others have not, and whether there is any link between these diseases is unresolved.

Clinical presentation

In one prospective study, symptoms of reactivation of pulmonary tuberculosis were cough in 78% patients, weight loss in 74%, fatigue in 68%, fever in 60% and night sweats in 55%.[38] Some patients have only mild feelings of nonspecific malaise. Hemoptysis occurs in about one-third of patients. It may be massive from either enlarged bronchial arteries around tuberculous cavities (Rasmussen's aneurysms) or more frequently from erosions involving other bronchial or pulmonary arteries. Dyspnea suggests extensive disease and is a late symptom. Pleuritic chest pain indicates inflammation in and possibly infection of adjacent pleura. Clinical examination may be misleading in the early stages of reactivation and radiologically apparent changes of consolidation and cavitation hard to detect. Noninfectious complications of tuberculosis may be present (see below). It is important to recognize that patients can present with advanced disease in acute respiratory failure progressing rapidly to the adult respiratory distress syndrome (ARDS).

Chest X-ray shows disease localized to apical and posterior segments of the upper lobes of the lung in over 85% of patients, with other sites often secondarily affected. The apical segment of the lower lobe is also frequently involved. Infiltration and cavitation secondary to caseous necrosis may be associated with air–fluid levels. On treatment most cavities heal completely leaving residual scarring, often calcific. Tuberculous chest X-rays frequently show fibrotic changes with lobar atelectasis, elevation of hilar nodes and deviation of the trachea. A wide range of less common findings are described, for example pneumonic consolidation (Fig. 30.8). It is notoriously difficult to distinguish early reactivation from chronic healed lesions without follow-up X-rays. CT scan findings include cavitation with scarring as well as characteristic nodules and branching linear structures sometimes referred to as a 'tree-in-bud pattern'.

Other investigations in pulmonary tuberculosis may reveal leukocytosis or more specifically a monocytosis. It is common for the leukocyte count to be normal and rare for it to be decreased. Anemia, generally normochromic and normocytic, is typical. An acute phase response is almost invariably present with elevated C-reactive protein (CRP) concentrations in plasma, raised erythrocyte sedimentation rate (ESR) and, in more chronic cases, decreased serum albumin. Hyponatremia occurs in about 10% of patients as a result of antidiuretic hormone-like activity. A much smaller percentage of patients will have hypercalcemia, probably caused by abnormal vitamin D processing by macrophages within granulomas (see Cadranel et al.[76])

Complications

The principal acute complications of pulmonary tuberculosis are hemoptysis, as discussed above, and pneumothorax. Bronchopleural fistulae may heal spontaneously but more often require tube drainage and sometimes surgery. Prognosis is good because of formation of scar tissue in tuberculosis. Chronic complications of lung tuberculosis relate to parenchymal damage and scarring. Aspergillomas may develop within healed cavitating lesions in up to 20% of cases;[39] patients usually present with hemoptysis. Localized bronchiectasis (see Chapter 2.26) may only become clinically significant many years later and is best defined by high-resolution CT scanning. Tissue destruction may be so great as to cause respiratory failure.

Pleural tuberculosis

Pleural tuberculosis classically occurs 3–6 months after primary disease but onset may be delayed and pleural disease may be the first sign of reactivation. Pleural disease may accompany lung infection or be the predominant feature. Tuberculosis and malignancy are the principal differential diagnoses of massive effusions that are exudates (protein concentration greater than 3g/dL). Effusions are usually straw colored but may be bloodstained and occasionally frankly bloody. Glucose concentrations in tuberculous effusions are frequently, but not always, below 40mg/dL (2.22mmol/L). Pleural fluid lysozyme, lactate and pH may be elevated in tuberculous effusions, as in bacterial infections. Elevated adenosine deaminase (ADA), derived from CD4 lymphocytes, is characteristic. Low ADA levels are against a diagnosis of tuberculosis but high concentrations are nonspecific. The leukocyte count of tuberculous effusions is usually raised and may be as high as 5000 cells/ml. Lymphocytes are generally the most prevalent cell type. Monocytes are also characteristic but mesothelial cells are scanty. Neutrophils may be present and may even predominate in acute disease.[40]

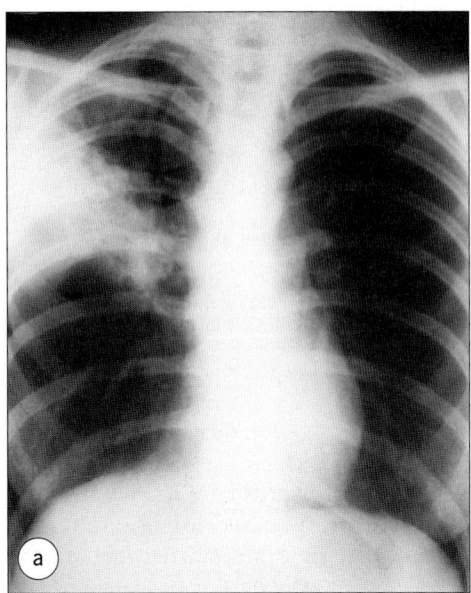
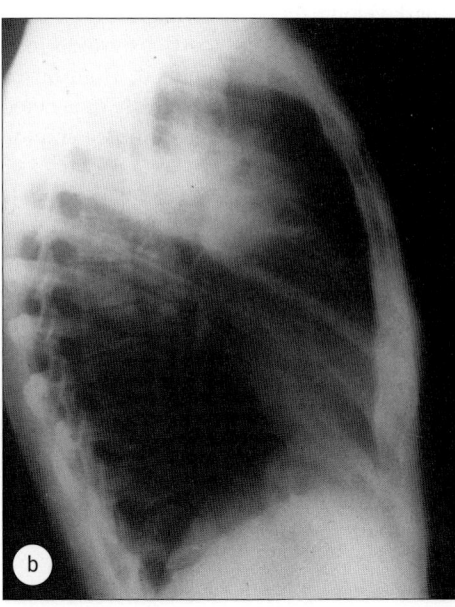

Fig. 30.8 Chest X-ray of pulmonary tuberculous pneumonia. (a) Posteroanterior and (b) lateral chest radiographs of a patient who has tuberculosis presenting as a consolidation. Courtesy of Dr W Lynn.

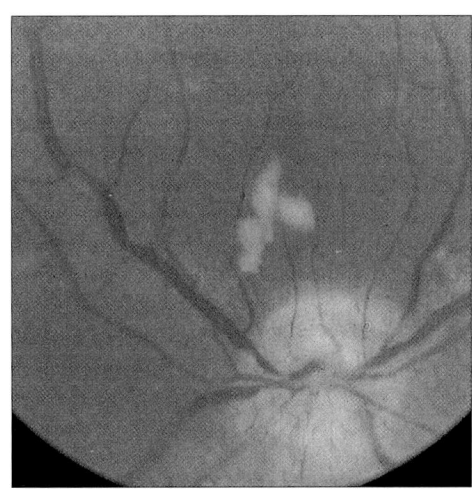

Fig. 30.9 Choroidal tuberculosis. Choroidal disease is a manifestation of tuberculosis that is very highly suggestive of miliary disease. With permission from James DG and Studdy PR.[73]

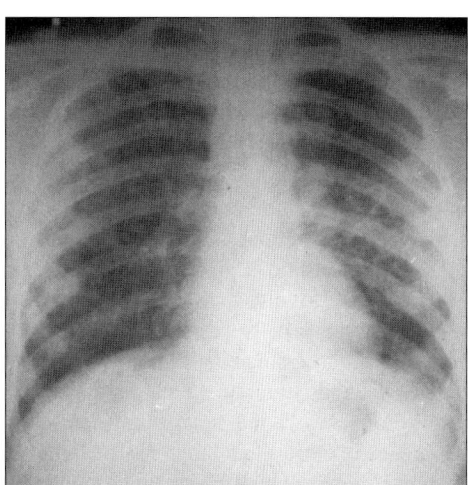

Fig. 30.10 Miliary tuberculosis. Chest X-ray of miliary tuberculosis showing characteristic mottled shadowing throughout both lung fields. Courtesy of Dr W Lynn.

Chest X-ray usually demonstrates a unilateral effusion, more often on the right. An effusion may be massive and bilateral effusions occur in approximately 10% of patients. Ultrasound may reveal loculated effusions containing fibrinous tissue, reflecting activation of the fibrinolytic system. Ultrasound and CT scanning are useful to document underlying disease and to aid diagnostic and therapeutic aspirations.

MILIARY TUBERCULOSIS

Miliary tuberculosis follows bloodborne dissemination of *M. tuberculosis* and thus clinical presentation is varied. Factors involved in development of miliary infection include decreased immune responses, mycobacterial virulence factors, mycobacterial load and the number of organisms able to gain entry to the bloodstream. At least 50% of patients who have miliary disease in developed countries are immunosuppressed, most commonly by alcohol. Diabetes, chronic renal failure, underlying malignancies and immunosuppressive drugs are other risk factors. Disseminated infection caused by *M. bovis*, BCG strain, may follow instillation of the organism into the bladder when it is used as an adjuvant to chemotherapy for malignancy.

Miliary tuberculosis may manifest as fever of unknown origin or with symptoms attributable to involvement of one or more organ systems. Commonly there are widespread pulmonary granulomas and central nervous system (CNS) disease and, occasionally, cardiac involvement (although pericardial, myocardial and endocardial manifestations all have been reported). Differential diagnosis is often wide and clinicians must be alert to the possibility of miliary tuberculosis. Acute miliary tuberculosis presenting with shock and ARDS has a mortality rate that may approach 90%. In chronic cases, cachexia is prominent and localizing features may be few. Widespread macular and papular skin lesions (tuberculosis miliaris disseminata) are suggestive of miliary infection. Choroidal tubercles, 0.5–3.0mm in diameter, are essentially diagnostic of miliary disease (Fig. 30.9).

The chest X-ray of miliary tuberculosis has well defined nodules less than 5mm in diameter throughout both lung fields (Fig. 30.10). X-ray changes may only develop after a patient has been admitted to hospital, so patients must be reassessed frequently. Larger nodules and a pulmonary focus occur in approximately one-third of patients. CT scanning, seldom of diagnostic value, may show smaller nodules not seen on X-ray. Ultrasound scanning may show increased echogenicity in the liver but is not diagnostic. Hematologic investigations are similar to those found in tuberculous pneumonia but a neutrophilia may be seen and should not put the diagnosis in doubt or cause empirical therapy to be restricted to antibacterials. Rarer abnormalities include disseminated intravascular coagulation and the hemophagocytic syndrome. Sterile pyuria and organisms in the absence of urinary leukocytes have been reported, but the exact frequency of such renal manifestations is uncertain. Delay in microbiologic diagnosis contributes to mortality.

EXTRAPULMONARY TUBERCULOSIS

This section reviews those forms of extrapulmonary tuberculosis not considered in detail elsewhere and refers readers to other key chapters where further information is to be found.

Lymph node disease

Lymphadenitis or scrofula or the 'King's evil' (so called because in Europe in the Middle Ages the royal touch was thought to be curative) is a very common extrapulmonary presentation of tuberculosis. In Europe, Australia and the USA, atypical mycobacteria (*Mycobacterium scrofulaceum* and *Mycobacterium avium-intracellulare* complex) are also a frequent cause of lymphadenitis in children,[41] unlike the situation in adults in whom *M. tuberculosis* predominates. Peripheral nodes are usually infected through hematogenous spread of *M. tuberculosis* from the lung. The commonest involved nodes are those in the cervical region, sometimes in association with axillary, inguinal or hilar lymphadenopathy. Patients may present with painless lymphadenopathy or with marked systemic symptoms. There may be associated sinuses and abscess formation. Hilar nodes may be associated with thoracic pain and, if untreated, may infrequently result in esophageal erosion or a bronchoesophageal fistula. Unusual symptoms such as obstructive jaundice have been reported in specific association with anatomically defined local lymph nodes

Tuberculosis of the head and neck

Aside from cervical node disease, tuberculosis of the head and neck is relatively uncommon and usually arises secondarily to pulmonary infection. Laryngeal tuberculosis may manifest with hoarseness, pain on speaking or swallowing, hemoptysis and respiratory obstruction. Cough may reflect lung disease or involvement of the superior laryngeal nerve. Untreated, widespread local tissue destruction may occur with secondary laryngeal stenosis. A plain chest radiograph may be suggestive, but in one series radiographic changes were minimal in two-thirds of patients (see Thaller *et al.*[74]) In this study from a specialist center, coexistent squamous cell carcinoma of the larynx was present in 10% of patients. Therefore, all laryngeal lesions should be biopsied to exclude malignancy.

Tuberculosis rarely involves the middle ear, where it may manifest with a local, painless discharge from which the organism may be cultured. There may be destruction of the ossicles, hearing loss and invasion of the facial nerve canal, sinuses and extension into the posterior cranial fossa. Secondary pyogenic infection may obscure the diagnosis. Tuberculosis of the nose, nasopharynx and adenoids is rare even in areas in which infection is endemic and symptoms such as epistaxis reflect local tissue damage. Tuberculosis in the oral cavity generally occurs as a solitary, often inflamed ulcer with irregular borders. There may be secondary infection of salivary glands.

Musculoskeletal infection

Vertebral infection (Pott's disease) is the commonest presentation of tuberculous osteomyelitis, accounting for about 50% of all bony tuberculosis (Fig. 30.11). The male to female ratio is approximately 2:1. The thoracic spine is the most frequently involved, followed by lumbar and then cervical regions. Presentation is usually with back or neck pain. Systemic symptoms tend to be less marked than in pulmonary disease. Neurologic symptoms, such as weakness, numbness and disturbances of gait, occur in about one-third of cases. Some patients have an associated flank mass or other evidence of extraspinal tuberculosis. In more advanced cases, vertebral body collapse and gibbus formation lead to kyphosis of the spine. Destructive lesions with invasion of the joint space and deformity may be seen on plain X-rays, although CT or ideally MRI scanning are better imaging modalities for spinal pathology.

Osteomyelitis is otherwise most frequently found in the metaphysis of long bones, although rib, pelvis and skull may be infected. In children in countries in which tuberculosis is prevalent, osteomyelitis is a significant cause of crippling deformity. Direct extension from the ribs to the lung is rare, as is meningitis or tuberculomas in patients in whom there is skull involvement. Bony tuberculosis may be accompanied by sinus tracts or soft tissue masses. Diagnosis may be difficult as lesions can appear osteolytic or sclerotic on X-ray and malignancy may be suspected first. Like X-rays, technetium-99 bone scans have no pathognomonic features. Trauma does not predispose to tuberculous osteomyelitis.

Tuberculous arthritis most frequently manifests in the hips and other weight-bearing joints, although any joint may be involved. Polyarticular disease occurs in less than 20% of patients, but evidence of tuberculosis elsewhere, generally the lung, is present in about 50% of cases. Synovial fluid is usually turbid with a high leukocyte count and up to 60% may be neutrophils rather than mononuclear cells.

Organisms are found in less than one-quarter of cases, although positive cultures are more frequent and ideally a synovial biopsy should be examined histologically and microbiologically. Prosthetic joints may be infected with *M. tuberculosis* after either hematogenous spread or contiguous reactivation of infection. Tenosynovitis is rare and generally associated with adjacent osteomyelitis.

Tuberculous abscesses may form in most soft tissues, including muscle (Fig. 30.12). This is usually secondary to contiguous spread of infection but may follow hematogenous dissemination. The classic abscess site is in the psoas muscle, and such an abscess can occur with or without localizing signs, therefore a high index of clinical suspicion is necessary for the appropriate imaging to be arranged in advance of diagnostic aspiration.

Abdominal infection

The abdomen is a frequent site of tuberculosis, especially in patients from the Indian subcontinent, where rates are up to 50 times higher than in Europe, and in those immunosuppressed with HIV. Disease is usually secondary to hematogenous spread of mycobacteria, but can be secondary to local invasion or ingestion of organisms. However, any infected person can present with disease in the abdomen and as tuberculosis frequently mimics other pathologies, such as gastrointestinal malignancy, diagnosis is often delayed. In the gut, tuberculosis most frequently affects the ileocecal region, then the small bowel and then the colon, with involvement of the duodenum occurring in less than 2.5% of cases and the stomach and esophagus in less than 1% of patients. Approximately one-third of patients have evidence of tuberculosis elsewhere, usually in the lung.

Symptoms reflect site of involvement but may be nonspecific with fever, weight loss, chronic abdominal pain, nausea and anorexia. Diarrhea occurs in less than 20% of cases and reflects either secondary overflow caused by obstruction or stimulation of the gastrointestinal tract by cytokines. Ileocecal tuberculosis may manifest as acute surgical abdomen secondary to obstruction of the bowel lumen or appendix, or after bowel perforation. Any tuberculous lesion, particularly those in the colon, may manifest with massive gastrointestinal

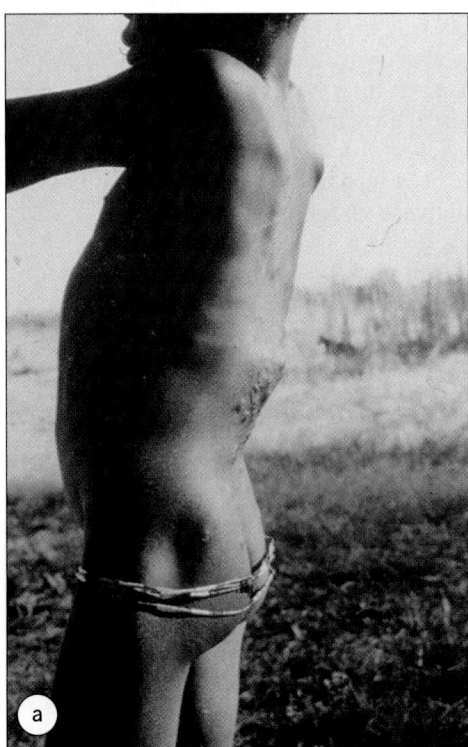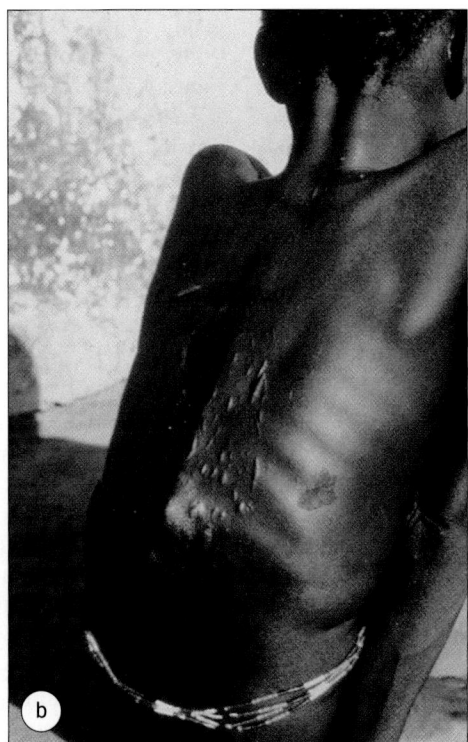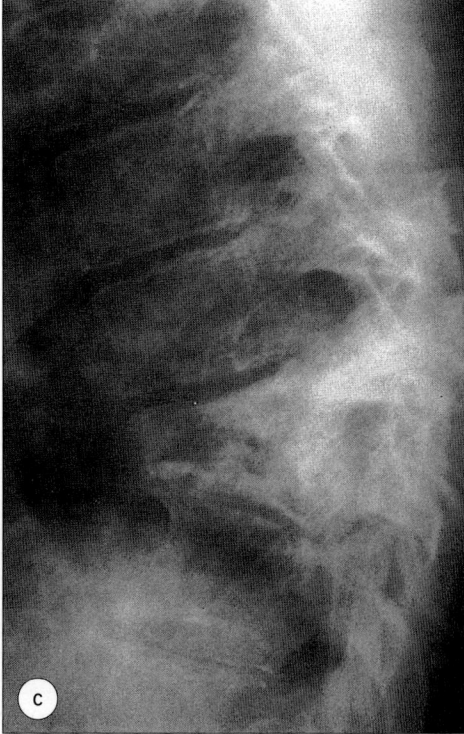

Fig. 30.11 Vertebral tuberculosis. Tuberculosis of the spine, or Pott's disease. Kyphosis is secondary to anterior destruction of vertebral bodies resulting in wedging of adjacent vertebrae and loss of disc space clearly seen by radiography. (a,b: Courtesy of Professor J Cohen; c: Courtesy of Dr A Wightman, with permission from Emond RTD, Rowland HAK, Welsby PD, Colour atlas of infectious diseases, 3E, London: Mosby, 1995).

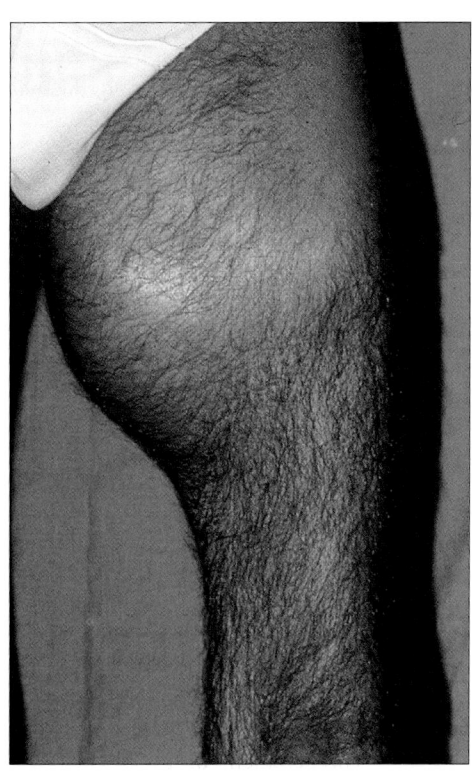

Fig. 30.12 Abscess formation in tuberculosis. This patient had multiple tuberculosis abscesses particularly affecting the psoas and quadriceps muscle groups.

bleeding, but this is rare. Lesions may be ulcerative or hypertrophic and can be associated with fistula, which are probably partly the result of secondary bacterial involvement. Unusual sites of intra-abdominal tuberculosis include the pancreas and the adrenal glands; in the latter, disease occurs very rarely as an adrenal crisis but more commonly with an insidious onset of symptoms that may be difficult to distinguish from those associated with infection. Tuberculous peritonitis is an important manifestation of disease and is discussed in Chapter 2.38. Hepatobiliary infection is considered in Chapter 2.37. Chapter 2.60 is a detailed review of urogenital tuberculosis.

Central nervous system and eye disease
Tuberculous meningoencephalitis and CNS tuberculomas are extremely important, carrying a high morbidity and mortality. These topics are further considered in Chapters 2.15 and 2.17, respectively.

Ocular tuberculosis is relatively uncommon but important because, if overlooked, blindness may result. The commonest manifestation is choroidal disease (Fig. 30.9) secondary to hematogenous spread in the context of miliary tuberculosis, which may rarely spread to the retina. Conjunctival tuberculosis may be caused by accidental self-inoculation by an infected person, spread from skin or very rarely by direct spread from another infected individual. Infection may be ulcerative or nodular, although occasionally focal tuberculomas, sometimes appearing polypoid, are seen. Tuberculosis of the sclera and cornea are rare, as is uveitis.

Pericardial infection
Tuberculous pericarditis is potentially fatal. A detailed description of the disease is to be found in Chapter 2.49.

Dematologic disease
Lupus vulgaris is the best documented manifestation of dermatologic tuberculosis. Details of the dermatologic manifestations of primary and miliary infection are to be found in Chapter 2.5.

CLINICAL MANIFESTATIONS IN HIV-POSITIVE PATIENTS
Tuberculosis is an AIDS-defining event in HIV-seropositive patients in the USA and a common secondary infection in HIV-seropositive patients living in countries in which tuberculosis is more prevalent.

The clinical manifestations of tuberculosis in HIV-seropositive and -seronegative patients are generally similar. However, tuberculosis may be more widespread, have more atypical features and is more often extrapulmonary in the former. Many unusual or rare presentations of tuberculosis have been reported, bronchoesophageal fistula being one example.[42] *Mycobacterium tuberculosis* bacteremia is much more frequent in HIV-seropositive patients.[43] In Africa, CNS and disseminated tuberculosis occur more often in patients who have peripheral CD4+ T-lymphocyte counts below 200/ml.

Making the correct diagnosis can be difficult when HIV and tuberculosis coexist. Nonspecific systemic features of tuberculosis, such as fever, malaise and a prolonged acute phase protein response, are also characteristic of HIV infection. In Africa, both HIV and tuberculosis contribute to the wasting entity recognized as Slim disease. Many opportunistic infections in HIV, including those caused by the *M. avium-intracellulare* complex, may cause similar symptoms to those of tuberculosis, adding to diagnostic confusion. In addition, low peripheral T-lymphocyte counts may secondarily reduce leukocyte counts in tuberculosis-infected pleural fluid, which may be diagnostically confusing.

NONINFECTIOUS COMPLICATIONS
Erythema nodosum is the most common noninfectious complication of primary tuberculosis, although it may occur in other granulomatous diseases (e.g. leprosy, sarcoidosis). It is particularly associated with primary disease. Arthritis occurs in up to 1% of patients who have acute infection and may also complicate reactivation. Poncet's disease is a reactive polyarthritis associated with tuberculosis, which resolves with antimycobacterial chemotherapy. Bazin's disease is a vasculitic skin reaction to tuberculosis that usually manifests as a purpuric rash on the lower extremities. Another important immunologic complication of tuberculosis is renal interstitial nephritis.

Bronchogenic carcinoma was thought for many years to be more frequent in patients who have tuberculosis, but this has not been borne out in careful studies. Hypertrophic pulmonary osteoarthropathy, principally associated with bronchogenic carcinoma, has been reported in tuberculosis,[44] although some attribute the finding to undiagnosed lung malignancy. Another report described clubbing in 21% of patients in a Nigerian hospital, but this figure is much higher than is the experience of most physicians.[45] The syndrome of inappropriate antidiuretic hormone secretion is more common in pulmonary and miliary disease.

DIAGNOSIS

CLINICAL APPROACH
The definitive diagnosis of tuberculosis requires identification of the mycobacterial pathogen in a patient's secretions or tissues. Therapy is often initiated before a definitive diagnosis has been made, but one should always be pursued. Identification of the organism is necessary for drug susceptibility testing, which guides local treatment policies and individual therapeutic regimens. Sputum examination has a high diagnostic yield, identifies the majority of infectious patients and is cheap to perform. Sputum should be collected on three separate occasions, but additional specimens are not cost-effective.[46] Induced sputums obtained in properly ventilated and isolated areas can be useful, but bronchoscopy with alveloar lavage has the best diagnostic yield.[47] Routine screening of induced sputums for tuberculosis in HIV-seropositive patients is not useful. *Mycobacterium tuberculosis* is seen infrequently on aspiration of pleural fluid and is cultured in under 50% of cases. However, pleural biopsy reveals granuloma or results in culture of the pathogen in over 90% of cases. Thoracoscopy may be indicated in exceptional circumstances because it allows visually guided biopsy of lesions.

In extrapulmonary or miliary infection, appropriate body fluids and/or tissues must be obtained for microbiologic and histologic examination, with the aid of ultrasound, CT or MRI scanning if available. Liver biopsy and bone marrow aspiration are useful investigations in disseminated or occult disease.[48] An acid-fast stain of buffy coat leukocytes may be diagnostic in immunosuppressed patients. For tuberculous lymphadenitis, fine needle aspiration is the initial investigation of choice because it is easy to perform, and has a high specificity and sensitivity when both microbiologic and cytologic specimens are collected. Fine needle aspiration does not preclude subsequent lymph node biopsy. Needle aspiration remains of value in countries in which tuberculosis is common but resources, including trained laboratory staff, are scarce.[49] It can also be used in other manifestations of suspected extrapulmonary disease such as tuberculous arthritis.

Specimens from potentially infected patients are normally analyzed in local laboratories, but drug sensitivity testing and more specialized facilities are ideally concentrated in centralized laboratories. All laboratories must be arranged to deal with hazardous, possibly drug-resistant pathogens. Safety measures include containment areas, approved safety cabinets, centrifuges, gowns, gloves, sinks and facilities for disposal of contaminated waste and treatment of spillages. Special training for the staff is essential.

Usual principles of microbiologic safety apply to collection of specimens into sterile containers. Tissue biopsies should be divided and a fresh specimen sent for microbiologic and one in formalin for histologic examination. Tissue is better for culture than necrotic material and old pus, which may contain acids toxic to mycobacteria, a fact to be considered when selecting biopsy sites. Blood and bone marrow specimens can be injected directly into blood culture bottles. Examination of cerebrospinal fluid for *M. tuberculosis* is usually an emergency investigation, with the clinician forewarning the laboratory. Specimens from gastric lavage should be rapidly transported to the laboratory because stomach acidity may kill mycobacteria. Feces are not useful in the diagnosis of *M. tuberculosis* in HIV-negative patients.

If no diagnostic results are forthcoming in patients in whom tuberculosis is a possibility, the clinician may reasonably resort to a trial of therapy. Improvement of symptoms and decrease in the acute phase response (monitored by ESR, CRP, etc.) are sufficient indication to move from the diagnostic trial to full therapy. Any diagnostic trial of therapy should last a minimum of 2 weeks and ideally 4.

MICROBIOLOGIC DIAGNOSIS

The standard method for staining clinical specimens for *M. tuberculosis* is that of Ziehl–Neelsen (Fig. 30.13), which requires application of heat, whereas a modification, the Kinyoun method, does not. Both methods utilize the fact that the stained cell wall is resistant to decolorization by acid-alcohol although the biochemical reason for this is unknown. Auramine staining has facilitated rapid screening of diagnostic specimens and has greater sensitivity (Fig. 30.14). Mycobacteria are often scanty and specimens should be reviewed by an experienced operator. Diagnostic microscopy is most successful in patients who have extensive disease and cavitation on chest X-ray and has an overall sensitivity of 50–90% depending on case mix.

Mycobacterium tuberculosis is traditionally cultured on egg and potato-based media such as Middlebrook 7H10/11. Such media are of limited value in analysis of clinical specimens because of overgrowth by more rapidly dividing commensal organisms. Selective media such as Lowenstein–Jensen or Petragnani are used, with Middlebrook being reserved for subcultures. Cultures must be maintained for up to 8 weeks. *Mycobacterium tuberculosis* is identified as slow-growing, rough, whitish colonies with a tendency to cord formation. More specific biochemical tests detect a range of characteristics, including the ability of the organism to produce niacin, reduce nitrate and produce a heat-sensitive catalase. To speed diagnosis, broth-based growth systems containing Middlebrook 7H12 with ^{14}C-labeled palmitic acid as the only carbon source are widely used. This is the BACTEC system, which detects release of radioactive [14]CO_2 from dividing mycobacteria and approximately halves the time to diagnosis in smear-positive and negative patients. The BACTEC system has been refined for specific identification of *M. tuberculosis*. Failure of a mycobacteria to grow in a BACTEC NAP vial (containing p-nitro-α-acetylamino-β-hydroxypropiophenone) indicates that it is either *M. tuberculosis*, *M. bovis* or *Mycobacterium africanum*. *Mycobacterium tuberculosis* can also be identified from a fatty acid profile obtained by high-performance liquid, gas–liquid or thin-layer chromatography. A novel colormetric diagnostic method is the mycobacteria growth indicator tube that contains 7H9 Middlebrook broth and an oxygen-sensitive fluorescent indicator that indicates bacterial growth. Once the indicator is positive, detection by genetic means is possible. Such

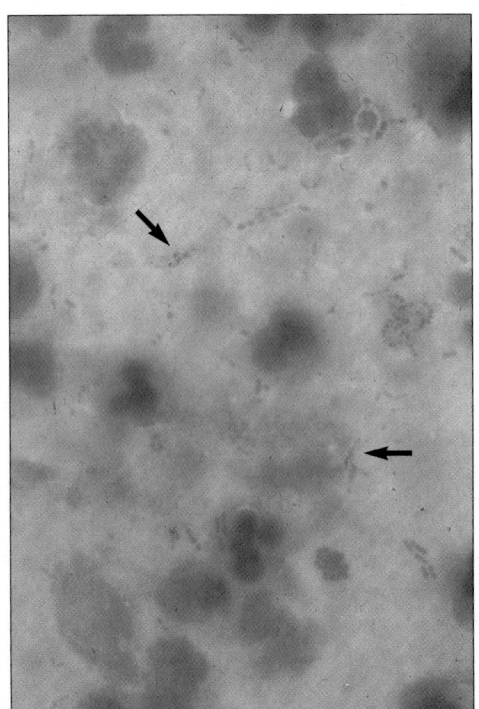

Fig. 30.13 Ziehl–Neelsen stain stained sputum specimens containing *Mycobacterium tuberculosis* (arrows). Courtesy of Dr F Ahmed.

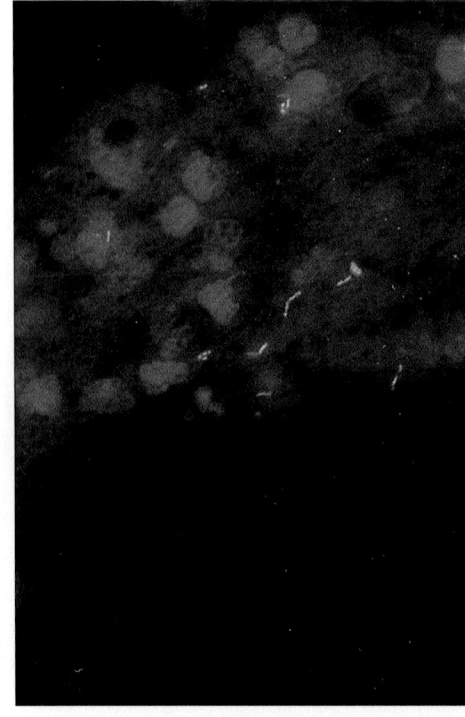

Fig. 30.14 *Mycobacterium tuberculosis* in sputum detected by Auramine staining. Courtesy of Mr M Croughan, with permission from Emond RTD, Rowland HAK, Welsby PD, Colour atlas of infectious diseases, 3E, London: Mosby, 1995.

methodology may have a particular role in rapid detection of drug-resistant organisms in clinical specimens.

There are four methods of susceptibility testing of *M. tuberculosis* that are intended to determine whether the majority of pathogens are sensitive to the drugs being prescribed. The absolute concentration method uses a series of cultures containing a graded range of dilutions of the drug being tested, as well as a control to determine the minimum amount of drug that inhibits growth of any isolate. The resistance ratio method, commonly used in the UK, is similar but results are related to the sensitivity of a known strain of *M. tuberculosis* such as H37-Rv. The proportion method, frequently employed in the USA, compares the number of colonies growing on a standard medium with the number on a drug-containing medium. However, in many countries, BACTEC bottles containing various drugs are now used as this is rapid and reliable. Pyrazinamide-sensitivity testing presents specific problems in that it must be carried out at pH5.5 and this degree of acidity can inhibit the growth of some strains of *M. tuberculosis* independently of drug action. An alternative approach has been to screen isolates for production of pyrazinamidase. In future, genetic techniques screening for relevant mutations are likely to have a role in rapidly identifying resistant organisms even though they will not detect novel mutations.

GENETIC TECHNIQUES

The polymerase chain reaction (PCR) has the potential to allow rapid detection of low levels of infection with the possibility of immediate probing for known drug resistance genes. The usual targets for amplification are the DNA insertion sequence IS6110, which is found in all the *M. tuberculosis* complex of organisms (*M. tuberculosis*, *M. bovis*, *M. africanum* and *Mycobacterium microti*) or rRNA. Considerable methodologic problems with PCR have been encountered. Several large scale studies have reported high sensitivity and specificity using culture positivity as the gold standard.[50] However, in one study only 70% of laboratories could make the diagnosis in samples containing 10,000 *M. tuberculosis* (lower limit for detection by microscopy) and 22% of laboratories identified the organism in negative control samples.[51] PCR is potentially of most use in smear-negative culture-positive disease, for which it should be able to identify over 50% of cases. Another problem is that PCR positivity in sputum may persist during treatment and after clinical cure.[52] It is likely that PCR will be useful in diagnosing extrapulmonary tuberculosis, but large studies of sensitivity are awaited. One interesting observation is that about 50% of patients are positive on blood-based PCR analysis for *M. tuberculosis*, which suggests that a blood test might be diagnostically useful.[53] Although PCR is likely to have a major role in the future, it has not yet replaced microscopy and culture and, in view of its cost, it is unlikely to do so soon in most areas of the world in which tuberculosis is prevalent.

The use of reporter phages encoding genes for luciferase from the firefly *Photinus pyralis* represents the main alternative genetic approach to diagnosis of tuberculosis. On introduction of a phage such as TM4 into mycobacteria in the presence of luciferin and ATP, oxidization results in generation of luciferyl-AMP and then oxyluciferin, which gives out 0.85 photons per molecule of substrate. This is measured in a luminometer, thus allowing detection of mycobacterial growth in a few hours. Subsequently, efficacy of drug activity can be rapidly screened within 48 hours by monitoring changes in luminescence.[54]

SERODIAGNOSIS

Serodiagnostic techniques are not in routine use in most laboratories. Enzyme-linked immunosorbent assays (ELISAs) have been developed to detect a number of mycobacterial proteins, such as the 16kDa hsp, the 30kDa antigen, the 38kDa antigens and LAM, but the sensitivity of antibody testing is not sufficiently high in ELISAs with adequate specificity to warrant their regular use. Local testing for antibodies at sites of infection, such as in pleural effusions, has not proved useful.

Antibody levels are also often low in culture-negative individuals in whom alternative diagnostic approaches are needed. Alterations in antibody levels over time are not a useful guide to clinical response to treatment. Finally, the impaired antibody response makes serology of negligible value in HIV-seropositive patients.

MANAGEMENT

FIRST-LINE ANTIMYCOBACTERIAL DRUGS AND THEIR TOXICITIES

This and the next section briefly outline the principal characteristics of the most important antituberculous drugs. More detail concerning mode of actin and dosage regimens can be found in Chapter 7.13.

Isoniazid

Isoniazid (INH or isonicotinic acid hydrazide: $C_6H_7N_3O$) is a bacteriocidal drug (MIC generally <0.1µg/ml), the biologic activity of which resides in a pyridine ring and a hydrazine group. Isoniazid is well absorbed, minimally bound to plasma proteins, has a half-life of 1–3 hours depending on patient acetylator status and is excreted into urine. Concentrations achieved in most tissues are similar to those in serum, with the important exception of the CNS in which concentrations are approximately 20% of those in serum. Thus, the drug is used at double the normal dose in CNS disease. Isoniazid enters *M. tuberculosis* by diffusion and by oxygen-dependent active transport where it inhibits mycolic acid synthesis and the nicotinamide adenine dinucleotide pathway and interacts with the catalase–peroxidase enzyme system. Mutations in the *kat* G gene encoding the catalase–peroxidase enzyme confer resistance to INH and account for approximately 25% of cases of drug resistance.[55] Mutations in the *inh* A gene, which encodes an enoylacyl carrier protein reductase probably involved in mycolic acid synthesis, appear important in drug resistance to INH and ethambutol in some mycobacteria but not *M. tuberculosis*.

The most important, potentially fatal, side effect of INH is hepatotoxicity, which is more common in patients older than 60 years, in the presence of coexisting liver disease and possibly in pregnancy. Asymptomatic, usually transient, rises in transaminases occur in about 20% of patients. A greater than threefold increase in enzyme levels above the normal range is an indication to discontinue therapy. In practice, it is often impossible to separate INH hepatotoxicity from that caused by rifampin or pyrazinamide but, interestingly, reintroduction of these drugs singly rather than in combination usually avoids a second episode of hepatotoxicity. The other major side effect is a peripheral and rarely optic neuritis caused by interference with niacin metabolism. This is prevented by concomitant administration of vitamin B6 (pyridoxine) 10mg daily. Less common side effects include nausea, vomiting and arthralgia and rarely hypersensitivity reactions, lupus-like reactions, cerebellar ataxia, convulsions, psychoses, hyperglycemia, agranulocytosis and in malnourished patients pellagra.

Rifampin

Rifampin is a bacteriocidal drug with excellent antituberculous activity. Rifampin undergoes first-pass metabolism in the liver where it is deacylated; it is excreted into bile and then into the gut where there is a minor degree of enterohepatic circulation. Rifampin is a potent inducer of hepatic enzymes and therefore has many clinically significant interactions with other drugs (Fig. 30.15). Rifampin targets the RNA polymerase β subunit, blocking initiation but not elongation of mRNA transcripts. Mutations in the *rpo* B gene, which encodes this subunit, are associated with drug resistance. A worrying development has been the emergence of rifampin-resistant tuberculosis through an *rpo* B mutation in a patient taking rifabutin prophylaxis for *M. avium-intracellulare* complex infection.[56]

Patients should be warned that rifampin turns all body secretions, including urine and tears, orange (Fig. 30.16). This is a useful side effect in terms of monitoring compliance. Rifampin may cause hepatic injury, particularly in the presence of pre-existing liver disease. Gastrointestinal side effects seldom necessitate stopping therapy and include anorexia, nausea, vomiting, abdominal pain and diarrhea. Pseudomembranous colitis caused by *Clostridium difficile* toxin production is occasionally described. Immune-mediated problems associated with rifampin include rashes, urticaria, conjunctivitis and rarely hemolysis or thrombocytopenic purpura. A 'flu-like'

DRUG INTERACTIONS WITH RIFAMPIN	
Drug category	Example
Antibacterials	Chloramphenicol
Antifungals	Fluconazole
Corticosteroids	Prednisolone
Anticoagulants	Warfarin
Analgesics	Methadone
Immunosuppressive therapy	Cyclosporin
Ulcer-healing drugs	Cimetidine
Respiratory drugs	Theophylline
Cardiac drugs	
Beta blockers	Propranolol
Calcium channel blockers	Diltiazem
Cardiac glycosides	Digitoxin (only member of class affected)
Antiarrhythmics	Disopyramide
Lipid-lowering drugs	Fluvastatin
CNS drugs	
Anti-epileptics	Phenytoin
Anxiolytics	Diazepam
Antidepressants	Tricyclic compounds
Antipsychotics	Haloperidol
Endocrine drugs	
Antidiabetics	Tolbutamide
Estrogens & progesterones	Combined & progesterone only contraceptive pill
Thyroid replacement	Thyroxine

Fig. 30.15 Drug interactions with rifampin. These are the principal classes of drugs the metabolism of which is increased (plasma concentration decreased) when taken with rifampin. The examples are not intended to be exhaustive and clinicians should check interactions with related drugs in appropriate formularies.

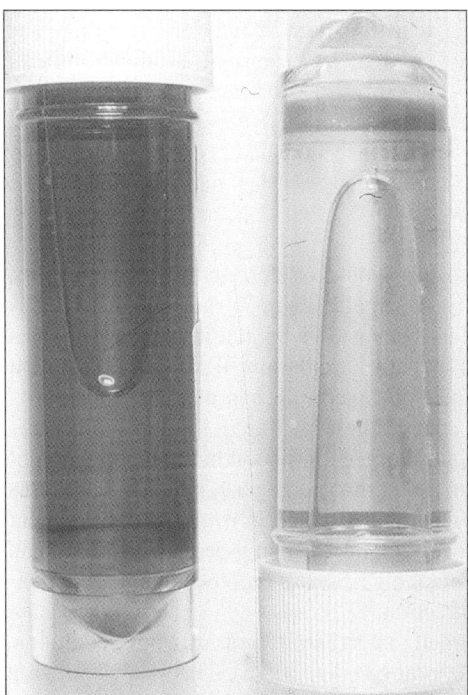

Fig. 30.16 Rifampin urine testing. Patients should be warned that rifampin turns urine and other body secretions orange (specimen on right is normal). This fact can be helpful in monitoring compliance with drug treatment. Courtesy of Dr W Lynn.

syndrome may be troublesome, particularly in intermittent therapy regimens, and very rarely may be severe with circulatory collapse and respiratory failure.

Pyrazinamide

Pyrazinamide, a structural analog of nicotinamide, is a bacteriocidal drug that is well absorbed via the gut and distributed widely, including in the CNS where concentrations are the same as those in serum in patients who have tuberculous meningitis. Serum half-life is about 10 hours and excretion is urinary. Pyrazinamide principally acts intracellularly at relatively acidic pH, although it may also have some cidal action on extracellular bacteria. The drug penetrates macrophages where an enzyme from *M. tuberculosis* converts it into active pyrazinoic acid. Little is known about mechanisms of drug resistance to pyrazinamide, although some strains of *M. tuberculosis* produce an enzyme called pyrazinamidase.

Hepatotoxicity ranging from elevation of liver transaminases to frank jaundice and liver failure is the principal side effect of pyrazinamide. More common are mild gastrointestinal problems and an arthralgia associated with raised serum urate concentrations secondary to inhibition of tubular secretion of uric acid by pyrazinamide; gout is rare. Sideroblastic anemia has been reported.

Ethambutol

Ethambutol is a bacteriocidal drug that is rapidly and well (over 80% of the dose) absorbed in the gut, with peak serum levels occurring 2 hours after a dose. It is then rapidly excreted in urine. Ethambutol appears to alter *M. tuberculosis* RNA synthesis and the transfer of mycolic acids into cell wall. Changes in cell wall lipids have been noted in organisms resistant to the drug.

The most important complication of ethambutol therapy is retrobulbar neuritis manifest by impaired visual acuity, color-blindness and restricted visual fields. Except in patients who have pre-existing ophthalmic disease, optic neuritis is extremely rare when ethambutol is used at standard doses (15mg/kg). In affluent countries, it is appropriate to have patients assessed by an ophthalmologist before treatment is begun, but lack of this facility should not prevent use of ethambutol. Patients should be warned to report symptoms of visual change immediately and ethambutol should generally be avoided in children. Very rarely ethambutol may cause a peripheral neuritis.

Streptomycin

Streptomycin, the first clinically useful drug discovered in the fight against tuberculosis, is an aminoglycoside that has to be given intramuscularly. Streptomycin penetrates cerebrospinal fluid and other remote tissues (e.g. prostate and eye) poorly. There is an immediate and a delayed pathway of excretion via the renal tract. The persistence of the drug at low doses is one factor in the development of side effects. Streptomycin binds to the 30S rRNA subunit, which results in decreased protein synthesis and misreading of mRNA. Mutations, including those in the 30S subunit, arise readily in response to isolated streptomycin therapy and lead to drug resistance. The principal side effects of aminoglycosides are ototoxicity and nephrotoxicity. Rarer ones are neuromuscular blockade and hypersensitivity reactions with maculopapular rashes, fever and eosinophilia.

SECOND-LINE DRUGS

Second-line agents are becoming increasingly important with the advent of multidrug resistant organisms. Information about these drugs is listed in Figure 30.17, although the use of many has not been confirmed in clinical trials. The value of proved efficacious drugs such as ethionamide is limited by toxicity. There is evidence to suggest that the role of other drugs such as imipenem in treatment of tuberculosis should be re-evaluated.[57] The potential second-line role of clofazamine, used in treatment of *M. leprae*, is also uncertain. It remains a poor reflection on the wealthier nations that thiacetazone,

SECOND-LINE THERAPY IN TUBERCULOSIS			
Drug (chemically closely related drug)	Mechanism of action	Toxicity	Usual initial adult dose
PAS	Competes with mycobacterial dihydropteroate synthetase	Gastrointestinal intolerance, hypersensitivity, hypothyroidism, crystaluria	12g/day (divided doses)
Ethionamide (Prothionamide)	Inhibits cell wall mycolic acid synthesis	Gastrointestinal intolerance, hepatitis, hypersensitivity, convulsions, depression, alopecia	0.5 - 1.0g/day (divided doses)
Ciprofloxacin (ofloxacin)	Inhibits topoisomerase II	Gastrointestinal intolerance, crystaluria, tremor, convulsions, rash, hepatitis, renal failure	750mg q12h
Capreomycin (viomycin)	Binds 30S and 50S ribosomes	Nephrotoxic, ototoxic, hypersensitivity	1g/day
Kanamycin	Binds 30S ribosome	Nephrotoxic, ototoxic, hypersensitivity	15mg q12h*
Amikacin	Binds 30S ribosome	Nephrotoxic, ototoxic, rash, neuromuscular blockade, eosinophilia	7.5mg/kg q12h*
Cycloserine	Competitive D-alanine analog	Seizures, psychoses, various CNS effects	250mg q12h/q8h
Thiacetazone	Bacteriostatic ?exact mechanism	Gastrointestinal intolerance, Stevens–Johnson syndrome bone marrow depression, ototoxic, hepatitis	150mg daily

* peak drug levels should be less than 3mg/dL (30mg/L) and trough less than 1mg/dL (10mg/L)

Fig. 30.17 Second-line therapy in tuberculosis. Second-line drugs used in treatment of tuberculosis are presented together with their mechanisms of action and toxicity.

which has a dangerous side-effect profile, continues to be widely used in developing countries because it is all that can be afforded. More details about these agents can be found in Section 7.

TREATMENT REGIMENS

Many trials, notably ones involving the British Medical Research Council, have established short-course chemotherapy as the preferred treatment of pulmonary, pleural, nodal and most other forms of tuberculosis. Such regimens are dependent on using the potent anti-tuberculous drugs isoniazid and rifampin throughout a 6-month course in addition to a 2-month initial treatment with pyrazinamide. An additional drug such as ethambutol or streptomycin is frequently used in the induction period and must be used if drug resistance is a possibility. Single drug resistance occurs at frequencies of up to 20% in West Africa and 10% in the USA.[58] The aim of therapy is to kill all *M. tuberculosis*, with multiple drugs countering the spontaneous emergence of drug-resistant mutants.

One standard treatment protocol is given in Figure 30.18. Alternative regimens are essential in the presence of drug resistance and are possible when drugs are in short supply. For example, 7 months isoniazid and ethambutol therapy can substitute for isoniazid and rifampin in the period after 2 months quadruple therapy. For sensitive organisms, drug therapy in compliant patients is very efficacious, with cure rates approaching 100%. However, it may be 2 weeks before clinical improvement becomes apparent, which is important in empiric trials of therapy and for appropriate patient expectations. Radiologic improvement lags further behind and it may take 3–5 months before all that remains is residual scarring on chest X-ray. Drug therapy must be linked with public health measures discussed above.

The necessary duration of treatment for extrapulmonary tuberculosis is debated. Limited trials in osteomyelitis, regarded as a difficult site to treat, indicate that 9 months' therapy is effective, providing both isoniazid and rifampin are used. In miliary disease, the 6-month regimens have been very successful. Complications may develop during treatment of disease, partly a result of influx of leukocytes. The consequences of this depend on the site of infection and include pneumothoraces, expansion of intracerebral granulomas or discharge from subcutaneous nodes.

Directly observed therapy

Compliance with therapy is critical for successful treatment and to limit development of drug-resistant strains. Many social, personal, public

SHORT–COURSE CHEMOTHERAPY REGIMENS FOR TUBERCULOSIS			
Drug	Adult dose (orally)	Duration of treatment	Modification of drug dose in renal failure
1. Isoniazid*	5 mg/kg (maximum 300mg)	6 months	No
2. Rifampin*	10 mg/kg (maximum 600mg)	6 months	No
3. Pyrazinamide*	30mg/kg (maximum 2.0g)	2 months	↓ dose or ↑ dosage interval
4. Ethambutol or	15mg/kg†	2 months	↓ dose or ↑ dosage interval
Streptomycin	15mg/kg im (maximum 1.0g)	2 months	↓↓ dose or ↑↑ dosage interval

* Isoniazid and rifampin are marketed as a single combination tablet ± pyrazinamide which may facilitate compliance
† Some authorities use ethambutol at 25mg/kg for 2 months only (longer courses should be at 15mg/kg)

Fig. 30.18 Short-course chemotherapy. Short-course chemotherapy regimen for treatment of tuberculosis and necessity for drug dose modifications in renal impairment.

health and economic factors influence patient noncompliance with treatments.[59] The WHO and others strongly advocate directly observed therapy, short-course (DOTS). When patients are in hospital, normal treatment regimens may be used, but for patients in the community intermittent therapy is preferred (Fig. 30.19). DOTS does not simply involve giving a patient tablets, but also actively monitoring their consumption and may be very effective in controlling tuberculosis.[60]

Treating multidrug-resistant organisms

Multidrug-resistant tuberculosis was first noted in HIV-seropositive patients in New York[61] but has since been widely reported. Resistance to second-line drugs has also emerged.[62] Multidrug resistance is caused by the sequential acquisition of single-drug resistance traits.[63] This has been a consequence of poor prescribing practice by doctors, patient noncompliance with treatment and the endogenous mutation rate of *M. tuberculosis*. Patients should never be prescribed less than three drugs initially and seldom less than four if there is any

INTERMITTENT CHEMOTHERAPY REGIMENS FOR TUBERCULOSIS		
Drug	3 times/week dose	2 times/week dose
1. Isoniazid	15mg/kg for 6 months (maximum dose 900mg)	15mg/kg for 6 months (maximum dose 900mg)
2. Rifampin	10mg/kg for 6 months (maximum dose 900mg)	10mg/kg for 6 months (maximum dose 900mg)
3. Pyrazinamide	50mg/kg for 2 months (maximum dose 3.0g)	70mg/kg for 2 months (maximum dose 4.0g)
4. Ethambutol or Streptomycin	30mg/kg for 2 months	50mg/kg for 2 months (some authorities reduce this dose by 5mg/kg)
	25mg/kg for 2 months (some authorities reduce this dose by 5mg/kg; maximum 1.5g dose)	30mg/kg for 2 months (some authorities reduce this dose by 5mg/kg; maximum 1.5g dose)

Fig. 30.19 Intermittent chemotherapy regimens for tuberculosis.

chance of resistance or a history of previous therapy, irrespective of the sensitivity of the organism initially isolated.

Treatment protocols for multidrug-resistant disease must be designed for the individual but the aim is to use as many of the first-line drugs as possible before adding second-line drugs. In view of the fact that at least four drugs and possibly more should be given, options are frequently limited. A second-line therapeutic regimen should be continued for 18–24 months after cultures are negative. It is critical that affected patients are adequately isolated. Adjunctive surgical therapy may have a role in circumscribed lesions. Treatment of multidrug-resistant tuberculosis can be difficult and response rates in HIV-seronegative patients vary from 56%[64] to 96%.[65]

In HIV-infected patients

HIV does not adversely influence the response to short-course chemotherapy in the absence of drug resistance.[59,66] The rate of relapse of tuberculosis treated with first-line drugs is below 5% in compliant patients but increases significantly if rifampin and isoniazid are not used. However, HIV-seropositive patients who have tuberculosis have a 5- to 14-fold increased risk of dying, although superinfection and disease caused by other opportunistic pathogens contribute to mortality. In HIV patients who have tuberculosis, four drugs should probably be given routinely in the induction phase of treatment. In contrast, the prognosis of patients who have multidrug-resistant disease is poor worse than that of HIV-seronegative patients. HIV-seropositive patients are more likely to have adverse reactions to antituberculous medication, particularly to thiacetazone but also to other drugs.[67]

The use of corticosteroids

Steroid therapy is often advocated but seldom proved to be of benefit in tuberculosis. In pericardial tuberculosis, corticosteroids have been shown to decrease acute mortality from pericarditis and reduce the need for pericardiocentesis.[68] Corticosteroids may have a role in pleural disease but further data are needed before they can be recommended.[69] Corticosteroids are used during treatment of CNS tuberculomas to limit their expansion caused by cellular influx and to prevent raised intracerebral pressure. Evidence in favor of using corticosteroids in tuberculous meningitis is conflicting but they are probably beneficial in severe infection and spinal disease.[70] Retrospective studies investigating the role of corticosteroids in miliary tuberculosis have shown no benefit. In all cases, steroid metabolism is increased by rifampin.

Pregnancy

Pregnancy probably does not increase the severity or reactivation rate of tuberculosis or responses to therapy.[71] However, there may be a significant increase in spontaneous abortions and labor difficulties. Congenital tuberculosis is very rare and usually presents with hepatosplenomegaly, respiratory distress and fever;[72] it carries a high mortality. Tuberculosis frequently requires treatment during pregnancy and this should not be deferred. Isoniazid, rifampin and ethambutol are not teratogenic but few data exist on pyrazinamide. Streptomycin is associated with fetal hearing loss and should be avoided. Little is known about second-line drugs in pregnancy except para-aminosalicyclic acid, which appears to be safe. The presence of antituberculous drugs in breast milk is seldom a problem unless both mother and child are on treatment, in which case up to 20% more isoniazid than indicated may be taken by the child and bottle feeding is preferable. Breast-feeding children of mothers taking isoniazid require pyridoxine supplementation.

SURGICAL THERAPY

Surgical techniques such as artificial pneumothoraces, phrenic nerve paralysis, plombage and thoracoplasty are part of the history of tuberculosis before the era of chemotherapy. Now surgeons are most often involved in diagnostic rather than therapeutic procedures relevant to tuberculosis. However, resection of tissue may be necessary in patients who have multidrug-resistant infection, massive hemoptysis (after embolization has failed) and in the management of tuberculous empyema, draining sinuses and bronchopleural fistulae. Surgery has been widely used in treatment of spinal tuberculosis but is only indicated for the presence of progressive neurologic abnormality, spinal instability and to drain large paravertebral abscesses in which CT-guided drainage is not possible. Surgery may be required after destructive tuberculosis involving weight-bearing joints. Surgery may have an adjuvant role in nodal tuberculosis if a fluctuant mass persists. In laryngeal infection, temporary tracheostomy may be necessary and a few patients may require complex surgery such as partial laryngectomy.

IMMUNOTHERAPY AND THE FUTURE

Drugs remain at the forefront in the treatment of tuberculosis but new compounds are urgently needed. The long-term aim must be to produce true short-course therapy of a few weeks' rather than months' duration. Novel approaches are required in the face of drug resistance. The cytokines interferon-γ and IL-2 have been used with success in *M. leprae* infection and such compounds have potential in tuberculosis. At present, it is only possible to speculate on other options such as encouraging cellular recruitment to areas of infection, but it remains vital that the necessary basic research is supported.

REFERENCES

1. Ravilione MC, Snider DE, Kochi A. Global epidemiology of tuberculosis: morbidity and mortality of a worldwide epidemic. JAMA 1995;273:220–6.
2. Sheldon CD, King K, Cock H, Wilkinson P, Barnes NC. Notification of tuberculosis: how many cases are never reported? Thorax 1992;47:1015–8.
3. Citron KM, Southern A, Dixon M. Out of the shadow. Crisis 1995.
4. Allen S, Batungwanayo J, Kerlikowske K, et al. Two-year incidence of tuberculosis in cohorts of HIV-infected and uninfected urban Rwandan women. Am Rev Respir Dis 1992;146:1439–44.
5. Perneger TV, Sudre P, Lundgren JD, Hirschel B, for the AIDS in Europe study group. Does the onset of tuberculosis in AIDS predict shorter survival? Results of a cohort study in 17 European countries over 13 years. Br Med J 1995;311:1468–71.
6. Hill AR, Premkkumar S, Brustein S, et al. Disseminated tuberculosis in the acquired immunodeficiency syndrome era. Am Rev Respir Dis 1991;144:1164–70.
7. Bhatti N, Law MR, Morris JK, Halliday R, Moore-Gillon J. Increasing incidence of tuberculosis in England and Wales: a study of the likely causes. Br Med J 1995;310:967–9.
8. Goletti D, Weissman D, Jackson RW, et al. Effect of Mycobacterium tuberculosis on HIV replication: role of immune activation. J Immunol 1996;157:1271–8.
9. Shattock RJ, Friedland JS, Griffin GE. Phagocytosis of Mycobacterium tuberculosis enhances HIV transcription in human monocytic cells. J Gen Virol 1994;75:849–56.
10. Zhang Y, Nakata K, Weiden M, Rom WN. Mycobacterium tuberculosis enhances Human Immunodeficiency Virus-1 replication by transcriptional activation of the long terminal repeat. J Clin Invest 1995;95:2324–31.
11. Edlin BR, Tokars JI, Grieco MH, et al. An outbreak of multidrug-resistant tuberculosis among hospitalized patients with the Acquired Immunodeficiency Syndrome. N Engl J Med 1992;326:1514–21.
12. Wheeler PR, Ratledge C. Metabolism of Mycobacterium tuberculosis. In: Bloom BR, ed. Tuberculosis: pathogenesis, protection and control. Washington DC: ASM Press; 1994:353–85.
13. Arruda S, Bomfin G, Knights R, Huima-Byron T, Riley LW. Cloning of an M. tuberculosis DNA fragment associated with entry and survival inside cells. Science 1993;261:1454–7.
14. Schlesinger LS. Macrophage phagocytosis of virulent but not attenuated strains of Mycobacterium tuberculosis is mediated by mannose receptors in addition to complement receptors. J Immunol 1993;150:2920–30.
15. Zhang Y, Broser M, Rom WN. Activation of the interleukin 6 gene by Mycobacterium tuberculosis or lipopolysaccharide is mediated by nuclear factors NF-IL6 and NF-kB. Proc Natl Acad Sci USA 1994;91:2225–9.
16. Kindler V, Sappino A, Grau GE, Piguet P, Vassalli P. The inducing role of Tumour Necrosis Factor in the development of bactericidal granulomas during BCG infection. Cell 1989;56:731–40.
17. Friedland JS, Remick DG, Shattock R, Griffin GE. Secretion of Interleukin-8 following phagocytosis of Mycobacterium tuberculosis by human monocyte cell lines. Eur J Immunol 1992;22:1373–8.
18. Molloy A, Laochumroonvorapong P, Kaplan G. Apoptosis but not necrosis of infected monocytes is coupled with killing of intracellular Bacillus Calmette–Guerin. J Exp Med 1994;180:1499–509.
19. Toossi Z, Gogate P, Shiratsuchi H, Young T, Ellner JJ. Enhanced production of TGF-β by blood monocytes from patients with active tuberculosis and presence of TGF-β in tuberculous granulomatous lung lesions. J Immunol 1995;154:465–73.

20. Barnes PF, Abrams JS, Lu S, et al. Pattterns of cytokine production by mycobacterium-reactive human T cell clones. Infect Immunol 1993;61:197–203.
21. Barnes PF, Lu S, Abrams JS, et al. Cytokine production at the site of disease in human tuberculosis. Infect Immunol 1993;61:3482–9.
22. Haregewoin A, Soman G, Hom RC, Finberg RW. Human γδ + T cells respond to mycobacterial heat-shock protein. Nature 1989;340:309–12.
23. Modlin RL, Pirmez C, Hofman FM, et al. Lymphocytes bearing antigen-specific γδ T-cell receptors accumulate in human infectious disease lesions. Nature 1989;339:544–8.
24. Flynn JL, Goldstein MM, Triebold KJ, Koller B, Bloom BR. Major histocompatibility complex class 1-restricted T cells are required for resistance to Mycobacterium tuberculosis infection. Proc Natl Acad Sci USA 1992;89:12013–7.
25. Sieling PA, Chatterjee D, Porcelli SA, et al. CD1-restricted T cell recognition of microbial lipoglycan antigens. Science 1995;269:227–30.
26. Rook GAW. The role of vitamin D in tuberculosis. Am Rev Respir Dis 1989;138:768–70.
27. Al-Arif LI, Goldstein RA, Affronti LF, Janicki BW. HLA-B15 and tuberculosis in a North American black population. Am Rev Respir Dis 1979;120:1275–8.
28. Vidal S, Malo D, Vogan K, Skamene E, Gros P. Natural resistance to infection with intracellular parasites: isolation of a candidate for bcg. Cell 1993;73:469–85.
29. Small PM, Shafer RW, Hopewell PC, et al. Exogenous reinfection with multidrug-resistant Mycobacterium tuberculosis in patients with advanced HIV infection. N Engl J Med 1993;328:1137–44.
30. ACCP/ATS Consensus conference. Institutional control measures for tuberculosis in the era of multiple drug resistance. Chest 1995;108:1690–710.
31. Gowan JE. Nosocomial tuberculosis: new progress in control and prevention. Clin Infect Dis 1995;21:489–505.
32. De Cock KM, Grant A, Porter JDH. Preventive therapy for tuberculosis in HIV-infected persons: international recommendations, research and practice. Lancet 1995;345:833–6.
33. Fine PEM. Variation in protection by BCG: implications of and for heterologous immunity. Lancet 1995;346:1339–45.
34. Karonga Prevention Trial Group. Randomised controlled trial of single BCG, repeated BCG, or combined BCG and killed Mycobacterium leprae vaccine for prevention of leprosy and tuberculosis in Malawi. Lancet 1996;348:17–24.
35. Stanford JL, Grange JM. New concepts for the control of tuberculosis in the twenty first century. J Roy Coll Phys 1993;27:218–23.
36. Tascon RE, Colston MJ, Ragno MJ, et al. Vaccination against tuberculosis by DNA injection. Nature Med 1996;2:888–92.
37. Auerbach O. Tuberculosis of the trachea and major bronchi. Am Rev Tuberc 1949;60:604–70.
38. Barnes PF, Verdegem TD, Vachom LA, Leedome JM, Overturf GD. Chest roentgenogram in pulmonary tuberculosis. New data on an old test. Chest 1988;94:316–20.
39. British Thoracic and Tuberculosis Society. Aspergilloma and residual tuberculosis cavities – the results of a resurvey. Tubercle 1970;51:227–45.
40. Epstein DM, Kline LR, Albelda SM, Miller WT. Tuberculous pleural effusions. Chest 1987;91:106–9.
41. Kwan KL, Stottmeier KD, Sherman IH, McCabe WR. Mycobacterial cervical lymphadenopathy: relation of etiologic agents to age. JAMA 1984;251:1286–8.
42. Porter JC, Friedland JS, Freedman AR. Tuberculous bronchoesophagela fistulae in patients infected with the Human Immunodeficiency Virus: three case reports and review. Clin Infect Dis 1994;19:954–7.

43. Barber TW, Craven DE, McCabe WR. Bacteremia due to Mycobacterium tuberculosis in patients with Human Immunodeficiency Virus infection: a report of 9 cases and review of the literature. Medicine 1990;69:375–83.
44. Webb JG, Thomas P. Hypertrophic osteoarthropathy and pulmonary tuberculosis. Tubercle 1986;67:225–8.
45. Macfarlane JT, Ibrahim M, Tor-Agbidye S. The importance of finger clubbing in pulmonary tuberculosis. Tubercle 1979;60:45–8.
46. Blair EB, Brown GL, Tull AH. Computer files and analysis of laboratory data from tuberculosis patients: analysis of six years' data on sputum specimens. Am Rev Respir Dis 1976;113:427–32.
47. Wilcox PA, Potgeiter PD, Bateman ED, Benatar SR. Rapid diagnosis of sputum negative miliary tuberculosis using the flexible fiberoptic bronchoscope. Thorax 1986;41:681–4.
48. Maartens G, Willcox PA, Benatar SR. Miliary tuberculosis: rapid diagnosis, hematologic abnormalities and outcome in 109 treated adults. Am J Med 1990;89:291–6.
49. Bem C, Patil PS, Elliott AM, et al. The value of wide-needle aspiration in the diagnosis of tuberculous lymphadenitis in Africa. AIDS 1993;7:1221–5.
50. Brisson-Noel A, Aznar C, Chureau C, et al. Diagnosis of tuberculosis by DNA amplification in clinical practice evaluation. Lancet 1991;338:364–6.
51. Nooedhoek GT, van Embden JDA, Kolk AHJ. Questionable reliability of the polymerase chain reaction in the detection of Mycobacterium tuberculosis. N Engl J Med 1993;329:2036.
52. Schluger NW, Kinney D, Harkin TJ, Rom WN. Clinical utility of the polymerase chain reaction in the diagnosis of infections due to Mycobacterium tuberculosis. Chest 1994;105:1116–21.
53. Condos R, McClune A, Rom WN, Schluger NW. Peripheral blood-based PCR assay to identify patients with active pulmonary tuberculosis. Lancet 1996;347:1082–5.
54. Jacobs WR, Barletta RG, Udani R, et al. Rapid assessment of drug susceptibilities of Mycobacterium tuberculosis by means of luciferase reporter genes. Science 1993;260:819–22.
55. Zhang Y, Heym B, Allen B, Young D, Cole S. The catalase-peroxidase gene and isoniazid resistance of Mycobacterium tuberculosis. Nature 1992;358:591–3.
56. Bishai WR, Graham NMH, Harrington S, et al. Brief report: rifampicin-resistant tuberculosis in a patient receiving rifabutin prophylaxis. N Engl J Med 1996;334:1573–6.
57. Chambers HF, Moreau D, Yajko D, et al. Can penicillins and other β-lactam antibiotics be used to treat tuberculosis? Antimicrob Agents Chemother 1995;39:2620–4.
58. Bloch AB, Caythen GM, Onorato IM, et al. Nationwide survey of drug-resistant tuberculosis in the United States. JAMA 1994;271:665–71.
59. Ackah AN, Coulibaly D, Digbeu H, et al. Response to treatment, mortality and CD4 lymphocyte counts in HIV-infected persons with tuberculosis in Abijan, Cote d'Ivoire. Lancet 1995;345:607–10.
60. Weis SE, Slocum PC, Blias FX, et al. The effect of directly observed therapy on the rates of drug resistance and relapse in tuberculosis. N Engl J Med 1994;330:1179–84.
61. Frieden TR, Sterling T, Pablos-Mendez A, et al. The emergence of drug-resistant tuberculosis in New York city. N Engl J Med 1993;328:521–6.
62. Sullivan EA, Krieswirth BN, Palumbo L, et al. Emergence of fluoroquinolone-resistant tuberculosis in New York City. Lancet 1995;345:1148–50.
63. Heym B, Honore N, Truffot-Pernot C, et al. Implications of multidrug resistance for the future of short-course chemotherapy of tuberculosis: a molecular study. Lancet 1994;344:293–8.

64. Goble M, Iseman MD, Madsen LA, *et al.* Treatment of 171 patients with pulmonary tuberculosis resistant to isoniazid and rifampicin. N Engl J Med 1993;328:527–32.

65. Telzak EE, Sepkowitz K, Alpert P, *et al.* Multidrug-resistant tuberculosis in patients without HIV infection. N Engl J Med 1995;333:907–11.

66. Perriens JH, St. Loius ME, Mukadi YB, *et al.* Pulmonary tuberculosis in HIV-infected patients in Zaire. N Engl J Med 1995;332:779–84.

67. Nunn P, Kibuga D, Gathua S, *et al.* Cutaneous hypersensitivity reactions due to thiacetazones in HIV-1 seropositive patients treated for tuberculosis. Lancet 1991;377:627–30.

68. Strang JIG, Kakaza HHS, Gibson DG, *et al.* Controlled clinical trial of complete open surgical drainage and of prednisolone in treatment of tuberculous pericardial effusion in Transkei. Lancet 1988;ii:759–64.

69. Musthuswamy P, Tzyy-Chyn H, Carasso B, Antonio M, Dandamudi N. Prednisolone as adjunctive therapy in the management of pulmonary tuberculosis. Chest 1995;107:1621–30.

70. Girgis NI, Farid Z, Kilpatrick ME, Sultan Y, Mikhail IA. Dexamethasone adjunctive treatment for tuberculous meningitis. Pediatr Infect Dis J 1991;10:179–83.

71. Espinal MA, Reingold AL, Lavandera M. Effect of pregnancy on the risk of developing active tuberculosis. J Infect Dis 1995;173:488–91.

72. Cantwell MF, Shehab ZM, Costello AM, *et al.* Brief report: congenital tuberculosis. N Engl J Med 1994;330:1051–4.

73. James DR, Studdy PR. In: Colour atlas of respiratory diseases, 2nd ed. London: Mosby; 1992.

74. Thaller SR, Gross JR, Pilch BZ, Goodman ML. Laryngeal tuberculosis as manifested in the decades 1963–1983. Laryngoscope 1987;97:848–50.

75. Newport MJ, Huxley CM, Huston S, *et al.* A mutation in the interferon-γ receptor gene and susceptibility to mycobacterial infection. N Engl J Med 1996;335:1941–9.

76. Cadranel J, Garabedian M, Milleron B, *et al.* Vitamin D metabolism by alveolar immune cells in tuberculosis: correlation with calcium metabolism and clinical manifestations. Eur Respir J 1994;7:1103–10.

Nontuberculosis Mycobacteria

David E Griffith

INTRODUCTION

The nontuberculous mycobacteria (NTM) encompass all mycobacterial species that are not included in the *Mycobacterium tuberculosis* complex. There are more than 50 species, most of which do not or only rarely cause human disease. A few NTM species, however, are important pathogens in both immunocompetent and immunocompromised hosts. In the past, patients with NTM disease were described as having 'atypical tuberculosis' regardless of the site of disease or the NTM species isolated. Because of the need for specific therapy directed at individual NTM species, 'atypical tuberculosis' has become an anachronistic and inappropriate label. Clinicians must now be knowledgeable about the virulence, sites of infection and treatment of individual NTM species.

Nontuberculous mycobacteria classification systems have generally not been helpful to the clinician. The most widely used classification scheme in the past, the Runyon system, was based on microbiologic characteristics of the organisms, such as rate of growth and colony pigment formation, and had little meaning from a clinical perspective. Familiarity with the Runyon system remains useful for presumptive identification of possible NTM pathogens; however, positive identification of NTM species is now largely based on biochemical and molecular biologic techniques. Classification of NTMs based on the organ system of primary involvement (lung, lymph node, disseminated, skin and soft tissue) is more useful to the clinician and is used in the following discussion.[1,2]

EPIDEMIOLOGY

The prevalence of NTM infection can only be estimated because NTM infections are not reportable and because the clinical significance of an NTM isolate is not always clear. There is evidence, however, that the prevalence of NTM disease is increasing, in both the AIDS and non-AIDS populations. Clues to the prevalence of NTM disease in the USA have been provided by two surveys of NTM isolates during the years 1979–1983.[3,4] Using combined data from these national surveillance studies, the prevalence of NTM disease, largely pulmonary, was estimated to be 1.8/100,000 population. *Mycobacterium avium* complex (MAC) accounted for 1.1/100,000 population, followed in frequency by '*M. fortuitum* complex' and *M. kansasii*. These prevalence figures are, at best, estimates as the surveys were not comprehensive and the authors could only estimate the number of clinically significant NTM isolates.

A more recent study from 1991 to 1992 demonstrated an apparent increase in the prevalence of NTM infection in the USA.[5] Despite the increase in *M. tuberculosis* isolates noted in the USA during these years, there were more isolates of MAC than of *M. tuberculosis* in this study. The emergence of disseminated NTM disease in AIDS patients probably had the greatest impact on the increased number of NTM isolates. Disseminated NTM infection, almost entirely due to MAC, is the most common bacterial infection in AIDS, occurring in 20–40% of AIDS patients.[6,7] Additional factors contributing to the increase in NTM isolates include:

- an increased total number of clinical specimens submitted for acid-fast bacilli (AFB) analysis (associated with the rise in tuberculosis incidence);
- better clinical recognition of NTM disease, especially chronic pulmonary disease, in immunocompetent patients; and
- improved laboratory techniques, which have made identification and isolation of NTM more accurate and rapid.

A bimodal age distribution in NTM isolates also emerged with peaks in young adults and in elderly patients, likely reflecting the age peaks in prevalence for disseminated and pulmonary NTM infections.[5]

Nontuberculous mycobacteria disease prevalence worldwide is also difficult to estimate, as no comprehensive surveys of NTM isolates or disease have been undertaken. A picture of NTM disease is emerging that suggests geographic clusters of disease caused by various NTM species. For instance, *Mycobacterium xenopi*, a rare pathogen in the USA, is the second most common cause of NTM lung disease in areas of Canada and the UK.[8] *Mycobacterium malmoense*, also a rare pathogen in the USA, is the second most common cause of NTM lung disease in Scandinavia and areas of Northern Europe.[9]

Although MAC disease has a worldwide distribution, disseminated MAC is rarely seen in people who have AIDS from central Africa, even though MAC can be recovered from that environment.[10] One possible explanation is that people who have AIDS in Africa may die from infection with other pathogens before developing disseminated MAC.

Important geographic clustering for NTM species is noted in Figure 31.3 describing NTM pathogens for specific organ systems. With heightened interest in mycobacterial disease as a result of worldwide AIDS and tuberculosis epidemics, a better understanding worldwide of NTM epidemiology will emerge.

PATHOGENESIS AND PATHOLOGY

Evidence is mounting to show that the environment is the source of most, if not all, human NTM infection. Nontuberculous mycobacteria are ubiquitous in the environment and have been isolated from water, soil, dust, domestic and wild animals, milk and food. It is now generally accepted, however, that water is the source of infection for most NTM infections in both immunocompetent and immunocompromised hosts.[2] The development of DNA fingerprinting by restriction fragment length polymorphism analysis has been especially useful for epidemiologic investigation (Fig. 31.1).

PULMONARY DISEASE

The evidence for environmental transmission of MAC in pulmonary disease is mostly circumstantial. It grows well in natural waters and is readily aerosolized above bodies of water.[11] *Mycobacterium avium* complex strains with plasmids, possibly associated with virulence, have been shown to be preferentially aerosolized.[12] Recovery rates of MAC from the environment in the USA are highest in the states bordering the Atlantic Ocean and Gulf of Mexico and this is also the area with the highest rates of MAC infection.[13] In a skin test survey performed on 275,000 naval recruits, each of whom had resided from birth in a single county, positive reaction to an MAC skin test antigen [purified protein

DNA FINGERPRINT PATTERNS OF AN *M. ABSCESSUS* OUTBREAK

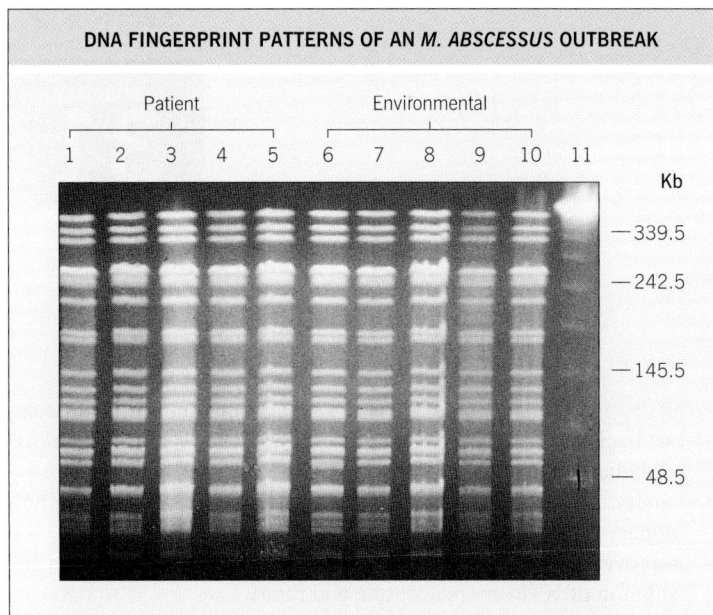

Fig. 31.1 Pulsed field gel electrophoresis (PFGE), DNA fingerprint patterns of 10 *Mycobacterium abscessus* isolates from an outbreak of *M. abscessus* infection in a hemodialysis center. Lanes 1–5 are identical *M. abscessus* strains recovered in blood cultures from 5 different patients, indicating a common source of infection. Lanes 6–10 are the same strain of *M. abscessus* recovered by sampling a water treatment system contaminated by *M. abscessus*, the source of the patients' *M. abscessus* isolates. Courtesy of Dr Yansheng Zhang and Dr Richard J Wallace Jr.

LYMPHOCYTE–MYCOBACTERIA-INFECTED MACROPHAGE INTERACTIONS

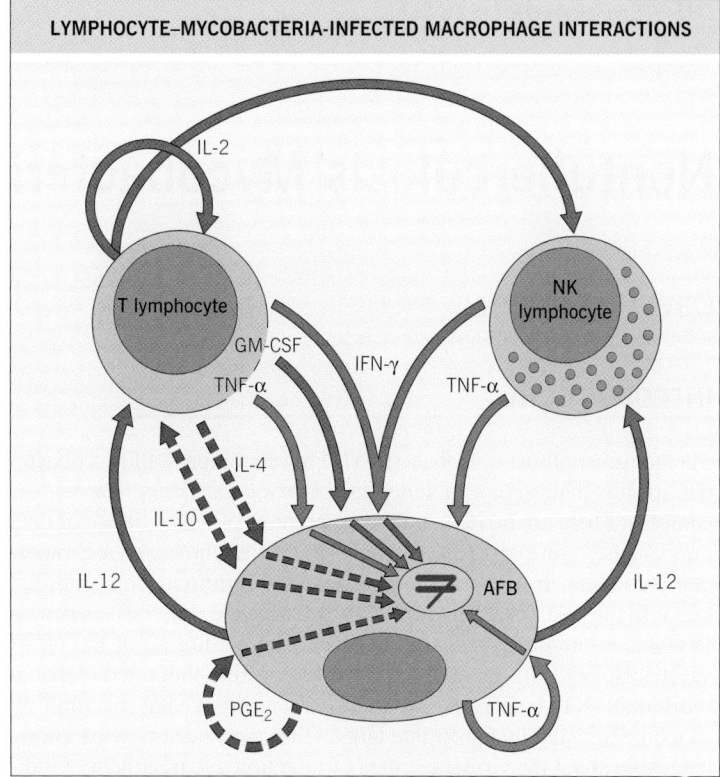

Fig. 31.2 Selected interactions between lymphocytes and mycobacteria-infected macrophages. Solid lines indicate activities that stimulate mycobacterial killing, whereas dashed lines indicate activities that inhibit it. Mycobacteria – acid-fast bacilli (AFB) – infect the macrophage and lead to the production of interleukin (IL)-12 to signal T and NK lymphocytes to produce interferon (IFN)-γ. The CD4+ T lymphocytes produce IFN-γ, which activates the macrophage to produce tumor necrosis factor (TNF)-α, kill intracellular bacteria and produce more IL-12. The CD4+ T lymphocytes also produce IL-2, which expands the number of T lymphocytes and NK lymphocytes available. Natural killer lymphocytes release granulocyte–macrophage colony stimulating factor (GM-CSF) and TNF-α,which also activate macrophages. Interleukin-10 is produced by macrophages and T lymphocytes to downregulate the effects of IFN-γ and TNF-α. PG, prostalgandin. Adapted with permission from Holland SM. Host defense against nontuberculous mycobacterial infections. Semin Respir Infect 1996;11:217–30.

derivative (PPD)/B] was heavily distributed among those who had lived along the Gulf Coast and Southern Atlantic states.[14] Although the skin test is not specific for MAC, these results support the correlation between geographic environmental exposure and infection in humans.

Pulmonary infection by *M. kansasii* also likely occurs via an aerosol route. Whereas MAC appears to be acquired in rural areas, *M. kansasii* is more likely acquired in urban environments.[15] *Mycobacterium kansasii* isolates of the same phage type as those isolated from patients have been recovered from urban drinking water distribution systems.[16] Clinical isolates and tap water isolates of the same genotype, determined by DNA fingerprinting, have also been identified.[17]

DISSEMINATED DISEASE
Environmental exposure in NTM by people who have AIDS also probably occurs from aqueous sources, resulting in gastrointestinal and/or pulmonary acquisition of NTM, usually MAC. Following ingestion of NTM there is direct tissue invasion, and at some point with a declining host immunity, NTM bacteremia. One study using DNA fingerprinting directly linked an environmental source of MAC (hospital tap water) with clinical disseminated MAC disease in some people who have AIDS who were exposed to this water source.[18]

LOCALIZED SKIN AND SOFT TISSUE INFECTIONS
Skin and soft tissue infections in immunocompetent patients are likely the result of direct exposure to contaminated water sources through inoculation after accidental trauma, surgery or injection. *Mycobacterium marinum* inhabits water and marine organisms. Infection in humans may be introduced into the skin:

- when cleaning fresh water fish tanks (fish tank granuloma);
- by scratches or puncture wounds from salt water fish, shrimp, fins, etc.; and
- through abrasions in nonchlorinated swimming pools (swimming pool granuloma).

Mycobacterium xenopi has been recovered from hot water taps within hospitals and in one study a clinical isolate and hospital water isolates were found to be identical by DNA fingerprint analysis.[19] Investigations

of nosocomial outbreaks caused by *M. fortuitum, M. chelonae* and *M. abscessus,* including the use of DNA fingerprinting, have demonstrated that tap water, ice prepared from tap water, processed tap water used for dialysis and distilled water used for preparing solutions are the source of these organisms in nosocomially acquired infection (see Fig. 31.1).[20,21]

TRANSMISSION
There is no firm evidence of human-to-human or animal-to-human transmission of NTM disease. Although family groupings of NTM infection have occasionally occurred in humans, these groupings have been assumed to be due to a common environmental exposure. *Mycobacterium avium* complex is an important cause of disease in poultry and swine, but recent DNA fingerprint studies have shown that strains infecting human and animals are different.[22,23]

HISTOPATHOLOGY
Nontuberculous mycobacteria disease is characterized histopathologically by the presence of caseating and noncaseating granulomatous inflammation, epithelial histiocytes and occasional giant cells. Nontuberculous mycobacterial infection cannot be differentiated histopathologically from tuberculosis. Poorly formed granulomas with histiocytic reactions are more commonly reported in immunodeficient, especially AIDS, patients, but can be seen in immunocompetent patients as not all NTM stimulate granuloma formation equally well.

INTERACTION BETWEEN NONTUBERCULOUS MYCOBACTERIA AND HOST DEFENSES

An understanding of the interaction between NTM and host defenses is only now emerging. The critical interaction that determines whether NTM infection is established, is between the mycobacterium and the macrophage. Mycobacteria are successful intracellular pathogens that not only penetrate host defense cells, but replicate within them. The mycobacterial cell wall, composed of glycopeptidolipids, including lipoarabinomannan, is probably a key element responsible for the survival and multiplication of NTM within the hostile intracellular environment of the macrophage.[24] Organisms engulfed by the macrophages are taken into intracellular vacuoles and the prevention of acidification of the intracellular vacuole may be an important mechanism of mycobacterial evasion of host defenses and a virulence factor.[25] If the organism persists and multiplies within the macrophage, then a lymphocyte-mediated immune response, including CD4+ T lymphocytes and natural killer (NK) cells, is triggered by the infected macrophage. The role of neutrophils in controlling NTM infection is not clear. The expanded immune response may result in augmented killing of intracellular mycobacteria by the macrophage or destruction of the infected macrophage itself by NK cells. The macrophage–lymphocyte interaction may result in granuloma formation and ultimately determines whether the NTM infection is limited (controlled) or progresses.

Infected macrophages and stimulated lymphocytes produce soluble factors, including cytokines and prostaglandins, that modulate a complicated immune interaction (Fig. 31.2). Important components of this immune response to mycobacteria include:

- tumor necrosis factor (TNF)-α,
- interferon (IFN)-γ,
- interleukins (IL) 2, 6, 10 and 12, and
- granulocyte–macrophage colony stimulating factor.

Tumor necrosis factor-α is produced by activated macrophages and NK cells and is probably the most important of the immunomodulators for controlling mycobacterial infection. Tumor necrosis factor-α has a significant additive effect on macrophage killing of MAC.[26] The release of TNF-α is stimulated by and is probably responsible for the antimycobacterial effects of IFN-γ.[26] Interleukin-2 greatly augments the capacity of NK cells to lyse MAC-infected monocytes and IL-2-stimulated NK cells also enhance intracellular monocyte killing of MAC, again, likely via TNF-α.[27] Interleukin-12 is a major stimulant for T lymphocytes and NK cells to produce IFN-γ and TNF-α and, in turn, IL-12 release is stimulated by IFN-γ and TNF-α.[28,29] Granulocyte–macrophage colony stimulating factor is produced by MAC-infected monocytes and NK cells and appears to augment mycobacterial killing.[30] In contrast, IL-6 and IL-10 downmodulate the inflammatory response, especially the effect of TNF-α, and are therefore permissive factors for proliferation of intracellular mycobacteria.[31,32]

These immune modulators act in a complicated fashion and it is difficult to isolate and measure in vivo any single aspect of the inflammatory cascade. Nevertheless, this line of investigation provides important clues to NTM disease pathogenesis. A practical application of this research is illustrated by a family with a monocyte defect in IL-12 production that was associated with disseminated MAC infection in the absence of HIV infection. This defect was overcome by exogenous administration of IFN-γ in addition to other antimycobacterial therapy, resulting in successful treatment of the disseminated MAC infection.[33,34]

Because most NTM are nonpathogenic and those NTM that are pathogens frequently cause disease in limited circumstances, there is intense interest in identifying virulence factors for NTM. Plasmids may encode virulence genes and are more common in MAC isolates from people who have AIDS than in environmental isolates.[35,36] Other potential virulence factors include:

- prevention of acidification of phagocytic vesicles;[25]
- prevention of phagosome–lysosome fusion;[37]
- delay in TNF secretion by infected host cells;[38] and
- catalase activity.[39]

Which factor or factors are most important and whether they can be favorably modified remains to be determined.

CLINICAL FEATURES

PULMONARY DISEASE

Chronic pulmonary disease in the most common clinical manifestation of NTM infection in the USA. It is unclear whether the increased numbers of respiratory NTM isolates recently observed is due to an increasing prevalence of disease or better recognition of existing disease.[4] Several NTM species can cause lung disease in the immunocompetent host (Fig. 31.3); however, MAC, *M. kansasii* and *M. abscessus* are the most common respiratory pathogens.[2] Whether these immunocompetent hosts have an unrecognized defect in host defences is unknown.

Signs and symptoms of NTM pulmonary disease are variable and nonspecific and include chronic cough, sputum production and fatigue. Malaise, dyspnea, fever, hemoptysis and weight loss can also occur, usually with advanced disease, but are less common than with tuberculosis.

Nontuberculous mycobacterial lung disease produces variable radiographic features, ranging from apical cavitary lung disease, typical of reactivation tuberculosis, to nodular disease associated with bronchiectasis. Although there are differences in the radiographic features of NTM lung disease compared with those of *M. tuberculosis,* there are no radiographic findings that discriminate with certainty between tuberculosis and NTM lung infection. Similarly, it is difficult to differentiate, on either a clinical or radiographic basis, between NTM species causing lung disease.

NONTUBERCULOUS MYCOBACTERIA THAT CAUSE PULMONARY DISEASE IN THE IMMUNOCOMPETENT HOST

Mycobacteria		Clinical comment
Common	*Mycobacterium avium* complex	Cavitary disease in male cigarette smokers with COPD; nodular/bronchiectatic disease in elderly nonsmoking women; southeast USA, worldwide
	Mycobacterium kansasii	Clinically and radiographically closely resembles tuberculosis; south central USA, UK, Europe
	Mycobacterium abscessus	Clinically resembles nodular/bronchiectatic form of MAC lung disease; southeast USA
Uncommon	*Mycobacterium fortuitum*	Single isolate usually not clinically significant; unusual lung pathogen except in the setting of gastroesophageal disease with chronic aspiration
	Mycobacterium xenopi	Canada, UK, Europe
	Mycobacterium simiae	Single isolate frequently not significant; southwest USA, Israel
	Mycobacterium szulgai	One culture positive specimen adequate for diagnosis
	Mycobacterium malmoense	One culture positive specimen adequate for diagnosis; Scandinavia, northern Europe
Rare	*Mycobacterium celatum*	
	Mycobacterium asiaticum	
	Mycobacterium shimodei	

Nontuberculous mycobacteria that usually represent contamination of respiratory specimens from immune competent hosts: *M. gordonae, M. genavense, M. smegmatis, M. nonchromogenicum, M. haemophilum, M. vaccae, M. thermoresistable, M. flavescens*

Fig. 31.3 Nontuberculous mycobacteria that cause pulmonary disease in the immunocompetent host. COPD, chronic obstructive pulmonary disease.

Mycobacterium avium complex infection

This is the most common cause of NTM lung disease. In the majority of patients in the USA, MAC lung disease is due to *M. intracellulare*; in other geographic areas *M. avium* infection is equally common.[40,41] Lung disease caused by MAC has traditionally been diagnosed in middle aged or older men, usually with a history of cigarette smoking and underlying lung disease such as chronic obstructive pulmonary disease, previous tuberculosis, pneumoconiosis or bronchiectasis.[15,42] The majority of these patients have cavitary changes on chest radiography (Fig. 31.4). This form of disease can be aggressive and cause extensive lung destruction.

It is now clear that MAC lung disease has a more heterogeneous clinical presentation, in particular in elderly women nonsmokers who have no known underlying lung disease.[43] These patients present radiographically with mid- and lower-lung field disease characterized by a combination of discrete, small (<5mm) pulmonary nodules and accompanying bronchiectasis, abnormalities that are especially apparent with high-resolution CT of the chest (Fig. 31.5).[44] Because this form of disease is radiographically atypical for mycobacterial disease, diagnosis may be delayed, even in patients who have persistent cough and progressive radiographic abnormalities. Disease progression is usually indolent; however, this form of MAC lung disease can be associated with significant morbidity and mortality.[43]

Mycobacterium kansasii infection

Mycobacterium kansasii produces pulmonary disease that most closely parallels clinical disease caused by *M. tuberculosis*. Patients with *M. kansasii* lung disease are characteristically older men from urban environments who are cigarette smokers with one or more underlying pulmonary diseases including chronic obstructive pulmonary disease, previous tuberculosis, bronchiectasis or pneumoconiosis.[15] The chest radiographic changes are also very similar to reactivated pulmonary tuberculosis with an upper lobe predilection and cavitation in approximately 90% of patients (Fig. 31.6). Not surprisingly, most patients with *M. kansasii* lung disease enter the health care system with suspected tuberculosis.

Mycobacterium abscessus infection

Patients who have *M. abscessus* lung disease are typically elderly female nonsmokers with no known underlying or predisposing lung disease.[45] This disease clinically and radiographically most closely resembles noncavitary (nodular bronchiectatic) pulmonary MAC disease. *Mycobacterium abscessus* and MAC are sometimes isolated concurrently or consecutively in some patients.[45]

LYMPHADENITIS

Mycobacterial lymphadenitis presents as an insidious, painless, unilateral process involving one or more nodes in a regional distribution with only rare associated systemic symptoms. Upper anterior cervical, submandibular, submaxillary and preauricular lymph nodes are the most commonly involved. Lymphadenitis is the most common disease manifestation of NTM in children. This presentation is most commonly due to MAC (60–80% of cases), whereas tuberculosis accounts for only 10–20% of mycobacterial lymphadenitis in this age group.[46] The predominance of MAC is a change from 20 years ago when most geographic areas reported *Mycobacterium scrofulaceum* as the most common etiologic agent.[46] In contrast, mycobacterial lymphadenitis in people over 12 years of age is due to *M. tuberculosis* in approximately 95% of cases. In children, and especially adults, the main differential diagnosis is therefore tuberculosis.

Nontuberculous mycobacterial adenopathy is not usually associated with a history of tuberculosis exposure: tuberculin skin testing in the patient and family are negative and the chest radiograph is normal. Confirming the diagnosis may be difficult because aspiration, biopsy and culture of the involved nodes yields positive cultures in only approximately 50% of the cases.[47] Other NTM that are uncommon causes of lymphadenitis include *M. malmoense*, *M. fortuitum*, *M. chelonae*, *M. abscessus*, *M. kansasii* and *M. haemophilum*.

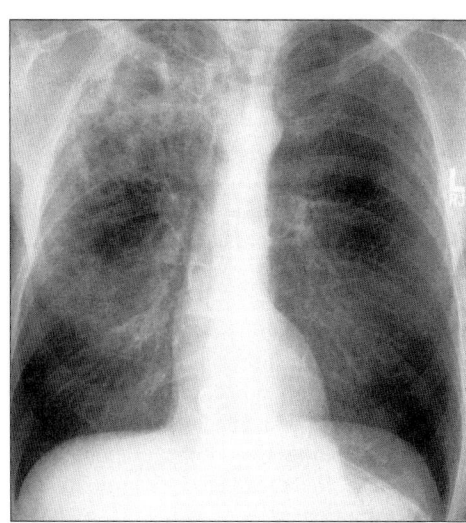

Fig. 31.4 Apical cavitary infiltrates similar to those caused by pulmonary tuberculosis in a 60-year old male cigarette smoker with *Mycobacterium avium* complex lung disease.

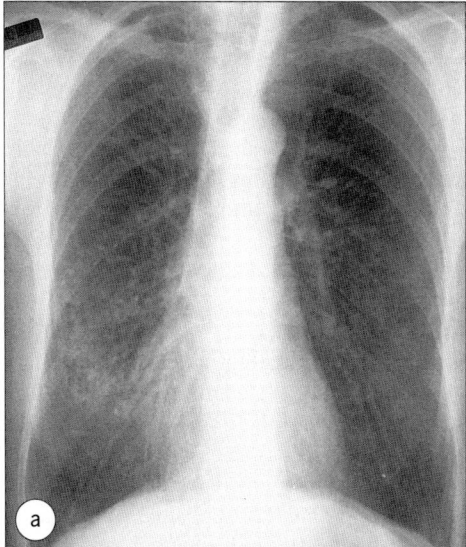

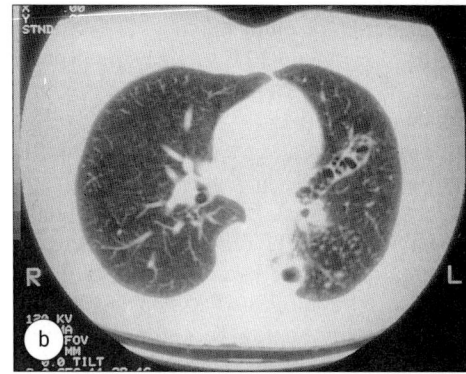

Fig. 31.5 *Mycobacterium avium* complex (MAC) lung disease. (a) Interstitial nodular midlung field infiltrates (right>left) in a 64-year old female with MAC lung disease. (b) Chest CT scan from a 52-year old female with MAC lung disease demonstrating three abnormalities common in MAC lung disease: bronchiectasis, a cavity and small (<5mm) nodules.

DISSEMINATED DISEASE

Disseminated NTM disease is the most common bacterial infection in people who have AIDS, but can also occur in people who have severe immunosuppression unrelated to AIDS, such as due to chronic corticosteroid use, organ transplantation or leukemia. More than 95% of disseminated NTM disease in people who have AIDS is due to isolates of MAC. In contrast to MAC pulmonary disease, 90% of MAC isolates in disseminated disease are *M. avium*.[41,48] Perhaps not surprisingly, polyclonal MAC infection in AIDS patients appears common and may occur in up to 20% of patients with disseminated MAC infection.[49] Other NTM species also produce disseminated disease, including *M. kansasii*, *M. chelonae*, *M. abscessus*, *M. xenopi*, *M. malmoense*, *M. genavense*, *M. conspicuum*, *M. gordonae* and *M. haemophilum*. Although disseminated MAC disease presents as a febrile wasting

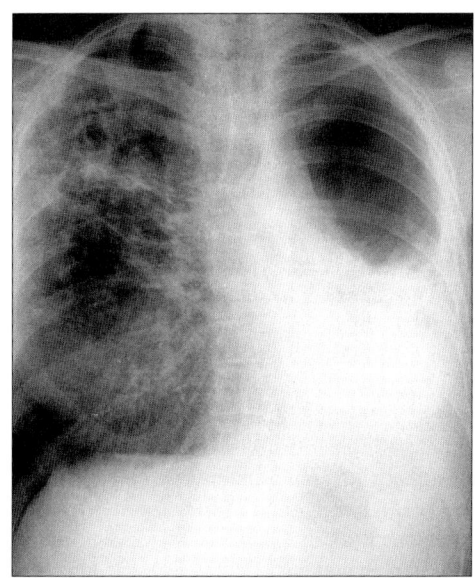

Fig. 31.6 Far-advanced *Mycobacterium kansasii* bilateral lung disease. A 42-year old male cigarette smoker with extensive cavitary destruction of the left upper lobe.

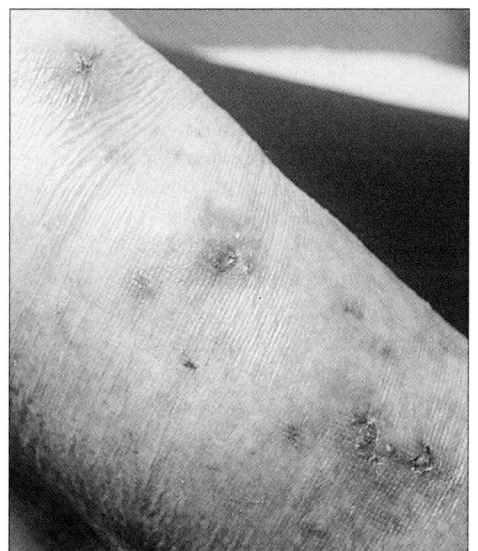

Fig. 31.7 Disseminated *Mycobacterium chelonae* disease. This is manifested by subcutaneous nodules on the lower extremities in an 81-year old female receiving high-dose corticosteroids for rheumatoid arthritis.

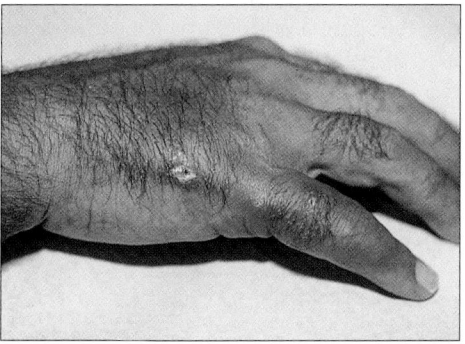

Fig. 31.8 Nodular lesions on the hand caused by *Mycobacterium marinum*. This 45-year old man contracted *M. marinum* after penetrating trauma while cleaning his boat in salt water.

prophylaxis, develop disseminated MAC at the rate of approximately 20%/year.[48] Presenting symptoms usually include several weeks of fever, sweats, diarrhea and wasting. Nausea, vomiting and intractable abdominal pain are indicative of the frequent gastrointestinal involvement. Physical findings include weight loss, hepatosplenomegaly and intra-abdominal lymphadenopathy. Worsening anemia and an elevated alkaline phosphatase out of proportion to hepatic transaminase elevation occur late with continuous bacteremia. Localized pulmonary disease due to MAC occurs in fewer than 5% of people who have AIDS with MAC infection.[50]

Mycobacterium kansasii infection in people who have AIDS, unlike MAC infection, frequently causes disease with the same symptomatology as in people who are immunocompetent.[51] It will disseminate in approximately 35% of AIDS patients who have the infection, usually in association with far-advanced pulmonary disease. Radiographic manifestations of *M. kansasii* pulmonary disease in people who have AIDS are somewhat atypical, with noncavitary changes in approximately 50% of patients. Clinical symptomatology is nonspecific and similar to that of disseminated MAC infection; however, disseminated *M. kansasii* may also present with multiple subcutaneous nodules. As in disseminated MAC disease, CD4+ lymphocyte counts average 24/mm³ in patients with disseminated *M. kansasii* disease, and not surprisingly, these patients may have co-existent disseminated MAC infection.

Differential diagnosis

Disseminated NTM disease must be differential from other infections that may be present in a similar way in patients with advanced AIDS. These include disseminated CMV, histoplasmosis and of course tuberculosis. Infections with *M. tuberculosis* tend to occur earlier in the course of AIDS than NTM infection, but there are no reliable clinical indicators to distinguish between disseminated NTM and disseminated tuberculosis. In general, a positive AFB specimen from a person who has AIDS must be assumed to be due to tuberculosis until proven otherwise.

Nontuberculosis mycobacteria rarely causes infection of the central nervous system (CNS) but the most common setting for NTM CNS involvement is as part of disseminated disease in a patient with severe immunocompromise, such as seen with advanced AIDS.[52] Nontuberculosis mycobacteria species that have been implicated in CNS infections in this setting are MAC, *M. kansasii*, *M. gordonae* and *M. genavense*. A very small number of cases of NTM CNS infections have been reported in nonimmunocompromised patients, especially due to *M. fortuitum* and associated with trauma, surgery, or chronic infections (otitis, mastoiditis). Presenting symptoms for NTM CNS infections are variable and may include neuropsychiatric symptoms, headaches, altered mental status, meningismus, cranial nerve abnormalities and problems with co-ordination. Not suprisingly these patients also sometimes have concomitant CNS infections caused by other pathogens. Treatment strategies for AIDS that decrease the number of patients with very severe immunocompromise should substantially reduce this problem.

LOCALIZED SKIN AND SOFT TISSUE INFECTION

Localized abscess formation after direct inoculation of organisms is most often due to *M. fortuitum*, *M. abscessus* or *M. chelonae*.[2] Nosocomial skin and soft tissue disease caused by these three species includes infections of long-term intravenous or peritoneal catheters, postinjection abscesses and surgical wound infections, including those after augmentation mammaplasty or cardiac bypass surgery. *Mycobacterium marinum*, MAC, *M. fortuitum*, *M. abscessus*, *M. chelonae* and *M. kansasii* have all been implicated in chronic granulomatous infection in tendon sheaths, bursae, joints and bones. *Mycobacterium haemophilum*, *M. nonchromogenicum* and *M. smegmatis* are rare causes of localized skin and soft tissue disease.

Mycobacterium marinum skin lesions usually appear as solitary papules on an extremity, especially on the elbows, knees and dorsa of the feet and hands, progressing subsequently to shallow ulceration and scar formation (Fig. 31.8). Occasionally, multiple 'ascending' subcutaneous lesions resembling sporotrichosis may develop.

illness, disseminated disease caused by *M. chelonae*, *M. abscessus* and *M. haemophilum* may present as diffuse subcutaneous nodules or abscesses (Fig. 31.7). Some NTM isolates that cause disseminated disease in people who have AIDS have been considered nonpathogenic when isolated from immunocompetent hosts (see Fig. 31.3); all NTM isolates from people who are severely immunocompromised, and especially from people who have AIDS, should therefore be regarded as potential pathogens, at least initially.

Disseminated MAC disease in people who have AIDS accompanies severe immunosuppression, with the average CD4+ lymphocyte count at the time of dissemination being approximately 25/mm³. Patients with fewer than 100 CD4+ lymphocytes/mm³, who are not receiving

Mycobacterium marinum requires low temperature incubation for isolation, so when a diagnosis of *M. marinum* infection is suspected, the laboratory should be notified. Disseminated infection by *M. marinum* has occurred in people who have AIDS and is presumably acquired in the same fashion as by immunocompetent hosts.

Mycobacterium ulcerans causes indolent necrotic lesions of the skin and underlying tissue. The lesions occur most commonly in children and young adults and can result in severe deformities of the extremities if left untreated. *Mycobacterium ulcerans* infections occur in tropical areas of the world, including Australia, but have not been reported in the USA (see Chapter 6.6).

DIAGNOSIS

The methods for handling clinical samples for recovery of *M. tuberculosis* and NTM are generally the same. All mycobacteria are 'acid fast' and the fluorochrome method (auramine stain) is the preferred method for microscopic recognition of NTM in clinical samples. The appearance of NTM by microscopy is sometimes indistinguishable from that of *M. tuberculosis*, therefore confirmation of the presence of NTM still requires cultures. Cultures should be inoculated onto one or more solid media (e.g. Lowenstein–Jensen and/or Middlebrook 7H10 or 7H11) and into a liquid medium as well, given the more rapid recovery of all mycobacteria in broth systems such as the BACTEC system. All skin or soft tissue samples should be incubated at two temperatures, 95°F and 82.4–89.6°F, because a number of pathogens that infect these tissues, including *M. haemophilum* and *M. marinum*, may grow only at the lower temperatures.

The majority of clinical and public health laboratories now use one or more rapid diagnostic methods for mycobacterial species identification. These rapid methods include high-performance liquid chromatography and commercial DNA probes, which are available for identifying isolates of *M. tuberculosis*, *M. gordonae*, *M. kansasii*, *M. avium* and *M. intracellulare*. These probes are highly sensitive and specific and can provide species identification using a culture directly from both media.

A variety of skin test reagents have been prepared from various species of NTM, including PPD-A from *M. avium* and PPD-B from *M. intracellulare*; however, they are not specific, lack standardization and are not clinically useful in the diagnosis of NTM disease. The use of NTM skin test reagents is currently confined to epidemiologic studies.

PULMONARY DISEASE

Unlike tuberculosis, a single positive NTM culture from a respiratory specimen, especially if it contains only a small number of organisms, is not always sufficient to diagnose NTM lung disease or initiate therapy. No single diagnostic algorithm is satisfactory for interpreting the clinical significance of all NTM respiratory isolates. For example, a single positive sputum culture for *M. kansasii* in the appropriate setting is diagnostic of lung disease caused by this organism. The same is probably true for *M. abscessus*, *M. szulgai* and *M. malmoense*, and possibly even MAC. For relatively nonvirulent pathogens, such as *M. fortuitum* and *M. simiae*, a single isolate from sputum is almost never adequate to confirm the diagnosis. Determining the significance of a respiratory NTM isolate requires knowledge of:
- the virulence of the NTM isolated;
- the frequency and quantity with which the NTM was isolated;
- the patient's symptoms, chest radiograph appearance, and comorbid conditions; and
- the rapidity of disease progression.

With increasing experience, the process will inevitably evolve to the point that diagnostic criteria will emerge for each NTM species, thereby eliminating the need for 'universal' NTM diagnostic criteria.

Diagnostic criteria for NTM lung disease in the past discriminated between patients with cavitary and noncavitary disease with more diagnostically rigorous criteria applied to noncavitary disease.[1]

Recently proposed diagnostic criteria are applicable to all patients with suspected NTM lung disease regardless of radiographic presentation (Fig. 31.9).[2]

The term 'colonization' has been used to describe the intermittent or occasional isolation of NTM from respiratory specimens. The significance of 'colonization' in this setting, with its implied benignity, has never been rigorously tested or validated. It may not be clear, for instance, whether a single isolate of an NTM from sputum is due to 'colonization' (superficial or noninvasive infection), slowly progressive or indolent infection, or contamination of the cultured specimen by an NTM from the environment of the patient or of the laboratory. For NTM species that are known to cause pulmonary disease, it is the responsibility of the patient's physician to ensure that a patient with slowly progressive disease is not misidentified as 'colonized' by the NTM. Isolation of a potential pulmonary NTM pathogen may require the clinician to follow the patient with serial sputum AFB analysis and periodic chest radiographs over a long period of time, perhaps years, in order to judge the significance of the isolated NTM. The worst mistake a clinician can make in managing a patient with NTM lung disease is not a short-term delay in starting therapy, but a failure to provide appropriate clinical and laboratory follow up for a patient who then has significant progression of NTM lung disease.

LYMPH NODE DISEASE
Nontuberculous mycobacteria disease in lymph nodes is diagnosed by culture of NTM infection in the presence of granulomatous inflammation found on biopsy of infected tissue. The use of fine-needle aspiration for obtaining diagnostic material is controversial because it will yield a positive culture in only 50% of cases.[47] Additionally, a simple diagnostic biopsy or incision and drainage of the involved lymph nodes can be followed by fistula formation with chronic drainage. Because complete excision of involved nodes constitutes adequate therapy for most NTM lymphadenitis, it may also be an appropriate diagnostic procedure.

DISSEMINATED DISEASE
Diagnosis of disseminated NTM infection in people who are immunocompromised, including those who have AIDS, is made by culture of organisms from sterile closed sites, such as blood, liver or bone marrow, or from biopsy of a skin lesion. A single positive blood culture is considered diagnostic of disseminated NTM in an AIDS patient. The isolation of MAC from the sputum or stool of a patient who has

---

PROPOSED DIAGNOSTIC CRITERIA FOR NTM PULMONARY DISEASE

Compatible clinical presentation based on symptoms, radiographic findings (chest radiograph or high-resolution CT scan) and exclusion of other diagnoses

Collection of at least three sputum and/or bronchial wash specimens

One culture-positive sputum or bronchial washing that is either heavily (2+ or greater) smear positive or heavily (2+ or greater) culture positive

or

One culture-positive sputum or bronchial washing associated with multiple smear-positive specimens

or

Multiple positive cultures (at least three) over 1 year, regardless of smear positivity

For unusual radiographic presentation or nondiagnostic sputum analysis, lung biopsy (bronchoscopy with transbronchial biopsy) demonstrating granulomatous inflammation or culture positive for NTM

Fig. 31.9 Proposed diagnostic criteria for nontuberculous mycobacterial pulmonary disease In questionable cases, obtain expert consultation. Adapted with permission from Wallace RJ Jr, *et al*.[2]

AIDS is not diagnostic for disseminated MAC infection; however, the presence of MAC in these specimens is a harbinger for disseminated MAC in that patient.[53]

The diagnosis of NTM CNS involvement is difficult, therefore, it is extremely important to suspect the diagnosis based on the clinical setting.[52] Nontuberculosis mycobacteria are rarely found on routine AFB smear analysis of cerebral spinal fluid (CSF) so that a positive AFB culture is usually required to make the diagnosis. The role of rapid diagnostic techniques applied to CSF, such as high performance liquid chromatography analysis, is unknown. The CSF in NTM disease usually shows an elevated white blood cell count with either a neutrophilic or lymphocytic predominance. Cerebral spinal fluid protein and glucose values may vary widely from within normal limits to far outside the normal range. Radiographic evaluation of NTM CNS involvement is usually not diagnostic and can be complicted by radiographic abnormalities caused by concomitant CNS infections due to other pathogens.

LOCALIZED SKIN AND SOFT TISSUE INFECTIONS

Diagnosis of NTM infection in skin, soft tissue, bones and joints is made by culture of the specific pathogen from drainage material or tissue biopsy. It is important from a therapeutic standpoint to differentiate between skin and soft tissue lesions related to penetrating injury and those associated with disseminated NTM infection.

MANAGEMENT

The recent introduction of agents such as clarithromycin, azithromycin and rifabutin has dramatically improved the treatment outcome for some NTM infections. Treatment recommendations for NTM diseases in both immunocompetent and immunocompromised hosts will likely continue to evolve at a relatively rapid rate; therefore, recommendations in this chapter may soon become outdated.

The treatment of NTM infections is complicated by the observation that response to therapy for some NTM infections does not correlate with in-vitro drug susceptibilities, especially to antituberculous drugs. Treatment of NTM infections is therefore not as simple or dependent on in-vitro drug susceptibilities as the treatment of tuberculosis; some familiarity with the treatment idiosyncrasies of each NTM is necessary. For instance, clinical response to multidrug antituberculous regimens for *M. kansasii* correlates only with in-vitro susceptibility to rifampin (rifampicin). Response of MAC disease to antituberculous drug regimens in the past frequently had no correlation with in-vitro drug susceptibilities. In contrast, there is a strong correlation between successful treatment of NTM infections, including MAC infection, with clarithromycin and azithromycin and the in-vitro macrolide susceptibility of the specific NTM. Patients with either pulmonary or disseminated MAC infection that is macrolide resistant will not respond favorably to macrolide-containing regimens.[40,54] Clarithromycin monotherapy for disseminated or pulmonary MAC disease is associated with a genetic mutation conferring resistance to macrolides and should therefore be avoided.[55]

Recommendations for treating NTM pulmonary disease are given in Figure 31.10. Potential toxicity and drug interactions of commonly used drugs are listed in Figure 31.11. Because of the duration of therapy required and potential toxicity of the medications, not all patients with NTM lung disease will benefit from therapy. For some patients, the treatment is in essence worse than the disease. Elderly patients who have few symptoms and minimal or very slowly progressive disease, or, alternatively, have severe comorbid conditions and limited life expectancy may not benefit from drug therapy directed at some NTM pathogens, especially MAC. These patients should be selected to receive treatment only after very careful evaluation.

TREATMENT RECOMMENDATIONS FOR SELECTED NTM CAUSING LUNG AND DISSEMINATED DISEASE			
NTM species	Suggested drug regimen	Duration of therapy	Comments
M. avium complex[56,57,61]	Clarithromycin 1g/day or azithromycin 500mg MWF plus rifabutin 300mg/day or rifampin 600mg/day plus ethambutol 15mg/kg/day	12 months of sputum AFB culture negativity for pulmonary disease, or lifetime therapy for disseminated disease unless immune status restored	Clarithromycin or azithromycin should not be used as monotherapy; consider surgical resection of limited pulmonary disease; add streptomycin initially (2–3 months) 500–1000mg im MWF or amikacin 400mg/day iv for severe disease; rifampin contraindicated with protease inhibitors (consider rifabutin 150mg/day with indinavir)
M. kansasii[1,2] (rifampin susceptible *in vitro*)	Rifampin 600mg/day plus INH 300mg/day plus ethambutol 25mg/kg/day for 2 months followed by 15mg/kg/day	18 months and 12 months of sputum AFB culture negativity for pulmonary disease or lifetime for disseminated disease unless immune status restored	Add streptomycin 500–1000mg im MWF or clarithromycin 1g/day initially (2–3 months) for advanced disease; treatment success with this regimen is dependent upon in-vitro rifampin susceptibility; PZA is not effective
M. kansasii (rifampin resistant *in vitro* or patient on protease inhibitor)	Clarithromycin 0.5g q12h plus ethambutol 25mg/kg/day for 2 months followed by 15mg/kg/day plus INH 900mg/day (B6 50mg/day) plus sulfamethoxazole 1.0g po q8h plus streptomycin 500–1000mg im MWF (initial 2–3 months)	12 months of sputum AFB culture negativity for pulmonary disease or lifetime for disseminated disease unless immune status restored	In-vitro rifampin resistance occurs as a consequence of treatment failure (noncompliance) for rifampin-susceptible *M. kansasii* lung disease; rifabutin 150mg/day can be used with indinavir
M. abscessus	Clarithromycin 1g/day or azithromycin 500mg MWF ± cefoxitin, imipenem, amikacin	12 months of sputum AFB culture negativity	No drug regimen of proven efficacy; surgical resection of limited pulmonary disease most effective therapy; first-line antituberculosis drugs not useful
M. fortuitum	Two agents including: ofloxacin 800mg/day or ciprofloxacin 1500mg/day; doxycycline 100mg q12h; sulfamethoxazole 1g q8h; clarithromycin 0.5g q12h	6 months	Therapy based on in-vitro antibiotic susceptibility; only 50% of *M. fortuitum* isolates susceptible to clarithromycin; for severe disease amikacin 400mg/day iv or cefoxitin 12g/day iv until favorable clinical response; first-line antituberculosis drugs not useful
M. chelonae	Clarithromycin 1g/day	6 months	Macrolide monotherapy effective in this clinical situation

Other NTM respiratory pathogens that likely would respond to macrolide-containing regimens: *M. xenopi, M. malmoense, M. simiae, M. szulgai*
Other disseminated NTM pathogens that likely would respond to macrolide-containing regimens: *M. gordonae, M. haemophilum, M. genavense*

Fig. 31.10 **Treatment recommendations for selected nontuberculous mycobacteria causing lung and disseminated disease.**
AFB, acid-fast bacilli; INH, isoniazid; PZA, pyrazinamide; MWF, Monday, Wednesday and Friday.

ADVERSE EVENTS AND DRUG INTERACTIONS ASSOCIATED WITH MEDICATIONS FOR NTM INFECTIONS		
Drug	Adverse events	Drug interactions
Clarithromycin	Bitter taste, nausea, vomiting, abnormal liver enzymes, hearing loss	Blocks cytochrome p450 enzyme metabolism of multiple agents including rifabutin; rifamycins (rifamycin, rifabutin) accelerate hepatic metabolism of clarithromycin
Azithromycin	Nausea, vomiting, diarrhea, abnormal liver enzymes, hearing loss	No known effect on cytochrome p450 enzymes or hepatic metabolism of other drugs
Rifabutin	Nausea, vomiting, abnormal liver enzymes, polyarthralgia, polymyalgia, leukopenia, thrombocytopenia, anterior uveitis	Promotes cytochrome p450 enzymes (less than rifampin) with increased hepatic metabolism of multiple drugs, including clarithromycin; severe side effects (uveitis) almost exclusively with combined clarithromycin therapy
Rifampin	Nausea, vomiting, abnormal liver enzymes, flu-like syndrome, thrombocytopenia, renal failure, hypersensitivity response	More potent cytochrome p450 enzyme promoter than rifabutin; increased hepatic metabolism of multiple drugs, including clarithromycin, protease inhibitors
Ethambutol	Optic neuritis with loss of red–green color discrimination, loss of visual acuity	

Fig. 31.11 Adverse events and drug interactions associated with medications commonly used to treat nontuberculous mycobacterial infections.

EFFECTIVE AGENTS FOR PROPHYLAXIS AGAINST DISSEMINATED MAC LUNG DISEASE		
Regimen	Dose	Comments
Rifabutin[63,64]	300mg/day	Rifamycin (rifampin) resistance can emerge with rifabutin monotherapy in patients with occult active tuberculosis; not compatible with some protease inhibitors
Clarithromycin[65]	1g/day	Well tolerated; clarithromycin resistance will emerge if monotherapy used for active disseminated MAC infection
Azithromycin[66]	1.2g/week	Well tolerated; macrolide (clarithromycin) resistance will emerge if monotherapy used for active disseminated MAC infection
Azithromycin[66] plus rifabutin	1.2g/week plus 300mg/day	Very effective prophylaxis regimen; high incidence of rifabutin toxicity

Fig. 31.12 Effective agents for prophylaxis against disseminated *Mycobacterium avium* complex lung disease in patients who have AIDS.

Patients undergoing therapy for NTM pulmonary disease require frequent follow-up:
- to evaluate symptomatic and objective response to therapy and medication toxicity; and
- to collect specimens for AFB analysis.

Serial sputum AFB analysis is the most important element of disease monitoring. The sputum analysis is a critical measure of medication efficacy and may provide evidence for treatment failure (possibly due to the emergence of selective drug resistance) or disease relapse. Additionally, the duration of therapy for some patients is determined by the duration of time sputum is AFB culture negative while on therapy. Patients who have NTM lung disease should not be placed on therapy for extended periods of time without routine sputum AFB evaluation. Although periodic chest radiographs are also helpful, the chest radiograph is likely to improve only very slowly.

Drug treatment is not successful for all patients with NTM lung disease. Surgical resection of limited disease remains an important option, although surgical morbidity and mortality dictates that the surgical approach should be undertaken only by surgeons experienced with mycobacterial disease.[58,59] Other approaches, such as cytokine therapy, are promising, but remain investigational.[33,60]

Recommendations for treating disseminated NTM disease in AIDS patients are listed in Figure 31.10. Survival of people who have AIDS and disseminated MAC is clearly shorter than that of patients who have comparable immunosuppression without disseminated MAC infection. Treatment of disseminated MAC results in clinical and bacteriologic improvement as well as increased survival. Treatment of these infections has recently been complicated by the introduction of protease inhibitors, which interact with rifamycins for the treatment of HIV infection.[62] For some patients it may be difficult to decide whether the highest priority is treatment of advancing HIV disease with a protease inhibitor or treatment of disseminated NTM infection with a rifamycin. Effective regimens for prophylaxis against disseminated MAC are outlined in Figure 31.12. The successful treatment of NTM CNS diseases is difficult because of the relative antibiotic resistance of the organisms, the poor CNS penetration of important agents, such as clarithromycin and the usually far advanced underlying disease of the host.[52]

Treatment of skin and soft tissue infections due to *M. fortuitum*, *M. abscessus*, or *M. chelonae* unrelated to disseminated disease involve regimens similar to those recommended for pulmonary or disseminated disease (see Fig. 31.10).[67,68] Surgical debridement is important for extensive or poorly responsive disease. Several regimens administered for 3 months are effective for the treatment of *M. marinum* infection, including:
- clarithromycin 500mg q12h;
- doxycycline 100mg q12h;
- trimethoprim–sulfamethoxazole (co-trimoxazole) 160/800mg q12h); and
- rifampin 600mg/day plus ethambutol 15mg/kg/day.

Again, surgical debridement may be necessary for extensive disease.

Complete surgical excision is the standard treatment for NTM lymphadenitis and is usually curative.[69] Antimycobacterial therapy is seldom necessary, except in patients who are immunocompromised. Regimens that contain the newer macrolides are effective for eradicating disease in patients who are unable to have surgery or who undergo incomplete excision of MAC lymphadenitis.[70]

REFERENCES

1. Wallace RJ Jr, O'Brien R, Glassroth J, Raleigh J, Dutt A. Diagnosis and treatment of disease caused by nontuberculous mycobacteria. Am Rev Respir Dis 1990;142:940–53.

2. Wallace RJ Jr, Glassroth J, Griffith DE, et al. Diagnosis and treatment of disease caused by nontuberculous mycobacteria. Am J Respir Crit Care Med 1997;156 (Suppl):1–25.

3. Good RC, Snider DE. Isolation of nontuberculous mycobacteria in the United States, 1980. J Infect Dis 1982;146:829–33.

4. O'Brien RJ, Geiter LJ, Snider DE. The epidemiology of nontuberculous mycobacterial diseases in the United States: results from a national survey. Am Rev Respir Dis 1987;135:1007–14.

5. Ostroff S, Hutwagner L, Collin S. Mycobacterial species and drug resistance patterns reported by state laboratories-1992 [Abstract U-9]. 93rd ASM General Meeting. 1992:170.

6. Nightingale SD, Byrd LT, Southern PM, Jockusch JD, Cal SX, Wynne BA. Incidence of Mycobacterium avium-intracellulare complex in human immunodeficiency virus-positive patients. J Infect Dis 1992;165:1082–5.

7. Hoover DR, Graham NMH, Bacellar H, et al. An epidemiologic analysis of Mycobacterium avium complex disease in homosexual men infected with human immunodeficiency virus type 1. Clin Infect Dis 1995;20:1250–8.

8. Beck A, Stanford JL. Mycobacterium xenopei: a study of sixteen strains. Tubercule 1968;47:226–34.

9. Henriques B, Hoffner SE, Petrini B, Juhlin I, Wåhlén P, Källenius G. Infection with Mycobacterium malmoense in Sweden: report of 221 cases. Clin Infect Dis 1994;18:596–600.

10. Okello, DO, Sewankambo N, Goodgame R, et al. Absence of bacteremia with Mycobacterium avium-intracellulare in Ugandan patients with AIDS. J Infect Dis 1990;163:208–10.

11. Gruft H, Falkingham JO, Parker BC. Recent experience in the epidemiology of disease caused by atypical mycobacteria. Rev Infect Dis 1981;3:990–6.

12. Meissner PS, Falkingham JO. Plasmid DNA profiles as epidemiologic markers for clinical and environmental isolates of Mycobacterium avium, Mycobacterium intracellulare, and Mycobacterium scrofulaceum. J Infect Dis 1986;153:325–31.

13. Falkingham JO III, Parker BC, Gruft H. Epidemiology of infection by nontuberculous mycobacteria: I. Geographic distribution in the eastern United States. Am Rev Respir Dis 1980;121:931–57.

14. Edwards LB, Acquaviva F, Livesay VT, Cross FW, Palmer CE. An atlas of sensitivity to tuberculin, PPD-B, and histoplasmin in the United States. Am Rev Respir Dis 1969;99:1–132.

15. Ahn CH, Lowell JR, Onstad GD, Shuford EH, Hurst GA. A demographic study of disease due to M. kansasii or M. intracellulare-avium in Texas. Chest 1979;75:120–5.

16. Engel HWB, Berwald LG, Havelaar AH. The occurrence of Mycobacterium kansasii in tap water. Tubercle 1980;61:21–6.

17. Picardeau M, Prod'holm G, Raskine L, LePennec MP, Vincent V. Genotypic characterization of five subspecies of Mycobacterium kansasii. J Clin Microbiol 1997;35:25–32.

18. von Reyn CF, Maslow JN, Barber TW, Falkingham JO III, Arbeit RD. Persistent colonization of potable water as a source of Mycobacterium avium infection in AIDS. Lancet 1994;343:1137–41.

19. Desplaces N, Picardeau M, Dinh V, et al. Spinal infections (SI) due to Mycobacterium xenopi after discectomies (DC) [Abstract J162]. San Francisco: 35th Interscience Conference on Antimicrobial Agents and Chemotherapy; 1995.

20. Hector JS, Pang Y, Mazurek GH, Zhang Y, Brown BA, Wallace RJ Jr. Large restriction fragment patterns of genomic Mycobacterium fortuitum DNA as strain-specific markers and their use in epidemiologic investigation of four nosocomial outbreaks. J Clin Microbiol 1992;30:1250–5.

21. Wallace RJ Jr, Zhang Y, Brown BA, Fraser V, Mazurek GH, Maloney S. DNA large restriction fragment patterns of sporadic and epidemic nosocomial strains of Mycobacterium chelonae and Mycobacterium abscessus. J Clin Microbiol 1993;31:2697–701.

22. Ahrens P, Giese SB, Klausen J, Inglis NF. Two markers, IS901-IS902 and p40, identified by PCR and by using monoclonal antibodies in Mycobacterium avium strains. J Clin Microbiol 1995;33:1049–53.

23. Guerro C, Bernasconi C, Burki D, Bodmer T, Telenti A. A novel insertion element from Mycobacterium avium, IS1245, is a specific target for analysis of strain relatedness. J Clin Microbiol 1995;33:304–7.

24. Chan J, Fan X, Hunter SW, et al. Lipoarabinomannan, a possible virulence factor involved in persistence of Mycobacterium tuberculosis within macrophages. Infect Immunol 1991;59:1755–61.

25. Sturgill-Koszycki S, Schlesinger PH, Chakraborty P, et al. Lack of acidification in Mycobacterium phagosomes produced by exclusion of the vesicular proton-ATPase. Science 1994;263:678–81.

26. Bermudez LEM, Young LS. Tumor necrosis factor, alone or in combination with IL-2, but not IFN-γ, is associated with macrophage killing of Mycobacterium avium complex. J Immunol 1988;140:3006–13.

27. Bermudez LEM, Young LS. Natural killer cell-dependent mycobacteriostatic and mycobactericidal activity in human macrophages. J Immunol 1991;146:265–70.

28. Flesch IEA, Hess JH, Huang S, et al. Early interleukin 12 production by macrophages in response to mycobacterial infection depends on interferon γ and tumor necrosis factor A. J Exp Med 1995;181:1615–21.

29. Bermudez LE, Wu M, Young LS. Interleukin-12-stimulated natural killer cells can activate human macrophages to inhibit growth of Mycobacterium avium. Infect Immunol 1995;63:4099–104.

30. Bermudez Le, Martinelli J, Petrofsky M, et al. Recombinant granulocyte–macrophage colony-stimulating factor enhances the effects of antibiotics against Mycobacterium avium complex (MAC) infection in the beige mouse model. J Infect Dis 1994;169:575–80.

31. Denis M. Interleukin-6 is used as a growth factor by virulent Mycobacterium avium: presence of specific receptors. Cell Immunol 1992;141:182–8.

32. Bermudez LE, Champsi J. Infection with Mycobacterium avium induces production of interleukin-10 (IL-10), and administration of anti-IL-10 antibody is associated with enhanced resistance to infection in mice. Infect Immunol 1993;61:3093–7.

33. Holland SM, Eisenstein EM, Kuhns DB, et al. Treatment of refractory nontuberculous mycobacterial infection with interferon gamma: a preliminary report. N Engl J Med 1994;330:1348–55.

34. Frucht DM, Holland SM. Defective monocyte costimulation for IFN-γ production in familial disseminated Mycobacterium avium complex infection. Abdominal IL-2 regulation. J Immunol 1996;157:411–6.

35. Crawford JT, Bates JH. Analysis of plasmids in Mycobacterium avium-intracellulare isolates from persons with acquired immunodeficiency syndrome. Am Rev Respir Dis 1986;134:659–61.

36. Jucker MT, Falkingham JO III. Epidemiology of infection by nontuberculous mycobacteria IX. Evidence for two DNA homology groups among small plasmids in Mycobacterium avium, Mycobacterium intracellulare and Mycobacterium scrofulaceum. Am Rev Respir Dis 1990;142:858–62.

37. Frehel C, de Chastellier C, Lang T, Rastogi N. Evidence for inhibition of fusion of lysosomal and prelysosomal compartments with phagosomes in macrophages infected with pathogenic Mycobacterium avium. Infect Immun 1986;52:252–62.

38. Furney SK, Skinner PS, Roberts AD, Appelberg R, Orme IM. Capacity of Mycobacterium avium isolates to grow well or poorly in murine macrophages resides in their ability to induce secretion of tumor necrosis factor. Infect Immun 1992;60:4410–3.

39. Steadham JE. High catalase Mycobacterium kansasii isolated from water in Texas. J Clin Microbiol 1980;11:496–8.

40. Wallace RJ Jr, Brown BA, Griffith DE, et al. Initial clarithromycin monotherapy for Mycobacterium avium-intracellular complex lung disease. Am J Respir Crit Care Med 1994;149:1335–41.

41. Guthertz LS, Damsker B, Bottone EJ, Ford EG, Midura TF, Janda JM. Mycobacterium avium and Mycobacterium intracellulare infections in patients with and without AIDS. J Infect Dis 1989;160:1037–41.

42. Anh CH, Anh SS, Anderson RA, Murphy DT, Mammo A. A four-drug regimen for initial treatment of cavitary disease caused by Mycobacterium avium complex. Am Rev Respir Dis 1986;134:438–41.

43. Prince DS, Peterson DD, Steinger RM, et al. Infection with Mycobacterium avium complex in patients without predisposing conditions. N Engl J Med 1989;321:863–8.

44. Hartman TE, Swensen SJ, Williams DE. Mycobacterium avium-intracellulare complex: evaluation with CT. Radiology 1993;187:23–6.

45. Griffith DE, Girard WM, Wallace RJ Jr. Clinical features of pulmonary disease caused by rapidly growing mycobacteria; an analysis of 154 patients. Am Rev Respir Dis 1993;1271–8.

46. Wolinsky E. Mycobacterial lymphadenitis in children: a prospective study of 105 nontuberculous cases with long-term follow-up. Clin Infect Dis 1995;20:954–63.

47. Joshi W, Davidson PM, Campbell PE, et al. Nontuberculous mycobacterial lymphadenitis in children. Eur J Pediatr 1989;148:751–4.

48. Horsburgh CR Jr, Selik RM. The epidemiology of disseminated nontuberculous mycobacterial infection in the acquired immunodeficiency syndrome (AIDS). Am Rev Respir Dis 1989;139:4–7.

49. Slutsky AM, Arbeit RD, Barber TW, et al. Polyclonal infections due to Mycobacterium avium complex in patients with AIDS detected by pulsed-field gel electrophoresis of sequential clinical isolates. J Clin Microbiol 1994;32:1773–8.

50. Kalayjian RC, Toossi Z, Tomashefski JR Jr, et al. Pulmonary disease due to infection by Mycobacterium avium complex in patients with AIDS. Clin Infect Dis 1995;20:1186–94.

51. Witzig RS, Fazal BA, Mera RM, et al. Clinical manifestations and implications of coinfection with Mycobacterium kansasii and human immunodeficiency virus type 1 [Review]. Clin Infect Dis 1995;21:77–85.

52. Cegielski JP, Wallace RJ Jr. Infections due to nontuberculous myobacteria. Infections of the central nervous system, 2nd ed. Philadelphia: Lippincott–Raven Publishers, 1997.

53. Chin DP, Hopewell PC, Yajko DM, et al. Mycobacterium avium complex in the respiratory or gastrointestinal tract and the risk of M. avium complex bacteremia in patients with human immunodeficiency virus infection. J Infect Dis 1994;169:289–95.

54. Chaisson RE, Benson CA, Dube MP, et al. Clarithromycin therapy for bacteremic Mycobacterium avium complex disease. Ann Intern Med 1994;121:905–11.

55. Meier A, Heifets L, Wallace RJ Jr, et al. Molecular mechanisms of clarithromycin resistance is Mycobacterium avium: observation of multiple 23S rDNA mutations in a clonal population. J Infect Dis 1996;174:354–60.

56. Wallace RJ Jr, Brown BA, Griffith DE, et al. Clarithromycin regimens for pulmonary Mycobacterium avium complex: the first 50 patients. Am J Respir Crit Care Med 1996;153:1766–72.

57. Griffith DE, Brown BA, Girard WM, Murphy DT, Wallace RJ Jr. Azithromycin activity against *Mycobacterium avium* complex lung disease in HIV negative patients. Clin Infect Dis 1996;23:983–9.

58. Pomerantz M, Brown JM. Surgery in the treatment of multidrug-resistant tuberculosis. Clin Chest Med 1997;18:123–30.

59. Parrot RG, Grosset JH. Post-surgical outcome of 57 patients with *Mycobacterium xenopi* pulmonary infection. Tubercle 1988;69:47–55.

60. Chatte G, Panteix G, Perrin-Fayolle M, Pacheoco Y. Aerosolized interferon gamma for *Mycobacterium avium* complex lung disease. Am J Respir Crit Care Med 1995;152:1094–6.

61. Shafran S, Singer J, Zarowny DP, *et al.* A comparison of two regimens for the treatment of *Mycobacterium avium* complex bacteremia in AIDS: rifabutin, ethambutol and clarithromycin versus rifampin, ethambutol, clofazimine, and ciprofloxacin. N Engl J Med 1996;335:377–83.

62. Centers for Disease Control and Prevention. Impact of HIV protease inhibitors on the treatment of HIV-infected tuberculosis patients with rifampin. MMWR Morb Mortal Wkly Rep 1996;45:921–7.

63. Nightengale SD, Cameron DW, Gordin FM, *et al.* Two controlled trials of rifabutin prophylaxis against *Mycobacterium avium* complex infection in AIDS. N Engl J Med 1993;329:828–33.

64. Bishai WR, Graham NMH, Harrington S, *et al.* Brief report: rifampin-resistant tuberculosis in a patient receiving rifabutin prophylaxis. N Engl J Med 1996;334:1573–6.

65. Pierce M, Crampton S, Henry D, *et al.* A randomized trial of clarithromycin as prophylaxis against *Mycobacterium avium* complex infection in patients with advanced acquired immunodeficiency syndrome. N Engl J Med 1996;335:384–91.

66. Havlir D, Dube M, Sattler F, *et al.* Prophylaxis against disseminated *Mycobacterium avium* complex with weekly azithromycin, daily rifabutin, or both. N Engl J Med 1996;335:392–8.

67. Wallace RJ Jr, Tanner D, Brennan PJ, Brown BA. Clinical trial of clarithromycin for cutaneous (disseminated) infection due to *Mycobacterium chelonae*. Ann Intern Med 1993;119:482–6.

68. Wallace RJ Jr. The clinical presentation, diagnosis, and therapy of cutaneous and pulmonary infections due to the rapidly growing mycobacteria, *M. fortuitum* and *M. chelonae*. Clin Chest Med 1989;10:419–29.

69. Schaad UB, Votteler TP, McCracken GH Jr, Nelson JD. Management of atypical mycobacterial lymphadenitis in childhood: a review based on 380 cases. J Pediatr 1979;95:356–60.

70. Berger C, Pfyffer GE, Nadal D. Treatment of nontuberculous mycobacterial lymphadenitis with clarithromycin plus rifabutin. J Pediatr 1996;128:383–6.

Practice Points

Aspiration of pleural fluid: pleural biopsy   *Wei-Shen Lim & John T Macfarlane*

INTRODUCTION

Pleural effusions result from diverse disorders ranging from malignancy to cardiac failure. In the context of infection, parapneumonic effusions (literally 'by the side of pneumonia') are common; they are present in up to 40% of cases of bacterial pneumonia. All such effusions of any significance should be sampled; one in 10 will need specific treatment such as tube drainage or a surgical procedure.

PATHOGENESIS

Pleural effusions are divided into transudates and exudates. Transudates occur when increased systemic or pulmonary capillary pressures (e.g. in cardiac failure) or reduced systemic oncotic pressures (e.g. in hypoalbuminemia or liver failure) result in pleural fluid formation exceeding removal.

Exudates usually result from disease of the pleural surfaces. Three suggested mechanisms are:
- an increase in protein production (e.g. parapneumonic effusions),
- a decrease in lymphatic absorption (e.g. in malignancy), and
- a decrease in pleural pressure caused by bronchial obstruction.

More than one of these mechanisms may operate simultaneously.

Parapneumonic effusions progress seamlessly through three stages. The exudative stage is characterized by the accumulation in the pleural space of sterile fluid with a high protein content. It occurs in response to pleural inflammation. In the fibropurulent stage, leukocytes and fibrin accumulate in the pleural space and loculations eventually develop. In the final stage of organization, fibroblasts invade and produce an inelastic pleural peel, which encases the affected lung.

MICROBIOLOGY

Empyema is defined as the presence of pus in the pleural fluid or a positive Gram stain or culture of the pleural fluid. Most empyemas (55%) develop as a complication of pneumonia; surgery and trauma account for the remainder of cases.

Pure aerobic infections account for 40–62% of empyemas, pure anaerobic infections for 15–30% and mixed aerobic and anaerobic infections for 8–20%. *Staphylococcus aureus, Streptococcus pneumoniae* and other *Streptococcus* spp. make up the majority of aerobic Gram-positive isolates, and *Pseudomonas* spp., *Escherichia coli* and *Klebsiella* spp. are the most common aerobic Gram-negative isolates. *Bacteroides* spp. are the most common anaerobic isolates, although microaerophilic streptococci may be isolated in up to 10% of anaerobic infections. In 28–43% of empyemas, multiple organisms are responsible (see Chapter 2.29).

The incidence of *Mycobacterium tuberculosis* as a cause of pleural effusion is related to local epidemiology.

CLINICAL FEATURES

Patients who have parapneumonic effusions may present with fever, chills, breathlessness or chest pain: symptoms very similar to those of pneumonia. The physical examination may be limited to findings of an effusion, which is sometimes not apparent on initial presentation and only develops later. An empyema should be suspected if there is a recrudescence or persistence of symptoms of infection after initial recovery from pneumonia. The patient may then also complain of malaise, weight loss, dull pleural pain and unresolving fever.

INVESTIGATIONS

The proper management of pleural effusions is crucially dependent on obtaining adequate samples for diagnosis. The analysis of both pleural fluid and pleural tissue is complementary in this regard.

Pleural aspiration

Large effusions can be safely aspirated at the bedside. Ultrasound guidance is useful when aspirating small or loculated effusions. The patient should be sitting comfortably, with arms stretched out in front and resting on a support. Aspiration is performed one interspace below the level of the effusion posteriorly or in the axilla using a 21 gauge needle attached to a 50ml syringe. The needle is passed perpendicular to the chest wall just above a rib, avoiding the neurovascular bundle. About 30ml of fluid should be aspirated for diagnostic purposes. Local anesthetic is not required if a single pass is successful. If large-volume aspiration is intended, the skin and chest wall should be infiltrated with local anesthetic and an 18 gauge cannula used and connected to a three-way tap after removal of the needle.

We recommend that pleural fluid be sent for measurement of protein content, lactate dehydrogenase (LDH) level and for cytologic and microbiologic analysis, including mycobacterial culture. A serum sample for measurement of protein and LDH should be taken simultaneously.

The value of other tests, including pH, glucose level and amylase, is limited to specific circumstances (Fig. 32.1). Samples for pH estimation need to be collected anaerobically in a heparinized syringe and analyzed promptly, the process being similar to arterial blood gas analysis.

Pleural biopsy

Pleural biopsy is a safe bedside procedure when performed by an experienced operator. It is important to obtain pleural biopsy specimens, if indicated, before complete removal of pleural fluid. The positioning of the patient and the approach is as for pleural aspiration. The use of an Abram's needle is described here, although a Cope's needle may also be used.

The biopsy site is cleaned and adequate local anesthetic infiltrated down to the pleural surfaces. A diagnostic pleural tap should be performed at this stage to confirm free entry into the pleural space and to avoid blood contamination after biopsy. A small vertical skin incision is made to allow easy passage of the Abram's needle through the skin.

PLEURAL FLUID EXAMINATION			
Investigation	Result	Possible causes	Comment
Visual inspection	Turbid (turbid supernatant)	Chylothorax, pseudochylothorax	Triglycerides >110mg/dl (1.2mmol/l), cholesterol >200mg/dl (5.2mmol/l)
	Pus	Empyema	
	Blood	Malignancy, tuberculosis, trauma, embolism	Pleural fluid hematocrit >50% of that of peripheral blood
Smell	Putrid	Empyema	Anaerobic infection
Protein	<3g/dl (30g/l)	Transudate (but also seen in malignancy, parapneumonic effusions)	See Light's criteria
	>3g/dl (30g/l)	Exudate, effusion in diuretic treated cardiac failure	See Light's criteria
Lactate dehydrogenase	Pleural fluid to serum ratio >0.6 Pleural fluid level >two-thirds upper limit normal serum level	Exudate	Indicates pleural inflammation
Amylase	Raised salivary amylase	Esophageal rupture, malignancy	
	Raised pancreatic amylase	Acute or chronic pancreatitis	
Glucose	<60mg/dl (3.3mmol/l)	Malignancy, tuberculosis, rheumatoid arthritis, parapneumonic	
pH	In parapneumonic effusions: >7.3	Uncomplicated parapneumonic effusion	
	>7.0 and <7.3	May progress to empyema	Requires close observation. Expert advice recommended
	<7.0	Empyema	Tube drainage recommended
Ultrasound	Loculations	Empyema	Consider tube drainage

Fig. 32.1 Pleural fluid examination.

With the side hole in the closed position, firm but controlled pressure is applied in a twisting movement until the pleural space is breached. There is usually a sudden 'give' when the parietal pleura is first penetrated. Care must be taken not to plunge the needle into underlying lung. A 20ml syringe is attached to the end of the needle and its positioning in the pleural space is confirmed by opening the side hole and aspirating pleural fluid. Keeping the side hole open, the needle is now withdrawn slowly, at an acute angle to the upper chest wall, until it 'catches' on the parietal pleura. While continuing to apply outward and lateral pressure in order to hold the pleura in the open side hole, the inner cylinder is rotated clockwise thus closing the side hole and cutting a biopsy of the pleura (Figs 32.2). (A common error is to fail to maintain outward pressure when closing the side hole.) The entire needle is then quickly removed and the biopsy site covered to minimize air entry while the biopsy is placed in a suitable container. The procedure is repeated with the side hole of the needle in different positions until adequate tissue has been obtained. A biopsy is not taken with the side hole at 12 o'clock so as to avoid damage to the neurovascular bundle running underneath each rib.

We recommend obtaining at least six good samples, five to be placed in formalin for histology and the sixth in sterile normal saline for microscopy and mycobacterial culture.

MANAGEMENT

Initial management of a pleural effusion is based on differentiating between transudates and exudates. Using a pleural protein level of >3.0g/dl (30g/l) alone to identify exudative effusions will miss some parapneumonic and malignant effusions as these effusions exhibit a wide range of protein levels. With Light's criteria (sensitivity 98%, specificity 77%, accuracy 95%), an exudate is identified by one or more of:
- pleural fluid to serum protein ratio >0.5,
- pleural fluid to serum LDH ratio >0.6, or

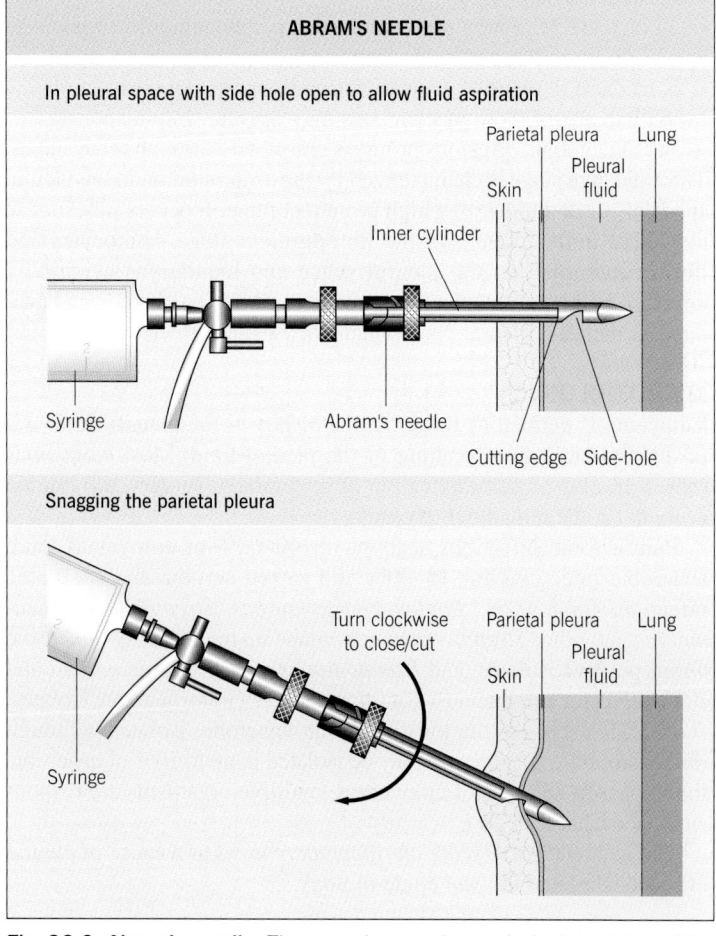

ABRAM'S NEEDLE

In pleural space with side hole open to allow fluid aspiration

Parietal pleura   Lung
Pleural fluid
Skin
Inner cylinder
Syringe
Abram's needle
Cutting edge   Side-hole

Snagging the parietal pleura

Turn clockwise to close/cut
Parietal pleura   Lung
Pleural fluid
Skin
Syringe

Fig. 32.2 Abram's needle. The curved arrow shows clockwise rotation of the inner cylinder to close the side hole.

- pleural LDH more than two-thirds the upper limit of normal serum LDH.

The management of parapneumonic effusions includes:
- sampling of the effusion to confirm the diagnosis and to determine whether it is complicated,
- deciding whether drainage is needed, and
- antibiotic therapy directed at likely or proven underlying infection.

Drainage is necessary in all cases of empyema or if loculations are seen on imaging. Where possible, ultrasound guided catheter placement is preferred. Ultrasound enables better visualization of loculations and small effusions, which enables better positioning and the use of smaller catheters, resulting in greater patient comfort. The effectiveness of tube drainage should be evident within 24 hours. Otherwise, the early use of intrapleural fibrinolytics should be considered before organization occurs.

Less evidence exists to aid the early identification of parapneumonic effusions that are likely to progress to empyema and hence require tube drainage. The pleural pH is of value in this situation. Sterile, nonpurulent effusions with pH >7.3 are very unlikely to develop a complicated course, whereas effusions with pH <7.0 are highly suggestive of empyema. Parapneumonic effusions with pH >7.0 but <7.3 fall in middle ground. Close observation with repeat thoracentesis according to clinical progress is a reasonable approach in some cases.

In all circumstances, antibiotic therapy should be guided by the underlying cause of pneumonia, if known. For ill patients in whom empiric therapy is required in the absence of positive microbiology, a second- or third-generation cephalosporin is recommended with the addition of metronidazole if anaerobic infection is suspected.

FURTHER READING

Hamm H, Light RW. Parapneumonic effusion and empyema. Eur Respir J 1997;10:1150–6.

Heffner JE, Brown LK, Barbieri C, DeLeo JM. Pleural fluid chemical analysis in parapneumonic effusions. A meta-analysis. Am J Respir Crit Care Med 1995;151:1700–8.

Light RW. Pleural diseases. Philadelphia: Lea and Febiger; 1983.

Sokolowski JW Jr, Burgher LW, Jones FL Jr, Patterson JR, Selecky PA. Guidelines for thoracentesis and needle biopsy of the pleura. Am Rev Respir Dis 1989;140:257–8.

Woodcock A, Viskum K. Pleural and other investigations. In: Brewis RAL, Corrin E, Geddes DM, Gibson GJ, eds. Respiratory medicine, vol 2, 2nd ed. London: WB Saunders; 1995:375–91.

Sternotomy wound infection

Lolita E Chiu

INTRODUCTION

Sternotomy infections are serious complications of cardiac surgery. These infections include cellulitis (the mildest form), subcutaneous tissue and fat necrosis, osteomyelitis and chondritis, and mediastinitis (the most severe form). Its incidence ranges from 0.4–5%, and the mortality rate may be as high as 80%. Early diagnosis and aggressive management are the important factors determining patients' survival.

RISK FACTORS

Previous clinical studies indicate that several clinical features may increase the risk of sternotomy wound infections. Some of the identified risk factors include obesity, diabetes mellitus, chronic obstructive lung disease or a history of heavy cigarette smoking, emergency surgery, skin shaving method, duration of surgery, reoperation for bleeding, and prolonged need for ventilatory support. Also, patients who preoperatively were known to be nasal carriers of *Staph. aureus* have a higher chance of developing *Staph. aureus* wound infections. The use of bilateral internal mammary artery grafting increases the chance of wound infection to five times that when saphenous vein grafting is used and three times that when single internal mammary artery grafting is used.

PATHOGENESIS

Most sternal wound infections are secondary to direct intraoperative contamination. The rest are due to hematogenous spread from indwelling catheters or other infection sites (the lungs, gastrointestinal tract, genitourinary tract or leg wounds).

Mechanical factors also play a role. Cardiopulmonary bypass impairs both cell-mediated and humoral immunity. Decreased blood supply to the sternum caused by internal mammary artery harvesting, the presence of hematomas or foreign bodies, and inappropriate timing of preoperative antibiotic prophylaxis all increase susceptibility to infections.

MICROBIOLOGY

About 90% of sternal wound infections are caused by *Staphylococcus* spp. – both *Staph. aureus* and coagulase-negative staphylococci. Other organisms that had been reported include *Enterococcus* spp., Gram-negative organisms (such as *Serratia* spp., *Escherichia* spp., *Pseudomonas* spp. and *Legionella* spp.), *Mycoplasma* spp., Bacteroides spp., *Mycobacterium fortuitum* and *Mycobacterium chelonae*, and *Candida* spp. A small percentage are polymicrobial.

CLINICAL FEATURES

The clinical presentation depends on the extent of the infection. Early signs and symptoms may be nonspecific, and may include fever, pain and leukocytosis. Patients often appear toxic, with poor recovery after cardiac surgery. Erythema, tenderness and serous discharge may also be present. Sternal instability with purulent discharge implies deeper tissue involvement.

DIAGNOSIS

Computed tomography is the 'gold-standard' imaging procedure for diagnosing sternotomy wound infections. It has a sensitivity of nearly 93% and a specificity of 82%.

Other diagnostic tests that may be helpful include:
- chest radiograph with lateral views, which may show air in the retrosternal space;
- blood cultures, which are positive in about half of patients with deep tissue involvement; and

- deep substernal aspirations, which should be sent for regular Gram staining and culture, acid-fast staining, and culture and fungal cultures.

However, the most important diagnostic modality is careful clinical observation.

TREATMENT

Aggressive surgical and medical management is needed for this type of infection. Surgery should include radical debridement of all necrotic tissues, adequate drainage, and removal of all foreign bodies. This is followed by open wound care, closed irrigation or flap reconstruction, depending on the extent of the infection.

Initial antibiotic therapy should provide broad-spectrum antimicrobial coverage, bearing in mind the organisms specific to the particular hospital environment, as well as their resistance patterns. Combination therapy with agents, such as vancomycin, gentamicin and rifampin (rifampicin), or single agents, such as imipenem, ticarcillin–clavulanate or piperacillin–tazobactam, may be used. Treatment can be narrowed down later once the causative organism is known. Duration of treatment ranges from 10–14 days for those with cellulitis, to 4–6 weeks for those with deeper tissue involvement.

FURTHER READING

Ger E, Stern D, Weiss J, *et al.* Clinical-radiological evaluation of poststernotomy wound infection. Plast Reconstr Surg 1998;101:348–55.

Gold JP, Isom OW. Infection in open heart surgery. In: Davis JM, Shikes GT, eds. Principles and management of surgical infections. Philadelphia: JB Lippincott; 1991:323–47.

Hazelrigg SR, Wellons HA Jr, Schneider JA, Kolm P. Wound complications after median sternotomy. Relationship to internal mammary grafting. J Thorac Cardiovasc Surg 1989;98:1096–9.

Kluytmans JA, Mouton JW, Ijzerman EP, *et al.* Nasal carriage of *Staphylococcus aureus* as a major risk factor for wound infections after cardiac surgery. J Infect Dis 1995;171:216–9.

Mossad SB, Serkey JM, Longworth DL, Cosgrove DM 3rd, Gordon SM. Coagulase-negative staphylococcal sternal wound infections after open heart operations. Ann Thorac Surg 1997;63:395–401.

Pett SB Jr. Post-sternotomy wound infections. In: Fry DE, ed. Surgical infections. Little, Brown; 1995:389–96.

Zacharias A, Habib RH. Factors predisposing to median sternotomy complications. Deep vs. superficial infection. Chest 1996;37:505–9.

The pros and cons of antibiotics for pharyngitis and otitis media

Jenifer Leaf Jaeger

Acute upper respiratory infections are the most common illnesses of humans and occur with greater frequency in children than adults. Sore throat is one of the most common complaints and otitis media is the leading indication for outpatient antibiotic use in the USA. Despite the frequency of these infections, controversy still exists regarding optimal treatment practices. Although most infections are relatively mild and resolve spontaneously, the data support the use of antimicrobial therapy for group A streptococcal (GAS) pharyngitis and acute otitis media (AOM). It has been found to be useful and often necessary to prevent suppurative and nonsuppurative complications. However, the lack of rigor in adhering to criteria for establishing these diagnoses leads to overdiagnosis and promotes selection of resistant bacteria.

PHARYNGITIS

Group A streptococci (*Streptococcus pyogenes*), the leading bacterial cause of pharyngitis, accounts for approximately 15% of all cases of pharyngitis. The majority of patients therefore have a nonstreptococcal illness and will not benefit from therapy. Accurate diagnosis of active infection is essential to adequately provide primary prevention of acute rheumatic fever (ARF), while minimizing the indiscriminant use of antibiotics. The considerable overlap in presentation among the various viral and bacterial illnesses and the presence of a carrier state for GAS makes clinical diagnosis less reliable.

Viruses are the most common causative agents identified in pharyngitis, accounting for up to 90% of all upper respiratory infections. Herpes simplex virus, Epstein–Barr virus, rhinovirus (usually in the setting of cough and coryza) and adenovirus infections commonly present as pharyngitis. Enteroviruses that are responsible for herpangina, lymphonodular pharyngitis and hand–foot–mouth disease are important in the differential diagnosis, as is the acute retroviral syndrome associated with

primary infection with HIV, which may present with pharyngitis.

Bacterial causes of pharyngitis other than GAS are rare. Non-group A streptococci, particularly groups C and G streptococci, cause pharyngitis in older children and will respond to antimicrobial therapy. These β-hemolytic streptococci can be isolated by throat culture but will not be identified by rapid antigen tests and have been associated with acute glomerulonephritis but not acute rheumatic fever. *Arcanobacterium* (formerly known as *Corynebacterium*) *haemolyticum* is an infrequent infection that may be indistinguishable from GAS infection. It may cause a scarlet fever-like rash, and it primarily infects adolescents and young adults. *Chlamydia pneumoniae* and *Mycoplasma pneumoniae* infections may present with pharyngitis with concurrent lower respiratory tract involvement.

Signs and symptoms suggestive of GAS infection, including sudden onset of sore throat, fever, headache, nausea, pharyngeal erythema with patchy exudate, and tender, enlarged anterior cervical chain lymph nodes, may be present in only 30–50% of patients. Antigen detection tests for GAS are highly specific (90–100%) but not as sensitive (55–90%) as throat culture. However, neither can distinguish between acute infection with GAS and the carrier state in people who have pharyngitis due to some other etiology.

The goals of therapy are straightforward:
- to hasten clinical recovery,
- to prevent transmission to others,
- to avoid suppurative complications, and
- to prevent development of rheumatic fever.

Strategies for achieving these goals are less clear.

The earlier in the course of the infection that antibiotics are begun, the greater the potential impact. Of patients treated appropriately 95% will become noninfectious within 24 hours, allowing an earlier return to work or school. However, early therapy may be associated with an increased recurrence rate as a result of an abortive antibody response. The development of protective, type-specific antibodies is slow and thus early treatment may interfere with the immunologic response. Local infections, such as retropharyngeal and peritonsillar abscess as well as invasive GAS disease, including streptococcal toxic shock syndrome, are known complications of GAS pharyngitis. However, there is no proven benefit of early treatment in decreasing the risk of these complications. Antibiotic therapy is effective in preventing rheumatic fever even if therapy is delayed up to 9 days after disease onset.

Indiscriminant use of throat culture or antigen tests contributes to excessive cost of health care, increases the likelihood of obtaining a 'false-positive' result (i.e. identifying a carrier), leads to substantial overuse of antibiotics and encourages development of resistant bacteria. Group A streptococci may be carried in the pharynx of untreated patients for several weeks or months and approximately 25% of patients who have been adequately treated become GAS carriers. Carriers are at low risk of developing invasive GAS disease or acute rheumatic fever and are unlikely to transmit GAS to contacts. Because most patients do not have a GAS infection, empiric therapy is not justified.

Surveillance of physician practices in the USA has revealed that 40% of physicians admit to continuing therapy despite negative culture results, and many acknowledge not following through with results. Therefore, it is reasonable to obtain a throat culture or antigen detection tests in patients who have an illness compatible with GAS infection and await results before starting therapy. A cost-effective strategy is the initial use of the antigen detection tests; a positive test allows prompt specific therapy, but a negative result must be followed by culture held for 48 hours.

Treatment of GAS pharyngitis is based on cost, efficacy. palatability and spectrum of activity. Penicillin remains the drug of choice in non-allergic patients. There have been no documented cases of penicillin-resistant GAS. Penicillin has a narrow spectrum of activity, and is safe, well tolerated and inexpensive. Amoxicillin is an acceptable alternative. It has the advantage of improved taste and is inexpensive. Although there are no data specifically assessing its efficacy in preventing rheumatic fever it is likely to be as effective as penicillin. The broader spectrum of activity of the aminopenicillins may exert greater selective pressure on the development of resistant bacteria. Macrolides are the drugs of choice for allergic patients in regions where resistance rates are low. Resistance rates to erythromycin as high as 40% have been reported in Japan and Finland. Decreasing availability of erythromycin in Finland has been associated with subsequent decreases in the number of resistant organisms. Clarithromycin and azithromycin appear to be as effective as erythromycin, have wider spectrums of activity and are more expensive, and thus their use is discouraged. Oral narrow-spectrum cephalosporins may be another alternative in penicillin-allergic patients, although cross-reactivity occurs in 15–20%. Cephalosporins are slightly more effective in eradicating the carrier state than penicillin, but given the benign nature of the carrier state therapy may not be worth the added expense. A 10-day course of therapy is effective in approximately 90% of children. Shorter courses of therapy are less effective, except for azithromycin, where a 5-day course is acceptable. A 5-day course of a cephalosporin has been suggested by some investigators but further study is necessary to confirm initial results. Whether use of a broader-spectrum drug for a shorter period will impede the development of resistant organisms remains to be demonstrated. This topic is reviewed in Chapters 2.24 and 8.14.

OTITIS MEDIA

Acute otitis media is one of the most frequent infections in childhood and accounts for more than one-quarter of all antibiotic prescriptions in the USA. Although there is considerable evidence supporting the use of antimicrobials in the treatment of AOM, the treatment effect is small. Tympanocentesis or needle aspiration of middle ear effusion has demonstrated a bacterial pathogen in only two-thirds of children who have AOM (*Strep. pneumoniae* accounts for 25–50% followed by nontypable *Haemophilus influenzae* in 15–30%), and two-thirds of patients improve

without intervention. However, there is no reliable method of determining which children require treatment. Overdiagnosis of AOM and unnecessary use of antibiotic therapy for otitis media with effusion (OME) contribute to the development of resistant organisms. Rigorous attention to distinguishing between AOM and OME and withholding antibiotics in the latter group alone would eliminate 6–8 million unnecessary prescriptions in the USA per year.

Acute otitis media is defined as the presence of fluid in the middle ear, with inflammation of the tympanic membrane in association with the rapid onset of signs and symptoms of local or systemic infection, whereas OME is characterized by an asymptomatic middle ear effusion in the absence of inflammation. Following appropriate therapy for AOM, middle ear effusion persists in 50% of patients at 1 month, and in 10% at 3 months. Thus, the presence of middle ear fluid in a child recently treated for AOM does not indicate treatment failure and does not warrant therapy.

Therapy should be reserved for those children who have effusion in the setting of new onset of illness or who have evidence of middle ear effusions accompanied by bilateral hearing loss for at least 3 months. These guidelines reflect the concern that persistent middle ear effusion may contribute to hearing impairment and subsequent language and cognitive deficits. A causal relationship between the modest conductive hearing impairment associated with otitis media and subsequent developmental deficits, however, has not been established. Moreover, there is a growing body of literature documenting an increased risk of infection and colonization with penicillin-resistant pneumococci in children receiving antimicrobial agents. Other disadvantages to therapy include cost and potential side effects of antimicrobial agents.

Antibiotic prophylaxis for control of recurrent AOM is indicated in the setting of three or more episodes in a 6-month period or four or more episodes in a 12-month period. Numerous studies have demonstrated that continuous treatment with low-dose amoxicillin or sulfisoxazole significantly reduces the number of new infections compared with placebo. The greatest benefit from this regimen is derived in those patients who have frequent recurrences, those under 2 years of age and in those attending day care. An alternative approach to antimicrobial prophylaxis is placement of tympanostomy tubes. Although tympanostomy tubes are somewhat less effective than antibiotics in reducing the number of recurrences, they are more effective in reducing the period during which an effusion is present. Their use is recommended in the context of hearing loss. Elimination of smoking in the household, encouragement of breast-feeding, removal of the child from day care, and vaccination against *H. influenzae* in infancy and pneumococci in children over the age of 2 years are additional strategies to consider. Otitis media is reviewed in detail in Chapter 2.25.

In summary, the evidence supports treating acute GAS pharyngitis and AOM. The injudicious use of antibiotics for those infections that are not likely to benefit from therapy and that often resolve spontaneously contributes greatly to the development of resistant bacteria. Understanding of the epidemiology and natural history of these infections is an essential component in the decision to treat.

FURTHER READING

Berman S. Otitis media in children. N Engl J Med 1995;332:1560–5.

Block SL, Harrison CJ, Hendrick JA, *et al*. Penicillin-resistant *Streptococcus pneumoniae* in acute otitis media: risk factors, susceptibility patterns and antimicrobial management. Pediatr Infect Dis J 1995;14:751–9.

Dajani A, Taubert K, Ferrieri P, Peter G, Shulman S, Committee on Rheumatic Fever, Endocarditis and Kawasaki Disease of the Council on Cardiovascular Disease in the Young, American Heart Association. Treatment of acute streptococcal pharyngitis and prevention of rheumatic fever: a statement for health professionals. Pediatrics 1995;96:758–64.

Dowel SF, Marcy M, Phillips WR, Gerber MA, Schwartz B. Otitis media – principles of judicioud use of antimicrobial agents. Pediatrics 1998;101:165–71.

Klein JO. Otitis media. Clin Infect Dis 1994;19:823–33.

Rosenfeld JO, Clarity G. Acute otitis media in children. Prim Care 1996;23:677–86.

Shulman ST. Streptococcal pharyngitis: clinical and epidemiologic factors. Pediatr Infect Dis J 1989;8:816–9.

When to use corticosteroids in noncentral nervous system tuberculosis

*Anur R Guhan &
John T Macfarlane*

INTRODUCTION

Tuberculosis, a chronic necrotizing infection, can involve any organ in the body. The clinical manifestations represent breakdown in local or systemic immunity against the causative organism, *Mycobacterium tuberculosis*. In this context, it might appear paradoxic that corticosteroids with their known immunosuppressive effects should even be considered in the treatment of tuberculosis. Indeed, this topic continues to be controversial.

Both cellular immunity and cytokines are involved in the pathogenesis of tuberculosis. Caseating granulomas, the pathognomonic lesions of the disease, represent the attempt by the immune system to contain the bacilli. Cytokines (tumor necrosis factor-α and interferon-γ) released by sensitized tissue macrophages and peripheral blood mononuclear cells are thought to be responsible for the necrosis of lesions, the tissue edema and the constitutional symptoms (such as fever, anorexia, weight loss and night sweats) that are seen in patients who have tuberculosis. Healing results in fibrosis, causing local architectural change, which may affect physiologic function.

The anti-inflammatory properties of corticosteroids have been used to modulate these harmful immune-mediated changes. Supported by case–control studies, the adjunctive use of corticosteroids with antituberculous medication was widely practiced in the 1950s and 1960s, especially with fulminant disease. However, the advent of short-course regimens containing rifampin (rifampicin) in the 1970s and the general decrease in the prevalence of tuberculosis in the Western world led to reduced need for adjuvant corticosteroid therapy except in selected situations.

With the resurgence of tuberculosis worldwide and the prospect of florid disease in the immunocompromised host, it is important to re-evaluate the adjuvant role of corticosteroids in the treatment of tuberculosis. The topic is discussed in this chapter basing recommendations on supporting evidence from the literature.

ADJUVANT ROLE OF CORTICOSTEROIDS

The anti-inflammatory properties of corticosteroids are well known, and their use in the treatment of tuberculosis is based on their known capacity to:
- control the systemic effects of cytokines and other immune mediators,
- reduce immune-mediated tissue edema that occurs before and with treatment,
- suppress the clinical manifestations of hypersensitivity to tubercular proteins, and
- reduce the extent of fibrosis associated with the healing process.

Corticosteroids should only be used together with effective antituberculous chemotherapy.

EVIDENCE OF EFFICACY

The strength of evidence supporting the adjuvant use of corticosteroids in the treatment of tuberculosis comes from a few prospective, randomized, placebo-controlled trials, several retrospective, case-controlled trials and numerous case reports. Most of these studies were conducted before the newer, more effective antituberculous medications became available. However, there is no reason why these results cannot be extrapolated to the newer drugs. Evidence from prospective placebo-controlled randomized trials is available for the following clinical situations.

Patients who have extensive pulmonary tuberculosis have shown a more rapid clinical improvement with corticosteroids, with faster normalization of body temperature, weight loss and other constitutional symptoms and earlier radiologic resolution of pulmonary cavities.

Conversely, other studies have shown no advantage from adjuvant corticosteroid therapy. A prospective randomized study of patients on short-course chemotherapy failed to show any benefit of additional prednisolone. However, it must be said that the dose of prednisolone used (20mg/day) was low considering the use of a rifampin-containing regimen.

Patients who had tubercular pericarditis who received prednisolone had significantly faster resolution of symptoms and effusion and significantly reduced acute mortality than those who received placebo. Similar results have been shown for tubercular pleural effusions.

Children who had tubercular mediastinal lymphadenopathy causing extrabronchial compression made significantly better recovery as judged by radiologic and bronchoscopic findings when treated with adjuvant prednisolone.

Risk of progressive tuberculosis with adjuvant corticosteroids

Studies have shown either a benefit or no benefit from adjuvant corticosteroids; there is no evidence of increased risk of disease progression when corticosteroids are given together with effective antituberculous chemotherapy. However, adjuvant corticosteroid therapy could have systemic side effects related to their influence on the metabolism of bone, protein and carbohydrate. Monitoring of blood sugar is important in patients who have diabetes mellitius as a comorbid condition.

USE OF ADJUVANT CORTICOSTEROIDS IN TUBERCULOSIS
Doses and regimen

There are no agreed standards on the corticosteroid dosage or the duration of adjuvant treatment. Most authors, including ourselves, use the regimen suggested by Crofton and Douglas for most clinical situations: prednisolone 30–40mg/day for 2 weeks, gradually tapered over 6 weeks. Rom and Gary suggest a higher initial dose for tuberculous pericarditis: prednisolone 60–80mg/day for 4 weeks, tapering over 8 weeks.

As rifampin increases the catabolism of exogenous corticosteroids by hepatic microsomal enzyme induction, the bioavailability of any administered dose of prednisolone would effectively be halved. It is important to bear this in mind, particularly during exogenous corticosteroid replacement for endogenous insufficiency.

The use of corticosteroids as adjuvant therapy in tuberculosis can be thought of under two headings:
- the adjuvant use of corticosteroids supported by evidence and general agreement (Fig. 32.3); and
- the adjuvant use of corticosteroids not supported by unequivocal evidence (Fig. 32.4).

The doses and duration of treatment suggested are what we would use in a particular clinical situation with a chemotherapy regimen that contains rifampin.

There is as yet insufficient information on the effects of adjuvant corticosteroids in patients who have HIV infection and tuberculosis. Coinfection with HIV and *M. tuberculosis* modifies the manifestations of clinical tuberculosis, making it difficult to extrapolate the results of trials on the use of adjuvant corticosteroids in the HIV-negative population to the HIV-positive population. However, evidence from cohort studies suggest that HIV-positive patients with all manifestations of tuberculosis fare better when receiving adjuvant corticosteroids compared with matched control groups. Further research is needed.

It is important to bear in mind that patients with AIDS may have other co-existing but unrecognized opportunistic infections, which may progress under corticosteroid cover unless specific therapy is instituted.

ADJUVANT USE OF CORTICOSTEROIDS SUPPORTED BY EVIDENCE AND GENERAL AGREEMENT		
Clinical situation	Aim and comments	Suggested regimen
Fulminant pulmonary tuberculosis with toxemia	Buy time for chemotherapy to take effect	Prednisolone 40mg/day until improvement in constitutional symptoms and erythrocyte sedimentation rate, then gradually taper by 2.5mg/day and stop
Miliary tuberculosis	Buy time for chemotherapy to take effect. Important to monitor for occult adrenal insufficiency	Prednisolone 40mg/day until improvement in constitutional symptoms and erythrocyte sedimentation rate, then gradually taper by 2.5mg/day and stop
Adrenal insufficiency	Corticosteroid replacement; monitor progress with short ACTH stimulation test	Prednisolone 60–80mg/day. Long-term maintenance therapy may be required
Tuberculous pericarditis and tamponade	Expedite fluid resolution, symptom control and improve acute survival	Prednisolone 60–80mg/day for 4 weeks, tapering over 8 weeks. Insignificant effect on need for later pericardectomy
Massive tuberculous effusion with toxemia	Expedite fluid resorption, temperature control and reduce risk of adhesions	Prednisolone 30–40mg/day for 2 weeks, tapering over 2 weeks
Extrabronchial compression or atelectasis caused by tuberculous mediastinal lymphadenopathy	Reduce lymph node enlargement and improve lumen and lobar aeration	Prednisolone 30–40mg/day until radiologic resolution of atelectasis, tapering over 6 weeks
Endobronchial tuberculosis	Reduce risk of post-treatment strictures	Prednisolone 30–40mg/day for 3 weeks, tapering over 12 weeks
Drug hypersensitivity reactions	Suppress manifestations of hypersensitivity while sequentially re-introducing antituberculous drugs. Dose and duration needs to be titrated to the individual. At least two effective antituberculous drugs must be introduced before corticosteroids are added	Prednisolone 20–30mg/day, while the suspected putative drug is re-introduced gradually in increasing doses. Cautious tapering of corticosteroid dose
Hypersensitivity phenomenon – tuberculides, episcleritis, scleritis, Eale's disease (retinal periphlebitis)	Modulate immunopathogenesis and reduce risk of scarring. Lesions are manifestations of hypersensitivity to tuberculoprotein and can occur with or without overt tuberculosis. Antituberculous chemoprophylaxis is required; in case of active tuberculosis, full-course chemotherapy is required	Ocular tuberculides, episcleritis and scleritis: topical corticosteroids Cutaneous tuberculides: topical corticosteroids; systemic corticosteroids occasionally needed Eale's disease: in consultation with an ophthalmologist, prednisolone 30–40mg/day for 3 weeks tapering over 8–12 weeks

Fig. 32.3 **Adjuvant use of corticosteroids supported by evidence and general agreement.**

CONCLUSION

Adjuvant corticosteroid therapy in related patients who have tuberculosis is effective, producing useful and faster clinical recovery from the disease. When used under cover of effective antituberculous chemotherapy there is no risk of disease progression. It should never be used when resistance to more than one drug is suspected. With rifampin-containing regimens, the recommended corticosteroid doses take into account increased hepatic metabolism and reduced bioavailability. Conversely, with regimens that do not contain rifampin the recommended doses should be halved.

Fig. 32.4 **Adjuvant use of corticosteroids not supported by unequivocal evidence.**

ADJUVANT USE OF CORTICOSTEROIDS NOT SUPPORTED BY UNEQUIVOCAL EVIDENCE		
Clinical situation	Aim and comments	Suggested regimen
Tuberculosis of the upper respiratory tract	Reduce risk of stricture formation after healing	Prednisolone 30–40mg/day for 3 weeks, tapering over 6 weeks. Endoscopic monitoring advisable
Tuberculous peritonitis	Expedite fluid resorption and reduce risk of adhesions	Prednisolone 30–40mg/day for 3 weeks tapering over 6 weeks
Tuberculosis of the genitourinary system	Reduce the risk of stricture formation and deformity	Prednisolone 30–40mg/day for 3 weeks tapering over 6 weeks
Tuberculosis and AIDS	Modulate the deleterious effects of cytokines and other immune mediators and buy time for chemotherapy to take effect	Similar to non-AIDS population. Prednisolone 40mg/day until improvement in constitutional symptoms and erythrocyte sedimentation rate, then gradually taper by 2.5mg/day and stop. Essential to be aware that AIDS patients may have coexisting cryptogenic opportunistic infections, which could progress under cover of corticosteroids

FURTHER READING

Barnes PF, Barrows SA. Tuberculosis in the 1990s. Ann Intern Med 1993;119:400–10.

Crofton J, Douglas A. Respiratory Diseases, 2nd ed. Oxford: Blackwell Scientific Publications; 1975.

Muthuswamy P, Hu TC, Carraso B, Antonio M, Dandamudi N. Prednisolone as adjunctive therapy in the management of pulmonary tuberculosis. Chest 1995;107:1621–30.

Rom WN, Garay S. Tuberculosis. Boston: Little, Brown and Company; 1996.

Senderovitz, Viskum K. Corticosteroids and tuberculosis. Respir Med 1994;88:561–5.

chapter
33

Orocervical and Esophageal Infection

Robert C Read

Infections of the oral cavity and neck include dental and periodontal infections, deep fascial space infections of the neck that are often odontogenic or caused by contiguous spread from pharyngeal foci, non-dental oral infections, including ulcerative and gangrenous stomatitis, and infections of the salivary glands. Infections of the esophagus mostly occur in the context of severe underlying disease.

DENTAL AND PERIODONTAL INFECTIONS

EPIDEMIOLOGY

Dental caries is the commonest infectious disease in humans. The incidence of the disease is closely related to the use of derivatives of cane sugar and began to take on epidemic proportions in Europe in the 19th century. Dental caries first becomes evident in infancy and is most noticeable on the chewing surfaces of the molar teeth. The likelihood of dental caries is increased by high sugar intake, poor oral hygiene and any factors that reduce salivary flow – notably drugs (e.g. antidepressants).[1]

Periodontal disease, including gingivitis, is mainly related to poor oral hygiene and increasing age. Increased incidence of periodontal disease is also evident in diabetics, and during hormonal disturbances, including puberty and pregnancy.[2] It is suspected that most periodontal disease arises from an inflammatory response to the accumulation of dental plaque in the gingival margin. Plaque contains mainly *Streptococcus spp.* and *Actinomyces* spp., which probably generate an early gingivitis leading ultimately to periodontitis.[3] These processes occur over many years with incremental destruction of periodontal tissue.[4]

PATHOGENESIS AND PATHOLOGY

The indigenous oral flora includes a large number of aerobic and anaerobic bacteria and varies by site within the oral cavity. There are of the order of 10^{11} micro-organisms per gram wet weight of oral secretions, with the majority being obligate anaerobes. *Streptococcus* spp., *Peptostreptococcus* spp., *Veillonella* spp., *Lactobacillus* spp., *Corynebacterium* spp., *Bacteroides* spp., *Prevotella* spp. and *Actinomyces* spp. form the majority of oral flora.[5]

Dental caries is characteristically polymicrobial with no fixed pattern of microbial etiology, except that *Streptococcus mutans* has emerged as the only organism consistently isolated from carious teeth compared with normal teeth. In contrast, gingivitis has characteristic microbial specificity; the normal flora of the periodontium (i.e. *Streptococcus sanguis* and *Actinomyces* spp.) is replaced by anaerobic Gram-negative rods, notably *Prevotella intermedia*. With chronic gingivitis there is ulceration of the mucosa, loss of attachment of periodontal tissue, loss of enamel and necrosis of the dental pulp, and an increase in complexity of microbial flora with a preponderance of anaerobic Gram-negative rods, including *Porphyromonas gingivalis*.[2] When abscesses form, for example periapical abscesses, the flora is always polymicrobial with species such as *Fusobacteria*, pigmented *Bacteroides*, *Peptostreptococcus*, *Actinomyces* and *Streptococcus*.

In healthy individuals teeth are protected from decay by the cleansing action of the tongue and buccal secretions, the buffering effect of saliva and the acquired pellicle – the fluid microenvironment of the tooth surface. With poor dental hygiene the acquired pellicle is colonized and replaced by plaque that contains bacteria, notably *S. mutans*. This process is accelerated by intermittent exposure to carbohydrates and simple sugars. The presence of subgingival plaque leads to inflammation of the gingival epithelium and to destruction of the periodontium.[5] The normal resident polymicrobial flora provides an important defense against invasion of gingival epithelium by pathogenic bacteria. Normal saliva also protects the epithelium by irrigating it with enzymes, including lysozyme and lactoperoxidase, and other antimicrobial substances such as lactoferrin. Secretory IgA provides additional protection by aggregating organisms and preventing bacterial adherence. The importance of intact phagocytic defenses is reflected by the high prevalence of periodontal infections in patients who have cyclic neutropenia and chronic granulomatous disease.[3] Some oral micro-organisms involved in periodontal disease secrete IgA proteases.[6] Host factors credited with leading to periodontitis include psychosocial stress, diet, smoking, alcoholism and intercurrent disease.[7]

The usual cause of deep-seated odontogenic infection is necrosis of the pulp of the tooth followed by bacterial invasion through the pulp chamber and into the deeper tissues.[8] If a pulp abscess is allowed to progress, infection will spread toward the nearest cortical plate (Fig. 33. 1).

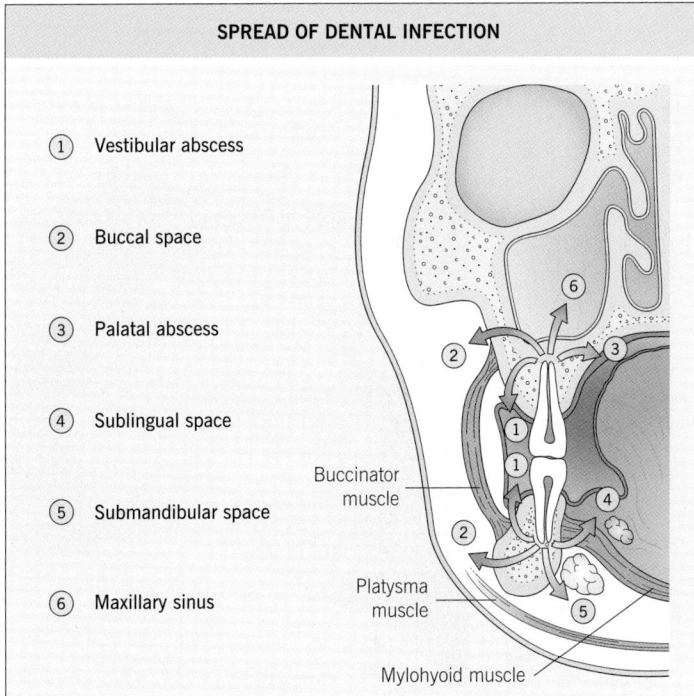

SPREAD OF DENTAL INFECTION

1. Vestibular abscess
2. Buccal space
3. Palatal abscess
4. Sublingual space
5. Submandibular space
6. Maxillary sinus

Buccinator muscle
Platysma muscle
Mylohyoid muscle

Fig. 33.1 Spread of dental infection. A spreading tooth abscess will encroach upon the nearest cortical plate and its subsequent spread depends on the relationship of that site to muscle attachment. Adapted from Peterson.[8]

PREVENTION

Prevention of dental and periodontal infections includes interference with transmission and suppression of *S. mutans* colonization once it has occurred. There is a strong correlation between maternal salivary *S. mutans* infection and the presence of this organism in children. Acquisition of *S. mutans* by infants has been prevented by aggressive treatment of *S. mutans* infection in mothers.[9] Existing infections can be suppressed by regular cleaning with agents that include fluoride and antimicrobial substances such as chlorhexidine. Periodontal disease can be prevented by good oral hygiene and regular rinsing with chlorhexidine. The use of controlled-release antibiotics is currently under investigation.[10]

CLINICAL FEATURES

Subgingival dental caries is asymptomatic, but destruction of enamel results in invasion of the pulp with subsequent necrosis eventually leading to a periapical abscess. The tooth becomes sensitive to temperature and pressure once the enamel is penetrated, and toothache results.

In simple gingivitis there is usually discoloration of the gum margin with occasional bleeding after brushing of the teeth. There may be halitosis. If gingivitis is allowed to become chronic there may be destruction of periodontal tissue with loosening of the teeth. This may be relatively asymptomatic or the patient may have itchy gums, temperature sensitivity and halitosis.

COMPLICATIONS

Dental pulp infections can lead to involvement of the maxillary and mandibular spaces (Fig. 33.1). Spread of infection from maxillary (upper) teeth most commonly leads to vestibular abscesses (Fig. 33.2). Erosion of canine pulp abscesses can lead to canine space abscesses if the abscess points above the insertion of the levator labii superioris. This results in swelling lateral to the nose, which usually obliterates the nasolabial fold. Buccal space abscesses can result when pulp abscesses of the molar teeth erode above or below the attachment of the buccinator muscle; these point below the zygomatic arch and above the inferior border of the mandible (Fig. 33.3).

When infection spreads from mandibular (lower) teeth the commonest result is again vestibular abscess. Deeper abscesses may point into the sublingual and submandibular spaces. The sublingual space lies underneath the oral mucosa and above the mylohyoid muscle (Fig. 33.1). Posteriorly, it communicates with the submandibular space. Infection within the sublingual space results in swelling of the floor of the mouth, which may spread to involve both sides and be sufficiently pronounced to lift the tongue. This space is involved if the infected tooth apex giving rise to the disease is superior to the insertion of the mylohyoid (e.g. premolars and first molars).

The submandibular space lies between the mylohyoid muscle and the skin. It becomes involved if the apex of the infected tooth is inferior to the insertion of the mylohyoid muscle (e.g. third molar). Clinically, infection in this space causes extraoral swelling (unlike sublingual space infections) that begins at the inferior lateral border of the mandible and extends medially to the digastric area. Occasionally the abscess may point spontaneously and rupture (Fig. 33.4).

Ludwig's angina refers to a severe cellulitis of the tissue of the floor of the mouth with involvement of the submandibular and sublingual spaces (Fig. 33.5). The source of infection is almost always the second and third mandibular molars. If the infection is allowed to continue there may be local lymphadenitis, systemic sepsis and extension of the disease to involve deep cervical fascia with a cellulitis that extends from the clavicle to the superficial tissues of the face. Other potential complications include asphyxia, aspiration and mediastinitis. The disease is almost always polymicrobial, including α-hemolytic streptococci and anaerobes such as *Peptostreptococci* spp., *Bacteroides melaninogenicus* and *Fusobacterium nucleatum*.[11]

Very rarely, spread of infection from maxillary teeth may cause orbital cellulitis or cavernous sinus thrombosis (see Chapter 2.17). The latter is distinguished by toxemia, venous obstruction within the eye and orbital tissues (Fig. 33.6), involvement of the III, IV and VI cranial nerves and meningismus.

MANAGEMENT

Treatment of dentoalveolar infections includes elimination of the diseased pulp and deep periodontal scaling or tooth extraction. Any dentoalveolar abscess present should be surgically drained. If drainage

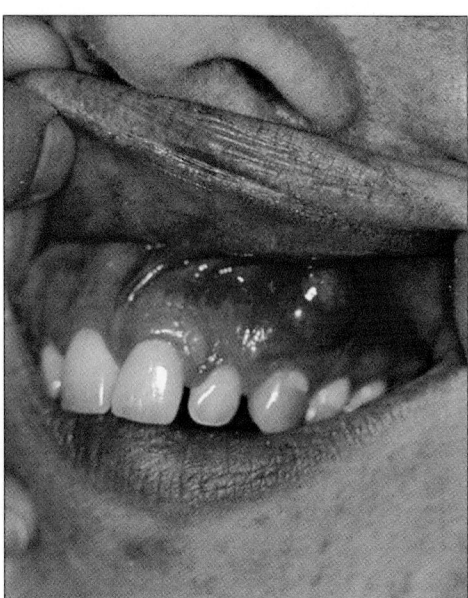

Fig. 33.2 Painful vestibular abscess. Courtesy of Professor I Brook.

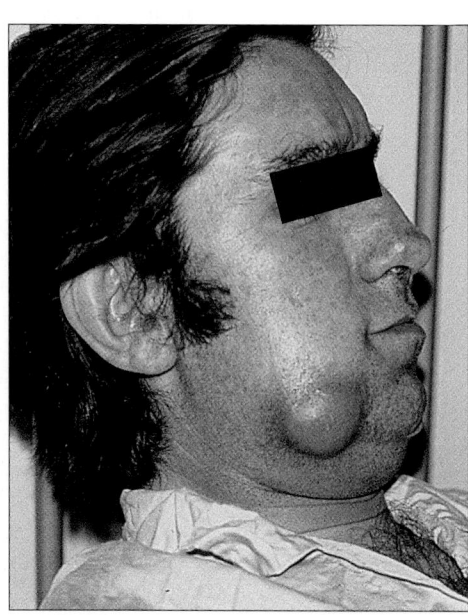

Fig. 33.3 Buccal space abscess originating from right lower molar infection. The buccal space lies between the buccinator muscle and the overlying skin and fascia. Courtesy of Professor I Brook.

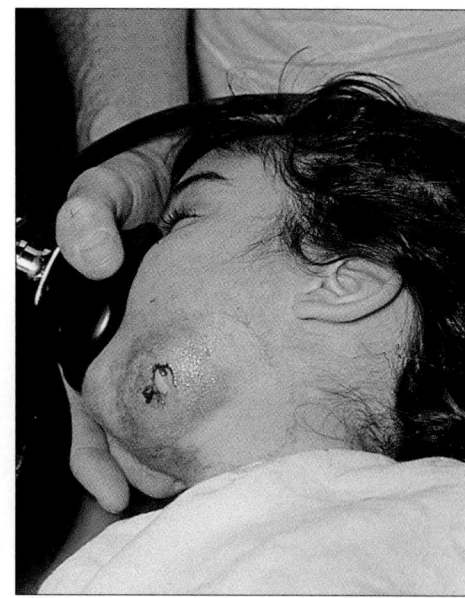

Fig. 33.4 Submandibular abscess originating from a 2nd molar tooth infection. Courtesy of University of Sheffield School of Dentistry, UK.

is not complete, antibiotic therapy is appropriate. Treatment of periodontal disease includes appropriate debridement and short-term antimicrobial therapy with oral metronidazole 400mg q8h or oral phenoxymethylpenicillin 500mg q6h. Periodontal and vestibular abscesses should be treated by drainage.

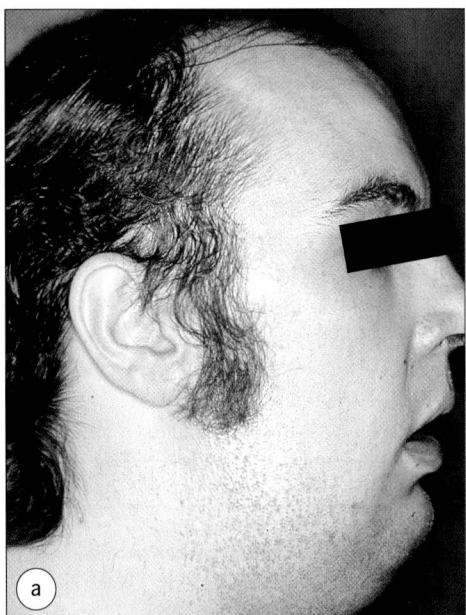

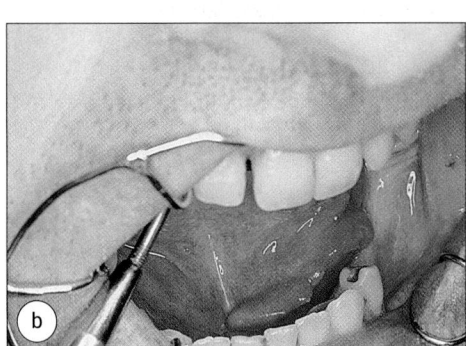

Fig. 33.5 Ludwig's angina. (a) This patient had painful cellulitis within the submandibular and sublingual spaces. (b) Brawny edema was present within the floor of the mouth, pushing the tongue upwards. Courtesy of University of Sheffield School of Dentistry, UK.

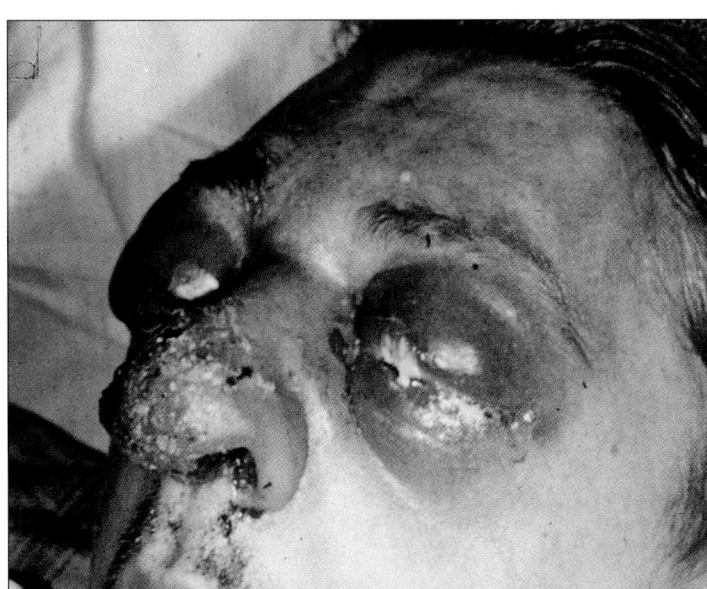

Fig. 33.6 Cavernous sinus thrombosis. A patient who displays evidence of severe orbital swelling caused by obstruction of orbital veins is shown. In this patient, the originating focus was infection of soft tissues of the nose. Courtesy of University of Sheffield School of Dentistry, UK.

Treatment of maxillary and submandibular space infections should always be by surgical drainage of pus. Ludwig's angina is a life-threatening condition and the first aim of treatment is protection of the airway, if necessary by emergency intubation or occasionally tracheostomy. Intravenous antibiotics should be administered. Benzyl-penicillin 1.2g q4h plus metronidazole 400mg q8h or clindamycin 450mg q8h are appropriate.

Management of cavernous sinus thrombosis is by surgical decompression and high-dose intravenous antibiotics, the choice of which is influenced by whether the originating focus is dental or within soft tissues.

DEEP CERVICAL SPACE INFECTION

Infections of the lateral pharyngeal space, the retropharyngeal space and the prevertebral space are uncommon but life-threatening problems. The lateral pharyngeal space is funnel-shaped, with its base at the sphenoid bone at the base of the skull and its apex at the hyoid bone. It is bounded by the medial pterygoid muscle laterally and the superior pharyngeal constrictor medially. Posteromedially it extends to the prevertebral fascia and communicates with the retropharyngeal space. The carotid sheath and cranial nerves are within the posterior compartment of the space. The retropharyngeal space lies posteromedial to the lateral pharyngeal space, between the superior constrictor muscle and the alar portion of the prevertebral fascia. Superiorly, it extends from the skull base of the pharyngeal tubercle down to the level of C7 where the superior pharyngeal muscle and the prevertebral fascia fuse.[8]

Unlike the lateral pharyngeal space it has few contents apart from lymph nodes, but its importance as a site of infection relates to its proximity to the airway and to the contents of the superior mediastinum. The prevertebral space extends from the skull base inferiorly to the diaphragm. It is bounded by the two layers of prevertebral fascia: the alar and prevertebral layers.

EPIDEMIOLOGY AND PATHOGENESIS

Parapharyngeal infections can complicate peritonsillar abscess (see Chapter 2.24), but a larger proportion of infections are odontogenic or secondary to intravenous drug abuse.[10] Rarer sources include parotitis, otitis and mastoiditis. The incidence of parapharyngeal infection has declined sharply in the antibiotic era and such infections now form less than 30% of all deep cervical infections.[11,12]

Infections of the retropharyngeal and prevertebral spaces most commonly result from lymphatic spread of infection in the pharynx or sinuses, with subsequent suppuration of the retropharyngeal lymph nodes. Retropharyngeal infections are therefore commonest in children mainly because retropharyngeal lymph nodes are more numerous.[13] Occasionally retropharyngeal infections may be caused by accidental perforation of the pharynx, for example during emergency intubation. The bacteriology of deep cervical space infections reflects the microbial flora of the originating source. Thus, infections arising from the pharynx are often caused by *Streptococcus pyogenes*, whereas odontogenic infections are polymicrobial and include *S. mutans* and anaerobic pathogens such as *F. nucleatum*, *B. melaninogenicus*, *Peptostreptococcus* spp., *Eikenella corrodens* and *Actinomyces* spp.

CLINICAL FEATURES

The characteristic feature of lateral pharyngeal space infection is severe trismus, which results from involvement of the pterygoid muscle and other muscles of mastication. There is also swelling of the lateral pharyngeal wall, which pushes the tonsil toward the midline. Occasionally there is lateral neck swelling below the angle of the mandible. The disease can be confused with peritonsillar abscess, although the latter should not produce trismus. The patient experiences fever, painful swallowing and pain that occasionally radiates to the ear. The infection tends to be severe and progresses rapidly. Posterior extension of the process into the carotid sheath can result in suppurative jugular thrombophlebitis, carotid artery erosion or interference with cranial nerves IX–XII. There is hyperacute sepsis, with rigors and high fever. There may be pain and swelling below the mandible, marked swelling of the lateral pharyngeal wall, torticollis and neck rigidity. There may be metastatic abscesses within the brain, lungs and bone. Suppurative thrombophlebitis of the internal jugular vein secondary to oropharyngeal infection was described by Lemierre and the syndrome bears his name.[14] The major organism associated with this complication is *Fusobacterium necrophorum*, which is usually obtained from blood cultures, but may require several days of anaerobic culture to grow.

Patients who have retropharyngeal abscess may present with fever and rigors that usually follow on from a streptococcal pharyngitis, but often there is no history of sore throat.[15] A child with a retropharyngeal abscess may be withdrawn and irritable. Adults may complain of sore throat, dysphagia, neck pain and dyspnea. The neck may be hyperextended, and there may be drooling and stridor. Examination of the throat by indirect laryngoscopy may reveal bulging of the posterior pharyngeal wall. Potential complications include upper airway obstruction as a result of anterior displacement of the posterior pharyngeal wall into the oropharynx, and spontaneous rupture of the abscess with aspiration pneumonia (which may complicate attempted insertion of an endotracheal tube). Other potential complications include purulent pleural effusion, pericardial effusion and posterosuperior mediastinitis.[16]

Patients who have AIDS, particularly intravenous drug users, have a higher incidence of deep neck infections, most commonly caused by *Staphylococcus aureus*, which is often methicillin resistant. In contrast to immunocompetent patients, there is often no leukocytosis.[17] Diabetics are also at increased risk of deep neck infections, and in addition to *S. aureus*, Gram-negative organisms, notably *Klebsiella* spp., may be isolated from these patients.[12]

DIAGNOSIS

If lateral pharyngeal space infection is suspected, the diagnosis is best confirmed by CT or MRI scanning. Plain radiographs are usually unhelpful. In contrast, a retropharyngeal space abscess can be diagnosed by a lateral radiograph of the neck (Fig. 33.7). The average width of the prevertebral soft tissue should be no more than 7mm (average 3.5mm) at C2 and no more than 20mm (average 14mm) at C6.[18] The neck should be fully extended during evaluation. The major clinical differential diagnosis of retropharyngeal abscess includes cervical

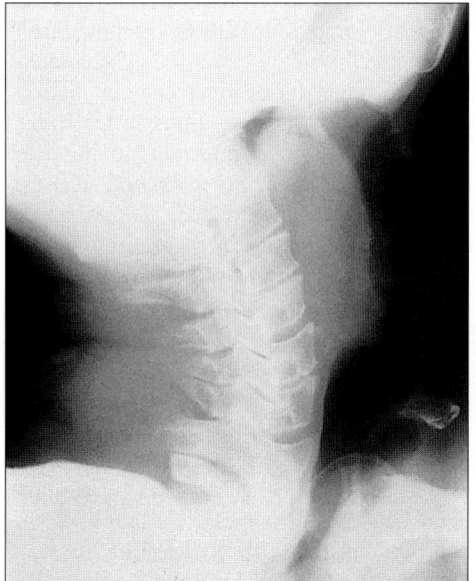

Fig. 33.7 Retropharyngeal abscess. Lateral radiograph of the neck in a patient who has a retropharyngeal abscess, showing gross expansion of prevertebral soft tissue. Courtesy of Mr R Bull.

osteomyelitis and meningitis. The latter can usually be discounted when there is obvious pharyngeal swelling, but cervical osteomyelitis may require MRI scanning of the cervical vertebral bodies for exclusion.

MANAGEMENT

In any patient with a suspected deep neck infection, maintenance of the airway is always the first consideration; about one-third of patients who have retropharyngeal abscess will require tracheostomy.[12] Incision and drainage of involved spaces and intravenous antibiotic therapy should be performed promptly in order to produce rapid and complete resolution of the infection with minimal likelihood of complications. Radiologic evidence of gas within soft tissues increases the urgency, because expansion of lesions containing anaerobes is usually rapid. Lateral pharyngeal and retropharyngeal abscesses can be drained by an incision along the anterior border of the sternocleidomastoid muscle followed by blunt dissection and drainage. Extensive surgery should be unnecessary if infections are treated promptly and high-dose intravenous antibiotics are used. Appropriate intravenous antibiotics include penicillin 1.2–1.8g q3h plus clindamycin 300–600mg q8h or metronidazole 400mg q8h, plus ceftriaxone 2g q12h.

CERVICAL NECROTIZING FASCIITIS

Cervical necrotizing fasciitis is a rare and extremely dangerous complication of odontogenic and deep cervical space infection. The disease is characterized by involvement of more than one neck space (usually bilaterally) and contiguously spreading necrosis of connective tissue, with cellulitis that extends below the hyoid bone to the chest wall, onto the face and into the mediastinum. Most cases are odontogenic, particularly after dental abscesses, but some cases follow on from tonsillar abscess or from surgical trauma to the oropharynx. Almost all cases are polymicrobial, often with a single aerobic isolate (e.g. *Streptococcus* spp.) plus two or more anaerobes (mostly *Prevotella melaninogenicus* and *F. nucleatum*), although any of the oral anerobes can be involved. The typical clinical presentation is usually with dental pain and submandibular swelling over a few days, followed by rapid evolution of fasciitis, which is extremely tender on palpation and usually associated with crepitus. Mediastinal extension can be clinically silent and detectable only by CT of the chest, but can lead to pericarditis, pneumonia or empyema. Predisposing conditions include diabetes mellitus, alcoholism and malignancy. Management includes surgical drainage via incision along the sternocleidomastoid muscle followed by blunt dissection of the neck. Appropriate intravenous antibiotic therapy is benzylpenicillin 1.2–1.8g q3h plus clindamycin 600mg q8h.[19]

ACTINOMYCOSIS

Actinomycosis is a chronic suppurative bacterial infection that principally affects the head and neck but can involve almost any system. It spreads directly through tissue, skin and bone, and therefore is able to form sinuses and fistulas.

EPIDEMIOLOGY AND PATHOGENESIS

The agents that cause actinomycosis are facultative anaerobic Gram-positive commensals of the mouth. *Actinomyces israelii* is the most common pathogen, but *Actinomyces naeslundii*, *Actinomyces viscosis*, *Actinomyces odontolyticus* and *Arachnia propionica* may also cause the disease. These agents commonly inhabit carious teeth, dental plaque and cavities and also the normal intestinal tract. Head and neck infection usually occurs in the context of dental disease or dentistry, during which the normal mucosal barriers are broken down. Thoracic involvement usually follows aspiration of infected oropharyngeal secretions in patients who have poor dentition. Lesions of actinomycosis consist of areas of acute inflammation surrounded by fibrosing granulation tissue. Such material contains 'sulfur granules' (colonies of organisms forming an amorphous center surrounded by a rosette of clubbed filaments); these usually contain associated organisms, including *Actinobacillus actinomycetemcomitans*, *Haemophilus* and *Fusobacterium* spp., which probably contribute to the pathogenesis of the disease.

Any age group can be infected, including infants and children. Males outnumber females by three to one.

CLINICAL FEATURES

The most common manifestation of actinomycosis is soft tissue swelling of the head, face or neck, usually over or underneath the mandible.[20] Occasionally the swelling is very extensive and waxes and wanes over many months, spreading to involve other parts of the head and neck, including the scalp, palate, eyes, larynx, salivary glands, middle ear and paranasal sinuses. Sinuses and tracts develop that open into the mouth and the skin (Fig. 33.8). Involvement of local bone (e.g. the mandible) can result in periosteal reaction or frank osteomyelitis.

DIAGNOSIS

The diagnosis is usually obvious in patients who have head and neck swelling, particularly in the context of poor dentition and discharging sinuses yielding sulfur granules. The granules can be trapped in gauze placed over the sinus opening or by injecting and aspirating saline from the sinus; by shaking the aspirate, the granules can be seen with the naked eye. Sulfur granules can also be seen in sputum on microscopic examination. Any material obtained can be cultured under anaerobic conditions. In formalin-fixed tissues, immunofluorescence can be used to identify species. There is no reliable serologic test; laboratory diagnosis depends on microscopy and culture of material from the patient.

MANAGEMENT

Most patients who have actinomycosis will respond to intravenous benzylpenicillin, 1.2–1.8g q3h for 3–6 weeks, followed by oral penicillin V, 2–4g/day for 6–12 months. Alternative treatments include intravenous amoxycillin or ampicillin, followed by oral amoxycillin. Chloramphenicol, erythromycin, tetracycline and clindamycin have also been used successfully. Prolonged treatment with penicillin results in complete resolution of the disease, although there may be some residual fibrosis or scarring (Fig. 33.8). Whilst intravenous benzylpenicillin has been the traditional treatment for this condition there have been reports of the use of intravenous agents that can be given in once daily dosing for home therapy, including ceftriaxone and imipenem.

INFECTIONS OF THE ORAL MUCOSA: GANGRENOUS STOMATITIS

Acute necrotizing ulcerative gingivitis, or trench mouth, is an ulcerative necrosis of the marginal gingivae. The disease may spread to other oral structures, including the tonsils or pharynx, to cause Vincent's disease, or may result in rapid necrosis and sloughing of facial structures producing the classic features of cancrum oris (noma).

EPIDEMIOLOGY

The disease is mostly seen in developing countries in the context of severe debilitation and malnutrition. In addition, poor oral hygiene, HIV infection, measles, local irritation from food impaction and smoking are associated factors.[21]

PATHOGENESIS

Necrotizing gingivitis may begin as an aseptic necrosis secondary to mucosal capillary stasis. In infections in which the disease spreads superficially to involve the pharynx, it is most likely secondary to a combination of *F. nucleatum* and Gram-negative anaerobic organisms (*Bacteroides* subsp. *intermedius*). If the disease spreads deeper into facial tissues to cause cancrum oris, fusospirochaetal organisms such as *Borrelia vincenti* and *F. nucleatum* are consistently cultured. *Prevotella melaninogenica* may also be present. Biopsies of any advancing lesion often reveal a mat of predominantly Gram-negative thread-like bacteria that cannot be positively identified.[22]

CLINICAL FEATURES

The earliest feature is a small painful red lesion that may be vesicular on the attached gingiva and often in the premolar or molar region of the mandible, with sudden onset of painful gums (Vincent's disease; Fig. 33.9). The disease may then progress rapidly to produce halitosis and gingival bleeding. If there is involvement of the tonsils and pharynx (Vincent's angina) there is searing pain in the pharynx with high fever, regional lymphadenopathy and anorexia. If the disease spreads into deeper tissues (noma) a necrotic ulcer rapidly develops with painful cellulitis of the lips and cheeks, which often sloughs exposing underlying bone, teeth and deeper tissues (Fig. 33.10).

DIAGNOSIS

Although the infection is usually polymicrobial, material should be obtained for Gram stain and aerobic and anaerobic culture. Debrided material is optimal for anaerobic culture. Gram stain may reveal fusospirochaetal Gram-negative organisms as well as Gram-positive cocci and Gram-negative rods.

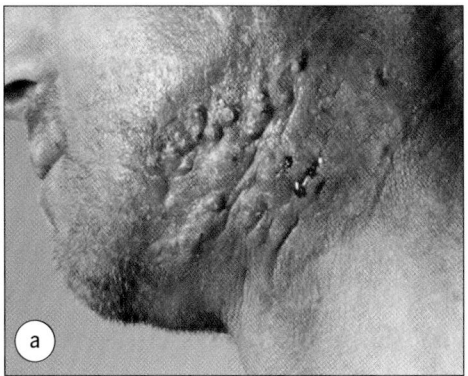
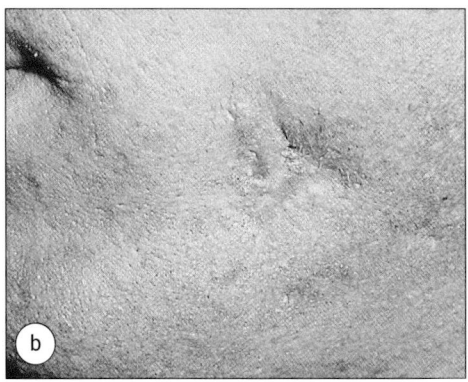

Fig. 33.8 Actinomycosis. (a) This patient had chronic disease over the mandible which (b) healed with several months of antibiotics, leaving a residual chronic sinus. Courtesy of Professor I Brook.

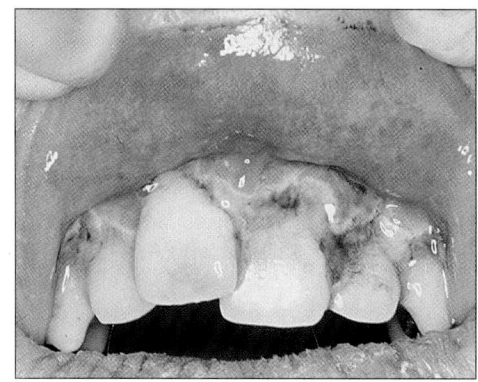

Fig. 33.9 Acute necrotizing gingivitis. Courtesy of Professor I Brook.

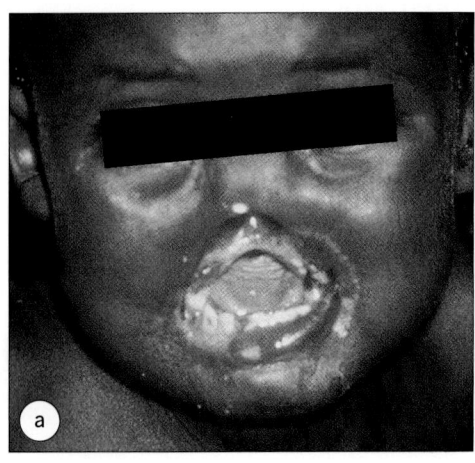
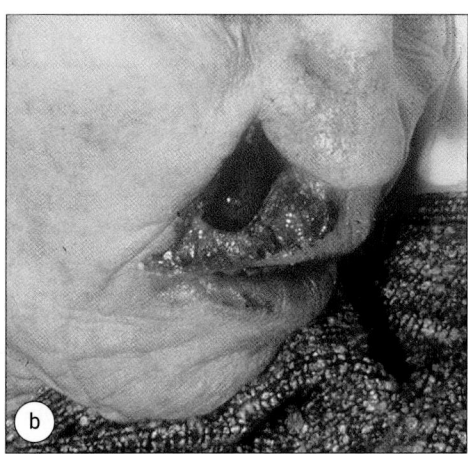

Fig. 33.10 Noma. This is a destructive process extending from oral structures, which is a sequel of necrotizing gingivitis and (a) is seen most commonly in patients in developing countries, although (b) occasionally it is seen in the elderly debilitated in developed countries. Courtesy of Professor I Brook.

MANAGEMENT

In early acute necrotizing ulcerative gingivitis (Vincent's infection), treatment with oral penicillin V 500mg q6h and metronidazole 400mg q8h is usually sufficient. In patients who have noma, high doses of intravenous penicillin and metronidazole are required, with the dose being dependent on the age and size of the patient. An antibiotic to treat aerobic Gram-negative rods, such as ceftriaxone may be necessary. Gangrenous tissues should be removed and loose teeth extracted. The patient should be carefully rehydrated. Once the infection has been controlled, reconstructive surgery is often necessary.

INFECTIONS OF THE ORAL MUCOSA: PRIMARY HERPETIC GINGIVOSTOMATITIS

EPIDEMIOLOGY

Herpes simplex virus (HSV)-1 and HSV-2 can cause a primary infection of the oral cavity, although type 1 is much more frequently responsible. The disease can occur in infants, although this is becoming increasingly uncommon. Oral lesions caused by HSV-2 are seen in sexual contacts of patients who have genital herpes and are clinically indistinguishable from those caused by HSV-1.

CLINICAL FEATURES

The disease may be very mild, with a few painful ulcers and no systemic features, or it may be more severe with fever, sore throat, malaise, headache and regional lymphadenopathy. Oral lesions tend to appear 1–2 days after the onset of pain and lead to a painful, red gingiva or palate. These symptoms generally persist for approximately 2 days. The vesicles occur as 2–4mm ulcers on a red background. When lesions coalesce they can resemble aphthous ulcers (Fig. 33.11). At this point the disease is highly infectious. The clinical course of unmodified primary herpetic gingivostomatitis usually lasts 2 weeks.

DIAGNOSIS

The clinical differential diagnosis of oral herpetic gingivostomatitis includes herpangina, varicella, herpes zoster and hand, foot and mouth disease. These diseases can usually be distinguished on the basis of concomitant cutaneous features. Primary herpes infection of the mouth can occasionally be recurrent, and several other recurrent diseases have similar oral lesions – these include minor aphthous ulcers, Behçet's syndrome, cyclical neutropenia and erythema multiforme. A laboratory diagnosis of herpes can be verified by direct immunofluorescence or viral culture of material obtained by swabbing the ulcers.

MANAGEMENT

In primary herpetic gingivostomatitis oral aciclovir 200–400mg q8h is appropriate therapy.

OTHER INFECTIONS OF THE ORAL MUCOSA

HERPANGINA

Herpangina produces characteristic oropharyngeal vesicles, generally at the junction of the hard and soft palates (Fig. 33.12). It primarily affects children and teenagers and generally occurs in epidemics during the summer. Several different Coxsackie viruses, notably Coxsackie virus A (types 1–10, 16 and 22), and less commonly Coxsackie virus B (types 1–5), have been associated with this disease. Other enteroviruses, including echovirus, have been implicated. Patients usually have mild disease, but they can complain of sudden fever, anorexia, neck pain, extremely sore throat and headache. The lesions are often more vesicular then herpetic lesions and consist of multiple, small, white papules with an erythematous base that appears less inflamed than that with herpetic lesions. These lesions usually spontaneously rupture within 2 or 3 days and seldom persist for more than 1 week. There may be cervical lymphadenopathy but this is unusual. A laboratory diagnosis can be obtained by culturing swabbed material from the lesions. Herpes simplex virus infection can usually be distinguished on clinical grounds, but can be rapidly excluded by direct immunofluorescence. Management consists of topical analgesia only.

HAND, FOOT AND MOUTH DISEASE

Hand, foot and mouth disease is caused by systemic infection with Coxsackie group A viruses (usually serotype 16) and primarily affects children, but occasionally adults. The disease consists of vesicular eruptions on the hands, wrists, feet and within the mouth. Lesions on the hands are almost always present, but oral lesions are present in 90% of patients and can occasionally be the only manifestation of the disease.[23] The oral vesicles are often on the palate, tongue and buccal mucosa and may range from a few isolated lesions to a marked stomatitis. In addition patients may suffer fever, malaise, conjunctival injection, headache and abdominal pain and occasionally diarrhea. The lesions on the feet and hands are flaccid, greyish vesicles, most often on the sides of the fingers, instep and toes.[24] If the disease is confined to the oral cavity it is almost indistinguishable from primary herpetic gingivostomatitis. Laboratory diagnosis of the disease can be confirmed by culture of feces or swabs obtained from the lesions. Management is symptomatic. The disease is usually self-limiting and rarely persists for more than 2 weeks.

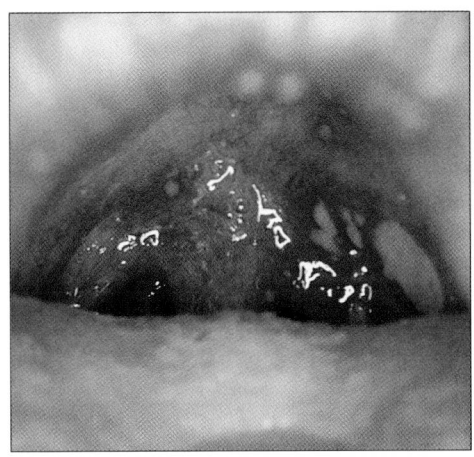

Fig. 33.11 Primary HSV-1 stomatitis.

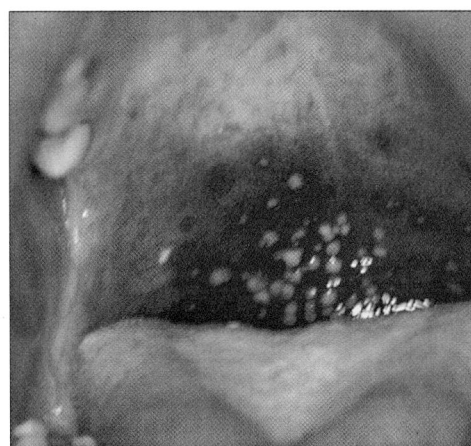

Fig. 33.12 Herpangina in a teenager with severe throat pain.

APHTHOUS STOMATITIS

The cause of aphthous ulceration is unknown but a number of infectious agents, including viruses, have been implicated. It usually manifests as small ulcers of the buccal and labial mucosa, often affecting the floor of the mouth or the inferolateral aspect of the tongue, almost always within the anterior part of the oral cavity; the palate and pharynx are rarely involved. The ulcers are characteristically exquisitely painful, particularly during eating, and in the most severe form can lead to anorexia. Humoral and cytotoxic T lymphocyte-mediated immune responses to oral mucosa have been demonstrated in some patients, suggesting an autoimmune process. The lesions are usually raised and appear greyish yellow, but in severe cases they may be herpetiform with secondary bacterial infection and cervical lymphadenopathy. Major aphthous ulcers may persist for months, but minor lesions usually heal over 2 weeks. They often recur, with periods of remission lasting as long as a few years. Culture of swabs from aphthous ulcers are negative on viral culture. Treatment is usually symptomatic with mouth washes and anesthetic lozenges. Oral prednisolone has been used in some patients but is generally unhelpful. Severe aphthous ulcers have been successfully treated with oral thalidomide. The risk of teratogenicity precludes the use of this drug in women of child-bearing potential. Ulcers are particularly severe in HIV infected patients.

PRIMARY SYPHILIS

Primary chancres can occur in the mouth approximately 3 weeks after oral sex. An ulcerating papule develops at the site of initial contact of *Treponema pallidum* with the oral mucosa. The papule is painless but is accompanied by significant regional cervical lymphadenopathy. At presentation patients are often seronegative, but darkground microscopy of material obtained from the ulcer may reveal spirochaetes, although care should be taken to avoid contamination of the material obtained with saliva because other *Treponema* species inhabit the mouth and may be easily mistaken for *T. pallidum*. Treatment is discussed in Chapter 2.64.

CANDIDA INFECTIONS OF THE MOUTH

Oral candidiasis is a common problem that usually signals local or generalized disturbance of host defenses.

EPIDEMIOLOGY

Most patients who have oral candidiasis are at the extremes of age, but any individual who has recently taken oral or inhaled steroids or broad-spectrum antibiotics is at risk. The disease is also seen in patients wearing dentures and patients who have diabetes mellitus.[25] Between 1980 and 1989, rates of oropharyngeal candidiasis in hospitalized patients increased from 0.34 to 1.6 cases per 1000, caused mainly by the HIV epidemic.[26]

PATHOGENESIS

Yeasts are common colonizers of the oral cavity of healthy individuals. *Candida albicans* is the most common of oral yeast isolates (up to 50%).[27] *Candida albicans* can adhere to complement receptors, various extracellular matrix proteins and carbohydrate residues on oral epithelial cells and oral micro-organisms.[28] The organism exists in yeast and hyphal forms. Invasion of tissue is probably related to secreted hydrolytic enzymes and hyphal formation; each of which is possibly initiated by contact with epithelial cells. The immunopathology of mucosal candida infections is unclear, although suppression of normal oral microflora by antibiotics probably permits proliferation of yeasts. Salivary antibodies inhibit bacterial adherence to buccal epithelial cells and are protective in animal models.[29] Saliva also contains a number of antifungal proteins, including histatins and calprotectin, that protect the mouth in concert with local antibody and cell-mediated defense. A disturbance of cell-mediated immunity is partly responsible for over-proliferation in patients who have HIV-1 infection and malignancy.

CLINICAL FEATURES

In patients using broad-spectrum antibiotics or who suffer candidiasis as a result of denture use, lesions are often erythematous with a burning sensation of the tongue, which displays diffuse redness of the entire dorsum. Most patients who have denture-related oral candidiasis are asymptomatic. Patients who have cell-mediated defects, (i.e. diabetics, those on oral steroids or immunosuppressed patients), mostly have the characteristic syndrome of thrush, a pseudomembranous form of the disease in which there is a layer of white curd-like flecks of material that can be wiped off to leave an erythematous surface, beneath which there may be bleeding points.

DIAGNOSIS

The diagnosis is usually clinically obvious in patients who have thrush, but in patients who have erythematous lesions diagnosis can be made by scraping the mucosa and identifying characteristic ovoid yeasts with hyphal forms on microscopy. The organism can be cultured on Sabouraud's agar, but culture alone is insufficient to make the diagnosis since the organism can be recovered from the mouth of approximately 10% of completely normal individuals with no symptoms.

MANAGEMENT

In normal individuals the disease can usually be terminated by removing the cause – either inhaled steroids or broad-spectrum antibiotics – or by removing dentures at night. If necessary, patients can use 7–14 days of topical antifungal therapy, such as nystatin or clotrimazole, which is usually quite sufficient to ablate the infection. Immunocompromised individuals, particularly those with advanced immunosuppression, may require systemic therapy. For a full discussion of candidiasis in patients who have AIDS see Chapter 5.9.

OTHER ORAL FUNGAL INFECTIONS

Histoplasma capsulatum is endemic in the midwestern USA and Central and South America. The organism is generally associated with lower respiratory tract infection, but oral lesions can occur, particularly in elderly, debilitated patients who have disseminated disease. The lesions tend to appear as erythematous areas that may ulcerate.[30] Biopsy is usually required to established a diagnosis. Because the infection is usually disseminated, systemic therapy with amphotericin B is generally required (see Chapters 7.16 & 8.27).

The dimorphic fungus *Paracoccidioides brasiliensis* is a major cause of systemic mycosis in Central America and South America and should be considered in patients originating from this region. Most patients have an oral mucosal ulcer with some surrounding edema. There may be perioral lesions that may be ulcerated or warty. Diagnosis can be made by smear and culture and treatment with oral imidazole compounds is generally sufficient (see Chapters 7.16 & 8.27).

ORAL LESIONS IN PATIENTS WHO HAVE MALIGNANCY

A common problem among cancer patients undergoing chemotherapy or radiotherapy is severe mucositis and stomatitis that occurs approximately 1 week after the onset of chemotherapy.[31] At this point, destruction of oral epithelium is at its height with an accompanying disturbance of immune surveillance of oral mucosal micro-organisms. This leads to opportunist bacterial[32] or fungal infection. Patients nearly always complain of pain and tenderness in the mouth with or without formation of a pseudomembrane. Symptoms can persist long after chemotherapy has been terminated. Management should include a vigorous search for a microbial etiology; a short course of metronidazole is sometimes helpful (see Chapter 4.9, Infections in patients with chronic lymphocytic leukemia) Some prevention can be achieved by careful oral hygiene and effective management of xerostomia associated with chemotherapy. Once there is established mucositis, topical therapy with antiseptic and anesthetic preparations is indicated. Aluminium hydroxide gel can be used to provide symptomatic relief of painful inflammation.

INFECTIONS OF THE SALIVARY GLANDS

The commonest cause of parotitis is mumps virus, but parotitis can occasionally be caused by bacteria or other viruses, including parainfluenza virus, Coxsackie virus, echovirus, Epstein–Barr virus and HIV.

EPIDEMIOLOGY

The incidence of mumps has markedly decreased in the era of childhood measles, mumps and rubella (MMR) vaccination, which confers lifelong immunity. Despite this, mumps virus remains the most common cause of parotitis. It is highly contagious by airborne droplet transmission. Mumps infections occur in late winter and early spring; enterovirus infections, including parotitis, are mostly seen in mid to late summer. Before the introduction of the MMR vaccine in the UK in 1988, the annual incidence of mumps was approximately 5 per 100,000 population, but in the post-vaccine era this has declined to less than 0.5 per 100,000.[33]

Most patients who have primary bacterial parotitis are over the age of 60 years and are frequently debilitated because of chronic illness or have underlying diseases such as diabetes. Patients who have dehydration, whatever the cause, are at greatest risk. Medications that lead to xerostomia include anticholinergic and occasionally diuretic agents. Poor oral hygiene increases the chances of reflux of bacteria into the salivary gland.[34]

PATHOGENESIS

Mumps virus is a paramyxovirus and gains entry via the respiratory tract. The subsequent viremia allows access of the virus to tissues for which it has tropism, including salivary gland tissue, gastrointestinal tissue such as pancreas, testicular tissue and the central nervous system. The incubation period is 18–21 days.

Bacterial infection of the salivary glands is normally prevented by constant salivary flow, which removes contaminants from the ductal systems. Dehydration, xerostomia or obstruction of the ducts can lead to bacterial proliferation within the salivary glands and subsequent parotitis.

CLINICAL FEATURES

The most common clinical manifestation is gradual onset of painful swelling of either one or both of the parotid glands, which occurs 14–21 days after contact with an infected individual. Pain within the parotid gland can be initiated by salivation during meals, and the glands are tender. Occasionally submandibular salivary glands are involved, but inflammation of sublingual glands is extremely rare. Orchitis is present in approximately 10–20% of individuals and is bilateral in 5%, but there is no firm evidence that it causes male sterility. Mumps meningoencephalitis may occur in concert with parotitis, but patients who have mumps meningitis often do not have parotitis. In the pre-MMR era mumps was a relatively common cause of viral meningitis in children less than 15 years old in whom permanent unilateral deafness was a recognized complication. Pancreatitis is rare. On examination there is smooth tender swelling that obliterates the angle of the jaw and may raise the pinna. Rarely, the outlet of Stensen's duct may be inflamed. There may be generalized symptoms, including fever, arthralgia, malaise and headache, that generally persist for up to a week. Culturable virus is present in the saliva for up to 1 week after gland enlargement. Management is essentially symptomatic.

Recurrent episodes of glandular swelling, particulary of the parotid gland, can occur in children with a history of mumps. Clinical features include recurrent parotid swelling with general malaise and pain frequently after a meal. Viridans streptococci are usually cultured from exudate from the Stensen's duct.

In primary bacterial parotitis there is usually rapid onset of pain, swelling and induration of the involved gland (Fig. 33.13). Manual palpation of the gland is exquisitely painful and can result in discharge of pus from the duct. In addition there are usually systemic features, including fever, rigors and a neutrophilia. The most frequently isolated organisms are *S. aureus, S. pyogenes,* viridans streptococci and *Haemophilus influenzae.*

HIV-associated salivary gland swelling most commonly occurs as a bilateral cystic enlargement of the parotid glands, occasionally in association with xerostomia, dry eyes and arthralgia. Salivary gland involvement can occur very early on in HIV infection but is most commonly seen in late disease. Histologically, there are numerous epithelium-lined cysts, some up to several centimeters in size, containing macrophages and lymphocytes. The commonest identified opportunist infection of salivary glands is CMV; about 15% of postmortem submandibular glands of all patients who have AIDS

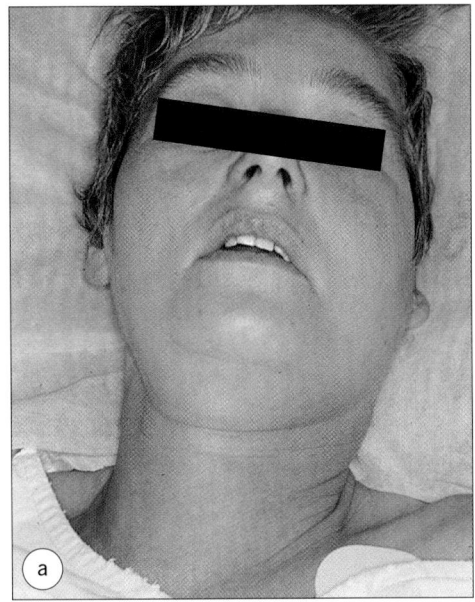
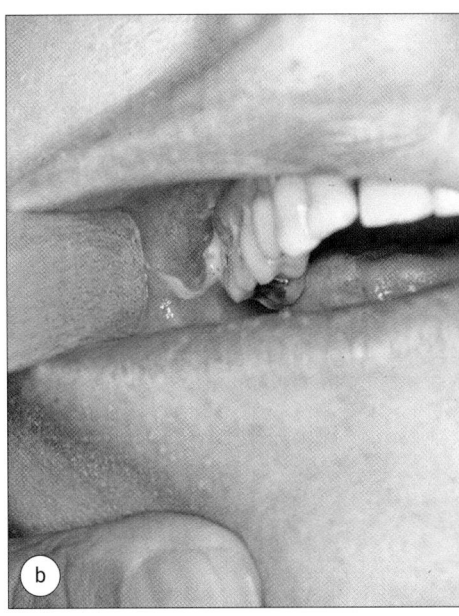

Fig. 33.13 Suppurative parotitis (a) in a diabetic patient who had a recent history of dehydration secondary to diabetic ketoacidosis. (b) Pus was manually expressed from Stensen's duct from which *Staphylococcus aureus* was cultured. Courtesy of Dr E Ridgway.

have evidence of CMV inclusion bodies.[35] In children, there is a strong association between HIV-parotid swelling and lymphocytic interstitial pneumonitis. Examination usually reveals smooth bilateral swelling. Uneven swelling should be biopsied because 10% of salivary gland disease in HIV-infected patients is caused by lymphoma.[36]

DIAGNOSIS

In mumps, this can be achieved by detection of salivary IgM or by culture of salivary washings or of viral throat swab. A convalescent rise in complement-fixing antibody occurs. In established viral parotitis there is elevation of serum salivary-type amylase. Rarely, there may be biochemical evidence of pancreatitis.

PREVENTION

The MMR vaccine consists of live attenuated measles, mumps and rubella viruses. Immunization provides protection for 90% of recipients for measles and mumps and over 95% for rubella. The antibody response to the mumps component is too slow for effective postexposure prophylaxis. After the first dose of MMR, malaise, fever or rash may occur about 1 week after immunization, although this syndrome usually self-terminates within 3 days. Febrile convulsions occur in approximately 0.1% of children between 1 and 2 weeks after administration of the vaccine (similar to the attenuated live measles vaccine), and by the fourth week parotid swelling is seen in approximately 1% of infants.[37]

MANAGEMENT

Management of viral parotitis is symptomatic. Bacterial parotitis can usually be managed by prompt fluid replacement and parenteral antibiotic therapy using amoxycillin/clavulanate 1.2g q8h or intravenous cefuroxime 750mg q8h. Drainage of the duct should be assisted by manual massage. Occasionally steroids are necessary to suppress inflammation and potentiate drainage. Surgical drainage of a salivary gland abscess is rarely necessary.

PAROTITIS CAUSED BY *MYCOBACTERIA* SPECIES

Nontuberculous mycobacterial infections of the parotid gland are now increasingly seen in children, in whom they present as unilateral painless indurated swellings that can be mistaken for neoplasm. Diagnosis can be made by fine needle aspiration with cytology and culture, which may reveal organisms such as *Mycobacterium scrofulaceum,*

Mycobacterium avium-intracellulare or *Mycobacterium malmoense*. Management is conservative. *Mycobacterium tuberculosis* infection of the parotid gland is rare, but is one of the differential diagnoses of parotid tumor, and should be rigorously excluded by histology of needle biopsy or fine needle aspiration cytology before unnecessary deforming surgery is undertaken.[38] The disease responds well to conventional antituberculous chemotherapy.

ESOPHAGEAL INFECTION

Normally there are relatively low numbers of micro-organisms within the esophagus; those present include α-hemolytic streptococci, lactobacilli, *Candida* spp. and low numbers of oral bacteria. Bacterial esophagitis is virtually unknown in the normal host, although occasionally the esophagus may be involved in generalized *M. tuberculosis* infection. Clinically important infections are fungal or viral and occur only in the context of immunosuppression or other underlying systemic diseases. The three most common causes of infective esophagitis in immunosuppressed patients are *Candida* spp. and, less commonly, HSV and CMV.

EPIDEMIOLOGY

Esophageal infection with *Candida* spp., HSV or CMV is generally seen in HIV-infected patients during the late stages of disease once the patient is profoundly immunodeficient, usually once the CD4+ count is less than 0.2×10^6 cells/ml. Each of these infections is an AIDS-defining illness in its own right. *Candida* esophagitis has been described in some patients during seroconversion illness as a result of the profound transient immunosuppression.[39] Patients who have solid tumors undergoing chemotherapy are at risk of *Candida* and HSV esophagitis. Mucositis caused by antineoplastic drugs predisposes patients to deep-seated candidiasis, including esophagitis. Solid organ transplant recipients are also susceptible to esophagitis caused by *Candida* spp., HSV and CMV.

PATHOGENESIS

Candida albicans is the predominant cause of superficial and deep-seated candidiasis, but other significant pathogens include *Candida tropicalis* (an important pathogen in neutropenic patients) and *Candida parapsilosis*. *Candida glabrata*, *Candida lusitaniae* and *Candida krusei* have also been associated with esophageal disease and noted to be resistant to certain antifungal drugs.[40] Deep-seated candidiasis can be seen in patients rendered neutropenic as a result of an underlying malignancy or its treatment, or with significant cell-mediated immune defects as seen in AIDS.

CLINICAL FEATURES

Patients who have infective esophagitis can experience dysphagia or retrosternal esophageal pain (odynophagia), or both. The clinical features of AIDS-related esophagitis associated with *Candida* spp., CMV and HSV are similar, but patients who have AIDS-related esophageal candidiasis often complain of dysphagia rather than pain, whereas odynophagia and retrosternal episodic pain without swallowing, in addition to dysphagia, are more commonly encountered in patients who have HSV esophagitis and CMV esophagitis.[41]

DIAGNOSIS

In the context of oral candidiasis, radiologic or endoscopic investigation of esophageal symptoms is not absolutely necessary, because a therapeutic trial with antifungal agents will suffice. Otherwise, endoscopy is indicated to exclude HSV or CMV infection and also rarer causes of esophageal symptoms in AIDS, particularly lymphoma,

Kaposi's sarcoma, mycobacterial infection, histoplasmosis or squamous cell carcinoma. The endoscopic appearance of *Candida* esophagitis ranges from diffuse mucosal hyperemia, with or without discrete white mucosal patches on the mucosa, to gross mucosal ulceration and perforation. In HSV and CMV disease there are usually discrete single ulcers of the distal third of the esophagus. With CMV disease these tend to be serpiginous, whereas in HSV they are small and punched out. These features can also be seen on barium studies of the esophagus; in candidiasis there is usually mucosal irregularity whereas in HSV disease ulcers can sometimes be seen in the distal third of the esophagus. At endoscopy, brushings are taken for detection of *Candida* spp. by direct microscopy or culture, for rapid diagnosis of HSV by direct immunofluorescence, and for viral culture of HSV and CMV. Biopsy of an ulcer edge may reveal cells with dense intranuclear inclusion bodies indicative of CMV disease, although their absence does not rule out the disease. Alternatively, esophageal biopsies may reveal epithelial cells with ballooning degeneration and occasional inclusion bodies suggestive of HSV infection.

MANAGEMENT

For a full discussion of treatment of eosophageal *Candida* spp., HSV and CMV infection (see Chapters 5.11, 5.12, 8.5 & 8.26).

REFERENCES

1. Shaw JH. Causes and control of dental caries. N Engl J Med 1987;317:996–9.
2. Tanner A, Stillman N. Oral and dental infections with anaerobic bacteria: clinical features, predominant pathogens, and treatment. Clin Infect Dis 1993;16(Suppl 4):S304–9.
3. Loesche WJ. Dental infections. In: Gorbach SL, Bartlett JG, Blacklow NR, eds. Infectious diseases. Philadelphia: WB Saunders:1992:415–23.
4. Goodson JM, Tanner ACR, Hassajee AD, et al. Patterns of progression and regression of advanced destructive periodontal disease. J Clin Periodontol 1982;9:472–7.
5. Chow AW. Infections of the oral cavity, neck and head. In: Mandell GL, Bennett JE, Dolin R, eds. Principles and practice of infectious disease, 4th ed. New York: Churchill Livingstone; 1994:593–606.
6. Kilian M. Degradation of immunoglobulins A1, A2 and G by suspected principle periodontal pathogens. Infect Immun 1982;34:757–64.
7. Clarke NA, Hirscu RS. Personal risk factors for generalized periodontitis. J Clin Periodontol 1995;27:136–45.
8. Peterson LJ. Odontogenic infections. In: Cummings CW, ed. Otolaryngology – head and neck surgery II, 2nd ed. St. Louis: Mosby Yearbook; 1993:1199–1215.
9. Kohler B, Andreen I, Jonsson B. The effect of caries-preventive measures in mothers on dental caries in the oral presence of the bacteria Streptococcus mutans and Lactobacilli in their children. Arch Oral Biol 1984;29:879–84.
10. Needleman IA, Pandya NV, Smith SR, Foyle DM. The role of antibodies in the treatment of periodontitis. Eur J Prosthodont Restorative Dent 1995;3:111–7.
11. Kuritzkes DR, Baker AS. Infections of head and neck spaces and salivary glands. In: Gorbach SL, Bartlett JG, Blacklow NR, eds. Infectious diseases. Philadelphia: WB Saunders; 1992:423–30.
12. Har-El G, Aroesty JH, Shaha A, Lucente F. Changing trends in deep neck abscess: a retrospective study of 110 patients. Oral Surg Oral Med Oral Pathol 1994;77:446–50.
13. Barratt GE, Koopmann CF, Coulthand SW. Retropharyngeal abscess: a ten year experience. Laryngoscope 1984;94:455–61.

14. Sinave CP, Hardy GJ, Fardy PW. Lemierre syndrome: suppurative thrombo-phlebitis of the internal jugular vein secondary to oropharyngeal infection. Medicine (Baltimore) 1989;68:85–9.
15. Thompson JW, Cohen SR, Reddix P. Retropharyngeal abscess in children: a retrospective and historical analysis. Laryngoscope 1988;98:589–97.
16. Colmenero Ruiz C, Labajo AD, Yanez Vilas I, Paniagua J. Thoracic complications of deeply situated serious neck infections. J Cranio-Maxillo-Facial Surg 1993;21:76-81.
17. Lee KC, Tami TA, Escavez M, Wildes TO. Deep neck infections in patients at risk for acquired immune deficiency syndrome. Laryngoscope 1990;100:915–9.
18. Wholey MH, Bruwer AJ, Baker HL. The lateral roentgenogram of the neck. Radiology 1958;71:350–9.
19. Mathieu D, Neviere R, Teillon C, et al. Cervical necrotizing fasciitis: clinical manifestations and management. Clin Infect Dis 1995;21:51–6.
20. Brown JR. Human actinomycosis: a study of 181 subjects. Hum Pathol 1973;4:319–30.
21. Enwonwu CO. Noma: a neglected scourge of children in sub-Saharan Africa. Bull WHO 1995;73:541–5.
22. Topazian RG. Uncommon infections of the oral and maxillofacial regions. In: Topazian RG, Golderberg MH, eds. Oral and maxillofacial infections, 2nd ed. Philadelphia: WB Saunders; 1987:317–29.
23. Adler JL, Mostow SR, Mellin H, Janney JH, Joseph JM. Epidemiological investigation of hand, foot and mouth disease. Am J Dis Child 1970;120:309–14.
24. Bendig JWA, Fleming DM. Epidemiological, virological and clinical features of an epidemic of hand, foot and mouth disease in England and Wales. Communicable Dis Rep 1996;6:R81-5.
25. Iacopino AM, Wathen WF. Oral candidal infection and denture stomatitis: a comprehensive review. J Am Dent Assoc 1992;123:46–51.
26. Fischer-Hoch SP, Hutwagner L. Opportunistic candidiasis. An epidemic of the 1980s. Clin Infect Dis 1996;21:897–904.
27. Samaranayake LB, Holmstrup P. Oral candidiasis in human immunodeficiency virus infection. J Oral Pathol Med 1989;18:554–64.

28. Cannon RD, Holmes AR, Mason AB, Monk BC. Oral candida: clearance, colonization, or candidiasis? J Dent Res 1995;74:1152–61.
29. Challacombe SJ. Immunological aspects of oral candidiasis. Oral Surg Oral Med Oral Pathol 1994;78:202–10.
30. Miller RL, Gould AR, Skolnick JL, Epstein WM. Localised oral histoplasmosis: a regional manifestation of mild chronic disseminated histoplamosis. Oral Surg 1982;53:367–74.
31. Epstein JB, Gangbear SJ. Oral mucosal lesions in patients undergoing treatment for leukemia. J Oral Med 1987;42:132–40.
32. Martin MJ. Irradiation mucositis: a reappraisal. Eur J Cancer 1993;29:1–2.
33. Measles, mumps, rubella. In: Salisbury DM, Begg NT, eds. Immunisation against infectious disease. London: HMSO; 1996:125–46.
34. Work WP, Hecht DW. Inflammatory diseases of the major salivary glands. In: Paperella MM, Schumrick DA, eds. Otolaryngology. Philadelphia: WB Saunders; 1980:2235–43.
35. Wagner RP, Tian H, McPherson MJ, Latham PS, Orestein JM. AIDS-associated infections in salivary glands: autopsy survey of 60 cases. Clin Infect Dis 1996;22:369–71.
36. Kane WJ, McCaffrey TV. Infections of the salivary glands. In: Cummings CW, ed. Otolaryngology – head and neck surgery II, 2nd ed. St. Louis: Mosby Yearbook; 1993:1008–17.
37. Balraj V, Miller E. Complications of mumps vaccines. Rev Med Virol 1995;5:219–27.
38. Weiner GM, Pahor AL. Tuberculosis parotitis: limiting the role of surgery. J Laryngol Otol 1996;110:96–7.
39. Polis MA. Esophagitis. In: Mandell, Douglas, Bennett, eds. Principles and practice of infectious diseases. Churchill Livingstone; 1995:962–5.
40. Richardson MD, Warnock DW. Fungal infection: diagnosis and management. Oxford: Blackwell; 1993.
41. Cello JP. Gastrointestinal tract manifestations of AIDS. In: Sande MA, Volberding PA, eds. The medical management of AIDS, 3rd ed. Philadelphia: WB Saunders; 1992:176–92.

chapter
34

Gastritis, Peptic Ulceration and Related Conditions

Andrew F Goddard & John C Atherton

INTRODUCTION

Until recently the inclusion of gastritis and peptic ulcer in a textbook of infectious diseases would have seemed incongruous. However, in 1983, Marshall and Warren described the bacterium now known as *Helicobacter pylori* (see Chapter 8.19) and suggested that it may be important in the pathophysiology of chronic active gastritis and peptic ulceration.[1] They were proved correct, and it is now accepted that *H. pylori* infection:

- causes chronic active gastritis;
- is the main cause of duodenal and gastric ulceration; and
- is an important risk factor for gastric adenocarcinoma and lymphoma.

This chapter focuses on this infection and on infection with the less common bacterium *Helicobacter heilmannii* (formerly *Gastrospirillum hominis*). The other (noninfective) causes of gastritis and peptic ulceration remain in the realm of a gastroenterology text and are not discussed.

The term 'gastritis' is often erroneously applied to the macroscopic appearance of 'inflamed' (erythematous) gastric mucosa seen at endoscopy (Fig. 34.1a). However, these appearances correlate poorly with histologic inflammation, for which the term gastritis should be reserved. Gastritis may be subtyped from the histologic appearance, which often indicates etiology (Fig. 34.2).

Peptic ulcers may be associated with some types of gastritis. A peptic ulcer is a macroscopic break in the gastric or duodenal mucosa with obvious depth and definite size (usually defined as greater than 0.5cm; Fig. 34.1a–c). Although gastric and duodenal ulcers share some characteristics, there are notable differences in their etiologies and pathogenesis (Fig. 34.3).

EPIDEMIOLOGY

PREVALENCE AND INCIDENCE

The age prevalence of *H. pylori* differs markedly between countries, but two broad patterns are found (Fig. 34.4).

- In group 1 countries (predominantly developing countries), there is a rapid rise in prevalence before 20 years of age, after which point prevalence stabilizes at above 80%, implying that *H. pylori* is acquired in childhood and persists throughout life.
- In group 2 (usually developed) countries, the prevalence of infection increases steadily with age at a rate of roughly 1%/year of life. Most epidemiologic evidence suggests that this is the result of a birth cohort effect.[3] According to this theory, about 30% of 30-year olds have acquired the infection in childhood, compared with 60% of 60-year olds, because of a changing incidence of infection in childhood over the past 60 years.

ASSOCIATIONS

Aside from associations with age and geographic area, *H. pylori* is closely associated with socioeconomic conditions, particularly in childhood. This may explain the different prevalences of infection found in different ethnic groups within the same geographic area.[4] Markers of childhood socioeconomic status that have been correlated with prevalence of infection include general level of hygiene, water supply and sanitation and level of crowding in the household.

Several associations suggest that *H. pylori* can sometimes be acquired in adulthood. Gastroenterologists and endoscopy nurses have a higher prevalence of infection than other medical professionals, presumably from exposure during their professional careers. A study comparing the prevalence of *H. pylori* in a German submarine crew with that in air force staff showed an increase in the submariners, suggesting that overcrowding and close contact are important.[5] Furthermore, a study of servicemen fighting in the Gulf war[6] showed an increase in prevalence over the course of the conflict, consistent with both acquisition of infection in adulthood and an

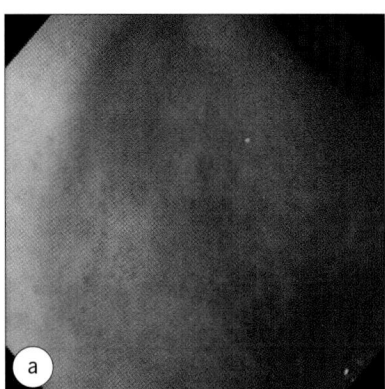

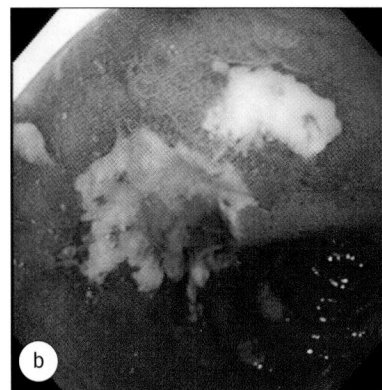

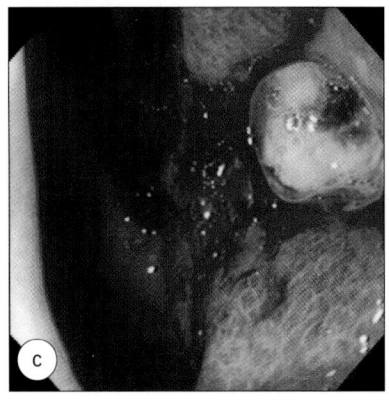

Fig. 34.1 Endoscopic pictures of the stomach and duodenum. (a) Erythema of the gastric antrum. This appearance correlates poorly with histologic gastritis and may be a normal finding. (b) Duodenal ulceration. (c) Gastric ulcer. Note the clot in the base indicating recent bleeding and high risk of rebleed and the endoscope entering the stomach through the cardia.

CLASSIFICATION OF CHRONIC GASTRITIS ACCORDING TO THE UPGRADED SYDNEY SYSTEM		
Type of gastritis		Etiologic factors
Nonatrophic		*Helicobacter pylori* Possibly other factors
Atrophic	Autoimmune	Autoimmunity
	Multifocal atrophic	*Helicobacter pylori* Dietary Other environmental factors
Special forms	Chemical	Chemical irritation (bile, NSAIDs/ aspirin, possibly other agents)
	Radiation	Radiation
	Lymphocytic	Idiopathic, overt or latent celiac disease, drugs (ticlopidine), possibly *Helicobacter pylori*
	Noninfectious granulomatous	Crohn's disease, sarcoidosis, vasculitides, foreign substances, idiopathic
	Eosinophilic	Food sensitivity, possibly other allergies
	Other infectious gastritides	Bacteria other than *Helicobacter pylori*, viruses, fungi, parasites

Fig. 34.2 Classification of chronic gastritis according to the upgraded Sydney system. Other infectious gastritides are very rare, usually occur in immunocompromised patients and are not discussed in this chapter. NSAID, nonsteroidal anti-inflammatory drug. Data from Dixon *et al.*, with permission.[2]

CAUSES OF DUODENAL AND GASTRIC ULCERATION (WITH ESTIMATED PROPORTIONS)			
Cause		Duodenal ulcer (% of cases)	Gastric ulcer (% of cases)
Infection	*Helicobacter pylori*	90	60–70
Drugs	Aspirin and NSAIDs	5–10	25–30
Neoplasms	Zollinger–Ellison syndrome	Rare	Rare
	Lymphoma	Rare	Rare
	Gastric adenocarcinoma	–	2–5
	Other adenocarcinoma	Rare	Rare
	Leiomyoma	–	Rare
Others	Crohn's disease	Rare	Rare

Fig. 34.3 Causes of duodenal and gastric ulceration (with estimated proportions). NSAIDs, nonsteroidal anti-inflammatory drugs.

important role for sanitation. Marital status is weakly associated with infection, but only when children are present in the household, suggesting that in normal life adults occasionally acquire the infection from children.

TRANSMISSION

It is unclear whether *H. pylori* is transmitted by the fecal–oral or oral–oral route of infection, or both. *Helicobacter pylori* DNA has been isolated from drinking water supplies in developing countries (although *H. pylori* has not been cultured from these sources) and the bacterium has been cultured with difficulty from the feces of people who have *H. pylori* infection in both developing and developed countries. *Helicobacter pylori* DNA has been found in dental plaque, but colonization has not been confirmed by culture. Transmission of *H. pylori* has been documented following insufficient sterilization of endoscopy equipment, although with adequate sterilization this is no longer a problem. Acute *H. pylori* infection by this route is thought to be the

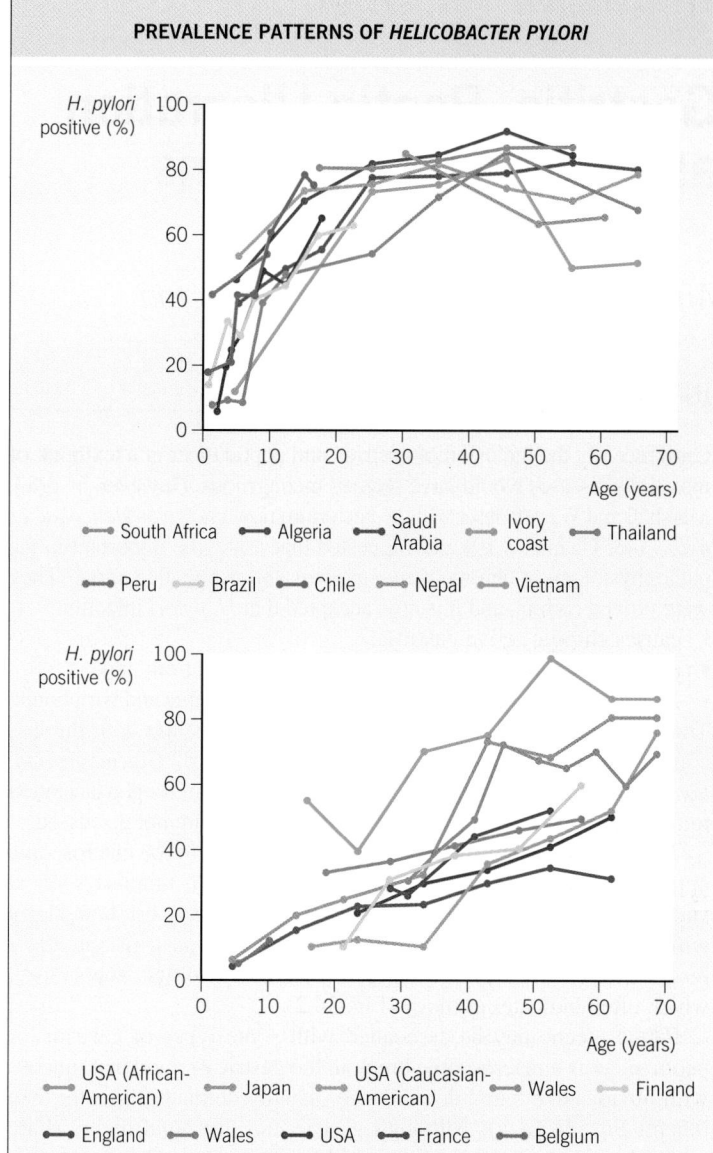

Fig. 34.4 Prevalence patterns of *Helicobacter pylori*. Prevalence of *H. pylori* infection in 10 developing countries (Group 1) and 10 developed countries (Group 2). Adapted with permission from Pounder and Ng, 1995.[3]

cause of epidemic acute hypochlorhydria[7] observed before the discovery of *H. pylori*.

HELICOBACTER HEILMANNII

Epidemiologic data regarding *H. heilmannii* is limited, there being no serologic markers of this infection. It has been estimated from endoscopic observational studies that 2–6% of the population of a developed country harbor the infection.[8] Bacteria identical in appearance are commonly found in a wide range of animals, and many consider the infection to be a zoonosis.[8]

PATHOGENESIS AND PATHOLOGY

Helicobacter pylori is primarily a gastric infection, although it may colonize areas of gastric metaplasia in the duodenum and oesophagus, and rarely heterotopic gastric tissue elsewhere in the gastrointestinal tract. In the stomach, infection causes chronic active gastritis characterized by continuing neutrophil and lymphocyte infiltration, epithelial damage and thinning of the mucus layer (Fig. 34.5a). This is in contrast to gastritis caused by chemical agents, including nonsteroidal anti-inflammatory drugs (NSAIDs), which is characterized by regenerative epithelial changes and a paucity of inflammatory cells (Fig. 34.5b). *Helicobacter pylori* gastritis is associated with several important pathologic conditions including:

- duodenal ulceration,
- gastric ulceration,
- gastric adenocarcinoma arising from the distal stomach, but not from the gastric cardia,
- gastric lymphoma, and
- a form of Ménétrier's disease.[9]

Duodenal ulceration is usually associated with an antral-predominant gastritis, whereas gastric ulceration and gastric adenocarcinoma are usually associated with a pangastritis. However, most people who have *H. pylori* infection do not develop any of these diseases in their lifetime. Where disease does develop, bacterial virulence, host susceptibility and environmental cofactors may all be important.

DUODENAL ULCER DISEASE

Approximately 90% of patients who have duodenal ulceration have *H. pylori* infection; the remaining 10% are aspirin or NSAID users, or have other rare conditions (Fig. 34.3). Few people now doubt that *H. pylori* causes ulcers; the best evidence is that eradication virtually abolishes ulcer relapse.[10,11]

Two characteristics are found more commonly in ulcer-associated than in nonulcer-associated *H. pylori* strains:

- production of a vacuolating cytotoxin; and
- presence of the *cag* (cytotoxin-associated gene) pathogenicity island for which the gene *cagA* is a marker.

The vacuolating cytotoxin is particularly suited to the stomach because it is activated by acid, then becoming acid and pepsin resistant.[12] Although only about 40% of strains isolated in the USA exhibit cytotoxin activity, all have *vacA*, the gene encoding the cytotoxin. However, only some *vacA* genotypes are associated with the toxigenic phenotype, and infection with strains of certain *vacA* genotypes is associated with increased severity of gastric inflammation and prevalence of peptic ulcer disease.[13] The *cag* island is a genetic region separate from *vacA* on the chromosome, containing over 20 genes; some of these encode proteins that cause enhanced inflammation.[14] About 70% of strains in the USA are *cag+*, and these strains colonize the gastric mucosa more densely and are more likely to be associated with ulcers than *cag−* strains.[15] Virtually all toxigenic strains are *cag+*, although the relative importance of the toxin and *cag*-encoded proteins is unclear. Other bacterial factors are thought to be important for pathogenesis such as the enzyme urease and the ability to adhere to gastric mucosa, but these are present in all strains, and so do not explain why only some strains cause ulcers.

Recently, the pathogenic link between infection in the stomach and ulceration in the duodenum has become better understood. Infection of the gastric antrum leads to a reduction in somatostatin-producing D-cells resulting in hypergastrinemia, as somatostatin inhibits gastrin production.[16] Interestingly, this hypergastrinemia is more marked in infection with *cagA+* strains. High gastrin levels lead to increased stimulated acid output from parietal cells in the gastric corpus, which is most marked when the corpus is relatively spared of infection. The

resulting increased acid load entering the duodenum leads to the formation of adaptive gastric metaplasia.[17] This can be colonized by *H. pylori*, and local inflammation and release of toxic bacterial products can lead to ulceration.

Specific host factors predisposing to duodenal ulceration have not been identified. However, environmental factors are important (e.g. smokers who have *H. pylori* infection are more likely to develop ulcers than nonsmokers who have the infection). Aspirin and NSAIDs can cause ulcers independently of *H. pylori* infection and further increase the risk of ulcers in people who have *H. pylori* infection.

GASTRIC ULCER DISEASE

Helicobacter pylori-associated gastric ulcers usually arise in junctional mucosa between antral- and corpus-type tissue, typically on the lesser curvature. They are not associated with increased stimulated acid output, and their pathogenesis is uncertain.

GASTRIC ADENOCARCINOMA

Based on seroepidemiologic data, the World Health Organization has classified *H. pylori* as a type 1 or causal carcinogen.[18] It is a risk factor for distal adenocarcinoma with a relative risk of 4–9, but is unrelated to carcinoma of the cardia, which is now the most common type of gastric carcinoma in the USA. Superficial gastritis caused by *H. pylori* is thought to progress through atrophy to intestinal metaplasia, dysplasia and ultimately carcinoma,[19] but factors governing progression are unknown: *cag+* strains are more likely to be associated with carcinoma than *cag−* strains. Young age at infection, smoking and dietary factors (high nitrosamines, low antioxidants) have also been associated with increased risk.

GASTRIC LYMPHOMA

There is an epidemiologic link between *H. pylori* infection and primary gastric lymphoma. Of particular interest are primary B-lymphocyte lymphomas arising in gastric mucosa-associated lymphoid tissue (MALT). They are thought to be driven by chronic stimulation by *H. pylori* antigens, and when histologically low grade, they regress following *H. pylori* eradication.[20]

HELICOBACTER HEILMANNII: ASSOCIATED PATHOLOGY

Like *H. pylori*, *H. heilmannii* infection is associated with a chronic superficial gastritis. In case reports it has been linked with peptic ulceration, gastric adenocarcinoma and gastric MALT lymphoma, but causality remains unproven.

PREVENTION

Prevention of *H. pylori* infection is difficult in view of our paucity of knowledge about its transmission, although improved living conditions, clean water and improved health should reduce the incidence in developing countries. In developed countries *H. pylori* incidence is falling steadily[3] and specific preventative measures may not be necessary.

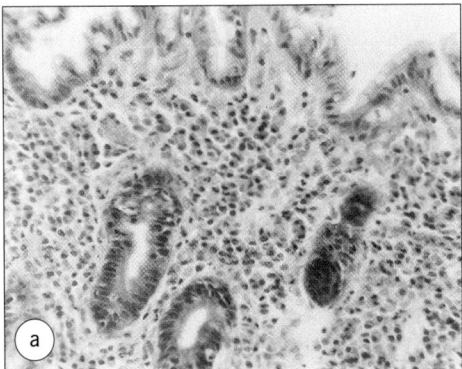
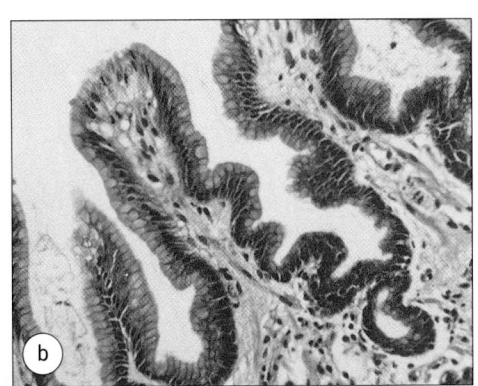

Fig. 34.5 Appearances of *Helicobacter pylori* and NSAID antral gastritis. (a) Antral gastritis in *H. pylori* infection with active (neutrophil) and chronic inflammation of the lamina propria and glands. The epithelial surface is typically ballooned. *Helicobacter pylori* are not readily apparent on a hematoxylin and eosin stain. (b) Antral gastritis associated with NSAID use. Foveolar hyperplasia with a mild chronic inflammatory infiltrate and smooth muscle cells are seen in the lamina propria. Courtesy of Dr MM Walker.

Helicobacter pylori vaccine research is ongoing, with encouraging early results in animal models. However, whether an effective human vaccine can be developed remains to be determined.

CLINICAL FEATURES

ACUTE *HELICOBACTER PYLORI* INFECTION

The clinical features of acute infection in the community are unknown. However, where high doses of cultured *H. pylori* have been self-administered, upper abdominal discomfort and pain occurred 3 days after dosing, followed by vomiting and finally a resolution of symptoms by the end of the week.[21,22] A similar pattern of symptoms was observed in patients with acute epidemic hypochlorhydria,[7] an illness that occurred in volunteers undergoing nasogastric intubation for acid secretion studies in the 1970s and presumed to be iatrogenic acute *H. pylori* infection.

CHRONIC *HELICOBACTER PYLORI* INFECTION

Chronic *H. pylori* infection is characterized by chronic active gastritis, but this condition is asymptomatic. Chronic infection is therefore only manifest symptomatically if complications develop, such as duodenal ulceration, gastric ulceration or gastric cancer. Nonulcer dyspepsia is a diagnosis of exclusion based upon negative results on investigation of dyspepsia. These patients frequently have *H. pylori* infection because of the high prevalence of both conditions, but there is no consistent correlation between symptoms and infection, and *H. pylori* treatment is not recommended.[23]

HELICOBACTER HEILMANNII INFECTION

Whether acute infection causes symptoms is unknown. Chronic infection with *H. heilmannii* appears to be asymptomatic, but there are case reports of the same associated conditions, as described for *H. pylori* infection.

DIAGNOSIS

Diagnosis of *H. pylori* infection can be by endoscopic biopsy-based tests[24] or by noninvasive tests.[25] Most patients require endoscopy to assess indications for treatment, so tests for *H. pylori* are usually performed at this time. The choice of endoscopic-based test depends upon the information required, cost and convenience; usually only a urease test on a mucosal biopsy is used. As infection is very likely in non-NSAID-associated duodenal ulcer, some regard testing for *H. pylori* in this context unnecessary. Our practice, however, is to make a positive diagnosis before prescribing potentially harmful multiple antibiotic treatment regimens. Nonendoscopic tests [the urea breath test (UBT) or serology] are useful in primary diagnosis only if a treatment indication already exists (e.g. in a patient with demonstrated previous ulcer).

Following *H. pylori* treatment, some consider retesting unnecessary due to the high efficacy of modern treatment regimens. We prefer to monitor treatment success or failure as a prognostic guide and as an aid to managing recurrent symptoms. Repeat endoscopy is usually unnecessary, and the UBT, which is well suited for assessing treatment success, is becoming more widely available. However, in situations where endoscopy is conventionally repeated (e.g. to check healing of gastric ulcers to exclude malignancy) biopsy-based tests are equally suitable. Tests must be delayed for at least 4 weeks after finishing treatment or false-negative results may occur; even in primary diagnosis, testing within 4 weeks of treatment with intercurrent antibiotics or bismuth compounds, or within 2 weeks of dosing with proton pump inhibitor may give false-negative results. Serologic tests are not suitable for checking the success of treatment as specific antibody levels fall only slowly.

ENDOSCOPIC TESTS

Endoscopic tests are based on mucosal biopsy specimens. Infection may be patchy, so at least two biopsies should be taken from the usually more uniformly infected antrum to minimize sampling error. In some situations, notably after treatment, during acid suppressive therapy, or when intestinal metaplasia and atrophy are likely (e.g. in the elderly) the infection may be more marked in the corpus, and at least two additional biopsies should be taken from there.

Culture

Helicobacter pylori can be cultured from gastric biopsies, although sensitivity is often low compared with that of other tests. Biopsies should be put into a sterile solution, preferably kept at 39.2°F, and transferred as soon as possible to the laboratory. Methods for culture and identification are discussed in Chapter 8.19. Cultured bacteria can be tested for antibiotic sensitivities and pathogenic potential.

Histology

Chronic superficial gastritis seen on standard hematoxylin and eosin staining is strongly indicative of *H. pylori* infection, but unless specialized stains are used [e.g. modified Giemsa, Gimenez (Fig. 34.6), Warthin–Starry or Genta] the infection may be missed. Histology is expensive, but sensitive, in experienced hands, may provide other useful information, such as the presence of epithelial dysplasia.

Biopsy urease test

In this test, two gastric biopsies are placed in a gel or solution containing urea and a pH indicator. If *H. pylori* is present, its urease enzyme catalyzes urea hydrolysis and a color change occurs. These tests can be performed in the endoscopy room, and are sensitive, specific, cheap, convenient and quick. A positive result can be obtained in a few minutes, although for most commercial tests a 24-hour wait is necessary to ensure that the test is negative.

NONENDOSCOPIC TESTS

Urea breath tests

Several protocols exist,[25] but in essence the patient drinks urea solution isotopically labeled with either stable ^{13}C or ultra-low dose radioactive ^{14}C. If *H. pylori* is present, the urea is hydrolyzed and labeled carbon dioxide can be detected in breath samples. Both isotopes are safe, although it is sensible to avoid ^{14}C in pregnant women and children. ^{13}C-UBT kits with centralized testing of breath samples are licensed in the USA and ^{14}C-UBT kits should soon follow. In Europe some hospitals run their own ^{14}C-UBT service, but ^{13}C-UBT kits are also available. The best UBT protocols are as specific as biopsy-based tests, and are perhaps more sensitive as sampling error is avoided.

Serology

Many commercial and in-house assays, usually enzyme-linked immunosorbent assays are available to test for specific IgG and IgA in serum. The best are as sensitive and specific as other tests, and serologic testing is more convenient and cheaper than even the UBT. This makes it the most suitable test for infection when there is a known indication for treatment and endoscopy is not required. A fall of over 40% in specific IgG titer 6 months after treatment accurately reflects treatment success, but testing paired pre- and 6 months post-treatment samples

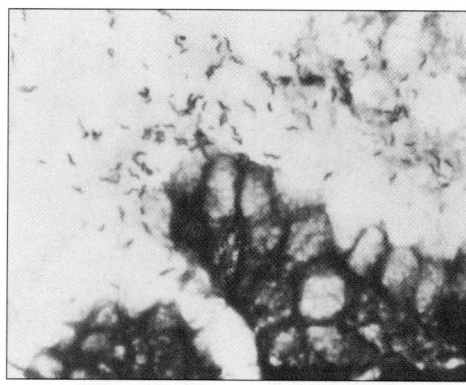

Fig. 34.6 *Helicobacter pylori* **(Gimenez stain).** Other special stains that can be used are the modified Giemsa stain or a silver stain such as Warthin–Starry stain. Courtesy of Dr MM Walker.

presents a storage problem and a long wait for results, and offers little cost advantage over the UBT. Rapid in-office tests for *H. pylori* are being heavily marketed to primary care physicians, but these usually perform poorly in independent studies and are not currently recommended.

DIAGNOSIS OF *HELICOBACTER HEILMANNII* INFECTION

Helicobacter heilmannii is usually diagnosed serendipitously at histology, when its characteristic long tight spiral morphology is easily recognized (Fig. 34.7). It is a very fastidious organism and culture has only recently been achieved. As *H. heilmannii* produces urease, biopsy urease tests and UBTs may be positive, although colonization density is generally low.

MANAGEMENT

The medical and surgical management of gastric adenocarcinoma are not within the context of this book. Here we address the management of *H. pylori*-associated peptic ulcer disease and infection.

PEPTIC ULCER DISEASE

Until recently, treatment of peptic ulcers was based upon acid-suppressing drugs. When the treatment was stopped, the ulcers often relapsed. However, eradication of *H. pylori* not only heals ulcers, but also prevents their recurrence. Therefore, once an ulcer is diagnosed by endoscopy or barium meal, *H. pylori* infection should be sought and if found, treated (Fig. 34.8). This is usually done immediately, but if there is a delay in performing diagnostic tests for *H. pylori*, ulcer healing can be started with acid-suppressing drugs and *H. pylori* treatment can be added when the infection has been confirmed.

Duodenal ulcers are virtually always benign, but gastric adenocarcinoma can present as gastric ulceration. Therefore, additional biopsies for histologic examination should be taken when there is gastric ulceration, with follow-up endoscopy performed 2–3 months after treatment to confirm healing.

HELICOBACTER PYLORI TREATMENT REGIMENS

The longest established treatment for *H. pylori*, so-called 'classic triple therapy'[26] – colloidal bismuth subcitrate, metronidazole and tetracycline (Fig. 34.9) – is still one of the most effective. However, the regimen is complex, side effects are common and compliance may be poor. Also, effectiveness is reduced in patients harboring metronidazole-resistant strains.[27] The more modern 'low-dose triple therapies' – omeprazole, amoxicillin and clarithromycin (OAC); omeprazole, clarithromycin and metronidazole (OCM); and omeprazole, amoxicillin and metronidazole (OAM) (see Fig. 34.10) – are as effective, use fewer tablets for a shorter time and have fewer side effects.[28] We recommend these as first-line treatments. Even simpler 'dual therapies' (a proton pump inhibitor or ranitidine–bismuth citrate plus either amoxicillin or clarithromycin) have been licensed for *H. pylori* eradication, but are less effective and we do not recommend them.

Knowledge of local antibiotic resistance patterns is helpful in choosing an optimal *H. pylori* treatment as regimens are less effective if *H. pylori* has *in vitro* resistance to a component antibiotic. Metronidazole-resistant *H. pylori* are common in:
- developing countries;
- in many ethnic populations within developed countries; and
- in individuals who have previously taken metronidazole for concurrent illnesses, even in the distant past.

Clarithromycin resistance is still rare, but increasing as the antibiotic becomes more commonly used for respiratory tract infections. Amoxicillin resistance does not appear to exist.

For any *H. pylori* treatment regimen, patients should be warned of the importance of compliance and potential side effects. Providing written instructions may be the most effective strategy. The success of treatment should be assessed by UBT or endoscopy, 4 weeks or more after treatment finishes.

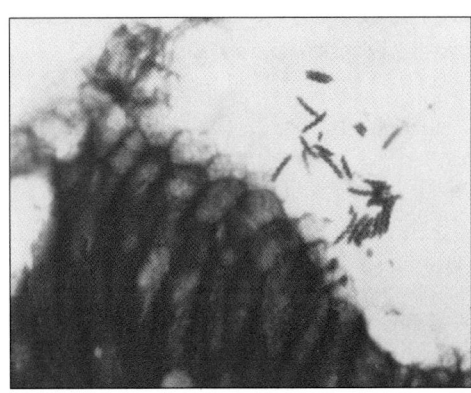

Fig. 34.7 *Helicobacter heilmannii* **(Gimenez stain).** Note the differing morphology from *H. pylori*. These bacteria have a tightly coiled appearance compared with the single curve of *H. pylori*. Courtesy of Dr MM Walker.

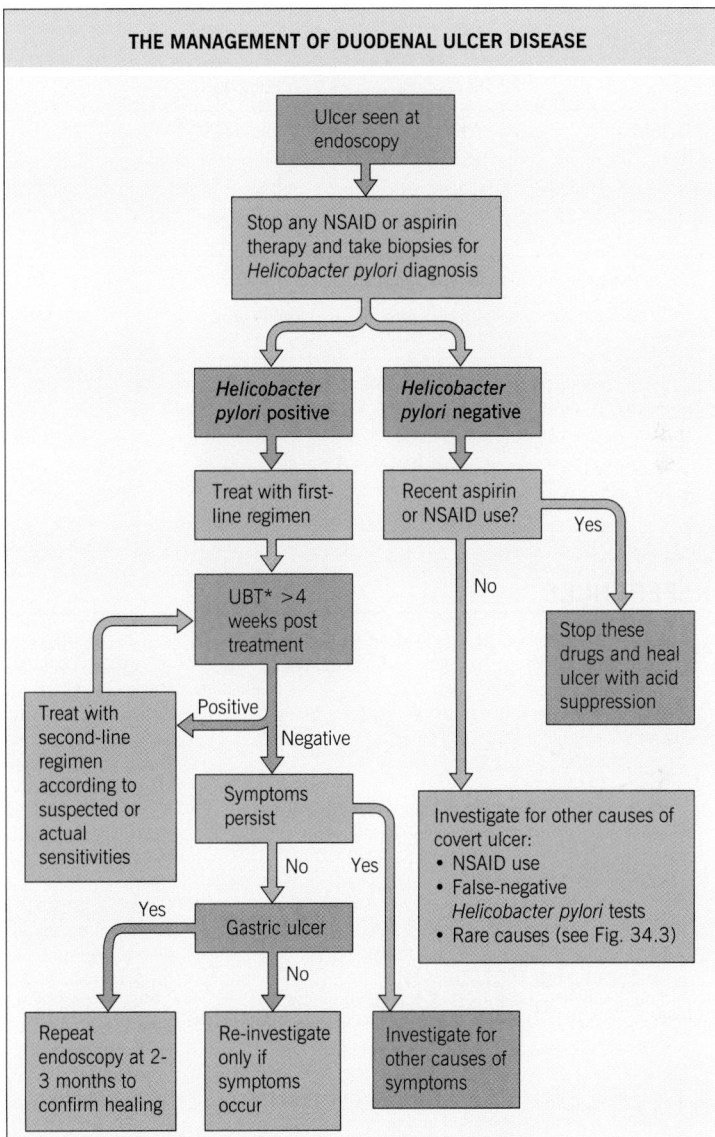

Fig. 34.8 Decision algorithm for the management of duodenal ulcer disease. *Or endoscopy if urea breath test (UBT) not available. NSAID, nonsteroidal anti-inflammatory drug.

FOR WHOM IS *HELICOBACTER PYLORI* ERADICATION JUSTIFIED?

Three groups of patients who have *H. pylori* infection should unequivocally receive eradication treatment:
- those with an active or previous duodenal ulcer;
- those with a nonmalignant gastric ulcer; and
- those with a MALT lymphoma, particularly if at an early stage.

In this last group, the need for additional chemotherapy will depend upon the grade of tumor.

HELICOBACTER PYLORI TREATMENT REGIMENS			
Abbreviation	Drugs	Dosage	Duration
OAC†	Omeprazole* Amoxicillin Clarithromycin	20mg q12h 1g q12h 500mg q12h	7 days
OCM†	Omeprazole Clarithromycin Metronidazole	20mg q12h 250mg q12h 500mg q12h	7 days
OAM	Omeprazole Amoxicillin Metronidazole	20mg q12h 1g q12h 500mg q12h	7 days
BMT‡	CBS§ Metronidazole Tetracycline	120mg q6h 500mg q8h 500mg q6h	14 days
OBMT	Omeprazole CBS§ Metronidazole Tetracycline	40mg q12h 120mg q6h 500mg q8h 500mg q6h	14 days

*Other proton pump inhibitors are equally effective.
†Recommended first-line treatments.
‡Acid suppression can be added to this regimen to speed up ulcer healing.
§Bismuth subsalicylate may be used instead of CBS.

Fig. 34.9 *Helicobacter pylori* treatment regimens. CBS, colloidal bismuth subcitrate.

The benefits of treating other groups of patients should be balanced against the potential risks of treatment.[29] These risks include:

- development of antibiotic resistance (both by *H. pylori* when treatment has failed, and by other organisms within the body);
- adverse drug reactions; and
- rarely, pseudomembranous colitis.

Patients for whom there is some evidence that *H. pylori* eradication may be beneficial include those with reflux esophagitis requiring long-term proton pump inhibition and those with high-grade gastric dysplasia. Recent evidence suggests that people in the former group have an increased risk of developing accelerated atrophic gastritis, which is thought to be an early step in the progression to adenocarcinoma.[30] However, whether the risk of gastric adenocarcinoma is increased and whether *H. pylori* eradication prevents this are both unknown. Until the situation is clear, it may be prudent to err on the side of caution and treat patients in this group. Outside these situations there is no accepted indication to treat *H. pylori* infection for the primary prevention of gastric malignancy, although many physicians treat the infection if there is a family history of gastric adenocarcinoma. Occasional patients with nonulcer dyspepsia make a good symptomatic response to *H. pylori* eradication. However, there is no method for selecting which patients will respond, and we do not recommend *H. pylori* treatment for this indication.

HELICOBACTER HEILMANNII INFECTION
Bismuth monotherapy has been used with apparent success in the treatment of *H. heilmannii* gastritis,[31] but no formal follow-up studies have been performed. We have used classic bismuth based triple therapy successfully.

REFERENCES

1. Marshall BJ, Warren JR. Unidentified curved bacilli in the stomach of patients with gastritis and peptic ulceration. Lancet 1983;i:1311–5.
2. Dixon MF, Genta RM, Yardley JH, et al. Classification and grading of gastritis. The updated Sydney system. Am J Surg Pathol 1996;20:1161–81.
3. Pounder RE, Ng D. The prevalence of Helicobacter pylori infection in different countries. Aliment Pharmacol Ther 1995;9(Suppl 2):33–9.
4. Graham DY, Malaty HM, Evans DG, et al. Epidemiology of Helicobacter pylori infection in an asymptomatic population in the United States. Effect of age, race, and socioeconomic status. Gastroenterology 1991;100:1495–501.
5. Hammermeister I, Janus G, Schamarowski F, et al. Elevated risk of Helicobacter pylori infection in submarine crews. Eur J Clin Microbiol Infect Dis 1992;11:9–14.
6. Smoak BL, Kelley PW, Taylor DN. Seroprevalence of Helicobacter pylori infection in a cohort of US Army recruits. Am J Epidemiol 1994;139:513–9.
7. Ramsey EJ, Carey KV, Peterson WL, et al. Epidemic gastritis with hypochlorhydria. Gastroenterology 1979;76:1449–57.
8. Heilmann KL, Borchard. Gastritis due to spiral shaped bacteria other than Helicobacter pylori: clinical, histological, and ultrastructural findings. Gut 1991;32:137–40.
9. Bayerdörffer E, Ritter MM, Hatz R, et al. Healing of protein losing hypertrophic gastropathy by eradication of Helicobacter pylori. Is Helicobacter pylori a pathogenic factor in Ménétrier's disease? Gut 1994;35:701–4.
10. Hentschel E, Brandstätter G, Dragosics B, et al. Effect of ranitidine and amoxicillin plus metronidazole on the eradication of Helicobacter pylori and the recurrence of duodenal ulcer. N Engl J Med 1993;328:308–12.

11. Forbes GM, Glaser ME, Cullen DJE, et al. Duodenal ulcer treated with Helicobacter pylori eradication: seven-year follow-up. Lancet 1994;343:258–60.
12. de Bernard M, Papini E, de Filippis V, et al. Low pH activates the vacuolating toxin of Helicobacter pylori, which becomes acid and pepsin resistant. J Biol Chem 1995;270:23937–40.
13. Atherton JC, Peek RM, Tham KT, et al. Clinical and pathological importance of heterogeneity in vacA, the vacuolating cytotoxin gene of Helicobacter pylori. Gastroenterology 1997;112:92–9.
14. Censini S, Lange C, Xiang Z, et al. cag, a pathogenicity island of Helicobacter pylori, encodes type I-specific and disease-associated virulence factors. Proc Natl Acad Sci USA 1996;93:14648–53.
15. Atherton JC, Tham KT, Peek RM, et al. Density of Helicobacter pylori infection in vivo as assessed by quantitiative culture and histology. J Infect Dis 1996;174:552–6.
16. El-Omar EM, Penman ID, Ardill JES, et al. Helicobacter pylori infection and abnormalities of acid secretion in patients with duodenal ulcer disease. Gastroenterology 1995;109:681–91.
17. Khulusi S, Badve S, Patel P, et al. Pathogenesis of gastric metaplasia of the human duodenum – role of Helicobacter pylori, gastric acid and ulceration. Gastroenterology 1996;110:452–8.
18. Moller H, Heseltine E, Vainio H. Working group on schistosomes, liver flukes and Helicobacter pylori. Int J Cancer 1995;60:587–9.
19. Correa P. Helicobacter pylori and gastric carcinogenesis. Am J Surg Pathol 1995;19(Suppl 1):37–43.
20. Bayerdörffer E, Neubauer A, Rudolph B, et al. Regression of primary gastric lymphoma of mucosa associated lymphoid tissue type after cure of Helicobacter pylori. Lancet 1995;345:1591–4.

21. Morris A, Nicholson G. Ingestion of Campylobacter pyloridis causes gastritis and raised fasting gastric pH. Am J Gastroenterol 1987;82:192–9.
22. Marshall BJ, Armstrong J, McGechie D, et al. Attempt to fulfil Koch's postulates for pyloric Campylobacter. Med J Aust 1985;142:436–9.
23. NIH Consensus Development Panel on Helicobacter pylori in Peptic Ulcer Disease. Helicobacter pylori in peptic ulcer disease. JAMA 1994;272:65–9.
24. Cohen H, Laine L. Endoscopic methods for the diagnosis of Helicobacter pylori. Aliment Pharmacol Ther 1997;11(Suppl 1):3–10.
25. Atherton JC. Non-endoscopic tests in the diagnosis of Helicobacter pylori infection. Aliment Pharmacol Ther 1997;11(Suppl 1):11–20.
26. Chiba N, Rao BV, Rademaker JW, et al. Meta-analysis of the efficacy of antibiotic therapy in eradicating Helicobacter pylori. Am J Gastroenterol 1992;87:1716–27.
27. Goddard AF, Logan RPH. Antimicrobial resistance and Helicobacter pylori. J Antimicrob Chemother 1996;37:639–43.
28. Goddard AF, Spiller RC. Helicobacter pylori eradication in clinical practice: one-week low-dose triple therapy is preferable to bismuth triple therapy. Aliment Pharmacol Ther 1996;10:1009–13.
29. Blaser MJ. Not all Helicobacter pylori strains are created equal: should all be eliminated? Lancet 1997;349:1020–2.
30. Kuipers EJ, Lundell L, Klinkenberg-Knol EC, et al. Atrophic gastritis and Helicobacter pylori infection in patients with reflux oesophagitis treated with omeprazole or fundoplication. N Engl J Med 1996;334:1018–22.
31. Yeomans ND, Kolt SD. Helicobacter heilmannii (formerly Gastrospirillum): association with pig and human gastric pathology. Gastroenterology 1996;111:244–59.

Enteritis, Enterocolitis and Infectious Diarrhea Syndromes

Roberto C Arduino & Herbert L DuPont

EPIDEMIOLOGY

Diarrheal illness is a public health problem for all populations. Figure 35.1 gives general estimates of the expected frequency of diarrhea development for a variety of populations. In most regions of the developing world, diarrheal diseases are second only to respiratory illnesses as causes of infectious morbidity. In many areas of the developing world, diarrhea is the most important cause of hospitalization among children.[1] The highest rates of illness in these areas occurs in infants under the age of 2 years. Recurrent episodes of diarrhea occur routinely in these regions; each child under the age of 5 years may experience up to six or more bouts of diarrhea on an annual basis.[2] In contrast, the average number of cases of diarrhea for children and adults in the USA is approximately 1–2 bouts per person.[3] In a subset of individuals in industrialized regions, the rate of diarrhea is substantially higher. These high risk persons include international travelers visiting tropical and semitropical regions, the elderly, gay men, infants in day-care centers, persons who receive antibiotic agents and immunocompromised persons, including patients who have advanced HIV infection (AIDS).

Although diarrhea is an important cause of morbidity worldwide, it is the association with excess mortality in children living in developing tropical and semitropical regions that makes diarrheal disease such an important public health problem worldwide. Nearly 5 million children succumb to the disease in the developing world each year.[4] Children younger than 2 years have a five times higher fatality rate than older children. Oral rehydration programs have successfully lowered the death rate associated with dehydration caused by diarrhea in most developing regions.[5] Many deaths still occur in developing tropical regions because of a number of factors, of which malnutrition is often primary. Figure 35.2 outlines a number of factors associated with death in patients who had diarrheal disease. The major factors that translate to a higher death rate associated with diarrhea include:

- malnutrition,
- complications of diarrhea, including dehydration, pneumonia, sepsis and the hemolytic–uremic syndrome,
- infection by an agent more likely to cause dehydration such as *Vibrio cholerae* and rotavirus,
- infection by an invasive pathogen such as *Shigella* spp., and
- failure to receive rehydration or antimicrobial therapy for illness requiring active intervention.

Although oral rehydration programs in developing countries have reduced mortality rates from diarrheal illness, they have not eliminated diarrhea as a cause of death in children. Two forms of enteric disease remain important as causes of fatal and potentially fatal illness. They include persistent diarrhea,[6] defined as illness lasting 14 days or longer, and invasive diarrhea often caused by *Shigella* spp., of which *Shigella dysenteriae* 1 is often the most serious.[7] The causes of persistent diarrhea are multiple, including infection by certain pathogens such as HEp-2 cell adherent *Escherichia coli*, *Shigella* spp. and enteric parasites, plus host factors including malnutrition and vitamin and micronutrient deficiency.

RATES OF ENDEMICITY OF DIARRHEA IN VARIOUS POPULATIONS	
Population	Prevalence/incidence of diarrhea
Infants (<2 years) in developing countries	3–6 bouts/person/year
Older children and adults in developing countries and all age children and adults worldwide	1–2 bouts/person/year
Travelers from industrialized regions during stays in developing tropical or semitropical areas	15–40% per trip
Patients who have AIDS: Africa	40%
North America	15%
Other high risk persons: elderly, gay men, infants in day-care centers, persons receiving antimicrobials	>1–2 bouts/person/year

Fig. 35.1 Rates of endemicity of diarrhea in various populations.

HOST, THERAPEUTIC AND MICROBIAL FACTORS PREDISPOSING TO DEATH IN DIARRHEAL DISEASE	
Host factors	Malnutrition
	Immunosuppression
Therapeutic factors	Failure to receive oral rehydration therapy for dehydrating illness
	Failure to receive antimicrobial therapy for invasive forms of diarrhea
Microbial factors	Rotavirus infection in infants
	Invasive organism (particularly *Shigella* spp.)
	Enterotoxigenic bacteria (particularly *Vibrio cholerae*)

Fig. 35.2 Host, therapeutic and microbial factors predisposing to death in diarrheal disease.

PATHOGENESIS AND PATHOLOGY

The pathogenesis of diarrhea illness caused by enteric pathogens in the gastrointestinal tract involves attachment or adherence to the intestinal mucosa, production of toxins and mucosal invasiveness (Fig. 35.3).

ADHERENCE TO THE INTESTINAL MUCOSA

Adherence is the ability of the organism to attach to and colonize the intestinal mucosa where the disease is caused. It is the first step for production of an infection, which can be followed by toxin production or invasion. Adherence capacity is defined by the bacteria exhibiting mannose-resistant adhesion to HeLa or HEp-2 tissue culture cells. Using these cell lines and varying the conditions of the adhesion assay, three distinct patterns of *E. coli* adherence have been observed.

Localized adhesion [localized adhering enteropathogenic *E. coli* (EPEC)] is characterized by tight clusters of organisms attaching onto

PATHOGENIC MECHANISMS OF DIARRHEA

Pathogenesis	Mode of action	Clinical presentation	Examples
Mucosal adherence	Attachment, colonization and effacement of intestinal mucosa	Secretory diarrhea	Localized adhering EPEC, enteroaggregative *E. coli*, diffuse adhering *E. coli*, ETEC
Toxin production:			
Neurotoxin	Action on the autonomous nervous system	Enteric symptoms	Staphylococcal enterotoxin b, *Clostridium botulinum*, *Bacillus cereus*
Enterotoxin	Fluid secretion without damage to the mucosa	Watery diarrhea	*Vibrio cholera*, ETEC, *Salmonella* spp., *Campylobacter* spp., *Clostridium difficile* toxin A, *Clostridium perfringens* type A
Cytotoxin	Damage to the mucosa	Inflammatory colitis, dysentery	*Shigella dysenteriae* serotype 1, *E. coli* O157:H7, *Clostridium difficile* toxin B, *Salmonella* spp., *Campylobacter* spp.
Mucosal invasiveness	Penetration into the mucosa and destruction of epithelial cells	Dysenteric syndrome	*Shigella dysenteriae* serotype 1, *Shigella sonnei*, *Shigella flexneri*, EIEC, *Campylobacter* spp., *Yersinia* spp.

Fig. 35.3 Pathogenic mechanisms of diarrhea.

the cell surface; diffuse adhesion (diffuse adhering *E. coli*) is characterized by organisms attaching in a scattered pattern onto the whole cell surface; and enteroaggregative adhesion (enteroaggregative *E. coli*) is characterized by clumps of organisms with a 'stacked brick' appearance that attach to cells and coverslips. EPEC adheres to the intestinal mucosa and produces a characteristic histopathologic lesion, named the attaching and effacing (A/E) lesion.[8,9] The A/E lesion is characterized by dissolution of the intestinal brush border, loss of microvillus structures (effacement) and F-actin polymerization beneath the site of bacterial attachment as a result of localized cytoskeletal breakdown.[10,11] The A/E lesion that appears to be a specific marker for EPEC and enterohemorrhagic *E. coli* (EHEC) can be detected by the fluorescent-actin staining reaction. The localized EPEC adherence property is mediated by bundle-forming pili, which cause bacterial aggregation to each other and to the microvilli. This inducible adherence property is conferred by 50–70mDa plasmids encoding the EPEC adherence factor.[12,13] The adhesion is followed by tyrosine phosphorylation of a 90kDa host protein and activation of protein kinases resulting in actin accumulation, effacement, alterations in ion permeability of the membrane (ion secretion or reduced ion absorption) and secretory diarrhea that is characteristic of EPEC infection.

Diffuse adhering *E. coli* is distinct from localized adhering EPEC because it does not hybridize with the EPEC adherence factor probe and is negative in the fluorescent-actin staining test.[14,15] The pathogenic capability and epidemiologic significance of diffuse adhering *E. coli* are controversial.[16]

Enteroaggregative *E. coli* does not hybridize with the EPEC adherence factor probe, is fluorescent-actin staining negative and does not produce A/E lesions. A lesion characterized by shortening of villi, hemorrhagic necrosis and mild inflammatory response of the submucosa is observed in rabbit and rat ileal loops.[17] Enteroaggregative *E. coli* possesses a 55–65mDa plasmid that encodes for fimbriae similar to bundle-forming pili of EPEC and mediates aggregative adhesion and hemagglutination.[18] Enteroaggregative *E. coli* was isolated from US travelers to Mexico and from Mexican and Indian children with protracted diarrhea.[19–21]

The HEp-2 adherence is also exhibited by enterotoxigenic *E. coli* (ETEC), and some salmonella and shigella. Enterotoxigenic *E. coli* produces a specific type of mannose-resistant pili that are important for the adherence and colonization of the mucosa. This adherence capacity is mediated by the production of bacterial surface adhesins called colonization factor antigens, which are genetically encoded by plasmids.

TOXIN PRODUCTION

The toxins produced by enteric bacteria causing diarrhea can be classified as neurotoxins, enterotoxins and cytotoxins.

Neurotoxins

These include staphylococcal enterotoxin b, *Clostridium botulinum* and *Bacillus cereus* emetic toxin. These toxins cause enteric symptoms, primarily because of their action on the autonomic nervous system.

Enterotoxins

These are bacterial products that act on the epithelial cells of the small intestine and produce a fluid secretion without any damage to the mucosa. *Vibrio cholerae* and ETEC produce toxins that are similar in structure and mode of action and are similar to the enterotoxins produced by other watery diarrhea-causing bacteria, such as *Salmonella* spp., *Campylobacter* spp., *Clostridium difficile* toxin A and *Clostridium perfringens* type A. Cholera toxin is a typical A–B subunit toxin. Cholera toxin binds via the B-subunit pentamer to the GM_1 ganglioside receptor on the membrane of the enterocyte. The A subunit enters the cell and is proteolytically cleaved to yield the A_1 and A_2 peptides. A_1 peptide activates adenylate cyclase via ADP-ribosylation of $G_{S\alpha}$, thereby increasing intestinal cAMP concentrations.[22,23] The cAMP activates a cAMP-dependent protein kinase that subsequently phosphorylates numerous substrates leading to inhibition of coupled influx of Na^+ and Cl^- across the brush border of the enterocyte. Cholera toxin also stimulates Cl^- secretion by gut crypt cells. The combination of oversecretion and underabsorption by the small intestine leads to the typical dehydrating diarrhea of cholera. In addition, prostaglandins, platelet-activating factor and the enteric nervous system appear to be involved in the secretory response to cholera toxin.[22,24]

Enterotoxigenic *E. coli* may produce one or two types of enterotoxins responsible for diarrheal illness, a heat-labile cholera-like enterotoxin (LT) and a low molecular weight, heat-stable enterotoxin (ST). The LT produces secretory and absorptive defects in the cells' mucosa, resulting in diarrhea via cAMP activation, after binding to ganglioside receptor GM_1, in the same manner as does cholera toxin. The entirely different STa, which contains 18–19 amino acids, binds to small bowel mucosa cells and activates cGMP, which leads to the secretory effect of enterotoxins. Another different type of enterotoxin produced by ETEC, STb, causes noncyclic nucleotide-dependent bicarbonate secretion in piglet loops, but its role in human disease remains unclear.[25] The genes controlling the production of LT and ST reside on transferable plasmids.

Cytotoxins

The cytotoxins are defined by their ability to produce damage to the mucosa that often results in inflammatory colitis, usually by inhibition of protein synthesis. The prototype of this group is the Shiga toxin, which is produced by *S. dysenteriae* serotype 1. This toxin is immunologically and structurally related to the cytotoxin produced by all strains of enterohemorrhagic *E. coli* O157:H7, an etiologic agent of hemorrhagic colitis and which is associated with hemolytic uremic syndrome. Using DNA hybridization and planned restriction patterns, this cytotoxin has also been shown for other *E. coli* serotypes.

These cytotoxins, also known as verotoxin or Shiga-like toxins, are composed of an enzymatically active A cytotoxic subunit and a B subunit pentamer that binds to the glycolipid globotriosyl ceramide Gb3 cell receptor. The A subunit cleaves the adenosine-4324 in the 28S rRNA of the 60S ribosomal subunit and permanently blocks protein synthesis by inhibiting elongation factor-1.[26] Histopathologic examination of human and animal tissues have suggested recently that vascular endothelial cells are a target for verotoxin. This finding is consistent with the capillary lesions of the gastrointestinal mucosa and renal glomerulus in the hemorrhagic colitis and hemolytic uremic syndrome, respectively.

Strains of *C. difficile* isolated from patients who have antibiotic-associated diarrhea produce a potent toxin that causes cellular damage in tissue cultures. *Clostridium perfringens* also produces a cytotoxin that displays a similar effect to Shiga-like toxin in HeLa cells and in animal models. *Salmonella* spp. elaborate an enterotoxin that activates cAMP and a cytotoxin that inhibits protein synthesis.

INVASIVENESS

Invasiveness is defined by the ability to penetrate into the intestinal mucosa and destroy the epithelial cells, causing a dysentery syndrome. Enteroinvasive *E. coli* (EIEC) and *Shigella* spp. are the prototypes of invasive enteric pathogens. The invasiveness of certain strains of *Shigella* and EIEC is demonstrated in the laboratory by the Séreny test. This test manifests destruction and invasion of the superficial corneal epithelium in guinea pigs. This property is mediated by proteins encoded by 120–140mDa plasmids found in *Shigella sonnei*, *Shigella flexneri* and EIEC[27,28] and appears to be dependent at least in part on additional chromosomally encoded products and a lipopolysaccharide structure.

PREVENTION

The major measure for the prevention of enteric infections is continuous vigilance over water supply and sanitation facilities. The morbidity caused by this type of illness has diminished notably in the USA with improvement in public health measures. The manufacture and distribution of nutritional products require extraordinary precautions from the food industry. Hand-washing is of vital importance, particularly after contact with animals or animal products or after contact with hospitalized patients.

Travelers to countries with higher risk of enteric infections may be able to reduce the probability of developing diarrheal illness by careful selection of food and beverages, use of prophylactic antimicrobial agents, use of prophylactic bismuth subsalicylate, or immunizations. The available evidence indicates that contaminated foodstuffs and water are the most important vehicles of diarrheal illness transmission in developing areas. Public restaurants and street vendors often fail to meet adequate food hygiene standards and food may be contaminated with ETEC, *Shigella*, *Campylobacter*, *Salmonella* and *Aeromonas* spp.[29] It is important to encourage the consumption of well-cooked food, pasteurized milk and potable or processed water or bottled drinks. Controlled studies have demonstrated that bismuth subsalicylate and antimicrobial prophylaxis are effective in preventing episodes of travelers' diarrhea. The protection, however, lasts only as long as the drug is being taken. There are several concerns about the use of antimicrobial agents, such as the risk of causing severe side-effects and the development of antibiotic resistance. Therefore, prophylaxis with antimicrobial agents is currently recommended only for travelers with concomitant serious medical illness, such as inflammatory bowel disease, AIDS, insulin-dependent diabetes mellitus and chronic renal failure, which are underlying conditions that might predispose to complications of dehydration or decreased gastric acidity, or for travelers in whom temporary incapacity is unacceptable.

The indiscriminate use of antimicrobial agents, particularly clindamycin, lincomycin, ampicillin and cephalosporins, increase the risk for developing pseudomembranous colitis in addition to promoting antibiotic resistance in bacteria.

Three typhoid vaccines are currently available. A parenteral heat-inactivated vaccine, an oral live-attenuated vaccine made from the Ty21a strain of *Salmonella typhi*, and a purified Vi capsular polysaccharide vaccine, Typhim Vi, for parenteral use. These vaccines have demonstrated overall efficacy of approximately 70%. Protection after vaccination with any of these three vaccines occurs 2 weeks after completion of the primary vaccine series; therefore, vaccination should not preclude meticulous attention to food and beverage hygiene precautions. The oral-killed B subunit/whole cell cholera vaccine has been demonstrated to give short-term protection against severe ETEC-associated diarrhea in mothers and children in endemic areas.[30] Although imperfect, protection has also been demonstrated in tourists traveling to endemic areas.[31]

CLINICAL FEATURES

Four pathophysiologic mechanisms that induce the production of infectious diarrhea have been described:[32]
- increased active intestinal secretion of electrolytes causing fluxes of water and ions, mediated by bacterial enterotoxins (watery diarrhea);
- malabsorption of nutrients and electrolytes secondary to the damage to the brush-border in either the small or the large intestine;
- increased intestinal osmolality secondary to saccharidase deficiency when the brush-border is damaged, with resultant lactose intolerance; and
- altered intestinal motility.

The first and second are the mechanisms most frequently involved in diarrhea. The role of alteration in intestinal motility is not clearly understood, and does not seem to be enough to produce a secretion of water and electrolytes.

On the basis of the clinical–pathologic features, acute infectious diarrhea can be classified as watery diarrhea, dysenteric syndrome, enteric fever (Fig. 35.4), travelers' diarrhea, diarrhea in homosexual men and diarrhea in HIV/AIDS patients.

WATERY DIARRHEA

This is a noninflammatory process that is confirmed by the absence of fecal leukocytes. There is usually a large volume of stool and a modest increase in the number of stools because the colonic reservoir is intact. This disorder is often manifested by nausea and vomiting, but other associated symptoms include cramping, abdominal pain, arthralgias, myalgias, chills and rarely fever. The diarrhea is mediated by bacterial enterotoxins that alter fluid and electrolyte transport (*V. cholera*,

MAJOR CLINICAL–PATHOLOGIC FEATURES AND CAUSES OF INFECTIOUS DIARRHEA			
Watery diarrhea		Cholera ETEC EPEC *Salmonella* gastroenteritis *Shigella* (initial phase) *Cryptosporidium* spp.	*Clostridium perfringens* *Bacillus cereus* *Giardia lamblia* Rotavirus Norwalk agent
Dysenteric syndrome	Acute dysentery	Shigellosis EIEC EHEC *Vibrio parahaemolyticus*	*Salmonella enteritidis* *Yersinia enterocolitica* *Campylobacter jejuni*
	Parasitic dysenteric-like illness	*Entamoeba histolytica* *Schistosoma japonicum* *Schistosoma mansoni*	*Trichinella spiralis* *Strongyloides stercoralis*
	Antibiotic-associated diarrhea	*Clostridium difficile* (pseudomembranous colitis)	
Enteric fever		*Salmonella typhi* *Salmonella paratyphi* A *Salmonella paratyphi* B (*Salmonella schottmuelleri*) *Salmonella paratyphi* C (*Salmonella hirschfeldii*)	
Enteric fever-like syndrome		*Yersinia enterocolitica* *Yersinia pseudotuberculosis* *Campylobacter jejuni*	

Fig. 35.4 Major clinical–pathologic features and causes of infectious diarrhea.

ETEC, EPEC, *Salmonella enteritidis*, *Salmonella typhimurium*, *Cryptosporidium* spp., *C. perfringens*, *B. cereus*) or organisms that characteristically affect the proximal small bowel (*Giardia lamblia*, rotavirus, Norwalk agent).

Cholera is the prototypic model of enterotoxigenic diarrhea. In any patient who has profuse watery diarrhea and severe dehydration, cholera should be considered. After an incubation period that varies from several hours to 5 days, the illness may begin with sudden onset of profuse, watery diarrhea or anorexia and abdominal discomfort followed by diarrhea. The stool has a characteristic 'rice water' appearance because of the mucus content, and a mild fishy smell. Tenesmus is absent and vomiting often occurs a few hours after onset of diarrhea.[33] Signs and symptoms of the cholera result from the severity of dehydration caused by the fluid and electrolyte losses from the intravascular and extracellular spaces into the gut lumen. Only 2–11% of patients infected with toxin-producing *V. cholera* O1 develop cholera gravis as a result of rapid fluid loss (500–1000ml/h). This leads to tachycardia, hypotension and severe hypovolemic shock.[34] Patients are typically afebrile, but low-grade fever occurs in up to 20% of the cases. Patients may experience abdominal pain, muscle cramps, nausea, vomiting, thirst and faintness as a result of the fluid loss. The electrolyte imbalance may also cause leg cramps. Most cholera complications are related to fluid and electrolyte losses and include altered consciousness, acidosis, hypoglycemia, hypokalemia (rarely resulting in intestinal ileus, weakness and cardiac arrhythmias), hypernatremia and renal failure.

Salmonella gastroenteritis is characterized by crampy abdominal pain, nausea, vomiting and diarrhea that begins 8–48 hours after ingestion of contaminated food. Diarrhea varies from cholera-like watery diarrhea to dysentery. Patients may have moderate fever. Approximately 1–4% of patients develop transient bacteremia. The most common serotypes that cause gastroenteritis are *S. typhimurium*, *S. enteritidis*, *Salmonella newport* and *Salmonella anatum*.

DYSENTERIC SYNDROME
Acute dysentery
This inflammatory or invasive process involves the colon and occasionally the distal small intestine. The finding of numerous leukocytes in feces indicates the diffuse colonic inflammation or invasion of the colonic mucosa. *Shigella dysenteriae* is the prototypic pathogen of bacillary dysentery. Elsewhere, other species may predominate, for example, *Shigella flexneri* in Mexico, South America and most other tropical countries, and *S. sonnei* in the USA. This condition is characterized clinically by fever, passage of low-volume stools that contain blood, mucus and leukocytes (dysentery), and variable degrees of fever, chills, abdominal cramping, tenesmus and vomiting. The patient feels the urge to defecate frequently, and may pass only small stools, flatus or mucus. This is caused by the colonic infection and decreased reservoir capacity of the colon.[35] Occasionally young infants with early shigellosis will have hyperpyrexia and febrile convulsions initially without enteric symptoms. *Shigella dysenteriae* 1 produces a more serious form of diarrhea and has been associated with hemolytic–uremic syndrome, disseminated intravascular coagulation and sepsis.

Enteroinvasive *E. coli* can cause a clinical illness that is indistinguishable from that produced by shigellosis. Enteroinvasive *E. coli* has been reported as causing diarrhea in 6% of travelers to Mexico and in 3% of US troops in the Middle East.[36,37]

A different form of dysentery that differs from that associated with EIEC is the bloody diarrhea (hemorrhagic colitis) caused by EHEC serotype O157:H7 and less commonly a variety of other serotypes O26:H11. This syndrome appears both as sporadic cases and in foodborne outbreaks characteristically associated with the consumption of undercooked ground beef in fast-food restaurants. *Escherichia coli* O157:H7 can cause asymptomatic infection, nonbloody diarrhea, hemorrhagic colitis, the hemolytic–uremic syndrome and thrombocytopenic

purpura. The disease begins with severe abdominal cramps and non-bloody diarrhea. By the second or third day of illness the individual may pass high-volume bloody stools. Nausea and vomiting are present in half of the patients. Unlike EIEC and shigellosis, high fever and fecal leukocytes are not a feature of *E. coli* O157:H7 infection. The hemolytic–uremic syndrome, which is a major cause of acute renal failure in children, develops in about 6% of patients and is usually diagnosed 2–6 days after onset of diarrhea.[38,39] The thrombocytopenic purpura, which is usually diagnosed in adults, has the clinical manifestations of the hemolytic–uremic syndrome, but the renal injury is less severe and the neurologic complications, including seizures, coma and hemiparesis, are more prominent. The clinical features of the hemorrhagic colitis can be confused with noninfectious diseases, such as ulcerative colitis, inflammatory bowel disease, intussusception, ischemic colitis, diverticulosis and appendicitis.

Other enterobacteria that cause dysentery syndrome are *Vibrio parahaemolyticus* and *C. difficile* (pseudomembranous colitis). *Salmonella enteritidis* and *Campylobacter jejuni* involve the small bowel and have the potential for developing acute inflammatory bowel disease. Some parasites may produce dysentery-like illness. Although *Entamoeba histolytica* is the best known pathogen, *Schistosoma japonicum*, *Schistosoma mansoni*, *Trichinella spiralis* and *Strongyloides stercoralis* infections may all result in bloody diarrhea during the acute phase of infection.

Pseudomembranous colitis
This illness is usually a complication of diarrhea associated with the administration of antimicrobial agents. Almost all antimicrobial agents have been reported in association with cases of pseudomembranous colitis. In the pre-antibiotic area, this disease was associated with intestinal obstruction, abdominal surgery, uremia, pneumonia, myocardial infarction and sepsis.[40] The onset of this form of antibiotic associated diarrhea is usually between 4 and 9 days after starting antibiotics. The clinical manifestations vary from mild watery or mucoid green diarrhea to dysenteric syndrome with bloody diarrhea, high fever, marked abdominal tenderness and the presence of fecal leukocytes. The pathogenesis of pseudomembranous colitis may involve the alteration of normal bowel flora by antimicrobial agents or the effect of surgery or debilitating diseases that allows an abnormal overgrowth of organisms. *Clostridium difficile* is documented in almost all cases. Colitis may result from cytotoxins produced by *C. difficile* that alter mucosal function and integrity. Sigmoidoscopy typically reveals the presence of small raised pseudomembranous nodules or plaques that may became confluent over an erythematous mucosa in the distal colon, sigmoid, or rectum. Complications of pseudomembranous colitis include hypovolemic shock, toxic megacolon, peritonitis, cecal perforation, hemorrhage and sepsis. This disorder should be suspected when bloody diarrhea develops in hospitalized patients who are receiving antibiotics. Inflammatory bowel disease, ischemic colitis, and other enteric pathogens such as *Salmonella* spp., *Shigella* spp., EIEC, *E. histolytica*, *Campylobacter*, *Yersinia* and *Strongyloides* spp. should always be considered in the differential diagnosis of pseudomembranous colitis.

ENTERIC FEVER
The enteric fever syndrome is an acute systemic illness characterized by fever, headache and abdominal discomfort. This syndrome is classically produced by *S. typhi* and referred to as typhoid fever; however, *Salmonella paratyphi* A, *paratyphi* B (*Salmonella schottmuelleri*) and *S. typhi* C (*Salmonella hirschfeldii*) may cause a similar but less severe clinical syndrome, referred to as paratyphoid fever. *Salmonella typhi* is a foodborne and waterborne organism for which humans are the only natural hosts. Salmonellae are ingested orally and must transverse the acid barrier of the stomach as well as the various pancreatic enzymes, bile and intestinal secretions, and secretory IgA, which are effective antimicrobial factors. The postgastrectomy state, hypochlorhydria, altered intestinal motility and prior antibiotic therapy are conditions

predisposing to salmonellosis. In addition, salmonella infection is a common occurrence in patients who have sickle-cell anemia, chronic liver disease and immunodeficiency of CD4 cell-mediated immunity accompanying neoplastic diseases and AIDS.

Salmonellae trancytose the intact distal small bowel mucosa, possibly via microfold cells over Peyer's patches. After replicating in the regional lymphatic nodules, organisms spread to the blood stream through the lymphatic route and replicate in reticuloendothelial cells in lymph nodes, liver, bone marrow and spleen. The presence of mononuclear cells in the stool examination when diarrhea is present indicates that the intestinal mucosa is not damaged. The incubation period varies from 5 to 21 days, depending on the inoculum and the immune status of the patient. The onset is insidious, characterized by nonspecific manifestations of remittent fever, headache and abdominal pain. Diarrhea is present in approximately 50% of patients. Physical findings of the patients who has typhoid fever include abdominal tenderness, splenomegaly, hepatomegaly, evanescent maculopapular rash on the upper abdomen and lower thorax ('rose spots'), relative bradycardia and mental confusion (at times delirium).[41] Complications of enteric fever occur during the third week of the illness and later as symptoms resolve. They may be related to recurrent bacteremia with dissemination of the organism, which may result in pneumonia, endocarditis, osteomyelitis, arthritis or meningitis; or related to local organ involvement, such as erosion of blood vessels in Peyer's patches, which may result in intestinal hemorrhage or perforation of the ileum.[42] The case fatality rate in the USA is approximately 2%.

Yersinia enterocolitica, *Yersinia pseudotuberculosis* and *C. jejuni* may also be responsible for an enteric fever-like syndrome indistinguishable from that of typhoid fever. This syndrome has frequently been reported in patients who have underlying diseases such as chronic liver disease, thalassemia, kwashiorkor and amyloidosis.[43,44]

TRAVELERS' DIARRHEA

Travelers' diarrhea is defined as the passage of three or more unformed stools per day in a resident of an industrialized country traveling in a developing nation. The onset of travelers' diarrhea usually occurs within the first 2 weeks after arrival in the foreign country, most often within the first week of travel. Approximately 30–50% of the travelers from industrialized countries that spend at least 3 weeks in a less developed area will experience diarrhea. The illness is more common among young travelers. Travelers' diarrhea is acquired through the ingestion of fecally contaminated food and/or water. A wide array of pathogens, including bacteria, viruses and protozoa, have been reported to cause travelers' diarrhea (Fig. 35.5).[45,46] Enterotoxigenic *E. coli* is the most commonly isolated organism, responsible for 40–70% of the cases of traveler's diarrhea in Latin America, Africa and Asia.[47] *Shigella* spp., *Salmonella* spp. and viruses (rotavirus and Norwalk agent) are each isolated in about 5–15% of patients who have traveler's diarrhea. *Entamoeba histolytica*, *G. lamblia*, *C. jejuni*, *Cryptosporidium*, *Vibrio*, *Aeromonas* and *Plesiomonas* spp. are other enteric pathogens responsible for travelers' diarrhea limited to certain geographic areas and seasons. Giardiasis and cryptosporidiosis watery diarrhea are frequently seen in travelers to Russia and national parks in the USA. *Cyclospora cayetanensis* has been associated with prolonged and intermittent, but eventually self-limiting diarrheal illness in travelers from Nepal, in staff physicians at a Chicago hospital, and in Peruvian infants and children living in the slums of Lima.[48,49]

Travelers' diarrhea is almost always a self-limiting illness, rarely lasting more than 5 days even when untreated. However, 30% of travelers with diarrhea will be confined to bed and another 40% will have to modify their travel plans.[50] The diarrhea is accompanied by abdominal pain and cramps in 20–60% of episodes. Nausea and vomiting are present in about 50% of the illnesses. Approximately 10% of patients develop fever. This clinical presentation is variable and depends on the etiologic agent, microbial virulence, size of the inoculum and host response. Travelers' diarrhea can be frequently separated

ETIOLOGIES OF TRAVELERS' DIARRHEA IN LATIN AMERICA, ASIA AND AFRICA

Organism	Latin America (%)	Asia (%)	Africa (%)
ETEC	40–70	20–34	36
Enteroadherent *E. coli*	?–12	?	?–33
EIEC	6	3	2
Shigella spp.	2–30	2–13	2–15
Salmonella spp.	0–16	11–15	0–4
Campylobacter jejuni	1–7	2–15	1–28
Aeromonas hydrophila	2	1–57	1–8
Rotavirus	4–36	18	0–6
Giardia lamblia	0–9	0–6	0
Undiagnosed	20–30	33–53	15–53

Fig. 35.5 Etiologies of travelers' diarrhea in Latin America, Asia and Africa. Highest rates of ETEC occur in rainy summertime; highest rates of *Campylobacter jejuni* occur in dry wintertime. (With permission from Arduino RC, DuPont HC. Travelers' diarrhea. In: Gracy M, Bouchier IAD, eds. Clinical gastroenterology: infectious diarrhea. London: Baillière Tindall; 1993;7:365.)

into four syndromes: noninflammatory or watery diarrhea (ETEC, *Salmonella* spp., *C. jejuni*, *Shigella* spp. and *V. cholera*), inflammatory or dysenteric diarrhea (*Shigella* spp., *C. jejuni*, nontyphi *Salmonella* spp., *E. histolytica*, *V. parahaemolyticus*, EIEC and *Aeromonas* spp.), vomiting out of proportion to diarrhea (*Staphylococcus aureus*, *B. cereus*, rotavirus and Norwalk agent) and persistent diarrhea lasting longer than 2 weeks (*Giardia*, *Entamoeba*, *Cryptosporidium* spp. and *C. cayetanensis*).

Diarrhea may also occur in travelers within days of their return to their country of origin. In 1–2% of travelers, diarrhea lasts for longer than 1 month. Bacterial pathogens such as *Shigella*, *Salmonella* and *Campylobacter* spp. are the most common causes of chronic diarrhea or remitting symptoms. In addition to parasites such as *G. lamblia*, the most common parasite acquired by travelers worldwide, *Cryptosporidium* spp., *C. cayetanensis* and *E. histolytica* can cause prolonged diarrhea.

DIARRHEA IN HOMOSEXUAL MEN

There is a high prevalence rate of acute rectal and enteric infections in homosexual men. This high prevalence varies widely depending on promiscuity, certain sexual practices and the incidence of asymptomatic and untreated infections. These enteric infections are often polymicrobial.[51] Oral–fecal contamination, which might occur during anal intercourse or oral–anal contact, appears to be the major risk factor for the transmission of enteric pathogens. In addition, anorectal infection with conventional venereal pathogens are caused by rectal intercourse. The predilection of these infections for certain segments of the gastrointestinal tract and the patient's symptoms allow division of the disease into four syndromes. Enteritis is an inflammation of the small intestine; patients may present with symptoms of diarrhea, abdominal cramps and bloating. Pathogens commonly associated with enteritis include *G. lamblia*, *Cryptosporidium* spp. and *Strongyloides stercoralis*. Proctocolitis refers to an inflammation throughout segments of the colon and rectum that causes diarrhea and lower abdominal cramps in addition to the symptoms of proctitis. Sigmoidoscopy is often abnormal beyond 15cm. Proctocolitis is associated with isolation of *Campylobacter* spp., *Shigella flexneri*, *Salmonella* spp., *E. histolytica*, *C. difficile* and *Chlamydia trachomatis* lymphogranuloma venereum serovar. Proctitis implies inflammation limited to the rectum that causes anorectal pain, mucopurulent anal discharge, constipation, tenesmus and rectal bleeding. Anoscopy is often abnormal and evidences rectal exudate, mucosal friability, ulceration and bleeding. Proctitis is commonly associated with *Neisseria gonorrhoeae*, herpes simplex virus, *C. trachomatis* and *Treponema pallidum*. The perianal disease is a dermatologic disorder involving the anus and perianal area that causes perianal discomfort, pruritus and external lesions such as those produced by syphilis, herpes simplex virus, chancroid, granuloma inguinale, condyloma acuminata and human papilloma virus.

DIARRHEA IN HIV/AIDS PATIENTS

Gastrointestinal symptoms are common in persons infected with HIV, and diarrhea is one of the most frequent complaints. It occurs in up to 50% of patients who have AIDS in the USA and Europe, and in up to 90% of those in developing countries.[52–55] A wide array of pathogens, including bacteria, viruses and protozoa, can be associated with diarrheal disease in HIV-infected patients. A pathogen can be identified in 50–80% of patients who have AIDS and diarrhea. Infection of the mucosa by HIV itself, infection with unrecognized or unidentified pathogens, dysregulation of the enteric immune system, fat malabsorption and small bowel bacterial overgrowth are potential causes of diarrhea and weight loss in some HIV-infected patients without detectable pathogens. Figure 35.6 shows the potential small and large bowel pathogens that cause diarrheal disease in relation to the absolute CD4+ lymphocyte count.

Cryptosporidium parvum enteritis is the most common cause of diarrhea in patients who have AIDS. It occurs in up to 20% of AIDS patients in the USA and 50% of patients in Africa and Haiti who have AIDS and diarrhea. *Cryptosporidium parvum* primarily causes a small-bowel disease characterized by chronic voluminous watery diarrhea. Patients may have anorexia, nausea, vomiting, crampy upper abdominal pain, low-grade fever and marked weight loss. Although *C. parvum* is generally restricted to the small bowel, it may involve the stomach and the colon, as well as the gallbladder, the pancreatic and biliary ducts, or the respiratory tract. *Isospora belli* occurs in fewer than 3% of AIDS patients in the USA, but it is an important cause of diarrhea in Haiti and Zaire. This parasite has also been reported in South America, Africa and Southeast Asia.[56] *Cyclospora cayetanensis* has been identified in stool specimens from HIV-infected patients who have chronic diarrhea in Haiti and Mexico,[57,58] but this pathogen is still rare among AIDS patients in the USA. *Enterocytozoon bieneusi* and to a lesser extent *Septata intestinalis* are two microsporidia species associated almost exclusively with AIDS patients. Prevalence rates of *E. bieneusi* among AIDS patients who have chronic diarrhea ranges from 7 to 50%. Enteritis is observed in patients who have CD4+ lymphocyte count below 100/ml. The clinical features of isosporiasis, cyclosporiasis and microsporiasis are indistinguishable from those seen in patients who have cryptosporidiosis. *Giardia lamblia*, *E. histolytica* and *Blastocystis hominis* are not significantly more frequently found among AIDS patients than among HIV-negative homosexual men.

Mycobacterium avium complex infection may present with fever, night sweats, abdominal pain, diarrhea, severe weight loss and anemia. *Salmonella* and *Shigella* spp. may cause protracted, severe and bacteremic infections in HIV-infected individuals despite relatively minor gastrointestinal symptoms. EPEC, enteroadherent *E. coli*, or both, have been found on colonic biopsy from AIDS patients who have chronic diarrhea, malabsorption and weight loss.[59]

Disseminated fungal infections, such as those caused by *Cryptococcus*, *Histoplasma* and *Aspergillus* spp., may also be accompanied by diarrhea. The colon is the site most commonly involved by *Histoplasma capsulatum*.

The colon is the gastrointestinal site most commonly involved by cytomegalovirus. The clinical presentation includes diarrhea with hematochezia, urgency, tenesmus, crampy abdominal pain and occasionally rebound tenderness. Fever, malaise, anorexia and weight loss frequently accompany the colitis. Herpes simplex virus is a common disease among HIV-infected patients, usually confined to the perianal region, rectum and esophagus. In addition to painful perianal ulcers, involvement of the distal rectum may result in low-volume bloody stools, constipation, painful defecation, inguinal lymphadenopathy, tenesmus and mucopurulent discharge that may be misinterpreted as

Absolute CD4+ lymphocyte count cells/ml	Pathogen	Small bowel pathogens	Large bowel pathogens
≥200	Protozoa	*Giardia lamblia*	*Entamoeba histolytica*
	Viruses	Rotavirus	Herpes simplex virus
		HIV	Adenovirus
	Bacteria	*Salmonella* spp.	*Shigella* spp.
		Enteroadherent *E. coli*	*Campylobacter* spp.
		EPEC	*Yersinia* spp.
		Mycobacterium tuberculosis	*Clostridium difficile*
	Fungi		*Histoplasma capsulatum*
≤100	Protozoa	*Cryptosporidium parvum*	
		Isospora belli	
		Cyclospora cayetanensis	
		Enterocytozoon bieneusi	
		Septata intestinalis	
		Microsporidia	
	Virus		Cytomegalovirus
	Bacteria	*Mycobacterium avium* complex	
		Enteroadherent *E. coli*	
		EPEC	
	Fungi	*Cryptococcus neoformans*	

CAUSES OF DIARRHEAL DISEASE IN RELATION TO THE ABSOLUTE CD4+ LYMPHOCYTE COUNT

Fig. 35.6 Diarrhea in HIV-positive patients: causes of diarrheal disease in relation to the absolute CD4+ lymphocyte count. (With permission from Arduino RC. HIV/AIDS: approach to the patient with diarrhea and/or wasting. In: Kelly WN, ed. Textbook of internal medicine, 3E. Philadelphia: JB Lippincott; 1996:1878–80.)

diarrhea. Rarely, extension to the sigmoid colon leads to proctocolitis and mild diarrhea. Rotavirus and adenovirus have also emerged as significant potential pathogens in patients who have AIDS and diarrhea.[60]

DIAGNOSIS

In the diagnostic approach to a patients who has diarrhea, the physician should obtain a careful exposure history and physical examination. Important diagnostic clues are history of antibiotic use, recent and remote travel, duration of diarrhea, weight loss, water supply, hobbies, pets, use of drugs that can cause diarrhea, other cases of diarrhea in the family and diet (e.g. lactose intolerance, intake of unpasteurized dairy products, raw or uncooked meat or fish). Once the context of the diarrheal illness is established, it is useful to distinguish between small- and large-bowel diarrhea. Large volume, and relatively infrequent or nocturnal diarrhea suggests small intestine involvement. It is often associated with bloating, gas and periumbilical pain. On the other hand, frequent small-volume stools with infraumbilical pain on either side and rebound tenderness suggest colonic involvement. Rectal symptoms such as tenesmus, incontinence and urgency occur with colonic and anorectal inflammation. Fever is common, indicating an inflammatory process. Fecal leukocytes and blood in the stool (dysentery) result from diffuse colonic mucosal inflammation. Patients who have colitis can develop severe weight loss, often as a complication of the pathogens causing diarrhea rather than malabsorption.

Laboratory tests for stool samples are time consuming and expensive. Final identification requires a battery of media that is not available in all clinical laboratories. Thus, in nonhospitalized patients who have mild to moderate diarrhea (five unformed stools or fewer without fever and/or cramps, pain, nausea and vomiting) routine stool culture is not justified from a cost–benefit point of view. Supportive treatment can be given. Fluid and electrolyte replacement and diet modification will usually be followed by spontaneous recovery. On the other hand, in patients who have more severe diarrhea (six unformed stools or more, presence of the

INDICATIONS FOR LABORATORY TESTS AND FINDINGS		
Test or procedure	Indications	Positive findings
Fecal leukocyte test	Fever and/or dysentery Moderate to severe diarrhea Hospitalized patients	Infectious: *Shigella, Salmonella, Campylobacter* spp.; less frequently, *Clostridium difficile, Yersinia enterocolitica, Vibrio parahaemolyticus, Aeromonas hydrophila,* EIEC, EHEC Noninfectious: ischemic colitis, Crohn's disease, ulcerative colitis, diverticulitis, pseudomembranous colitis, necrotizing enterocolitis
Stool culture	Fever and/or dysentery Moderate to severe diarrhea Hospitalized patients or hospital admission Diarrhea and dehydration Diarrhea >1 week in duration Patients with immunodeficiency diseases Diarrhea outbreak	*Shigella, Salmonella, Campylobacter* spp.
Parasitic examination	Diarrhea >2 weeks in duration Bloody stool with few leukocytes Recent travel to developing countries, Russia, or Rocky Mountains Diarrhea in homosexual men or in infants in day-care centers	*Giardia lamblia, Entamoeba histolytica, Cryptosporidium* spp.
Proctosigmoidoscopy	Chronic diarrhea Severe antibiotic-associated diarrhea with equivocal test for *C. difficile* toxin Amebiasis Idiopathic inflammatory bowel disease HIV-positive with large-bowel diarrhea or acute proctitis History of anal manipulation	White-yellowish plaques in pseudomembranous colitis, selective sampling of ulcers in amebiasis, biopsy to rule out other pathologies
Gastroduodenoscopy	HIV-positive patients who have small-bowel diarrhea	*Giardia lamblia, Cryptosporidium parvum, Enterocytozoon bieneusi, Septata intestinalis, Mycobacterium tuberculosis, Mycobacterium avium* complex

Fig. 35.7 Indications for laboratory tests and findings. (With permission from Arduino RC, DuPont HL. Diarrhea in the critically ill: causes and treatment in five clinical settings. J Crit Illness 1992;6:715–24.)

aforementioned clinical symptoms and/or positive fecal leukocytes), protracted diarrhea (lasting >2 weeks), dehydration, requiring admission to hospital, who are very young, debilitated or with immunodeficiency diseases, or during an outbreak, laboratory tests can offer invaluable help in diagnosis and management (Fig. 35.7).

DIRECT EXAMINATION

Microscopic examination of fecal smears can give rapid and useful information at a low cost. This test should be done in any patients who has moderate to severe diarrhea. One drop of stool, preferably including blood and mucus, is mixed with two drops of methylene blue on a glass slide, and a coverslip is placed. The finding of numerous polymorphonuclear leukocytes, using high power magnification (×40), indicates diffuse colonic inflammation (involvement of the mucosa) caused by an invasive enteric pathogen, but does not specify the etiology. Mononuclear leukocytes may predominate in patients who have typhoid fever or amebic dysentery. The most common enteric pathogens that cause positive fecal leukocytes are *Shigella*, *Salmonella* and *Campylobacter* spp. Other disorders associated with feces containing leukocytes are *C. difficile*, *Y. enterocolitica*, *Aeromonas hydrophila*, *V. parahaemolyticus*, EIEC and EHEC. The finding of numerous fecal leukocytes is an indication for performing stool culture and giving antibiotic treatment. The examination of feces on saline wet mount preparations by dark-field or phase-contrast microscope for motility can reveal *Campylobacter* or *Vibrio* spp., which show 'darting motility'.

Examination for parasites is indicated in all patients who have diarrhea lasting longer than 2 weeks, diarrhea acquired while traveling to the Rocky Mountains, Russia, or developing countries, persons in day-care centers, male homosexual patients or HIV-infected patients. Wet mounts can be performed using a drop of iodine solution. With low power magnification (×10) eggs, larvae, cysts and trophozoites can be detected. Special stains which are used when trophozoites of amoeba are suspected. *Giardia lamblia* is missed in half of these cases. If *G. lamblia* is suspected but the examination is negative, it is recommended to continue by collecting a small bowel fluid sample, performing a small bowel biopsy, using the nylon string test, or treating the patient empirically (see Chapter 8.3).

Modified Kinyoun's acid-fast stain and trichrome staining of stool should be done, particularly in immunocompromised patients, for cryptosporidiosis, isosporiasis and microsporidiosis. The oocytes stain red against a blue background with these stains. Stool concentration techniques and duodenal aspirates increase the sensitivity of examination for parasites. *Microspora* spores can be demonstrated in stool by light microscopy using Gram, Weber chromotrope-based, Giemsa or chitin-binding fluorochrome stains. However, small-bowel aspirates or jejunal biopsy may be required for identification of these organisms (see Chapter 8.32). Electron microscopy is a valuable adjunct for the identification and taxonomy of microsporidia in infected tissues and fluids.

Monoclonal-based immunofluorescence stains and enzyme-linked immunosorbent assay (ELISA) have been developed for the direct detection of *Isospora*, *Giardia*, *Cryptosporidium* spp. and *E. histolytica* antigens in feces.

Diagnosis of cyclosporiasis can be improved by concentrating oocysts from fecal samples without the use of formalin, to allow them to sporulate at room temperature in 5% potassium dichromate, and visualizing the sporocysts by auto-fluorescence using ultraviolet light or by modified acid-fast stain.

STOOL CULTURE

Bacteria cause 15–50% of cases of diarrhea in adults, depending upon the severity and duration of illness when studied. Clinical laboratories are able to identify the most commonly recognized invasive pathogens, such as *Shigella*, *Salmonella* and *Campylobacter* spp. Routine use of media for the isolation of other pathogens varies depending on the geographic location and patient history. For example, history of exposure to coastal areas and seafood should prompt culture for vibrios (*V. cholera, V. parahaemolyticus* and others). These organisms require a selective thiosulfate citrate bile salt sucrose agar. Culture of *Y. enterocolitica* may require the selective process of cold enrichment, alkali treatment, or selective cefsulodin–irgasan–novobiocin agar, but these methods are not cost-effective for routine diagnosis of diarrhea.

Unfortunately, there are no specific biochemical tests that are useful to detect any one of the different groups of diarrheagenic *E. coli* in stool. The ETEC, EPEC, EIEC, enteroaggregative *E. coli* and EHEC belong to different serotypes based on their O and H antigens. Although certain serotypes have been associated with these different types of *E. coli*, routine serotyping in sporadic cases is of limited value. Immunospecific tests including ELISA, receptor ELISA, latex and coagglutination have been developed to detect both STa and LT. Unlike most other *E. coli* serotypes, O157:H7 does not ferment sorbitol rapidly; here, sorbitol-containing MacConkey agar can be used as a culture medium for stool for patients who have bloody diarrhea, non-bloody diarrhea who may have been exposed to the organism, or the hemolytic–uremic syndrome. Sorbitol-negative colonies that agglutinate with O157 antiserum can be presumptively identified as *E. coli* O157:H7. Commercial testing reactions are available to detect *E. coli* which produces shiga-like toxin. Diagnostic DNA probes from genes encoding virulence factors have been developed to find complementary sequences of DNA by hybridization, and to identify the different groups of diarrheagenic *E. coli*.

Stool cultures for *C. difficile* or tests for the presence of its toxins in stools are indicated in patients who have diarrhea and history of prior antibiotic use. Detection of *C. difficile* toxin A or B can be performed by ELISA or tissue culture cytotoxicity assay, respectively.

BLOOD CULTURE

Blood cultures are recommended in patients ill enough to require hospitalization, in those in whom typhoid fever or bacteremia is suspected, or in those with systemic enteric infections, nosocomially acquired diarrhea or who are immunocompromised.

ENDOSCOPIC EXAMINATION

Proctosigmoidoscopy may be very helpful in the differential diagnosis of patients who have bloody diarrhea, prior antibiotic use, history of anal manipulation, who are HIV-positive with large-bowel diarrhea or acute proctitis. It is valuable in diagnosing pseudomembranous colitis (characterized by whitish yellow plaques), amebiasis (selective sample of ulcers) and idiopathic inflammatory bowel disease.

In HIV-positive patients who have no pathogen identified in stool and/or blood, gastroduodenoscopy is important in establishing the diagnosis in those with small-bowel diarrhea, colonoscopy in those with symptoms suggesting colitis, or both, when it is not possible to differentiate between small- and large-bowel diarrhea. Examination of small-bowel biopsies from the distal duodenum or proximal jejunum should include light and electron microscopy, viral (i.e. cytomegalovirus) and mycobacterial cultures, and special stains for acid-fast bacteria, viral inclusions, fungi and parasites. Examination of colonic biopsies includes light and electron microscopy, mycobacterial and viral cultures (i.e. cytomegalovirus, adenovirus, herpes simplex virus) and special stains for viral inclusion, acid-fast bacteria and fungi.

MANAGEMENT

There are four perspectives in the management of patients who have acute diarrhea: fluids and electrolytes, diet, symptomatic drugs, and antimicrobial agents.

FLUIDS AND ELECTROLYTES

Fluid and electrolyte replacement is the cornerstone of therapy for acute diarrhea.[61] It may be life-saving for infants and the elderly with dehydrating illness. For severe cholera-like diarrhea, fluid therapy has two phases: rehydration over the first few hours of treatment and then maintenance to match continuing losses. Patients who have severe dehydration are ordinarily treated with intravenous fluids and electrolytes. Ringer's lactate is the preferred intravenous solution. For most patients who have diarrhea oral rehydration solution can be used for both phases of fluid therapy. For patients who have intense cholera-like diarrhea, the oral therapy should consist of one of the higher sodium-containing solutions (approximately 90mmol/l sodium) and plain water. For less intense diarrhea not associated with moderate or severe dehydration the solutions with lower sodium content (30–60mmol/l sodium) may be used. Close monitoring of fluid intake, output of urine and vomitus, and hydration status are required for all patients.

DIET ALTERATION

During a bout of illness the diet should be modified.[61] The intestinal tract may have difficulty absorbing certain food items. Milk other than breast milk for an infant should be withheld during the early stages of illness. To facilitate enterocyte renewal, calories should be taken in during a bout of acute diarrhea. For infants breast milk or lactose-free formula may be administered. For older children and for adults the foods to take include boiled starches and cereals such as potatoes, noodles, rice, wheat and oats with some salt added. Crackers, yogurt, bananas, soup and boiled vegetables may also be eaten. When stools are formed, diet may return to normal.

SYMPTOMATIC THERAPY

Although the major objective of therapy for diarrhea in young infants and in the elderly is amelioration of complications of illness such as dehydration, in most older children and nonelderly adults an important objective of therapy is amelioration of morbidity and suffering.[62] Symptomatic drugs do play a role in reducing the number of stools passed and duration of illness in most forms of diarrhea. Nonspecific therapy may be employed where improvement in symptoms is the objective. Figure 35.8 offers a perspective on the use of three common agents used to improve symptoms of diarrhea. These drugs can be useful in nondehydrated patients to ameliorate unpleasant symptoms of enteric illness, helping to return patients to school, work or leisure activities. These drugs do not cure illness and they are not indicated for infants with diarrhea, particularly in developing regions.[63]

ANTIMICROBIAL THERAPY

Although antimicrobial therapy is primarily used for the treatment of pathogen-specific illness, these drugs can be used in one of several clinical syndromes in which an etiologic agent is suggested by the resultant illness.[64] Patients living in industrialized regions with febrile dysentery (presence of fever and passage of bloody stools) often have enteric infection caused by an invasive enteric bacterial pathogen, such as *Shigella* spp. and *C. jejuni*. Empiric therapy in this setting is appropriate. Figure 35.9 lists recommended drugs and dosage for children and adults. For adults one of the fluoroquinolones is recommended. For children trimethoprim–sulfamethoxazole (co-trimoxazole) in combination with erythromycin is recommended. The same drugs are used for adults and children with moderate to severe travelers' diarrhea, in which a variety of bacterial pathogens may be encountered. A single drug, furazolidone, may be used in children with travelers' diarrhea.[65] When diarrhea persists for 2 weeks or longer, a work-up for the etiology should be undertaken. Many would use empiric anti-*Giardia* therapy for such patients, usually metronidazole given for 7 days. For young children furazolidone is preferred because a pediatric suspension form of the drug is available.

In Figure 35.10, specific recommendations for therapy are provided according to the etiologic agent identified. It is advisable to treat all patients who have proven shigellosis in view of the potential for transmission of the infecting organism to susceptible contacts. In the case of intestinal *Salmonella* spp. infection, the decision to use

SYMPTOMATIC THERAPY OF OLDER CHILDREN AND ADULT PATIENTS WITH ACUTE DIARRHEA		
Pharmacologic agent	Dose	Comment
Bismuth subsalicylate	30ml or two tablets each 30 minutes for eight doses for no more than 48 hours	Will turn stools and tongues black; is 50% effective in reducing number of stools passed
Loperamide	4mg initially, then 2mg after each unformed stool, not to exceed 8mg/day (over the counter dosage) or 16mg/day (prescription dosage) for no more than 48 hours	This agent is 80% effective in reducing number of stools passed; the drug may rarely worsen invasive forms of diarrhea and may produce post-treatment constipation
Attapulgite	1.2g initially followed by the same dose after each unformed stool passed not to exceed 8.4g/day	Will make stools more formed; probably the safest form of antidiarrheal compound

Fig. 35.8 Symptomatic therapy of older children and adult patients who have acute diarrhea.

EMPIRIC THERAPY OF ACUTE DIARRHEAL DISEASE		
Clinical syndrome	Adults	Children
Febrile dysenteric diarrhea in industrialized regions or moderate to severe travelers' diarrhea	Norfloxacin 400mg, ciprofloxacin 500mg or ofloxacin 200mg q12h for 3–5 days	Trimethoprim–sulfamethoxazole 5–25 mg/kg/day in two equally divided doses for 3–5 days plus erythromycin 40 mg/kg/day in four divided doses for 5 days; or in travelers' diarrhea furazolidone alone may be given 7mg/kg/day in four equally divided doses for 5 days
Persistent diarrhea (≥14 days in duration) in industrialized countries	Consider anti-Giardia therapy: metronidazole 250mg q8h for 7 days	Consider anti-Giardia therapy: metronidazole 20mg/kg/day in three divided doses for 7 days; use furazolidone in dose given above for 7 days for infants

Fig. 35.9 Empiric therapy of acute diarrheal disease.

antimicrobials often depends on the severity of clinical illness together with the presence of certain host conditions known to predispose to more serious infection by the organism. Indications for treating intestinal salmonellosis include presence of high fever and systemic toxicity suggesting bacteremic illness, or one of the conditions known to predispose to bacteremic illness and higher risk for fatal illness. These conditions include the following: age greater than 65 years or less than 3 months, malignancy, inflammatory bowel disease, hemodialysis, uremia, renal transplantation, aortic aneurysm and patients who have AIDS. For these patients, treatment is given for 10–14 days. Other patients who have less severe cases of salmonellosis without underlying medical conditions need not be treated with antimicrobial agents. Other enteric infections where specific therapy may be given include C. jejuni diarrhea, diarrhea caused by diarrheagenic E. coli other than enterohemorrhagic E. coli (in which case antimicrobials may predispose to the hemolytic–uremic syndrome[66]), Aeromonas and Plesiomonas diarrhea, yersiniosis, giardiasis, amebiasis, isosporiasis and cyclosporiasis. Patients who have cryptosporidiosis are usually not treated, although patients who have advanced HIV infection may benefit from suppressive treatment with paromomycin.[67]

TREATMENT OF PATHOGEN-SPECIFIC DIARRHEA		
Pathogen-specific diarrhea	Drug therapy for adults	Drug therapy for children
Shigellosis	Acquired in industrialized areas: TMP–SMX 160–800mg q12h for 3–5 days; if in developing regions treat as travelers' diarrhea (see Fig. 35.9)	Acquired in industrialized areas: TMP–SMX 5–25 mg/kg/day in two equally divided doses for 3–5 days; if in developing regions or resistance suspected treat with cefixime, ceftriaxone or cefotaxime (see Fig. 35.9)
Salmonellosis	For a healthy person with mild illness or asymptomatic, no antimicrobial therapy; with underlying illness (see text) use norfloxacin 400mg, ciprofloxacin 500mg or ofloxacin 200mg q12h for 5–7 days depending upon speed of clinical improvement	If ≤3 months old, use ceftriaxone 50mg/kg once daily iv; if >3 months of age and healthy with mild illness or asymptomatic, no antimicrobial therapy; with underlying illness (see text) use ceftriaxone 50mg/kg once daily iv (not to exceed 2g/day)
Campylobacteriosis	Erythromycin stearate 500mg q12h for 5 days	Erythromycin stearate 40 mg/kg/day in four divided doses for 5 days
Enterotoxigenic, enteropathogenic or enteroinvasive E. coli diarrhea	Same as empiric therapy for febrile dysentery and travelers' diarrhea (see Fig. 35.9)	Same as shigellosis
Enterohemorrhagic (Shigatoxin and Shiga-like toxin producing) E. coli	The role of antimicrobial therapy is unclear	The role of antimicrobial therapy is unclear
Aeromonas and Plesiomonas diarrhea	Same as empiric therapy for febrile dysentery and travelers' diarrhea (Fig. 35.9)	Same as empiric therapy for febrile dysentery and travelers' diarrhea (Fig. 35.9)
Yersiniosis	Same as empiric therapy for febrile dysentery and travelers' diarrhea (Fig. 35.9); for severe cases use ceftriaxone 1g once daily iv for 5 days	Ceftriaxone 50mg/kg once daily for 5 days
Giardiasis	Metronidazole 250mg q8h for 7 days	For infants furazolidone 7mg/kg/day in four divided doses for 7 days; for older children give metronidazole 20mg/kg/day in three divided doses for 7 days
Amebiasis	Metronidazole 750mg po q8h for 5 days plus diiodohydroxyquin 650mg q8h for 20 days	Metronidazole 50mg/kg/day in three divided doses iv plus diiodohydroxyquin 40mg/kg/day in three divided doses for 20 days
Cryptosporidiosis	None; consider paromomycin 500mg q8h for 7 days for severe cases; in those with AIDS give for 14–28 days then q12h indefinitely	None
Isosporiasis	TMP–SMX 160–800mg q12h for 7 days; in those with AIDS give 320–1600mg q12h for 2–4 weeks then 160–800mg once daily indefinitely	TMP–SMX 10–50 mg/kg/day in two divided doses for 7 days
Cyclosporiasis	TMP–SMX 160–800mg q12h for 7 days; in those with AIDS give the same dose for 10 days then once three times a week indefinitely	TMP–SMX 10–50 mg/kg/day in two divided doses for 7 days

Fig. 35.10 Treatment of pathogen-specific diarrhea. (TMP–SMX: trimethoprim–sulfamethoxazole.)

REFERENCES

1. Black RE, Brown KH, Becker S, Alim AR, Huq I. Longitudinal studies of infectious diseases and physical growth of children in rural Bangladesh. II. Incidence of diarrhea and association with known pathogens. Am J Epidemiol 1982;115:315–24.

2. DuPont HL. Diarrheal diseases in the developing world. Infect Dis Clin North Am 1995;9:313–24.

3. Glass RI, Lew JF, Gangarosa RE, LeBaron CW, Ho MS. Estimates of morbidity and mortality rates for diarrheal diseases in American children. J Pediatr 1991;118:S27–33.

4. Snyder JD, Merson MH. The magnitude of the global problem of acute diarrhoeal disease: a review of active surveillance data. Bull World Health Organ 1982;60:605–13.

5. Impact of the National Control of Diarrhoeal Diseases Project on infant and child mortality in Dakahlia, Egypt. National Control of Diarrhoeal Diseases Project. Lancet 1988;2:145–8.

6. Schorling JB, Wanke CA, Schorling SK, et al. A prospective study of persistent diarrhea among children in an urban Brazilian slum. Patterns of occurrence and etiologic agents. Am J Epidemiol 1990;132:144–56.

7. Gangarosa EJ, Perera DR, Mata LJ, et al. Epidemic Shiga bacillus dysentery in Central America. II. Epidemiologic studies in 1969. J Infect Dis 1970;122:181–90.

8. Moon HW, Whipp SC, Argenzio RA, Levine MM, Giannella RA. Attaching and effacing activities of rabbit and human enteropathogenic Escherichia coli in pig and rabbit intestines. Infect Immun 1983;41:1340–51.

9. Taylor CJ, Hart A, Batt RM, McDougall C, McLean L. Ultrastructural and biochemical changes in human jejunal mucosa associated with enteropathogenic Escherichia coli (O111) infection. J Pediatr Gastroenterol Nutr 1986;5:70–3.

10. Rothbaum R, McAdams AJ, Giannella R, Partin JC. A clinicopathologic study of enterocyte-adherent Escherichia coli: a cause of protracted diarrhea in infants. Gastroenterology 1982;83:441–54.

11. Finlay BB, Rosenshine I, Donnenberg MS, Kaper JB. Cytoskeletal composition of attaching and effacing lesions associated with enteropathogenic Escherichia coli adherence to HeLa cells. Infect Immun 1992;60:2541–3.

12. Levine MM, Nataro JP, Karch H, et al. The diarrheal response of humans to some classic serotypes of enteropathogenic Escherichia coli is dependent on a plasmid encoding an enteroadhesiveness factor. J Infect Dis 1985;152:550–9.

13. Baldini MM, Kaper JB, Levine MM, Candy DCA, Moon HW. Plasmid-mediated adhesion in enteropathogenic Escherichia coli. J Pediatr Gastroenterol Nutr 1983;2:534–8.

14. Nataro JP, Scaletsky IC, Kaper JB, Levine MM, Trabulsi LR. Plasmid-mediated factors conferring diffuse and localized adherence factor of enteropathogenic Escherichia coli. Infect Immun 1985;48:378–83.

15. Knutton S, Baldwin T, Williams PH, McNeish AS. Actin accumulation at sites of bacterial adhesion to tissue culture cells: basis of a new diagnostic test for enteropathogenic and enterohemorrhagic Escherichia coli. Infect Immun 1989;57:1290–8.

16. Girón JA, Jones T, Millán-Velasco F, et al. Diffuse-adhering Escherichia coli (DAEC) as a putative cause of diarrhea in Mayan children in Mexico. J Infect Dis 1991;163:507–13.

17. Vial P, Robins-Browne R, Lior H, et al. Characterization of enteroadherent-aggregative Escherichia coli, a putative agent of diarrheal disease. J Infect Dis 1988;158:70–9.

18. Baudry B, Savarino SJ, Vial P, Kaper JB, Levine MM. A sensitive and specific DNA probe to identify enteroaggregative Escherichia coli, a recently discovered diarrheal pathogen. J Infect Dis 1990;161:1249–51.

19. Bhan MK, Raj P, Levine MM, et al. Enteroaggregative Escherichia coli associated with persistent diarrhea in a cohort of rural children in India. J Infect Dis

20. Cravioto A, Tello A, Navarro A, et al. Association of Escherichia coli HEp-2 adherence patterns with type and duration of diarrhoea. Lancet 1991;337:262–4.

21. Mathewson JJ, Johnson PC, DuPont HL, et al. A newly recognized cause of travelers' diarrhea: enteroadherent Escherichia coli. J Infect Dis 1985;151:471–5.

22. Kaper JB, Morris JG Jr, Levine MM. Cholera. Clin Microbiol Rev 1995;8:48–86.

23. Guerrant RL, Chen LC, Sharp GWG. Intestinal adenyl-cyclase activity in canine cholera: correlation with fluid accumulation. J Infect Dis 1972;125:377–81.

24. Peterson JW, Ochoa LG. Role of prostaglandins and cAMP in the secretory effects of cholera toxin. Science 1989;245:857–9.

25. Weikel CS, Nellans HN, Guerrant RL. In vivo and in vitro effects of a novel enterotoxin, STb, produced by Escherichia coli. J Infect Dis 1986;153:893–901.

26. Endo Y, Tsurugi K, Yutsudo T, et al. Site of action of a Vero toxin (VT2) from Escherichia coli O157:H7 and of Shiga toxin on eukaryotic ribosomes. RNA N-glycosidase activity of the toxins. Eur J Biochem 1988;171:45–50.

27. Sansonetti PJ, Kopecko DJ, Formal SB. Involvement of a plasmid in the invasive ability of Shigella flexneri. Infect Immun 1982;35:852–60.

28. Harris JR, Wachsmuth IK, Davis BR, Cohen ML. High-molecular-weight plasmid correlates with Escherichia coli enteroinvasiveness. Infect Immun 1982;37:1295–8.

29. Wood LV, Ferguson LE, Hogan P, et al. Incidence of bacterial enteropathogens in foods from Mexico. Appl Environ Microbiol 1983;46:328–32.

30. Clemens JD, Harris JR, Sack DA, et al. Field trial of oral cholera vaccines in Bangladesh: results of one year of follow-up. J Infect Dis 1988;158:60–9.

31. Peltola H, Siitonen A, Kyrönseppä H, et al. Prevention of travellers' diarrhoea by oral B-subunit/whole cell cholera vaccine. Lancet 1991;338:1285–9.

32. Mentec H, Leport C, Leport J, et al. Cytomegalovirus colitis in HIV-1-infected patients: a prospective research in 55 patients. AIDS 1994;8:461–7.

33. Cash RA, Music SI, Libonati JP, et al. Response of man to infection with Vibrio cholera. I. Clinical, serologic, and bacteriologic responses to a known inoculum. J Infect Dis 1974;129:45–52.

34. Pierce NF, Mondal A. Clinical features of cholera. In: Barua D, Burrows W, eds. Cholera. Philadelphia: W. B. Saunders Co.; 1974:209–20.

35. DuPont HL, Hornick RB, Dawkins AT, Snyder MJ, Formal SB. The response of man to virulent Shigella flexneri 2a. J Infect Dis 1969;119:296–9.

36. Hyams KC, Bourgeois AL, Merrell BR, et al. Diarrheal disease during operation Desert Shield. N Engl J Med 1991;325:1423–8.

37. Wanger AR, Murray BE, Echeverria P, Mathewson JJ, DuPont HL. Enteroinvasive Escherichia coli in travelers with diarrhea. J Infect Dis 1988;158:640–2.

38. Boyce TG, Swerdlow DL, Griffin PM. Escherichia coli O157:H7 and the hemolytic–uremic syndrome. N Engl J Med 1995;333:364–8.

39. Karmali MA, Petric M, Lim C, et al. The association between idiopathic hemolytic uremic syndrome and infection by verotoxin-producing Escherichia coli. J Infect Dis 1985;151:775–82.

40. Goulston SJ, McGovern VJ. Pseudo-membranous colitis. Gut 1965;6:207–12.

41. Hoffman TA, Ruiz CJ, Counts GW, Sachs JM, Nitzkin JL. Waterborne typhoid fever in Dade County, Florida. Clinical and therapeutic evaluation of 105 bacteremic patients. Am J Med 1975;59:481–7.

42. Rowland HAK. The complications of typhoid fever. J Trop Med Hyg 1961;64:143–52.

43. Rabson AR, Hallett AF, Koornhof HJ. Generalized Yersinia enterocolitica infection. J Infect Dis 1975;131:447–51.

44. Schmidt U, Chmel H, Kaminski Z, Sen P. The clinical spectrum of Campylobacter fetus infection: report of 5 cases and review of the literature. Q J Med 1980;49:431–42.

45. Black RE. Pathogens that cause travelers' diarrhea in Latin America and Africa. Rev Infect Dis 1986;8(suppl 2):131–5.

46. Taylor DN, Echeverria P. Etiology and epidemiology of travelers' diarrhea in Asia. Rev Infect Dis 1986;8(suppl 2):136–41.

47. Gorbach SL, Kean BH, Evans DG, Evans DJ Jr, Bessudo D. Travelers' diarrhea and toxigenic Escherichia coli. N Engl J Med 1975;292:933–6.

48. Ortega YR, Sterling CR, Gilman RH, Cama VA, Díaz F. Cyclospora species – a new protozoan pathogen of humans. N Engl J Med 1993;328:1308–12.

49. Centers for Disease Control. Outbreaks of diarrheal illness associated with cyanobacteria (blue-green algae)-like bodies – Chicago/Nepal, 1989 and 1990. MMWR Morb Mort Wkly Rep 1991;40:325–7.

50. Gorbach SL. Travelers' diarrhea. N Engl J Med 1982;307:881–3.

51. Quinn TC, Stamm WE, Goodell SE, et al. The polymicrobial origin of intestinal infections in homosexual men. N Engl J Med 1983;309:576–82.

52. Smith PD, Lane HC, Gill VJ, et al. Intestinal infections in patients with the acquired immunodeficiency syndrome (AIDS). Etiology and response to therapy. Ann Intern Med 1988;108:328–33.

53. René E, Marche C, Regnier B, et al. Intestinal infections in patients with acquired immunodeficiency syndrome. A prospective study in 132 patients. Dig Dis Sci 1989;34:773–80.

54. Colebunders R, Francis H, Mann JM, et al. Persistent diarrhea strongly associated with HIV infection in Kinshasa, Zaire. Am J Gastroenterol 1987;82:859–64.

55. Smith PD. Infectious diarrheas in patients with AIDS. Gastroenterol Clin North Am 1993;22:535–48.

56. DeHovitz JA, Pape JW, Boncy M, Johnson WD Jr. Clinical manifestations and therapy of Isospora belli infection in patients with the acquired immunodeficiency syndrome. N Engl J Med 1986;315:87–90.

57. Pape JW, Verdier RI, Boncy M, Boncy J, Johnson WD Jr. Cyclospora infection in adults infected with HIV. Clinical manifestations, treatment, and prophylaxis. Ann Intern Med 1994;121:654–7.

58. Sifuentes-Osornio J, Porras-Cortés G, Bendall RP, et al. Cyclospora cayetanensis infection in patients with and without AIDS: biliary disease as another clinical manifestation. Clin Infect Dis 1995;21:1092–7.

59. Kotler DP, Orenstein JM. Chronic diarrhea and malabsorption associated with enteropathogenic bacterial infection in a patient with AIDS. Ann Intern Med 1993;119:127–8.

60. Janoff EN, Orenstein JM, Manischewitz JF, Smith PD. Adenovirus colitis in the acquired immunodeficiency syndrome. Gastroenterology 1991;100:976–9.

61. Duggan C, Santosham M, Glass RI. The management of acute diarrhea in children: oral rehydration, maintenance, and nutritional therapy. Centers for Disease Control and Prevention. MMWR Morb Mort Wkly Rep 1992;41:1–20.

62. DuPont HL. Commentary: the diarrhea burden in industrialized regions. Infect Dis Clin Pract 1995;4:386–8.

63. The rational use of drugs in the management of acute diarrhoea in children. Geneva: World Health Organization; 1990:1–71.

64. DuPont HL. Nonfluid therapy and selected chemoprophylaxis of acute diarrhea. Am J Med 1985;78(suppl 6B):81–90.

65. DuPont HL, Ericsson CD, Galindo E, et al. Furazolidone versus ampicillin in the treatment of traveler's diarrhea. Antimicrob Agents Chemother 1984;26:160–3.

66. Pavia AT, Nichols CR, Green DP, et al. Hemolytic–uremic syndrome during an outbreak of Escherichia coli O157:H7 infections in institutions for mentally retarded persons: clinical and epidemiologic observations. J Pediatr 1990;116:544–1.

67. White AC Jr, Chappell CL, Hayat CS, et al. Paromomycin for cryptosporidiosis in AIDS: a prospective, double-blind trial. J Infect Dis 1994;170:419–24.

Whipple's Disease

Andrew M Veitch & Michael JG Farthing

EPIDEMIOLOGY

Whipple's disease was originally described by George Whipple in the Johns Hopkins Medical Bulletin in 1907.[1] The disease is rare, with fewer than 1000 validated cases reported in the literature, although it has been estimated that two to three unpublished cases may exist for each one reported. The majority of cases have occurred in the USA, the UK, Europe, Australia, South America and South Africa, with a small number of additional cases from Japan, India and China.

The largest review to date, published in 1970, reported 19 patients who had Whipple's disease, and reviewed the literature from 1950 to 1969.[2] A further 114 patients were identified, of whom 88% were male. All 114 patients were white, with the exception of one native American and three black patients. Of the 19 patients reported, 18 were male and all were white. The mean age at diagnosis was 48 years (range 33–62 years). Other studies have confirmed this demographic distribution.

PATHOGENESIS AND PATHOLOGY

Whipple's disease is a multisystem disorder. It most commonly affects the small intestine and its lymphatic drainage, but the pathologic features of the disease have been demonstrated in most organs (Fig. 36.1). In the small intestinal mucosa the presence of numerous macrophages that stain strongly with periodic acid Schiff (PAS) is pathognomonic (Fig. 36.2). Whipple noted the presence of a great number of rod-shaped organisms in affected tissues but these were only identified as bacilli in 1961, when Whipple's disease tissue was examined using electron microscopy.[3] The bacilli are rod-shaped and approximately 0.2mm wide by 1.5–2.5mm long, with cell walls that consist of a trilaminar membrane (Fig. 36.3). These cell walls reflect the PAS-positive material within macrophages in affected tissues seen under light microscopy. Despite repeated efforts, these bacteria have never been cultured successfully; however, they have been identified and classified phylogenetically using molecular genetic techniques.

PATHOLOGIC FEATURES OF WHIPPLE'S DISEASE	
System	Feature
Gastrointestinal tract	Transmural involvement of the esophagus, stomach, intestine and colon
	PAS-positive macrophages concentrated in lamina propria
Central nervous system	PAS-positive macrophages present throughout the brain
	Occasional microinfarcts reported as a result of microvascular occlusion
Cardiovascular system	PAS-positive macrophages in endocardium, myocardium and pericardium
	Fibrosis of heart valves
	Lymphocytic myocarditis
Respiratory system	PAS-positive macrophages predominantly in intra-alveolar septa and pleura of lungs
	Occasionally granulomatous 'sarcoid-like' reaction in tissues
Genitourinary tract	Few PAS-positive macrophages noted
Lymphoreticular system	PAS-positive macrophages in spleen and lymph nodes throughout body
Eyes	Uveitis
	PAS-positive macrophages in vitreous humor
Bone marrow	Focal collections of PAS-positive macrophages

Fig. 36.1 Pathologic features of Whipple's disease.

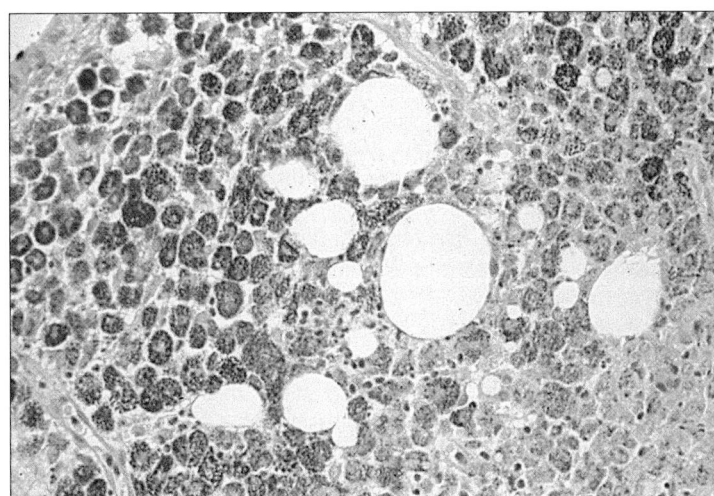

Fig. 36.2 Section from a PAS-stained duodenal biopsy. Numerous (pink-staining) PAS-positive macrophages in the lamina propria are shown.

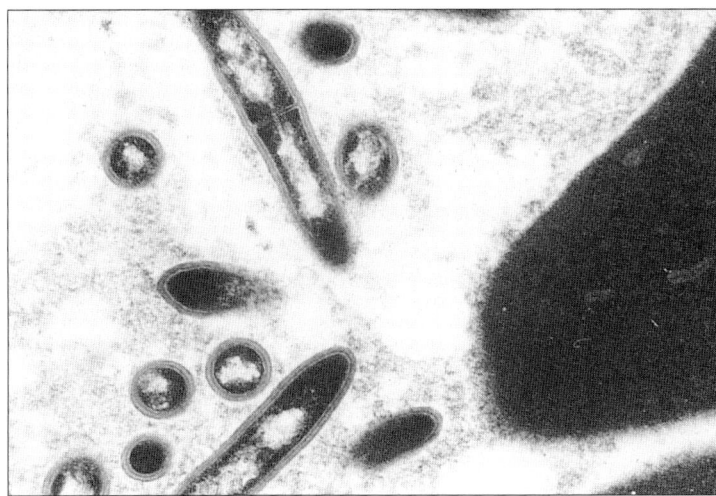

Fig. 36.3 Electron micrograph of small intestinal mucosa, demonstrating the typical appearance of the Whipple's disease bacillus. Courtesy of Professor H Hodgson.

Bacteria can be identified by amplification of the bacterial small subunit (16S) rRNA sequence from infected tissue. rRNA is present in all living cells and is highly conserved. All genetic sequences accumulate mutations with time; the evolutionary distance between species is proportional to the number of nucleotide differences between two copies of the same gene and can be inferred from the number of rRNA sequence differences between them, thereby allowing a phylogenetic classification. The phylogenetic classification of an unknown organism can be determined by comparing its 16S rRNA with a catalog of rRNA sequences from known organisms. The polymerase chain reaction (PCR) is used to amplify and sequence minute quantities of rRNA from infected tissue. In 1991 this technique was applied to a small bowel specimen from a patient who has Whipple's disease.[4] On the basis of its16S rRNA sequence the organism was found to be most closely related to *Rhodococcus*, *Arthrobacter* and *Streptomyces* spp. (see Chapter 8.15). In 1992 a unique 1321-base bacterial 16S rRNA sequence was identified in a patient who has Whipple's disease; from this sequence specific PCR primers that enabled detection of this bacillus in four other patients were designed.[5] The organism was not detectable in tissue from 10 control patients. Analysis of the 1321-base 16S rRNA sequence revealed the organism to be a previously uncharacterized bacterium belonging to the subdivision of Gram-positive bacteria known as actinomycetes (Fig. 36.4). This newly characterized organism has been named *Tropheryma whippelii*. Using a similar technique, a second, distinct bacterium related to the nocardioforms has been identified, but this has only been reported in a single patient who has Whipple's disease.[6]

Whipple's disease bacillus has been identified using light or electron microscopy (EM) in all tissues affected by the disease. However, the pathogenesis of the disease is unknown. EM studies of infected intestinal mucosa have demonstrated extensive epithelial cell invasion by bacilli;[7] the route of invasion appears to be from the lamina propria rather than the intestinal lumen. There is evidence of ultrastructural damage to the infected epithelial cells, but no signs of injury were seen in macrophages, polymorphonuclear leukocytes, plasma cells, mast cells or intraepithelial lymphocytes containing the bacilli.

Several attempts have been made to investigate whether there is a host immune defect in patients who have Whipple's disease. No abnormalities of humoral immunity have been demonstrated, but subtle defects of cell-mediated immunity have been noted, with a reduction in the number of circulating lymphocytes and a decreased response to mitogens. It is not possible to distinguish a primary immunologic defect from those that might arise as a consequence of nutritional deficiency. A decreased response to skin test antigens has been described, which persists after treatment. In addition there is a greater association with the HLA B27 haplotype in Whipple's disease patients than in controls.[8] In a recent immunohistochemical study, major histocompatibility complex (MHC) class I expression on small intestinal epithelial cells was normal, but MHC class II was markedly reduced compared with controls.[9] This defect was restored to normal after treatment, suggesting that the observed immune changes in the intestinal mucosa may occur as a result of infection rather than as a primary defect.

The characteristic pathologic appearances of Whipple's disease are seen in the small intestine. Macroscopically the mucosa is often normal, although it may appear erythematous, with a friable mucosa and small erosions or yellow–white plaques. Microscopically the villi may be normal, reduced in height or flattened in severe cases. Enterocyte height is reduced and some show vacuolization of the cytoplasm. PAS-positive macrophages within the lamina propria and other infected tissues are characteristic but not specific. PAS-positive staining may persist after successful treatment as a result of bacterial cell wall remnants within the macrophages.

PREVENTION

The origin of the bacterium presumed to be the etiologic agent of Whipple's disease is unknown, as are any possible environmental factors or host characteristics. To date there are no known preventative measures for this disease.

CLINICAL FEATURES

In Whipple's original description of this disease he identified most of the important clinical and pathologic features.[1] The patient described in the original case initially presented with recurrent attacks of arthritis, progressive weakness and weight loss. This was followed by a cough and mild fever, then persistent diarrhea. The abdomen was swollen with a mass below the umbilicus and the skin was pigmented. The patient was found to be severely anemic and examination of stools revealed an excess of fat. At laparotomy, the mesenteric lymph nodes were enlarged and the diagnosis was considered to be tuberculosis. The patient died. At autopsy there was deposition of fat in the intestine and mesenteric glands, the heart was also enlarged and the aortic valve affected. The serosa of the heart, lungs and abdomen was affected and microscopy revealed extensive tissue infiltration by macrophages.

The most common symptoms and signs reported in Whipple's disease are listed in Figure 36.5. The onset is often insidious and several years may pass before a diagnosis of Whipple's disease is made. Intermittent arthralgia, low-grade fever and weight loss are common and a rheumatologic cause is often sought initially. Arthralgia may predate other symptoms by many years; in the series reported in 1970, 14 of the 19 patients suffered from arthralgia for more than 10 years before developing other symptoms.[2] Arthralgia is usually migratory, and largely involves the ankles, knees, shoulders or wrists. The joints may become swollen and inflamed, but a chronic deforming arthropathy is rare. Weight loss may be the only presenting feature and may be profound.

Diarrhea may be watery or steatorrheic. Edema secondary to hypoalbuminemia may occur, and less commonly ascites. Tetany

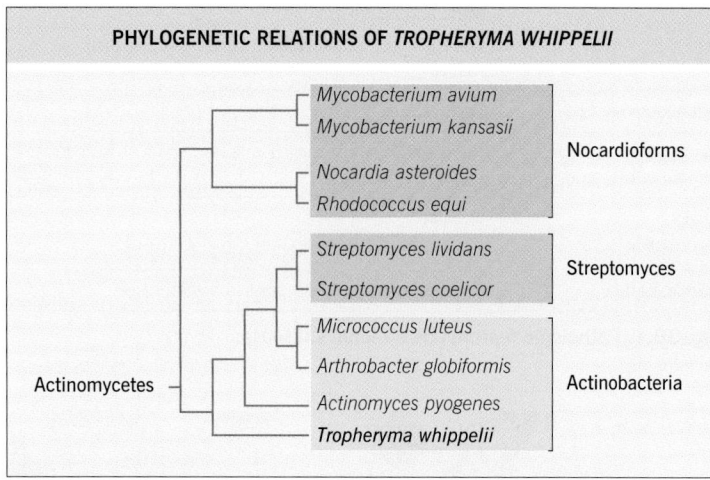

Fig. 36.4 Phylogenetic relations of the Whipple's disease bacterium, *Tropheryma whippelii*.

COMMON CLINICAL FEATURES OF WHIPPLE'S DISEASE

Symptoms	Signs	
Weight loss	Weight loss	Glossitis
Diarrhea	Hypotension	Abdominal tenderness
Arthralgia	Lymphadenopathy	Abdominal mass
Abdominal pain	Skin pigmentation	Ascites
Gastrointestinal bleeding	Fever	Splenomegaly
Central nervous system manifestations	Edema	Abnormal neurologic signs

Fig. 36.5 Common clinical features of Whipple's disease (in order of decreasing frequency of occurrence).

caused by hypocalcemia has been described, but not osteomalacia or bony fractures. Scurvy may occur. Occult gastrointestinal bleeding is common and may occasionally become frank. Five patients who had intestinal bleeding have been described; three presented with overt bleeding and the others with microcytic anemia and positive fecal occult blood tests; two showed an erythematous friable duodenal mucosa that bled on contact at endoscopy.[10] Small intestinal and rectosigmoid ulceration have also been described.

Neurologic features usually manifest late, occasionally in the absence of other symptoms, and may even develop after apparently successful treatment for other features of Whipple's disease. Central nervous system (CNS) manifestations include personality change, apathy, dementia and encephalopathy. Hypothalamic symptoms of insomnia, hypersomnia, hyperphagia and polydipsia may occur. Clonic movements, spastic paresis and hyperactive reflexes with extensor plantar responses are also described. Ocular manifestations include papilledema, nystagmus and gaze pareses. Isolated bilateral uveitis has also been described.[11]

Symptomatic cardiac involvement is rare at presentation, but congestive cardiac failure is a common terminal event in untreated disease. Sudden death caused by dysrhythmia may occur in up to 20% of patients. At autopsy PAS-positive macrophages have been demonstrated in heart valves, endocardium, myocardium and pericardium. Lymphocytic myocarditis has been reported.[12] Cardiomyopathy in the absence of gastrointestinal symptoms has also been reported, although doudenal biopsy was diagnostic of Whipple's disease.[13] Endomyocardial biopsy failed to show the presence of PAS-positive macrophages, but electron microscopy revealed the presence of Whipple's bacteria within the endothelium of myocardial capillaries. Atrial tachycardia with right bundle branch block was observed. Treatment with antibiotics was associated with a recovery of cardiac function and a return to sinus rhythm.

Skin involvement in Whipple's disease is characterized by hyperpigmentation, most commonly in exposed areas and in scars. Various skin rashes have also been described. Lymphadenopathy is common and enlarged intestinal lymph nodes may occasionally result in a palpable abdominal mass.

DIFFERENTIAL DIAGNOSIS

The differential diagnosis of Whipple's disease is extensive because of the multisystem nature of the disease and the variable way in which symptoms may occur. An initial presentation of fever, weight loss and arthralgia would be compatible with a diagnosis of rheumatoid arthritis or seronegative arthropathy. The combination of these symptoms together with skin rashes, cardiac or neuropsychiatric features may suggest a connective tissue disease such as systemic lupus erythematosus. When pulmonary manifestations are prominent, sarcoidosis may be suspected. A granulomatous inflammatory reaction with poor or absent PAS-staining may occasionally occur in Whipple's disease infected tissues, further confusing the diagnosis with sarcoidosis. Hyperpigmentation necessitates exclusion of Addison's disease. The combination of any of the above features with diarrhea, with or without frank malabsorption, should alert the clinician to the possibility of Whipple's disease. When diarrhea is the predominant symptom the differential diagnosis would include celiac disease, giardiasis or inflammatory bowel disease.

DIAGNOSIS

When the diagnosis of Whipple's disease is suspected a small bowel biopsy is the initial diagnostic investigation of choice and is usually obtained by endoscopic biopsy of the second part of the duodenum. Examination of formalin-fixed paraffin-processed biopsies stained with hematoxylin and eosin may demonstrate nonspecific enteropathic changes. However, PAS staining will demonstrate the presence of multiple PAS-positive macrophages within the lamina propria and is

highly suggestive of Whipple's disease, but not specific. Systemic *Mycobacterium avium intracellulare* (MAI) infection associated with AIDS may mimic Whipple's disease clinically, with weight loss, fever and malabsorption, and histopathologically as a result of PAS-positive macrophages within an enteropathic small bowel.[14] PAS-positive macrophages may also be found in the intestinal mucosa in histoplasmosis and macroglobulinemia, although other pathologic features may differ. The finding of Whipple's bacilli by EM of affected tissues is diagnostic.

Recently, the diagnosis of Whipple's disease has become possible by applying the molecular phylogenetic techniques described above.[4,5] PCR detection of *T. whippelii* 16S rRNA has been successfully applied diagnostically in peripheral blood,[15] cerebrospinal fluid[16] and vitreous fluid.[11] A simplified PCR protocol has been developed.[17] Modified primers and a specific hybridization probe were designed and tested against a wide range of bacterial control strains and in paraffin-embedded intestinal biopsy material from patients with and without Whipple's disease. The specificity and sensitivity of the technique were extremely good. PCR became negative about 1 year after treatment; however, in three patients who had negative intestinal PCR after treatment, cerebral Whipple's disease developed. The technique is therefore of more value in diagnosis than as a marker of response to treatment. Diagnostic PCR for the detection of *T. whippelii*, however, is a very promising technique, and is cheaper, faster and potentially more readily available than EM. This technique is also likely to be particularly valuable in Whipple's disease patients without intestinal involvement, in whom the diagnosis is more difficult to establish.

Because the Whipple's bacillus has not been cultured to date, microbiologic techniques serve only to exclude other infective differential diagnostic causes. Anemia is present in the majority of patients, with hemoglobin concentrations of <8g/dl in one-quarter of patients.[2] The anemia is usually microcytic and may be related to chronic gastrointestinal blood loss.[10] Megaloblastic anemia is rare. Serum vitamin B12 is usually normal, but serum folate is often reduced. The erythrocyte sedimentation rate is usually raised. Hypoalbuminemia is common and is likely to result from a combination of increased intestinal loss, decreased hepatic synthesis and protein malabsorption. Stool examination in the majority of patients will reveal an excess of fat.

Small bowel contrast radiology is abnormal in the majority of patients. The findings are nonspecific but include coarsening and thickening of the duodenal and jejunal folds and occasional dilatation.

MANAGEMENT

Whipple's disease was inevitably fatal until clinical improvement was noticed in patients treated with antibiotics in the 1950s.

A number of antibiotic regimens have been used for the treatment of Whipple's disease with variable success. The antibiotic treatment and outcome of 88 patients with Whipple's disease was reviewed retrospectively;[18] of the 57 patients who responded to treatment [mean follow-up 8.2 years (range 18 months to 27 years)], 31 (54%) relapsed [mean time to relapse 4.2 years (range 2 months to 20 years)]. There were no significant differences in sex or age at diagnosis between those who relapsed and those who did not. Of those who relapsed 21 out of 31 were treated with tetracycline alone. Two patients who relapsed were treated with parenteral penicillin and streptomycin followed by oral tetracycline, but the latter drug was given for only 2 weeks. CNS relapse was common, occurring in 11 out of 31 patients. All occurred late, 9 out of 11 occurred in patients treated with tetracycline alone and none in patients treated with antibiotics that penetrate the blood–brain barrier. Treatment of CNS relapse was ineffective when using drugs with poor CNS penetration. A combination of parenteral and oral penicillin and chloramphenicol followed by oral trimethoprim–sulfamethoxazole (co-trimoxazole) was effective. In a more recent review of treatment, trimethoprim–sulfamethoxazole (co-trimoxazole) was more efficacious than tetracycline in inducing remission (92 versus 59%) and resulted in fewer CNS relapses.[19]

However, 40% of patients with cerebral Whipple's disease did relapse after treatment with trimethoprim–sulfamethoxazole (co-trimoxazole) alone. CNS relapse has been treated successfuly with oral chloramphenicol, although one case of CNS relapse occurring on long-term trimethoprim–sulfamethoxazole (co-trimoxazole) has been successfully treated with oral cefixime (400mg q12h) after failure of oral chloramphenicol. In two further cases, intravenous ceftriaxone (2g q12h) resulted in improvement of cerebral symptoms.[20] No randomized prospective trial of alternative treatment regimens has been published.

We would recommend intravenous benzylpenicillin (2.4g daily) and streptomycin (1g daily, reduced to 0.5–0.75g daily if the patient is elderly or has a body weight <50kg) for 2 weeks followed by oral trimethoprim–sulfamethoxazole (co-trimoxazole) (960mg q12h) for 1 year (Fig. 36.6). Patients allergic to penicillin and those with prominent CNS involvement at presentation should be treated with intravenous ceftriaxone (2g q12h) and streptomycin for 2 weeks, followed by oral trimethoprim–sulfamethoxazole (co-trimoxazole) (960mg q12h) for 1 year. The duration of treatment remains empiric and relapse may occur after apparently successful treatment. Relapse may be confirmed by demonstrating the presence of Whipple's bacilli by EM in biopsy samples. The persistence of PAS-positive macrophages after treatment is common and is not diagnostic of relapse. CNS relapse on treatment should be treated with oral chloramphenicol (500mg q6h) for at least 1 year; a third-generation cephalosporin with good CNS penetration is the alternative.

In addition to specific antibiotic therapy, various symptomatic treatments and supportive measures may be required, depending upon the clinical manifestations of the disease. Pain caused by arthropathy may be treated with simple analgesics or nonsteroidal anti-inflammatory drugs. Diarrhea and malabsorption may necessitate nutritional support with protein-calorie enteral supplementation and vitamins. Antidiarrheal agents such as codeine or loperamide may provide symptomatic relief. Cardiac involvement with cardiac failure may require diuretic and angiotensin converting enzyme inhibitor therapy. Antidysrhythmics may also be required. Occasionally mitral or aortic valve replacement has been required for those with advanced valvular involvement. The wide range of neurologic manifestations may require nursing support, physiotherapy and neurorehabilitation. Recovery may not be complete.

CURRENT RECOMMENDED TREATMENT REGIMENS FOR WHIPPLE'S DISEASE

Indication	Antibiotic regimen	Duration
No clinical CNS involvement at presentation	Benzylpenicillin 2.4g daily iv + streptomycin 15mg/kg daily iv then trimethoprim– sulfamethoxazole 960mg q12h po	2 weeks 1 year
Penicillin allergy or CNS symptoms at presentation	Ceftriaxone 2g q12h iv + streptomycin daily iv then trimethoprim–sulfamethoxazole 960mg q12h po	2 weeks 1 year
CNS relapse on treatment	Chloramphenicol 2g daily po	1 year

Fig. 36.6 Current recommended treatment regimens for Whipple's disease. Streptomycin dose should be monitored and reduced as needed in patients who have impaired renal function, especially the elderly.

REFERENCES

1. Whipple GH. A hitherto undescribed disease characterised anatomically by deposits of fat and fatty acids in the intestinal mesenteric lymphatic tissues. Bull Johns Hopkins Hosp 1907;18:382–91.
2. Maizel H, Ruffin JM, Dobbins WO. Whipple's disease: a review of 19 patients from one hospital and a review of the literature since 1950. Medicine 1970;49:175–205.
3. Chears WC Jr, Ashworth CT. Electron microscopic study of the intestinal mucosa in Whipple's disease: demonstration of encapsulated bacilliform bodies in the lesions. Gastroenterology 1961;41:129–38.
4. Wilson KH, Blitchington R, Frothingham R, Wilson JAP. Phylogeny of the Whipple's-disease-associated bacterium. Lancet 1991;338:474–5.
5. Relman DA, Schmidt TM, MacDermott RP, Falklow S. Identification of the uncultured bacillus of Whipple's disease. N Engl J Med 1992;327:293–301.
6. Harmsen D, Heesesmann J, Brabletz T, Kirchner T, Muller-Hermelink HK. Heterogeneity among Whipple's-disease-associated bacteria. Lancet 1994;343:1288.
7. Dobbins WO, Kawanishi H. Bacillary characteristics

in Whipple's disease: an electron microscopic study. Gastroenterology 1980;80:1468–75.
8. Dobbins WO. Is there an immune deficit in Whipple's disease. Dig Dis Sci 1981;26:247–52.
9. Ectors NL, Geboes KJ, de Vos RM et al. Whipple's disease: a histological, immunocytochemical, and electron microscopic study of the small intestinal epithelium. J Pathol 1994;172:73–9.
10. Feldman M, Price G. Intestinal bleeding in patients with Whipple's disease. Gastroenterology 1989;96:1207–9.
11. Rickman LS, Freeman WR, Green WR et al. Uveitis caused by Tropheryma whippelii (Whipple's bacillus). N Engl J Med 1995;332:363–6.
12. Pelech T, Fric P, Huslarova A, Jirasek A. Interstitial lymphocytic myocarditis in Whipple's disease. Lancet 1991;337:553–4.
13. de Takats PG, de Takats DLP, Iqbal TH, et al. Symptomatic cardiomyopathy as a presentation in Whipple's disease. Postgrad Med J 1995;71:236–9.
14. Gillin JS, Urmacher C, West R, Shike M. Disseminated Mycobacterium avium intracellulare infection in aquired immunodeficiency syndrome mimicking Whipple's disease. Gastroenterology 1983;85:1187–91.

15. Lowsky R, Archer GL, Fyles G et al. Diagnosis of Whipple's disease by molecular analysis of peripheral blood. N Engl J Med 1994;331:1343–6.
16. Cohen L, Berthet K, Dauga C, Thivart L, Pierrot-Deseilligny C. Polymerase chain reaction of cerebrospinal fluid to diagnose Whipple's disease. Lancet 1996;347:329.
17. Von Herbay A, Ditton HJ, Maiwald M. Diagnostic application of a polymerase chain reaction assay for the Whipple's disease bacterium to intestinal biopsies. Gastroenterology 1996;110:1736–43.
18. Keinath RD, Merrell DE, Vliestra R, Dobbins WO. Antibiotic treatment and relapse in Whipple's disease. Long-term follow up of 88 patients. Gastroenterology 1985;88:1867–73.
19. Feurle GE, Marth T. An evaluation of antimicrobial treatment for Whipple's disease. Tetracycline versus trimethoprim-sulphamethoxazole. Dig Dis Sci 1994;39:1642–8.
20. Schnider PJ, Reisenger EC, Gerschlager W et al. Long-term follow-up in cerebral Whipple's disease. Eur J Gastroenterol Hepatol 1996;8:899–903.

chapter
37

Parasitic Infections of the Gastrointestinal Tract

Andrew D Mackay & Peter L Chiodini

INTRODUCTION

This chapter examines the parasitic causes of gastrointestinal infection in the nonimmunocompromised host. The organisms involved are a very heterogeneous group of protozoa and helminths. They vary in size from microsporidia, which are barely visible using light microscopy, to long multicellular organisms such as *Taenia saginata*, which can reach 25m in length (Fig. 37.1). The clinical approach is emphasized here because the parasites themselves are discussed elsewhere (see Chapters 8.31, 8.32, 8.33, 8.35), and diagnosis is covered in Chapter 6.10. Parasitic gastrointestinal infections in HIV infection are discussed in Chapter 5.13. The parasites discussed in this chapter are listed in Figure 37.2.

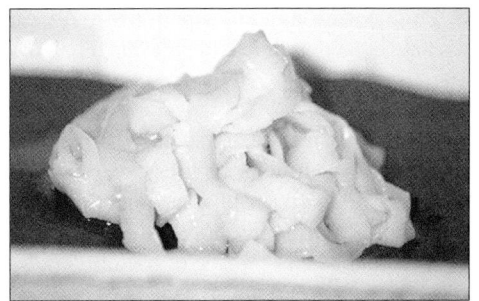

Fig. 37.1 Adult beef tapeworm (*Taenia saginata*) passed in a patient's feces.

EPIDEMIOLOGY

In the developed world, parasitic infections appear to be uncommon causes of gastrointestinal illness. Certain populations are particularly likely to be affected these include:
- returned travelers,
- day care workers and patients,
- immigrant workers, and
- homosexual men.

The most common causes of parasitic gastrointestinal infection are *Giardia lamblia* and *Cryptosporidium parvum*.

In developing countries the impact of parasitic infections is of much greater significance in relation to morbidity, mortality and economic impact. Their epidemiology is varied and their control presents a complex sociopolitical problem. The most important infections are *Entamoeba histolytica*, *G. lamblia*, hookworms, *Ascaris* spp. and tapeworms.

GEOGRAPHIC DISTRIBUTION OF PARASITES
The distribution of a parasite depends upon:
- human behavior,
- the physical environment, and
- the biologicical environment.

Human behavior
Behavioral factors are often dominant but the distribution of vectors, intermediate hosts and reservoir hosts is also to some extent under

Fig. 37.2 Gastrointestinal parasites.

GASTROINTESTINAL PARASITES		
Intestinal protozoa	Amebae	*Entamoeba histolytica; Entamoeba dispar* Commensals *Entamoeba coli* *Entamoeba hartmanni* *Endolimax nana* *Iodamoeba butschlii* *Blastocystis hominis*
	Flagellates	*Giardia lamblia* *Dientamoeba fragilis*
	Ciliate	*Balantidium coli*
	Coccidia	*Cryptosporidium parvum* *Cyclospora cayetanensis* *Isospora belli*
	Microsporidia	*Enterocytozoon bieneusi* *Encephalitozoon intestinalis* (formerly *Septata intestinalis*)
Intestinal helminths	Nematodes (round worms)	*Ascaris lumbricoides* *Enterobius vermicularis* Hookworms: *Ancylostoma duodenale* *Necator americanus* *Trichuris trichiura* *Strongyloides stercoralis*
	Trematodes (flukes)	*Fasciolopsis buski* *Heterophyes heterophyes*
	Cestodes (tapeworms)	*Taenia solium* *Taenia saginata* *Hymenolepis nana* *Diphyllobothrium latum*

human control. Some parasites are worldwide in their distribution, such as *E. histolytica* and *G. lamblia*, whereas others are very localized.

Physical environment

The physical environment also affects the distribution of parasites. Temperature and humidity affect the viability of parasites in the external environment; viability is lost in cold or over-hot temperatures and most parasites require moist, aerobic conditions. Examples of parasites for which these factors are critical include:

- the cysts of protozoa with direct lifecycles, such as *E. histolytica*, *G. lamblia*, *Balantidium coli* and the various gut commensal species (*Entamoeba coli*, *Entamoeba hartmanni*, *Endolimax nana*, *Iodamoeba butschlii*);
- the oocysts of *Isospora belli*;
- the eggs and larvae of soil-transmitted nematodes [*Ascaris* spp., hookworm[1] and *Strongyloides stercoralis* (see Fig. 37.5)];
- the eggs of trematodes (*Fasciolopsis buski* and *Heterophyes heterophyes*) and cestodes before their entry into the aquatic environment; and
- the eggs of cestodes before their ingestion by the intermediate hosts (*Taenia solium* and *Taenia saginata*).

Temperature and humidity also affect sporulation of oocysts, the rates of embryonation of nematode, cestode and trematode eggs and the development times for hookworm and *Strongyloides* larvae. Parasites that have a soil stage are affected by the particular physical properties of the soil, including its particle size and water-holding capacity, and by factors such as rainfall. Susceptibility to anaerobic conditions is important for some parasites when 'night soil' (human feces) is used raw or after composting as a fertilizer.

The aquatic environment is important in the lifecycle of many parasites. In the trematodes, the cercariae of *Heterophyes* spp. must survive long enough to infect the fish or shrimp and the metacerariae of *F. buski* must survive long enough to infect the human or pig hosts. *Strongyloides* larvae live in the capillary water films in soil and on low vegetation.

Biologic environment

The biologic environment also affects the epidemiology of these gastrointestinal parasites. The distribution in nature of appropriate vectors, intermediate hosts and reservoir hosts can obviously affect the distribution of parasites. Examples of animal reservoirs are *F. buski* in dogs, pigs or rabbits; *B. coli* in pigs; *C. parvum* in domestic animals, particularly cattle; and *H. heterophyes* in fish-eating mammals. Secondary hosts include snails for *F. buski* and freshwater fish for *H. heterophyes*. An important biologic factor is the presence of dung beetles that take the parasitic ova or larvae underground to a more favorable physical environment.

HUMAN FACTORS
Population density and urbanization

The agricultural revolution in developing countries has produced large resident human populations with the potential for direct person-to-person spread of infection and greater environmental contamination by feces. In addition, animal husbandry has created other cycles for parasite transmission, for example *Cryptosporidium* spp. in calves. Rapid urbanization, especially in the tropics, is often associated with increased poverty, poorer housing and unsanitary conditions. The result is that people may be living in a more fecally polluted environment than in rural areas, encouraging such diseases as amebiasis and giardiasis. Epidemics, such as outbreaks of cryptosporidiosis, may occur when public water supplies become fecally contaminated. The soil-transmitted nematodes *Ascaris lumbricoides* and *Trichuris trichiura*[2] are often more common in towns and cities. Overcrowding favors direct transmission of *Hymenolepis nana* and *Enterobius vermicularis*, especially in children when levels of hygiene and sanitation are poor.[3]

Population movements

Population changes associated with mining, political unrest or industrialization may cause people to move into at risk areas; travelers may also visit such areas.

Dams and irrigation

Development programs in the tropics frequently involve irrigation projects, where contaminated water supplies reach greater numbers of people and larger water-borne outbreaks may occur. Irrigation and poor drainage supplies favor the breeding of flies that may have a role in spreading fecal material.

AGRICULTURE

Cattle raising may be complicated by bovine cysticercosis (*T. saginata*), which renders carcasses unsaleable, and calves may be a source of human infection. Pigs can allow *T. solium*, the pork tapeworm, to be spread and *F. buski*, the intestinal fluke, to prosper. *Balantidium coli* is also acquired from close contact with pigs. Fish farms in which water plants such as water calthrop are grown transmit *F. buski*, especially if human or pig feces are used as fertilizer.

DOMESTIC ENVIRONMENT

Sanitation, water supplies and domestic customs in hygiene and food preparation are all very important. Children are at risk of parasitic infections because of poor hand washing after defecation, finger sucking and playing with soil. Local dietary behavior is critical for parasite transmission. Ingestion of certain fish, crustacea, molluscs and aquatic vegetation can lead to fluke infection. Tapeworms are contacted by ingestion of undercooked pork or beef (*Taenia* spp.) or certain fish (*Diphyllobothrium* spp.). People who have occupations involving sewage, water or soil contact are at increased risk of parasitic infection.

HOST SUSCEPTIBILITY

Host susceptibility is affected by many factors such as nutritional status, intercurrent disease, pregnancy, immunosuppressive drugs and malignancy. Previously mild or clinically inapparent infections can produce dangerous disease when host immunity falls, such as occurs in strongyloidiasis, in which the parasite is capable of multiplying by autoinfection within its host, and fatal amebiasis that may occur if corticosteroids are administered in error.

Some protective immunity is usually acquired by the host but its effectiveness is variable. The absence of symptomatic giardiasis in adults in places where the infection is common is good evidence for acquired immunity. Re-infection and superinfection, possibly by different gastrointestinal parasite strains, is certainly common in areas of endemic infection. Immunodeficiency associated with HIV infection is of paramount importance in some of the more recently recognized gastrointestinal parasitic diseases such as cryptosporidiosis and microsporidiosis (see Chapter 5.13).

PATHOGENESIS AND PATHOLOGY

Gastrointestinal parasites cause disease in a variety of ways. Most are present in the lumen of the gut or attached to the mucosa of the gut wall and are not capable of invasion. The coccidian parasites such as cryptosporidia can invade the epithelial cells of the small bowel. Others, such as *E. histolytica*, *S. stercoralis* and occasionally *B. coli*, do invade the mucosa (Fig. 37.3).

GASTROINTESTINAL PROTOZOA
Amebiasis

Amebic ulcers mostly develop in the cecum, appendix or adjacent ascending colon, although the sigmoidorectal region can be involved.[4] Amebic ulcers are formed on the mucosa. They are usually flask shaped with a small, raised opening and a larger area of mucosal destruction below. The mucosa between abscesses is normal but lesions can be confluent.

Pathogenic amebae are able to resist complement-mediated lysis and they possess other virulence factors such as attachment lectins, cysteine proteases and other enzymes.[5] Amebae have tissue-lysing enzymes on their surfaces that can be released from lysosomes or after amebic rupture.

Giardiasis

The histopathology of the upper small bowel varies from normal to subtotal villous atrophy in giardiasis. *Giardia* spp. seem unable to penetrate the mucosal wall in humans but are able to attach to the mucosa of the small bowel. In symptomatic cases there is increased mucus secretion and dehydration.[6] *Giardia lamblia* may undergo antigenic variation, thereby evading the human immune response.[7] Giardiasis is more common in the immunodeficiency syndromes, particularly in common variable hypogammaglobulinemia, although there is no particular increase in incidence among the HIV-infected population.

Balantidium coli

The trophozoite of *Balantidium coli* causes mucosal inflammation and ulceration, invading the distal ileal and colonic mucosa. Invasion may be enhanced by hyaluronidase produced by the parasite. Other products liberated by the parasite as well as host factors, such as the recruitment of mucosal inflammatory cells, may also be important.[8]

Cryptosporidiosis

Cryptosporidium parvum, a coccidian parasite, infects the intracellular, extracytoplasmic area of host epithelial cells of the small bowel. The intracellular stage of *C. parvum* resides within a parasitophorous vacuole in the microvillus region of the host cell. Oocysts undergo sporogony while in the host cells. Approximately 20% of the oocysts do not form the usual environmentally resistant oocysts but are released as sporozoites that are capable of penetrating the microvillus regions of other cells within the intestine. This explains the ability of *C. parvum* to cause severe diarrhea in some patients, particularly in the immunocompromised. The infection leads to destruction of the microvilli. The exact mechanism for the diarrhea is unknown.[9]

Cyclosporiasis

The mechanism of diarrhea production has not been clearly established for *Cyclospora cayetanensis*. The organism is found within enterocytes. There is reduction in villus height with associated mucosal inflammation and increased numbers of intraepithelial lymphocytes, which suggests a direct effect on the intestinal mucosa.[10]

Isosporiasis

Mild to subtotal villus atrophy occurs in *I. belli* infection. Histologically there may be infiltration of the lamina propria with eosinophils, neutrophils and round cells.

Microsporidiosis

Intestinal microsporidia infect enterocytes in the small bowel and undergo sporogony, which leads to enterocyte degeneration, vacuolation and loss of the brush border. These cells are sloughed off and the spores are capable of infecting further enterocytes.[11]

GASTROINTESTINAL HELMINTHS
Nematode infections

Ascariasis (roundworm infection). The embryonated eggs of *A. lumbricoides* are ingested and hatch in the stomach and duodenum, from where the larvae penetrate the intestinal wall (Fig. 37.4). They are carried to the lungs in the circulation and usually cause no symptoms unless there are a large number of larvae, in which case pneumonitis can ensue. The larvae then break out of the lung tissue and may cause some bronchial epithelial damage. Intense tissue reaction with infiltration of eosinophils, macrophages and epithelioid cells occurs.[12]

Ancylostomiasis (hookworm infection). Hookworm disease is caused by *Ancylostoma duodenale* and *Necator americanus*. Vesiculation and

pustules can occur on the skin at the site of entry of the filariform larvae. Asthma and bronchitis occur during migration through the lungs, with small hemorrhages into the alveoli and infiltration of eosinophils and leukocytes. Adult hookworms attach firmly to the small bowel mucosa; *A. duodenale* does this by means of well-developed mouth parts and *N. americanus* by means of cutting plates. There tends to be chronic blood loss at the site where the worm attaches. ***Trichuriasis (whip worm).*** The egg of the nematode *T. trichiura* hatches in the small intestine and the larva penetrates the villi causing no pathologic reaction. It re-emerges after 1 week and migrates to the cecum and colorectum. When few worms are present there is little damage, but with heavy infections there is hemorrhage, mucopurulent stools and symptoms of dysentery, sometimes with rectal prolapse (the *Trichuris* dysentery syndrome).[13]

Strongyloidiasis. The lifecycle of *S. stercoralis* is complex (Fig. 37.5). Human infection is acquired when filariform larvae in the soil penetrate the skin. This can cause petechial hemorrhages, congestion and edema at the site of entry. The larvae migrate into cutaneous blood vessels and are carried to the lungs, where they break out of the pulmonary capillaries and sequentially enter the alveoli, trachea, pharynx and then the mucosa of the duodenum and upper jejunum. There can be pathologic findings similar to those of bronchopneumonia with lobar

ANATOMIC LOCATION OF GASTROINTESTINAL PARASITES		
Lumen only	Small bowel (normally)	*Ascaris lumbricoides*
	Large bowel	*Entamoeba histolytica/dispar* *Balantidium coli* *Enterobius vermicularis*
Mucosal attachment	Small bowel	*Giardia lamblia* Tapeworm Hookworm *Fasciolopsis buski* *Heterophyes heterophyes*
	Large bowel	*Trichuris trichiura*
Epithelial cell invasion	Small bowel	*Isospora belli* *Cyclospora cayetanensis* *Cryptosporidium parvum* Microsporidia
Mucosal invasion	Small bowel	*Strongyloides stercoralis*
	Large bowel	*Entamoeba histolytica* *Balantidium coli*

Fig. 37.3 Anatomic location of gastrointestinal parasites.

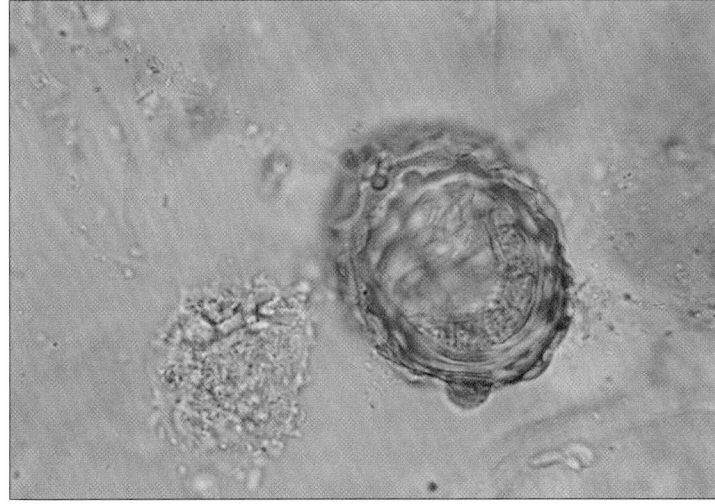

Fig. 37.4 *Ascaris lumbricoides* ovum in feces. The ovum measures 50–70μm × 40–50μm and is elliptical. The rough albuminous coat gives it a mammillated appearance.

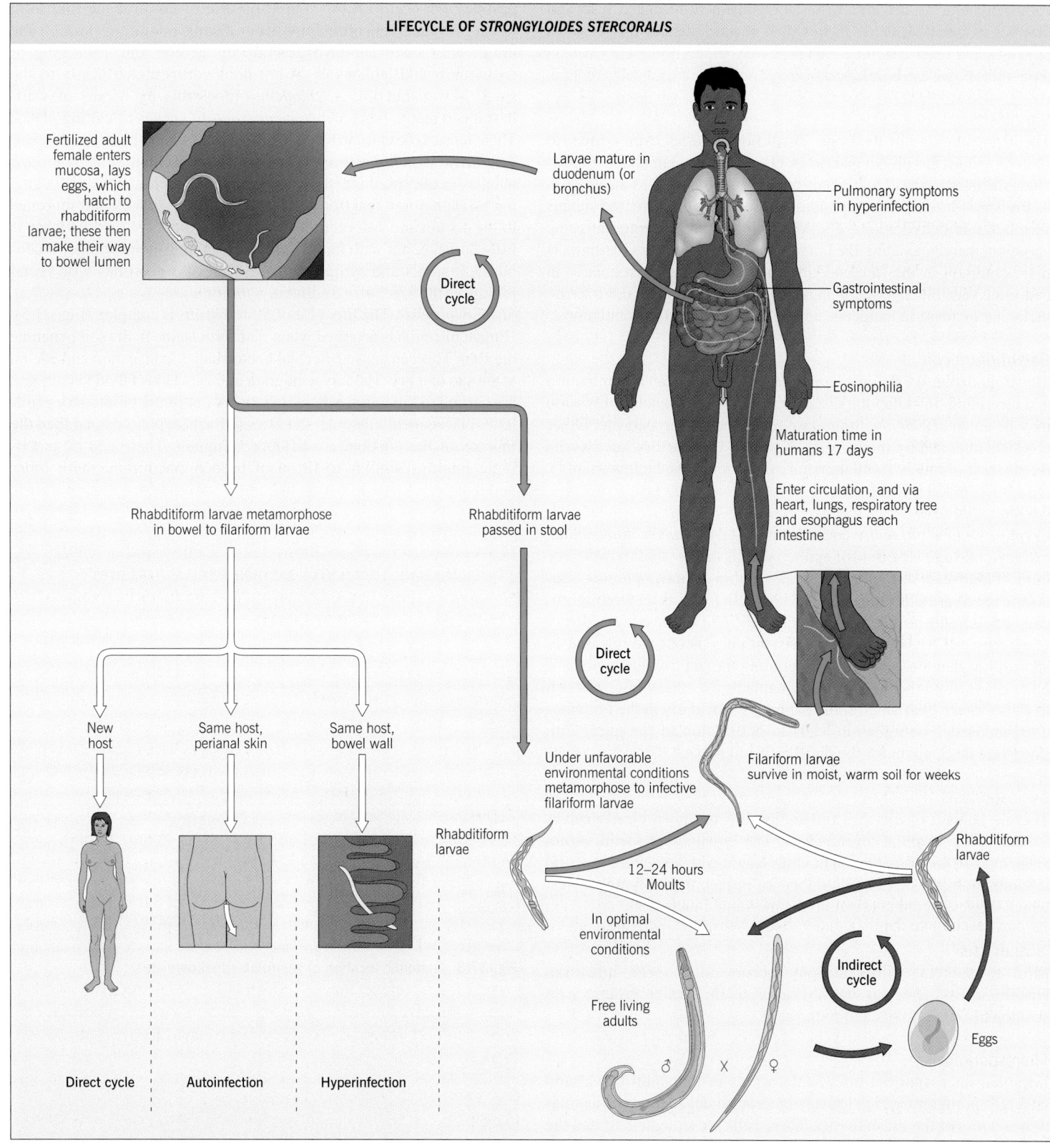

Fertilized adult female enters mucosa, lays eggs, which hatch to rhabditiform larvae; these then make their way to bowel lumen

Larvae mature in duodenum (or bronchus)

Pulmonary symptoms in hyperinfection

Gastrointestinal symptoms

Direct cycle

Eosinophilia

Maturation time in humans 17 days

Enter circulation, and via heart, lungs, respiratory tree and esophagus reach intestine

Rhabditiform larvae metamorphose in bowel to filariform larvae

Rhabditiform larvae passed in stool

Direct cycle

New host

Same host, perianal skin

Same host, bowel wall

Under unfavorable environmental conditions metamorphose to infective filariform larvae

Filariform larvae survive in moist, warm soil for weeks

Rhabditiform larvae

Rhabditiform larvae

12–24 hours Moults

In optimal environmental conditions

Indirect cycle

Free living adults

♂   X   ♀

Eggs

Direct cycle | Autoinfection | Hyperinfection

Fig. 37.5 Lifecycle of *Strongyloides stercoralis*.

consolidation. The females mature in the intestine, invade the tissues of the bowel wall and lay their eggs, which hatch and release first-stage (rhabditiform) larvae in the feces. In certain situations, the rhabditiform larvae mature in the intestine to the filariform stage, and these parasites bore into the wall of the duodenum and jejunum and initiate another cycle of infection, which eventually results in there being more adult worms in the small bowel. Filariform larvae that penetrate the bowel wall can spread throughout the lymphatic system to the mesenteric lymph glands and can enter the general circulation and hence the liver, lungs, kidneys and gallbladder. They can cause granulomas in the

gastrointestinal tract and mesenteric glands. There are abscesses in the lungs and there may be granuloma in the liver. Migrating larvae may cause the patient to die from sepsis arising from the normal intestinal bacterial flora.

Trematode infections (flukes)

Fasciolopsis buski *infection*. The giant intestinal fluke *F. buski* is contracted by humans and pigs through eating metacercariae attached to water plants. The parasite excysts and attaches to the mucosa of the jejunal and duodenal wall causing mechanical injury and inflammation, which can lead to ulcers, bleeding or abscesses. There may be a mild anemia and low levels of serum vitamin B12, owing to the parasite's competition for the vitamin or impairing its absorption.

Heterophyes heterophyes *infection.* *Heterophyes heterophyes* is a trematode that infects humans and is found mainly in Asia. The pathology depends on the degree of infection acquired through ingestion of pickled or raw fish. The metacercariae excyst and attach to the walls of the small intestine. The adults may cause only a mild inflammatory reaction. Eggs may enter the circulation because the adults are attached deeply into the intestinal wall. Ectopic eggs can provoke granuloma formation, especially if they lodge in the heart or brain.[14]

Cestodes infections (tapeworms)

Taenia solium *and* **Taenia saginata.** The pork tapeworm (*T. solium*) and the beef tapeworm (*T. saginata*)[15] are acquired by the human host by ingestion of poorly cooked meat that contains the encysted larvae (cysticerci). The larva is digested in the stomach and the head of the tapeworm evaginates in the upper small intestine, attaches via the scolex to the intestinal mucosa and feeds by absorbing nutrients from the bowel. The scolex of *T. solium* has four suckers and a rostellum that contains a double row of hooks; *T. saginata* has the suckers only. Very little pathology is caused by these well-adapted adult worms, which may reach 7m and 25m in length respectively. The pathologically significant stage for humans is the cysticercus of *T. solium*. The eggs passed in feces are ingested and hatch when they are exposed to gastric juice. The oncospheres that are released penetrate the intestinal wall and are carried via the bloodstream and can potentially form a cysticercus in any organ. The cysticercus is an ovoid, milky-white bladder with the parasite head invaginated inside. The pathology is described in detail in Chapter 6.28.

Dwarf tapeworm (**Hymenolepis nana**)*.* Once the ova of the dwarf tapeworm *H. nana* are ingested they encyst in the small intestinal villus mucosa. The adult worm reaches a length of 3–4cm and begins egg production. Heavy infections of more than 100 worms can cause some symptoms, and the competition for nutrients has been linked with growth retardation in children, although this may be more the result of insanitary conditions, poverty and malnutrition.

Fish tapeworm (**Diphyllobothrium latum**)*.* The fish tapeworm *D. latum* has a lifecycle involving a first intermediate host of tiny aquatic invertebrates, a second intermediate host of fish and a definitive host that includes humans, other terrestrial mammals and marine mammals. The tapeworm attaches to the small intestinal mucosa by means of two longitudinal slit-like suckers (bothria). Infections are commonly multiple and may reach more than 100 individual worms, each measuring up to 10m in length. The pathology is minimal from the local effects. Tapeworm anemia has been described exclusively in Finland and has now all but died out as a result of control measures. The anemia is caused by vitamin B12 deficiency, with worms competing for the limited dietary vitamin B12, and it is strongly associated with gastritis and achlorhydria; there is probably a genetic predisposition to this condition.

PREVENTION

The prevention and control of parasitic gastrointestinal disease can be achieved through improvement of living standards, personal hygiene and better sanitary conditions.[16] In immunocompromised patients, different recommendations need to be considered (see Chapter 5.9).

PUBLIC HEALTH HYGIENE MEASURES

Disposal of human sewage and waste water is fundamental to the control of parasitic gastrointestinal infections. Fecal material contaminates agricultural food crops or water supplies if it is passed promiscuously in the fields or close to habitation or if it is deliberately used unprocessed on fields as fertilizer ('night soil'). Any of the gastrointestinal parasites can be transferred in this way. Following rain, fecal material is washed into rivers and pools. Giardia cysts are found in surface water in many parts of the world.

The provision of latrines can reduce these sources of environmental contamination but, unfortunately, unless they are well constructed and maintained, latrines can themselves become important foci of infection. The prevalence of *Ascaris* infection is often higher among urban latrine users than among rural non-users. The eggs of *A. lumbricoides* and also those of *T. trichiura* are very often resistant and can remain viable in the latrine environment for long periods. In addition, the moist soil around a latrine favors the survival of hookworm larvae[17] and the free-living cycle of *S. stercoralis*.

Domestic waste water (and the excreta that it accompanies) when used for irrigation puts crops and workers at risk. Sewage may enter lakes, rivers and ponds and the water then be used for drinking or irrigation. *Cryptosporidium* oocysts are particularly difficult to eliminate from water and require an efficient filtration system. Boiling water is the most reliable method of killing oocysts.

Composting is another reliable way of killing the infective forms of parasites. This takes 3–4 months. Cysts, eggs and larvae are quite rapidly killed at temperatures of 131°F (55°C) and die within a few days at 113°F (45°C). The compost heap needs turning and good maintenance, or the periphery may become an intense transmission focus. Chemical treatment of excreta has been used, for example 12–24 hours in ammonium sulfate, but proper control is important to maintain efficacy and avoid toxicity to fish and plant life. Solid waste from sewage treatment plants is used as agricultural fertilizer and can contain viable parasites if inadequately processed. Sewage treatment removes or destroys parasites by sedimentation and the creation of completely anaerobic conditions. The eggs of *Taenia* spp. and *A. lumbricoides* are notoriously resistant and they sometimes survive in the solid wastes taken from sedimentation tanks or ponds.

PERSONAL HYGIENE MEASURES

Most gastrointestinal diseases could be prevented if it were easy to modify human behavior. In practice this is often very difficult, but health education can be very effective and it can take many forms. Schools can be targeted or the local press used for a health awareness campaign. The fecal–oral route of transmission is very important, especially for intestinal protozoa. For example, infected food handlers are disseminators of *G. lamblia* and *E. histolytica* cysts. There is high prevalence of infection in institutions for children or the mentally subnormal, where personal hygiene is poor. Those intestinal helminths whose lifecycles can lead to fully embryonated eggs being released or formed very soon after entry into the environment (*H. nana* and *E. vermicularis*) are also spread in this way. Microsporidia are probably spread by the fecal–oral or urinary–oral routes. Simple hand washing before preparing and eating food prevents transmission of these infections. The soil-to-skin route of infection can be inhibited by wearing shoes.[18] Infective forms of hookworm and *Strongyloides* larvae will be stopped from entering the skin. Persons dealing with composted human feces must use boots and gloves.

Good food hygiene is essential. Prevention of most of the parasites transferred by the fecal–oral route can be achieved by washing all salad vegetables and fruit before consumption. Kitchen utensils and hands should be washed frequently. Avoidance of wild-grown watercress and other water plants prevents *F. buski* infections. Proper cooking of meat and fish removes the risk of flesh-derived parasites such as *H. heterophyes* and tapeworms. Problems arise when cultural preferences dictate consuming these products raw, undercooked, salted, dried or pickled. The inspection of meat can detect the presence of cysticerci in the carcasses and allow infected meat to be condemned. Stopping the consumption of fish that is raw, pickled or salted is often impossible if it is part of a deep cultural tradition. Deep freezing of meat and fish at temperatures colder than –4°F (–20°C) for 24–48 hours kills all these parasites.

PREVENTION BY CHEMOTHERAPY

The treatment of these gastrointestinal parasites with appropriate chemotherapy is helpful in the prevention of further cases. This is particularly so in developed parts of the world. In areas where parasitic disease is endemic, generally only symptomatic patients are treated. Patients that are asymptomatic, those in whom the diagnosis is incidental and those who do not have heavy infections are usually not treated, as re-infection is probably inevitable. Mass chemotherapy has been used in amebiasis, soil-transmitted nematodes (*A. lumbricoides*,[19] hookworm, *T. trichiura*) and tapeworms (*T. saginata, T. solium* and *D. latum*).[20] Success depends upon several factors:

- the chemotherapeutic agent used should have a broad spectrum of activity and be given annually as a single oral dose;
- the drugs should be cheap to purchase and administer; and
- the drugs should have few side effects.

In the past, mass chemotherapy was used in an attempt to eradicate amebiasis but, because treatment required a prolonged course of luminal amebicides, compliance was poor and re-infection in endemic areas was high. *Fasciolopsis buski* infection in Indonesia has been treated by community-based praziquantel treatment but rapid re-infection followed. Selective or targeted chemotherapy may be of more use. *Enterobius vermicularis* infection in one child requires treatment not only of that child but also all family contacts together with education in personal hygiene.

VACCINES

As yet no vaccines have been used in humans for the control of gastrointestinal parasitic diseases.[21]

ROLE OF PROPHYLAXIS

There is no evidence for prophylactic use of chemotherapy being helpful in prevention of these gastrointestinal parasitic diseases.

Advice for travelers on preventive measures is discussed in Chapters 6.2 and 6.3.

CLINICAL FEATURES

The symptoms produced by gastrointestinal parasites are diverse. The most common presentation is of poorly localized abdominal pain; less commonly there is nonspecific diarrhea (Fig. 37.6). The severity varies from asymptomatic carriage to life-threatening gastrointestinal disease, as occurs in amebiasis and cryptosporidiosis. It is important to emphasize that the identification of an infection by stool microscopy does not necessarily imply that it is the cause of a patient's symptoms. This is particularly so in the case of light helminth infections, which are often completely symptomless. Other pathologies should be excluded before attributing the patient's symptoms to the gut parasite. Some of

these infections present with extraintestinal manifestations, such as iron-deficiency anemia, wasting or (in the case of hookworm infection) growth retardation.

GASTROINTESTINAL DISEASE CAUSED BY PROTOZOA

Amebiasis (*Entamoeba histolytica*)

It is now recognized that there are two species of amebae that were formerly termed pathogenic and nonpathogenic *E. histolytica*.[22] Methods used to separate these include biochemical, immunologic and genetic data. These are now called *Entamoeba histolytica* and *Entamoeba dispar*. Only *E. histolytica* is capable of causing disease. Asymptomatic cyst carriers may excrete cysts for a variable length of time, usually only a few weeks.

Amebic intestinal disease

The incubation period of invasive amebiasis varies from a few days to 1–4 months. There is a good correlation with the presence of *E. histolytica* trophozoites containing ingested red blood cells. Patients may be asymptomatic or present with colicky abdominal pain, frequent bowel movements and tenesmus. Amebic dysentery is characterized by blood-stained stools with mucus occurring up to 10 times a day. The duration of the dysentery can be very variable and may last for only a few days or for several months with concomitant weight loss and debility. The symptoms may be confused with inflammatory bowel disease. In acute cases the clinical picture may mimic appendicitis, cholecystitis, intestinal obstruction or diverticulitis.

Amebic extraintestinal disease

Amebic dysentery progresses to invasive amebic disease in between 2 and 8% of patients. Symptoms can be gradual in onset, with right upper quadrant pain and fever (see Chapter 6.4). Weakness, weight loss, dry cough and sweating are less common. Tender hepatomegaly is often seen with liver function tests that are normal or only slightly abnormal. Jaundice is very unusual. The site most commonly involved is the upper right lobe of the liver, and abscesses are mostly solitary. A raised right diaphragm may be found on chest radiograph. The abscess is visualized by ultrasound, CT or MRI. Hematogenous spread to the brain (see Chapter 6.19), lung (see Chapter 6.10), pericardium and other sites is possible. Serologic tests are valuable in cases of suspected amebic abscess. The indirect fluorescent antibody test is positive in over 95% of cases after 14 days, but it should be confirmed by the cellulose acetate precipitin test.

Giardiasis (*Giardia lamblia*)

The clinical spectrum of giardiasis ranges from asymptomatic infection, through acute gastrointestinal infection to severe chronic diarrhea[23] with intestinal malabsorption.[24] The avergae incubation period is 9 days and the acute infection is self-limiting.[25] Common symptoms include nausea, diarrhea, flatulence and upper abdominal cramps with distention and nausea. Weight loss is common and there can be signs of malabsorption (steatorrhea, disaccharidase deficiency and vitamin B12 deficiency).

Blastocystis infection (*Blastocystis hominis*)

There is controversy surrounding *B. hominis*; it is unclear whether it causes gastrointestinal disease or not. When large numbers are found in stool in the absence of other parasites, bacteria or viruses it may be the cause of diarrhea, cramps, nausea, fever, vomiting and abdominal pain. Data from Canada indicate that, although it is commonly seen in stools, it is not pathogenic.[26] It is possible that a small subset of *B. hominis* organisms have virulence factors that are missing in most.[27]

Dientamoeba fragilis infection

Like *Blastocystis*, the pathogenicity of *Dientamoeba fragilis* is uncertain. It has been associated with a wide range of symptoms. In

GASTROINTESTINAL PARASITES ASSOCIATED WITH DIARRHEA	
Diarrhea and fever	*Entamoeba histolytica* *Cryptosporidium parvum* *Isospora belli* *Cyclospora cayetanensis* (occasionally)
Diarrhea with blood in stool	*Entamoeba histolytica* *Trichuris trichiura* *Strongyloides stercoralis* (rarely)
Chronic diarrhea	*Entamoeba histolytica* *Giardia lamblia* *Cryptosporidium parvum* *Isospora belli* *Cyclospora cayetanensis* Microsporidia *Trichuris trichiura* Hookworm (*Necator americanus* and *Ancylostoma duodenale*) *Strongyloides stercoralis*

Fig. 37.6 Gastrointestinal parasites associated with diarrhea.

children, symptoms may include intermittent diarrhea, abdominal pain, nausea, anorexia, malaise, fatigue, poor weight gain and unexplained eosinophilia.[28]

Cryptosporidiosis (*Cryptosporidium parvum*)

The incubation period of *Cryptosporidium parvum* infection averages 3–6 days. Symptoms include a flu-like illness, diarrhea, malaise, abdominal pain, anorexia, nausea, flatulence, malabsorption, vomiting, mild fever and weight loss. Oocyst excretion generally occurs for 3–30 days (average 12 days) and occurs at the same time as the symptoms. Generally the symptoms are self-limiting, and prolonged disease in uncommon.[29] In immunocompromised patients the situation is different and there can be intractable, profuse, life-threatening diarrhea[30] (see Chapter 5.13).

Cyclosporiasis (*Cyclospora cayetanensis*)

There is epidemiological evidence that *Cyclospora cayetanensis* is the cause of persistent diarrhea in immunocompetent patients as well as in immunocompromised patients. Initially, the clinical findings do not distinguish cyclosporal diarrhea from other causes of diarrhea. Other common symptoms are abdominal pain, nausea, vomiting and anorexia. Cyclospora infection can last for 1–8 weeks.[10]

Isosporiasis (*Isospora belli*)

The predominant clinical symptom is diarrhea, which may last for months or even years. Stools are watery, soft, foamy and offensive, which may suggest malabsorption. There is associated weight loss, abdominal pain and fever.[31] In HIV-infected patients, chronic infection occurs (see Chapter 5.13).

Microsporidiosis

Microsporidia may cause acute self-limiting diarrhea in immunocompetent persons[11] and in patients who have immunodeficiency other than AIDS. In HIV infection (see Chapter 5.13), chronic diarrhea and wasting are common.[32] *Enterocytozoon bieneusi* is one of the most important intestinal pathogens in severely immunodeficient HIV-infected patients; it is present in 7–50% of those who have otherwise unexplained chronic diarrhea. There are also increasing reports of intestinal microsporidial infections in immunocompetent people.[33] *Encephalitozoon intestinalis* (formerly *Septata intestinalis*) is a less commonly recognized cause of chronic diarrhea. *Encephalitozoon cuniculi* intestinal infection has been reported. These are covered in Chapters 5.13 and 8.32.

Balantidiasis (*Balantidium coli*)

Balantidium coli, the largest and least common of the human protozoan pathogens, is capable of causing an infection resembling amebic colitis. It is particularly prevalent among people living in close association with pigs in South America, Iran, Papua New Guinea and the Philippines. Up to 80% of persons carrying the organism are asymptomatic carriers.[8] Acute diarrhea with blood and mucus begins abruptly and is associated with nausea, abdominal discomfort and marked weight loss. There can be inflammatory changes and ulceration in the proctosigmoid region but the rectum is usually spared. Peritonitis and colonic perforation can progress rapidly to death. A chronic infection occurs with intermittent diarrhea and infrequent bloody stools.

HELMINTHIC GASTROINTESTINAL DISEASE
Ascariasis (*Ascaris lumbricoides*)

Most cases of ascariasis are asymptomic; symptomatic infections are more common in children than adults. When large numbers of larvae migrate to the lungs in a short time period, *Ascaris* pneumonitis can result. This is the clinical picture of Löffler's syndrome, which is characterized by dyspnea, dry cough, wheezing or coarse rales, fever up to 104°F (40°C), transient eosinophilia and a chest radiograph that

is suggestive of viral pneumonia and that resolves within a couple of weeks. In addition, eosinophils, Charcot–Leyden crystals and larvae may rarely be found in the sputum. Symptoms of asthma and urticaria may continue during the intestinal phase of ascariasis. The adult worms occasionally migrate from the small bowel and cause biliary or hepatic ascariasis. Rarely, adult worms migrate into the biliary tree with secondary sepsis and abscess formation. Pancreatitis may result from migrating ascarids that obstruct the pancreatic duct. In people who have large numbers of adult worms intestinal obstruction can occur owing to the sheer bulk of worm bodies. Adult worms migrate more in the presence of a stimulus such as a fever of over 102°F (38.9°C) or the use of a general anesthetic, and they may block the bile duct or pancreatic duct or enter the liver or peritoneal cavity. In children, nutritional deficiencies such as kwashiorkor (protein-energy malnutrition) and vitamin A deficiency are related to the burden of the adult worms.[34]

Enterobiasis (*Enterobius vermicularis*)

Infection with *Enterobius vermicularis* (threadworm or pinworm) causes few or no symptoms in the vast majority of people. The predominant symptom is nocturnal pruritus ani, caused by migration of the female worms from the anus to the perianal skin in the process of laying their eggs. Scratching may be intense and secondary infection may ensue. Pruritus vulvi caused by pinworms entering the vulva is occasionally seen. In children, insomnia, loss of appetite, loss of weight, emotional instability, enuresis and irritability may also be found.[34]

Ancylostomiasis (hookworm infection, *Ancylostoma duodenale*, *Necator americanus*)

Hookworm causes ground itch, a moderate-to-severe pruritus of the skin, usually of the feet, as the hookworm larvae penetrate. Secondary infection can occur if the vesicular lesions are excoriated by scratching. A pneumonitis, caused by alveolar migration of larvae, is less common, less severe and causes less sensitization than that seen with *Ascaris* or *Strongyloides* infection. Symptoms of the intestinal phase are fatigue, nausea, vomiting, abdominal pain, diarrhea with occult bleeding, and weakness. Heavy worm burdens may have serious sequelae in young children.[35] This is particularly problematic with *A. duodenale* infection. Eosinophilia is usually present. According to the degree of worm burden, chronic infection leads to an iron deficiency anemia[17] and hypoproteinemia with pallor, edema of the face and feet, listlessness, koilonychia, cardiomegaly, heart failure and rarely mental retardation.

Trichuriasis (*Trichuris trichiura*)

This common, ubiquitous infection rarely causes any symptoms. In heavy infection (more than 10,000 eggs per gram of feces), epigastric pain, vomiting, distention, flatulence, anorexia and weight loss may occur. Rarely the *Trichuris* dysentery syndrome may occur, with blood and mucus in the stools and, in heavy infections, prolapse of the rectum. The diagnosis is made when numerous worms are seen on the rectal mucosa. A 'honeycomb' effect of the small intestine has appearances similar to Crohn's disease. There may be deformity of the proximal colon and also the ileum or appendix.

Strongyloidiasis (*Strongyloides stercoralis*)

Strongyloides stercoralis largely causes asymptomatic infection of the small intestine, which can last for 30 years or longer.[36] The prepatent period from infection through the skin to the appearance of rhabditiform larvae in the stools is 1 month or more. Symptoms only develop with high intestinal worm loads, which can be the result of several factors. In people debilitated by concurrent disease or malnutrition, there may be massive invasion of the tissues by *S. stercoralis*. Treatment with immunosuppressive drugs in a patient harboring *S. stercoralis* can also lead to the same effect.[37] Infection with human T-cell leukemia virus 1 is important in predisposing to massive infection

2

37.7

by *S. stercoralis*. Infection with HIV is not a common cause of the *Strongyloides* hyperinfection syndrome (see Chapter 5.13). Symptoms include watery mucous diarrhea, with the severity depending on the intensity of the infection. Sometimes diarrhea alternates with constipation. Malabsorption of fat and vitamin B12 with a chronic diarrhea and protein-losing enteropathy has also been described and is rapidly reversed by treatment.

There are two types of skin rash. The first is larva currens, which occurs on the trunk or near the anus and is a linear eruption in which the larvae migrate under the skin causing an itchy, nonindurated wheal with a red flare that moves rapidly and disappears in a few hours (see Chapter 6.34). This contrasts to the indurated and persistent track of nonhuman hookworm larvae (cutaneous larva migrans). The second type of rash is urticaria.

Features of the strongyloidiasis hyperinfestation syndrome (see Fig. 37.5) include severe diarrhea, malabsorption, edema, hepatomegaly and paralytic ileus. Gram-negative sepsis is a recognized complication. In very severe cases encephalopathy and even secondary pyogenic meningitis have been described.

Fasciolopsis buski infection
Fasciolopsis buski is confined to Asian countries, particularly Thailand. Symptoms are more frequent in children than adults owing to their greater exposure to water plants while at play. Like many other intestinal parasites, the majority of infected people have very minor symptoms or none at all. In heavier infections, symptoms can include diarrhea, abdominal pain, vomiting, flatulence, poor appetite, eosinophilia and fever. In very severe cases there may be ascites, edema of the face, abdomen and legs, anemia, anorexia, weakness and even intestinal obstruction. Intestinal ulceration may cause malabsorption and lead to malnutrition and wasting.[14]

Heterophyes heterophyes infection
Heterophyes heterophyes causes few symptoms unless the infection is heavy, which is dependent on the quantities of pickled or uncooked fish eaten in endemic areas (mostly the Middle and Far East). The adult worms produce abdominal pain, diarrhea with mucus and ulceration of the intestinal wall.

Beef and pork tapeworm infection (*Taenia saginata* and *Taenia solium*)
The clinical features of *T. saginata*, the beef tapeworm, and *T. solium*, the pork tapeworm, are similar. The adult worms in the gastrointestinal phase of both organisms usually cause no symptoms, but carriers can sometimes feel a proglottid emerging from the anus; the motile proglottid may be upsettingly obvious in the feces. Other associated symptoms, such as abdominal pain and distension, nausea and anorexia have been attributed to the tapeworm. There is occasionally a mild eosinophilia but there is no anemia, even in long-term infection. Cysticercosis complicates infection with *T. solium* only. Ingestion of *T. solium* eggs leads to the dissemination of oncospheres in the bloodstream; these can become lodged anywhere in the subcutaneous and intramuscular tissues,[38] where they become cysticerci; symptoms depend on the particular body site involved. The clinical findings of neurocysticercosis are discussed in detail in Chapter 6.28.

Dwarf tapeworm infection (*Hymenolepis nana*)
As with other tapeworms, there are usually few symptoms in *H. nana* infection. Symptoms that may occur include abdominal pain, anorexia, irritability and headache. Eosinophilia is common. Symptoms are more common in heavy infections and may cause growth retardation in children.

Fish tapeworm infection (*Diphyllobothrium latum*)
There are few if any symptoms from infection with *D. latum*. Symptoms including diarrhea, headache and nonspecific malaise all appear to be

somewhat more common than in uninfected people. Tapeworm-associated anemia is probably related to vitamin B12 deficiency caused by competition for the vitamin between the tapeworm and a genetically predisposed host; however, this is now exceedingly rare.

DIAGNOSIS

Microscopic examination of the stool is fundamental to the diagnosis of all the gastrointestinal infections (see Chapter 6.10). A minimum of three stool specimens, examined by trained personnel using a concentration and a permanent stain technique, should be used.

Amebiasis is often suspected on clinical grounds but confirmation is always required by demonstrating cysts and trophozoites in the stools or trophozoites from the bowel mucosa. Fresh stools examined within 20 minutes for the presence of trophozoites containing ingested red blood cells enables *E. histolytica* to be distinguished from the nonpathogenic *E. dispar*. *Entamoeba hartmanni*, *Entamoeba coli*, *Iodamoeba butschlii* and *Endolimax nana* are nonpathogenic amebae, the cysts of which can be distinguished by their size and morphology (see Chapter 6.25). Material aspirated or scraped from mucosal surfaces at sigmoidoscopy needs microscopic examination. Culture of amebae is possible and allows zymodeme pattern analysis (a reference standard to diagnose and distinguish between *E. histolytica* and *E. dispar*). The polymerase chain reaction (PCR) can also distinguish *E. histolytica* from *E. dispar*. Monoclonal antibodies and DNA probes for this purpose are available in research centres. A recent rapid stool antigen enzyme-linked immunosorbent assay (ELISA) kit, based on antilectin antibodies, is 80% sensitive and 99% specific in diagnosing *Entamoeba* infection; another commerical test is 95% sensitive and 93% specific in distinguishing between *E. histolytica* and *E. dispar* when compared with culture and zymodeme analysis.[39] If this becomes widely accepted it may be useful in the management of asymptomatic carriers, because it would allow discrimination between pathogenic and nonpathogenic strains and avoid unnecessary treatment. Serologic diagnosis of invasive amebiasis is discussed below.

Giardial cysts and sometimes trophozoites are seen in fecal specimens. Multiple fecal specimens are required. A duodenal aspirate, biopsy or string test may sometimes be positive in the presence of negative stool microscopy. Giardial antigens can be detected in feces by a commercially available ELISA with reported sensitivity and specificity of 87–100% compared with microscopy; research laboratories can offer DNA probes or PCR diagnosis. An indirect immuno-fluorescence test using a cyst-specific anti-*Giardia lamblia* monoclonal antibody has been reported to detect twice the number of positive stool specimens than light microscopy.[40] This may allow more accurate diagnosis from fewer stool samples and obviate the need for biopsy or endoscopy.

Diagnosis of *Cryptosporidium*, *Cyclospora* and *Isospora* infections relies on identification of the oocysts in feces or on intestinal biopsy. For cryptosporidia, three staining methods are used: auramine, modified Ziehl–Neelsen and immunofluoresence using monoclonal antibodies to the oocysts.[41] Cryptosporidial antigen detection in feces and PCR techniques are research tools at present. Serologic tests are of limited diagnostic use. *Cyclospora* and *Isospora* spp. can be seen by light microscopy and identified by transmission electron microscopy. *Isospora* oocysts are stained by modified Ziehl–Neelsen and they fluoresce with phenol auramine stain under ultraviolet light.

Microsporidia are so small that they are hard to detect in stool, but a modified trichrome stain or fluorescent chromotrope stain makes this possible. Histologists are able to visualize the spores in small bowel sections with Giemsa and other stains, but electron microscopy is needed for species identification. The parasitology is covered in detail in Chapter 8.32.

The diagnosis of the gastrointestinal helminths depends on the finding and identification of ova, proglottids, larvae or worms in the feces on light microscopy (Fig. 37.7). Eggs are never uniformly distributed, so a fecal sample should be mixed well before examination. The deposit made by a concentration method is usually used and examined by light microscopy at magnifications of 100 and 400. Chapter 6.10 discusses methods used in detail. The parasites are identified by appearance and size. Culture can be undertaken for *S. stercoralis*.

Serologic tests for the intestinal protozoa and helminths are helpful only in the diagnosis of amebiasis, strongyloidiasis, invasive giardiasis and cysticercosis (but not intestinal tapeworm infection). The amebic immunofluorescent antibody test is positive in 95% of cases of amebic abscess by the end of the first 14 days of illness. However, there are some false-positive results in nonamebic liver disease, so a cellulose acetate precipitin test is done to confirm the diagnosis. Anticysticercal antibodies have a useful role in the diagnosis of neurocysticercosis (see Chapter 6.28).

An ELISA for *Strongyloides* is useful in screening patients who have suggestive symptoms or eosinophilia. Cross-reactions occur occasionally with ascariasis and filarial infection. The filarial ELISA cross-reacts in some cases of strongyloidiasis. Serum antigiardial antibody detection is not clinically useful in highly endemic areas because people may be seropositive from past infection. The giardial immunofluorescent antibody test gives good titers if the disease has caused mucosal damage, and it is helpful in the investigation of parasite-associated malabsorption.

MANAGEMENT

GASTROINTESTINAL PROTOZOA

The management of gastrointestinal protozoa is summarized in Figure 37.8. Treatment regimens are discussed in detail in Chapter 7.17.

Entamoeba histolytica

Treatment of *E. histolytica* infection is divided into two types. Luminal amebicides, such as diloxanide furoate, act on organisms in the intestinal lumen and are not effective against organisms in tissue. Tissue amebicides, such as metronidazole and tinidazole are effective in treating invasive amebiasis but less effective in the treatment of organisms in the bowel lumen.

There is some controversy about treating asymptomatic patients. Ideally, any amebic cysts should be tested to identify whether it is *E. histolytica* (in which case the infection should be treated to avoid the risk of developing invasive disease and to prevent secondary spread) or *E. dispar* (which does not require any treatment). However, until

TREATMENT OF GASTROINTESTINAL PROTOZOAL INFECTION

Condition	Drug	Dosage
Amebiasis Asymptomatic carrier of intestinal cysts		
1st choice	Diloxanide furoate	500mg q8h for 10 days
2nd choice	Paromomycin (aminosidine)	500mg q8h for 10 days
Intestinal infection (amebic dysentery or ameboma)	Metronidazole or	750–800mg q8h for 5 days
	Tinidazole followed by	2g daily for 2–3 days
	Diloxanide furoate or	500mg q8h for 10 days
	Paromomycin	500mg q8h for 10 days
Amebic liver abscess	Metronidazole or	400–500mg q8h for 5–10 days
	Tinidazole followed by	2g daily for 3–5 days
	Diloxanide furoate	500mg q8h for 10 days
Giardiasis 1st choice	Tinidazole or	2g single dose
	Metronidazole	2g daily for 3 days
2nd choice	Albendazole	400mg daily for 5 days
3rd choice	Mepacrine	100mg q8h for 5–7 days
***Balantidium coli* infection** 1st choice	Tetracycline	500mg q6h for 10 days
Alternatives	Ampicillin, metronidazole, or paromomycin	
***Cyclospora cayetanensis* infection**	Trimethoprim–sulfamethoxazole	960mg q12h for 7 days
***Isospora belli* infection** 1st choice	Trimethoprim–sulfamethoxazole (co-trimoxazole)	960mg [160mg (TMP)/800mg (SMX)] q12h for 7–10 days (q6h in immunosuppressed patients)
2nd choice (if intolerant to sulfonamides):	Furazolidone	100mg q6h for 10 days

Fig. 37.8 Treatment of gastrointestinal protozoal infection. All treatments are adult dosage and given orally unless stated otherwise.

newer ELISA or monoclonal antibody tests become widely available it will continue to be usual to treat asymptomatic patients in nonendemic areas with diloxanide furoate 500mg orally q8h for 10 days (see Fig. 37.8). When asymptomatic cyst carriage persists after treatment for amebic dysentery or liver abscess, further treatment with a luminal amebicide is mandatory, otherwise relapse is frequent. The treatment of asymptomatic cyst carriers in endemic areas is of questionable value because of the high rate of re-infection. A second choice intraluminal amebicide is paromomycin 500mg orally q8h for 10 days.[42]

Proven amebic dysentery should always be treated. Drugs of choice are metronidazole (750–800mg orally q8h for 5 days) or tinidazole (2g daily for 2–3 days) followed by diloxanide furoate (see Fig. 37.8). Amebic liver abscess is treated with metronidazole, 400–500mg orally q8h, followed by diloxanide furoate as above. Tinidazole (2g daily orally for 3–5 days) is an alternative; chloroquine (150mg base q6h for 2 days then 150mg base q12h for 19 days) can also be used.

Giardia lamblia

Treatment is often unnecessary because most healthy, immunocompetent patients have a self-limiting disease and recover by their own natural host defense mechanisms. Treatment of symptomatic patients reduces the duration and severity of symptoms. The treatment of asymptomatic cyst carriers is controversial in endemic areas.

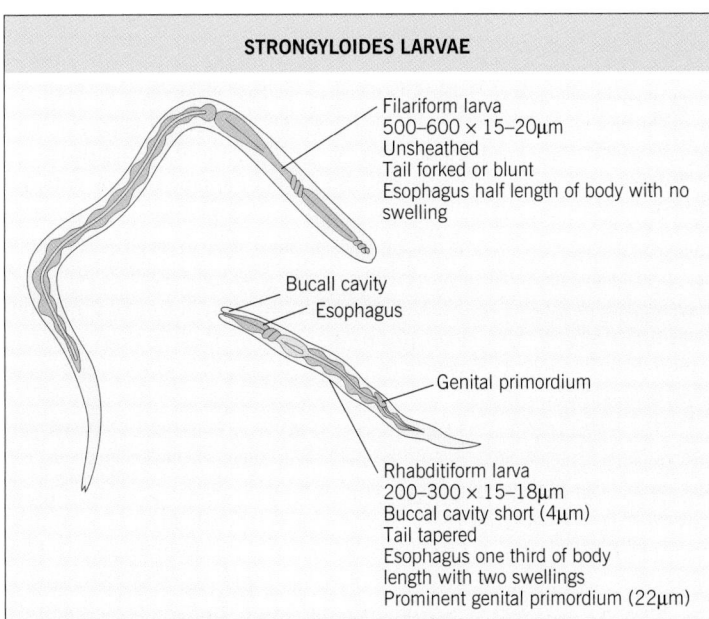

STRONGYLOIDES LARVAE

Filariform larva
500–600 × 15–20µm
Unsheathed
Tail forked or blunt
Esophagus half length of body with no swelling

Bucall cavity
Esophagus

Genital primordium

Rhabditiform larva
200–300 × 15–18µm
Buccal cavity short (4µm)
Tail tapered
Esophagus one third of body length with two swellings
Prominent genital primordium (22µm)

Fig. 37.7 Strongyloides larvae.

Generally, in a nonendemic area, asymptomatic *Giardia* cyst carriers are treated. The 5-nitroimidazole derivatives metronidazole or tinidazole are the treatment of choice and can be used in short courses.[25] Albendazole, 400mg daily for 5 days, has been shown to have useful antigiardial activity. Mepacrine, an acridine dye, has a similar efficacy but is generally less well tolerated with an incidence of 1.5% of acute psychosis. Furazolidone, a nitrofuran, has lower efficacy but is well tolerated. In-vitro and in-vivo resistance of *G. lamblia* has been demonstrated, although rarely, to conventional therapy, particularly to the 5-nitroimidazoles such as metronidazole and tinidazole.[43]

Blastocystis hominis
If *B. hominis* is present in the stool, the physician must not stop looking for another cause of diarrhea. Whether any treatment is required is controversial. Metronidazole seems to be the most appropriate drug.

Dientamoeba fragilis
In adults infected with *D. fragilis*, improvement can be seen with tetracycline; in children, metronidazole is appropriate.

Balantidium coli
Tetracycline, 500mg four times a day for 10 days, is effective against *B. coli*. Other drugs to which *B. coli* is sensitive are ampicillin, metronidazole and paromomycin. Surgery may be required for fulminant disease with perforation or abscess formation.

Cryptosporidium parvum
Cryptosporidium parvum infection is self-limiting in those who have normal immunity. It presents a severe problem when it occurs in patients who have AIDS as no treatment regimen has a reliable effect other than HAART (highly active anti-retroviral therapy).[30]

Cyclospora cayetanensis
Many cases of *C. cayetanensis* infection are self-limiting. When treatment is felt to be necessary trimethoprim–sulfamethoxazole (cotrimoxazole) 960mg (160gm TMP/800mg SMX) q12h for 7 days has been found to be effective, eradicating the oocysts from 94% of 16 patients in 7 days compared with 12% of 17 patients who received placebo.[44] Relapse is common in the immunocompromised but responds to a second course of treatment.

Isospora belli
Treatment of *I. belli* infection may be necessary in the immunocompromised, when oral trimethoprim–sulfamethoxazole [960mg (160gm TMP/800mg SMX) q6h daily for 7–10 days] eliminates the parasite in most cases; relapse is common but retreatment is usually effective. Prophylactic trimethoprim–sulfamethoxazole may then be necessary. Pyrimethamine–sulfonamide combinations have also been proved to be effective. If the patient is intolerant to sulfonamides, furazolidone 100mg 4 times daily for 10 days is an alternative.

Microsporidia
The treatment of microsporidiosis in the immunocompetent is not required. Evidence and experience in treating these infections comes from HIV-infected patients (see Chapter 5.13) where albendazole has been shown to be useful with some species of microsporidia.

GASTROINTESTINAL HELMINTHS
The management of gastrointestinal helminths is summarized in Figure 37.9 (see Chapter 7.17).

Ascaris lumbricoides
Treatment is effective only against the adult worm. It is usual to treat any established infection. The drugs used are albendazole (400mg, single dose), mebendazole (100mg q12h for 3 days), levamisole (150mg, single dose) or piperazine in a single adult dose of 4g of piperazine phosphate or 4.5g of piperazine hydrate, or pyrantel pamoate in a single dose of 10mg/kg. *Ascaris* pneumonitis responds dramatically to prednisolone therapy, and anthelmintics should be given for 2 weeks after lung involvement. Surgery is sometimes required for bowel perforation or obstruction.

Enterobius vermicularis
Enterobius vermicularis infection is treated with mebendazole (100mg, single dose, which is repeated if necessary after 2–3 weeks), piperazine phosphate (4g, single adult dose repeated after 14 days) or pyrantel pamoate (10mg/kg, single dose). The whole family should be treated simultaneously, fresh bed linen and night clothes should be provided and the nails kept short and scrubbed. Repeat treatment may be required because recurrence is common.

Hookworm
Hookworm infection is treated by eliminating the adult worms and treating anemia if present; these treatments can be carried out concurrently. In endemic countries where re-infection is inevitable, light infections are treated only in children, not in adults. Mebendazole (100mg q12h for 3 days) or albendazole (400mg, single dose) are effective against both *A. duodenale* and *N. americanus*. In a single-dose comparison of albendazole and mebendazole, albendazole gave better cure and egg reduction rates.[45] Levamisole (150mg orally, single dose) is less effective against *N. americanus*, and pyrantel pamoate (10mg/kg orally) is preferred.

TREATMENT OF GASTROINTESTINAL HELMINTHIC INFECTION

Condition	Drug	Dosage
Nematodes Round worms *Ascaris lumbricoides*	Albendazole Mebendazole	400mg, single dose 100mg q12h for 3 days
	Levamisole Piperazine hydrate	150mg, single dose 4.5g, single dose
Enterobius vermicularis	Mebendazole Piperazine phosphate Pyrantel pamoate	100mg, single dose 4g, single dose 10 mg/kg, single dose
Hookworms *Ancylostoma duodenale* *Necator americanus*	Mebendazole Albendazole Levamisole	100mg q12h for 3 days 200mg q24h for 3 days 150mg, single dose (less effective against *N. americanus*)
Trichuris trichiura	Pyrantel pamoate Mebendazole	10mg/kg, single dose 100mg q12h for 3 days or 600mg, single dose
Strongyloides stercoralis	Albendazole Ivermectin Albendazole	400mg, single dose 200µg/kg, single dose 400mg q12–24h for 3 days
	Thiabendazole	25mg/kg (max 1.5g) q12h for 3 days
Trematodes (flukes) *Fasciolopsis buski* *Heterophyes heterophyes*	Praziquantel Praziquantel	15mg/kg, single dose 10–20mg/kg, single dose
Cestodes (tapeworms) *Taenia solium* *Taenia saginata* *Hymenolepis nana*	Praziquantel Niclosamide Praziquantel Niclosamide	10mg/kg, single dose 2g, single dose 20mg/kg, single dose 2g on day 1 then 1g/day for 6 days
Diphyllobothrium latum	Praziquantel Niclosamide	10mg/kg, single dose 2g, single dose

Fig. 37.9 Treatment of gastrointestinal helminthic infection. All treatments are adult dosage and given orally unless stated otherwise.

Trichuris trichiura

In symptomatic patients and in asymptomatic carriers who have high numbers of eggs, trichuriasis is treated with mebendazole (100mg q12h for 3 days or 600mg, single dose) or albendazole (400mg, single dose). In undernourished children who have moderate infection intensities in Jamaica, albendazole treatment also resulted in improvement in some tests of cognitive ability and in school attendance and school performance, even after controlling for socioeconomic status.[46]

Strongyloides stercoralis

Strongyloides stercoralis infection should be treated in both symptomatic and asymptomatic people because of its ability to cause hyperinfection if immunosuppression occurs. Ivermectin is the drug of choice (200μg/kg orally, single dose). This regimen has proven very effective in a prospective randomized trial comparing the efficacy of ivermectin and thiabendazole in Cambodian refugees who had symptomatic chronic strongyloidiasis.[47] Ivermectin also looks very promising in HIV-positive patients infected with *S. stercoralis* (see Chapter 5.13). Albendazole, 400mg once or twice daily for 3 days is also effective. Thiabendazole, 25mg/kg (maximum 1.5g) orally twice daily for 3 days, is effective but often poorly tolerated.

Fasciolopsis buski

Fasciolopsis buski infection is treated with praziquantel (15mg/kg orally), which is highly effective. Niclosamide (2g orally, single dose) has also been used.

Heterophyes heterophyes

Heterophyes heterophyes infection is treated with a single dose of praziquantel (10–20mg/kg orally). Niclosamide is an alternative.

Taenia solium and Taenia saginata

Patients who have *T. solium* infection should be evaluated for the presence of cerebral cysticercosis before commencing therapy against the intestinal tapeworm. Praziquantel (10mg/kg, single dose) is effective therapy for the adult worm. Niclosamide (2g, single dose) has also been widely used.

Hymenolepis nana

Hymenolepis nana infection can be treated with a single oral dose of praziquantel (20mg/kg). Niclosamide (2g on day 1, then 1g daily for 6 days) is also successful.

Diphyllobothrium latum

Diphyllobothrium latum infections are treated with praziquantel (10mg/kg, single dose). Niclosamide (2g, single dose) was extensively used in the past.

REFERENCES

1. Pritchard DI. The survival strategies of Hookworms. Parasitol Today 1995;11:255–9.
2. Warren KS. Helminthic diseases endemic in the United States. Am J Trop Med Hyg 1974;23:723–30.
3. Vermund SH, Macleod S. Is pinworm a vanishing infection? Am J Dis Child 1988;142:566–8.
4. Garcia LS, Bruckner DA. Intestial protozoa: amoebae. In: Garcia LS, Bruckner DA, eds. Diagnostic medical parasitology, 3rd ed. Washington, DC: American Society for Microbiology; 1997:6–33.
5. Reed SL. New concepts regarding the pathogenesis of amebiasis. Clin Infect Dis 1995;21 (Suppl 2):182–5.
6. Farthing MJ. Diarrhoeal disease: current concepts and future challenges. Pathogenesis of giardiasis. Trans R Soc Trop Med Hyg 1993;87(Suppl 3):17–21.
7. Nash TE, Herrington DA, Levine MM, Conrad JT, Merritt JW Jr. Antigenic variation of *Giardia lamblia* in experimental human infections. J Immunol 1990;144:4362–9.
8. Farthing MJG, Cevallos A, Kelly P. Intestinal protozoa. In: Cook GC, ed. Manson's tropical diseases, 20th ed. London: WB Saunders; 1996:1255–98.
9. Phillips AD, Thomas AG, Walker-Smith JA. *Cryptosporidium*, chronic diarrhoea and the proximal small intestinal mucosa. Gut 1992;33:1057–61.
10. Bendall RP, Lucas S, Moody A, Tovey G, Chiodini PL. Diarrhoea associated with cyanobacterium-like bodies: a new coccidian enteritis of man. Lancet 1993;341:590–2.

11. Weber R, Bryan RT. Microsporidial infections in immunodeficient and immunocompetent patients. Clin Infect Dis 1994;19:517–21.
12. Pawlowski ZS. Ascaris. In: Pawlowski ZS, ed. Intestinal helminthic infections, vol. 12, no.3. London: Bailliere Tindall; 1987:595–615.
13. Gilman RH, Chong YH, Davis C, *et al*. The adverse consequences of heavy *Trichuris trichiura* infection. Trans R Soc Trop Med Hyg 1983;77:432–8.
14. Haswell-Elkins MR, Elkins DB. Food-borne trematodes. In: Cook GC, ed. Manson's tropical diseases, 20th ed. London: WB Saunders; 1996:1456–76.
15. Baily GG, Intestinal Cestodes. In: Cook GC, ed. Manson's tropical diseases, 20th ed. London: WB Saunders; 1996:1477–85.
16. World Health Organization. Prevention and control of intestinal parasitic infections. WHO Technical Report Series no 749. Geneva: World Health Organization; 1987.
17. Pawlowski ZS, Schad GA, Stott GJ. Hookworm infection and anemia approaches to prevention and control. Geneva: World Health Organization; 1991.
18. Conway DJ, Lindo JF, Robinson RD, Bundy DAP. Towards effective control of *Strongyloides stercoralis*. Parasitol Today 1995;11:420–4.
19. Guyatt HL, Chan MS, Medley GF, Bundy DAP. Control of Ascaris infection by chemotherapy: which is the most cost-effective option? Trans R Soc Trop Med Hyg 1995;89:16–20.
20. Bundy DAP, Guyatt HL. Anthelmintic chemotherapy: the individual and the community. Curr Opin Infect Dis 1995;8:466–72.

21. Bundy DAP, Chan MS, Guyatt HL. The practicality and sustainability of vaccination as an approach to parasite control. Parasitology 1995;110(Suppl):51–8.
22. Diamond LS, Clark CG. A redescription of *Entamoeba histolytica* Schaudinn, 1903 (Emended Walker, 1911) separating it from *Entamoeba dispar* Brumpt, 1925. J Eukaryotic Microbiol 1993;40:340–4.
23. Lengerich EJ, Addiss DG, Juranek DD. Severe giardiasis in the United States. Clin Infect Dis 1994;18:760–3.
24. Babb RR. Giardiasis. Taming this pervasive parasitic infection. Postgrad Med 1995;98:155–8.
25. Hill DR. Giardiasis. Issues in diagnosis and management. Dis Clin North Am 1993;7:503–25.
26. Shlim DR, Hoge CW, Rajah R, Rabold JG, Echeverria P. Is *Blastocystis hominis* a cause of diarrhea in travelers? A prospective controlled study in Nepal. Clin Infect Dis 1995;21:97–101.
27. Logar J, Andlovic A, Poljsak-Prijatelj M. Incidence of *Blastocystis hominis* in patients with diarrhoea. J Infect 1994;28:151–4.
28. Spencer MJ, Garcia LS, Chapin MR. *Dientamoeba fragilis*: an intestinal pathogen in children? Am J Dis Child 1979;133:390–3.
29. Chappell CL, Okhuysen PC, Sterling CR, DuPont HL. *Cryptosporidium parvum*: intensity of infection and oocyst excretion patterns in healthy volunteers. J Infect Dis 1996;173:232–6.
30. Hoepelman AI. Current therapeutic approaches to cryptosporidiosis in immunocompromised patients. J Antimicrob Chemother 1996;37:871–80.
31. Soave R, Hohnson WD Jr. *Cryptosporidium* and *Isospora belli* infections. J Infect Dis 1988;15:225–9.

32. Bryan RT. Microsporidiosis as an AIDS-related opportunistic infection. Clin Infect Dis 1995;21 (Suppl 1):62–5.

33. Desportes-Livage I. Human microsporidioses. Curr Opin Infect Dis 1998;11:177–81.

34. Gopinath R, Keystone JS. Ascariasis, Trichuriasis and Enterobiasis. In: Blaser MJ, Smith PD, Ravdin HI, et al., eds. Infections of the gastrointestinal tract. Philadelphia: Raven Press; 1995:1167–78.

35. Hotez PJ. Hookworm disease in children. Pediatr Infect Dis J 1989;8:516–20.

36. Raffalli J, Friedman C, Reid D, et al. Diagnosis: disseminated Strongyloides stercoralis infection. Clin Infect Dis 1995;21:1377.

37. Liu LX, Weller PF. Strongyloidiasis and other intestinal nematode infections. Infect Dis Clin North Am 1993;7:655–92.

38. Tsang VCW, Wilson M: Taenia solium cysticercosis: an under-recognized but serious public health problem. Parasitol Today 1995;11:124–6.

39. Haque R, Neville LM, Hahn P, Petri WA Jr. Rapid diagnosis of Entamoeba infection by using Entamoeba and Entamoeba histolytica stool antigen detection kits. J Clin Microbiol 1995;33:2558–61.

40. Winiecka-Krusnell J, Linder E. Detection of Giardia lamblia cysts in stool samples by immunofluorescence using monoclonal antibody. Eur J Clin Microbiol Infect Dis 1995;14:218–22.

41. Tee GH, Moody AH, Cooke AH, Chiodini PL. Comparison of techniques for detecting antigens of Giardia lamblia and Cryptosporidium parvum in faeces. J Clin Pathol 1993;46:555–8.

42. Reed SL. Amoebiasis: an update. Clin Infect Dis 1992;14:385–93.

43. Upcroft JA, Upcroft P. Drug resistance and Giardia. Parasitol Today 1993;9:187–190.

44. Hoge CW, Shlim DR, Ghimire M, et al. Placebo-controlled trial of co-trimoxazole for Cyclospora infections among travellers and foreign residents in Nepal. Lancet 1995;345:691–3.

45. Albonico M, Smith PG, Hall A, Chwaya HM, Alawi KS, Savioli L. A randomised controlled trial comparing mebendazole and albendazole against Ascaris, Trichuris and hookworm infections. Trans R Soc Trop Med Hyg 1994;88:585–9.

46. Simeon DT, Grantham-McGregor SM, Callender JE, Wong MS. Treatment of Trichuris trichiura infection improves growth, spelling scores and school attendance in some children. J Nutr 1995;125:1875–83.

47. Gann PH, Neva FA, Gam AA. A randomized trial of single and two-dose ivermentin versus thiabendazole for treatment of strongyloidiasis. J Infect Dis 1994;169:1076–9.

Peritonitis, Pancreatitis and Intra-abdominal Abscesses

Bo Brismar, Svante Sjöstedt & Carl Erik Nord

INTRODUCTION

Despite advances in diagnosis, antimicrobial therapy, operative and intensive care, generalized peritonitis and intra-abdominal abscesses remain serious and life-threatening conditions.

The abdominal cavity can, for practical purposes, be divided in a supracolonic and an infracolonic part, and these parts can be further subdivided. These sites may all be the location of intra-abdominal abscesses.

The right subphrenic space is situated between the diaphragm and the right liver lobe. The right subhepatic space (Morison's pouch) is located under the right lobe of the liver and the gallbladder. The left subphrenic space is found between the diaphragm, the left liver lobe, the stomach and the spleen. The left subhepatic space is often called the lesser omental sac.

The intercolonic space is the space between the ascending, transverse and descending colon. The paracolonic space is along the outside of and lateral to the ascending and descending colon. The retroperitoneal space is the space containing the duodenum, the pancreas and the kidneys.

PERITONITIS

PATHOGENESIS
Primary bacterial peritonitis
Spontaneous bacterial peritonitis is seen typically in patients who have liver disease and ascites. Its incidence in patients who have liver cirrhosis and ascites is reported to be 4–12%.[1] The pathogenesis has the following sequence:
* translocation of micro-organisms into the mesenteric lymph node,
* bacteremia arising from the lymphatic system,
* growth of bacteria in ascites secondary to bacteremia, and
* growth of bacteria in opsonin-deficient ascites.[2–4]

The same micro-organisms are found in the blood and the ascites of approximately 50% of patients who have liver cirrhosis and culture-positive ascites.[5] The incidence of bacterial peritonitis is high in patients who have cirrhosis and impaired reticuloendothelial system phagocyte activity[6] and susceptibility to bacterial peritonitis is probably higher in patients if there is decreased opsonin activity in the ascites.[7] Direct translocation of micro-organisms from the intestinal mucosa to ascitic fluid is not of major importance.[7]

Microbiologic findings. Escherichia coli is most frequently isolated from the ascites, followed by *Klebsiella pneumoniae,* pneumococci, streptococci and enterococci. *Staphylococcus aureus* is not often found in primary peritonitis. Anaerobic bacteria are isolated in 5% of patients. Primary peritonitis is rarely caused by *Chlamydia pneumoniae, Neisseria gonorrhoeae* and *Mycobacterium tuberculosis.* Primary peritonitis due to pneumococci used to be observed as a complication of nephrotic syndrome in children but is now seldom seen.

Secondary bacterial peritonitis
Secondary bacterial peritonitis is most often caused by perforation of the intestine resulting in spillage of intestinal contents into the abdominal cavity. The magnitude of bacterial contamination depends upon several factors such as the site of the perforation, the cause of the perforation and the local defense system limiting the infection. Another type of secondary bacterial peritonitis is iatrogenic peritonitis caused by peritoneal dialysis.

The introduction of micro-organisms into the abdominal cavity starts different pathogenic processes.[8] About 80% of the micro-organisms are cleared via the lymphatic system of the peritoneal membranes. The rest are phagocytosed following the release of opsonins by polymorphonuclear leukocytes and macrophages in the peritoneum. Vascular permeability is increased and, as a result, plasma containing fibrinogen and thromboplastin are released into the abdominal cavity.[9]

If the immune defense system is not capable of killing the micro-organisms, an abscess develops. A diffuse peritonitis results if the infectious process cannot be contained. Contamination with blood, feces, foreign bodies and necrotic tissue increases the risk of abscess formation and peritonitis.

Microbiologic findings. The number and types of micro-organisms depend upon the site of gastrointestinal perforation. When the stomach is perforated, rather few types of acid-resistant micro-organisms such as lactobacilli, streptococci and *Candida* spp. are recovered. The proximal small intestinal microflora also contains relatively fewer micro-organisms, whereas the number of microbial species is greater in the distal ileum. Perforation of the upper small intestine leads to the isolation of lactobacilli, streptococci, enterococci and clostridia are isolated.

When the large intestine perforates many different microbial species are spilled into the peritoneal cavity. In most cases when an infection develops, five types of pathogenic bacteria predominate:
* *E. coli,*
* enterococci,
* *Bacteroides fragilis,*
* anaerobic Gram-positive cocci, and
* clostridia.

In animal experiments it has been shown that *E. coli* is responsible for early sepsis and death whereas *B. fragilis* is responsible for late abscess formation. With colonic perforation, *E. coli* is the most frequently recovered aerobic micro-organism and *B. fragilis* is the most frequently isolated anaerobic micro-organism. Severely ill hospitalized patients may have an altered lower intestinal microflora with increased numbers of *Pseudomonas aeruginosa, Enterobacter* spp., and multidrug-resistant nosocomial pathogens such as *Enterococcus faecium, E. faecalis,* and *Candida* spp. These micro-organisms in turn can be recovered from intrabdominal sepsis when colonic perforations occur in these compromised patients.

CLINICAL FEATURES
Abdominal trauma
Blunt abdominal trauma can induce peritonitis. For example, the abdomen can be compressed by the seat belt during a car accident resulting in rupture of the small intestine or separation of the mesentery and subsequent intestinal gangrene. Penetrating injuries of the abdomen are also a cause of secondary peritonitis. Injuries produced by knives can sometimes be treated conservatively with antimicrobial agents, but gunshot injuries usually require operative treatment.[10]

Iatrogenic bacterial peritonitis

Bacterial peritonitis is an iatrogenic complication of continuous peritoneal dialysis. Improvements in the techniques of peritoneal dialysis such as plastic bags, titanium adapters and Y-sets have decreased the incidence of peritonitis to 0.5 episodes/patient per year.[11] Contamination by *Staphylococcus epidermidis* has significantly decreased, but catheter infections by *S. aureus* remain a clinical problem.

MANAGEMENT
Primary bacterial peritonitis

Because most cases of primary peritonitis are caused by Enterobacteriaceae and Gram-positive cocci, the antimicrobial treatment should be directed against these micro-organisms. The third-generation cephalosporins are effective in the treatment of primary peritonitis. Other antimicrobial agents include broad-spectrum penicillins (ticarcillin and piperacillin), beta-lactam/beta-lactamase inhibitor combinations (ampicillin–sulbactam, ticarcillin–clavulanate and piperacillin–tazobactam) and carbapenems (imipenem and meropenem). Aminoglycosides should be avoided due to their potential renal toxicity and slow penetration into infected tissues.

Monobactams, trimethoprim–sulfamethoxazole (co-trimoxazole) and quinolones such as ciprofloxacin should not be used because their activities against Gram-positive cocci are low. Short courses (5 days) of treatment have been shown to be as effective as long courses (10 days).

Secondary bacterial peritonitis

Operative management. The goals of operative management are to:
- eliminate the source of bacterial contamination,
- minimize the bacterial contamination in the peritoneal cavity, and
- protect against relapsing infections.[12]

The traditional operative approach includes laparatomy by midline incision to identify the cause of infection. Laparoscopic techniques have introduced new diagnostic and therapeutic possibilities for acute appendicitis and cholecystitis. For inflammatory processes that are likely to progress, a resection is recommended, whereas a primary closure can be performed for perforations resulting in localized peritoneal contamination. The inflammatory process can in some cases be self-limiting, for example in Crohn's disease or when an ischemic but viable intestinal loop is detached after an ileus.

The perforation of extraperitoneal organs such as the duodenum and rectum can sometimes cause operative difficulties. Severe inflammation of intraperitoneal organs such as perforated diverticulitis and acute gangrenous cholecystitis can also present operative problems. In these situations, drainage and antimicrobial treatment may be the first choice of treatment and resection carried out as a secondary procedure.
Antimicrobial treatment. Both operative and antimicrobial therapy are required for severe intra-abdominal infections. Use of antimicrobial agents against both aerobic and anaerobic bacteria is recommended. Agents active against aerobic bacteria are aminoglycosides, third-generation cephalosporins, monobactams and fluoroquinolones, whereas agents active against anaerobic bacteria are clindamycin and nitroimidazoles. These two groups of aerobic and anaerobic agents should be combined in the treatment of intra-abdominal infections. Monotherapy with antimicrobial agents active against both aerobic and anaerobic bacteria is provided by the carbapenems and the beta-lactam/beta-lactamase inhibitor combinations. The duration of antimicrobial treatment is usually 5–7 days, but depends upon the severity of infection and clinical response. A short treatment of 24 hours is recommended for sterile peritonitis. The need for antimicrobial treatment of enterococci or yeasts, mainly *Candida albicans,* in intra-abdominal infections is controversial but is generally recommended if found in significant numbers in the peritoneal space.

INTRA-ABDOMINAL ABSCESS

PATHOGENESIS
Local deposition of fibrin plays an important role in limiting an abdominal infection, but also plays a role in abscess formation. Without such limitation, micro-organisms can proliferate without being phagocytosed. Fibrin can also cover the micro-organisms and so hinder opsonization of the micro-organisms.[13] Experimental investigations have shown that intraperitoneal fibrinolysis improves phagocytosis, such that abscess development can be avoided in rats when plasminogen activators are given.[14]

Microbiologic findings
The micro-organisms recovered from intra-abdominal abscesses are similar to those isolated in secondary bacterial peritonitis. When the large intestine is involved, *E. coli* is the dominant aerobic bacterial species and *B. fragilis* is the dominant anaerobic bacterial species. Experimental investigations in animals have showed that *B. fragilis* is involved in abscess formation. The polysaccharide capsule and cell wall lipopolysaccharide of *B. fragilis* contribute to abscess development. In abscesses of the upper small intestine, streptococci, enterococci and *Candida* spp. are recovered.

CLINICAL FEATURES
Intra-abdominal abscesses are intraperitoneal, retroperitoneal or involve the viscera. In 50% of cases intraperitoneal abscesses are localized to the lower right quadrant of the abdomen.[15] They may also be localized in the lower left quadrant or subphrenic or subhepatic spaces. Retroperitoneal abscesses often originate from the kidneys or pancreas.

Appendicitis and diverticulitis are responsible for more than 25% of all intra-abdominal abscesses. Spontaneous leakage secondary to a gastrointestinal tumor, pancreatitis or intestinal gangrene are other important causes. Intra-abdominal abscesses are also seen as a complication in 2–3% of cases of penetrating abdominal trauma.[16] Increased age, perforation of the left colon, a large loss of blood and multiple organ injuries increase the risk of developing an abscess.[17]

The time lapse between diagnosis and treatment is an important factor in the resulting mortality rate, which varies between 30% for patients managed operatively and 100% for those managed conservatively.[18]

DIAGNOSIS
Intra-abdominal abscesses are diagnosed on the basis of the medical history and clinical findings. Radiologic methods such as CT, ultrasound and gallium scintigraphy can be used to make the diagnosis. Computed tomography is the most accurate (92%)[19] and allows simultaneous percutaneous drainage of the abscess.[20] Successful outcome of percutaneous drainage requires good collaboration between the surgeon and the radiologist.

Ultrasonography also allows percutaneous drainage, but the success rate is lower (75–82%) than in CT-guided drainage.[21,22] Ultrasound is most suitable for abscesses in the upper right quadrant, retroperitoneum and pelvis, when it has a diagnostic sensitivity of 90%.[23] The sensitivity of gallium scintigraphy is low and it is seldom used to diagnose an intra-abdominal abscess.

For patients with septic features and a suspected infectious focus, scanning with [111]indium-labeled white blood cells can be used to localize an abscess. A diagnostic sensitivity of 90% has been reported. However, usually CT or ultrasound investigations are preferred.[24]

MANAGEMENT
Operative management
An intra-abdominal abscess requires both operative drainage and antimicrobial therapy. Diseased organs must be repaired, excised or exteriorized to avoid further peritoneal contamination.

Several methods can be used to minimize the risk for further local infection and secondary sepsis. Lavage of the intra-abdominal cavity with normal saline that contains antimicrobial agents has been proposed, whereas the value of peritoneal lavage through catheters has been questioned.[25] An alternative approach is to leave the abdominal cavity open after operation for daily inspection of the infection. All fluid, pseudomembranes and exudates should be removed and the cavity washed with saline.[26] The abdominal cavity is covered with sterile dressings and run-through steel sutures are inserted to facilitate secondary closure of the abdomen after 48–72 hours. By leaving the abdominal cavity open, any purulent material can drain during this early postoperative period.[27]

Antimicrobial treatment

Antimicrobial agents that are active against both aerobic and anaerobic bacteria should be used in combination with operative management in the treatment of intra-abdominal abscess. Suitable agents are the aminoglycosides, third-generation cephalosporins, monobactams and fluoroquinolones against aerobic bacteria, and clindamycin and nitroimidazoles against anaerobic bacteria. Monotherapy with carbapenems or beta-lactam/beta-lactamase inhibitors can also be used. Usually a course of 5–7 days is sufficient.

PANCREATITIS

PATHOGENESIS

Infection complicating necrotizing pancreatitis is common and potentially lethal. The risk of infection is related to the duration and extent of necrosis. In the early phase the necrotic tissue is sterile, but later about 40% of the patients develop infection.[28] Micro-organisms may spread in the following ways:[29]
- as a result of direct penetration from the colon,
- via lymph vessels from the gallbladder or colon, and
- by infected bile via the pancreatic duct.

Microbiologic findings

Acute pancreatitis is seldom caused by micro-organisms, It is usually a sterile process induced by chemical autodigestion of the pancreas complicating alcoholism, trauma or biliary disease.

Infected necrotizing pancreatitis occurs in 3–6% of patients who have acute pancreatitis. *Escherichia coli* is the most common isolate, followed by enterococci, streptococci, *Klebsiella* spp., *Enterobacter* spp., *Proteus* spp. and *Pseudomonas* spp. *Staphylococcus aureus* is recovered less often. Anaerobic bacteria have been reported in 6–16%

of cases with *B. fragilis* as the dominant species. The microbiolgy of necrotizing pancreatitis and pancreatic pseudocysts are similar.

CLINICAL FEATURES

The clinical findings of infected necrotizing pancreatitis do not differ from those of sterile pancreatitis. The clinical diagnosis is, however, important because the two diseases have different prognoses. The mortality rate is high for infected necrotizing pancreatitis. Computed tomography with percutaneous needle aspiration is the most accurate diagnostic tool.[30] Pancreatic or peripancreatic fluid does not necessarily indicate abscess formation and may result from a pseudocyst, previous bleeding or sterile fluid. The diagnosis of 'infected necrotizing pancreatitis' can only be confirmed by culture of material obtained by percutaneous needle aspiration. Ultrasound is of less diagnostic value because the pancreatitis often causes secondary bowel distension and ileus, thus limiting the value of this investigation.

MANAGEMENT
Operative management

Patients who have infected necrotizing pancreatitis must undergo laparotomy with debridement of necrotic pancreatic tissue and removal of all devitalized and purulent material. Percutaneous drainage, which is well established in the treatment of other intra-abdominal abscesses, is not a reliable method in the treatment of pancreatic abscesses, which are usually multiple and contain pus, debris and necrotic material that frequently obstructs the drainage tubes. Percutaneous drainage of an infected pseudocysts is usually safe and effective. Continuous drainage must be established. In about 30% of the patients a further laparotomy is required due to persistent infection.[31] The operative management must always be combined with antimicrobial treatment.

Antimicrobial treatment

Antimicrobial agents are always necessary for patients who have necrotizing pancreatitis and pancreatic abscesses. Whenever possible, selection should be based on sensitivity testing of isolated micro-organisms. Drugs that achieve therapeutic levels in the pancreas are cefotaxime, ciprofloxacin, trimethoprim–sulfamethaxozole, clindamycin, metronidazole and imipenem.

REFERENCES

1. Wilcox C, Dismukes W. Spontaneous bacterial peritonitis. A review of pathogenesis, diagnosis and treatment. Medicine 1987;66:447–56.
2. Pollock A. Nonoperative anti-infective treatment of intra-abdominal infections. World J Surg 1990;14:227–30.
3. Arroyo V, Navasa M, Rimola A. Spontaneous bacterial peritonitis in liver cirrhosis: treatment and prophylaxis. Infection 1994;22(Suppl 3):167–75.
4. Bhuva M, Ganger D, Jensen D. Spontaneous bacterial peritonitis: an update on evaluation, management, and prevention. Am J Med 1994;97:169–75.
5. Llach J, Rimola A, Navasa M, et al. Incidence and predictive factors of first episode of spontaneous bacterial peritonitis in cirrhosis with ascites: relevance of ascitic fluid concentration. Hepatology 1992;16:724–7.
6. Rimola A, Solu R, Bory F, Arroyo V, Piera C, Ronés J. Reticuloendothelial systemic phagocytic activity in cirrhosis and its relation to bacterial infections and prognosis. Hepatology 1984;4:53–8.

7. Runyon BA. Patients with deficient ascitic fluid opsonic activity are predisposed to spontaneous bacterial peritonitis. Hepatology 1988;8:632–5.
8. Gallinaro R, Polk H. Intra-abdominal sepsis: the role of surgery. Baillière's Clin Gastroenterol 1991;5:611–37.
9. Rotstein OD. Role of fibrin deposition in the pathogenesis of intra-abdominal infection. Eur J Clin Microbiol Infect Dis 1992;11:1064–8.
10. De Lacey AM, Pera M, Garcia Valdecasas JC. Management of penetrating abdominal stab wounds. Br J Surg 1988;75:231–3.
11. Piraino B. Research directions in peritoneal dialysis infections. Blood Purif 1995;13:171–9.
12. Nathens A, Rotstein OD. Therapeutic options in peritonitis. Surg Infect 1994;74:677–92.
13. Whitnack E, Beachey EH. Inhibition of complement-mediated opsonization and phagocytosis of *Streptococcus pyogenes* by D fragments of fibrinogen and fibrin bound to cell surface M protein. J Exp Med 1985;162:1983–97.

14. Rotstein OD, Kao J. Fibrinolysis using recombinant tissue plasminogen activator prevents intra-abdominal abscesses. J Infect Dis 1988;158:766–72.
15. Altemeier WA, Culbertson WR, Fullen WD. Intra-abdominal abscesses. Am J Surg 1973;125:70–9.
16. Gibson DM, Feliciano DV, Mattox KL. Intra-abdominal abscess after penetrating abdominal trauma. Am J Surg 1981;142:699–703.
17. Nichols R. The treatment of intra-abdominal infections in surgery. Diagn Microbiol Infect Dis 1989;12:195S–9S.
18. Mueller PR, Simeone JF. Intra-abdominal abscesses. Diagnosis by sonography and computed tomography. Radiol Clin North Am 1983;21:425–43.
19. Saini S, Kellum JM, O'Leary MP, et al. Improved localization and survival in patients with intra-abdominal abscesses. Am J Surg 1983;145:136–41.

20. Gerzof SG, Robbins AH, Johnsson WC, Birkett DH, Nabseth DC. Percutaneous catheter drainage of abdominal abscesses: five-year experience. N Engl J Med 1981;305:653–7.

21. Knochel JQ, Koehler PR, Lee TG, Welch DM. Diagnosis of abdominal abscesses with computed tomography, ultrasound, and 111 In. leukocyte scans. Radiology 1980;137:425–32.

22. Dobrin PB, Gully PH, Greenlee HB. Radiologic diagnosis of an intra-abdominal abscess: do multiple tests help? Arch Surg 1986;121:41–6.

23. Ferruci JT Jr, van Sonneberg E. Intra-abdominal abscess: radiological diagnosis and treatment. JAMA 1981;246:2728–33.

24. McClean KL, Sheehan GJ, Harding GKM. Intra-abdominal infection: a review. Clin Infect Dis 1994;19:100–16.

25. Leiboff AR, Soroff HS. The treatment of generalized peritonitis by closed postoperative peritoneal lavage – a critical review of the literature. Arch Surg 1987;122:1005–10.

26. Hudspeth AS. Radical surgical debridement in the treatment of advanced generalized peritonitis. Arch Surg 1975;110:1233–6.

27. Steinberg D. On leaving the peritoneal cavity open in acute generalized suppurative peritonitis. Am J Surg 1979;137:216–20.

28. Beger HG, Bittner R, Block S, Büchler M. Bacterial contamination of pancreatic necrosis: a prospective clinical study. Gastroenterology 1986;91:433–8.

29. Bittner R. Clinical significance and management of pancreatic abscess and infected necrosis complicating acute pancreatitis. Ann Ital Chir 1995;66:217–222.

30. Aldridge MC. Diagnosis of pancreatic necrosis. Br J Surg 1988;75:99–100.

31. Widdison AL, Alvarez C, Reber HA. Surgical intervention in acute pancreatitis: when and how. Pancreas 1991;6:44–51.

Viral Hepatitis

Stephen D Ryder

INTRODUCTION

The clinical syndrome of acute hepatitis has been recognized since antiquity and is characterized by jaundice, usually after a prodromal illness. Acute hepatitis may cause severe sequelae, including fulminant hepatitis, but the major impact on human health is chronic liver disease and hepatocellular carcinoma resulting from chronic infection.

The nomenclature of the hepatitis viruses is somewhat eclectic, being based on the time of discovery of new or putative agents rather than on any consideration of modes of transmission or clinical problems associated with that agent. There are at present five primary human hepatotropic viruses, A, B, C, D and E, which are well characterized and known to account for approximately 90% of acute and 95% of chronic viral hepatitis. Other viruses, F and G, may cause human disease.

EPIDEMIOLOGY

HEPATITIS A VIRUS

Hepatitis A virus (HAV) is distributed throughout the world and causes outbreaks of infection, usually in association with direct fecal–oral contact[1] or contaminated water supplies.[2] Most food-related outbreaks of HAV infection are sporadic and due to poor food hygiene measures, but contamination of shellfish caused by sewage contamination is well described[3] and represents a continuing problem because molluscs are able to retain and concentrate viruses from water. Homosexual men and those working with newly imported nonhuman primates are high-risk groups for HAV infection. In the 1980s the proportion of cases of hepatitis A spread by blood contact increased to 19% of reported cases in the USA; this appears to have been due to intravenous drug use.[4]

In the developed world, the proportion of people who have immunity to HAV has declined over the past 2 decades, owing to improved sanitary conditions in childhood. Travelers from low-risk geographic areas to high-risk areas are at substantial risk of acquiring HAV infection.[5] In the developing world, infection rates are as high as 95% by the age of 16 years. Early infection usually produces a less severe clinical illness and immunity to future infection. The incubation period is short, ranging from 15 days to 50 days (mean 30 days).

HEPATITIS B VIRUS

Hepatitis B virus (HBV) is one of the most common chronic viral infections in the world, with estimates of approximately 170 million chronically infected people.[6] Hepatitis B virus infection is relatively rare in developed countries, with an incidence of 1 per 550 population in the UK and North America. Up to 20% of the population of South East Asia and sub-Saharan Africa have evidence of previous infection.[7] A major mode of spread in high-endemicity areas is vertical transmission from carrier mother to child, and this may account for 40–50% of all HBV infections in such areas.[8] This mode of transmission is highly efficient; more than 95% of children of carrier mothers are infected and develop chronic viral infection themselves. In low-endemicity countries, the mode of spread is predominantly by sexual transmission or blood-borne transmission through intravenous drug use. Only 5–10% of these groups of infected patients develop chronic viral infection. Certain groups in the western world are known to be at higher risk of HBV exposure; these include intravenous drug users, hemodialysis patients, homosexual men and institutionalized people, particularly those with mental handicap. Males are more likely to become chronic HBV carriers than females, for reasons that are unclear. The incubation period ranges from 28 days to 160 days (mean 80 days).

HEPATITIS C VIRUS

Hepatitis C virus (HCV) infection is common, with an estimated 500 million cases worldwide. Unlike infection with HBV, this infection is not confined to the developing world, with 0.3–0.7% of the UK population infected. The virus is spread almost exclusively by blood contact. Of cases in northern Europe 35% have a past history of blood transfusion and a further 40% have used intravenous drugs. Sexual transmission does occur, but it is unusual. Less than 5% of long-term sexual partners becoming infected.[9] Vertical transmission also occurs, but again it is unusual. It is certainly not the predominant mode of spread of HCV, with the frequency of infection in children of viremic mothers less than 5%.[10] The rate of infection in children of infected parents may rise in the first 10 years of life but it seems relatively difficult to acquire this viral infection from close household contact.

This leaves a substantial minority of those identified in whom no specific risk factor is present. This proportion may be up to 20% of cases. It has been postulated that this group may have acquired the infection from medical interventions. This is based on the high prevalence of infection in areas such as southern Italy, where military vaccination programs were undertaken in the period immediately after the Second World War, and in Egypt, where up to 20% of the population have HCV markers in certain geographic areas and treatment for diseases such as schistosomiasis are commonly given by injection. Hospitalization for whatever reason appears to be a risk factor for HCV infection. The incubation period varies between 14 and 60 days (mean 50 days).

HEPATITIS D VIRUS

Hepatitis D virus (HDV) or delta virus is an incomplete RNA virus that uses hepatitis B surface antigen (HBsAg) to enable replication and transfer from cell to cell. Hence, its epidemiology is closely linked to that of HBV. There are, however, considerable differences in the frequency of delta infection or superinfection in different patient groups. Intravenous drug users have a relatively high incidence of HDV infection whereas homosexual men, a high-risk group for the sexual spread of HBV, have a low incidence of delta infection. The reason for this epidemiologic paradox is unknown. Transmission of HDV is parenteral,[11] either via transfusion or close personal contact. Screening of blood products for HBsAg effectively excludes HDV-positive donors. The commonest risk factor for the acquisition of HDV infection in the western world is intravenous drug use, with between 17 and 90% of HBsAg-positive addicts also testing positive for HDV.[12] In developing countries, HDV infection generally parallels HBV infection, although there are exceptions, particularly in areas of Asia, where HDV is rare despite a high level of HBV carriage. In general, approximately 5% of people with chronic HBsAg carriage will be co-infected with HDV, giving an estimated worldwide figure in excess of 10 million. The incubation period is quite variable.

HEPATITIS E VIRUS

Hepatitis E virus is transmitted by the fecal–oral route. Its epidemiology correlates with the presence of contaminated water. It is responsible for outbreaks of epidemic-type hepatitis in the Indian subcontinent, but sporadic cases are seen throughout the world (Fig. 39.1). The incubation period is short, ranging between 15 and 45 days (mean 40 days).

HEPATITIS F VIRUS

Hepatitis F virus was described as the cause of a fulminant giant cell hepatitis. Its pathogenicity in humans is controversial, and if it does cause human disease it is rare.

HEPATITIS G VIRUS

Hepatitis G virus has only recently been described and its potential role as a pathogen and its epidemiology are largely unknown. In the USA and Europe, initial studies suggest that up to 1% of blood donors are viremic.

PATHOGENESIS AND PATHOLOGY

The molecular structure of the hepatitis viruses is considered in Chapter 8.4. The mechanisms of pathogenicity of the hepatitis viruses are complex and involve viral and host immune factors. The basis of any hepatitis is hepatocyte death, usually immunologically mediated in order to eliminate infected cells and to prevent further viral replication. It is highly likely that the mechanisms involved vary depending on the virus. Further differences in either the virus or the host response are involved in the development of chronic infection with HBV or HCV. Because these are the major cause of liver disease, these two viruses are considered in detail in this chapter.

HEPATITIS B VIRUS

Hepatitis B virus enters the hepatocyte by binding of determinants that are present on HBsAg. The virus replicates mainly in the hepatocyte (Fig. 39.2), although HBV DNA has been found in extrahepatic tissues, including skin, pancreas, kidneys, bone marrow and peripheral blood mononuclear cells. Hepatitis B virus has a highly unusual genetic structure, with a circular, partially ssDNA genome. When internalized in the hepatocyte, the genome is released and the negative strand is converted by ligation to a closed circular supercoiled form.[13] This form is present in the hepatocyte nucleus and forms the template for HBV RNA synthesis. Hepatitis B virus is almost unique in that its DNA is synthesized via an RNA intermediate; the same molecules are therefore used for protein synthesis and for reverse transcription to DNA.

The HBV RNA template is encapsulated in hepatitis B core antigen (HBcAg) particles and reverse transcribed to produce negative-strand DNA. This is then used to synthesize an incomplete positive DNA strand and the virion is encapsulated with HBsAg before excretion from the cell.

There are a number of host mechanisms deployed to prevent initial infection and then to remove infected hepatocytes. Hepatitis B virus is not thought to be directly cytopathic except in highly specific circumstances, such as fibrosing cholestatic hepatitis seen in re-infection of liver grafts, when the host is immunosuppressed. Liver cell damage in both acute and chronic HBV infection is thought to be immunologically mediated.

Cell-mediated and humoral immune responses occur in HBV infection, and both are probably important in limiting and eliminating infection. There is invariably a humoral immune response directed against HBcAg and usually against HBsAg,[14] but this response alone is not the cause of hepatitis as evidenced by liver disease in agammaglobulinemic patients. The responses of HLA class I restricted

cytotoxic T lymphocytes are thought to be the major mechanism of liver cell injury.[15] The fact that patients with production of HBsAg alone in hepatocytes usually have little inflammatory liver disease suggests that the target of this attack is likely to be core antigen.

Acute HBV infection can be self-limiting with complete clearance of the virus, or it can develop into chronic infection with the potential for the development of cirrhosis and primary liver cell cancer.

Chronic HBV infection can be thought of as occurring in phases, depending on the degree of immune response to the virus. This is

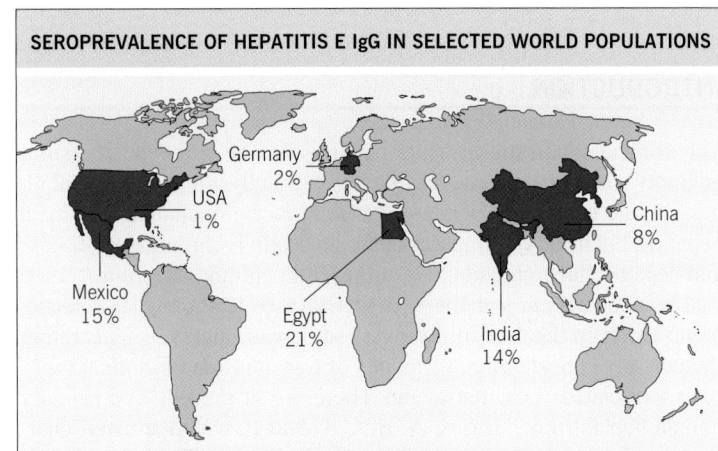

Fig. 39.1 Seroprevalence of hepatitis E IgG in selected world populations.

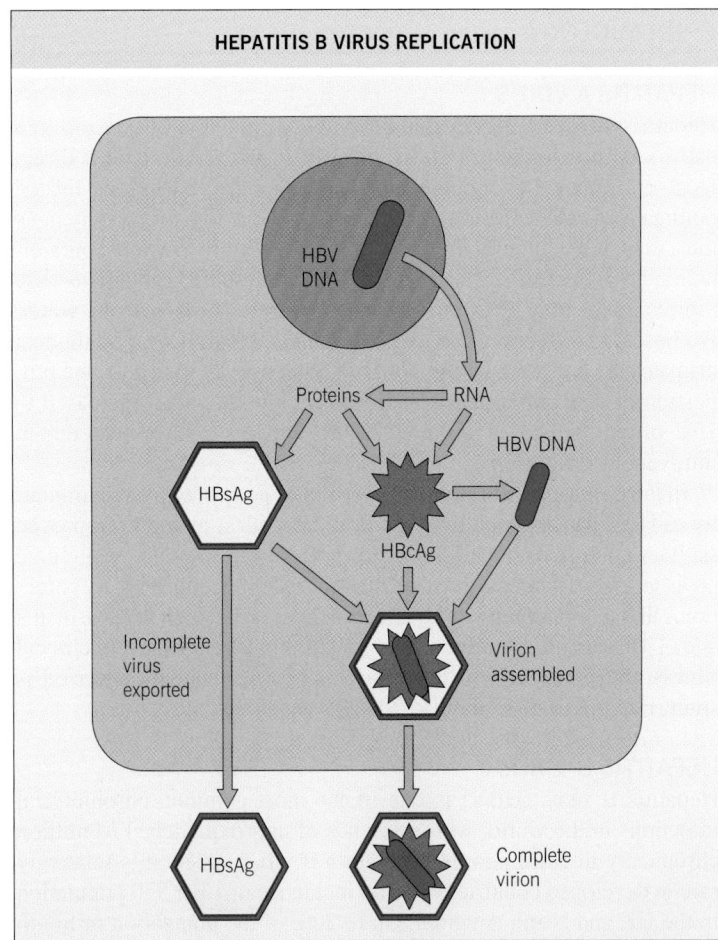

Fig. 39.2 Hepatitis B virus replication. Viral DNA present in the nucleus is transcribed to RNA, which then acts both as a template for protein synthesis (viral coat-HBsAg and viral proteins essential for infectivity and replication-HBcAg). Viral particles are then assembled and secreted from the cell cytoplasm. For every complete virion a large number of incomplete particles derived from HBsAg alone are exported. HBV, hepatitis B virus; HBsAg, hepatitis B surface antigen; HBcAg, hepatitis B core antigen.

particularly true of patients infected in the first few weeks of life. If infected when the immune response is 'immature', there is initially little or no immune response to HBV. The levels of HBV DNA in serum are very high and the hepatocytes contain abundant HBsAg and HBcAg, but little or no ongoing hepatocyte death is seen on a liver biopsy because of the defective immune response. This state persists for a variable period of time; usually the degree of immune recognition increases over some years. When immune recognition starts to occur, the level of HBV DNA tends to fall and the liver biopsy shows increasing inflammatory liver disease. This inflammation and hepatocyte death produces hepatic fibrosis. Once this phase of infection is initiated there are two major possible outcomes: either the immune response is adequate and the virus is inactivated and then removed from the system or the attempt at removal results in extensive fibrosis, distortion of the normal liver architecture and death from the complications of cirrhosis.

HEPATITIS C VIRUS

Chronic HCV infection has a long natural history, with most patients discovered in the presymptomatic stage. In the UK, most patients are now screened because of an identifiable risk factor (previous intravenous drug use or blood transfusion) or because of abnormal liver biochemistry.

The mechanism by which HCV causes human disease is unclear. A very high proportion (80%) of acute infections go on to become chronic, and the prognosis from chronic infection is very variable. Some infected people have normal liver histology,[16] which indicates that HCV is not directly cytopathic for hepatocytes. Immune mechanisms are again thought to be important in determining outcome.

Hepatitis C virus is an RNA virus. It is highly variable, with six major genotypes[17] Genotypes are frequently geographically restricted, such as type 4 in the Middle East, or may vary with time and mode of spread. This has been seen in Europe with genotype 1 occuring in older transfused individuals, with type 3 in younger drug users. There is some evidence that viral factors are important in the outcome of HCV infection. More severe fibrotic disease has been found in patients infected with genotype 1a or 1b than in those infected with other genotypes.[18] This is somewhat controversial as there are confounding factors, such as duration and mode of transmission, that make interpretation difficult.[19] The variability of the infecting HCV has also been postulated to affect outcome. The number of quasispecies present, a measure of genetic variability within a viral population, has been suggested as an important factor in evading the host immune response. Furthermore, quasispecies variability has been shown to be associated with increasing severity of liver disease,[20] whereas the number of quasispecies present in serum is higher in acute infection than in chronic infection.[21] More severe outcome appears to be correlated with selection of single species in the infecting HCV, which are presumably better adapted to survive in that particular immune environment.[22]

The level of viremia in a patient with HCV infection can be estimated using quantitative polymerase chain reaction (PCR) methods or branched chain DNA technologies, although these are somewhat less sensitive. High levels of viremia have been found to correlate with severity of liver disease.[23]

Evidence suggests that the host immune response is important in determining the outcome of HCV infection. There are HLA associations with viral clearance as evidenced by positive antibodies and negative tests for circulating viral genome (using PCR). In addition, patients with combined HCV and HIV infections and patients who were infected with HCV as a result of contaminated immunoglobulin given for hypogammaglobulinemia have more severe and more rapidly progressive liver disease.

PREVENTION

HEPATITIS A

Primary prevention mechanisms are the avoidance of water contaminated by human urine or feces. As water purification has improved, the seroprevalence of HAV infection has fallen. In countries with a low seropositivity for HAV infection, protective immunization is recommended for certain groups at high risk (see Chapter 8.4). It should be remembered that the severity of the acute illness caused by HAV increases with age of exposure. Approximately 5% of those over the age of 65 years who are infected will develop fatal acute fulminant hepatitis.

HEPATITIS B

The prevention of HBV infection is covered in Chapter 8.4.

HEPATITIS C

There is at present no effective vaccine against HCV infection. The difficulties in developing such a vaccine are numerous: the virus is highly variable, the mutation rate is high and the development of antibodies does not protect against re-infection with the same strain of HCV. The production of a clinically useful vaccine is likely to take many years.

HEPATITIS D

No specific vaccine for HDV exists. In patients known to carry HBsAg, prevention is restricted to avoidance of risk factors. In populations at risk, the high level of effectiveness of HBV vaccination will also protect against HDV infection.

HEPATITIS E

Prevention is restricted to avoidance of contaminated water. No vaccine is available.

CLINICAL FEATURES

ACUTE HEPATITIS
Anicteric disease
A large proportion of infections with any of the hepatitis viruses are asymptomatic or anicteric illnesses. Hepatitis A virus typically causes a minor illness in childhood, with more than 80% of infections being asymptomatic. In adult life infection is more likely to produce clinical symptoms, although only 30% of a cohort exposed to contaminated water experienced icteric illness.[2] Infections with HBV, HCV and HDV can also be asymptomatic. With HBV infection this again depends on the mode and time of transmission. Vertical transmission of infection from mother to child is almost always asymptomatic, although it produces chronic infection in the child. Transmission of HBV by other routes is much more likely to produce a symptomatic illness; about 30% of cases transmitted by intravenous drug use are icteric.

Clinically apparent acute hepatitis
Acute hepatitis presents with jaundice or elevated liver enzymes, usually preceded by a prodromal illness. The clinical features give little indication as to the likely etiologic agent. A history from patients who are suspected to have an acute hepatitis should be aimed at identification of specific risk factors for viral or other liver disease (Fig. 39.3).

IMPORTANT POINTS IN THE HISTORY OF A PATIENT WHO HAS SUSPECTED VIRAL HEPATITIS

- Contacts with jaundiced patients
- Intravenous drug use
- History of blood transfusion
- Surgery or hospitalizations
- Family history of chronic liver disease
- Occupation

Fig. 39.3 Important points in the history of a patient who has suspected viral hepatitis.

Common symptoms in the pre-icteric phase include myalgia, nausea, vomiting, fatigue and malaise. There is often a change in the sense of smell or taste, and right upper abdominal pain is common. Coryza, photophobia and headache are often seen, and cough may be prominent in hepatitis A. Diarrhea with transient pale stools and dark urine may occur.

A serum sickness-like illness occurs in about 10% of patients who have acute HBV infection and in 5–10% of patients who have acute HCV infection.[24] This is characterized by an urticarial or maculopapular rash and arthralgia, typically affecting the wrist, knees, elbows and ankles. This illness is due to immune complex formation and rheumatoid factor is frequently positive. It is almost always self limiting and usually settles rapidly after the onset of jaundice.

Viral hepatitis may produce other clinical or subclinical problems. Acute hepatitis B is rarely associated with clinical pancreatitis in the acute phase of the illness, although elevation of amylase is present in up to 30% of patients and autopsy studies in patients who have fulminant hepatitis B show histologic changes of pancreatitis in up to 50%. Myocarditis, pericarditis, pleural effusion, aplastic anemia, encephalitis and polyneuritis have all been reported.

Physical examination in the pre-icteric phase is usually normal although mild hepatomegaly (10%), splenomegaly (5%) and lymphadenopathy (5%) may be seen. Stigmata of chronic liver disease should not be present in patients who have an acute illness, and their detection suggests either that the episode causing presentation is the direct result of chronic liver disease or that there has been an acute event superimposed on a background of chronic liver disease, as for example in HDV superinfection in a HBV carrier (Fig. 39.4).

Biochemical confirmation of acute hepatic injury was seen with an elevated transaminase level. These may reach 100 times normal.[25] No other biochemical test has been shown to be a better indicator of acute liver injury. There are a number of other laboratory tests that may be abnormal in patients who have acute viral hepatitis. Leukopenia is common, and in 10% of patients the white cell count may fall below 5000/mm³.[26] Both anemia and thrombocytopenia are described. Immunoglobulin levels may be nonspecifically elevated in viral hepatitis, with levels usually returning to normal within 2 weeks. In a small proportion of patients who have acute viral hepatitis, a profound cholestatic illness may occur. This is most frequently seen in patients who have hepatitis A and it may be prolonged, with occasional patients remaining jaundiced for up to 8 months.

Death from acute viral hepatitis is usually due to the development of fulminant hepatitis. This is usually defined as hepatic encephalopathy with an onset within 8 weeks of symptoms or within 2 weeks of onset of jaundice.[27] The risk of developing fulminant liver failure is generally low but there are groups with higher risks. Pregnant women with acute HEV infection have a risk of fulminant liver failure of around 15%, with a mortality of 5%.[28] The risk of developing fulminant liver failure in HAV infection increases with age[29] and with preexisting liver disease.[30] Fulminant hepatitis B is seen in adult infection but it is relatively rare.

The primary clinical features of acute liver failure are encephalopathy and jaundice. Jaundice almost always precedes encephalopathy in acute liver failure, and the onset of confusion or drowsiness in a patient who has acute viral hepatitis is always a sinister development. The degree of the rise in transaminase values does not correlate with the risk of developing liver failure. Prolongation of coagulation is the biochemical hallmark of liver failure; it is caused by lack of synthesis of liver-derived clotting factors. Prolongation of the prothrombin time in acute hepatitis, even if the patient is clinically well without signs of encephalopathy, should be regarded as sinister and monitored closely. Hypoglycemia is seen only in fulminant liver disease, when it can be profound.

CHRONIC HEPATITIS

The agents that cause chronic hepatitis are HBV, HCV and HDV. Chronic hepatitis has been defined as abnormality of transaminase values persisting for more than 6 months. This has generally been a useful concept in patients who present with an acute illness. In clinical practice, the vast majority of patients will present with either an asymptomatic biochemical or serologic abnormality or the complications of cirrhosis, and it is reasonable to assume chronicity in these clinical settings at the time of initial presentation. Chronic viral hepatitis is characterized by the presence of inflammatory infiltrates in the liver associated with hepatocyte death.

The risk of developing chronic infection varies greatly with the virus implicated. Hepatitis A virus never causes chronic viremia or chronic liver disease. Hepatitis B virus causes chronic liver disease in a proportion of infected patients; this rate varies depending on the mode of transmission. Patients who are infected at or around the time of birth via a chronic carrier mother have infection rates of almost 100%, with the vast majority becoming chronic carriers of the virus and therefore at risk of long-term liver damage.[31] If HBV is acquired in later life, the risk of chronic infection falls considerably, with only 5% of such patients remaining HBsAg positive at 5 years.[32] The difference in the rate of chronic infection is probably related to the maturity of the host immune response.

Infection with HCV has, overall, the highest risk of chronicity. Post-transfusion studies indicate that at least 50% of patients with icteric disease develop chronically abnormal transaminase values, and some studies have suggested that up to 80% of acutely infected people remain viremic.[33]

Hepatitis D virus can cause chronic liver damage, and there is evidence to suggest that the combination of HBV and HDV carries a particularly poor outlook.

Most patients who have chronic viral hepatitis either present with a complication of their viral liver disease or are detected by screening, either for viral serology or for abnormal biochemistry.

Symptoms

The majority of patients who have chronic viral hepatitis are asymptomatic and patients are often unaware of the infection. In HCV infection a number of symptoms are frequently reported by patients in the absence of severe liver disease. These include lethargy, inability to concentrate and pain over the liver. It is unclear if these symptoms are the direct result of the viremia or are related to depression as a result of the diagnosis. These symptoms, whatever their origin, contribute to a reduced quality of life for patients with hepatitis C compared to patients with chronic hepatitis B.[34] Other symptoms are either due either to associated diseases affecting organs other than the liver or to end-stage liver disease.

Extrahepatic manifestations. Chronic hepatitis B can be associated with polyarteritis nodosa, with vasculitic rash, fever and polyarthralgia. Circulating HBsAg and anti-HBs complexes can be demonstrated, as can cryoproteins and HBsAg in blood vessel walls.[35] Cyclophosphamide appears to be effective.

Glomerulonephritis is now known to occur with both HBV[36] and HCV infections.[37] This is a relatively rare association thought to be

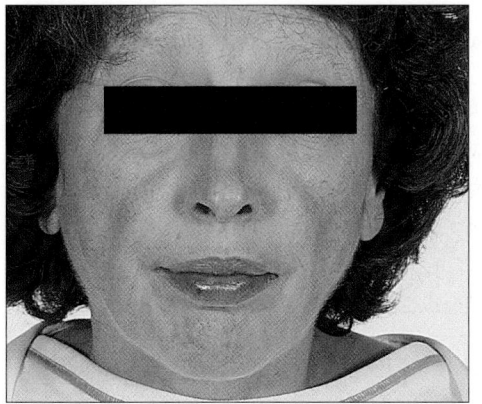

Fig. 39.4 Facial stigmata of chronic liver disease. This woman presented with serologically proven acute hepatitis A virus infection. She has multiple stigmata of chronic liver disease including facial spider nevi and was shown to have pre-existing cirrhosis.

mediated by the deposition of immune complexes. There are reports of improvement of the renal lesion on treatment of the responsible virus.

Up to 60% of patients who have mixed essential cryoglobulinemia are anti-HCV positive;[38] the condition is again thought to be the result of immune complex formation and antigen–antibody deposition in the vasculature (Fig. 39.5). Successful therapy of the underlying hepatitis C may produce remission.

Porphyria cutanea tarda is strongly associated with HCV infection, with up to 76% of Italian patients with porphyria cutanea tarda having antibodies to HCV.[39] Lichen planus is also associated with HCV infection.

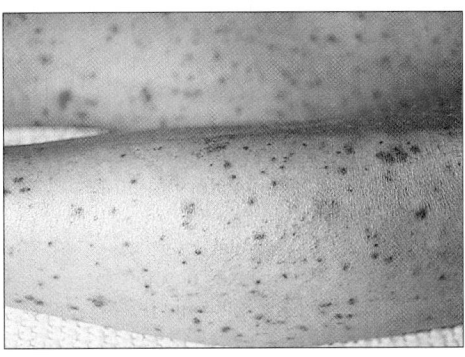

Fig. 39.5 Vasculitic rash in a patient who has mixed cryoglobulinemia.

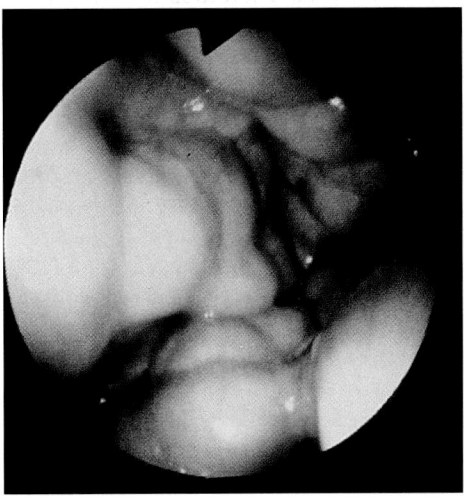

Fig. 39.6 Endoscopic view of esophageal varices.

Clinical signs

Patients who have decompensated cirrhosis caused by viral agents present with jaundice, encephalopathy, ascites or gastrointestinal bleeding as a result of portal hypertension (Fig. 39.6).

Cutaneous stigmata of chronic liver disease, spider naevi, leukonychia, gynecomastia, testicular atrophy and loss of body hair may be present. A late complication of chronic liver disease caused by HBV, HCV or HDV is hepatocellular carcinoma (Figs 39.7 & 39.8).

Hepatocellular carcinoma may present as a sudden decompensation of previously stable chronic liver disease or as pain in the right upper quadrant of the abdomen, or there may be distant metastatic disease, with pulmonary or bone metastases being most common. Alpha-fetoprotein is often raised, although this is normal in up to 60% of small hepatomas.

All of these clinical signs occur late in the course of these viral infections and for most of the duration of infection no abnormal clinical signs will be present and the patient will be asymptomatic.

DIAGNOSIS

ACUTE HEPATITIS
Hepatitis A
Infection with HAV can be reliably diagnosed by the presence of anti-HAV IgM. This test has very high sensitivity and specificity.[40] Very occasional false-positive results can be seen in liver disease of other etiologies where very high levels of immunoglobulin are present but the clinical context usually makes this obvious.

Hepatitis B
Infection with HBV is usually characterized by the presence of HBsAg. In acute HBV infection the serology can be difficult to interpret. The reason that an acute hepatitis develops is the immune recognition of infected liver cells, which results in T-lymphocyte-mediated hepatocyte killing. Active hepatocyte regeneration then occurs to replace those hepatocytes that have been lost. As well as a cell-mediated immune response, a humoral immune response develops, and this is probably important in removing viral particles from the blood and thus preventing re-infection of hepatocytes. Because of the immune response attempting to eradicate HBV, at the time of presentation with acute hepatitis B, viral replication may already have ceased and the patient may be HBsAg positive, hepatitis B e antigen (HBeAg) negative, e antigen being a surrogate marker of HBV replication.

It is difficult in this situation to be certain that a patient's illness was due to acute hepatitis B and that the serology does not imply past infection unrelated to the current episode. To enable a clear diagnosis to be made, most reference centers now report the level of IgM

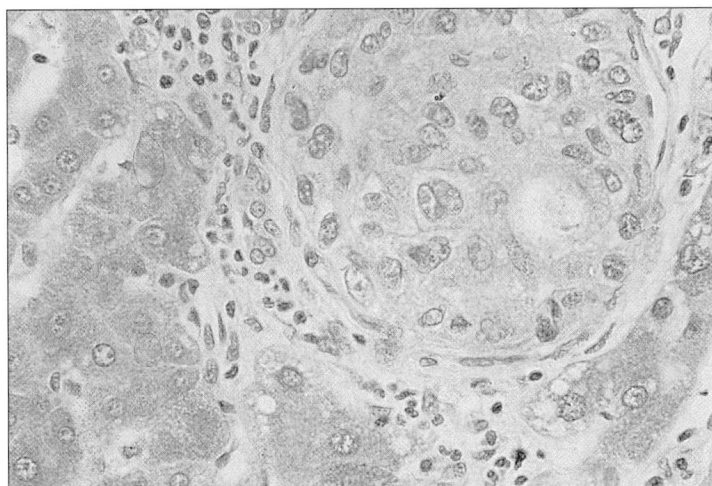

Fig. 39.7 Surgical histology of a nodule of hepatocellular carcinoma in a patient undergoing liver transplantation for hepatitis C cirrhosis.

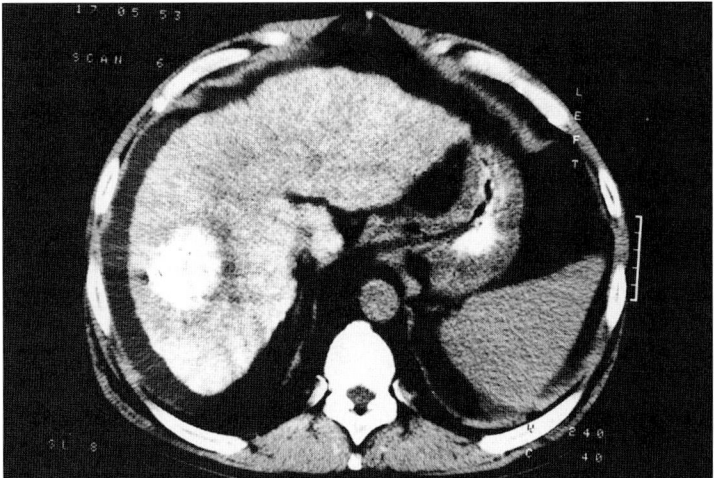

Fig. 39.8 Computed tomography scan following lipiodol injection into the hepatic artery showing hepatocellular carcinoma in the cirrhotic liver of a hepatitis B virus-positive male. Lipiodol is selectively retained in the tumor.

antibody to HBcAg (IgM anti-core; Fig. 39.9). As core antigen does not appear at any time in serum, this implies an immune response against HBV within liver cells and has been shown to represent a sensitive and specific marker of acute HBV infection.[41]

Rarely, the immune response to HBV infection is sufficiently brisk that even HBsAg has been cleared from serum by the time of presentation with jaundice. This may be more frequent in patients who develop severe acute liver disease and has been reported in up to 5% of patients who have fulminant hepatitis in whom the diagnosis was made by an appropriate pattern of antibody response.

Diagnosing past HBV infection or establishing immunity to vaccine is easy serologically. If the virus is cleared after infection with HBV, antibodies to all viral antigens can be detected. The levels of most of these in blood, however, decline with time. This is particularly true of anti-HBsAg: after 1 year, most patient's level of antibody has fallen below the level of detection in most commercially available assays. Despite this low level, immunity is still sufficient to prevent re-infection.

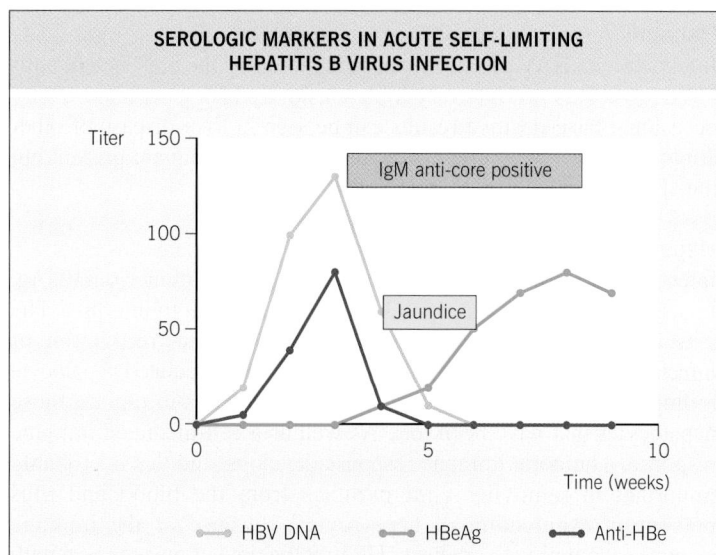

Fig. 39.9 Serologic markers in acute self-limiting hepatitis B virus infection. HBV, hepatitis B virus; HBeAg, hepatitis B e antigen. Measurements in arbitary units.

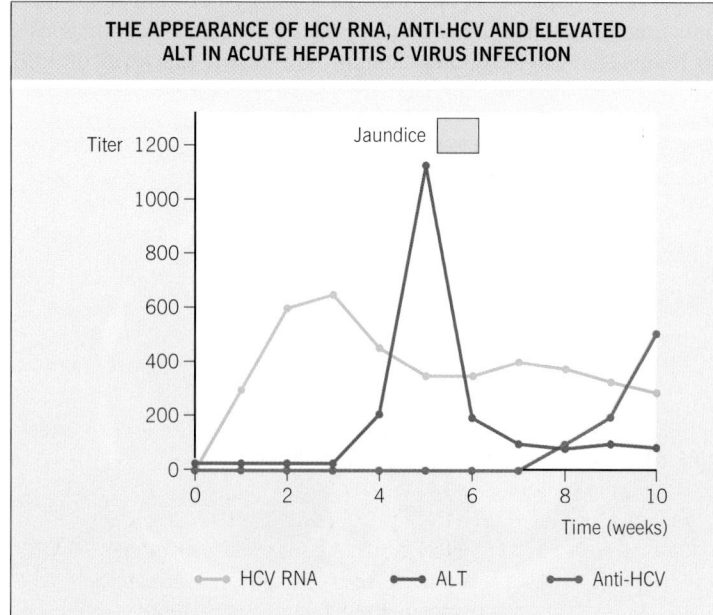

Fig. 39.10 The appearance of hepatitis C virus RNA, anti-hepatitis C virus and elevated ALT in acute hepatitis C virus infection. HCV, hepatitis C virus; ALT, alanine transaminase. Measurements in arbitary units.

Natural immunity is proven by the presence of IgG antibodies to HBcAg. These are a highly reliable marker of past infection and remain at detectable levels for a long period. Vaccine-induced immunity is directed purely against HBsAg epitopes, and hence a vaccinated person will have detectable levels of anti-HBsAg but no anti-HBcAg.

Hepatitis C

Screening tests for HCV infection are enzyme-linked immunosorbent assay (ELISA) techniques that use recombinant viral antigens and patient's serum. Acute hepatitis C cannot be reliably diagnosed by antibody tests because these frequently do not become positive for up to 3 months (Fig. 39.10).

Hepatitis C virus used to be the cause of more than 90% of all post-transfusion hepatitis in Europe and North America[42], acute HCV infection is now most commonly seen in intravenous drug users. Antibodies to HCV appear relatively late in the course of acute infection and therefore, if clinical suspicion is high and risk factors are present, testing of the patient's serum for HCV RNA is the only means of establishing the diagnosis (see Fig. 39.10). Identification of cases of acute HCV infection is important because there is strong evidence that early treatment with interferon alfa may reduce the risk of chronic infection with HCV. The apparent rate of chronicity in untreated patients is approximately 80%; with interferon therapy this falls to less than 50%.

Hepatitis D

As HDV requires the presence of HBsAg for infectivity, it occurs only in patients who are infected with HBV either previously (superinfection) or simultaneously (co-infection). Co-infection is usually relatively benign; the determining factor for severity of illness is the HBV infection. As this is usually self-limiting, with loss of HBsAg after a relatively short interval, chronic infection with HDV is rare (about 2%).

Superinfection with HDV, by contrast, is a much more severe disease. The presence of large amounts of HBsAg allows rapid replication of the HDV and establishment of both acute and chronic infection. Chronic infection is common in this setting because the continued production of HBsAg allows the delta agent to continue replication.

Diagnosis of delta hepatitis is not easy: the encapsulation of HDV by HBsAg masks much of the HDV antigenemia, and assays for the detection of delta RNA in serum are not widely available and are not always reliable. Conventional solid-phase immunoabsorbent tests for the detection of delta antigen in serum are only positive early in the infection, before the development of delta antibodies, which complex with antigen. Immunoblot assay is now more widely available and does not have the same drawback because it is independent of antidelta antibody. The IgG antidelta antigen antibody is not protective and elevated levels correlate with continued infection.[43]

A number of other viruses can cause hepatitis (Fig. 39.11). In the main, liver involvement is incidental and other features of the illness will suggest a diagnosis other than primary hepatitis. The exceptions are yellow fever, and disseminated herpes simplex and varicella-zoster infections in immunosuppressed patients, which in both cases may be associated with a severe hepatitis.

CHRONIC VIRAL LIVER DISEASE

Chronic viral liver disease may present with abnormal liver biochemistry, by serologic testing in at-risk groups without symptoms or as a result of the complications of cirrhosis. Abnormal liver biochemistry in viral hepatitis is usually a sustained elevation of transaminases. In contrast to the situation in acute infection, the rise in the transaminase values is modest, characteristically only two or three times the upper limit of normal. In HCV infection, the γ-glutamyl transpeptidase values are also often elevated. The degree of abnormality of transaminases has little relevance to the degree of underlying hepatic inflammation. This is particularly true of HCV infection, in which the transaminase values are often normal despite active liver inflammation.

VIRAL INFECTIONS THAT MAY BE ASSOCIATED WITH HEPATITIS

Virus	Comment
EBV, CMV	Both these viruses cause an acute mononucleosis type syndrome in the normal host. Mild elevations of the liver transaminases may be seen but are usually of little consequence
HSV, VZV, CMV	All may cause hepatitis in the immunosuppressed host as part of a disseminated infection. CMV is the least severe
Flaviviruses	Yellow fever causes severe hepatitis
Measles, rubella, rubeola, coxsackie B adenovirus	Mild hepatitis occurs occasionally

Fig. 39.11 Viral infections that may be associated with hepatitis. EBV, Epstein–Barr virus; CMV, cytomegalovirus; HSV, herpes simplex virus; VZV, varicella-zoster virus.

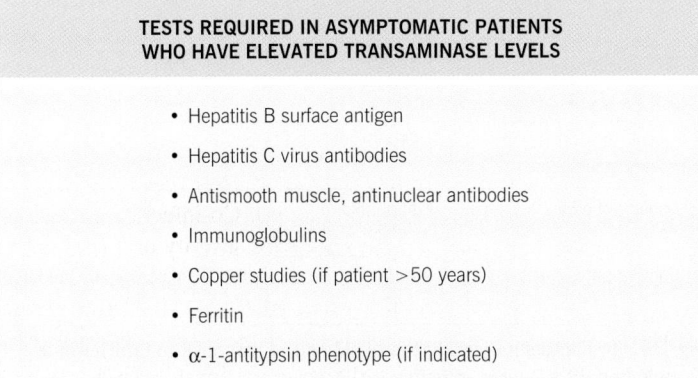

TESTS REQUIRED IN ASYMPTOMATIC PATIENTS WHO HAVE ELEVATED TRANSAMINASE LEVELS

- Hepatitis B surface antigen
- Hepatitis C virus antibodies
- Antismooth muscle, antinuclear antibodies
- Immunoglobulins
- Copper studies (if patient >50 years)
- Ferritin
- α-1-antitypsin phenotype (if indicated)

Fig. 39.12 Tests required in asymptomatic patients who have elevated transaminase levels.

TESTS REQUIRED FOR DIAGNOSIS IN HEPATITIS B VIRUS INFECTION

- Hepatitis B surface antigen
- Hepatitis B e antigen
- Hepatitis B anti-core antibody (HB total anti-core)
- Hepatitis B DNA
- Hepatitis B IgM anti-core

Fig. 39.13 Tests required for diagnosis in hepatitis B virus infection.

Further investigation in patients who have a positive serologic test for a hepatotrophic virus is to exclude other concomitant liver disease and assess the severity of liver damage induced by the hepatotropic virus. The risk of development of serious liver pathology is increased in the presence of multiple pathologies. Figure 39.12 shows the required baseline serologic tests required. In HCV infection, autoantibodies are frequently positive, antismooth muscle antibodies being detected in about 10% of patients and low-titer antinuclear antibodies in 15–20%. These autoantibodies do not appear to play a part in pathogenesis and would only alter management if a high titer were present with a raised IgG, suggesting a primary autoimmune hepatitis, in which interferon therapy may be contraindicated.

Chronic hepatitis B

The vast majority of patients who have hepatitis B will be HBsAg positive. There are viral mutants that do not produce HBsAg detectable by

PRODUCTION OF HEPATITIS B CORE ANTIGEN AND HEPATITIS B E ANTIGEN AND THE GENERATION OF E ANTIGEN-NEGATIVE MUTANTS

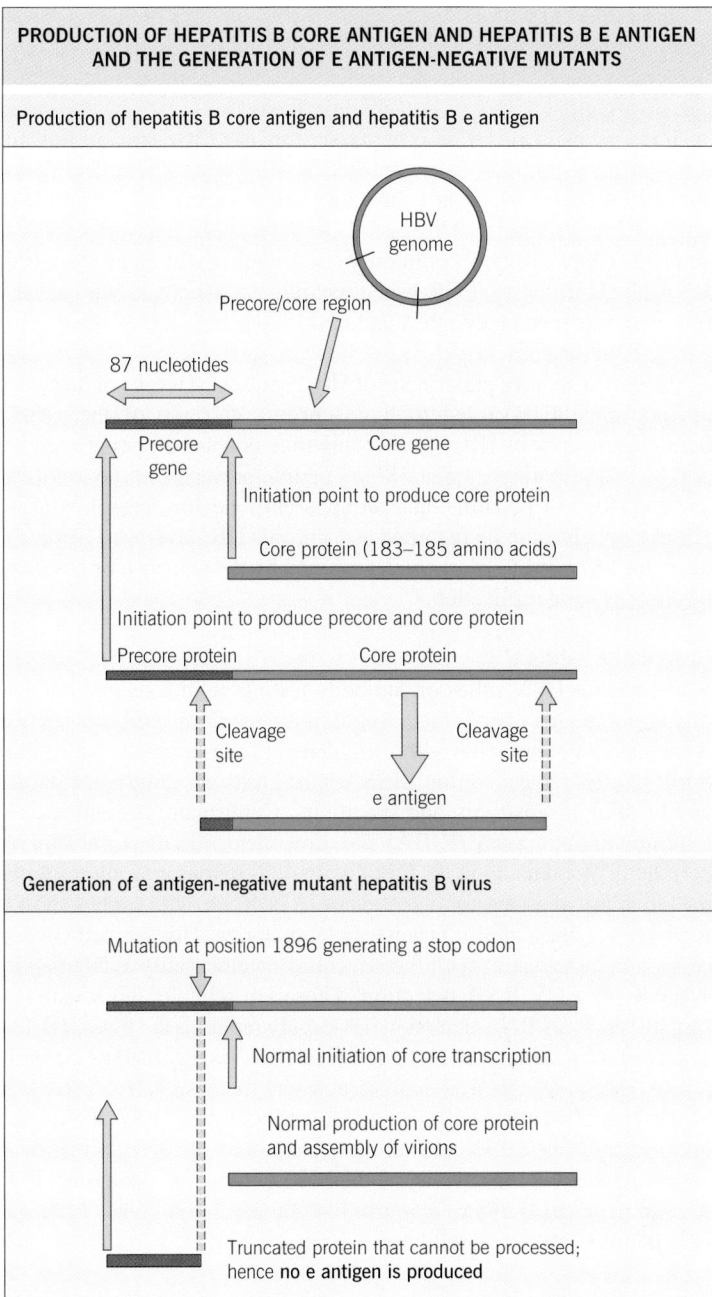

Fig. 39.14 Production of hepatitis B core antigen and hepatitis B e antigen and the generation of e antigen-negative mutants. Hepatitis B virus (HBV) has a closed circular genome that contains insufficient bases to produce all its required proteins. It therefore uses different start points for transcription, enabling it to use the same base sequence to produce different proteins. Two important proteins, e antigen and core antigen, are produced by transcription of the same region with overlap; e antigen is produced from the core protein by cleavage at a specific site.

the usual serologic tests (Fig. 39.13), but these are very rare except in patients treated with interferon or after liver transplant.

The traditional classification of those individuals who have chronic hepatitis B has been based on the presence of HBeAg. All patients who have HBsAg can be regarded as infected but HBeAg has been regarded as a marker of infectivity. Hepatitis B e antigen is produced as a truncated version of core protein (Fig. 39.14).

In the wild-type virus, HBcAg and HBeAg are transcribed together using overlapping bases. Hence HBeAg is an indirect marker of viral replication. The exact function of HBeAg is unclear but it appears to be involved in the downregulation of the T-lymphocyte response to HBV infection and may play a pivotal role in the development of the long phase of relative immunologic tolerance seen in chronic HBV-infected carriers who acquire their infection in childhood. It has been shown that children infected with HBeAg-negative viral mutants do not have the immune tolerance that is almost universal in wild-type HBV transmission; most infected infants develop severe hepatic inflammation and cases of fulminant liver failure are described.

The discovery of HBeAg-negative mutant viruses has produced the need for a more specific marker of viral replication. The measurement of HBV DNA now provides direct detection of the circulating HBV genome.[44] This is the most sensitive measure of viral activity. There are two commonly used methods to estimate HBV DNA levels in serum: PCR-based techniques, which are very sensitive, and branched chain DNA technology, which is rather cheaper to perform but less sensitive.

Patients who have persistence of HBsAg after 20 weeks of an acute episode can be assumed to have chronic carriage of the virus. Spontaneous loss of HBsAg after this time is unusual, being seen in only 1–2% of patients a year. Many people present with no obvious acute episode of hepatitis, and an apparently healthy person who is HBsAg positive can be regarded as a chronic HBV carrier. The prognosis for that person is largely determined by the presence or absence of ongoing viral replication.

Chronic hepatitis C

Screening for HCV relies on antibody testing, with a second confirmatory test usually performed. Initial first-generation antibody assays were relatively unreliable with a high rate of false-positive results, but third- and fourth-generation ELISA-based tests are readily available and have high sensitivity and specificity. Confirmatory tests include radioimmunoblot assay (RIBA) and direct detection of viral RNA in peripheral blood using PCR. Initially there were major problems with the reliability of assays for detection of HCV RNA, with studies showing large variation in results between laboratories. This has been overcome to a large extent with the advent of commercially available kit systems for HCV RNA detection. These are reliable and sensitive. Hepatitis C virus RNA detection has largely replaced the use of RIBA testing in most centers. Detection of HCV RNA is regarded as the best test to determine infectivity and response to therapy.

Patients presenting with detectable antibodies to HCV should be investigated (Fig. 39.15) to exclude other causes of chronic liver disease and to assess the severity of their HCV infection. Assessment of the severity of liver disease requires liver biopsy. Liver biopsy findings in hepatitis C are discussed later.

Chronic hepatitis D

Chronic infection with HDV has a high risk of producing severe liver disease. In the vast majority of cases of chronic infection, the HBV infection is nonreplicative as evidenced by HBeAg negativity and absence of HBV DNA.[45] This viral interference is seen in many combined viral infections (e.g. HBV and HCV infections) and it is rare to find patients with two replicating hepatotropic viruses. However, if the accompanying HBV is replicating, the prognosis is very poor with rapid progression to cirrhosis over as little as 2 years.[45]

Diagnosis of chronic HDV infection is usually by antibody testing in serum, where both IgM and IgG antidelta antigen antibodies are usually present in high titer, or by delta antigen staining on liver biopsy. For patients who have chronic infection, delta antigen staining in liver biopsy material remains the most definitive diagnostic test.[46]

MANAGEMENT

HEPATITIS B

Assessment of chronic hepatitis B virus infection

Any patient who has detectable levels of HBsAg is chronically infected. Assessment of a patient who has chronic HBV infection should include more detailed HBV serology, including measurement of HBV DNA levels. In patients who have no evidence of viral replication and normal liver enzyme levels and a normal liver

INVESTIGATIONS REQUIRED IN ANTI-HEPATITIS C VIRUS-POSITIVE PATIENTS	
Tests to assess hepatitis C virus	Tests to exclude other liver diseases
PCR for hepatitis C virus RNA	Ferritin
Viral load	Autoantibodies and immunoglobulins
Genotype	Hepatitis B serology
	Liver ultrasound

Fig. 39.15 Investigations required in anti-hepatitis C virus-positive patients.

FACTORS INDICATING THE LIKELIHOOD OF RESPONSE TO INTERFERON IN CHRONIC HEPATITIS B VIRUS INFECTION		
Factor	High probability of response	Low probability of response
Age	<50 years	>50 years
Sex	Female	Male
Hepatitis B DNA level	Low	High
Activity of liver inflammation	High	Low
Country of origin	Europe, North America, Australasia	Asia
Coinfection with HIV	Absent	Present

Fig. 39.16 Factors indicating the likelihood of response to interferon in chronic hepatitis B virus infection. PCR, polymerase chain reaction.

ultrasound, liver biopsy is not usually required. Such patients have a very low risk of developing symptomatic liver disease or hepatocellular carcinoma. Reactivation of HBV replication has been described and patients who are HBsAg positive should be followed with yearly serology and liver enzyme estimations. The low risk of hepatocellular carcinoma does not justify screening in this group. In patients who have abnormal liver biochemistry (even without detectable HBV DNA) or an abnormal liver texture on ultrasound, a liver biopsy is probably required, because such patients may either have superinfection with HDV or have had ongoing replication of HBV in the past, sustaining substantial liver damage in the process. It is estimated that around 5% of patients in developed countries who have only HBsAg carriage at presentation will have a posthepatitic cirrhosis on liver biopsy. This finding is important because they are at risk of developing the complications of cirrhosis including variceal bleeding and hepatocellular carcinoma.

Assessment of patients who have HBV replication is carried out by assessing the degree of liver inflammation and the stage of the underlying liver disease. Patients who are still in the tolerant phase of their infection usually have normal transaminase levels and high serum levels of HBV DNA (in excess of 250pg/ml). As immune recognition increases, the HBV DNA levels fall, the degree of hepatic damage increases and the transaminases become abnormal. This is important in the selection of patients for therapy. Patients who have viral replication and abnormal transaminases should have a liver biopsy. The need for liver biopsy in a patient who have high levels of HBV DNA and repeatedly normal transaminases is less clear because it is very unlikely that the biopsy will show advanced liver disease or considerable inflammatory activity.

COMMON SIDE EFFECTS OF INTERFERON-α THERAPY FOR VIRAL HEPATITIS	
Side effect	Frequency (%)
Flu-like syndrome	80
Depression	20
Local inflammation at injection sites	25
Hypothroidism	10
Arthralgia or arthritis	10
Hair loss	10

Fig. 39.17 Common side effects of interferon-α therapy for viral hepatitis.

	Full blood count	Liver function tests	Hepatitis B virus DNA	Hepatitis B surface antigen and e antigen
	MONITORING OF INTERFERON THERAPY IN HEPATITIS B VIRUS INFECTION			
Before treatment	+	+	+	+
Week 1	+	+	−	−
Week 2	+	+	−	−
Week 4	+	+	+	+
Week 8	+	+	−	−
Week 12	+	+	+	+
Week 16	+	+	+	+
Week 20	+	+	+	+

Fig. 39.18 Monitoring of interferon therapy in hepatitis B virus infection.

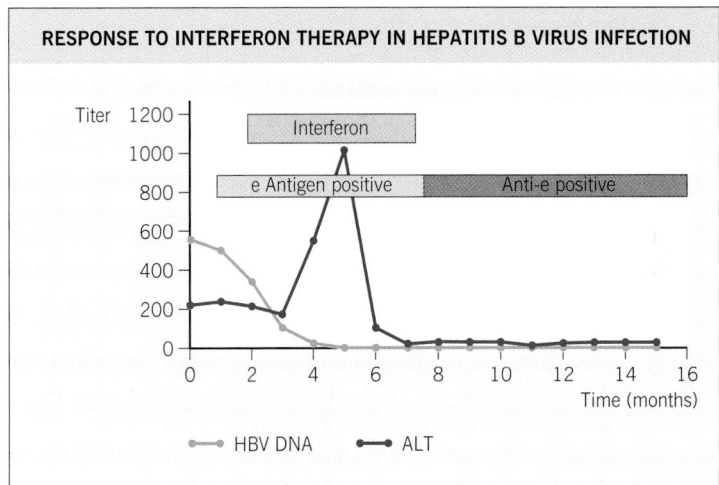

Fig. 39.19 Response to interferon therapy in hepatitis B virus infection. HBV, hepatitis B virus; ALT, alanine transaminase. Measurements in arbitary units.

Interferon therapy

Interferon-α was first shown to be effective for some patients who have HBV infection in the 1980s and it remains the mainstay of therapy.[47] There are a number of commercially available variants of interferon-α, natural interferon, recombinant interferons and consensus interferons. In HBV infection there is little evidence that the type of interferon used has any substantial difference in effect or side-effect profile.

There are a number of factors that can help predict the likelihood of response to treatment and these help in selection of patients who have the best chance of response to therapy (Fig. 39.16).

Overall, the probability of response to interferon therapy in chronic hepatitis B is between 25 and 40%. A response to therapy is the cessation of viral replication; only a small number of patients lose all markers of infection with HBV and HBsAg usually remains in the serum. There is now good evidence that successful therapy with interferon, which renders the HBV nonreplicative, produces a sustained improvement in liver histology and a decrease in the risk of developing end-stage liver disease. The risk of developing hepatocellular carcinoma also appears to be reduced but it is not abolished in those who remain HBsAg positive.

Interferon therapy has a number of drawbacks: it is not effective in many patients, it is expensive and it has a large number of side effects (Fig. 39.17). In general, about 15% of patients on interferon therapy have no side effects, 15% cannot tolerate therapy and the remaining 70% experience side effects but are able to continue therapy. Most patients are able to continue at work during therapy but many require substantial support. Depression can be a major problem and both suicide and admissions with acute psychosis are well described. Early use of antidepressants and close monitoring are essential, especially if there is a preceding history of depression.

Treatment of hepatitis B in patients who have severe liver disease is rewarding because they have a relatively high probability of response and have most to gain from cessation of viral replication. Many patients have a substantial improvement in liver function if viral replication is stopped, but treatment in such patients does carry an increased risk. Interferon therapy produces viral clearance by inducing immune-mediated killing of infected hepatocytes, and hence a transient hepatitis can cause severe decompensation requiring liver transplantation.

The optimal dose and duration of interferon for hepatitis B remains somewhat contentious, but most clinicians use 8,000,000–10,000,000 units three times a week for 4–6 months. Monitoring therapy is intensive, and appropriate schedules are shown in Figure 39.18.

Patterns of response and special situations. The most frequent pattern of response to interferon-α is shown in Figure 39.19. The HBV DNA level falls rapidly after initiation of interferon therapy. This is followed by a marked rise in transaminase values. This represents immune-mediated clearance of virus, and HBV DNA levels quickly fall to undetectable levels. This is then followed within a few weeks by seroconversion to HBeAg-negative, HBeAb-positive status with complete normalization of transaminases. This type of response is seen in

25% of treated patients. Hepatitis B surface antigen usually remains positive, with a small proportion of patients clearing all markers of viral infection either during interferon therapy (2%) or many months after it (6%). A further proportion of patients show a late seroconversion after therapy (Fig. 39.20).

In such patients there is often an initial fall in HBV DNA levels but these remain detectable throughout therapy together with persistently abnormal transaminase values. After the end of treatment there is then a progressive fall in HBV DNA and normalization of transaminases. Seroconversion from HBeAg to anti-HBeAb follows after a few weeks or months of HBV DNA negativity. Such delayed responses to therapy occur in 10–15% of treated patients and this emphasizes the need to persevere with therapy once the decision to undertake treatment has been made.

There are a number of specific situations in which the above treatment protocols may change. In Greece and Italy, the proportion of patients with HBeAg-negative mutant virus infection is relatively high, and this situation is also encountered elsewhere. There is compelling evidence that, although such patients show a good rate of initial response to interferon with disappearance of HBV DNA from serum, patients very frequently relapse after cessation of treatment (Fig. 39.21). There is now evidence that giving interferon therapy for longer in such patients may improve the rate of loss of viral replication. A regimen of 6,000,000 units three times a week for 24 months has been shown to produce a loss of viral replication in 30% of patients.[48]

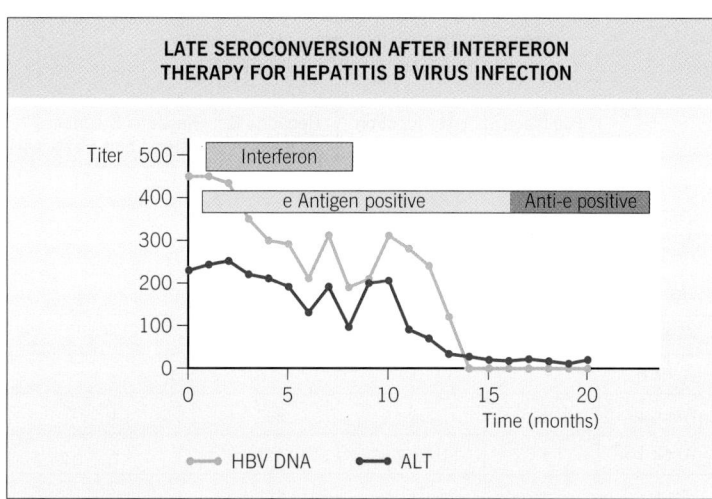

Fig. 39.20 Late seroconversion after interferon therapy for hepatitis B virus infection. HBV, hepatitis B virus; ALT, alanine transaminase. Measurements in arbitary units.

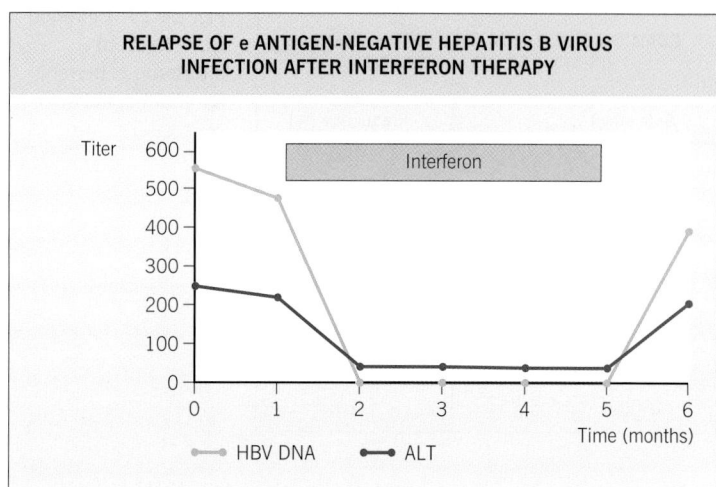

Fig. 39.21 Relapse of eAg-negative hepatitis B virus after interferon therapy. HBV, hepatitis B virus; ALT, alanine transaminase. Measurements in arbitary units.

Lamivudine therapy

Lamivudine, a nucleoside analog, is a potent inhibitor of HBV DNA replication. Lamivudine has a good safety profile and has now been widely tested in patients who have chronic HBV infection. It was initially shown to produce a rapid fall in HBV DNA levels in short-term trials, mainly in post-transplant, recurrent HBV infection. In this setting, it produces marked improvement in liver function and histology and there is little doubt that this agent represents a major improvement in the therapy of post-transplant hepatitis B.

Both in the post-transplant setting and when given in short-term trials in patients who have chronic HBV in their own livers (Fig. 39.22), lamivudine has been shown to produce rapid inhibition of HBV DNA production, but this rapidly returns when therapy is stopped. With a 6-month period of therapy, 80% of patients who have chronic HBV became HBV DNA negative.[49] In about 14% of transplant patients a breakthrough was seen in which viral replication started again despite continuation of therapy. This phenomenon has also been seen in patients treated in the nontransplant setting with similar frequency (14% at 1 year),[50] and has been shown to be due to selection of a mutation in the YMDD locus of the HBV polymerase gene,[51] which allows viral replication in the presence of lamivudine.

In longer-term trials in patients of Asian origin, who have a relatively low probability of response to interferon therapy, almost all treated patients showed prompt inhibition of HBV DNA and, if therapy was continued for 12 months, a sustained inhibition of replication was seen in 35% with seroconversion to HBeAg negativity. This was associated with an improvement of inflammation and a reduction in progression of fibrosis on liver biopsy. Side effects of treatment are generally mild. Breakthrough occurred in 6% of treated patients.

A trial in Hong Kong looking at combination therapy with interferon and lamivudine failed to show any additional benefit from combining therapy. Lamivudine monotherapy, however, may have an important role in the treatment of HBV.

HEPATITIS C
Natural history of hepatitis C virus infection

In order to assess the need for treatment in a patient who has hepatitis C it is important to have a clear understanding of the natural history of this infection and of the factors that may predispose to more severe outcome. In general, our knowledge is limited because of the relatively recent discovery of HCV. It is however clear that HCV-related liver disease is usually slowly progressive, taking many years to produce significant hepatic fibrosis. The most definitive studies to date suggest that the average time from infection to the development of cirrhosis is 33 years.[52] The rate of progression is, however, very

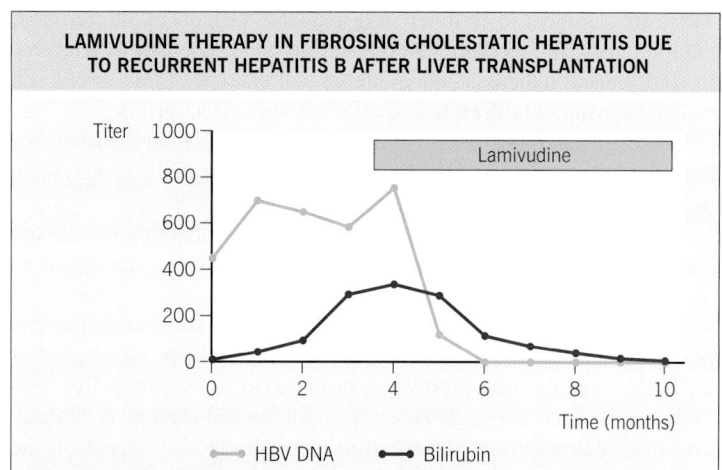

Fig. 39.22 Lamivudine therapy in fibrosing cholestatic hepatitis due to recurrent hepatitis B after liver transplantation. HBV, hepatitis B virus. Measurements in arbitary units.

variable with some 'rapid fibrosers' progressing to cirrhosis 11 years after infection and other 'slow fibrosers' who would take more than 40 years to progress to cirrhosis. The major factors associated with increased risk of progressive liver disease were age over 40 years at infection, high alcohol consumption and male sex (Fig. 39.23). Viral genotype may be important in progression but the data are controversial. This is illustrated by the epidemiology of HCV infection in Italy, which can be regarded as two separate outbreaks. The first outbreak, which involved HCV genotype 1, was spread by blood transfusion, infected older people and produced severe liver disease. The second, later outbreak was spread by intravenous drug use and was predominantly due to HCV genotype 3; it appeared to be associated with less severe liver disease. This emphasizes the difficulty of extracting single risk factors for progression of liver disease from epidemiologic studies because patients infected via transfusion are older as well as being infected by a different viral genotype.

In general, virologic factors have not proved as significant in predicting rates of progression; high viral load and genotype 1 have been proposed as markers of more serious liver disease but evidence that they are directly related to rapid progression of liver disease is lacking.

Management of the patient is usually based on the degree of liver damage as assessed by biopsy.

Liver biopsy

Assessing the need for therapy in hepatitis C is difficult. This is a disease which has a long natural history and an uncertain outcome. Liver

FACTORS INFLUENCING THE PROGRESSION OF HCV INFECTION	
Risk factor	Time from infection to cirrhosis (years)
Age <50 years	12
Age >50 years	35
Alcohol <50g/day	31
Alcohol >50g/day	24
Male	26
Female	36

Fig. 39.23 Factors influencing the progression of hepatitis C virus (HCV) infection. From Poynard et al.[52]

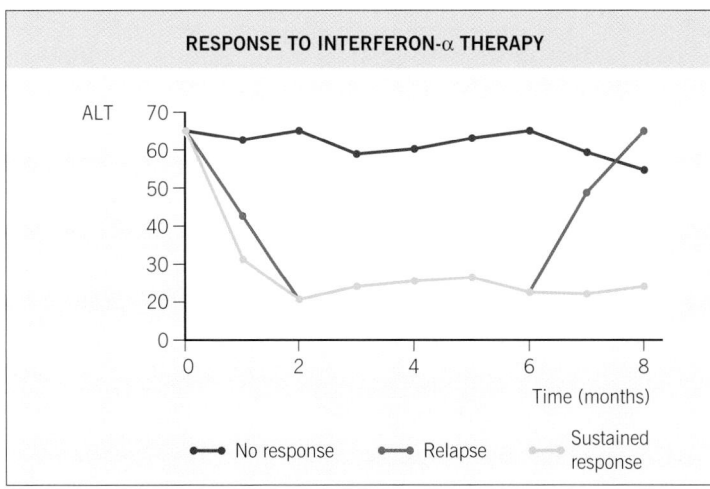

Fig. 39.24 Response to interferon-α therapy. The three main possible outcomes of treatment are shown. ALT, alanine transaminase.

biopsy is the only method of directly assessing the degree of inflammation in the liver and the stage of liver disease (fibrosis). All patients who are viremic with abnormal transaminases need assessment by liver biopsy. There is a small group of patients who have documented viremia who have persistently normal transaminase levels. In this group, the incidence of serious disease on biopsy appears low.[53] However, the degree of elevation of alanine transaminase (ALT) in HCV infection is often minor and it fluctuates. Hence many patients with an initial normal ALT level will have abnormal values if they are followed carefully. In general it seems sensible to have liver biopsy evidence of the stage of disease in all viremic patients.

Assessment of liver biopsies. There are two important features in the histologic assessment of hepatitis C. The first is disease stage (fibrosis); the second is the degree of necroinflammatory change. In order to improve the reproducibility of assessment there are a number of scoring systems that have been used to quantify viral hepatitis: the most widely used are the Knodell score[54] and a modification of this, the Ishak score.[55] These scores combine the two elements of assessment of chronic viral liver disease, fibrosis stage and inflammation. The difference between the Ishak and Knodell score is that Ishak expanded the stage score to allow more discrimination of minor degrees of fibrosis.

Interferon-α therapy

The only licensed treatment for hepatitis C is interferon-α. It is possible to predict response rates in patient populations, but wide variations are seen between patient groups.

Response to therapy is defined by measurement of two parameters, serum transaminases and the detection of HCV RNA in serum. Many studies have also examined the effect of interferon therapy on the histologic progression of liver disease.

Interferon-α was first used to treat non-A, non-B hepatitis in the 1980s. Since the identification of HCV in 1989, a large amount of information has become available about the effectiveness of interferon therapy in HCV infection and its drawbacks. There is some evidence that the natural interferons may have slightly more antiviral effect than the recombinant interferons in HCV infection. This difference is, however, marginal at best and in practice there is little difference in effectiveness or side effects with any of the commercially available variants.

Defining response to therapy. There are three potential responses to interferon therapy in patients who have HCV infection:

- no response in either biochemical or virologic markers (non-responders),
- a suppression of HCV RNA and normalization of ALT on therapy but relapse after cessation of therapy (relapsers), or

- a disappearance of HCV RNA and normalization of ALT that is maintained after stopping therapy (sustained responders).

Overall, the chance of sustained response in HCV infection is approximately 20%.[56]

Predicting response to therapy. The response to interferon-α therapy in chronic HCV infection is highly variable. A number of factors, relating both to the stage of liver disease and to the virus, have been identified as carrying an altered probability of response to therapy (Fig. 39.24).

The most important predictive factors of a poor response to interferon are the presence of cirrhosis, in which response fall to around 8%, and the presence of genotype 1a or 1b, where response rates are approximately 10%. Male sex and advancing years are other factors predictive of a poor response.

Treatment regimens for hepatitis C. Compelling data exist that the dose and duration of therapy for hepatitis C are different from those used in HBV infection. Initial regimens used 3,000,000 units of interferon-α three times a week with a 6-month duration of therapy. It has been shown that increasing the duration of therapy to 12 months produces a significant increase in the probability of a sustained response.[53] Subsequent studies have shown that a dose–response effect is seen but that the increase in cost and side effects of 6,000,000 units compared with 3,000,000 units three times a week led the authors to recommend 3,000,000 units three times a week as the initial dose.[57]

Ribavirin (1-β-D-ribofuranosyl-1H-1,2,4-triazole-3-carboxamide) is an oral nucleoside analogue which inhibits replication of a number of viruses. Initial studies in hepatitis C infection showed a biochemical response to monotherapy with ribavirin but no virological response. Experience with other RNA viruses and this initial encouraging data led to trials of interferon in combination with oral ribavirin. A randomized study of 100 patients treated with either interferon alpha alone at a dose of 3 million units thrice weekly versus ribavirin at a dose of 1000 to 1200mg per day in combination with interferon.[58] With six months therapy the sustained virological response rates were 36% in the combination therapy group compared with 18% of the interferon monotherapy group. This data suggests that combination therapy is likely to be significantly better at producing a sustained loss of HCV RNA in blood. It is likely that a combination of drugs will be the way forward in hepatitis C therapy.

HEPATITIS D

Treatment of hepatitis D virus infection

Interferon alfa therapy has been studied in HDV infection with only limited success. Response rates to treatment are probably seen in only 15% of patients. There are emerging data to suggest that longer treatment regimens may be more effective.

REFERENCES

1. Benenson MW, Takafuji ET, Bancroft WH, et al. A military community outbreak of hepatitis type A related to transmission in a child care facility. Am J Epidemiol 1980;112:471–7.

2. Morse LJ, Bryan JA,Hurley JP, et al. The Holy Cross College football team hepatitis outbreak. JAMA 1972;219:706–12.

3. Dismukes WE, Bisno AL, Katz S, et al. An outbreak of gastroenteritis and infectious hepatitis attributed to raw clams. Am J Gastroenterol 1969;85:555–60.

4. Centers for Disease Control. Hepatitis A among drug users. MMWR Morb Mortal Wkly Rep 1988;37:297–310.

5. Frame JD. Hepatitis among missionaries in Ethiopia and Sudan: susceptibles at high risk. JAMA 1967;203:389–94.

6. Szmuness W. Hepatocellular carcinoma and the hepatitis B virus: evidence for a causal association. Prog Med Virol 1978;24:40–8.

7. Szmuness W, Harley EJ, Ikran H, et al. Sociodemographic aspects of the epidemiology of hepatitis B. In: Vyas GN, Cohen SN, Schmidt R, eds. Viral hepatitis. Philadelphia: Franklin Institute Press; 1978:297–319.

8. Stevens CE, Beasley RP, Tsui V, et al. Vertical transmission of hepatitis B antigen in Taiwan. N Engl J Med 1975;292:771–7.

9. Bresters D, Mauser-Bunschoten EP, Reesink HW, et al. Sexual transmission of hepatitis C virus. Lancet 1993;342:210–2.

10. Ohto H, Terazawa S, Sasaki N, et al. Transmission of hepatitis C virus from mother to infants. N Engl J Med 1994;330:744–6.

11. Rizzetto M, Verme G, Gerin J, Purcell R. Hepatitis delta virus disease. New York: Grune and Stratton; 1986;VIII:417–31.

12. Rizzetto M, Ponzetto A, Forzani I. The hepatitis delta virus as a global health problem. Vaccine 1990;8(suppl 1):S10–4.

13. Seegar C, Ganem D, Varmus HE. Biochemical and genetic evidence for the hepatitis B virus replication strategy. Science 1986;232:477–9.

14. Lambert PH, Tribolet E, Celada A, et al. Quantitation of immunoglobulin associated HBsAg antigen in patients with acute and chronic hepatitis, in healthy carriers and in polyarteritis nodosa. J Clin Lab Immunol 1980;3:1–7.

15. Naumov N, Mondelli M, Alexander GMJ, et al. Relationship between expression of hepatitis B virus antigens in isolated hepatocytes and autologus lymphocyte cytotoxicity in patients with chronic hepatitis B virus infection. Hepatology 1984;4:13–21.

16. Brillanti S, Foli M, Gaiani S, et al. Persistent hepatitis C viraemia without liver disease. Lancet 1993;431:464–5.

17. Simmons P, Alberti A, Alter HJ, et al. A proposed system for the nomenclature of hepatitis C viral genotypes. Hepatology 1994;19: 1321–4.

18. Dusheiko G, Schmilovitz WH, Brown D, et al. Hepatitis C virus genotypes: an investigation of type-specific differences in geographic origin and disease. Hepatology 1994; 19:13–8.

19. Nousbaum JB, Pol S, Nalpas B, et al. Hepatitis C virus type 1b (II) infection in France and Italy. Ann Intern Med 1995;122:161–8.

20. Honda M, Kaneko S, Sakai A, et al. Degree of diversity of hepatitis C virus quasispecies and progression of liver disease. Hepatology 1994;20:1144–51.

21. Yamaguchi K, Tanaka E, Higashi K, et al. Adaptation of hepatitis C for persistent infection in patients with acute hepatitis. Gastroenterology 1994;106:1344–8.

22. Kumar U, Monjardino J, Thomas HC. Hypervariable region of hepatitis C envelope glycoprotein (E2/NS1) in an agammaglobulinaemic patient. Gastroenterology 1994;106: 1072–5.

23. Kato N, Yokosuka O, Hosoda K, et al. Quantification of hepatitis C virus RNA in serum of asymptomatic blood donors and patients with type C chronic liver disease. Hepatology 1993;17:545–50.

24. Fernandez R, McCarty DJ. The arthritis of viral hepatitis. Ann Intern Med 1971;74:207–11.

25. Clermont RJ, Chalmers TC. The transaminase tests in liver dsease. Medicine 1967;46:197–202.

26. Kivel RM. Hematologic aspects of acute viral hepatitis. Am J Dig Dis 1961;6:1017–1020.

27. Bernuau J, Rueff B, Benhamou JP. Fulminant and subfulminant liver failure: definitions and causes. Semin Liver Dis 1986;6:97–113.

28. Nanda SK, Yalcinkaya K, Panigrahi AK, et al. Etiological role of hepatitis E virus in sporadic fulminant hepatitis. J Med Virol 1994;42:133–7.

29. Fagan EA, Williams R. Fulminant viral hepatitis. Br Med Bull 1990;46:462–9.

30. Akriviadis EA, Redeker AG. Fulminant hepatitis A in intravenous drug users with chronic liver disease. Ann Intern Med 1989;110:838–42.

31. Beasley RP, Trepo C, Stevens CE, et al. The e antigen and vertical transmission of hepatitis B surface antigen. Am J Epidemiol 1977;105:94–102.

32. Krugman S, Overby LR, Mushahwar IK, et al. Viral hepatitis type B. Studies on natural history and prevention reexamined. N Engl J Med 1979;300:101–5.

33. Pham D, Walshe D, Montgomery J. Seroepidemiology of hepatitis B and C in an urban VA medical center. Hepatology 1994;20(suppl 1):236A.

34. Foster GR, Goldin RD, Thomas HC. Chronic hepatitis C virus infection causes a significant reduction in quality of life in the absence of cirrhosis. Hepatology 1998;27:209–12.

35. Michelak T. Immune complexes of hepatitis B surface antigen in the pathogenesis of polyarteritis nodosa. Am J Pathol 1978;90:619–23.

36. Knecht GL, Chisari FV. Reversibility of hepatitis B virus-induced glomerulonephritis and chronic active hepatitis after spontaneous clearance of hepatitis B surface antigen. Gastroenterology 1978;75:1152–8.

37. Johnson RJ, Gretch DR, Yamabe H, et al. Membranoproliferative glomerulonephritis associated with hepatitis C infection. N Engl J Med 1993;328:465–9.

38. Lunel F, Mosset L, Cacoub P, et al. Cryoglobulinemia in chronic liver disease: role of hepatitis C virus and liver damage. Gastroenterology 1994;106:1291–6.

39. Fargion S, Piperno A, Cappellini MD, et al. Porphyria cutanea tarda and hepatitis C virus infection. Hepatology 1992;16:1322–6.

40. Roggendorf M, Frosner GG, Deinhardt F, et al. Comparison of solid phase test systems for demonstrating antibodies against hepatitis A virus (anti-HAV) of the IgM class. J Med Virol 1980;5:47–51.

41. Hoofnagle JH. Type B viral hepatitis: virology, serology and clinical course. Semin Liver Dis 1981;1:7–22.

42. Alter MJ, Margolis HS, Krawczynski K, et al. The natural history of community acquired hepatitis C in the United States. N Engl J Med 1992;327:1899–903.

43. Aragona M, et al. Serological response to the hepatitis delta virus in hepatitis D. Lancet 1987;i:478–80.

44. Bonino F, Hoyer B, Moriarty A, et al. Hepatitis B virus DNA in the sera of HBsAg carriers: a marker of active HBV replication in the liver. Gastroenterology 1980;79:1009–12.

45. Rizzetto M, Alberti M, et al. Chronic HBsAg hepatitis with intrahepatic expression of Delta antigen. An active and progressive disease unresponsive to immunosuppressive treatment. Ann Intern Med 1983;98:437–41.

46. Smedlie DL. Diagnosis of delta virus infection. Hepatology 1986;6:1297–9.

47. Hoofnagle JH, Peters M, Mullen KD, et al. Randomized, controlled trial of recombinant human alpha-interferon in patients with chronic hepatitis B. Gastroenterology 1988;95:1318–22.

48. Lampertico P, De Ninno E, Manzin A, et al. A randomized, controlled trial of a 24-month course of interferon alpha 2b in patients with chronic hepatitis B who had hepatitis B virus DNA without hepatitis B e antigen in serum. Hepatology 1997;26:1621–5.

49. Nevens F, Main J, Honkoop P, et al. Lamivudine therapy for chronic hepatitis B: a six month randomized dose-ranging study. Gastroenterology 1997;113:1258–63.

50. Leung NWY, Lai CL, Liaw YF, et al. Lamivudine (100mg) for one year significantly inproves necroinflammatory score and reduces progression in fibrosis stage: results of a placebo-controlled multicenter study in Asia of Lamivudine for chronic hepatitis B infection. Hepatology 1997;26 (suppl 1):357.

51. Bartholomew MM, Jansen RW, Jeffers LJ, et al. Hepatitis B virus resistance to lamivudine given for recurrent infection after orthotopic liver transplantation. Lancet 1997;349:20–2.

52. Poynard T, Bedossa P, Opolon P, et al. Natural history of liver fibrosis progression in patients with chronic hepatitis C. Lancet 1997;349:825–32.

53. Knodell RG, Ishak K, Black C, et al. Formulation and application of numerical scoring system for activity in asymptomatic chronic active hepatitis. Hepatology 1981;1:431–3.

54. Ishak KG. Chronic hepatitis. Morphology and nomenclature. Mod Pathol 1994;7:690–696.

55. Davis GL, Balart LA, Schiff ER, et al. Treatment of chronic hepatitis C with recombinant interferon alfa. A multicenter randomized, controlled trial. N Engl J Med 1989;321:1501–6.

56. Poynard T, Bedossa P, Chevallier M, et al. A comparison of three interferon alpha-2b regimens for the long term treatment of chronic non-A, non-B hepatitis. N Engl J Med 1995;332:1457–62.

57. Poynard T, Leroy V, Cohard M, et al. Meta-analysis of interferon randomized trials in the treatment of viral hepatitis C: effect of dose and duration. Hepatology 1996;24:778–90.

58. Reichard O, Nokrans G, Fryden A, et al. Randomized, double-blind, placebo controlled trial of interferon α-2b with and without ribavirin for chronic hepatitis C. Lancet 1998;351:83–7.

Hepatobiliary Infections

Janice Main

LIVER ABSCESSES

PYOGENIC ABSCESS

PATHOGENESIS AND PATHOLOGY

Bacteria can reach the liver via the portal vein, the systemic circulation, the biliary tree or directly (after trauma or transhepatic procedures such as liver biopsy). Pyogenic liver abscesses are usually associated with biliary tree obstruction or gastrointestinal tract infection such as occurs in missed appendicitis, diverticulitis, perforated peptic ulcers, colonic carcinoma or after colonic surgery. The usual organisms are therefore from the gastrointestinal tract or biliary tree. Liver abscesses are often polymicrobial, with Enterobacteriaceae, enterococci and anaerobic bacteria predominating. *Streptococcus milleri* is increasingly seen in liver abscesses, and staphylococci are not uncommon. *Actinomyces* spp.,[1] *Bartonella henselae*[2] and *Capnocytophaga* spp.[3] are more unusual isolates; in immunosuppressed patients nocardial infections[4] mycobacterial infections[5] and fungal infections, in particular *Candida* spp., can occur. Abscesses can be solitary or multiple and they range in size from several centimeters in diameter to microabscesses that must be identified histologically.

CLINICAL FEATURES

Pyogenic liver abscesses are classically seen in elderly patients who have underlying gastrointestinal disease. The patient may complain of right hypochondrial discomfort that is insidious in onset or the patient may present more acutely with fever or confusion. Interventions such as transarterial embolization for hepatocellular carcinoma can be complicated by liver abscess[6] and the diagnosis of pyogenic liver abscess may be missed because fever and discomfort are not uncommon after such procedures. The differential diagnoses include cholecystitis and pyelonephritis.

DIAGNOSIS

Abdominal ultrasound is the simplest way of making the diagnosis. Single or multiple abscesses may be present and the ultrasound may also help identify the original source of the sepsis, such as an obstructed biliary tree. Smaller abscesses that are undetected by ultrasound may be visible on CT scanning.[7] Aspiration of the abscess yields useful microbiologic material and is an important part of therapy. Cytologic examination of smears from the abscess are important to exclude underlying malignancy.

Blood cultures are sometimes positive. The leukocyte count is usually elevated and the liver function tests may be deranged, with elevation of the alkaline phosphatase. Iron overload syndromes should be considered in patients when *Yersinia* spp. are identified.[8]

MANAGEMENT

Drainage of the abscess is important and the favored approach is needle aspiration under ultrasound guidance. This may need to be repeated on several occasions, particularly if there are multiple lesions. Percutaneous catheter drainage is another approach but this is generally only practical if there is one large and accessible abscess.

Abscesses are often polymicrobial, and broad-spectrum intravenous antibiotics are generally recommended. If the abscesses are thought to have occurred as a result of biliary sepsis, it is advisable to give antibiotics that achieve good concentrations in bile. Positive blood cultures and cultures from the abscess should help direct antimicrobial chemotherapy. The combination of gentamicin and amoxycillin–clavulanic acid or ticarcillin–clavulanic acid are useful regimens and should be given with metronidazole to broaden the anaerobic cover and also if there is concern about possible amebic infection. Piperacillin–tazobactam and the carbapenems are also useful.[9]

AMEBIC LIVER ABSCESS

PATHOGENESIS AND PATHOLOGY

Entamoeba histolytica reaches the liver via the portal vein and causes necrosis of the liver parenchyma. Infection is a complication in up to 10% of cases of amebic colitis. The necrosis leads to liquefaction of the liver and the characteristic thick reddish brown pus, which is said to resemble anchovy sauce. On microscopy, hepatocytes, neutrophils and red blood cells are evident. Secondary bacterial infection can occur and this can complicate the clinical picture and cause confusion with pyogenic liver abscess.

CLINICAL FEATURES

Clinical features of amebic and pyogenic abscesses are compared in Figure 40.1. An amebic abscess can develop many years after travel to tropical areas and this latency has not been adequately explained. Cases have been described 30 years after the initial bowel infection. The patient may complain of right hypochondrial pain and fever. Lesions near the diaphragm can cause referred right shoulder discomfort. Low-grade fever may be present. More acute presentations with rigors have been reported. An abscess that is encroaching on the biliary tree may cause some biliary obstruction and mild jaundice, but deep jaundice is unusual. Right hypochondrial tenderness may be present and rarely a swelling may be evident in the epigastrium or the right hypochondrium. There may be elevation of the right hemidiaphragm or a pleural effusion and so reduced expansion, dullness to percussion and reduced air entry may be present. Rarely, an abscess can rupture within the lung or pericardium.

DIAGNOSIS

An ultrasound, CT or MRI examination will demonstrate the presence of an abscess, which is typically large and located in the right lobe of the liver. Smaller abscesses may be present. Aspiration may reveal the characteristic 'anchovy sauce' appearance and although it is unusual to demonstrate amebae on microscopy, microscopy and culture are important in order to exclude a pyogenic liver abscess or secondary infection of an amebic abscess. A bleed into an underlying malignant lesion can mimic the symptoms of an amebic abscess. Cytology can also demonstrate the presence of malignant cells and point to the diagnosis of an underlying metastatic lesion or primary hepatocellular carcinoma.

The liver function tests may be normal or show elevation of alkaline phosphatase and bilirubin, and a large abscess can have a compressive effect on the intrahepatic biliary tree.

FEATURES OF PYOGENIC AND AMEBIC LIVER ABSCESSES		
	Pyogenic liver abscesses	Amebic liver abscesses
Patients	Elderly Underlying gastrointestinal or biliary tract disease	Males much more commonly affected than females
Imaging	Single or multiple abscesses	Solitary abscess right lobe
Pathogens	Polymicrobial Enterobacteriaceae, enterococci	*Entamoeba histolytica*
Other tests	Blood cultures	Amebic immunofluorescent antibody test
Treatment	Broad-spectrum antimicrobials Aspiration	Metronidazole + diloxanide ± aspiration

Fig. 40.1 Features of pyogenic and amebic liver abscesses.

MAJOR CAUSES OF GRANULOMATOUS LIVER DISEASE	
Bacteria Mycobacteria (*Mycobacterium tuberculosis, Mycobacterium avium-intracellulare, Mycobacterium leprae*) *Brucella* spp. *Listeria monocytogenes* *Tropheryma whippelii* *Yersinia* spp. *Treponema pallidum*	Protozoa *Leishmania* spp.
	Helminthic parasites *Schistosoma* spp. *Toxocara gondii*
	Fungal infections Histoplasmosis Coccidioidomycosis
Viruses Cytomegalovirus Epstein–Barr virus Hepatitis A virus, hepatitis C virus	Drugs
	Primary liver disease (e.g. primary biliary cirrhosis)
Rickettsiae *Coxiella burnetti* *Rickettsia conori, Rickettsia typhi*	Neoplasms (e.g. lymphoma)
	Diseases of unknown cause (e.g. sarcoidosis, inflammatory bowel disease)

Fig. 40.2 Major causes of granulomatous liver disease.

TREATMENT

Metronidazole is the treatment of choice followed by diloxanide to remove luminal amebic cysts from the gastrotintestinal tract. In patients who have large amebic abscesses aspiration in conjunction with metronidazole hastens recovery.[10]

DIFFUSE PARENCHYMAL INVOLVEMENT OF THE LIVER

The liver may be involved in many systemic infections. Viral infection is described in Chapter 2.39, but acute hepatitis has been described with several bacterial pathogens including meningococci, *Listeria* spp., *Campylobacter* spp., *Salmonella typhi*, *Borrelia* spp. and *Brucella* spp.[11,12] Sepsis and other causes of circulatory collapse can also cause hepatic ischemia, which can be associated with high transaminase values.[13] Infections account for many of the main causes of granulomatous liver disease (Fig. 40.2). Liver involvement and symptoms of liver disease can be a major part of:

• mycobacterial infections,
• syphilis, and
• leptospirosis.

MYCOBACTERIAL INFECTION

TUBERCULOSIS OF THE LIVER

The liver is generally involved in miliary tuberculosis and the liver biopsy may help establish a diagnosis of tuberculosis in a patient who has unexplained fever.

Pathology

Tuberculosis of the liver may present as an abscess[5] or more diffuse disease. Liver biopsy may reveal nonspecific hepatitis or granulomatous liver disease. Rarely there may be tuberculomas or enlarged intra-abdominal lymph nodes that cause compression of the biliary tree, and the patient presents with features of biliary tract obstruction.

Clinical features

Fever and weight loss are the usual symptoms. The patient may appear wasted. Hepatomegaly may be evident but massive hepatomegaly is unusual. In severe tuberculosis the patient may present with liver failure.

Diagnosis

Elevated alkaline phosphatase levels are usually present and the serum albumin levels may be low if the disease has been longstanding. Anemia and elevation of the erythrocyte sedimentation rate and C-reactive protein are common. A chest radiograph is important to exclude active pulmonary disease, which is evident in a minority of

cases.[14] An abdominal ultrasound may demonstrate intrabdominal lymphadenopathy or evidence of peritoneal involvement. Liver biopsy may be diagnostic, but caseating granulomas with acid-fast bacilli are demonstrable in less than 10% of cases on histologic examination. The appearances may be nonspecific and it is important to culture some of the liver biopsy material. It is hoped that rapid diagnostic methods such as polymerase chain reaction will facilitate diagnosis in the future.[15]

Treatment

Standard antimycobacterial therapy should be given (see Chapters 2.30 & 7.13). Liver function tests should be monitored as with standard therapy. As the patient improves the elevated alkaline phosphatase gradually returns to normal. Elevation in the transaminase level may be a sign of drug toxicity. Fever may persist for several weeks but if the patient fails to improve the possibilities of resistant *Mycobacterium tuberculosis* or atypical mycobacteria have to be considered.

ATYPICAL MYCOBACTERIA

Atypical mycobacterial infection of the liver is usually seen in the setting of immunosuppression, particularly underlying HIV infection[16] or congenital immunodeficiency. Again, culture of the biopsy material is important to establish the diagnosis, but the appearance of many organisms with poorly formed granulomas may be an important clue to atypical mycobacterial infection in an immunocompromised host.

SYPHILIS

The liver is involved with congenital syphilis, secondary syphilis and later stages of syphilis. The standard screening tests usually confirm the diagnosis of congenital infection but the diagnosis should also be considered in the setting of undiagnosed acute hepatitis in young adults.[17] This is discussed in detail in Chapters 2.64 and 8.18.

LEPTOSPIROSIS

EPIDEMIOLOGY

Several *Leptospira* spp. are associated with human disease but *Leptospira icterohaemorrhagiae* is specifically associated with Weil's disease. The main source of this pathogen is rat urine and it is therefore a hazard for farm and sewage workers and those who use contaminated waters for recreational purposes (see Chapters 6.34 & 8.19).

PATHOLOGY

The liver demonstrates cholestasis with swelling of hepatocytes but very little necrosis. In classic Weil's disease there is renal disease with acute tubular necrosis. There may be evidence of multifocal hemorrhage, particularly within skeletal and cardiac muscle.

PREVENTION

The use of protective clothing can help prevent occupational exposure and it has been recommended that sewage workers carry cards to remind clinicians of the possibility of leptospirosis should they become ill. Prophylactic antimicrobials such as doxycycline[18] have been suggested for those at greatest risk of exposure through work or leisure activities such as canoeing, although this practice is not generally recommended.

CLINICAL FEATURES

The patient's occupation or leisure activities may point to the diagnosis.

In common with other spirochetal infections there are several characteristic stages of the disease process. The severity varies from a minor influenza-type illness to life-threatening multisystem failure. The incubation period ranges from 2 to 17 days.

The first (septic) stage is of a multisystem disease. It is abrupt in onset. Features may include:

- high fever;
- myalgia, which is often severe;
- abdominal pain;
- nausea;
- vomiting;
- severe headache and meningitis, and analysis of the cerebrospinal fluid may show leukocytosis and an elevated protein level;
- pneumonitis;
- conjunctivitis, which is a frequent feature;
- hepatomegaly, and jaundice is an ominous sign; and
- bleeding, which is thought to be related mainly to capillary damage and which leads to ecchymoses, gastrointestinal bleeding and, on occasion, intracerebral bleeding.

Urinalysis reveals proteinuria and bilirubinuria. The white count is usually elevated (it may be as high as 30,000/mm³) with mainly polymorphonuclear cells. Thrombocytopenia may be present. The liver function tests demonstrate elevated levels of bilirubin and alkaline phosphatase. In contrast to fulminant viral hepatitis, the transaminase values may be normal or moderately elevated.

During the second or 'immune' stage the pyrexia generally resolves but life-threatening disease may be evident. There may be signs of myocardial involvement with dysrhythmias and nonspecific changes on the electrocardiogram. Blood tests confirm deteriorating liver function with evidence of muscle damage (elevated muscle enzymes). Worsening renal function is also a feature, with elevations in the serum creatinine and proteinuria.

In the third (convalescent) stage, a steady clinical and biochemical improvement occurs with resolution of the liver and renal failure and improved myocardial function. Minor relapses of symptoms can occur at this stage with further episodes of myalgia and spikes of fever.

DIAGNOSIS

During the early phase of the disease leptospira may be found on examination of the blood film or grown from blood with suitable media. Leptospira may be evident on urine microscopy but the diagnosis is more likely to be made from the serologic tests for antileptospiral antibodies, which are found in increasing titers in the convalescent phase of the disease.

At the time of the initial presentation, the symptoms and jaundice may suggest a viral hepatitis but the high fever and leukocytosis would be unusual for a viral etiology. However, similar hepatitic illnesses with or without renal failure have been described with hantaviruses (see Chapter 8.11).[19,20]

MANAGEMENT

Most patients with leptospirosis are not seriously ill, but for the small proposition with Weil's disease and multi-organ involvement full supportive care is required, often in the intensive care unit, with hemodialysis. High-dose intravenous penicillin is the treatment of choice but the dose may need modification according to the renal function. With antibiotic therapy, a febrile reaction similar to the Jarisch–Herxheimer reaction can occur.

HELMINTHIC PARASITES OF THE LIVER

SCHISTOSOMIASIS

Schistosomal ova can reach the liver via the mesenteric veins and portal system (see Chapter 6.27). Liver involvement is particularly seen with *Schistosoma japonicum* and *Schistosoma mansoni*, but it can also occur with *Schistosoma haematobium*. In the early stages a granulomatous reaction is seen but over years, if untreated, extensive collagen deposition can lead to portal fibrosis with the development of portal hypertension and splenomegaly (Fig. 40.3).

The diagnosis of schistosomal liver disease may come to light only when the patient presents with features of portal hypertension and, for example, has a variceal bleed.

DIAGNOSIS

The diagnosis may be made from the schistosomal enzyme-linked immunosorbent assay or from the histologic appearances of the granulomatous liver disease in the early stages and the fibrosis in the later stages. In the early stages a peripheral eosinophilia may be evident.

MANAGEMENT

Praziquantel is the treatment of choice. Patients should be warned that an influenza-like illness can follow therapy. Supportive therapy is required for the patient who has severe fibrosis, and liver transplantation may be required in advanced cases.

HYDATID INFECTION

Hydatid cysts can follow infection with the *Echinococcus* tapeworm.

EPIDEMIOLOGY

The disease is widespread and humans are infected by close contact with dogs that have become infected by the consumption of eggs from infected meat. Echinococcal infection is endemic in the main sheep-farming areas of the world and is a particular concern throughout much of Europe, the Mediterranean littoral, Asia, South America and Kenya (see Chapter 6.29).

PATHOLOGY

The liver is the most frequent site for hydatid cysts.

The ova enter the liver via the portal vein and lead to cyst formation within the liver parenchyma, classically involving the right lobe of the liver on the inferior surface (Fig. 40.4). Rupture of a cyst, either spontaneously or after trauma or surgical procedures, can lead to a state of cardiovascular collapse. This is thought to be an inappropriate immune response to released hydatid antigens. Rupture of the cysts can also lead to infection in the biliary tree, the peritoneum, the lungs or the pleura.

CLINICAL FEATURES

Hydatid disease may be asymptomatic and liver cysts found incidentally on ultrasound examination, as calcified lesions on plain abdominal radiographs or as an incidental finding at autopsy. Hepatomegaly may be present. The cyst may be diagnosed after it ruptures or if secondary infection of the cyst occurs. Cysts may also be found within the brain, lungs, kidney, heart and spine (see Fig. 40.4).

DIAGNOSIS

The hydatid serologic test is particularly useful, although false-positive and false-negative results can occur. There may be a peripheral eosinophilia. Several radiologic features can be helpful in making the diagnosis:

- plain abdominal radiographs may reveal calcified spheric structures within the liver;
- ultrasound examination can often detect several forms of the cysts which can be single, multiple, thin-walled or thick-walled; and
- CT scanning can detect smaller lesions and the presence of calcification.

It may difficult to differentiate a single cystic lesion from a tumor. Biopsy or aspiration of the cysts may be dangerous in view of the risk of antigen leakage and immune response, and this should be performed only when there is appropriate backup to treat circulatory collapse and laryngeal edema.

MANAGEMENT

The management of hepatic hydatidosis remains controversial and many approaches have been tried. It is recognized that by itself antimicrobial therapy with albendazole, mebendazole or praziquantel is generally ineffective and should be combined with a drainage procedure. Percutaneous drainage has the advantage of avoiding major surgery, but in open surgical procedures peritoneal contamination is thought to be minimized by packing the surgical field with povidone–iodine swabs, decompressing the cysts by aspiration and then removing the cyst contents. Some surgeons advocate injecting formalin or hypertonic saline into the cysts after decompression. In one study[21] 50 patients with hepatic hydatidosis were randomized to receive either percutaneous aspiration and albendazole or cystectomy. Similar efficacies were demonstrated in both treatment groups but the open surgical procedure was associated with greater morbidity.

LIVER FLUKES

Liver flukes are thought to invade the liver from the peritoneal cavity and migrate through the liver parenchyma to the biliary tree, where an inflammatory reaction develops (see Chapter 8.35).

CLONORCHIS SINENSIS

Infection with *Clonorchis sinensis* is usually associated with the consumption of raw or undercooked fish in Asia. The flukes live within capillaries of the biliary tree and the inflammatory reaction can

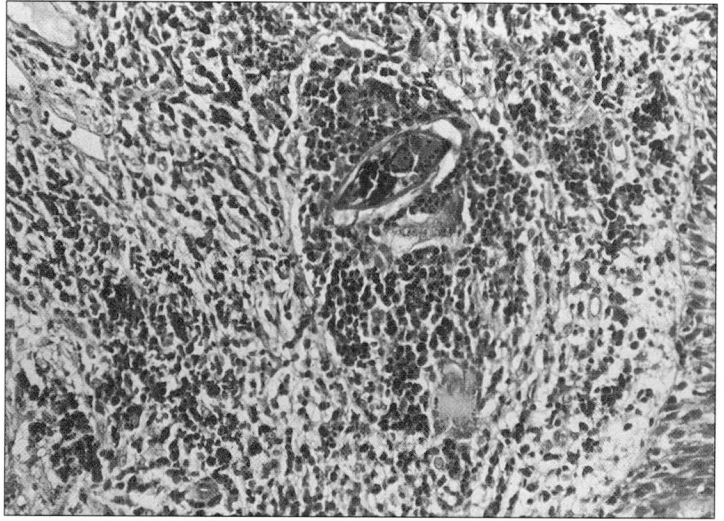

Fig. 40.3 Schistosomiasis of the liver. A refractile schistosome ova, located in a portal tract, associated with an eosinophil rich, granulomatous inflammatory reaction.

cause obstruction and encourage cholelithiasis. Cholangitis is a common complication, and the ongoing inflammation and fibrotic reaction is thought to predispose the patient to the development of cholangiosarcoma.[22]

DIAGNOSIS

Flukes may be evident on imaging techniques such as percutaneous transhepatic cholangiography or ERCP. This diagnosis must be borne in mind when atypical cholangiopathy is diagnosed in patients from the Far East. The diagnosis is confirmed by the finding of the ova on stool microscopy.

MANAGEMENT

Praziquantel is the treatment of choice. Surgical or endoscopic approaches may be required to deal with associated cholelithiasis and biliary obstruction.

FASCIOLA HEPATICA

Infection with *Fasciola hepatica*, a common sheep fluke, can follow consumption of contaminated watercress and is recorded throughout Europe, South America, the Caribbean, Africa and China.

PATHOLOGY

The picture is usually of biliary tract infection and obstruction, but hepatic granulomatous reactions can also occur.

CLINICAL FEATURES

In the early stages of infection, the patient may complain of fever and right hypochondrial pain. Hepatomegaly may be present. The migration of the flukes within the biliary tree can lead to inflammatory and fibrotic reactions. Cholelithiasis can occur and the clinical picture may be of a bacterial cholangitis. In common with bacterial cholangitis the alkaline phosphatase may be elevated but the presence of an eosinophilia should point to the possibility of a fluke infection.

DIAGNOSIS

The diagnosis may be suggested by a history of watercress consumption and features of cholangitis and an eosinophilia. Praziquantel is the therapy of choice and surgical and endoscopic intervention may be required to deal with biliary tree obstruction.

PROTOZOAL INFECTIONS OF THE LIVER

LEISHMANIASIS

Visceral leishmaniasis or kala azar can lead to massive hepatosplenomegaly (see Chapters 6.32 & 8.31).

EPIDEMIOLOGY

Leishmanial infection is transmitted by sandflies and is reported particularly around the Mediterranean basin, in South America and in Asia.

PATHOLOGY

Host factors are thought to be important in determining the disease outcome after leishmanial infection. It is not known why some patients develop only localized lesions and others develop more serious systemic disease. Underlying HIV infection is associated with multisystem disease and reactivation of previous infections, and this is being increasingly recognized in AIDS patients.[23]

CLINICAL FEATURES

The patient may present with fever or anemia. Massive hepatosplenomegaly may be present.

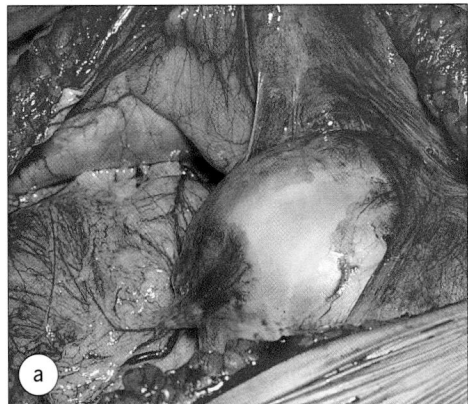

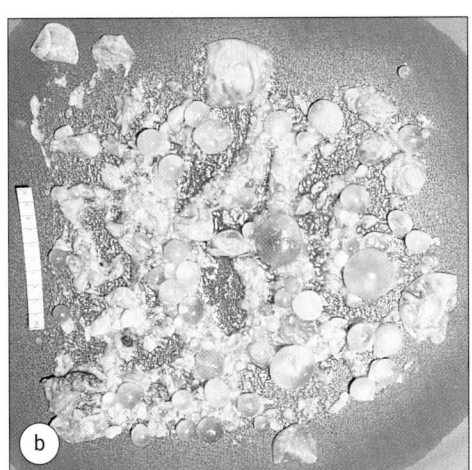

Fig. 40.4 **Hydatid disease.** (a) Hydatid cyst of the liver. (b) Hydatid 'daughter cysts'.

Fig. 40.5 Other parasitic causes of liver disease.

DIAGNOSIS

The presence of organisms may be detected by bone marrow examination, liver biopsy or splenic aspirate. Hypergammaglobulinemia is often present. Serologic tests are often useful but antibody tests are often negative in patients who have HIV infection.

MANAGEMENT

Therapy of leishmaniasis is somewhat limited by the toxicity of many of the antimicrobial agents. Antimonial compounds, for example, can cause pancreatitis. Liposomal and other preparations of amphotericin B are being increasingly used with success. In the setting of immunosuppression, maintenance regimens are often required with regular administration of amphotericin B or intravenous pentamidine. Other parasites that may occasionally involve the liver are shown in Figure 40.5.

FUNGAL INFECTIONS OF THE LIVER

The liver may be involved as part of a systemic fungal infection in a patient who has candidemia.[24] Cryptococcal infection, histoplasmosis and pneumocystosis of the liver are mainly seen in patients who have HIV infection.

Aspergillus infection of the liver with abscess formation is mainly seen in patients who have neutropenia as a result of chemotherapy.

BILIARY TREE INFECTIONS

ACUTE CHOLECYSTITIS

PATHOLOGY

Gallbladder infections are usually the results of gallstone formation and impaction within the cystic duct;[25] consequent impaired biliary drainage leads to infection, edema and compressive effects on the local blood supply, which can cause gangrene of the gallbladder. Suppuration within the gallbladder can lead to bacteremia, sepsis, cholangitis and liver abscess formation. Acalculous cholecystitis can follow infection with *Salmonella* spp. or *Campylobacter* spp. or can occur in acutely ill patients after major surgery or burns. In the setting of HIV infection, infection with *Salmonella* spp. or *Campylobacter* spp. may be implicated or the gallbladder disease may be a feature of HIV cholangiopathy,[26] which is often associated with cytomegalovirus, cryptosporidiosis, microsporidiosis or lymphoma.

CLINICAL FEATURES

The patient may describe right hypochrondrial discomfort, which can occur in waves. Radiation to the right shoulder is common. Fever or rigors can occur and the patient may develop bacteremia and sepsis. Right hypochondrial tenderness is usually present and the gallbladder is palpable in one-third of cases. A degree of jaundice may be present according to the extent of biliary tree obstruction.

DIAGNOSIS

The diagnosis is usually made clinically, but ultrasound of the liver and gallbladder may demonstrate gallstones with thickening of the gallbladder wall or dilatation of the biliary tree in the presence of obstruction. Laboratory findings include an elevated leukocyte count, hyperbilirubinemia and elevated levels of serum alkaline phosphatase. There may be modest elevations of the transaminase values. Impaired biliary drainage because of pancreatic carcinoma can also cause dilatation of the biliary tree and ERCP may be required to delineate the anatomy and to facilitate drainage if required.

MANAGEMENT

The priorities are to facilitate drainage of the biliary tree and to treat infection. Open cholecystectomy has a high mortality rate in elderly septic patients, and ERCP can be both lifesaving and diagnostic; stones are removed endoscopically by sphincterotomy, basket or balloon, or by stent insertion. Where ERCP is not available or in cases when it is not technically feasible, percutaneous biliary drainage can be performed.

Elective cholecystectomy can generally be performed subsequently, but emergency surgery may be required if the situation is complicated by a gangrenous gallbladder or poor response to antimicrobial therapy.[27]

Antimicrobial therapy should cover Gram-negative bacilli, enterococci and anaerobes. Cephalosporins and quinolones do not adequately cover enterococcal infection and, if they are used, they should be combined with amoxycillin, piperacillin or ticarcillin. Alternative regimens include ticarcillin or piperacillin in combination with an aminoglycoside and metronidazole. Aminoglycosides must be used carefully in this setting because there is a high incidence of renal impairment in patients who have sepsis of the biliary tree. Antimicrobial prophylaxis is also advised for procedures involving an obstructed biliary system.

CHOLANGITIS

PATHOLOGY

Gall stones within the cystic duct lead to acute cholecystitis, but if gallstones reach the common bile duct the obstruction and inflammation can lead to ascending cholangitis.

CLINICAL FEATURES

The symptoms and signs are generally similar to acute cholecystitis but the patient may have no history of abdominal pain and may present with sepsis.

DIAGNOSIS

Bacteremia has been reported in half the cases of cholangitis. Blood cultures are important. Alkaline phosphatase and bilirubin levels are usually elevated. An ultrasound may show dilatation of the biliary tree with stones, or it may be normal. Once the patient has been stabilized, ERCP is useful for diagnosis.

MANAGEMENT

As with cholecystitis the priorities are supportive care for the patient, with the appropriate antimicrobial chemotherapy, and drainage of the obstructed biliary system. The mortality when endoscopic sphincterotomy is used is less[28] than with conventional surgical techniques

REFERENCES

1. Sugano S, Matuda T, Suzuki T, et al. Hepatic actinomycosis: case report and review of the literature in Japan. J Gastroenterol 1997;32:672–6.
2. Dunn MW, Berkowitz FE, Miller JJ, Snitzer JA. Hepatosplenic cat-scratch disease and abdominal pain. Paediatr Infect Dis J 1997;16:269–72.
3. Weber G, Abu-Shakra M, Hertanu Y, Borer A, Sukenik S. Liver abscess caused by Capnocytophaga species. Clin Infect Dis 1997;25:152–3.
4. Elliot MA, Tefferi A, Marshall WF, Lacy MQ. Disseminated nocardiosis after allogeneic bone marrow transplantation. Bone Marrow Transplant 1997;20:425–6.
5. Yeoh KG, Yap I, Wong ST, Wee A, Gaun R, Kang JY. Tropical liver abscess. Postgrad Med J 1997;73:89–92.
6. Chen C, Chen PJ, Yang PM, et al. Clinical and microbiological features of liver abscess after transarterial embolization for hepatocellular carcinoma. Am J Gastroenterol 1997;92:2257–9.
7. Saini S. Imaging of the hepatobiliary tract. N Engl J Med 1997;336:1889–4.
8. Beeching NJ, Hart HH, Synek BJ, Bremner DA. A patient with hemosiderosis and multiple liver abscesses due to Yersinia enterocolitica. Pathology 1985;17:530–2.
9. Huang CJ, Pitt HA, Lipsett PA, et al. Pyogenic hepatic abscess. Changing trends over 42 years. Ann Surg 1996;223:600–7.
10. Tandon A, Jain AK, Dixit VK, Agarwal A K, Gupta JP. Needle aspiration in large amoebic liver abscess. Trop Gastroenterol 1997;18:19–21.
11. Yu VL, Miller WP, Wing EJ, et al. Disseminated listeriosis presenting as acute hepatitis. Case reports and review of hepatic involvement in listeriosis. Am J Med 1982;73:773–7.
12. Dan M, Bar-Meir S, Jedwab M, Shibolet S. Typhoid hepatitis with immunoglobulins and complement deposits in bile canaliculi. Arch Intern Med 1982;142;148–9.
13. Hawker F. Liver dysfunction in critical illness. Anaesth Intens Care 1991;19:165–81.
14. Essop AR, Posen JA, Hodkinson J, Segal I. Tuberculous hepatitis; a clinical review of 96 cases. Q J Med 1984;53:465–77.
15. Alcantara-Payawal DE, Matsumara M, Shiratori Y, et al. Direct detection of Mycobacterium tuberculosis using polymerase chain reaction assay among patients with hepatic granuloma. J Hepatol 1997;27:620–7.
16. Schneiderman DJ, Arensen DM, Cello JP, et al. Hepatic disease in patients with the acquired immune deficiency syndrome (AIDS). Hepatology 1987;5:925–30.
17. Schlossberg D. Syphilitic hepatitis: a case report and review of the literature. Am J Gastroenterol 1987;82:552–3.
18. Takafuji ET, Kirkpatrick JW, Miller RN, et al. An efficacy trial of doxycycline chemoprophylaxis against leptospirosis. N Engl J Med 1984;310:498–500.
19. Glass GE, Watson AJ, LeDuc JW, Childs JE. Domestic cases of hemorrhagic fever with renal syndrome in the United States. Nephron 1994;68:48–51.
20. Meng G, Lan Y, Nakagawa M, et al. High prevalence of hantavirus infection in a group of Chinese patients with acute hepatitis of unknown aetiology. J Viral Hepar 1997;4:231–4.
21. Khuroo MS, Wani NA, Javid G, et al. Percutaneous drainage compared with surgery for hepatic hydatid cysts. N Engl J Med 1997;337:881–7.
22. Chan CW, Lam SK. Diseases caused by liver flukes and cholangiocarcinoma. In: Gyr KE, ed. Bailliere's clinical gastroenterology. Tropical gastroenterology, vol 1. London: Bailliere Tindall; 1987:297–318.
23. Montalban C, Calleja JL, Erice A, et al. Visceral leishmaniasis in patients infected with human immunodeficiency virus. Co-operative Group for the Study of Leishmaniasis in AIDS. J Infect 1990;21:261–70.
24. Lewis JH, Patel HR, Zimmerman HJ. The spectrum of hepatic candidiasis. Hepatology 1982;2:479–87.
25. Strasberg, SM. Cholelithiasis and acute cholecysytitis. Baillieres Clin Gastroenterol 1997;11:643–61.
26. Cello JP. Human immunodeficency virus-associated biliary tract disease. Semin Liver Dis 1992;12:213–8.
27. McCarron B, Love WC. Acalculous nontyphoidal salmonellal cholecystitis requiring surgical intervention despite ciprofloaxin therapy: report of three cases. Clin Infect Dis 1997;24:707–9.
28. Leese T, Neoptolemos JP, Baker AR, Carr-Locke DL. Management of acute cholangitis and the impact of endoscopic sphincterotomy. Br J Surg 1986;73:988–92.
29. Adams DB, Tarnasky PR, Hawes RH, et al. Outcome after laparoscopic cholecystectomy for chronic acalculous cholecystitis. Ann Surg 1998;64:1–5.

Practice Points

Proper use of stool microscopy for ova and parasites

J Wendi Bailey &
Nicholas J Beeching

The cost-effective use of examination of fecal specimens for parasites requires close co-operation between the clinician and the laboratory. Adequate clinical details should be provided on the request form, together with a direct clinical question. The geographic setting influences both the level of expertise available in the laboratory and the range of parasites that may be expected, and the diagnostic approach to screening a population of apparently asymptomatic people, such as refugees, should be very different to that used for screening a traveler who has chronic diarrhea, for example.

The key issues that have to be addressed when selecting the appropriate diagnostic laboratory pathway are outlined. The balance of how these are dealt with sometimes differs among European and North American laboratories. Laboratory staff in industrialized nations often have less experience of recognizing parasites than their counterparts in less resourced countries, and in this situation, where staff costs are relatively high, 'hi-tech' approaches may be appropriate to supplement or replace conventional parasitologic techniques. In the resource-poor setting, nothing is more guaranteed to overload the laboratory and to demoralize staff than the common practice, particularly on pediatric wards, of routinely sending stool specimens from all inpatients for 'parasitology'. Such requesting behavior has no proven clinical benefit.

CLINICAL APPROACH
The clinician should decide whether requests are for general population screening, for screening of an individual patient for specific parasites, or for patient-oriented diagnostic purposes. This decision should be based on assessment of the behavior and location of the patient together with details of symptoms, concurrent illnesses and treatment that will influence the choice of tests (Fig. 41.1). It is rarely useful to search for a parasitologic cause for diarrhea of less than 1 week's duration in the general practice setting, and it is inappropriate to initiate a series of parasitologic examinations in a patient who develops diarrhea after 3 or 4 days in hospital, until other causes such as *Clostridium difficile* have been excluded, or unless a specific nosocomial outbreak is suspected.

The clinician should be clear in his or her own mind about how clinical management will be influenced by establishing a parasitological diagnosis. This applies particularly in the identification of parasites of controversial clinical significance such as *Blastocystis hominis*, or to the differentiation of morphologically similar parasites such as *Entamoeba histolytica* and *Entamoeba dispar* before possible treatment of asymptomatic cyst excretors. Specific clinical situations may require extra tests, such as searches for microsporidia in an HIV-positive patient with prolonged watery diarrhea, and in such situations a larger number of stool samples than usual may need to be examined.

CLINICAL DATA OF VALUE IN THE ASSESSMENT OF STOOL MICROSCOPY FOR OVA AND PARASITES	
Clinical data	Specific points
Purpose of test	Screening for all parasites (e.g. food handlers, population survey, refugees)
	General diagnostic test in an ill patient (testing for all parasites may be needed)
	Specific parasite suspected clinically (e.g. *Entamoeba histolytica*), hence parasite-directed tests as sole test or adjunctive test
	Pretreatment exclusion (e.g. strongyloidiasis before transplantantation)
	Outbreak investigation
	Evaluation of antiparasite chemotherapy or other need for quantitative rather than qualitative diagnosis
Geography	Location of laboratory (in endemic area or not)
	Patient travel to high-risk area, lifestyle while there, how long ago?
Duration of diarrhea	Acute or chronic or none
Type of diarrhea	Watery, bloody, presence of mucus, steatorrhea
Other symptoms	Fever, perianal itching (*Enterobius* spp.), hematuria (schistosomiasis), cutaneous larva currens (*Strongyloides stercoralis*), visible worm segments in stool
Other laboratory findings	Eosinophilia (helminths and cestodes)
	Findings on relevant serologic tests (e.g. for *Schistosoma* spp. or *Strongyloides* spp.)
	Findings on fecal culture, fecal electron microscopy or virus antigen tests
	Findings on endoscopy with or without histology
Patient characteristics	Child or adult
	Potential contact risk (e.g. water exposure, animal contact)
	Behavior (delusions of parasitosis)
	Setting [(e.g. overcrowding, mental institution, other potentially infected family members, (e.g. with giardiasis)]
	Immunocompromised (e.g. HIV infection, cytotoxic therapy, tumors, transplant)
	Hospitalized patient or outpatient
	Other illnesses (e.g. inflammatory bowel disease, psychiatric problems)
	Previous treatment for parasites
	Current or recent antibiotic treatment that might suppress parasites

Fig. 41.1 Clinical data required for appropriate use and interpretation of stool microscopy for ova and parasites.

SPECIMEN COLLECTION

Patients must be given the appropriate specimen collection device and instructions on how to use it; specimen pots (of all descriptions) frequently arrive in our laboratory containing totally inadequate amounts of feces. If serial stool specimens are required, the patient must understand that samples of feces passed on different occasions should be delivered, rather than multiple aliquots of the same stool. For unpreserved samples in which macroscopically visible parasites are expected (e.g. threadworms, roundworms, tapeworms, proglottids), colored plastic rather than transparent pots are useful. If *Enterobius vermicularis* is the main parasite suspected, a nocturnal perianal scotch-tape or saline swab specimen is preferable to a fecal specimen, and the patient or carer of the patient will need instructions on how to collect this. If microsporidia are to be sought with calcofluor stains, the specimen should be fixed in 10% formol–saline as soon as possible. Timed specimens may be needed for quantitative tests (e.g. 2–24-hour excretion of cryptosporidia), particularly in clinical trial situations.

DIRECT SMEARS

There are two distinct approaches to the examination of fecal specimens for parasites. In the UK, stools are usually received without the addition of a fixative. If the sample is received on the day that it is passed, a direct saline smear (for trophozoites) is examined, followed by a concentration technique, typically modified formol–ethyl acetate (FEA), for which commercial concentrators such as 'Evergreen' or 'ParaSep' are useful. In other countries it is more common for the laboratory to receive fecal specimens in a preservative, usually sodium–acetate acetic acid–formalin (SAF), and the advantages and disadvantages of this are discussed below.

Formed stools rarely contain trophozoites of clinical significance, and direct smears from these are unlikely to be useful. Stains for cryptosporidia may be indicated if initial direct smears of liquid stools are negative. Most parasite trophozoites die within hours of the fecal specimen being passed, although it may be possible to see active trichomonas or giardial trophozoites on the following day, so routine practice is to omit direct examination of smears from specimens more than 24 hours old.

Bloody stools with mucus may contain *E. histolytica* trophozoites, which are best detected in a 'hot stool' and examined within 30 minutes of being produced [or kept at 98.6°F (37°C) for up to 1 hour], preferably on site, for amebae with engulfed erythrocytes. The presence of inflammatory cells or bacteria on direct examination is more suggestive of a bacterial cause. The clinical effectiveness of using the presence of fecal leukocytes as a screening tool for bacterial pathogens is now being questioned in the USA. It is doubtful whether the common practice of examining direct smears routinely for parasites is clinically useful either, except in the genuine 'hot stool' or after staining for specific pathogens such as cryptosporidia or microsporidia.

PRESERVATIVES OR NOT?

The value of conventional microscopy for parasites, which is time-consuming, depends on the experience and salary costs of the staff. In our specialist practice, only 10 minutes are needed to examine direct and concentrated smears from an unpreserved stool, stained with iodine if necessary, which will identify the majority of clinically relevant parasites apart from cryptosporidia and microsporidia. Introduction of routine stains such as trichrome on fixed material would add unacceptably to the time taken to process specimens with little extra yield. However, in many countries, fixed fecal material is routinely received by the laboratory. This has the advantage that everything is preserved and can be processed at leisure. Fixation and staining specifically identifies *Dientamoeba fragilis* (rarely seen in unfixed specimens), but this is of questionable clinical importance. Apart from possible delays incurred in processing and staining fixed fecal material, the major disadvantage is that it is unsuitable for

culture for bacteria or parasites, for which separate specimens are needed. This is specifically relevant in the diagnosis of *Strongyloides* spp., for which fecal culture methods have at least twice the detection rates of staining procedures. Nevertheless, the diagnostic yield of examination of specimens preserved with SAF is better than unpreserved specimens in some hands, and it is probably safer to transport preserved specimens than unpreserved specimens.

NUMBER OF SPECIMENS

How many specimens should be processed, given the intermittent excretion rates of many parasites? It is generally accepted that no more than three specimens are required, except in specific situations such as searches for scanty *Schistosoma mansoni*, when up to five stools may need to be examined using specialized techniques such as digestion or Kato concentration. In some settings a single stool examination can detect more than 90% of parasites, but in most circumstances, especially if more than one parasite is likely, multiple specimens should be processed. There is good evidence that pooling of three specimens from an individual patient increases the diagnostic yield and saves time and money, and this is one of the major advantages of receiving fixed fecal material that may be stored for batch processing.

NEW TECHNOLOGY

Conventional approaches to fecal parasitology may soon be replaced in routine clinical practice by the newer techniques that are rapidly being introduced, particularly for protozoa. Many of these methods are expensive but can be shown to have better diagnostic yields for specific parasites, particularly in areas where technicians are relatively inexperienced. Introduction of many of the parasite-specific detection methods needs prospective evaluation of cost-effectiveness, including their use for 'office-based' patient screening. This requires a more focused clinical approach to decide which parasite or parasites are being sought, since the positive yield for specific pathogens may be increased at the expense of not screening for other parasites that may be present but not detected.

Antigen detection systems have many potential advantages. For the diagnosis of giardiasis, in which cyst or trophozoite excretion is notoriously intermittent, use of a coproantigen enzyme-linked immunosorbent assay (ELISA) on one specimen gives a similar yield to microscopic examination of three specimens, and several commercial assays are now available for this purpose; similar assays are also available for the detection of cryptosporidia. The yield of microscopy for giardia and cryptosporidia can also be improved by the use of direct fluorescence staining and is now preferred in many laboratories. Further refinements, such as flow cytometry of stained fecal material, will have to be shown to be cost-effective before they are widely adopted. Both direct fluorescence staining and ELISA methods are better performed on fresh, unpreserved stools (within 24 hours of being passed) than on specimens preserved in formol–saline; these methods are less effective, but they can be used in SAF preserved samples.

New techniques have revolutionized our approach to the diagnosis of amebic infections, because light microscopy does not distinguish between *E. histolytica* and *E. dispar* and axenic culture and isoenzyme analysis is not performed in routine diagnostic practice. Assays for *E. histolytica* adhesins are clinically useful, and a number of commercial enzyme immunoassay kits are currently being assessed. Some provide better correlation than others compared with nested polymerase chain reaction (PCR) on fecal samples. These are important both for improved detection of parasites and for species verification, because *E. dispar* is not pathogenic.

Finally, PCR-based systems are showing considerable promise in the technically difficult area of screening feces for microsporidia. There is considerable variation between laboratories in the interpretation of results of staining feces with (for example) Uvitex 2B or Weber's trichome stains, and clinically useful primers for the most common fecal pathogens, *Enterocytozoon bieneusi* and *Encephalitozoon intestinalis*, are now available. This seems likely to become a useful clinical diagnostic test in the near future. Both PCR-based and antigen-detection assays are likely to find a place in assessing cure after treatment for specific pathogens, although the microscopic gold standard for evaluating their performance in this regard will be difficult to establish.

In summary, traditional approaches to fecal parasitologic examination have differing advantages and disadvantages. Both will be radically altered in the next few years by technologic advances. These will necessitate a clarification of the clinical questions that should accompany the fecal specimen, as parasite-specific tests will be more expensive, especially if several are used on one specimen. In the resource-poor setting, the old-fashioned labor-intensive methods are likely to hold sway for many years and these traditional skills will still be needed to validate the newer technology based methods in developed countries and to identify the new pathogens that will inevitably emerge.

FURTHER READING

Goodgame RW, Genta RM, White AC Jr, Chappell CL. Intensity of infection in AIDS-associated cryptosporidiosis. J Infect Dis 1993;167:704–9.

Haque R, Ali IKM, Akther S, Petri WA Jr. Comparison of PCR, isoenzyme analysis and antigen detection for diagnosis of *Entameba histolytica* infection. J Clin Microbiol 1998;36:449–52.

Hiatt RA, Markell EK, Ng E. How many stool examinations are necessary to detect pathogenic intestinal protozoa? Am J Trop Med Hyg 1995;53:36–9.

Hines J, Nachamkin I. Effective use of the clinical microbiology laboratory for diagnosing diarrheal diseases. Clin Infect Dis 1996;23:1292–301.

Ligoury O, David F, Sarfati C, *et al*. Diagnosis of infections caused by *Enterocytozoon bieneusi* and *Encephalitozoon intestinalis* using polymerase chain reaction in stool specimens. AIDS 1997;11:723–6.

Mank TG, Zaat JO, Blotkamp J, Polderman AM. Comparison of fresh versus sodium acetate acetic acid formalin preserved stool specimens for diagnosis of intestinal protozoal infections. Eur J Clin Microbiol Infect Dis 1995;14:1076–81.

Mayer HB, Wanke CA. Diagnostic strategies in HIV-infected patients with diarrhea. AIDS 1994;8:1639–48.

Valdez LM, Dang H, Okhuysen PO, Chappell CL. Flow cytometric detection of *Cryptosporidium* oocysts in human stool samples. J Clin Microbiol 1997;35:2013–17.

Management of an outbreak of gastroenteritis   *WTA Todd*

The World Health Organization defines food poisoning or 'food-borne disease' as 'any disease of an infectious or toxic nature caused by or thought to be caused by the consumption of food or water'.

The term 'outbreak' has recently replaced 'epidemic' in the parlance of infectious diseases. The two are strictly synonymous and can be defined either as 'two or more linked cases of the same illness' or 'the occurrence of any disease clearly in excess of normal expectancy'. Three types of outbreak are commonly recognized:
- point source, involving exposure to a single source of infection at a defined time point (e.g. consumption of contaminated food at a social function); all exposed people will develop symptoms at or around the expected incubation period for that illness;
- common source outbreak, involving exposure to a single source of infection over a period of time (e.g. an asymptomatic carrier of infection in a retail food outlet); spread through national or international food distribution networks has expanded the scope of this type of outbreak in recent years and large numbers of people may be exposed over prolonged periods of time through this means; and
- person-to-person outbreak, in which the chain of transmission is from one infected person to another by direct contact (e.g. a child infected at a birthday party infecting family members or school friends); this type of spread maintains the outbreak with clusters of infection separated by the incubation period of the infection.

After recognition of an outbreak of food-borne infection there must be:
- a clear definition of the problem,
- investigation of the source,
- establishment of control plans, and
- a concomitant formulation of practical arrangements to deal with cases.

There is a need for clear communication with care providers, the public at large and the media.

The management of any outbreak falls into two distinct areas:
- the public health control of the condition, comprising the recognition of the problem, elucidation of the source and the establishment of adequate control measures; and
- the clinical management of infected cases with the required re-organization of clinical services to cope with the numbers of cases.

COMMON CAUSES OF FOOD-BORNE OUTBREAKS OF GASTROENTERITIS.

Details of the common causes of food-borne outbreaks of gastroenteritis are given in Chapter 2.35, but Figures 41.2 and 41.3 collate details of these conditions that are especially relevant to the management of outbreaks.

IDENTIFICATION OF AN OUTBREAK

The clustering of cases that heralds an outbreak may first be recognized by public health clinicians or epidemiologists by way of formal national notification systems or through clinicians, laboratory personnel or the general public. There should be clear communication channels to the designated local or national body that has the authority to declare that an outbreak is occurring and to initiate investigation, control and containment measures. This process is best effected by the formation of an outbreak control team (OCT). The key members of the team will be:
- a senior consultant who has public health responsibility,
- a senior environmental health officer,
- a consultant microbiologist, and
- secretarial support staff.

In addition the team should have the ability to co-opt other appropriate members (e.g. consultants in infectious diseases, local press officers, infection control nurses, primary care representatives, national surveillance center representatives, toxicologists, government representatives). Full notes and records of all meetings and decisions should be made and stored.

EPIDEMIOLOGIC INVESTIGATION

The OCT must initiate appropriate investigations of the source and nature of the outbreak using recognized epidemiologic methodology and establish a case definition appropriate to the condition involved. Thereafter it must act rapidly to control further risk to the public and make appropriate arrangements for the care of patients.

PRACTICAL ARRANGEMENTS

A skeleton plan of local arrangements must be agreed before the recognition of any outbreak situation. This is best achieved as an addition to the major incident plan of the hospital or community. An outbreak of food-borne disease constitutes a major medical incident differing from a trauma, radiation or fire incident in the potentially protracted presentation of cases, and the cumulative and prolonged disruption it may cause to clinical services.

Once the causative organism is known and the type of outbreak has been identified, a realistic prediction of the time scale of disruption can be made. In addition, the potential for the development of complications, even in a small proportion of cases, should be recognized because this may produce an additional burden on resources.

A point source outbreak produces disruption to normal working practice similar to that produced by a major trauma incident; common source or person-to-person outbreaks constitute a much more extended disruption with a cumulative effect on clinical resources. The time scale of this will be a function of the incubation period of the illness and the expected duration of symptoms. All of these elements of disruption will be compounded if there is an ongoing need for adequate isolation of sufferers. The OCT should take cognizance of these features from the outset (see Fig. 41.3).

Bed availability

Hospitals and primary care facilities should agree a stepwise plan for the utilization of clinical areas. There may be also be a need for resources in neighboring hospitals or health authority areas, and such possibilities should also have been rehearsed.

TYPES OF FOOD POISONING			
Infection	Incubation period	Major symptoms	Outbreak pattern
Clostridium perfringens	18–36 hours	Watery diarrhea and colicky abdominal pain	1
Norwalk agent (small round-structured viruses)	24–48 hours	Vomiting, diarrhea, myalgias, headache	1, 2, 3
Scombrotoxic poisoning	1–4 hours	Histamine poisoning (headache, flushing, urticaria, swelling, tingling lips)	1
Diarrhetic shellfish poisoning	<1 day	Acute diarrhea (severity proportional to dose of toxin)	1, 2
Paralytic shellfish poisoning	4–6 hours (?)	Bradycardia, parasthesia, muscle weakness	1, 2
Salmonellosis	18–36 hours	Diarrhea, vomiting	1, 2, 3
Bacillus cereus toxin (rapid)	1–6 hours	Nausea, precipitant vomiting	1, 2
Bacillus cereus toxin (late)	10–12 hours	Abdominal pain, profuse watery diarrhea, nausea	1, 2
Clostridium botulinum	24–48 hours	Cranial nerve palsy followed by general paralysis	1
Bean hemagglutinins	Minutes after ingestion	Severe vomiting, profuse diarrhea	1
Shigellosis	1–3 days	Fever prodrome, colic and diarrhea, occasional hyperpyrexia in children	2, 3
Escherichia coli O157, varo-toxin producing *E. coli* organisms	1–2 days (up to 5 days)	Brisk watery diarrhea, bloody stools, abdominal pain	1
Food-poisoning *Vibrio* spp.	5–92 hours	Watery diarrhea and colicky abdominal pain	1, 2
Yersinia enterocolitica	3–7 days	Mild-to-moderate gastroenteritis, aching abdominal pain	1, 2
Staphylococcal toxin	30 minutes to 6 hours	Nausea, precipitant vomiting	1
Campylobacter spp.	2–4 days (maximum 8–9 days)	Diarrhea, vomiting, abdominal pain, blood *per rectum*	1, 2, 3

Fig. 41.2 Types of food poisoning. Outbreak patterns: 1, point source; 2, common source; 3, person-to-person.

COMPLICATIONS OF FOOD POISONING			
Infection	Complications	Patients who have complications (%)	Isolation needed
Bacillus cereus toxin (rapid)	Dehydration, occasional shock	Unusual	No
Bacillus cereus toxin (late)	No direct complications	–	No
Bean hemagglutinins	Dehydration, shock	Rare	No
Campylobacter spp.	Prolonged symptom, potential for relapse, bacteremia, focal sepsis, rarely Guillain–Barré syndrome	10–20% ill for >1 week, 5–10% relapse, bacteremia in <1%	Yes
Clostridium botulinum	Full requirement for respiratory support	50–80%	No
Clostridium perfringens	Dehydration occasional shock	Elderly and compromised	Yes
Diarrhetic shellfish poisoning	No complications	–	No
Escherichia coli O157, varo-toxin producing *E. coli* organisms	Hemolytic–uremic syndrome, thrombotic thrombocytopenic purpura	2–8%	Yes
Food-poisoning *Vibrio* spp.	No complications	–	Yes
Norwalk agent (small round-structured viruses)	Not recorded	–	Yes
Paralytic shellfish poisoning	Death	Rare	No
Salmonellosis	Sepsis, reactive arthritis, distant focal collection, osteomyelitis in sickle cell disease, meningitis in infants	5% sepsis, 2% reactive arthritis	Yes
Scombrotoxic poisoning	Hypotensive crisis	<1%	No
Shigellosis	Osteomyelitis in sickle cell disease	rare	Yes
Staphylococcal toxin	Shock, occasional death	<1%	No
Yersinia enterocolitica	Postinfectious arthritis, erythema nodosum	Arthritis 10–30%, erythema nodosum 30%	Yes

Fig. 41.3 Complications of food poisoning.

Staffing

Plans should recognize the need for additional staffing (e.g. medical staff, nursing staff, including infection control personnel, managerial and administrative staff, counselors, public interface and media link personnel, support staff, catering staff and laboratory personnel).

The possible prolonged disruption to normal working practice, such as on-call arrangements and regular clinics, requires administrative staff to re-organize these features of normal health care. Clinical staff involved in the care of outbreak cases are not available for normal duties for the duration of an outbreak. A major feature of any prolonged outbreak is the considerable stress engendered by this departure from normal routine. Planners do well to recognize this in advance and prepare to provide a staff counseling service at an early stage in the procedure.

COMMUNICATION

At all stages in an outbreak regular and quality communication is essential. At the earliest possible opportunity in the planning process, appropriate cascades of personnel should be constructed for the following contingencies:

- initial notification of the outbreak,
- convening of the OCT, and
- contacting of key staff (see below) and alerting of appropriate personnel.

A cascade system allows nominated people to hold contact details for a number of staff. Once alerted, each nominated person is then responsible for contacting the next available person on the list, so freeing switchboard and other personnel from a very time-consuming occupation.

These cascades should be updated at regular intervals (e.g. junior medical staff every 6 months) and regularly tested to ensure that the hospital switchboard does not become jammed with outgoing calls. People must be reminded of their cascade responsibilities. A central record should be held of the different cascades to assist during the emergency. A typical list of essential contacts would include:

- executives of the health authority and any clinical establishments involved or likely to become so;
- clinicians involved or likely to become so;
- laboratory staff involved or likely to become so;
- primary care providers and those who will have first clinical contact with cases; and
- government and local authorities.

Health authority personnel, clinicians and laboratory staff should be notified by the appropriate cascade system, which is initiated either by switchboard operators or by individual members of the OCT.

Primary care providers (including out-of-hours and locum services), accident and emergency departments and local pharmacies should be notified early by a special general circular, preferably disseminated electronically. This should be updated regularly and should contain summary information on the likely presentation, complications and simple management of clinical cases. This information should not assume familiarity with the condition.

Effective communication with the public is vital in any outbreak. Anxieties must be addressed and appropriate questions must be answered in an accurate and comprehensible manner. Jargon, complex medical terminology and patronizing attitudes must be avoided. A central telephone 'helpline' is a very effective means of providing this service.

An early decision will be required as to how to handle the media. Undue exposure of clinical staff in this extremely stressful activity must be avoided. A single media contact with experience in dealing with the press should be centrally appointed and all communications directed through that person.

Political interest, both local and national, cannot be underestimated. There will be a regular demands for accurate and timely information. A data-gathering facility should be constructed such that clinical staff are not distracted from patient care to provide such information. It is far more practical to provide such information at the end of each working day than at the beginning.

RESEARCH AND THE FURTHERANCE OF KNOWLEDGE

Outbreaks of any type present unique opportunities to extend our knowledge of infection, its epidemiology, control and management. It is vital not only that accurate records are kept during the episode and communicated to the wider scientific community, but also that time is allowed from the outset to consider the research opportunities and the related requirements afforded by the epidemic. It is recommended that relevant academics are involved as early as possible to work with local clinical staff in this essential element of outbreak management.

FURTHER READING

Investigation and control of outbreaks of foodborne disease in Scotland. Edinburgh: Scottish Office Department of Health Advisory Group on Infection; 1996.

Management of outbreaks of foodborne illness. Guidance produced by a Department of Health Working Group. Heywood, Lancashire: BAPS Health Publication Centre; 1994

Tauxe RV. Emerging foodborne diseases: an evolving public health challenge. Emerg Infect Dis (special issue) 1997;3:425–34.

Kok-Ann Gwee &
Michael W McKendrick

Management of persistent postinfectious diarrhea

INTRODUCTION

The presence of diarrhea beyond 2 weeks of a confirmed or presumed infectious exposure is a useful working definition of persistent diarrhea as this helps to exclude most common acute bacterial and viral infections, although protozoal infections may persist for longer. Patients who have persistent diarrhea who have recently returned from a tropical or developing country can also be considered as having postinfectious diarrhea.

PATHOGENESIS AND CLINICAL FEATURES

Postinfectious irritable bowel syndrome

In a prospective study, we found that 25% of previously healthy patients developed a diarrhea-predominant type of irritable bowel syndrome (IBS) (Fig. 41.4) after an episode of acute infectious diarrhea. Psychologic disturbances such as anxiety and stressful recent life events were important

predictors for the development of IBS. Other potential pathogenic factors are lactose malabsorption, alterations in colonic motility and sensitivity, changes in the colonic microflora and bile acid malabsorption.

Inflammatory bowel disease

Some patients who have inflammatory bowel disease (IBD) in their initial presentation have a positive microbial finding. However, symptoms may persist or recur despite the eradication of the inciting organism. Commonly implicated pathogens are *Entamoeba histolytica*, *Shigella* spp., *Salmonella* spp., *Aeromonas* spp. and *Clostridium difficile*. Possible explanations for this association include bacterial infection added on to previously unrecognised IBD, and the precipitation of IBD by an altered intestinal microflora or by an immunopathogenic effect of bacterial products of inflammation.

POINTS TO NOTE IN THE HISTORY AND PHYSICAL EXAMINATION OF PATIENTS WHO HAVE PERSISTENT DIARRHEA

- Onset of diarrhea in relation to confirmed or presumed infectious illness
- Travel to or residence in tropics or developing countries
- Weight loss
- Nature of the stools: frequency, consistency, estimated volume, steatorrhea
- Bowel symptoms suggesting irritable bowel syndrome: abdominal pain relieved by defecation, constipation, passage of mucus, feeling of incomplete evacuation, bloating
- Other abdominal symptoms: flatulence (suggesting giardiasis, lactose malabsorption), blood in the stool (suggesting colitis, dysentery)
- Risk factors for HIV if appropriate
- Examination for evidence of weight loss, anemia, malabsorption, abdominal masses, lymph nodes

Fig. 41.4 Points to note in the history and physical examination of patients who have persistent diarrhea.

Human immunodeficiency virus-associated enteropathy

HIV-associated enteropathy may present with chronic diarrhea and significant weight loss or malabsorption. It is believed that in the majority of HIV-infected patients who have chronic diarrhea, a potential pathogen can be detected.

Postinfective malabsorption

Tropical sprue presents with chronic gastrointestinal symptoms and malabsorption following an acute diarrheal episode that is usually contracted in a tropical country (although it has also been described in travelers to the Mediterranean area). Although a specific microbial agent has not been identified, the typical response to broad-spectrum antibiotics suggests an infectious pathogenesis. Intestinal infections with parasites, especially *Giardia lamblia*, may also present similarly.

Persistent intestinal infections

Occasionally infective colitis associated with *E. histolytica*, *Campylobacter jejuni* or *Salmonella* spp. may persist beyond 6 weeks (Fig. 41.5). The clinical spectrum of *G. lamblia* infection ranges from asymptomatic cyst excretion through chronic diarrhea with marked flatulence to intestinal malabsorption. *Cyclospora cayetanensis* is a newly recognized protozoal parasite that causes prolonged watery diarrhea even in immunocompetent patients. Although cases of chronic diarrhea associated with *Blastocystis hominis*, *Aeromonas* spp. and *Plesiomonas shigelloides* have been reported, their pathogenic potential remains uncertain.

DIAGNOSIS

Patients can be stratified to an appropriate level of testing on the basis of the points listed in Figure 41.4.

Level 1 tests are:
- stool studies – microscopy, culture, ova, cysts and parasites, and tests for *C. difficile* toxin;
- blood studies – full blood count, erythrocyte sedimentation rate, biochemistry (electrolytes, protein, albumin, thyroid hormones) and studies for the detection of HIV antibodies; and
- sigmoidoscopy.

In a patient who has no history of travel to or residence in a tropical or developing country and no significant weight loss or blood in the stools, level 1 tests would usually be sufficient. To optimize the yield from stool examinations, three specimens, preferably when stools are loose, should be collected on separate days and processed rapidly. Sigmoidoscopy and rectal biopsy help to exclude colitis, although biopsies taken late in an infective colitis often show changes that are hard to distinguish from IBD. When there is doubt about the diagnosis, a follow-up biopsy 6–8 weeks later is helpful, as infective colitis

ORGANISMS THAT MAY BE INVOLVED IN CHRONIC DIARRHEA AND THEIR ANTIBIOTIC TREATMENT

Organism		Antibiotic	Suggested dosage
Bacteria	*Shigella* spp.	Quinolones, e.g. ciprofloxacin, norfloxacin	500mg q12h for 5 days
	Salmonella spp.		400mg q12h for 5 days
	Campylobacter spp.		
	Aeromonas spp.		
	Plesiomonas shigelloides		
	Spirochetes	Metronidazole	400mg q8h for 10 days
Protozoa	*Giardia lamblia*	Metronidazole	2g q24h for 3 days
		Tinidazole	2g once daily for 1 day
	Entamoeba histolytica	Metronidazole	800mg q8h for 5 days
		Tinidazole	1g q12h for 3 days
	Cyclospora cayentensis	Trimethoprim–sulfamethoxazole	2 tablets q12h for 7 days
	Isospora belli	Trimethoprim–sulfamethoxazole	2 tablets q6h for 14 days
Helminths	*Strongyloides stercoralis*	Thiabendazole	25mg/kg (maximum 1.5g) q12h for 3 days
		Albendazole	400mg q12h for 3 days (repeat at 3 weeks if required)
	Trichuris trichiura	Mebendazole	100mg q12h for 3 days
	Capillaria philippinensis	Mebendazole	100mg q6h for 20–30 days
	Mixed infection	Mebendazole	200mg q12h for 5 days
		Albendazole	400mg q24h for 3 days
Tropical sprue		Tetracycline plus folic acid	250mg q6h for 30 days (minimum)
			5mg q12h for 90 days

Fig. 41.5 Organisms that may be involved in chronic diarrhea and their antibiotic treatment.

usually reverts spontaneously to normal. In the absence of proctitis, a rectal biopsy can still provide an indication of mild but significant forms of proximal colitis. The decision to test further should be based on clinical indications and the results of the level 1 tests. For instance, in the presence of relevant exposure, or the finding of lymphopenia, the issue of testing for HIV should be addressed.

Level 2a tests are:
- a lactose hydrogen breath test or a 2-week trial of dietary exclusion; and
- Selenium-75 labelled homotaurocholic acid test (SeHCAT) of bile malabsorption or trial of cholestyramine.

For patients whose presentation is consistent with IBS (see Fig. 41.4), level 2a tests can be considered, depending on the clinical circumstances and the facilities available. Level 2b test are:
- tests for malabsorption (serum folate, vitamin B12, iron and xylose absorption tests),
- enterotest (string test), and
- a small bowel biopsy.

If there is a suspicion of malabsorption, evidence for this should be obtained as indicated in level 2b. Where there is positive evidence, and if stools are negative, further tests should be done to explain the malabsorption. Duodenal fluid obtained either by aspiration or an enterotest can be examined for *Giardia* spp. In the enterotest, the patient swallows a gelatin capsule to which a nylon thread is attached. After 4–6 hours the string is retrieved and sent to the laboratory, and the bile-stained distal end is smeared on a microscopic slide. Some investigators recommend jejunal biopsy combined with an impression smear of the jejunal mucosa.

Level 3 test are:
- radiologic examinations (barium studies of the small and large bowel); and
- colonoscopy.

If the diagnosis remains uncertain, level 3 tests help to exclude Crohn's disease, colonic tumors, small intestinal diverticula (which may give rise to bacterial overgrowth) and intestinal lymphoma.

MANAGEMENT

If malabsorption or weight loss is present and a specific infective diagnosis can be made, the indication for antimicrobial therapy is clear. If the diagnosis remains uncertain after thorough investigation, a chemotherapeutic trial of metronidazole or tetracycline appears justified. In the presence of HIV, a persistent search for an enteric pathogen is important because it is recognized that a potentially treatable pathogen can often be detected. Nutritional supplements may occasionally be required.

Patients who have a positive stool isolate but no malabsorption, weight loss or dysenteric stools pose a therapeutic dilemma. Many of these patients are persistent excretors or carriers of the organism and are suffering from postinfectious IBS; antibiotic treatment will either not improve the diarrhea or will produce a temporary improvement, possibly as a nonspecific effect of antibiotics on colonic flora. However, occasionally bacterial pathogens may give rise to protracted diarrhea and, as long as the pathogenic potential of an organism remains uncertain, a trial of antimicrobial chemotherapy can be justified. Repeated courses of antibiotics should not be pursued if the patient shows no improvement.

In patients who have postinfectious IBS, treatment with a lactose-free diet, loperamide, cholestyramine and antispasmodic agents may be helpful, although the condition may be extremely resistant to any therapeutic intervention. Some patients give a history of intolerance to specific foods or drinks or eating at a particular time of day; in these patients, a lifestyle or diet modification may be helpful. The pronounced urgency, perhaps one of the most troublesome symptoms, is very difficult to treat but usually improves with time. Sometimes, it may be necessary to consider admission to hospital for observation of stool frequency and weight stability. In IBS, despite frequent defecation, stool weight typically remains within the normal range (<200g/day).

FURTHER READING

Anand AC, Reddy PS, Saiprasad GS, Kher SK. Does non-dysenteric intestinal amebiasis exist? Lancet 1997;349:89–92.
Cook GC. Persisting diarrhea and malabsorption. Gut 1994;35:582–6.
Dickinson RJ, Gilmour HM, McClelland DB. Rectal biopsy in patients presenting to an infectious disease unit with diarrheal disease. Gut 1979;20:141–8.
Gwee KA, Graham JC, McKendrick MW, et al. Psychometric scores and persistence of irritable bowel after infectious diarrhea. Lancet 1996;347:150–3,617–8,1267.
McKendrick MW, Geddes AM, Gearty J. Campylobacter enteritis: a study of clinical features and rectal mucosal changes. Scand J Infect Dis 1982;14:35–8.
Smith PD, Quinn TC, Strober W, Janoff EN, Masur H. Gastrointestinal infections in AIDS. Ann Intern Med 1992;116:63–77.
Stewart GT. Post-dysenteric colitis. Br Med J 1950;405–9.

Antibiotics in infectious gastroenteritis or diarrhea
Richard Yu

INTRODUCTION

Diarrhea is one of the most common manifestations of infectious diseases in the world. It is characterized by an increase in the frequency of bowel movements and a change in the character of the stools from formed to liquefied. It is a major cause of morbidity and mortality in childhood in developing nations. In the USA, it has been estimated that approximately 8 million patients seek medical attention for diarrhea on an annual basis. Up to 25,000 of these require hospitalization.

PATHOGENESIS

Transmission of the disease is through fecally contaminated food and water, poor personal hygiene and sanitation, and homosexual activity. Risk is high among:
- children and workers in day care centers,
- the elderly in nursing home facilities,
- the immunocompromised (e.g. caused by chemotherapy, corticosteroid therapy, HIV infection), and
- those who have prior antibiotic use.

The most common causes are viruses and, to a lesser extent, bacteria and parasites. In bacterial diarrhea, mechanisms of disease include adherence of the organism to intestinal mucosal cells (with or without mucosal damage and invasion) and production of enterotoxins and cytotoxins.

DIAGNOSIS

The clinical presentation is of the utmost importance in the evaluation of the patient who has diarrhea. Evaluation should include a comprehensive history of food and water intake, recent traveling or camping, recent antibiotic use, sexual practices, close contacts with similar signs and symptoms, exposure to day care centers or nursing home facilities and the duration of diarrhea. A thorough physical examination should take into account the state of the patient's hydration (mucous membranes, blood pressure, heart rate, urine output), fever, tenesmus, abdominal pain and tenderness, and character of the stools (bloody, mucoid).

The disease is self-limiting in most cases. If the diarrheal illness is of limited duration without signs of dysentery or patient toxicity, no further diagnostic work-up is indicated. Supportive care, oral rehydration therapy and observation should be given. In patients who have evidence of systemic toxicity, abdominal pain, tenesmus, protracted or bloody diarrhea or immunocompromised states, further work-up for an etiologic diagnosis should be pursued. Treatment is reserved for selected, invasive bacterial or parasitic infections for which specific therapy is available and proven to be effective (see Chapter 2.35).

ANTIBIOTIC THERAPY

Initially, after reviewing the history, physical examination and the preliminary laboratory findings, a decision must be made as to whether antimicrobial agents should be used. The need for antimicrobial agents should be based on the potential pathogen and whether there is clinical data to prove efficacy for antimicrobial therapy. The patient's clinical examination should be considered along with the patient's underlying medical problems. The presence of blood, mucus or polymorphonuclear leukocytes in the stools make a stronger case for antibiotic therapy. Suspected viral agents should not be treated unless specific therapy is available (e.g. for cytomegalovirus colitis in AIDS).

Infectious agents that respond favorably to specific antimicrobial therapy include *Shigella* spp., *Vibrio cholerae*, *Clostridium difficile*, *Entamoeba histolytica*, *Giardia lamblia* and *Isospora belli*. Enteric pathogens for which the clinical indication for antimicrobial use is less clear include enteropathogenic *Escherichia coli*, enterohemorrhagic *E. coli*, nontyphoidal *Salmonella* spp., *Campylobacter jejuni* and *Yersinia enterocolitica*. Proctitis caused by sexually transmitted diseases such as herpes simplex virus (the most common), *Chlamydia trachomatis*, and *Neisseria gonorrhoeae* require specific therapy. A longer course of therapy with chronic suppressive treatment may be needed for immunocompromised patients. In some cases, antibiotic therapy may prolong excretion of the pathogen and may facilitate the development of resistance. Suggested treatment regimens are given in Figures 41.6 and 41.7.

FURTHER READING

Cheney CP, Wong RK. Acute infectious diarrhea. Med Clin North Am 1993;77:1169–96.

Dupont HL. Guidelines on acute infectious diarrhea in adults. Am J Gastroenterol 1997;92:1962–75.

Fekety R. Guidelines for the diagnosis and management of *Clostridium difficile*-associated diarrhea and colitis. Am J Gastroenterol 1997;92:739–50.

Goodgame RW. Understanding intestinal spore-forming protozoa: cryptosporidia, microsporidia, isospora, and cyclospora. Ann Intern Med 1996;124:429–41.

Park SI, Giannella RA. Approach to the adult patient with acute diarrhea. Gastroenterol Clin North Am 1993;22:483–97.

PARASITIC CAUSES OF DIARRHEA AND RECOMMENDED THERAPY	
Protozoa	Antimicrobial therapy
Blastocystis hominis	No therapy shown to be effective; consider metronidazole 750mg po for 10 days, trimethoprim–sulfamethoxazole
Cryptosporidium parvum	No effective therapy; consider paromomycin 500mg po q6h for 2 weeks, 500mg q12h for chronic suppression
Cyclospora cayentensis	Trimethoprim–sulfamethoxazole 160/800mg po q12h for 7 days, consider suppressive therapy in patients who have AIDS
Entamoeba histolytica	Metronidazole 750mg po q8h for 10 days or tinidazole 1g po q12h for 3 days with diloxanide furoate 500mg q8h for 10 days or paromomycin 500mg q8h for 10 days
Giardia lamblia	Metronidazole 250mg po q8h for 5 days or tinidazole 2g po for 1 dose
Isospora belli	Trimethoprim–sulfamethoxazole 160/800mg po q6h for 10 days then q12h for 3 weeks
Microsporidia	Albendazole 200–400mg po q12h for 1 month; chronic suppressive therapy in patients who have AIDS (metronidazole 500mg po q8h, or atovaquone 750mg po q8h)

Fig. 41.6 Parasitic causes of diarrhea and recommended therapy.

BACTERIAL PATHOGENS THAT CAUSE DIARRHEA AND RECOMMENDED THERAPY	
Bacterial pathogen or associated clinical condition	Antimicrobial agents, comments
Fever with dysentery with leukocytes or blood in stool	Empiric therapy with a quinolone for 3–5 days
Traveler's diarrhea	Empiric therapy if moderate to severe: quinolone for 3–5 days; trimethoprim–sulfamethoxazole 160/800mg for 3–5 days for suspected enterotoxigenic *Escherichia coli* infection
Aeromonas hydrophilia	Trimethoprim–sulfamethoxazole or a quinolone
Campylobacter jejuni	Ciprofloxacin 500mg po q12h or norfloxacin 400mg po q12h or erythromycin stearate 500mg po q12h for 5 days
Clostridium difficile	Metronidazole 250mg po q6h or vancomycin 125–250mg po q6h or bacitracin 25,000U po q6h
Enterohemorrhagic *Escherichia coli*	Antimicrobials not generally effective
Enteroinvasive *Escherichia coli*	No placebo-controlled therapeutic trials; trimethoprim–sulfamethoxazole or ciprofloxacin are used
Enteropathogenic *Escherichia coli*	Neomycin 25mg/kg per day po q6h or colistin 3.75mg/kg per day q6h or trimethoprim–sulfamethoxazole (effective in placebo-controlled trials) or oral gentamicin
Listeria monocytogenes	Ampicillin 200mg/kg iv q6h or trimethoprim–sulfamethoxazole 160/800mg po q8h for 7 days (in immunocompromised or pregnant patients)
Plesiomonas shigelloides	A quinolone or trimethoprim–sulfamethoxazole or tetracycline
Shigella spp.	Ciprofloxacin 500mg po q12h for 3 doses or trimethoprim–sulfamethoxazole 160/800mg (3 doses)
Salmonella spp.	No therapy in mild to moderate disease in the healthy host; in severe disease or in immunocompromised patients, trimethoprim–sulfamethoxazole or a quinolone for 3–7 days (10 days in immunocompromised patients)
Vibrio cholerae	Ciprofloxacin 1g po (single dose), norfloxacin 400mg po q12h for 3 days or tetracyline 500mg po q6h for 3 days or doxycycline 300mg po (single dose)
Vibrio parahaemolyticus	Tetracycline, quinolone (but antibiotic therapy has not been shown to shorten the course of the disease)
Yersinia enterocolitica	A quinolone or trimethoprim–sulfamethoxazole or doxycycline; ceftriaxone g iv q24h for 5 days for severe cases (efficacy not confirmed)

Fig. 41.7 Bacterial pathogens that cause diarrhea, associated clinical findings and recommended therapy.

Infective and Reactive Arthritis

Douglas R Osmon & James M Steckelberg

Infective arthritis is an inflammation of the joint space caused by invasion by one or more of a multitude of different micro-organisms. The incidence of infective arthritis in adults caused by bacteria other than *Neisseria gonorrhoeae* is relatively low, but these infections can cause major morbidity as a result of pain, immobility and loss of joint function. Successful treatment requires prompt drainage of the joint, using multiple arthrocenteses or open arthrotomy, and prolonged antimicrobial therapy to achieve sterilization of the joint space as well as a satisfactory functional result. This chapter discusses infective arthritis in adults, with the major emphasis on bacterial infective arthritis. Viral and reactive arthritis are discussed briefly. Infective arthritis caused by *Borrelia burgdorferi* is discussed in Chapter 2.45 and mycobacterial arthritis in Chapter 2.30.

BACTERIAL ARTHRITIS

EPIDEMIOLOGY

In 1993, according to the Centers for Disease Control and Prevention, there were an estimated 20,000 cases of pyogenic arthritis in the USA, or 7.8 cases per 100,000 person/years; 56% of the patients were male, and 45% were 65 years of age or older.[1] The mean duration of hospitalization of the 11,000 patients who had a primary diagnosis of pyogenic arthritis was 11.5 days. These data are in agreement with other published incidence rates of bacterial arthritis in the general population.[2,3] Disseminated gonococcal infection with associated gonococcal infective arthritis is the leading cause of hospital admission due to infective arthritis in the USA, with an estimated incidence rate of 2.8 per 100,000 person/years (Chapter 8.16).[4]

RISK FACTORS

Rheumatoid arthritis, diabetes mellitus, malignancy, old age and HIV infection alone or through their treatment suppress the immune system and, as such, are risk factors for acquiring bacterial arthritis.[5–8] Local abnormalities of host defenses caused by previous joint damage or surgery also predispose the joint to infection, as do situations that increase the risk of bacteremia, such as injection drug use, indwelling intravenous catheters and skin infection, and situations that allow direct inoculation of micro-organisms, such as intra-articular injection or arthroscopy.

Disseminated gonococcal infection is more common among sexually active, menstruating women, although it can also occur during pregnancy and the peripartum period.[4] The male:female ratio is approximately 1:4. Often the microbiologic etiology of infective arthritis can be predicted based on the specific risk factor predisposing to infection (Fig. 42.1).[9]

PATHOGENESIS

Nongonococcal bacterial arthritis most often results from hematogenous seeding of the joint space as a result of bacteremia. Synovial tissue has a rich vascular supply but no basement membrane, factors that favor ingress of blood-borne organisms.[8,9] The bacteremia can be primary or secondary to an infection elsewhere in the body (e.g. pneumonia,

cellulitis) or to injection drug use.[5] An identifiable focus of infection can be found in approximately 50% of cases.[8,10]

Direct inoculation of micro-organisms into the joint space because of trauma, arthrotomy, arthroscopy or diagnostic and therapeutic arthrocenteses is another mechanism of infection. The risk of septic arthritis after arthrocentesis has been reported to be 0.002–0.007%; after arthroscopy it is reported to be 0.04–0.4%.[11] Infection of the joint space as a result of contiguous soft tissue infection or periarticular osteomyelitis is much less common.

Once bacteria have entered the joint space there is ingress of polymorphonuclear leukocytes, which results in hydrolysis of proteoglycans and collagen through stimulation of locally synthesized cytokines and release of enzymes.[11] If left untreated, destruction of the articular cartilage eventually occurs, leading to irreversible joint damage.[12–14]

Staphylococcus aureus is the most common etiologic agent of infective arthritis in adults (see Fig. 42.2).[8,15–18] In young sexually active persons, *N. gonorrhoeae* is the predominant pathogen. Infection in patients who have rheumatoid arthritis is due to *S. aureus* in as many as 80% of patients. Group B streptococcal infection is more likely to occur in patients who have diabetes mellitus. Coagulase-negative staphylococci may cause infection following arthroscopy and other medical procedures, including intra-articular injections. Infective arthritis due to Gram-negative bacilli is more common in the elderly and in patients who have comorbid illnesses.[19]

EPIDEMIOLOGIC AND CLINICAL FEATURES ASSOCIATED WITH SPECIFIC ETIOLOGIC AGENTS OF INFECTIVE ARTHRITIS	
Clinical or epidemiologic setting	Likely etiologic agent
Rheumatoid arthritis	*Staphylococcus aureus*
Injection drug use	*Staphylococcus aureus*, *Pseudomonas aeruginosa*
After arthroscopy	*Staphylococcus aureus*, coagulase-negative staphylococci, Enterobacteriaceae, *Pseudomonas aeruginosa*
Menstruation, pregnancy, multiple skin lesions, age <30 years	*Neisseria gonorrhoeae*
More than 100 skin lesions	*Neisseria meningitidis*
Human bite	Usual oral flora (e.g. *Eikenella corrodens*)
Cat or dog bite	*Pasteurella multocida*, oral anaerobes from animal's oral flora
Rat bite	*Streptobacillus moniliformis*
Hypogammaglobulinemia	*Mycoplasma* spp.
Tick exposure	*Borrelia burgdorferi*
Trauma in aquatic environment	*Mycobacterium marinum*
Rose thorn injury or splinter injury acquired from moist soil	*Sporothrix schenckii*

Fig. 42.1 **Epidemiologic and clinical features associated with specific etiologic agents of infective arthritis.** Data from Smith and Piercy.[9]

ETIOLOGIC AGENTS OF NONGONOCOCCAL BACTERIAL ARTHRITIS IN ADULTS	
Micro-organisms	Cases (%)
Staphylococcus aureus	68
Streptococci (including β-hemolytic streptococci, viridans group streptococci and Streptococcus pneumoniae)	20
Haemophilus influenzae	1
Aerobic Gram-negative bacilli	10
Polymicrobial and miscellaneous	1
Unknown	<1

Fig. 42.2 Etiologic agents of nongonococcal bacterial arthritis in adults. Data from Roberts and Mock.[18]

COMPARISON OF CHARACTERISTICS OF GONOCOCCAL AND NONGONOCOCCAL BACTERIAL ARTHRITIS		
Characteristic	Gonococcal arthritis	Other bacterial arthritis
Patient profile	Young, healthy, sexually active, female	Elderly, immunocompromised host, rheumatoid or other systemic arthritis
Initial presentation	Migratory polyarthralgia, tenosynovitis, dermatitis	Hot, swollen painful joint
Polyarticular (% of cases)	40–70	10–20
Recovery of bacteria	<50% from synovial fluid, <10% from blood	>90% from synovial fluid, 50% from blood
Response to antibiotics	Within a few days	Takes weeks, and joint drainage must be adequate
Functional outcome	Excellent	Often poor

Fig. 42.3 Comparison of characteristics of gonococcal and nongonococcal bacterial arthritis. Data from Goldenberg.[8]

Anaerobic infection is uncommon except in the setting of septic arthritis occurring after human or animal bite injuries or diabetic foot infections. Among injection drug users, *Pseudomonas aeruginosa* and *S. aureus* are common pathogens.[20,21] Hypogammaglobulinemia is a risk factor for infective arthritis due to *Mycoplasma* spp.[22]

PREVENTION

Prevention of infective arthritis is obviously preferable to treatment of established infection. Examples of efforts to decrease the incidence of infective arthritis include the promotion of public health measures to prevent the acquisition of *N. gonorrhoeae*, measures to decrease the incidence of animal bites, prophylactic foot care in patients who have diabetes mellitus and eradication of injection drug use. Rapid and effective treatment of antecedent infections that may cause joint infections, such as catheter-associated bacteremia due to *S. aureus* or skin and soft tissue infection in patients who have rheumatoid arthritis and diabetes mellitus, as well as the administration of vaccines against *Haemophilus influenzae* and *Streptococcus pneumoniae*, are also effective preventive measures.[23]

CLINICAL FEATURES

NONGONOCOCCAL INFECTIVE ARTHRITIS

Nongonococcal infective arthritis is typically monoarticular and has an acute presentation. Patients complain of pain and limitation of motion in over 90% of cases.[9] In one study, fever was present in 78% of patients within 24 hours of hospitalization, although it was rarely above 102°F (39°C).[14] Chills were uncommon. Physical examination usually reveals a large effusion and a marked decrease in active and passive range of motion of the joint. However, these findings may be minimal or absent in those patients who have rheumatoid arthritis, and they may be difficult to discern in infections of the hip or shoulder.

The knee is the most commonly involved native joint in adults. In a recent case series from The Netherlands, the percentage of cases involving a particular joint was: knee 55%, ankle 10%, wrist 9%, shoulder 7%, hip 5%, elbow 5%, sternoclavicular joint 5%, sacroiliac joint 2% and foot joint 2%.[3] Sacroiliac or sternoclavicular joint infection is more common among injection drug users and may be difficult to diagnose. Polyarticular infection occurs in approximately 15% of patients and is often due to *S. aureus*.[24] Thus, a polyarticular presentation does not always imply the presence of gonococcal, viral, reactive or noninfectious arthritis. It is more common among patients with rheumatoid arthritis and patients who have other comorbid illnesses.

The case-fatality rate for patients with nongonococcal bacterial arthritis is estimated to be between 10 and 16%, and as many as 50% of patients who survive their infection will have some degree of permanent loss of joint function.[8,15–17] Morbidity and mortality is dependent on a number of factors, including age, presence of rheumatoid arthritis, infection in the hip or shoulder, duration of symptoms before treatment, the presence of polyarticular arthritis, persistently positive joint fluid cultures after appropriate therapy, the presence of bacteremia and the virulence of the infecting organism.[2,8,25,26]

GONOCOCCAL ARTHRITIS

Disseminated gonococcal infection presents with two distinct clinical entities.[4] Early after dissemination from mucosal surfaces such as the cervix or urethra the patient presents with bacteremia, fever, polyarthralgia, tenosynovitis (typically of the hands and fingers) and multiple maculopapular, pustular, vesicular or necrotic skin lesions (Fig. 42.3). Asymmetric joint involvement is common. The knee, elbow, wrist, metacarpalphalangeal and ankle joints are the most commonly involved joints. This presentation accounts for 60% of patients who present with disseminated gonococcal disease, and it has been described as the dermatitis–arthritis syndrome. If left untreated, the patient will present later with monoarticular arthritis, usually without tenosynovitis or skin lesions. Coinfection with HIV often leads to infection of unusual joints and an aggressive course.[27]

The outcome of disseminated gonococcal infection is almost always excellent (see Chapter 8.16).

DIAGNOSIS

Although the history and physical examination can lead to a high index of suspicion for infection, a synovial fluid culture that yields a causative micro-organism is the only definitive method for diagnosing bacterial arthritis. Fever and rigors in the setting of an inflammatory arthritis have a low positive predictive value for bacterial arthritis and have been reported in crystal-induced arthropathy.[11] The erythrocyte sedimentation rate (ESR), C-reactive protein and leukocyte counts are elevated in the majority of cases, although again the positive predictive value of these tests in the setting of a monoarticular inflammatory arthritis is low. A rise in the ESR may help in the differential diagnosis of new joint pain and effusion in those patients who have rheumatoid arthritis.[9,28] Blood cultures are positive in up to 70% of all patients, and more often than this in patients who have polyarticular involvement.[17,24]

In disseminated gonococcal infection the majority of patients have an elevated ESR, and only 50% will have an abnormal leukocyte count. Anemia and abnormal liver function tests also may occur but these findings are usually transient.[4]

In approximately 80% of patients who have disseminated gonococcal arthritis there is a positive culture or *N. gonorrhoeae* DNA can be identified by polymerase chain reaction or ligase chain reaction in samples from the cervix, urethra, rectum, pharynx or urine. Skin lesions yield *N. gonorrhoeae* in 30% of cases, and blood cultures in 5%.

The diagnostic procedure of choice for bacterial arthritis is an arthrocentesis. This should be done immediately once the the diagnosis of joint infection is suspected so as not to delay appropriate medical or surgical therapy. If synovial fluid cannot be obtained by blind needle aspiration (e.g. in the case hip joint infection), then aspiration should be done with the help of a radiologist. If necessary, an open arthrotomy should be performed to make a definitive diagnosis.

Synovial fluid is often cloudy or purulent in appearance. The synovial fluid should be routinely examined for uric acid and calcium pyrophosphate crystals, and a leukocyte count and differential should be obtained on each specimen. The leukocyte count is usually greater than 50,000/mm³ and often greater than 100,000/mm³, with more than 75% polymorphonuclear leukocytes. These findings can also be seen in patients who have inflammatory arthritis and crystal deposition arthritis. The sensitivity and specificity of a synovial fluid leukocyte count of >2×10⁹ for the presence of inflammatory arthritis have been estimated to be 84% and 84%.[29] For a differential count of >75% polymorphonuclear leukocytes the sensitivity and specificity are 75% and 92%. Although many clinicians order synovial fluid glucose and protein levels, the results of these tests have been shown to be less informative than the leukocyte count and differential.[29] The synovial fluid lactic acid and lactate dehydrogenase levels are often elevated in patients who have infective arthritis, but elevation of these tests can be seen in other inflammatory joint disorders as well.[8]

Synovial fluid should be cultured for both aerobes and anaerobes and other organisms, depending on the clinical circumstances. The synovial fluid culture will be positive in 90% of cases of nongonococcal arthritis assuming that antibiotic therapy has not been started before the sample has been collected.[14] The Gram stain is positive in 50% of patients.[8]

In patients who have disseminated gonococcal infection, the synovial fluid cultures are positive in 25–30% of all patients and 50% of patients who present with monoarticular arthritis. The role of the polymerase chain reaction in detecting bacterial pathogens in patients who have infective arthritis has not yet been defined, although the technique seems a promising tool for the detection of infectious arthritis due to *N. gonorrhoeae*. Polymerase chain reaction can help to distinguish disseminated gonococcal infection from other inflammatory arthropathies such as Reiter's syndrome.[30]

Synovial tissue cultures are indicated only for chronic infective arthritis when mycobacterial or fungal arthritis is suspected or when synovial fluid cultures cannot be obtained by less invasive techniques.

Periarticular soft tissue swelling is the most common abnormality seen on plain radiography in patients who have bacterial arthritis. Periarticular erosions and osteoporosis as well as joint space narrowing due to cartilage destruction do not occur for several weeks. Thus plain radiographs are not usually helpful in making a diagnosis of bacterial arthritis. Occasionally, in longstanding infection, periarticular osteomyelitis will be visible on plain radiograph (Fig. 42.4). It is often difficult to distinguish infection from inflammatory arthritis using radiographic methods in the setting of rheumatoid arthritis, but the development of a rapid destructive arthritis in one or two joints suggests infection. Computed tomography scans and MRI are more useful than plain radiographs for identifying concomitant periarticular osteomyelitis, soft tissue abscesses and joint effusions, but they are expensive and most often are not necessary (Fig. 42.5). Sacroiliac or sternoclavicular joint disease is optimally evaluated with these modalities as well as with radionuclide studies. ¹¹¹Indium scans may be useful for identifying relatively asymptomatic septic arthritis in immunocompromised patients who have one or more known septic joints in whom there is a high index of suspicion for polyarticular infection.

In adults, the differential diagnosis for patients with an acute onset of fever, chills and an inflammatory arthritis of one or more joints includes bacterial arthritis, gout, pseudogout, rheumatic fever, reactive arthritis and rheumatic illnesses such as rheumatoid arthritis and psoriatic arthritis. Gout and pseudogout are the most common noninfectious inflammatory arthritides that need to be differentiated from bacterial arthritis.[8] They should be suspected when there is a history of previous episodes or there is chondrocalcinosis on plain film. Synovial fluid analysis using polarized light microscopy is the most useful diagnostic test for gout or pseudogout.

The articular manifestations of rheumatic fever occur in approximately 75% of first episodes, last for several weeks and do not cause permanent joint damage. Typically there is development of a migratory polyarthritis involving the knees, elbows, ankles and wrists that occurs within 1–5 weeks of the antecedent streptococcal pharyngitis. Joint symptoms can range from arthralgia without obvious physical findings to inflammatory arthritis that is indistinguishable from infective polyarthritis.

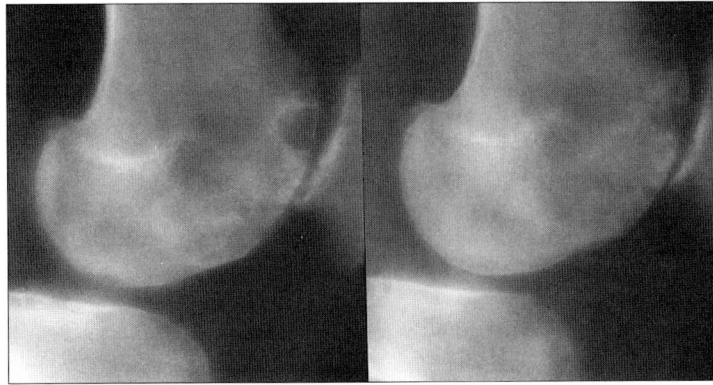

Fig. 42.4 Tomogram of right knee of a patient who has *Staphylococcus aureus* septic arthritis and periarticular osteomyelitis. Note the mixed sclerosis and lytic changes suggestive of osteomyelitis.

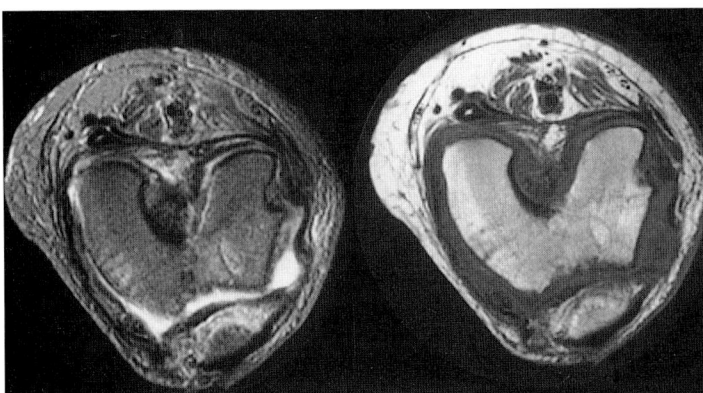

Fig. 42.5 MRI scan of right knee of a patient who has *Staphylococcus aureus* septic arthritis. Note the soft tissue inflammation and a joint effusion.

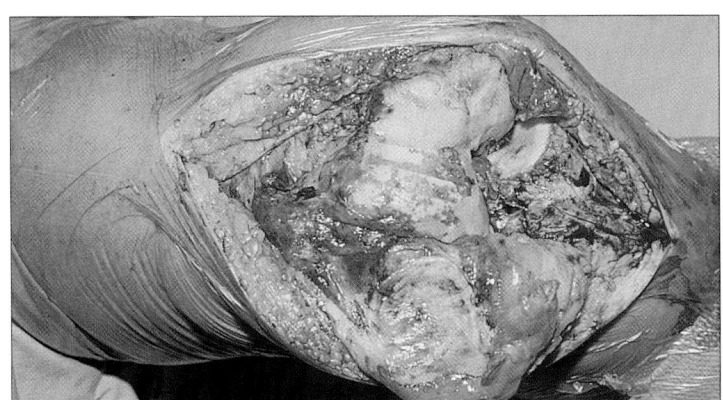

Fig. 42.6 Intraoperative photograph of right knee of a patient who has *Staphylococcus aureus* septic arthritis. Note the damaged joint and dark brown, boggy and hyperemic synovium.

ANTIBIOTIC THERAPY OF INFECTIVE ARTHRITIS IN ADULTS FOR SELECTED MICRO-ORGANISMS		
Micro-organisms	Antibiotic therapy	Alternative therapy
Staphylococcus aureus Methicillin-sensitive strains	Nafcillin or oxacillin 1.5–2.0g iv q4h *or* Cefazolin (or other first-generation cephalosporins in equivalent dosages) 1g iv q8h	Vancomycin 15mg/kg iv q12h, not to exceed 2g in 24h unless serum levels are monitored
Methicillin-resistant strains	Vancomycin 15mg/kg iv q12h, not to exceed 2g in 24h unless serum levels are monitored	Consult a specialist in infectious diseases
Penicillin-sensitive streptococci or pneumococci with an MIC≤0.1µg/ml	Aqueous crystalline penicillin G 20×10⁶U per 24 hours iv either continuously or in six equally divided doses *or* Ceftriaxone 2g iv or im q24h *or* Cefazolin 1g iv q8h	Vancomycin 15mg/kg iv q12h, not to exceed 2g in 24h unless serum levels are monitored
Enterococci or streptococci with an MIC ≥0.5µg/ml or nutritionally variant streptococci (all enterococci causing infection must be tested for antimicrobial susceptibility in order to select optimal therapy)	Aqueous crystalline penicillin G, 20×10⁶U per 24h iv either continuously or in six equally divided doses, plus gentamicin sulfate, 1mg/kg iv or im q8h *or* Ampicillin sodium 12g per 24h iv either continuously or in six equally divided doses	Vancomycin 15mg/kg iv q12h, not to exceed 2g in 24h unless serum levels are monitored
Neisseria gonorrhoeae	Ceftriaxone 1g im or iv q24h for 24–48h after clinical improvement followed by Cefixime 400mg po q12h for 1 week *or* Ciprofloxacin 500mg po q12h for 1 week *or* Ofloxacin 400mg po q12h for 1 week	Ciprofloxacin 400mg iv q12h for 24–48h after clinical improvement *or* Ofloxacin 400mg iv q12h for 24–48h after clinical improvement *or* Spectinomycin 2g im q12h for 24–48h after clinical improvement *followed by* Ciprofloxacin 500mg po q12h for 1 week *or* Ofloxacin 400mg po q12h for 1 week
Enterobacteriaceae *Pseudomonas aeruginosa, Enterobacter* spp.	Ceftriaxone 2g iv q24h *or* Ciprofloxacin 750mg po q12h (based on in-vitro susceptibility)	Levofloxacin 500mg po q12h

Fig. 42.7 Antibiotic therapy of infective arthritis in adults for selected bacterial micro-organisms.
Dosages recommended are for patients who have normal renal function.

Often more than six joints are affected. The diagnosis of rheumatic fever is dependent on satisfying the updated Jones criteria (see Chapter 8.14).[31]

Bacterial arthritis should be suspected in those patients at increased risk of infection. Fungal and mycobacterial infection is usually monoarticular but their presentation is usually over weeks to months instead of hours to days. Diseases that must be distinguished from disseminated gonococcal infection include viral and reactive arthritis, rheumatic fever and secondary syphilis.

MANAGEMENT

The keys to the management of infective arthritis are:
- drainage of the purulent synovial fluid,
- debridement of any concomitant periarticular osteomyelitis, and
- administration of appropriate parenteral antimicrobial therapy.

Experimental models of septic arthritis suggest that early drainage and antimicrobial therapy prevent cartilage destruction.[32] Local antimicrobial therapy is unnecessary and may cause a chemical synovitis.[8] Joint immobilization and elevation is useful for symptomatic relief of pain early in the course of the disease, but early active range of motion exercises are beneficial for ultimate functional outcome.

SYNOVIAL FLUID DRAINAGE

The optimal method of drainage of an infected joint remains controversial, in part because no well-controlled randomized trials exist to guide therapy and because the therapy of each patient should be individualized.[33] Most adults who have septic arthritis have been managed with repeated joint aspirations instead of surgical debridement.[14]

Patients who have disseminated gonococcal infection rarely require repeat joint aspirations, arthroscopy or arthrotomy.[4]

The use of arthroscopy has expanded in recent years because of the minimal morbidity of the procedure and the improved ability of athroscopy to adequately drain purulent material from the joint compared with joint aspiration.[34–39] Large multicenter, randomized trials are needed to evaluate the comparative efficacy of these modalities.

DEBRIDEMENT

Recommended indications for surgical debridement have included effusions that fail to resolve with 7 days of conservative therapy and inability to adequately drain the infected joint by aspiration or arthroscopy either because of location (hip and shoulder) or loculations of pus[8,9] (see Fig. 42.6).

ANTIMICROBIAL THERAPY

There are no randomized studies to help guide the clinician in the antimicrobial therapy of septic arthritis. Initial antimicrobial therapy should be based on the results of the Gram stain and the specific clinical and epidemiologic setting. If no micro-organisms are seen on the Gram-stain, then empiric therapy for *S. aureus*, streptococci and gonococci (in young sexually active adults) should be given. Most experts administer 2–4 weeks of intravenous antimicrobial therapy for the treatment of septic arthritis.[8,9] In most cases this therapy can be administered on an outpatient basis after an initial period of hospitalization.

Suggested antimicrobials for specific pathogens causing infective arthritis are shown in Figure 42.7.

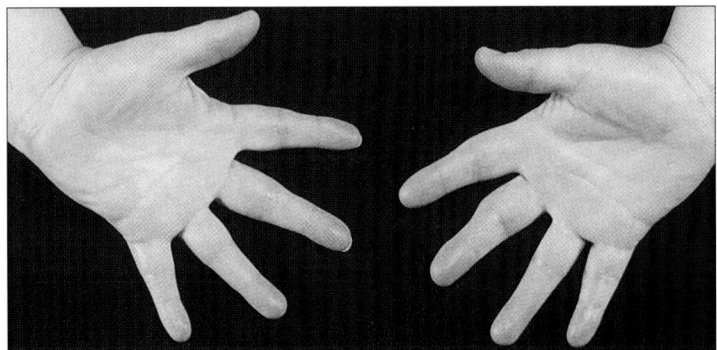

Fig. 42.8 Polyarticular arthritis due to parvovirus B19. Note the inflammation of the small joints of both hands. Courtesy of KD Moder.

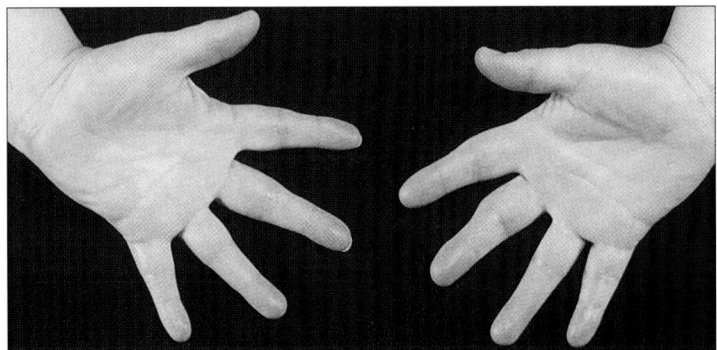

Oral antimicrobial therapy with an effective agent with excellent bioavailability, such as ciprofloxacin or trimethoprim–sulfamethoxazole (cotrimoxazole), is also acceptable, particularly if the patient has rapidly improved on intravenous therapy.

Current treatment guidelines for gonococcal septic arthritis recommend ceftriaxone as the initial drug of choice, followed by oral therapy with a cephalosporin or a quinolone after initial clinical improvement (Fig. 42.7).

VIRAL ARTHRITIS

Arthritis is a common complication of infections with hepatitis B virus, parvovirus B19, rubella and alphaviruses, and is relatively rare with mumps virus, enteroviruses, adenoviruses and herpesviruses. The most common mechanism by which viruses cause arthritis is by invasion of the joint during the period of viremia. Other postulated mechanisms include immune complex deposition, insertion of the viral genome into the host DNA thus promoting autoimmunity through an 'altered self' and direct viral infection of the immune system thus altering the immune response.[40–43]

Typically, viral arthritis occurs during the prodromal stages of viral infection and is associated with a rash. Polyarticular involvement, including the small joints of the hands is typical (Fig. 42.8). There is no specific pattern of joint involvement that is unique to a given viral etiology. Diagnosis is based on historic and clinical clues (Fig. 42.9) and diagnostic testing specific for each individual virus, the details of which are discussed in the relevant chapters. Viral arthritis is usually self-limiting but may progress to a chronic arthropathy in certain instances. It is important that viral arthritis should be distinguished from rheumatic fever and the initial presentation of autoimmune disorders, including rheumatoid arthritis (see Chapters 8.2, 8.4, 8.10 & 8.11).

Treatment is discussed in the chapters devoted to specific viruses. Prevention of viral arthritis is dependent on vaccination against the specific pathogen causing arthritis (e.g. mumps virus, rubella, hepatitis A virus, hepatitis B virus and varicella-zoster virus).

REACTIVE ARTHRITIS

Reactive arthritis describes the acute onset of an inflammatory arthritis soon after an infection elsewhere in the body in which micro-organisms cannot be cultured from the synovial fluid. However, genetic material may be found in the joint using molecular diagnostic techniques. Reiter's syndrome (the classic triad of arthritis, urethritis and conjunctivitis) is a common example of reactive arthritis. Many patients who develop reactive arthritis are HLA-B27-positive. The micro-organisms that have been associated with reactive arthritis are detailed in Figure 42.10.[44]

CLINICAL OR EPIDEMIOLOGIC FEATURES OF INFECTIVE ARTHRITIS CAUSED BY SELECTED VIRUSES

Viral agent	Characteristics of patients or country of origin
Rubella (including rubella vaccine)	Adult females with tenosynovitis. Additive symmetric arthritis, usually involving the metacarpal and proximal phalangeal joints; may precede, coincide with or follow rash; generally lasts a few weeks but occasionally persists longer or recurs
Parvovirus B19	Adult females with erythema infectiosum. Severe polyarticular arthritis of sudden onset; occurs in 60% of adult patients; rare in children; usually temporary but may persist for years
Mumps	Adult males. Involvement of large joints 1–2 weeks after parotid gland swelling; rare in children; usually lasts about 2 weeks
Hepatitis A virus	Arthralgia and rash during acute phase in 10–14% of cases
Hepatitis B virus	Severe arthritis of sudden onset, usually symmetric and polyarticular; morning stiffness is considerable; occurs in 20–25% of cases; typically resolves during the preicteric phase. Arthritis may persist with chronic hepatitis B virus infection
Hepatitis C virus	Acute arthralgia and myalgia of sudden onset rapidly progressing to arthritis; joint pain often disproportionate to physical findings; few inflammatory signs
HIV	Arthralgia, painful monoarticular or oligoarticular syndrome, which may mimic gout, HIV arthropathy
Human T-lymphocyte leukemia virus 1	Chronic oligoarticular arthritis involving large and small joints
Enteroviruses, adenoviruses	Joint involvement accompanying upper respiratory tract infection or gastroenteritis in some cases of coxsackie virus and adenovirus infection
Varicella-zoster virus	Arthritis similar to that occurring with mumps; associated bacterial arthritis may develop if organisms spread from an infected skin lesion
Lymphocytic choriomeningitis virus	Adults who have aseptic meningitis
Arthropod-borne alpha-virus infection	
Chikungunya	East Africa, India, South East Asia, Philippines
O'nyong-nyong	East Africa
Ockelbo agent	Sweden
Ross River agent	Australia, New Zealand
Barmah Forest virus	Australia

Fig. 42.9 Clinical or epidemiologic features of infective arthritis caused by selected viruses. Data from Smith and Piercy,[9] Siegel and Gall.[40]

Typically, reactive arthritis begins several weeks after an antecedent infection. The initial clinical presentation is usually an asymmetric oligoarticular arthritis without prominent constitutional symptoms. The syndrome also occurs without any identifiable symptom of infections, however, particularly in the case of *Chlamydia trachomatis*. In the case of Reiter's syndrome, extra-articular manifestations are also present.

Laboratory abnormalities are nonspecific and include mild elevations in the leukocyte count, ESR and C-reactive protein. Radiographs usually show only soft tissue swelling in early disease, but juxta-articular osteoporosis and erosion may also be seen.

Reactive arthritis is normally a self-limited disease, but chronic arthritis and sacroiliitis can occur in up to 15–30% of patients. Treatment is with anti-inflammatory agents. The role of antibacterial therapy is controversial although it may be effective for acute reactive arthritis, particularly if it is due to *Chlamydia* spp.[45] Prevention of infection is reliant on effective prevention and treatment of precipitating antecedent infections.

MICRO-ORGANISMS ASSOCIATED WITH REACTIVE ARTHRITIS					
Definite association			Possible association		
Genitourinary tract	Gut	Genitourinary tract	Gut	Other	
Chlamydia trachomatis	Shigella flexneri	Neisseria gonorrhoeae	Enteropathogenic Escherichia coli	Borrelia burgdorferi	
	Salmonella enteritidis	Ureaplasma urealyticum	Cryptosporidia	Streptococci spp.	
	Salmonella typhimurium	Gardernella vaginalis	Entamoeba histolytica	Mycobacterium tuberculosis	
	Yersinia enterocolitica		Giardia lambia	Blastocystis hominis	
	Yersinia pseudotuberculosis		Clostridium difficile	Chlamydia psittaci	
	Campylobacter jejuni		Shigella sonnei	Brucella abortus	
			Strongyloides stercoralis	Chlamydia pneumoniae	
			Taenia saginata	Staphylococcus aureus	
			Helicobacter cinaedi	Coagulase-negative staphylococci	
			Hafnia alvei		
			Campylobacter lari		
			Plesiomonas shigelloides		
			Leptospira icterohaemorrhagica		

Fig. 42.10 Micro-organisms associated with reactive arthritis. Data from Hughes and Keat.[44]

REFERENCES

1. Graves E. Detailed diagnoses and procedures, national hospital discharge survey. Vital Health Stat [13] 1993;122:61–113.
2. Cooper C, Cawley MI. Bacterial arthritis in an English health district: a 10 year review. Ann Rheum Dis 1986;45:458–63.
3. Kaandorp CJ, Dinant HJ, van de Laar MA, Moens HJ, Prins AP, Dijkmans BA. Incidence and sources of native and prosthetic joint infection: a community based prospective survey. Ann Rheum Dis 1997;56:470–5.
4. Cucurull E, Espinnoza LR. Gonnococcal arthritis. Rheum Dis Clin North Am 1998;24:305–322.
5. Esterhai JL, Jr., Gelb I. Adult septic arthritis. Orthop Clin North Am 1991;22:503–14.
6. Kaandorp CJ, Van Schaardenburg D, Krijnen P, Habbema JD, van de Laar MA. Risk factors for septic arthritis in patients with joint disease. A prospective study. Arthritis Rheum 1995;38:1819–25.
7. Saraux A, Taelman H, Blanche P, et al. HIV infection as a risk factor for septic arthritis. Br J Rheumatol 1997;36:333–7.
8. Goldenberg DL. Septic arthritis. Lancet 1998;351:197–202.
9. Smith JW, Piercy EA. Infectious arthritis. Clin Infect Dis 1995;20:225–30.
10. Cunningham R, Cockayne A, Humphreys H. Clinical and molecular aspects of the pathogenesis of Staphylococcus aureus bone and joint infections. J Med Microbiol 1996;44:157–64.
11. Pioro MH, Mandell BF. Septic arthritis. Rheum Dis Clin North Am 1997;23:239–58.
12. Gauger M, Mohr W. Cartilage destruction in septic arthritis – electron microscopy and historical considerations. Z Rheumatol 1995;54:241–9.
13. Subimal R, Bhawan J. Ultrastructure of articular cartilage in pyogenic arthritis. Arch Pathol 1975;99:44–7.
14. Goldenberg DL, Reed JI. Bacterial arthritis. N Engl J Med 1985;312:764–71.
15. Morgan DS, Fisher D, Merianos A, Currie BJ. An 18 year clinical review of septic arthritis from tropical Australia. Epidemiol Infect 1996;117:423–8.
16. Le Dantec L, Maury F, Flipo RM, et al. Peripheral pyogenic arthritis. A study of one hundred seventy-nine cases. Rev Rheum 1996;63:103–10.
17. Ryan MJ, Kavanagh R, Wall PG, Hazleman BL. Bacterial joint infections in England and Wales: analysis of bacterial isolates over a four year period. Br J Rheumatol 1997;36:370–3.
18. Roberts NJ, Mock DJ. Joint infections. In: Reese RE, Betts RF, eds. A practical approach to infectious diseases. Boston, Massachusetts: Little, Brown and Company; 1996:578–605.
19. McGuire NM, Kauffman CA. Septic arthritis in the elderly. J Am Geriatr Soc 1985;33:170–4.
20. Roca RP, Yoshikawa TT. Primary skeletal infections in heroin users: a clinical characterization, diagnosis and therapy. Clin Orthop 1979;144:238–48.
21. Gifford DB, Patzakis M, Ivler D, Swezey RL. Septic arthritis due to pseudomonas in heroin addicts. J Bone Joint Surg [Am] 1975;57:631–5.
22. Furr PM, Taylor-Robinson D, Webster AD. Mycoplasmas and ureaplasmas in patients with hypogammaglobulinaemia and their role in arthritis: microbiological observations over twenty years. Ann Rheum Dis 1994;53:183–7.
23. Peltola H, Kallio MJ, Unkila-Kallio L. Reduced incidence of septic arthritis in children by Haemophilus influenzae type-b vaccination. Implications for treatment. J Bone Joint Surg [Br] 1998;80:471–3.
24. Dubost JJ, Fis I, Denis P, et al. Polyarticular septic arthritis. Medicine 1993;72:296–310.
25. Kaandorp CJ, Krijnen P, Moens HJ, Habbema JD, van Schaardenburg D. The outcome of bacterial arthritis: a prospective community-based study. Arthritis Rheum 1997;40:884–92.
26. Yu LP, Bradley JD, Hugenberg ST, Brandt KD. Predictors of mortality in non-post-operative patients with septic arthritis. Scand J Rheumatol 1992;21:142–4.
27. Anaya JM, Joseph J, Scopelitis E, Espinoza LR. Disseminated gonococcal infection and human immunodeficiency virus. Clin Exp Rheumatol 1994;12:688.
28. Gardner GC, Weisman MH. Pyarthrosis in patients with rheumatoid arthritis: a report of 13 cases and a review of the literature from the past 40 years. Am J Med 1990;88:503–11.
29. Shmerling RH, Delbanco TL, Tosteson AN, Trentham DE. Synovial fluid tests. What should be ordered? JAMA 1990;264:1009–14.
30. Liebling MR, Arkfeld DG, Michelini GA, et al. Identification of Neisseria gonorrhoeae in synovial fluid using the polymerase chain reaction. Arthritis Rheum 1994;37:702–9.
31. Dajani A, Ayoub E, Bierman F, al el. Guidelines for the diagnosis of rheumatic fever: Jones criteria, updated 1992. Circulation 1993;87:302–7.
32. Riegels-Nielsen P, Frimodt-Moller N, Sorensen M, Jensen JS. Synovectomy for septic arthritis. Early versus late synovectomy studied in the rabbit knee. Acta Orthop Scand 1991;62:315–8.
33. Broy SB, Schmid FR. A comparison of medical drainage (needle aspiration) and surgical drainage (arthrotomy or arthroscopy) in the initial treatment of infected joints. Clin Rheum Dis 1986;12:501–22.
34. Jarrett MP, Grossman L, Sadler AH, Grayzel AI. The role of arthroscopy in the treatment of septic arthritis. Arthritis Rheum 1981;24:737–9.
35. Jackson RW. The septic knee – arthroscopic treatment. Arthroscopy 1985;1:194–7.
36. Ivey M, Clark R. Arthroscopic debridement of the knee for septic arthritis. Clin Orthop 1985;199:201–6.
37. Broy SB, Stulberg SD, Schmid FR. The role of arthroscopy in the diagnosis and management of the septic joint. Clin Rheum Dis 1986;12:489–500.
38. Smith MJ. Arthroscopic treatment of the septic knee. Arthroscopy 1986;2:30–4.
39. Thiery JA. Arthroscopic drainage in septic arthritides of the knee: a multicenter study. Arthroscopy 1989;5:65–9.
40. Siegel LB, Gall EP. Viral infection as a cause of arthritis. Am Fam Physician 1996;54:2009–15.
41. Phillips PE. Viral arthritis. Curr Opin Rheumatol 1997;9:337–44.
42. Schnitzer TJ, Penmetcha M. Viral arthritis. Curr Opin Rheumatol 1996;8:341–5.
43. Naides SJ. Viral infection including HIV and AIDS. Curr Opin Rheumatol 1994;6:423–8.
44. Hughes RA, Keat AC. Reiter's syndrome and reactive arthritis: a current view. Semin Arthritis Rheum 1994;24:190–210.
45. Lauhio A, Konttinen YT, Salo T, et al. Placebo-controlled study of the effects of three-month lymecycline treatment on serum matrix metalloproteinases in reactive arthritis. Ann N Y Acad Sci 1994;732:424–6.

chapter
43

Acute and Chronic Osteomyelitis

Carl W Norden

EPIDEMIOLOGY

The character of osteomyelitis changed with the advent of antibiotics, evolving from a disease of high mortality to a disease with high morbidity. Certain trends are apparent. Bone and joint tuberculosis has become less common in the developed world, although the advent of HIV-related disease may bring about a reversal in that trend. An increasing number of chronic bone infections are now associated with trauma, surgery and joint replacement rather than being secondary to hematogenous spread. Nosocomial osteomyelitis is no longer rare.

The epidemiology of acute hematogenous osteomyelitis has been detailed.[2] The incidence is higher in males and it varies among geographic areas (Fig. 43.1). The male-to-female ratio increases with age from 1.25 in the 0–4-year age group to 3.69 in the 13–19-year age group. There is also a seasonal trend, with peaks in the late summer in New Zealand and Australia, and peaks in October in Scotland and Canada. There are also racial differences in incidence, with substantially higher rates in Maori children from New Zealand and Aboriginal children from Western Australia compared both with European children and with white children living in New Zealand and Australia. These differences are probably socioeconomic in origin, but biologic and hereditary factors cannot be excluded.

The demographics and economic consequences of foot infections (frequently osteomyelitis) in elderly diabetic patients are well documented.[2] There are an estimated 11 million people in the USA with either known or undiagnosed diabetes; from 1979 to 1981, 53% of diabetic people were aged 60 years or older compared with only 25% of the general population. The most dramatic statistic is that 25% of people with diabetes will have a foot problem at one time or another and that 1 in 15 will require limb amputation. Foot problems have been estimated to be responsible for 15% of hospital admissions of diabetic patients and to account for about one-quarter of all hospital days. The annual hospital costs for limb amputations that are related to diabetes amount to more than US$350 million.

PATHOGENESIS AND PATHOLOGY

MICROBIAL FACTORS

Adhesion is the initial event in the localization of infection.[3] The initial loose adhesion to bone is potentially reversible. However, if the solid phase offers a configuration that is acceptable to the receptors of the micro-organisms, a more permanent adhesion occurs. *Staphylococcus aureus* strains possess receptors for collagen, fibrinogen, fibronectin, bone sialoprotein and heparin sulfate.[4,5] It is possible that trauma or injury may expose binding sites for strains of *S. aureus*. Following adhesion, firm attachment occurs. For *S. aureus*, the polysaccharide pseudocapsule forms strong links between the bacterial cell and bone. The synthesis of capsular polysaccharide (glycocalyx) produces a 'biofilm' within which bacteria can form microcolonies that are connected to the surrounding environment and to each other by this matrix of glycocalyx material (Figs 43.2 & 43.3). The glycocalyx may act to protect the organisms from host defense mechanisms and also from antibiotics.[6] Glycocalyx may serve a protective function for bacteria by interfering with phagocytosis, by covering the teichoic acid moiety which enhances opsonization, and by consuming or covering and altering the configuration of complement.

Prostaglandins are potent bone resorption agents that enhance osteoclast activity and collagen synthesis. It was noted in studies of human bone, as well as in studies of experimental osteomyelitis in animals, that increased production of prostaglandin E2 (the most potent prostenoid in the resorption of bone) was present.[7]

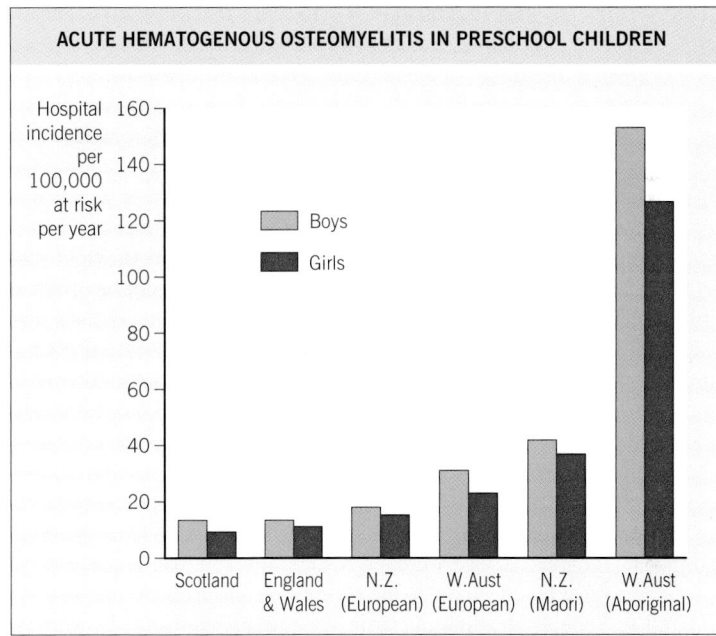

ACUTE HEMATOGENOUS OSTEOMYELITIS IN PRESCHOOL CHILDREN

Hospital incidence per 100,000 at risk per year

Boys
Girls

Scotland | England & Wales | N.Z. (European) | W.Aust (European) | N.Z. (Maori) | W.Aust (Aboriginal)

Fig. 43.1 Acute hematogenous osteomyelitis in preschool children. Data from Gillespie.[1]

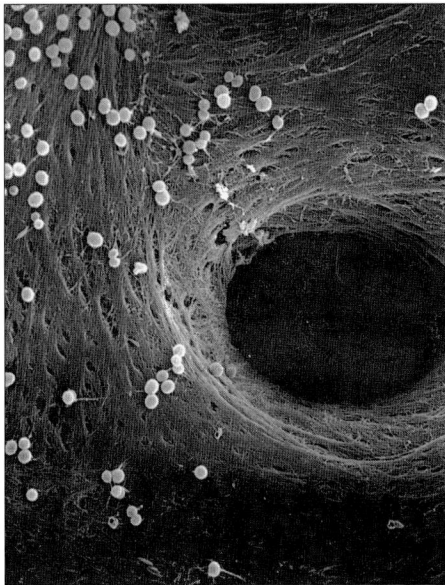

Fig. 43.2 Endosteum of bone showing staphylococci near the endosteal haversian canal. In-vitro incubation of bone chips with *Staphylococcus aureus* interrupted at 48 hours. (Scanning electromicrograph). From Norden CW, Gillespie WJ, Nade S. Infections in bones and joints. Blackwell Scientific Publications; 1994, with permission.

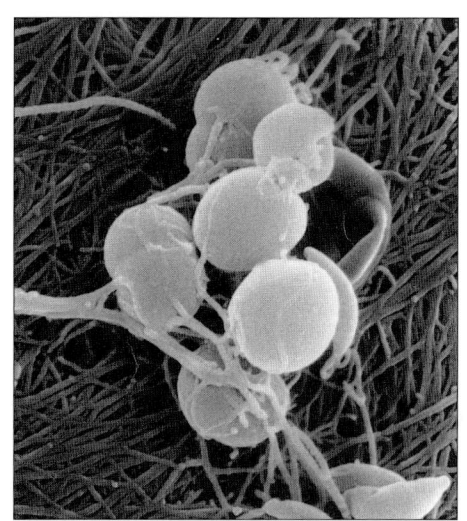

Fig. 43.3 Staphylococci enmeshed in glycocalyx near the haversian osteum. In-vitro incubation of bone chips with *Staphylococcus aureus* interrupted at 48 hours. (Scanning electromicrograph). From Norden CW, Gillespie WJ, Nade S. Infections in bones and joints. Blackwell Scientific Publications; 1994, with permission.

ANATOMIC CLASSIFICATION OF OSTEOMYELITIS IN ADULT LONG BONES

Stage 1 (medullary osteomyelitis)

Necrosis limited to medullary contents and endosteal surfaces
Etiology: hematogenous
Treatment: early: antibiotics, host alteration
late: unroofing; intramedullary reaming

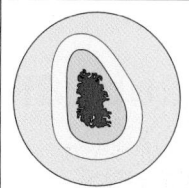

Stage 2 (superficial osteomyelitis)

Necrosis limited to exposed surfaces
Etiology: contiguous soft tissue infection
Treatment: early: antibiotics, host alteration
late: superficial debridement, coverage; possible ablation

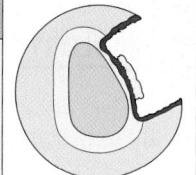

Stage 3 (localized osteomyelitis)

Well marginated and stable before and after debridement
Etiology: trauma; evolving stages 1 and 2; iatrogenic
Treatment: antibiotics, host alteration; debridement, dead space management; temporary stabilization, bone graft optional

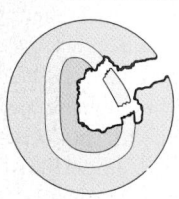

Stage 4 (diffuse osteomyelitis)

Circumferential and/or permeative; unstable before and after debridement
Etiology: trauma; evolving stages 1 and 2 and 3; iatrogenic
Treatment: antibiotics, host alteration; stabilization (open reduction and internal fixation), external fixation (Ilizarov); debridement, dead space management; possible ablation

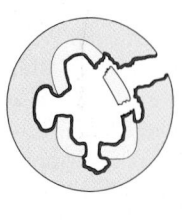

Fig. 43.4 Anatomic classification of osteomyelitis in adult long bones. Adapted with permission from Mader and Calhoun, 1995.[11]

The role of cytokines is just beginning to be understood. A careful study of patients with acute post-traumatic osteomyelitis demonstrated significantly higher levels of interleukin (IL)-8, IL-6, tumor necrosis factor-α, IL-1β, and leukotriene B_4 in acute osteomyelitis than in either controls or patients with chronic osteomyelitis.[8] Those cytokines that were significantly increased are derived from macrophages or leukocytes, whereas arachidonic acid products such as thromboxane B_2 and 6-keto-prostaglandin-F1α were not significantly increased.

PATHOLOGY

As in most organs, an insult to bone is followed by vascular and cellular responses. However, in bone this process is modified by the rigid wall of bone cortex because the increased tissue pressure cannot be diffused into soft tissue. With increased intramedullary pressure, sinuses and capillaries are compressed in the marrow, producing infarction. At the infarction edge, there is reactive hyperemia, which is associated with increased osteoclastic activity. This in turn produces loss of bone and localized osteoporosis. An inflammatory process begins at the margin of the infarcted area and penetrates through the cortex into the subperiosteal area. Because there are few anchoring fibers in the periosteum of infants and children, the periosteum is readily stripped from the bone surface by the increased periosteal pressure. This can result in disruption of the periosteal blood supply to the cortex, and this leads to cortical bone infarction, bone death and sequestrum formation. Sequestrum formation is usually followed by a rim of reactive new bone (the involucrum), formed by the periosteum around the sequestrum.[9]

CLASSIFICATION SYSTEMS FOR OSTEOMYELITIS

The most frequently used classification system is that of Waldvogel *et al*.[10] In this classification, infections are classified as either hematogenous or secondary to a contiguous focus of infection. A second classification system, developed by Mader and Calhoun,[11] combines four stages of anatomic disease and three categories of physiologic host (Fig. 43.4). This classification may be useful in terms of approaches to treatment and is amenable to study. The host categories include the following: A, normal except for osteomyelitis; B, systemic or local compromise; and C, treatment would be worse than the disease.

CAUSATIVE AGENTS OF OSTEOMYELITIS

In acute hematogenous osteomyelitis in children, *S.aureus* accounts for more than half of the organisms isolated.[12] The next most frequent group of isolates are streptococci. In puncture wounds to the foot, *Pseudomonas aeruginosa* is isolated frequently and is associated with the wearing of sneakers. The organism is found in the sole of the sneaker and is presumably carried into the foot by the puncturing nail.[13] *Salmonella* spp., although an infrequent overall cause, are more common in patients with sickle cell disease. In diabetic patients with foot infections, *S. aureus*, *Staphylococcus epidermidis*, enterococci, other streptococci and *Corynebacterium* spp. are among the most frequent aerobic organisms that are isolated. Anaerobic organisms are also frequently isolated, with *Peptostreptococcus* spp. being most common. In one recent series, it was reported that diabetic patients with methicillin-resistant coagulase-negative staphylococcal osteomyelitis frequently had a prior history of treatment with ciprofloxacin.[14] Fungi, mycoplasma, mycobacteria, brucella, treponema, and parasites have also been associated with osteomyelitis.

PREVENTION

There is no known effective method of preventing the development of acute hematogenous osteomyelitis. There is also no proven effective means of preventing the development of chronic osteomyelitis secondary to bacterial seeding from an infected focus, such as an intravenous catheter. In such instances, removal of the catheter and treatment for up to 6 weeks with an antimicrobial agent effective against the organism producing the bacteremia has not uniformly prevented the development of osteomyelitis at a remote site.[15]

Antibiotic prophylaxis has been used successfully to prevent wound infections following surgery for noncompound hip fractures, and it has also been used successfully in the placement of total hip and knee prostheses.[16] The end point of these studies has been wound infections, but it is reasonable to presume that a certain number of patients who develop wound infections could go on to develop infection of the underlying bone, and therefore antibiotic prophylaxis may play some role in preventing osteomyelitis. Finally, it should be stressed that meticulous surgical technique is of major importance in preventing wound infections and subsequent complications.

CLINICAL FEATURES

ACUTE HEMATOGENOUS OSTEOMYELITIS

An early sign in children, particularly infants, is failure to move the affected extremity and pain on passive movement. These findings in an infant with an acute febrile illness should lead to suspicion of skeletal infection. Soft tissue changes of swelling, redness and heat occur late in osteomyelitis; if found early in the course of illness, one should suspect cellulitis. In older children, the diagnosis is often easier, but it may be difficult to distinguish between bone and joint infection. Most radiographs do not show evidence of infection until at least 10–14 days after the onset, but they may show soft tissue changes.

In a large series,[12] about 3% of children developed chronic infection as a complication. However, most of these represented failure to treat adequately with antibiotics or significant delays in treatment. Pathologic fractures are rare. If infection involves the growth plate, the risk of one limb becoming shorter than the other is a possibility. In general, the outcome of acute osteomyelitis in pediatric patients is good, as long as patients are seen within 7–10 days of the onset of illness and treatment is begun and continued for at least 3 weeks.

CHRONIC OSTEOMYELITIS IN LONG BONES

Chronic osteomyelitis in long bones usually occurs as a result of trauma, or less frequently as a complication of acute hematogenous osteomyelitis. Patients usually have few systemic symptoms but are commonly troubled by persistent pain and drainage through sinus tracts. The fundamental problem is the prolonged persistence of viable pathogens. The process involves the consequences of continuing necrosis, such as sequestrum and sinus formation, versus repair with new bone formation and scar (Figs 43.5 & 43.6).

Potential complications of chronic osteomyelitis include secondary amyloidosis, which is a relatively rare occurrence (one series reported an incidence of about 1%).[17] A second complication, long recognized, is the development of squamous cell carcinoma in scar tissue. Again, the incidence is low (probably less than 1%) and those cases that have been reported occurred after an average of 27 years of osteomyelitis

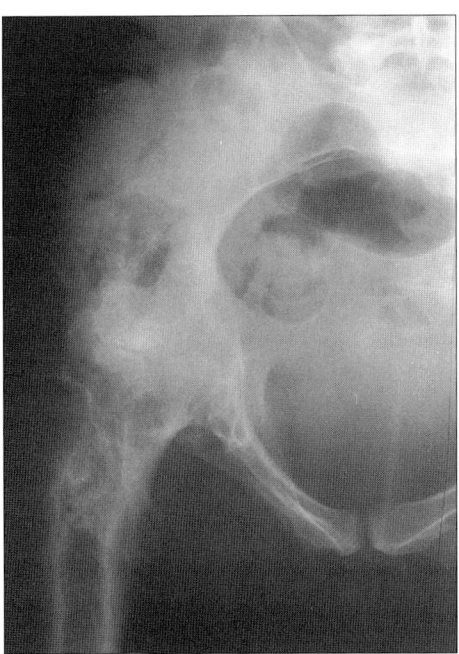

Fig. 43.5 Chronic osteomyelitis. The patient is a 30-year old man who was born in Pakistan and who, as a child, had chronic osteomyelitis caused by *Staphylococcus aureus*. He is asymptomatic now except for occasional pain in the hip and a limp. The radiograph shows destruction of the femoral head and acetabulum, chronic changes in the femoral shaft and fusion of the right hip joint. Courtesy of Dr Joseph Mammone.

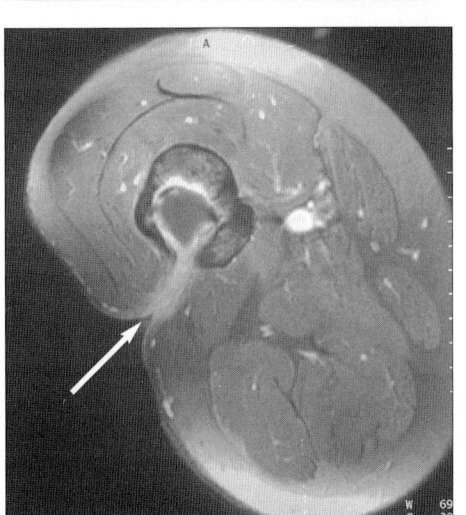

Fig. 43.6 Chronic active osteomyelitis in the femur. This case of osteomyelitis was secondary to a fracture and open reduction and internal fixation 30 years before. This axial, contrast-enhanced, fat-suppressed T1-weighted MRI shows cortical thickening and a focal intraosseous fluid collection with an enhancing rim, communicating via a sinus tract to the surface of the thigh (arrow).

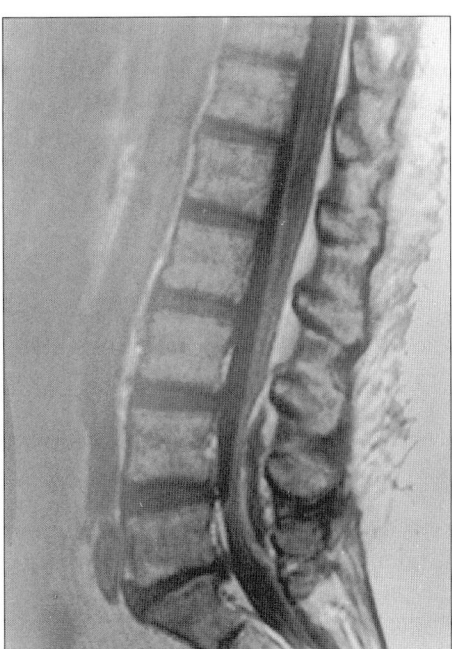

Fig. 43.7 Vertebral osteomyelitis. A sagittal, contrast-enhanced convential spin echo MRI (T1) demonstrates a posteriorly located epidural abscess at the L4–L5 vertebral level with an enhancing rim and displacement of the nerve roots anteriorly. Courtesy of Dr Joseph Mammone.

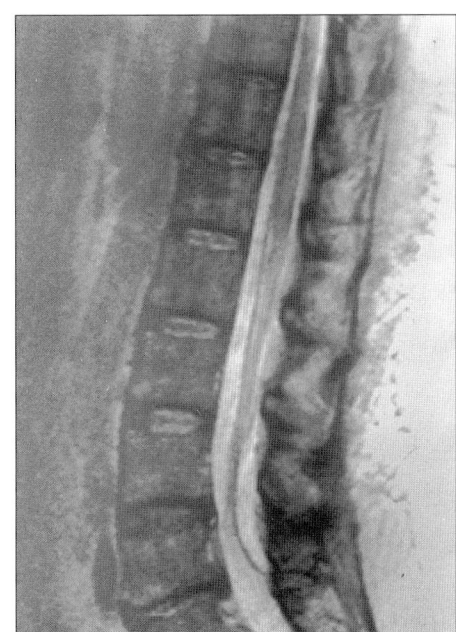

Fig. 43.8 Vertebral osteomyelitis. A sagittal, turbo spin echo MRI (T2) from the same patient as the scan in Figure 43.7. Courtesy of Dr Joseph Mammone.

with drainage. The clinical features that are characteristic of malignancy include increased pain, increased drainage, odor and a mass. There was usually more X-ray evidence of bone destruction than is seen in patients with uncomplicated osteomyelitis.

VERTEBRAL OSTEOMYELITIS

The most typical presentation of vertebral osteomyelitis is back pain. The pain is increased by motion and relieved by rest and may seem out of proportion to the examination. In about 10% of patients, symptoms may be present for less than 1 week and the illness appears more severe with fever, night sweats and other systemic signs of infection. In such patients, blood cultures are usually positive. The majority have a subacute presentation with symptoms of back pain that are present for anywhere from 2 weeks to 2 years before diagnosis. Generally, only about half the patients will be febrile on initial evaluation.

The major complications of vertebral osteomyelitis are neurologic symptoms, usually due to an associated epidural abscess.[18] The classic clinical progression goes from spinal ache to root pain to weakness, followed by paralysis. Careful and repeated examination of patients with vertebral osteomyelitis is critical; if such symptoms begin, they should be investigated rapidly with radiologic studies (particularly MRI; Figs 43.7 & 43.8). Urgent surgical decompression is often needed.[19] Unfortunately, the neurologic complications of epidural abscess are not always reversible, so the goal of management should be detection at the earliest stage (Fig. 43.9).

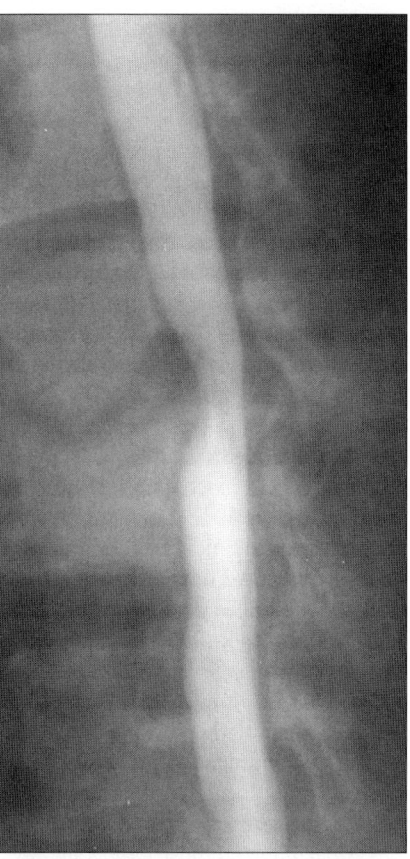

Fig. 43.9 Vertebral osteomyelitis. A myelogram showing posterior compression of the spinal cord by an inflammatory mass. Note the involvement of adjacent vertebral end-plates and the intervertebral disc. Courtesy of Dr Joseph Mammone.

BONE INFECTIONS THAT UNDERLIE PRESSURE SORES

Confirming the diagnosis of osteomyelitis beneath a pressure sore can be difficult. Radiographic or nuclear imaging and soft tissue cultures can be abnormal in the area of a pressure sore and may suggest osteomyelitis when none is present. Such misdiagnosis can lead to prolonged and potentially toxic courses of antimicrobial agents.

A careful study[20] of bone infections and pressure sores made several valuable points:

- the diagnosis of underlying bone infection should be considered whenever a pressure sore does not heal;
- clinical evaluation of depth of the sore or its duration is not helpful in determining whether bone infection is present;
- failure of the sore to close after pressure is removed is helpful in determining whether there is underlying osteomyelitis;
- nuclear scans are generally useful only if negative – the negative predictive value was high;
- Gram-negative bacilli, anaerobes, and streptococci are most often cultured from infected bone; and
- bone biopsy histology and culture are the gold standard in diagnosing osteomyelitis; the procedure is rarely associated with complications.

SPECIAL PATIENT POPULATIONS
Diabetic patients

The suspicion of osteomyelitis should be raised in diabetic patients with soft tissue infections or skin ulcerations that have been present for 1 week or more, especially if the skin infections or ulcers are over bony prominences. Unfortunately, less-than-adequate evaulations are frequently performed and critical tests are omitted.[21] Generally, patients with diabetic foot infections have no fever and may show relatively little evidence of inflammation of the ulcer. A few clinical findings are predictive of the presence of osteomyelitis. The larger and deeper the skin ulceration is, the more likely osteomyelitis is. If bone can be seen or probed through an ulcer, there is a high probability of underlying osteomyelitis.[22] Large amounts of pus may be clinically undetected in the planes and spaces of the foot; probing with blunt dissection may uncover unexpected pus. Frank destruction of bone may be seen on radiograph (Fig. 43.10).

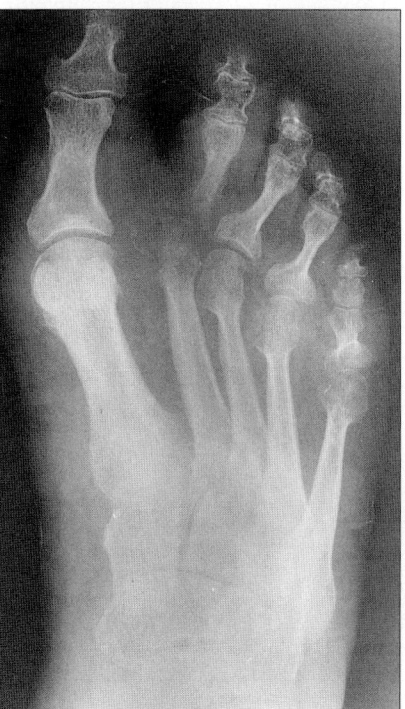

Fig. 43.10 Osteomyelitis in a diabetic patient. Diabetic patient with osteomyelitis and destruction of proximal second phalanx and metatarsal as well as second metatarsal-phalangeal joint. Courtesy of Dr Joseph Mammone.

Patients undergoing hemodialysis

In hemodialysis patients who present with bony pain or fractures, there must be a high index of suspicion of bone infections. Bone biopsy is necessary to make the diagnosis and identify the infecting agent because the clinical signs, X-ray picture and symptoms can mimic those of renal osteodystrophy.[23] The usual infecting organisms are staphylococci (either *S. aureus* or *S. epidermidis*) or *P. aeruginosa*.

Intravenous drug abusers

Although septic arthritis is more common than osteomyelitis in intravenous drug abusers, the diagnosis must be suspected if bone pain is present. Pain and tenderness are common. In general, the organisms isolated from bone appear to parallel the distribution of organisms in patients with bacteremia. Among this population, staphylococci, streptococci and *P. aeruginosa* are the most frequently recovered bacteria.

DIAGNOSIS

The diagnosis of osteomyelitis requires clinical suspicion, a consistent history and physical examination, and supportive laboratory studies (both radiographic and microbiologic). Certain conditions mimic osteomyelitis, and these differential diagnoses are reviewed briefly later.

ACUTE OSTEOMYELITIS

The diagnosis of acute hematogenous osteomyelitis is essentially a clinical one assisted by some of the studies discussed below. In the absence of a clear cause, limping or pain in an extremity should raise the suspicion of infection of bone. The sedimentation rate and C-reactive protein are frequently elevated in the presence of osteomyelitis, but normal values do not exclude this diagnosis.[24] Indeed, in one series, the sedimentation rate was less than 15mm/h in 42% of children tested; it was less commonly elevated in children over 2 years of age. Plain radiographs may show soft tissue swelling

but are otherwise usually normal because it takes anywhere from 10 to 14 days to destroy 50% of the bone (which is the amount of destruction required to show up as a lesion on conventional radiograph).

TESTS FOR OSTEOMYELITIS				
	Sensitivity (%)	Specificity (%)	Positive predictive value (%)	Negative predictive value (%)
Three-phase bone scan	95	33	53	90
Gallium scan	81	69	71	80
Indium-labeled white blood cell scan	88	85	86	87
MRI	95	88	93	92

Fig. 43.11 Tests for osteomyelitis. Sensitivity, specificity, positive predictive values and negative predictive values of tests used to diagnose infection of bone. Adapted from White *et al.*, 1995.[28]

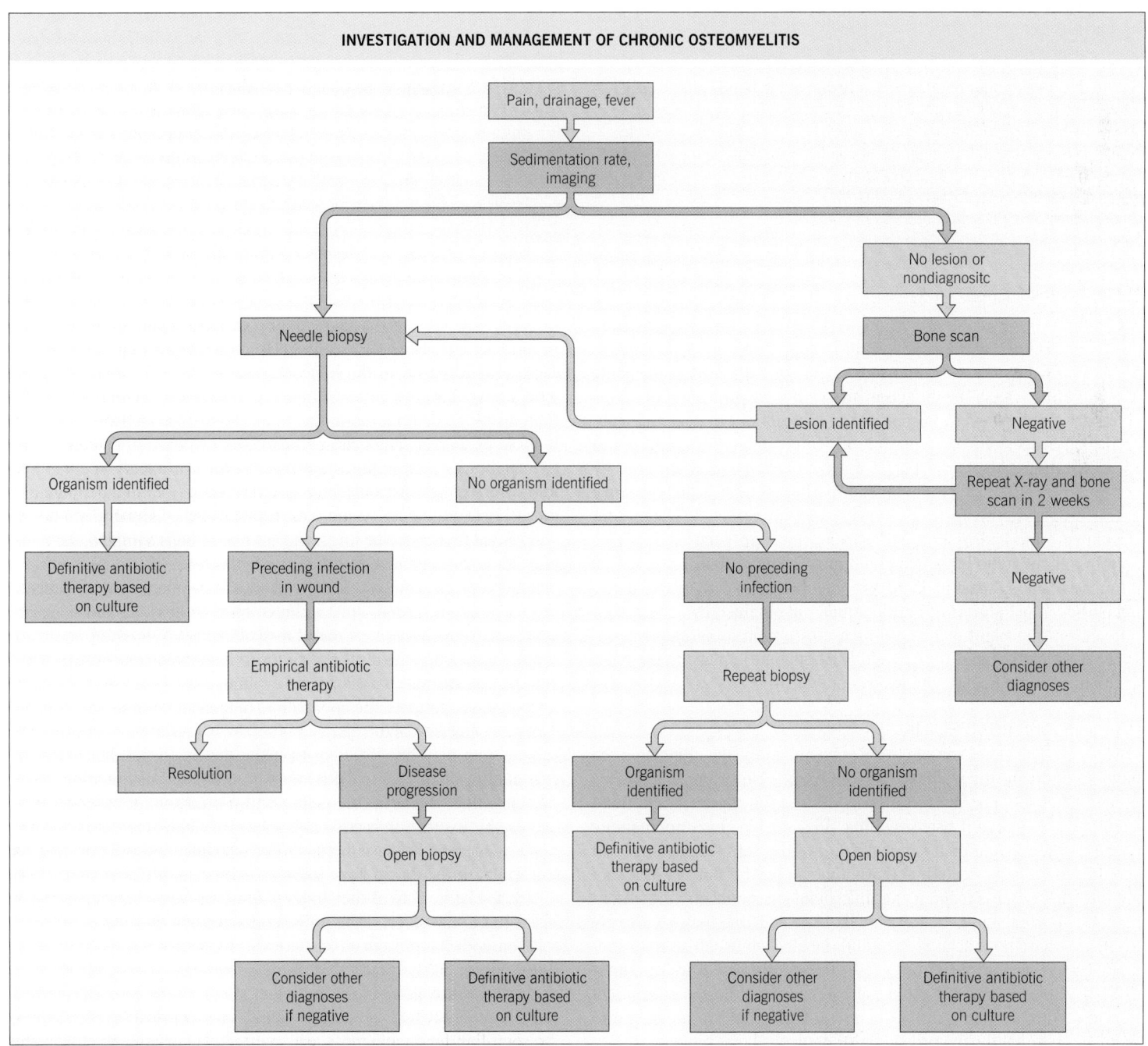

INVESTIGATION AND MANAGEMENT OF CHRONIC OSTEOMYELITIS

Fig. 43.12 Investigation and management of chronic osteomyelitis.

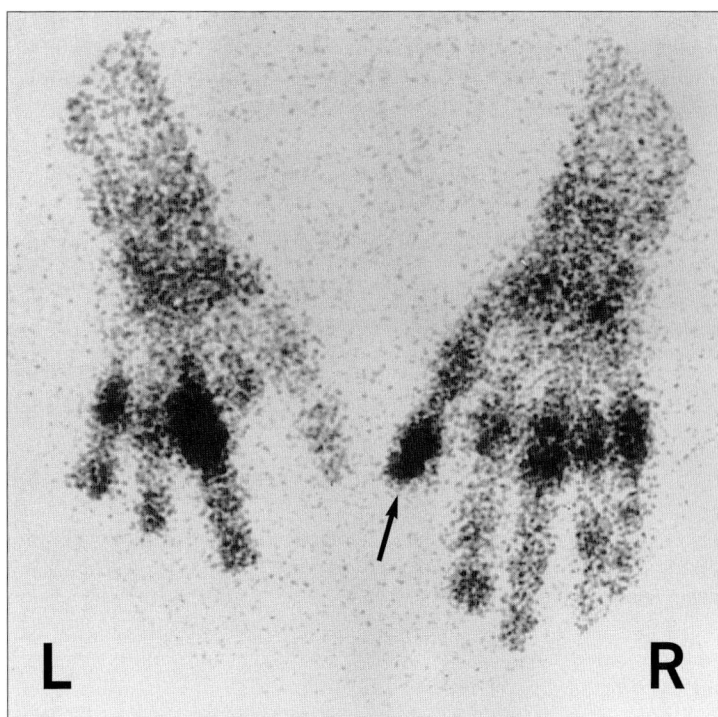

Fig. 43.13 Twenty-four hour bone scintigram of the hands. The patient is a 50-year old diabetic with a draining ulcer at the top of the right thumb (arrow). A biopsy grew *Staphylococcus aureus*. There is intense uptake in distal first phalanx and in multiple neuropathic joints. With permission from Jacobson AF, Harley J, Kipsky B, Pecoraro R. Diagnosis of osteomyelitis in the presence of soft tissue infection and radiologic evidence of osseous abnormalities. Am J Roentgenol 1991;157:807–12.

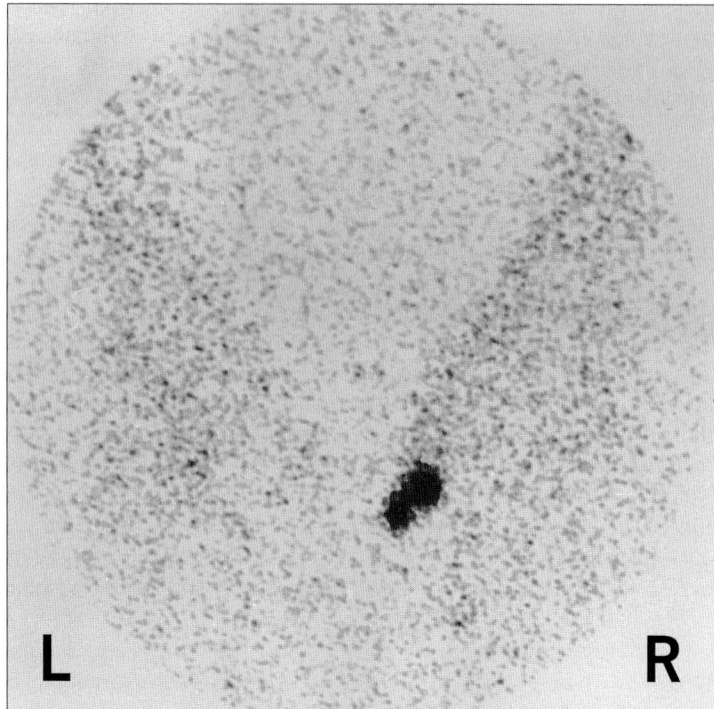

Fig. 43.14 Leukocyte scintigram of the hands. This scan is from the same patient as the scan in Figure 43.13. Again there is intense uptake in distal first phalanx, but there is no accumulation of leukocytes in the multiple neuropathic joints. With permission from Jacobson AF, Harley J, Kipsky B, Pecoraro R. Diagnosis of osteomyelitis in the presence of soft tissue infection and radiologic evidence of osseous abnormalities. Am J Roentgenol 1991;157:807–12.

Technetium bone scans are exquisitely sensitive and are generally positive before lesions appear on radiograph; however, false-negative bone scans have been reported when the diagnosis of acute osteomyelitis has been confirmed by aspiration of pus. Ultrasonography has been reported to be successful in detecting subperiosteal abscess in the presence of acute osteomyelitis; deep soft tissue swelling is the earliest sign of acute osteomyelitis, followed by periosteal elevation and a thin layer of periosteal fluid, which, in some cases, progresses to form a subperiosteal abscess.[25,26] These later stages were marked by cortical erosion; this sign generally appears only in patients who have had symptoms for more than 1 week. The ultimate diagnostic test in acute osteomyelitis is growth of the infecting pathogen in cultures of purulent material obtained by needle aspiration from the painful infected area. Tests such as indium-labeled white blood cell scan, CT scan and MRI have little place in the management of acute hematogenous osteomyelitis.

CHRONIC OSTEOMYELITIS

Given a clinical suspicion of chronic osteomyelitis, the clinician has a plethora of diagnostic studies to choose from.[27] Unfortunately, none is perfect (Fig. 43.11). An algorithm is offered for approach and management of suspected osteomyelitis (Fig. 43.12). In a nondiabetic patient, if the conventional radiograph is positive for osteomyelitis, one should generally proceed directly to bone biopsy for determination of the infecting organism and its antimicrobial susceptibility. If the radiograph is normal and osteomyelitis is suspected, one may go directly to a three-phase bone scan or to indium-labeled white cell scan. In general, CT scan and MRI are less frequently used to diagnose osteomyelitis, but they are often used to determine the extent of infection and whether there are collections of pus that are amenable to drainage. Ultimately, the procedure of choice is bone biopsy.

Bone biopsy is often referred to as the 'gold standard' for osteomyelitis. The test is easily done, but false negatives are reported in some series to be as high as 65%. Because osteomyelitis has a patchy disease distribution in the bone, it may be that CT-guided biopsies would have a higher positive yield. All specimens should be sent for both histology and microbiology. In one well-done study, in which 16 biopsy specimens demonstrated histologic evidence of osteomyelitis, only eight were also culture-positive.[28] In the same study, if either histology or culture was considered a positive criterion for osteomyelitis, the positive predictive value was 100% and the negative predictive was 66%. Obviously, the larger the amount of bone sampled, the more biopsies taken, and the better the imaging guidance, the more likely one is to get a positive biopsy. Finally, it should be noted that, in diagnosing osteomyelitis, sinus tract cultures have little value and correlate poorly with the organisms found in specimens taken in the operating room.[29] Therefore, the results of cultures of draining sinuses should not be relied on to identify the causative pathogen.

In diabetic patients, the approach to diagnosing osteomyelitis in the foot (the usual site of the disease) is somewhat different. Conventional radiographs may be sufficient to make the diagnosis, but it can be extremely difficult to distinguish diabetic osteopathy from osteomyelitis. Because osteopathy will not respond to antimicrobial agents, this distinction is critical. Nuclear medicine scans are often difficult to interpret because there is soft tissue infection and it is difficult to localize infection to bone as opposed to a soft tissue ulcer (Figs 43.13 & 43.14). One of the simplest tests is to take a steel probe and insert it into the ulcer; if the probe contacts bone, this has a high correlation with the presence of osteomyelitis. If the probe does not hit bone, the negative predictive value of the test is not adequate to exclude osteomyelitis; in this instance, MRI should be used because it has an extremely high predictive value for osteomyelitis (Fig. 43.15). An algorithm for the diagnosis and management of osteomyelitis in the diabetic patient with infection of the foot is given in Figure 43.16.

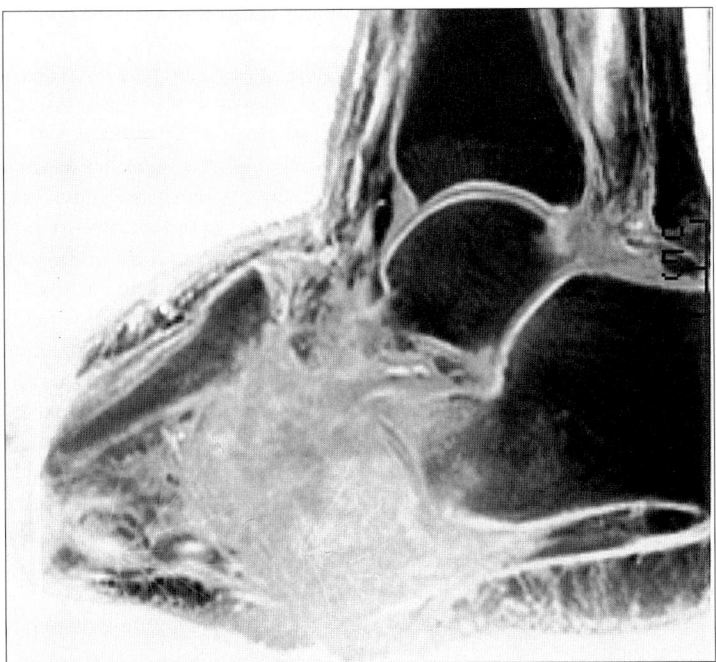

Fig. 43.15 T1-weighted image of the foot. The scan reveals forefoot amputation and a normal signal in distal tibia, talus, and posterior calcaneus. The interior portion of the calcaneus has edema. The remainder of the tarsal bones have been destroyed and replaced by a pale, heterogeneous inflammatory mass.

DIFFERENTIAL DIAGNOSIS
Chronic multifocal osteomyelitis

The syndrome of chronic multifocal osteomyelitis generally occurs in female children. They may have months to years of malaise, painful lesions, arthralgia and painful swelling of adjacent joints. The onset is usually insidious and may be associated with skin disorders such as pustular rashes. X-ray and isotope scans reveal multiple skeletal lesions that are well demarcated and osteolytic and that cannot be distinguished from pyogenic osteomyelitis. The key to making this diagnosis correctly is the failure to recover organisms on bone biopsy. Management of these children is difficult because of persisting symptoms, but it is critical to remember that this disease is self limiting and one should not give repeated courses of antibiotics in the face of negative cultures.[30]

Histiocytosis X (eosinophilic granuloma)

Eosinophilic granulomas may present as one of several destructive foci within the skeleton, often without any constitutional indications of illness. The lesions generally respond to curettage or low-dose irradiation.

Gaucher's disease

Gaucher's disease is a hereditary metabolic disturbance in which cerebrosides accumulate in reticuloendothelial cells. The disease occurs mainly in Ashkenazi Jews. Constitutional symptoms include fatigue, weakness, weight loss, abdominal discomfort, hepatomegaly and splenomegaly. Bone symptoms include pain and limitation of motion, primarily of the hips and the knees. Vascular infarcts can mimic acute osteomyelitis; pathologic fractures may occur. The combination of necrosis of bone and subsequent repair produces an appearance on radiograph similar to that of bone infection.

MANAGEMENT

ACUTE HEMATOGENOUS OSTEOMYELITIS

In the management of acute osteomyelitis, the experience of Nelson *et al.* is invaluable.[12] Optimal surgical management is controversial. In general, if frank pus is found in a diagnostic aspiration, surgical decom-

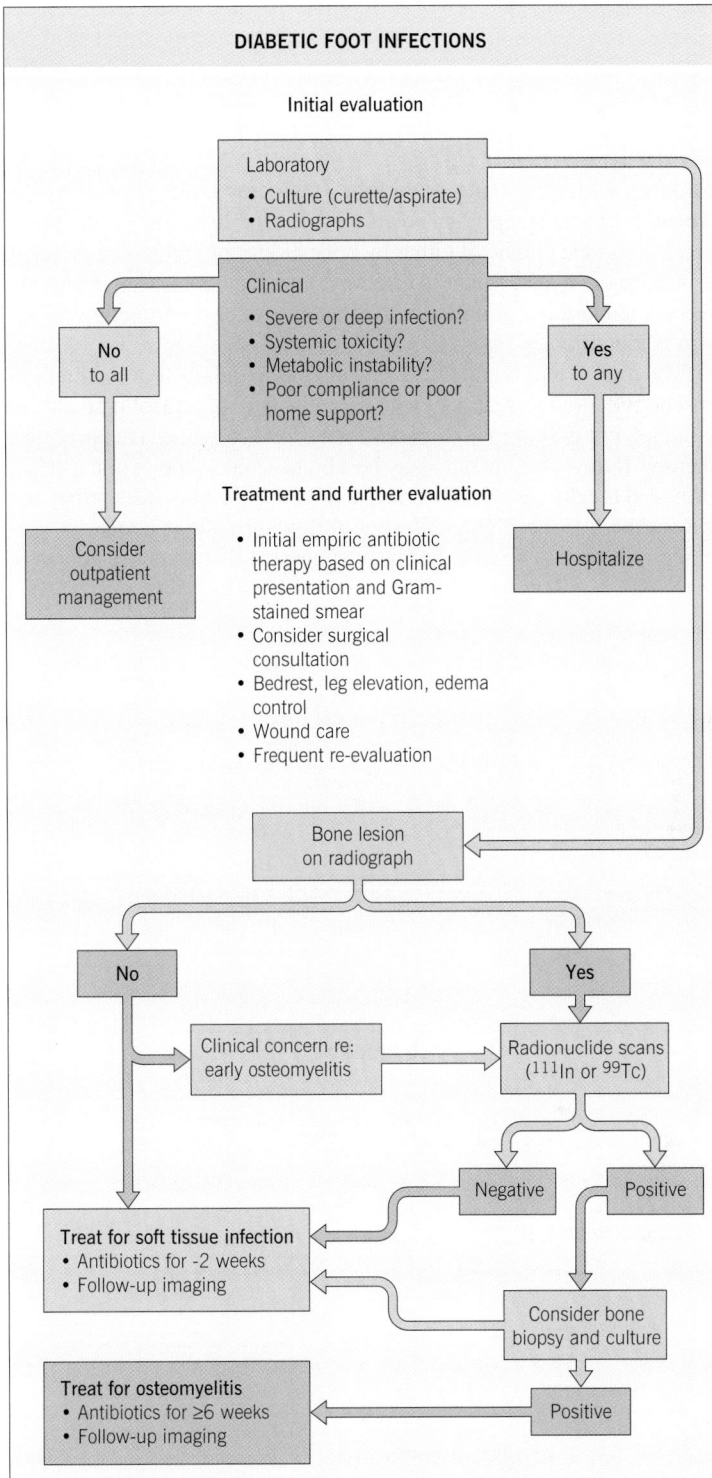

Fig. 43.16 Diabetic foot infections. Algorithmic approach to diagnosis and management. Adapted with permission from Lipsky, *et al.*, 1990.[2]

pression is usually done. If the tap produces only bloody material, medical therapy will generally be sufficient. The choice of initial antibiotic agent can be guided by the results of Gram-stained specimens and modified if necessary after the results of culture are available. If the Gram stain is unrewarding, therapy must be empiric, based on the age of the patient and the most likely pathogen in that age group. The data obtained by Nelson *et al.* indicate that when patients are treated for a minimum of 3 weeks for infections caused by staphylococci or Gram-negative bacilli, the response is excellent and chronic osteomyelitis does not ensue. Longer periods of therapy may be necessary if the clinical response is slow or the erythrocyte sedimentation rate remains elevated. Oral antibiotics may be given after a short course of parenteral therapy, provided that the patient and family are compliant, the drug is well absorbed and the organism is sensitive to the antibiotic.

CHRONIC OSTEOMYELITIS
Patients with long bone or vertebral osteomyelitis

Antimicrobial therapy. As noted earlier, establishment of an appropriate etiologic diagnosis either by bone biopsy or by blood cultures is critical to the management of osteomyelitis. Figure 43.17 indicates my recommendations for antimicrobial therapy once the infecting organism is identified.

The most common infecting organism is *S. aureus*. For methicillin-susceptible strains, treatment with nafcillin 2g q6h, cefazolin 1g q8h, or clindamycin 600mg q6–8h parenterally for 4–6 weeks is appropriate therapy. Intravenous therapy may be administered at home; oral therapy, provided the drug is well absorbed and the organism is susceptible, has been shown to be highly effective following a short course of parenteral therapy. A few studies have suggested that an entire course of

oral therapy will be as effective as parenteral therapy, but these studies have involved relatively few patients.

For osteomyelitis caused by methicillin-resistant strains of *S. aureus*, vancomycin remains the drug of choice. However, this agent has not always been effective, and rifampin (rifampicin) or rifampin plus gentamicin have been used in addition to vancomycin. Controlled studies are lacking in this area. For less common causes of osteomyelitis, including Gram-negative organisms, therapy is based on sensitivities of the infecting organism. Recommendations for duration of therapy for either Gram-negative or Gram-positive osteomyelitis are not based on controlled data, but I recommend a minimum of 4 weeks' therapy.

Quinolones have been used with increasing frequency in the treatment of chronic osteomyelitis. Unfortunately, most of the studies to date with quinolones have been open, not prospective and noncomparative. In two randomized trials, ciprofloxacin[31] or ofloxacin[32] was compared with parenteral antibiotics in the treatment of osteomyelitis. Overall success rates were 74% for ofloxacin, 77% for ciprofloxacin, and 79 and 86%, respectively, for parenteral therapy in the two trials. Because of the relatively small size of the studies, there was insufficient power to exclude a true difference, but these results are encouraging.

It is possible to draw certain conclusions regarding quinolones in osteomyelitis:[33,34]

- the published success rate in osteomyelitis due to Enterobacteriaceae is sufficiently high (92%) to eliminate the need for further trials;
- for osteomyelitis caused by *P. aeruginosa* or *S. aureus*, success rates of 72 and 75% suggest a need for further comparative trials with larger sample sizes before quinolones can be recommended with confidence to treat these pathogens[33];
- development of resistance to quinolones has been observed with disturbing frequency among strains of *S. aureus*;
- the combination of rifampin and quinolones appears to offer promise; further studies are required in this area as well; and
- as newer quinolones with increased activity against gram-positive organisms are developed, they may play an increasing role in the treatment of osteomyelitis due to *S. aureus*.

Complications of antimicrobial therapy. Among the potential complications of parenteral antibiotic therapy with high serum concentrations (particularly of aminoglycosides) are toxic reactions involving the kidneys, hearing, and vestibular function. In theory, these potentially adverse effects of systemic antibiotic therapy can be avoided by releasing antibiotics locally into the wound in high concentrations through either antibiotic impregnated cement or antibiotic impregnated beads.[35,36] The biggest issue and problem with the beads has been the elution of antibiotics at a constant rate. Although the peak levels achieved with beads may be very high, they have been erratic and sometimes not predictable. Another issue has been the ability of the antibiotic to be eluted. Aminoglycosides have been most commonly used; however, because of their poor spectrum of activity against Gram-positive organisms, their use is still relatively limited. What is needed in this area are antibiotics that have good activity against Gram-positive organisms (the most common pathogens in osteomyelitis) and a consistent rate of elution so that concentrations of drug in the local area are constant and predictable.

Surgery. Surgery plays a major role in the management of osteomyelitis of long bones. The presence of dead bone or sequestra makes eradication of infection exceedingly difficult because the dead bone is usually avascular, and antibiotic is rarely delivered to an avascular site. Thus, the goal of surgical management is to debride sufficiently to remove as much dead bone as is feasible while still preserving stability and functional union.

In vertebral osteomyelitis, surgery is generally not needed except to drain epidural or paravertebral abscesses. In the case of epidural abscesses, neurologic compromise frequently occurs. This is a dreaded complication because it may not always be reversible even with surgery. Scanning with MRI and CT are valuable tools in diagnosing epidural abscess, but clinical suspicion and careful observation of

ANTIMICROBIAL THERAPY FOR INFECTIONS OF BONE AND JOINTS		
	Antimicrobial agent of choice	
Organism	Agent	Alternative agents
Staphylococcus aureus (methicillin-sensitive)	Nafcillin or oxacillin 2g q6h iv	Cefazolin, vancomycin, clindamycin
Staphylococcus aureus (methicillin-resistant)	Vancomycin 1g q12h iv	Trimethoprim–sulfamethoxazole plus rifampin
Streptococcus pneumoniae	Penicillin G 5 x 10⁶ U q6h iv*	Cefazolin, vancomycin, clindamycin
Group A beta-hemolytic streptococci	Penicillin G 5 x 10⁶ U q8h iv	Cefazolin, vancomycin, clindamycin
Enterococci	Ampicillin 2g q4h iv†	Vancomycin
Haemophilus influenzae (beta-lactamase-negative)	Ampicillin 2g q4h iv	Trimethoprim–sulfamethoxazole, ceftriaxone
Haemophilus influenzae (beta-lactamase-positive)	Ceftriaxone 1g q12h iv	Trimethoprim–sulfamethoxazole
Klebsiella pneumoniae	Ceftriaxone 1g q12h iv	Ciprofloxacin, piperacillin, imipenem
Escherichia coli	Cefazolin 1g q8h iv	Ciprofloxacin, ceftriaxone, imipenem
Pseudomonas aeruginosa	Ciprofloxacin 400mg q12h iv or ceftazidime 1g q8h iv	Pipercillin plus aminoglycoside, aztreonam
Serratia marcescens	Ceftriaxone 1g q12h iv	Imipenem, trimethoprim–sulfamethoxazole, ciprofloxacin
Salmonella spp.	Depends on sensitivity test; choose between ampicillin, ceftriaxone, imipenem, ciprofloxacin	
Bacteroides spp.	Clindamycin 600mg q8h iv	Imipenem, metronidazole

* If susceptible or intermediate resistance. If high level resistance, use ceftriaxone 1g q24h or vancomycin 1g q12h.

† If susceptible. If ampicillin resistant but vancomycin susceptible, use vancomycin. If resistant to both, check susceptibility to tetracyclines, chloramphenicol or experimental agents.

Fig. 43.17 Antimicrobial therapy for infections of bone.

patients with vertebral osteomyelitis are critical to allow early detection by these sensitive imaging techniques.

Hyperbaric oxygen therapy. Hyperbaric oxygenation (HBO) has been proposed frequently as a treatment modality or adjunct therapy for chronic osteomyelitis. Experimentally, there is evidence that increasing intramedullary oxygen tensions allows increased effectiveness of leukocytes in killing staphylococci. Increased oxygen tensions may also improve wound healing. Several clinical trials have reported improvement with the use of hyperbaric oxygen in the outcome of patients with chronic osteomyelitis who were refractory to prior therapy. However, there is currently no compelling controlled clinical evidence to support the use of HBO, and it probably has little to add to the treatment of osteomyelitis when adequate debridement produces a well-vascularized wound. However, in patients where this condition is not met, HBO may be of some therapeutic value. The need for controlled studies in this area is obvious.[37]

Foot infections in diabetic patients

It is particularly difficult to treat osteomyelitis in diabetic patients because peripheral vascular disease is common and blood flow is often limited. Surgical treatment of infected areas by an experienced surgeon, with resection or debridement down to living bone, is of critical importance. Selection of antimicrobial agents to treat such infection should be based on culture of bone. If therapy must be empiric, one pathogen that should be covered is *S. aureus*. Beta-lactam agents, clindamycin, or vancomycin are most frequently used. For methicillin-resistant *S. aureus*, rifampin has been added to vancomycin, but there is little data to support the additional efficacy of a second drug. Quinolones may be useful, but the currently available agents have minimal activity against anaerobes and are not optimal for some aerobic Gram-positive cocci because of the development of resistance.

The role of anaerobic bacteria is not always clear, but it is stated that anaerobes are less common pathogens in diabetic osteomyelitis than in soft tissue infection. Features that are associated with anaerobic bone infections include increased severity of infection, longer duration of infection, failure of prior antimicrobial therapy, presence of necrotic material and foul odor. In such cases, clindamycin or metronidazole should be part of the therapy.

The optimal duration of therapy is not known. It has been noted that antimicrobial therapy, especially if given parenterally for at least 1 week and for a total duration of at least 2 weeks, combined with adequate debridement of infected bone may cure many if not most cases of osteomyelitis in the feet of diabetic patients; others treat for a minimum of 4 weeks. In my opinion, the most critical element is frequent and adequate debridement, and the duration of antibiotic therapy (provided it is at least 2 weeks) is less important.

The need for an aggressive surgical approach now appears to be well documented. Early surgical intervention has been shown to be associated with a lower rate of above-the-ankle amputation and a shorter duration of hospitalization then delayed or less aggressive surgical intervention.[38]

Surgical resection of infected bone may be helped by delineating the area of infection. In one series of 35 patients, 21 underwent surgical resection of infected bone. In 13 of these, the surgery was limited to the specific region of infection demonstrated at MRI. In all patients, the surgical margin encompassed the region of bone with abnormal MRI signal intensity, and there were no recurrences at the surgical margins with an average follow-up of 9 months.[39]

REFERENCES

1. Gillespie WJ. Epidemiology in bone and joint infection. Infect Dis Clin North Am 1990;4:361–76.
2. Lipsky BA, Pecoraro RE, Wheat LJ. The diabetic foot. Soft tissue and bone infection. Infect Dis Clin North Am 1990;4:409–32.
3. Gristina AG, Oga M, Webb LX, Hobgood CD. Adherent bacterial colonization in the pathogenesis of osteomyelitis. Science 1985;228:990–3.
4. Buxton TB, Rissing JP, Horner JA, et al. Binding of a *Staphylococcus aureus* bone pathogen to type I collagen. Microb Pathog 1990;8:441–8.
5. Herrmann M, Vaudlaux PE, Pittet D, et al. Fibronectin, fibrinogen and laminin act as mediators of adherence of clinical staphylococcal isolates to foreign material. J Infect Dis 1988;158:693–701.
6. Buxton T, Horner J, Hinton A, Rissing J. *In vitro* glycocalyx expression by *Staphylococcus aureus* phage type 52/52A/80 in *S. aureus* osteomyelitis. J Infect Dis 1987;156:942–6.
7. Plotquin D, Dekel S, Katz S, Danon A. Prostaglandin release by normal and osteomyelitic human bones. Prostaglandins, leukotrienes and essential fatty aids 1991;43:13–5.
8. Klosterhalfen B, Peters KM, Tons C, Hauptmann S, Klein CL, Kirkpatrick CJ. Local and systemic inflammatory mediator release in patients with acute and chronic posttraumatic osteomyelitis. J Trauma Injury Infect Crit Care 1996;40:372–8.
9. Fallon MD, Schwamm H. Metabolic and other nontumorous disorders of bone. In: Kissane JM, ed. Anderson's pathology. St. Louis; Mosby: 1990:1929–2017.
10. Waldvogel F, Medoff G, Swartz MN. Ostoemyelitis: a review of clinical features, therapeutic considerations and unusual aspects. N Eng J Med 1970;282:198–206.
11. Mader JT, Calhoun J. Osteomyelitis. In: Mandell G, Bennett J, Dolin R, eds. Infectious diseases. New York: Churchill-Livingstone; 1995:1039–52.
12. Nelson J. Acute osteomyelitis in children. Infect Dis Clin North Am 1990;4:513–22.
13. Fisher MC, Goldsmith JF, Gilligan PH. Sneakers as a source of *Pseudomonas aeruginosa* in children with osteomyelitis following puncture wounds. J Pediatr 1985;106:607–9.
14. Armstrong DG, Lanthier J, Lelievre P, Edelson GW. Methicillin-resistant coagulase-negative staphylococcal osteomyelitis and its relationship to broad spectrum oral antibiosis in a predominantly diabetic population. J Foot Ankle Surg 1995;34:563–6.
15. Corso F, Shaul DB, Wolfe BM. Spinal osteomyelitis after TPN catheter-induced septicemia. J Parenter Enter Nutr 1995;19:291–5.
16. Norden C. Prevention of bone and jont infections. Am J Med 1985;78:229–31.
17. Alabi ZO, Ojo OS, Odesanmi WO. Secondary amyloidosis in chronic osteomyelitis. Int Orthop 1991;15:21–2.
18. Baker AS, Ojemann RG, Swartz MN, Richardson EP Jr. Spinal epidural abscess. N Eng J Med 1975;293:463–8.
19. Baker AS, Ojemann RG, Baker RA. To decompress or not to decompress – spinal epidural abscess. Clin Infect Dis 1992;15:28–9.
20. Sugarman B. Pressure sores and underlying bone infection. Arch Intern Med 1987;147:553–5.
21. Edelson GW, Armstrong DG, Lavery LA, Calceo G. The acutely infected diabetic foot is not adequately evaluated in an inpatient setting. Arch Intern Med 1996;156:2373–8.
22. Grayson ML, Gibbons GW, Balogh K, Levin E, Karchmer AW. Probing to bone in infected pedal ulcers. A clinical sign of underlying osteomyelitis in diabetic patients. JAMA 1995;273:721–3.
23. Leonard A, Comty CM, Shapiro FL, Raij L. Osteomyelitis in hemodialysis patients. Ann Intern Med 1973;78:651–8.
24. Perry M. Erythrocyte sedimentation rate and C reactive protein in the assessment of suspected bone infection – are they reliable indices. J R Coll Surg Edinb 1996;41:116–9.
25. Kaiser S, Rosenborg M. Early detection of subperiosteal abscesses by ultrasonography. Pediatr

Radiol 1994;24:336–9.

26. Mah ET, Lequesne GW, Gent RJ, Paterson DC. Ultrasonic features of acute osteomyelitis in children. J Bone Joint Surg [Br] 1994;76B:969–74.

27. Schauwecker DJ. The scintigraphic diagnosis of osteomyelitis. Am J Roentgenol 1992;158:9–18.

28. White LM, Schweitzer ME, Deely DM, Gannon F. Study of osteomyelitis: utility of combined histologic and microbiologic evaluation of percutaneous biopsy samples. Radiology 1995;197:840–2.

29. Mackowiak PA, Jones SR, Smith JW. Diagnostic valve of sinus-tract cultures in chronic osteomyelitis. JAMA 1978;239:2772–5.

30. Kozlowski K, Masel J, Harbison S, Yu J. Multifocal chronic osteomyelitis of unknown etiology. Pediatr Radiol 1983;13:130–6.

31. Gentry LO, Rodriguez-Gomez G. Oral ciprofloxacin compred with parenteral antibiotics in the treatment of osteomyelitis. Antimicrob Agents Chemother 1990;34:40–3.

32. Gentry L, Rodriguez-Gomez G. Ofloxacin versus parenteral therapy for chronic osteomyelitis. Antimicrob Agents Chemother 1991;35:538–41.

33. Lew D, Waldvogel FA. Quinolones and osteomyelitis: state-of-the-art. Drugs 1995;49:100–11.

34. Wispelwey B, Scheld WM. Ciprofloxacin in the treatment of *Staphylococcus aureus* osteomyelitis. Diagn Microbiol Infect Dis 1990;13:169–71.

35. Henry SL, Seligson D, Margino P, Popham GJ. Antibiotic-impregnated beads. Orthop Rev 1991;20:242–7.

36. Wininger DA, Fass RJ. Antibiotic-impregnated cement and beads for orthopedic infections. Antimicrob Agents Chemother 1996;40:2675–9.

37. Mader JT, Adams KR, Wallace WR, Calhoun JH. Hyperbaric oxygen as adjunctive therapy for osteomyelitis. Infect Dis Clin North Am 1990;4:433–40.

38. Tan JS, Friedman NM, Hazelton-Miller C, Flanagan JP, File TM Jr. Can aggressive treatment of diabetic foot infections reduce the need for above-ankle amputation? Clin Infect Dis 1996;23:286–91.

39. Morrison WB, Schweitzer ME, Wapner KL, Hecht PJ, Gannon FH, Behm WR. Osteomyelitis in feet of diabetics: clinical accuracy, surgical utility, and cost-effectiveness of MR imaging. Radiology 1995;196:557–64.

Infections of Prosthetic Joints and Related Problems

Anthony R Berendt

INTRODUCTION

Infections of orthopaedic devices are paradigms of device-related infection, with skin commensals of low virulence often behaving as important pathogens. This affects both treatment and microbiologic diagnostic tests, which must be performed and interpreted with care to avoid misleading results. Surgery to infected orthopaedic devices is usually necessary, to remove infected foreign material and necrotic tissue, to restore skeletal integrity and soft tissue cover and, in some cases, to obtain diagnostic specimens. Antibiotics are used along with surgery or to suppress infection when further surgical intervention cannot be contemplated – hence the role of the specialist in infection is to help the orthopaedic surgeon to perform and interpret microbiologic tests appropriately and to choose and use antimicrobials rationally.

EPIDEMIOLOGY

Reported infection rates for hip and knee replacements are approximately 0.5–1% and 1–2%, respectively.[1,2] Most infection presents within the first 5 years of implantation, but all prosthetic joints are at a continuing low lifelong risk of infection. This risk probably rises if the joint begins to fail mechanically. Thus, rates of infection depend on the duration and diligence of follow up and also on the criteria used for diagnosis. Risk factors include delayed wound healing, rheumatoid arthritis and revision surgery, because revision operations tend to be long and technically difficult.

Rates of fracture-fixation infection vary widely depending on the site and the method of fixation adopted. Infection rates for closed fractures undergoing internal fixation by incisions through healthy soft tissue, for example, by intramedullary nailing, should be comparable to those of other 'clean' surgical procedures. Compound fractures are at higher risk, depending on the extent of environmental contamination, soft tissue injury and vascular injury.[3] In addition, delay in wound debridement and soft-tissue closure leads to greatly increased infection rates.

The treatment of scoliosis or spinal instability with modern posterior spinal instrumentation systems involves the exposure of large areas of bone beneath the paraspinal muscles, followed by the insertion of complex implants (bilateral longitudinal rods held in place with hooks, cross-links and sublaminar wires). Published rates of early infection for these lengthy operations are surprisingly similar to those of other clean operative procedures at approximately 1–2%, but there have been accounts of delayed infection occurring with a much higher frequency, approaching 10%.[4]

PATHOGENESIS AND PATHOLOGY

PATHOGENESIS

Infection commences with the adhesion of bacteria to host tissues or biomaterials, either directly or via host plasma proteins, such as fibronectin, deposited on the biomaterial surface.[5] Bacteria express numerous structures to enhance adhesion, including proteinaceous cell-wall-associated adhesins and capsular polysaccharide adhesins.

Furthermore, the surfaces of many bacteria are relatively hydrophobic, enhancing initial interactions mediated by Van der Waals forces.

Adherent micro-organisms frequently produce exocellular polysaccharides that enmesh the bacteria. The resulting consortium of adherent bacteria is called a biofilm, which may be monomicrobial or polymicrobial. Compared with the same organisms cultured in liquid media, bacteria in biofilms are exceedingly difficult to kill with antibiotics or biocides or by host defenses. The possible mechanisms for this resistance include alterations in the growth rate of organisms within the biofilm and adherence-dependent differential gene expression. It does not appear to be due to impaired antibiotic access. It is not clear whether biofilm formation is as relevant to the chronic nature of orthopaedic implant infections as it is to infections of vascular access devices and other catheters. However, recent advances in the understanding of the molecular genetics of exopolysaccharide formation by coagulase-negative staphylococci[6] should shortly allow the role of biofilm formation to be examined in animal models. In human disease, the relationship between adherence to plastic or elaboration of exopolysaccharide and the clinical manifestations caused by isolates has been studied, with inconclusive results.

Host responses are impaired in the vicinity of biomaterials. Neutrophils show defective phagocytosis, partly owing to the concentrations of metal ions or to the presence of monomeric or polymerized methacrylate (bone cement). In addition, bacterial exocellular polysaccharide may inhibit phagocytosis and other elements of the immune response.[7] Abnormalities of host defense in the region of an implant were first recognized in the classic observations of Elek and Conen, who showed that the inoculum of *Staphylococcus aureus* required to cause a skin infection in human volunteers was dramatically reduced in the presence of a skin suture.[8]

PATHOLOGY

Once the organisms have established an association with the surface of the biomaterial, chronic infection ensues with two major pathologic features:

- an acute inflammatory response develops around the prosthetic material, giving some or all of the classical signs of infection; and
- activation of osteoclasts and recruitment of monocyte-derived bone-resorbing cells as a result of this response, leading to bone loss at the interface with the implant.[9]

The normally thin layer of poorly vascularized fibrous tissue between the host and the implant or its anchoring cement, generally termed the 'membrane' by orthopaedic surgeons, becomes markedly thickened and more vascular. Frank granulation tissue may be produced alongside the implant and eventually free pus is formed. In prosthetic joint infection, these processes exaggerate the pathologic mechanisms operating in aseptic loosening, in which a chronic inflammatory response is produced in response to wear particles derived from acrylic cement and polyethylene.[10] This chronic inflammation, associated with mononuclear cells and giant cells, also leads to bone resorption (Fig. 44.1). A key feature of infection is thus the presence of an acute inflammatory infiltrate, but it may be superimposed on chronic inflammation (Fig. 44.2).[11]

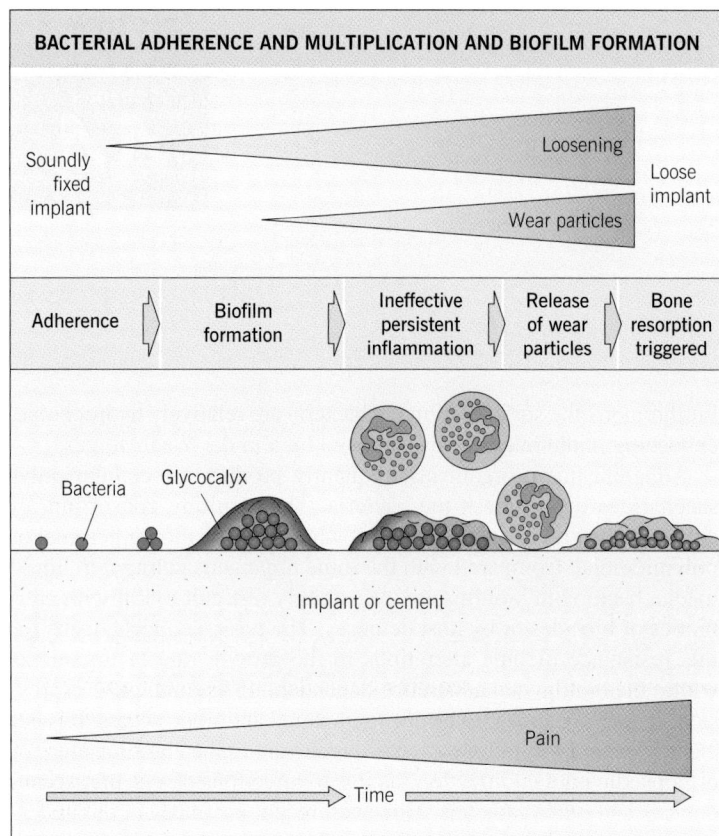

BACTERIAL ADHERENCE AND MULTIPLICATION AND BIOFILM FORMATION

Fig. 44.1 Bacterial adherence to the implant, bacterial multiplication on the surface and biofilm formation. An ineffective host response triggers bone resorption, contributing to loosening, which is accelerated by wear particles and the host response to them.

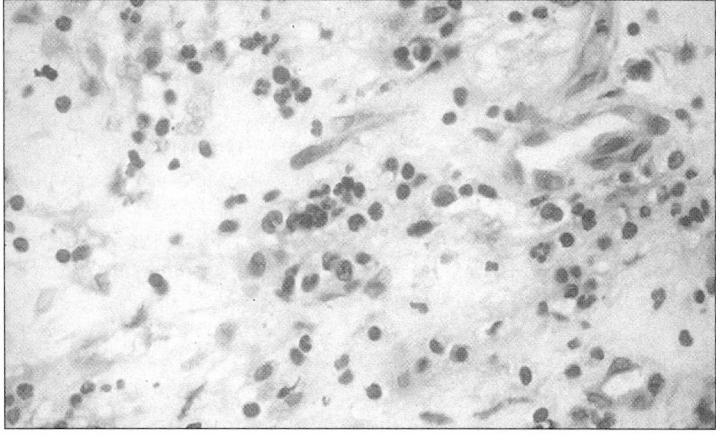

Fig. 44.2 Histologic features of infection. Periprosthetic tissue from a clinically infected total hip replacement from which multiple specimens grew an indistinguishable organism. Numerous neutrophils are present in the tissue.

MICROBIOLOGY

Orthopaedic implant infections are classified as early, delayed and late (Fig. 44.3).

Early infections usually manifest (and may sometimes begin) as wound infections. They tend to be caused by higher-grade pathogens able to exploit postoperative hematomas and breaches in the skin. *Staphylococcus aureus*, including methicillin-resistant strains, and aerobic Gram-negative rods predominate in such cases.

Delayed infections, in which pain and swelling develop in the context of a healed wound, are more often caused by coagulase-negative staphylococci and other skin commensals. This is presumably because, as lower virulence pathogens, they take longer to reach the critical number of organisms needed to produce clinical symptoms.

BACTERIA ASSOCIATED WITH INFECTED IMPLANTS PRESENTING AT DIFFERENT STAGES	
Early infection (up to 1 month)	*Staphylococcus aureus* Aerobic Gram-negative rods Coagulase-negative staphylococci
Delayed infection (2–12 months)	Coagulase-negative staphylococci Other skin commensals
Late infection, including hematogenous seeding (more than 12 months)	Coagulase-negative staphylococci Other skin commensals *Staphylococcus aureus* Aerobic Gram-negative rods Anaerobes

Fig. 44.3 Bacteria associated with infected implants presenting at different stages.

Late infections, which present more than 12 months postoperatively, are mostly caused by Gram-positive skin commensals but also include cases of hematogenous seeding with organisms capable of causing bacteremia.

Irrespective of the time of presentation, mixed infections are relatively common (accounting for approximately 20% of cases), with a variable proportion of aerobic Gram-negative rods, fastidious anaerobes and culture-negative cases.[12] False-negative cultures may be due to a number of factors. Prior antibiotic therapy may drop the bacterial load below the limits of detection of the test used, and improper specimen collection (e.g. sending too few specimens or sending swabs instead of tissue) may lead to negative results through sampling error. Some rare pathogens, such as *Mycoplasma* spp., L-forms (cell-wall-deficient bacteria), *Campylobacter* spp., *Mycobacterium tuberculosis* and the atypical mycobacteria, as well as more common pathogens may be present in exceedingly low densities or in non-culturable states and so cannot be isolated using standard techniques.

PREVENTION

Prevention of all infections of orthopaedic devices depends to a great extent on good surgical technique and operating room discipline. The transit of theater staff should be minimized and obsessive attention should be paid to skin preparation, sterile technique and the handling of soft tissues. Diathermy should be used judiciously, surgical dead space and tissue trauma minimized and operating time kept to a minimum. Ultraclean air in theaters reduces infection rates, as do prophylactic antibiotics. In most centers, one to three doses of a first- or second-generation cephalosporin are used;[13] where methicillin-resistant *S. aureus* is endemic, glycopeptide prophylaxis may be necessary. Surgeons may need to be reminded of the need to give repeat doses of antibiotic during the procedure if it is prolonged or accompanied by excessive blood loss. There is insufficient evidence to be certain whether three doses of prophylactic antibiotic are superior to one and it is more important to ensure that adequate levels are present throughout the time that the wound is open.

For joint replacement, specialized theater apparatus may also be used, including total body exhaust suits and the Charnley–Howarth sterile air enclosure, a plastic hood that excludes most of the operating theater environment from the vicinity of the surgical field. For prevention of fracture-fixation infection, energetic wound debridement and early soft tissue closure are essential, with initial stabilization by external fixation before proceeding to internal fixation once the soft tissues have recovered from the initial trauma. Free tissue transfer using myocutaneous flaps and microvascular anastomosis allows debridement to be radical, removing all devitalized and contaminated tissue and replacing it with healthy tissue at the fracture site.

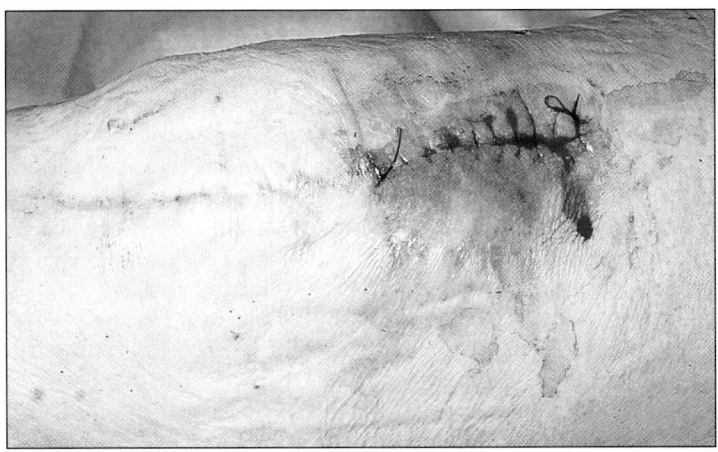

Fig. 44.4 An acutely infected knee replacement. The site was washed out but the infection failed to resolve. At re-operation the implant was found to be loose and it needed to be removed. *Staphylococcus aureus* was grown from deep specimens.

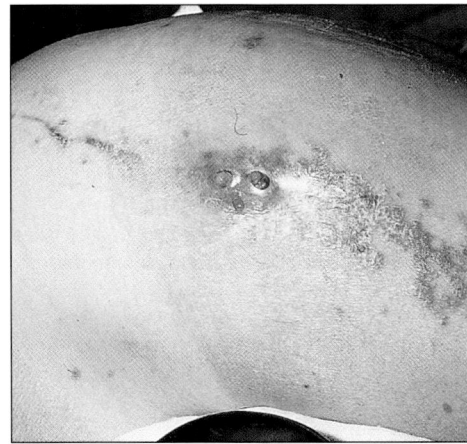

Fig. 44.5 A sinus tract discharging from an infected total hip replacement. *Staphylococcus aureus* was grown from deep specimens. Note the Koebner phenomenon; this patient's psoriasis was probably a significant risk factor for infection.

LATE PROPHYLAXIS

The risk of hematogenous infection of prosthetic joints must be considered when planning procedures that are known to cause transient bacteremia. The risk is unclear, but the routine use of antibiotic prophylaxis for all procedures liable to cause bacteremia in all patients with prosthetic joints is probably not justified on risk–benefit or economic criteria. Patients at particular risk are likely to be those with newly implanted or loose prostheses and those with active infection elsewhere, including dental infection, and it may be reasonable to offer prophylaxis in these situations[13] using protocols similar to those used for the prevention of infective endocarditis.

CLINICAL FEATURES

Orthopaedic implant infections are almost always associated with pain, which may be mild at first but which usually becomes severe. 'Infection pain' is often distinguishable from other pains, even at the same site, but it does not have pathognomonic features. It is commonly present to some extent as soon as the infection is active. Even if presentation is delayed, many patients give a history that the implant was 'never right', that is, that it never became comfortable. Pain is due to inflammation but is also caused by loosening of the implant. The characteristics of pain due to loosening, particularly with prosthetic joints, are of 'start-up' pain, initially severe following rest (and therefore especially in the morning) but subsequently easing off with use of the joint. As loosening worsens, however, use of the joint or limb becomes increasingly painful at all times, and night pain and unpredictable spasms develop.

Early infections are generally also associated with fever and marked inflammation in the operative wound. There may be purulent discharge (Fig. 44.4) or frank wound breakdown with skin necrosis when high-grade pathogens are involved. Rarely, sepsis results; this is also often a feature in hematogenous late infections. If infection with less virulent pathogens presents early, the clinical features may be less florid, with a wound that continues to drain in a patient who is systemically well. In either case, inadequate treatment will lead to the formation of a sinus tract, which is also often seen with delayed and late infections (Fig. 44.5). It is not unusual for patients to give histories of recurrent wound infections, treated with repeated short courses of oral antibiotics because the underlying deep infection was not addressed. By the time such infections present to the specialist, the implant has usually loosened. A proportion of delayed and late infections simply present with rapid loosening and do not show any signs of local or systemic inflammation, although they do cause pain.

DIAGNOSIS

Diagnosis of infection requires clinical suspicion and appropriate investigation. When wounds develop purulence, spreading cellulitis, persistent erythema or persistent drainage (even with serosanguinous fluid), the implant should be considered infected until proved otherwise. Unless there are convincing alternative explanations, the same approach should be adopted for any implant that fails early or is persistently painful.

EARLY INFECTIONS

Early infections are generally accompanied by fever and an elevated erythrocyte sedimentation rate (ESR), C-reactive protein (CRP) and white blood cell count. The exception to this are early infection with low virulence pathogens or freely draining (and hence decompressed) wounds, when fever may be absent. Blood cultures may demonstrate a bacteremia. Ultrasound of the implant may reveal a fluid collection or a hematoma; if so, this should be aspirated for microscopy and culture. If unexplained fever is present, aspiration of the joint space or the region of the fracture should be considered. Plain radiographs are of little value in early infection, but they serve as a useful baseline for subsequent change.

Of central importance in making the diagnosis is exploration, which should be performed before starting antibiotic therapy if the overall condition of the patient and the state of the soft tissues permit it. Multiple deep tissue specimens should be taken for culture and for histology; surgeons should be discouraged from sending swabs, because air trapped in the interstices of the cotton may kill obligate anaerobes; superficial material is also unsuitable. The interpretation of a positive culture result from a single specimen (even if deep) is very difficult if a skin commensal is obtained, because such an organism may be a contaminant or a true pathogen. To a lesser extent, this problem extends even to the isolation of *S. aureus* or an aerobic Gram-negative rod because of changes in skin flora on hospitalization and after surgery. By contrast, if multiple specimens obtained with separate instruments yield the same organism, it is highly likely to be of clinical significance.[14]

LATE INFECTIONS

These are accompanied by systemic features only in the small minority of patients in whom bacteremia or abscess formation occurs. The white blood cell count, ESR and CRP may all be normal. Plain radiographs usually demonstrate loosening (Fig. 44.6), although this may be hard to see with spinal instrumentation. Additional features, such as periosteal reaction and endosteal erosion (with intramedullary implants), may be seen.

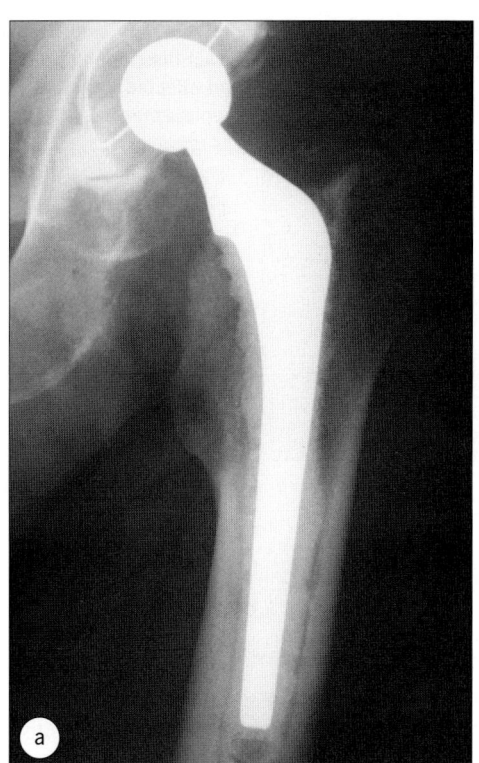

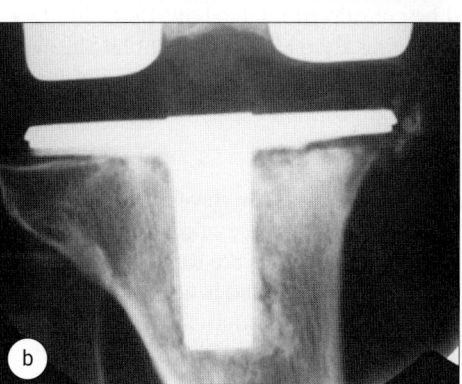

Fig. 44.6 Implant loosening in late infection.
(a) Radiograph of the infected hip shown in Figure 44.5. There is an obvious radiolucent line at the bone–cement interface. This implant required revision.
(b) Radiograph of a loose knee replacement, showing resorption of bone beneath the tibial component, a cause of instability. Coagulase-negative staphylococci were grown from multiple deep specimens.

inflammation. This variability, which was also observed in experimental studies of infected prosthetic joints in dogs, is probably due to infection with very low numbers of micro-organisms in a patchy distribution.[16,17] Frozen sections can be used to make the diagnosis during surgery, again using as criteria the presence of neutrophils.[18–20]

If there is sinus tract drainage, the diagnosis of infection is effectively beyond doubt. However, because sinus tracts commonly acquire a complex mixed flora of both commensals and pathogens, including *S. aureus*, aerobic Gram-negative rods, enterococci and anaerobes, it has long been recognized that the predictive value of sinus tract cultures is poor. Such cultures should be discouraged except for the purpose of infection control in hospitals, where attempts are made to identify cases of methicillin-resistant *S. aureus*.

Aspiration for microscopy and culture is frequently performed, but published sensitivities and specificities vary widely. This may be explained by differences in techniques of aspiration, in sample handling and processing, and in the criteria used for the final diagnosis of infection when evaluating the test. One recent study of prosthetic joint infection, in which the preoperative and intraoperative protocols and final diagnostic criteria are carefully documented, showed a sensitivity of 92% and a specificity of 97%.[21]

Definitive microbiologic diagnosis requires culture of periprosthetic tissue samples. For maximum diagnostic yield, deep specimens should be obtained from multiple areas around the implant at debridement or excision and transported to the laboratory without delay. The surgeon must use separate instruments to prevent cross-contamination of samples, and these should be processed in a laminar flow cabinet to avoid contamination in the laboratory. Enrichment cultures are essential. Unfortunately, criteria for the diagnosis of infection based on operative samples are nonstandardized, ranging from the isolation of organisms in four out of five or five out of six specimens to diagnosing infection on the basis of a single positive direct culture or on two or more positive enrichment cultures.[22–24] A prospective study found that if three or more independent specimens of periprosthetic tissue yielded indistinguishable micro-organisms, infection could be confidently diagnosed. The same study recommended that five or six samples be sent for maximum sensitivity and specificity.[14]

MANAGEMENT

EARLY INFECTIONS OF PROSTHETIC JOINTS
These should be considered to be emergencies, for two reasons:
- infection may lead to bacteremia or soft tissue loss or both; and
- some cases of early infection have good long-term outcomes if aggressive debridement is combined with appropriate antibiotic therapy, whereas there is evidence that delay worsens outcome.[25,26]

Hence, early infections should be managed by urgent exploration, debridement of infected and devitalized tissue, and inspection of the prosthesis. If the implant is soundly fixed, salvage may be possible; if loose, the prosthesis should be removed. After specimens have been taken, intravenous broad-spectrum antibiotics should be given; these should be such as to include activity against methicillin-resistant staphylococci and aerobic Gram-negative rods. Antibiotic treatment can be rationalized according to culture results.

Many authors recommend treatment with intravenous antibiotics for 6 weeks. Outpatient intravenous therapy may make this more acceptable to the patient and the surgeon and to health economists. It is unclear whether prolonging antibiotics beyond this point affects the natural history. When long-term antibiotics are opted for (e.g. when revision surgery would carry a high risk), patients need careful supervision because of potential drug allergies and other side effects.

A similar protocol is recommended for acute presentations of hematogenous seeding. In all cases, the key features associated with a good outcome appear to be:
- the carrying out of a thorough debridement early after the onset of infection;

The clinical context is helpful in interpreting plain film changes, as infection is generally associated with early failure and with more rapid loosening. For prosthetic joints, arthrography combined with aspiration for microscopy and culture may be useful for determining the extent of loosening and it may even detect loosening that is not apparent on the plain radiograph. If pain is immediately relieved by the installation of local anesthetic, the prosthesis is likely to be loose. More elaborate methods of imaging have been disappointing. Metal artifact renders CT scanning and MRI of little value. Technetium scanning is sensitive but not specific and although indium-labelled white cells, gallium citrate or labelled immunoglobulin scans all have their supporters, there is no widely applicable and robust test with high sensitivity and specificity.[12,13,15]

Molecular diagnosis, using the polymerase chain reaction to detect bacterial DNA, offers the advantage of speed, but has not be validated as a diagnostic test and does not provide antibiotic sensitivities, even if bacterial DNA is detected.

Pathology has a useful role to play in the analysis of tissue specimens when these can be obtained. In the absence of inflammatory joint disease, the presence of neutrophils is indicative of infection. Different authors have set different limits for an abnormal number of neutrophils, ranging from 5 cells per high power field to 1 cell per high power field, averaged over at least 10 fields. Often, however, the histologic changes are focal, with some specimens negative and others showing unequivocal early

- infection with a sensitive organism (poorer outcomes occur with *S. aureus* and aerobic Gram-negative rods);
- the absence of a draining sinus; and
- a soundly fixed prosthesis.

If wound breakdown is a feature, implant salvage will also require the prompt restoration of soft tissue cover to prevent secondary colonization with other, more resistant flora. Plastic surgery may be necessary to cover large defects with free or rotational flaps, which obliterate the dead space generated by debridement and provide a mechanism for systemic antibiotics to reach to the site of infection.

In all situations of early infection, there is a need for randomized trials to address the question of whether long-term antibiotic therapy improves outcomes and, if it does, at what cost. In addition, identification of the subgroups that should proceed to immediate revision surgery would save some patients from prolonged and ineffective attempts at salvage treatment.

DELAYED AND LATE INFECTIONS OF PROSTHETIC JOINTS
Excision arthroplasty
If the prosthesis is loose, revision surgery is usually needed. The simplest option is excision arthroplasty, which has a high cure rate provided that the debridement of cement and dead tissue is adequate. In the hip, where a Girdlestone's pseudarthrosis is the result, function is generally very much poorer than with a successfully re-implanted hip. The affected leg is short, requiring a substantial shoe raise, the patient walks with a limp and at least one stick for life and function is particularly poor in patients of above average weight. Excision arthroplasty alone is rarely employed for prosthetic knee infections because it leaves the knee flail and the limb unstable, with the result that an external support is needed for life. Nonetheless, in certain cases where limited demands are placed on the leg and poor bone stock makes re-implantation or fusion unlikely to succeed, this may still be preferable to an above-knee amputation. In the hip, excision arthroplasty is an option in cases where attempted reconstruction is technically unrealistic or poses unacceptable risks of re-infection, other major morbidity or death.

One-stage revision
In one-stage procedures, the excision is followed by immediate re-implantation. Although systemic antibiotics may also be administered, in the largest published experiences of this method, great reliance was placed on a meticulous debridement and the use of gentamicin-impregnated bone cement. The high prevalence of gentamicin resistance among hospital-acquired coagulase-negative staphylococci has led to a decline in the popularity of this strategy.

It should, however, be noted that the benefits to the patient of a successful one-stage revision are enormous, making this a technique that would justify renewed efforts to improve its success. Published success rates vary, depending both on the skill of the surgeon and on the completeness of the follow up, but in the most reliable and largest series, approximately 80–85% of treated implants show no signs of recurrence at 7 years.[27,28]

One-stage revision can still be considered for patients for whom a staged procedure carries unacceptable anesthetic risks and there is prior knowledge of a highly sensitive pathogen. It is less successful if there are resistant organisms involved; furthermore, few surgeons would happily perform this operation in the presence of extensive bone loss, for which bone allografting is often used in reconstruction.

Two-stage revision
In two-stage revision, an excision arthroplasty is combined with intensive antibiotic treatment, often for 6–12 weeks, followed by re-implantation of a new prosthesis. Antibiotics may be administered systemically (intravenously or orally) or locally using antibiotic-impregnated cements. For technical reasons, antibiotic-impregnated cement spacers are usually used in the knee for the maintenance of length and to allow weight bearing; they are less common in the treatment of infected hips but they have been used to allow improved function over a Girdlestone's pseudarthrosis while the patient waits for re-implantation.

Comparative studies between local or systemic routes of antibiotic administration are not available. Local delivery offers obvious advantages of convenience to patient and surgeon without the complications of systemic therapy, but it is necessary to know the infecting flora and antibiotic sensitivities in advance of the excision arthroplasty, and this may necessitate an additional diagnostic procedure. Although again variable, the best results for two-stage revision of both hips and knees appear superior (90% success or greater) to one-stage revision, but these are in noncomparative, nonrandomized studies.[12,24,29] Of the many studies needed, perhaps the most important is to put these two different surgical strategies to the test of a randomized, controlled, multicenter trial, using robust end points including health economic analyses.

Arthrodesis and amputation
The quality of bone stock at the distal femur and proximal tibia or the state of the soft tissues (including the extensor mechanism) may preclude an attempt at re-implantation of a functioning knee prosthesis. In these situations the options are external bracing (see above), a fusion or an above-knee amputation. In all series, a proportion of cases progress to these unsatisfactory outcomes and this proportion rises if the revision implant itself becomes infected.[30] Therefore, the risks should be discussed openly with all patients before knee revision surgery is embarked upon.

Suppressive therapy
For a small group of patients, the pursuit of radical cure and the surgery necessary to achieve it is inappropriate. This group includes the medically unfit patient in whom the risk of an anesthetic and an operation is unacceptable, patients with obvious infection (e.g. with sinus tract drainage or early infection) but a pain-free, mechanically sound implant, and patients in whom excision of a prosthesis would lead to an unreconstructable defect. Such cases may be suitable for long-term antibiotic suppression, particularly when infected with organisms that are sensitive to safe and well-tolerated antibiotics. An advance in this regard may be the recognition that combinations of a 4-quinolone and rifampin (rifampicin) show excellent killing activity inside abscesses, inside cells and in experimental models of biofilms or infected foreign devices. There are encouraging reports of this combination as an adjunct to surgery in the treatment of infections in orthopaedic devices in humans for the salvage of implants.[31,32]

INFECTIONS OF FRACTURE FIXATIONS AND SPINAL INSTRUMENTATION
These pose related but different problems. Internal fixation devices are designed to stabilize the skeleton until mechanical strength is restored biologically by fracture healing or by the incorporation of bone graft. Infection may impair these processes, leading to nonunion, but mechanical instability also appears to play an important role in this. For the purposes of obtaining union or fusion, a stable but infected fracture (with implant retained) may be preferable to an unstable, uninfected fracture, and it is definitely preferable to an unstable, infected fracture. Thus the goal of obtaining radical cure of infection may have to take second place to the need to allow the implant to perform its function (ideally with infection controlled), after which it may be removed and the infection treated definitively.

It follows that the key factor in management is whether or not union or fusion has occurred. Irrespective of the time of presentation, exploration and debridement should be carried out. If the fracture has not united but the implant is mechanically sound, the device can be retained, provided the organisms cultured are sensitive to a suitable antibiotic, the bone at the fracture or fusion site appears viable and soft tissue cover can be obtained. If the implant is loose or substantial amounts of dead bone are present, in which case fracture healing is unlikely, the implant should be removed and stability ensured, preferably with an external fixator. Once multiple samples have been obtained, an empiric antibiotic regimen can be commenced and refined according to results. Infections that are well established before the onset of suppression are liable to relapse once antibiotics are discontinued, whereas success may sometimes be possible if very early infections are treated promptly. Elective implant removal and final debridement of poor-quality tissue once union has occurred has the advantage that the soft tissues (and the patient) are in an optimal state for the procedure while infection is suppressed. Oral suppression need not be stopped before removal of implants (assuming the diagnosis is known). Depending on whether organisms are cultured at the time of implant removal, definitive antibiotic treatment may be offered, but this should include at least 1 month of therapy in order to protect bone wounded by the debridement.

If the fracture or fusion has united, the implant should be removed unless there are compelling reasons not to undertake this, because the likelihood of cure with antibiotics alone is low. Duration of antibiotic therapy following debridement should be as for established chronic osteomyelitis.

REFERENCES

1. Malchau H, Herberts P, Ahnfelt L. Prognosis of total hip replacement in Sweden. Follow-up of 92,675 operations performed between 1978–1990. Acta Orthop Scand 1993;64:497–506.
2. Wymenga AB, van Horn JR, Theeuwes A, Muytjens HL, Sloogg TJJH. Perioperative factors associated with septic arthritis after arthroplasty. Prospective multicenter study of 362 knee and 2651 hip operations. Acta Orthop Scand 1992;63:665–71.
3. Gustilo RB, Anderson JT. Prevention of infection in the treatment of one thousand and twnety five open fractures of long bones: Retrospective and prospective analyses. J Bone Joint Surg [Am] 1976;58A:453–8.
4. Theiss SM, Lonstein JE, Winter RB. Wound infections in reconstructive spinal surgery. Orthop Clin North Am 1996;27:105–10.
5. Christensen GD, Baldassarri L, Simpson WA. Colonization of medical devices by coagulase-negative staphylocci. In: Bisno AI, Waldwogel FA, eds. Infections associated with indwelling medical devices. ASM Press; 1994:45–78.
6. Heilmann C, Schweitzer O, Gerke C, Vanittanakom N, Mack D, Götz F. Molecular basis of intercellular adhesion in the biofilm-forming Staphylococcus epidermidis. Mol Microbiol 1996;20:1083–91.
7. Schurman DJ, Smith RL. Bacterial biofilm and infected biomaterials, prostheses and artificial organs. In: Esterhai JL, Gristina AG, Poss R, eds. Musculoskeletal infection. Park Ridge, II: American Academy of Orthopaedic Surgeons; 1992:133–47.
8. Elek SD, Conen PE. The virulence of Staphylococcus pyogenes for man: a study of the problems of wound infection. Br J Exp Pathol 1957;38:573–86.
9. Panday R, Quinn J, Joyner C, Murray DW, Triffit JT, Athanasou NA. Arthroplasty implant biomaterial particle associated macrophages differentiate into lacunar bone resorbing cells. Ann Rheum Dis 1996;55:388–95.
10. Charosky CB, Bullough PG, Wilson PD. Total hip replacement failures. J Bone Joint Surg [Am] 1973;55A:49–58.
11. Mirra JM, Marder RA, Amstutz HC. The pathology of failed joint arthroplasty. Clin Orthop 1982;170:504–46.
12. Steckelberg JM, Osmon DR. Prosthetic joint infections. In: Bisno AI, Waldwogel FA, eds. Infections associated with indwelling medical devices. ASM Press; 1994:259–90.
13. Gillespie WJ. Prevention and management of infection after total joint replacement. Clin Infect Dis 1997;25:1310–7.
14. Atkins BL, Athanasou N, Deeks JJ, et al. Prospective evaluation of criteria for microbiolgical diagnosis of prosthetic-joint infection at revision arthroplasty. J Clin Microbiology 1998;36(10):2932–9.
15. Spangehl MJ, Younger ASE, Masri BA, Duncan CP. Diagnosis of infection following total hip arthroplasty. Instr Course Lect. Rosemont, Il: American Academy of Orthopaedic Surgeons; 1998;47:285–95.
16. Petty W, Spanier S, Shuster JJ, Silverthorne C. The influence of skeletal implants on incidence of infection. J Bone Joint Surg [Am] 1985;67A:1236–44.
17. Petty W, Spanier S, Shuster JJ. Prevention of infection after total joint replacement. J Bone Joint Surg [Am] 1988;70A:536–9.
18. Fehring TK, McAlister JA. Frozen histologic section as a guide to sepsis in revision joint arthroplasty. Clin Orthop 1994;304:229–37.
19. Athanasou NA, Pandey R, de Steiger R, Crook D, McLardy-Smith P. Diagnosis of infection by frozen section during revision arthroplasty. J Bone Joint Surg [Br] 1995;77B:28–33.
20. Feldman DS, Lonner JH, Desai P, Zuckerman JD. The role of intraoperative frozen sections in revision total joint arthoplasty. J Bone Joint Surg (Am) 1995;77:1807–13.
21. Lachiewicz PF, Roger GD, Thomason HC. Aspiration of the hip joint before revision total joint arthroplasty. J Bone Joint Surg (Am) 1996;78:749–54.
22. Kristinsson KG, Hope PG, Norman P, Elson RA. Deep infection of cemented total hip arthroplasties caused by coagulase negative staphylococci. J Bone Joint Surg [Br] 1989;71B:851–5.
23. Kamme C, Lindberg L. Aerobic and anaerobic bacteria in deep infections after total hip arthroplasty. Clin Orthop 1981;154:201–7.
24. Tsukayama DT, Estrada R, Gustilo RB. Infection after total hip arthroplasty. J Bone Joint Surg [Am] 1996;78A:512–23.
25. Schoifet SD, Morrey BF. Treatment of infection after total knee arthroplasty by debridement with retention of the components. J Bone Joint Surg [Am] 1990;72A:1383–90.
26. Brandt CM, Sistrunk WW, Duiffy MC, et al. Staphylococcus aureus prosthetic joint infection treated with debridement and prosthesis retention. Clin Infect Dis 1997;24:914–9.
27. Buchholz HW, Elson RA, Engelbrecht E, Lodenkamper H, Rottger J, Siegel A. Management of deep infection of total hip replacement. J Bone Joint Surg [Br] 1981;63B:342–53.
28. Raut VV, Siney PD, Wroblewski BM. One-stage revision of total hip arthroplasty for deep infection. Clin Orthop 1995;321:202–7.
29. McDonald DJ, Fitzgerald RH, Ilstrup DM. Two-stage reconstruction of a total hip arthroplasty because of infection. J Bone Joint Surg [Am] 1989;71A:828–34.
30. Hanssen AD, Trousdale RT, Osmon DR. Patient outcome with reinfection following reimplantation for the infected total knee arthroplasty. Clin Orthop 1995;321:55–67.
31. Widmer AF, Gaechter A, Ochsner PE, Zimmerli W. Antimicrobial treatment of orthopaedic implant-related infections with rifampin combinations. Clin Infect Dis 1992;14:1251–3.
32. Drancourt M, Stein A, Argenson JN, Zannier A, Curvale G, Raoult D. Oral rifampin plus ofloxacin for treatment of Staphylococcus aureus-infected orthopaedic implants. Antimicrob Agents Chemother 1993;37:1214–8.

chapter
45

Lyme Disease

Daniel W Rahn

HISTORY

The early elucidation of Lyme disease by Allen Steere and his colleagues at Yale is one of the most fascinating stories of clinical and epidemiologic investigation in recent years. In November 1975, a resident of Old Lyme, Connecticut, informed the Connecticut State Health Department that 12 children from that rural community of 5000 residents had been diagnosed as having juvenile rheumatoid arthritis. Almost concurrently, a second mother from Old Lyme informed physicians at the Yale Rheumatology Clinic that she, her husband, two of their children and several neighbors had all developed arthritis.[1] A surveillance system organized by Dr Steere, Dr Malawista and others revealed that 51 people (39 children and 12 adults) in three contiguous rural communities had developed arthritis between July 1972 and May 1976. Most had recurrent brief attacks of pain and swelling (median 1 week) involving one large joint or a few. The knee was the joint most predominantly affected. In 55% of cases, the first attack of arthritis occurred between June and September, and 13 (25%) had noted a peculiar, expanding, erythematous skin lesion a median of 4 weeks before the onset of arthritis. One recalled being bitten by a tick at the site of the skin lesion. The skin lesion was suspected of being erythema chronicum migrans (EM), which had been described by Afzelius in 1910 and was known to occur in Europe, where it had been associated with the bite of the sheep tick, *Ixodes ricinus*[2] and was suspected of being caused by infection with a transmissible agent.[3]

In addition, new features of the illness uncovered included self-limited cardiac conduction abnormalities and a variety of neurologic abnormalities, including Bell's palsy, sensory radiculopathy and lymphocytic meningitis. Cardiac abnormalities had not been previously associated with EM but neurologic abnormalities were well documented. In 1922 Garin-Bujadoux had reported sensory radiculitis with meningeal signs following EM,[4] and in 1944 Bannwarth had described patients with pain, paresthesia, Bell's palsy and lymphocytic pleocytosis following a tick bite and EM.[5] The new name Lyme disease was coined, recognizing the multisystem nature of the illness.

In subsequent reports, the cardiac conduction abnormalities and neurologic manifestations of Lyme disease were characterized more fully.[6,7] Epidemiologic studies revealed an ixodid tick, *Ixodes scapularis*, a newly described member of the *I. ricinus* complex in the region where cases of Lyme disease were occurring,[8,9] strengthening the tick vector hypothesis. Antibiotic trials demonstrated that EM resolved faster and that later manifestations were usually prevented in people who were given penicillin or tetracycline,[10] suggesting a bacterial agent transmitted by the tick vector. Subsequently, in 1982, Burgdorfer *et al.* reported the isolation of a spirochete from *Ixodes dammini* ticks collected on Shelter Island, an area known to be endemic for Lyme disease.[11] This organism, subsequently characterized as a *Borrelia* sp. and named *Borrelia burgdorferi*, was cultured from *I. scapularis* ticks in Connecticut and from skin lesions, blood and meningitic cerebrospinal fluid of Lyme disease patients in Connecticut. It was also linked serologically to the disease.[12] These data collectively established it definitively as the cause of Lyme disease.

EPIDEMIOLOGY

Lyme disease is the commonest vector-borne disease in the USA[13] and occurs widely throughout Europe and the former Soviet Union.[14] The infecting organism, *B. burgdorferi*, is maintained in and transmitted by ticks of the *I. ricinus* complex, including *I. scapularis* in north-east and north–central USA, *Ixodes pacificus* on the west coast of the USA, *I. ricinus* in Europe and the western Soviet Union, and *Ixodes persulcatus* in Asia (see Chapter 2.4).

The illness is increasing in both incidence and recognition, with more than 110,000 cases reported in the USA between 1982 and 1997. The known endemic range is expanding, but the precise incidence and geographic spread are uncertain due to difficulties in diagnosis and disagreement regarding diagnostic criteria. A National Surveillance Case Definition was adopted in the USA in 1990, to establish uniform diagnostic criteria for surveillance (see Fig. 45.1). Cases have been reported from 48 states in the continental USA. However, despite this apparent wide geographic spread, over 90% of cases have been reported from 100 counties in 10 states in the north-east, upper midwest and Pacific coastal regions.[13] Even within these endemic states, the regional distribution is highly variable. The recent upsurge in cases in the USA may be explained by the reforestation of land used for farming a generation ago, creating environments suitable for deer (for *I. scapularis*, at least, deer are important for maintenance of the tick lifecycle),[15] and outward migration of residential areas from cities into these rural areas.

There are no known racial or sexual predilections but most cases have occurred in whites. Although cases have occurred at all ages, individuals who are active outdoors in spring and summer months are at greatest risk.[4,16] In north-east and north–central USA, where *I. scapularis* is the primary vector, most cases begin in summer with the occurrence of EM. Those people who do not manifest this marker of disease onset may come to medical attention months later with one or more symptoms of disseminated disease.

The seasonal variation of onset in temperate climatic zones is explained by the ecology of the predominant tick vectors. Among the ixodid tick vectors, the lifecycle and feeding habits of *I. scapularis* are best understood (see Figs 45.2 & 45.3). This tick has a three-stage lifecycle (larva, nymph and adult) that spans 2 years. Larvae hatch from fertilized eggs in late spring and feed once for 2 or more days in midsummer. Preferred hosts include a broad range of small mammals. The next spring they molt into nymphs, and feed again for 3 or 4 days, with the same host range. After this second blood meal, the nymphs molt into adults. Adult *I. scapularis* has a narrower host range, with a preference for deer. Mating occurs on deer, and the female deposits her eggs and the cycle begins anew.[17] In endemic areas, 30% or more of nymphs may be infected with *B. burgdorferi*; the rate of infection in adult ticks may be even higher, but infection rates in unfed larvae are less than 1%,[18] a pattern suggesting that ticks acquire *B. burgdorferi* from a reservoir host in the environment rather than from congenital transmission. The white-footed mouse, *Peromyscus leucopus*, is the primary reservoir host for *I. scapularis*.[19]

An enzootic cycle of infection is maintained through passage of *B. burgdorferi* back and forth between ticks and their hosts. Infected nymphal

Fig. 45.1 Lyme disease: a summary of the US National Surveillance case definition.

LYME DISEASE: US NATIONAL SURVEILLANCE CASE DEFINITION	
Definition	A systemic, tick-borne disease with protean manifestations: dermatologic, rheumatologic, neurologic and cardiac abnormalities. The initial skin lesion, erythema migrans, is the best clinical marker (occurs in 60–80% of patients)
Case definition	1. Erythema migrans present *or* 2. At least one late manifestation and laboratory confirmation of infection
General definitions	
1. Erythema migrans (EM)	• Skin lesion typically beginning as a red macule/papule and expanding over days or weeks to form a large round lesion, often with partial central clearing • A solitary lesion must measure at least 5cm; secondary lesions may also occur • An annular erythematous lesion developing within several hours of a tick bite represents a hypersensitivity reaction and does not qualify as erythema migrans • The expanding EM lesion is usually accompanied by other acute symptoms, particularly fatigue, fever, headache, mildly stiff neck, arthralgias and myalgias, which are typically intermittent • Diagnosis of EM must be made by a physician • Laboratory confirmation is recommended for patients with no known exposure
2. Late manifestations These include any of the opposite *when an alternative explanation is not found*	**Musculoskeletal system** • Recurrent, brief attacks (lasting weeks or months) of objective joint swelling in one or a few joints, sometimes followed by chronic arthritis in one or a few joints • Manifestations not considered to be criteria for diagnosis include chronic progressive arthritis not preceded by brief attacks, chronic symmetric polyarthritis, or arthralgias, myalgias or fibromyalgia syndromes alone **Nervous system** • Lymphocytic meningitis, cranial neuritis, particularly facial palsy (may be bilateral), radiculoneuropathy or, rarely, encephalomyelitis alone or in combination • Encephalomyelitis must be confirmed by evidence of antibody production against *Borrelia burgdorferi* in cerebrospinal fluid (CSF), shown by a higher titer of antibody in the CSF than in serum • Headache, fatigue, paresthesia or mildly stiff neck alone are not accepted as criteria for neurologic involvement **Cardiovascular system** • Acute-onset, high-grade (2nd- or 3rd-degree) atrioventricular conduction defects that resolve in days to weeks and are sometimes associated with myocarditis • Palpitations, bradycardia, bundle-branch block or myocarditis alone are not accepted as criteria for cardiovascular involvement
3. Exposure	• Exposure to wooded, brushy or grassy areas (potential tick habitats) in an endemic county no more than 30 days before the onset of erythema migrans • A history of tick bite is not required
4. Endemic county	• A county in which at least two definite cases have been previously acquired or in which a tick vector has been shown to be infected with *B. burgdorferi*
5. Laboratory confirmation	• Isolation of the spirochete from tissue or body fluid *or* • Detection of diagnostic levels of IgM or IgG antibodies to the spirochete in the serum or the CSF *or* • Detection of an important change in antibody levels in paired acute and convalescent serum samples • States may separately determine the criteria for laboratory confirmation and diagnostic levels of antibody • Syphilis and other known biologic causes of false-positive serologic test results should be excluded, when laboratory confirmation is based on serologic testing alone

ticks transmit *B. burgdorferi* to mice, which serve as a reservoir from which uninfected larvae may acquire infecting organisms. In this manner, a high rate of infection can be maintained in the tick population once the organism, ticks, mice and deer are all present in the environment.

The establishment and maintenance of an enzootic cycle requires a competent reservoir host in addition to a tick vector. Variation in vector–host relationships provide the primary explanation for wide regional variation in the rate of infection in the tick population in California,[20] the south-east USA[21] and the north-east USA.

Lyme disease occurs when an infected tick (most often a nymph) feeds on a susceptible individual and transmits the causative spirochete.[16] As yet unknown factors influence the risk of developing Lyme disease after a bite by an infected tick. In published studies, the risk of developing Lyme disease after a bite by an infected tick has been less than the rate of infection in the tick vectors alone would predict. The low risk of transmission after a known tick bite may relate to the duration of tick attachment before removal.[22,23] A tick attached for less than 24 hours has a low likelihood of transmitting *B. burgdorferi*.

Other modes of transmission have been postulated including transfusion of infected blood products[24] and biting flies,[25,26] but evidence strongly favors ixodid ticks as the primary and, most likely, exclusive vector of Lyme disease. Congenital transmission has been reported,[27,28] but the evidence regarding clinical disease resulting from transplacental transfer is inconclusive.

CLINICAL FEATURES

LOCALIZED EARLY DISEASE

Lyme disease begins with the appearance of a characteristic skin lesion, EM, at the site of a tick bite, although most patients are unaware of

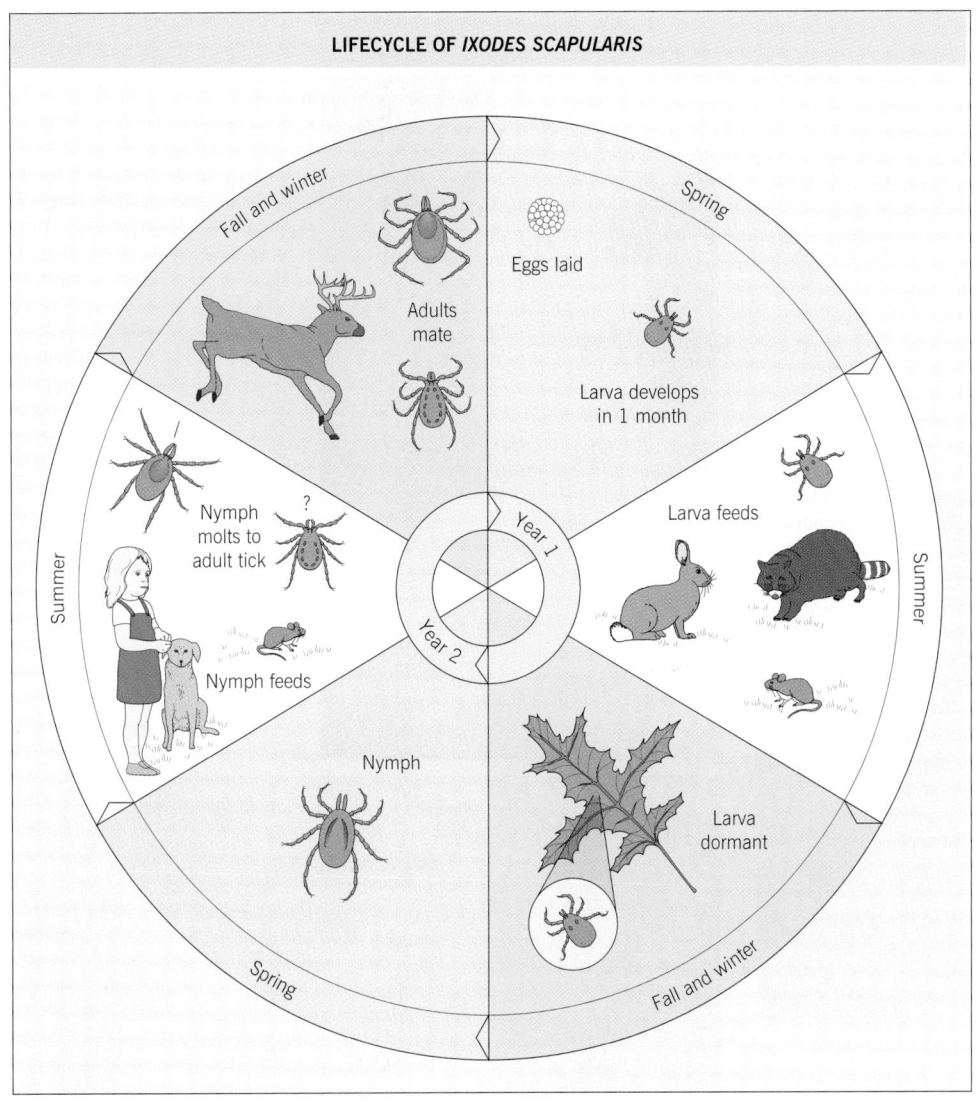

LIFECYCLE OF *IXODES SCAPULARIS*

Fig. 45.2 Lifecycle of *Ixodes scapularis* (also known as *I. dammini*). The lifecycle spans 2 years. Eggs hatch in the spring; six-legged larvae develop and feed once in the summer, acquiring *Borrelia burgdorferi* from their preferred host, the white-footed mouse. Next spring, the larvae molt into eight-legged nymphs, which feed once: mice are the preferred host, humans not being necessary for the ticks' lifecycle. The nymphs molt into adult male and female ticks; mating often occurs while the female feeds on a deer, and the male may remain on the deer, the female falling off and then laying eggs. Adapted, with permission, from an illustration by Nancy Lou Makris in Rahn and Malawista.[29]

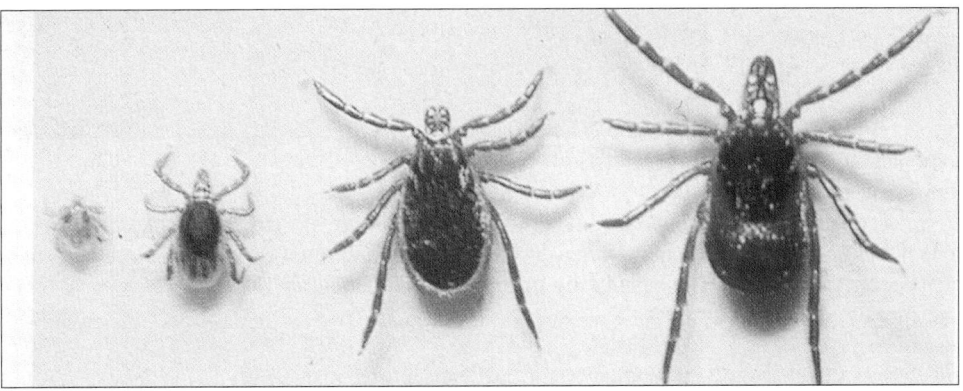

Fig. 45.3 *Ixodes scapularis.* Larva, nymph, adult male and adult female. Courtesy of Pfizer Central Research.

being bitten (Figs 45.4–45.7). In perhaps one-third of cases, however, this skin lesion is missed or absent and patients present with symptoms of later, disseminated disease. The interval between tick bite and appearance of EM varies from a few days to a month (median 7 days). The lesion begins as an erythematous papule and expands over several days to achieve a median diameter of 15cm; favored sites are the groin, buttock, popliteal fossa and axilla. Erythema migrans lesions are generally annular with a sharply demarcated outer border and an erythematous or bluish hue. They are warm to the touch, flat and minimally or not tender. Lesions may show partial central clearing but may also be indurated or even necrotic. This cutaneous lesion is the best clinical marker of Lyme disease.[16] An annular erythema following a tick bite is insufficient evidence for a definitive diagnosis of Lyme disease, however, especially in nonendemic areas. Thorough study of possible early Lyme disease in Missouri and North Carolina has revealed that many

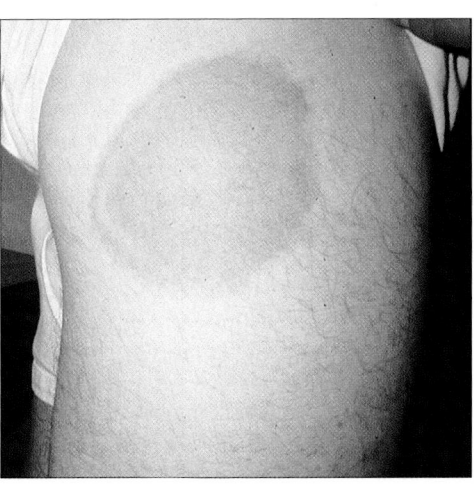

Fig. 45.4 Erythema migrans. A typical annular, flat, erythematous lesion with a sharply demarcated border and partial central healing. Courtesy of Dr Steven Luger.

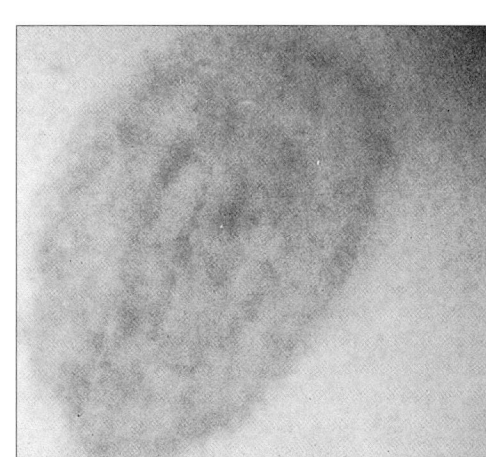

Fig. 45.5 Erythema migrans. A lesion with variation in color and a target-like appearance. The bite site is visible in the center. Courtesy of Dr Steven Luger, Old Lyme, Connecticut, USA.

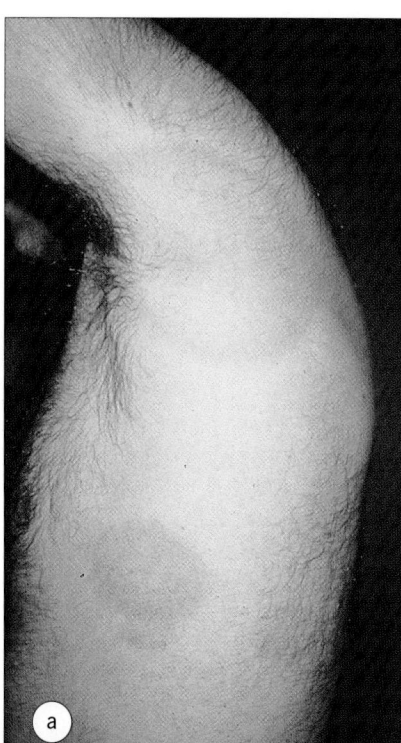

Fig. 45.7 Multiple erythema migrans lesions. Lateral (a) and posterior (b) views of the same patient with multiple erythematous macules of EM. Secondary lesions result from hematogenous spread. They may occur anywhere in the body. Secondary lesions are usually of uniform color and lack in duration. Courtesy of Dr Steven Luger.

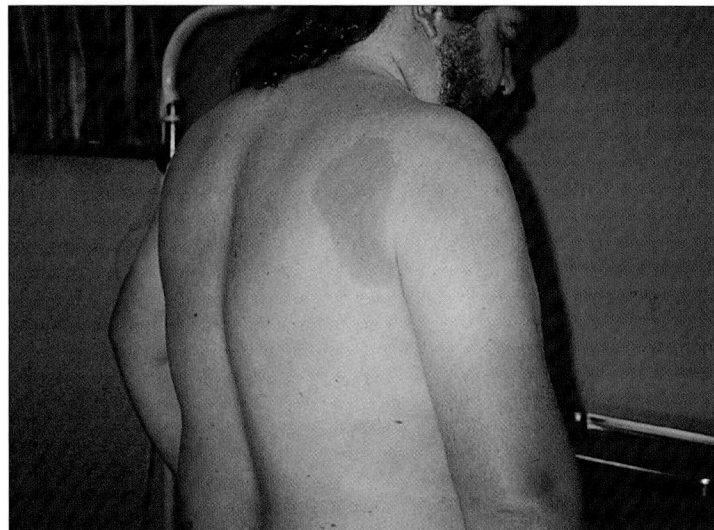

Fig. 45.6 Erythema migrans. A lesion with a dusky center, a common variant. Courtesy of Dr Steven Luger.

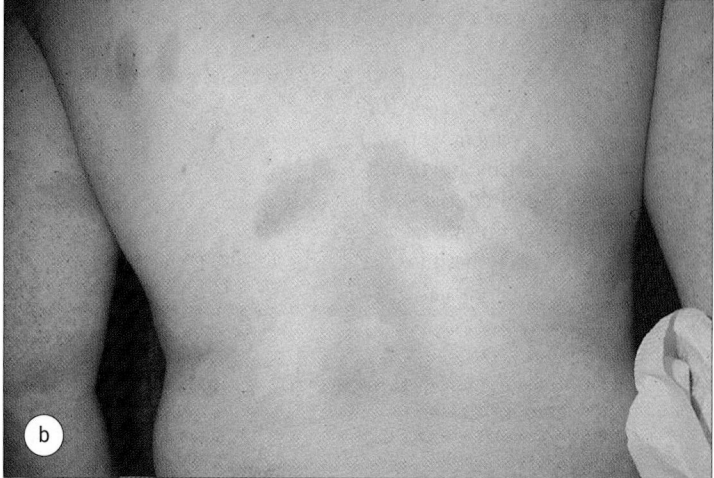

annular rashes associated with tick-bite in these regions are not due to *B. burgdorferi*.[30,31]

EARLY DISSEMINATED DISEASE

Within several days of the appearance of EM, many patients develop evidence of dissemination of their infection by the appearance of prominent systemic symptoms, the occurrence of multiple secondary skin lesions, or both. Malaise, fatigue, lethargy, headache, fever and chills, arthralgia and myalgia are particularly common, each occurring in one-half or more of patients. Symptoms may fluctuate rapidly and vary from a flu-like syndrome to a meningitis-like illness from day to day.

Secondary skin lesions resemble primary lesions but they are usually smaller, show less expansion with time and lack indurated centers. They may occur anywhere on the body, but the palms and soles are generally spared. These manifestations of early disseminated infection appear to be more common in the USA than in Europe and may reflect biologic differences in infecting organisms. Erythema migrans, secondary skin lesions and associated symptoms resolve, even without antibiotic therapy, a median of 28 days after onset, but recurrent crops of evanescent lesions may occur, and fatigue, intermittent musculoskeletal pain and headaches may persist for months.

DISSEMINATED DISEASE

After resolution of the signs and symptoms of early disease, some patients (20% in one series)[32] experience a long-lasting spontaneous remission, which may reflect cure. Most, however, subsequently develop other disease manifestations, with predominant involvement of the heart, nervous system and joints, although case reports have described involvement of multiple organs, including the liver,[33]

subcutaneous tissue,[34] muscle,[35] eye structures[36] and spleen.[37] More than one organ system may be (and often is) affected simultaneously or sequentially in an individual patient.

Carditis

Fewer than 10% of patients with untreated early Lyme disease develop carditis, generally a few weeks to a few months after EM.[8] However, palpitations from an arrhythmia or unexplained syncope from high-degree atrioventricular block may be the presenting manifestation of Lyme disease.[38] The primary clinical manifestation of Lyme carditis is heart block, which may fluctuate from first-degree to complete heart block over minutes to hours and generally resolves spontaneously in a few weeks or sooner, even in untreated patients.[6] Although temporary pacing is frequently required, permanent pacing is rarely needed.[38]

Much less commonly, congestive heart failure has been linked to Lyme disease. A case report suggested that Lyme carditis might be a cause of chronic dilated cardiomyopathy.[39] Endomyocardial biopsy and electrophysiologic testing have revealed direct spirochetal invasion of cardiac muscle and widespread abnormalities of cardiac conduction.[40]

Neurologic manifestations

Neurologic abnormalities were recognized as being associated with ixodid tick bites and EM in Europe many years before the initial description of Lyme disease in the USA.[4,5] In the early series of Lyme disease cases described in the USA, frank neurologic abnormalities, including cranial neuropathy, meningitis, radiculoneuropathy, myelopathy and encephalopathy, occurred in 15% of patients. Neurologic symptoms generally began a few weeks after EM (median 4 weeks), although some patients presented with neurologic manifestations alone.[7,16] Subtle neurologic complaints without objective deficits (headache, irritability, paresthesias, photophobia and lethargy) may accompany early disease dissemination and represent the mildest end of the spectrum of neurologic Lyme disease. Multiple neurologic abnormalities may coexist or occur sequentially but, for clarity, they are described here as distinct syndromes.

The characteristic features of Lyme meningitis were described in a series of 38 patients from Connecticut. The usual clinical picture includes headache, neck stiffness and lymphocytic pleocytosis in cerebrospinal fluid (CSF).[41] Peripheral or cranial neuropathy (particularly Bell's palsy) occurred in 32% and 50% of these cases, respectively. As is the case for idiopathic Bell's palsy, residual facial weakness occurs in some cases of facial palsy associated with Lyme disease.[42]

Peripheral nerve abnormalities may involve sensory and motor nerve roots, plexi and both motor and sensory nerve fibers.[3,43,44] Meningitis and radiculoneuropathy often wax and wane for weeks to months but ultimately resolve spontaneously.

Before elucidation of the bacterial cause of Lyme disease, corticosteroids were used with some success to treat the symptoms associated with meningitis, cranial neuropathy and radiculoneuropathy, suggesting that the clinical features associated with these syndromes result from a reversible inflammatory mechanism rather than direct tissue destruction by *B. burgdorferi*. *Borrelia burgdorferi* has been isolated from the CSF of a patient whose only complaint was tinnitus,[45] and has been demonstrated by polymerase chain reaction (PCR) in patients with symptoms limited to headache, Bell's palsy or paresthesia, indicating that the symptoms associated with central nervous system (CNS) infection may be minimal.[46] The emergence of subtle neurologic manifestations years after onset of Lyme disease also supports the possibility of latent persistent infection in the CNS (see 'Late neurologic syndromes').

Rarely, cases of demyelinating encephalopathy mimicking multiple sclerosis have been reported.[47,48]

Arthritis

Most people who have untreated Lyme disease develop arthritis. Brief, intermittent attacks of migratory musculoskeletal pain commonly begin while EM is present and may persist for months before the appearance of overt arthritis. Frank arthritis occurs in 60% of patients in the USA, at a median of 6 months after EM, but, as with other symptoms of disseminated disease, arthritis may be the presenting manifestation of Lyme disease.[49] Although the clinical expression varies, patients most often experience brief recurrent attacks of monoarticular or oligoarticular inflammatory arthritis involving large joints, particularly the knee.[1,32,50] Effusions may be massive (100ml or more), causing popliteal cysts, which may rupture and result in a pseudothrombophlebitis syndrome. Attacks last a few days to a few weeks and over time (months to years) decrease in severity, frequency and duration.[32] Arthritis has been reported to be milder in children than in adults.[51,52] Polyarthritis is decidedly uncommon. Synovitis becomes chronic in 20% of cases (see 'Chronic arthritis').

LATE (PERSISTENT) DISEASE

After the disseminated stage of Lyme disease during which multiorgan involvement occurs and symptoms are often changing and self-limited, inflammation may become chronic and persistent in some tissues. This has been been called 'late Lyme disease'. Late Lyme disease may involve the CNS, the joints and (particularly in Europe) the skin. Information is still emerging on this patient group. It is as yet unclear whether the clinical manifestations of late Lyme disease result from persistent infection in all cases.

Late neurologic syndromes

Both a mild, predominantly sensory, peripheral neuropathy and subtle encephalopathy may occur months to years after onset of Lyme disease.[44,53,54] Peripheral nerve complaints may be limited to paresthesia and require careful electrodiagnostic studies for documentation. The diagnosis of encephalopathy hinges on the presence of cognitive deficits involving primarily short-term memory and concentration. Chronic fatigue, headaches and sleep disturbance may accompany these abnormalities, but these are not sufficient, without a documented neurologic deficit, to support the diagnosis of neurologic Lyme disease. Rarely, severe encephalomyelopathy has occurred with impairment of higher cortical function, seizures and spinal cord lesions.

Chronic arthritis

Arthritis becomes chronic in 20% of patients who have untreated Lyme disease, resulting in a syndrome that is clinically indistinguishable from other forms of monoarticular or oligoarticular inflammatory arthritis. However, chronic Lyme arthritis is preceded by recurrent brief attacks of joint inflammation in most cases. The knee is by far the most commonly affected joint. Immunogenetic factors, particularly HLA, may predict which people are at highest risk of developing chronic Lyme arthritis.[55] Even chronic Lyme arthritis may eventually remit spontaneously. Only a minority of patients develop radiographic evidence of erosions of cartilage or bone.[56] There have been no unequivocal cases of symmetric, peripheral, polyarticular, inflammatory arthritis with joint destruction resulting from Lyme disease. Differentiation from rheumatoid arthritis is rarely a problem.

Chronic skin involvement

Chronic skin involvement (acrodermatitis chronicum atrophicans) as a late manifestation of Lyme disease occurs primarily in Europe.[57] It usually occurs on the acral portion of an extremity and is characterized by violaceous discoloration and swelling of involved skin, often at a site where EM occurred years earlier. The lesion eventually becomes atrophic (see Fig. 45.8). Acrodermatitis chronicum atrophicans is thought to result from local persistence of *B. burgdorferi*, which has been isolated from a lesion 10 years after onset.[58] Morphea-like lesions have also been described.[57]

INVESTIGATIONS

It is often difficult to diagnose Lyme disease definitively because of the variation in clinical presentation and course, and because of the limitations of currently available diagnostic assays. The National Surveillance Case Definition of Lyme disease developed in the USA (see Fig. 45.1) requires either the presence of EM or a definite late manifestation of Lyme disease combined with laboratory confirmation of infection in a person who has had opportunity to be exposed to the causative agent. Definitive laboratory confirmation requires isolation of the causative organism from clinically involved tissue, but this is rarely achievable in clinical practice. Demonstration of specific serologic immune responsiveness against *B. burgdorferi* has been accepted as a substitute for bacteriologic isolation. Because the sensitivity and specificity of many tests has been poor,[59–61] Western blot confirmation of all positive and equivocal results is recommended.[62] The key to diagnosing Lyme disease rests with recognition of the characteristic clinical features of the illness. Laboratory testing should only be used for confirmation.

The laboratory abnormalities associated with early Lyme disease reflect the inflammatory nature of the illness. When the infection is localized to a single skin lesion, blood tests are typically normal. As the infection spreads, with development of systemic symptoms and secondary skin lesions, there may be a mild leukocytosis, anemia,

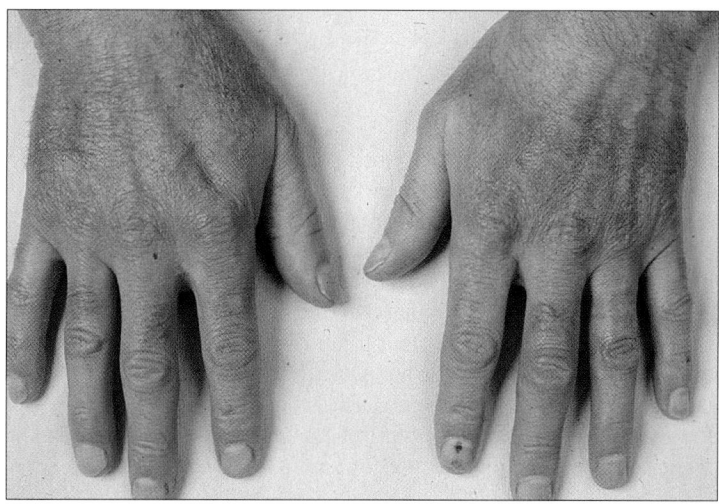

Fig. 45.8 Acrodermatitis chronicum atrophicans. Typical inflammatory bluish-red lesions of acrodermatitis chronicum atrophicans. Lesions usually occur on acral portions of extremities. Courtesy of Dr Eva Asbrink.

elevation in the erythrocyte sedimentation rate, microscopic hematuria, elevation in liver enzymes and elevation in total serum IgM (which mirrors the specific IgM immune response).[16] These abnormalities resolve spontaneously when this phase of illness remits.

Subsequent localization of inflammation to specific target organs results in abnormalities of organ-specific tests. Patients who have carditis have fluctuating atrioventricular block and occasionally more generalized repolarization abnormalities, including ST-segment and T-wave changes on electrocardiogram.[6] If carditis affects ventricular performance, the chest radiograph may reveal cardiomegaly, and cardiac ultrasonography and radionuclide ventriculography may reveal impaired ventricular performance.

The laboratory hallmark of Lyme meningitis is a lymphocytic pleocytosis (generally a few to a few hundred cells)[43] in the CSF; the CSF protein may be elevated and, in protracted cases, the ratio of IgG to albumin may be elevated and oligoclonal bands may be present, reflecting the immunologic component of the inflammatory process within the CNS.[44]

Attacks of arthritis result in the accumulation of inflammatory joint fluid containing a few hundred to 50,000 white blood cells, mostly polymorphonuclear, elevation in protein and normal glucose.[50] Radiographs of affected joints most often show only soft tissue swelling but, when joint inflammation has persisted for many months, there may be pannus formation and erosions of underlying cartilage and bone.[56] Some patients develop enthesopathy with calcifications of tendon and ligament attachment sites.

Cognitive deficits associated with late neurologic involvement may be quantified by neuropsychologic testing, a very helpful modality in the formal assessment of cognitive complaints.[53,54] A depressive overlay is often present, but findings should also reveal an organic encephalopathy primarily affecting short-term memory. Peripheral neuropathy and radiculoneuropathy cause abnormalities on electromyography and, less often, abnormalities of peripheral nerve conduction;[44,54] sensory fibers are more frequently affected than motor fibers. Although these findings on tests of central and peripheral nervous system function are not specific for Lyme disease, abnormal findings indicate a definite disorder of the nervous system, and the combination of central and peripheral nerve abnormalities characteristic of Lyme disease is uncommon in other diseases.

Specific laboratory confirmation may be sought through either direct or indirect means. Efforts at direct confirmation have included culture of affected tissue, employing PCR on skin, urine, joint fluid, blood or CSF to amplify specific gene sequences unique to *B. burgdorferi*, and antigen testing of urine.[63] Although the causative organism has been cultured from affected skin,[12,58,64] blood,[65,66]

CSF[12,45] and joint fluid,[67] the rarity with which it has been isolated limits the usefulness of culture. Polymerase chain reaction has been validated as a means of identifying the presence of *B. burgdorferi* both *in vitro*[68] and in tick vectors[69] using a variety of primers. Work on human tissues and fluids is in progress,[70–74] but PCR cannot be considered a routine diagnostic test for Lyme disease at present.

Detection of a specific immune response to *B. burgdorferi* remains the best means of confirming the diagnosis of Lyme disease. The first immune response in Lyme disease is mediated by T lymphocytes and is directed against a variety of epitopes.[75,76] This T-lymphocyte response subsequently localizes preferentially to involved tissues.[75,77] Unfortunately, tests to measure this response are not standardized, are technically demanding, require live cells and have varied in sensitivity and specificity.[78] For these reasons, measurement of the T-lymphocyte response cannot be recommended routinely for diagnosis.

The serologic response to *B. burgdorferi* has been well characterized[12,79] (Fig. 45.9). Specific IgM antibody, directed initially primarily against the flagellae of the organism, is detectable a few weeks after disease onset. The response broadens to include additional antigens over time and peaks by 3–6 weeks. Generally IgM antibody falls to within the normal range by 6 months but occasionally it may remain elevated for much longer. Specific IgG antibody is detectable a few weeks after IgM but it may not peak until many months after disease onset. The IgG response is also initially directed primarily against flagellin and broadens with time to include an array of antigens on the outer surface of the organism.

Both immunofluorescence and enzyme-linked immunosorbent assay (ELISA) have been used to detect this antibody response; in general, ELISA is preferable because of better sensitivity, objectivity and reproducibility and because of its adaptability to automated systems. Serology results may be falsely positive or negative for various reasons, so the diagnosis of Lyme disease cannot be made by serologic test results alone. Either immunofluorescence or ELISA may yield false-positive results because of epitopes in the test antigen preparations that are crossreactive with other bacteria.[61] False-positive results may also occur in conditions associated with polyclonal B lymphocyte activation. Specificity is increased by a two-step approach in which all positive or equivocal results are confirmed by Western immunoblotting. This two-step approach was recommended by participants in a national conference on Serologic Diagnosis of Lyme disease held in 1994 under the sponsorship of the Centers for Disease Control and Prevention.[62] A true positive ELISA is associated with immunoreactivity against polypeptides specific for *B. burgdorferi*, reactivity that is absent in the

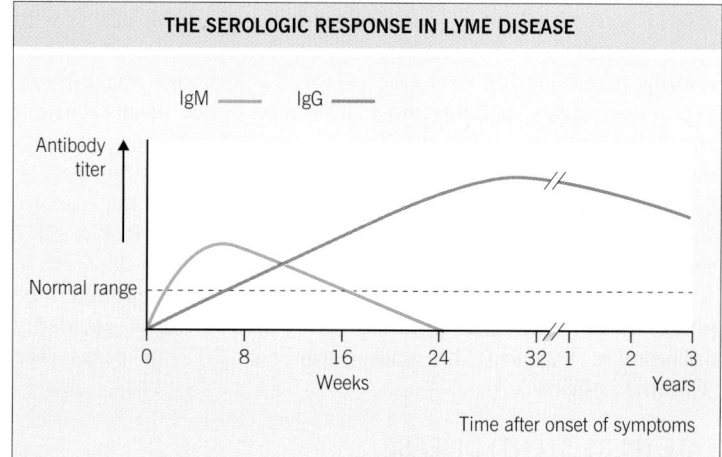

Fig. 45.9 The usual serologic response in Lyme disease. Specific IgM becomes detectable 1–2 weeks after symptom onset and the appearance of erythema migrans. The later appearance of IgG is frequently concurrent with systemic manifestations. IgG is nearly always elevated with late disease. Typically, and even in untreated patients, IgM falls over 4–6 months; persistence for longer than this predicts later manifestations.

various conditions associated with false-positive ELISA results. The currently recommended criteria for a positive Western blot are given in Figure 45.10.

One special circumstance deserves mention. Antibiotic therapy administered early in the course of Lyme disease may result in a negative serology by curing the infection and eliminating antigen before systemic immune challenge.[80] One series indicated, however, that infection may persist after early antibiotic therapy despite persistently negative serologies.[76] These limitations notwithstanding, the greatest problem with serologic testing for Lyme disease results from interlaboratory variation. Standardization of procedures and performance as recommended by the Centers for Disease Control and Prevention is essential before serologic response can be used reliably as a screening tool for Lyme disease. At best, serologic testing can only indicate immunologic exposure, not ongoing infection.

Measurement of immunoreactivity in CSF is a useful adjunct in the diagnosis of CNS Lyme disease.[81,82] To have diagnostic value, a CSF index should be calculated comparing the ratios of specific antibody to total immunoglobulin in CSF and serum. A specific antibody response in CSF is not found uniformly in cases meeting other clinical criteria for CNS Lyme disease in the USA, but it is helpful if positive.

Until more specific serologic tests based on recombinant antigens are developed,[83] culture techniques are improved, or tests based on the PCR or antigen detection are available routinely, caution must be exercised in the use of diagnostic tests for Lyme disease. Serologic testing should be ordered only when the diagnosis is suspected from suggestive clinical data; in this circumstance, a positive serology and Western blot performed in a laboratory with high performance standards should be considered confirmatory of the diagnosis. As a corollary, a negative result should lead to serious doubt of the diagnosis. If testing is ordered indiscriminantly, many false-positive results must be expected, thus diminishing the predictive value of a positive test.

DIFFERENTIAL DIAGNOSIS

Erythema migrans is the classic skin lesion of Lyme disease and, in its typical appearance, can be confused with little else. However, atypical presentations may lead to confusion.[84] Not all annular erythemas associated with tick bites are indicative of Lyme disease, so particular caution must be exercised in nonendemic areas.[30,31]

Lesions with indurated centers may be confused with cellulitis, and those with necrotic centers may look like spider bites, but EM lesions are generally minimally tender or nontender. Secondary skin lesions may be confused with erythema multiforme, but mucosal lesions do not occur and palms and soles are generally spared in Lyme disease. Secondary skin lesions may also have an urticarial appearance. Erythema migrans lesions are generally nonpruritic, however, and other features of disseminated early Lyme disease aid in distinguishing it from a generalized allergic reaction or a systemic condition associated with generalized urticaria, such as the prodromal phase of hepatitis B.

An EM-like illness has recently been described in Missouri and North Carolina. The skin lesions in this illness are always single and are associated with *Amblyomma americanum*, a tick not known to transmit Lyme disease. Patients do not develop immunoreactivity against *B. burgdorferi*, and skin biopsy specimens have been negative for *B. burgdorferi* in culture and by PCR.[30,31] The importance of this syndrome is that it demonstrates that EM-like skin lesions alone occurring in a patient in a nonendemic region are not sufficient to support a diagnosis of Lyme disease.

In later stages, Lyme disease may mimic a variety of cardiac, neurologic and arthritic disorders. Carditis can be confused with subacute bacterial endocarditis or acute rheumatic fever, but valvular lesions do not occur in Lyme disease. Blood cultures are negative.

The most helpful diagnostic feature of neurologic Lyme disease is the frequent simultaneous or sequential involvement of multiple levels of the CNS and peripheral nervous system. Bell's palsy caused by Lyme disease is indistinguishable from idiopathic Bell's palsy, but Lyme disease is one of very few causes of bilateral Bell's palsy (a helpful clue if present) and, by this stage of disease, patients are typically seropositive. Lyme meningitis presents a clinical picture similar to that of viral meningitis, but there is often an antecedent history of EM, the course is more protracted and Lyme meningitis is characterized by relapses and remissions. The peripheral neuropathy associated with chronic neurologic Lyme disease mimics other predominantly sensory neuropathies; a history of previous non-neurologic involvement is usually present, however. The rare patients who have demyelinating encephalopathy must be distinguished from patients who have multiple sclerosis; positive serology (particularly if present in CSF) combined with an exposure history is very helpful in this rare circumstance.

The typical Lyme arthritis patient who has monoarticular inflammatory arthritis of a knee has a clinical appearance similar to that of reactive arthritis or septic arthritis. At initial presentation, bacterial infection must always be excluded. The pattern of brief, recurrent attacks is more common in Lyme disease than in either reactive or septic arthritis. Furthermore, patients who have Lyme arthritis are virtually always seropositive.

Patients who have chronic fatigue and nonspecific symptoms (headaches, musculoskeletal pain, back pain, sleep disturbance and mood swings) have often been presumptively diagnosed as having Lyme disease with little or no substantiation of this diagnosis. The diagnosis of Lyme disease should not be made on the basis of nonspecific complaints unsubstantiated by either objective neurologic deficits or inflammation of joints in a pattern known to be due to this illness, particularly if serologic confirmation is lacking. It is particularly important to differentiate fibromyalgia from chronic Lyme disease, as prognosis and response to therapy are quite different.[85]

PATHOGENESIS AND PATHOLOGY

Borrelia burgdorferi has been unequivocally established as being the cause of Lyme disease. Clinical isolates differ in their outer surface protein expression[86,87] and genetic composition.[88] Three different genospecies have been described: *B. burgdorferi* itself, *Borrelia garinii* and *Borrelia afzelii*. All three genospecies have been isolated from patients who have Lyme disease and from ticks of the *I. ricinus* complex. There is some evidence that disease expression in humans may vary depending upon the genospecies of the infecting organism, but this is preliminary at present.

Unlike *Treponema pallidum*, *B. burgdorferi* can be grown in culture

---

WESTERN BLOT CRITERIA

- All serum specimens found to be positive or equivocal by a sensitive enzyme immunoassay or immunofluorescent assay should be tested by a standardized Western blot procedure

- When Western immunoblot is used in the first 4 weeks of illness, both IgM and IgG procedures should be performed

- After the first 4 weeks of illness, IgG alone should be performed

- An IgM blot is considered positive if two of the following three bands are present: 24kDa (OspC), 39kDa (BmpA) and 41kDa (Fla)

- An IgG blot is considered positive if five of the following 10 bands are present: 18, 21 (OspC), 28, 30, 39 (BmpA), 41 (Fla), 45, 58, 66 and 93kDa

Recommendations of the Second National Conference on Serologic Diagnosis of Lyme Disease sponsored by the Centers for Disease Control and Prevention, the Association of State and Territorial Public Health Laboratory Directors and the Michigan Department of Health

Fig. 45.10 Western blot criteria. Centers for Disease Control and Prevention Working Group recommendations for Western blot positivity. Osp, outer surface protein; Fla, flagella.

although specialized medium is required.[11,12] Serial passage in culture alters surface protein expression with loss of pathogenicity in mice,[88] but the specific factors conferring pathogenicity have not yet been identified. *Borrelia burgdorferi* can penetrate endothelial monolayers and survive intracellularly in cultured fibroblasts.[89] The implications for human infection of this intracellular persistence *in vitro* are unclear. Work in progress is providing insight into the mechanisms enabling the organism to cause persistent infection in humans despite a vigorous immune response.

Borrelia burgdorferi has been recovered from tissues or fluids of patients who have Lyme disease. It is most readily isolated by biopsy and culture of EM lesions,[64] but this is rarely indicated clinically. Later in the disease, organisms are scant in histologic sections[90] and have been recovered by culture only in research settings.

Borrelia burgdorferi is transmitted to the skin of the host by an infected tick. The organism may evade eradication through an initially delayed and ineffective immune response. It disseminates preferentially to certain target organs where it engenders an immunologically mediated inflammatory response, with tissue injury occurring as a result of the inflammatory response. Why this lesion becomes persistent in some people and whether live organisms persist in all cases of chronic disease remain to be elucidated.

An important question is how *B. burgdorferi* avoids destruction in the presence of the vigorous specific T-lymphocyte and B-lymphocyte responses that are usually apparent within a few weeks of onset of disease. In humans, the early immune response is directed primarily against a flagellar antigen. Vaccine studies in mice have shown that specific antibodies against this antigen do not protect against subsequent infection. Vaccination with outer surface protein (Osp) A, an immunodominant surface antigen, antibodies to which appear much later in human disease, is protective.[91] It may be that, in human Lyme disease, *B. burgdorferi* is able to establish infection because of an ineffective initial immune response focused primarily against flagellae. Later, when the immune response broadens, infection may be already established and disease may be perpetuated through other mechanisms.

Immunogenetic studies have suggested that HLA-DR4 predisposes to the development of chronic Lyme arthritis and that DR4 is associated with lack of response to antibiotics.[55] Patients who are HLA-DR4 positive and who have treatment-resistant Lyme arthritis also have been shown to have a strong immune response to an epitope on OspA that cross reacts with human lymphocyte function antigen-1 (LFA-1), which may serve as an autoantigen.[92] This evidence suggests a possible autoimmune mechanism for chronic Lyme arthritis through a mechanism involving molecular mimicry between OspA and LFA-1 in HLA DR4 positive individuals. No predictors of chronic neurologic disease have been described as yet. A third potential mechanism through which organisms may evade antibiotic and immune-mediated destruction is by entering human cells.[89]

Histologic studies of affected tissues have provided evidence for immunologically mediated inflammation. Stains of EM lesions reveal a perivascular mononuclear infiltrate and fibrin deposition in the dermis, without epidermal changes except at the site of the bite.[49] Endomyocardial biopsies have revealed similar changes in the heart, with a focal perivascular infiltrate of mononuclear cells and fibrin deposition in both the endocardium and myocardium.[41] Biopsies of affected nerves, although few in number, have shown inflammatory infiltrates around endoneurial and perineurial vessels without vessel necrosis.[93] Both myelinated and unmyelinated fibers may be affected. Hematoxylin and eosin stains of synovium from arthritic joints have revealed synovial lining cell hyperplasia and hypertrophy, vascular proliferation and lymphocytic infiltration of the subsynovial areas. The intensity of the infiltrate varies, and fibrin deposition may be pronounced. Aggregates of T lymphocytes and B lymphocytes, often with lymphoid follicle formation, are common and may be concentrated in perivascular areas with obliteration of vessels but without vessel necrosis.[90] Levels of

interleukin-1,[94] prostaglandin E_2 and collagenase[95] in joint fluid are elevated similar to the situation in rheumatoid arthritis.

Spirochetes have been visualized in skin lesions,[12] heart tissue[39–41] and synovium,[90] but not in peripheral nerves, where an autoimmune mechanism has been postulated to account for the inflammatory lesions.[96]

MANAGEMENT

The primary goals of therapy for Lyme disease are the control of inflammation and the eradication of the infection. Lyme disease is most responsive to antibiotic therapy early in the course of the disease. As with syphilis, some later disease manifestations do not seem to improve after administration of antibiotics.

Treatment regimens are based in part on data from controlled clinical trials and in part on clinical experience.[97] In-vitro antibiotic sensitivity testing does not reliably predict clinical response. Loose criteria for diagnosis accepted without critical review have led to widespread antibiotic use for presumptive Lyme disease in patients who almost certainly have other explanations for their symptoms. In one report, the leading reason for failure to respond to antibiotic therapy for Lyme disease was incorrect diagnosis.[98] In addition, the appropriate end point of antibiotic therapy is often not clear because of the difficulty of proving when the infection has been eradicated and because of the common persistence of symptoms long after treatment. Current treatment recommendations (Fig. 45.11) represent a distillation of available evidence and will no doubt be refined in time.

EARLY LOCALIZED OR EARLY DISSEMINATED DISEASE

If antibiotic therapy is initiated early in the course of Lyme disease, EM typically resolves promptly and later stage disease is prevented.[99,100] Early localized infection, limited to a single skin lesion, with mild or no systemic symptoms, is uniformly responsive to short-course oral antibiotic therapy with a number of agents. Of the antibiotics studied to date, amoxicillin (500mg q8h), doxycycline (100mg q12h) or cefuroxime axetil (500mg q12h) have been the most effective for this stage of disease.[100,101] Although the optimal duration of therapy is unknown, most clinicians currently recommend 2 to 3 weeks for both early localized and early disseminated disease.

The appearance of systemic symptoms (fever, arthralgias, fatigue) and secondary skin lesions reflects dissemination of the organism beyond the site of inoculation. As long as no neurologic symptoms are present, 3 weeks of oral therapy is sufficient for this group of patients as well. In a recent study, 10% of patients with a single EM lesion and no systemic symptoms had a positive PCR on blood. This was interpreted as demonstrating that clinically silent bloodstream invasion may be relatively common early in the course of infection.[72]

Some experts have recommended the addition of probenecid to amoxicillin, but this combination has been associated with a relatively high frequency of rashes and is not known to be superior to amoxicillin alone. The pediatric dose range of amoxicillin is 30–40mg/kg per day in three divided doses. Herxheimer-like reactions, with intensification of fever and arthralgias, may occur shortly after initiation of therapy. If possible, doxycycline should be avoided in children under the age of 9 years and during pregnancy, because of the possibility of staining of the teeth. Tetracyclines must be used with caution during summer in all patients because they may predispose the patient to sun-sensitive rashes or severe sunburn. Penicillin-allergic young children can be treated with cefuroxime or erythromycin, but results with macrolide antibiotics have been less satisfactory than those with penicillin, amoxicillin or tetracyclines.[99] Azithromycin has been studied systematically and found to be less effective than amoxicillin.[102]

Regardless of which agent is chosen, some patients experience delayed resolution of systemic symptoms (headache, musculoskeletal pain, fatigue), which may persist as long as 3 months after completion of therapy. These symptoms usually resolve spontaneously and do

SUGGESTED ANTIBIOTIC REGIMENS FOR LYME DISEASE	
Early disease	• Doxycycline, 100mg po, q12h for 21 days, or • Amoxicillin (with or without probenecid) 500mg, q8h for 21 days, or • Erythromycin, 250–500mg po, q6h for 21 days, or • Azithromycin 500mg daily for 7 days, or • Cefuroxime axetil, 500mg po, q12h for 21 days Shorter courses (14 days) may suffice for localized early disease. Erythromycin and azithromycin less effective than other choices
Lyme arthritis	Initial treatment: • Doxycyline, 100mg po, q12h for 30 days, or • Amoxicillin and probenecid, 500mg each po, q6h for 30 days If initial treatment fails: • Penicillin G, 20×10^6 IU, daily in divided doses for 14 days, or • Ceftriaxone sodium, 2g iv, daily for 14 days
Neurologic manifestations	For facial nerve paralysis alone: • Doxycycline, 100mg po, q12h for 21–30 days, or • Amoxicillin, 500mg po, q8h for 21–30 days
Additional signs (e.g. Lyme meningitis, radiculopathy, encephalitis)	• Ceftriaxone, 2g iv, daily for 30 days, or • Penicillin G, 20×10^6 IU iv, daily in divided doses for 30 days Possible alternatives: • Cefotaxime sodium, 2g iv, q8h for 30 days, or • Doxycycline, 100mg po, q12h for 14–30 days, or • Chloramphenicol, 1g iv, q6h for 14–30 days
Lyme carditis	• Ceftriaxone, 2g iv, daily for 14 days, or • Penicillin G, 20×10^6 iv, daily in divided doses for 14 days Possible alternatives: • Doxycycline, 100mg po, q12h for 21 days, or • Amoxicillin, 500mg po, q8h for 21 days
During pregnancy	Localized, early disease: • Amoxicillin, 500mg po, q8h for 21 days Other manifestations: • Penicillin G, 20×10^6 IU iv, daily in divided doses for 14–30 days, or • Ceftriaxone, 2g, daily for 14–30 days

Fig. 45.11 Suggested antibiotic regimens for Lyme disease.

not indicate continued infection requiring further antibiotic therapy.[100] A seemingly self-perpetuating fibromyalgia syndrome may develop as a sequel of Lyme disease; this too is unresponsive to antibiotic therapy.[103] The likelihood of delayed resolution of symptoms is greatest in patients who have prominent systemic symptoms or delay in diagnosis before institution of antibiotics.[99]

DISSEMINATED DISEASE

With the possible exception of arthritis, which usually responds to oral therapy (see 'Arthritis'), disseminated infection with target organ involvement other than skin should generally be treated with intravenous antibiotics. Carditis, meningitis, cranial neuropathy and radiculoneuropathy, and arthritis are discussed separately.

Carditis

Although carditis resolves spontaneously, observational data suggest that resolution of heart block may be hastened by treatment with salicylates, corticosteroids, oral penicillin, oral tetracyclines and intravenous ceftriaxone and penicillin.[6,38] This response to either anti-inflammatory therapy or antibiotics suggests that the proximate cause of the heart block is the inflammatory reaction engendered by the Lyme spirochete rather than direct tissue destruction resulting from the infection. Control of the inflammatory response leads to resolution of clinical manifestations.

Heart block caused by carditis may progress suddenly, necessitating a temporary pacemaker, but permanent pacing is rarely necessary. Hospitalization with cardiac monitoring is prudent while antibiotic therapy is instituted. Although no comparative trials have been conducted, treatment with intravenous penicillin or a third-generation cephalosporin for a minimum of 2 weeks to eradicate systemic spirochetal infection is recommended. Salicylates or nonsteroidal anti-inflammatory agents may hasten symptom resolution. Systemic corticosteroids may be dramatically effective in reversing heart block, but they may be best avoided during antibiotic therapy if possible.

Neurologic manifestations

Data on treatment of neurologic manifestations are derived primarily from clinical experience. The tendency for spontaneous resolution of Bell's palsy, the fluctuating course of meningitis, the clinical variation of neurologic syndromes and the delayed emergence of the subtle deficits associated with late neurologic Lyme disease must all be considered in evaluating the clinical response to antibiotic therapy.[41,44,54] The emergence of chronic neurologic impairment years after remission of acute neurologic symptoms highlights the danger of complacency about the potential consequences of incomplete eradication of CNS infection.

Bell's palsy. Historically, Lyme facial palsy has been treated with oral antibiotics, whereas other neurologic syndromes have been treated intravenously. It is unclear whether this distinction is warranted. Facial palsy itself resolves completely or nearly completely in nearly all patients (121 of 122 patients in one series).[42] Patients who have facial palsy should undergo a careful neurologic evaluation, including a CSF examination. Cerebrospinal fluid invasion has been demonstrated by PCR in patients who have minimal CNS complaints and facial palsy, most of whom have had clinically silent CSF pleocytosis.[46,74] If facial palsy is the only clinical abnormality and CSF is normal, current practice is to administer oral antibiotics for 21–30 days, a practice that has resulted in favorable outcomes. Long-term follow-up of this group is important and, if CSF examination is not possible, the preferred course at present is to administer intravenous antibiotics.

Meningitis. Intravenous penicillin for 10 days has been shown in clinical trials to be effective for treatment of meningitis. In one small series, intravenous ceftriaxone for 14 days was superior to a 10-day course of penicillin.[104] Most experts prefer a 30-day course of treatment, however, because of the occasional occurrence of late neurologic relapses after shorter courses of therapy. It is not necessary to document clearing of all CSF abnormalities before discontinuation of therapy, because clearing of inflammation may lag behind bacteriologic cure. The co-occurrence of encephalopathy or encephalomyelopathy does not change this approach.

Radiculoneuropathy. Radiculoneuropathy is less clearly responsive to antibiotic therapy. Intravenous penicillin has not been shown to hasten resolution, and the response to ceftriaxone is unpredictable.[43,44] Current practice is to administer intravenous antibiotic therapy, however, based on favorable long-term outcome with this approach and the belief that radiculoneuropathy is driven by systemic infection.

Resolution of neuropathy may be very gradual (taking place over months) and, with chronic involvement, this response may be incomplete. Doxycycline has been used orally and intravenously as an alternative to ceftriaxone or penicillin, but experience with this agent is limited.[105] One patient who had severe neurologic involvement, unresponsive to penicillin, responded favorably to chloramphenicol.[106]

Arthritis

Arthritis may respond to either oral[107] or parenteral[91,97,108,109] antibiotic therapy, but antibiotic failures occur with either approach. Amoxicillin plus probenecid given orally for 4 weeks cures the majority of patients and those who fail oral therapy do not appear to respond to intravenous therapy. In a carefully done PCR study, there were no PCR-positive joint fluids in patients who had received at least 8 weeks of antibiotic therapy. The optimal duration of therapy is unknown but an initial course for 4 weeks is recommended. The role for parenteral therapy for Lyme arthritis is unclear. Patients who have concurrent neurologic involvement should receive intravenous treatment. In one randomized study, intramuscular benzathine penicillin given weekly for 3 weeks cured less than one half of patients, but intravenous penicillin for 10 days cured a higher percentage.[109] Ceftriaxone given for 14 days has been found more effective than 10 days of penicillin.[106] The primary reason for selection of intravenous therapy is concurrent neurologic involvement, in which case ceftriaxone or cefotaxine for 2–4 weeks are probably the agents of choice.

Resolution is commonly delayed, with synovitis persisting for months after completion of antibiotic therapy before eventually resolving. Administration of intra-articular corticosteroids during or before antibiotic therapy has been suspected to increase the risk of antibiotic failure but a single intra-articular injection after completion of antibiotic therapy may hasten resolution. Failures with a first course of therapy may respond to a repeat course, but there is no known rationale for a course of longer than 8 weeks. Adjunctive treatment measures should include evacuation of large effusions and limitation of weight-bearing during acute attacks. Chronic inflammatory arthritis may occur through an autoimmune mechanism rather than as a result of persistent infection.

LATE LYME DISEASE

Late Lyme disease, a designation reserved for those patients who have symptoms that persist for longer than 1 year, generally involves persistent inflammation in the CNS, joints or skin (acrodermatitis chronicum atrophicans). Generally, patients who have acrodermatitis chronicum atrophicans respond to oral penicillin. Late neurologic and arthritic involvement, however, are less predictably responsive. In one report, only one-half of patients who had late neurologic symptoms showed either resolution or sustained improvement after 6 months of follow-up after a 2-week course of ceftriaxone.[54] Those who did not respond, however, did not show progressive worsening. Long-term follow-up of this patient group is essential. In a European trial ceftriaxone and penicillin for 2 weeks were both effective for late neurologic involvement.[110]

Persistent arthritis after antibiotic therapy occurs most often in HLA-DR4 positive people.[55] They are usually PCR negative and may be treated satisfactorily with arthroscopic synovectomy after failing to respond to either oral or intravenous antibiotics, suggesting that the pathogenesis of antibiotic-resistant arthritis may involve mechanisms other than persistent infection.[111] A recent study has provided strong evidence of an autoimmune mechanism for chronic Lyme arthritis.[92] Comparative trials of different antibiotics and varying durations of therapy are currently in progress for the treatment of late manifestations of Lyme disease, but there are no controlled data involving treatment periods longer than 4 weeks.

PREGNANCY

Lyme disease acquired during pregnancy represents a special category because the health of the fetus must also be considered. Case reports have provided convincing evidence that *B. burgdorferi* can cross the placenta. Stillbirth[112,113] and neonatal death[27,28] have been attributed to *B. burgdorferi* transmitted from mother to fetus *in utero* but the evidence to support this conclusion is still incomplete. The vast majority of pregnancies complicated by maternal Lyme disease have normal outcomes. *Borrelia burgdorferi* has not been linked statistically to congenital anomalies,[100] and no increased risk of an adverse outcome of pregnancy has been associated with asymptomatic seropositivity[114] or history of previous Lyme disease. It is appropriate to maintain a lower threshold for institution of aggressive antibiotic therapy for suspected Lyme disease during pregnancy, but women should be reassured that no cases of fetal Lyme disease have occurred with currently recommended antibiotic regimens.

PREVENTION

If possible, it is preferable to prevent Lyme disease by personal protection and the use of vaccine than to treat it. One obvious issue with regard to prevention is whether an individual with a known ixodid tick bite in a Lyme disease endemic area should be treated prophylactically with antibiotics. This question has been studied in a Lyme disease endemic area in Connecticut. A randomized, double-blind trial of amoxicillin therapy for tick bites[23] showed that, although the tick infection rate approached 15%, the risk of Lyme disease in untreated people was so low – 1.2% (95% CI 0.1–4.1%) – that prophylactic therapy (although probably effective) was not warranted. Personal protection measures, including the wearing of protective clothing, the use of insect repellant containing N,N-diethyl-meta-toluamide (DEET) and the prompt removal of ticks, all reduce the risk of Lyme disease.

Another area of active research involves efforts to develop a Lyme disease vaccine. A recombinant vaccine based on OspA has been shown to induce active immunity in mice[115] with some cross-strain protection. Two OspA-based vaccines have been tested in large, multicenter clinical trials in adults in the USA.[116,117] Both vaccines have been administered in a three-dose regimen at months 0, 1 and 12. Efficacy has been reported to be 79%[116] and 92%[117] after three doses. No serious side-effects have been associated with vaccine administration, with over 10,000 individuals receiving vaccine in the two trials. One Lyme vaccine has received FDA approval for uses in individuals over the age of 15 years. Adults at high risk of exposure should be considered for vaccine. Protection is not optional until after a three dose regimen over 12 months.

REFERENCES

1. Steere AC, Malawista SE, Snydman DR, *et al*. Lyme arthritis: An epidemic of oligoarticular arthritis in children and adults in three Connecticut communities. Arthritis Rheum 1977;20:7–17.
2. Afzelius A. Verhandlungen der Dermatologischen Gesellschaft zu Stockholm on October 29, 1909. Arch Dermatol Syph 1910;101:404.
3. Sonck CE. Erythema chronicum migrans with multiple lesions. Acta Derm Venereol (Stockh) 1965;45:34–6.
4. Garin-Bujadoux C. Paralysie par les tiques. J Med Lyon 1922;71:765–7.
5. Bannwarth. A Zur Klinik und pathogenese der Ôchronischen lymphozytaren meningitis'. Arch Psychiat Nervenkr 1944;117:161–85.
6. Steere AC, Batsford WP, Weinberg M, *et al*. Lyme carditis: cardiac abnormalities of Lyme disease. Ann Intern Med 1980;93:8–16.
7. Reik L, Steere AC, Bartenhagen NH, Shope RE, Malawista SE. Neurologic abnormalities of Lyme disease. Medicine 1979;58:28.
8. Steere AC, Broderick TE, Malawista SE. Erythema chronicum migrans and Lyme arthritis: Epidemiologic evidence for a tick vector. Am J Epidemiol 1978;108:312–21.
9. Steere AC, Malawista SE. Cases of Lyme disease in the United States; locations correlated with distribution of *Ixodes dammini*. Ann Intern Med 1979;91:730–3.
10. Steere AC, Malawista SE, Newman JH, Spieler PN, Bartenhagen NH. Antibiotic therapy in Lyme disease. Ann Intern Med 1980;93:1–8.
11. Burgdorfer W, Barbour AG, Hayes SGF, Benach JL, Grunwalt E, David JP. Lyme disease – A tick borne spirochetosis? Science 1982;216:1317–19.
12. Steere AC, Grodzicki RL, Kornblatt AN, *et al*. The spirochetal etiology of Lyme disease. N Engl J Med 1983;308:733–40.
13. Lyme Disease – United States, 1996. Morb Mortal Wkly Rep 1997;45:531–5.
14. Dekonenko EJ, Steere AC, Berardi CP, Kravchuk LN. Lyme borreliosis in the Sovient Union. A cooperative US–USSR report. J Infect Dis 1988;158:748–53.
15. Burgdorfer W. Vector/host relationships of the Lyme disease spirochete, *Borrelia burgdorferi*. Rheum Dis Clin North Am 1989;15:775–87.
16. Steere AC, Bartenhagen NH, Craft JE, *et al*. The early clinical manifestations of Lyme disease. Ann Intern Med 1983;99:76–82.
17. Spielman A, Wilson ML, Levine JF, Piesman J. Ecology of *Ixodes dammini*-born human babesiosis and Lyme disease. Ann Rev Entomol 1985;30:439–60.
18. Rahn DW, Craft J. Lyme disease. Rheum Dis Clin North Am 1990,16:601–15.
19. Mather TN, Wilson ML, Moore SI, Riberio JMC, Spielman A. Comparing the relative potential of rodents as reservoirs of the Lyme disease spirochete (*Borrelia burgdorferi*). Am J Epidemiol 1989;130:143–50.
20. Brown RN, Lane RS. Lyme disease in California: A novel enzootic transmission cycle of *Borrelia burgdorferi*. Science 1992;256:1439–42.
21. Oliver JH, Chandler FW, Luttrell MP, *et al*. Isolation and transmission of the Lyme disease spirochele from the southeastern United States. Proc Natl Acad Sci USA 1993;90:7371–5.
22. Costello CM, Steere AC, Pinkerton RE, Feder HM. A prospective study of tick bites in an endemic area for Lyme disease. J Infect Dis 1989;159:136–9.
23. Shapiro ED, Gerber MA, Holabird NB, *et al*. A controlled trial of antimiocrobial prophylaxis for Lyme disease after deer-tick bites. N Engl J Med 1992;327:1769–73.
24. Badon SJ, Fister RD, Cable RG. Survival of *Borrelia burgdorferi* in blood products. Transfusion 1989;29:581–3.
25. Magnarelli LA, Anderson JF, Barbour AG. The etiologic agent of Lyme disease in deer flies, horse

flies and mosquitoes. J Infect Dis 1986;154:355–8.
26. Luger SW. Lyme disease transmitted by a biting fly. N Engl J Med 1990;322:1752.
27. Schlesinger PA, Duray PH, Burke BA, Steere AC. Maternal–fetal transmission of the Lyme disease spirochete, *Borrelia burgdorferi*. Ann Intern Med 1985;103:67–8.
28. Weber K, Bratzke HJ, Neubert U. *Borrelia burgdorferi* in a newborn despite oral pencillin for Lyme borreliosis during pregnancy. Pediatr Infect Dis 1988;7:286–9.
29. Rahn DW, Malawista SE. Clinical judgement in Lyme disease. Hosp Pract 1990;25:39–56.
30. Campbell, GL, Paul WS, Schriefer ME, Craven RB, Robbins KE, and Dennis DT. Epidemiologic and diagnostic studies of patients with suspected early Lyme disease, Missouri, 1990–1993. J Infect Dis 1995;172:470–80.
31. Kirkland KB, Klimbo TB, Meriwether RA, *et al*. Erythema migrans-like rash illness at a camp in North Carolina: a new tick-borne disease? Arch Intern Med 1997;157:2635–41.
32. Steere AC, Schoen RT, Taylor E. The clinical evolution of Lyme arthritis. Ann Intern Med 1987;107:725–31.
33. Goellner MH, Agger WA, Burgess JH, Duray PH. Hepatitis due to recurrent Lyme disease. Ann Intern Med 1988;108:707–8.
34. Kramer N, Rickert RR, Brodkin RH. Rosenstein ED. Septal panniculitis as a manifestaiton of Lyme disease. Am J Med 1986;81:149–52.
35. Atlas E, Novak SN, Duray PH, Steere AC. Lyme myositis: muscle invasion by *Borrelia burgdorferi*. Ann Intern Med 1988;109:24–6.
36. Steere AC, Duray PH, Kauffman DJ, Wormser, GP. Unilateral blindness caused by infection with the Lyme disease spirochete, *Borrelia burgdorferi*. Ann Intern Med 1985;103:382–4.
37. Rank EL, Dias SM, Hasson J, *et al*. Human necrotizing splenitis caused by *Borrelia burgdorferi*. Am J Clin Pathol 1989;91:493–8.
38. McAlister HF, Klementowicz PT, Andrews C, Fisher JD, Feld M, Furman S. Lyme carditis: An important cause of reversible heart block. Ann Intern Med 1989;110:339–45.
39. Stanek G, Kelin J, Bittner R, Globar D. Isolation of *Borrelia burgdorferi* from the myocardium of a patient with longstanding cardiomyopathy. N Engl J Med 1990;322:249–52.
40. Van der Linde MR, Crijns HJGM, de Koning J, *et al*. Range of atrioventricular conduction disturbances in Lyme borreliosis: a report of four cases and review other published reports. Br Heart J 1990;63:162–8.
41. Steere AC, Pachner AR, Malawista SE. Neurologic abnormalities of Lyme disease: successful treatment with high-dose intravenous pencillin. Ann Intern Med 1983;99:767–72.
42. Clark JR, Carlson RD, Casaki CT, Pachner AR, Steere AC. Facial paralysis in Lyme disease. Laryngoscope 1985;95:1341–5.
43. Pachner AR, Steere AC. The triad of neurologic manifestations of Lyme disease, meningitis, cranial neuritis, and radiculoneuritis. Neurology 1985;35:47–53.
44. Halperin JJ, Little BW, Coyle PK, Dattwyler RJ. Lyme disease, a cause of a treatable peripheral neuropathy. Neurology 1987;1700–6.
45. Pfister HW, Preac-Mursic V, Wilske B, Einhaupl KM, Weinberger K. Latent Lyme neuroborreliosis. Presence of *Borrelia burgdorferi* in the cerbrospinal fluid without concurrent inflammatory signs. Neurology 1989;39:1118–20.
46. Luft BJ, Steinman CR, Neimark HC, *et al*. Invastion of the central nervous system by *Borrelia burgdorferi* in acute disseminated infection. JAMA 1992;267:1364–7.
47. Reik L Jr, Smith L, Kan A, Nelson W. Demyelinating encephalopathy in Lyme disease. Neurology 1985;35:267–9.

48. Pachner AR, Duray P, Steere AC. Central nervous system manifestations of Lyme disease. Arch Neurol 1989;46:790–5.
49. Steere AC, Malawista SE, Hardin JA, Ruddy S, Askenase PW, Andiman WA. Erythema chronicum migrans and Lyme arthritis. The enlarging clinical spectrum. Ann Intern Med 1977;86:685–98.
50. Steere AC, Gibofsky A, Pattarroyo ME, Winchester RJ, Hardin JA, Malawista SE. Chronic Lyme arthritis: Clinical and immunogenetic differentiation from rheumatoid arthrits. Ann Intern Med 1979;90:286–91.
51. Eichenfeld AH, Goldsmith DP, Banache JL, *et al*. Childhood Lyme arthritis: experience in an endemic area. J Pediatr 1986:109:753–8.
52. Huppertz H, Karch H, Suschke H, *et al*. Lyme Arthritis in European children and adolescents. Arthritis Rheum 1995;38:361–8.
53. Halperin JJ, Luft BJ, Anand AK, *et al*. Lyme neuroborreliosis: central nervous system manifestations. Neurology 1989;39:753–9.
54. Logigian EL, Kaplan RF, Steere AC. Chronic neurologic manifestations of Lyme disease. N Engl J Med 1990;323:1438.
55. Steere AC, Dwyer E, Winchester R. Association of chronic Lyme arthritis with HLA-DR4 and HLA-DR2 alleles. N Engl J Med 1990;323:219–23.
56. Lawson JP, Rahn DW. Lyme disease and radiologic findings in Lyme arthritis. Am J Radiol 1992;158:1065–9.
57. Weber K, Schierz G, Wilske B, Preac-Mursic V. European erythema migrans disease and related disorders. Yale J Biol Med 1984;57:464–71.
58. Asbrink E, Hovmark A. Successful cultivation of spirochetes from skin lesions of patients with erythema chronicum migrans Afzelius and acrodermatitis chronica atrophicans. Acta Pathol Microbiol Immunol Scand Sect B 1985;93:161–3.
59. Schwartz BS, Goldstein MD, Riberiro JMC, Schultz TL, Shahied SI. Antibodiy testing in Lyme diseae. JAMA 1989;262:3431–4.
60. Luger SW, Krauss E. Serologic tests for Lyme disease: interlaboratory variability. Arch Intern Med 1990;150:761–3.
61. Magnarelli LA, Miller JN, Anderson JF, Riviere GR. Cross-reactivity of nonspecific treponemal antibody in serologic tests for Lyme disease. J Clin Microbiol 1990;28:1276–9.
62. Centers for Disease Control. Lyme disease surveillance summary 1995;6:1–12.
63. Hyde FW, Johnson RC, White TJ, Shelbourne CE. Detection of antigens in urine of mice and humans infected with *Borrelia burgdorferi*, etiologic agent Lyme disease. J Clin Microbiol 1989;27:58–61.
64. Berger BW, Kaplan MH, Rothenberg IR, Barbour AG. Isolation and characterization of the Lyme disease spirochete from the skin of patients with erythema chronicum migrans. J Am Acad Dermatol 1985;3:44–9.
65. Benach JL, Bosler EM, Hanrahan JP, *et al*. Spirochetes isolated from the blood of two patients with Lyme disease. N Engl J Med 1983;308:740–2.
66. Nadelman RB, Pavia CS, Magnarelli LA, Worsmer GP. Isolation of *Borrelia burgdorferi* from the blood of seven patients with Lyme disease. Am J Med 1990;88:21.
67. Snydman DR, Schenkein DP, Beradi CP, Lastavica CC, Pariser KM. *Borrelia burgdorferi* in joint fluid in chronic Lyme arthritis. Ann Intern Med 1986;104:798–800.
68. Rosa PA, Schwan TG. A specific and sensitive assay for the Lyme disease spirochete *Borrelia burgdorferi* using the polymerase chain reaction. J Infect Dis 1989;160:6006–15.
69. Persing DH, Telford SR, Spielman A, Barthold SW. Detection of *Borrelia burgdorferi* infection in *Ixodes dammini* ticks by using the polymerase chain reaction. J Clin Microbiol 1990;28:566–72.

70. Persing DH, Rys PN, Van Blaricom G, *et al*. Multi-target detection of *B. burgdorferi*-associated DNA sequences in synovial fluids of patients with Lyme arthritis. Arthritis Rheum 1990;33(Suppl):36.

71. Goodman JL, Jurkovich P, Kramber JM, Johnson RC. Molecular detection of persistent *Borrelia burgdorferi* in the urine of patients with active Lyme disease. Infect Immun 1991;59:269–78.

72. Goodman JL, Bradley JF, Ross AE, *et al*. Bloodstream invasion in early Lyme disease: Results from a prospective, controlled, blinded study using the polymerase chain reaction. Am J Med 1995;99:6–12.

73. Nocton JJ, Dressler F, Rutledge BJ, Rys PN, Persing DH, Steere AC. Detection of *Borrelia burgdorferi* DNA by polymerase chain reaction in synovial fluid from patients with Lyme arthritis. N Engl J Med 1994;330:229–34.

74. Keller TL, Halperin JJ, Whitman M. PCR detection of *Borrelia burgdorferi* DNA in cerebrospinal fluid of Lyme neuroborreliosis patients. Neurology 1992;42:32–42.

75. Sigal L, Steere AC, Freeman DH, Dwyer JM. Proliferative responses of mononuclear cells in Lyme disease. Arthritis Rheum 1986;29:761–9.

76. Dattwyler RJ, Volkman DJ, Luft BJ, Halperin JJ, Thomas J, Golightly MG. Dissociation of specific T- and B-lymphocyte responses to *Borrelia burgdorferi*. N Engl J Med 1989;319:1441–6.

77. Pachner AR, Steere AC, Sigal LH, Johnson CJ. Antigen-specific proliferation of CSF lymphocytes in Lyme disease. Neurology 1985;35:1642–4.

78. Zoschke DC, Skemp AA, Defosse DL. Lymphoproliferative responses to *Borrelia burgdorferi* in Lyme disease. Ann Intern Med 1991;114:285–9.

79. Craft JE, Grodzicki RL, Steere AC. Antibody response in Lyme disese: evaluation of diagnostic tests. J Infect Dis 1984;149:789–95.

80. Shrestha M, Grodzicki RL, Steere AC. Diagnosing early Lyme disease. Am J Med 1985;78:235–40.

81. Steere AC, Berardi VP, Weeks KE, Logigian EL, Ackerman R. Evaluation of the intrathecal antibody response to *Borrelia burgdorferi* as a diagnostic test for Lyme neuroborreliosis. J Infect Dis 1990;161:1203–9.

82. Wilske B, Schierz G, Preac-Mursic V, *et al*. Intrathecal production of specific antibodies against *Borrelia burgdorferi* in patients with lymphocytic meningoradiculitis (Bannwarth's syndrome). J Infect Dis 1986;153:304–14.

83. Berland R, Fikrid E, Rahn D, Hardin J, Flavell RA. Molecular characterization of the humoral response to the 41-kD flagellar antigen of *Borrelia burgdorferi*, the Lyme disease agent. Infect Immun 1991;59:3531–5.

84. Feder HM, Whitaker DL. Misdiagnosis of erythema migrans. Am J Med 1995;99:412–419.

85. Steere AC, Taylor E, McHugh GL, Logigian EL. The overdiagnosis of Lyme disease. JAMA 1993;269:1812–16.

86. Wilske B, Preac-Mursic V, Gobel UB, *et al*. An OspA serotyping system for *Borrelia burgdorferi* based on reactivity with monoclonal antibodies and OspA sequence analysis. J Clin Microbiol 1993;31:340–350.

87. Barantan G, Postic D, Girons IS, *et al*. Delineation of *Borrelia burgdorferi* sensu stricto, *Borrelia garinii* sp. nov., and Group VS461 associated with Lyme borreliosis 1992;42:378–83.

88. Schwan TG, Burgdorfer RW, Garon CF. Changes in infectivity and plasmid profile of the Lyme disease spirochete, *Borrelia burgdorferi* as a result of *in vitro* cultivation. Infect Immun 1988;56:1831–6.

89. Klempner MS, Noring R, Rogers RA. Invasion of human skin fibroblasts by the Lyme disease spirochete, *Borrelia burgdorferi*. J Infec Dis 1993;167:1074–81.

90. Steere AC, Duray PH, Butcher EC. Spirochetal antigens and lymphoid cell surface markers in Lyme synoviits. Arthritis Rheum 1988;31:487–95.

91. Fikrig E, Barthold SW, Kantor FS, Flavell RA. Protection of mice against Lyme disease agent by immunizing with recombinant OspA. Science 1990;250:553–6.

92. Gross DM, Forsthuber T, Tary-Lehmann M, *et al*. Identification of LFA-1 as a candidate autoantigen in treatment-resistant Lyme arthritis. Science 1998;281:703–6.

93. Vallet JM, Hugon J, Lubeau M, *et al*. Tick-bite meningoradiculoneuritis: clinical, electrophysiological, and histologic findings in 10 cases. Neurology 1987;37:749–53.

94. Habicht GS, Beck G, Benach JL, Coleman JL, Leichtling KD. Spirochetes induce human and murine interleukin-1 production. J Immunol 1985;134:3147–54.

95. Steere AC, Brinckerhoff CE, Miller DJ, Drinker H, Harris ED Jr, Malawista SE. Elevated levels of collagenase and prostaglandin E_2 from synovium associated with erosion of cartilage and bone in a patient with chronic Lyme arthritis. Arthritis Rheum 1980;23:591–9.

96. Sigal L, Tatum AH. Lyme disease patients' serum contains IgM antibodies to *Borrelia burgdorferi* that cross-react with neuronal antigens. Neurology 1988;38:1439–42.

97. Rahn DW, Malawista SE. Lyme disease: recommendations for diagnosis and treatment. Ann Intern Med 1991;114:472–81.

98. Sigal LH. Summary of the first 100 patients seen at a Lyme disease referral center. Am J Med 1990;88:577–81.

99. Steere AC, Hutchinson GJ, Rahn DW, *et al*. Treatment of the early manifestations of Lyme disease. Ann Intern Med 1983;99:22–6.

100. Dattwyler RJ, Volkman DJ, Connaty SM, *et al*. Amocxycillin plus probenecid versus doxcycline for treatment of erythema migrans borreliosis. Lancet 1990;336:1404–6.

101. Nadelman RB, Luger SW, Frank E, *et al*. Comparison of cefuroxime axetil and doxycycline in the treatment of early Lyme disease. Ann Intern Med 1992;117:273–80.

102. Massarotti EM, Luger SW, Rahn DW, *et al*. Treatment of early Lyme disease. Am J Med 1992;92:396–403.

103. Dinerman H, Steere AC. Lyme disease associated fibromyalgia. Ann Intern Med 1992;117:281–5.

104. Dattwyler RJ, Volkman DJ, Halperin JJ, Luft BJ. Treatment of late Lyme borreliosis – randomized comparison of ceftraxone and penicillin. Lancet, 1988;331:1191–4.

105. Dotevall L, Alestig K, Hanner P, Norfrans G, Hagberg L. The use of doxycycline in nervous sytem *Borrelia burgdorferi* infection. Scand J Infect Dis 1988;53:74–9.

106. Diringer MN, Halperin JJ, Dattwyler RJ. Lyme meningoencephalitis; report of a severe, pencillin-resistant case. Arthritis Rheum 1987;30:705–8.

107. Steere AC, Levin RE, Molloy PJ, *et al*. Treatment of Lyme arthritis. Arthritis Rheum 1994;37:878–88.

108. Roberts ED, Bohm RP, Cogswell FB, *et al*. Chronic Lyme disease in the Rhesus monkey. Laboratory Investigation 1995;72:146–60.

109. Steere AC, Green J, Schoen RT, *et al*. Successful parenteral antibiotic therapy of established Lyme arthritis. N Engl J Med 1985;312:869–74.

110. Hassler D, Zoller L, Haude M, *et al*. Cefotaxime versus pencillin in the late stage of Lyme disease-prospective, randomized therapeutic study. Infection 1990;18:16–20.

111. Schoen RT, Aversa JM, Rahn DW, Steere AC. Treatment of refractory chronic Lyme arthritis with arthroscopic synovectomy. Arthritis Rheum 1991;34:1056–60.

112. Macdonald AB, Benach JL, Burgdorfer W. Stillbirth following maternal Lyme disease. N Y State J Med 1987;87:615–16.

113. Markowitz LE, Steere AC, Benach JL, Slade JD, Broome CV. Lyme disease during pregnancy. JAMA 1986;255:3394–6.

114. Williams CL, Benach JL, Curran AS, Spierling P, Medici F. Lyme disease during pregnancy: a cord blood serosurvey. Ann N Y Acad Sci 1988;539:504–6.

115. Fikrig E, Barthold SW, Kantor FS, Flavell RA. Long-term protection of mice from Lyme disease by vaccination with OspA. Infection and Immunity 1992;60:773–7.

116. Steere AC, Sikand VK, Meurice F, *et al*. Vaccination against Lyme disease with recombinant *Borrelia Burgdorferi* outer-surface lipoprotein A with adjuvant. N Engl J Med 1998;339:209–15.

117. Sigal LH, Zahradnik JM, Lavin P, *et al*. A vaccine consisting of recombinant *Borrelia Burgdorferi* outer-surface protein A to prevent Lyme disease. N Engl J Med 1998;339:216–22.

Practice Points

Fever and arthralgia

Molly Stenzel

INTRODUCTION

Arthralgia, with or without objective arthritis, is a component of many febrile syndromes. The differential diagnosis is therefore quite broad, and includes a number of infectious and noninfectious entities. It is incumbent upon the clinician to assess the probability of a serious underlying cause of fever and arthralgia because potentially life-threatening infections may present in this manner. It is often helpful to categorize patients who have fever and arthralgia on the basis of the pattern of presenting signs and symptoms. Clinical groups include:
*   acute monoarticular arthritis,
*   oligoarticular arthritis,
*   polyarticular arthritis, and
*   fever and arthralgia or arthritis with associated skin eruption.

The common etiologic agents within each category are listed in Figure 46.1. Major causes of fever and arthritis, and an approach to their diagnosis, are listed in Figure 46.2. The topic of septic arthritis is reviewed in detail in Chapter 2.42.

INVESTIGATIONS

In this, as in other syndromes for which the differential diagnosis is quite broad, there is no substitute for a thorough history and physical examination. Historic information requiring particular emphasis includes severity and duration of symptoms, occupational and leisure activities, travel history, dietary history (ingestion of raw or under-cooked meat or of unpasteurized dairy products), sexual activity, potential exposures to wild and domesticated animals and arthropod vectors, immunization status, previous blood and blood product transfusions, and recent exposures to others who have acute illness. As fever and arthritis may be immune-mediated sequelae of infection, information should be elicited about past illnesses that may have seemed trivial or unrelated to current symptoms, such as flu-like syndromes, bouts of diarrhea or sexually transmitted disease.

Physical examination should include a thorough examination of the joints, including the sacroiliac region and axial skeleton, in search of objective signs of inflammation. As many of the entities typified by arthralgia and fever are associated with characteristic dermatologic findings (see Fig. 46.1), skin and mucous membranes should be inspected carefully for ulcerations, rash, and signs of vasculitis or psoriasis.

Standard initial investigation includes a complete blood count with differential leukocyte count, blood urea nitrogen, creatinine, urinalysis, hepatic enzymes, total bilirubin and lactate dehydrogenase. If an inflamed joint is identified, diagnostic arthrocentesis should be performed. Synovial fluid analysis should include at least a Gram stain and culture, a cell count with differential, and examination for crystals. Blood for routine cultures should be obtained. Additional specific testing should be guided by the clues gathered through interview and examination of the patient. This might include cultures of oropharynx,

genital secretions or stool, serum titers of antibodies directed against specific viral or bacterial pathogens, rheumatologic serologies or biopsy of associated skin lesions. In some instances, the simultaneous determination of acute and convalescent antibody titers can be

CAUSES OF FEVER AND ARTHRALGIA	
Monoarticular arthritis	**Polyarticular arthritis**
Septic arthritis	Viral infections
Tuberculosis	Hepatitis B virus
Bacterial endocarditis	Hepatits C virus
Calcium pyrophosphate dihydrate deposition disease	HIV
	Cytomegalovirus
Gout	Epstein–Barr virus
	Arboviruses
Oligoarticular arthritis	Rheumatic fever
	Rheumatoid arthritis
Disseminated gonococcal infection	Relapsing fever
Brucellosis	Whipple's disease
Fungal infections	Giardiasis
Histoplasmosis	*Loa loa* infection
Coccidioidomycosis	Toxoplasmosis
Sporotrichosis	Paraneoplastic syndromes
Reactive arthritis	Atrial myxoma
Salmonella spp. infection	Fluoroquinolone-induced
Shigella spp. infection	Familial Mediterranean fever
Campylobacter spp. infection	
Yersinia spp. infection	**Arthralgia or arthritis with skin eruption**
Chlamydial infection	
Lymphogranuloma venereum	Lyme disease
Bacterial endocarditis	Disseminated gonococcal infection
Rheumatic	Chronic meningococcemia
Still's disease	Syphilis
Inflammatory bowel disease	Rocky Mountain spotted fever
Psoriatic arthritis	Rat-bite fever (streptobacillary form)
Ankylosing spondylitis	Murine typhus
	Parvovirus
Paraneoplastic syndromes	HIV
Serum sickness	Rubella (natural or vaccine)
Sarcoidosis	Dengue fever
Strongyloidiasis	Systemic lupus erythematosus
	Systemic vasculitis
Dracunculiasis	Mixed cryoglobulinemia

Fig. 46.1 Causes of fever and arthralgia.

CLINICAL FINDINGS AND DIAGNOSTIC STRATEGIES IN SELECTED DISEASES THAT CAUSE FEVER AND ARTHRALGIA

Disease	Etiologic agent(s)	Associated clinical findings	Diagnostic strategy
Bacterial endocarditis	*Staphylococcus aureus*, coagulase-negative staphylococci, viridans streptococci, other organisms	Cardiac murmur, splenomegaly, Osler's nodes, splinter hemorrhages, petechiae	Blood cultures, echocardiography
Lyme disease	*Borrelia burgdorferi*	History of tick exposure, erythema migrans, headache, myalgia, malaise, fatigue	Acute disease: characteristic rash; chronic disease: serology, confirmed by Western blotting
Disseminated gonococcal infection	*Neisseria gonorrhoeae*	History of sexual exposure, pustular or necrotic skin lesions in acral and juxta-articular distribution, more common in women and associated with menses	Confirmatory culture from urethra, endocervix, rectum, pharynx, or involved joint; characteristically prompt resolution of symptoms with antibiotic therapy
Rheumatic fever	*Streptococcus pyogenes*	History of recent pharyngitis, cardiac murmur, erythema marginatum	Throat culture or streptococcal antigen assay; anti-streptolysin O titer, anti-DNAse B, anti-hyaluronidase; Jones criteria
Parvovirus	Parvovirus B19	Erythema infectiosum ('slapped-cheek' rash) or reticular recrudescent rash, mild-to-severe pancytopenia	Parvovirus IgM and IgG antibody titers
Reactive arthritis (Reiter's syndrome)	*Salmonella* spp., *Shigella* spp., *Yersinia* spp., *Campylobacter* spp., *Chlamydia* spp.	History of diarrheal illness or previous sexually transmitted disease, conjunctivitis, urethritis, dactylitis, enthesopathy, oral ulceration	No specific diagnostic test, haplotyping for HLA-B27 provides supportive evidence for diagnosis
HIV-associated arthropathy	HIV	Arthralgia, which may occur at any stage of disease, including acute seroconversion, may be severe and refractory to analgesics ('painful articular syndrome'), increased susceptibility to other forms of arthritis such as Reiter's arthritis and psoriatic arthritis	Testing for HIV antibodies; in acute infection, HIV RNA testing by PCR
Rubella	Rubella virus (wild-type and live-attenuated vaccine strains)	Erythematous, macular rash, spreading from face to trunk, which may occur 2–4 weeks after vaccination, particularly in adults	Viral isolation from throat swab or blood, four-fold rise in IgG antibodies from acute to convalescent period
Hepatitis B	Hepatitis B virus	In acute infection, immune-complex-mediated serum sickness associated with malaise, anorexia, maculopapular rash, urticaria preceding onset of jaundice by about 10 days; in chronic infection, mixed cryoglobulinemia with associated palpable purpura, urticaria, hepatosplenomegaly and glomerulonephritis	In acute infection, hepatitis B surface antigen, elevated hepatic enzymes and bilirubin; in chronic infection, hepatitis B surface antigen, core antigen, anti-hepatitis B core antigen, anti- hepatitis B surface antigen
Septic arthritis	*Staphylococcus aureus*, streptococci	History of pre-existing arthritis or injury, injection drug use is a risk factor	Arthrocentesis revealing high white blood cell count with polymorphonuclear predominance; Gram stain and culture of synovial fluid
Brucellosis	*Brucella melitensis*	History of contact with livestock or ingestion of unpasteurized dairy products, typically a unilateral sacroiliitis	Culture of blood and synovial fluid, serologic testing (standard tube agglutinin test)
Crystal-induced arthritis	Urate crystals (gout), calcium pyrophosphate dihyrate crystals (pseudogout)	Tophi, first episode frequently involves the metatarsophalangeal joint of the first toe; recurrence generally polyarticular	Arthrocentesis with identification of crystals in the synovial fluid

Fig. 46.2 Clinical findings and diagnostic strategies in selected diseases that cause fever and arthralgia.

diagnostic. Setting aside a serum sample at the time of presentation preserves the opportunity for additional testing later, and is recommended.

MANAGEMENT

Treatment is dependent on identification of the underlying etiology. Initiation of empiric antibiotics, except in patients who are critically ill, should be avoided. Likewise, every attempt shoud be made to rule out the possibility of acute infection before starting a course of corticosteroids as presumptive treatment of rheumatologic disease.

FURTHER READING

Bocanegra TS. Musculoskeletal manifestations of parasitic diseases. In: Maddison PJ, Isenverg DA, Woo P, Glass DN, eds. Oxford textbook of rheumatology. Oxford: Oxford University Press; 1993.

Carsons SE. Fever in rheumatic and autoimmune disease. Infect Dis Clin North Am 1996;10:67–84.

Pinals RS. Polyarthritis and fever. N Engl J Med 1994;330:769–74.

Andrew R Murry &
Robert J Fass

How long should osteomyelitis be treated?

INTRODUCTION

Bone infections vary considerably in their pathogenesis, microbiology and clinical presentation. They are usually classified as acquired by hematogenous or contiguous spread and as acute or chronic. The transition from acute to chronic evolves over a period of weeks to months. The antimicrobial treatment of osteomyelitis needs to be tailored to the characteristics of the individual infection.

PATHOGENESIS

Hematogenous osteomyelitis is most common in infants, children and the elderly. Bone involvement may become obvious during the acute illness or as recrudescent disease after the bacteremia has cleared. The preceding bacteremia may be inapparent, with osteomyelitis presenting as an isolated finding. Most cases of acute osteomyelitis in adults do not result from bacteremia, but are a consequence of contiguous spread from infected wounds, teeth, sinuses, ulcers, open fractures or implanted prosthetic devises. Early, vigorous antimicrobial treatment of acute bone infections reduces the risk of progression to chronicity. Chronic osteomyelitis is associated with devitalized bone, fibrosis, sinus tract formation and clinical recrudescence. Chronic infections are much more difficult to cure, particularly in the presence of diabetes mellitus, vascular disease or any condition that impairs host defenses.

MICROBIOLOGY
The pathogens most associated with various types of osteomyelitis are shown in Figure 46.3.

CLINICAL FEATURES
Acute infections may be associated with local symptoms and signs, including pain and local inflammation with or without fever, chills and other constitutional manifestations of infection. In those infections acquired by contiguous spread, the presence of bone involvement may be indeterminate by clinical criteria. Findings may be more vague in chronic infection, with only nonspecific pain and few constitutional symptoms. Vertebral osteomyelitis commonly presents with dull, constant back pain, spasm of the paravertebral muscles and tenderness over the involved vertebrae. Infected prosthetic joints may become painful. Sinus tracts may develop or increase their drainage.

INTERVENTIONS
The presence of osteomyelitis can often be confirmed by plain radiographs of the suspected area, although abnormalities may not be apparent for about 2 weeks. Radiographs may be difficult to interpret when there are soft tissue infections, fractures or noninfectious skeletal diseases. Radionuclide scans, CT axial or MRI can be helpful early in the disease. They do not need to be obtained routinely if treatment is initiated on the basis of clinical suspicion, and follow-up plain radiographs will be subsequently performed. Computed tomography and MRI are particularly useful when planning surgery.

A specific microbiologic diagnosis is most helpful in choosing antimicrobial therapy. Bone biopsy, although not through infected soft tissues, provides the most reliable specimen for microbiologic study. Although the results from cultures of sinus tracts, ulcers or wounds are somewhat unreliable, they may be useful for antibiotic selection if a single pathogen is consistently found or when a biopsy cannot be performed. Blood cultures should be obtained when appropriate.

MANAGEMENT
Acute osteomyelitis may be treated with antibiotics alone, but chronic infection often requires surgery to drain abscesses, resect fistulae, debride ulcers or necrotic devascularized bone, remove foreign bodies (including prostheses), manage dead space, provide stability or restore vascular supply as well as for reconstruction. Optimization of host factors such as control of diabetes mellitus is also important.

Initial antimicrobial therapy is based on the known or probable pathogens as determined by the nature of the infection and the available culture and susceptibility test results. The antimicrobial agents most commonly used to treat osteomyelitis are shown in Figure 46.4. Preferred drugs include the beta-lactams, clindamycin and the fluoroquinolones. Vancomycin, trimethoprim–sulfamethoxazole (co-trimoxazole) and metronidazole have more limited indications. Rifampin (rifampicin) may be used with a beta-lactam to treat staphylococcal infections but there is more favorable experience using clindamycin alone. Aminoglycosides may be used with a beta-lactam for Gram-negative infections but they are toxic and ineffective when used alone. Macrolides and tetracyclines are not very effective and should be avoided.

Osteomyelitis has traditionally been treated with relatively high doses of intravenous antimicrobial agents for 4–6 weeks, although shorter courses of treatment have proven adequate in some children who have acute infection. Children who have acute infection caused by *Haemophilus influenzae*, *Neisseria* spp. or streptococci should be treated for at least 10–14 days and infections caused by *Staphylococcus aureus*, Enterobacteriaceae or *Pseudomonas aeruginosa* for at least 3 weeks.

For acute infections in adults and chronic infections in patients of any age, the recommended duration of treatment of 4-6 weeks should be considered a minimum unless the infected bone is completely removed by debridement. If this is accomplished, treatment can probably be abbreviated and, in patients undergoing amputation of an infected limb, treatment may be discontinued postoperatively if there is no residual soft tissue infection. For patients who have chronic, recalcitrant osteomyelitis that can not be completely debrided, treatment with an appropriate agent for 3–12 months may be beneficial. Such infections may 'burn out' over a prolonged period of time with continued antimicrobial suppression.

Prolonged intravenous treatment has proved to be problematic because of hospitalization costs and the inconvenience and complications of long-term intravenous lines. The availability of highly active, predictably absorbed oral antimicrobial agents has provided an alternative mode of therapy. The first experiences with oral therapy, usually a penicillin, cephalosporin or clindamycin, after about 5–10 days of initial intravenous therapy, were in children. Intravenous, and then oral, ampicillin–sulbactam was subsequently used successfully. Switching from intravenous to oral therapy has also been successfully accomplished in adults using those drugs or trimethoprim–sulfamethoxazole. Ciprofloxacin (and to a lesser extent other fluoroquinolones) initially available only orally, has been extensively used to treat skeletal infections successfully.

When using oral treatment, either after an initial course of intravenous treatment or from the start, it is necessary to have a predictably absorbed drug that is highly active against the pathogen being treated. Although beta-lactams are often considered the preferred drugs for the treatment of skeletal infections, oral derivatives may not be predictably absorbed and do not yield serum concentrations as high as parenteral derivatives, even at high doses with probenecid. Serum

COMMON PATHOGENS IN OSTEOMYELITIS			
	Contiguous spread		
Hematogenous spread	Acute skin and soft tissue infections	Orofacial and dental infections	Diabetic foot and pressure sores
Staphylococcus aureus *Streptococcus* spp. *Haemophilus influenzae* * Enterobacteriaceae † *Staphylococcus epidermidis* ‡,§ *Candida* spp. § *Pseudomonas aeruginosa* ** *Salmonella* spp. ††	*Staphylococcus aureus* *Streptococcus agalactiae* *Streptococcus pyogenes*	*Streptococcus* spp. Anaerobic cocci *Fusobacterium* spp. *Prevotella melaninogenicus* *Pasteurella multocida* ‡‡ *Eikenella corrodens* §§	*Staphylococcus aureus* *Staphylococcus epidermidis* *Streptococcus* spp. Enterobacteriaceae *Pseudomonas aeruginosa* *Enterococcus faecalis* Anaerobic cocci *Bacteroides* spp. *Clostridium* spp.
* Infants and unimmunized children † Elderly and neonates	‡ Bone and joint prostheses § Intravenous devices	** Injection drug use and foot puncture wounds †† Hemoglobinopathies	‡‡ Dog and cat bites §§ Human bites

Fig. 46.3 Common pathogens in osteomyelitis.

COMPARISON OF INTRAVENOUS AND ORAL ANTIMICROBIAL REGIMENS TO TREAT OSTEOMYELITIS IN ADULTS

		Intravenous				Oral	
Drug		Dose	Approximate peak serum concentration (mg/l)	Usual MIC (mg/l) of appropriate pathogens	Drug	Dose	Approximate peak serum concentration (mg/l)
Beta-lactams	Penicillin G	1–2mU q4–6h	10–20 (U/ml)	≤0.12	Penicillin V	500mg q6h	5
	Ampicillin	1–2g q4–6h	20–50	≤0.12, 0.5–2*	Amoxicillin	500mg q8h	5–10
	Ampicillin–sulbactam	1.5–3g q6h	50–150	≤2, 2–8†	Amoxicillin–clavulanate	500mg q8h	5–10
	Nafcillin	1–2g q4–6h	40–80	≤0.5	Dicloxacillin	0.5–1g q6h	10–25
	Cefazolin	1–2g q8h	80–150	≤2	Cephalexin‡	0.5–1g q6h	15–25
	Ceftriaxone	1–2g q24h	100–250	≤4	Cefixime§	400mg q6h	4
Non-beta-lactams	Clindamycin	600mg q8h	8	≤0.5	Clindamycin	300mg q6h	5
	Trimethoprim–sulfamethoxazole	160/800mg q8h	6/120	≤0.5/9.5	Trimethoprim–sulfamethoxazole	160mg/800mg q8h	4/100
	Ciprofloxacin	400mg q8–12h	4	≤0.25, 0.06–2**	Ciprofloxacin	500–750mg q12h	3–4
	Metronidazole	500mg q6h	15–25	≤4	Metronidazole	500mg q6h	12
	Vancomycin	1g q12h	40	≤2	No oral equivalent is available††		

* MIC ≤0.12mg/l for most susceptible organisms; 0.5–2mg/l for *Enterococcus faecalis*

† MIC ≤2mg/l for beta-lactamase-positive *Haemophilus influenzae*; 2–8mg/l for susceptible Enterobacteriaceae

‡ Cephalexin is four–fold less active than cefazolin against *Staphylococcus aureus*

§ Cefixime is for Gram-negative organisms only

** MIC ≤0.25mg/l for Enterobacteriaceae; 0.06–2mg/l for susceptible *Pseudomonas aeruginosa*

†† Trimethoprim–sulfamethoxazole or clindamycin may be active against methicillin-resistant staphylococci

Fig. 46.4 Comparison of intravenous and oral antimicrobial regimens to treat osteomyelitis in adults.

concentrations after both intravenous and oral clindamycin far exceed those necessary to inhibit most staphylococci and streptococci. Serum concentrations of trimethoprim–sulfamethoxazole after intravenous and oral administration are virtually identical and far exceed those necessary to inhibit most staphylococci and Enterobacteriaceae. Careful studies have shown oral ciprofloxacin to be equivalent to intravenous ciprofloxacin and serum concentrations with either route of administration far exceed those needed to inhibit most Enterobacteriaceae and *P. aeruginosa*. Serum concentrations of metronidazole after intravenous and oral administration are nearly equivalent and exceed those needed to inhibit most anaerobes.

Appropriate follow-up is necessary to evaluate adherence to the therapeutic regimen and to monitor for clinical improvement and radiographic healing. Determination of serum antibiotic concentrations or performing serum bactericidal tests may be helpful in drug regimens that might be marginal, but these tests are usually not necessary.

Normalization of the erythrocyte sedimentation rate (ESR) is reassuring. If the ESR has fallen but not normalized, further treatment might be appropriate, and a persistently elevated ESR often predicts relapse within months of discontinuing antimicrobial agents.

FURTHER READING

Black J, Hunt TL, Godley PJ, Matthew E. Oral antimicrobial therapy for adults with osteomyelitis or septic arthritis. J Infect Dis 1987;155:968–72.

Fass RJ. Bone and joint infections. In: O'Grady F, Lambert HP, Finch RG, Greenwood D, eds. Antibiotic and chemotherapy: anti-infective agents and their use in therapy, 7th ed. Edinburgh: Churchill Livingstone; 1997:760–7.

Gentry LO. Oral antimicrobial therapy for osteomyelitis (editorial). Ann Intern Med. 1991;114:986–7.

Hass DW, McAndrew MP. Bacterial osteomyelitis in adults: evolving considerations in diagnosis and treatment. Am J Med. 1996;101:550–61.

Jensen AG, Espersen F, Skinhøj P, Frimodt-Møller N. Bacteremic *Staphylococcus aureus* spondylitis. Arch Intern Med. 1998;158:509–17.

Mader JT, Oritz M, Calhoun JH. Update on the diagnosis and management of osteomyelitis. Clin Pediatr Med Surg 1996;13:701–24.

Management of chronic infection in prosthetic joints

Jonathan Cohen

INTRODUCTION

Joint replacement is one of the surgical success stories of recent years. Hips, knees, shoulders and elbows are all amenable to this approach. The major complication is infection, which occurs in 1–5% of cases. Acute infection of a prosthetic joint is unmistakable: there is pain, fever and physical signs of inflammation around the joint. However, a common and often more difficult problem is the patient who presents with features consistent with chronic prosthetic joint infection (PJI).

PATHOGENESIS

Most PJIs are caused by exogenous infection by organisms that gain entry at the time of operation, and this is reflected in the type of organisms isolated from these cases (see Chapter 2.44), which are typically low-grade pathogens associated with skin contamination. However, prosthetic joints can become infected by the hematogenous route, and this is more common in late infections, more than 2 years after operation.

MICROBIOLOGY

About 80% of infections are associated with a single organism, 10% are mixed infections and 10% are sterile. Gram-positive bacteria are the commonest isolates, particularly coagulase-negative staphylococci (Fig. 46.5). It is of note that about 10% of cases are said to be caused by anaerobic bacteria, typically peptococci and peptostreptococci, which are part of the mouth flora.

CLINICAL FEATURES

The dominant complaint is of pain. It is usually aching in character, may be continuous or intermittent and is not necessarily of great severity. Local signs of inflammation are often absent, but there may be some erythema, induration or swelling. The finding of a sinus is very helpful; it may discharge very little material, and only intermittently. General systemic features of infection (fever, malaise, shaking chills) are very uncommon in chronic PJI.

The principal differential diagnosis is joint loosening without infection. Laboratory investigations are not very helpful (see below); the diagnosis can be established only by joint aspiration and isolation of the causative organism.

INVESTIGATIONS

Establishing the microbiologic diagnosis is of great importance in managing these infections. Isolation of the causative organism will not only confirm the diagnosis of infection, but will also be crucial in guiding the choice of antimicrobial therapy. In this context, interpreting the microbiologic findings from a discharging sinus can present difficulties. While it may seem 'logical' to use this as a surrogate for direct joint aspiration (particularly as both the patient and the physician may be reluctant to do a further surgical procedure), there are pitfalls. The most obvious is that bacteria such as *Staphylococcus epidermidis* are common causes of PJI, but they are also common skin commensals and likely to be isolated from sinus swabs. On the other hand, isolation of *Staphylococcus aureus*, *Proteus* spp. or *Pseudomonas* spp. from such a sinus is a very good indication of the likely cause of the underlying infection. A reasonable approach is to require:

- that the organism should be repeatedly isolated from the sinus, and
- that the organism is identical on each occasion by techniques such as antibiograms and, where appropriate, other more sophisticated forms of bacterial typing.

If there is any doubt, and in particular in cases where a patient presents after one failed course of therapy, joint aspiration should be done.

The laboratory should be forewarned, and anaerobic cultures should be included in the processing of the specimen.

Measurement of the C-reactive protein (CRP) is particularly helpful in gauging the response to treatment. It is nonspecific, but in my experience it is not significantly elevated in noninfected joints (even if they are loose and painful). Failure of the CRP to normalize is a reliable sign of persistent infection. Other investigations are less useful. The leukocyte count is rarely elevated in chronic PJI. Radiologic investigations have been particularly disappointing. Plain radiographs do not generally distinguish between infection and an uninfected loose joint. Scintigraphic investigations using gallium, technetium or indium are neither sensitive nor specific enough to be of real clinical value, particularly in the patient who has a low-grade, chronic infection. Ultrasound is useful for identifying collections that may be susceptible to surgical drainage, and it deserves further evaluation in chronic infections.

MANAGEMENT

Lasting cure almost always requires removal of all prosthetic material and extensive local debridement. The procedure of choice is a two-stage revision. First, the infected joint is removed and the patient is given 6 weeks of antimicrobial therapy based on the susceptibility pattern of the causative organism. In the second stage, a replacement joint is fitted. An alternative approach is a single-stage procedure involving removal of the infected prosthesis and immediate replacement with the new joint using antibiotic-impregnated bone cement.

A detailed discussion of the surgical aspects of the treatment can be found in orthopedic textbooks, but for the infectious diseases practitioner there are a number of difficult and unresolved questions.

Duration of antibiotic treatment

The advice to use 6 weeks of treatment is based on clinical experience rather than comparative clinical trials; it is probably no coincidence that endocarditis was traditionally treated with 6 weeks of antibiotics. A practical consequence of this is that the regimen chosen should either be available as oral agents, or else offered as part of a home-antibiotic treatment program.

Choice of regimen

Despite the fact that there are a number of antibiotics that have been used quite extensively in these infections, there are no good clinical trials that rigorously compare different regimens. For instance, there is no agreement as to whether one or two drugs should be used; many UK orthopaedic surgeons favor the combination of flucloxacillin and fusidic acid, whereas in North America single-agent therapy is more common. Another issue is whether there is any merit in parenteral therapy; is high-dose oral therapy just as good?

MICROBIAL CAUSES OF PROSTHETIC JOINT INFECTION

Pathogen	Proportion of infected joints (%)
Staphylococci	50
Coagulase-negative staphylococci	25
Staphylococcus aureus	25
Streptococci	20
Gram-negative aerobic bacilli	20
Anaerobes	10

Fig. 46.5 Microbial causes of prosthetic joint infection.

DRUGS FOR THE TREATMENT OF PROSTHETIC JOINT INFECTIONS

Antibiotic	Spectrum	Preparation used	Comments
Vancomycin	Gram-positive bacteria; used particularly for coagulase-negative staphylococci	Only as a parenteral agent	A single daily infusion is suitable for HAI therapy Nephrotoxic
Teichoplanin	Gram-positive bacteria; used particularly for coagulase-negative staphylococci Do not assume that vancomycin and teichoplanin have interchangeable susceptibility patterns	Only as a parenteral agent	Given as a single daily infusion is suitable for HAI therapy Nephrotoxic potential
Isoxazolyl penicillins: nafcillin, flucloxacillin and related compounds	Gram-positive bacteria, particularly *Staphylococcus aureus* Most coagulase-negative staphylococci are resistant	Both oral and parenteral preparations	
Fusidic acid (not available in USA)	*Staphylococcus aureus* and many strains of coagulase-negative staphylococci	Oral (intravenous also available)	Excellent record in bone infections, generally used in combination with flucloxacillin Parenteral preparation has significant hepatotoxicity; avoid if at all possible
Clindamycin	*Staphylococcus aureus* and some strains of coagulase-negative staphylococci Has activity against some strains of anaerobic bacteria	Both oral and parenteral formulations	A large body of successful experience in bone and joint infections Care in elderly people because of risk of antibiotic-associated colitis
Rifampin	*Staphylococcus aureus* and many strains of coagulase-negative staphylococci	Most useful as an oral agent	Little published experience in this setting, but widely used in tuberculosis
Cephalosporins	Broad activity which may include *Staphylococcus aureus* and many aerobic Gram-negative bacilli, depending on the particular agent chosen Not active against coagulase-negative staphylococci	Both oral and parenteral formulations	Most useful when the microbiology is unknown and it is necessary to treat empirically with broad-spectrum agents Long-acting drugs such as ceftriaxone are useful for HAI
Ciprofloxacin (and other quinolones)	Wide activity including *Staphylococcus aureus* and many aerobic Gram-negative bacilli Not active against coagulase-positive staphylococci	Oral and parenteral formulations	Very valuable agents in mixed infections, known Gram-negative infection, patients with beta-lactam hyper-sensitivity, or as second-line agents
Trimethoprim–sulfamethoxazole	Broad spectrum includes many strains of *Staphylococcus aureus* and Gram-negative aerobic bacilli Not active against coagulase-negative staphylococci	Oral and parenteral formulations	Often forgotten; a useful reserve agent particularly in patients who have beta-lactam hypersensitivity

Fig. 46.6 Drugs for the treatment of prosthetic joint infections. HAI, home antibiotic infusion.

In the absence of adequate data, the following recommendations are suggested, based on my experience; they will need modifying in the light of individual circumstances:
- for proven or presumed Gram-positive infection with coagulase-negative staphylococci, 6 weeks of parenteral vancomycin (or teicoplanin) plus oral rifampin (rifampicin);
- for proven or presumed *S. aureus* infection: 2 weeks of high-dose (2–4g/day) intravenous flucloxacillin (or nafcillin) plus oral fucidic acid (where available), followed by 4 weeks of oral therapy;
- for proven or presumed Gram-negative infection, 6 weeks of ciprofloxacin;
- for mixed infections or infections of uncertain etiology, the combination of vancomycin plus ciprofloxacin is useful;
- reserve agent for Gram-positive infection: clindamycin; and
- reserve agent for Gram-negative infection: trimethoprim–sulfamethoxazole (co-trimoxazole).

Specific antianaerobic agents may be needed, depending on the microbiologic findings; penicillin, clindamycin and metronidazole are all useful for this purpose. The treatment of pseudomonal infections is particularly difficult; there may be benefit in adding gentamicin to ciprofloxacin, but the dangers of a long course of an aminoglycoside, particularly in the elderly, are such that this should only be done after very careful consideration.

FURTHER READING

Norden C, Gillespie WJ, Nade S. Infections in bones and joints. Boston, Massachusetts: Blackwell Scientific Publications; 1994.

Sepsis

William A Lynn

This chapter examines the pathophysiologic consequences of the systemic effects of infection. This is broadly referred to as sepsis and is a heterogeneous syndrome resulting from a complex interaction between host defenses and invading pathogens. In this chapter, I describe the pattern of disease seen in sepsis and detail a logical approach to therapy.

EPIDEMIOLOGY

DEFINITION AND NOMENCLATURE

For many years physicians recognized that infection could lead to generalized circulatory collapse and death. The association of bloodstream infection with severe systemic illness was generally referred to as septicemia, and in the 1960s the work of McCabe *et al.* described in detail, for the first time, the spectrum of disease associated with Gram-negative bacteremia, including septic shock.[1,2] Although sepsis and septic shock are terms that most practitioners recognize, if asked to define bacteremia, sepsis, septicemia and septic shock a considerable range of views would emerge. Driven by the need to adopt a common currency of terms, Bone[3] initiated a debate that continues to provoke much discussion. Bone suggested that 'sepsis' be used for the systemic response to infection according to specific clinical criteria (Fig. 47.1). Furthermore, he introduced the concept of the sepsis syndrome, which refers to sepsis plus impaired organ perfusion, and recognized that an identical syndrome could occur with noninfective inflammatory stimuli.[3] In response to this initiative a consensus conference was convened by the American College of Chest Physicians and American Society of Critical Care Medicine (ACCP/ASCCM) to discuss the terminology of sepsis in detail.[4] They accepted much of what Bone suggested but introduced the term the systemic inflammatory response syndrome (SIRS). The terminology of sepsis is defined in Figure 47.1; although these terms have gained general acceptance, some authors have criticized SIRS for being nonspecific and encompassing too wide a range of disease processes.[5] Thus, although these concepts have helped to improve our understanding of the pathophysiology of sepsis, it is important to remember that all different infections may not behave the same way in all patients.

There is no single classification system that will satisfy the requirements of clinicians and researchers alike, but the current definitions can be used as a basis for recognizing patients who have sepsis and directing both therapies and clinical resources. These processes are best considered as a continuum, with localized inflammation at one end and a severe generalized inflammatory response leading to multiorgan failure at the other.[6,7] Patients may present at either end of this spectrum or alternatively may visibly progress from early sepsis, through severe sepsis, to refractory shock and death. The challenge for physicians is to recognize the onset of sepsis and intervene early to try to prevent progression along this continuum, because once shock and organ failure are established the mortality remains high despite intensive therapy.[7]

INCIDENCE AND PREVALENCE OF SEPSIS

For a number of reasons, there are few precise data available to calculate the incidence of sepsis. Many host and environmental factors interact in the development of sepsis, making it a heterogeneous condition with varying rates in different patient populations. Furthermore, sepsis is not a notifiable disease and measurement of the incidence of sepsis and SIRS has been further confounded by the failure of multi-center studies of novel therapeutic agents to include all patients fulfilling the definition of sepsis or SIRS. However, it is clear that sepsis is a major cause of hospital morbidity and mortality and has been increasing in prevalence over the past 30 years, presumably due to increased numbers of critically ill patients at risk of hospital-acquired infection.[7–9]

Bacteremia is responsible for approximately 7–12/1000 hospital admissions and it has been estimated that within the USA the annual incidence of sepsis is of the order of 400,000 cases/year, with 200,000

DEFINITIONS OF SEPSIS, BACTEREMIA AND RELATED DISORDERS	
Disorder	**Definition**
Infection	Presence of organisms in a normally sterile site that is usually, but not necessarily, accompanied by an inflammatory host response
Bacteremia	Bacteria present in blood, as confirmed by culture; may be transient
Sepsis	Clinical evidence of infection, plus evidence of a systemic response manifested by two or more of the following conditions: • Temperature >110.4°F (38°C) or <96.8°F (36°C) • Heart rate >90 beats/min • Respiratory rate >20 breaths/min or arterial CO_2 tension <32mmHg (<4.3kPa) • WBC >12,000 cells/mm^3, <4000 cells/mm^3, or >10% immature (band) forms
Hypotension	A systolic blood pressure of <90mmHg or a reduction of >40mmHg from baseline in the absence of other causes of hypotension
Severe sepsis	Sepsis associated with organ dysfunction: • Hypotension • Lactic acidosis • Oliguria • Confusion • Hepatic dysfunction
Septic shock	Severe sepsis with hypotension despite adequate fluid resuscitation
Refractory septic shock	Septic shock that lasts for more than 1h and does not respond to fluid administration or pharmacologic intervention
Systemic inflammatory response syndrome	Response to a wide variety of clinical insults, which can be infectious, as in sepsis, but can be noninfectious in etiology (e.g. burns, pancreatitis)

Fig. 47.1 Definitions of sepsis, bacteremia and related disorders. Adapted from Bone *et al.*[4]

cases of septic shock and at least 100,000 deaths.[8,10] In a recent study in a Dutch teaching hospital, Kieft *et al.*[11] measured the attack rate for SIRS at 13.6/1000 hospital admissions and septic shock at 4.6/1000 hospital admissions.[11] In a study of 11,828 consecutive patients in France, SIRS was present in 9/100 intensive care unit (ICU) admissions.[12] Once in the ICU the prevalence of SIRS is high, and in one recent study fully 68% of 3708 patients in intensive care fulfilled the criteria for SIRS at some time during their ICU stay.[6]

MORBIDITY/MORTALITY

The mortality of SIRS/sepsis varies both between countries and between different patient groups, possibly because of variations in case definition, ICU facilities and patient populations.[13,14] In an analysis of four large sepsis trials, 14-day mortality averaged 26% and 28-day mortality 42%.[15] The mortality rate is related to the degree of organ dysfunction, with reported mortality rates of 10–20% for bacteremia, 20–30% for sepsis rising to around 50% in patients who have severe sepsis or shock, and over 80% in patients who have multiorgan failure. Factors associated with early death include the number of organ systems involved, low arterial blood pH, shock and an unfavorable SAPS or APACHE score. Later deaths (within 28 days) are associated with the underlying disease process, pre-existing cardiac or liver disease, hypothermia, thrombocytopenia and multiple sources of infection. *Pseudomonas aeruginosa, Candida* spp. and mixed infections have a higher attributable mortality than other infectious agents.[7] Thus the overall mortality from sepsis and SIRS is 40–60% and sepsis remains the single most important cause of death in the ICU setting. Patients who have sepsis often have serious underlying medical or surgical problems that contribute to mortality, but even when this is taken into account the attributable mortality from sepsis has still been measured as at least 25%.[7] Furthermore, a recent long-term follow-up of patients enroled in the Veterans Affairs co-operative study of corticosteroids in systemic sepsis performed in the early 1980s revealed a significant reduction in survival persisting for at least five years after the episode of sepsis.[10] Thus there are many potentially avoidable/recoverable deaths from sepsis annually.

RISK FACTORS FOR SEPSIS

Broadly speaking, risk factors for sepsis are those factors that weaken/breach host defenses, increasing the likelihood of bacterial invasion of otherwise sterile tissue:

- hospitalization and duration of hospital stay;
- type of hospitalization (rates higher on ICUs);
- operative procedures, particularly nonsterile ('dirty') surgery;
- indwelling urinary catheter;
- indwelling intravascular devices; and
- underlying chronic medical/surgical conditions.

PATHOGENESIS AND PATHOLOGY

ETIOLOGIC AGENTS OF SEPSIS

Bacteria are the commonest underlying pathogens in patients presenting from the community and in hospital-acquired sepsis. Classic studies in the early 1960s by McCabe *et al.*[1] identified Gram-negative bacteria as the predominant cause of septic shock at that time. Over the past decade, however, there has been a shift in the etiology of nosocomial infections, with increased infection due to Gram-positive bacteria.[16] This is also reflected in the pattern of underlying infections in patients who have sepsis (Fig. 47.2). Staphylococci, *Escherichia coli* and enterococci remain the most commonly isolated pathogens.

Although it remains true that bacterial infections continue to be frequent, there has been a growing awareness that a wide range of nonbacterial pathogens may induce the pathologic responses necessary to lead to sepsis. This includes fungi (e.g. *Candida* spp.), rickettsia (e.g. *Rickettsia rickettsii* – Rocky Mountain spotted fever), protozoa (including *Plasmodium falciparum*) and certain viruses (e.g. those that cause dengue fever). Furthermore, as mentioned in Figure 47.1, a variety of noninfectious insults can also trigger the onset of a physiologic response identical to sepsis, including pancreatitis, trauma, chemical toxins and burns.

As with other aspects of infectious diseases, the occurrence of sepsis is due to the combination of host and environmental factors. Thus the organisms responsible will vary geographically; for example, melioidosis due to *Burkholderia pseudomallei* is a common cause of community-acquired sepsis in South East Asia. Also there are large differences between specific patient groups, with certain pathogens occurring more frequently in vulnerable hosts, for example pneumococcal sepsis in asplenic patients.

BACTERIAL PRODUCTS INVOLVED IN SEPSIS

Bacteria produce a variety of extracellular products (exotoxins) and endogenous cell wall products that have the capacity to induce proinflammatory responses *in vitro* that may culminate in sepsis *in vivo* (Fig. 47.3). Such products are released by bacteria during local or systemic infection and, in turn, may have local or distant proinflammatory effects. Thus, it is possible for a localized infection to induce the full inflammatory response leading to sepsis without the infecting organism itself actually disseminating. The most commonly recognized

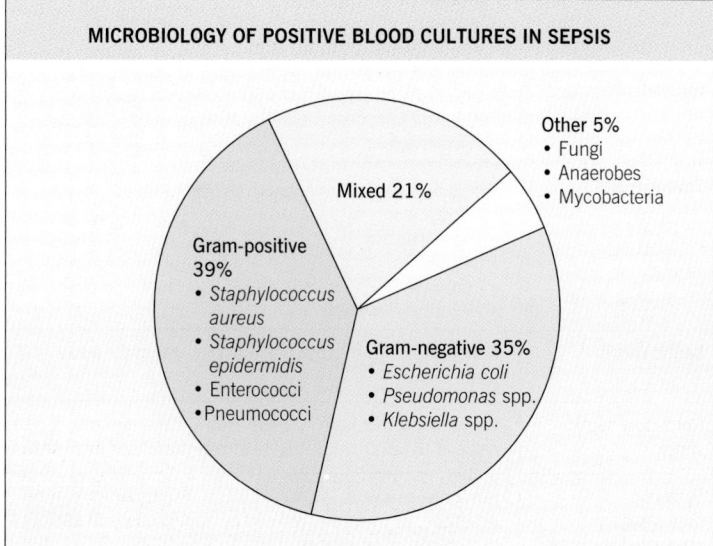

MICROBIOLOGY OF POSITIVE BLOOD CULTURES IN SEPSIS

Other 5%
- Fungi
- Anaerobes
- Mycobacteria

Mixed 21%

Gram-positive 39%
- *Staphylococcus aureus*
- *Staphylococcus epidermidis*
- Enterococci
- Pneumococci

Gram-negative 35%
- *Escherichia coli*
- *Pseudomonas* spp.
- *Klebsiella* spp.

Fig. 47.2 Microbiology of positive blood cultures in sepsis. Adapted from Brun-Buisson *et al.*[12]

BACTERIAL COMPONENTS IN THE PATHOGENESIS OF SEPTIC SHOCK

Bacterial component	Source	Examples
Endotoxin (LPS, lipid A)	All Gram-negative bacteria	*E. coli* septicemia Meningococcemia
Peptidoglycan	All bacteria	
Lipoteichoic acid	Gram-positive bacteria	
Pore-forming exotoxins	*S. aureus* *S. pyogenes* *E. coli* *Aeromonas* spp.	α-hemolysin Streptolysin-O *E. coli* hemolysin Aerolysin
Superantigens	*S. aureus* *S. pyogenes*	Toxic shock syndrome toxin 1 Enterotoxins A–F Pyrogenic exotoxins A + C, SPE
Enzymes	*S. pyogenes* *Clostridium perfringens*	IL-1β convertase Phospholipase C

Fig. 47.3 Bacterial components in the pathogenesis of septic shock. SPE, streptococcal pyrogenic exotoxin.

bacterial products are outlined in Figure 47.3 (there are undoubtedly numerous others yet to be discovered or defined) and it is important to recognize that they may be additive or synergistic in their proinflammatory actions. For two bacterial toxins, namely endotoxin and toxic shock syndrome toxin 1 (TSST-1), considerable progress has been made in the understanding of their molecular and cellular interactions and these are discussed in some detail here.

Cellular activation by endotoxin

The central role of endotoxin [lipopolysaccharide (LPS)] in pathogenesis has been recognized for many years.[17,18] Lipopolysaccharide is found only in Gram-negative bacteria, where it forms part of the outer leaflet of the bacterial cell wall (Fig. 47.4). It consists of a polysaccharide domain covalently bound to a unique di-glucosamine-based phospholipid, lipid A (see Fig. 47.5), which is the key toxic moiety of LPS; when injected into experimental animals purified lipid A induces lethal shock.[17] Lipid A and LPS induce a wide range of both proinflammatory and counter-regulatory responses *in vitro* and *in vivo* (Fig. 47.6). These include release of cytokines from macrophages and neutrophils, activation of the complement cascade, and upregulation of the adhesive capacity of neutrophils and endothelial cells.[7] In human volunteers, administration of small amounts of endotoxin induces fever

and release of cytokines including tumor necrosis factor (TNF)-α, interleukin (IL)-1 and IL-6.[19] That LPS alone can initiate severe sepsis in humans was reported in dramatic style in 1993 when a laboratory worker developed septic shock after deliberate self-administration of *Salmonella minnesota* endotoxin.[20]

So how does this lipid exert such widespread effects on a variety of cell types? It is now apparent that the interaction of LPS with cells is complex, involving both serum LPS-binding proteins and cell-bound and soluble LPS receptors.[21] When released from bacteria, LPS interacts with serum proteins that may either enhance or negate its bioactivity. One of these, LPS-binding protein (LBP) binds LPS with high affinity and presents it to LPS acceptor molecules including CD14, a glycosphatidyl-inositol (GPI) anchored protein on the surface of monocyte/macrophages and neutrophils.[22] In 1990 Wright and coworkers recognized the crucial role of LBP and CD14 in cellular responses to LPS.[23,24] Subsequent studies have shown that LBP acts as a 'shuttle' in transferring free LPS to CD14, leading to both cellular activation and LPS clearance.[25] A surprising finding was that some cell types that do not express surface CD14, such as endothelial cells, responded to LPS in a LBP/CD14-dependent manner. The explanation for this came from the discovery that CD14 is, in addition to being anchored to neutrophils and monocyte/macrophages, also present in human serum

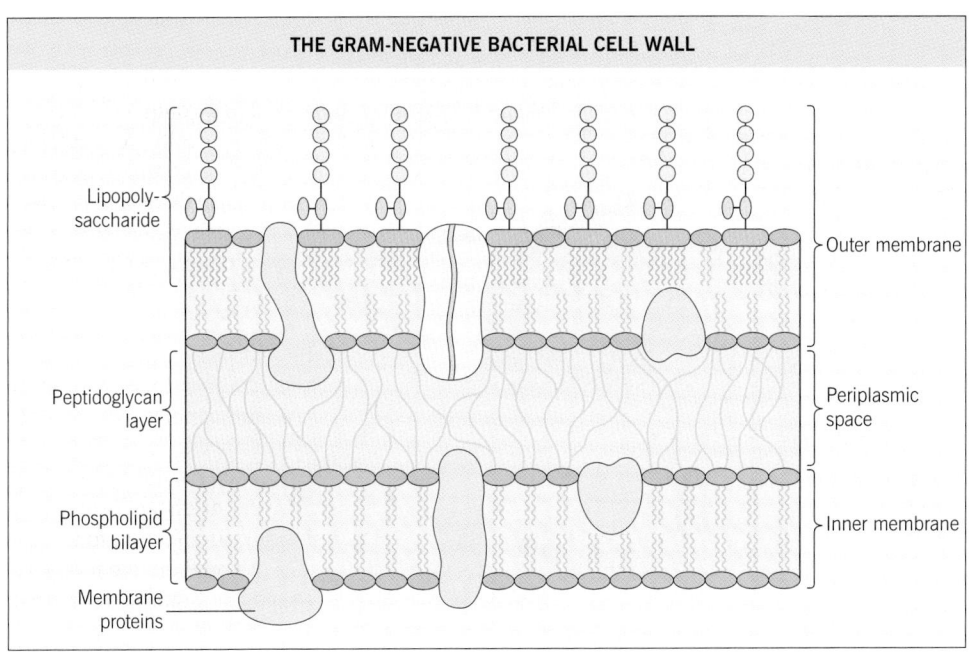

Fig. 47.4 The Gram-negative bacterial cell wall. In the cell wall of a Gram-negative bacteria such as *Escherichia coli*, the inner membrane is composed of phospholipids and membrane proteins and is separated from the outer membrane by the periplasmic space and peptidoglycan. Lipopolysaccharide is found only in the outermost leaflet of the outer membrane with the lipid A moiety in the membrane and the polysaccharide (O) side chain directed outwards. Adapted from Raetz *et al.*[17]

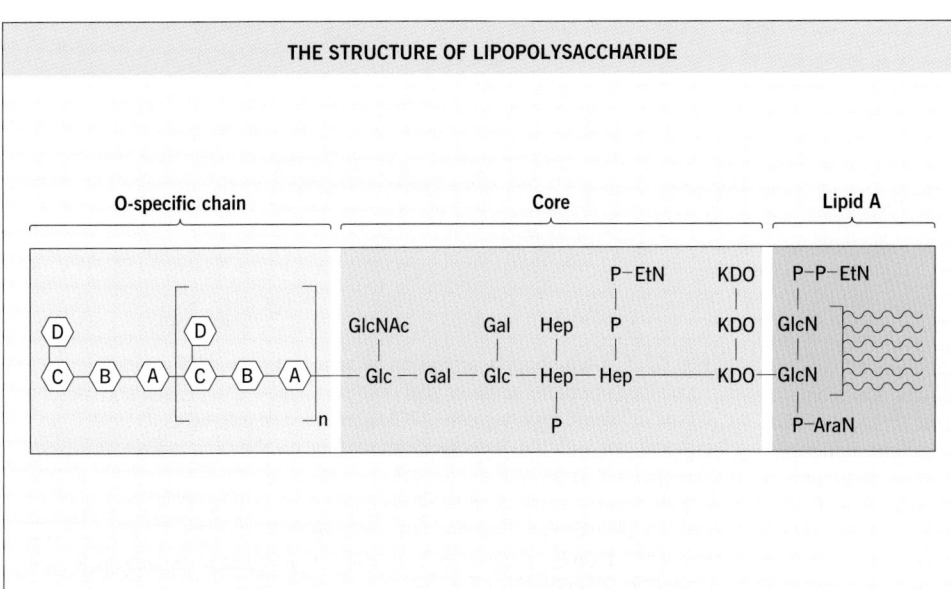

Fig. 47.5 The structure of lipopolysaccharide. Lipid A is highly conserved across Gram-negative bacteria and consists of a phosphorylated diglucosamine backbone decorated with six or seven acyl side chains. Dephosphorylation or deacylation of lipid A abrogates its toxicity. Lipid A is covalently linked to an inner core of sugar residues that is relatively well conserved across species and antibodies directed against the core may protect against challenge with heterologous Gram-negative bacilli. The core is followed by an outer polysaccharide chain, of repeating sugar residues, that varies between different of bacterial strains (O antigen). Antibodies directed against the O antigen will only protect against challenge with that individual bacterial strain. KDO, 3-deoxy-D-manno-octuylosonic acid; Hep, L-glycero-D-manno-heptose; Glc, D-glucose; Gal, D-galactose; GlcNAc, N-acetyl-D-glucosamine.

and that this soluble form of CD14 can complex with LPS and LBP to activate endothelial cells.[26] The precise mechanisms leading to cell signaling after CD14 binding have yet to be elucidated but recent data suggests that CD14 interacts with a member of the Toll-2 family of cell surface receptors.[27] Several other LPS receptors have been identified and their interrelationships remain to be elucidated.[21] Following receptor binding there is rapid activation of a number of second-messenger pathways, including nuclear factor-κB (NF-κB), protein kinase C and tyrosine kinases, leading to activation of many genes.

A protein closely related to LBP is bactericidal/permeability-increasing protein (BPI), which is stored in neutrophil secondary granules. On neutrophil activation, for example by released LPS, BPI is both secreted and expressed on the neutrophil cell surface.[28] Bactericidal/permeability-increasing protein binds LPS with a higher affinity than LBP and then neutralizes LPS. It is intriguing that there are endogenous proteins that both enhance and neutralize the effects of LPS, and this reinforces the central role of LPS in the interaction of Gram-negative bacilli and the immune system.

More recently it has been recognized that CD14 is also involved in the recognition of molecules from non-Gram-negative pathogens, including molecules from mycobacteria, yeasts and Gram-positive bacteria.[21] Thus, it has been proposed that CD14 is acting as a 'sentinel' receptor of the immune system, being able to respond to many bacterial challenges. Although the details of how this occurs have yet to be elucidated the available data would place CD14 at the heart of the early events triggering the cellular responses that lead to sepsis from many different organisms.[21,29]

Superantigens and toxic shock

Superantigenic bacterial toxins can cause profound hypotension, organ failure and inflammation.[30] It is postulated that strains of *Staphylococcus aureus* and *Streptococcus pyogenes* that are able to express these toxins (see Fig. 47.3) are the causal agents of staphylococcal and streptococcal toxic shock.[31] The principle behind immune activation by superantigens is outlined in Figure 47.7. Essentially, the bacterial toxin is capable of bypassing the normal highly antigen-specific mechanisms of T-lymphocyte activation by directly linking major histocompatability complex (MHC) II on antigen-presenting cells to the Vβ subunit of the T-lymphocyte receptor. Whether an individual infected with a superantigen-producing organism develops toxic shock will therefore depend both on microbial factors, (i.e. amount of toxin produced), and on the genetically determined composition of the individual's MHC molecules and T-lymphocyte repertoire of Vβ subunits. The interaction of these factors was clearly demonstrated in outbreaks of staphylococcal toxic shock epidemiologically linked to tampon use in the USA in the 1970s. Toxin-producing strains of staphylococci were presumably already present in the community, but the use of a particular type of superabsorbent tampon allowed proliferation and increased toxin production by staphylococci in the vagina, leading to a marked increase in cases of menstruation-associated cases of toxic shock syndrome.[30]

ROLE OF SPECIFIC PROINFLAMMATORY MEDIATORS IN SEPSIS
Cytokines

The evidence that proinflammatory cytokines such as TNF-α and IL-1 play a causative role in sepsis stems from several lines of research. First, IL-1 and TNF-α can induce features of septic shock in experimental animals, and inhibitors of these cytokines can prevent the onset

INFLAMMATORY MEDIATORS IN SEPSIS			
Targets	Proinflammatory mediators	Modulating mediators	Anti-inflammatory mediators
Monocyte/ macrophage	TNF-α, IL-1, IL-8, IFN-γ tissue factor, prostanoids, leukotrienes, PAF, NO (rodents)	IL-6 IL-12	IL-1Ra sTNFr TGF-β
Neutrophils	Integrin expression, superoxide, TNF-α, IL-1		BPI, CAP 57, defensins, acyloxyacylhydrolase
Lymphocytes	IFN-γ, TNF-β	IL-2	IL-4, IL-10 sIL-2r
Endothelial cells	Selectins, VCAM, ICAM, NO, tissue factor		
Platelets	Serotonin, prostanoids	PDGF	
Plasma components	Coagulation cascade, complement activation, bradykinin	CRP, LBP	

Fig. 47.6 Inflammatory mediators in sepsis. BPI, bacterial/permeability-increasing protein; CRP, C-reactive protein; ICAM, intercellular adhesion molecule; IFN-γ, interferon γ; IL-1Ra, interleukin-1 receptor antagonist; LBP, lipopolysaccharide-binding protein; NO, nitric oxide; PAF, platelet-activating factor; PDGF, platelet-derived growth factor; sIL-2r, soluble IL-2 receptor; sTNFr, soluble TNF receptor; TGF-β, transforming growth factor-β; TNF, tumor necrosis factor; VCAM, vascular cell adhesion molecule.

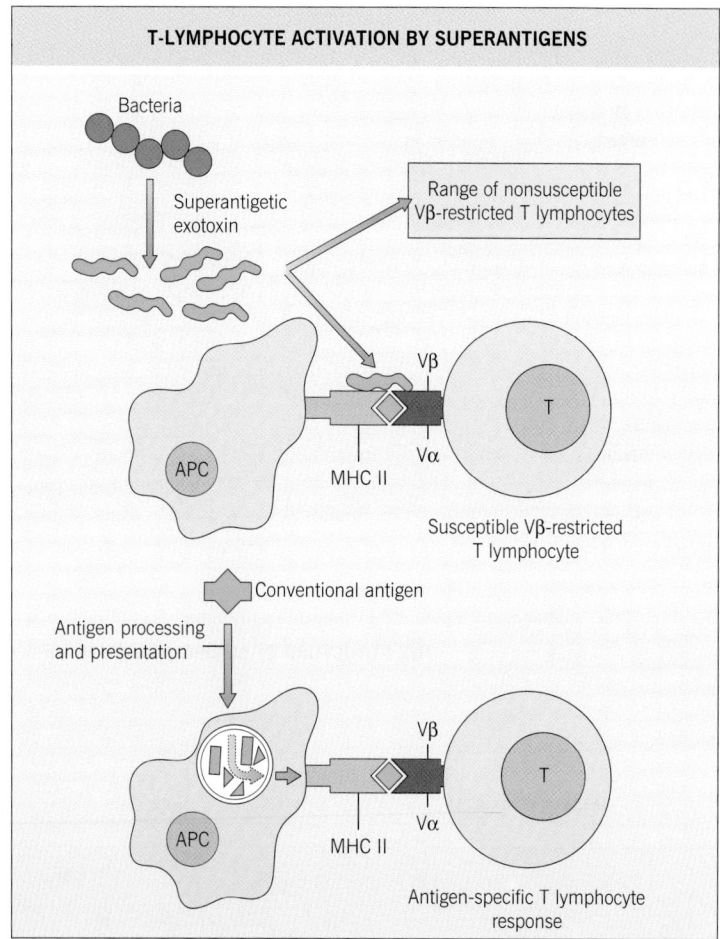

T-LYMPHOCYTE ACTIVATION BY SUPERANTIGENS

Bacteria

Superantigetic exotoxin

Range of nonsusceptible Vβ-restricted T lymphocytes

Vβ

T

APC

MHC II

Vα

Susceptible Vβ-restricted T lymphocyte

Conventional antigen

Antigen processing and presentation

Vβ

T

APC

MHC II

Vα

Antigen-specific T lymphocyte response

Fig. 47.7 T-lymphocyte activation by superantigens. In the conventional response to bacterial antigens (bottom) the antigen is processed and presented by the antigen-presenting cell (APC) in association with MHC II. Only T lymphocytes with the correct antigen recognition site can then be activated (i.e. this is a highly antigen-specific process). Superantigens (top) are able to bypass this process by bridging between MHC II and the Vβ subunit of the T-lymphocyte receptor. Thus the entire population of T lymphocytes expressing that particular Vβ subunit can be activated; this can be up to 20% of the total T-lymphocyte population. Adapted from Sriskandan and Cohen.[31]

of sepsis in these models.[32] Furthermore, mice deficient in the genes encoding receptors for TNF-α are resistant to septic shock induced by endotoxin. Finally, these cytokines are elevated in human sepsis, and high levels of cytokines correlate with a poor outcome.[33] Tumor necrosis factor-α is released early in response to LPS challenge,[19] and the cooperative effects of TNF-α, IL-1 and interferon (IFN)-γ in producing inflammatory responses have made these three cytokines prime targets for experimental intervention in sepsis.[32]

Arachidonic acid metabolites

Thromboxane A_2 and prostaglandins are released via the cyclo-oxygenase pathway and leukotrienes through the action of lipoxygenases. Lipopolysaccharide and other mediators can activate increased synthesis and release of cyclo-oxygenase and lipoxygenase products in sepsis.[34] Broadly speaking, prostaglandins (PGs), particularly PGE_1 and PGI_2, have beneficial effects in sepsis by reducing procoagulant activity and improving tissue perfusion. Thromboxane and leukotrienes, however, are largely deleterious and have been particularly implicated in the pathogenesis of adult respiratory distress syndrome (ARDS). In the complicated setting of septic shock it is difficult to assess the contribution of individual arachidonic acid metabolites to the overall clinical picture.

Platelet-activating factor

Platelet-activating factor (PAF) is a potent phospholipid mediator produced by a variety of cell types – monocytes, neutrophils, platelets and endothelial cells – during severe sepsis. It enhances neutrophil chemotaxis, primes neutrophils for superoxide release and increases thromboxane synthesis in the lung. In animal models, infusion of PAF leads to a sepsis-like state and in particular can cause the pathophysiologic changes of ARDS. Increased levels of PAF can be detected in sepsis, and experimental strategies directed against PAF have been developed.[34]

Complement

The complement system exists to provide an immediate and nonspecific host response to a variety of invading pathogens. Activation of complement leads to a proteolytic cascade resulting in the liberation of molecules that can act as opsonins, chemoattractants and also mediate bacterial lysis. Lipopolysaccharide and other bacterial products activate complement by the alternative pathway. Massive local activation of complement during sepsis will fuel the inflammatory response by recruiting neutrophils, and through the activation of kinins and histamine will contribute to increased endothelial permeability and capillary leakage.[35] In addition, complement-mediated lysis of bacteria, by

releasing endotoxin and other bacterial products, can exacerbate the septic response to infection.[36]

Coagulopathy

Widespread activation of the coagulation pathways leading to disseminated intravascular coagulation (DIC) is a serious consequence of severe sepsis.[7,37] Endotoxin and other bacterial products may directly activate some components of the coagulation system and also indirectly activate them via activation of tissue factor on endothelial surfaces and release of kinins. In addition to the direct effects of DIC, the widespread activation of coagulation factors and damage to the microvasculature further impairs endothelial function and exacerbates capillary leak.

Nitric oxide

Nitric oxide (NO) may be involved in the pathophysiology of sepsis through a number of mechanisms.[38] First, NO is a free radical and has the ability to kill phagocytosed organisms in rodents, although the importance of this action in humans is not clear. Second, NO is a potent vasodilator and a basal level of NO is required for the maintenance of normal arteriolar tone. Synthesis of NO is increased by a number of bacterial products, including LPS and cytokines. In particular, TNF-α, IL-1 and IFN-γ appear to increase NO synthesis synergistically. Sepsis is characterized by widespread peripheral vasodilatation and loss of the normal regulation of tissue blood flow. There is considerable experimental evidence in animals to suggest that the vasodilatation in sepsis is mediated by increased NO levels. In humans, elevated urinary nitrite levels are found in sepsis/SIRS, implying increased NO synthesis. Inhibitors of NO synthase increase peripheral vascular resistance and blood pressure, but at the expense of reducing tissue perfusion and cardiac output.

Neutrophil–endothelial cell interactions

An early response to the local production of cytokines and other inflammatory mediators is the upregulation of adhesion molecules on endothelial cells and the release of chemokines, leading to recruitment of neutrophils and other inflammatory leukocytes to the site of infection (Fig. 47.8). This is a key event in the successful containment of infection; for example, patients who have leukocyte adhesion deficiency have neutrophils that cannot cross the endothelium and, as a result, they suffer from severe recurrent bacterial infections.[39] Furthermore, exposure of neutrophils to LPS and some cytokines enhances the ability of neutrophils to release further inflammatory molecules and primes neutrophils for the generation of oxygen radicals and release of proteolytic enzymes. These mechanisms enable

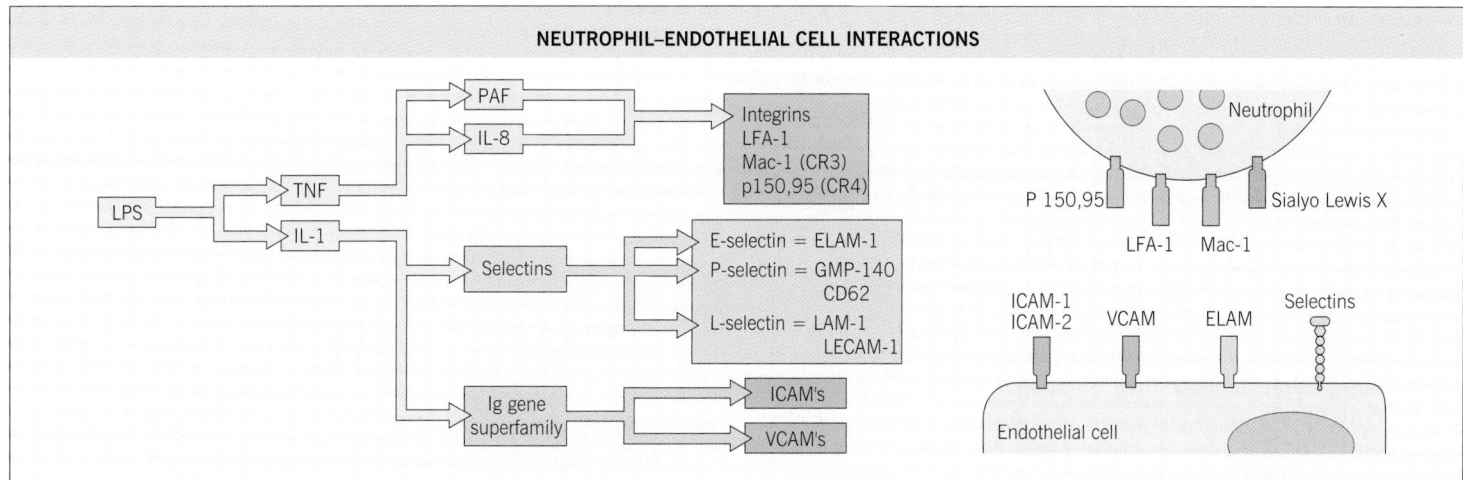

Fig. 47.8 Neutrophil–endothelial cell interactions. A number of different adhesion molecules are involved in neutrophil transmigration across the endothelium. ELAM, endothelial leukocyte adhesion molecule; GMP, granule membrane protein; ICAM, intercellular adhesion molecule; LAM, leukocyte adhesion molecule; LECAM, leukocyte endothelial cell adhesion molecule; LFA, lymphocyte function-associated molecule.

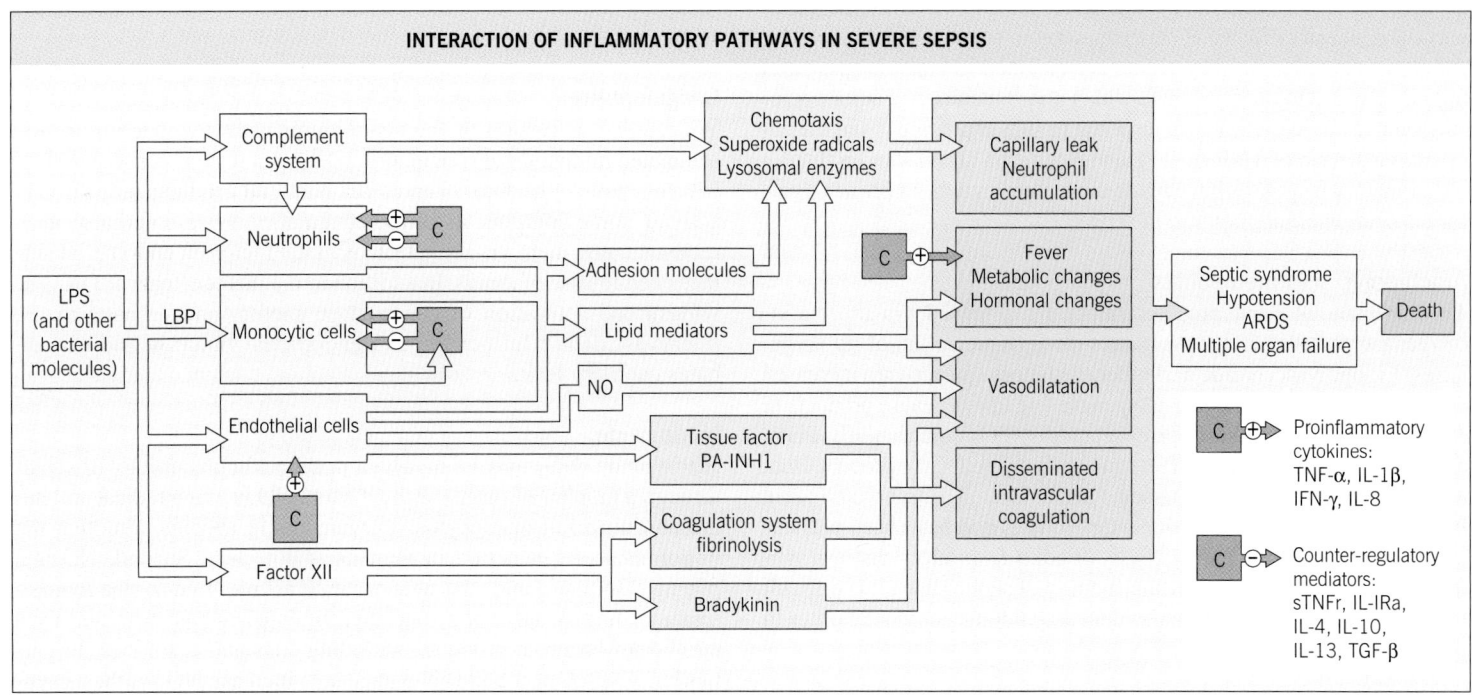

Fig. 47.9 Interaction of inflammatory pathways in severe sepsis. IL-1Ra, interleukin-1 receptor antagonist; TGF-β, transforming growth factor-β; sTNFr, soluble TNF receptor.

neutrophils to survive longer in an inflammatory environment and to kill more bacteria, but excessive activation of endothelial adhesion may result in the migration of primed activated neutrophils into sites distant from infection. The ensuing tissue damage stimulates a vicious cycle of re-recruitment of inflammatory cells, ultimately leading to organ damage and failure.[40]

ENDOGENOUS ANTI-INFLAMMATORY MEDIATORS IN SEPSIS
In addition to the large number of proinflammatory mediators induced during severe sepsis there are a growing number of counter-regulatory mediators being discovered. They have specific actions and may neutralize or detoxify bacterial products, block the synthesis or release of cytokines, or downregulate cell responses to inflammatory stimuli. The most important molecules identified to date are given in Figure 47.6.

INTERACTION OF MEDIATORS IN SEPSIS
As already discussed, LPS and other bacterial products are potent activators of the host defenses. There has been an intense search for the 'central mediator' of septic shock and attention has focused in turn on complement, prostaglandins, PAF, TNF and other cytokines, NO, and other mediators (see Fig. 47.6). What has become clear is that there is no single central mediator, but rather there is a complex network of inflammatory responses to infection, which can in certain circumstances result in sepsis as depicted in Figure 47.9. Once activated, these mediators induce further inflammatory responses in what has been referred to as the 'sepsis cascade', leading to tissue damage and eventually death. However, these same inflammatory processes release another complicated network of counter-regulatory or anti-inflammatory mediators, such as the IL receptor antagonist (IL-1Ras) and soluble TNF receptors. Thus, it is the balance between these opposing mechanisms that will determine whether inflammation is successful in eliminating the infection and then 'shutting down', or progressing so that healthy tissues are damaged at sites distant from the infective source and become victims of 'friendly fire'. In sepsis it is not always correct to assume that more inflammation is 'bad'. A recent study of severe sepsis found that a high IL-10/TNF ratio correlated more closely with mortality than TNF levels alone.[41]

PATHOPHYSIOLOGIC EVENTS LEADING TO ORGAN FAILURE IN SEPSIS
How do the complicated and often confusing inflammatory responses outlined above actually lead to tissue damage and eventually multiorgan failure? At the cellular level, the end result of the inflammatory process is cell death. In the whole organism the key to organ damage lies in the breakdown of normal vascular homeostasis, leading

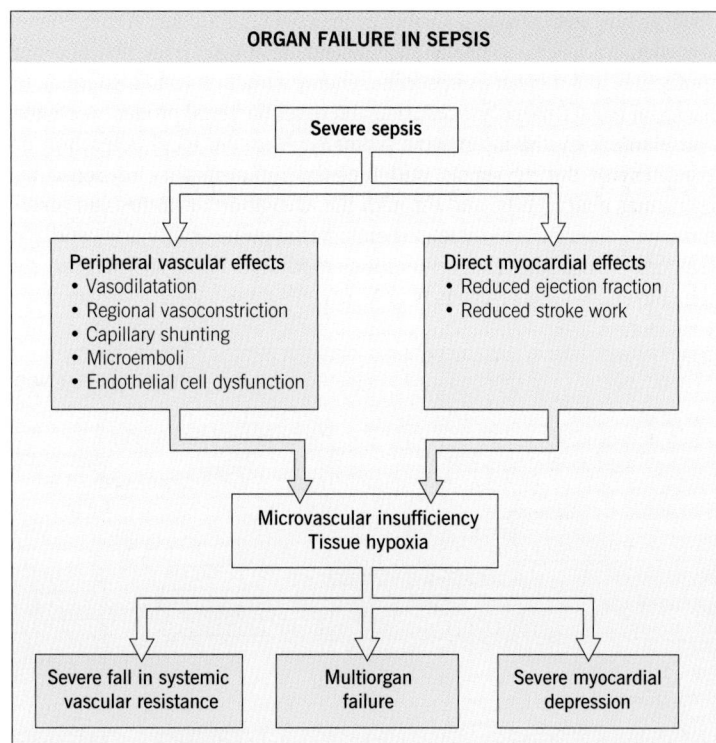

Fig. 47.10 Organ failure in sepsis. In sepsis inflammatory mediators have direct and indirect effects upon both the myocardium and peripheral vasculature. The net effect of these is microvasculature shunting, hypotension and hypoxia. The combination of these leads to a failure of tissue oxygenation resulting in acidosis and further decline in vascular function. Eventually this process leads to multiorgan failure and death.

PATHOGENESIS OF MULTIORGAN FAILURE IN SEPTIC SHOCK

Organ/tissue	Clinicopathologic features	Mechanism
Peripheral vasculature	Vasodilatation Refractory hypotension Shunting Coagulopathy (DIC) Fibrin deposition	Endothelial NO Smooth muscle NO Tissue factor expression and procoagulant activity Neutrophil migration
Myocardium	Myocardial depression and arrhythmias	Altered calcium influx Decreased contractility
Lung	Adult respiratory distress syndrome	Increased endothelial permeability Neutrophil activation/migration
Kidney	Acute tubular necrosis	Renal hypoperfusion
Liver	Zonal necrosis, hepatic failure	Hypoperfusion Acidosis
Gut	Breach of epithelial integrity	Hypoperfusion Acidosis
Brain	Encephalopathy	Hypoperfusion Acidosis

Fig. 47.11 Pathogenesis of multiorgan failure in septic shock. Adapted from Sriskandan and Cohen.[31]

HEMODYNAMIC CHANGES IN SEVERE SEPSIS

Parameter	Normal range	Changes in severe sepsis
Heart rate (HR)	72–88 beats/min	Sinus tachycardia
Mean arterial pressure (MAP)	70–105mmHg	Hypotension <60mmHg
Cardiac output (CO)	4–8l/min	Increased but not enough to compensate for low SVR
Systemic vascular resistance (SVR)	800–1500dyne/s/cm^2	Reduced (<600 if no pressor agents)
Oxygen delivery (Do_2)	520–720ml/min/m^2	Decreased
Oxygen consumption (Vo_2)	100–180ml/min/m^2	Typically increased

$CO = SV \times HR$, $SVR = (MAP - CVP)/CO \times 79.92$
$Do_2 = CI \times$ arterial oxygen $\times 10$, $Vo_2 = CI \times$ (arterial $-$ venous oxygen) $\times 10$

Fig. 47.12 Hemodynamic changes in sepsis. CI, cardiac index (CO/m^2 surface area); CVP, central venous pressure; SV, stroke volume.

to tissue hypoxia as described in Figure 47.10. The consequences of these events are shown in Figure 47.11; the three most important factors are depressed myocardial function, alterations in the peripheral vasculature and failure of oxygen exchange in the lung.

Cardiac function

Initially when peripheral vasodilatation occurs in sepsis there is a compensatory rise in cardiac output (Fig. 47.12). However, the increase in cardiac output is often less than that predicted and it is recognized that most patients who have severe sepsis have impaired myocardial function. Cumulative evidence suggests that the impairment of myocardial contractility seen in sepsis is a consequence of circulating cytokines. Tumor necrosis factor-α directly reduces myocyte contractility and is also implicated in the pathogenesis of myocardial dysfunction in dilated cardiomyopathy. In addition induction of myocardial NO synthesis by cytokines also impairs myocardial function.

Peripheral vasculature

The hallmark of severe sepsis is widespread peripheral vasodilatation and, in refractory septic shock, it may resist all attempts at pharmacologic intervention. As mentioned earlier, this is largely the consequence of increased NO production in response to cytokines. The most serious consequence of the vasodilatation is the loss of homeostatic regulation of tissue blood flow. Thus, much of the circulating blood volume is shunted through capillary beds, bypassing deep tissues and reducing the opportunity for oxygen extraction. This in turn exacerbates tissue hypoxia and helps to drive the metabolic acidosis that is one of the prominent features of severe sepsis. Further local impairment of perfusion may occur as the result of aggregation of platelets and activation of coagulation in the microcirculation.

Respiratory failure

The lung is one of the most vulnerable organs in sepsis, and TNF-α, PAF, C5a, IL-8 and thromboxane appear to play prominent roles in the development of ARDS, increased neutrophil adherence to and migration across the pulmonary endothelium being the key pathophysiologic mechanism. The passage of neutrophils across the endothelium and subsequent degranulation in the lung interstitium leads to further impairment of endothelial integrity and the accumulation of fluid and inflammatory cells in the alveolar spaces. Impaired gas exchange inevitably produces hypoxia, which further worsens the situation. The combination of hypoxia and increased pulmonary thromboxane synthesis increases pulmonary vascular resistance, in contrast to the fall in systemic vascular resistance. Thus the end result of the pulmonary events in sepsis is the development of interstitial edema and pulmonary hypertension, the hallmarks of ARDS.

PREVENTION

The morbidity, mortality and hospital costs associated with sepsis demand that strenuous efforts must be made to reduce the incidence of this serious disease. These can be divided into three main areas:

- assiduous infection control for high risk patients;
- the use of prophylactic antibiotic therapies; and
- possibly, in the future, immunomodulation.

Details of infection control policies are outlined elsewhere (see Chapters 3.9, 3.10 & 7.3), but it is worth re-emphasizing that many cases of sepsis are acquired in hospital, particularly in the ICU, and that nosocomial sepsis has a much higher mortality than community-acquired sepsis. It has been estimted that up to one-third of cases of nosocomial infections are preventable and a multidisciplinary approach to infection control can lead to significant reductions in ICU pneumonia and sepsis.[42,43]

The principles of antibiotic prophylaxis are covered elsewhere (see Chapter 1.4), but it is worth noting here that, particularly when performing invasive procedures, it is important to recognize patients who have risk factors for developing sepsis, for example manipulation of the urinary tract in the presence of active infection, and to administer appropriate antimicrobial therapy.

In animal models, it is possible to manipulate the immune system by a variety of methods to limit the 'septic response' to infection. As yet there are no agents in routine clinical use, but some (e.g. recombinant bactericidal/permeability-increasing proteins, an endotoxin antagonist) are in clinical trials.[44] However, many other 'immunotherapies' have not been successful in large clinical trials.[45]

CLINICAL FEATURES

A rigorous history, physical examination and directed investigations are essential to arrive at the correct diagnosis of any infectious disease. However, severe sepsis and shock is a medical emergency and therefore full assessment may have to be delayed until resuscitation and empiric antimicrobial therapy have been commenced. The aims of clinical evaluation are to establish the diagnosis of sepsis, estimate disease severity and prognosis, and elucidate the underlying cause. Although sepsis has many features common to most cases, the exact presentation will depend on the site of infection, the nature of the infecting organism, the host response and co-existent illness. Therefore, in the elderly and other immunocompromised groups the physical signs and some of the laboratory parameters that suggest sepsis may be absent; in this group it is important to consider sepsis in the differential diagnosis of any unexplained illness.

HISTORY AND SYMPTOMATOLOGY

Symptoms that suggest the onset of sepsis are often nonspecific and include sweats, chills or rigors, breathlessness, nausea and vomiting or diarrhea, and headache. Confusion may be found in 10–30% of patients, especially the elderly.[46] There may be specific symptoms to suggest the underlying pathology, such as cough, dysuria or meningism, but in many cases there are no clues. Other important points to elicit that may give an indication of the diagnosis or help in choosing empiric therapy include recent travel, contact with animals, local infectious disease outbreaks, recent surgical procedures, indwelling prosthetic devices, prior antibiotics, underlying pathology and immunosuppressive illness or medication. For the critically ill patient such details are often unavailable, and it may be helpful to speak to relatives or the patient's primary care physician.

PHYSICAL SIGNS ON EXAMINATION

In its simplest form sepsis simply refers to the physiologic response to infection. With progression to severe sepsis and shock there is increasing evidence of organ dysfunction; the key physical signs and physiologic changes indicating this are encapsulated in the ACCP/ASCCM guidelines (see Fig. 47.1). One of the most important clinical points to remember is that sepsis is a dynamic evolving clinical picture, and therefore frequent evaluation and careful monitoring of the patient is essential.

The characteristic patient who has severe sepsis is febrile, tachypneic, tachycardiac with warm peripheries and often a bounding arterial pulse, hypotensive, disoriented and oliguric. The observation chart of one such patient is shown in Figure 47.13, but many patients have a much more subtle presentation necessitating a high index of suspicion to recognize early disease. Although most patients are febrile, severe sepsis may present with hypothermia. A detailed physical examination is vital and it is important to examine the skin, all wounds and the fundi, and to perform full ear, nose and throat, and rectal and vaginal examinations as these sites are often overlooked and may hold valuable clues as to the diagnosis (e.g. a retained vaginal tampon in the toxic shock syndrome). In the hospitalized patient and the ICU patient who develops sepsis, it is necessary to pay particular attention to indwelling intravenous/intra-arterial lines, insist on exposing and examining all wounds, and carefully review the pressure areas as these are frequently neglected sources of infection. Occasionally, the physical examination

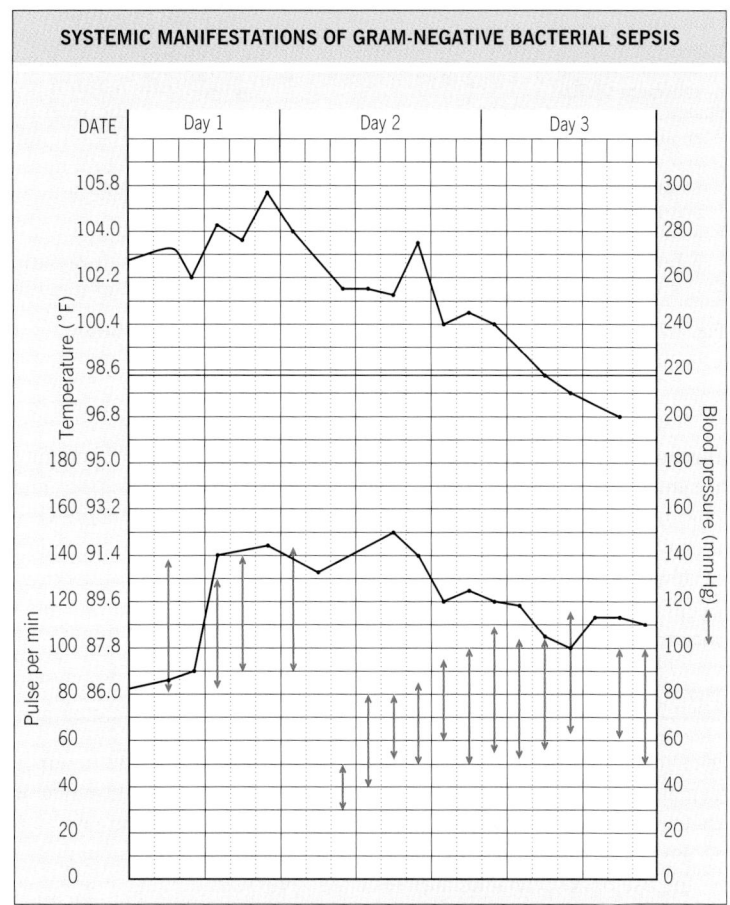

Fig. 47.13 Systemic manifestations of Gram-negative bacterial sepsis. Observation chart of a 49-year old woman admitted to hospital with a suspected drug fever. For the first 24 hours she was observed without antimicrobial chemotherapy and demonstrated a persistent fever and tachycardia (sepsis). At this point she suddenly became confused, hypotensive and oliguric indicating the development of severe sepsis. The underlying cause was an *Escherichia coli* bacteremia from an unsuspected urinary tract infection. She responded to fluid replacement and antibiotics and made a full recovery.

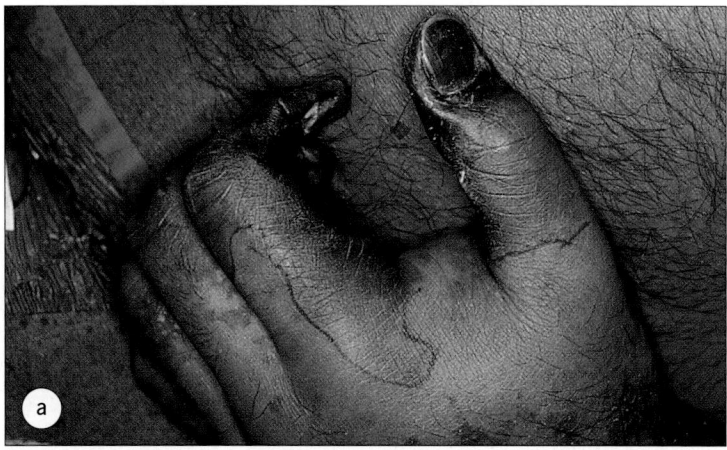

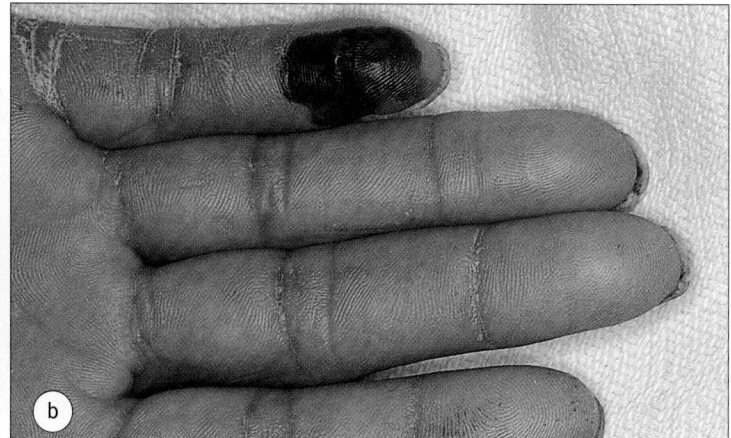

Fig. 47.14 Cutaneous changes in severe sepsis. (a) The confluent purpuric rash and severe peripheral gangrene that may be seen in severe sepsis due to meningococcal infection. (b) Much more localized tissue necrosis suggestive of an embolic phenomenon; in this case the patient was found to have underlying *Staphylococcus aureus* endocarditis. Courtesy of Jonathan Cohen, London.

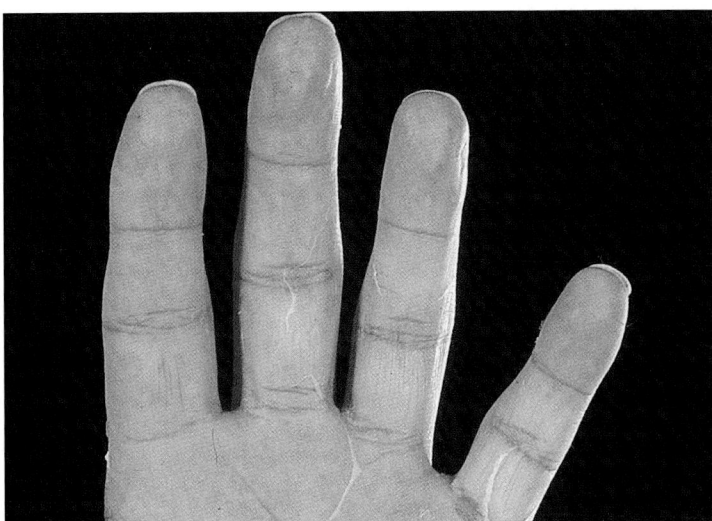

Fig. 47.15 Desquamation of the palms following an episode of **staphylococcal toxic shock.** Courtesy of M Jacobs.

will directly establish the diagnosis; helpful signs include the purpuric rash or peripheral gangrene of meningococcemia (Fig. 47.14a), peripheral emboli in endocarditis (Fig. 47.14b), the erythematous rash or desquamation in staphylococcal or streptococcal toxic shock (Fig. 47.15), ecthyma gangrenosum in patients who have neutropenia and *P. aeruginosa* bacteremia, or the retinal lesions of *Candida* endophthalmitis. Focal physical signs may help to identify the site of infection, for example renal angle tenderness, pulmonary consolidation, cardiac murmur or finding an intra-abdominal mass, but in many cases the site of the infection remains uncertain.

If the patient is hypotensive, other causes of shock such as cardiac dysfunction (including myocardial infarction and cardiac tamponade), hypovolemia, and redistributive shock from pancreatitis and physical injuries need to be considered. Invasive physiologic measurements are often used to distinguish between these (see below), but it is important to remember that the hypotension seen in sepsis is often multifactorial and sepsis may complicate or co-exist with other causes of shock. Thus such invasive measurements must not be interpreted in isolation but should be reviewed in the context of the whole clinical picture.

DIAGNOSIS

LABORATORY INVESTIGATIONS

These can broadly be divided into those that help to confirm that the patient has sepsis and detect and follow complications such as organ failure, and those that establish the underlying cause.

Hematologic and biochemical evaluation in sepsis

Full blood count and blood film. Look for leukopenia or a neutrophil leukocytosis. Leukopenia in sepsis is generally associated with a worse prognosis. The blood film may suggest bacterial infection with toxic granulation of neutrophils even when the white cell count is within the normal range. Leukopenia at presentation is a poor prognostic sign. Low platelet count suggests DIC and evidence of a microangiopathic hemolysis may be visible. In patients who have traveled to an endemic area, three separate thick and thin films for malaria parasites are required.

Coagulation screen. Look for evidence of DIC – prolonged prothrombin or activated partial thromboplastin time, low fibrinogen and elevated markers of fibrinolysis (fibrin degradation products or D-dimer levels).

Electrolytes and renal function. It is essential to monitor renal function closely; markedly elevated potassium may indicate rhabdomyolysis, which can occasionally complicate severe sepsis.

Liver function tests. Minor abnormalities are very common in patients who have bacteremia and sepsis, and do not necessarily signify a hepatic source of infection. Rises in bilirubin, alkaline phosphatase or transaminases of two to three times the normal level may be seen in up to 30–50% of patients.[47] These are generally transient and not of prognostic importance. More markedly abnormal liver function suggests the possibility of underlying hepatic or biliary tract infection, particularly if the pattern of liver enzymes suggests biliary obstruction. Progressively deteriorating liver function in patients who have sepsis suggests hepatocellular damage or acalculous cholecystitis, which may occur as complications of severe sepsis.

Plasma albumin. In patients who have severe sepsis an acute fall in albumin, to as low as 1.5–2.0g/dl over 24 hours, may occur as a result of widespread endothelial damage and capillary leakage of protein. In patients who have chronic underlying illness or prolonged infection, the albumin falls as a result of poor nutrition and a switch in hepatic metabolism towards acute-phase proteins.

C-reactive protein. This is an acute-phase reactant that rises within a few hours of bacterial infection. High levels are detectable in patients who have septic shock and sequential values are useful in monitoring the response to therapy, although a raised CRP does not reliably distinguish septic from nonseptic causes of shock. Procalcitonin levels are also elevated in bacterial infections and may be a more sensitive marker than CRP, but this test is not yet widely available.[48]

Blood glucose. Hypoglycemia may occur in severe sepsis. In patients who are diabetic, normalization of blood glucose is essential in helping to control the infection.

Plasma lactate. This is often increased three- to five-fold in severe sepsis (normal 1.0–2.5mmol/l) and relates to the degree of tissue hypoxia. Lactate estimations may be helpful both in confirming the diagnosis and in monitoring the response to therapy.

Arterial blood gases. Typically a respiratory alkalosis occurs early and metabolic acidosis late. The degree of acidosis is a marker of the severity of illness. The onset of hypoxia indicates severe disease and a high risk of ARDS. Measurement of venous and arterial oxygen content allows calculation of oxygen delivery and consumption (see below).

Other biochemical investigations. Amylase, creatinine phosphokinase, calcium and magnesium levels should be measured at baseline.

Endotoxin or cytokine levels. In some but not all studies, the level of endotoxemia has been correlated with outcome of Gram-negative sepsis.[49-51] Technical difficulties with the collection and analysis of plasma endotoxin and the often intermittent appearance of endotoxin in the blood makes routine testing impractical at present.

Microbiologic investigations in sepsis

Ideally, cultures should be taken before initiating antibiotic therapy, but treatment is urgent and should not be unduly delayed.[52] For example, studies have clearly shown that the administration of antibiotics to cases of suspected meningococcal sepsis before transfer to hospital improves outcome.

Blood cultures are the most important microbiologic investigation. Two or three separate blood cultures, from a total of 20–30ml of blood, should be inoculated into one of the standard commercial blood culture media. It is important to stress that culturing an inadequate volume of blood is the most common reason for not detecting bacteremia.[53] The bottles should be incubated aerobically and anaerobically at 98°F (37°C), preferably agitated, for 7 days. Where there is a high risk of underlying fungal infection then additional cultures inoculated into specific fungal media may be helpful.[54]

Sputum and urine microscopy and culture should be performed in all cases. All wounds should be swabbed and sterile body sites such as cerebrospinal fluid (CSF), joint or pleural fluid sampled as indicated. In cases in which toxic shock syndrome is suspected, wound, nose, throat and vaginal swabs should be taken. If staphylococci or streptococci are isolated in cases of toxic shock then the appropriate reference laboratories can assay the isolate for toxin production. Cultures should be repeated as directed by previous results and the condition of the patient.

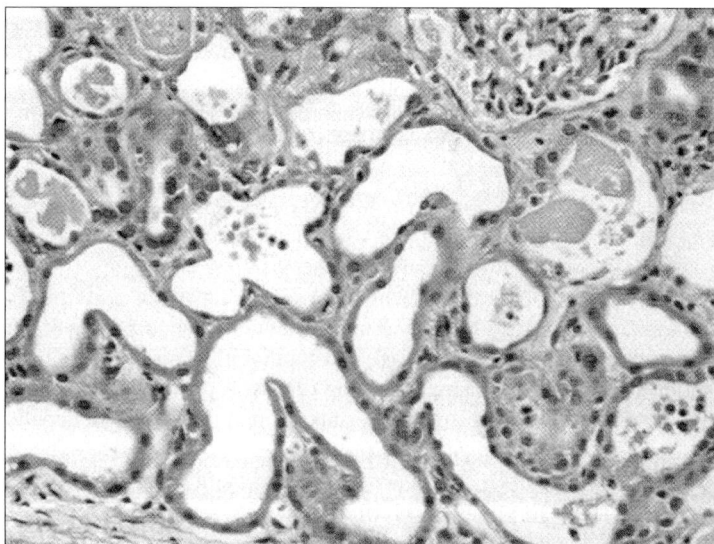

Fig. 47.16 **Acute tubular necrosis.** The tubules are dilated with flattened epilithial cells, and contain debris; the glomerulus is not greatly affected. Haematoxylin and eosin. With permission from Williams JD *et al.*, Clinical atlas of the kidney. London: Mosby.

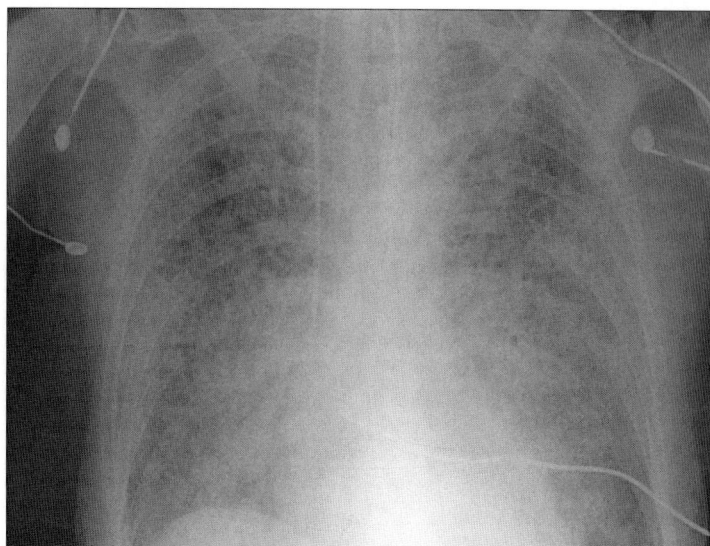

Fig. 47.18 **Chest radiograph showing multilobar consolidation due to severe ARDS complicating acute pancreatitis.**

Histopathologic changes in sepsis

The organ pathology in sepsis is due to the combined effects of hypoxia, local impairment in tissue perfusion and severe acidosis. In the lung the changes are those of ARDS, with early findings of interstitial and alveolar edema, fibrosis developing at a later stage. The kidneys may show acute tubular necrosis that is generally reversible (Fig. 47.16). Hepatic changes are of an ischemic zonal necrosis and some cases may develop an acalculous cholecystitis. In the brain there may be areas of focal ischemia or hemorrhage. In severe cases of septic shock associated with *Neisseria meningitidis* there may be peripheral gangrene due to severe impairment of perfusion (see Fig. 47.14) and hemorrhage into the adrenal glands (Fig. 47.17). The gut is also affected by ischemia and may show mucosal ulcerations and areas of infarction.

RADIOLOGIC INVESTIGATIONS

Chest radiography is necessary in all cases and may show signs of ARDS (Fig. 47.18); other studies may be indicated. Radiologic investigations can be of great help in identifying occult sites of infection, and close liaison with the diagnostic radiology department is

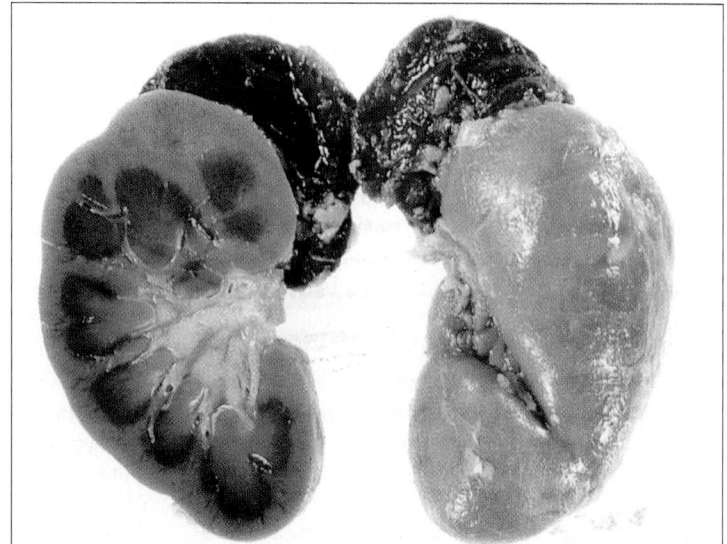

Fig. 47.17 **Acute hemorrhagic necrosis of the adrenal glands (Waterhouse-Friderichsen syndrome).** Both adrenal glands of a child with meningococcal septicemia show hemorrhagic necrosis leading to acute adrenal failure. With permission from Stevens A, Lowe J. Pathology. London: Mosby; 1995.

vital. Ultrasound and CT are particularly useful when trying to detect deep abscesses; in selected cases nuclear medicine techniques may pinpoint the site of infection. In recent years, the interventional radiologist's contribution, through percutaneous sampling/drainage of sites of infection, has grown.

MANAGEMENT

Mortality from sepsis and multiorgan failure remains high and some authors have been very pessimistic about attempts to treat patients who have severe sepsis. However, it would be incorrect to assume that medical care has little to offer for this condition. Although recent studies defining the epidemiology and natural history of sepsis show that many patients do indeed progress from early sepis to shock and organ failure,[6] by early recognition and prompt therapeutic intervention many patients can be prevented from progressing down this path. There are four therapeutic goals:
- to treat underlying infection,
- to preserve vital organ perfusion,
- to maintain tissue oxygenation, and
- to avoid complications.

ANTIBIOTIC CHEMOTHERAPY

Clinical studies of patients who have sepsis/SIRS have identified the use of inappropriate empiric antibiotics (i.e. the infecting organisms were resistant to the antibiotics used) as being associated with a higher mortality.[55,56] In general it is accepted that the regimen used in severe sepsis should be bactericidal rather that bacteriostatic. There has been considerable debate regarding the use of monotherapy or combination therapy regimens in a number of infections, including sepsis. The arguments in favor of combination treatment, generally with a beta-lactam plus an aminoglycoside, include improved antimicrobial spectrum, decreased potential for resistance and possible synergistic activity. However, in studies of sepsis/SIRS in which appropriate empiric therapy has been employed it has been hard to demonstrate that any particular antibiotic or combination of antibiotics is superior. The decision regarding antibiotic choice should, therefore, be made on the same principles as for any serious infection. For example, the choice of antibiotic for pyelonephritis is not influenced by whether the patient is septic, but rather by the likely microbiology of the infection, the potential for antibiotic resistance and the need to use a drug that penetrates into renal tissue.

POSSIBLE EMPIRIC ANTIBIOTIC CHOICE IN SEVERE SEPSIS	
Suspected site of infection	Antibiotic

Pneumonia
  Community-acquired
  Hospital-acquired
	Cefotaxime + erythromycin
	Cefotaxime/ceftazidime alone
	  or ureidopenicillin + aminoglycoside

Urinary tract
  Community-acquired
 	
  Hospital-acquired
	Amoxicillin + clavalunic acid (co-amoxiclav)
	  or cefotaxime
	Ceftazidime alone
	  or ureidopenicillin + aminoglycoside

Skin and soft tissue
  Community-acquired
  Hospital-acquired
	Benzyl-penicillin + nafcillin (flucloxacillin)
	Cefotaxime + nafcillin
	  or cefotaxime + vancomycin

Intra-abdominal	Cefotaxime + metronidazole
	  or ureidopenicillin + aminoglycoside
	  or imipenem monotherapy

Biliary tract	Ureidopenicillin + aminoglycoside
Neutropenic	Ureidopenicillin + aminoglycoside or ceftazidime monotherapy

Fig. 47.19 Possible empiric antibiotic choice in severe sepsis.

If the infecting organism has been identified and drug sensitivities determined, then the choice of antibiotics is comparatively easy. However, in most clinical situations empiric choice of the appropriate antibiotic(s) needs to be made before laboratory results are available. Figure 47.19 provides a useful guide to antibiotic choice for the more common causes of sepsis, but it is not possible to recommend specific antibiotic regimens for all cases because of variations in infecting pathogens and antimicrobial resistance between hospitals. The principles underlying the selection are outlined below.

Factors in empiric antibiotic choice

Site of infection. This is the most influential factor in determining the likely microbiology of the infection and hence in directing antimicrobial therapy; for example, penetrating abdominal trauma requires cover for Gram-negative bacilli, anaerobic bacteria and possible enterococci. It is also important to choose antibiotics that penetrate to the site of infection; for example, aminoglycosides are very effective for *E. coli* urinary tract sepsis, but are less effective in abscesses or meningitis, because of poor penetration.

Environmental exposure. This is a crucial factor, particularly in nosocomial infections and in individuals who have recently traveled. Penicillin currently remains the antibiotic of choice for presumed pneumococcal sepsis in the UK, for example, but isolation of penicillin-resistant pneumococci is increasing worldwide, particularly in southern Europe, South Africa and some parts of the USA, and alternative agents are required as empiric therapy for presumed pneumococcal disease in these countries. An up-to-date knowledge of the local antimicrobial resistance patterns and prompt detection of resistance problems within the hospital are vital in ensuring correct therapy.

Immunosuppression. Impaired host response alters the range of pathogens and the presentation of disease, due to increased host susceptibility and decreased ability of the host to clear certain pathogens. Typical examples include overwhelming pneumococcal sepsis in an individual without a functional spleen, increased rates of bacterial sepsis in alcoholics and fungal sepsis in trauma patients on intensive care.

Drug allergy. Although most empiric regimens for sepsis are based on beta-lactam antibiotics (penicillins and cephalosporins), it is important to have suitable alternative choices for those patients who have a history of severe penicillin allergy (see Fig. 47.19).

Reviewing empiric therapy. The antibiotic regimen should be reviewed, and if necessary amended, every 24 hours in the light of the clinical situation and available microbiology data.

Antibiotic-induced endotoxin release.

As discussed earlier (see above), endotoxin has been identified as the major factor in the pathogenesis of shock due to Gram-negative bacteria. In experimental models, and some limited situations in humans, release of endotoxin from bacteria has been shown to increase the inflammatory response and different antibiotics vary in their capacity to induce endotoxin release from bacteria.[57] Thus, a school of thought has developed to suggest that antibiotics should be chosen on the basis of their potential to cause endotoxin release. However, beyond a handful of small studies there are few clinical data to support a major role for this hypothesis in sepsis. At present, antibiotics should therefore be selected on the basis of efficacy for the specific clinical picture, rather than on the theoretic risk of endotoxin release.

DETECTION AND REMOVAL OF INFECTED MATERIAL

In addition to antimicrobial therapy it is essential to drain/remove all possible infective foci as these are often the cause for treatment failure. Thus, abscesses should be drained, dead tissue resected and infected foreign material, such as an infected central venous catheter, removed. The critically ill patient on intensive care may have repeated episodes of sepsis; locating the underlying focus often requires considerable determination and patience and sometimes repeated discussions with surgical colleagues.

SUPPORTIVE THERAPY

The central goal of supportive therapy is to try to maintain tissue oxygen delivery, a concept advanced by Shoemaker and others through the 1970s.[58] A full discussion of advanced techniques to preserve organ function in the critically ill patient is beyond the scope of this chapter, but the principles underpinning successful care are discussed here.

Ideally, patients who have sepsis should be closely monitored in an intensive therapy or high-dependency unit. Indeed a review of 41 patients who had septic shock revealed increased mortality when patients were managed outside of the intensive therapy unit, 70% versus 39%, even though the patients had less severe illness.[14] Minimal requirements for safe management would include facilities for measurement of blood pressure, continuous cardiac monitoring, central venous pressure recording, rapid arterial blood gas analysis, continuous oxygen and facilities for mechanical ventilation or dialysis when required.

Invasive monitoring is useful in excluding other causes of shock such as hypovolemia and in directing supportive therapy. However, invasive monitoring is not a substitute for careful examination and assessment of the patient. Many factors such as cardiovascular disease, hypovolemia or inotropic drugs can confound monitoring data; results must be interpreted in the context of the clinical situation. Normal values and the typical ranges for hemodynamic parameters in severe sepsis are given in Figure 47.12.

In hemodynamic management of sepsis, the aim is to achieve sufficient arterial blood pressure for organ perfusion. This does not require normalization of blood pressure and generally can be achieved with a mean arterial pressure of 50–60mmHg. Sepsis is characterized by vasodilatation and widespread capillary leak.[59] There may be significant depletion of intravascular volume, in which case correction of hypovolemia should be performed immediately. There is continuing debate about the ideal fluid replacement, some preferring crystalloid and others preferring different types of colloid. There has been some concern over the saftey of human albumin preparations as volume replacement and until this debate is resolved albumin is best avoided.[60] It is probably best to avoid dextrans in sepsis, due to because of the risk of bleeding. In practice, a balance must be kept between early aggressive fluid replacement, which is required to maintain tissue perfusion and organ function, and fluid overload, which may increase the risk of

ARDS and should be avoided.[61] Therefore, most clinicians use both colloid and crystalloid during the care of patients who have severe sepsis; monitoring of central venous pressure and preferably pulmonary capillary wedge pressure is essential to achieve the correct balance. Pulmonary capillary wedge pressure measurements were routinely used but there has been some doubt over the saftey and utility of pulmonary artery catheters in the critically ill patient. As a result many intensive therapy units have reduced their use of pulmonary catheters and monitor cardiac output and pulmonary artery pressure noninvasively. Blood transfusion is required in the event of hemorrhage or severe anemia (Hb < 9g/dl) but probably does not improve oxygen delivery in patients who have Hb > 10g/dl.

If there is an inadequate response to volume replacement the use of inotropic/pressor agents is required. In addition to vasodilatation in sepsis there is often also associated myocardial suppression. This may be due to a number of factors, including the effects of bacterial toxins and cytokines on the myocardium. Impaired myocardial contractility responds to dobutamine (2–25µg/kg/min) or epinephrine (adrenaline, 2–8µg/min). However, it may be necessary to add pressor agents such as norepinephrine (noradrenaline, 2–8µg/min) or dopamine (2–25µg/kg/min) to raise peripheral resistance and increase blood pressure.[62] No single regimen is effective for all patients and there is no consensus as to the optimal combination or dosage of inotropic and pressor agents. Patients are best managed by repeated observation of response to different therapeutic measures.[63]

In established shock with multiorgan failure, poor perfusion and oxygenation of tissue is a major cause of treatment failure and death. Patients require supplemental oxygen, and may need mechanical ventilation to maintain arterial oxygen saturation. Tissue hypoxia increases lactic acidosis and will further impair cardiac and other functions. Experimental methods of extracorporeal oxygenation have been tried but none are in routine use.[61]

Measurement of oxygen delivery (DO_2) and oxygen consumption ($\dot{V}O_2$) are also employed in some intensive care units to monitor the response to treatment. In patients who have severe sepsis, $\dot{V}O_2$ is increased and therefore a high DO_2 is required to maintain tissue oxygenation. In patients with sepsis, DO_2 is generally inadequate and often is referred to as an 'oxygen debt'.[64] If DO_2 and $\dot{V}O_2$ are calculated then fluids, inotropes and oxygenation can be adjusted to attempt to achieve optimal oxygen delivery. Tissue hypoxia can also be measured directly by using tonometry to follow gastric pH, by hepatic venous oxygen measurement and by muscle needle probes, but it is not clear whether routine use of these measurements will improve patient outcome.

MANAGEMENT OF COAGULOPATHY
Currently there is no universally accepted approach to the management of DIC in patients who have sepsis. Some authors have advocated anticoagulation with heparin, and there are animal data and anecdoatal reports of improvement to support this view. However, to date, there have been no large clinical trials and the routine use of anticoagulation cannot be supported. For patients who have severe DIC, replacement of clotting factors with fresh frozen plasma or cryoprecipitate may be required to combat bleeding. However, it must be remembered that plasma also contains potentially proinflammatory components, such as complement, and that replacing the clotting factors may simply fuel the processes leading to DIC. Indeed, one case–control study has suggested that the routine use of blood products in meningococcal disease increases morbidity and mortality.[65] Thus, patients should be treated with clotting factors not simply because of abnormal laboratory parameters but rather when there is a clear clinical indication. Other modulators of coagulation are protective in experimental models of sepsis[32,37] and antithrombin III concentrates are the subject of clinical trials.[66]

NUTRITION
Patients who have severe sepsis are extremely catabolic and it is very important to plan nutritional support and supplementation at an early stage. Unless there is a contraindication to oral feeding, nutrition should be given by the enteral route. Enteral feeding may help to protect the gut mucosa from ischemic damage in sepsis and to reduce bacterial translocation from the gut, which is thought to be involved in some episodes of sepsis. Parenteral nutrition increases the rate of secondary infections, particularly bacterial and fungal intravenous catheter infections, and so should be avoided if the gut is functional.

CORTICOSTEROIDS IN SEPSIS
There has been considerable controversy surrounding the use of corticosteroids in severe sepsis. In animal models pretreatment with corticosteroids protected against endotoxemia, and initial promising reports in humans lead to the widespread use of high-dose corticosteroids in sepsis. Subsequently two large multicenter trials failed to show benefit and recent meta-analyses of all suitable trials confirmed that the use of corticosteroids in sepsis is not of benefit and may actually be deleterious by increasing rates of secondary infection.[67]

EXPERIMENTAL THERAPY FOR SEPSIS
Despite all the therapies available, the mortality of established septic shock and organ failure remains high.[10] The concept that organ damage in sepsis is the result of the host inflammatory response has lead to an enormous research effort to understand and intervene in this process.[32,45] Many therapeutic strategies have been investigated in the laboratory setting and the past decade has seen large randomized clinical trials of some of the more promising agents. This has highlighted the difficulties inherent in performing interventional studies in sepsis and initial results have often been conflicting and disappointing.[45] However, our understanding of the pathophysiologic processes underlying sepsis continues to increase and suggests that it will be possible to intervene positively in severe sepsis in the near future.

REFERENCES

1. McCabe WR, Jackson GG. Gram-negative bacteremia I. Etiology and ecology. Arch Intern Med 1962;110:847–55.
2. McCabe WR, Jackson GG. Gram-negative bacteremia II. Clinical, laboratory, and therapeutic observations. Arch Intern Med 1962;110:856–64.
3. Bone RC. Sepsis, the sepsis syndrome, multi-organ failure: a plea for comparable definitions. Ann Intern Med 1991;114:332–3.
4. Bone RC, Balk RA, Cerra FB, et al. Definitions for sepsis and organ failure and guidelines for the use of innovative therapies in sepsis. Chest 1992;101:1644–55.
5. Vincent J-L. The 'at risk' patient population. In: Sibbald WJ, Vincent J-L, eds. Update in intensive care and emergency medicine: clinical trials for the treatment of sepsis. Berlin: Springer-Verlag; 1995:71–85.
6. Rangel-Frausto MS, Pittet D, Costigan M, Hwang T, Davis CS, Wenzel RP. The natural history of the systemic inflammatory response syndrome (SIRS). A prospective study. JAMA 1995;273:117–23.
7. Wenzel RP, Pinsky MR, Ulevitch RJ, Young L. Current understanding of sepsis. Clin Infect Dis 1996;22:407–12.
8. Wenzel RP. The mortality of hospital-acquired blood stream infections: need for a new vital statistic. Int J Epidemiol 1988;17:225–7.
9. Glauser MP, Heumann D, Baumgartner JD, Cohen J. Pathogenesis and potential strategies for prevention and treatment of septic shock: an update. Clin Infect Dis 1994;18:S205–16.
10. Quartin AA, Schein RM, Kett DH, Peduzzi PN. Magnitude and duration of the effect of sepsis on survival. JAMA 1997;277:1058–63.
11. Kieft H, Hoepelman AI, Zhou W, Rozenberg-Arska M, Struyvenberg A, Verhoef J. The sepsis syndrome in a Dutch university hospital. Clinical observations. Arch Intern Med 1993;153:2241–7.
12. Brun Buisson C, Doyon F, Carlet J. Bacteremia and severe sepsis in adults: a multicenter prospective survey in ICUs and wards of 24 hospitals. Am J Respir Crit Care Med 1996;154:617–24.
13. Sands KE, Bates DW, Lanken PN, et al. Epidemiology of sepsis syndrome in 8 academic medical centers. JAMA 1997;278:234–40.
14. Lundberg JS, Perl TM, Wiblin T, et al. Septic shock: an analysis of outcomes for patients with onset on hospital wards versus intensive care units. Crit Care Med 1998;26:1020–4.
15. Bone RC. Towards an epidemiology and natural history of SIRS (systemic inflammatory response syndrome). JAMA 1992;268:3452–5.
16. Vincent JL, Bihari DJ, Suter PM, et al. The prevalence of nosocomial infection in intensive care units in Europe. Results of the European Prevalence of Infection in Intensive Care (EPIC) Study. JAMA 1995;274:639–44.
17. Raetz CRH, Ulevitch RJ, Wright SD, Sibley CH, Ding A, Nathan CF. Gram-negative endotoxin: an extraordinary lipid with profound effects on eukaryotic signal transduction. FASEB J. 1991;5:2652–60.

18. Rietschel ET, Brade H. Bacterial endotoxins. Sci Am 1992;267:26–31.
19. Michie HR, Manogue KR, Spriggs DR, et al. Detection of circulating tumor necrosis factor after endotoxin administration. N Engl J Med 1988;318:1481–6.
20. DaSilva AMT, Kaulbach HC, Chuidian FS, Lambert DR, Suffredini AF, Danner RL. Shock and multiple-organ dysfunction after self-administration of salmonella endotoxin. N Engl J Med 1993;328:1457–60.
21. Fenton MJ, Golenbock DT. LPS-binding proteins and receptors. J Leukoc Biol 1998;64:25–32.
22. Zeigler-Heitbrock HWL, Ulevitch RJ. CD14: cell surface receptor and differentiation marker. Immunol Today 1993;14:121–5.
23. Wright SD, Ramos RA, Tobias PS, Ulevitch RJ, Mathison JC. CD14, a receptor for complexes of lipopolysaccharide (LPS) and LPS-binding protein. Science 1990;249:1431–3.
24. Schumann RR, Leong SR, Flaggs GW, et al. Structure and function of lipopolysaccharide binding protein. Science 1990;249:1429–31.
25. Wurfel MM, Hailman E, Wright SD. Soluble CD14 acts as a shuttle in the neutralization of lipopolysaccharide (LPS) by LPS-binding protein and reconstituted high density lipoprotein. J Exp Med 1995;181:1743–54.
26. Pugin J, Ulevitch RJ, Tobias PS. Activation of endothelial cells by endotoxin: direct versus indirect pathways and the role of CD14. Prog Clin Biol Res 1995;392:369–73.
27. Yang RB, Mark MR, Gray A, et al. Toll-like receptor-2 mediates lipopolysaccharide-induced cellular signalling. Nature 1998;395:284–8.
28. Weersink AJL, vanKessel KPM, vandenTol ME, et al. Human granulocytes express a 55-KDa lipopolysaccharide-binding protein on the cell surface that is identical to the bactericidal/permeability-increasing protein. J Immunol 1993;150:253–63.
29. Wright SD, Kolesnick RN. Does endotoxin stimulate cells by mimicking ceramide? Immunol Today 1995;16:297–302.
30. Schlievert PM. Role of superantigens in human disease. J Infect Dis 1993;167:997–1002.
31. Sriskandan S, Cohen J. The pathogenesis of septic shock. J Infect 1995;30:201–6.
32. Lynn WA, Cohen J. Adjunctive therapy for septic shock: a review of experimental approaches. Clin Infect Dis 1995;20:143–58.
33. Casey LC, Balk RA, Bone RC. Plasma cytokine and endotoxin levels correlate with survival in patients with the sepsis syndrome. Ann Intern Med 1993;119:771–8.
34. Bone RC. Phospholipids and their inhibitors: a critical evaluation of their role in the treatment of sepsis. Crit Care Med 1992;20:884–90.
35. Bone RC. Inhibitors of complement and neutrophils: a critical evaluation of their role in the treatment of sepsis. Crit Care Med 1992;20:891–8.

36. Lehner PJ, Davies KA, Walport MJ, et al. Meningococcal septicaemia in a C6-deficient patient and effects of plasma transfusion on lipopolysaccharide release. Lancet 1992;340:1379–81.
37. Bone RC. Modulators of coagulation: a critical appraisal of their role in sepsis. Arch Intern Med 1992;152:1381–9.
38. Moncada S, Palmer RMJ, Higgs EA. Nitric oxide: physiology, pathophysiology, and pharmacology. Pharmacol Rev 1991;43:109–42.
39. Hogg N. The leukocyte integrins. Immunol Today 1989;10:111–4.
40. Weiss SJ. Tissue destruction by neutrophils. N Engl J Med 1989;320:365–76.
41. van Dissel JT, van Langevelde P, Westendorp RGJ, Kwappenberg K, Frolich M. Anti-inflammatory cytokine profile and mortality in febrile patients. Lancet 1998;351:1125–8.
42. Widmer AF. Infection control and prevention strategies in the ICU. Intensive Care Med 1994;20:S7–11.
43. Haley RW, Culver DH, White JW, et al. The efficacy of infection surveillance and control programs in preventing nosocomial infections in US hospitals. Am J Epidemiol 1985;121:182–205.
44. Giroir BP, Quint PA, Barton P, et al. Preliminary evaluation of recombinant amino-terminal fragment of bactericidal/permeability-increasing protein in children with severe meningococcal sepsis. Lancet 1997;350:1439–43.
45. Vincent J-L. Search for effective immunomodulating strategies against sepsis. Lancet 1998;351:922–3.
46. Sprung CL, Peduzzi PN, Shatney CH, Wilson MF, Hinshaw LB. The impact of encephalopathy on mortality and physiologic derangements in the sepsis syndrome. Crit Care Med 1988;16:398–405.
47. Sikuler E, Guetta V, Keynan A, Neumann L, Schlaeffer F. Abnormalities in bilirubin and liver enzyme levels in adult patients with bacteremia. Arch Intern Med 1989;149:2246–8.
48. Whang KT, Steinwald PM, White JC, et al. Serum calcitonin precursors in sepsis and systemic inflammation. J Clin Endocrinol Metab 1998;83:3296–301.
49. Danner RL, Elin RJ, Hosseini JM, Wesley RA, Reilly JM. Endotoxemia in human septic shock. Chest 1991;99:169–75.
50. Dofferhoff AS, Bom VJ, de-Vries-Hospers HG, et al, Patterns of cytokines, plasma endotoxin, plasminogen activator inhibitor, and acute-phase proteins during the treatment of severe sepsis in humans. Crit Care Med 1992;20:185–92.
51. Goldie AS, Fearon KC, Ross JA, et al. Natural cytokine antagonists and endogenous antiendotoxin core antibodies in sepsis syndrome. JAMA 1995;274:172–7.
52. Lynn WA, Cohen J. Microbiological requirements for studies of sepsis. In: Sibbald WJ, Vincent J-L, eds. Update in intensive care and emergency medicine: clinical trials for the treatment of sepsis. Berlin: Springer-Verlag; 1995:141–56.

53. Washington J. Blood cultures: principles and techniques. Mayo Clin Proc 1975;50:91–7.
54. Burhard KW. Fungal sepsis. Infect Dis Clin North Am 1992;6:677–92.
55. Ziegler EJ, Fisher CJ, Sprung CL, et al. Treatment of Gram-negative bacteremia and septic shock with HA-1A human monoclonal antibody against endotoxin. N Engl J Med 1991;324:429–36.
56. Kreger BE, Craven DE, McCabe WR. Gram-negative bacteremia IV. Re-evaluation of clinical features and treatment in 612 patients. Am J Med 1980;68:344–55.
57. Hurley JC. Antibiotic-induced release of endotoxin. A therapeutic paradox. Drug Saf 1995;12:183–95.
58. Shoemaker WC, Mohr PA, Printen KJ, et al. Use of sequential physiologic measurements for evaluation and therapy of uncomplicated septic shock. Surg Gynecol Obstet 1970;131:245–54.

59. Parillo JE, Parker MM, Natanson C, et al. Septic shock in humans. Advances in the understanding of pathogenesis, cardiovascular dysfunction, and therapy. Ann Intern Med 1990;113:227–41.
60. Cochrane Injuries Group Albumin Reviewers. Human albumin administration in critically ill patients: systematic review of randomised controlled trials. Br Med J 1998;317:235–40.
61. Temmesfeld-Wollbruck B, Walmrath D, Grimminger F. Prevention and therapy of the adult respiratory distress syndrome. Lung 1995;173:139–64.
62. Meier-Hellmann A, Reinhart K. Influence of catecholamines on regional perfusion and tissue oxygenation in septic shock. In: Reinhart K, Eyrich K, Sprung C, eds. Update in intensive care and emergency medicine: current perspectives in pathophysiology and therapy. Berlin: Springer-Verlag; 1994:274–91.

63. Shoemaker WC, Appel PL, Kram HB, Bishop MH, Abraham E. Sequence of physiologic patterns in surgical septic shock. Crit Care Med 1993;21:1876–89.
64. Shoemaker WC, Appel PL, Kram HB. Tissue oxygen debt as a determinant of lethal and nonlethal postoperative organ failure. Crit Care Med 1988;16:1117–20.
65. Busund R, Straume B, Revhaug A. Fatal course in severe meningococcemia: clinical predictors and effect of transfusion therapy. Crit Care Med 1993;21:1699–705.
66. Inthorn D, Hoffmann JN, Hartl WH, Muhlbayer D, Jochum M. Antithrombin III supplementation in severe sepsis: beneficial effects on organ dysfunction. Shock 1997;8:328–34.
67. Lefering R, Neugebauer EAM. Steroid controversy in septic shock: a meta-analysis. Crit Care Med 1995;23:1294–303.

Infections Associated with Intravascular Lines, Grafts and Devices

Alan L Bisno & Gordon M Dickinson

INFECTIONS OF VASCULAR ACCESS DEVICES

Vascular access devices are among the most versatile and useful implements used in medical therapy. There are multiple designs available from many commercial sources. They may be constructed from a variety of materials, including polypropylene, polyethylene, polyurethane or silicone; most catheters used in the USA are made of either polyurethane or silicone.

A simple steel needle (the 'butterfly') suffices to provide temporary venous access of a few minutes to a day or so; short catheters (3.8–5cm) or mid-length catheters (7.6–20.3cm) provide better stability for short-term access and are the catheters most widely used for peripheral venous access. More elaborate catheters, composed of polyurethane or silicone elastomer and often of a length sufficient to reach the vena cava, are used when central venous access through jugular, subclavian or femoral veins is needed. Relatively large-bore, double-lumen dialysis catheters have been developed specifically for dialysis or apheresis when permanent arteriovenous shunts or grafts are not available. Surgically implanted catheters designed to remain in place for months may be either located subcutaneously with a reservoir and diaphragm or tunneled subcutaneously with the distal end externalized. These catheters often have a polyester cuff into which fibroblasts invade to form a further barrier to pathogens. The central venous catheters and the surgically implanted catheters may have two or three separate lumens to allow multipurpose, simultaneous access. Arterial catheters for monitoring hemodynamic pressures and partial pressures of arterial blood gases are frequently used in intensive care settings, and arterial lines are used to deliver regional chemotherapy.

EPIDEMIOLOGY

Among hospitalized patients, venous catheters have long been recognized as a major contributor to nosocomial bacteremia; vascular devices may be responsible for as many as 82% of these infections.[1] The reported rates of infectious complications vary widely, reflecting the influence of many factors. Surveillance of intensive care units in hospitals participating in the National Nosocomial Infection Surveillance System of the US Centers for Disease Control and Prevention, October 1986 to December 1990, found bacteremia rates ranging between 2.1 and 11.4 per 1000 days of central catheter placement. In burns units, however, the rate was 30.2 per 1000 days.[2] The rates observed for peripheral catheters ranged from as low as zero in some coronary, medical and medical–surgical intensive care units to 2.0 per 1000 days in trauma units.

The higher rates of infection associated with central catheters have been attributed to the longer indwelling time of these devices; furthermore, central catheters tend to be placed in sicker patients. Factors generally accepted as contributing to the increased risk of infection include surgical cutdowns for insertion, breaks in sterile technique during insertion, improper manipulation of the device once in place and, for simple venous catheters, extended duration of use. Composition of the catheter also may influence the rate of infection:

peripheral catheters composed of polytetrafluoroethylene or polyurethene are less prone to infection than those made with polyethylene.[3]

For many years indwelling venous catheters were used primarily in hospitalized patients. They have become indispensable for delivery of fluids and medication as well as for frequent monitoring of partial pressure of arterial blood gases, pulmonary artery pressure and systemic vascular resistance in critically ill patients. However, over the past two decades there has been increased emphasis on delivery of medical care, including intravenously administered fluids and medications, in the outpatient setting. Outpatients, whose lines arguably receive less expert care, also face a significant risk of infection and bacteremia related to indwelling intravenous catheters.[4,5]

PATHOGENESIS AND PATHOLOGY

Intravascular catheters provide a direct route through the skin and into the bloodstream, with potential dissemination of pathogens to distant foci. It is this circumvention of natural barriers that is presumably the single most important factor contributing to the risk for infection.

There are several routes that pathogens may potentially follow in the development of catheter-associated infection (Fig. 48.1). Invasion from the surface of the skin along the external surface of the catheter, either at the time of insertion or during subsequent use, is probably the

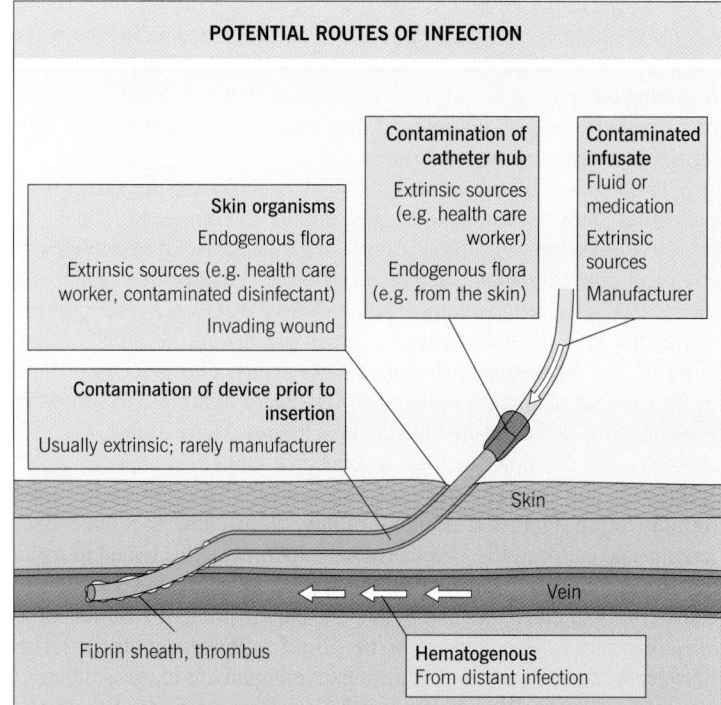

POTENTIAL ROUTES OF INFECTION

Skin organisms
Endogenous flora
Extrinsic sources (e.g. health care worker, contaminated disinfectant)
Invading wound

Contamination of catheter hub
Extrinsic sources (e.g. health care worker)
Endogenous flora (e.g. from the skin)

Contaminated infusate
Fluid or medication
Extrinsic sources
Manufacturer

Contamination of device prior to insertion
Usually extrinsic; rarely manufacturer

Skin

Vein

Fibrin sheath, thrombus

Hematogenous
From distant infection

Fig. 48.1 Potential routes of infection. Sources of micro-organisms and potential routes of invasion for catheter-associated infection. Adapted with permission from Maki.[6]

major route. The importance of this route of invasion is suggested by the predominance of skin flora as causative pathogens and the success of subcutaneous tunneling of cuffed catheters in reducing infection. On the other hand, there is a growing body of data to suggest that contamination of the hub with spread through the catheter lumen is also important. Contamination of the hub or connecting site presumably plays a greater role when catheters are in place for more than 10 days.[7] On occasion, catheters undoubtedly become colonized by bacteria reaching the bloodstream from a distant site (translocation). Contamination of the infusate itself, either on-site or during commercial preparation, has been well documented, and may give rise to clusters of infection involving patients in one institution or in more than one. Fortunately, appreciation of this risk has led to improved quality control.

As might be expected from infections associated with a cutaneous focus, the causative pathogens are frequently *Staphylococcus* spp. (*Staphylococcus aureus* or coagulase-negative staphylococci, usually *S. epidermidis*). Many other micro-organisms have also been implicated. Endemic flora within medical facilities, influenced by local antibiotic prescribing practices, often provide a source of other pathogens. For example, vancomycin-resistant enterococci, Gram-negative bacilli and *Candida* spp. are frequent causes of bacteremia in some medical centers. Rare pathogens and micro-organisms that are generally considered of low virulence for humans have also emerged as potential culprits (Fig. 48.2). Some of these are characterized by an ability to replicate in nutrient-poor solutions (e.g. *Enterobacter* spp.) or to thrive in hyperalimentation solutions (e.g. *Malessezia furfur*, *Candida* spp.). When identified in blood cultures, these organisms suggest possible contamination of infusates.

All indwelling vascular devices constitute a foreign substance within the body, and as such they elicit some degree of inflammatory response. Furthermore, in experimental animal models, phagocytic and bactericidal capacities of polymorphonuclear cells are decreased in the presence of foreign bodies such as implanted plastic capsules.

Even though they appear smooth to the naked eye, many indwelling devices contain microscopic pits and crevices on their surfaces that serve as niduses to which micro-organisms preferentially adhere. Moreover, the host seeks to 'humanize' the intruding foreign body by covering its surface with a rich layer of host-derived proteins such as albumin, fibrinogen, fibronectin, collagen, laminin, vitronectin and immunoglobulins. Although some of these components may retard microbial adherence, others may serve as efficient binding sites for bacteria. If infection ensues, micro-organisms and their products, including bacterial glycocalyceal material (see below), are incorporated on to the surface. This complex of host constituents, bacteria and bacterial products constitutes a biofilm.

The processes by which micro-organisms colonize the surfaces of indwelling intravascular devices are complex and remain the subject of intensive investigation. Initial events are thought to involve physicochemical characteristics, such as electrostatic charges that result in a weak association of the micro-organism with the device. In order to persist in the face of hemodynamic forces present in the bloodstream, however, the organisms must adhere more firmly. This is accomplished by attachment of surface molecules (ligands or adhesins) to receptors present on the device or on adherent host tissues. Many strains of *S. epidermidis*, for example, express a substance known as capsular polysaccharide adhesin. This mediates adherence to foreign bodies, and immunization against it protects rabbits from catheter-related bacteremia and endocarditis.[8] Furthermore, experimentally created mutants that are deficient in capsular polysaccharide adhesin adhere to silastic catheter tubing much less avidly than the parent strains do. Strains of *S. aureus* express surface proteins that bind at the molecular level to fibronectin and fibrinogen. Gram-negative organisms express filamentous surface organelles, known as pili. The distal portions of these pili contain epitopes that bind specifically to mannose or other carbohydrate moieties. Other examples could be cited, and indeed it is likely that individual microbes use multiple adhesins to mediate adherence.

MICRO-ORGANISMS ASSOCIATED WITH INFECTIONS OF INTRAVASCULAR DEVICES	
Common	*Staphylococcus aureus*
	Coagulase-negative staphylococci
	Enterococci
	Candida spp.
Uncommon	*Enterobacter* spp.
	Acinetobacter spp.
	Serratia marcescens
	Pseudomonas spp.
	Malassezia furfur

Fig. 48.2 Micro-organisms associated with infections of intravascular devices. Some of the organisms listed as being uncommon may be associated with contaminated infusate.

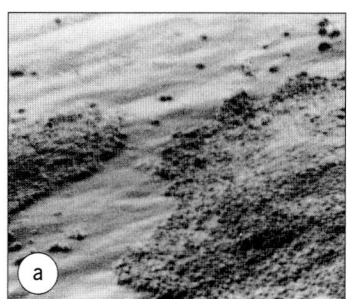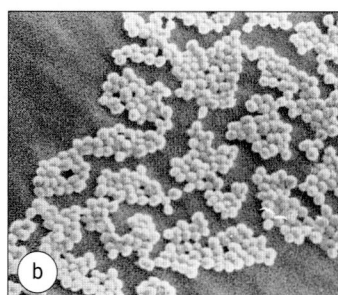

Fig. 48.3 Slime-producing coagulase-negative staphylococci. Scanning electron micrograph of the surface of an intravascular catheter incubated *in vitro* with (a) slime-producing and (b) nonslime-producing strains of *Staphylococcus epidermidis*. With permission from Christensen.[9]

Micro-organisms elaborate a variety of complex polysaccharides. In some cases these may remain tightly adherent to the bacterial cell to form the bacterial capsule, although sometimes they are more loosely associated with the cell, diffusing into the extracellular milieu to form a so-called slime layer. Many strains of coagulase-negative staphylococci are exuberant slime producers (Fig. 48.3). Elaboration of slime is not believed to play a role in the initial process of bacterial adherence to biomaterials, but this complex polysaccharide may be critical in the formation of biofilms and microbial persistence. Slime promotes intercellular adhesion, facilitates capture of nutrients and protects micro-organisms from antimicrobial agents. There is also experimental evidence to suggest that slime attenuates host defenses. These effects include decreased cellular responses to chemotactic stimuli, decreased phagocytosis and impaired T-lymphocyte function. The relative importance of these host, bacterial and foreign-body influences on the development and perpetuation of catheter-associated infection is still to be elucidated.

PREVENTION

Measures aimed at decreasing the incidence of catheter-associated infection include alterations in the composition of the device, refinements in the insertion process or in the care of the device, and more stringent guidelines for frequency of change of the catheter components or their attachments. Most peripheral catheters in use today are composed of polyurethane or polytetrafluoroethylene, materials that provoke less phlebitis and are associated with fewer infectious complications.[3] Further endeavors along this line have included manufacture of catheters impregnated or coated with antibiotics or with antiseptics such as silver sulfadiazine and chlorhexidine.[3] In the opinion of the authors, conclusive evidence that these coated catheters warrant the expense is not yet available.

Because most infections arise from contamination of the device during insertion or subsequent colonization at the site of insertion with spread along the external surface of the catheter, considerable attention has focused on the details of insertion and care of the device once in place. Many centers have dedicated intravenous teams to ensure a high level of expertise and uniformity of catheter care. Strict adherence to protective precautions and, in the case of central venous catheters, the use of barrier precautions (gown, masks, sterile gloves and large drapes) reduce the incidence of infection.[10,11]

The insertion site should be selected to ensure immobilization of the device and avoidance of contamination by indigenous flora. For example, catheters placed in the femoral or jugular veins carry a greater risk of subsequent infection than catheters in the subclavian veins.[3] Preparation of the insertion site with cleansers and antiseptics has received considerable attention. Tincture of iodine is among the most effective antiseptics but it frequently causes skin irritation. Povidone-iodine, a slow-release formulation of iodine, and aqueous chlorhexidine are effective and are now widely used, not only because they are less irritating to the skin, but also because they provide residual antimicrobial activity. However, povidone-iodine must be left in place for at least 2 minutes to achieve maximal antisepsis.[12]

A number of antiseptic and antimicrobial ointments have been proposed as a means to preventing colonization at the insertion site, and there are varying degrees of enthusiasm for their use.[3,13] Whereas some studies have indicated significant benefit, micro-organisms resistant to the active ingredient may be found in increased numbers at the site.[14,15]

The choice of protective dressing has also been an area of intensive research. Clear polyurethane dressings firmly anchor the catheter and allow visual inspection of the insertion site. Their effect on infection rates has been controversial.[16,17] Some of these dressings retain moisture and may nurture growth of micro-organisms.[18-20] The weight of evidence suggests that these dressings do not increase the rate of infection, although they do reduce the frequency of changes and allow continuous inspection of the insertion site.

The incidence of phlebitis and infection associated with peripheral catheters increases dramatically after 72 hours. The current standard of care is to replace these catheters every 48–72 hours. Nontunneled central catheters can be maintained for extended periods, although the cumulative risk for infection rises with these devices, too. There is no universal standard regarding frequency of change for these devices as there is for peripheral catheters. Because insertion of nontunneled central lines carries a risk of hemorrhage, pneumothorax (in the case of subclavian lines) and considerable discomfort, it is common practice to change an existing line over a guidewire at the same site. If the catheter is replaced according to a protocol and not for suspected or known infection, this may be safely done. However, if catheter infection is already present, the involved catheter should be removed and a new one inserted at another site.[3]

The proper frequency of change of administration sets and stopcocks depends on the infusate. Nutrient solutions such as lipid emulsions represent greater risk than normal saline and therefore require daily replacement of the external tubing. Lines used only for administration of saline or inert medications or antibiotics can generally be used for 48–72 hours without undue risk.

Despite the best of efforts, vascular devices will never be free of the potential for infectious complications, and clinicians must never become cavalier about their use.

CLINICAL FEATURES

Infections associated with vascular catheters may be localized to the insertion site, involve the lumen of the vessel (septic phlebitis) or invade the bloodstream (Fig. 48.4).

Infection at the site of catheter insertion characteristically produces swelling, induration and erythema with varying amounts of suppuration and tenderness. Occasionally there is phlebitis of the involved vein. For surgically implanted tunneled catheters these may be further categorized:

- exit site infections are localized to the first 2cm from the point of insertion;
- tunnel infections extend along the subcutaneous track of the catheter; and
- septic thrombophlebitis is a frank infection with suppurative changes in the substance of the vein itself.

Infections involving the subcutaneous track of externalized semipermanent surgically implanted catheters, so-called 'tunnel infections', are manifest by tenderness and induration along the track of the catheter and are usually clinically obvious. Patients with totally implantable ports may develop infection in the surgically created pocket into which the reservoir has been inserted. Here again, infection may be obvious, owing to local swelling, induration, erythema, tenderness and fluctuance, or even to extrusion of the port through the skin.

The onset of catheter-associated bacteremia is typically heralded by the nonspecific findings of fever, malaise, tachycardia and varying degrees of prostration. The virulence of the causative organism and the status of the host defenses contribute to the picture. For example, Gram-negative bacteremia in the neutropenic patient is typically a rapidly progressive process, which, if untreated, may evolve into full-blown septic shock. On the other hand, some infections may produce no more than an intermittent fever. The sudden onset of new fever is typical of catheter-associated infection and often occurs in the absence of any discernible abnormality around the device.

Apart from the consequences of an uncontrolled bacteremia, the most serious complication of catheter infections is septic thrombophlebitis. This entity was first described among burns patients with peripheral catheters. Septic thrombophlebitis may cause profound inflammation over the involved section of the vein with considerable swelling and woody induration, but in some cases these signs are

DEFINITIONS OF CATHETER-RELATED INFECTION	
Type of infection	Definition
Colonized catheter	Growth of 15 cfu (semiquantitative culture) or >10³ cfu (quantitative culture) from a proximal or distal catheter segment in the absence of accompanying clinical symptoms
Exit-site infection	Erythema, tenderness, induration and/or purulence localized to the first 2cm from the point of insertion
Pocket infection	Erythema and necrosis of the skin over the reservoir of a totally implantable device, or purulent exudate in the subcutaneous pocket containing the reservoir
Tunnel infection	Erythema, tenderness and induration in the tissues overlying the catheter and more than 2cm from the exit site
Catheter-related bacteremia	Isolation of the same organism (i.e. identical species, antibiogram) from a semiquantitative or quantitative culture of a catheter segment and from the blood (preferably drawn from a peripheral vein) of a patient with accompanying clinical symptoms of bacteremia and without another apparent source of infection. In the absence of laboratory confirmation, defervescence after removal of an implicated catheter from a patient with bacteremia may be considered indirect evidence of catheter-related bacteremia
Infusate-related bacteremia	Isolation of the same organism from infusate and from separate percutaneous blood cultures, with other identifiable source of infection

Fig. 48.4 Definitions of catheter-related infections. Adapted from Pearson.[3]

minimal or absent. Septic thrombophlebitis complicating surgically implantable catheters in the subclavian or jugular vein is typically associated with spiking fever, toxicity and positive blood cultures. The involved vein may be occluded, resulting in distal edema; swelling of the head, shoulder and upper extremities suggest the presence of central venous obstruction.

Less commonly encountered complications are metastatic foci of infection seeded from catheter-associated bacteremia or fungemia.[21] These often involve the lungs and present with nodular or localized peripheral infiltrates (Fig. 48.5). Disseminated metastatic foci, distant in time as well as location, also may occur. Candidal osteomyelitis may develop months after an apparently innocuous catheter-associated fungemia.

DIAGNOSIS

The diagnosis of localized catheter-associated infection is usually obvious on physical inspection. Exit site infections are often truly local processes with no systemic symptomatology. Phlebitis, a frequent manifestation of peripheral catheter infection, can also represent a sterile inflammatory reaction to the infusate or the catheter itself. Because sterile phlebitis may predispose to infection, the catheter should be removed promptly as soon as local signs are detected; this maneuver generally resolves the problem and no further studies are necessary. Any suppuration found at the insertion site should be cultured at the time of catheter removal. Persistence of phlebitis and fever is an indication for aspiration of the lumen of the involved vein for microscopy and culture.

Exudate at the exit site of surgically implanted catheters should be submitted for smear and culture. Tunnel infections, in the absence of frank abscess formation, usually provide no material for direct microbiologic examination but blood cultures may be positive. So-called pocket infections, involving the tissue around subcutaneous ports, should be aspirated for microscopy and culture.

Bloodstream infections arising from catheters are often indistinguishable from those arising from other sources. The challenge is not only to diagnose the bacteremia but also to determine whether it emanates from the catheter or from another site. Local manifestations at the catheter insertion site or vein may implicate the catheter but are frequently absent. A number of methods have been described to differentiate catheter-associated bacteremia from that arising from other sources (Fig. 48.6).[22] None of these methods combines a high degree of sensitivity and specificity, and each has advantages and disadvantages. The qualitative and quantitative catheter segment methods all require removal of the catheter and involve various levels of technical skill and time. The semiquantitative 'roll plate' method of Maki et al. has been widely used.[23] This involves removing the catheter, placing a 5cm distal segment onto the surface of blood agar and rolling the segment across the plate. Colonies of growth are counted after 18–24 hours of incubation. A count of 15 colonies or more is indicative of colonization of the catheter per se, whereas fewer colonies are consistent with contamination during removal. An obvious disadvantage of this method is the need for removal of the catheter.

Because an estimated 80–90% of febrile episodes occurring in persons with a venous catheter are unrelated to the catheter,[24,25] removal of each catheter may be unnecessary and, indeed, not always practical. Replacement of surgically implanted devices, for example, is an invasive measure. Culture of blood, on the other hand, is performed without prior removal of the catheter. A blood specimen collected by peripheral venepuncture does not indicate the source of any pathogen isolated. Furthermore, culture of a single specimen aspirated through the catheter is relatively nonspecific, albeit quite sensitive. The paired quantitative blood culture method involves collection of two blood specimens, one by venepuncture at a distant site and one through the catheter. The specimens are transported immediately to the laboratory where quantitative cultures to provide colony counts are performed. A ratio of catheter-to-venepuncture specimen colony counts exceeding 3:1 to 5:1 is considered to be indicative of catheter-associated bacteremia. This method is intuitively attractive, although data to support its efficacy in differentiating catheter-associated from other causes of bacteremia are limited.[22] Moreover, many clinical laboratories are not able to perform quantitative blood cultures. Nevertheless, when the catheter in question is a surgically implanted device, the difficulty and cost of catheter replacement may well justify the expense of the paired quantitative method.

MANAGEMENT

The management of a catheter-associated infection depends on the type of catheter, the nature of the infection and the circumstances of the particular patient. For peripheral catheters, prompt removal with adjunctive antibiotics is the mainstay of treatment. In general, peripheral

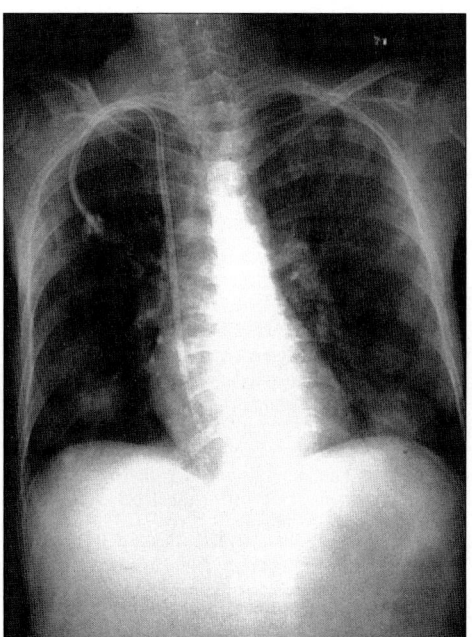

Fig. 48.5 Septic pulmonary emboli. Multiple nodular pulmonary infiltrates secondary to a dialysis catheter-associated infection. The patient presented with high fevers, cough and pleuritic chest pain. *Staphylococcus aureus* was isolated from multiple blood specimens.

SENSITIVITY AND SPECIFICITY OF METHODS USED FOR THE DIAGNOSIS OF CATHETER-RELATED BLOODSTREAM INFECTION		
Method	Pooled sensitivity (%)	Specificity (%)
Qualitative catheter segment culture	39/41 (95)	654/867 (75)
Semiquantitative catheter culture	109/128 (85)	2688/3152 (85)
Quantitative catheter segment culture	65/69 (94)	620/674 (92)
Unpaired qualitative catheter blood culture	54/59 (91)	569/660 (86)
Unpaired quantitative catheter blood culture	40/51 (78)	395/412 (96)
Paired quantitative blood culture	58/73 (79)	160/170 (94)

Fig. 48.6 Compilation of data from studies evaluating the sensitivity and specificity of methods used for the diagnosis of catheter-related bloodstream infections. Adapted with permission from Siegman-Igra.[22]

catheters should be replaced; visible phlebitis with any type of catheter is a reason for its removal, as is the development of severe sepsis.

The replacement of central venous catheters and dialysis catheters, however, has more serious implications. Nevertheless, pulmonary artery catheters and nonsurgically implanted central lines should be changed if there are signs of insertion site infection. Replacing a catheter over a guidewire decreases the risk of mechanical complications. In the presence of infection, however, the risk of contamination of the new catheter dictates replacement with a device inserted at a new site.

In circumstances in which the catheter-associated infection is suspected but not clinically obvious, the physician may choose to maintain the device while first attempting antimicrobial treatment. Obviously, many bacteremias are unrelated to the device.[24,25] Moreover, some catheter-associated infections do respond to systemic antimicrobials, but this approach should be undertaken with recognition that control of the infection may not be achieved or that relapse may occur.

Infections with certain pathogens are unlikely to respond to systemic antimicrobial therapy. Among these are infections caused by fungi and by micro-organisms that are highly resistant to antimicrobial agents, such as vancomycin-resistant enterococci.

Similar considerations pertain to the management of febrile patients with surgically implanted devices but no obvious local inflammation.[13,26–28] If the patient is treated with the device left in place, a clinical and microbial response should be seen within the first 48–72 hours. In the absence of response, the device should be removed at that point.

A presumptive diagnosis of catheter-associated bacteremia is grounds for empiric antimicrobial therapy. Once material for culture has been collected, therapy should be initiated. Given the extensive array of organisms that may be associated with catheter-related infections, no single agent will treat all potential pathogens. Because of the relative importance of Gram-positive cocci, particularly *S. aureus* and coagulase-negative staphylococci, the selection of antimicrobials should include an agent active against these organisms. A first- or second-generation cephalosporin, such as cefazolin or cefuroxime, or a penicillinase-resistant penicillin, such as oxacillin, may be administered as initial treatment, but in certain circumstances an antibiotic with a broader spectrum of activity may be appropriate. Knowledge of resistant pathogens among the current hospital flora may be helpful in guiding the selection of initial therapy, especially when the patient is located in an intensive care unit or has been hospitalized for a long period of time. The rise in incidence of infections caused by methicillin-resistant staphylococci[5] (both *S. aureus* and coagulase-negative staphylococci) followed by the dramatic spread of vancomycin-resistant enterococci has posed a dilemma. The use of vancomycin clearly facilitates the spread and persistence of vancomycin-resistant enterococci, but a growing proportion of catheter-related bacteremias are due to methicillin-resistant staphylococci. Thus, the initial choice of empiric antimicrobial therapy must be individualized. One approach is to reserve empiric treatment with vancomycin for those patients who appear septic and for patients known to be colonized with these organisms before the onset of the bacteremia. In general, an antifungal agent does not need to be administered as part of the initial empiric regimen; it can await microbiologic confirmation. A patient receiving broad-spectrum antimicrobial therapy for 1–2 weeks or more before the onset of a suspected bacteremia may be an exception to this, especially if the patient is known to be colonized by fungi.

Once the identity and susceptibility of the infecting organism are known, therapy should be adjusted to be as specific as possible. The duration of antimicrobial treatment of catheter-associated bacteremia is not well defined, but most authorities agree that between 10 days and 2 weeks is appropriate.[29–31] If significant metastatic foci of infection have occurred or secondary endocarditis is suspected, then the duration should be lengthened to 4–6 weeks.

INFECTIONS OF VASCULAR GRAFTS

EPIDEMIOLOGY

The experiments of Alexis Carrel[32] in the early years of the 20th century laid the groundwork for the surgical replacement of large arterial vessels, but bypass surgery came into general use only with the availability of synthetic graft materials in the 1950s. Vascular occlusive disease is the major indication for vascular graft surgery, with repair of aneurysms accounting for most of the remaining cases. According to the *National Hospital Discharge Survey*[33] of short-stay hospitals in the USA, 115,000 abdominal aorta bypasses and peripheral artery bypasses (primarily in the lower limb) were performed in 1993. Today most prosthetic bypass grafts are composed of either woven or knitted polyethylene terephthalate (Dacron) or polytetrafluoroethylene. Polyethylene terephthalate is preferred for aortic bypass because of its resilience, whereas polytetrafluoroethylene is preferred in lower extremity procedures. Many surgeons use venous autogenous grafts, if available, for lower extremity bypass because they are less prone to occlusion and infection. Composite grafts with polytetrafluoroethylene or polyethylene terephthalate for the proximal portion and autogenous veins for the smaller distal section are frequently used when insufficient venous material is available.

The reported risk of infection complicating arterial graft implantation in the thorax or abdomen is approximately 1%,[34,35] whereas the rates for procedures involving the groin are considerably higher. In a review of 2411 vascular graft reconstructions performed in the years 1978–1981, infections were found in 62 (2.6%) cases, all of which had occurred after surgery involving the groin.[36] The rates of postoperative wound infections not involving the graft are still higher.[37]

Published rates of infection may be misleading because the infection may not present until several years after the procedure. Factors associated with an increased risk for infection include advanced age and impaired health of the patient, prolonged duration of surgery, surgery performed under emergency conditions and presence of pre-existing infection in the anatomic area. Surgery in the groin is associated with special risk for subsequent infection.[34,36] Proximity to the perineum and colonization with bowel flora, overlying tissue folds that trap moisture, compromise of lymphatic drainage of the lower extremities, and the propensity for frequent motion through the incision site all are thought to contribute to the high risk of infection in this region. Whenever possible, surgeons avoid placing an incision in this area.

The causative organisms encountered are predominantly Gram-positive cocci, with coagulase-negative staphylococci and *S. aureus* accounting for the majority of vascular graft-associated infections. However, other organisms, including Enterobacteriaceae, *Pseudomonas aeruginosa* and, on occasion, fungi such as *Candida* spp. or *Aspergillus* spp., have been implicated. Polymicrobial infections occur in some cases, especially in abdominal aortic graft infection.

PATHOGENESIS AND PATHOLOGY

The inciting event for most vascular graft infections is contamination at the time of implantation. This may occur because of pre-existing infection (e.g. when the surgery is for replacement of an infected graft or repair of a mycotic aneurysm). More commonly it is related to contamination of the prosthesis during surgery. In some cases, a postoperative wound infection spreads contiguously to involve the graft. Abdominal aortic grafts placed in proximity to the gastrointestinal tract may erode through the wall of a viscus and become infected with gastrointestinal flora.

The newly implanted graft presents a niche to which bacteria may adhere. Some micro-organisms elaborate an exopolysaccharide (slime) that forms a protective cover, which shields them from antibodies and phagocytes. Some bacteria of low virulence, such as coagulase-negative staphylococci, produce inflammation that is minimal. More virulent micro-organisms (e.g. *S. aureus* and *P. aeruginosa*) tend to elicit a vigorous host response with local suppuration and systemic toxicity. Often the graft-associated infection involves the anastamotic site, with rupture or formation of a pseudoaneurysm (Fig. 48.7). Deposition of fibrin, thrombin, platelets and other substances at the site of infection may lead to thrombotic vascular occlusion or embolism.

PREVENTION

The catastrophic effect of infection associated with a vascular prosthesis and the difficulty of its management have heightened efforts at prevention. Vascular surgery should be postponed whenever possible until any local or systemic foci of infection have resolved, although this may prove difficult in cases in which arterial insufficiency is contributing to persistence of the infection.

Although most vascular repair operations are considered to be clean surgery, pre-operative prophylactic antimicrobials are recommended as the standard of care because of the ominous consequences of infection. A drug that is effective against both staphylocci and Gram-negative bacilli is desirable. For this reason, a first-generation cephalosporin such as cefazolin is often used. The emergence of methicillin-resistant strains of *Staphylococcus aureus* and coagulase-negative staphylococci in many centers, however, has compromised the efficacy of regimens widely used for the past two decades. Although vancomycin is the only antimicrobial agent with predictable activity against these methicillin-resistant micro-organisms, the specter of vancomycin resistance (e.g. vancomycin-resistant enterococci) is a cause for concern. Because methicillin-resistant staphylococci are largely nosocomial micro-organisms, prophylaxis with vancomycin might be reserved for patients with recent hospitalization or a prolonged hospital (or nursing home) stay before surgery.

It has not been proved that smooth-walled grafts such as those constructed of polytetrafluoroethylene are more resistant to infection than the netted or woven polyethylene terephthalate grafts, but there are experimental data to suggest this.[38] Autologous tissue and allografts are less prone to infection than synthetic grafts. Refinements in surgical techniques have also improved results. For example, placement of abdominal aorta grafts away from the fixed section of the duodenum has minimized the development of enteroaortic fistulae. Similarly, placing the graft well away from subcutaneous tissue and using flaps of muscle to cover grafts lessen the chances of erosion and subsequent infection.

CLINICAL FEATURES

The clinical presentation of infection associated with a vascular prosthesis depends on the vessel involved, the causative organisms, certain host factors and events related to surgery.

The infection may present with predominantly systemic symptoms, particularly when it is caused by virulent pathogens or is associated with bacteremia. Conversely, the infection may present with focal signs at the surgical incision site with minimal systemic symptoms. Indeed, complications of graft-associated infection may occur in the absence of either local or systemic signs of inflammation. These include development of an aneurysm at the anastomotic site, rupture of the anastomotic site and graft occlusion. Abdominal aorta grafts may erode into a viscus, or a fistula communicating with the gut may develop. Often these present with gastrointestinal hemorrhage in the absence of traditional signs and symptoms of infection. Grafts placed superficially under the skin (e.g. axillofemoral grafts or grafts placed in the lower extremity) may erode and be extruded.

Postoperative wound infections, especially in the groin area, range from superficial stitch abscesses to infections that extend to and encompass the graft. The following grading system for infections associated with vascular graft implantation procedures in the immediate postoperative period has been proposed:[39]

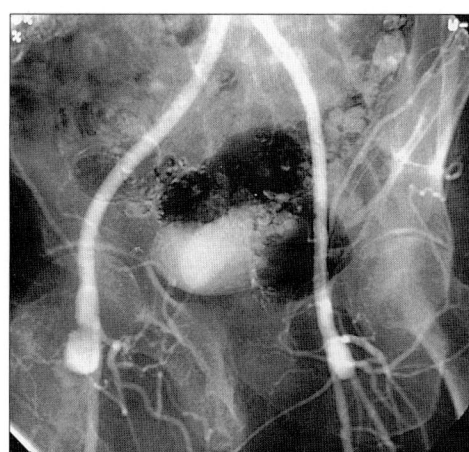

Fig. 48.7
Pseudoaneurysm. A pseudoaneurysm at the distal anastomosis of the right limb of an aortobifemoral polyethylene terephthalate graft secondary to *Pseudomonas aeruginosa* infection. Courtesy of M Tabbara, MD.

- grade I, infection extending only to the dermal layer;
- grade II, infection extending into the subcutaneous tissue not surrounding the graft; and
- grade III, infection surrounding and in contact with the graft.[40]

Other classification systems have been proposed to subclassify grade III infections.

DIAGNOSIS

The diagnosis of vascular graft infection is established by demonstration of anatomic abnormalities related to the graft and by isolation of a causative pathogen. Such abnormalities include local inflammation, a pulsatile mass, wound dehiscence, a draining sinus and externalization of the graft.

Although the diagnosis may be obvious from the signs and symptoms, in some instances it may be difficult to demonstrate abnormalities at the graft site or to distinguish them from noninfectious causes when abnormalities are present. Computed tomography and MRI are noninvasive procedures that provide a detailed view of the graft, showing patency, inflammatory changes or collections around the graft and the presence of sinus tracts (Fig. 48.8).

In the early postoperative period, sterile fluid collections that have not yet resolved must be distinguished from infection. Serial scans can help clarify which collections represent an infectious process; sterile fluid gradually resolves as the graft is incorporated into the surrounding tissue.[41] Computed tomography scans may also be used to guide aspiration and culture of perigraft tissue or fluid (Fig. 48.9). Indium[111] radioisotope scans have been used with some success and may identify a graft-associated inflammatory process indicative of infection.[42]

Isolation and identification of a causative pathogen are critical not only for diagnosis but also for guiding selection of antimicrobial therapy. Blood cultures should always be collected, although in many cases they will be negative. Aspiration of collections in the area of the graft should be performed before therapy is initiated. Failure of a graft to become incorporated into surrounding tissue is highly suggestive of infection, but it may be due to sterile seromas of unclear etiology. Seromas can only be distinguished from infection by aspiration; unfortunately, the causative organism may be closely adherent to the graft and not be identified by microscopy or culture of perigraft collections. Only further observation will reveal the infectious nature of the process. If a draining sinus is present, a deep specimen should be collected, but this method may be limited by external contamination with colonizing micro-organisms. Lymphoceles may occur in the groin when the surgery has disrupted the lymphatic vessels. These are sterile collections similar to seromas but they are prone to becoming infected.

Most postoperative wound infections remain limited to the superficial tissue, but it is necessary to demonstrate that such an infection does

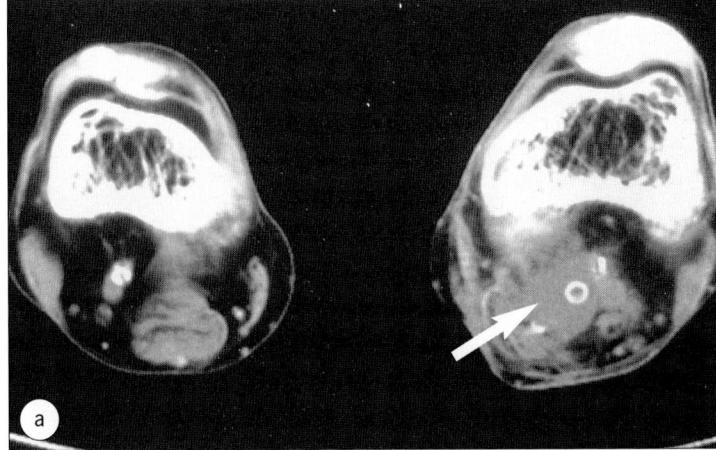

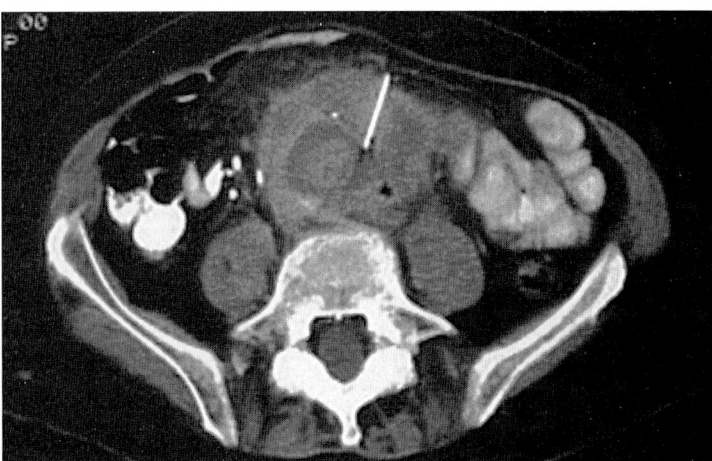

Fig. 48.9 Computed-tomography-guided needle aspiration. A large collection anterior to the lower abdominal aortic graft is readily defined for introduction of a needle. Courtesy of J Casillas, MD.

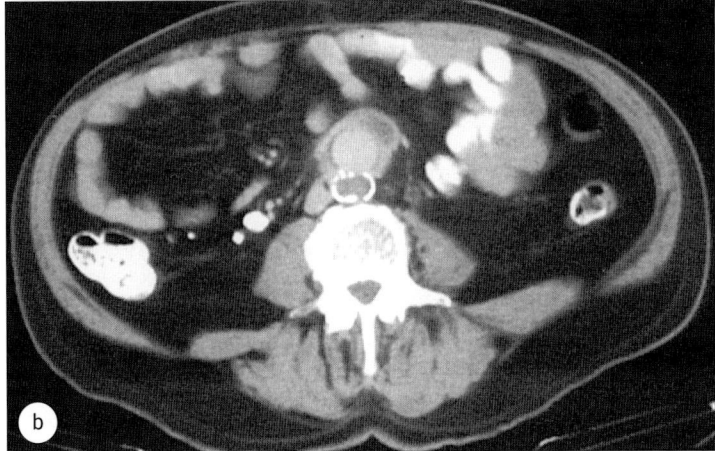

Fig. 48.8 Computed tomography scan showing perigraft collection. (a) A collection (arrowed) around a femoral-popliteal graft in the left leg. The right leg graft is not involved. Courtesy of M Tabbarra, MD. (b) Collection encircling a polyethylene terephthalate graft placed anterior to the calcified abdominal aorta which is seen just anterior to the vertebral body. Courtesy of J Casillas, MD.

not extend down to the graft. This may require surgical re-exploration. One form of graft infection deserves special note. Slime-producing coagulase-negative staphylococci may be tightly adherent to the graft and thus not identified when specimens are processed in the usual manner. When infection is suspected, submitting a resected specimen of graft to ultrasound may disrupt the shielding biomatrix and allow isolation of these bacteria from specimens that would otherwise appear sterile.[42]

MANAGEMENT

The management of graft infection has two goals:
• eradication of the infection; and
• preservation of the blood flow into the distal arterial bed.

To achieve the first goal, conventional wisdom has held that removal of the involved graft *en bloc* together with ectopic bypass is necessary – measures that often preclude achievement of the second goal. Removal of the aortic component of the graft is major, difficult surgery with a significant mortality rate, especially if renal or mesenteric arteries are involved.

In the face of daunting morbidity and mortality, some surgeons have reported approaches that minimize the extent of surgery. These include staged operations with an extra-anatomic bypass to maintain perfusion to the distal extremity before the infected graft is removed, resection of the graft with in-situ placement of autologous vein graft, subtotal resection of only the involved portion of the graft, debridement of surrounding tissue without removal of the graft or a combination of these. In general, these approaches are associated with lower rates of mortality and amputation but with higher rates of relapse. If the infection is caused by Gram-negative bacilli or by fungi, the patient is 'septic' or an enteroaortic fistula is present, total excision is mandatory. Infections that involve polyethylene terephthalate grafts usually require total excision too. Infrapopliteal grafts with distal implantation to tibial or fibular arteries are particularly challenging because of insufficient distal vascular tissue necessary for reconstruction.

Antibiotics, selected on the basis of susceptibility studies, should be administered for 4–6 weeks. A bactericidal regimen should be chosen. For selected patients in whom there is reason to suspect a persistent focus of infection, indefinite administration of suppressive antimicrobial therapy may be offered if curative surgery is not an option. All patients should be closely observed for relapse, especially if the involved graft was not excised *in toto*. The long-term success of management of infections associated with vascular grafts is overshadowed by the relatively poor long-term survival rates attributed to underlying cardiovascular disease.

REFERENCES

1. Bisno AL, Dickinson GD. Infections associated with indwelling devices: concepts of pathogenesis. Infections associated with intravascular devices. Antimicrob Agents Chemother 1989;33:597–601.
2. Jarvis WR, Edwards JR, Culver DH, et al. Nosocomial infection rates in adult and pediatric intensive care units in the United States. Am J Med 1991;91:185S–91S.
3. Pearson ML, Hierholzer WJ Jr, Garner JS, et al. Special guidelines for prevention of intravascular device-related infections. Am J Infect Control 1996;24:262–93.
4. Graham DR, Keldermans MM, Klemm LW, Semenza NJ, Shafer ML. Infectious complications among patients receiving home intravenous therapy with peripheral, central, or peripherally placed central venous catheters. Am J Med 1991;91:95S–100S.
5. Steinberg JP, Clark CC, Hackman BO. Nosocomial and community-acquired *Staphylococcus aureus* bacteremias from 1980 to 1993: impact of intravascular devices and methicillin resistance. Clin Infect Dis 1996;23:255–9.
6. Maki DG. Infections due to infusion therapy. In: Bennett JV, Brachman PS, Sanford JP, eds. Hospital infections, 3rd ed. Boston: Little, Brown; 1992:849–98.
7. Raad I, Costerton W, Sabharwal W, Sacilowski M, Anaissie E, Bodey GP. Ultrastructural analysis of indwelling vascular catheters: a quantitative relationship between luminal colonization and duration of placement. J Infect Dis 1993;168:400–7.

8. Takeda S, Pier GB, Kojima Y, *et al*. Protection against endocarditis due to *Staphylococcus epidermidis* by immunization with capsular polysaccharide/adhesion. Circulation 1991;84:2539–46.

9. Christensen GD, Simpson WA, Bisno AL, Beachey EH. Adherence of slime-producing strains of *Staphylococcus epidermidis* to smooth surfaces. Infect Immun 1982;37:318–26.

10. Maki DG. Yes, Virginia, aseptic technique is very important: maximal barrier precautions during insertion reduce the risk of central venous catheter-related bacteremia. Infect Control Hosp Epidemiol 1994;15:227–30.

11. Raad II, Hohn DC, Gilbreath BJ, *et al*. Prevention of central venous catheter-related infections by using maximal sterile barrier precautions during insertion. Infect Control Hosp Epidemiol 1994;15:231–8.

12. Maki DG, Ringer M, Alvarado CJ. Prospective randomised trial of povidone-iodine, alcohol, and chlorhexidine for prevention of infection associated with central venous and arterial catheters. Lancet 1991;338:339–43.

13. Raad II, Bodey GP. Infectious complications of indwelling vascular catheters. Clin Infect Dis 1992;15:197–210.

14. Zinner SH, Denny-Brown BC, Braun P, Burke JP, Toala P, Kass EH. Risk of infection with indwelling intravenous catheters: effect of application of antibiotic ointment. J Infect Dis 1969;120:616–9.

15. Maki DG, Band JD. A comparative study of polyantibiotic and iodophor ointment in prevention of vascular catheter-related infection. Am J Med 1981;70:739–44.

16. Maki DG, Ringer M. Evaluation of dressing regimens for prevention of infection with peripheral intravenous catheters. Gauze, a transparent polyurethane dressing, and an iodophor-transparent dressing. JAMA 1987;258:2396–403.

17. Hoffmann KK, Weber DJ, Samsa GP, Rutala WA. Transparent polyurethane film as an intravenous catheter dressing: a meta-analysis of the infection risks. JAMA 1992;267:2072–6.

18. Craven DE, Lichtenberg A, Kunches LM, *et al*. A randomized study comparing a transparent polyurethane dressing to a dry gauze dressing for peripheral intravenous catheter sites. Am J Infect Control 1985;6:361–6.

19. Conly JM, Grieves K, Peters B. A prospective, randomized study comparing transparent and dry gauze dressings for central venous catheters. J Infect Dis 1989;159:310–9.

20. Powell C, Regan C, Fabri PJ, Ruberg RL. Evaluation of Op-site catheter dressings for parenteral nutrition: a prospective, randomized study. JPEN J Parenter Enteral Nutr 1982;6:43–6.

21. Arnow PM, Quimosing EM, Beach M. Consequences of intravascular catheter sepsis. Clin Infect Dis 1993;16:778–84.

22. Siegman-Igra Y, Anglim AM, Shapiro DE, Adal KA, Strain BA, Farr BM. Diagnosis of vascular catheter-related bloodstream infection: a meta-analysis. J Clin Microbiol 1997;35:928–36.

23. Maki DG, Weise CE, Sarafin HWA. A semiquantitative culture method for identifying intravenous-catheter-related infection. N Engl J Med 1997;296:1305–9.

24. Ryan JA, Abel RM, Abbott WM, *et al*. Catheter complications in total parenteral nutrition: a prospective study of 200 consecutive patients. N Engl J Med 1974;290:757–61.

25. Sitzmann JV, Townsend TR, Siler MC, Bartlett JG. Septic and technical complications of central venous catheterization: a prospective study of 200 consecutive patients. Ann Surg 1985;202:766–70.

26. Capdevila JA, Segarra A, Planes AM, *et al*. Successful treatment of haemodialysis catheter-related sepsis without catheter removal. Nephrol Dial Transplant 1993;8:231–4.

27. Jones GR, Konsler GK, Dunaway RP, Lacey SR, Azizkhan RG. Prospective analysis of urokinase in the treatment of catheter sepsis in pediatric hematology-oncology patients. J Pediatr Surg 1993;28:350–5; [discussion] 355–7.

28. Riikonen P, Saarinen UM, Lahteenoja KM, Jalanko H. Management of indwelling central venous catheters in pediatric cancer patients with fever and neutropenia. Scand J Infect Dis 1993;25:357–64.

29. Raad II, Sabbagh MF. Optimal duration of therapy for catheter-related *Staphylococcus aureus* bacteremia: a study of 55 cases and review. Clin Infect Dis 1992;14:75–82.

30. Jernigan JA, Farr BM. Short-course therapy of catheter-related *Staphylococcus aureus* bacteremia: a meta-analysis. Ann Intern Med 1993;119:304–11.

31. Malanoski GJ, Samore MH, Pefanis A, Karchmer AW. *Staphylococcus aureus* catheter-associated bacteremia. Minimal effective therapy and unusual infectious complications associated with arterial sheath catheters. Arch Intern Med 1995;155:1161–6.

32. Carrel A. Ultimate result of aortic transplantation. J Exp Med 1912;15:389–98.

33. Graves EJ. Detailed diagnoses and procedures, National Hospital Discharge Survey, 1993. Hyattsville, Maryland: Department of Health and Human Services; 1995:13.

34. O'Hara PJ, Hertzer NR, Beven BG, Krajewski LP. Surgical management of infected abdominal aortic grafts: review of a 25-year experience. J Vasc Surg 1986;3:725–31.

35. Wengerter KR, Marin ML, Veith FJ. Femoropopliteal occlusive disease. In: Ritchie WP, Steele G, Dean RH, eds. General surgery. Philadelphia: JB Lippincott; 1995:655–69.

36. Lorentzen JE, Nielsen OM, Arendrup H, *et al*. Vascular graft infection: an analysis of sixty-two graft infections in 2411 consecutively implanted synthetic vascular grafts. Surgery 1985;98:81–6.

37. Risberg B, Drott C, Dalman P, *et al*. Oral ciprofloxacin versus intravenous cefuroxime as prophylaxis against postoperative infection in vascular surgery: a randomised double-blind, prospective multicentre study. Eur J Vasc Endovasc Surg 1995;10:346–51.

38. Schmitt DD, Bandyk DF, Pequet AJ, Towne JB. Bacterial adherence to vascular prostheses. A determinant of graft infectivity. J Vasc Surg 1986;3:732–40.

39. Thomas P, Forstrom L. In-111 labeled purified granulocytes in the diagnosis of synthetic vascular graft infections. Clin Nucl Med 1994;19:1075–8.

40. Olson ME, Lam K, Bodey GP, King EG, Costerton JW. Evaluation of strategies for central venous catheter replacement. Crit Care Med 1992;20:797–804.

41. Szilagyi DE, Smith RF, Elliot JT, *et al*. Infection in arterial reconstruction with synthetic grafts. Ann Surg 1972;176:321.

42. Spartera C, Morettini G, Petrassi C, *et al*. Role of magnetic resonance imaging in the evaluation of aortic graft healing, perigraft fluid collection, and graft infection. Eur J Vasc Surg 1990;4:69–73.

chapter

49

Myocarditis and Pericarditis

W Garrett Nichols & G Ralph Corey

MYOCARDITIS

EPIDEMIOLOGY

The term myocarditis applies to a variety of disease states that produce inflammation of the myocardium. In its acute form, myocarditis ranges from an asymptomatic illness with reversible changes to fulminant myocardial necrosis and death. In its chronic form, lymphocytic infiltration of the myocardium may cause subacute deterioration of cardiac function; indeed, chronic myocarditis may predate the development of 'idiopathic' dilated cardiomyopathy (IDC). The possible association between viral myocarditis and IDC is intriguing and potentially important. Although frequently ascribed to inflammation caused by an infectious agent, myocarditis may also be seen in allergic reactions, drug reactions, and in association with systemic inflammatory disease. A diagnosis of acute infectious myocarditis is suggested when unexplained heart failure or malignant arrhythmias occur in the setting of a systemic febrile illness or after symptoms of an upper respiratory tract infection.

The incidence of infectious myocarditis in the general population is unknown. In a prospective study of Finnish military recruits conducted over several years, a mean annual incidence of 0.02% was found.[1] Within immunosuppressed patients, myocarditis is more prevalent, affecting approximately 50% of AIDS patients at autopsy.[2]

PATHOGENESIS AND PATHOLOGY

In myocarditis, damage to cardiac myocytes appears to involve one or more of four possible mechanisms:
- direct cytopathic effects of an infectious agent;
- cellular injury secondary to circulating exogenous or bacterial toxins;
- specific cell-mediated or humoral immunologic response to the inciting agent or induced neoantigens;
- nonspecific cellular injury caused by generalized inflammation.

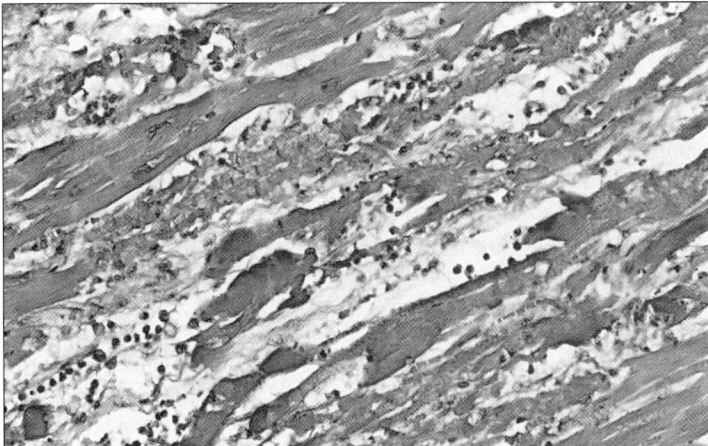

Fig. 49.1 Acute viral myocarditis, with a characteristic mononuclear infiltrate.

Histologically, both myocyte necrosis and infiltration by inflammatory cells in the absence of ischemia are pathognomonic of the disease. The infiltrate may be composed of a variety of cell types, including neutrophils, lymphocytes, macrophages, plasma cells, eosinophils and/or giant cells (Fig. 49.1).

The pathologic abnormalities, location, severity and changes over time span a wide range depending on the etiologic agent and individual host response involved. Coxsackievirus, for example, appears to infect cardiac myocytes directly, and can cause either focal or widespread inflammatory infiltration and cellular necrosis. Infection with hepatitis B virus and varicella-zoster virus appears to involve vascular endothelium, and thus can produce a different histologic pattern. Analysis of endomyocardial biopsy specimens obtained during infection with different agents shows considerable overlap, however. Thus, an histologic diagnosis of myocarditis usually does not indicate the agent responsible.

BACTERIA

Bacteria may cause myocarditis by a variety of mechanisms. Bacteremia caused by a wide variety of species may result in metastatic foci within the myocardium. Myocarditis has been noted in association with streptococcal and staphylococcal bacteremia, meningococcemia, brucellosis and Legionnaire's disease. However, the resulting myocardial dysfunction is only clinically significant in some patients who have overwhelming infections. In contrast, myocardial involvement in bacterial endocarditis is more common, and is often clinically significant. Bacteria (especially *Staphylococcus aureus*) may directly invade the myocardium from infected valves to cause abscesses, valvular failure and conduction abnormalities, or may embolize throughout the myocardium to cause global ventricular dysfunction. Cardiac infections caused by salmonella are particularly serious; mural involvement responds poorly to antimicrobial agents, and without surgical therapy mortality is 100%.

Bacterial toxin production can also be clinically significant. Subtle evidence of myocarditis can be detected in as many as two-thirds of patients who have diphtheria, with 10–25% of patients developing clinical cardiac dysfunction that is in direct proportion to the severity of the respiratory tract infection.[3] The virulence of *Corynebacterium diphtheriae* does not result from direct invasion of myocardium but from the effect of its potent exotoxin, which inhibits protein synthesis. Thus, evidence of cardiac toxicity may occur 1–2 weeks after onset of diphtheria, often when the oropharyngeal manifestations are improving. Patients who have electrocardiogram (ECG) changes of myocarditis have a mortality rate three to four times that of patients who have normal tracings, with atrioventricular nodal and left bundle branch block carrying a mortality rate of 60–90%.[4]

Spirochetes

Spirochetes such as *Borrelia burgdorferi,* the etiologic agent of Lyme disease, are important causes of myocarditis. The cardiac manifestations of Lyme disease may occur in an isolated manner, or coincident with other features such as erythema chronicum migrans or neurologic abnormalities. Within several weeks of infection, about 8% of patients will develop cardiac manifestations.[5] The most prevalent abnormality is fluctuating atrioventricular block, but some patients have evidence of more diffuse myopericardial involvement. Indeed, organisms have occasionally been demonstrated in endomyocardial biopsy tissue both premortem[6] and at autopsy,[7] providing supportive evidence for direct spirochetal invasion.

Rickettsiae

Rickettsiae produce systemic vasculitis by endothelial invasion, which not infrequently involves the myocardium. Rocky Mountain spotted fever (caused by *R. rickettsii*) and scrub typhus (caused by *R. tsutsug-amushi*) infections may cause transient cardiac dysfunction in severe illness, which invariably clears with disease resolution.

PARASITES

Many parasites are known to cause chronic myocarditis and sustained myocardial dysfunction, primarily in the developing world. Chagas' disease, which is widely distributed in Central and South America, is caused by the protozoan *Trypanosoma cruzi*, which enters the human host via the bite of the reduviid bug. Rarely, patients develop fever myalgias, hepatosplenomegaly and myocarditis during acute infection; far more common is the development of biventricular failure from chronic myocarditis, which occurs in 30% of infected individuals. Residence in Central or South America should increase clinical suspicion for this pathogen.

Epidemiologic exposure is also essential for the diagnosis of *Trichinella spiralis*, an important parasite with worldwide distribution that has been linked to fatal myocarditis. Myocarditis generally develops in severe infections, in which the cardinal features of periorbital edema, myositis, fever and eosinophilia are present. Recent consumption of poorly cooked pork enhances the likelihood of this diagnosis.

VIRUSES

Although any infectious agent may produce inflammation within the myocardium (Fig. 49.2), viruses are thought to cause the majority of cases of acute infectious myocarditis in the Western world. Historically, outbreaks of mumps, influenza, measles, poliomyelitis and enterovirus-associated pleurodynia were commonly associated with classic findings of myocardial involvement. In the present era of widespread immunization, the enteroviruses (e.g. echovirus, Coxsackie A and Coxsackie B virus) have been most commonly implicated in clinically significant myocarditis.

Until recently, evidence of a causal link between enterovirus infection and myocarditis was primarily circumstantial. For example, many individuals with acute myocarditis present with flu-like symptoms; in one prospective study of patients who had biopsy-proved myocarditis, over 50% had experienced an antecedent viral syndrome in the previous 3 months.[8] Observations of increased enteroviral antibody titers or a fall in convalescent titers have been offered as further evidence that enteroviruses are the causative agents. Unfortunately, these infections are common in the general population, and it has been difficult temporally to associate serologic changes with changes in cardiac function. In one study it was found that 34% of patients who had IDC had coxsackievirus B titers of 1:40, but the same incidence was found in control individuals.[9] However, if a cut-off antiviral titer of 1:1024 was used, 30% of patients who had IDC were abnormal compared with 2% of control individuals.[10] Viral culture from myocardial biopsies has not been revealing.

Given the lack of confirmatory culture or serologic data, animal models of viral myocarditis have been constructed to demonstrate the pathogenicity of the enteroviruses. Murine models of Coxsackie B virus-induced myocarditis have been extensively studied, and have shed light on the possible immunopathogenesis of infection. In this model, acute viral infection is characterized by viral attachment, myocyte penetration and subsequent viral replication, with resulting scattered foci of cellular necrosis. This initial phase terminates with viral clearance by mononuclear cells.[11] The chronic phase of infection is characterized by the presence of macrophages and T lymphocytes, not virus, within myocardial tissue. Interestingly, depletion of T lymphocytes prevents the later stages of myocardial injury. Further cellular injury or scars do not form, although replicating virus persists within the myocardium. These experiments highlight the importance of T lymphocytes in the perpetuation of myocardial injury. The antigens to which they are directed, however, remain unknown. Segments of the viral genome itself have not been shown to induce chronic immune activation. Rather, it appears that autoimmune reactivity to a novel tissue antigen induced by infection may be involved.[12] In addition, circulating autoantibodies against mitochondrial, contractile and adrenergic receptor proteins have recently been demonstrated in humans,[13] although their role in the pathogenesis of myocardial damage remains unclear.

These findings have led to the hypothesis that acute viral myocarditis may predate chronic inflammation within the myocardium. The resulting chronic myocarditis may be the final common pathway to IDC, which accounts for 25% of cases of heart failure in the USA. Recent studies using molecular techniques suggest that 18–53% of patients who have myocarditis or IDC may have persistent enteroviral infection.[14] In a representative study, enteroviral RNA was detected in 6 out of 19 patients who had IDC; no RNA could be detected in a control group of 21 patients who had other cardiac disorders.[15] Histologic evidence of myocarditis and persistence of enteroviral genomic sequences, however, often appear as independent variables in many studies, and the findings correlate poorly with one another. A recent study using nested polymerase chain reaction demonstrated enteroviral sequences in only 7% of the patient sample; sequence analysis of the amplified products casts doubt on the true positivity of even these samples.[16] Moreover, the isolation of intact replicating virus from 'infected' tissue remains elusive, suggesting that any detected sequences are viral fragments that may merely be markers of previous infection. Whether these fragments result in antigenic persistence, forming a nidus for chronic autoimmunity, remains to be determined.

IMMUNOCOMPROMISED PATIENTS

Immunocompromised patients are subject to the same infections as the immunocompetent; however, they are uniquely at risk for unusual pathogens. In end-stage AIDS, as many as 10% of patients will have clinically significant cardiomyopathy.[17] In a study of 33 patients infected with HIV who underwent cardiac biopsy, specific DNA hybridization demonstrated HIV in 5 out of 33 patients and cytomegalovirus (CMV) in 16,

INFECTIOUS CAUSES OF MYOCARDITIS		
	Normal host	Immunocompromised host
Common and/ or important	Coxsackie A virus Coxsackie B virus Echovirus Cytomegalovirus (CMV) Epstein–Barr virus (EBV) Infectious endocarditis Lyme disease American trypanosomiasis Trichinosis Diphtheria	CMV Toxoplasmosis HIV Disseminated fungal infections EBV Herpes simplex virus ? Varicella-zoster virus
Uncommon	Staphylococcus Streptococcus Meningococcus Clostridia Rickettsia	Brucellosis Mycoplasma Psittacosis Tuberculosis
Rare in developed world	Poliovirus Mumps Rubella Rubeola Arenaviruses	Rabies Chikungunya Ebola virus Leptospirosis African trypanosomiasis

Fig. 49.2 Infectious causes of myocarditis.

NONINFECTIOUS CAUSES OF MYOCARDITIS	
Connective tissue disorders	Systemic lupus erythematosus, rheumatoid arthritis, systemic sclerosis, dermatomyositis, polymyositis
Idiopathic inflammatory/ infiltrative disorders	Kawasaki disease, sarcoidosis, giant cell myocarditis
Insect and arachnid stings	Wasp, scorpion, spider stings
Medications	Cocaine, ethanol, arsenic, cyclophosphamide, daunorubicin, adriamycin, sulfonamides, tetracycline, methyldopa
Post-irradiation myocarditis	
Peripartum myocarditis	
Pheochromocytoma	
Thrombotic thrombocytopenic purpura	
Thyrotoxicosis	

Fig. 49.3 Noninfectious causes of myocarditis.

suggesting that cardiotropic viral infections may be important in pathogenesis.[18] Both *Cryptococcus neoformans*[19] and *Toxoplasma gondii*[20] have also been reported in the setting of HIV disease. Disseminated fungal or viral infections such as herpes simplex virus or varicella-zoster virus may also present with myocarditis in the immunocompromised patient, but can usually be identified by associated findings. Cytomegalovirus is an important pathogen in solid organ and bone marrow transplant recipients with myocarditis. The role of CMV in myocarditis of immunocompetent patients is also particularly intriguing; a recent study found intramyocyte CMV DNA in 14% of patients who had myocarditis but none in control individuals.[21]

A wide variety of other diseases may cause myocardial inflammation. Important noninfectious causes of myocarditis are listed in Figure 49.3.

CLINICAL FEATURES

The clinical expression of acute myocarditis ranges from an asymptomatic state to rapidly progressive myocardial dysfunction and death. Complaints on presentation may include fever, fatigue, malaise, chest pain, dyspnea and palpitations; arthralgias and upper respiratory tract symptoms are more frequently associated with viral myocarditis, but are nonspecific. Chest pain may be vague, pleuritic (suggesting pericardial involvement) or angina-like. The majority of patients, however, have no precordial discomfort. Indeed, mild aymptomatic myocardial involvement diagnosed by serial electrocardiographic changes was present in over 1% of military conscripts with acute viral syndromes.

Physical examination may reveal tachycardia out of proportion to the height of fever or degree of heart failure. Cardiac auscultation may be unrevealing, or may demonstrate muffled heart sounds, extra beats, transient murmurs or loud ventricular gallops; friction rubs are uncommon and indicate pericardial involvement. In severe cases, signs of congestive heart failure (CHF) are present, and pansystolic apical pulses may be palpated.

The electrocardiographic manifestations of myocarditis are usually transient, and occur far more frequently than clinical myocardial involvement. ST-segment elevation and T-wave inversions are seen acutely, and reflect the focal nature of the myocardial inflammation. These changes usually return to normal within 2 months. Atrial and ventricular arrhythmias are common. Atrioventricular nodal or intraventricular conduction defects denote involvement of the conduction system, and suggest more widespread disease or specific etiologies (e.g. Lyme carditis). Although usually transient and without sequelae, complete heart block may cause sudden death in these patients. Routine radiologic examination demonstrates cardiomegaly and pulmonary vascular congestion in severe cases.

DIAGNOSIS

The clinical diagnosis of myocarditis is often difficult, and requires a high index of suspicion. When unexplained heart failure or malignant arrhythmias occur in the setting of an acute febrile illness, the clinical diagnosis of infectious myocarditis is suggested. Heart failure of recent onset mandates that the physician first consider ischemic, valvular, primary pulmonary or congenital disease in the differential diagnosis. Other causes of acute myocardial dysfunction, such as rheumatologic disease, endocrinopathies, electrolyte disturbances and toxin exposure (e.g. ethanol, cocaine and heavy metals), must also be ruled out.

Electrocardiogram changes are important ancillary findings, but given the high incidence of nonspecific ST-segment and T-wave changes seen in acute viral syndromes, they alone are often nondiagnostic. Similarly, laboratory abnormalities such as leukocytosis and an elevated erythrocyte sedimentation rate are also nonspecific. Serum creatinine phosphokinase (CPK) elevations, on the other hand, do signify acute myocardial injury and thus are very important. Unfortunately, these elevations do not differentiate the cause of that injury (i.e. ischemic versus inflammatory). Myocardial enzyme release parallels myocyte necrosis, as in small-to-moderate myocardial infarctions. However, in contrast to ischemic necrosis in which CPK levels return to normal with 72 hours, elevated CPK levels may persist for 6 days in myocarditis.[22] The CPK-MB is elevated in 70% of patients who have myocarditis and ST-segment elevation on ECG, but is usually normal if only T-wave changes are present. Although serum assays for troponin T (a cardiac contractile protein) offer greater specificity for myocardial damage and persist for 2–3 days longer than CPK-MB determinations, they also are not specific for myocarditis.

Echocardiography is a valuable tool in the initial evaluation of the patient and in follow-up. Echocardiograms in myocarditis commonly show variable degrees of cardiac dysfunction, often with striking focal wall motion abnormalities. Dyskinesia or akinesia is most often biventricular. Furthermore, the test may eliminate other anatomic causes of CHF, and may demonstrate the presence of ventricular thrombi or pericardial effusions. Echocardiographic changes generally resolve within a few days in parallel with the clinical course; if progressive ventricular dysfunction is demonstrated, chronic myocarditis may be suggested.

Many other imaging modalities have been evaluated in acute myocarditis. Gallium scanning may demonstrate inflammation within the myocardium; the sensitivity and specificity of this test, however, is unknown. Antimyosin scans have been shown to identify the degree of myocyte necrosis, but this finding does not help in determining the cause of this necrosis. Magnetic resonance imaging is sensitive to the alterations in the water content of tissue that occur in the inflammatory response. Although this modality has shown promise in children with myocarditis,[23] it has not been evaluated in adults.

Despite advances in imaging techniques, the definitive diagnosis of myocarditis can only be made by endomyocardial biopsy. Because the inflammation involves both ventricles, a transvenous approach is generally utilized in order to obtain a biopsy of the right ventricular septum. In experienced hands the procedure is relatively safe, although deaths have occurred. Biopsy studies in acute disease have generally been carried out in cases of fulminant myocarditis. Studies using serial biopsies have demonstrated findings similar to those seen in the murine model. In the majority of cases, histologic evidence of myocarditis has resolved 3–4 weeks after the onset of symptoms.[24] Late biopsy is thus unhelpful. Furthermore, due to the focal nature of the disease, many practitioners have recommended obtaining four or five biopsies from different sites at initial catheterization. Repeat biopsies and/or left heart catheterization with biopsy have sometimes been necessary to establish the diagnosis firmly.

Disagreement among pathologists regarding interpretation of specimens has also been problematic. Recently, a working standard, termed the Dallas criteria, was established; these guidelines are now used by the majority of investigators to define the disease.[24]

- Active myocarditis is defined as 'an inflammatory infiltrate of the myocardium with necrosis and/or degeneration of adjacent myocytes not typical of the ischemic damage associated with coronary heart disease.'
- Borderline myocarditis is present when infiltration is sparse, or when cardiac myocytes are infiltrated with leukocytes, but associated myocyte necrosis is not present; myocarditis cannot be diagnosed in the absence of inflammation.
- The absence of myocarditis indicates normal myocardium or pathologic changes of a noninflammatory nature (fibrosis, atrophy, hypertrophy).

The adoption of the Dallas criteria has led to 90% concordance among experienced pathologists. Application of the criteria in the Multicenter Treatment Trial for Myocarditis (MTT) suggests that the prevalence of 'active myocarditis' in patients who have recent onset (<12 months) CHF is approximately 10%;[25] a recent study demonstrated identical findings.[26] However, these patients are qualitatively different from those with acute infectious myocarditis in which fever and acute ECG changes are present. They are best characterized as having IDC with myocardial inflammation.

The rationale for the development of the Dallas criteria was to identify patients prospectively who were likely or unlikely to benefit from immunosuppressive therapy. Given the results of the MTT (see below), many physicians have called into question the utility of the endomyocardial biopsy. In selected cases, however, the biopsy can provide valuable clinical data. Rarely, a biopsy will identify specific disease processes (i.e. toxoplasmosis, CMV, Lyme carditis, Chagas' disease, trichinosis, sarcoidosis) for which specific therapy is available, or for which a prognosis can be given (i.e. systemic lupus erythematosus, Pompe's disease, amyloidosis). Nevertheless, the approach for the patient who has acute myocarditis should focus on the management of CHF and its complications (see below). We believe that in many cases, endomyocardial biopsy is unnecessary; transplant recipients and those with AIDS are notable exceptions. A thorough history (with attention to epidemiologic detail) and physical examination will unearth the majority of nonviral etiologies, in which signs and symptoms other than CHF frequently dominate the clinical picture. In the febrile patient, blood cultures should be obtained. The routine use of acute and convalescent enteroviral titers adds little to the management of these patients in the acute setting. Given their lack of specificity, their use in retrospective diagnosis is also suspect. Perhaps future advances in virology or molecular biology will allow a more precise definition of the etiology of myocarditis; for now, however, the majority of cases remain classified as 'idiopathic'.

MANAGEMENT

The natural history of acute infectious myocarditis is quite variable, although the majority of cases run a benign, self-limited course. Acute cardiac dysfunction does not predict chronic impairment, as most of these individuals demonstrate normalization of laboratory, echocardiographic and histologic parameters within one month of symptom onset. For this reason, supportive care in lieu of aggressive, invasive procedures is of primary importance.

General measures target CHF, arrhythmias and other derangements associated with myocarditis. Animal models have demonstrated that exercise during viral myocarditis is associated with higher mortality and more extensive histologic damage; thus, bedrest may be important. Conventional therapy has included oxygen, diuretics, digoxin and sodium restriction, as for any patient who has CHF. Most practitioners recommend anticoagulation for all patients who have documented intracardiac thrombi, and for those with severely depressed myocardial function in order to prevent thromboembolic complications. In the murine model, early treatment with the angiotensin converting enzyme inhibitor captopril decreased left ventricular mass and myocardial necrosis, suggesting benefits above and beyond afterload reduction.[27]

Randomized trials in humans have yet to be conducted, although afterload reduction appears safe and effective in other settings. Rarely, fulminant heart failure requires the use of inotropic support, intra-aortic balloon pumps or ventricular assist devices as a bridge to the resumption of cardiac function. Unfortunately, there are no clinical or laboratory indicators to identify those patients who will spontaneously recover. For those that do not respond, cardiac transplantation is an option; however patients who have myocarditis before transplantion have a significantly higher incidence of rejection and death in the first year.

As significant arrhythmias are probably associated with the majority of deaths in acute myocarditis, all hospitalized patients should be monitored on telemetry. Premature beats are common and do not require therapy. Supraventricular tachycardia, however, worsens heart failure and should be electrically converted. The use of anti-arrhythmic agents for high-grade ventricular ectopy has not been studied. Care should be exercised with any anti-arrhythmic agent (including digoxin, which has a low threshold for toxicity in these patients), but sustained ventricular arrhythmias may be cautiously treated, as in ischemic heart disease. Complete heart block is an indication for temporary venous pacing. The condition often resolves without a need for permanent pacemaker placement.

Contrary to expectations, anti-inflammatory therapy and immunosuppression have not favorably influenced outcome. Nonsteroidal anti-inflammatory drugs (NSAIDs)[28] and cyclosporine[29] have been associated with more severe histologic damage when used in the acute stage of murine viral myocarditis. Late stage immunosuppression has also been disappointing. In the MTT, the largest clinical trial of immunosuppressive therapy for myocarditis to date, 111 patients who had biopsy-proved myocarditis and CHF for less than 2 years were randomized to receive placebo or combination therapy with prednisone/cyclosporine or prednisone/azathioprine. At 28 weeks, left ventricular ejection fraction improved in both groups from 0.25 to 0.34; there was no significant difference in mortality between the two groups at 1 year (20% in all patients) and 4.3 years (56%). Interestingly, markers of effective immune response were associated with a more favorable outcome.[30] It is also worth noting that more than 2000 patients underwent biopsy to find 111 with sufficient inflammation to warrant inclusion in the study group. If there exists a subgroup within this population that may benefit from these drugs, it is a small one indeed.

Prognosis in myocarditis appears to be more intimately linked to clinical parameters than to histologic findings of inflammation. The endomyocardial biopsies of patients who have CHF of recent duration were retrospectively reviewed at the Duke University Medical Center; 380 patients were identified over a 7-year period (1984–1991), and follow-up for an average of 3 years was provided (unpublished data). Most of the cohort had nonspecific pathologic findings; 2% had active and 20% had borderline myocarditis by the Dallas criteria. Four variables were found to be independent predictors of mortality: increased age, worse CHF functional class, decreased serum concentration of sodium and the presence of cardiac amyloidosis (found in 5% of cases). Histologic findings of T-lymphocyte infiltrates, myofibril loss, or myocyte hypertrophy were not independent predictors of mortality.

PERICARDITIS

EPIDEMIOLOGY

Interest in the pericardium dates to antiquity. The writings of Homer and Maximus relate the history of the 'hairy hearts of heroes' such as Aristomenes, the legendary Messinian warrior; his heart was cut out in battle and found to be 'stuffed with hair', probably the first recorded case of fibrinous pericarditis. Significant understanding of the etiology and pathophysiology followed, from Galen's first pericardial resection in the 2nd century AD to Lower's classic description of tamponade, constrictive pericarditis and pulsus paradoxus in the 17th century.

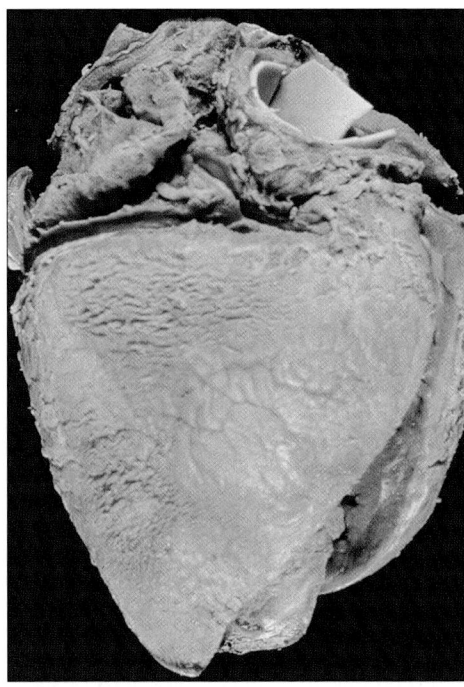

Fig. 49.4 Heart at autopsy of a patient who had acute suppurative pericarditis. The parietal pericardium has been stripped from the specimen, revealing a 'bread and butter' appearance.

INFECTIOUS CAUSES OF PERICARDITIS	
Viruses	**Mycobacteria**
Cytomegalovirus	*Mycobacterium tuberculosis*
Herpes simplex virus	*Mycobacterium chelonae*
Coxsackie A virus	*Mycobacterium avium* complex
Coxsackie B virus	**Spirochetes**
Echovirus	
Adenovirus	*Borrelia burgdorferi*
Influenza	
Mumps	**Mycoplasma**
Varicella–zoster virus	*Mycoplasma pneumoniae*
Epstein–Barr virus	*Ureaplasma urealyticum*
HIV	*Mycoplasma hominis*
Bacteria	**Fungi**
Streptococcus pneumoniae	*Histoplasma capsulatum*
Streptococcus spp.	*Coccidioides immitis*
Staphylococcus aureus	*Cryptococcus neoformans*
Neisseria meningitidis	*Blastomyces dermatiditis*
Listeria monocytogenes	*Candida* spp.
Haemophilus influenzae	*Aspergillus fumigatus*
Francisella tularensis	
Brucella melitensis	**Parasites**
Enteric Gram-negative rods	*Toxoplasma gondii*
Actinomyces spp.	*Entamoeba histolytica*
Nocardia asteroides	*Echinococcus granulosus*
Legionella pneumophila	*Schistosoma* spp.
Tropheryma whippelii	
Salmonella spp.	
Campylobacter spp.	

Fig. 49.5 Infectious causes of pericarditis.

Medical advances in antibiotic therapy, surgical technique, antineoplastic therapy and hemodialysis have substantially altered the spectrum and prognosis of pericardial disease in the 20th century. Imaging modalities have also made a significant impact; since the advent of echocardiography in 1955, pericardial effusions are now readily diagnosed. The etiologic determination of pericardial disease, however, remains difficult. Timely, directed therapy depends in large part on the diligence of the clinician.

The incidence of pericardial inflammation detected in several autopsy series ranges from 2–6%, whereas pericarditis is diagnosed clinically in only about 1 out of 1000 hospital admissions. The relative frequency of each etiologic process depends upon the clinical setting. Thus, viral or idiopathic pericarditis often presents in the outpatient clinic, whereas malignant or uremic effusions are more frequently seen in referral centers.

PATHOGENESIS AND PATHOLOGY

The human pericardium forms a strong flask-shaped sac that encloses the heart and the origins of the great vessels. It is composed of a fibrous outer layer and an inner serous membrane formed by a single layer of mesothelial cells. This membrane is attached to the surface of the heart to form the visceral pericardium; it reflects upon itself, lining the inside of the collagen-based fibrous layer to form the parietal pericardium. The visceral pericardium continuously produces a clear pericardial fluid that serves as a lubricant; it is also the source of excess fluid in disease states. The human pericardium normally contains up to 50ml of this fluid, which drains via the thoracic and right lymphatic duct into the central circulation.

Pericardial effusion may develop in response to pericardial injury (as in pericarditis) or may be secondary to other processes that alter the secretion and drainage of pericardial fluid. The pathologic changes seen in acute pericarditis are those of nonspecific inflammation with cellular infiltration, fibrin deposition and the outpouring of pericardial fluid. These changes may resolve spontaneously over time, or may organize with fibrous adhesions between the epicardium and visceral pericardium, the visceral and parietal pericardium, or the pericardium and adjacent sternum and pleura (Fig. 49.4). Thus, inflammation, fluid exudation, and fibrin organization account for the cardinal manifestations of pericarditis: chest pain, pericardial effusion, and constriction.

NONINFECTIOUS CAUSES OF PERICARDIAL DISEASE
Idiopathic
Connective tissue disorders
Acute rheumatic fever, SLE, RA, scleroderma, mixed connective tissue disease, Wegener's granulomatosis, polyarteritis nodosa, temporal arteritis
Metabolic
Uremia, hypothyroidism
Malignancies
Lung cancer, breast cancer, leukemia, lymphoma, others
Acute myocardial infarction
Post-myocardial infarction syndrome (Dressler syndrome)
Dissecting aortic aneurysm
Traumatic
Chest trauma, post-surgical hemopericardium, pacemaker insertion, cardiac catheterization, esophageal rupture, pancreatic-pericardial fistula
Post-irradiation
Idiopathic infiltrative/inflammatory disorders
Sarcoidosis, amyloidosis, inflammatory bowel disease, Behçet disease
Medications
Procainamide, hydralazine, isoniazid, phenylbutazone, dantrolene, doxorubicin, dilantin, methysergide

Fig. 49.6 Noninfectious causes of pericardial disease.

The causes of this pericardial inflammation are numerous, including both infectious (Fig. 49.5) and noninfectious (Fig. 49.6) etiologies.

NONINFECTIOUS AGENTS

The three most prevalent noninfectious causes of pericardial disease are malignancies, uremia and connective tissue disorders.

- *Neoplasms* may cause pericarditis or effusions by direct involvement of the pericardium (in which malignant cells are usually demonstrated within pericardial fluid) or by obstruction of the pericardial lymphatic drainage (with resulting 'benign' effusions).
- *Uremic pericarditis*, which affects up to 20% of patients on chronic hemodialysis, is characterized by the appearance of a shaggy, fibrinous exudate without cellular infiltration.
- *Collagen vascular diseases* (most commonly systemic lupus erythematosus) are notable for their propensity to involve the pericardium; immune complex deposition is thought to be primary in the pathogenesis of pericardial disease.

INFECTIOUS AGENTS

A variety of microbes have been reported to cause pericarditis. Chief among these are viruses, which can produce a clinical syndrome of myopericarditis, but often infectious agents are also implicated.

Viruses

Coxsackievirus and echovirus type 8 have been most commonly identified. As is the case for myocarditis, these viruses have only rarely been isolated from pericardial fluid or tissue (see above); as such, evidence for viral causation of pericardial inflammation is primarily based upon isolation of virus from other sites, such as stool, or by demonstration of a four-fold rise in serum antibody titers. Historic evidence, however, favors a viral etiology for the majority of community acquired 'idiopathic' pericarditis. For example, epidemic pleurodynia (Bornholm disease), caused by coxsackievirus infection, has long been noted to be epidemiologically associated with outbreaks of self-limited pericarditis. In addition, most cases of idiopathic pericarditis seem to cluster in the spring and fall, coincident with outbreaks of enteroviral infections.

Many other viruses have been associated with pericarditis (see Fig. 49.5). For example, CMV has been pathologically confirmed as a cause of pericardial disease in the immunocompetent patient who has the CMV mononucleosis syndrome. One series reported five cases of culture-proved CMV infection in patients who had large pericardial effusions. In four of these CMV cases, the patients were not immunosuppressed at the time of diagnosis.[31] In addition, CMV may be a common pathogen in HIV-infected patients. Herpes simplex pericarditis has also been documented both in patients who have AIDS and in patients who have uremia.

Bacteria and other infectious agents

Bacteria may cause pericarditis by a number of different mechanisms. Hematogenous seeding of the pericardium may occur during the course of bacteremia caused by a variety of organisms. In the pre-antibiotic era, most cases of purulent pericarditis were seen as complications of bacteremia or pneumonia. Today, extension of infection from a contiguous focus within the chest is seen as a postoperative or post-traumatic complication. Subdiaphragmatic abscesses may also cause pericardial infection by direct extension. Highly invasive bacterial infections within the heart, such as acute staphylococcal endocarditis, may erode into the pericardium from a perivalvular abscess to cause purulent pericarditis. Pericardial effusions in patients who have subacute infective endocarditis provide another mechanism by which bacterial infection can lead to pericardial disease. Pathologic changes in the pericardium are caused by immune complex deposition, resulting in sterile exudates. Although common, these effusions are not associated with prognosis, and most resolve without specific therapy.

The microbiology of bacterial pericarditis continues to evolve (see Fig. 49.5). Before antibiotics, uncontrolled pneumococcal, streptococcal or staphylococcal pulmonary infections were most frequently implicated. Streptococci and staphylococci remain important pathogens today (particularly in traumatic and post-thoracotomy pericarditis), with Gram-negative bacilli and atypical bacteria assuming important roles. Pericardial involvement has also been documented in the course of such illnesses as tularemia, brucellosis, salmonellosis, Legionellosis and meningococcal disease. Local infection with anaerobes has also been reported. In children, bacteria cause proportionately more cases of pericarditis than is the case in adults; *S. aureus* and *Haemophilus influenzae* are the most common etiologic agents.

Mycoplasma *spp.* Pericarditis caused by *Mycoplasma* spp. deserves special mention. Although pericarditis has been recognized in the course of mycoplasma disease since 1944, culture of the organism has proved difficult. Therefore, autoimmune phenomena have been invoked to explain the association. Recently *Mycoplasma pneumoniae*, *Mycoplasma hominis* and *Ureaplasma urealyticum* were isolated from culture of pericardial fluid and/or tissue in five patients who had large pericardial effusions.[32] Treatment with doxycycline after drainage of the effusions resulted in complete resolution in all five cases. Pericarditis caused by *Mycoplasma* spp. is thus probably more common than previously recognized, and fluid obtained for culture should always be analyzed for the presence of these organisms.

Mycobacteria. Mycobacteria continue to be important causes of acute pericarditis, pericardial effusion and constrictive pericarditis, particularly in the Third World. The incidence of tuberculous pericarditis among patients who have pulmonary tuberculosis ranges from about 1–8%.[33] In Transkei, South Africa, tuberculous pericarditis with secondary constriction is the second most common cause of 'heart failure' after rheumatic disease.[34]

Histoplasma capsulatum. *Histoplasma capsulatum* is the most common cause of fungal pericarditis; in large outbreaks, pericarditis was noted in 6% of patients who have symptomatic histoplasmosis. It most commonly develops as a noninfectious inflammatory response that resolves spontaneously without therapy. Occasionally, seeding of the pericardium occurs in the course of disseminated infection. In contrast, pericarditis has only rarely been reported in cases of severe coccidiomycosis. In the severely immunosuppressed or post-thoracotomy patient, infection caused by *Candida* spp., *Aspergillus fumigatus* or *Cryptococcus neoformans* has occasionally resulted from either fungemia or direct inoculation.

Pericarditis in AIDS

In contrast to other immunocompromised states, pericardial disease in patients who have AIDS is quite common. Effusions are frequently noted in end-stage AIDS (occurring in 16–40% of patients) and are associated with a poor prognosis. Etiologies include a variety of pathogens (including viruses, bacteria, fungi and mycobacteria) though in the majority of cases no causative agent can be defined. Malignant effusions secondary to lymphomatous involvement of the pericardium have also been noted. Furthermore, although extrapericardial disease suggested specific infectious or malignant etiologies in 55% of patients who have pericardial effusions in one trial, these assumptions proved incorrect for all those in whom pericardiocentesis was performed.[35]

CLINICAL FEATURES

Acute pericarditis is most often recognized by its chief presenting manifestation: chest pain. The pain is usually precordial or retrosternal, often with radiation to the trapezius ridge or neck; it is exacerbated by lying supine, coughing or deep inspiration, with relief upon sitting upright or forward. The patient's discomfort may be caused by inflammation of the adjacent pleura, accounting for the pleuritic component that often accompanies the pain. This pain is distinguished from the pain of myocardial ischemia by its quality, its duration (pain may last for days without therapy) and the absence of associated factors (i.e. pain is unchanged with exertion or rest). Patients may also report that splinting reduces the pleuritic discomfort.

A pericardial friction rub is the pathognomonic physical finding of acute pericarditis. Characterized as scratchy or grating, it is best appreciated along the left sternal border with respirations suspended and the patient leaning forward. The classic friction rub has three components, corresponding to atrial systole, ventricular systole and the rapid ventricular filling phase of early diastole, although one or more of these phases may be absent. Of note, the friction rub frequently waxes and wanes in intensity, and may disappear altogether with the accumulation of fluid within the pericardial sac. The pericardial rub may again become prominent in tamponade, in which the pericardium rubs against the adjacent pleura.

Pericardial effusions range from the asymptomatic to those causing cardiac tamponade. The rate of fluid accumulation is a major determinant in physiologic manifestations. When the effusion develops slowly, the pericardium may stretch to accumulate as much as 2 liters of fluid. The normal pericardium, however, can accommodate the rapid accumulation of only 100–200ml of fluid before signs and symptoms of tamponade develop. Patients may then complain of dyspnea or a dull retrosternal ache, and examination will reveal jugular venous distension, the most common physical finding in acute tamponade. A 10mmHg or greater fall in systolic blood pressure during inspiration (the pulsus paradoxus) is recognized as a hallmark of critical cardiac tamponade, although it may be absent if hypotension is already present.

Enlargement of the cardiac silhouette on routine X-ray usually does not occur until at least 250ml of fluid have accumulated in the pericardial space. Other findings on chest X-ray (CXR), such as a 'water bottle' heart (Fig. 49.7) or a prominent fat stripe sign, are found only in large pericardial effusions; their absence does not rule out the presence of a hemodynamically significant effusion. Chest radiographs may also provide etiologic clues for pericardial disease, such as pneumonic infiltrates or mediastinal adenopathy.

Electrocardiographic changes in acute pericarditis imply inflammation of the pericardium. Thus, in uremic or neoplastic pericardial effusions, characteristic ECG changes are often absent. Cardiac arrhythmias are uncharacteristic in isolated pericardial disease; their presence implies myocardial involvement. The ECG typically evolves through four stages during acute pericarditis.

- *Diffuse ST-segment elevation (usually concave up) with reciprocal ST depression in aVR and V1* accompanies the onset of chest pain, and is virtually diagnostic of pericarditis; these findings are present in 50% of patients who have acute pericarditis.[36] PR depression in the inferolateral leads is frequently seen in this stage (Fig. 49.8).
- *ST and PR segments normalize*, typically several days later.

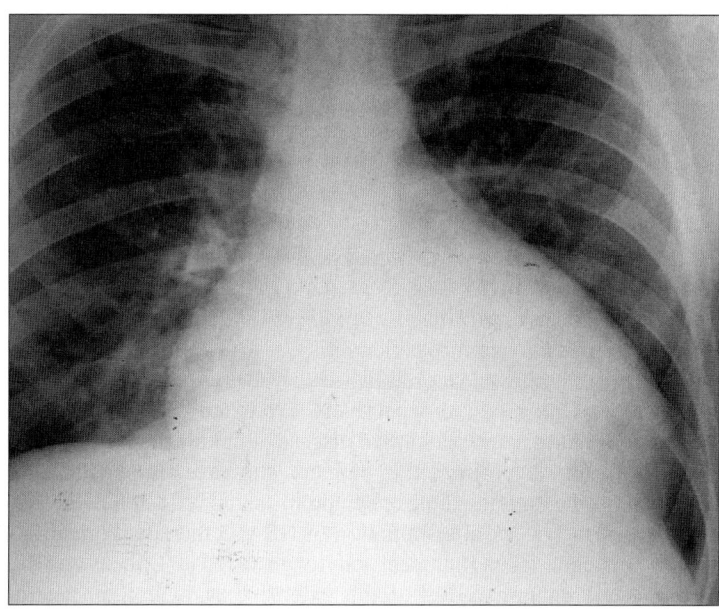

Fig. 49.7 Cardiomegaly in a patient who has pericarditis. The presence of a 'water-bottle' heart on this plain film suggests a large pericardial effusion.

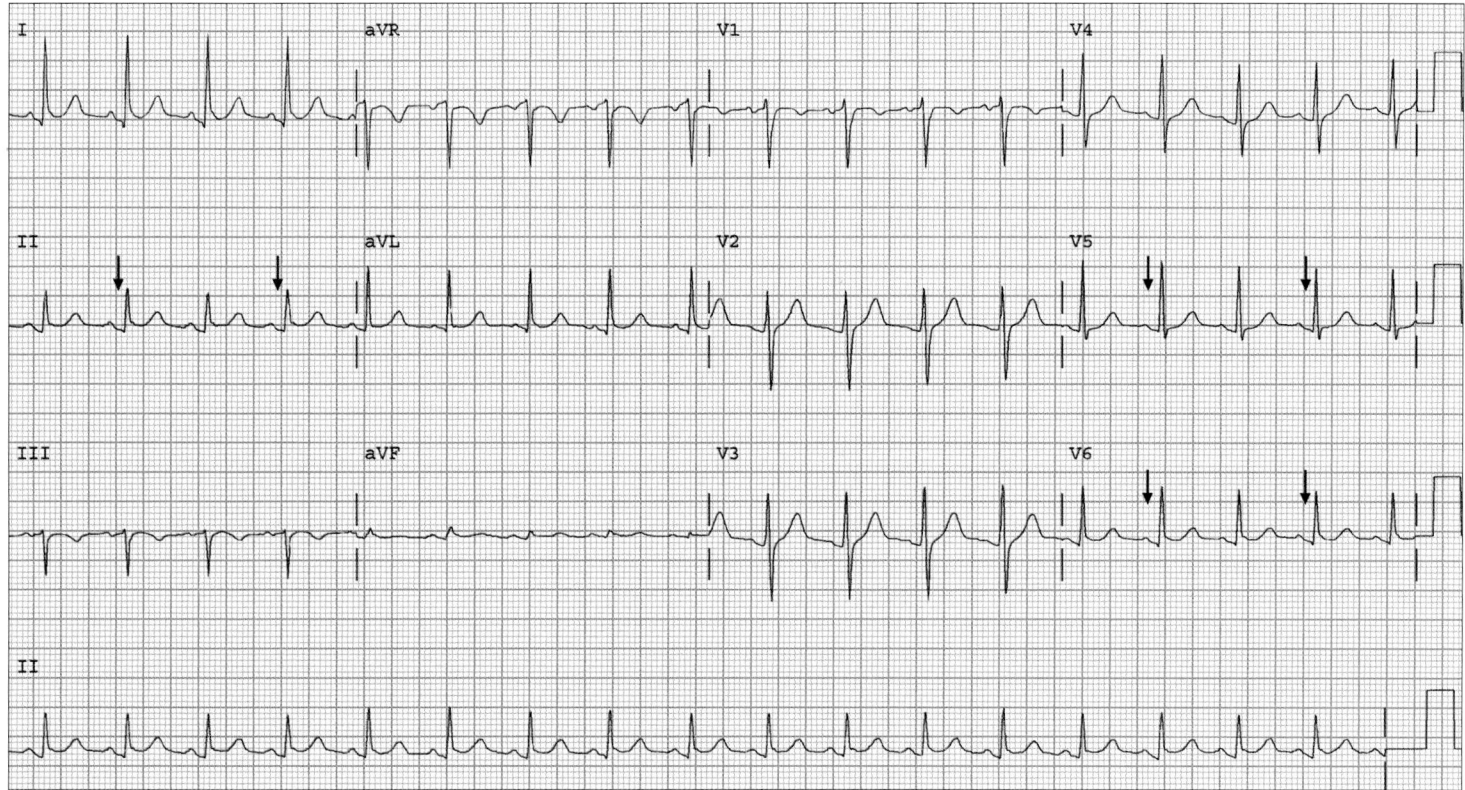

Fig. 49.8 Electrocardiogram of a patient who has early acute pericarditis. Note the presence of diffuse ST- segment elevation and PR depression in the inferolateral leads (arrows). 25mm/sec; 10.0mm/mV; F–W 0.05–100

ETIOLOGY OF LARGE PERICARDIAL EFFUSIONS

Etiology	% of 75 diagnoses
Malignancy	27
Viral	16
Collagen–vascular disease	14
Radiation	11
Uremia	11
Mycobacterial	5
Mycoplasma	3
Bacterial	1
Idiopathic	5
Other	8

Fig. 49.9 Etiology of large pericardial effusions.

- *Diffuse T-wave inversions develop*, generally after ST segments become isoelectric.
- *Electrocardiograph changes normalize*; long-term inversion of T waves suggests 'chronic' pericarditis.

A number of studies have established the utility of using a stepped approach.[37] One study prospectively evaluated 231 consecutive patients who have acute pericardial disease of unknown cause.[38] Pericardiocentesis was performed in patients who have tamponade, suspicion of purulent pericarditis, or symptoms and/or effusion persisting for more than 1 week after initiation of NSAID therapy. Pericardial biopsy was undertaken if clinical activity persisted at 3 weeks and the etiology was unknown. Despite this extensive evaluation, a specific diagnosis was confirmed in only 32 patients: neoplasia in 13, tuberculosis in 9, rheumatic disease in 4, purulent pericarditis in 2, toxoplasmosis in 2, and viral pericarditis in 2. Diagnostic yield was substantial when pericardiocentesis or biopsy were performed to relieve tamponade, but poor when used solely for diagnostic purposes. Over a mean follow-up of 31 months, no patient diagnosed with idiopathic pericarditis and treated with NSAIDs showed signs of recurrent or chronic pericardial disease.

Because of the recent interest in subxiphoid pericardial biopsy and drainage of pericardial effusions, we recently undertook a prospective nonrandomized trial of all patients who have large pericardial effusions hospitalized at our institution. These patients underwent a similar stepped preoperative approach, with subsequent subxiphoid pericardial biopsy and drainage of their effusions.[39] Diligent handling and extensive microbiologic analysis (including cultures for aerobic and anaerobic bacteria, viruses, chlamydiae, mycoplasma, fungi and mycobacteria) of pericardial fluid and tissue allowed specific diagnoses to be established in 53 out of 57 patients, confirming prior reports of high diagnostic yield when stepped algorithms are used for large effusions. More than one-third of the patients had malignancy or a history of irradiation to the thorax for malignancy. Infections (mostly viral), collagen–vascular disease and uremia were also frequently implicated (Fig. 49.9). Unexpected pathogens included CMV in 3 patients, herpes simplex virus 1 in 1, *Mycoplasma pneumoniae* in 2, *Mycobacterium avium–intracellulare* in 1, and *Mycobacterium chelonei* (see Fig. 49.5) in 1 patient. No patient showed evidence of Coxsackie A or B viral infection.

A comparison of diagnostic yield between pericardial fluid and biopsy demonstrated that fluid analysis was far more sensitive for malignancy; tissue provided additional information only in infected patients in whom fluid was not available for analysis. Previous studies demonstrated similar utility of pericardial fluid analysis; in a retrospective study of 93 cases of malignant effusion with both pericardial fluid and tissue analysis, cytology was correct in 87 cases (diagnostic accuracy 94%) with 100% specificity.[40]

In summary, acute pericarditis is most often viral or idiopathic in etiology; as such, invasive work-ups are usually not necessary. For the patient who has large effusions, tamponade, or presentation suggestive of purulent pericarditis, early and aggressive intervention will often yield diagnostic and therapeutic rewards.

DIAGNOSIS

As noted previously, a wide variety of infectious and noninfectious agents can cause acute pericarditis and/or pericardial effusions. For the patient presenting with acute chest pain, initial evaluation should focus on identifying conditions that may be rapidly fatal. Thus, myocardial infarction, aortic dissection, purulent pericarditis and cardiac tamponade should be systematically ruled out. An appropriate work-up includes a thorough history and physical examination, ECG and CXR (to rule out intrathoracic malignancy, tuberculosis, or a widened mediastinum suggestive of aortic dissection), and routine laboratory studies including complete blood counts, serum chemistries, serial CPK with MB fraction determination, thyroid function tests, rheumatoid factor and antinuclear antibodies; blood cultures should be obtained for the febrile patient. Due to the serious consequences of untreated tuberculous pericarditis, a tuberculin skin test with appropriate controls should be placed as well.

For the majority of individuals, a specific etiology will not be apparent, and a diagnosis of acute viral or idiopathic pericarditis will be made. Because either entity typically follows a brief and benign course, a full diagnostic evaluation is not appropriate. The confirmation of a particular viral agent is not necessary, as serologic titers and/or viral cultures are quite nonspecific, the work-up is costly and a retrospective diagnosis is usually not helpful in management. Because significant pericardial effusions may accumulate even in idiopathic disease, however, all patients should be carefully evaluated for their presence; hemodynamic compromise on physical examination, cardiac enlargement on CXR, or significant effusions on echocardiography necessitate rapid intervention. For patients who have large effusions, and for those in whom another diagnosis is suggested, a more thorough work-up includes pericardial drainage with or without pericardial biopsy.

As noted above, noninvasive diagnosis of pericardial disease in patients who have AIDS is extremely difficult. Because specific etiologic diagnosis often has important treatment ramifications, pericardial effusions in these patients should be managed on an individualized basis, with invasive diagnostic testing employed in those whose baseline health would benefit from aggressive therapeutic measures. Patients who have large pericardial effusions may demonstrate electric alternans, reflecting swinging of the heart within the pericardium.

Echocardiography has largely replaced other methods for the detection of pericardial fluid. With experience, operators can detect as little as 20ml of excess fluid posterior to the left ventricle. Echocardiography can also provide ancillary data in assessing the patient who has an effusion. Increased respiratory flow variation across the mitral valve with Doppler echocardiography is characteristic of cardiac tamponade. In addition, other etiologies of myocardial dysfunction such as right ventricular infarction can be ruled out. Finally, the echocardiogram can direct attempts at pericardiocentesis by identifying the location of pericardial fluid.

Computed tomography scans of the chest are primarily helpful in the diagnosis of pericardial thickening. Significant effusions are also readily demonstrated (Fig. 49.10). In addition, CT scans are more sensitive for the demonstration of small parenchymal nodules and mediastinal lymphadenopathy than is conventional roentgenography, and thus have clinical utility in the diagnosis of malignant pericarditis.

Cardiac catheterization is reserved for patients in whom pericardial constriction is believed to play a role in symptomatology. In those with chest pain of undetermined etiology, catheterization is also useful for ruling out myocardial ischemia as a confounding diagnosis.

MANAGEMENT

Nearly all patients who have acute pericarditis should be hospitalized for relief of symptoms, diagnostic evaluation and observation for complications. Specific medical therapy is tailored to the cause of pericarditis. Aspirin, at doses of 2–6g/day or other NSAIDs are effective in reducing symptoms of pericarditis, and are the agents of choice for idiopathic or viral pericarditis. Corticosteroids should be reserved for symptomatic nonresponders. Prednisone, however, is the drug of choice in pericarditis associated with connective tissue disease.

Idiopathic or viral pericarditis generally follows a benign, self-limited course, but the occasional patient will present after resolution with recurrent pericardial pain. Treatment for recurrences generally begins with NSAIDs; corticosteroids have been used successfully for NSAID-resistant cases. Colchicine has shown promise as a steroid-sparing agent in a number of small trials.[41] Pericardiectomy for recurrent pericarditis should be reserved for those who fail medical therapy. Interestingly, only one-third of patients will respond.[42]

Targeted intravenous antibiotics and surgical drainage of the pericardium remain the mainstays of therapy for purulent pericarditis. Pericardiocentesis urgently performed for the critically ill patient does not obviate the need for complete drainage and irrigation; fluid may reaccumulate rapidly, and sequelae such as constriction may develop in hours. There is no rationale for intrapericardial antibiotic administration, as pericardial penetration of antibiotic is excellent.

Tuberculous pericarditis remains a diagnostic and therapeutic challenge. Clinical features are nonspecific, the disease course is confusing and laboratory evaluation is often nondiagnostic, particularly in low prevalence settings and in patients who have localized disease. For example, although large effusions are more likely to be tuberculous, up to 50% of tuberculous effusions resolve spontaneously despite ongoing tissue infection. The tuberculin skin test may be negative in up to 30% of patients as a result of cutaneous anergy, yet may be positive in the patient who has acute idiopathic pericarditis and benign natural history. Suggestive, but not diagnostic, findings include a recent history of pulmonary tuberculosis, a positive sputum smear or culture, or a high pericardial fluid adenosine deaminase level (>45U/l). Even granulomatous inflammation of the pericardium is not diagnostic, as this may be demonstrated in pericardial disease from other causes, such as histoplasmosis, sarcoidosis and rheumatoid arthritis. Additionally, a negative biopsy of the pericardium does not rule out tuberculous pericarditis, as removal of the entire pericardium may be necessary to

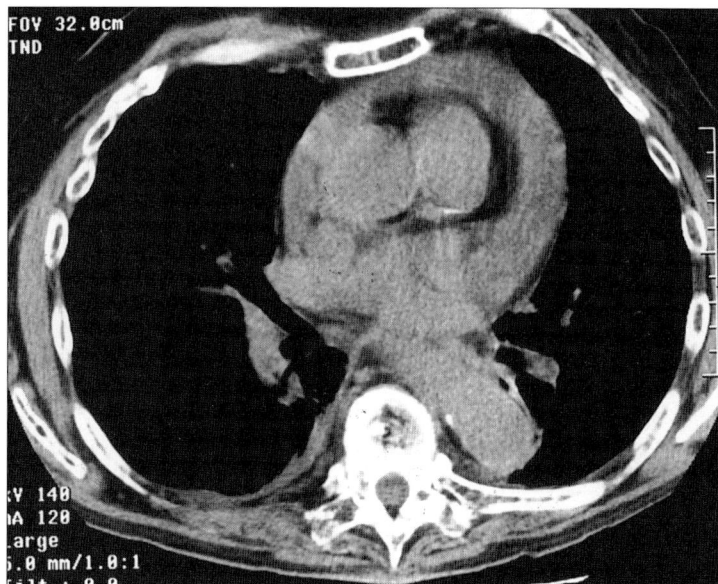

Fig. 49.10 Chest CT of a patient who has large, crescent-shaped pericardial effusion.

demonstrate clear-cut evidence of tuberculosis.[44]

Definitive diagnosis rests upon the demonstration of the tubercle bacillus in pericardial fluid and/or tissue. However, the need for early therapy demands that treatment often be undertaken based upon a presumptive diagnosis. Initial treatment should consist of four drugs including isoniazid and rifampin (rifampicin) until sensitivities are known. The use of concomitant prednisone (at doses of 60mg/day initially) to reduce pericardial inflammation is supported by two large controlled trials in Transkei, South Africa. Clinical improvement occurred more rapidly, 2-year mortality was lower (4 versus 11) and pericardiectomy was required less often (21% versus 30%) compared with those treated with four-drug therapy alone.[45] These data also highlight the incidence of constrictive complications in this disease. Complete pericardiectomy is advocated for those with recurrent effusions or cardiac compression with constrictive physiology after 4–6 weeks of oral therapy. Such early pericardiectomy is associated with a good outcome; mortality is substantially higher in patients who undergo pericardiectomy at the late stage of calcific pericardial constriction.[46]

REFERENCES

1. Karjalainen J, Heikkila J, Nieminen M, et al. Etiology of mild acute infectious myocarditis. Relation to clinical features. Acta Med Scand 1983;213:65–73.
2. Friman G, Wesslen L, Fohlman J, Karjalainen J, Rolf C. The epidemiology of infectious myocarditis, lymphocytic myocarditis and dilated cardiomyopathy. Eur Heart J 1995;16:36–41.
3. Morgan BC. Cardiac complications of diphtheria. Pediatrics 1963;32:549.
4. Ledbetter MK, Cannon AB, Costa AF. The electrocardiogram in diphtheric myocarditis. Am Heart J 1964;68:599–611.
5. Steere AC, Batsford WP, Weinberg M, et al. Lyme carditis: cardiac manifestations of Lyme disease. Ann Intern Med 1980;93:8.
6. Resnick JW, Braunstein DB, Walsch RL, et al. Lyme carditis. Electrophysiologic and histopathologic study. Am J Med 1986;81:923.
7. Marcus LC, Steere AC, Duray PH, et al. Fatal pancarditis in a patient with coexistent Lyme disease and babesiosis: demonstration of spirochetes in the heart. Ann Intern Med 1985;103:374.

8. Sahi T, Karjalainen J, Viitasalo MT, et al. Myocarditis in connection with viral infections in Finnish conscripts. Ann Med Milit Fenn 1982;57:198–203.
9. Fletcher GF, Coleman MT, Feorino PM, et al. Viral antibodies in patients with primary myocardial disease. Am J Cardiol 1968;21:6–10.
10. Cambridge G, MacArthur CGC, Waterson AP, et al. Antibodies to coxsackie B viruses in congestive cordiomyopathy. Br Heart J 1979;41:692–6.
11. Woodruff JF. Viral myocarditis: a review. Am J Pathol 1980;101:427–79.
12. Lange LG, Schreiner GF. Immune mechanisms of cardiac disease. N Engl J Med 1994;330:1129–35.
13. Neumann DA, Burke CL, Baughman KL, et al. Circulating heart-reactive antibodies in patients with myocarditis or cardiomyopathy. J Am Coll Cardiol 1990;16:839.
14. Tracy S, Wiegand V, McManus B, et al. Molecular approaches to enteroviral diagnosis in idiopathic cardiomyopathy and myocarditis. J Am Coll Cardiol 1990;15:1688–94.

15. Schwaiger A, Umlauft F, Weyrer K, et al. Detection of enteroviral ribonucleic acid in myocardial biopsies from patients with IDC by polymerase chain reaction. Am Heart J 1993;126:406.
16. Giacca M, Severini, GM, Mestroni L, et al. Low frequency of detection by nested PCR of enterovirus RNA in endomyocardial tissue of patients with idiopathic cardiomyopathy. J Am Coll Cardiol 1994;24:1033–40.
17. Kinney EL, Brafman D, Wright RT. Echocardiographic findings in patients with AIDS and ARC. Cath Cardiovasc Diagn 1989;16:182–5.
18. Herskowitz A, Wu T, Willoughby S, et al. Myocarditis and cardiotropic viral infection associated with severe LV dysfunction in late stage infection with HIV. J Am Coll Cardiol 1994;24:1025–32.
19. Lafont A, Wolff M, Marche C, Clair B, Regnier B. Overwhelming myocarditis due to Cryptococcus neoformans in an AIDS patient. Lancet 1987;2:1145–6.

20. Adair OV, Randive N, Krasnow N. Isolated toxoplasma myocarditis in AIDS. Am J Med 1986;81:19–23.

21. Maisch B, Schonian U, Crombach M, et al. CMV-associated inflammatory heart muscle disease. Scand J Infect Dis 1993; (Suppl 88):135–48.

22. Karjalainen J. Clinical diagnosis of myocarditis and dilated cardiomyopathy. Scand J Infect Dis 1993;(Suppl 88):33–43.

23. Gagliardi MG, Bevilacqua M, Di Renzi P, Picardo S, Passariello R, Marcelletti C. Usefulness of MRI for diagnosis of acute myocariditis in infants and children, and comparision with endomyocardial biopsy. Am J Cardiol 1991;68:1089–91.

24. Aretz HT, Billingham ME, Edwards WD, et al. Myocarditis: a histopathological definition and classification. Am J Cardiovasc Pathol 1990; 15:283.

25. Mason JW. Incidence and clinical characteristics of myocarditis. Circulation 199;(Suppl 8):2.

26. Herskowitz A, Campbell S, Deckers J, et al. Demographic features and prevalence of idiopathic myocarditis in patients undergoing endomyocardial biopsy. Am J Cardiol 1993;71:982–6.

27. Rezkalla S, Kloner RA, Khatib G, Khatib R. Effect of delayed captopril therapy on left ventricular mass and myonecrosis during acute coxsackievirus murine myocarditis. Am Heart J 1990;120:1377.

28. Rezkalla S, Khatib G, Khatib R. Coxsackievirus B3 murine myocarditis: deleterious effects of NSAIDs. J Lab Clin Med 1986;107:393.

29. O'Connell JB, Reap EA, Robinson JA. The effects of cyclosporine on acute murine coxsackie B3 myocarditis. Circulation 1986;73:353.

30. Mason JW, O'Connel JB, Herskowitz A, et al. A clinical trial of immunosuppressive therapy for myocarditis. N Eng J Med 1995;333:269–75.

31. Campbell PT, Li JS, Wall TC, et al. Cytomegalovirus pericarditis: a case series and review of the literature. Am J Med Sci 1995;309:229–34.

32. Kenney RT, Li JS, Clyde WA, et al. Mycoplasmal pericarditis: evidence of invasive disease. Clin Infect Dis 1993;(Suppl 17):58–62.

33. Larneu AJ, Tyers GF, Williams EH, Derrick JR. Recent experience with tuberculous pericarditis. Ann Thorac Surg 1980;29:464.

34. Strang JIG. Tuberculous pericarditis in Transkei. Clin Cardiol 1984;5:667.

35. Hsia J, Ross AM. Pericardial effusion and pericardiocentesis in HIV infection. Am J Cardiol 1994;74:94–6.

36. Lorell BH, Braunwald E. Pericardial disease. In: Braunwald F, ed. A textbook of cardiovascular medicine, 4th ed. Philadelphia: WB Saunders; 1992:1465–515.

37. Zayas R, Anguita M, Torres F et al. Incidence of specific etiology and role of methods for specific etiologic diagnosis of primary acute pericarditis. Am J Cardiol 1995;75:378–82.

38. Permanyer-Miralda G, Sagrista-Salueda J, Soler-Soler J. Primary acute pericardial disease: prospective series of 231 consecutive patients. Am J Cardiol 1985;56:623–30.

39. Corey GR, Campbell PT, Van Tright P, et al. Etiology of large pericardial effusions. Am J Med 1993;95:209–13.

40. Meyers DG, Bouska DJ. Diagnostic usefulness of pericardial fluid cytology. Chest 1989;95:1142–3.

41. Adler Y, Zandman-Goddard G, Ravid M, et al. Usefulness of colchicine in preventing recurrences of pericarditis. Am J Cardiol 1994;73:916–17.

42. Fowler NO. Pericardial disease. Heart Dis Stroke 1992;2:85–94.

43. Cheitlin MD, Serfos LJ, Sbar SS, Glosser SP. Tuberculous pericarditis: is limited pericardial biopsy sufficient for diagnosis? Am Rev Respir Dis 1968;98:287.

44. Martinez Vasquez JM, Ribera E, et al. ADA activity in tuberculous pericarditis. Thorax 1986;41:888.

45. Strang JI, Gibson DG, Mitchinson DA, et al. Controlled clinical trial of complete open surgical drainage and of prednisone in treatment of tuberculous pericardial effusion in Transkei. Lancet 1988;2:759–63.

46. Fennell WMP. Surgical treatment of constrictive tuberculous pericarditis. S Afr Med J 1982;62:353.

Endocarditis and Endarteritis

Philippe Moreillon

INTRODUCTION

This chapter reviews infective endocarditis (IE) and other endovascular infections in the context of their evolving epidemiology, diagnostic tools and therapeutic strategies. These diseases were invariably lethal in the pre-antibiotic era.[1] Fifty years ago, the introduction of penicillin followed by other antibiotics revolutionized the treatment and prognosis of IE. More recently, developments in clinical microbiology and the availability of improved imaging techniques, especially transthoracic and transesophageal echocardiography, have led to new, more accurate diagnostic criteria.[2] In industrialized countries, despite improvements in health care and the sharp decrease in the incidence of chronic rheumatic heart disease, IE has not disappeared and has even increased in some populations.[2–5] New at-risk groups have emerged, including intravenous drug users (IVDUs), elderly people with sclerotic cardiac valves and patients who have intravascular prostheses.

EPIDEMIOLOGY

Studies of the epidemiology of IE have been hampered by several factors: IE is a relatively rare disease, it is not officially a reportable disease and a precise case definition is lacking. This lack of a precise case definition is an important problem because it may be difficult to make a clinical diagnosis of IE with certainty. Therefore, many former studies were based on autopsy series. Fortunately, newer diagnostic criteria now allow a better assessment of IE in live patients.[2]

Overall, the incidence of IE ranges between 2 and 6 per 100,000 population per year.[2–5] Men and women are more or less equally affected, with some variations.[6] Although antibiotics have dramatically decreased the mortality and morbidity of endocardial infections, the disease has not disappeared; it may even be increasing, according to recent reports from Europe and the USA.[2–5]

The risk factors and the infecting micro-organisms have both changed over time. Chronic rheumatic heart disease, which was a prime risk factor in up to 75% of cases in the pre-antibiotic era,[7] is now rare in industrialized countries.[8] Classic pathogens such as pneumococci and gonococci have become uncommon, whereas there is an increasing number of cases due to *Staphylococcus aureus* and *S. epidermidis*.[2,4,5] These micro-organisms occur frequently in the newer risk groups of IVDUs, elderly people and patients who have prosthetic valves or pacemakers.

Infective endocarditis is commonly classified in four categories, which are discussed below:
- native valve IE,
- prosthetic valve IE,
- IE in IVDUs, and
- nosocomial IE.

NATIVE VALVE INFECTIVE ENDOCARDITIS

Risk factors for native valve IE include congenital heart disease and acquired abnormalities such as chronic rheumatic heart disease and degenerative heart disease. People who have cardiac abnormalities that result in high-to-low pressure gradients are at greater risk of infection.

Turbulent blood flow may provoke damage or peeling of the endothelium and formation of vegetation. Circulating bacteria tend to adhere on the low-pressure side of such Venturi-like systems. These observations explain why left-sided valves and left-to-right ventricular or arterial shunts are the most common sites of IE.

Congenital heart disease

Congenital heart disease is a lifelong risk factor. It is a major risk factor in children, in whom it accounts for 30–40% of IE.[8] It is a less frequent risk factor in adults, but it still represents about 5% of cases.[9] This includes all of the cardiac abnormalities associated with turbulent blood flow. Tetralogy of Fallot carries the highest risk for IE, followed by bicuspid aortic valve, coarctation of the aorta and ventricular septal defect. In contrast, secundum atrial septum defects rarely put the patient at risk, probably because they result in a low-pressure shunt.

Surgical or medical closure of a patent ductus arteriosus usually eliminates the risk of endovascular infection. However, surgical correction does not exclude the risk of IE in patients suffering major congenital heart disease, such as tetralogy of Fallot. Importantly, the type of surgical correction may influence the risk of subsequent infection in this situation. In a long-term survey[10] involving 1142 patient-years of observation, IE occurred in 23% of patients treated with anastomotic operations but in only 9% of patients treated with pulmonary valvulotomy or infundibular resection or both. Because vascular anastomoses are likely to generate turbulent blood flow, this observation underlines the importance of hydrodynamic disturbances in promoting endovascular infections.

Rheumatic heart disease

Rheumatic heart disease was the most frequent acquired cardiac anomaly leading to IE in the pre-antibiotic era. In one series, the frequency of chronic rheumatic heart disease in patients who had developed IE decreased from approximately 22% between 1933 and 1952 to less than 1% between 1963 and 1972.[7] Although the prevalence of the disease has decreased to less than 10 per 100,000 population per year in industrialized countries, it remains up to 50 times more common in certain developing countries. Moreover, recent clusters of rheumatic fever have been described in the USA,[11] suggesting a possible resurgence of the disease. Thus, rheumatic heart disease remains an important risk factor for IE.

Mitral valve prolapse

Mitral valve prolapse predisposes to endocarditis, primarily when there is associated regurgitation with a systolic murmur. A recent prospective study suggests that patients with mitral valve prolapse may have a 10- to 100-fold increased risk of developing IE compared with the general population.[12] Mitral valve prolapse is a common problem, especially in young women, in whom it was found in up to 20% of patients. Because it is related to body leanness, mitral valve prolapse is even more common in ballet dancers – 59% of women and 36% of men, compared with only 14% of control women and 4% of control men[13] – and anorexic patients. Mitral valve prolapse may be especially important in children and in patients over the age of 50 years because these groups seem to carry a higher risk of developing IE.[14]

Degenerative valve lesions

Degenerative valve lesions are present in up to 25% of patients aged over 40 years and in 50% of patients over age 60 years with IE.[15] Degenerative valve lesions leading to senile aortic stenosis or mitral regurgitation are frequent in patients aged over 70 years. Thus, elderly people should be carefully examined for clinical evidence of valve dysfunction.

PROSTHETIC VALVE INFECTIVE ENDOCARDITIS

Prosthetic valve endocarditis (PVE) occurs in 1–5% of cases, or 0.32–1.2% per patient-year.[16] The issue of whether mechanical or bioprosthetic valves are more prone to infection remains unresolved. Prosthetic valve endocarditis is usually classified as either early infection or late infection, depending on whether the symptoms of infection occur within 60 days after surgery or later. The risk of PVE peaks during the 2 months after valve implantation; thus infection probably results from perioperative contamination.[17] Early PVE is often due to *S. epidermidis,* and less frequently to *S. aureus*, organisms that are commonly found on the skin and are frequently introduced into the heart or bloodstream during or soon after surgery. Progressive endothelialization of the prosthetic material over 2–6 months eventually reduces the susceptibility of the implanted valve to infection. This is

reflected in a change in the predominant pathogens over time. *Staphylococcus epidermidis* causes PVE most often during the first year after a valve implantation; later, this organism is replaced by streptococci and sometimes Gram-negative bacteria of the so-called HACEK group, including *Haemophilus* spp., *Actinobacillus actinomycetem comitans*, *Cardiobacterium hominis*, *Eikenella corrodens*, and *Kingella kingae*. Patients with a prosthetic valve implanted during active IE also have a greater risk (up to seven times) of subsequent PVE than patients undergoing elective valve replacement, although the infection may be due to a different organism.

INFECTIVE ENDOCARDITIS IN INTRAVENOUS DRUG USERS

Intravenous drug users constitute a special risk group constituted of relatively young people, with a median age of about 30 years.[18] Men are more often affected than women. The prevalence of IVDUs among patients with IE depends on the study population, representing up to 40% of cases of IE in San Francisco, but less than 1% in Olmsted County, Minnesota, USA.[19] Right-sided IE is common in this population, most often involving the tricuspid valve. It has been suggested that repeated injections of impure drugs and particulate material might produce microtrauma to the tricuspid leaflets, thus facilitating microbial colonization and infection. However, 20–40% of IVDUs suffering IE have pre-existing cardiac lesions, often caused by previous valve infection. The tricuspid valve is infected in more that 50% of cases, followed by the aortic valve in 25% and the mitral valve in 20%, with mixed right-sided and left-sided IE in a few cases. The responsible bacteria often originate from the skin, which explains the predominance of *S. aureus* infections (Fig. 50.1), but streptococci and other microorganisms are also encountered; some pathogens, such as *Pseudomonas aeruginosa* and fungi, may produce severe forms of IE. Infection with HIV is not itself a risk factor for IE, except in rare cases caused by *Bartonella* spp. Nevertheless, the mortality of IE is higher in patients with AIDS, especially in advanced cases, than in other patients.[20]

NOSOCOMIAL INFECTIVE ENDOCARDITIS

Nosocomial IE is another growing category of patients. In a recent series, over 10% of cases were of nosocomial origin, most often in patients over 60 years of age.[21] Many of these patients had underlying cardiac diseases. In more than 95% of these cases a potential source of infection that may produce transient bacteremia, such as intravenous lines or invasive procedures, could be identified. Accordingly, the pathogens usually originated from the skin or the urinary tract: staphylococci and enterococci were the most common. Right-sided IE is also increasingly recognized in association with central venous catheters and pulmonary artery catheters, as well as pacemakers. Possible right-sided IE was reported in 5% of bone marrow transplant recipients who had central venous catheters.

Thus, although IE can develop in people in apparently normal health, susceptible patients often can be identified on the basis of specific risk factors. Until recently, these were primarily intrinsic anomalies of the heart. Today we must consider other lesions provoked by extrinsic interventions, such as prosthetic valves, and transient or permanent intravascular catheters or devices. Any procedure producing transient bacteremias represents some degree of risk for susceptible patients. Such considerations are important for appropriate prophylaxis and accurate diagnosis of IE.

PATHOGENESIS, PATHOLOGY AND INFECTING MICRO-ORGANISMS

The key issues in the pathogenesis of IE, discussed below, are:
- the predisposing host factors,
- the characteristics of the infecting micro-organisms,
- the role of transient bacteremia, and
- the inability of the immune system to eradicate micro-organisms once they are located on the endocardium.

MICROBIOLOGY OF INFECTIVE ENDOCARDITIS IN THE GENERAL POPULATION AND IN INTRAVENOUS DRUG USERS

Pathogens	Number (% total) of cases in non-IVDU patients*	Number (%) of cases in IVDU patients†
Staphylococci	152 (42.1)	45 (61)
S. aureus	128 (35.4)	45 (61)
Coagulase-negative staphylococci	24 (6.6)	0 (0)
Streptococci	125 (34.6)	10 (13.5)
Oral streptococci	81 (22.4)	NS
Strep. pneumoniae	3 (0.8)	NS
Strep. agalactiae (group B)	15 (4.1)	NS
Strep. pyogenes (group A)	1 (0.3)	NS
Strep. bovis	12 (3.3)	NS
Unspecified	13 (3.6)	NS
Enterococci	29 (8.0)	2 (2.7)
Enterococcus faecalis	14 (3.9)	NS
Enterococcus durans	1 (0.3)	NS
Unspecified	14 (3.9)	NS
Other organisms	31 (8.6)	17 (23)
Haemophilus spp.	10 (2.7)	NS
Pseudomonas spp.	3 (0.8)	11 (14.9)
Escherichia coli	1 (0.3)	NS
Candida spp.	1 (0.3)	NS
Unspecified	13 (3.6)	NS
Polymicrobial	3 (0.8)	6 (8.1)
Culture-negative infective endocarditis‡	24 (6.6)	0 (0)
Total episodes	361 (100)	74 (100)

*Includes 53 (14.6%) prosthetic valve infection and 4 (1.1%) IE in IVDUs[2,4,5]
†Includes 27 methicillin-susceptible and 18 methicillin-resistant *S. aureus*[18]
‡Etiology not specified

Fig. 50.1 Microbiology of infective endocarditis in the general population and in intravenous drug users. IVDU, intravenous drug user; NS, not specified.[2,4,5]

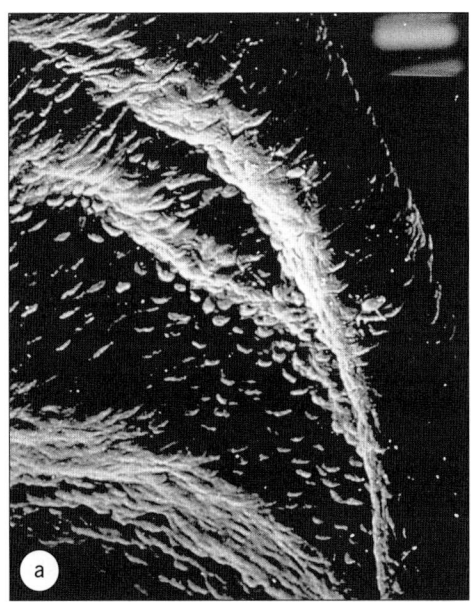

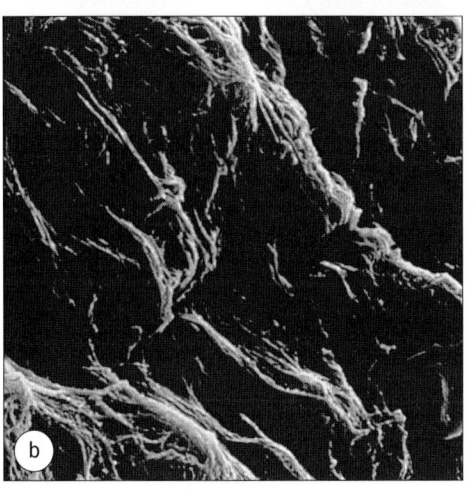

Fig. 50.2 Scanning electron microscopy of a rabbit aortic valve leaflet. (a) A normal valve, covered by a monolayer of endothelial cells. (b) The meshwork of fibrin and platelets covering a damaged valve. Mechanical lesions of the valve were created by inserting a catheter through the right aortic carotid and across the aortic valve.

COLONIZATION AND INFECTION OF AN ENDOTHELIAL LESION BY *STAPHYLOCCUS AUREUS*

Pathogen		Host	
Clumping factor		Platelet	
Coagulase		Fibrin/fibrinogen	
Fibronectin binding protein		Fibronenctin	

Staphylococcus aureus

Platelet factors

Coagulation

Tissue factor

Endothelium

Matrix proteins

Fig. 50.3 Colonization and infection of an endothelial lesion by *Staphylococcus aureus*. Exposure of the subendothelial matrix triggers the deposition of platelet–fibrin clots and other plasma-soluble and matrix proteins, including fibrinogen, fibrin, fibronectin and thrombospondin. Triggering of the coagulation cascade is also mediated by tissue factor, which contributes to platelet activation and the constitution of a nonbacterial thrombotic vegetation. *Staphylococcus aureus* is equipped with a wealth of surface determinants that may promote binding and colonization of nonbacterial thrombotic vegetations. The best known of these are fibrinogen-binding protein (or clumping factor), fibronectin-binding protein and coagulase. These factors are likely to mediate direct or indirect attachment to vascular lesions and promote infection.

PREDISPOSING HOST FACTORS

The importance of host factors is indicated by the fact that IE most often develops on pre-existing lesions of the layer of endothelial cells covering the valve or endovascular surfaces. Normally, this endothelium is resistant to colonization by circulating bacteria, but damage to this delicate protective layer increases the susceptibility to bacterial colonization by several orders of magnitude (Fig. 50.2). Exposure of the underlying extracellular matrix proteins and the local production of tissue factors trigger the deposition of platelets and fibrin as a normal host response initiating the healing process. Such a platelet–fibrin meshwork, referred to as nonbacterial thrombotic endocarditis (NBTE), is a favorable nidus for bacterial colonization during transient bacteremias.[22]

Endothelial damage may occur in several ways. Congenital cardiac abnormalities may cause turbulent blood flow, which in turn may provoke peeling of the endothelium. Valve scarring and calcification following rheumatic carditis or in the sclerotic valves of elderly patients results in endothelial lesions. Extrinsic intervention, such as prosthetic valve replacement or indwelling electrodes or catheters, also promote endothelial lesions. Recently, the presence of *Chlamydia pneumoniae* or cytomegalovirus in endovascular locations has been linked to arteriosclerosis.[23] Whether these organisms also promote endothelial lesions that promote IE remains to be demonstrated.

CHARACTERISTICS OF THE MICRO-ORGANISMS

The pathogens most frequently responsible for IE are also those that have the greatest ability to adhere to and colonize damaged valves.[24] Together, *S. aureus*, *Streptococcus* spp. and enterococci are responsible for more than 80% of all cases of IE (see Fig. 50.1).[2,4,5] These Gram-positive organisms have the greatest capacity to adhere to NBTE

in vitro and i*n vivo*,[24,25] for they are well equipped with surface determinants that mediate adherence to the endocardium. Figure 50.3 presents a likely scenario in the case of IE due to *S. aureus*. These organisms possess several surface ligands that mediate attachment to proteins that are present in the milieu of endothelial lesions. Fibrinogen-binding protein (also called clumping factor) is involved in valvular colonization.[26] The role of other bacterial ligands, such as fibronectin-binding protein and coagulase, is currently being investigated. In streptococci, production of exopolysaccharides is an additional factor that promotes adherence to NBTE. Thus, bacteria causing IE possess an abundance of surface adhesins, which promote colonization of the target tissues.

Although bacterial colonization of pre-existing NBTE is a leading mechanism for establishment of IE, direct invasion of endothelial cells may also occur under certain circumstances. A few cases of IE are due to intracellular pathogens such as *Coxiella burnetii* (the agent of Q fever), *Chlamydia* spp., *Legionella* spp. and *Bartonella* spp.[27] Infection by these pathogens may occur by direct or indirect invasion of the cardiac endothelium. Direct invasion of endothelial cells has been demonstrated *in vitro* with *S. aureus*.[28] During infection, general or local production of cytokines or other inflammatory mediators induces endothelial cells to express integrins, which in turn promote adherence and local extravasation of monocytes and granulocytes. These events may be important in the pathogenesis of endovascular inflammation.

THE ROLE OF TRANSIENT BACTEREMIA

Infective endocarditis has been modeled in rats and rabbits with catheter-induced valvular lesions. These experiments have allowed the determination of a hierarchy of the infectivity of the various pathogens.

Bacterial adherence is a critical factor and the magnitude and duration of the bacteremia after inoculation are also important determinants.[29]

Medical and surgical procedures in nonsterile anatomic sites may provoke transient invasion of the bloodstream with bacteria from the local flora. Such bacteremia is usually low grade and of short duration (e.g. 1–100 cfu/ml of blood for less than 10 minutes in the case of dental extraction).[30] Depending on the characteristics of the circulating bacteria, even these transient bacteremias may put patients with pre-existing cardiac lesions at greater risk of developing IE. In the case of dental procedures, postextraction bacteremia is more important in patients suffering from gingivitis than in individuals with a healthy gingivodental status. This was simulated in rats with catheter-induced aortic NBTE.[31] Animals suffering from gingivitis were at a much greater risk of postextraction endocarditis than those with healthy gingivae. Most interestingly, although all the rats developed polymicrobial bacteremias during a dental procedure, only two types of organisms – group G streptococci and *S. aureus* – colonized the valves to cause IE. This correlates with the ability of these bacteria to attach to NBTE.[32]

Transient bacteremias occur spontaneously during chewing, toothbrushing and other normal activities. These spontaneous bacteremias provide the likely explanation for the fact that most cases of IE are not preceded by medical or surgical procedures. Moreover, because streptococci are normal inhabitants of the mouth, spontaneous bacteremias arising from the mouth during chewing may explain why these bacteria are a predominant cause of IE. Thus, proper prophylactic measures during specific medical interventions will only marginally affect the overall frequency of IE.[33] Simple prevention strategies such as good dental hygiene provide the best method of prophylaxis in this context.

THE ROLE OF HOST DEFENSES

Infective endocarditis is most often due to Gram-positive organisms, and rarely to Gram-negative bacteria (see Fig. 50.1). The reason for this is probably multifactorial. Differences in bacterial adherence to NBTE may be one explanation. However, differences in the susceptibility of Gram-positive and Gram-negative bacteria to serum-induced killing may also account for these variations. The C5b–C9 membrane-attack complex of complement kills Gram-negative bacteria by perforating their outer membrane. In contrast, complement does not kill Gram-positive bacteria. Moreover, their plasma membrane is protected from the membrane-attack complex of complement by the surrounding peptidoglycan.

The importance of serum was demonstrated in experimental IE induced by serum-susceptible *Escherichia coli*.[34] These organisms were spontaneously cleared from the vegetations even after infection with very large inocula. Nevertheless, some Gram-negative bacteria may carry thick capsules or other modifications of their outer membrane that helps them resist complement-induced killing. An important subgroup of cases of IE are caused by Gram-negative bacteria, including microorganisms of the HACEK group, as well as *P. aeruginosa* in IVDUs.[18]

Although Gram-positive bacteria are resistant to complement, they may be the target of another nonspecific immune factor, the platelet microbicidal proteins (PMPs).[35] Platelet microbicidal proteins are peptides produced by activated thrombocytes that kill bacteria by a mechanism that is as yet incompletely understood. Indirect evidence for the protective role of PMPs in IE came from experiments in which thrombocytopenic rabbits demonstrated greater bacterial densities in their vegetations than rabbits with normal platelet counts. Likewise, microorganisms recovered from patients with IE were consistently resistant to PMP-induced killing, whereas similar bacteria recovered from patients with other types of infection were susceptible to PMP. Therefore platelets, which are a major component of the vegetations, may be key players in the nonspecific defense against IE.

Humoral and cellular immunity seem to play only a limited role in defense against IE. In animal studies, immunization against the challenging pathogen protected against IE to some extent.[36] On the other hand, administration of granulocyte colony-stimulating factor did not influence the course of infection.[37] Infective endocarditis is not notice-

ably more frequent in immunocompromised patients than in those without immune defects. In established infection, bacteria are clustered in amorphous platelet–fibrin clots (the vegetations), permitting little access to professional phagocytes to remove the bacteria (Fig. 50.4). This explains why successful treatment of IE relies primarily on the ability of antibiotics rather than host defenses to kill bacteria *in situ* in the vegetation.

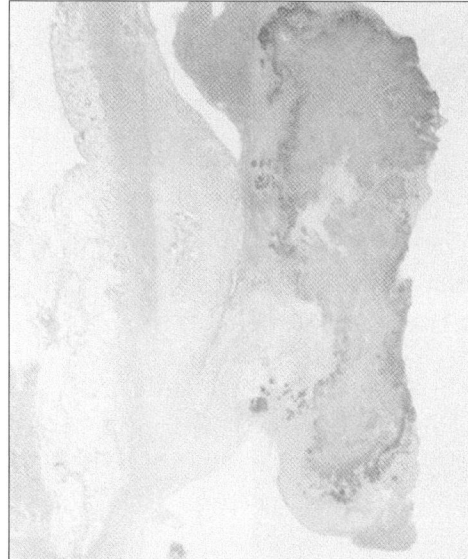

Fig. 50.4 Microscopic appearance of a vegetation from experimental infective endocarditis caused by *Streptococcus sanguis*. The purple area represents clusters of streptococci packed within a fibrin–platelet meshwork. Professional phagocytes are essentially absent from the lesion.

PRE-EXISTING CONDITIONS ASSOCIATED WITH AN INCREASED RISK OF ENDOCARDITIS	
Endocarditis prophylaxis recommended	
High-risk patients	Prosthetic cardiac valves, including bioprosthetic and homograft valves
	Previous infectious endocarditis
	Complex cyanotic congenital heart disease (e.g. single ventricular states, transposition of the great arteries, tetralogy of Fallot)
	Surgically constructed systemic pulmonary shunts or conduits
Moderate-risk patients	Most other congenital cardiac malformations (other than above and below)
	Acquired valve dysfunction (e.g. rheumatic heart disease)
	Hypertrophic cardiomyopathy
	Mitral valve prolapse with valve regurgitation or thickened valve leaflets
Endocarditis prophylaxis not recommended	
Low-risk patients (risk similar to that in the general population)	Isolated secundum atrial septal defect
	Surgical repair of atrial septal defect, ventricular septal defect, or patent ductus
	Previous coronary artery bypass
	Mitral valve prolapse without valve regurgitation
	Functional heart murmur
	Previous Kawasaki disease without valve dysfunction
	Previous rheumatic fever without valve dysfunction
	Cardiac pacemaker (intravascular or epicardial) and implanted defibrillator

Fig. 50.5 Pre-existing conditions associated with an increased risk of developing endocarditis. Adapted from recommendations in Europe[38] and the USA.[39]

PREVENTION

Because of its severity, it is generally agreed that IE should be prevented whenever possible. Choice of appropriate prophylactic measures requires:
- identification of patients at risk,
- determination of the procedures or circumstances that may result in bacteremias,
- choice of an appropriate antimicrobial regimen, and
- balancing of the known risks against the possible benefits of intervention.

In many countries, recommendations for prophylaxis have been established, based on underlying cardiac conditions and distinguishing between high-risk and low-risk situations depending on the anatomical defects and the medical or dental procedure in question (Fig. 50.5).[38,39]

The practice of IE prophylaxis is not based on the results of randomized studies because these would require too many patients and raise difficult ethical issues. Therefore, antibiotic regimens used in humans are based upon their proven efficacy in animal models of IE. In contrast to therapy, successful prophylaxis does not require bactericidal antibiotics. The key factor is the period of time during which serum levels of antibiotics remain above the MIC for the circulating pathogen. For amoxicillin, this optimal duration is more than 10 hours.[40] Therefore, prophylactic antibiotics are given in large single doses or in repeated doses, or both, in order to ensure the prolonged presence of the drug in the serum.

Antibiotics are chosen in relation to the most probable pathogens circulating in the blood during a given procedure (Fig. 50.6). For oropharyngeal manipulation, antibiotic prophylaxis should be aimed at streptococci. For gastrointestinal or urogenital manipulations, it should be aimed at enterococci. Indeed, although gastrointestinal procedures are more likely to produce Gram-negative bacteremia, these organisms are rarely responsible for IE. For drainage of skin or other infected lesions, it should be aimed at the most likely infecting organism present in the lesion and, as a minimum, it should cover staphylococci. It is noteworthy that, during dental manipulation, the risk of bacteremia correlates with the status of dental hygiene; patients with healthy gums are at lower risk than those with severe gingivitis. In cases of severe gingivitis, the local application of an antiseptic wash using chlorhexidine may be a useful additional measure.

CLINICAL FEATURES

Infective endocarditis may follow an acute or subacute course. The general clinical features (Fig. 50.7) are not usually specific.

ACUTE INFECTIVE ENDOCARDITIS

Acute IE is most frequently caused by *S. aureus*, followed by enterococci and certain streptococci, such as *Streptococcus milleri*. Infective endocarditis caused by *S. aureus* and other primary, invasive pathogens can be devastating. Bacterial production of proteases and other exoproteins contributes to rapid destruction of valve leaflets and the development of abscesses located in the valve ring and the myocardium. Myocarditis and pericardial effusions are frequent. Patients are prostrate and have a high fever. Hypotension and shock may occur, caused both by the septic state and by cardiac failure. Cardiac vegetations may vary from a few millimeters in diameter to more than 1cm. Large vegetations are frequent in acute staphylococcal and fungal IE (Fig. 50.8) and are more likely to detach and give rise to septic emboli.

PRINCIPAL PROCEDURES REQUIRING PROPHYLAXIS AND RECOMMENDED REGIMENS			
Type of procedure	Procedure	Recommended prophylaxis	
Oropharyngeal procedures	Dental extractions	Oral route, standard	Amoxicillin 2g (children 50mg/kg) 1 hour before procedurei
	Periodontal procedures such as surgery, scaling, root planing, probing and maintenance	Oral route, allergic to penicillin	Clarithromycin 500mg (children 15mg/kg) 1 hour before procedure
	Placement of dental implant and re-implantation of avulsed teeth		Azithromycin 500mg (children 15mg/kg) 1 hour before procedure
	Root canal instrumentation or surgery (only beyond apex)		Clindamycin 600mg (children 20mg/kg) 1 hour before procedure
	Subgingival placement of antibiotic fibers or strips		
	Initial placement of orthodontic bands (but not brackets)	Parenteral route, standard	Ampicillin 2g (children 50mg/kg) im or iv 30 minutes before procedure
	Intraligamentary local anesthetic injections		
	Prophylactic cleaning of teeth or implants involving bleeding	Parenteral route, allergic to penicillin	Vancomycin 1g (children 20mg/kg) iv over 1–2 hours, with infusion completed within 30 minutes of starting procedure
	Tonsillectomy, adenoidectomy and surgical procedures involving the respiratory mucosa		
Respiratory tract procedures	All surgical procedures involving the respiratory mucosa		
Gastrointestinal tract procedures	Sclerotherapy of esophageal varices		
	Esophageal stricture dilatation		
Gastrointestinal tract procedures	Endoscopic retrograde cholangiography with biliary obstruction	Moderate-risk patients	Amoxicillin or ampicillin as above
	Biliary tract surgery		Vancomycin 1g iv over 1–2 hours, with infusion completed within 30 minutes of starting procedure (for penicillin-allergic patients) (adapt doses for children)
	Surgical procedures involving the intestinal mucosa		
Genitourinary tract procedures	Prostatic surgery	High-risk patients, allergic to penicillin	Ampicillin 2g im or iv plus gentamicin 1.5mg/kg im or iv 30 minutes prior to procedure, plus ampicillin 1g im or iv or amoxicillin 1g orally 6 hours later (adapt doses for children)
	Cystoscopy		
	Urethral dilatation		Vancomycin 1g iv over 1–2 hours, with infusion completed within 30 minutes of starting procedure, plus gentamicin 1.5mg/kg im or iv 30 minutes before procedure (adapt doses for children)

Fig. 50.6 Principal procedures requiring prophylaxis and recommended regimens. Adapted from recommendations in Europe[38] and the USA.[39] Moderate-risk and high-risk patients are defined as in Figure 50.5.

GENERAL SYMPTOMS AND SIGNS OF INFECTIVE ENDOCARDITIS	
General symptoms	Frequency of occurrence (%)
Fever	90
Fatigue	50
Dyspnea	40
Myalgia	28
Gastrointestinal symptoms	22
Cough	20
Nausea	16
Thoracic pain	15
Mental deterioration	15
Skin lesions	10
Arthralgia	9
Edema	9
Weight loss	8
Hepatomegaly	8
Night sweat	5
Splenomegaly	<5

Fig. 50.7 General symptoms and signs in infective endocarditis. The figures relate to 98 prospective episodes of infective endocarditis.[4] Note that 97% of patients with *Staphylococcus aureus* endocarditis had fever with body temperature over 102°F (39°C), compared to 57% of patients with streptococcal endocarditis.

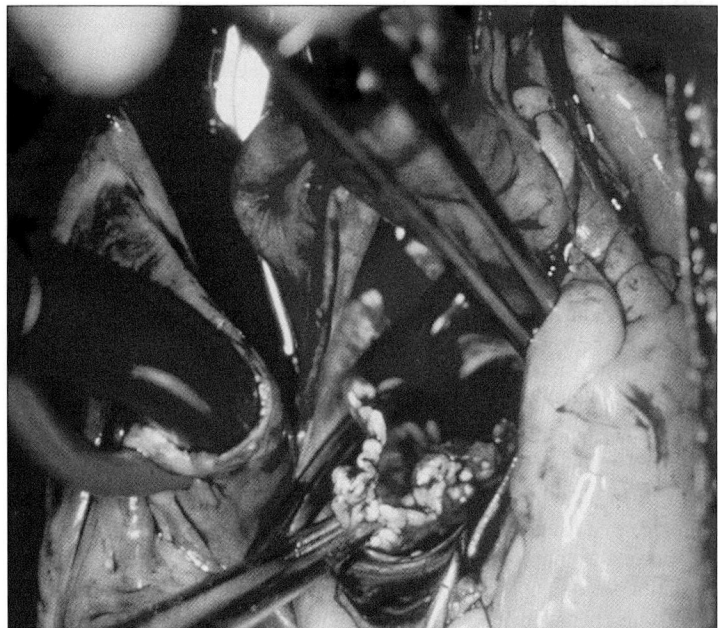

Fig. 50.8 Aortic valve of a patient undergoing emergency valve replacement for acute endocarditis caused by *Staphylococcus aureus*. In this patient, emergency valve replacement was mandatory because of multiple embolizations and acute heart failure. Here, the aorta has been opened and the valve is viewed from its upper side. The lower tweezers are holding a valve leaflet covered with vegetations. Next to the upper tweezers, a portion of a cuspid with a normal appearance can be distinguished.

Complications in peripheral organs mainly result from embolic lesions; these may include skin abscesses and retinal emboli (Fig. 50.9) and cerebral abscesses and splenic lesions (Fig. 50.10).

Major indications for urgent valve replacement include refractory cardiac failure due to valve destruction and persistent sepsis related to myocardial abscesses. A defect in atrioventricular conduction is often an early sign of septal invasion by a contiguous valve ring abscess, which usually requires urgent surgery.

SUBACUTE INFECTIVE ENDOCARDITIS

Subacute IE is not usually due to *S. aureus*, but it may be due to any of the organisms listed in Figure 50.1. The course of subacute IE can mimic chronic wasting diseases. The duration between an identifiable event producing bacteremia (e.g. dental procedure) and the diagnosis of IE can vary from a few days to 5 weeks or more. Fever is almost always present (see Fig. 50.7). Physical signs reflect the existence of cardiac or peripheral complications. These include a new or changing heart murmur and evidence of embolic events.

Immunologic stimulation during subacute IE causes hyperproduction of gammaglobulin. Rheumatoid factor is present in up to 50% of patients after 6 weeks of subacute infection; its level decreases after effective treatment. Immune phenomena may be the cause of petechiae, splinter hemorrhages, Osler nodes and Roth spots, arthritis and glomerulonephritis. Osler nodes are small and painful nodular lesions on the pads of the fingers or toes or on the thenar or hypothenar eminences (Fig. 50.11). They are caused by an allergic vasculitis. Although classic, they are not pathognomonic of subacute IE. Roth spots are rounded retinal hemorrhages with a white center. Focal or diffuse glomerulonephritis is present in most of the cases. Because these phenomena follow stimulation of the immune system, they are less common in acute IE.

VASCULAR COMPLICATIONS

Embolic lesions result from vegetation fragments breaking off the valve and lodging in arteries serving peripheral organs. Other types of vascular manifestations are the consequence of immune-related vasculitis. Mycotic aneurysms are found in up to 15% of cases, and are especially common in staphylococcal IE. They may arise either from direct invasion

of the arterial wall by the infecting organisms, from septic embolization of the vasa vasorum or from the deposition of immune complexes that may trigger local inflammation and weakening of the arterial wall. Mycotic aneurysms tend to be located at the bifurcation points of vessels. They may either heal during antibiotic therapy or become clinically evident later, even months after the clinical cure of the disease. Therefore, the true incidence of mycotic aneurysms during IE is probably underestimated. In right-sided IE, embolization occurs in the pulmonary circulation and gives rise to pulmonary infiltrates and lung abscesses.[41]

NEUROLOGIC COMPLICATIONS

Neurologic manifestations occur in up to 40% of cases.[42] However, because patients without neurologic symptoms do not undergo specific investigations, the true incidence of neurologic events during IE may be underestimated. Anatomic alterations include cerebral infarction, arteritis, abscesses, mycotic aneurysms, intracerebral or subarachnoid hemorrhage, encephalomalacia, cerebritis and meningitis. Such complications occur most often in staphylococcal or streptococcal IE, but they are not restricted to IE caused by these pathogens.

The management of IE patients with cerebral complications is aimed at controlling the infection, decreasing the risk of embolization and dealing with the complications. When large vegetations are present, surgical vegetectomy or valve replacement is necessary. This decision may be difficult because anticoagulation during extracorporeal circulation and after valve replacement puts the patients at an increased risk of secondary intracerebral hemorrhage. Therefore, the tendency is often to postpone emergency surgery and wait for the patient to stabilize. On the other hand, ongoing studies suggest that earlier intervention may be beneficial in such patients. The best approach to these challenging issues needs continuing investigation.

DIAGNOSIS

Whether acute or subacute, IE may result in life-threatening complications. Therefore, precise clinical and microbiologic diagnosis is mandatory in order to guide therapy. Infective endocarditis combines both persistent bacteremia and anatomic lesions of the valves. Clinical

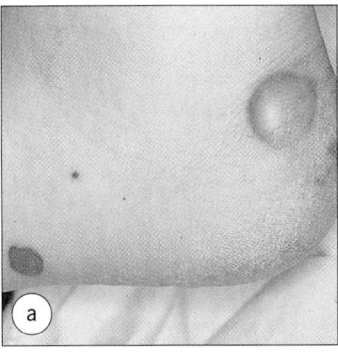
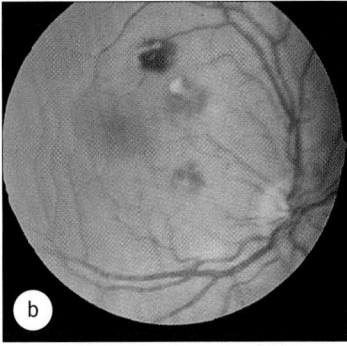

Fig. 50.9 Skin lesions on the foot (a) and septic emboli of the retina (b), the result of peripheral emboli in acute endocarditis caused by *Staphylococcus aureus*. These occurred in the patient described in Figure 50.8 and were present on admission to hospital.

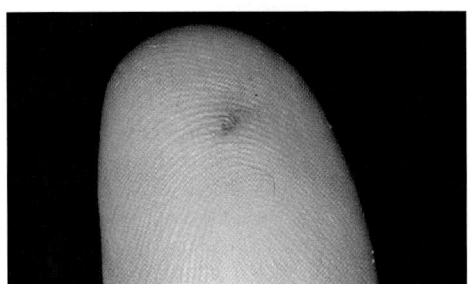

Fig. 50.11 Osler node on the thumb during subacute endocarditis. This was a rounded, tender, inflamed mass about 5mm in diameter.

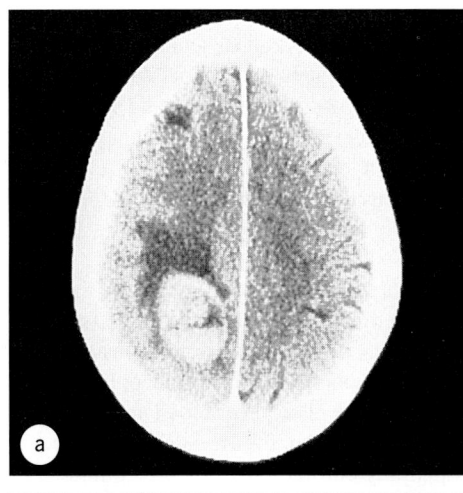

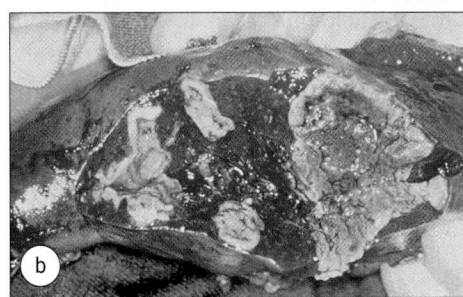

Fig. 50.10 A cerebral abscess (a) and multiple abscesses and ischemic necroses of the spleen (b), the result of peripheral emboli in acute endocarditis caused by *Staphylococcus aureus*. Again, these occurred in the patient described in Figure 50.8 and developed after admission to hospital.

diagnosis of IE can be difficult when blood cultures remain negative or when changes in the valve status cannot be assessed owing to lack of information on pre-existing cardiac lesions.[2,6]

THE DUKE CRITERIA

Recently, new diagnostic criteria based on clinical and laboratory information relying on noninvasive techniques were proposed (Fig. 50.12).[2] These criteria, which are referred to as the Duke criteria, take advantage of both microbiologic data and imaging of cardiac lesions by transthoracic or transesophageal echocardiography in order to achieve greater sensitivity and specificity than previous criteria.[2,6] Today, nearly all patients suspected of having IE should undergo at least one echocardiographic evaluation, including transesophageal echo in selected cases.

BLOOD CULTURES

Blood cultures are of primary importance because they reveal the infecting organism and thus guide antibiotic therapy. For the main etiologic agents, the first two blood cultures will be positive in more than 90% of cases. However, certain micro-organisms may be difficult to isolate. Variables affecting isolation include the volume of blood cultured, the number of blood cultures obtained before antimicrobial therapy is started, the type of micro-organism involved and the techniques of blood culture.

The volume of blood cultured is critical because persistent bacteremia in IE often is of low level, representing only 1–100 bacteria/ml of blood. For each culture, 8–12ml of venous blood should be drawn with careful antiseptic precautions and distributed into a two-bottle system for incubation. Blood for culture should be drawn on two or three separate occasions over a 24-hour period. If possible, the interval between each culture should be at least 30–60 minutes.

Culture-negative IE deserves special attention. The most common situation in which blood cultures remain negative is in patients who have taken antibiotics within the previous 2 weeks. In such patients, it may be necessary to obtain additional blood cultures and to use media supplemented with beta-lactamase when appropriate. Some pathogens require special media, so it is important that the clinician gives adequate information to the microbiology laboratory when ordering the test. Negative cultures should be incubated for 2–3 weeks

THE DUKE CRITERIA FOR DIAGNOSIS OF INFECTIVE ENDOCARDITIS

Criteria	Major	1. Blood culture Positive blood cultures (≥2/2) with typical infective endocarditis micro-organisms (viridans streptococci, *Streptococcus bovis*, HACEK group, or community-acquired *Staphylococcus aureus* or enterococci in the absence of a primary focus). Persistently positive blood cultures (>12h or ≥3/3) with organisms compatible with infective endocarditis 2. Endocardial involvement Indicated by a new regurgitation murmur or a positive echocardiogram for infective endocarditis (oscillating mass, abscess, new dehiscence of prosthetic valve)
	Minor	1. Predisposing cardiac condition or intravenous drug use 2. Fever 3. Vascular phenomena: emboli, mycotic aneurysms, petechiae 4. Immunologic phenomena: glomerulonephritis, Osler nodes, Roth spots, rheumatoid factor 5. Echocardiogram consistent with infective endocarditis but not meeting major criteria 6. Positive blood cultures but not meeting major criteria; serologic evidence of active infection with plausible micro-organisms
Diagnosis	Definite	Pathology or bacteriology of vegetations, or 2 major criteria, or 1 major and 3 minor criteria, or 5 minor criteria
	Possible	Neither 'definite' nor 'rejected'
	Rejected	Firm alternative diagnosis, or Resolution on ≤4 days of antibiotics

Fig. 50.12 The Duke criteria for diagnosis of infective endocarditis. HACEK group includes *Haemophilus* spp., *Actinobacillus actinomycetemcomitans*, *Cardiobacterium hominis*, *Eikenella corrodens* and *Kingella kingae*. Adapted from Durack, Lukes, Bright and the Duke Endocarditis Service.[2]

to allow sufficient time for fastidious organisms to grow.

If cultures remain negative, it is important to search for serologic evidence of active infection with organisms such as *Brucella* spp., *Chlamydia* spp., *Coxiella burnetii*, *Legionella* spp. and *Bartonella* spp.[27] in order to detect these rare causes of IE. Newer techniques, such as broad-range polymerase chain reaction, are being developed to improve diagnosis under these circumstances.[43]

OTHER TESTS

Although many laboratory findings may be abnormal, most of them are nonspecific. The erythrocyte sedimentation rate and the C-reactive protein are elevated in 90–100% of cases. Acute IE may be accompanied by high or low leukocyte counts with increased polymorphonuclear cells and immature forms, as well as other blood and chemistry abnormalities related to an active infection. In subacute IE, nonspecific laboratory findings accompanying chronic infection are common but not universal. These findings include mild anemia with low serum iron concentration and low iron-binding capacity and thrombocytosis; as well as leukocytosis, hypergammaglobulinemia and the presence of circulating immune complexes. Urinalysis often reveals proteinuria and microscopic hematuria. Although none of these tests can prove the diagnosis of IE, their return to normal values during treatment is an indirect marker of therapeutic success.

MANAGEMENT

Successful treatment of IE relies primarily on antibiotic therapy. Combined medical and surgical treatment is needed in up to one-third of cases. Both experimental and clinical studies have indicated the importance of using bactericidal drugs in order to cure IE. For instance, 2 weeks penicillin treatment for streptococcal IE was insufficient to prevent relapses, whereas 2 weeks of the synergistic combination of penicillin plus an aminoglycoside successfully cured patients. Combination of bactericidal drugs is even more important against enterococcal IE, where the association of beta-lactams and aminoglycosides is mandatory to ensure treatment success.

Therapeutic schemes recommended for the most common pathogens are presented in Figures 50.13 and 50.14. High concentrations of antibiotic in the serum are desirable to ensure penetration into vegetations. Moreover, prolonged treatment is mandatory to kill dormant bacteria clustered in the infected foci (see Fig. 50.4). Therefore, prolonged parenteral therapy is recommended.

The choice of an optimal therapeutic regimen is based on antibiotic susceptibility testing. Minimal inhibitory concentrations of the principal drugs for the infecting pathogens should be determined. More sophisticated tests, such as MBC or serum inhibitory and bactericidal concentrations during drug therapy, are not usually needed, although they may be useful when the therapeutic response is inadequate. In such cases, it is important to exclude other causes of treatment failure, such as inadequate antibiotic administration, antibiotic resistance or the presence of a surgically removable focus.

Resistant pathogens may fail to respond to standard therapy. The three most problematic organisms in this respect are penicillin-resistant streptococci, methicillin-resistant staphylococci and multiple-drug-resistant enterococci.

PENICILLIN-RESISTANT STREPTOCOCCI

Streptococci are becoming increasingly resistant to penicillin and other beta-lactams, owing to a decreased affinity of their membrane-bound penicillin-binding proteins (PBP). Penicillin-resistant streptococci are classified as having either intermediate resistance (MIC of 0.1–1mg/l) or high resistance (MIC over 2mg/l).

Intermediately resistant streptococci may respond to standard therapy because the drug concentrations in the serum produced by intravenous beta-lactams are up to one or two orders of magnitude greater than the MIC for these bacteria (Fig. 50.13). For instance, peak serum levels of

SUGGESTED TREATMENT FOR NATIVE VALVE ENDOCARDITIS CAUSED BY STREPTOCOCCI, ENTEROCOCCI AND HACEK MICRO-ORGANISMS				
Antibiotic		Dosage and route	Duration (weeks)	Comments
Penicillin-susceptible viridans streptococci and *Streptococcus bovis*	Penicillin G	2–3 million U q4h iv	4	Preferred in patients older than 65 years or with impaired renal function
	Ceftriaxone	2g/day iv or im	4	
	Penicillin G with gentamicin	2–3 million U q4h iv 1mg/kg q8h iv or im	2 2	Studies suggest that gentamicin once daily might be adequate
	Ceftriaxone with netilmicin	2g/day iv or im 4mg/kg/day iv	2 2	
	Vancomycin	15mg/kg q12h iv	4	Recommended for beta-lactam allergic patients
Intermediate penicillin-resistant (MIC 0.1–1mg/l) viridans streptococci and *Streptococcus bovis*	Penicillin G with gentamicin	3 million U q4h iv 1mg/kg q8h iv or im	4 2	Studies suggest that gentamicin once daily might be adequate
	Vancomycin	15mg/kg q12h iv	4	Recommended against highly resistant strains
Enterococcus spp.	Penicillin G with gentamicin	3–5 million U q4h iv 1mg/kg q8h iv or im	4–6 4–6	6 weeks' therapy recommended for patients with symptoms for more than 3 months
	Ampicillin with gentamicin	2g q4h iv 1mg/kg q8h iv or im	4–6 4–6	Studies suggest that gentamicin once daily might be adequate
	Vancomycin with gentamicin	15 mg/kg q12h iv 1mg/kg q8h iv or im	4–6 4–6	Monitor drug serum levels and renal function
Micro-organisms of the HACEK group	Ceftriaxone	2g/day iv or im	4	
	Ampicillin with gentamicin	2g q4h iv 1mg/kg q8h iv or im	4 4	Studies suggest that gentamicin once daily might be adequate

Fig. 50.13 Suggested treatment for native valve endocarditis caused by streptococci, enterococci and HACEK micro-organisms. The regimens with ceftriaxone are preferred for outpatient treatment. Treatment of endocarditis caused by vancomycin-resistant enterococci requires a careful assessment of susceptibility to alternative antibiotics, including the new streptogramin combination quinupristin–dalfopristin. Adapted from Francioli *et al.*,[46] Wilson *et al.*,[47] and Francioli *et al.*[48]

penicillin G, amoxicillin or ceftriaxone are of the order of 100mg/l, compared with MICs of these drugs, which vary between 0.1 and 1mg/l. Nevertheless, a beta-lactam should preferably be combined with an aminoglycoside in such situations.

Against highly resistant streptococci, on the other hand, alternative drugs must be considered. These include vancomycin, to which streptococci are still largely susceptible. In the future, newer quinolones with activity against Gram-positive bacteria or injectable streptogramins, such as the quinupristin–dalfopristin combination, may prove useful.

Antibiotic	Dosage and route		Duration	Comments
SUGGESTED TREATMENT FOR NATIVE VALVE AND PROSTHETIC VALVE INFECTIVE ENDOCARDITIS CAUSED BY STAPHYLOCOCCI				
Native valves				
Methicillin-susceptible staphylococci	Flucloxacillin, or oxacillin, or nafcillin with gentamicin (optional)	2g q4h iv 1mg/kg q8h iv or im	4–6 weeks 3–5 days	The benefit of adding gentamicin has not been demonstrated
	Cefazolin (or other first-generation cefalosporins) with gentamicin (optional)	2g q8h iv 1mg/kg q8h iv or im	4–6 weeks 3–5 days	Alternative for patients allergic to penicillins (not in case of immediate-type penicillin hypersensitivity)
	Vancomycin	15mg/kg q12h iv	4–6 weeks	Recommended for beta-lactam allergic patients
Methicillin-resistant staphylococci	Vancomycin	15mg/kg q12h iv	4–6 weeks	Recommended for beta-lactam allergic patients
Prosthetic valves				
Methicillin-susceptible staphylococci	Flucloxacillin, or oxacillin, or nafcillin with rifampin and gentamicin	2g q4h iv 300mg q8h po 1mg/kg q8h iv or im	≥6 weeks ≥6 weeks 2 weeks	Rifampin increases the hepatic metabolism of numerous of drugs, including warfarin
	Vancomycin with rifampin and gentamicin	15mg/kg q12h iv 300mg q8h po 1mg/kg q8h iv or im	≥6 weeks ≥6 weeks 2 weeks	Recommended for beta-lactam allergic patients
Methicillin-resistant staphylococci	Vancomycin with rifampin and gentamicin	15mg/kg q12h iv 300mg q8h po 1mg/kg q8h iv or im	≥6 weeks ≥6 weeks 2 weeks	

Fig. 50.14 Suggested treatment for native valve and prosthetic valve infective endocarditis caused by staphylococci. Note that rifampin (rifampicin) plays a special role in prosthetic device infection, because it helps kill bacteria attached to foreign material. Rifampin should never be used alone, because it selects for resistance at a high frequency (about 10^{-6}). Adapted from Wilson *et al*.[47]

METHICILLIN-RESISTANT STAPHYLOCOCCI

Staphylococci resistant to methicillin carry a new, low-affinity PBP called PBP 2A. This protein allows cell wall assembly when normal PBPs are blocked by beta-lactams. Penicillin-binding protein 2A confers cross-resistance to most beta-lactam drugs. In addition, methicillin-resistant staphylococci are usually resistant to most other drugs, leaving only vancomycin to treat severe infections.

Vancomycin resistance has emerged among many strains of enterococci, and can be transferred experimentally to *S. aureus* via a transposable genetic element. Moreover, both *S. aureus* and coagulase-negative staphylococci with intermediate resistance to vancomycin have recently emerged in Japan and in the USA. The mechanism of resistance in these bacteria is different from that in enterococci, being mediated by chromosomal mutations affecting the synthesis of the cell wall.[44]

Treatment of infections caused by vancomycin-resistant staphylococci will require new drugs. At the present time, few alternatives are available besides older beta-lactams with relatively good affinity to PBP 2A and the new injectable streptogramin, quinupristin–dalfopristin.

MULTIPLE-DRUG-RESISTANT ENTEROCOCCI

These organisms are of major concern because they have become resistant to most available drugs, including vancomycin. Today, treatment of such organisms often relies on the combination of multiple drugs and the use of experimental antibiotics. Treatment of such infections requires precise determination of antibiotic susceptibilities, testing for bactericidal activity and sometimes determination of serum inhibitory and bactericidal titers, and monitoring drug levels in the serum. Importantly, although aminoglycoside resistance is usually present, these antibiotics may still be synergistic with cell-wall inhibitors provided that the MIC for the aminoglycosides is 1000mg/l or less. Depending on the mechanism of resistance, streptomycin is worth testing because it may be active against enterococci that are resistant to other aminoglycosides.

SURGERY

The leading indications for surgery are:
- refractory cardiac failure caused by valvular insufficiency;
- persistent sepsis caused by a surgically removable focus or a valvular ring or myocardial abscess; and
- persistent life-threatening embolization.

The decision when to operate on an unstable patient is difficult and requires a multidisciplinary assessment of the situation.

ENDARTERITIS AND MYCOTIC ANEURYSMS

Endarteritis is the inflammation of the arterial wall. The term mycotic aneurysm was coined by Osler[1] to define a nonsyphilitic aneurysm resulting from infective endarteritis. Arterial infection may result from:
- microembolization of bacteria in the vasa vasorum,
- hematogenous seeding of the arterial intima or of thrombi lining atherosclerotic plaques during bacteremia,
- extension from contiguous infected foci, or
- arterial trauma with direct bacterial contamination.

The first two mechanisms are most important during IE. Other risk factors include pre-existing endarterial lesions (e.g. congenital malformations such as patent ductus arteriosus and aortic coarctation, atherosclerosis of large vessels, vascular prosthesis and sometimes depressed host immunity due to diabetes, cirrhosis or corticosteroid therapy). Infected aneurysms represent 2.6% of all aneurysms, with a male-to-female ratio of about 3:1.[45]

MICROBIAL PATHOGENS AND CLINICAL MANIFESTATIONS

In the context of IE, the pathogens of endarteritis follow the pattern shown in Figure 50.1. In the absence of IE, on the other hand, Gram-negative bacteria are found more frequently. *Salmonella* spp., *E. coli* and other enterobacteria are isolated in more than 50% of cases of abdominal aortitis.[45] *Salmonella choleraesuis* and *Salmonella typhimurium* seem to have a particular tropism for atherosclerotic arteries. It was proposed that all patients over 50 years of age who develop *Salmonella* bacteremia should undergo abdominal imaging to detect possible aortic lesions. *Staphylococcus aureus* is the organism most often associated with extra-abdominal lesions and infections of vascular prosthesis, and it has been reported in about 30% of endarteritis overall. Other pathogens, including fungi, are occasionally reported.

Signs and symptoms depend on the anatomic site of the disease. Local signs include pain, erythema, manifestations due to compression of contiguous organs, and distal ischemia or embolization. Fever and leukocytosis are almost always present.

DIAGNOSIS AND MANAGEMENT

Diagnosis requires a high degree of clinical suspicion. Microbiologic documentation is essential. Blood cultures and cultures of surgical specimens should be performed, if possible before starting antibiotic treatment. Otherwise, special culture media should be used by the laboratory to inactivate antimicrobial drugs present within the samples. Ultrasonography, CT, MRI and gallium- or indium-labeled leukocyte scans are helpful to delineate the lesions. None of these techniques will distinguish between sterile and infected fluids; however, they may guide more invasive diagnostic procedures such as percutaneous needle aspiration of the affected area.

Appropriate antibiotic therapy and surgical resection of the infected vessel with extensive local debridement is mandatory. The material should be carefully examined by both the pathologist and the microbiologist. Whenever possible, autologous vascular graft and bypass in uninfected tissue should be performed in order to decrease the risk of re-infection. Antibiotics should be given for at least 4–6 weeks. Certain situations are so complicated that therapeutic strategies must be adapted for each particular case. Sometimes, patients are kept on antibiotics for much longer periods of time, even for life. Despite antibiotic treatment, the morbidity of vascular infections remains high. Infections of lower extremities arteries result in amputation in as many as 20% of cases.[49] Moreover, the mortality rate of patients with infected aneurysms that are diagnosed late may exceed 70%.[50]

REFERENCES

1. Osler W. The Gulstonian lectures on malignant endocarditis. Br Med J 1885;1:467–70.
2. Durack DT, Lukes AS, Bright DK et al. New criteria for diagnosis of infective endocarditis: utilization of specific echocardiographic findings. Duke endocarditis service. Am J Med 1994;96:200–9.
3. Berlin JA, Abrutyn E, Strom BL, et al. Incidence of infective endocarditis in the Delaware valley, 1988–1990. Am J Cardiol 1995;76:933–6.
4. Hogevic H, Olaison L, Andersson R, et al. Epidemiologic aspects of infective endocarditis in an urban population. Medicine 1995;74:324–39.
5. Benn M, Hagelskjaer LH, Tvede M. Infective endocarditis, 1984 through 1993: a clinical and microbiological survey. J Intern Med 1997;242:15–22.
6. von Reyn CF, Levy BS, Arbeit RD, et al. Infective endocarditis: an analysis based on strict case definitions. Ann Intern Med 1981;94:505–18.
7. Johnson DH, Rosenthal A, Nadas AS. A forty-year review of bacterial endocarditis in infancy and childhood. Circulation 1975;51:581–8.
8. Normand J, Bozio A, Etienne J, et al. Changing patterns and prognosis of infective endocarditis in childhood. Eur Heart J 1995;16(Suppl B):28–31.
9. Rose AG. Infective endocarditis complicating congenital heart disease. South Afr Med J 1978;53:739–43.
10. Deuchar D, Lopez Bescos L, Chakorn S. Fallot's tetralogy: a 20 year surgical follow-up. Br Heart J 1972;34:12–22.
11. Mason T, Fisher M, Kujala G. Acute rheumatic fever in West Virginia. Arch Intern Med 1991;151:133–6.
12. Zuppiroli A, Rinaldi M, Kramer-Fox R, et al. Natural history of mitral valve prolapse. Am J Cardiol 1995;75:1028–32.
13. Cheng TO. Mitral valve prolapse: an overview. J Cardiol 1989;19(Suppl XXI):3–21.
14. Kim S, Kuroda T, Nishinaga M, et al. Relation between severity of mitral regurgitation and prognosis of mitral valve prolapse: Echographic follow-up study. Am Heart J 1996;132:348–55.
15. McKinsey DS, Ratts TE, Bisno AL. Underlying cardiac lesions in adults with infective endocarditis. Am J Med 1987;82:681–8.
16. Douglas JL, Cobbs CG. Prosthetic valve endocarditis. In Kaye D, ed. Infective endocarditis. New York: Raven Press; 1992:375–96.
17. Ivert TS, Dismukes WE, Cobbs CG, et al. Prosthetic valve endocarditis. Circulation 1983;69:223–32.
18. Levine DP, Crane RL, Zervos MJ. Bacteremia in narcotic addicts at the Detroit Medical Center. II. Infectious endocarditis: a prospective comparative study. Rev Infect Dis 1986;8:374–96.
19. Steckelberg JM, Melton LJ, Ilstrup DM, et al. Influence of referral bias on the apparent clinical spectrum of infective endocarditis. Am J Med 1990;88:582–8.
20. Pulvirenti JJ, Kerns E, Benson C, et al. Infective endocarditis in injection drug users: importance of human immunodeficiency virus serostatus and degree of immunosuppression. Clin Infect Dis 1996;22:40–5.
21. Terpenning MS, Buggy BP, Kaufman CA. Hospital-acquired infective endocarditis. Arch Intern Med 1988;148:1601–3.
22. Gould K, Ramirez-Ronda CH, Homes RK, et al. Adherence of bacteria to heart valves in vitro. J Clin Invest 1975;56:1364–70.
23. Maass M, Bartels C, Engel PM, et al. Endovascular presence of viable Chlamydia pneumoniae is a common phenomenon in coronary artery disease. J Am Coll Cardiol 1998;31:827–32.
24. Baddour LM. Virulence factors among gram-positive bacteria in experimental endocarditis. Infect Immun 1994;62:2143–8.
25. Crawford J, Russell C. Comparative adhesion of seven species of streptococci isolated from the blood of patients with sub-acute bacterial endocarditis to fibrin-platelet clots in vitro. J Appl Bacteriol 1986;60:127–33.
26. Moreillon P, Entenza JM, Francioli P, et al. Role of Staphylococcus aureus coagulase and clumping factor in pathogenesis of experimental endocarditis. Infect Immun 1995;63:4738–43.
27. Raoult D, Fournier PE, Drancourt M, et al. Diagnosis of 22 new cases of Bartonella endocarditis. Ann Intern Med 1996;125:646–52.
28. Beekhuizen H, van de Gevel JS, Olsson B, et al. Infection of human vascular endothelial cells with Staphylococcus aureus induces hyperadhesiveness for human monocytes and granulocytes. J Immunol 1997;158:774–82.
29. Glauser MP, Bernard JP, Moreillon P, et al. Successful single dose amoxicillin prophylaxis against experimental endocarditis: evidence for two mechanisms of protection. J Infect Dis 1983;147:568–75.
30. Hall G, Hedstrom SA, Heimdahl A, et al. Prophylactic administration of penicillins for endocarditis does not reduce the incidence of postextraction bacteremia. Clin Infect Dis 1993;17:188–94.
31. Malinverni R, Overholser CD, Bille J, et al. Antibiotic prophylaxis of experimental endocarditis after dental extraction. Circulation 1988;77:182–7.
32. Moreillon P, Overholser CD, Malinverni R, et al. Predictors of endocarditis in isolates from cultures of blood following dental extractions in rats with periodontal disease. J Infect Dis 1988;157:990–5.
33. Van der Meer JT, Van Wijk W, Thompson J, et al. Efficacy of antibiotic prophylaxis for prevention of native-valve endocarditis. Lancet 1992;339:135–9.
34. Yersin B, Glauser MP, Guze PA, et al. Experimental Escherichia coli endocarditis in rats: role of serum bactericidal activity and duration of catheter placement. Infect Immun 1988;56:1273–80.
35. Dankert J, Van den Werff J, Zaat SAJ, et al. Involvement of bactericidal factors from thrombin-stimulated platelets in clearance of adherent viridans streptococci in experimental infective endocarditis. Infect Immun 1995;63:663–71.
36. Durack DT, Gilliland BC, Petersdorf RG. Effect of immunization on susceptibility to experimental Streptococcus mutans and Streptococcus sanguis endocarditis. Infect Immun 1978;22:52–6.
37. Vignes S, Fantin B, Elbim C, et al. Critical influence of timing of administration of granulocyte-stimulating factor on antibacterial effect in experimental endocarditis due to Pseudomonas aeruginosa. Antimicrob Agents Chemother 1995;39:2702–7.
38. Leport C, Horstkotte D, Burckhardt D, et al. Antibiotic prophylaxis for infective endocarditis from an international group of experts towards a European consensus. Eur Heart J 1995;16(Suppl B):126–31.
39. Dajani AS, Taubert KA, Wilson W, et al. Prevention of bacterial endocarditis, recommendations by the american heart association. JAMA 1997;277:1794–801.
40. Fluckiger U, Francioli P, Blaser J, et al. Role of amoxicillin serum levels for successful prophylaxis of experimental endocarditis due to tolerant streptococci. J Infect Dis 1994;169:1397–400.
41. Hecht SR, Berger M. Right-sided endocarditis in intravenous drug users. Ann Intern Med 1992;117:560–6.
42. Salgado AV, Furlan AJ, Keys TF, et al. Neurologic complications of endocarditis: a 12-year experience. Neurology 1989;39:173–8.
43. Goldenberger D, Kunzli A, Vogt P, et al. Molecular diagnosis of bacterial endocarditis by broad-range PCR amplification and direct sequencing. J Clin Microbiol 1997;35:2733–9.
44. Hiramatsu K, Aritaka N, Hanaki H, et al. Dissemination in Japanese hospitals of strains of Staphylococcus aureus heterogeneously resistant to vancomycin. Lancet 1997;350:1670–3.
45. Kearny RA, Eisen HJ, Wolf JE. Nonvalvular infection of the cardiovascular system. Ann Intern Med 1994;121:219–30.
46. Francioli P, Etienne J, Hoigne R, et al. Treatment of streptococcal endocarditis with a single daily dose of ceftriaxone sodium for 4 weeks. Efficacy and outpatient treatment feasability. JAMA 1992;267:264–7.
47. Wilson WR, Karchmer AW, Dajani AS, et al. Antibiotic treatment of adults with infective endocarditis due to streptococci, enterococci, staphylococci, and HACEK microorganisms. JAMA 1995;274:1706–13.
48. Francioli P, Ruch W, Stamboulian D, et al. Treatment of streptococcal endocarditis with a single daily dose of ceftriaxone and netilmicin for 14 days: a prospective multicenter study. Clin Infect Dis 1995;21:1406–10.
49. Johnson JR, Ledgerwood AM, Lucas CE. Mycotic aneurysm. New concepts in therapy. Arch Surg 1983;118:577–82.
50. Ben-Haim S, Seabold JE, Hawes DR, et al. Leukocyte scintigraphy in the diagnosis of mycotic aneurysm. J Nucl Med 1992;33:1486–93.

Practice Points

Role of white cell scans for deep-seated sepsis

Verka Beric

INTRODUCTION

White blood cell scans are performed in the nuclear medicine department and are used to locate areas of pyogenic infection or acute inflammation.

The neutrophil is the active component of the radiolabeled leukocyte preparation used during the scan. Lymphocytes play no part in the investigation as they are damaged by radioactive labeling; similarly, monocytes fail to respond to the labeling technique. In pyogenic infections, neutrophils are mobilized from their resting positions, along the margins of blood vessels, in order to migrate specifically to inflamed tissues. This migratory activity is most vigorous during the acute illness and it is this phenomenon that is exploited by the white cell scan. White cell scans have, however, a limited role in the investigation of chronic sepsis and inflammation, in which neutrophil migratory activity is reduced. Unless secondary pyogenic infection exists, a negative result is seen in viral, mycobacterial, fungal and parasitic infections because of the relative lack of neutrophil activity.

TECHNIQUE

Mixed leukocytes from the patient and labeled *in vitro* with a chelated radioactive gamma-emitting isotope. ^{111}Indium-oxine (^{111}In-oxine) remains the gold standard radiopharmaceutical used for labeling purposes but ^{99m}technetium-hexamethylpropylene amine oxime (^{99m}Tc-HMPAO) is now preferred in certain clinical situations. The labeled leukocytes are then injected intravenously. The sites within the body to which the radioactive neutrophils migrate are detected by imaging the distribution of the isotope with a gamma camera. Sites of focal infection and acute inflammation appear as areas of abnormally increased isotope uptake.

The normal physiologic distribution of ^{111}In-oxine immediately after injection is the blood pool, lungs, liver and spleen, with activity decreasing over time. ^{99m}Tc-HMPAO has a similar distribution but has the disadvantage of additional renal and intestinal clearance. Renal, bladder, gallbladder and bowel activity may be seen within the first hour and are usually seen by 4 hours.

Despite the above limitation, ^{99m}Tc-HMPAO is less costly, more readily available, imparts a lower radioactive dose to the patient and yet provides images of superior quality than ^{111}In-oxine. The relatively short half-life of ^{99m}Tc-HMPAO means that sensitivity is near maximal at 60 minutes. Indeed, the study may be completed by 2–4 hours, thereby allowing abdominal imaging to be performed before signs of bowel clearance occur. By virtue of its longer half-life, ^{111}In-oxine usually requires a 24-hour image for maximal sensitivity, which in turn becomes advantageous in situations in which the rate of neutrophil migration and turnover is reduced. With both agents, in order to limit errors in interpretation, serial images are acquired at approximately 1 hour, 3 hours and 24 hours. Despite such precautions, false-positive and false-negative results may be found in certain clinical conditions (Fig. 51.1).

The decision to use the white cell scan and the choice between using ^{99m}Tc and ^{111}In for a particular clinical situation are both confusing and controversial issues. Suggested guidelines based upon current use and literature are outlined below.

Abdominal sepsis

The white cell scan is the next investigation of choice for the patient who has suspected abdominal or pelvic sepsis after an inconclusive ultrasound or CT scan.

Despite the normal physiologic uptake of ^{99m}Tc-HMPAO in the bowel, it is the preferred agent for imaging the abdomen in most situations, particularly when rapid diagnosis is required. Indeed, the main clinical role of ^{99m}Tc-HMPAO in some centers is to detect acute relapses of inflammatory bowel diseases such as ulcerative colitis and Crohn's disease.

For the diagnosis of abdominal abscesses that communicate with bowel (typically seen in diverticular disease, Crohn's disease and as a result of pancreatitis), ^{111}In-oxine is preferred for its lack of physiologic bowel excretion. Early images demonstrate focal abscess activity that declines with time as the abscess decompresses and discharges into the bowel. As a result, the isotope is first detected within the bowel lumen on the 24-hour image.

^{111}In-oxine is also preferred for the diagnosis of abscesses close to the liver and spleen, where they may be obscured by the intense physiologic uptake of these organs on early images. The abscess is identified by its increase in activity with sequential images over 24 hours, whereas the activity in the liver and spleen either reduces or remains constant during this period.

FALSE-NEGATIVE AND FALSE-POSITIVE WHITE CELL SCAN RESULTS

False-negative results

Chronic low-grade infection
Parasitic, fungal, mycobacterial and viral infections
Encapsulated nonpyogenic abscess
Acute vertebral osteomyelitis
Intrahepatic or intrasplenic abscess
Abnormal neutrophil function caused by chemotherapy or corticosteroid use
Appropriate antibiotic use

False-positive results

Drug-induced pneumonitis
Graft-versus-host disease
Inflammatory bowel disease
Hematoma and gastrointestinal hemorrhage
Pseudoaneurysm
Swallowed labeled leukocytes from oropharynx, esophagus or lungs
Surgical wounds, enterostomy or catheter sites

Fig. 51.1 False-negative and false-positive white cell scan results.

Thoracic sepsis

The white cell scan has no place in the routine investigation of pulmonary sepsis. It is usually negative for lobar pneumonia. Rarely, the white cell scan is used to determine the degree of inflammatory activity present in cavities thought to represent pulmonary abscesses or in a region of lung known to be bronchiectatic.

White cell scans are almost always negative for bacterial endocarditis and valvular vegetations. The investigation is only justified in these cases when pyrexia develops with associated positive blood cultures, thereby raising suspicion of septic emboli or metastatic abscesses.

Musculoskeletal and soft tissue infection

Acute osteomyelitis has traditionally been diagnosed with the combination of a ^{99m}Tc-methylene diphosphonate (^{99m}Tc-MDP) bone scan and plain radiography. The ^{111}In-oxine white cell scan is preferred for suspected acute relapses of chronic osteomyelitis or suspected prosthetic joint infection where plain radiography and the bone scan may appear abnormal, even in the absence of acute infection. In this situation, a map of the normal physiologic marrow uptake of neutrophils must be obtained in order to differentiate the areas of abnormal inflammatory uptake seen with the white cell scan. Normal marrow uptake is depicted by the 1-hour ^{111}In-oxine image or by a separate ^{99m}Tc-colloid scan.

Similarly, the combination of a ^{99m}Tc-MDP bone scan with a ^{111}In-oxine white cell scan may be used to determine whether soft tissue infection, such as a diabetic foot ulcer, has extended to involve the underlying bone. The scans are acquired simultaneously and super-imposed to determine the precise anatomic relationship between focal neutrophil activity and the 'bone map' provided by the bone scan. Neutrophil activity overlying the bone scan image is taken to represent osteomyelitis. The combination of scans is required because the bone scan alone may be abnormal in the absence of osteomyelitis, owing to the effects of local hyperemia from the soft tissue infection.

Prosthetic vascular graft infection is associated with high morbidity and mortality rates if delay in diagnosis occurs. A high index of suspicion is required because the only indication may be a low-grade fever, although aortofemoral or iliofemoral graft infections may additionally present with groin pain or local soft tissue infection. White cell scans are particularly useful for demonstrating the extent of infection along the graft and for imaging abdominal grafts. ^{111}In-oxine is the preferred agent for detecting chronic graft infections.

Undiagnosed fever

In this situation, the white cell scan is used simply to locate the pathology causing the fever so that a diagnosis may be made with more conventional means. Determining the characteristics of the undiagnosed fever and using the white cell scan only if appropriate may optimize the yield of positive results.

A true 'fever of unknown origin' is defined as a fever of at least 3 weeks' duration where at least 1 week of in-hospital investigation has failed to reach a diagnosis. Most causes of fever of unknown origin are due to nonpyogenic infection, malignancy or connective tissue disease. Pyogenic infection is seen in only 10–20% of cases.

Any infection associated with an occult fever is likely to be subacute or chronic with reduced neutrophil migration and, therefore, the ^{111}In-oxine white cell scan is preferred for its superior 24-hour images.

Neutropenic patients and HIV-positive patients may have fever and infection without localizing signs. Because the low neutrophil count will produce a suboptimal result with the white cell scan, fresh cross-matched donor leukocytes may be used instead and are often preferred in HIV-positive patients in order to avoid risk of contamination to staff handling the blood.

DISCUSSION

The role of the white cell scan in deep-seated sepsis may be solely to localize or to confirm the presence of a pyogenic infection. A specific diagnosis is often regarded as a bonus. It is important to realize that this investigation may not be the most appropriate in chronic and non-pyogenic infections such as fever of unknown origin, sarcoidosis, tuberculosis and *Pneumocystis carinii* pneumonia. In these situations, more general inflammatory markers, such as ^{67}Gallium and the newer agents, ^{99m}Tc- or ^{111}In-labeled human polyclonal immunoglobulin may be more suitable. Further, other imaging modalities may be more appropriate in certain clinical situations for example, MRI scanning in musculoskeletal infections. Advice from an imaging specialist should be sought in all but the most straightforward cases.

FURTHER READING

Peters AM. Development of radiolabelled white cell scanning. Scand J Gastroenterol 1994;(Suppl)203:28–31.

Peters AM. The utility of Tc-99m-HMPOA labeled leukocytes for imaging infection. Semin Nucl Med 1994;24:110–27.

Spinelli F, Milella M, Sara R, et al. The 99mTc-HMPOA leukocyte scan: an alternative to radiology and endoscopy in evaluating the extent and the activity of inflammatory bowel disease. J Nucl Biol Med 1991;35:82–7.

Lipman BT, Collier BD, Carrera GF, et al. Detection of osteomyelitis in the neuropathic foot: nuclear medicine, MRI and conventional radiography. Clin Nucl Med 1998;23:77–82.

Peters AM. The use of nuclear medicine in treating infections. Br J Radiol 1998;71:252–61.

Peters AM. The choice of an appropriate agent for imaging inflammation (editorial). Nucl Med Commun 1996;17:455–8.

Becker W. The contribution of nuclear medicine to the patient with infection. Eur J Nucl Med 1995;22:1195–211.

Should infected intravascular lines be removed?

John S Cheesbrough &
Amanda J Barnes

INTRODUCTION

Long-term intravascular access is a critical component of many current medical treatments, including total parenteral nutrition (TPN), hemodialysis and chemotherapy for malignant disease. Infection and blockage are the main causes of premature line removal. The risk of infection is related to the type of line and the demands placed upon it. Dedicated lines for TPN have a low rate of infection at around 0.05 per 100 catheter days, whereas rates for multipurpose lines used in patients who have malignant disease range from 0.4 per 100 catheter days for Hickman and Broviac cuffed lines to 0.1 per 100 catheter days for totally implantable devices (see Chapter 2.48).

PATHOGENESIS

Micro-organisms gain access to the catheter by three principal routes:
- by ingress from the exit site and tracking around the exterior of the catheter into the subcutaneous tissues,
- via the lumen of the catheter from manipulation of the hub or contamination of infusate, and
- by hematogeneous seeding from a distant focus of infection.

Although the relative importance of each route remains controversial, in the case of tunneled and totally implantable devices, intraluminal contamination is generally accepted as the major route of infection.

MICROBIOLOGY

Gram-positive organisms, notably coagulase-negative staphylococci, *Staphylococcus aureus*, streptococci and diphtheroids, are the most common cause of infection; staphylococci account for two-thirds of episodes of bacteremia. Among the Gram-negative organisms, *Klebsiella* spp., *Enterobacter* spp. and *Serratia* spp. are common and their presence suggests contamination of infusate. Yeasts are relatively more common among patients on TPN. Virtually any organism listed in a textbook of medical microbiology can cause infection of an intravascular catheter.

CLINICAL FEATURES

Clinical features vary depending on the site of infection, the virulence of the organism and the immunocompetence of the host. Intraluminal infection with coagulase-negative staphylococci, the most common situation, is characterized by low-grade fever without hypotension, although rigors may occur, most often after line manipulation. Exit-site infection with coagulase-negative staphylocci are usually indolent with local erythema and mild tenderness at the exit site. In contrast, *S. aureus* infections are often associated with frank sepsis and more rapidly extending cellulitis involving the subcutaneous catheter tunnel. Metastatic foci of infection are most common with *S. aureus* and yeasts, and are occasionally the presenting feature: endophthalmitis secondary to *Candida* spp. and endocarditis following *S. aureus* infection are well recognized.

INVESTIGATION

Cultures of blood taken via the line and from a peripheral vein and a swab from the exit site are essential. Because the most common causes of line-related infection are members of the normal skin flora and are frequently encountered as blood culture contaminants, it is essential to exercise care in ascribing clinical relevance to coagulase-negative staphylococci or diphtheroids isolated from patients who have lines. Similarly, swab culture results must be interpreted in the context of the clinical appearance of the exit site: a heavy growth of any organism should be regarded as indicative of local infection only when definite inflammation is present.

In the case of multilumen catheters, a set of cultures should ideally be drawn from each lumen to ensure complete sampling. Positive cultures from a single bottle or set with coagulase-negative staphylocci or diphtheroids that are not accompanied by a similar organism in peripheral blood should be regarded as being of doubtful significance. Growth from further sets of blood cultures will usually clarify the situation.

A reasonable approach in a stable patient who has a single bottle growing coagulase-negative staphylococci or diphtheroids is to repeat blood cultures both centrally and peripherally, and to withhold any treatment pending results.

Comparison of quantitative blood cultures from the catheter lumen and peripheral blood can be helpful: an eight-fold higher colony count in catheter-derived blood confirms bacteremia of line origin. However, quantitative cultures are technically demanding and few laboratories routinely offer this service. Alternatively a substantially shorter (at least 2 hours) 'time to signal' in central-line blood compared with peripheral blood when blood cultures are processed by a continuous monitoring system (BacT/Alert or Bactec 9000) strongly supports the line being the origin of the bacteremia. This can provide useful data only if samples are collected within a few minutes of each other, labeled appropriately and placed in the machine without pre-incubation. An alternative approach to sampling catheter microbial flora is the intraluminal brush. This is a promising development and, although its role is yet to be fully established, it would appear to be both more sensitive (95%) and specific (84%) than the traditional catheter tip roll culture for the diagnosis of catheter-related sepsis. A rapid diagnosis can sometimes be gained by acridine orange staining of blood aspirated from the line.

MANAGEMENT

The traditional approach to the infected line is to remove it immediately and give appropriate antibiotics for patients who have clinical sepsis. This is an appropriate approach for patients who have short-term, easily resited lines, but for patients who have 'precious' lines that are critical to their further care, a trial of treatment with the line *in situ* is usually warranted. This certainly applies to lines with Dacron cuffs or totally implantable devices, the resiting of which requires a substantial invasive procedure, and to any line the resiting of which would pose technical problems. The factors to be considered are shown in Figure 51.2.

Circumstances in which a trial of treatment, assuming a suitable antimicrobial agent is available, is not appropriate are:
- severe sepsis, especially if it is due to *Streptococcus pyogenes*, in which any delay to optimal bacterial clearance may be life threatening;
- infection due to *Enterobacteria*, *Pseudomonas* sp. or *Candida* sp.; and
- extensive tunnel infection, in which success is very unlikely.

The most common problem, intraluminal infection with coagulase-negative staphylococci, responds in about 90% of cases, and success is also common with localized exit-site infections caused by these organisms. Although successful clearance of *S. aureus* has been obtained, the risk of metastatic sepsis demands careful observation and a low threshold for line withdrawal if response is not prompt and confirmed by clearance of bacteremia (Fig. 51.3). Antibiotic-absorbing blood culture bottles can be helpful in this circumstance. Infected lines with impaired flow caused by clot may respond to antibiotics accompanied by clot lysis with a urokinase lock.

FACTORS TO BE CONSIDERED WHEN TREATING AN INFECTED LINE *IN SITU*

Factor	Outcome		Increased risk of metastatic focus
	Success likely	Success unlikely	
Infecting organism	Coagulase-negative staphylococci Diphtheroids	Fungi *Streptococcus pyogenes* Multiresistant organism (e.g. glycopeptide-resistant *Enterococcus* spp.) *Stenotrophomonas maltophilia*	*Staphylococcus aureus* *Candida* spp.
Site of infection	Intralumenal Local exit site	Extensive tunnel infection Frank pus from exit site	
Line factors	Line functioning well	Impaired flow Unable to aspirate	
Host factors	Minimal evidence of systemic sepsis	Severe systemic sepsis	Abnormal or prosthetic heart valves

Fig. 51.2 Factors to be considered when treating an infected line *in situ*.

CHOICE OF ANTIBIOTIC

The choice of antibiotic depends on results of testing *in vitro*. Empiric treatment for line-related infection must cover the most serious causes, and failure to cover coagulase-negative staphylococci rarely has major adverse consequences. Inclusion of a glycopeptide is therefore not essential unless the patient is known or suspected to be colonized with methicillin-resistant *S. aureus*. Reasonable empiric treatment should cover virulent pathogens and depends on the underlying disease. Blood culture will usually confirm line-related infection, and treatment can then be modified accordingly.

When systemic infection has resolved or is not marked and metastatic infection is not suspected, intraluminal infection can be managed with a high success rate and a low risk of adverse drug reaction by using an antibiotic lock technique. The dead space of the catheter is filled with a concentrated solution of antibiotic that is left *in situ* for as long as possible, at least 8–12 hours/day. This approach exposes the infecting organisms to a very high level of antibiotic and has succeeded in some cases when conventional infusion via the line has failed (Fig. 51.4)

The duration of antimicrobial therapy depends on clinical response. Line-related bacteremia caused by coagulase-negative staphylococci will often settle with 5–7 days' treatment, whereas *S. aureus* bacteremia warrants a minimum of 10 days' treatment. Prolonged treatment lasting 4–6 weeks is required in patients who have *S. aureus* bacteremia, and risk factors for endocarditis and candidemia is another indication for prolonged (4–6 weeks) therapy.

PRACTICE POINTS

- Most line infections will respond to antibiotics without removal.
- Antibiotics must be given via the infected line if intraluminal infection is suspected.
- Confirmation of diagnosis requires central and peripheral blood cultures. Distinguishing contaminants from genuine infection with coagulase-negative staphylococci can be difficult and may require numerous sets of blood cultures. In practice two positive sets will often warrant a trial of therapy.
- A low threshold for line removal is essential with *S. aureus*, yeasts and multiresistant organisms.
- Antibiotic lock techniques show promise and may be the treatment of choice for intraluminal infection with organisms other than *S. aureus*.

FURTHER READING

Elliott TSJ. Line-associated bacteraemias. Communicable Disease Report, CDR Review 1993;3:R91–5.
Jones GR, Konsler GK, Dunaway RP, Lacey SR, Azizkhan RG. Prospective analysis of urokinase in the treatment of catheter sepsis in pediatric hematology-oncology patients. J Pediatr Surg 1993;28:350–7.
Kite P, Dobbins BM, Wilcox MH, *et al.* Evaluation of a novel endoluminal brush method for *in situ* diagnosis of catheter related sepsis. J Clin Pathol 1997;50:278–82.
Messing B, Peitra-Cohen S, Debure A, Beliah M, Bernier JJ. Antibiotic-lock technique: A new approach to optimal therapy for catheter-related sepsis in home-parenteral nutrition patients. J Parenter Enter Nutr 1987;12:185–9.
Quilici N, Audibert G, Conroy MC, *et al.* Differential quantitative blood cultures in the diagnosis of catheter-related sepsis in intensive care units. Clin Infect Dis 1997;25:1066–70.

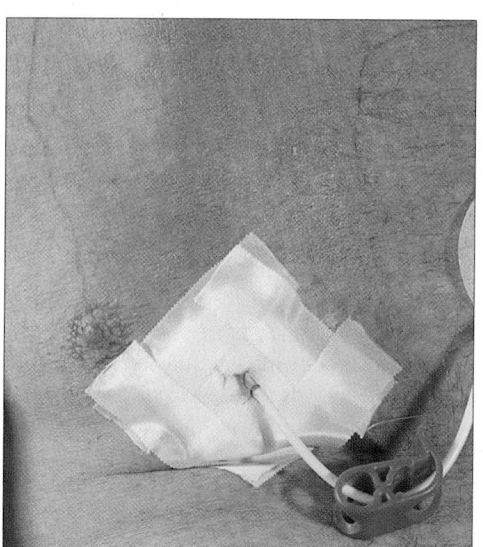

Fig. 51.3 Severe subcutaneous tunnel infection with *Staphylococcus aureus* in a patient who has a Hickman catheter. The extending cellulitis (maximum extent shown by black marker pen line) has responded but the local tunnel infection persists and mandates line removal.

ANTIOBIOTICS THAT HAVE BEEN REPORTED IN LINE LOCK TECHNIQUES	
Agent	Concentrations used (mg/ml)
Vancomycin	1–5
Amikacin	1.5–2
Amphotericin B	2–2.5 (minimum 14 days)
Ampicillin	2
Gentamicin	2–5
Minocycline	0.2
Mezlocillin	2
Teicoplanin	120

Fig. 51.4 Antibiotics that have been reported in line lock techniques. The minimum dwell time is 8–12 hours, and the usual duration of treatment is 1 week.

Vaginitis, Vulvitis and Cervicitis

Jack D Sobel

VAGINITIS

Vaginal symptoms are extremely common, and vaginal discharge is among the 25 most common reasons for consulting physicians in private office practice in the USA. Vaginitis is found in more than one quarter of women attending sexually transmitted disease (STD) clinics. Not all women with vaginal symptoms have vaginitis; approximately 40% of women with vaginal symptoms will have some type of vaginitis (Fig. 52.1).

EPIDEMIOLOGY

Bacterial vaginosis is the most common cause of vaginitis in women of child-bearing age. It has been diagnosed in 17–19% of women seeking gynecologic care in family practice or student health care settings.[1] The prevalence increases considerably in symptomatic women attending STD clinics, reaching 24–37%. Bacterial vaginosis has been observed in 16–29% of pregnant women. *Gardnerella vaginalis* has been found in 10–31% of virgin adolescent girls but is found significantly more frequently among sexually active women, reaching a prevalence of 50–60% in some at-risk populations.

Evaluation of epidemiologic factors has revealed few clues of the cause of bacterial vaginosis. Use of the intrauterine device and douching was found to be more common in women with bacterial vaginosis. Bacterial vaginosis is significantly more common among African-American and sexually active women including lesbians.

PATHOGENESIS AND PATHOLOGY

Bacterial vaginosis is the result of massive overgrowth of mixed flora, including peptostreptococci, *Bacteriodes* spp., *G. vaginalis*, *Mobiluncus* spp., and genital mycoplasma.[2] There is little inflammation, and the disorder represents a disturbance of the vaginal microbial ecosystem rather than a true infection of tissues. The overgrowth of mixed flora is associated with a loss of the normal *Lactobacillus* spp. dominated vaginal flora. No single bacterial species is responsible for bacterial vaginosis. Experimental studies in human volunteers and studies in animals indicate that inoculation of the vagina with individual species of bacteria associated with bacterial vaginosis (e.g. *G. vaginalis*), rarely results in bacterial vaginosis. In support of the role of sexual transmission is the higher prevalence of bacterial vaginosis among sexually active young women than among sexually inexperienced women, and the observation that bacterial vaginosis-associated micro-organisms are more frequently isolated from the urethras of male partners of females with bacterial vaginosis.[1]

The cause of the overgrowth of anaerobes, *Gardnerella*, *Mycoplasma*, and *Mobiluncus* spp. is unknown. Theories include increased substrate availability, increased pH and loss of the restraining effects of the predominant *Lactobacillus* spp. flora. It has been reported that normal women are colonized by hydrogen-peroxide-producing strains of lactobacilli, whereas women with bacterial vaginosis have reduced population numbers of lactobacilli, and the species present lack the

CAUSES OF VAGINITIS IN ADULT WOMEN	
Common infectious vaginitis	Bacterial vaginosis (40–50%)
	Vulvovaginal candidiasis (20–25%)
	Trichomonal vaginitis (15–20%)
Uncommon infectious vaginitis	Atrophic vaginitis with secondary bacterial infection
	Foreign body with secondary infection
	Desquamative inflammatory vaginitis (clindamycin responsive)
	Streptococcal vaginitis (group A)
	Ulcerative vaginitis associated with *Staphylococcus aureus* and toxic shock syndrome
	Idiopathic vulvovaginal ulceration associated with HIV
Noninfectious vaginitis	Chemical/irritant
	Allergic, hypersensitivity and contact dermatitis (lichen simplex)
	Traumatic
	Atrophic vaginitis
	Postpuerperal atrophic vaginitis
	Desquamative inflammatory vaginitis (corticosteroid responsive)
	Erosive lichen planus
	Collagen vascular disease, Behçet's syndrome, pemphigus syndromes
	Idiopathic

Fig. 52.1 Causes of vaginitis in adult women.

ability to produce hydrogen peroxide.[3] The hydrogen peroxide produced by lactobacilli may inhibit the pathogens associated with bacterial vaginosis, either directly by the toxicity of hydrogen peroxide, or as a result of the production of hydrogen-peroxide halide complex in the presence of natural cervical peroxidase.

Accompanying the bacterial overgrowth in bacterial vaginosis is the increased production of amines by anaerobes, facilitated by microbial decarboxylases. Volatile amines in the presence of increased vaginal pH produce the typical fishy odor, which is also produced when 10% potassium hydroxide is added to vaginal secretions. Trimethylamine is the dominant abnormal amine in bacterial vaginosis. It is likely that bacterial polyamines together with the organic acids found in the vagina in bacterial vaginosis (acetic and succinic acid) are cytotoxic, resulting in exfoliation of vaginal epithelial cells and creating the vaginal discharge. *Gardnerella vaginalis* attaches avidly to exfoliated epithelial cells, especially at the alkaline pH found in bacterial vaginosis. The adherence of *Gardnerella* organisms results in the formation of the pathognomonic clue cells.

PREVENTION

Because the pathogenesis of bacterial vaginosis is obscure, preventive measures have not been forthcoming. Although not typically sexually transmitted, barrier contraception may reduce occurrence and avoiding douching is recommended.

CLINICAL FEATURES

As many as 50% of women with bacterial vaginosis may be asymptomatic. An abnormal malodorous vaginal discharge, often described as fishy, that is infrequently profuse and often appears after unprotected coitus, is usually described. Pruritus, dysuria and dyspareunia are rare. Examination reveals a nonviscous, grayish-white adherent discharge.

Bacterial vaginosis has been considered to be largely of nuisance value only. There is now considerable evidence of serious obstetric and gynecologic complications of bacterial vaginosis, including asymptomatic bacterial vaginosis diagnosed by Gram stain. Obstetric complications include chorioamnionitis, pre-term labor, prematurity and postpartum fever.[4] Gynecologic sequelae are as follows: postabortion fever, posthysterectomy fever, cuff infection and chronic mast cell endometritis. A more recent association is reported between untreated bacterial vaginosis and cervical inflammation and low grade dysplasia.[5]

DIAGNOSIS

Signs and symptoms are unreliable in the diagnosis of bacterial vaginosis (Fig. 52.2). The clinical diagnosis can reliably be made in the presence of at least three of the following objective criteria:
- adherent, white, nonfloccular homogeneous discharge;
- positive amine test, with release of fishy odor on addition of 10% potassium hydroxide to vaginal secretions;
- vaginal pH >4.5; and
- presence of clue cells on light microscopy.

These features are simple and reliable, and tests for them are easy to perform. The presence of clue cells is the single most reliable predictor of bacterial vaginosis. Clue cells are exfoliated vaginal squamous epithelial cells covered with *G. vaginalis*, giving the cells a granular or stippled appearance with characteristic loss of clear cell borders. Of observed epithelial cells, diagnostic significance is indicated by 20% clue cells. Occasionally, clue cells covered exclusively by curved Gram-negative rods belonging to *Mobiluncus* spp. can be demonstrated. The offensive fishy odor may be apparent during the physical examination or may become apparent only during the amine test. Gram strain of vaginal secretions is extremely valuable in diagnosis, with a sensitivity of 93% and specificity of 70%.

Although cultures for *G. vaginalis* are positive in almost all cases of bacterial vaginosis, *G. vaginalis* may be detected in 50–60% of women who do not meet the diagnostic criteria for bacterial vaginosis. Accordingly, vaginal culture has no part in the diagnosis of bacterial vaginosis.

MANAGEMENT

Poor efficacy has been observed with triple sulfa creams, erythromycin, tetracycline, acetic acid gel and povidone–iodine vaginal douches.[6]

Only moderate cure rates have been obtained with ampicillin (mean 66%) and amoxicillin. The most successful oral therapy remains metronidazole. Most studies using multiple divided-dose regimens of 800–1200mg/day for 1 week achieved clinical cure rates in excess of 90% immediately, and of approximately 80% at 4 weeks. Although single-dose therapy with 2g metronidazole achieves comparable immediate clinical response rates, higher recurrence rates have been reported. The beneficial effect of metronidazole results predominantly from its anti-anaerobic activity and because *G. vaginalis* is susceptible to the hydroxymetabolites of metronidazole. Although *Mycoplasma hominis* is resistant to metronidazole, the organisms are usually not detected at follow-up visits of successfully treated patients. Similarly, *Mobiluncus curtisii* is resistant to metronidazole but usually disappears after therapy.

Topical therapy with 2% clindamycin once daily for 7 days or metronidazole gel 0.75% administered twice daily for 5 days have both been shown to be as effective as oral metronidazole, without any of the side effects of the latter.

DIAGNOSTIC FEATURES OF INFECTIOUS VAGINITIS					
		Normal	*Candida* vaginitis	Bacterial vaginosis	*Trichomonas* vaginitis
Symptoms		None or physiologic leukorrhea	Vulvar pruritus, soreness, increased discharge, dysuria, dyspareunia	Malodorous moderate discharge	Profuse purulent discharge, offensive odor, pruritus, and dyspareunia
Discharge	Amount	Variable, scant to moderate	Scant to moderate	Moderate	Profuse
	Color	Clear or white	White	White/gray	Yellow
	Consistency	Floccular nonhomogenous	Clumped but variable	Homogenous, uniformly coating walls	Homogenous
	'Bubbles'	Absent	Absent	Present	Present
	Appearance of vulva and vagina	Normal	Introital and vulvar erythema, edema and occasional pustules, vaginal erythema	No inflammation	Erythema and swelling of vulvar and vaginal epithelium (strawberry cervix)
	pH of vaginal fluid	<4.5	<4.5	>4.7	5.0–6.0
	Amine test (10% potassium hydroxide)	Negative	Negative	Positive	Occasionally present
	Saline microscopy	Normal epithelial cell Lactobacilli predominate	Normal flora, blastospores (yeast) 40–50% pseudohyphae	Clue cells, coccobacillary flora predominate, absence of leukocytes, motile curved rods	PMN's +++ Motile trichomonads (80–90%), no clue cells, abnormal flora
10% potassium hydroxide microscopy		Negative	Positive (60–90%)	Negative (except in mixed infections)	Negative

Fig. 52.2 Diagnostic features of infectious vaginitis.

In the past, asymptomatic bacterial vaginosis was not treated, especially because patients often improve spontaneously over several months. However, the growing evidence linking asymptomatic bacterial vaginosis with numerous obstetric and gynecologic upper tract complications has caused reassessment of this policy, especially with additional convenient topical therapies.[4,7] Asymptomatic bacterial vaginosis should be treated before pregnancy, in women with cervical abnormalities and before elective gynecologic surgery. Routine screening for and treatment of asymptomatic bacterial vaginosis in pregnancy remains controversial, pending the outcome of studies proving that therapy of bacterial vaginosis reduces pre-term delivery and prematurity.[8]

Despite indirect evidence of sexual transmission, no study has documented reduced recurrent rates of bacterial vaginosis in women whose partners have been treated with a variety of regimens, including metronidazole. Accordingly, most clinicians do not routinely treat male partners.

After therapy with oral metronidazole, approximately 30% of patients initially responding experience recurrence of symptoms within 3 months.[1] Reasons for recurrence are unclear, including the possibility of re-infection, but recurrence more likely reflects vaginal relapse, with failure to eradicate the offending organisms and re-establishes the normal protective *Lactobacillus* spp. dominant vaginal flora. Management of bacterial vaginosis relapse includes oral or vaginal metronidazole, or topical clindamycin, usually prescribed for 14 days. Maintenance antibiotics regimens have been disappointing and new approaches include exogenous *Lactobacillus* spp. recolonization using selected bacteria-containing suppositories.

TRICHOMONIASIS

EPIDEMIOLOGY

Studies estimate that 2–3 million American women contract trichomoniasis annually, with a worldwide distribution of approximately 180 million annual cases.[1] The prevalence of trichomoniasis correlates with the overall level of sexual activity of the specific group of women under study, being diagnosed in about 5% of women in family-planning clinics, in 13–25% of women attending gynecology clinics, in 50–75% of prostitutes, and in 7–35% of women in STD clinics. In many industrialized countries, recent surveys indicate a decline in the incidence of trichomoniasis.

PATHOGENESIS AND PATHOLOGY

Sexual transmission is the dominant method of introduction of *Trichomonas vaginalis* into the vagina.[1] Trichomonas vaginalis was identified in the urethra of 70% of men who had had sexual contact with infected women within the previous 48 hours. There is also a high prevalence of gonorrhea in women with trichomoniasis, and both of these are significantly associated with use of nonbarrier methods of contraception.

Recurrent trichomoniasis is common and is indicative of lack of significant protective immunity. Nevertheless, an immune response to *Trichomonas* spp. does develop, as indicated by low titers of serum antibody, but this is insufficient for diagnostic serology. Anti-trichomonal IgA has been detected in vaginal secretions, but a protective role is not defined.

Delayed hypersensitivity in natural infection can also be demonstrated. The predominant host defense response is provided by the numerous polymorphonuclear leukocytes (PMNs), which respond to chemotactic substances released by trichomonads and are capable of killing *T. vaginalis* without ingesting trichomonads. *Trichomonas vaginalis* destroys epithelial cells by direct cell contact and cytotoxicity. The urethra and Skeene's glands are infected in the majority of patients, and organisms are occasionally isolated from bladder urine.

PREVENTION

Sexual transmission of trichmonads is efficiently prevented by use of barrier contraception. Spermicidal agents such as nonoxynol-9 also reduce transmission. Re-infection of women is common, hence the mandatory requirement of treatment, preferably simultaneously, of all sexual partners with metronidazole.

CLINICAL FEATURES

Infection with *Trichomonas* spp. in women ranges from an asymptomatic carrier state to severe acute inflammatory disease.[9,10] Vaginal discharge is reported by 50–75% of women diagnosed with trichomoniasis; however, the discharge is not always described as malodorous. Pruritus occurs in 25–50% of patients and is often severe. Other infrequent symptoms include dyspareunia, dysuria and, rarely, frequency of micturition. Lower abdominal pain occurs in fewer than 10% of patients and should alert the physician to the possibility of concomitant salpingitis caused by other organisms. Symptoms of acute trichomoniasis often appear during or immediately after menstruation. Although controversial, the incubation period has been estimated to range from 3 to 28 days.

Physical findings represent a spectrum depending on the severity of disease. Vulvar findings may be absent, but are typically characterized in severe cases by diffuse vulvar erythema (10–33%), edema and a copious, profuse and malodorous vaginal discharge, which is often described as being yellow-green and frothy, but is frequently grayish-white.[10] Frothiness is seen in a minority of patients and is more commonly seen in bacterial vaginosis.

The vaginal walls are erythematous and in severe cases may be granular in appearance. Punctate hemorrhages (colpitis macularis) of the cervix may result in a strawberry-like appearance that, although apparent to the naked eye in only 1–2% of patients, is present in 45% of cases on colposcopy.[10]

The clinical course of trichomoniasis in pregnancy is identical to that seen in the nonpregnant state, and when untreated it is associated with premature rupture of membranes and prematurity. Trichomoniasis is reported to facilitate HIV transmission.

DIAGNOSIS

None of the clinical features of vaginitis caused by *Trichomonas* spp. are sufficiently specific to allow a diagnosis of trichomonal infection based on signs and symptoms alone (Fig. 52.2).[9] Definitive diagnosis requires the demonstration of the organism. Vaginal pH is markedly elevated, almost always above 5.0, and not infrequently 6.0. On saline microscopy, an increase in number of PMNs is almost invariably present. The ovoid parasites are slightly larger than PMNs and are best recognized by their motility. The wet mount is positive in only 40–80% of cases. Gram stain is of little value because of its inability to differentiate PMNs from nonmotile trichomonads, and use of Giemsa, acridine orange and other stains has no advantage over saline preparations. Although trichomonads are often seen on Papanicolaou smears, this method has a sensitivity of only 60–70% when compared with saline preparation microscopy, and false-positive results are not infrequently reported.

Several equivalent culture medium methods are available, and growth is usually detected within 48 hours. Culture is now recognized as the most sensitive method for detecting the presence of trichomonads (95% sensitivity) and should be considered in patients with vaginitis in whom an elevated pH, PMN excess, absence of motile trichomonads and clue cells are found. Several new rapid diagnostic kits using DNA probes are under investigation.

MANAGEMENT

Therapy consists of administering the 5-nitroimidazole group of drugs – metronidazole, tinidazole and ornidazole, which are all of similar efficacy.[6] Oral therapy as opposed to topical vaginal therapy, is preferred, because of the frequency of infection of the urethra and periurethral glands, which provide sources for endogenous recurrence.

Treatment consists of oral metronidazole, 500mg q12h for 7 days, which has a cure rate of 95%. Comparable results have been obtained with a single oral dose of 2g metronidazole, achieving cure rates of 82–88%. The latter cure rate increases to greater than 90% when sexual partners are treated simultaneously. The advantages of single-dose therapy include better patient compliance, lower total dose, shorter period of alcohol avoidance and possibly decreased incidence of subsequent vaginitis caused by Candida spp. A disadvantage of single-dose therapy is the need to insist on simultaneous treatment of sexual partners.

The 5-nitroimidazoles are not in themselves trichomonacidal, but low-redox proteins reduce the nitro group, resulting in the formation of highly cytotoxic products within the organisms. Aerobic conditions interfere with this reduction process and decrease the antianaerobic activity of the 5-nitroimdazoles. Most strains of T. vaginalis are highly susceptible to metronidazole, with MICs of 1mg/l.

Patients not responding to an initial course often respond to an additional standard course of 7-day therapy. Some patients are refractory to repeated courses of therapy even when compliance is assured and sexual partners are known to have been treated. If re-infection is excluded, these rare patients may have strains of T. vaginalis that are resistant to metronidazole, which can be confirmed in vitro. Increased doses of metronidazole and longer duration of therapy are necessary to cure these refractory patients. The patients should be given maximal tolerated dosages of oral metronidazole of 2–4g/day for 10–14 days. Rarely, intravenous metronidazole, in dosages as high as 2–4g/day, may be necessary, with careful monitoring for drug toxicity. Considerable success has been observed in treating resistant infections with oral tinidazole; however, the drug is not readily available and the optimal dose to be used is unknown. Most investigators use high-dose tinidazole 1–4g/day for 14 days. Rare patients not responding to nitroimidazoles can be treated with topical paramomycin.

Side effects of metronidazole include an unpleasant or metallic taste. Other common side effects include nausea (10%), transient neutropenia (7.5%) and a disulfiram-like effect when alcohol is ingested. Caution should be taken when 5-nitroimidazoles are used in patients taking warfarin. Long-term and high-dose therapy increases the risk of neutropenia and peripheral neuropathy. In experimental studies, metronidazole has been shown to be mutagenic for certain bacteria, indicating a carcinogenic potential, although cohort studies have not established an increase in cancer morbidity. Thus, the risk to humans of short-term low-dose metronidazole treatment is extremely small. Superinfection with Candida spp. is by no means uncommon.

Treatment of trichomoniasis in pregnancy is unsatisfactory.[6] Metronidazole readily crosses the placenta, and because of concern for teratogenicity some consider it prudent to avoid its use in the first trimester of pregnancy. More recently investigators have become more comfortable with the use of metronidazole throughout pregnancy. Topical clotrimazole and povidone–iodine jelly offer minimal benefit.

VULVOVAGINAL CANDIDIASIS

EPIDEMIOLOGY

Data from the UK reveal a sharp increase in the incidence in vulvovaginal candidiasis (VVC). In the USA, Candida spp. are now the second commonest cause of vaginal infections.[11,12]

It is estimated that 75% of women experience at least one episode of VVC during their child-bearing years, and approximately 40–50% experience a second attack. A small subpopulation of women of undetermined magnitude, probably less than 5% of adult females, suffers from repeated, recurrent, often intractable episodes of Candida vaginitis.[12]

Point-prevalence studies indicate that Candida spp. may be isolated from the genital tract of approximately 20% of asymptomatic, healthy women of child-bearing age. The natural history of asymptomatic colonization is unknown, although animal and human studies suggest that vaginal carriage continues for several months and perhaps years. Several factors are associated with increased rates of asymptomatic vaginal colonization with Candida spp., including pregnancy (30–40%), use of oral contraceptives, uncontrolled diabetes mellitus, and frequency of visits to STD clinics (Fig. 52.3). The rarity of isolation of Candida spp. in premenarchial girls, the lower prevalence of Candida vaginitis after menopause and the possible association with hormone replacement therapy emphasize the hormonal dependence of VVC.

PATHOGENESIS AND PATHOLOGY

THE ORGANISM

Between 85 and 90% of yeast isolated from the vagina are Candida albicans strains. The remainder are other species, the commonest of which are Candida glabrata and Candida tropicalis. Non-albicans Candida spp. are capable of inducing vaginitis and are often more resistant to conventional therapy. Recent surveys indicate an increase in VVC caused by non-albicans Candida spp., particularly C. glabrata.[12,13]

Germination of Candida spp. enhances colonization and facilitates tissue invasion. Factors that enhance or facilitate germination (e.g. estrogen therapy and pregnancy) tend to precipitate symptomatic vaginitis, whereas measures that inhibit germination (e.g. bacterial flora and local mucosal cell-mediated immunity) may prevent acute vaginitis in women who are asymptomatic carriers of yeast.

Candida organisms gain access to the vaginal lumen and secretions predominantly from the adjacent perianal area. This finding is borne out by epidemiologic typing studies. Candida vaginitis is seen predominantly in women of child-bearing age, and only in the minority of cases can a precipitating factor be identified to explain the transformation from asymptomatic carriage to symptomatic vaginitis in individual patients.

HOST FACTORS

Host factors associated with increased asymptomatic vaginal colonization by Candida spp. and with Candida vaginitis are outlined in Figure 52.3. During pregnancy, the vagina is more susceptible to vaginal infection, resulting in higher incidences of vaginal colonization, vaginitis and lower cure rates. The clinical attack rate is maximal in the third trimester, and symptomatic recurrences are also more common throughout pregnancy. The high levels of reproductive hormones result in a higher glycogen content in the vaginal environment, which

HOST FACTORS ASSOCIATED WITH INCREASED ASYMPTOMATIC VAGINAL COLONIZATION BY CANDIDA AND WITH CANDIDA VAGINITIS		
Genetic		
Blood group antigen/secretor status		
Acquired		
Biologic		Pregnancy Uncontrolled diabetes mellitus Corticosteroids/immunosuppressive therapy Antimicrobial therapy (systemic, topical) HIV infection
Behavioral (sexual)		Oral contraceptives Intrauterine device/contraceptive sponge Nonoxynol-9 spermicide Receptive oral–genital sex Coital frequency (?)

Fig. 52.3 Host factors associated with increased asymptomatic vaginal colonization by Candida and with Candida vaginitis.

provides an excellent carbon source for growth and germination of *Candida* spp. A more common mechanism is where estrogens enhance vaginal epithelial cell avidity for *Candida* spp. adherence, and a yeast cytosol receptor or binding system for female reproductive hormones has been documented. These hormones also enhance yeast mycelial formation. Several studies have shown increased VVC associated with oral contraceptive use,[14] and uncontrolled diabetes mellitus. Glucose tolerance tests have been recommended for women with recurrent VVC; however, the yield is low, and testing is not justified in otherwise healthy premenopausal women.

Symptomatic VVC is frequently observed during or after courses of systemic antibiotics. Although no antimicrobial agent is free of this complication, broad-spectrum antibiotics, such as tetracycline, and beta-lactams are mainly responsible and are thought to act by eliminating the normal protective vaginal bacterial flora. The natural flora provides a colonization-resistance mechanism and prevents germination of *Candida* spp. The provider of this protective function has been singled out to be *Lactobacillus* spp.[15] *Lactobacillus–Candida* interaction includes competition for nutrients, steric interference with adherence of *Candida* spp. and elaboration of bacteriocins that inhibit yeast proliferation and germination.

Other factors that contribute to an increased incidence of *Candida* vaginitis include the use of tight, poorly ventilated clothing and nylon underclothing, which increases perineal moisture and temperature.

Candida spp. may cause cell damage and resulting inflammation by direct hyphal invasion of epithelial tissue. It is possible that proteases and other hydrolytic enzymes facilitate cell penetration with resultant inflammation, mucosal swelling, erythema and exfoliation of vaginal epithelial cells, The characteristic nonhomogenous vaginal discharge consists of a conglomerate of hyphal elements and exfoliated nonviable epithelial cells with few PMNs. *Candida* spp. may also induce symptoms by hypersensitivity or allergic reactions, particularly in women with idiopathic recurrent VVC (see Noninfectious vaginitis and vulvitis, below).[16]

Oral and vaginal thrush correlates well with depressed cell-mediated immunity in debilitated or immunosuppressed patients.[16] This is particularly evident in patients who have chronic mucocutaneous candidiasis and AIDS.

PATHOGENESIS OF RECURRENT AND CHRONIC *CANDIDA* VAGINITIS

Careful evaluation of women with recurrent vaginitis usually fails to reveal any precipitating or causal mechanism.[17] In the past, investigators attributed frequent episodes to repeated fungal re-inoculation of the vagina from a persistent intestinal source or to sexual transmission.

The intestinal theory is based on the report of recovery of *Candida* spp. on rectal culture in almost 100% of women with VVC. Typing of simultaneously obtained vaginal and rectal isolates almost invariably reveals identical strains. This theory has been criticized in the past few years because of lower concordance between rectal and vaginal cultures in patients with recurrent VVC. Moreover, long-term therapy with oral nonabsorbable nystatin is not effective in preventing recurrences.

Although sexual transmissions of *Candida* organisms occurs via vaginal intercourse and orogenital contact, the role of sexual reintroduction of yeast as a cause for recurrent VVC is doubtful. Recurrent VVC frequently occurs in celibate women and only a minority of male partners of women who have recurrent VVC are colonized with *Candida* spp. Although most studies aimed at treating male partners have not reduced the frequency of recurrent episodes of vaginitis, reduction was achieved in recurrent vulvovaginal candidiasis by treating colonized male partners.[17]

Vaginal relapse implies that incomplete eradication or clearance of *Candida* spp. from the vagina occurs after antimycotic therapy. Organisms persist in small numbers in the vagina and result in continued carriage of the organisms, and when host environmental conditions permit, the colonizing organisms increase in number and undergo mycelial transformation, resulting in a new clinical episode.

Whether recurrence is caused by vaginal re-infection or relapse, women with recurrent VVC differ from those with infrequent episodes in their inability to tolerate small numbers of *Candida* organisms re-introduced or persisting in the vagina. On the basis of typing of organisms, women with recurrent and infrequent infection have the same distribution frequency of *Candida* strains as do women without symptoms.

Host factors responsible for frequent episodes are not clearly delineated, and more than one mechanism may be operative. There is no evidence of complement, phagocytic cells, or immunoglobulin deficiency in these patients. Recurrent VVC is rarely caused by drug resistance.[18] Current theories about the pathogenesis of recurrent VVC include qualitative and quantitative deficiency in the normal protective vaginal bacterial flora and an acquired, often transient antigen-specific deficiency in T-lymphocyte function that similarly permits unchecked yeast proliferation.[16,19] Another theory is that of an acquired acute hypersensitivity reaction to *Candida* antigen, which is accompanied by elevated vaginal titers of *Candida* antigen-specific IgE. This theory has a clinical basis in that patients with recurrent VVC often present with severe vulvar manifestations (rash, erythema, swelling and pruritus) with minimal exudative vaginal changes, little discharge, and lower numbers of organisms. Allergic responses to *Candida* spp. have been reported to involve the male genitalia immediately after coitus with a woman infected with *Candida* spp. and are characterized by the acute onset of erythema, edema, severe pruritus and irritation of the penis. As yet, only a minority of women with recurrent VVC have been shown to have elevated *Candida*-specific vaginal IgE. Limited studies using *Candida* antigen desensitization have been found to be helpful in reducing the frequency of recurrent episodes of vaginitis.

Women who are HIV seropositive have higher vaginal colonization rates than do seronegative women, but the attack rate of symptomatic VVC appears similar. Reports of chronic, severe recurrent VVC are largely unsubstantiated. Recurrent VVC in the absence of other risk factors for HIV is not an indication for HIV testing.[12]

PREVENTION

In women with confirmed recurrent VVC linked to frequent courses of systemic antibiotics, prophylactic antimycotics are justified. A useful regimen is fluconazole 100mg once weekly for the duration of antibiotic therapy. No other dietary or alternative method has stood the test of time in preventing VVC. In women prone to VVC, avoiding use of oral contraceptives, intrauterine devices and the contraceptive sponge is prudent.

CLINICAL FEATURES

The most frequent symptom of VVC is vulvar pruritus, because vaginal discharge is not invariably present and is frequently minimal.[12] Although described as typically cottage cheese-like in character, the discharge may vary from watery to homogeneously thick. Vaginal soreness, irritation, vulvar burning, dyspareunia and external dysuria are commonly present. Odor, if present, is minimal and nonoffensive. Examination frequently reveals erythema and swelling of the labia and vulva, often with discrete pustulopapular peripheral lesions. The cervix is normal and vaginal mucosal erythema with adherent whitish discharge is present. Characteristically, symptoms are exacerbated in the week before the onset of menses, with some relief with the onset of menstrual flow.

DIAGNOSIS

The relative lack of specificity of symptoms and signs precludes a diagnosis that is based only on history and physical examination. Most patients with symptomatic VVC may be readily diagnosed on the basis of simple microscopic examination of vaginal secretions. A wet mount or saline preparation has a sensitivity of 40–60%. The 10% potassium hydroxide preparation is more sensitive in diagnosing the presence of germinated yeast. A normal vaginal pH (4.0–4.5) is found in *Candida* vaginitis, and the finding of a pH in excess of 4.5 should suggest the possibility of bacterial vaginosis, trichomoniasis or a mixed infection.[12]

Although routine fungal cultures are unnecessary, vaginal culture should be performed in the presence of negative microscopy. The Papanicolaou smear is unreliable, being positive in only about 25% of cases. There is no reliable serologic technique for the diagnosis of *Candida* vaginitis.

MANAGEMENT

TOPICAL AGENTS FOR ACUTE *CANDIDA* VAGINITIS

Antimycotics are available for local use as creams, vaginal tablets, suppositories and coated tampons (Fig. 52.4). There is little to suggest that the formulation of the topical antimycotic influences clinical efficacy.[20] Extensive vulvar inflammation dictates local vulvar application of cream.

The average mycologic cure rate of 7- and 14-day courses of nystatin is 75–80%. Azoles appear to achieve slightly higher clinical

THERAPY FOR VAGINAL CANDIDIASIS		
Topical Agents		
Drug	Formulation	Dosage regimen
*Butoconazole	2% cream	5g/day for 3 days
*Clotrimazole	1% cream 100mg vaginal tablets 100mg vaginal tablets 500mg vaginal tablets	5g/day for 7–14 days 1 tablet/day for 7 days 2 tablets/day for 3 days 1 tablet, single dose
*Miconazole	2% cream 100mg vaginal suppository 200mg vaginal suppository 1200mg vaginal suppository	5g/day for 7 days 1 suppository/day for 7 days 1 suppository/day for 3 days 1 suppository, single dose
Econazole	150mg vaginal tablet	1 tablet/day for 3 days
Fenticonazole	2% cream	5g/day for 7 days
*Tioconazole	2% cream 6.5% cream	5g/day for 3 days 5g, single dose
Terconazole	0.4% cream 0.8% cream 80mg vaginal suppository	5g/day for 7 days 5g/day for 3 days 80mg/day for 3 days
Nystatin	100,000U vaginal tablets	1 tablet/day for 14 days

Fig. 52.4 Therapy for vaginal candidiasis — topical agents. *Drugs available over the counter, without prescription.

CLASSIFICATION OF VULVOVAGINAL CANDIDIASIS	
Uncomplicated	Complicated
Candida albicans + Infrequent episodes + Vaginitis mild-to-moderate + Normal host	Non-*albicans Candida* spp. Resistant *Candida albicans* (rare) or History of recurrent VVC or Severe VVC or Abnormal host, for example, uncontrolled diabetes, pregnancy, immunocompromised

Fig. 52.5 Classification of vulvovaginal candidiasis.

mycologic cure rates than do the polyenes (nystatin): 85–90%. Although many studies have compared the clinical efficacies of the various azoles, there is little evidence that any one azole agent is superior to others.[20] Topical azoles are remarkably free of local and systemic side effects; nevertheless, the initial application of topical agents is not infrequently accompanied by local burning and discomfort.

There has been a major trend toward shorter treatment courses with progressively higher antifungal doses, culminating in highly effective single-dose topical regimens. Although short-course regimens are effective for mild and moderate vaginitis, cure rates for severe and complicated vaginitis are lower.

Oral systemic azoles available for the treatment of VVC include ketoconazole 400mg q12h for 5 days, itraconazole 200mg/day for 3 days (or q12h single-day regimen) and, finally, fluconazole 150mg single-dose.[21] All the oral regimens achieve clinical cure rates in excess of 80%; however, only fluconazole is approved for use in the USA. Oral regimens are generally preferred by women because of convenience and lack of local side effects. None of the systemic regimens should be prescribed during pregnancy and the potential for systemic side effects and toxicity exists. In particular, hepatotoxicity with ketoconazole precludes its widespread use in VVC.[20]

Vulvovaginal candidiasis is classified as uncomplicated or complicated on the basis of the likelihood of achieving clinical and mycologic cure with short-course therapy (Fig. 52.5). Uncomplicated VVC represents by far the most common form of vaginitis seen, is caused by highly sensitive *C. albicans* and, provided that the severity is mild-to-moderate, patients respond well to all topical or oral antimycotics, including single-dose therapy. In contrast, patients who have complicated VVC have an organism, a host factor or a severity of infection that dictates more intensive and prolonged therapy lasting 7–14 days. Most non-*albicans Candida* infections respond to conventional topical or oral antifungals provided they are administered for sufficient duration. However, vaginitis caused by *C. glabrata* often fails to respond to azoles and may require treatment with vaginal capsules of boric acid 600mg/day for 14 days.[22]

TREATMENT OF RECURRENT VULVOVAGINAL CANDIDIASIS

The management of women who have recurrent VVC aims at control rather than cure. The clinician should first confirm the diagnosis of recurrent VVC. Uncontrolled diabetes mellitus must be controlled and use of corticosteroids, or other immunosuppressive agents, should be discontinued where possible. Unfortunately, in the majority of women with recurrent VVC, no underlying or predisposing factor can be identified. Recurrent vulvovaginal candidiasis requires long-term maintenance with a suppressive prophylactic regimen. Because of the chronicity of therapy, the convenience of oral treatment is apparent, and the best suppressive prophylaxis has been achieved with weekly oral fluconazole at a dosage of 100mg. An effective topical prophylactic regimen consists of weekly vaginal suppositories of clotrimazole 500mg.[12]

ATROPHIC VAGINITIS

Clinically significant atrophic vaginitis is actually quite rare, and the majority of women with mild-to-moderate atrophy are asymptomatic. Because of reduced endogenous estrogen, the epithelium becomes thin and lacking in glycogen, which contributes to a reduction in lactic acid production and an increase in vaginal pH. This change in the environment encourages the overgrowth of nonacidophilic coliform organisms and the disappearance of *Lactobacillus* spp. Despite these major but usually gradual changes, symptoms are mostly absent, especially in the absence of coitus.

With advanced atrophy, symptoms include vaginal soreness, dyspareunia and occasional spotting or discharge. Burning is a frequent complaint and is often precipitated by intercourse. The vaginal mucosa is thin, with diffuse redness, occasional petechiae, or ecchymoses with few or no vaginal folds. Vulvar atrophy may also be apparent and discharge may be serosanguinous, thick or watery, and the pH of the vaginal secretions ranges from 5.5 to 7.0. The wet smear frequently shows increased number of PMNs associated with small, round epithelial cells. The latter parabasal cells represent immature squamous cells, which have not been exposed to sufficient estrogen. The *Lactobacillus* spp. dominated flora is replaced by mixed flora of Gram-negative rods. Bacteriologic cultures in these patients are unnecessary, and can be misleading.

The treatment of atrophic vaginitis consists primarily of topical vaginal estrogen. Nightly use of half or all the contents of an applicator for 1–2 weeks is usually sufficient to alleviate the atrophic vaginitis.

NONINFECTIOUS VAGINITIS AND VULVITIS

Women frequently present with acute or chronic vulvovaginal symptoms caused by noninfectious etiologies. Symptoms are indistinguishable from those of infectious syndromes, but are most commonly confused with those of acute *Candida* vaginitis, including pruritus, irritation, burning, soreness and variable discharge. Noninfectious causes include the following: irritants [physical (e.g. minipads) or chemical (e.g. spermicides, betadyne, topical antimycotics, soaps and perfumes, topical 5-fluorouracil etc.)]; and allergens, which are responsible for immunologic acute and chronic hypersensitivity reactions, including contact dermatitis (e.g. latex condoms, antimycotic creams). An enormous list of topical factors responsible for local inflammatory reactions and symptoms exist and many more have yet to be defined. Depending on the site of contact, symptoms may be vaginal or vulvar. A noninfectious mechanism may co-exist with or follow an infectious process, and should be considered when the three common infectious causes and hormone deficiency are excluded and in the presence of a normal vaginal pH, normal saline and potassium hydroxide microscopy, and, ultimately, a negative yeast culture. Unfortunately, given the anticipated 20% colonization rates in normal asymptomatic women, occasionally a positive yeast culture in a symptomatic patient reflects the presence of an innocent bystander and not the cause of the vulvovaginal symptoms. The only logical way of establishing the role of *Candida* spp. in this context is to treat with an oral antifungal agent and assess the clinical response.

Once a local chemical irritant or allergic reaction is suspected, a detailed inquiry into possible causal factors is essential. Offending agents or behaviours should be eliminated wherever possible, including avoiding chemical irritants and allergens (e.g. soaps, detergents etc.). The immediate management of severe vulvovaginal symptoms of noninfectious etiology should not rely on topical corticosteroids, which are rarely the solution and frequently high potency corticosteroid creams cause intense burning. Local relief measures include sodium bicarbonate sitz baths, oral antihistamines, etc.

A syndrome of hyperacidity of the vagina causing overgrowth of lactobacilli has been described but not confirmed. Rebound increase in population numbers of lactobacilli is thought to occur after completion of topical antimycotics and is alleged to suppress population numbers of healthy resident flora. The proposed syndrome of cytolytic vaginosis is characterized by vulvovaginal burning, irritation, soreness and dyspareunia and is usually incorrectly diagnosed as vulvovaginal candidiasis. The finding of large numbers of lactobacilli on wet count and low pH, together with extensive squamous epithelial cell cytolysis is said to confirm the diagnosis. Recommended therapy for cytolytic vaginosis is daily alkaline douching using sodium bicarbonate to elevate the low vaginal pH and suppress growth of lactobacilli.

VULVITIS

Most of the important causes of vulvitis have been described in the section on vaginitis. Human papillomavirus and genital herpes are described in Chapters 2.66 and 2.65 respectively. Bacterial vulvitis due to streptococci, anaerobes and Gram-negative rods occurs infrequently and should be diagnosed by clinical features and bacterial culture. Specific antimicrobial treatment is indicated for patients with the diagnosis of bacterial vulvitis. Occasionally a Bartholin's abscess creates a painful swelling in the vulva. This can be due to *N. gonorrhoeae* or to a variety of pathogens, particularly Gram-positive organisms. A Bartholin cyst infection should be treated with appropriate antibiotics and occasionally may require drainage.

CERVICITIS

EPIDEMIOLOGY

The presence of a purulent exudate in the cervical os has been highly associated with cervical infection with *Chlamydia trachomatis, Neisseria gonorrhoeae*, Herpes simplex virus and cytomegalovirus. Infection with *Trichomonas vaginalis* correlates with colpitis macularis and inflammatory changes of the ectocervix.[23,24] Not infrequently, mucopurulent endocervitis or ectocervicitis (MPC) are seen in the absence of these pathogens, indicating that additional, as yet unrecognized causes exist. A role for disruption of vaginal flora, specifically overgrowth of anaerobes in causing cervical inflammation has been proposed. Rare causes of cervicitis include *Mycobacterium tuberculosis* and *Actinomyces israelii*, the latter almost invariably in the presence of intrauterine devices. Although the most important and prevalent infection of the cervix is undoubtedly human papilloma virus, this virus does not cause cervicitis and is discussed in Chapter 8.6.

The prevalence of genital chlamydial infection ranges from 8 to 40%.[25] Risk factors include young age, unmarried status, lower socioeconomic conditions, number and recent change of sexual partner, ectopy, oral contraceptive use and concurrent gonococcal infection; the latter may reactivate latent chlamydial infection and increases shedding of chlamydia from endocervix.[25] Risk factors for gonococcal mucopurulent cervicitis are identical to those of *Chlamydia* spp. but also include urban dwelling, prostitution, illicit drug use and minority racial status. Up to 60% of women with *N. gonorrhoeae* have co-infection with chlamydia.[25] Herpetic cervicitis is rare in the absence of genital lesions and is most commonly associated with first-episode, primary disease with an 80% viral isolation rate.[24] Cytomegalovirus is thought to be responsible for approximately 5% of cases of cervicitis, is usually asymptomatic and when it is isolated from cervical secretions, the detection may not imply a causal relationship with present pathology.

CLINICAL FEATURES

Cervicitis is frequently asymptomatic and is detected on routine pelvic examination. Alternatively cervical inflammation is recognized because of signs and symptoms of concomitant infection (e.g. vaginal trichomoniasis, genital herpes or salpingitis). Mucopurulent cervicitis (MPC) may result in a purulent vaginal discharge in its own right. Accordingly cervical speculum evaluation should be an essential part of vaginal examination in women with an abnormal discharge. Mucopurulent endocervicitis results in swelling and erythema of the zone of ectopy associated with friability, contact bleeding, spotting and a yellow or a green endocervical exudate. The purulent discharge is best appreciated by obtaining an endocervical swab specimen and observing the latter against a white background.

Trichomoniasis is associated with ectocervical squamous epithelial mucosal inflammation giving the cervix a 'strawberry' appearance due to microscopic focal patchy petechiae (colpitis macularis) in 5–20% of patients.[12] Primary herpes cervicitis may be associated with severe necrosis that is reminiscent of cervical cancer. Most commonly, primary herpetic cervicitis is characterized by increased surface vascularity, and micro- and macro-ulcerations with and without necrotic areas. Asymptomatic shedding of herpesvirus occurs in the absence of cervical lesions.

DIAGNOSIS

MPC is confirmed when a Gram–stained specimen of green or yellow endocervical exudate reveals more than 30 PMNs per high power field. Microscopic examination of cervical mucus from a patient with mucopurulent endocervicitis reveals an overabundance of inflammatory cells, obliterating the background ferning pattern. A similar excess of inflammatory cells can be found from Papanicolaou smear. These two microscopic studies are not reliable in identifying the underlying cause of MPC. For diagnosis of *C. trachomatis* cervicitis, culture techniques to identify the obligate intraparasites served as the gold standard in the past. Now the development of the more widely available enzyme-linked immunosorbent assay antigen detection tests has been replaced by the highly sensitive DNA amplification techniques, particularly ligase chain reaction, allowing diagnosis not only from cervical specimens, but also by screening urine specimens. Gram stain of cervical mucus may reveal intracellular Gram-negative diplococci, but has low sensitivity and specificity in the diagnosis of gonococcal cervicitis. Diagnosis relies mainly upon culture of the endocervix utilizing a modified Thayer–Martin medium; however, diagnostic methodologies now include use of DNA probes, especially for screening purposes, given the high sensitivity of these newer techniques.

Although Papanicolaou smears in herpetic cervicitis are useful in revealing multinucleated giant cells, viral culture and fluorescein-conjugated monoclonal antibodies are the mainstay of clinical diagnosis; polymerase chain reaction is used for monitoring asymptomatic viral shedding in a research context.

The clinical differentiation of the various causes of cervicitis is not possible, but requires the aforementioned diagnostic tests, recognizing that frequently more than one etiologic agent may be present simultaneously, because many of the pathogens share risk factors and behavior. The most important diagnostic problem is that of overdiagnosis of cervicitis. All too frequently physiologic changes in the appearance of the cervix, in spite of the use of colposcopy, are interpreted as reflecting pathological cervicitis. Regrettably, after failed attempts to identify pathogenic micro-organisms, patients are needlessly treated with cervical ablative techniques. Cervical ectopy is often mistaken for cervicitis, with eversion of endocervical columnar cells, and is commonly seen in women on oral contraceptives.[26] Other physiologic changes related to childbirth and dilatation of the cervical canal are mistakenly diagnosed as cervicitis. Equally important is the failure to recognize that a friable, abnormal cervix may reflect dysplasia and neoplasia. If the Papanicolaou smear reports inflammatory cells with or without atypia, the presence of atypical squamous cells of undetermined significance (ASCUS) should be considered in the differential diagnosis between a benign change in reaction to a stimulus and low grade squamous intraepithelial lesion. Accordingly, women with a Papanicolaou smear showing ASCUS should have their smears repeated. Persistence of an ASCUS smear should prompt colposcopy.

MANAGEMENT

Antimicrobial regimens for infectious cervicitis are shown in the chapters on gonorrhea and chlamydial infections and pelvic inflammatory disease (see Chapters 2.53, 2.63 & 8.25).

REFERENCES

1. Holmes KK. Lower genital tract infections in women: cystitis, urethritis, vulvovaginitis, and cervicitis. In: Holmes KK, Mardh P-A, Sparling PF, et al. eds. Sexually transmitted diseases, 2nd ed. New York: McGraw Hill; 1990:527–47.
2. Hill GB. Microbiology of bacterial vaginosis. Am J Obstet Gynecol 1969;169:450–4.
3. Eschenbach DA, Davick PR, Williams BL, et al. Prevalence of hydrogen peroxide producing *Lactobacillus* species in normal women and women with bacterial vaginosis. J Clin Microbiol 1989;27:251–6.
4. Hillier SL, Krohn MA, Cassen E, et al. The role of bacterial vaginosis and vaginal bacteria in amniotic fluid infection in women in preterm labor with intact fetal membranes. Clin Infect Dis 1995;20(Suppl 2):276–8.
5. Platz-Christensen JJ, Sundstrom F, Larsson PG. Bacterial vaginosis and cervical intraepithelial neoplasia. Acta Obstet Gynecol Scand 1994; 73:586–8.
6. Centers for Disease Control and Prevention: 1993 Sexually Transmitted Diseases Treatment guidelines. MMWR Morb Mortal Wkly Rep 1993;42:1–46.
7. Hillier SL, Nugent RP, Eschenbach DA, et al. Association between bacterial vaginosis and preterm delivery of a low birth-weight infant. N Engl J Med 1995;333:1737–42.
8. Hauth JC, Goldenberg RL, Andrews WW, DuBard MD, Copper RC. Reduced incidence of preterm delivery with metronidazole and erythromycin in women with bacterial vaginosis. N Engl J Med 1995;333:1732–6.

9. Spence MR, Hollander DH, Smith J, et al. The clinical and laboratory diagnosis of *Trichomonas vaginalis* infection. Sex Transm Dis 1980;7:168–71.
10. Wolner-Hanssen P, Krieger JN, Stevens CE, et al. Clinical manifestations of vaginal trichomoniasis. JAMA 1989;261:571–6.
11. Kent HL. Epidemiology of vaginitis. Am J Obstet Gynecol 1991;165:1168–76.
12. Sobel JD. Candidal vulvovaginitis. Clin Obstet Gynecol 1993;36:153–65.
13. Spinillo A, Capuzzo E, Egbe TO, et al. *Torulopsis glabrata* vaginitis. Obstet Gynecol 1995;85:993–8.
14. Foxman B. Epidemiology of vulvovaginal candidiasis: Risk factors. Am J Public Health 1996;80:329–31.
15. Hooton TM, Roberts PL, Stamm WF. Effects of recent sexual activity and use of a diaphragm on the vaginal microflora. Clin Infect Dis 1994;19:274–8.
16. Fidel PL Jr, Sobel JD. Immunopathogenesis of recurrent vulvovaginal candidiasis. Rev Clin Microbiol 1996;9:335–48.
17. Spinillo A, Carrato L, Pizzoli G. Recurrent vulvovaginal candidiasis: results of a cohort study of sexual transmission and intestinal reservoir. J Reprod Med 1992;37:353–47.
18. Lynch ME, Sobel JD. Comparative in vitro activity of antimycotic agents against pathogenic yeast isolates. J Med Vet Mycol 1994;32:267–74.
19. Fidel PL Jr, Lynch ME, Redondo-Lopez V, Sobel JD, Robinson R. Systemic cell-mediated immune reactivity in women with recurrent vulvovaginal candidiasis. J Infect Dis 1993;168:1458–65.

20. Reef S, Levine WC, Mneil MM, et al. Treatment options for vulvovaginal candidiasis, background paper for development of 1993 STD treatment recommendations. Clin Infect Dis 1995;29(Suppl):580–90.
21. Sobel JD, Brooker D, Stein GE, et al. Single oral dose fluconazole compared with clotrimazole topical therapy of *Candida* vaginitis. Fluconazole Vaginitis Study Group. Am J Obstet Gynecol 1955;172:1263–8.
22. Sobel JD, Chaim W. Treatment of *Candida glabrata* vaginitis: a retrospective review of boric acid therapy. Clin Infect Dis 1997;24:649–52.
23. Kiviat NB, Paavonon JA, Wolner-Hanssen P, et al. Histopathology of endocervical infection caused by *Chlamydia trachomatis*, herpes simplex virus, *Trichomonas vaginalis* and *Neisseria gonorrhoeae*. Hum Pathol 1990;21:831–7.
24. Wald A, Zeh J, Selke S, et al. Virologic characteristics of subclinical and symptomatic genital herpes infections. N Engl J Med 1995;333:770–5.
25. Cates W, Wasserheit JN. Genital chlamydial infections: epidemiology and reproductive sequelae. Am J Obstet Gynecol 1991;164:1771–8.
26. Critchlow CW, Wolner-Hanssen P, Eschenbach DA, et al. Determinants of cervical ectopia and of cervicitis: age, oral contraceptives, specific cervical infection, smoking, and douching. Am J Obstet Gynecol 1995;173:534–43.

Infections of the Female Pelvis Including Septic Abortion

Gina Dallabetta, Munkolenkole C. Kamenga & Mary Lyn Field

Infections of the female pelvis constitute a diverse group. This chapter considers three groups of infections: pelvic inflammatory disease (PID), postpartum and postabortal infections (including postpartum endometritis and cesarean section, episiotomy infections and post-abortion sepsis) and postsurgical gynecologic infections.

PELVIC INFLAMMATORY DISEASE

EPIDEMIOLOGY

Pelvic inflammatory disease refers to an acute clinical syndrome that results when vaginal or cervical organisms ascend into upper tract structures of the female reproductive tract unrelated to pregnancy or surgery.[1,2] The term PID includes the following: endometritis, parametritis, salpingitis, oophoritis, pelvic peritonitis, tubo-ovarian abscess, periappendicitis, perihepatitis (Fitz-Hugh–Curtis syndrome) and perisplenitis.

Pelvic inflammatory disease and sexually transmitted diseases (STDs) share many of the same risk factors and, in the USA, 40–80% of PID is attributed to STDs. Bacterial vaginosis may be an antecedent vaginal condition.[3] The identified risk factors for PID include younger age, unmarried status, lower socioeconomic status, sexual behavior (number of sexual partners, age of sexual debut, rate of acquiring new partners), substance abuse, poor health care behavior (treatment-seeking and compliance with treatment instructions), douching and intrauterine device insertion.[1,4] In studies from the USA and Europe, about three-quarters of women with PID were under 25 years of age, and about one-half had never been pregnant.[2] Oral contraceptive users tend to have clinically and laparoscopically milder infection than do nonusers and oral contraceptives appear to protect against chlamydial PID.[5]

PATHOGENESIS AND PATHOLOGY

The vast majority of PID cases result from a direct canalicular spread of organisms from the endocervix to the mucosa of the endometrium and fallopian tubes although the precise mechanisms are poorly understood. Postinfectious scarring (e.g. intratubal adhesions, tubal occlusion, peritubal scarring and damaged fimbrial ostia) results in the long-term sequelae of PID.

Occurrence of PID is described only among sexually active women and its risk is associated with the numbers of sexual partners and the frequency of sexual acts among women with only one sexual partner. Multiple organisms have been implicated as etiologic agents of PID (Fig. 53.1). The rates of isolation of these organisms are variable. They may vary with geographic regions, duration of infection and the sites of sampling (i.e. cervix, fallopian tubes, or endometrium). The most commonly recovered organisms are *Neisseria gonorrhoeae* and *Chlamydia trachomatis,* followed by other aerobic and anaerobic bacteria associated with bacterial vaginosis (e.g. *Gardnerella vaginalis, Mycoplasma hominis,* and *Proventella* and *Peptostreptococcus* spp.). Rates of isolation of 10–20% in the upper genital tract and as high as 85% (5–27% in studies from Europe versus 44–70% in those from

COMMON MICRO-ORGANISMS IDENTIFIED AS ETIOLOGIC AGENTS IN PELVIC INFLAMMATORY DISEASE	
Aerobic bacteria	*Neisseria gonorrhoeae* *Chlamydia trachomatis* *Gardnerella vaginalis* *Escherichia coli* *Streptococcus* spp. *Haemophilus influenzae*
Anaerobic bacteria	*Bacteroides* spp. *Peptostreptococcus* spp. *Peptococcus* spp. *Prevotella* spp.
Mycoplasmas	*Mycoplasma hominis*

Fig. 53.1 Common micro-organisms identified as etiologic agents in pelvic inflammatory disease.

North America) in the lower genital tract have been reported for *N. gonorrhoeae.* For *C. trachomatis,* rates of 1.2–31% in the upper genital tract and 31% in the lower genital tract have been reported.[2,3,6] It is estimated that between 10 and 40% of women with untreated gonococcal or chlamydial cervical infection will develop acute upper tract infection. However, PID is a polymicrobial infection, even in the setting of gonococcal or chlamydial cervicitis. It has been suggested that in many cases of PID, STD organisms initiate the inflammation of the tubal mucosa and this process facilitating the invasion of the mucosa by organisms endogenous to the lower genital tract.[2]

PREVENTION

Prevention is directed at reducing a woman's risk of acquiring an STD, and the detection and treatment of lower genital tract infections. A recent study showed that women screened and treated for asymptomatic chlamydial infection were nearly 60% less likely than unscreened women to develop PID.[7] Prompt and correct treatment of upper tract infections will ameliorate some of the long-term sequelae.

CLINICAL FEATURES

The most common clinical complaint in a woman with PID is bilateral lower abdominal or pelvic pain. Gonococcal PID tends to have an abrupt, fulminant presentation within 1 week of the onset of menses. Chlamydial PID is characterized by a subacute course with mild symptoms, often described as a dull pain. It is not unusual for a woman with chlamydial PID to be unaware of her infection and to present as a contact of a male with urethritis, with right upper quadrant pain or with other genitourinary complaints, such as dyspareunia, dysuria, dysmenorrhea, menorrhagia or abnormal vaginal discharge. Chlamydial PID represents the diagnostic challenge as uterine and adnexal tenderness may be very mild. The clinician should be alert to adnexal masses or fullness as the major signs of chlamydial infection. Women with HIV infection and PID may present with more clinically severe disease.[8]

These traditional clinical signs and symptoms of PID, however, are neither sensitive nor specific for the syndrome. Laparoscopy confirms salpingitis in 45–89% of women with clinical PID. Of women with acute clinical PID, 6–45% have normal fallopian tubes and 5–33% have other conditions, including ectopic pregnancy, appendicitis, hemorrhagic ovarian cysts, endometritis, pelvic adhesions and torsion of an adnexal structure.[6,9] False-negative clinical diagnoses for PID range from 16 to 47%.[9] The diagnoses prior to laparoscopy in women with laparoscopically confirmed PID included ectopic pregnancy, ovarian cyst, hemorrhagic ovarian cyst, endometriosis, fibroids, ovarian tumor, appendicitis, unclear diagnosis and pyelonephritis.

The common complications and sequelae of PID include ectopic pregnancy, tubal infertility, recurrent PID, chronic abdominal pain, tubo-ovarian abscesses and pelvic adhesions. A woman's risk of ectopic pregnancy increases seven- to ten-fold after an episode of PID. The number of episodes of PID, the woman's age and the severity of tubal inflammation determined at laparoscopy influences the fertility prognosis of PID (Fig. 53.2). It appears that PID caused by chlamydial infection may result in more infertility than PID caused by gonococcal infection. Recurrent pelvic infections will develop in up to one-third of women with PID. Chronic abdominal pain lasting more than 6 months occurs in 15–18% of women after PID. Pyosalpinx, tubo-ovarian abscesses and pelvic adhesions occur in 15–20% of women with PID and often require surgical intervention. Mortality from acute PID is rare. The most common cause of death from PID is a ruptured tubo-ovarian abscess with subsequent peritonitis. The mortality rate from this complication of PID is 6–8%.

DIAGNOSIS

The clinical diagnosis of PID is imprecise. Laparoscopy can be used to obtain a more accurate diagnosis, but is neither readily available in most cases nor justifiable in clinically mild disease.

Women with lower abdominal tenderness, adnexal tenderness, and cervical motion tenderness should be treated for PID if there is no other diagnosis that should be considered.[10] Additional tests to document an inflammatory and infectious process in the lower genital tract should be used to increase the sensitivity of the clinical signs.

A ratio of more than one white blood cell to epithelial cell on vaginal wet mount or an endocervical Gram stain, obtained after cleaning the ectocervix, showing Gram-negative intracellular diplococci or 30 or more polymorphonuclear leukocytes per 1000× field is highly supportive of the diagnosis of PID in women with appropriate clinical criteria. Tests (culture or antigen) for the detection of *N. gonorrhoeae* and *C. trachomatis* are useful in supporting the diagnosis but not in the decision to start therapy. A pregnancy test should be done. Erythrocyte sedimentation rate, C-reactive protein and complete white blood cell count may also be useful. Pelvic and endovaginal ultrasound can detect findings consistent with severe PID, including tubo-ovarian abscesses, dilated fallopian tubes and cul-de-sac fluid. Ultrasound is less useful in mild or atypical clinical presentations. Computed tomography shares the same limitations with ultrasound. However, in severe cases of PID with atypical ultrasound findings CT can be useful.[11] For example, spiral CT scanning optimizes identification of small air bubbles that are specific for abscess.[12] More research is needed in the use of this relatively new imaging technique in the diagnosis of PID.

Endometrial biopsy documenting plasma cell endometritis confirms the diagnosis but requires at least 24 hours for processing. Purulent material from the peritoneal cavity obtained by culdocentesis, a painful procedure, may support the diagnosis of PID but may also occur with other intra-abdominal infections, such as appendicitis. Laparoscopy is the gold standard for the diagnosis and staging of acute PID. The minimum criteria for visual confirmation of PID include hyperemia of the tubal surface, edema of the tubal wall and a sticky exudate on the tubal surface and from the fimbriated end when patent.[13]

MANAGEMENT

Management of a patient with PID includes therapy, education, careful follow-up and partner management. The goal is to cure the patient, prevent recurrences and, ultimately, to preserve fertility. Empiric treatment should be instituted as soon as the diagnosis is suspected. Based on the polymicrobial nature of PID, therapy must provide broad-spectrum coverage. Several antimicrobial regimens have proven to be highly effective in achieving a clinical cure of PID, but there are few data on the efficacy of recommended or tested regimens on preventing the late sequelae.[14] Studies from the pre-antibiotic era documented infertility rates after PID of 60–70%, indicating that prompt institution of antimicrobial therapy does influence the fertility outcome.[2]

Pelvic inflammatory disease should always be treated with at least two antibiotics for at least 10–14 days (Fig. 53.3). The combination regimen of an extended-spectrum parenteral cephalosporin plus doxycycline provides good coverage for all potential pathogens, including beta-lactamase-producing strains. There are no data on the use of oral cephalosporins for the treatment of PID. An alternative parenteral in-patient regimen is the combination of clindamycin plus an aminoglycoside. Although this combination provides coverage against gonococcal and chlamydial infections, it is inferior to the cephalosorin–doxycycline combination for these pathogens. The combination of ofloxacin and clindamycin or metronidazole also provides excellent coverage.

Many experts recommend that all PID patients should be hospitalized to receive optimal therapy, although this is not always possible. Hospitalization is recommend for women with an uncertain tolerance or compliance with outpatient regimens, factors that complicate treatment, severe illness, or an uncertain diagnosis (Fig. 53.4).

Supportive therapy includes hydration, bedrest in the semi-Fowler position to localize the infection to the pelvis, pelvic rest and pain relief. Intrauterine devices should be removed. The patient should abstain from sexual intercourse until test-of-cure studies and resolution of signs and symptoms. All sexual partners in the previous 30 days should be evaluated and presumptively treated for gonococcal and chlamydial infection. Explicit and clear patient education cannot be overemphasized in the treatment of PID, especially in the context of outpatient management.

The incidence of PID among pregnant women is unknown but is believed to be rare.[15] However, given the high-risk of miscarriage and pre-term delivery associated with PID, pregnant women with PID must be hospitalized and given parenteral antibiotics therapy.[10]

Women with tubo-ovarian abscesses should be hospitalized and begun on broad-spectrum antibiotics (aminoglycoside plus clindamycin or metronidazole). The vast majority of abscesses with a diameter of 4–6cm respond to antibiotics alone, whereas only 40% of those that are 10cm or larger respond to medical therapy alone.[16] Increasing abscess size or failure to defervesce 72 hours after administration of antibiotics suggests medical failure and requires surgical intervention (e.g. percutaneous or transvaginal drainage under sonographic guidance, laparoscopic drainage

Number and severity of episodes of salpingitis	Age 15–24 years	Age 25–34 years	Total
0	0	0	0
1	9.4	19.2	11.4
Mild	3.5	7.8	6.1
Moderate	10.8	22.0	13.4
Severe	27.3	40.0	30.0
2	20.9	31.0	23.1
≥3	51.6	60.0	54.3

Fig. 53.2 Prevalence of tubal infertility after salpingitis, Lund, Sweden, 1960–1979.[2]

or laparotomy). Leaking or ruptured abscesses require immediate laparotomy after stabilization of the patient. Extensive surgery such as complete hysterectomy is rarely indicated except in life-threatening complications such as extensive necrotic myometrium.

POSTPARTUM ENDOMETRITIS AND CESAREAN SECTION

EPIDEMIOLOGY

Postpartum endometritis, an infection of the uterus, is the most common cause of maternal postpartum fever and includes the inflammatory conditions of endometritis, endomyometritis and endoparametritis. It can be categorized into early infection, i.e. onset within 48 hours of delivery, and late infection, i.e. onset 2 days to 2 weeks after delivery. The most significant risk factor for postpartum endometritis is cesarean section. The incidence of postpartum endometritis after vaginal delivery is 2–5% whereas the rate after cesarean section ranges from 20 to 55%.[17] Postpartum upper tract infections following vaginal delivery are about 10 times more common in developing countries than in developed countries as a result of unclean delivery practice, traditional birth practices and the high prevalence of STDs in some populations.[18]

PATHOGENESIS AND PATHOLOGY

Early postpartum endometritis usually is associated with nonelective cesarean section and is probably the result of direct uterine contamination by organisms in the amniotic cavity. This is in direct contrast to women who develop late postpartum endometritis, who usually deliver vaginally. The timing of these late infections suggest an ascending infection similar to the mechanisms for PID. Wound infections after cesarean section appear to be a result of a direct contamination of the wound by organisms in the endometrium at the time of surgery.

Postpartum endometritis is a mixed aerobic–anaerobic infection (Fig. 53.5). *Ureaplasma urealyticum* and *Mycoplasma hominis* have also been isolated from the endometrium and blood but their clinical significance is not clear. *Chlamydia trachomatis* is associated with the late form of postpartum endometritis.[19] Group A β-hemolytic streptococcal endometritis is rare and clustered cases are probably related to a common source, often a care-giver. Bacteremia occurs in 10–20% of patients and most common blood isolates are group B streptococci, *Gardnerella vaginalis* and *Peptostreptococcus* spp.[20]

PREVENTION

The timely diagnosis and treatment of lower tract syndromes during pregnancy, especially bacterial vaginosis, would prevent some postpartum endometritis. Prophylactic antibiotic use for patients requiring a nonelective cesarean section after labor or rupture of membranes of any duration greatly reduces the incidence of postcesarean endometritis.[16,21]

CLINICAL FEATURES

Risk factors for postpartum endometritis include duration of labor, length of time membranes remain ruptured, presence of STDs, presence of bacterial vaginosis, the number of vaginal examinations, the use of internal fetal monitoring and socioeconomic status.[20,22,23]

Postpartum endometritis should be suspected in any woman who develops significant fever [oral temperature 101.3°F (38.5°C) or higher in the first 24 hours after delivery or 100.4°F (38°C) or higher for at least 4 consecutive hours, 24 hours or more after delivery]. The diagnosis of postpartum endometritis can be made on the basis of clinical features of fever and when signs on physical examination suggest an endometrial inflammatory process including abdominal pain, uterine tenderness, foul lochia, and uterine subinvolution. Late onset endometritis tends to have a mild, subacute clinical presentation.

RECOMMENDED TREATMENT OF PELVIC INFLAMMATORY DISEASE		
Oral treatment		
Regimen A	Either	Cefoxitin 2g im plus probenecid 1g po in a single dose concurrently, or
		Ceftriaxone 250mg im, or
		Other parenteral third-generation cephalosporin (e.g. ceftizoxime or cefotaxime)
	Plus	Doxycycline 100mg po q12h for 14 days
	Plus	Metronidazole 500mg po q8h for 7 days
Regimen B		Ofloxacin 400mg po q12h for 14 days
	Plus either	Clindamycin 450mg po q6h for 14 days, or
		Metronidazole 500mg po q12h for 14 days
Parenteral treatment		
Regimen A	Either	Cefoxitin 2g iv q6h, or
		Cefotetan 2g iv q12h
	Plus	Doxycycline 100mg iv or po q12h
This regimen should be continued for 48 hours after substantial clinical improvement. Doxycycline 100mg orally q12h should then be administered for a total of 14 days.		
Regimen B		Clindamycin 900mg iv q8h
	Plus	Gentamicin loading dose iv or im (2mg/kg body weight) followed by a maintenance dose of 1.5mg/kg q8h
This regimen should be continued for 48 hours after substantial clinical improvement. Doxycycline 100mg po q12h or clindamycin 450mg po q6h should then be administered for a total of 14 days.		

Fig. 53.3 Recommended treatment of pelvic inflammatory disease.[10]

RECOMMENDATIONS FOR HOSPITALIZATION OF PATIENTS WITH PELVIC INFLAMMATORY DISEASE	
Uncertain tolerance or compliance with outpatient regimen	Adolescents
	Substance abusers
	Nausea and vomiting
	Follow-up at 72 hours after starting antibiotic treatment is problematic
Complicating factors	Pregnancy
	HIV infection
	Intrauterine device use
	Suspected pelvic or tubo-ovarian abscess
	Recent history of intrauterine instrumentation
Severe illness	Temperature over 101°F (38.3°C)
	White blood cell count greater than 15,000/ml
	Peritoneal signs
	Septic
Uncertain diagnosis	Failure to respond clinically to outpatient treatment
	Inability to exclude surgical emergencies (ectopic pregnancy, appendicitis)

Fig. 53.4 Recommendations for hospitalization of patients with pelvic inflammatory disease.

Acute complications of postpartum endometritis include pelvic abscess and puerperal ovarian vein thrombophlebitis. Puerperal ovarian vein thrombophlebitis is an acute thrombosis of one or both ovarian veins postpartum and is usually associated with postpartum endometritis with an onset of 2–4 days after delivery. The reported incidence is 1 in 2000 deliveries.[24] Chronic complications and sequelae result from postinfectious scarring.

DIAGNOSIS

Blood cultures should be obtained from all patients before starting therapy. Tests for the detection of cervical infection with *N. gonorrhoeae* and *C. trachomatis* should be obtained from all women at risk of STDs (in women failing initial therapy). Quantitative endometrial cultures obtained using a triple lumen catheter, which minimizes contamination, provides useful information. A complete white blood cell count should be done. If an adnexal mass is felt on examination, ultrasound or CT can be used to confirm the diagnosis.

MANAGEMENT

Mild to moderately severe postpartum endometritis is commonly treated parenterally with broad-spectrum antibiotics, including the second generation cephalosporins (cefoxitin or cefotetan) or the extended-spectrum penicillins (ticarcillin–clavulanate or sulbactam–ampicillin).[23] In more severe illness, an aminoglycoside plus clindamycin is a good regimen to use. Women should continue to receive parenteral therapy until fever has resolved, uterine tenderness and abdominal pain are gone and white blood cell count has normalized. Subsequent oral antibiotic therapy with erythromycin or doxycycline need only be given to women with documented chlamydial infection for a total of 10–14 days. Reasons for failure to respond to antimicrobial therapy include inappropriate antibiotics (enterococcal infection or resistant anaerobic infection), pelvic or wound abscess, or ovarian vein thrombophlebitis. When postpartum septic pelvic thrombophlebitis is suspected heparin should be given.[25] Late postpartum endometritis can be managed in the same way as PID (Fig. 53.3).

EPISIOTOMY INFECTIONS

EPIDEMIOLOGY

Episiotomy infections are rare. The rate of infection of episiotomies is 0.1% overall but increases to 1–2% of episiotomies complicated by third- or fourth-degree extensions. Episiotomy infections, however, can have severe and even fatal consequences.

PATHOGENESIS AND PATHOLOGY

Episiotomy infections have been classified into four categories based on the depth of infection in the soft tissue: simple infection, superficial fascial infection, superficial fascial necrosis and myonecrosis.[26]

Bacteria implicated in episiotomy infections include skin pathogens, streptococci and staphylococci, and bacteria associated with vaginal flora, Enterobacteriaceae and anaerobic bacteria, including *Bacteroides fragilis*. *Clostridium perfringens* and *Clostridium sordellii* are likely if myonecrosis is present.

COMMON ENDOGENOUS MICRO-ORGANISMS IDENTIFIED AS POTENTIAL ETIOLOGIC AGENTS IN POSTOPERATIVE PELVIC INFECTIONS	
Aerobic bacteria	*Streptococcus* spp. *Enterococcus faecalis* *Staphylococcus aureus* *Staphylococcus epidermidis* *Escherichia coli* *Klebsiella mirabilis* *Gardnerella vaginalis*
Anaerobic bacteria	*Bacteroides* spp. *Peptostreptococcus* spp. *Prevotella bivia* *Prevotella disiens* *Fusobacterium* spp.
Mycoplasmas	*Mycoplasma hominis* *Ureaplasma urealyticum*

Fig. 53.5 Common endogenous micro-organisms identified as potential etiologic agents in postoperative pelvic infections.

PREVENTION

Treatment standards should be introduced that reduce the liberal or routine use of episiotomies, as they appear to increase the risk of third- and fourth-degree tears.

CLINICAL FEATURES

The simple wound infection is a local infection limited to incision site in the skin and the superficial fascia. Clinically there is edema and erythema only along the incision. A superficial fascial infection involves two layers of the superficial fascia and resembles a cellulitis with erythema, edema and pain. This superficial infection is indistinguishable on the basis of skin appearance from an early superficial fascial infection with necrosis (necrotizing fasciitis). Necrotizing fasciitis involves all layers of the superficial fascia (and may involve the deep fascia). Skin anesthesia may precede the skin breakdown caused by involvement of nerves. As nutrient vessels are occluded the skin may turn dusky, and develop bullae and then frank necrosis. Subcutaneous gas may be present with the mixed infection. These patients often have evidence of marked toxicity out of proportion to the clinical findings. In myonecrosis, pain is often the dominant feature. Patients are extremely toxic, restless, and confused or disoriented.

DIAGNOSIS

Prompt diagnosis is of paramount importance because necrotizing fasciitis and myonecrosis are rapidly progressive. Frozen section examination of full depth biopsy specimens has been helpful in the diagnosis of necrotizing faciitis.[27] However, surgical exploration is warranted if necrotizing fasciitis or myonecrosis are suspected.

MANAGEMENT

Management of a simple episiotomy wound infection includes opening of the incision and exploration to ensure that there is no accumulated blood or a rectovaginal opening. Any superficial fascial infection should be managed with broad-spectrum antibiotic coverage (e.g. ampicillin–gentamicin–metronidazole or ampicillin–gentamicin–clindamycin) and observed closely. Surgical exploration should be undertaken if:
- erythema and edema extend beyond the incision site;
- there is no improvement in 24–48 hours after the start of antibiotics or if the patient deteriorates; or
- the patient has severe systemic manifestations.

In the case of necrotizing fasciitis the superficial fascia will separate easily from the deep fascia with a probe or finger (this does not occur in healthy tissue), the incisions will be bloodless and the exudate will be serosanguineous rather than purulent. Surgical debridement of all necrotic and pale tissue should be performed promptly and broad-spectrum antibiotic therapy should be instituted. The wound should be left open after debridement. A second-look procedure is often necessary after 24 hours.

Myonecrosis is an extremely rare event that is usually caused by *C. perfringens* or *C. sordellii* but may result from an extension of necrotizing fasciitis through the deep fascia to the muscle. Therapy includes high-dose penicillin and urgent surgical debridement. Hyperbaric oxygen therapy remains controversial and should be considered only as an adjunctive therapy.

POSTABORTION SEPSIS

EPIDEMIOLOGY

Postabortion sepsis is an ascending infection of the female pelvis after spontaneous or induced abortions. Inflammatory conditions associated with infectious complications of abortions are similar to those for PID, but can be complicated by retained, poorly perfused tissue and uterine or bowel trauma. The mortality from abortions in developed countries is low (an estimated 0.6 per 100,000 cases), and abortion accounts for 5% of all maternal mortality in the USA. Infection is the major cause when mortality does result from abortion complications. In a review of 107 deaths caused by abortion in the USA between 1975 and 1977, 33% were caused by sepsis.[28] In developing countries the World Health Organization estimates that illegal abortion accounts for 25–50% of the 500,000 maternal deaths that occur each year.

PATHOGENESIS AND PATHOLOGY

The bacteria associated with postabortion sepsis are similar to those associated with PID. However, the potential of direct uterine or bowel injury, and retention of the products of conception after an abortion may result in injured and poorly vascularized tissue and an enlarged spectrum of enteric organisms, including *C. perfringens*. In developing countries, tetanus is a cause of mortality after abortion.

PREVENTION

Prevention measures include providing effective and acceptable contraception and appropriate medical management of abortion. Prophylaxis for cervical and vaginal infections before voluntary termination of pregnancy, has been suggested as a preventive measure but there are few data to support this practice. Prompt diagnosis and effective treatment of endometritis after the procedure is extremely important as delayed treatment is a common feature in cases of death from septic abortion.

CLINICAL FEATURES

The diagnosis of septic abortion should be considered in any woman with a temperature of 100.4°F (38°C) or higher on two occasions more than 24 hours after an abortion and in any woman of reproductive age who presents with fever, abdominal pain and bleeding. Additionally, details of the procedure, including microbiologic studies and pathology of the aborted tissues, should be obtained. Physical examination findings typically include uterine tenderness, foul or purulent cervical discharge and products of conception at the cervical os. In more severe infections the patient may be hypotensive or in shock. The presence of cervical or vaginal lacerations should be assessed. Women with clostridial infection may have severe disseminated intravascular hemolysis.

Acute complications are seen in advanced stages of the disease process and include the respiratory distress syndrome, septic shock, renal failure, abscess formation, septic pelvic vein thrombophlebitis and septic emboli, and disseminated intravascular coagulopathy; death may also occur. The chronic complications are similar to those of PID and include infertility, chronic pelvic pain and ectopic pregnancy.

DIAGNOSIS

Except for women with mild, early, uncomplicated postabortion endometritis, all women should have blood and cervical cultures as well as a complete white blood cell count and urinalysis. Upright and flat abdominal and pelvic radiographs should be done to assess the presence of air in the abdominal cavity, dilated bowel and gas in the uterus. Pelvic ultrasound can determine the presence of retained tissue and other fluid collections, and the disruption of the myometrium by fluid or gas. Computed tomography is useful in assessing the entire abdomen. Laparoscopy can be used to examine the uterus for perforation but is suboptimal for a detailed examination of the bowel.[29]

MANAGEMENT

Any woman with an incomplete or failed abortion or retained clotted or liquid blood (hematometra) should undergo immediate re-evacuation.[30] This tissue serves as a nidus for infection. The recommended treatment of PID (Fig. 53.3) is appropriate for a woman with early, uncomplicated postabortion infection limited to the endometrial cavity. The patient should be evaluated 48 hours after institution of therapy. If fever or pain persist the patient should be hospitalized and evaluated as above.

Women with more severe illness should be hospitalized and begun on broad-spectrum antibiotics such as ampicillin, gentamicin and clindamycin. If clostridial infection is suspected, high dose penicillin therapy should be used. These patients should be monitored closely and aggressively evaluated for uterine perforation and bowel injury. Laparotomy with possible hysterectomy should be performed if there is failure to respond to uterine evacuation and medical therapy, uterine perforation with necrotic myometrium or suspected bowel injury, pelvic and adnexal abscesses, or clostridial myometritis. Indications for a total hysterectomy with removal of adnexae include a discolored, woody appearance of the uterus and adnexae, clostridial sepsis, pelvic tissue crepitation and gas in the uterine wall on radiographs.

POSTOPERATIVE GYNECOLOGIC INFECTIONS

EPIDEMIOLOGY

Hysterectomy is the most frequently performed elective surgical procedure among women of reproductive age in the USA.[31] The spectrum of postoperative infections after hysterectomy include vaginal cuff cellulitis, pelvic cellulitis, vaginal cuff abscess, phlegmon, pelvic abscess and wound infections.[21] Rates of infection after abdominal hysterectomy without antibiotic prophylaxis ranged from 11 to 38% and from 4 to 8% with antibiotic prophylaxis. For vaginal hysterectomies without antibiotic prophylaxis infection rates varied between 12 and 64% and with prophylaxis from 0 to 10%.[32] Risk factors for postoperative infection include duration of surgery, younger age, lower socioeconomic status and the presence of bacterial vaginosis.

PATHOGENESIS AND PATHOLOGY

Bacterial contamination of the operative site with flora of the lower reproductive tract occurs at the vaginal incision. The exposure in a vaginal hysterectomy occurs from the initial vaginal incision throughout the procedure and the exposure in an abdominal hysterectomy occurs near the end of the procedure. Hospitalization itself, regardless of whether antimicrobial prophylaxis is given, changes the vaginal flora, resulting in an increase in colony counts of *Escherichia coli*, *Enterococcus faecalis* and *Bacteroides* spp. and a decline in *Staphylococcus epidermidis* and *Streptococcus* and *Peptostreptococcus* spp.

Postoperative infections involve a mix of aerobic and anaerobic bacteria from the lower reproductive tract (Fig. 53.5). *Bacteroides fragilis* and *Fusobacteria* spp. are more common in infections than when they are found in normal vaginal flora.

PREVENTION

Patients undergoing elective hysterectomy should be screened and, if needed, treated for bacterial vaginosis several weeks before surgery. Preoperative single-dose antibiotic prophylaxis substantially reduces the rate of postoperative febrile morbidity in these procedures.[21,32]

CLINICAL FEATURES

Postoperative fever itself does not indicate infection but should prompt the clinician to evaluate the patient for one. In pelvic cellulitis symptoms usually occur 2–3 days after surgery and include fever [temperature over 100.4°F (38°C)] and complaints of increasing abdominal and pelvic pain that may not be symmetric.[33] Parametrial tenderness without palpable mass is found on bimanual examination. Histologic vaginal cuff cellulitis will develop in all women postoperatively as part of the normal healing process and most cases resolve without antibiotic therapy. Women with more severe cellulitis will complain of increasing central or lower abdominal pain, increasing vaginal discharge or low grade fever, usually within the first 2 weeks postoperatively. Bimanual pelvic examination may show only mild suprapubic tenderness to deep palpation without masses. Speculum examination will show a tender, indurated, hyperemic vaginal surgical margin. In a vaginal cuff abscess patients typically have fever 2 or 3 days postoperatively and may report vaginal fullness. On examination a tender, palpable collection will be found above the vaginal surgical margin. A phlegmon would be diagnosed if a tender mass were felt in one or both parametrial areas and if no abscess could be identified on radiographic studies. Pelvic abscesses are a late postoperative complication that present many weeks after surgery and most have palpable mass in the pelvis. Wound infections are characterized by pain, marginal cellulitis and purulent exudate.

Septic pelvic vein thrombophlebitis and osteomyelitis pubis are both rare complications of gynecologic surgery.

DIAGNOSIS

Microbiologic cultures obtained from drained abscesses are useful in guiding therapy. Cultures of the vaginal cuff are likely to be contaminated with vaginal flora. Abdominal and pelvic ultrasound and CT scans are useful to confirm the presence of a fluid collection when pelvic abscesses are suspected.

MANAGEMENT

Patients who have pelvic cellulitis should be treated with a broad-spectrum parenteral antibiotic regimen, such as a second-generation cephalosporin (cefoxitin or cefotetan), extended-spectrum penicillin (ticarcillin–clavulanate or sulbactam–ampicillin), or an aminoglycoside plus clindamycin, for 24–36 hours after the patient becomes afebrile. Cuff abscesses should be managed similarly and the abscess should be drained. Vaginal cuff cellulitis can be managed on an outpatient basis with oral antibiotics such as amoxicillin–clavulanic acid, but patients should have a follow-up evaluation 72 hours after starting therapy. Medical therapy that covers Gram-negative aerobes and Gram-negative anaerobes (aminoglycoside–clindamycin or aminoglycoside–metronidazole) is often successful in treating postoperative pelvic abscesses that are inaccessible to drainage. Patients who fail to respond to medical therapy alone (no defervescence in 72 hours or enlarging abscess) will require laparotomy and drainage, or excision. Abscesses accessible from a cutaneous surface should be drained. Patients should be treated with parenteral antibiotics until all signs and symptoms have resolved. Some clinicians give postdischarge outpatient treatment with metronidazole and amoxicillin for a week after discharge in those patients who responded to medical management. All patients with pelvic abscesses should be re-evaluated 2 weeks after discharge to ensure no recurrence of the abscess has occurred.

REFERENCES

1. Centers for Disease Control and Prevention. Policy guidelines for prevention and management of pelvic inflammatory disease. MMWR Morb Mortal Wkly Rep 1991;40:1–25.
2. Weström L, Märdh P-A. Acute pelvic inflammatory disease (PID). In: Holmes KK, Märdh P-A, Sparling PF, Wiesner PJ, eds. Sexually transmitted diseases. New York: McGraw-Hill; 1990:593–613.
3. Sweet RL. Role of bacterial vaginosis in pelvic inflammatory disease. Clin Infect Dis 1995;20(Suppl 2):271–5.
4. Farley TMM, Rosenberg MJ, Rowe PJ, Chen JH, Meirick O. Intrauterine devices and pelvic inflammatory disease: an international perspective. Lancet 1992;339:785–8.
5. Wolner-Hanssen P, Eschenbach DA, Paavonen J, et al. Decreased risk of chlamydial pelvic inflammatory disease associated with oral contraceptive use. JAMA 1990;263:54–9.
6. Cates W, Rolfs RT, Aral SO. Sexually transmitted diseases, pelvic inflammatory disease and infertility. An epidemiologic update. Epidemiol Rev 1990;12:199–220.
7. Scholes D, Stergachis A, Heidrich FE, et al. Prevention of pelvic inflammatory disease by screening for cervical chlamydial infection. N Engl J Med 1996;334:1362–6.
8. Sweet RL, Landers DV. Pelvic inflammatory disease in HIV-positive women. Lancet 1997;349:1265–6.
9. Sellors J, Mahony J, Goldsmith C, et al. The accuracy of clinical findings and laparoscopy in pelvic inflammatory disease. Am J Obstet Gynecol 1991;164:113–20.
10. Centers for Disease Control and Prevention. Guidelines for treatment of sexually transmitted diseases. Pelvic inflammatory disease. MMWR Morb Mortal Wkly Rep 1997;47:79–86.
11. Taourel P, Pradel J, Fabre JM, et al. Role of CT in the acute nontraumatic abdomen. Sem Ultrasound CT MRI 1995;16:151–64.

12. Urban BA, Fishman EK. Spiral CT of the female pelvis: clinical applications. Abdom Imaging 1995;20:9–14.
13. Soper DE. Diagnosis and laparoscopic grading of acute salpingitis. Am J Obstet Gynecol 1991;164:1370–6.
14. Dodson MG. Antibiotic regimens for treating acute pelvic inflammatory disease: an evaluation. J Reprod Med 1994;39:285–96.
15. Brunham RC, Holmes KK, Embree JE. Sexually transmitted diseases in pregnancy. In: Holmes KK, Märdh P-A, Sparling PF, Wiesner PJ, eds. Sexually transmitted diseases. New York: McGraw-Hill; 1990:771–801.
16. Amstey MS, Sweet R. Definition of pelvic abscess. Am J Obstet Gynecol 1993;168:740–1.
17. Faro S, Martens MG, Mannill HA, et al. Antibiotic prophylaxis: is there a difference? Am J Obstet Gynecol 1990;162:900–9.
18. Meheus A. Women's health: importance of reproductive tract infections, pelvis inflammatory disease and cervical cancer. In: Germain A, Holmes KK, Piot P, Wasserheit JN, eds. Reproductive tract infections: global impact and priorities for women's reproductive health. New York: Plenum Press; 1992:61–91.
19. Hoyme UB, Kivian N, Eschenbach DA. The microbiology and treatment of late postpartum endometritis. Obstet Gynecol 1986;68:226–32.
20. Watts DH, Eschenbach DA, Kenny GE. Early postpartum endometritis: The role of bacteria, genital mycoplasmas, and Chlamydia trachomatis. Obstet Gynecol 1989;73:52–60.
21. Hemsell DL. Prophylactic antibiotics in gynecologic and obstetric surgery. Rev Infect Dis 1991;13(Suppl 10):821–41.
22. Newton ER, Prihoda TA, Gibbs RS. A clinical and microbiologic analysis of risk factors for puerperal endometritis. Obstet Gynecol 1990;75:402–6.

23. Watts DH, Krohn MA, Hillier SL, Eschenbach DA. Bacterial vaginosis as a risk factor for post-cesarean endometritis. Obstet Gynecol 1990;75:52–8.
24. Duff P, Gibbs RS. Pelvic vein thrombophlebitis: diagnostic dilemma and therapeutic challenge. Obstet Gynecol Surv 1983;38:365–73.
25. Hamadeh G, Dedmon C, Mozley P. Post partum fever. Am Fam Physician 1995;52:531–8.
26. Shy KK, Eschenbach DA. Fatal perineal cellulitis from an episiotomy site. Obstet Gynecol 1979;54:292–8.
27. Stamenkovic I, Lew PD. Early recognition of potentially fatal necrotizing fasciitis: Use of frozen-section biopsy. N Engl J Med 1984;310:1689–93.
28. Grimes Da, Cates W Jr. Complications from legally induced abortion: a review. Obstet Gynecol Surv 1979;34:177–91.
29. Grimes DA, Cates W Jr, Selik RM. Fatal septic abortion in the United States, 1975–1977. Obstet Gynecol 1981;57:739–44.
30. Chow AW, Marshall JR, Guze LB. A double-blind comparison of clindamycin with penicillin plus chloramphenicol in treatment of septic abortion. J Infect Dis 1977;135(Suppl):35–9.
31. Dicker RC, Greenspan JR, Strauss LT, et al. Complications of abdominal and vaginal hysterectomy among women of reproductive age in the United States. Am J Obstet Gynecol 1982;144:841–8.
32. Polk BF. Antimicrobial prophylaxis to prevent mixed bacterial infection. J Antimicrob Chemother 1981;8(Suppl D):115–29.
33. Hemsell DL, Nobles B, Heard MC. Recognition and treatment of post-hysterectomy pelvic infections. Infect Surg 1988;7:47–68.

Complications of Pregnancy: Maternal Perspectives

chapter
54

Marleen Temmerman

EPIDEMIOLOGY

Medical progress, such as effective antibiotics and vaccines, in combination with improved living conditions have modified the sequelae of infections, yet infectious morbidity in pregnancy remains a serious problem.

Any acute or chronic infection may occur before conception, during pregnancy or during the puerperium and may have serious consequences for the mother, the fetus and the neonate. Some microorganisms are known to cause congenital infections and are discussed in Chapter 2.55. Others primarily influence the health of pregnant women and are described below.

The problem of maternal infections during pregnancy is addressed with emphasis on organ systems, including genitourinary tract infections respiratory tract infections, gastrointestinal infections, puerperal

sepsis, wound infection, mastitis, thrombophlebitis, endocarditis and meningitis. The infectious etiology of pre-term birth, premature pre-term rupture of membranes (pPROM) and chorioamnionitis deserves special attention. In addition, the implications of specific infections, including malaria, listeriosis, Lyme disease, varicella-zoster, HIV and other sexually transmitted diseases (STDs), are summarized in Figures 54.1 and 54.2.

The topic of infections in pregnancy is too wide to summarize in a single chapter. The interested reader will find excellent reviews by Sweet and Gibbs, Ledger, Hurley and Charles.[1-4]

INCIDENCE AND PREVALENCE

Genital micro-organisms, particularly sexually transmitted organisms, are important in poor pregnancy outcome, including pre-term birth,

IMPLICATIONS OF SPECIFIC INFECTIONS ON PREGNANCY			
	Impact on mother and child	Prevention	Management
Malaria	• More frequent, more severe in pregnancy, especially in nonimmune women; increased risk of hypoglycemia in the mother • LBW, IUGR, pre-term birth, abortion and stillbirth increased • Congenital malaria (fever, hepatosplenomegaly, jaundice, anemia)	Chemoprophylaxis in travelers to endemic areas If no *Plasmodium falciparum* resistance, chloroquine phosphate 500mg/week po In case of resistance proguanil 200mg/day + chloroquine 500mg/week po Avoid exposure	Prompt treatment with chloroquine or quinine according to resistance patterns Similar treatment regimens to those in nonpregnant women
Listeriosis	• Mild maternal infection, but increased susceptibility • Serious impact on the fetus: amnionitis, pre-term birth, septic abortion, stillbirth, fatality rate 3–50%	Early diagnosis in any febrile illness in pregnancy, cervical and blood cultures for *Listeria monocytogenes* Avoid implicated foods, e.g. unpasteurized cheese	Ampicillin 2g q6h iv + gentamicin 2mg/kg q8h for 1 week
Lyme disease	• Erythema migrans in the mother, risk of transmission unknown, probably low • Pre-term birth, stillbirth, syndactyle, cortical blindness,rash	Protective clothes in tick-infected areas (rural forest); remove ticks	Early treatment with amoxicillin 500mg q6h po for 10–30 days or ceftriaxone 2g iv for 14 days
Varicella-zoster	• Rare in adults, fever, malaise followed by rash, 20% risk of varicella pneumonia • Risk of abortion, stillbirth • Congenital varicella (limb hypoplasia, cortical atrophy, retardation, IUGR, cutaneous scars, microphthalmia)	IgG testing if exposed If no IgG: varicella-zoster immunoglobulin 125U/10kg, max 625 U im, <96h after exposure	In cases of pneumonia: admission, respiratory support, aciclovir 10–15mg/kg for 7days Ultrasound assessment of the fetus
Measles	• Increased maternal mortality secondary to pneumonia • Risk of prematurity • Developmental abnormalities (e.g. congenital heart disease, cleft lip, cerebral leukodystrophy and cyclopia have been reported)	Passive immunization in susceptible exposed women with pooled immunoglobulins 0.25ml/kg within 6 days of exposure Avoid measles vaccine in pregnancy	Symptomatic
Group B streptococci	Sepsis in 1–3/1000 neonates, high mortality rates	No consensus Antenatal case detection and treatment, or intrapartum treatment of women at risk?	Ampicillin 2g q4h iv in labor

LBW, low birth weight; IUGR, intrauterine growth retardation

Fig. 54.1 Implications of specific infections on pregnancy.

IMPLICATIONS OF SOME SEXUALLY TRANSMITTED INFECTIONS ON PREGNANCY			
	Impact on mother and child	Prevention	Management
Neisseria gonorrhoeae	Ophthalmia nenatorum, pre-term delivery, puerperal infections	Silver nitrate 1% or tetracycline eye ointment	Spectinomycin 2g im, ceftriaxone 250mg im, or standard antimicrobial treatment
Chlamydia trachomatis	Ophthalmia neonatorum, puerperal infections, pre-term delivery	Tetracycline eye ointment	Erythromycin 500mg for 4–7 days
Bacterial vaginosis	Risk of pre-term birth	Case detection and treatment is still under study	Metronidazole 250mg for 3–7 days or erythromycin base 333mg for 3–14 days
Trichomonas vaginalis	Risk of pre-term birth	Case detection and treatment no proven effect	Metronidazole 2g single dose
Condylomata acuminata	Risk of respiratory papillomatoses 1/80–1/1500	Case detection and treatment	Topical trichloroacetic acid (85%)/surgery
Herpes simplex	• Neonatal herpes 50% in mother with primary herpes at delivery	History from pregnant woman, careful inspection of the genital tract on the day of delivery	In cases of active lesions, cesarean section or vaginal delivery under aciclovir 200–400 mg q8h (under study)
HIV	• Transmission in 25–45% • Risk of abortion, pre-term delivery, puerperal infections	Zidovudine from 14 weeks –>6 weeks postpartum	Avoid long labor, rupture of membranes >4h Treat neonate with zidovudine

Fig. 54.2 Implications of some sexually transmitted diseases on pregnancy.

pPROM, spontaneous abortion, perinatal morbidity and mortality, and maternal infections.[5–12] Recent publications confirm the role of *Neisseria gonorrhoeae* in low birth weight and in spontaneous abortion, of bacterial vaginosis in pre-term birth, and of genital mycoplasmas in pPROM and in postpartum febrile infections in women and neonates. Bacterial vaginosis has received renewed attention because of its role in pre-term delivery, and because it is possibly prone to interventions. The prevalence of bacterial vaginosis varies between 15 and 25%. Group B streptococci (GBS), which are known to be a risk factor for neonatal infections and pre-term birth, also contribute to spontaneous abortion. The reported rates of GBS colonization in the genital tract range from 5 to 40%, with an average transmission rate to the neonate of 60%. The rates of early-onset GBS infection in the neonate, especially in pre-term and low birth weight babies, can be as high as 3 in 1000.

Prevalence rates of HIV in pregnant women are increasing all over the world, but have reached endemic proportions in developing countries, where over 25% of pregnant women in some urban areas are HIV seropositive. The impact of maternal HIV infection on pregnancy outcome is still debated but most data from large studies of pregnant women who do not use drugs show an increased risk of adverse obstetric outcome, including abortion, prematurity, low birth weight and stillbirth, with perinatal HIV transmission rates of 15–40%.

Urinary tract infections (UTIs) are the most common infections in pregnancy, with or without clinical signs or symptoms. Asymptomatic bacteriuria is found in 4–7% of pregnant women, of whom 25–30% will develop pyelonephritis later in pregnancy.

Upper respiratory tract infections are common but of limited consequences for mother and child. In contrast, pneumonia is a serious illness for a pregnant woman.

Gastrointestinal infections caused by viruses are usually mild with no harm to the pregnancy and no need for specific medication. Meningitis is rare except for areas in which HIV and cryptococcal meningitis are endemic. Bacterial endocarditis is also uncommon and incidence rates vary from 1 in 4000 to 1 in 16,000 deliveries.

Febrile illness at delivery is uncommon in uncomplicated term pregnancies. Common underlying causes are chorioamnionitis, pyelonephritis, influenza and listeriosis.

The overall incidence of postpartum infections varies between 1 and 10% depending on definitions used, particularly for mastitis and postpartum endometritis. Postpartum infections consist of genital tract infections, puerperal mastitis, pelvic thrombophlebitis, UTIs, wound infections, complications of anesthesia and other infectious complications.

Genital tract infections of the uterus are the most common cause of puerperal infection and are categorized as endometritis, endomyometritis or endoparametritis depending on the extent of the infection. Wound and episiotomy infections occur frequently. After cesarean section wound infection defined as erythema, positive discharge and/or positive wound cultures varies between 5 and 10%, with emergency cases at higher risk of infection.

Septic thrombophlebitis is a rare complication of pregnancy with reported incidence rates of 1 in 2000 deliveries. The incidence of puerperal mastitis is estimated at around 1% in lactating women. Most have a mild disease.

BURDEN OF DISEASE, MORBIDITY AND MORTALITY

In the general population the attributable risk of infections for adverse pregnancy outcome depends on the prevalence rates of infections in the population as well as on the socioeconomic and cultural factors that influence health, health behavior and health-seeking behavior. All infections that manifest with fever increase the risk of pre-term birth because of the release of pyrogens that increase myometrial activity.

Intra-amniotic infection diagnosed on clinical criteria occurs in 1–5% of pregnancies, with or without ruptured membranes. Consequences are pre-term birth, pPROM and postpartum and neonatal infections. The mother and the fetus are put at risk with pPROM, as it is associated with pre-term birth and frequent infectious morbidity. Ascending infections, either the cause or the result of pPROM, may lead to intra-amniotic infection, chorioamnionitis, placentitis and fetal infections, including pneumonia and bacteremia.

The impact of asymptomatic UTI on pregnancy complications such as hypertension, anemia and poor obstetric outcome remains controversial. In contrast, ascending UTIs clearly play a role in the etiology of pre-term delivery and neonatal death.

Lower respiratory tract infections, meningitis and bacterial endocarditis are all life-threatening conditions for the mother and should be treated without delay.

Although postpartum infections are seldom life threatening, sepsis remains an important cause of maternal death worldwide. Maternal mortality rates of 1–5 per 100,000 live births are registered in the western world, whereas 100–600 per 100,000 pregnant or child-bearing women in developing countries die as a consequence of reproduction.

In addition, for every woman who dies in childbirth another 30 women suffer from injuries, infections and disabilities. Overall, 25% of maternal mortality is considered to be caused by infections and this number can be lowered substantially by better health services and prompt treatment. A number of reports estimating the role of infections in maternal death are summarized in Figure 54.3. Few etiologic studies have been carried out in developing countries, but the role of infections is likely to be more important. My own personal observations from Nairobi, Kenya indicate that infections play a role in up to 40% of mothers dying in childbirth. The silent tragedy of maternal death should receive more attention from the international community, and also from the research world, because a substantial proportion of maternal deaths as a result of infections, bleeding and eclampsia is avoidable and interventions have to be tested to lower this unacceptable consequence of giving birth.

Postpartum genital infections may lead to chronic pain and discomfort, bleeding irregularities and infertility caused by ascending infections. Wound infections may increase pain and discomfort, and prolong hospital stay. Pelvic vein thrombophlebitis may lead to serious complications such as septic pulmonary emboli.

RISK FACTORS

Poverty is the most important risk factor for maternal infections during pregnancy. Poor women are more susceptible to malnutrition, infections, including STDs, less adequate sanitary conditions and lower access to preventive and curative health care than those who are financially better off.

Risk factors for UTI in pregnancy include sexual activity, older age, history of UTIs, lower socioeconomic status, diabetes mellitus, sickle-cell disease and specific bacterial factors such as the serotype and the virulent determinants of the micro-organisms.

Risk factors for lower respiratory disease include low socio-economic status and HIV infection, particularly for infections with *Streptococcus pneumoniae*. Bacterial endocarditis has been reported more often in urban settings and among drug users.

Risk factors for puerperal genital infections include socio-economic variables, anemia, STD, obstetric factors such as length of rupture of membranes, pre-term delivery, cesarean section and number of vaginal examinations. Puerperal fever caused by group A β-hemolytic streptococci, once one of the most striking examples of iatrogenic infections in the 19th century, is a rare event in modern obstetrics, although sporadic outbreaks have been reported. A toxic-shock-like syndrome can occur caused by the release of pyrogenic exotoxins from streptococcal isolates.

Factors known to increase the risk for wound infections are age, obesity, bacterial contamination, operating time and duration of pre-operative hospitalization, emergency procedures, number of vaginal examinations, duration of internal fetal monitoring, length of labor and underlying maternal disease. Puerperal mastitis can be related to poor nursing techniques and lack of strict hygienic measures.

PATHOGENESIS AND PATHOLOGY

PATHOGENESIS

The pathogenesis of most infections is similar in pregnant and non-pregnant women except for possible alterations in the immune system as noted below. Of specific interest is the role of infectious agents in the onset of labor or, more importantly, of pre-term labor. Although the exact mechanism of the onset of labor is still part of the human parturition puzzle, there is convincing evidence for the role of prostaglandins in the initiation of parturition. Arachidonic acid, one of the precursors of prostaglandins, is made available for prostaglandin synthesis by the enzyme phospholipase A_2. This enzyme, produced by many micro-organisms but especially by anaerobes, might be one of the mechanisms of pre-term initiation of labor. Micro-organisms can stimulate the release of cytokines, such as interleukins and tumor necrosis factor, that stimulate prostaglandin precursors thus leading to uterine contractions.

CASES OF MATERNAL DEATH FROM INFECTIONS		
	Date of study	%
Michigan	1950–1971	23
Iowa	1926–1980	56
	1950–1980	16
South Carolina	1970–1984	14
Oklahoma	1950–1979	7

Fig. 54.3 Cases of maternal death from infections. Data from Sweet and Gibbs.[1]

In theory, the amniotic cavity is sterile, protected by the placental membranes, with the cervical mucus serving as an effective barrier in preventing micro-organisms from entering the uterine cavity. With the onset of labor and the rupture of membranes, bacteria may ascend and result in an amniotic infection. Pathogens may also gain access to the amniotic cavity through intact membranes or after invasive procedures such as amniocentesis, chorion villus sampling, umbilical blood sampling and cervical cerclage.

Urinary tract infections are caused by organisms that are part of the normal fecal flora, with *Escherichia coli* responsible for 80–90% of infections. Others are facultative Gram-negative bacteria, including *Klebsiella*, *Proteus*, *Enterobacter* and *Pseudomonas* spp., and Gram-positive bacteria such as staphylococci and GBS. Symptomatic UTIs are more frequent in pregnancy for several reasons, including decreased ureteric muscle tone and activity, dilatation of the ureter and renal pelvis because of the progesterone effect and mechanical obstruction caused by an enlarging uterus, changes of the bladder and alterations in the properties of urine during pregnancy. Bacteriuria is of concern because of the increased risk of pyelonephritis associated with pre-term labor caused by pyrogens, ureteric contractions leading to reflex myometrial contractions, the release of bacterial enzymes that may weaken the membranes and bacterial products that stimulate prostaglandin synthesis.

The most common organisms causing pneumonia in pregnant women are *S. pneumoniae*, *Haemophilus influenzae*, group A β-hemolytic streptococci and coagulase-positive streptococci.

Postpartum endometritis seems to be a mixed infection with aerobic and anaerobic bacteria from the genital tract. Sexually transmitted diseases, including *Chlamydia trachomatis* and *N. gonorrhoeae*, are important risk factors for ascending infections. Cesarean section is the single most important predisposing factor for pelvic infection. Wound infections are determined by the surgical techniques used, the amount of bacterial contamination and the resistance of the patient. An adequate blood supply is necessary to avoid acidosis in the wound. Organisms involved are *Streptococcus faecalis*, *E. coli*, *Staphylococcus aureus*, *Staphylococcus epidermidis*, *Proteus* spp. and anaerobes. Predisposing factors for septic pelvic thrombophlebitis include changes in coagulation factors, alterations in the vein wall and stasis of blood flow.

In most cases of mastitis, *S. aureus* is the responsible organism, although *S. epidermidis* and viridans streptococci may also be isolated. Sporadic mastitis, usually the result of a poor nursing technique, manifests as a cellulitis of the breast, primarily involving the inter-lobular connective tissue by which the pathogens gain entry via a cracked or fissured nipple. In epidemic mastitis, however, infection occurs via the ductal system and spreads throughout the entire breast, resulting in mammary adenitis.

IMMUNITY

The normal course of pregnancy is associated with a variety of changes in humoral and cellular immunity, such as a loss in CD4 lymphocytes and other alterations in T-lymphocyte subsets.[13–16] Reports on T-lymphocyte subsets during pregnancy have been conflicting. Some studies have found a progressive fall in the CD4 count throughout pregnancy, from a mean of 950 cells/ml before 18 weeks to 720 cells/ml at term. Others have either reported a U-shaped CD4 cell count profile during pregnancy, with a minimum at approximately 32 weeks of gestation (CD4 of 30% and a CD4 count of 876 cells/ml), or have found stable CD4 levels and CD4:CD8 ratios during pregnancy with a rise (rebound) afterwards. Such differences may be attributable to different methodology (manual fluorescence microscopy versus automated flow cytometry), to differences in study populations or to the fact that blood was taken at different times during pregnancy. The altered immune status of pregnant women may also alter the response of the host to infectious agents.

Despite conflicting laboratory data most studies agree that the humoral immune response in pregnancy is similar to that in non-pregnant women, but that the cellular immune response is diminished. Mortality rates of, for example, pneumococcal pneumonia, malaria or influenza have been found to be higher in pregnant than in nonpregnant women.

PREVENTION

Elimination of poverty and improvement of antenatal care attendance in deprived groups of society are primary prevention strategies to adverse pregnancy outcome. The challenge of identifying women at risk of adverse obstetric outcome is still a subject of intensive research. Early markers of infectious illness in pregnant women are needed to identify a subset of the population at risk who could benefit from antimicrobial therapy. The finding of mucopurulent cervicitis defined by >30 polymorphonuclear cells per high-power field has been identified as a predictor of poor pregnancy outcome.[17] Elevated reproductive tract phospholipase A_2 concentrations were detected in pregnant women colonized with bacterial vaginosis, *Trichomonas vaginalis* or *C. trachomatis*.[18] Phospholipase A_2 is an enzyme that leads to prostaglandin synthesis and is important in the physiology of human parturition. Randomized controlled trials, identifying and treating women at risk of pre-term birth by measuring phospholipase A_2 concentration in vaginal fluids, are needed to assess the value of this test. Fetal fibronectin in cervical secretions was found to be a poor predictor of pre-term birth in low-risk women.[19]

Case detection through screening and treatment of pregnant women for common genitourinary infections such as bacterial vaginosis, trichomoniasis, GBS and others, depending on the prevalence of infectious agents in the population, is a generally recommended policy. Recent intervention studies have provided convincing evidence of the benefit of identifying and treating bacterial vaginosis in pregnancy.[8,9] However, more studies are needed to examine the feasibility, the effect and the cost–benefit of screening for bacterial vaginosis in populations with low prevalence rates. Screening for GBS in pregnant women is still a subject of debate. Between 10 and 30% of pregnant women are colonized with GBS, an important source of perinatal morbidity and mortality. Recently, the Centers for Disease Control and Prevention have issued recommendations for the active prevention of GBS, which have been adopted by the American College of Obstetricians and Gynecologists.[22] A risk strategy based on either late prenatal cultures or clinical and historic factors, followed by intrapartum treatment with penicillin or other broad-spectrum antibiotics is recommended. Others argue that routine antimicrobial treatment with a broad-spectrum antibiotic is optimal for pregnant women at high risk of adverse pregnancy outcome in order to reduce the incidence of infectious complications such as pre-term birth, neonatal infections and maternal infectious morbidity.[20] Risk may be based solely on laboratory findings or on clinical and obstetric factors (bad obstetric history, clinical signs and symptoms). However, many questions remain unanswered, especially the benefit of screening and treating low-risk groups and the ideal antimicrobial regimen. The existing evidence is hampered by methodologic weaknesses such as small numbers, use of combination of antibiotics and differences in populations studied. Before definitive practice guidelines can be established it is essential to prove that

the costs and the benefits associated with screening and treating genital infections in pregnant women outweigh the potential risks and effects. Only prospective, randomized and blinded clinical trials with large study populations can determine the effect of antimicrobial therapy on infectious morbidity and mortality in pregnancy.

Intercourse during pregnancy has been implied as a risk factor for pre-term birth. This could be because of the effect of STDs or because of increased myometrial activity and cervical ripening caused by the prostaglandins in sperm. After correcting for STDs, there is little evidence of a causal relation between sexual intercourse and pre-term birth. Randomized trials of condom use versus unprotected sex in high-risk groups for poor pregnancy outcome have not been carried out to date.

Detection and treatment of maternal bacteriuria in early pregnancy, preferably around 16 weeks, can reduce the risk of pyelonephritis, pre-term delivery and neonatal mortality.

Routine examination of stools for pathogens is not useful in pregnant women, except in populations with high rates of anemia and malnutrition.

Prevention of puerperal infections is a major concern in obstetrics. Antenatal detection and treatment of STDs and hygienic standards during delivery decrease the risk for puerperal infection. The indications for cervical cerclage have to be carefully weighed against the risks, and antibiotic prophylaxis should be given. Active management of labor, including shorter labor, fewer vaginal examinations and reduced cesarean section rates, help to prevent genital infections. Antibiotic prophylaxis in cases of long, complicated or operative deliveries is effective, although resistance is a limiting factor.

Mastitis can be prevented through good nursing techniques, including strict hygienic measures.

CLINICAL FEATURES

Infections in pregnancy can be asymptomatic but usually manifest with symptoms similar to those in nonpregnant individuals.[1–4] The course of the infection may be worse because of alterations in immune response and because of the potential hazards for the outcome of pregnancy and the well-being of the fetus.

The clinical diagnosis of intra-amniotic infection is based upon fever, uterine tenderness, fetal tachycardia, leukocytosis and elevated C-reactive protein, with or without ruptured membranes.

Urinary tract infections are the most common infectious complications of pregnancy, and can be asymptomatic or manifest with signs of cystitis such as frequency, urgency and dysuria. Fever, flank pain and chills occur with ascending UTIs.

Lower respiratory tract infections manifest with cough, fever and chest pain.

Gastrointestinal infections appear as diarrhea and are usually self-limiting and without complications. If the diarrhea persists beyond 24 hours, a stool specimen should be obtained for culture. Acute appendicitis can be a diagnostic dilemma as the clinical presentations differ from those seen in nonpregnant women because of the large uterus and the altered immune response. Appendicitis may manifest as upper right quadrant pain with nausea and vomiting, without leukocytosis or fever, and should be differentiated from acute cholecystitis and amebic liver diseases.

Meningitis should be considered in every patient with headache, malaise, nausea, vomiting and fever. The diagnosis of bacterial endocarditis in pregnant women should be considered in any febrile, lethargic patient with no signs of localizing infection. Cutaneous lesions and heart murmurs should be sought. Blood cultures are required for diagnosis.

Diagnostic criteria for postpartum endometritis include fever, uterine and/or adnexal tenderness, purulent or foul lochia and leukocytosis in the absence of other signs of infection within the first 5 days after delivery. Late postpartum endometritis may occur weeks after delivery. Retention of placental products has to be excluded.

Early wound infection starts usually within 48 hours postpartum, and manifests with fever and cellulitis or edema of the wound. Early wound infection is often caused by group A or group B streptococci, or *Clostridium perfringens*. In clostridial infection, wound cellulitis is associated with a watery discharge and a bronze appearance of the skin. Late-onset wound infections occur about 4–8 days after surgery, and manifest with fever and an erythematous, draining wound.

Early recognition of life-threatening complications such as necrotizing fasciitis is crucial. Cutaneous findings can be minimal and include cellulitis, edema and sometimes crepitations. The patient, however, may be critically ill and require prompt treatment. A surgical exploration of the wound may be necessary to make the diagnosis.

Puerperal mastitis occurs with breast engorgement and milk stasis often in the second or third week after delivery. The onset of sporadic mastitis is rather sudden, with breast tenderness, chills, fever, malaise and headache mimicking a flu-like syndrome. The breast may show foci of local infection characterized by erythema, tenderness and warmth. The development of a breast abscess is rare in lactating women.

Patients with ovarian vein thrombophlebitis, which is more frequently present on the right, usually have distinct clinical findings. They present with fever and lower abdominal pain, and on examination are acutely ill with tachycardia and tachypnea and may be in respiratory distress. Abdominal examination usually shows direct tenderness, guarding and a tender abdominal mass. Pelvic pain thrombophlebitis without pulmonary emboli manifests less dramatically and has a more rapid response to therapy. These patients are more often not as critically ill, and just have fever and tachycardia.

DIAGNOSIS

Most infections that manifest with clinical signs and symptoms do not give rise to diagnostic difficulties, as they are related to specific infections of the urinary or reproductive tract, or to common infections in the community. Outlining a complete scheme of investigations is beyond the scope of this chapter, but a summary of the most important diagnostic leads and laboratory tests is presented in Figure 54.4.

Rapid and inexpensive tests for the early detection of intra-amniotic infection in patients in pre-term labor, including amniotic fluid Gram stain, leukocyte esterase, amniotic fluid glucose concentration and the Limulus amebocyte lysate assay, have been tested in women admitted with pPROM or pre-term birth. The greatest sensitivity for predicting infection was demonstrated by a low glucose level in amniotic fluid, but none of the tests had sufficient accuracy to allow clinical decisions.[20,21] For women with cervical dilatation in the mid-trimester of pregnancy, amniocentesis to determine the microbiologic characteristics of the amniotic cavity should be considered before placing a cerclage because of the poor prognosis in women with microbial invasion of the amniotic cavity.

The diagnosis of UTI is based on quantitative cultures with >100,000cfu/ml clear-voided urine (midstream) in asymptomatic patients, or >100cfu/ml in symptomatic patients. Direct suprapubic

bladder aspiration is a better technique for obtaining uncontaminated urine but is less readily accepted by patients and/or physicians. To avoid screening all pregnant women with expensive and time-consuming urine cultures, rapid screening tests such as leukocyte esterase dipstick, microscopy for pyuria, nitrite tests and enzymatic screening tests have been developed. The rapid enzymatic test seems to be a reliable alternative to culture screening with a sensitivity of 100%, a specificity of 81% and a negative predictive value of 100%.[23]

The key to the care of lower respiratory tract infections is an early diagnosis, with careful clinical evaluation and examination, if possible, of a sputum sample and a blood culture. One should not hesitate to take a chest X-ray, as well as an arterial Po_2 in pregnant women if a serious lower respiratory tract infection is suspected. In patients with meningitis, a spinal tap with Gram stain, culture and chemical analysis of the cerebrospinal fluid is usually indicated.

Postpartum endometritis is a clinical diagnosis supplemented by a cervical swab for aerobic culture to identify pathogens that may require additional measures besides the antibacterial therapy. Isolation of group A streptococci should lead to isolation of the patient whereas that of GBS should prompt further action in relation to the neonate. Culturing techniques of the endometrium with double- and triple-lumen devices have been hampered by vaginal and cervical contamination and are not used routinely.

The diagnosis of early wound infection is made clinically and confirmed by a Gram stain. Gram-positive rods are highly suggestive of clostridia, and Gram-positive cocci indicate the presence of group A streptococci or *S. aureus*.

The diagnosis of mastitis is a clinical diagnosis. Mammography and ultrasound can be useful in the early diagnosis of an abscess and to differentiate infection from a breast malignancy. However, this technique is rarely used because of pain and discomfort to the patient.

Pelvic vein thrombophlebitis is a difficult clinical diagnosis often confused with acute appendicitis, torsion of an adnexa, urolithiasis, pyelonephritis, leiomyoma and pelvic abscess. In case of clinical suspicion of a pelvic vein thrombophlebitis, additional examinations such as venography, computed axial tomography and sonography have to be performed.

MANAGEMENT

A number of interventions with proven value in the management of morbidity related to infection during pregnancy are discussed. The serologic screening and subsequent management of viral infections, including rubella, toxoplasmosis, cytomegalovirus, HIV and others, is discussed in Chapter 2.55.

Although the initiating mechanism of labor, and particularly pre-term labor, is unknown, the potential role of inflammation is clear. Consequently, attempts to prolong gestation and improve pregnancy outcome using antimicrobials have been made. A number of prospective, randomized clinical trials with antibiotics have been reviewed. There is evidence that antibacterial therapy of women at risk of pre-term delivery on the basis of vaginal bacteriologic studies are effective in women with bacterial vaginosis. In addition, the use of antibiotics in women with pre-term labor or with pPROM significantly prolongs the interval to delivery and improves neonatal outcome in those with pPROM.[24,25] Despite some controversy, the evidence that antibiotics contribute to the prevention of pre-term labor is convincing. However, improved diagnostic methods are needed to identify those patients who will benefit most from antimicrobial therapy during pregnancy or delivery.

As bacteriuria predisposes the pregnant woman to pyelonephritis with potential hazards for mother and fetus, screening and management in pregnancy is justified. Antimicrobial treatment options of UTIs include 3-day courses of amoxicillin 500mg q8h, nitrofurantoin 100mg q6h, cephalexin 500mg q6h, or trimethoprim–sulfamethoxazole (co-trimoxazole) 160/800mg q12h. The latter regimen should be avoided in the third trimester because sulfonamides cross the placenta and compete

CLINICAL AND LABORATORY CRITERIA IN THE DIAGNOSIS OF INFECTION IN PREGNANCY	
History	Signs, symptoms, onset, specific localization, additional signs such as pain, rash, uterine tenderness, leakage of amniotic fluid, exposure to infections, pets, occupation, hobbies, travel, place of residence, history of infections
Clinical examination	Auscultation of heart and lungs, assessment of the uterus and cervix, examination of the breasts, detection of masses, enlargement of spleen, liver, lymph nodes, signs of thrombophlebitis
Laboratory tests	White blood cell count and differential, C-reactive protein, serum enzymes, blood smears, blood cultures, throat and vaginal swabs, specific antibodies, urine culture

Fig. 54.4 Clinical and laboratory criteria in the diagnosis of infection in pregnancy.

with bilirubin in the fetus. Trimethoprim is a folate antagonist and should be combined with folinic acid if given in high doses. In view of the high rate of recurrence of bacteriuria in pregnancy, suppressive therapy is recommended until 2 weeks postpartum in women with recurrent UTIs. Pregnant women with acute pyelonephritis require admission for parenteral administration of antibiotics and careful monitoring.

Penicillin is the drug of choice in women with lower respiratory tract infections caused by pneumococci. The fever may cause premature contractions. Because of possible cardiopulmonary complications, β-mimetic tocolytic drugs should be avoided or, if necessary, administered with caution.

Treatment of gastrointestinal infections is usually not necessary during pregnancy except when the problems persist and interfere with the mother's health. Metronidazole should be prescribed for *Entamoeba histolytica* infection. Pregnant women with acute appendicitis should undergo surgical exploration by the obstetrician together with the surgeon, and antibiotics should be prescribed.

Treatment of postpartum genital infection includes appropriate antibiotics with good anaerobic coverage. After cesarean section the desired results have been obtained with a combination of clindamycin and gentamicin. Newer antibiotics such as the monobactams may replace gentamicin in combination with clindamycin, and the newer cephalosporins with a wide spectrum of activity are increasingly used. Intravenous antibiotics should be continued for 24–48 hours after the patient has become afebrile, and can be stopped without changing to oral antibiotics unless a staphylococcal infection is present. The treatment of early wound infections may require excision of the necrotic tissue and aggressive antibiotic treatment with a cephalosporin or clindamycin. In late-onset (after 5 days) wound infection incision of the wound and drainage is required. If the patient does not become afebrile after 24 hours, antibiotics should be prescribed. Open wounds can be allowed to close spontaneously by granulation after wound debridement and packing. Surgical closure of cesarean section has been shown to be successful and requires less healing time. The procedure may be carried out under general or local anesthesia, and antibiotic prophylaxis

is generally used. Episiotomy incisions should not be resutured but given time to heal by granulation, unless the sphincter muscle or the rectal mucosa is involved. In rare complications such as necrotizing fasciitis or clostridial gas gangrene, treatment must be aggressive, including high doses of broad-spectrum antibiotics and extensive drainage and debridement

Therapy of mastitis includes continuation of lactation and treatment with a penicillinase-resistant penicillin or a cephalosporin, given orally except in the case of a severely sick patient. Ice packs, breast support, analgesics and regular emptying of the infected breast may help to prevent abscesses. In case of abscess formation, surgical incision and drainage should be performed.

Treatment of pelvic vein thrombophlebitis includes broad-spectrum antibiotics, heparin for 7–10 days intravenously, followed by long-term anticoagulation with oral anticoagulants. Surgery, including bilateral ovarian vein and inferior vena cava ligation, may be required for patients who do not respond to treatment. Hysterectomy is seldom required.

CONCLUSIONS

Infectious diseases are important risk factors for maternal and neonatal morbidity and mortality and can be detected early with improved outcomes or prevented entirely. Maternal mortality due to infections is an unbearable tragedy and must be addressed by improved access to modern obstetric care for all pregnant women. This care must be affordable, even in resource-limited countries, and should be a priority for governments and international agencies.

Preventing pre-term birth is a global issue, including industrialized countries. A substantial portion of pre-term births can be prevented with improvements in the detection and management of infections during pregnancy. Further research is required to identify women and babies at risk, to develop preventive, diagnostic and management strategies to enhance care with maximal benefits at minimal costs and adverse effects.

REFERENCES

1. Sweet RL, Gibbs RS. Gynecologic and obstetric infections. In: Sweet RL, Gibbs RS, eds. Infectious diseases of the female genital tract, 3rd ed. Baltimore: Williams and Wilkins; 1995:429–617.
2. Ledger W. Maternal infections during pregnancy. In: Reece EA, Hobbins JC, Mahoney MJ, Petrie RH, eds. Medicine of the fetus and mother. Philadelphia: JB Lippincott; 1992:1183–236.
3. Hurley R. Fever and infectious diseases. In: de Swiet M, ed. Medical disorders in obstetric practice, 3rd ed. Oxford: Blackwell Science; 1995:552–67.
4. Charles D. Obstetric and perinatal infections. In: Sanford JP, Tyrrell DAJ, Weller TH, Wolff SM, eds. Handbook of infectious diseases. St Louis, MO: Mosby Year Book; 1993:29–251.
5. Brunham RC, Holmes KK, Embree JE. Sexually transmitted diseases in pregnancy. In: Holmes KK, Mardh P-A, Sparling PF, et al. eds. Sexually transmitted diseases, 2nd ed. New York: McGraw-Hill; 1990;64:771–801.
6. Temmerman M, Plummer FA, Mirza NB, et al. Infection with human immunodeficiency virus (HIV) as a risk factor for adverse obstetrical outcome. AIDS 1990;4:1087–93.
7. Temmerman M, Lopita M, Sinei S, et al. Sexually transmitted infections as risk factors for spontaneous abortion. Int J STD AIDS 1992;3:418–22.
8. Hillier SL, Nugent RP, Eschenbach DA, et al. Association between bacterial vaginosis and preterm delivery of a low-birth-weigth infant. N Engl J Med 1995;333:1737–42.
9. Hauth JC, Goldenberg RL, Andrews WW, DuBard MB, Copper RL. Reduced incidence of preterm delivery with metronidazole and erythromycin treatment in women with bacterial vaginosis. N EnglJ Med 1995;333:1732–6.

10. McDonald HM, O'Loughlin JA, Jolley P, Vignesrwaran R, McDonald PJ. Prenatal microbiological risk factors associated with preterm birth. Br J Obstet Gynaecol 1992;99:190–6.
11. Meis PJ, Goldenberg RL, Mercer B, et al. The preterm prediction study: significance of vaginal infections. Am J Obstet Gynecol 1995;173:1231–5.
12. Neman-Simha V, Renaudin H, de Barbeyrac B, et al. Isolation of genital mycoplasmas from blood of febrile obstetrical-gynecological patients and neonates. Scand J Infect Dis 1992;24:317–21.
13. Siegel I, Gleicher N. Changes in peripheral mononuclear cells in pregnancy. Am J Reprod Immunol 1981;1:154–5.
14. Sridama V, Pacini F, Yang SL, et al. Decreased levels of helper T cells: a possible cause of immunodeficiency in pregnancy. N Engl J Med 1982;307:352–6.
15. Vanderbeeken Y, Vlieghe MP, Delespesse G, Duchateau J. Characterization of immunoregulatory T cells during pregnancy by monoclonal antibodies. Clin Exp Immunol 1982;48:118–20.
16. Biggar RJ, Pahwa S, Minkoff H, et al. Immunosuppression in pregnant women infected with human immunodeficiency virus. Am J Obstet Gynecol 1989;161:1239–44.
17. Nugent RP, Hillier S. Mucopurulent cervicitis as a predictor of chlamydial infection and pregnancy outcome. Sex Transm Dis 1992;19:198–202.
18. McGregor JA, French JI, Jones W, et al. Association of cervicovaginal infections with increased vaginal fluid phospholipase A_2 activity. Am J Obstet Gynecol 1992;167:1588–94.

19. Hellemans P, Gerris J, Verdonck P. Fetal fibronectin detection for prediction of preterm birth in low risk women. Br J Obstet Gynaecol 1995;102:207–12.
20. Romero R, Gonzalez R, Sepulveda W, et al. Infection and labor. VIII. Microbial invasion of the amniotic cavity in patients with suspected cervical incompetence: prevalence and clinical significance. Am J Obstet Gynecol 1992;167:1086–91.
21. Gauthier DW, Meyer WJ. Comparison of Gram stain, leukocyte esterase activity, and amniotic fluid glucose concentration in predicting amniotic fluid culture results in preterm premature rupture of membranes. Am J Obstet Gynecol 1992;167:1092–5.
22. ACOG Committee Opinion. Prevention of early-onset group B streptococcal disease in newborns. Int J Gynecol Obstet 1996;54:197–205.
23. Hagay Z, Levy R, Miskin A, et al. Uriscreen, a rapid enzymatic urine screening test: useful predictor of significant bacteriuria in pregnancy. Obstet Gynecol 1996;87:410–3.
24. Kirschbaum T. Antibiotics in the treatment of preterm labor. Am J Obstet Gynecol 1993;168:1239–46.
25. Mercer BM, Arheart KL. Antimicrobial therapy in expectant management of preterm premature rupture of membranes. Lancet 1995;346:1271–9.

Implications for the Fetus of Maternal Infections in Pregnancy

E Lee Ford-Jones & Greg Ryan

The nature of congenital infections is changing rapidly with new opportunities to link pathogens to untoward events through advances in molecular technology [e.g. polymerase chain reaction (PCR)] and wider availability of intrauterine diagnostic testing (e.g. maternal serum α-fetoprotein screening, ultrasound, amniocentesis, fetal blood sampling). Congenital infection in pregnancy may come to clinical attention through:

- a history of maternal risk factors,
- known exposure,
- documented acute maternal infection,
- laboratory screening,
- detection of fetal abnormalities on clinical examination or ultrasonography,
- suggestive findings in the neonate, and
- suggestive findings in the child.

Depending on the scenario, one or a range of infections must be considered in the differential diagnosis.

Fortunately, the vast majority of maternal infections have no effect on the fetus, either because there is no transmission to the intrauterine site or because the fetal infection is asymptomatic. Fear and poor understanding of risk on the part of the parents or physician can lead to unnecessary termination of pregnancy.

EPIDEMIOLOGY

Although many micro-organisms are known to cause congenital (intrauterine) infection (Fig. 55.1),[1] only more common agents are discussed (see below). A brief summary of infections transmitted primarily at the time of delivery are discussed at the end of the chapter.

Because the use of appropriate diagnostic testing is highly variable and because many of these diseases are not reportable to public health departments, there are few data on incidence. Actual rates are highly variable and depend on the presence of specific risk factors; estimates are provided in Figure 55.2.

GEOGRAPHIC

There is considerable geographic variation in risk of exposure. Although some variation is related directly to the presence of the pathogen (e.g. *Plasmodium* spp., *Trypanosoma cruzi*), in others it may be related to other practices (e.g. breast-feeding). Maternal toxoplasmosis exposure reflects culinary practices, including handling and ingestion of fresh raw meat.[3]

OTHER FACTORS ASSOCIATED WITH INFECTION

Annual seroconversion rates to cytomegalovirus (CMV) for health care workers, usually in the range of 2–4%, are generally lower than rates in day care workers or susceptible parents of children in day care (12–45%).[4] Syphilis in pregnancy generally affects women who are young, unmarried, of low socioeconomic status and who receive inadequate prenatal care. Factors associated with maternal–fetal infection are summarized in Figure 55.3.

INFECTIOUS AGENTS KNOWN TO CAUSE CONGENITAL INFECTION	
Viruses	Herpesviruses: cytomegalovirus, herpes simplex virus, varicella-zoster virus
	Parvovirus B19
	Rubella virus
	Measles virus
	Enteroviruses: coxsackie B virus, echovirus, poliovirus
	HIV-1 and HIV-2 viruses
	Lymphocytic choriomeningitis virus
	Hepatitis B virus
	Vaccinia
	Smallpox
	Adenovirus
	Western equine encephalomyelitis virus
	Venezuelan equine encephalomyelitis virus
Bacteria	*Treponema pallidum*
	Mycobacterium tuberculosis
	Listeria monocytogenes
	Campylobacter fetus
	Salmonella typhosa
	Borrelia burgdorferi
Protozoa	*Toxoplasma gondii*
	Plasmodium spp.
	Trypanosoma cruzi

Fig. 55.1 Infectious agents known to cause congenital infection. Adapted with permission from Guerina.[1]

PATHOGENESIS AND PATHOLOGY

Infections occurring in the neonate may be acquired in the following ways:

- transplacentally *in utero* (congenital or intrauterine) by direct blood flow to the amniotic fluid or from the genital tract via the cervical amniotic route, during pregnancy or just before delivery. The placenta can be infected and even act as a repository for pathogen growth;
- at the time of birth (perinatal) through vaginal secretions and blood; and
- after birth but during the neonatal period (postnatal), from the mother, her breastmilk, or other sources.

Adverse effects include abortion, stillbirth, premature delivery, physical defects, intrauterine growth restriction [e.g. rubella, enterovirus, herpes simplex virus (HSV)] and postnatal persistence of infection (e.g. rubella, CMV, HSV). Association of these findings, particularly early gestational loss, with particular pathogens has been hampered by the lack of availability of molecular diagnostic testing of macerated and hydrolyzed fetal tissues.

General associations of the following sites of infection with adverse effects, exist:

GENERAL RATES OF SELECTED CONGENITAL AND PERINATAL INFECTIONS

Infection	Rate/live births
Group B streptococcus	1–5/1000
Cytomegalovirus	2–24/1000 (10–20% have disease)[4]
HSV (intrauterine)	1–2/200,000
HSV (perinatal)	1/2000–5000 USA; 1/33,000 UK[2]
Toxoplasma	0.1–3.5/1000
Syphilis	0.05–6.1/1000 (varies with definition)

Fig. 55.2 General rates of selected congenital and perinatal infections.

- embryo: malformations, spontaneous abortion;
- fetus: stillbirth, neurologic sequelae; and
- placenta: preterm birth, stillbirth, neonatal death.

FACTORS AFFECTING FETAL DISEASE
Pathogen
The greater virulence of some microbes in the fetus and infant is probably caused by the hematogenous route of exposure and inoculum size, as well as the status of the immune response derived from the infant and passively derived maternal antibody and postnatally, immunocompetent cells in colostrum and breast milk.[5] Primary mechanisms of damage include cell death, abnormalities of cell growth (mitotic inhibition), direct cytoxic effect (chromosomal injury, cell necrosis) and secondary inflammatory responses.

Certain organisms have a propensity for certain stages of organogenesis. Rubella virus inhibits cell growth and thus causes structural damage. Enterovirus, CMV, toxoplasma and HSV may also be associated with intrauterine growth restriction. The inflammatory response to HSV infection leads to intrauterine infection rather than any particular developmental anomalies. There is a receptor for parvovirus B19 on the red blood cell (p antigen), with the result that at the time of the rapid increase in erythrocye numbers during the second trimester, anemia and hydrops occur. Postnatal persistence of infection and some further damage can occur with rubella, CMV, HSV and varicella-zoster virus (VZV) infections.

Maternal immunity
Before conception. Usually maternal antibody in the immunocompetent host is protective to the fetus. Exceptions include viruses with known latency, such as CMV and occasionally HSV, and rarely rubella, for which maternal immunity has waned, and untreated *Treponema pallidum*.

The rate of intrauterine transmission is 30–40% after primary maternal CMV infection, with approximately 15% of affected infants ultimately developing clinically significant disease during childhood. Although fetal infection can follow recurrent maternal CMV infection, clinical symptoms in infants are rare. For example, primary maternal infection is associated with bilateral sensorineural hearing loss in 8% of cases and intelligence quotient below 70 in 13%, while following recurrent maternal infection, neither occurs.[6]

Fetal disease follows both symptomatic and asymptomatic maternal infection. Immunosuppressive disorders and immunosuppressive therapy will alter the risk of fetal disease (e.g. HIV-1 infection facilitates the transmission of toxoplasma).
During pregnancy and before delivery. The length of time before conception during which infection may occur without causing later fetal damage is not known. In the immunocompetent mother, it is advisable to have an interval of 7–9 months between *Toxoplasma gondii* acquisition and conception. Over 50% of infants born to mothers with primary or secondary syphilis will have congenital infection, decreasing to 40% with early latent syphilis and 10% with late latent

FACTORS ASSOCIATED WITH MATERNAL–FETAL INFECTION

Association	Pathogen
Seasonality (in North America)	Parvovirus B19 (winter, spring) Rubella (winter, spring) Enterovirus (summer, autumn)
Handling/ingestion of uncooked, previously unfrozen meat	*Toxoplasma gondii*
Children: Day care School Household	 CMV, parvovirus Parvovirus CMV, parvovirus
Exposure in travel to certain geographic regions	*Toxoplasma gondii, Mycobacterium tuberculosis, Plasmodium* spp., *Trypanosoma cruzi, Borrelia burgdorferi*, hepatitis B virus
Kitten/cat feces within 21 days of primary infection (handling animals, kitty litter, gardening)	*Toxoplasma gondii*
Number of sexual partners, sex industry worker/partner, illicit drug use	*Treponema pallidum*, herpes simplex virus, hepatitis B virus
Sexually active adolescents	CMV, herpes simplex virus, hepatitis B virus
Unimmunized (e.g. immigrant from developing world; World Health Organization Expanded Program of Immunization does not include rubella)	Rubella

Fig. 55.3 Factors associated with maternal–fetal infection.

infection.[7] Although the risk of intrauterine syphilis increases during gestation and is particularly high in late pregnancy, it can occur at any time during pregnancy.

In some infections the mother may develop immunity to an infection, but the fetus is delivered before transplacental transmission of this protection. Essentially the infant experiences a massive viremia, but with cutting of the umbilical cord is left without protection. For example, the risk of acquiring maternal varicella in the 5 days before delivery, is associated with a 30% risk of congenital infection in the neonate.

Placenta
Placental infection is more common than fetal infection for a variety of infections, including rubella, malaria and tuberculosis. This may be because of specific placental immunologic defense, antimicrobial properties (e.g. interferon production), placental phagocytic capacity, or a nonspecific physical barrier function. In early gestation, the small developing placenta effectively excludes most pathogens. As the placenta matures, with expansion of the maternal–fetal interface, this barrier becomes more porous, rendering transplacental transmission more likely. Placental dysfunction may also be associated with hypoxia, fever, toxins, thrombosis and placentitis and result in fetal injury or death indirectly.[5]

Stage of fetal gestation
Fetal disease may result from many pathogens at any time during gestation. In general, however, transplacental transmission (via umbilical blood flow or direct spread to the amniotic fluid) is less likely early in gestation, but the results of infection, if it occurs, are more likely to be severe. The deficiencies in immune function of the young fetus both in humoral and in cellular function contribute to tissue damage, organ dysfunction, and teratogenicity. Detectable IgM is rarely produced before 20–24 weeks of gestation. Certain pathogens are associated

with producing particular effects at certain stages of cell development. For example, maternal rubella infection in pregnancy after 16 weeks is not associated with defects.[8]

Congenital varicella syndrome occurs almost exclusively before 20 weeks of gestation; in five studies of varicella infection in pregnancy, 4 out of 145 babies had congenital anomalies. After 20 weeks of gestation early, childhood zoster is the presenting finding, occurring after maternal infections between 17 and 24 weeks in 0.8% of cases and after infection between 25 and 36 weeks in 1.7%.[10] While transmission of toxoplasmosis occurs in only about 15% of first trimester infections, severe disease occurs in about 40% of infected infants. In the third trimester the reverse is true with 60% transmission, but the disease is generally milder or asymptomatic.

PREVENTION

Prevention of maternal infection in pregnancy requires a combination of approaches: education, immunization, screening and intervention (Fig. 55.4).

PRENATAL PREVENTION THROUGH IMMUNIZATION AND EDUCATION

Certain preventive efforts should antecede pregnancy including documentation of rubella immunity and preventive education regarding optimal food handling practices (i.e. toxoplasma, enteric bacterial pathogens, *Listeria* spp.). All women should also be immune to measles, mumps, tetanus, diphtheria and poliomyelitis, either by natural infection or by vaccination. Hepatitis B virus, influenza and pneumococcal immunization are recommended for women who are at high-risk of infection. Immune globulin or specific immune globulin may be indicated on exposure to measles, hepatitis A or B virus, tetanus, varicella, or rabies, and in the case of certain travel, to poliomyelitis, yellow fever, typhoid and hepatitis B virus.[11] Although inactivated vaccines are generally considered safe, some physicians wait until after the first trimester to administer them. Live viral or bacterial vaccines should be avoided during pregnancy. However, the risk of congenital rubella syndrome after administration of vaccine to a pregnant woman, is very low.

The efficacy of education regarding toxoplasmosis has been demonstrated. All women who are planning pregnancy should be given general information. The following should be included in the general information for women planning pregnancy.
- Keep all adult immunizations up to date.
- Ensure that you are immune to rubella by blood test. If you are not, you require immunization.
- Follow simple procedure to reduce the risk of infection with *Toxoplasma* spp. (Fig. 55.5).[1]
- Minimize the risk of other food-borne infections (Fig. 55.6).
- If you are exposed to erythema infectiosum (fifth disease, human parvovirus B19), chickenpox or shingles during pregnancy, inform your physician promptly.
- If your partner is diagnosed with an infection other than a cold or flu, inform your physician.
- There is currently no effective strategy to prevent the complications of CMV or enterovirus during pregnancy. Although women who regularly handle the respiratory secretions or diapers of young children may wish to be tested for CMV immunity before pregnancy, the only current preventive strategy for susceptible women is good hygiene when they are with young children in their home or in the group child care environment.[12]
- Symptoms of genital herpes may occur years after the original infection; it is usually the first infection, which may occur without any symptoms (asymptomatic primary), that affects the infant; such infections are very rare and cannot be identifed.
- In pregnancy, your doctor routinely tests for rubella immunity, hepatitis B virus and syphilis infection.

SUMMARY OF PREVENTIVE ANTENATAL STRATEGIES

Pathogen	Education/ Immunization	Routine screen	Selective screen	Maternal–fetal intervention
CMV	Yes		Day care workers (pre-pregnancy only)	Handwashing after handling respiratory secretions and urine
Parvovirus B19			Exposure, epidemic	Intrauterine transfusion(s)
Rubella	Yes	Yes	Exposure	If susceptible, postpartum immunization before discharge
VZV	Yes		Exposure	If susceptible, some experts recommend varicella-zoster immune globulin ≤ 96 hours after exposure
Treponema pallidum	Yes	Yes	If high risk, third trimester delivery	Penicillin, HIV testing, monthly serologic follow-up
Toxoplasma gondii	Yes	Only if recommended by regional authority	If ingestion of raw, previously unfrozen meat; handling of kitten or litter	Spiramycin or pyrimethamine/ sulfadiazine/folinic acid with monitoring

Fig. 55.4 Summary of preventive antenatal strategies.

MEASURES TO REDUCE THE RISK OF INFECTION WITH *TOXOPLASMA* SPP.

Source of infection	Preventive measure
Meat	Avoid eating undercooked meat in pregnancy; previously frozen meat is free of toxoplasma
	Wash hands thoroughly after handling; keep cooking utensils thoroughly cleaned
Cats	Avoid contact with materials potentially contaminated with cat excrement
	Avoid kitty litter boxes; infectious toxoplasma may be present if in use more than 24 hours
	Disinfect with boiling water for 5 minutes; avoid aerosolization
	(Even indoor cats may be in contact with mice and fresh, raw meats)
Vegetables	Wash raw fruit and vegetables thoroughly before eating; wash hands after handling
Gardening	Wear gloves

Fig. 55.5 Measures to reduce the risk of infection with *Toxoplasma* spp.

MEASURES TO REDUCE THE RISK OF FOOD-BORNE INFECTIONS OTHER THAN TOXOPLASMA

- Wash hands thoroughly before eating and before and after food preparation
- Use separate or thoroughly cleaned surfaces for foods to be served raw and cooked
- Avoid unpasteurized milk or cheese
- Avoid soft cheese (e.g. Brie, Camembert)
- Reheat leftovers and pre-cooked foods until piping hot
- Wash and scrub raw vegetables before eating
- Use foods before the expiry date

Fig. 55.6 Measures to reduce the risk of food-borne infections other than toxoplasma.

SCREENING FOR INFECTION DURING PREGNANCY

Rubella screening in pregnancy alerts the physician to which mothers require postpartum immunization. Also, if the susceptible woman has known exposure or disease, the physician can confirm acute infection through study of a second sera. Antenatal screening for syphilis is cost-effective at an incidence as low as 5 in 100,000 population.[13] Hepatitis B virus screening allows for preventive management of the infant of the hepatitis B surface antigen (HBsAg)-positive mother.

The interpretation of other serology in pregnancy in the absence of seroconversion is fraught with difficulty as the acuity of the infection often cannot be determined. A woman at high-risk of CMV infection (e.g. a day care worker) would therefore be advised to establish her immune status before pregnancy.

Screening for toxoplasma requires testing teach trimester to document seroconversion and to allow for prompt treatment before transplacental transmission has occurred. *Toxoplasma*-specific IgM antibody persists for more than a year in about one-third of infections. Screening is costly in populations where 80–90% of the population is susceptible, but may be worthwhile if the incidence of primary maternal infection exceeds 1.1 per 1000. Practitioner-based testing for acute toxoplasmosis in the absence of a community-based program should be discouraged.

CLINICAL AND ULTRASOUND FINDINGS

Clinical and ultrasound findings may provide an additional opportunity to make diagnoses in the fetus.

Maternal illness

Rash in pregnancy should always suggest syphilis, rubella, parvovirus B19 or enterovirus infection. Arthritis occurs with parvovirus B19 infection as well as with rubella. In the presence of acute mononucleosis-like symptoms of fatigue and lymphadenopathy, CMV, *Toxoplasma* and HIV infection must be considered.

Fetal ultrasonography

Ultrasound findings of in-utero infection are provided in Clinical features, below. For toxoplasmosis identified ultrasonographically, maternal antimicrobial therapy with spiramycin before 18 weeks of gestation and pyrimethamine and sulfadiazine therafter may reduce the severity of disease. In nonresolving fetal hydrops caused by parvovirus B19 infection, intrauterine transfusion may be used to treat severe fetal anemia.

CLINICAL FEATURES

FETAL

The features of in-utero infections are summarized in Figure 55.7. Some fetal abnormalities detected on antenatal ultrasonography may be caused by infection. However, no ultrasonographic findings are pathognomonic for a particular agent. Postnatal follow up of infants, including ophthalmologic examination, cranial neuro-imaging (i.e. CT, MRI), and head growth and developmental progress over the first 2 years of life is important in identifying affected infants, particularly with CMV and *Toxoplasma* infections. Ophthalmologic examination and cranial neuroimaging studies are abnormal in 40–50% of apparently normal, but *Toxoplasma*-infected infants at birth.[16]

PREMATURITY AND LOW BIRTHWEIGHT

Routine investigation of these infants for congenital infection is unlikely to yield positive results. Prematurity is typical of congenital syphilis and common in perinatal HSV infection. Intrauterine growth occurs with rubella, CMV infections, toxoplasmosis and, occasionally, enteroviral infection.

SPONTANEOUS ABORTION AND STILLBIRTH

Pregnancy loss has been associated with infection with CMV, enterovirus, HSV, HIV, parvovirus B19, rubella, *T. pallidum* and *T. gondii*. Fetal loss occurring with any maternal viral infection requires

CLINICAL FEATURES OF IN-UTERO INFECTION	
General	Intrauterine growth retardation: all etiologies
	Hydrops fetalis: parvovirus B19, CMV, syphilis, *Toxoplasma*, HSV, Coxsackie B3 virus[14]
	Placentamegaly: CMV, syphilis
Head and neck	Hydrocephalus: CMV, *Toxoplasma*, enterovirus
	Microcephalus: CMV, *Toxoplasma*, rubella, varicella, HSV
	Intracranial calcifications: CMV, *Toxoplasma*, HSV, rubella, HIV
Heart	Congestive heart failure: parvovirus B19, syphilis, CMV, *Toxoplasma*
	Pericardial effusion: parvovirus B19, syphilis, CMV, *Toxoplasma*
	Cardiac defects: rubella, parvovirus B19, mumps (not proved)
	Myocarditis: enterovirus
Lungs	Pleural effusion: parvovirus B19, syphilis, CMV, *Toxoplasma*
	Pulmonary hypoplasia: CMV
Abdomen	Hepatosplenomegaly: CMV, rubella, *Toxoplasma*, HSV, syphilis, enterovirus, parvovirus B19
	Hypoechogenic bowel: CMV, *Toxoplasma*[15]
	Hepatic calcifications: CMV, *Toxoplasma*
	Meconium peritonitis: CMV, *Toxoplasma*
	Ascites: parvovirus B19, CMV, *Toxoplasma*, syphilis
Extremities	Limb reduction, restriction: VZV

Fig. 55.7 Clinical features of in-utero infection.

RATIO OF NEONATAL INFECTION TO NEONATAL AND POSTNATAL SYMPTOMS			
Micro-organism	Infected fetuses/ neonates with clinical manifestations (%)	Additional percentage with late-onset manifestations	Late-onset manifestations
CMV	10%	5–15%	At ≤2 years sensorineural hearing loss, microcephaly, motor defects, mental retardation, chorioretinitis, dental defects >2 years hearing loss
Rubella	First 16 weeks, decreasing from 90% to 24%	>20%	Hearing loss, visual defects, multiple endocrinopathies, panencephalitis
Treponema pallidum	30%[17] (30–40% stillborn)	Unknown	Hearing loss, visual defects; abnormal dentition, bones and joints, CNS
Toxoplasma gondii	Severe organ damage in 20% of infants of untreated mothers and in 2% in treated mothers	Subclinical infection in 41% of infants of untreated mothers and in 17% in treated mothers	>85% have chorioretinitis

Fig. 55.8 Ratio of neonatal infection to neonatal and postnatal symptoms.

comprehensive pathologic and microbiologic evaluation to determine the role of the infection in pathogenesis.

SYNDROMES OF CONGENITAL INFECTION
General
The majority of infected infants have no symptoms at birth although some will develop sequelae later in childhood (Fig. 55.8). The clinical findings in congenital infection are summarized in Figure 55.9.

Sepsis-like illness
Herpes simplex virus acquired just before delivery or intrapartum occasionally presents similarly to perinatal disease, without skin lesions, as neonatal sepsis or pneumonitis, with one of the earliest laboratory clues being abnormal liver enzymes. Shock, coagulopathy, fulminant hepatitis and, often, skin lesions, follow.

Hepatitis
Enterovirus, HSV and *Toxoplasma* can cause overwhelming acute neonatal liver failure in the first week of life. Other infections including CMV[20] and parvovirus B19[21] can also present with hepatic findings.

Central nervous system
Central nervous system (CNS) involvement may occur with all of the congenital infections (as well as with perinatally acquired HSV and enteroviral infections), although initial findings may be very subtle. Occult findings in congenital neurosyphilis have led to general recommendations that neurosyphilis be assumed with any CSF abnormality.[22] With newer molecular techniques, CNS involvement may be better recognized (i.e. PCR detection of CMV DNA in the CSF). Clinical findings may be preceded by ophthalmologic and neuroimaging findings. Central nervous system involvement in congenital toxoplasmosis may be manifest only on neuroimaging at birth.[14] As opposed to the poorer prognosis of cranial calcifications in CMV infection, the cranial calcifications of toxoplasmosis may disappear during therapy in infancy or persist, with normal cognitive development.

Cardiac
Rubella infection causes structural defects including patent ductus arteriosus; parvovirus B19 may cause intrauterine congestive heart failure with resulting prenatal closure of the foramen ovale and Epstein's anomaly.[23] Viral myocarditis is characteristically caused by coxsackie B virus or other enteroviruses.

Ophthalmologic
Ophthalmologic abnormalities are seen in a variety of congenital infections (Fig. 55.9).[5]

Deafness
Deafness is a common sequela of CMV and rubella infection, as well as of untreated *Toxoplasma* and syphilis infections. One-third of sensorineural hearing loss is caused by congenital CMV infection. Of rubella-infected infants, 80% or more may have deafness, often as the only significant consequence. Given the progressive nature of impairment, serial hearing evaluations to age 6–9 years are recommended for CMV-infected infants.

SPECIFIC INFECTIONS
Cytomegalovirus
Up to 10% of CMV-infected infants will have typical findings of petechiae, hepatosplenomegaly, jaundice, microcephaly, inguinal hernia in males, chorioretinitis or other, atypical findings. Symptomatic infants are at high-risk of significant neurologic and developmental dysfunction, particularly if abnormalities are noted on cranial CT or chorioretinitis exists. Cerebral calcifications tend to be periventricular. Infants with asymptomatic infection have a 5–15% risk of hearing loss, mental retardation, motor spasticity and microcephaly evolving in the early years.

Enteroviruses (Coxsackieviruses, echovirus)
Although high rates of maternal infection in pregnancy (up to 25%) have been reported, disease is limited to case reports or series of infected infants with a variety of entities including growth retardation, CNS malformations, blueberry muffin rash, hepatic necrosis, myocarditis or pericarditis.

Herpes simplex virus
Intrauterine HSV infection is characterized by the triad of skin vesicles or scarring, eye lesions, and microcephaly or hydranencephaly. It may

CLINICAL FINDINGS IN CONGENITAL INFECTION	
Prematurity	Syphilis, HSV
Intrauterine growth retardation	All etiologies
Anemia with hydrops	Parvovirus B19, syphilis, CMV, *Toxoplasma*
Bone lesions	Syphilis, rubella
Cerebral calcification	*Toxoplasma* (widely distributed) CMV and HSV (usually periventricular) Parvovirus B19, rubella, HIV
Congenital heart disease	Rubella, parvovirus B19, mumps (not proved)
Hepatosplenomegaly	CMV, rubella, *Toxoplasma*, HSV, syphilis, enterovirus, parvovirus B19
Hydrocephalus	*Toxoplasma*, CMV, syphilis, possibly enterovirus
Hydrops, ascites, pleural effusions	Parvovirus B19, CMV, *Toxoplasma*, syphilis
Jaundice	CMV, *Toxoplasma*, rubella, HSV, syphilis, enterovirus
Limb paralysis with atrophy and cicatrices	Varicella
Maculopapular exanthem	Syphilis, measles, rubella, enterovirus
Microcephaly	CMV, *Toxoplasma*, rubella, varicella, HSV
Ocular findings (see below)	CMV, *Toxoplasma*, rubella, HSV, syphilis, enterovirus, parvovirus B19
Progressive hepatic failure and clotting abnormalities	Echovirus, Coxsackie B, enterovirus, HSV, *Toxoplasma*
Pseudoparalysis	Syphilis
Purpura (usually appears on first day)	CMV, *Toxoplasma*, syphilis, rubella, HSV, enterovirus, parvovirus B19[18]
Vesicles	HSV, syphilis, varicella, CMV, parvovirus B19, enterovirus
Cataracts	Rubella, HSV, VZV, parvovirus B19, *Toxoplasma*, syphilis
Chorioretinitis	HSV, VZV, rubella, CMV, *Toxoplasma*
Optic atrophy	HSV, VZV, rubella, CMV, *Toxoplasma*, syphilis
Microphthalmia	Rubella, HSV, parvovirus B19, *Toxoplasma*, CMV
Coloboma	CMV
Keratoconjunctivitis	HSV
Pigment retinopathy	Rubella
Glaucoma	Rubella, toxoplasmosis, syphilis
Iritis	HSV, rubella, syphilis
Anophthalmia	CMV
Peter's anomaly	CMV
Horner syndrome	VZV

Fig. 55.9 Clinical findings in congenital infection.[5,19]

LABOR ATORY EVIDENCE OF CLINICALLY SIGNIFICANT MATERNAL INFECTION		
Micro-organism	Detection by culture, PCR (site)	Serology
CMV		Seroconversion Possibly CMV IgM capture enzyme-linked immunosorbent assay
Enterovirus	Yes (stool, throat, other)	Seroconversion
HSV	Yes (vesicle)	Seroconversion Research laboratory required to differentiate between HSV-1 and HSV-2
Parvovirus B19	Yes (blood)	Seroconversion Parvovirus B19-specific IgM
Rubella		Seroconversion Rubella-specific IgM
VZV	Yes (vesicle)	Seroconversion
Treponema pallidum	Yes (lesion, dark field)	Venereal Disease Research Laboratory/rapid plasma reagin ≥1/8 and positive treponemal test
Toxoplasma gondii		Seroconversion Toxoplasma-specific IgM with confirmatory timing of infection in reference laboratory

Fig. 55.10 Laboratory evidence of clinically significant maternal infection.

follow primary or recurrent, symptomatic or asymptomatic, HSV-1 or HSV-2 maternal infection at any stage of gestation. Acquisition just before delivery can lead to disease identical to that acquired at delivery, except that it occurs within the first 48 hours of life.

Parvovirus B19

The spectrum of infection in the fetus and neonate continues to expand and includes spontaneous abortion, nonimmune hydrops fetalis, stillbirth, congenital liver damage (portal fibrosis), transfusion-dependent congenital anemia, neutropenia and thrombocytopenia, prenatal closure of the foramen ovale, and a syndrome of anemia, blueberry muffin rash and hepatomegaly.

The vast majority of maternal infections, both symptomatic and asymptomatic, are followed by delivery of a healthy term infant, perhaps in most cases because the fetus is not infected. Whereas the exact rate of loss in early and late pregnancy remains to be determined, there appears to be an excess loss in the second trimester. The absolute risk of fetal loss after maternal parvovirus B19 infection has been reported to be in the order of 5–9%.

Rubella

The clinical features of congenital rubella syndrome (CRS) can be divided into the categories of transient, in newborns and infants; permanent at birth or during the first year of life; and delayed, occurring in 10–20% of patients, usually in the second decade of life. In rare cases, re-infection with maternal rubella has resulted in CRS.

Varicella-zoster virus

The congenital varicella syndrome including cicatricial skin lesions, eye abnormalities, and hypoplastic limbs with or without CNS abnormalities occurs almost exclusively with maternal varicella infection acquired before 20 weeks of gestation, although cases have been reported at 26–28 weeks of gestation. Generally, after 20 weeks manifestations include skin scars, as with postnatal VZV infection, and childhood shingles.

Treponema pallidum

Most commonly physicians are required to investigate the asymptomatic infant whose mother had positive serologic testing for syphilis. Of the diverse findings, bone lesions are the most frequently encountered abnormality, occurring in 20% of symptom-free infected infants. Cerebrospinal fluid examination is required and some experts believe that milder abnormalities in the CSF should be considered to indicate neurosyphilis. These include leukocyte counts of 5mm^3 or more and protein concentrations of 100mg/dl or greater.[24]

Toxoplasma gondii

The diversity of findings may be classified according to timing of symptomatology as symptomatic neonatal disease; disease in the first months of life, usually with neurologic and ophthalmologic findings; sequela of previously undiagnosed infection (i.e. chorioretinitis later in childhood); and subclinical disease. Of asymptomatic infected infants, half will have abnormalities on cranial imaging or ophthalmologic examination. Among 23,000 mothers and infants in the Collaborative Perinatal Project, infants of IgG *Toxoplasma* antibody-positive mothers had a two-fold increase in hearing loss, a 60% increase in the incidence of microcephaly and a 30% increase in the occurrence of low intelligence quotient (<70).[25]

Other

Intrauterine adenovirus infection has been associated with fetal myocarditis, pneumonia and encephalitis. Measles infection in pregnancy increases the risk of prematurity in the first 2 weeks after rash.

DIAGNOSIS

DIAGNOSIS OF FETAL INFECTION

Attribution of adverse outcome to a particular micro-organism in early fetal life requires molecular diagnostic testing (e.g. DNA detection by PCR) and well-controlled studies. Detection of micro-organism-specific IgM is hampered not only by the testing method, but also by the failure of the fetus to reliably produce IgM-specific antibody before 22–24 weeks. Fetal infection may follow maternal infection by at least 4–6 weeks, providing false reassurance if fetal diagnosis, through direct detection or antibody production, is attempted too soon after maternal infection.

Antenatal diagnosis of fetal infection requires a multidisciplinary approach to exclude noninfectious causes and to undertake maternal–fetal studies. Follow-up of the infant at birth and in the ensuing few months is also required to determine the presence, extent and damage, if any, resulting from the infection. Efforts to establish the presence of fetal disease with a positive clinical history or the cause of ultrasonographically detected abnormalities antenatally in the absence of a positive clinical history may well provide a diagnosis.[26]

In the absence of fetal disease, the prenatal diagnosis of fetal infection is not warranted because the predictive values of positive and negative results should not be used as a basis for management decisions.[27] For example, in contrast to the prenatal diagnosis of genetic diseases for which the outcome is reasonably certain, most infants with congenital CMV infection are asymptomatic and do not suffer sequelae.

MATERNAL TESTING

Most maternal infections are asymptomatic and all infections, symptomatic or otherwise can pose a risk to the fetus. Laboratory tests are listed in Figure 55.10. Routine broad screening of a single serum is unlikely to be helpful and is rarely indicated. The diagnosis of a primary CMV infection can be made by demonstration of seroconversion of CMV-specific IgG antibodies from negative to positive, but not by boosting of a titer, as this may occur with recurrent infection. Differentiation of the serofast state from inadequately treated syphilis can be challenging. Although a serofast patient has been considered as having a titer of ≤1:4, it is not unusual to find titers as high as 1:8.[28]

MATERNAL HISTORY RELEVANT TO CONGENITAL INFECTIONS

Woman's history

Underlying illness and medications

Previous history of sexually transmitted disease (HSV, syphilis, chlamydia, gonorrhea, HIV)

Drug or alcohol use, current and previous

Travel during pregnancy (consider culinary practices and other factors in region traveled)

Occupation
- Working with children wearing diapers or who have disabilities (CMV)
- Working with elementary school children (parvovirus, rubella)
- Working with animals or raw meat products (*Toxoplasma*)
- Working in the sex trade industry (HIV, syphilis, tuberculosis, hepatitis B virus, hepatitis C virus).

Household exposure to young children (CMV)

During her pregnancy
- Has she eaten raw meat or tasted it while cooking? (toxoplasmosis)
- Has she consumed unwashed vegetables? (food-borne pathogens, *Toxoplasma*)
- Has she changed kitty litter without wearing gloves? (*Toxoplasma*)
- Has she worked in soil/garden without wearing gloves? (*Toxoplasma*)
- Has she had any illness she might not have mentioned until now?
- Cold sore? (HSV)
- Dysuria, burning, itching? (HSV)
- Profound fatigue? (CMV, *Toxoplasma*, HIV)
- Swollen glands? (CMV, *Toxoplasma*, HIV)
- Arthritis? (rubella, parvovirus B19)
- Rash? (rubella, parvovirus B19, syphilis, enterovirus)

Has her husband/partner had any particular illness?
- Skin sores anywhere? (HSV, syphilis, HIV)

Routine serologic testing

Hepatitis B surface antigen, rubella-specific antibody, syphilis serology (Venereal Disease Research Laboratory, rapid plasma reagin)
- First trimester
- If high risk, repeat third trimester, delivery

Antenatal care

- If absent, see Figure 55.18

Fig. 55.11 Maternal history relevant to congenital infections.

Maternal symptoms and their likelihood

Although fetal disease follows both symptomatic and asymptomatic maternal infection and most maternal infections are asymptomatic, the following symptoms should suggest a search for these micro-organisms: flu, an acute mononucleosis syndrome-like illness (CMV, *Toxoplasma*, HIV); and arthritis or rash (parvovirus B19, rubella, *T. pallidum*).

FETAL TESTING

Detection of the micro-organism by culture or DNA by PCR amplification and product detection in amniotic fluid or fetal blood is promising, but should generally not be undertaken in the absence of fetal abnormalities because of the uncertain sensitivity and specificity. After week 18 of gestation, and at least 4 weeks after maternal infection, PCR testing of the amniotic fluid will detect 97% of toxoplasmosis-infected fetuses.[29] Fetuses infected with CMV are likely to have positive amniotic fluid cultures after 20–22 weeks of gestation because fetal kidney infection is common. Other sites such as effusions may also be cultured and tested by PCR; there are case reports of positive enteroviral cultures.[30]

EVALUATION OF NEONATE WITH SUSPECTED CONGENITAL INFECTION

Clinical	Physical examination (gestational age, height, weight, head circumference) to identify prematurity, intrauterine growth retardation, microcephaly
	Measure liver/spleen size
	Ophthalmologic examination (pediatric expert)
Laboratory	Complete blood count and smear
	Platelet count
	Liver transaminase levels
	Bilirubin level, direct and indirect
	CSF examination (cells, protein, with pertinent antibody, detection; see Fig. 55.13)
	Laboratory testing [detection of agent, maternal and infant (not cord) serology
	Immunoglobulin determinations
	Hold pretransfusion blood for possible additional tests
Other	Cranial CT scan with enhancement
	Long-bone radiographs (if syphilis, rubella likely)
	Placental pathology
	Audiology assessment
	Multidisciplinary follow-up

Fig. 55.12 Evaluation of the neonate with suspected congenital infection.

Other indirect evidence of infection may be obtained through hematologic and biochemical profiles including hepatic enzymes and in the future, through study of lymphocyte subclass populations and cytokine production.

NEONATAL TESTING

In evaluating the neonate with suspected congenital infection at birth, it is necessary to:
- review the maternal history including serologic screening (Figs 55.10 & 55.11);
- review ultrasonography undertaken in pregnancy (Fig. 55.7);
- evaluate the infant (Figs 55.9 & 55.12);
- attempt detection of the pathogen in the neonate; and
- undertake judicious maternal and infant serologic testing pertinent to the most likely diagnoses.

Detection of the micro-organism in the neonate

The best evidence for infection with CMV, enterovirus, HSV, parvovirus B19, rubella, syphilis and *Toxoplasma* comes from detection of the agent in the neonate (see below).

Maternal and infant testing pertinent to the most likely diagnoses

Diagnostic tests are summarized in Figure 55.13. Over- and under-diagnosis of congenital infection has arisen as a result of failure to:
- submit maternal serology for documentation of a source of infection;
- detect the organism in the infant through culture (or newer methods of antigen detection);
- sequentially test the infant serologically; and
- appreciate the enormous rate of false-positive and false-negative test results obtained through IgM-specific testing and use of cord blood.

False-negative IgM tests in infants are extremely common. An exception is the rubella-specific IgM test, which is highly sensitive and specific. Parvovirus IgM is frequently negative when virus is detected by PCR.

Serologic documentation of maternal infection and acute and

LABORATORY INVESTIGATION AND FOLLOW-UP OF NEONATE WITH SUSPECTED CONGENITAL INFECTION			
Infection	Mother at birth	Neonatal (not cord blood)	Follow-up of infant
CMV	Antibody	Virus detection in urine, saliva, blood leukocytes, CSF IgM capture ELISA and radioimmunoassay Antibody	Repeated antibody testing to 6–12 months; passive maternal antibody disappears at 4–9 months; negative infant and maternal antibody rules out infection, although intrapartum cervical and postpartum breast milk transmission is common
Enterovirus	Virus detection in stool, throat, blood, of mother of infant with suspected congenital enteroviral infection Bank serum	Virus detection in stool, throat, CSF, nose, blood, other Bank birth and 2nd serum at 2–4 weeks	Selective testing of paired infant and maternal sera appropriate to infant, maternal, or community isolates
HSV	Antibody	Virus detection in skin vesicles, throat, CSF, urine, nose, conjunctiva, rectal swab Antibody	Repeated antibody testing to 6–12 months (cannot differentiate between type 1 and type 2 viruses) Negative infant and maternal antibody rules out infection
Parvovirus B19	IgM and IgG antibody Detection of DNA (e.g. by PCR) in blood	Detection of DNA (e.g. by PCR) in blood, bone marrow Parvovirus-IgM	Repeated antibody testing to 6–12 months Infected infants and their mothers may lack IgM antibody
Rubella	Rubella-specific IgG and IgM antibody	Rubella-specific IgM antibody Virus detection in urine, nasopharynx, CSF, blood CSF rubella-specific IgM antibody	Repeated antibody testing to 6–12 months Negative infant antibody at 6–12 months usually rules out infection
VZV	Antibody	Virus detection in skin lesions Antibody	Antibody testing 6–12 months postnatally Intrauterine infection commonly manifest only as persistent antibody and childhood zoster
Toxoplasma gondii	Toxoplasma-specific IgM and IgG antibody To determine acuity of infection in IgM positive mother, need reference laboratory testing Seroconversion or four-fold rise in Toxoplasma-specific IgG in pregnancy	Reference laboratory testing of Toxoplasma-specific: IgM-ISAGA, DS-IgM-ELISA, IgE-ELISA, IgE-ISAGA, IgA-ELISA or Blood culture (Toxoplasma-specific IgM falsely positive and negative) Culture and histopathology of the placenta	Repeated antibody testing to 6–12 months Negative infant antibody at 6–12 months usually rules out congenital infection
Treponema pallidum	Quantitative Venereal Disease Research Laboratory (VDRL). Rapid plasma reagin (RPR) Treponemal antibody (e.g. fluorescent treponemal antibody absorption) If positive, maternal HIV status	Detection of treponemes in nasal secretions, skin lesions, etc. by dark-field examination Quantitative VDRL, RPR Serum treponemal antibody [e.g. fluorescent treponemal antibody absorbed (FTA) test]	Repeated quantitative VDRL and treponemal antibody testing to 12–15 months No test at birth can differentiate between the asymptomatic infected and uninfected neonate Passively transferred antibody disappears at 6 months (VDRL, RPR) and 12–15 months (treponemal)

Fig. 55.13 Laboratory investigation and follow-up of neonate with suspected congenital infection.

follow-up serology of the infant over the first months or year of life can be diagnostic, albeit not sufficiently quickly to facilitate decisions about therapy. Passively transferred antibody will disappear in the first 6–12 months, whereas antibody persists or rises in the infected infant. Follow-up serology is more complicated in the case of congenital CMV as infection may also be acquired at birth or postnatally through breast-milk or other contact.

Cord blood is not acceptable for specific antibody testing for syphilis, Toxoplasma or CMV because of false-positive and -negative results. Total cord IgM levels may be falsely elevated through contamination by maternal blood. Cases of congenital syphilis have been reported in which both mothers' and neonates' titers were negative at birth but the infants subsequently developed clinical syphilis at 3–14 weeks of age with strongly positive titers.[31]

The futility of a single serologic [syphilis, toxoplasmosis, other agents, rubella, CMV, herpes virus (STORCH)] screen is well known and a more directed approach is required. In preference to a single serum (STORCH titer), every effort should be made to recover the organism from the neonate and test booking and follow-up maternal and infant blood (Fig. 55.14).

DEFINITIONS OF SELECTED CONGENITAL INFECTIONS

Because of delayed onset and/or recognition of signs infection as well as the varied availibility of diagnostic tests, definitions have been developed that take into consideration the likelihood of infection (Fig. 55.15).

MANAGEMENT

GENERAL

A through understanding of the consequences of infection in pregnancy is required to counsel parents regarding risks to the fetus and possible courses of action.

Selected maternal infections should be followed by ultrasonography to identify adverse effects. Antenatal diagnosis is generally attempted only if fetal abnormalities are present. After delivery, additional information about contagiousness, breast-feeding, and risk of transmission in subsequent pregnancies should be conveyed. Comprehensive long-term pediatric follow-up is required to identify and manage the spectrum of cognitive, motor, visual, hearing and other impairments that may be imparted by some of these infections.

APPROPRIATE SPECIMENS TO DIAGNOSE CONGENITAL INFECTION		
Specimen	Tests	Interpretation
Urine	Viral culture/detection (CMV, HSV, rubella)	Urine for CMV must be obtained at ≤2 weeks of age Positive is diagnostic
Throat swab	Viral culture (CMV, HSV, rubella, enteroviruses)	Positive is diagnostic
Blood	Agent detection (CMV, parvovirus B19)	Positive is diagnostic
Neonatal serum (single specimen)	Rubella-specific IgM	Positive is diagnostic, although determination of status at 10–12 months is confirmatory
Sequential neonatal, infant sera over 6–12 months	All	Passive maternal antibody in uninfected infant disappears at 4–9 months for CMV (unless peri-, postnatal transmission); 8 months for *Toxoplasma gondii*; 6 months VDRL, rapid plasma reagin; 12–15 months (treponemal) Positive specific antibody at 8–12 months suggests congenital toxoplasmosis, parvovirus B19, rubella, VZV infection
Single maternal serum at delivery	*Toxoplasma*-specific IgM	If IgM-specific antibody positive, reference laboratory testing of maternal, infant sera and placenta
Serology of both mother and infant	All	Negative maternal serology rules out source of infection Serial infant serology identifies passive maternal antibody (titers fall) and active infection (titers remain the same, rise over months)
CSF culture, detection	Detection of CMV, enteroviruses, HSV, *Toxoplasma* (reference laboratory), parvovirus B19 Rubella-specific IgM antibody VDRL	
Skin lesions culture, detection	If active/vesiculated at birth: herpes, enteroviruses VZV Syphilis dark-field	
Nasopharyngeal secretions	Syphilis dark-field	
Stool cultures	Enteroviruses	
Placenta	Variable	

Fig. 55.14 Appropriate specimens to diagnose congenital infection.[19]

SPECIFIC INFECTIONS
Cytomegalovirus
Neurologic outcome cannot be reliably predicted until the infant is 2 or 3 years of age, during which head growth is monitored and achievement of developmental milestones is documented. Infants with abnormal cranial imaging are more likely to have cognitive and other deficits in follow-up.[32] Progression of existing retinal lesions or delayed development of chorioretinitis during childhood has been reported in about 20% of children, whereas hearing loss will evolve in about 30% of children, as late as school age.[33,34]

The highly variable, unpredictable course of congenital CMV infection make randomized controlled trials of therapy such as ganciclovir imperative before widespread use. Infants with CNS disease at birth have already sustained enormous damage. Theoretically, therapy might be of some use because infection is active at birth and damage appears to continue for up to 2.5 years.[35] Prevention through vaccination is urgently needed.

Herpes simplex virus
As intrauterine infection is rare, infected women should be assured that maternal infection is common, but that the risk of fetal infection is essentially negligible.

Parvovirus B19
After maternal exposure and documented infection, serial ultrasonography for 1–14 weeks will identify the hydropic fetus. For the fetus with nonimmune hydrops fetalis and a low hematocrit and reticulocyte count, one or more intravascular fetal transfusions of packed erythrocytes until marrow aplasia resolves, has been used with good results. Hydropic fetuses with an intermediate hemoglobin and a high reticulocyte count, in whom the process is resolving spontaneously, need not be transfused and show no sequelae. The management of the neonate who has sustained red cell aplasia through a 'hit and run' effect of the virus on the bone marrow may respond to immunoglobulin and corticosteroids. There is no medical indication for termination of the pregnancy complicated by parvovirus B19 infection.[36]

Rubella
Infected infants should be considered infectious for the first year of life unless repeated nasopharyngeal and urine cultures are negative. Long-term follow-up will identify progressive hearing loss and visual deterioration, endocrinopathies and subacute sclerosing panencephalitis.

Treponema pallidum
All infected women should receive penicillin therapy appropriate to their stage of disease to minimize or eliminate the risk of transmission to the fetus. If serology has been positive for less than 1 year, the patient may be treated with benzathine penicillin G 2.4 million units intramuscularly (IM) as a single dose. If the patient has been seropositive for 1 year or more, benzathine penicillin G 2.4 million units IM in a single dose weekly for 3 successive weeks is required. Maternal CSF examination (protein, cell count, CSF-VDRL) is required only if neurosyphilis is suspected; it is not routinely required in patients with infectious syphilis if the CNS examination is negative. Retreatment during pregnancy is unnecessary if titers followed monthly continue to fall. In the presence of penicillin allergy, desensitization is the preferred management; any other therapy will necessitate treatment of the infant after birth. All women with positive serology require HIV testing and testing of their recent sexual contacts, as well as repeat testing in the third trimester and at birth. Cord blood should not be used for rapid

DEFINITIONS OF SELECTED CONGENITAL INFECTIONS

CMV	Confirmed	Detection of CMV in the first 2–3 weeks of life from urine, throat, or other sources in newborn with one or more of: • Small for gestational age • Hematologic findings (petechiae, purpura, splenomegaly, jaundice at birth) • Neurologic findings (microcephaly, chorioretinitis, neurologic abnormality, intracranial calcifications, hearing impairment) • Laboratory findings (direct hyperbilirubinemia >3mg/dl), thrombocytopenia (platelet count <75,000/ml), liver function abnormality (alanine aminotransferase >100 mg/dl)
	Possible	As for Confirmed, except viral detection only after 3 weeks of age and other diseases ruled out
HSV	Congenital	Detection of HSV within 24 hours of birth or stable positive titer over 3 months in infants with one or more of skin, eye, and brain lesions
	Perinatal	Detection of HSV after 24 hours and in first 6 weeks of life further characterized by clinical and laboratory findings as one of: • Disseminated • CNS • Skin, eye, mouth disease
Rubella	Confirmed	Defects of congenital rubella syndrome present and one or more of: • Virus detected • Positive rubella-specific IgM antibody • Positive infant serology after disappearance of passively transferred maternal antibodies at 3–12 months
	Compatible	Insufficient laboratory data for confirmation of diagnosis but any two complications from (a) or one from (a) and one from (b): (a) Cataracts or congenital glaucoma, congenital heart disease, hearing loss, pigmentary retinopathy (b) Purpura, splenomegaly, jaundice, radiolucent bone disease, meningoencephalitis, microcephaly, mental retardation
	Possible	Presence of some compatible clinical findings, but insufficient criteria for either the Confirmed or Compatible categories
Syphilis	Confirmed	Identification of *Treponema pallidum* in nasal or skin lesions
	Presumptive	One or more of: • Infant born to mother with untreated or inadequately treated syphilis • Treated with drug other than penicillin and/or • <30 days to 3 months before delivery • Infant has reactive treponemal test with findings of one or more of abnormal physical examination, long bone radiographs, CSF (including reactive CSF-VDRL and/or a leukocyte count of 20ml or greater or a protein concentration of 100mg/dl or greater), four-fold higher VDRL than mother signs • Infant has documented four-fold rise in titers and positive treponemal test • Infant has reactive treponemal test that does not revert by 12–15 months
Toxoplasma gondii	Confirmed	• *Toxoplasma*-specific IgM (or if available, Sabin-Feldman Dye test >300 IU) in maternal sera with infant findings of chorioretinitis, cerebral calcifications or hydrocephalus in the absence of CMV infection • Positive antibody in infant at 8–10 months (after disappearance of passively transferred maternal antibody) with or without clinical findings
	Compatible	• Chorioretinitis with positive *Toxoplasma*-specific antibody after 8–10 months of age • Cerebral calcifications and/or hydrocephalus with positive *Toxoplasma*-specific antibody after 8–10 months of age in the absence of CMV infection
Parvovirus B19		Detection of parvovirus B19 by: • Direct electron microscopy or nucleic acid in blood and/or tissue obtained within the first 3 weeks of life in the presence of fetal or neonatal findings of hydrops and anemia • Parvovirus B19-specific IgM in the first 3 weeks or persistent IgG beyond 3–12 months with either documented maternal infection or fetal/neonatal findings of hydrops/anemia
Varicella		One or more of: • Anomalies of congenital varicella syndrome (skin, eye, limb, neurologic) • Acute varicella at birth with viral detection • Herpes zoster in the first year of life with viral detection • VZV-specific IgM at birth, persistent IgG to 12 months, or detection of specific lymphocyte transformation in response to VZV virus antigen

Fig. 55.15 Definitions of selected congenital infections.

plasma reagin/VDRL testing as it may be falsely negative or positive.[37] Long bone radiographs and usually CSF examination are required.

Indications for treatment include:
• symptomatic disease;
• inadequate maternal treatment (i.e. not documented, inadequate or unknown), use of a drug other than penicillin, treatment within 4 weeks of delivery (or last trimester, according to some experts);
• uncertain follow-up; and
• secondary or latent syphilis in the mother within one year of delivery.

Therapy with aqueous crystalline penicillin G 100,000–150,000 IU/kg (given every 8–12 hours) intravenously for 10–14 days is recommended. After the second week of life, or with confirmed neurosyphilis or severe disease, aqueous penicillin 200,000–250,000 U/kg per day may be used.[22] A preliminary study suggests that selected asymptomatic infants may be treated with benzathine penicillin 50,000 U/kg IM once, provided that there are no signs of congenital syphilis on physical examination, CSF cell count or VDRL, X-ray studies of the long bones of the lower extremities, platelet counts or liver function tests.[38] Follow-up of all infants is required up to 1 year or beyond to ensure that the appropriate falls in titers have occurred and that treatment or retreatment is not

TREATMENT OF TOXOPLASMOSIS OF THE FETUS AND INFANT			
Manifestation of disease	Medication	Dosage	Duration of therapy
In pregnant women with acute toxoplasmosis	Spiramycin	1g every 8 hours without food	Until fetal infection documented or excluded at 18–20 weeks; if documented, in alternate months with pyrimethamine, leukovorin, and sulfadiazine until term (France)
If fetal infection confirmed after week 17 of gestation or if maternal infection acquired in last few weeks of gestation	Pyrimethamine and	Loading dose: 100mg/day in two divided doses for 2 days then 50mg/day	Until term (leukovorin is continued 1 week after pyrimethamine is discontinued)
	Sulfadiazine	Loading dose: 75mg/kg per day in two divided doses (maximum 4g/day) for 2 days then 100mg/kg per day in two divided doses (maximum 4g/day)	
	Leukovorin (folinic acid)	10–20mg/day	
Congenital *Toxoplasma* infection in the infant	Pyrimethamine and	Loading dose: 2mg/kg per day for 2 days, then 1mg/kg per day for 2–6 months, then this dose every Monday, Wednesday and Friday	1 year
	Sulfadiazine and	100mg/kg per day in two divided doses	1 year
	Leukovorin	10mg 3 times a week	1 year
	Corticosteroids (prednisone) have been used when CSF protein is ≥1g/dl and when active chorioretinitis threatens vision	1mg/kg per day in two divided doses	Until resolution of elevated (≥1 g/dl) CSF protein level or active chorioretinitis that threatens vision

Fig. 55.16 **Treatment of toxoplasmosis of the fetus and infant.** Adapted with permission from Hohlfeld *et al.*[39] and Remington *et al.*[3]

required. Nontreponemal antibody titers, followed at 1, 2, 4, and 6 months, should be nonreactive at 6 months. At 12–15 months treponemal titers, if negative, rule out infection.

Toxoplasma gondii

If acutely infected women can be identified and treated in pregnancy through organization of a regional system of screening, the outcome is very good. In comparison with historical controls, only 2% of infants with first or second trimester fetal infection whose mothers received treatment developed disease, compared to 20% of those whose mothers did not.[39]

Although maternal spiramycin therapy reduces the rate of transmission to the fetus, the combination of pyrimethamine and sulfadiazine is required once infection is established to improve fetal outcome. The regimen currently recommended for treatment in North America is given in Figure 55.16.

In the absence of antenatal diagnosis and fetal therapy,[40] the results of a 1-year course of therapy in infants in whom therapy was initiated within 2.5 months of birth have been reported in the Chicago Collaborative Treatment Trial.[41] Developmental, audiologic and visual performance was adequate for normal function in 75% of treated children in follow-up of 33 months. The single most important predictor of poor outcome was hydrocephalus. Evidence of hydrocephalus must be actively sought and the condition managed aggressively. When infants are not treated or receive 1 month of pyrimethamine and sulfadiazine, late sequelae after subclinical disease include active chorioretinitis in 85%, including some cases of blindness or impaired vision, developmental delay in 20–75% and moderate hearing loss in 10–30%.

PERINATAL INFECTIONS

These occur as a result of ascending infection and premature rupture of the membranes or through intrapartum transmission. Their management and prevention are summarized in Figure 55.17.

Specific infections

Enterovirus. Enteroviruses are among the commonest pathogens encountered by the newborn in the first months of life. The most common symptoms are undifferentiated fever and aseptic meningitis. No specific therapy is available. Given the likelihood that an infected infant has received no passive maternal antibody, high-dose intravenous immune globulin may be reasonable in the acutely ill infant, although efficacy has not been demonstrated.[42]

Herpes simplex virus. Because it is the primary infection, rather than recurrent infection in pregnancy that is a risk to the fetus, transmission cannot be eliminated despite the best obstetric care. Primary infection is characterized by cervical infection in 80% of cases, protracted shedding for a mean of 11 days, and a 33% risk of transmission to the newborn if shedding occurs at delivery. Conversely, in recurrent infection, there is only a 13% risk of cervical shedding, 2–4 days of shedding, and a 3% risk of transmission if there is shedding at delivery.

Neither a positive nor a negative clinical history will predict the neonatal risk for HSV infection. Of women with no previous history of genital HSV, 0.2% will have positive genital cultures at delivery.[43] Because viral shedding at the time of delivery cannot be predicted by third trimester cultures, screening is not recommended.

Women with recurrent disease should be reassured. With a risk of asymptomatic shedding of about 2% and a transmission rate of 3%, the risk of neonatal infection in this situation is about 1 in 2000 births. Cesarian section is generally recommended for women with active lesions at birth or a clinical primary infection during pregnancy, particularly in the last half of gestation; infection may occur in spite of cesarian section. Fetal scalp monitors should be avoided. Viral cultures should be obtained from the maternal cervix as well as from the infant at birth. Infant cultures should be repeated at 24 hours and the child carefully observed for symptoms of neonatal HSV requiring therapy.

Herpes simplex virus commonly presents without skin lesions as

PREVENTIVE STRATEGIES AND INTRAPARTUM MANAGEMENT			
Micro-organism	Clinical situation	Preventive management	Comment
Enterovirus	Active maternal enteroviral infection (i.e. fever, abdominal pain) at delivery	Attempt to defer delivery	May allow transmission of antibody
Hepatitis B virus	Maternal HBsAg status unknown	Neonatal immunization	Many experts recommend universal neonatal immunization
HSV	Maternal lesions at delivery	Active observation of neonate for signs of infection	See detailed guidelines Cesarian section for active lesions or primary infection in (late) pregnancy
HIV-1	HIV-positive mother	Single or combination antiviral therapy of infant	Antenatal screening and therapy is advisable
Rubella	High risk, no antenatal care, no serology at delivery	Postpartum immunization of susceptibles before hospital discharge	
VZV	Maternal lesion within 1 week before or after delivery	Varicella-zoster immune globulin ± aciclovir therapy of neonate	
Treponema pallidum	High risk, no antenatal care, no serology at delivery		In high-risk women repeat screen in third trimester, delivery

Fig. 55.17 Preventive strategies and intrapartum management.

neonatal sepsis or pneumonitis, with one of the earliest clues being abnormal liver enzymes. Shock, coagulopathy, fulminant hepatitis and skin lesions follow. Prematurity is extremely common, occurring in about 26% of infected infants. Infected infants may have progressive deterioration over the first year, especially with a history of multiple episodes of recurrent skin lesions in the first 6 months, suggesting that CNS relapse may be common and that involvement of the CNS, not initially evident, may occur. The role of prophylactic oral antiviral therapy in infected infants is under study.

Therapy is indicated for the infant who is unwell, especially if liver function tests are abnormal, if surface cultures are positive after 48 hours, or if the CSF is abnormal, with possible prematurity if there is prolonged rupture of the membranes, interventions (e.g. scalp monitoring, forceps) or primary infection near birth.

Aciclovir therapy is provided at a dosage of 30mg/kg per day intravenously q8h for 14 days,[44] although higher doses are being used in research trials. While outcome is certainly improved, mortality remains at approximately 20%, depending on the clinical presentation. The progression of cutaneous to CNS disease can be halted by antiviral therapy in the majority of cases. Emergence of resistant organisms may be expected in the future. Isolation of the infant with lesions is required.

Varicella-zoster virus. A neonate whose mother has developed varicella 5 days before delivery to 48 hours after delivery should receive a dose of 125U (1.25ml or 1 vial) of zoster immune globulin as soon as possible. These infants carry a 30% risk of infection without the protection of passive maternal antibody and are at grave risk of serious disease. Aciclovir at a dose of 1500mg/m^2 per day is used to treat symptomatic neonates,[45] with dose adjustments for liver and renal failure or prematurity.[46] Separation of an infected and contagious mother from the child may be advisable. Isolation of the exposed hospitalized infant is required.

HIV-1. There is evidence for both early and late in-utero transmission, including two-fold higher infection rates in the first-born than second-born twin. Fetal diagnostic testing may result in iatrogenic infection of the fetus and is generally contraindicated.

Prevention of transmission is achievable through antiretroviral therapy with zidovudine. During delivery, the mother should receive 2mg/kg intravenously over 1 hour and then 1 mg/kg per hour for the duration of labor and throughout the delivery. The infant should be washed, given vitamin K and provided with zidovudine at 2mg/kg per dose, q6h orally in liquid form within 8–12 hours after birth, continued for 6 weeks. The possibility of a 30–50% reduction in transmission with cesarean section requires further study. Non-breastfed

infants of infected mothers can be accurately diagnosed by 3 months of age.[47]

Hepatitis B virus. In four studies of over 33,000 pregnant women in North America, a prevalence of HBsAg carriage of 0.8% was documented; 52% of women acknowledged no known risk factors. The risk of perinatal infection is greater if the maternal infection was acquired in the third trimester (80–90% versus less than 10% in the first trimester). If HBsAg positivity is accompanied by e-antigen positivity, the neonate is both more likely to become infected (70–90% versus 20–25%) and is more likely to become a chronic carrier (85% versus 5%). The strongest predictor of transmission may be maternal hepatitis B virus DNA load.

Infants of carrier mothers should receive 0.5ml hepatitis B immune globulin within 12 hours of birth and either 5µg of the Merck hepatitis B vaccine (Recombivax HB) or 10µg of the SmithKline Beecham hepatitis B vaccine (Engerix-B). The second dose of vaccine is given at 1–2 months of age and the 3rd dose at 6 months of age. Infants born to mothers of unknown status should receive either 5µg of Recombivax HB or 10µg of Engerix-B. The second dose of vaccine is given at 1–2 months of age and the third dose at 6 months of age.

Hepatitis C virus. In 20 studies the risk of perinatal transmission of hepatitis C virus was 14%, being 21% in infants born to HIV-infected mothers (65 out of 309), 10% in infants born to HIV-negative mothers (50 out of 495), 14% in those born to hepatitis C virus RNA-positive mothers and 2% in those born to hepatitis C virus RNA-negative mothers (Delages G, personal communication).

Group B streptococcus. Two alternative approaches to the prevention of group B streptococcal disease have been developed in the USA.[48] According to the screening-based approach, all pregnant women should be screened at 35–37 weeks' gestation for anogenital group B streptococcus colonization. Intrapartum antibiotics are offered to all culture-positive women, regardless of risk factors. If the results of cultures are not known at the time of labor, intrapartum antibiotics are used in the presence of risk factors, which include the following: less than 37 weeks' gestation; more than 18 hours of membrane rupture; temperature higher than 100.4°F (38°C). The alternative approach is based on risk factors alone. Also, women with a previously infected infant and women with group B streptococcus bacteriuria during pregnancy are treated with intrapartum antibiotics. In geographic regions with differing epidemiologic data, this approach is not appropriate.

Absence of antenatal care. For women in whom there has been inadequate antenatal care, detection of infection is required at delivery, as summarized in Figure 55.18.

BREAST-FEEDING
Breast-feeding during an active infection
Contaminated milk has been implicated in neonatal infection with *Staphylococcus aureus,* group B streptococci, *Mycobacterium* spp. and possibly *Salmonella* spp.

Although viral contamination of milk by rubella, HSV, hepatitis B virus and CMV has been reported, serious sequelae have not generally occurred. Mothers with herpetic lesions on their breasts should refrain from breast-feeding. They should cover other active lesions and wash hands before breast-feeding.

Breast-feeding is estimated to confer an additional risk of 14% over transmission of HIV-1 *in utero* or at delivery.[47]

Breast-feeding and drug therapy
The American Academy of Pediatrics recommends that breast-feeding be discontinued while a nursing mother is being treated with metronidazole and warns about the use of nitrofurantoin and sulfa drugs, which can cause hemolysis in glucose-6-phosphatase-deficient infants.[49] Although it would be unusual for an effective maternal medication to be contraindicated because of risks to the infant through breast milk, physicians should be aware of information specific to agents being used. Frequent feeding exposes the infant to more drug than feeding at 4-hour intervals. Mothers can be encouraged to avoid frequent feedings to reduce drug exposure and the consequent changes in the infant's gastrointestinal flora and risk of oropharyngeal candidiasis.

WOMEN WITH LIMITED OR NO ANTENATAL CARE	
Mother	• Genital examination for findings suggestive of STDs
	• Cultures for *Chlamydia trachomatis*, *N. gonorrheae*
	• Serologic testing for HBsAg, hepatitis C virus, HIV, syphilis (nontreponemal and treponemal testing), rubella
	• Adequate follow-up
Infant	• Prophylactic eye care
	• Serologic testing for HBsAg, hepatitis C virus, HIV, syphilis (nontreponemal and treponemal testing)
	• First dose of hepatitis B vaccine
	• Adequate follow-up

Fig. 55.18 Women with limited or no antenatal care.

REFERENCES

1. Guerina N. Management strategies for infectious diseases in pregnancy. Semin Perinatol 1994;18:305–20.
2. Greenough A. The TORCH screen and intrauterine infections. Arch Dis Child 1994;70:F163–5.
3. Remington J, McLeod R, Desmonts G. Toxoplasmosis. In: Remington JS, Klein J, ed. Infectious diseases of the fetus and newborn. Philadephia: WB Saunder;, 1995:140–267.
4. Stagno S. Cytomegalovirus. In: Remington JS Klein J, ed. Infectious diseases of the fetus and newborn infant. Philadelphia: WB Saunders; 1995:312–53.
5. Pass R. Viral infections in the fetus and neonate. In: Long S, Pickering LK Prober C, ed. Principles and practice of pediatric infectious disesases. New York: Churchill Livingstone; 1997:614–8.
6. Fowler KB, Stagno S, Pass RF. The outcome of congenital CMV in relation to maternal antibody status. N Engl J Med 1992;326:663–7.
7. Fiumara N, Fleming WL, Downing JG, et al. The incidence of prenatal syphilis at the Boston City Hospital. N Engl J Med 1952;247:48–52.
8. Miller E, Cradock-Watson JE, Ridehalgh MKS, et al. Consequences of confirmed maternal rubella at successive stages of pregnancy. Lancet 1982;2:782–4.
9. Pastuszak AL, Levy M, Schick B, et al. Outcome after maternal varicella infection in the first 20 weeks of pregnancy. N Engl J Med 1994;330:901–5.
10. Enders G, Miller E, Cradock-Watson J, et al. Consequences of varicella and herpes zoster in pregnancy: prospective study of 1739 cases. Lancet 1994;343:1548–50.
11 American College of Obstetricians and Gynecologists. Immunization during pregnancy. ACOG Tech Bull 1991;160.

12. Demmler G. Congenital cytomegalovirus infection and disease. Adv Pediatr Infect Dis 1996;11:134–62.
13. Stray-Pedersen B. Economic evaluation of maternal screening to prevent congenital syphilis. Sex Transm Dis 1983;10:167–72.
14. Barron SD, Pass RF. Infectious causes of hydrops fetalis. Semin Perinatol 1995;19:493–501.
15. Stringer M, Thornton JG, Mason GC. Hyoechogenic fetal bowel. Arch Dis Child 1996;74:F1–2.
16. Guerina N, Meissner HC, Maguire J, et al. Neonatal serologic screening and early treatment for congenital *Toxoplasma gondii* infection. N Engl J Med 1994;330:1858–63.
17. Ikeda MK, Jenson HB. Evaluation and treatment of congenital syphilis. J Pediatr 1990;117:843–52.
18. Silver M, Hellmann J, Zielenska M, et al. Anemia, blueberry-muffin rash, and hepatomegaly in a newborn infant. J Pediatr 1996;128:579–86.
19. Greenough A. Paediatric problems. In: Greenough A, Osborne J, eds. Congenital, perinatal, and neonatal infections. Edinburgh: Churchill Livingstone; 1992:17.
20. Tarr P, Haas JE, Christie DL. Biliary atresia, cytomegalovirus and age at referral. Pediatrics 1996;97:828–31.
21. Metzman R, Anand A, DeGuilio PA, Knisely AS. Hepatic disease associated with intrauterine parvovirus B19 infection in a newborn premature infant. J Pediatr Gastroenterol and Nutr 1989;9:112–4.
22. Glaser J. Centers for Disease Control and Prevention guidelines for congenital syphilis. J Pediatr 1996;129:488–90.
23. Silver MM, Zielenska M, Perrin D, MacDonald JK. Association of prenatal closure of the foramen ovale and fetal parvovirus B19 infection in hydrops fetalis. Cardiovasc Pathol 1995;4:103–9.

24. Centers for Disease Control and Prevention. Case definitions for public health surveillance. MMWR Morb Mortal Wkly Rep 1990;39:36–8.
25. Sever JL, Ellenberg JH, Ley ACX, et al. Toxoplasmosis: maternal and pediatric findings in 23,000 pregnancies. Pediatrics 1988;82:181–92.
26. Weiner CP, Grose CF, Naides SJ. Diagnosis of fetal infection in the patient with an ultrasonographically detected abnormality but a negative clinical history. Am J Obstet Gynecol 1993;168:6–11.
27. Pass R. Is there a role for prenatal diagnosis of congenital CMV infection? Pediatr Infect Dis J 1992;11:608–9.
28. Risser W, Lu-Yu H. Problems in the current case definitions of congenital syphilis. J Pediatr 1996;129:499–505.
29. Hohlfield P, Daffos F, Costa JM, et al. Prenatal diagnosis of congenital toxoplasmosis with a polymerase-chain reaction test on amniotic fluid. N Engl J Med 1994;331:695–9.
30. Abzug M. Perinatal enterovirus infections. In: Rotbart H, ed. Human enterovirus infections. Washington: American Society for Microbiology; 1995:221–38.
31. Dorfman DH, Glaser JG. Congenital syphilis presenting in infants after the newborn period. N Engl J Med 1990;323:1299–302.
32. Boppana SP, Fowler KB, Vaid Y, et al. Neuroradiologic findings in the newborn period and long-term outcome in children with symptomatic congenital cytomegalovirus infection. Pediatrics 1997;99:409–14.
33. Fowler KB, McCollister FP, Dahle AJ, Boppana S, Britt WJ, Pass RF. Progressive and fluctuating sensorineural hearing loss in children with asymptomatic congenital cytomegalovirus infectin. J Pediatr 1997;130:624–30.

34. Connolly PK, Jerger S, Williamson DW, *et al.* Evaluation of higher level auditory function in children with asymptomatic congenital cytomegalovirus infection. Am J Otol 1992;13:185–93.

35. Nigro G, Scholz H, Bartman U. Ganciclovir therapy for symptomatic congenital cytomegalovirus infection in infants: a two-regimen experience. Pediatrics 1994;124:318–22.

36. Gratacos E, Torres P-J, Vidal J, *et al.* The incidence of human parvovirus B19 infection during pregnancy and its impact on perinatal outcome. J Infect Dis 1995;171:1360–3.

37. Chabra RS, Brion LP, Castro M, *et al.* Comparison of maternal sera, cord blood, and neonatal sera for detecting presumptive congenital syphilis: relationship with maternal treatment. J Pediatr 1993;91:88–91.

38. Zenker PN, Berman SB. Congential syphilis trends and recommendations for evaluation and management. Pediatr Infect Dis J 1991;10:515–20.

39. Hohlfeld P, Daffos F, Thulliez P, *et al.* Fetal toxoplasmosis; outcome of pregnancy and infant follow-up after in utero treatment. J Pediatr 1989;115:765–9.

40. Daffos F, Forrestier R, Capella-Pavlovsky M, *et al.* Prenatal management of 746 pregnancies at risk for congenital toxoplasmosis. N Engl J Med 1988; 318:271–5.

41. McAuley JM, Boyer KM, Patel D, *et al.* Early and longitudinal evaluations of treated infants and children and untreated historical patients with congenital toxoplasmosis: The Chicago Collaborative Treatment Trial. Clin Infect Dis 1994;18:38–72.

42. Johnston J, Overall JC. Intravenous immunoglobulin in disseminated neonatal echovirus 11 infection. Pediatr Infect Dis J 1989;8:254–6.

43. Prober C. Use of routine viral cultures at delivery to identify neonates exposed to herpes simplex virus. N Engl J Med 1988;318:887–91.

44. Whitley R, Arvin A, Prober C, *et al.* A controlled trial comparing vidarabine with acyclovir in neonatal HSV infection. N Engl J Med 1991;324:444–9.

45. Bakshi S, Miller TC, Kaplan M, *et al.* Failure of VZIG in modifcation of severe congenital varicella. Pediatr Infect Dis J 1986;5:699–702.

46. Englund J, Fletcher CV, Balfour HH. Acyclovir therapy in neonates. J Pediatr 1991;119:129–135.

47. Scarlatti G. Paediatric HIV infection. Lancet 1996;348:863–8.

48. Prevention of prenatal group B streptococcal disease: a public health perspective. MMWR Morb Mortal Wkly Rep 1996;45(RR-7):1–24

49. American Academy of Pediatrics. 1994 Red Book; Report of the Committee on Infectious Diseases. Elk Grove Village, Illinois: American Academy of Pediatrics; 1994.

chapter
56

Practice Points

Management of an HIV-positive pregnant woman with a positive VDRL test from an area endemic for *Treponoma* infection

Naiel N Nassar &
Justin D Radolf

INTRODUCTION

Infections with HIV and syphilis are significantly interrelated. As sexually transmitted diseases, each poses a risk for the other, and syphilitic lesions (chancres) probably facilitate the transmission of HIV. Also, the immunologic abnormalities associated with HIV infection may alter the natural history of syphilis, albeit in a minority of patients. In persons coinfected with syphilis and HIV, there may be reactivation of latent syphilis, decrease in the latent period before the onset of neurosyphilis, enhanced severity of clinical manifestations and altered serologic responses. Furthermore, associated HIV infection may render conventional antisyphilitic therapy inadequate. Nevertheless, most HIV-infected patients with early syphilis have clinical manifestations comparable to those observed in HIV-uninfected people and respond appropriately to the currently recommended regimens.

SEROLOGIC TESTING FOR TREPONEMAL INFECTIONS

Serologic tests for syphilis are a mainstay of diagnosis and are particularly important in diagnosing infection in patients who either lack clinical manifestations or whose manifestations are not readily apparent. Two different kinds of serologic tests are used in the diagnosis of syphilitic infection. The first type, represented by the Venereal Disease Research Laboratory (VDRL) test and the rapid plasma reagin (RPR) test, detect antibodies to a defined mixture of cardiolipin, lecithin and cholesterol. These tests have traditionally been designed as 'nontreponemal', based upon the belief that the antibodies being detected are induced by lipoidal antigens of host origin. Nontreponemal tests (NTTs) are used as screening tests in syphilis because they are easy to

perform and have reasonably high sensitivity. Because they are titratable and decline in parallel with disease activity, they are also used to monitor response to therapy. The term 'biologic false-positive' is used to signify false positivity of the NTTs, which may occur in a variety of conditions (see Chapter 2.64, Fig. 64.15). False-positive tests are usually of lower titer (<1:8). Although pregnancy is a recognized cause of NTT false-positivity, one must exercise great caution in labeling a reactive NTT in a pregnant patient as a false-positive result.

The second type of diagnostic test, represented by the fluorescent treponemal antibody-absorption test and the microhemagglutination *T. pallidum* treponemal tests, detect antibodies that are directed against *T. pallidum* antigens and are therefore designated as treponemal tests. Treponemal tests are used to confirm that reactivity in a NTT is indeed due to syphilitic infection. Because they are more difficult and expensive to perform than NTTs, treponemal tests may not always be available in underdeveloped countries.

Both treponemal and nontreponemal serologic tests for syphilis are reliable for diagnosis and management of most patients who are coinfected with *T. pallidum* and HIV. However, HIV-infected patients who have syphilis may show higher than expected NTT titers, false-negative treponemal or nontreponemal tests, or delayed seroreactivity. In the rare instances when clinical findings in an HIV-infected patient are consistent with a diagnosis of syphilis but serologic tests are non-reactive, alternative tests, such as biopsy of lesions with darkfield examination of direct fluorescent antibody staining, may be useful. Nonvenereal endemic treponematoses are impossible to differentiate serologically from syphilis.

NONVENEREAL TREPONEMAL INFECTIONS					
Disease	Organism	Endemic areas	Primary lesion	Secondary lesions	Tertiary lesions
Yaws	*Treponema pallidum* subsp. *pertenue*	Rural areas of Africa, Central and South America, the Caribbean, equatorial islands of South East Asia, and remote parts of India and Thailand	Papule Papilloma Ulcer	Diffuse papules, papillomas and ulcers Osteitis Dactylitis	Destructive gummas of skin and bone
Pinta	*Treponema carateum*	Underdeveloped rural areas of Mexico and northern South America	Erythematous papule	Scaly papules Areas of altered skin pigmentation	Areas of altered skin pigmentation Hyperkeratosis
Bejel	*Treponema pallidum* subsp. *endemicum*	West Africa, small foci in Zimbabwe, Botswana, Arabian peninsula and central Australia	Oral mucosal ulcer	Oral and pharyngeal ulcers Mucous patches Condyloma lata Periostitis	Gummas of skin, bone and joints

Fig. 56.1 **Nonvenereal treponemal infections**.

It is estimated that of all pregnant women who have untreated syphilis, only 20% will both carry the fetus to term and deliver a normal child. Complications include stillbirth (30%), neonatal death (10%) and mental handicap (40%). Because of the seriousness of these complications, pregnant women should be screened serologically for syphilis early in pregnancy. For patients at high risk, serologic testing should be done again at 28 weeks and at delivery. Women who are seropositive should be examined carefully for evidence of syphilitic infection. Pregnant women who are seropositive but who lack clinical manifestations should be considered infected unless an adequate treatment history is clearly documented and sequential serologic antibody titers have declined appropriately. Given the inability to distinguish between venereal and nonvenereal treponematoses on the basis of serodiagnostic tests, syphilis should be the presumed diagnosis in all asymptomatic seropositive pregnant patients from areas that are endemic for the nonvenereal treponematoses (see Fig. 56.1).

TREATMENT

Penicillin, in a regimen appropriate for the stage of syphilis, is the antimicrobial of choice in the treatment of syphilis and other treponematoses during pregnancy (Fig. 56.2). The present consensus is that alternative regimens are potentially too harmful to the fetus (e.g. tetracycline), lack efficacy because of the inability of the drug to cross the placenta (e.g. erythromycin) or are insufficiently studied (e.g. ceftriaxone).

Because penicillin is clearly the preferred treatment, penicillin skin testing is recommended for reportedly penicillin-allergic pregnant women who have syphilis. If the penicillin allergy is confirmed, desensitization can be accomplished using incremental doses of oral penicillin V over 4–6 hours. A Jarisch–Herxheimer reaction, which presents with fever, headache and myalgia, can occur within hours of initiation of penicillin therapy in early syphilis. Women treated for syphilis during the second half of pregnancy may also experience self-limited uterine contractions, decreased fetal activity and fetal heart rate abnormalities after penicillin treatment, but premature labor or fetal distress are rare. Women should be warned of the symptoms of the Jarisch–Herxheimer

TREATMENT OF SYPHILIS DURING PREGNANCY IN HIV-INFECTED WOMEN	
Primary or secondary syphilis	Benzathine penicillin G 2.4MU im (single dose)
Early latent syphilis	Benzathine penicillin G 2.4MU im (single dose)
Late latent syphilis or latent syphilis of unknown duration	Benzathine penicillin G 7.2MU in three doses each of 2.4MU im at 1-week intervals
Tertiary syphilis	Benzathine penicillin G 7.2MU in three doses each of 2.4MU im at 1-week intervals
Neurosyphilis	Aqueous crystalline penicillin G 18–24MU a day, administered as 3–4MU iv q4h for 10–14 days

Fig. 56.2 Treatment of syphilis during pregnancy in HIV-infected women.

reaction and be instructed to use acetaminophen (paracetamol) to control these symptoms and to self-monitor uterine and fetal activity during the first 48 hours after penicillin therapy. Ultrasound signs of fetal syphilis (hepatomegaly, hydrops fetalis) indicate a greater risk to fetal health; such cases should be managed in consultation with specialists in high-risk obstetrics.

FURTHER READING

Centres for Disease Control and Prevention. 1998 guidelines for the treatment of sexually transmitted diseases.

Radolf JD, Isaacs RD. Nonvenereal treponematosis: yaws, pinta, and endemic syphilis. In: Kelley WN, ed. Textbook of internal medicine, 3rd ed. Philadelphia: Lippincott-Raven.

Radolf JD et al. Congenital syphilis. In: Holmes KK et al., eds. Sexually transmitted diseases, 3rd ed. New York: McGraw–Hill; 1999.

Ray JG. Lues-lues: maternal and fetal considerations of syphilis. Obstet Gynecol Surv 1995;50:845–50.

Tramont EC. Syphilis in adults: from Christopher Columbus to Sir Alexander Fleming to AIDS. Clin Infect Dis 1995;21:1361–9.

Treatment of a positive *Toxoplasma* titer in pregnancy

William R Bowie

INTRODUCTION

Clinically recognized toxoplasmosis is infrequent, but serologic evidence of toxoplasmosis is frequent. In immunologically competent people, even symptomatic toxoplasmosis is usually of minimal clinical significance. The exception is when symptomatic or asymptomatic infection is acquired just before or during pregnancy. *Toxoplasma gondii* readily crosses the placenta to infect the fetus, with immense clinical and financial implications. It is estimated that in North America, approximately 1 pregnancy in 1000 is affected. Because early treatment of the mother decreases the risk of infection of the fetus and diminishes the sequelae in infected fetuses, appropriate management of the mother is critical.

Because most infected women are either asymptomatic or have nonspecific and transient symptoms, the diagnosis is rarely made clinically. Rather, the health care provider and the woman are typically faced with a positive serologic test without clear information on when the infection was acquired. 'Positive' serology with routine tests does not reliably determine the acuteness of infection, which is what determines the management. Inappropriate response may result in unwarranted psycyhologic distress, unnecessary evaluations and treatments, and even unnecessary termination of pregnancy.

PATHOGENESIS

The definitive hosts of *T. gondii* are felines, and people are infected by direct or indirect contact with oocysts excreted by cats. Oocysts, spread for example in cat litter or soil or sand contaminated by cat feces, are highly infective. When ingested by animals or humans, they ultimately result in cysts in tissues. These also infect humans when uncooked or inadequately cooked meat containing viable cysts are ingested. Rarely, humans can also be infected by blood transfusions (see Chapter 2.55).

During acute infection of humans, toxoplasmosis is disseminated widely. Infection acquired immediately before conception or during pregnancy carries with it the risk of spread to the fetus. The risk of transmission is lowest in the first trimester (10–15%), but the consequences then are the most devastating (severe disease or death). By the second trimester, there is 25–40% transmission with usually nonfatal sequelae. By the third trimester, over 60% of fetuses are infected, with typically mild or asymptomatic manifestations.

The classic triad of clinical features in severely infected infants who survive includes hydrocephalus, intracranial calcifications and chorioretinitis. Asymptomatically infected infants are typically not recognized at birth, but many if not most are thought to be at risk of developing chorioretinitis, hearing loss or subtle neurologic manifestations.

The economic impact of congenital toxoplasmosis is substantial, and screening programs to detect infection in pregnancy or at birth have been considered. In the USA, routine screening for toxoplasmosis in pregnancy is rarely recommended, but in some other countries screening is repeated serially in pregnancy, particularly in France.

INVESTIGATION AND MANAGEMENT

The focus of this practice point is on immunocompetent pregnant women who have had a 'positive' test for antibody to *T. gondii*. This will usually have been performed as a screening test rather than a diagnostic one. Depending on the laboratory, this will be either a positive IgG titer, or possibly a positive titer for both IgG and IgM. Unless timing was fortuitous, even with repetition titers are likely to be stable rather than rising or falling.

Difficulties in interpretation of serologic results

There are several substantial problems in the interpretation of results. First, there are problems with sensitivity, and more frequently specificity of many of the commercially available tests. Second, potential markers of acuteness of infection, such as IgM and IgA, may persist long after the risk of transmission to the fetus ends, so that although positive IgM and IgA results may be true positive results, they do not by themselves establish acuteness of infection. Thus, when the IgM is reported as being 'positive', it can be a false positive (with the rate of false positives dependent on the test and the laboratory), a true positive indicative of recent infection, or a true positive but simply reflecting persistence of IgM antibody. Third, history and physical examination only rarely aid in the ascertainment of infection.

Negative anti-*Toxoplasma gondii* immunoglobulin G and IgM

Unless it is very early in infection, this indicates absence of previous infection. Women with such results are susceptible to infection. Primary prevention messages should be reinforced. Subsequent repeat testing is required if one wishes to exclude infection later on in the pregnancy.

Immunoglobulin G titer only available, and it is positive

An IgM test should be requested on the same or a new serum specimen because a single positive IgG titer provides no information about acuteness of infection. The presence of IgG antibody with a negative IgM antibody excludes recent infection. If performed early in pregnancy, no further investigation is required for toxoplasmosis. If performed late in pregnancy, there is an outside possibility that acute infection may have arisen in pregnancy, with subsequent disappearance of IgM. Because of long-term persistence of IgM this is unlikely, but if there is any clinical concern of toxoplasmosis, the infant should be screened at birth.

Initial negative immunoglobulin G titer with positive or equivocal immunoglobulin M titer

When the IgG titer is negative, it is highly likely that the IgM titer is falsely positive. However, because the woman could be in the process of seroconverting, testing should be repeated in parallel on a second sample that is collected approximately 3 weeks after the first. If the IgG titer remains negative, then the result is probably falsely positive. Unless there are other features suggesting active infection, no further investigation is needed. If the IgG titer becomes positive or there is a significant increase in the IgM titer, this strongly suggests recent acquisition of infection.

Initial or subsequent positive immunoglobulin G titer, and immunoglobulin M titer is positive

Unless there is seroconversion or a significant increase in titers, interpretation at this stage is much more difficult because this information by itself does not establish acuteness of infection. This requires further clinical assessment and serologic and other studies in the mother and potentially in the fetus.

History and examination of the mother. Although symptoms are usually absent or so nonspecific as to be unhelpful, a careful history and examination might detect symptoms that provide a clue to the onset of the disease. Most helpful would be development of lymphadenopathy, typically involving one node or a few nodes. A physical examination should be performed, looking in particular for abnormal lymphadenopathy and ocular disease.

Serologic studies in the mother. Pregnant women are often screened for a variety of processes (e.g. rubella, HIV). Prior stored serum should be tested for antibody to *T. gondii*. The results may help in determining the chronicity of infection.

Additional testing is required on available or newly acquired serum. If repeat testing on specimens run in parallel (that is, testing is performed on all specimens at the same time) shows or has shown seroconversion or a four-fold or greater rise, infection is acute. Usually titers are stable, and further testing is required in specialized or reference laboratories. A battery of tests is usually performed to assess acuteness of infection. Results should be interpreted in consultation with the reference laboratory. The two tests most often employed to assess acuteness of infection are IgG avidity and differential agglutination testing. If these are consistent with acute infection or if they do not exclude acute infection, the woman should be managed as below.

Studies diagnostic of or consistent with acute infection in pregnancy or immediately before conception

Management is in part determined by the time when infection was acquired. If results are consistent with infection immediately before or just after conception, the risk of delivering an infected baby is low. Either the fetus is not infected or if it is infected it is likely to abort. When infection occurs later, the risk of having a viable but affected infant is much greater.

The mother should immediately be started on treatment (see below) for the duration of pregnancy and the fetus should be assessed by ultrasound. Amniocentesis for polymerase chain reaction (PCR) should be strongly considered.

Fetal ultrasound may show features consistent with infection, especially increased size of the ventricles. Negative studies do not exclude fetal involvement and studies may need to be performed serially.

With or without fetal abnormalities, amniocentesis should be considered at 18 weeks or later. If performed, as a minimum the amniotic fluid should be tested by PCR. Although this can be falsely positive or falsely negative, if it is positive treatment of the mother should be switched to pyrimethamine and sulfadiazine.

Some authorities also sample fetal blood to detect the parasite or a fetal immunologic response, but PCR on amniotic fluid is probably safer.

Treatment of the mother

Initial treatment is with spiramycin 1g orally q8h. Spiramycin reduces the incidence and severity of fetal infection, but when the fetus is known to be infected, pyrimethamine and sulfonamides are more active than spiramycin. Hence, ultrasound or amniotic fluid findings suggestive of fetal involvement should prompt a change of treatment to pyrimethamine and a sulfonamide. A variety of dosage regimens have been used, but currently suggested is pyrimethamine 25mg/day and sulfadizine 2g orally q12h, with supplemental folinic acid 5mg/day. When treatment of the mother is initiated, it should be continued for the duration of the pregnancy.

Spiramycin is a macrolide with possible adverse reactions including nausea, vomiting, anorexia and diarrhea. Sulfadiazine has typical adverse reactions associated with sulfonamides, including concerns of kernicterus. The major adverse reaction to pyrimethamine is dose-related bone marrow suppression. To assess hematologic abnormalities, testing is recommended at least once weekly to detect anemia, leukopenia and thrombocytopenia.

Although other drugs have been used to treat toxoplasmosis, there is minimal experience with them in the context of pregnancy and fetal infection.

Termination of pregnancy

Many women with 'positive' serology for toxoplasmosis have had inappropriate termination of pregnancy. Positive IgG and IgM serology is not of itself an indication for termination. Most of these women will not have infected fetuses, but even if the fetus is infected, with appropriate long-term treatment the infants often do well. Termination should only be considered when there is documented evidence of fetal involvement, especially if infection was acquired early in the first trimester. However, even most of these infants who survive have done well with treatment of the mother followed by treatment of the infant.

Initial management of the infant at birth

If clinical, serologic or other testing suggests congenital toxoplasmosis, the infant should be treated for 1 year. On this treatment, even infants who have clinically apparent manifestations such as intracranial calcifications, meningitis or chorioretinitis are highly likely to have a favorable outcome.

HIV AND TOXOPLASMOSIS IN PREGNANCY

In contrast to immunocompetent women, women who have HIV infection whose antibody to *T. gondii* is IgG positive and IgM negative are at risk of transmitting HIV to the fetus. Appropriate management is unclear. Important variables probably include the degree of immunosuppression, concurrent *Pneumocystis carinii* prophylaxis with trimethroprim–sulfamethoxazole (co-trimoxazole), *Mycobacterium avium-intracellulare* treatment or prophylaxis with macrolides, *T. gondii* treatment or suppression, and infection acquired in pregnancy. Acute infection with *T. gondii* in pregnancy should be managed aggressively, probably with pyrimethamine and sulfadiazine, whether or not there is objective evidence of fetal involvement (see Chapter 5.20).

OTHER CONSIDERATIONS

Pregnant women who have possible or proven toxoplasmosis are likely to feel guilty that they did something that put their fetus at risk. It is prudent for women who are or might be pregnant to avoid direct or indirect contact with cats or raw or inadequately cooked meat. However, most people with toxoplasmosis are totally unaware of when or how they became infected. Care should be taken to avoid adding guilt to the stress that women who have 'positive' serology undergo.

FURTHER READING

Beaman MH, McCabe RE, Wong SY, Remington JS. *Toxoplasma gondii*. In: Mandell GL, Bennett JE, Dolin R, eds. Principles and practice of infectious diseases, 4th ed. New York: Churchill Livingstone; 1995:2455–75.

Berrebi A, Kobuch WE, Bessieres MH, *et al*. Termination of pregnancy for maternal toxoplasmosis. Lancet 1994;344:36–9.

Boyer K. Diagnosis and treatment of congenital toxoplasmosis. Adv Pediatr Infect Dis, vol 11. St. Louis: Mosby–Year Book; 1996.

Dannemann BR, Vaughan WC, Thulliez P, Remington JS. Differential agglutination test for diagnosis of recently acquired infection with *Toxoplasma gondii*. J Clin Microbial 1990;28:1928–33.

Lappalainen M, Kosela P, Koskiniemi M, *et al*. Toxoplasmosis acquired during pregnancy: improved serodiagnosis based on avidity of IgG. J Infect Dis 1993;167:691–7.

McAuley J, Boyer KM, Patel D, *et al*. Early and longitudinal evaluations of treated infants and children and untreated historical patients with congenital toxoplasmosis: The Chicago Collaborative Treatment Trial. Clin Infect Dis 1994;18:38–72.

Wong SY, Remington JS. Toxoplasmosis in pregnancy. Clin Infect Dis 1994;18:853–62.

A pregnant patient with a previous pregnancy complicated by group B streptococcal disease
Upton Allen

INTRODUCTION

The group B streptococcus (GBS, *Streptococcus agalactiae*) remains an important cause of invasive disease in neonates and pregnant women. Among neonates, premature infants are at greatest risk of an adverse outcome from GBS infection. These premature infants account for 25% of the cases of GBS disease among neonates. In these infants, the disease manifests itself as an early-onset form (<7 days after birth) and a late-onset form (≥7 days after birth). Disease among infants usually presents as bacteremia, pneumonia and meningitis. However, they may experience other syndromes, including soft tissue and bone infection. The fatality rate ranges from 5 to 20% among neonates, an improvement in recent years that is attributed to advances in neonatal care (see Chapter 8.14).

EPIDEMIOLOGY

The organism colonizes the gastrointestinal tract of humans, with the genitourinary tract being the most common site for secondary spread. Colonization rates vary widely among different ethnic groups, geographic areas and age groups. These rates generally indicate that from 10 to 30% of pregnant women have vaginal or rectal colonization with GBS. Approximately 1–2% of all infants born to colonized women develop early-onset GBS disease. Data from a multistate population-based study in the USA indicate that early-onset disease accounts for about 80% of neonatal GBS disease.

The incidence of early-onset disease is higher in babies born to women less than 20 years of age and in those who are of black race in the USA. Intrapartum risk factors include premature onset of labor (at <37 weeks' gestation), prolonged rupture of membranes (≥18 hours) and intrapartum fever [over 100.4°F (38°C)]. Additional risk factors include heavy vaginal colonization with GBS, previous delivery of an infant with GBS disease and the presence of low maternal levels of anti-GBS capsular antibody. Women who have GBS bacteriuria are at an increased risk of delivering an infected baby with early-onset disease. This is related in part to the fact that women who have GBS bacteriuria are usually heavily colonized with GBS. Bacteriuria caused by GBS is associated with an increased risk of preterm labor. Antibiotic therapy of women who have GBS bacteriuria reduces the risk of preterm labor, although it does not necessarily eliminate vaginal colonization.

MICROBIOLOGY

Group B streptococci are represented by several serotypes, including Ia, Ib/c, Ia/c, II, III, IV, V, VI and VII. All serotypes may cause disease in humans, but serotype III is the main cause of early-onset meningitis as well as of late-onset GBS disease among neonates.

In the determination of the GBS carrier status of a pregnant woman, culture techniques that maximize the recovery of GBS are essential. The optimal method for GBS screening involves collection of a single vaginal–anorectal swab or two separate swabs from the vagina and rectum. Swabs should be placed in a transport medium if the bacteriology laboratory is off-site and subcultured on to selective broth medium. After overnight incubation, the specimen is subcultured on to solid blood agar. Slide agglutination tests or other tests used to detect GBS antigen may be used to enable specific identification of GBS.

PREVENTION

Although research is being carried out to develop vaccines that could be administered to pregnant women to prevent GBS disease in neonates, this modality has not yet evolved as a preventive strategy. However, chemoprophylaxis has evolved as a useful preventive strategy. In this regard, because the majority of newborns who have GBS disease acquire infection *in utero*, the administration of antibiotics to

ESTIMATED IMPACT OF GROUP B STREPTOCOCCAL PREVENTION STRATEGIES		
Strategy	Early onset GBS disease prevented (%)	Deliveries receiving IAP (%)
Recommended screening-based strategy: Culture at 35–37 weeks; IAP for preterm deliveries and all GBS carriers	86.0	26.7
Recommended risk-factor-based strategy: No prenatal cultures; IAP for all women who have intrapartum risk factors	68.8	18.3
Previous strategy recommended by the American Academy of Pediatrics: Culture at 26–28 weeks; IAP for GBS carriers who develop risk factors	50.7	3.4

Fig. 56.3 Estimated impact of group B streptococcal prevention strategies. The figures are derived from the Morbidity and Mortality Weekly Report (1996;45 No RR-7:1–24) and Rouse, et al., (1994). Boyer and Gotoff (1985) found that the proportion of deliveries among women who had positive prenatal cultures and who went on to develop intrapartum risk factors was 4.6%. GBS, group B streptococcus; IAP, intrapartum antimicrobial prophylaxis.

RISK FACTORS FOR WHICH INTRAPARTUM CHEMOPROPHYLAXIS IS RECOMMENDED

Preterm labor (<37 weeks' gestation)

Term labor (≥37 weeks' gestation) if there is:
- prolonged rupture of membranes (chemoprophylaxis should be given if labor is likely to continue beyond 18 hours; neonatal benefits are optimally achieved if antibiotics are given at least 4 hours before delivery)
- maternal fever during labor [100.4°F (38°C) taken orally]

Previous delivery of a newborn with GBS disease regardless of current GBS colonization status

Previously documented GBS bacteriuria

Fig. 56.4 Risk factors for which intrapartum chemoprophylaxis is recommended. GBS, group B streptococcus. Modified from Centers for Disease Control and Prevention (1996).

neonates (postnatal prophylaxis) will not prevent the majority of GBS disease. Intrapartum chemoprophylaxis (administration of antibiotic during labor) has the potential of preventing neonatal as well as maternal GBS disease.

Guidelines based on intrapartum chemoprophylaxis have been established by various groups. However, it should be noted that many countries do not have specific recommendations for prophylaxis against GBS disease. Recent guidelines are based on collective evidence that shows a beneficial effect of intrapartum prophylaxis in preventing early-onset GBS sepsis. The most widely accepted recommendations are those proposed by the US Centers for Disease Control and Prevention. These recommendations follow.
- Obstetric practitioners, in conjunction with supporting laboratories and labor and delivery facilities, should adopt a strategy for the prevention of early-onset GBS disease.
- Women who have symptomatic or asymptomatic GBS bacteriuria detected during pregnancy should be treated at the time of diagnosis; because such women are usually heavily colonized with GBS, they should also receive intrapartum chemoprophylaxis.
- Women who have previously given birth to an infant with GBS disease should receive intrapartum chemoprophylaxis; prenatal screening is not necessary for these women.

Based on the current state of knowledge, two approaches are appropriate; a screening-based and a risk-factor-based approach. As shown in Figure 56.3, in the recommended screening-based strategy, in which women are cultured at 35–37 weeks' gestation and intrapartum antimicrobial prophylaxis (IAP) offered to those who have preterm deliveries and all GBS carriers, an estimated 86% of GBS disease is prevented. The trade-off is that proportionally more women receive antibiotics (26.7%) than they would with a risk-factor-based approach (18.3%).

Screening-based approach

All pregnant women should be screened at 35–37 weeks' gestation for anogenital GBS colonization. Patients should be informed of the screening results and of the potential benefits and risks of intrapartum antimicrobial prophylaxis for GBS carriers. Information systems should be developed and monitored to ensure that prenatal culture results are available at the time and place of delivery. Intrapartum prophylaxis should be offered to all pregnant women identified as GBS carriers by culture at 35–37 weeks' gestation.

If the result of GBS culture is not known at the time of labor, intrapartum antimicrobial prophylaxis should be administered if one of the following risk factors is present:
- <37 weeks' gestation,
- duration of membranes ruptured ≥18 hours, or
- body temperature ≥100.4°F (38°C).

Culture techniques that maximize the likelihood of GBS recovery should be used. Because lower vaginal and rectal cultures are recommended, cultures should not be collected by speculum examination.

Laboratories should report results to both the anticipated site of delivery and the health care provider who ordered the test. Ideally, laboratories that perform GBS cultures will ensure that clinicians have continuous access to culture results.

Risk-factor approach

A prophylaxis strategy based on the presence of intrapartum risk factors alone [e.g. <37 weeks' gestation, duration of membrane rupture ≥18 hours, or temperature ≥100.4°F (38°C)] is an acceptable alternative (Fig. 56.4).

The above recommendations are accompanied by a suggested approach to the management of neonates born to mothers who received IAP (Fig. 56.5). This approach is based on the gestation age of the neonate, the presence or absence of symptoms and signs of sepsis and whether sufficient time had elapsed between IAP and delivery. Antibiotics must be administered at least 4 hours prior to delivery to allow for adequate antibiotic levels in amniotic fluid.

SUMMARY OF THE MANAGEMENT OF A PREGNANT WOMAN WITH A PREVIOUS GBS-AFFECTED NEWBORN

A woman who has lost an infant as a result of GBS disease requires the usual understanding and support given to any woman who has lost an infant during the neonatal period. Intrapartum prophylaxis is recommended regardless of screening cultures because of the previous delivery of a baby with GBS disease. Routine vaginal–rectal screening for GBS is not necessary in this setting. However, it would be appropriate to obtain urine cultures at different antenatal visits to determine whether GBS bacteriuria is present. As indicated above, the presence of symptomatic or asymptomatic GBS bacteriuria is an indication for antibiotics at the time the diagnosis is made.

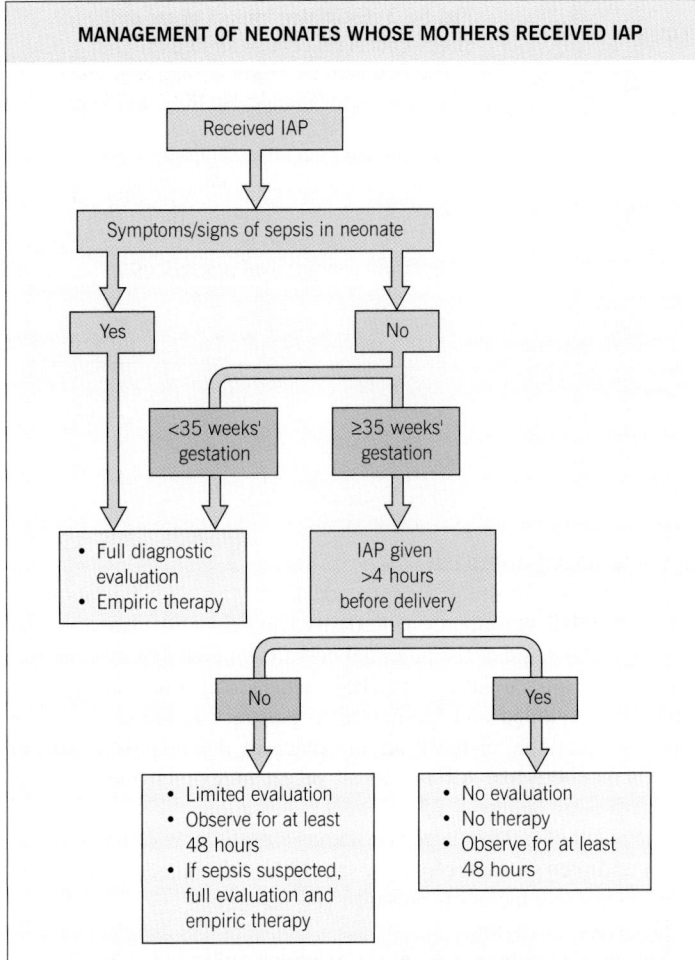

Fig. 56.5 Management of neonates born to mothers who have received IAP as prophylaxis for early-onset GBS disease. Full diagnostic evaluation includes full blood count and differential white cell count, blood culture and chest radiograph. A lumbar puncture is performed at the discretion of the clinician. Limited evaluation includes full blood count and differential white cell count plus blood culture. GBS, group B streptococcus; IAP, intrapartum antimicrobial prophylaxis.

Penicillin G (5MU intravenous initially followed by 2.5MU intravenous q4h) should be given until delivery. Ampicillin (2g intravenous initially and then 1g intravenous q4h until delivery) is an acceptable alternative. Penicillin G is preferred because it has a narrow spectrum and is thus potentially less likely to select out resistant bacteria. Women who are allergic to penicillin should receive clindamycin or erythromycin.

Group B streptococci are associated with various maternal infectious disease complications during various stages of pregnancy. These include septic abortion, urinary tract infections, chorioamnioitis, wound infection and endometritis. Although intrapartum antimicrobial prophylaxis may have a beneficial effect on endometritis, an assessment is necessary in the immediate postpartum period in order to guide further antibiotic therapy directed at the mother.

The newborn infant of a mother who has received intrapartum prophylaxis requires a special management approach. The guidelines in Figure 56.5 may be used as a guide to the management of neonate. However, if the infant is believed to have invasive GBS disease, the following apply.

- Penicillin G or ampicillin plus an aminoglycoside is the initial treatment. Penicillin G may be given alone when GBS is proven as the etiologic agent and clinical and microbiologic responses have been documented.
- In cases of meningitis, a second lumbar puncture at 24 hours after the start of treatment is recommended by some experts; this may have prognostic significance.
- Bacteremia without a defined focus should be treated for a minimum of 10 days.
- Uncomplicated meningitis should be treated for 14–21 days (longer periods of treatment are needed in infants who have complicated courses).
- Osteomyelitis should be treated for a minimum of 4 weeks.
- There is a high incidence of co-infection among twins, and the twin of an index case should be observed or evaluated for sepsis as clinically indicated.

FURTHER READING

Allen UD, Navas L, King SM. Effectiveness of intrapartum penicillin prophylaxis in preventing early-onset group B streptococcal infection: results of a meta-analysis. Can Med Assoc J 1993;149:1659–65.

American Academy of Pediatrics. Group B streptococcal infections. In: Peter G, ed. 1997 red book: report of the Committee on Infectious Diseases, 24th ed. Elk Grove Village, Illinois, USA: American Academy of Pediatrics; 1997:494–501.

Baker CJ, Edwards MS. Group B streptococcal infections. In: Remmington J, Klein JO, eds. Infectious diseases of the fetus and newborn infant, 4th ed. Philadelphia: WB Saunders; 1995:980–1054.

Boyer KM, Gotoff SP. Prevention of early-onset group B streptococcal disease with selective intrapartum chemoprophylaxis. N Engl J Med 1986;314:1665–9.

Boyer KM, Gotoff SP. Strategies for chemoprophylaxis of GBS early-onset infections. Antibiot Chemother 1985;35:267–80.

Centers for Disease Control and Prevention. Prevention of perinatal group B streptococcal disease: a public health perspective. MMWR Morb Mortal Wkly Rep 1996;45(No RR-7):1–24.

Jafari HS, Schuchat A, Hilsdon R, et al. Barriers to prevention of perinatal group B streptococcal disease. Pediatr Infect Dis J 1995;14:662–7.

Rouse DJ, Goldenberg RL, Cliver SP, et al. Strategies for the prevention of early-onset neonatal group B streptococcal sepsis: a decision analysis. Obstet Gynecol 1994;83:483–94.

Schuchat A, Wenger JD. Epidemiology of group B streptococcal disease: risk factors, prevention strategies and vaccine development. Epidemiol Rev 1994;16:374–402.

Zangwill KM, Schuchat A, Wenger JD. Group B streptococcal disease in the United States, 1990: report from a multistate surveillance system. In: CDC surveillance summaries (November 20). MMWR Morb Mort Weekly Rep 1992;41:25–32.

Cystitis and Urethral Syndromes

Stephen T Chambers

Urinary tract infections (UTIs) are the second most common infectious cause for consultation and prescription of antibiotics among family physicians and are a common cause of morbidity in institutional care. Most are limited to the lower urinary tract but may cause pyelonephritis and bacteremia. The global incidence is estimated to be 2–3%, or about 150 million cases per annum, costing billions of dollars annually.[1]

ACUTE CYSTITIS

EPIDEMIOLOGY

Quantitative bacterial counts have provided a useful means of determining the frequency of UTIs, defining risks and studying the natural history because the prevalence in surveys mirrors that of clinical UTIs. In the first 3 months of life UTIs are about three times more common in males than females, but thereafter infections occur more frequently in females. The prevalence in preschool- and school-aged girls is about 1.2%, which is 30 times higher than that in boys. About 5–6% of girls will have had at least one episode of bacteriuria during their school-age years. Thereafter the prevalence of significant bacteriuria among females increases at about 1% per decade (Fig. 57.1). Men have low rates of bacteriuria until advanced age when rates rise dramatically.[2]

Asymptomatic bacteriuria during childhood identifies a population at risk of developing UTIs when they become sexually active. Previous symptomatic UTI is also a risk factor with at least 20% of women developing a recurrent infection within 6 months of the first.

Acute cystitis in young women is clearly associated with sexual activity. Studies of university women found the relative risk of UTI increased nine-fold for women who had intercourse seven times during the preceding week compared with those who had not been sexually active. More than two-thirds of acute episodes may be attributable to intercourse in this age group.[3] Other risk factors include use of diaphragm and spermicide. Less is known about the relationship between intercourse and UTI in older age groups, including post-menopausal women.[4]

Asymptomatic bacteriuria occurs in 4–7% of pregnant women. It is important as acute pylenonephritis may develop (in 15–40% of cases) during the third trimester or in the puerperium. This is preventable in most cases and up to 20% of patients will have significant abnormalities of the urinary tract. Bacteriuria of pregnancy has also been associated with increased risk of pre-eclampsia, lowered fetal birth weight, prematurity and increased perinatal mortality.[5]

Urinary tract infection in males is commonly associated with abnormalities of the urinary tract. There is also a higher incidence in uncircumcised males, homosexual men and those with AIDS. In the latter the risk increased with a lowered CD4+ count.[6]

In the elderly, both disease of the urinary tract and concurrent medical conditions contribute to the high prevalence. Instrumentation is associated with a risk of 1% in ambulatory patients but at least 10% in hospitalized patients and is an important cause of UTI in this group. Other contributing factors are shown in Figure 57.2.

PREVALENCE OF BACTERIURIA IN DIFFERENT AGE GROUPS		
	Group	Prevalence (%)
Females	Schoolgirls	1.2
	Sexually active young women	2–4
	Women	
	>60 years	6–8
	70 years	5–10
	80 years	20
	Institutionalized elderly	30–50
Males	Childhood to middle age	<1
	Men	
	60–65	1–3
	>80 years	>10
	Institutionalized elderly	20–30

Fig. 57.1 Prevalence of bacteriuria in different age groups.

RISK FACTORS FOR LOWER URINARY TRACT INFECTION			
Young adults	Women	Past history of UTI	Parity
		Sexual intercourse	Diabetes (women)
		Diaphragm use	Primary biliary cirrhosis
		Spermicide	Sickle cell anemia (pregnancy)
			Instrumentation
	Men	Lack of circumcision	Homosexual activity
		AIDS	
Elderly people	Women	Loss of estrogen effect	Abnormalities of urinary tract
		Incomplete emptying of bladder	Rectoceles
			Urethroceles
			Bladder diverticula
	Men	Strictures	Prostatic disease
		Instrumentation	Benign enlargement
			Calculi
			Loss of bactericidal secretions
	Both sexes	Neurologic disease	
		Alzheimer's disease	Cerebrovascular disease
		Parkinson's disease	

Fig. 57.2 Risk factors for lower urinary tract infection.

PATHOGENESIS

INFECTING ORGANISMS

In uncomplicated cystitis more than 95% of infections are caused by a single organism. The most common pathogen is *Escherichia coli* (80–90% of cases) and *Staphylococcus saprophyticus* accounts for 10–20% of

ORGANISMS ASSOCIATED WITH URINARY TRACT INFECTIONS		
Common organisms	*Escherichia coli* *Staphylococcus saprophyticus*	
Less common organisms	*Klebsiella* spp. *Enterobacter* spp. *Proteus* spp. *Morganella* spp. *Citrobacter* spp. Group B streptococcus Group D streptococcus Enterococci	*Pseudomonas aeruginosa* *Acinetobacter* spp. *Serratia* spp. Yeasts *Corynebacterium urealyticum*
Rare infections	*Haemophilis influenzae* *Mycobacterium tuberculosis* Anaerobes	*Salmonella* spp. *Shigella* spp. Adenovirus (type 11)
Unproven causes	*Gardinerella vaginalis* *Ureaplasma urealyticum* *Mycoplasma hominis*	

Fig. 57.3 Organisms associated with urinary tract infections.

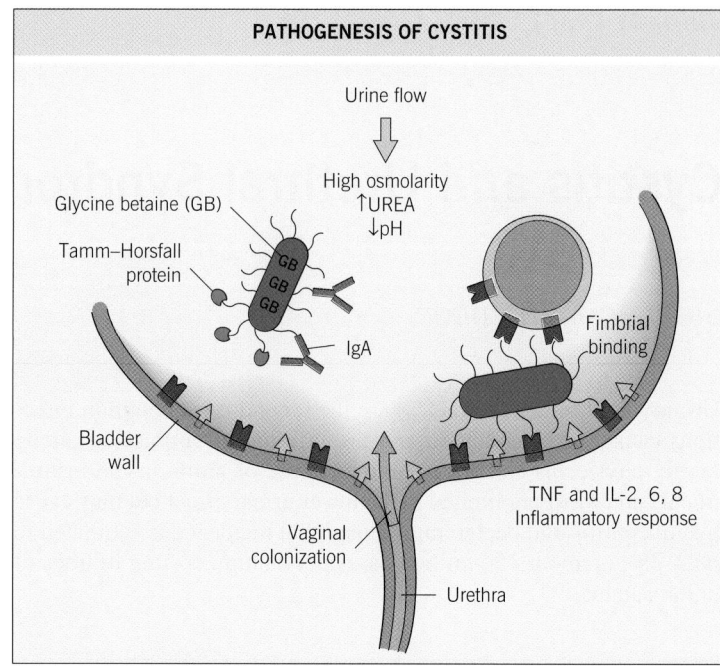

Fig. 57.4 Pathogenesis of cystitis. Factors favouring bacterial persistence and infection include bacterial binding to bladder mucosa (fimbriae), and high bacterial growth rates despite high osmolarity and urea concentrations and low pH. Factors favouring bacterial elimination include high urine flow rate, high voiding frequency, bactericidal effects of bladder mucosa, secreted proteins which bind to fimbrial adhesins and the inflammatory response.

cases in young women during late summer and autumn.[7] Other enteric Gram-positive cocci occasionally cause infection (Fig. 57.3).[8]

Complicated infections and those in the institutionalized elderly are more often polymicrobial (30% of cases), particularly when stones are present. There is an increased incidence of resistant *E. coli, Klebsiella* spp., *Enterobacter* spp., *Proteus* spp., group B and D streptococci, as well as *Pseudomonas aeruginosa,* coagulase-negative staphylococci and yeasts.[9]

Infections caused by urease-producing organisms *(Proteus, Providentia,* and *Morganella* spp.)* leads to the conversion of urea to ammonia, which activates complement (fourth component), and raises the pH of urine. This promotes precipitation of struvite crystals $(MgNH_4PO_4.6H_2O)$ and stone formation.

MECHANISMS

Cystitis is almost always caused by ascending infection. The mechanisms of acquisition and progression of cystitis and production of symptoms depends on a series of complex, interdependent host–parasite interactions that determine colonization of the periurethral area from the bowel, ascent into the bladder, growth in urine, tissue invasion and immune response (Fig. 57.4).

Colonization

The region between the anus and urethra has distinct ecologic niches that are normally colonized with specialized flora. Some women with recurrent UTI have an increased susceptibility to colonization with enteric organisms. Colonization of the periurethral zone precedes infection and persists between episodes.[10] *Escherichia coli* adheres more to buccal and vaginal epithelial cells from these patients than from those of controls. Blood group antigens may be involved as lectins or inhibitors of adhesion as nonsecretors; those with Lewis blood group [Le(a+b-)] and recessive [Le(a-b-)] phenotypes are at greater risk of recurrent UTI.[11] Likewise, *E. coli* which carry DNA sequences for P fimbriae, colonize the intestine in patients who have the P blood group.[12]

Other factors that promote vaginal colonization with Gram-negative enteric bacteria include the use of diaphragms and spermicides for contraception,[13] estrogen deficiency, which discourages the growth of lactobacilli, and an overgrowth of enteric organisms.[14]

Ascent

Bacteria normally enter the bladder by ascending along the mucosal sheath. This may be introduced mechanically by instrumentation or sexual activity. The mechanisms are poorly understood but presumably include Brownian motion augmented by motile flagella and, possibly, adherence by extracellular glycocalyx.

Fimbriae: roles in mucosal adherence and inflammation

Symptomatic bacteriuria is highly correlated with the presence of bacteria that mediate attachment to urothelial cells. Type I (mannose-sensitive) fimbriae are important in initiating colonization of the bladder, but once the organisms attach to the bladder wall they undergo phase variation and no longer express the fimbriae. This may prevent binding to Tamm–Horsfall protein and IgA, and decrease recognition by phagocytic cells.[15] Type II fimbrial attachment (mannose-resistant) is mediated by P fimbriae (Gal-Gal), which are associated with pyelonephritis, and attach to a variety of receptors associated with the globose series of glycolipids, including Gal-Gal and Globo A structures.[16] Attachment of bacteria to the mucosa and cell wall components, such as lipid A, activate an inflammatory response, including production of tumor necrosis factor, interleukin (IL)-2, IL-6 and IL-8, and attraction of inflammatory cells. Phagocytic cells have a major role in elimination of infection.[17]

In contrast, asymptomatic bacteriuria is usually caused by organisms that do not possess fimbriae, and do not excite an inflammatory response unless tissue invasion occurs. The molecular mechanism by which they reach the urine and maintain colonization of the bladder, despite the host protective mechanisms, is unknown.[18]

Urodynamics

Normal structure and function are of primary importance in eliminating bacteria from the urinary tract. Efficient function depends on urine flow rate, frequency of voiding and residual bladder volume.[19] Complete voiding eliminates free floating organisms and the bladder mucosa can kill organisms on contact. Small amounts of residual urine allow organisms to escape and perpetuate the infection. Similarly there is a critical rate of flow of urine in relation to the volume of the upper tract and doubling time of bacteria that can wash out free organisms. Compromise of these factors by reflux, neurologic disease, diabetes, debility and anatomic changes is likely to be critical in the high rates of infection in groups such as the elderly.

Growth in bladder urine
The ability of organisms to grow in urine is essential for their invasion of the urinary tract. Gonococci, anaerobes and urethral commensals are inhibited by urine, whereas aerobic bacteria that cause infection grow well. These organisms are inhibited by extremes of pH (<5.5 and >7.5), and by high tonicity, and urea and organic acid concentrations. Bacteria counter the inhibitory effects of high osmotic forces by increasing their internal osmolarity by the accumulation of osmolytes.[20] The most important are glycine betaine and proline betaine, which are present in large amounts in urine, and are taken up via specific transporters. These serve a secondary function in counteracting the toxicity of urea and low pH by stabilizing macromolecular structure. Osmotic pressure also influences expression of bacterial fimbriae genes but the importance of this in pathogenesis is uncertain. Cranberry juice has a slight antibacterial effect attributable to the formation of hippuric acid from quinic acid contained in the juice. Enteric bacteria aromatize the quinic acid to benzoic acid which is converted to hippuric acid in the liver.

Immune response
Locally produced urinary antibodies produced in response to febrile UTI (monomeric and dimeric IgA and IgG) decrease adherence by interference with adhesion receptors and agglutination of bacteria. Hyperimmunisation can protect animals against experimental UTI.[21]

PREVENTION

NORMAL URINARY TRACT
Women who suffer recurrent or closely spaced symptomatic UTI suffer considerable morbidity and anxiety. When no cause is found, advice is often given to empty their bladder completely, maintain a high fluid intake, including at night, and void after intercourse. Application of antiseptic cream (e.g. 0.5% cetrimide w/w) appears to help. Those who use a diaphragm and spermicide should consider alternative methods of contraception. Postmenopausal women with recurrent UTI have been shown to benefit from application of estriol vaginal cream (0.5mg/day for 2 weeks then twice weekly).[14]

DRUG REGIMENS FOR PROPHYLACTIC THERAPY ADMINISTERED AS A SINGLE DOSE AT NIGHT	
Drug	Dose
Nitrofurantoin	50mg
Trimethoprim	100mg
trimethoprim–sulfamethoxazole (co-trimoxazole)	480mg
Norfloxacin	200mg
Cephalexin	125mg
Hexamine hippurate	1.0g

Fig. 57.5 **Drug regimens for prophylactic therapy administered as a single dose at night.**

If these measures fail, chemoprophylaxis should be considered (Fig. 57.5). Low-dose antibiotics are effective if taken nightly, three times weekly or after intercourse.[22] Efficacy continues for up to 5 years. Nitrofurantoin is an excellent agent in part because it does not alter the fecal flora, and resistance occurring during treatment is rare. Trimethoprim and norfloxacin penetrate the vaginal mucosa, which may eliminate colonization of invasive clones.

ABNORMAL URINARY TRACT
It is essential that, where possible, any lesions in the urinary tract should be corrected. Urologic referral is essential. Large residual volumes and high pressure may require intermittent self-catheterization. Low-dose chemoprophylaxis is often effective.

VACCINE
There is no vaccine currently available, although there has been interest in development of vaccines directed against type I and type II pili.[21] These are more likely to be useful for prevention of pyelonephritis than cystitis, but anatomic and functional abnormalities make ithem unlikely to be widely applicable.

CLINICAL FEATURES

SYMPTOMATIC INFECTION
The dominant complaint in cystitis is usually of painful micturition (dysuria), which may be associated with frequency, urgency, strangury, initial and terminal hematuria, suprapubic discomfort and passing small amounts of turbid urine. Low grade fever may occur but is usually absent. Pyuria and/or microscopic hematuria are almost always present and the diagnosis is confirmed by the presence of significant numbers of bacteria in the urine. Elderly patients usually present in a similar manner but occasionally present with deterioration in continence, smelly urine or epididymo-orchitis in males.[23] Hemorrhagic cystitis is less often associated with UTI in the elderly.

Dysuria caused by bacterial cystitis should be distinguished from that caused by vulvitis and urethritis (see Chapter 2.52). In vulvitis there is often discomfort of the labia as the stream of urine is passed. Genital herpes and candidiasis are common causes. In urethritis there may be a history of a new sex partner, prolonged symptoms with chlamydia (>6 days), urethral discharge, mucopurulent cervicitis, or bartholinitis. *Chlamydia trachomatis,* and *Neisseria gonorrhoeae* are the usual causes.

ASYMPTOMATIC BACTERIURIA
Asymptomatic bacteriuria is very common in elderly patients. It may occasionally cause vague systemic symptoms, poor appetite and urinary incontinence. Similarly, symptoms such as frequency, dysuria and hesitancy, which may be caused by infection are common and nonspecific and often fail to respond to treatment of co-existing bacteriuria.[24] Asymptomatic UTIs have not been shown to have increased morbidity or mortality in the elderly.

DIAGNOSIS

A secure diagnosis of UTI requires a urine culture. This is essential in all suspected UTIs in men, children and infants. However, clinicians may elect to treat without obtaining a urine specimen in selected circumstances, such as in women with an isolated episode of cystitis.

PYURIA
The preferred method for assessment of pyuria is microscopic examination of uncentrifuged fresh urine using a hemocytometer, although counts per microscopic field are reasonably reliable in the clinical laboratory. Urine from adult patients who have symptomatic UTI almost always (>96%) contains more than 10 leukocytes/ml. Pyuria is a less reliable indicator of infection in asymptomatic bacteriuria of pregnancy (50% positive) and the elderly (90% positive).

CONDITIONS ASSOCIATED WITH PYURIA BUT WITHOUT CULTURABLE BACTERIA USING STANDARD BACTERIAL ISOLATION TECHNIQUES

Recent treatment of UTI	
Organism not culturable on usual bacterial media	*Myobacterium tuberculosis*
	Fungal infections
	Chlamydia trachomatis
	Neisseria gonorrhoeae
	Anaerobes
	Leptospirosis
	Adenovirus
	Herpes simplex
Noninfectious causes	Tubulointerstitial disease
	Stones
	Foreign bodies
	Transplant rejection
	Trauma
	Neoplasms
	Glomerulonephritis
	Vaginal contamination
	Cyclophosphamide therapy

Fig. 57.6 Conditions associated with pyuria but without culturable bacteria using standard bacterial isolation techniques.

VALUE OF QUANTITATIVE URINE CULTURE IN DIAGNOSIS OF URINARY TRACT INFECTION WITH GRAM-NEGATIVE BACILLI IN WOMEN

	Number of specimens	Organisms/ml of urine	Sensitivity	Specificity
Asymptomatic women	two	$>10^5$	>95%	>80%
Symptomatic women with pyuria	one	$>10^5$	51%	99%
	one	$>10^3$	80%	90%
	one	$>10^2$	95%	85%

Fig. 57.7 Value of quantitative urine culture in diagnosis of UTI with Gram-negative bacilli in women.

DRUG TREATMENT REGIMENS FOR A 3-DAY COURSE OF ORAL THERAPY FOR BACTERIAL CYSTITIS

Drug	Dose
Trimethoprim	300mg q24h
trimethoprim–sulfamethoxazole (co-trimoxazole)	960mg q12h
Nitrofurantoin	50mg q8h
Nalidixic acid	500mg q8h
Norfloxacin	400mg q12h
Ciprofloxacin	250mg q12h
Lomefloxacin	400mg q24h
Fleroxacin	400mg q24h
Cephalexin	250mg q8h
Cephradine	250mg q8h
Sulfamethizole	1g q8h
Pivmecillinam	200mg q8h
Amoxicillin	250mg q8h
Amoxicillin/clavulanate	500/125mg q12h

Fig. 57.8 Drug treatment regimens for a 3-day course of oral therapy for bacterial cystitis.

Pyuria in the absence of bacteriuria is not a reliable predictor of infection. Specimens from women with vaginitis often contain white cells and there are many other causes of inflammation within the urinary tract (Fig. 57.6)

Urine dipsticks using esterase provide a simple inexpensive method for detecting pyuria at the bedside. A positive test indicates a minimum of eight white blood cells/high power field and has a sensitivity of 88–95% and specificity of 94–98% compared with the counting chamber method. The presence of blood, rifampin (rifampicin), nitrofurantoin, bilirubin and ascorbic acid may result in a false-negative test, whereas trichomonads, imipenem and amoxicillin/clavulanate may give a false-positive test.[25]

DETECTION OF BACTERIA

The presence of bacteria on microscopy of urine correlates well with culture results. Experienced laboratories can reliably detect 10^8 organisms/per liter in unstained specimens. Chemical methods of detecting bacteria such as the nitrite test are unreliable, except for Gram-negative bacilli in first morning urines. This is because prolonged incubation in the bladder is required to allow reduction of nitrate to nitrite.

Midstream urine specimens

The simplest and most widely used method for obtaining urine for culture is to collect a clean specimen of freshly voided urine. The confounding effects of contamination are minimized by avoiding the first 10ml and performing quantitative culture. The sensitivity and specificity of this technique is highly dependent on the clinical state of the patient and the presence of pyuria. It was shown that, in asymptomatic women, two colony counts, 24 hours apart, of more than 10^5/ml of Gram-negative bacilli in pure culture with or without pyuria had a sensitivity of up to 80% and specificity of greater than 95% for diagnosis of UTI. A single count of 10^4–10^5/ml had a 95% chance of representing contamination. Unfortunately, a bacterial count of more than 10^5/ml became misapplied to other clinical circumstances.[26]

The presence of symptoms and pyuria (>10 white blood cells/ml) radically alters the probability that a UTI is present. In carefully conducted studies a single count of more than 10^5/ml in women with uncomplicated cystitis had a very high specificity (>99%) but a low sensitivity (51%).[27] Routine application of such criteria would fail to diagnose one-third of women with acute bacterial cystitis (Fig. 57.7). Specimens from males are less likely to be contaminated and lower counts (>10^3/ml) are highly predictive of infection. Gram-positive bacteria and yeast in urine tend to have lower counts than do Gram-negative bacilli.

This has raised a problem as to how results should be processed and reported in routine laboratories, as specimens are often poorly collected and delays in processing allow bacterial multiplication. A recent international working party has suggested that, in the presence of pyuria, a bacterial count greater than 10^3/ml is a reasonable criterion for a routine laboratory, bearing in mind that this represents 10 organisms on a plate if a 0.01ml loop is used. Others argue that >10^4/ml is more realistic in these circumstances and specimens with lower counts should be repeated.

False-positive culture results are caused by delays in processing without refrigeration. False-negatives can occur in the presence of obstruction, antimicrobial agents and, possibly, diuresis.

Suprapubic aspiration

Suprapubic aspiration of urine from a distended bladder is an efficient means of diagnosis. Any bacteria identified can be regarded as significant as the technique avoids contamination. In most infected specimens bacteria can be seen microscopically, and so treatment can be started promptly. Provided the patient has a full bladder it is safe and acceptable to patients.

Catheter specimens

The main justification for catheterization specifically for a urine culture in adults is an inability to co-operate to obtain uncontaminated mid-stream urine, or to hold urine in the bladder for a suprapubic aspiration. Catheterization rarely leads to false-positive results but may introduce bacteria into the bladder. Straight plastic catheter or Alexa bag techniques are satisfactory.

IMAGING OF THE URINARY TRACT

All men, children and infants need investigations of their urinary tract if they have a UTI, regardless of clinical features at presentation. This is not cost-effective in women unless there is some evidence of an unusual clinical pattern,[28] such as urinary infection as a child, treatment failure, and persistent microscopic hematuria or pyuria at follow-up. A careful ultrasound examination including postmicturition bladder volumes plus a plain abdominal radiograph, including the kidneys, ureters and bladder, or an intravenous urogram, is adequate in most instances. Cystoscopy rarely yields useful information in women with acute cystitis.

MANAGEMENT

The goal of treatment is to eradicate the infection, and to reduce morbidity caused by relapse or recurrence with minimum toxicity, inconvenience and distress for the patient. It is essential to relieve anxiety about sexual activity, perceived long-term consequences, and advice offered by family and the popular press.

The cornerstone of management is effective antimicrobial therapy (Fig. 57.8). Drinking large amounts of fluids may decrease bacterial counts and improve symptoms, but rarely eliminates the infection and adds little to effective antimicrobial therapy. Likewise alkalinizing agents may decrease symptoms somewhat but do not influence bacterial eradication.

Follow-up visits at 7–14 days after completion of therapy are required to obtain urine cultures and discuss the importance of the diagnosis.

ACUTE UNCOMPLICATED BACTERIAL CYSTITIS

Short-course therapy has now become the standard for treatment in clinical practice, although 7–10 days is still used by some investigators in clinical trials. Short-course therapy is contraindicated in complicated infections, diabetes, structural abnormalities, or for patients in whom follow-up is likely to be poor. Advantages of short-course therapy include better compliance, lower cost, fewer side effects and decreased likelihood of the emergence of resistant strains. Both single-dose and 3-day courses are highly effective and have strong advocates[29,30]. A treatment algorithm is given in Figure 57.9.

Single-dose therapy

Single-dose therapy is essentially 1 day of treatment given in a single dose that produces inhibitory concentrations of antibiotic over a 12–24-hour period. It is most suitable for cystitis in sexually active women and for younger patients who have normal urinary tracts and a short history (<7 days) (Fig. 57.10).

Amoxicillin was the first drug promoted for single-dose therapy but proved less effective than either trimethoprim–sulfamethoxazole (co-trimoxazole) or trimethoprim alone and is no longer recommended in single-dose regimens. Fluoroquinolones are very effective, although they may be less effective against *S. saprophyticus* than Gram-negative bacilli. Fosfomycin trometamol has proved highly effective and has been marketed specifically for single-dose therapy.

Those who fail to respond to single-dose therapy have an increased risk of abnormalities within the urinary tract.[31]

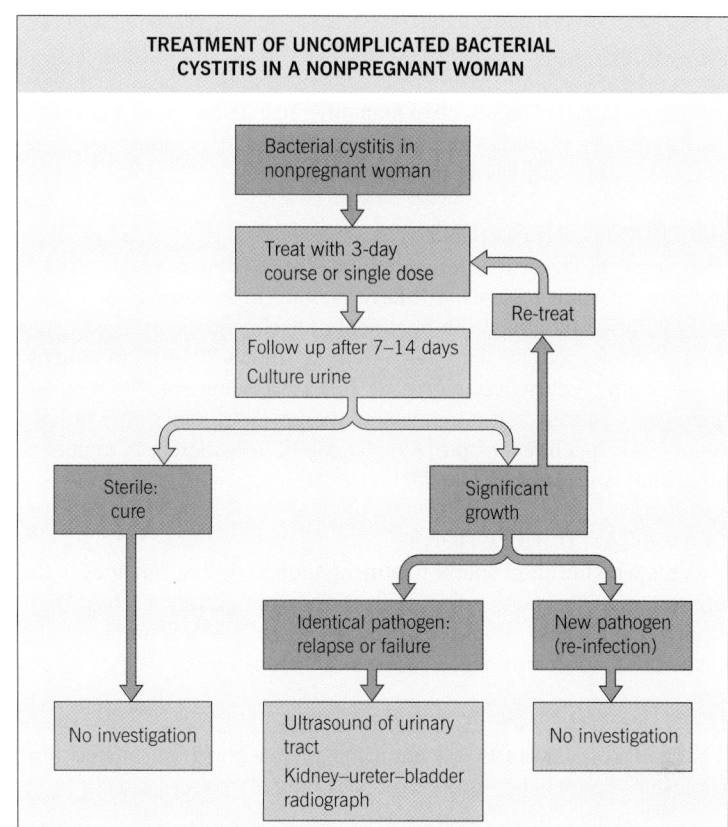

Fig. 57.9 Treatment of uncomplicated cystitis in a nonpregnant woman.

SUGGESTED DRUG TREATMENT REGIMENS FOR SINGLE-DOSE THERAPY	
Drug	Dose
Trimethoprim	600mg
Trimethoprim–sulfamethoxazole (co-trimoxazole)	1.92g
Norfloxacin	800mg
Ciprofloxacin	500mg
Fleroxacin	400mg
Fosfomycin trometamol	3g

Fig. 57.10 Suggested drug treatment regimens for single-dose therapy.

Three-day therapy

This provides many of the advantages of short course therapy and may have a higher rate of success particularly in the older women. It is often preferred by patients as it may take 3 days for symptoms to abate (Fig. 57.8).

THERAPEUTIC AGENTS

Both trimethoprim–sulfamethoxazole (co-trimoxazole) and trimethoprim alone are highly effective, but trimethoprim has fewer side effects, especially in the elderly, and there is no evidence the combination with sulfamethoxazole prevents emergence of resistance. Nitrofurantoin is ineffective against *Proteus mirabilis*. The side effects of nausea and vomiting can be minimized by treating with 50mg q8h without loss of efficacy, rather than 100mg q6h. The fluoroquinolones have essentially superseded nalidixic acid and oxolinic acid. All of these agents are extremely active and effective against most pathogens including many hospital pathogens. Norfloxacin is the most cost-effective fluorquinolone for treatment of cystitis in many countries.[32]

Amoxicillin is the treatment of choice for treating *Streptococcus faecalis* but increasing resistance has limited its usefulness against other uropathogens. Combinations of beta-lactam with beta-lactamase inhibitors may be less effective than other agents and have a high rate of diarrhea. Cephalosporins such as cephalexin, cephradine and cefaclor are useful particularly in renal failure.

RECURRENT INFECTIONS

The major problem with uncomplicated infections is recurrence. A majority of adult females will have another infection within 1 year, most within 3 months. With treatment of each episode most will stop having recurrences at some stage. In large studies 20–30% of patients cease having recurrences with each course of treatment.[33] If episodes are closely spaced, self-administered therapy, preferably after obtaining a urine specimen, or prophylaxis can be considered. A treatment algorithm is given in Figure 57.11.

COMPLICATED INFECTIONS

Patients who fail short course treatment often have abnormalities of the urinary tract (e.g. stones, diverticulae, strictures, chronic bacterial prostatitis, etc.). These should be corrected where possible and infection treated with more prolonged courses of therapy.

URINARY TRACT INFECTIONS IN PREGNANCY

The risks of symptomatic infection and pyelonephritis during the third trimester of pregnancy in mothers and prematurity in infants can be prevented by early detection and eradication of asymptomatic bacteriuria. In the first instance single-dose or a 3-day course of therapy are appropriate (Fig. 57.12). If relapse or re-infection occurs then the patients should be retreated. At that stage the simplest strategy is to institute prophylaxis (e.g. nitrofurantoin 50mg or cephalexin 250mg at night), although some prefer close surveillance with repeated cultures and prompt treatment of each episode. All such patients need evaluation of the urinary tract with ultrasonography and plain abdominal radiograph after delivery.

There is probably no absolute contraindication to any antimicrobial agent during pregnancy but caution is urged with some agents.[34] The antifolic acid activity of trimethoprim and trimethoprim–sulfamethoxazole is minimal in short courses and probably safe between 16 and 30 weeks of gestation (Fig. 57.13).

MALES

Lower UTI in males may be complicated by infection of prostatic fluid, even if there is no clinical prostatitis.[35] For this reason there is reluctance to treat men with short regimens and studies of single-dose therapy in elderly men have been disappointing.[36] Long-term prophylaxis may be helpful.

ASYMPTOMATIC BACTERIURIA

Asymptomatic bacteriuria is often best left untreated except in pregnancy. In elderly patients it is extremely common and there is no convincing evidence that treatment benefits the patient either in terms of

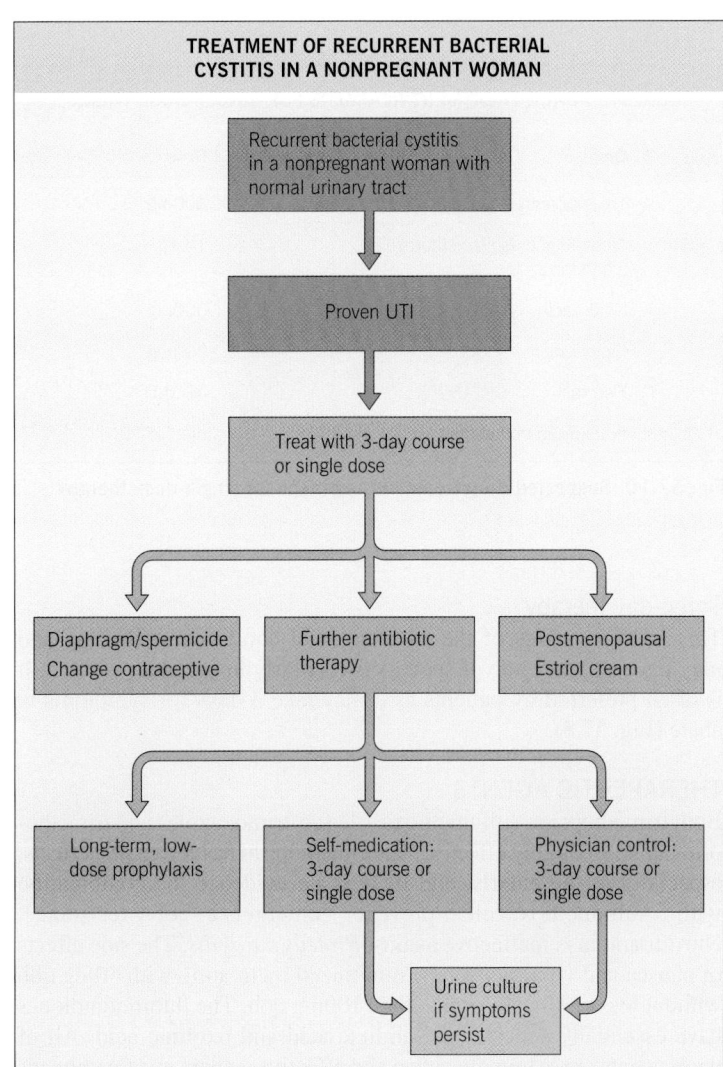

Fig. 57.11 Treatment of recurrent bacterial cystitis in a nonpregnant woman.

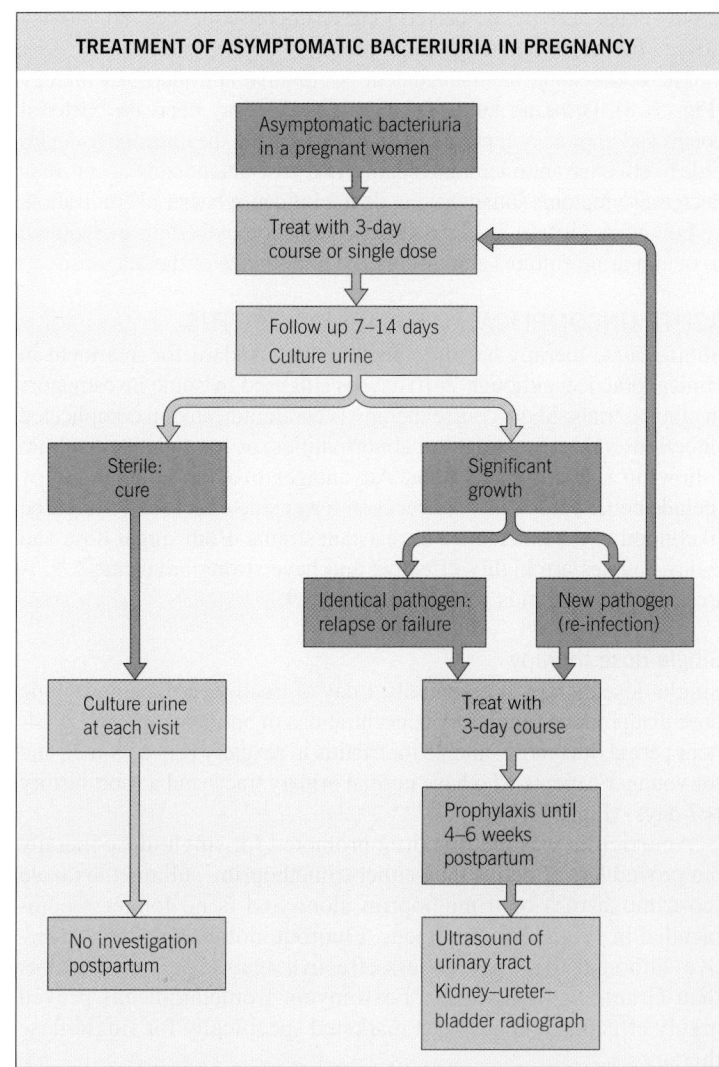

Fig. 57.12 Treatment of asymptomatic bacteriuria in pregnancy.

POSSIBLE TOXICITIES OF ANTIMICROBIAL AGENTS IN PREGNANCY	
Agent	Toxicity
Trimethoprim sulfonamides	Antifolate activity and megaloblastic anemia
Sulfonamides (protein bound)	Kernicterus of newborn
Sulfonamides/nitrofurantoin	Hemolytic anemia in G6PD deficiency
Tetracycline	Fatty liver/hepatic necrosis in mother, stained teeth in baby
Fluoroquinolones	Not approved

Fig. 57.13 Possible toxicities of antimicrobial agents in pregnancy.

recurrent symptomatic episodes or mortality. Antimicrobial therapy is associated with adverse effects, potential for development of resistant strains, and financial cost.[9]

INVASIVE PROCEDURES

Asymptomatic bacteriuria should be treated if the patient is to undergo an invasive procedure of the genitourinary tract. Mucosal trauma may cause postprocedural bacteremia and occasionally septic shock and death. The antimicrobial agent should be selected on the basis of the sensitivity of the infecting organism.[37] Likewise, it is prudent to treat any urinary infections before the insertion of permanent indwelling devices, particularly prosthetic joints.

TREATMENT IN THE PRESENCE OF RENAL FAILURE

If treatment is truly indicated, drugs that achieve adequate urine concentrations in the presence of renal failure should be used. The best levels may be achieved with penicillin and cephalosporins. Trimethoprim and fluoroquinolones will probably achieve adequate concentrations, whereas nitrofurantoin, sulfamethoxazole and doxycycline are present in very low concentrations when creatinine clearance falls below about 0.16ml/s.

INFECTIONS WITH *CANDIDA* SPP.

Infections with *Candida* spp. may occur either from hematogenous spread or via the ascending route. There is an increased risk in those with diabetes, prolonged antimicrobial therapy and instrumentation of the urinary tract. The natural history has not been well-defined but most infections are asymptomatic, limited to the lower urinary tract and may resolve in otherwise normal patients. Occasionally pyelonephritis, papillary necrosis or bezoars occur, especially in patients who have diabetes mellitus, obstructive uropathy or renal transplantation. Those at increased risk should be treated, but it is less clear for other patients. The

treatment of choice for those without a catheter is oral fluconazole (50–100mg/day), although some species such as *Candida krusei* may be resistant.[38] A single dose of intravenous amphotericin B (0.3mg/kg) is usually effective, presumably because of prolonged renal excretion. Oral flucytosine and alteration of urinary pH are ineffective. If a catheter is present, bladder washouts with amphotericin B may be used but are of questionable efficacy.

URETHRAL SYNDROMES

PATHOGENESIS AND CLINICAL FEATURES

Following the introduction of quantitative bacterial counts, it was observed that about half of adult women with acute symptoms of UTI did not have significant ($>10^5$cfu/ml) numbers of bacteria in their urine. These were said to have acute urethral syndrome or dysuria–pyuria syndrome. Many women with acute urethral syndrome had periurethral colonization with uropathogenic organisms and low numbers of *E. coli*, *S. saprophyticus* and enteric Gram-negative organisms present in their urine. Furthermore many such patients responded to antibiotic therapy, suggesting that this was essentially a UTI. It has therefore been suggested that a low count of bacteria ($>10^2$cfu/ml) form the basis of diagnosis of UTI.[26] These patients probably have urethritis with little infection of the bladder and the diagnosis may not be made by routine laboratories because of the low numbers of organisms present.

There remains a group with similar symptoms who do not have low counts of bacteria in their urine. It is possible that symptoms are caused by infection confined to the proximal urethra, especially if there is pyuria, but it is very difficult to diagnose. Various agents, including organisms that commonly cause UTIs (especially in women who suffer recurrent UTI), *Ureaplasma urealyticum*, *C. trachomatis* and other sexually transmitted pathogens, are possible pathogens. Multiple other causes have been suggested, including infection of the female paraurethral glands, lactobacilli, chemicals (e.g. bubble baths and deodorants), and traumatic and psychologic factors, but none is supported by convincing evidence.

MANAGEMENT

Management of the urethral syndrome is difficult. A pelvic examination should be done to exclude herpes simplex, gonorrhea and vaginitis. The symptoms usually settle in a few days although some patients appear to benefit from a high fluid intake. Antimicrobial therapy is helpful if pyuria is present, presumably reflecting bacterial urethritis or chlamydial infection. Antibiotics useful for treatment of UTI are often prescribed in the first instance. If these fail, doxycycline (100mg q12h) for 10 days may be effective.[39]

REFERENCES

1. Harding GKM, Ronald AR. The management of urinary infections: what have we learned in the past decade? Int J Antimicrob Ag 1994;4:83–8.
2. Kunin CM. Detection, prevention and management of urinary tract infections, 5th ed. Baltimore: Williams and Wilkins: 1997;128–64.
3. Hooton TM, Scholes D, Hughes JP, et al. A prospective study of risk factors for symptomatic urinary tract infection in young women. N Engl J Med 1996;335:468–74.
4. Hooton TM, Fihn SK, Johnson C, Roberts PL, Stamm WE. Association between bacterial vaginosis and acute cystitis in women using diaphragms. Arch Intern Med 1989;149:1932–6.
5. Schultz R, Read AW, Straton JA, et al. Genitourinary tract infections in pregnancy and low birth weight: Case control study in Australian aboriginal women. Br Med J 1991;303:1369–73.

6. Hopelman AIM, Van Buren M, Van den Broek J, et al. Bacteriuria in men infected with HIV-1 is related to their immune status (CD4+ cell count). AIDS 1992;6:179–84.
7. Latham RH, Running K, Stamm WE. Urinary tract infections in young women caused by Staphylococcus saprophyticus. JAMA 1983;250:3063–6.
8. Gould JC. The comparative bacteriology of acute and chronic urinary tract infections. In: O'Grady F, Brumfitt W, eds. Urinary tract infections. London: Oxford University Press; 1968:43–50.
9. Nicolle LE, Mayhew WJ, Bryan L. Prospective randomised comparison of therapy and no therapy for asymptomatic bacteriuria in institutionalised elderly women. Am J Med 1987;83:27–33.

10. Stamey TA, Timothy M, Millar M, Mihara G. Recurrent urinary infections in adult women. The role of introital enterobacteria. Calif Med 1971;115:1–19.
11. Sheinfeld J, Schaffer AJ, Corrdon-Cardo C, Rogatko A, Fair WR. Association of Lewis blood group phenotype with recurrent urinary tract infections in women. N Engl J Med 1989;320:773–7.
12. Johnson JR. Virulence factors in Escherichia coli urinary tract infections. Clin Microbiol Rev 1991;4:80–128.
13. Hooton TM, Hillier S, Johnson PL, Stamm WE. Escherichia coli bacteriuria and contraceptive method. JAMA 1991;265:64–9.
14. Raz R, Stamm WE. A controlled trial of intravaginal estriol in postmenopausal women with recurrent urinary tract infections. N Engl J Med 1993;329:753–6.

15. Orskov I, Ferenc A, Orskov F. Tamm-Horsfall protein orosomucoid is the normal urinary slime that traps type I fimbriated *Escherichia coli*. Lancet 1980;1:887.

16. Lindstedt R, Baker N, Falk P, *et al.* Binding specificities of wild-type and cloned *Escherichia coli* strains recognising globo-A. Infect Immun 1989;57:3389–94.

17. Andersson P, Egberg I, Lidin-Jansson G, *et al.* Persistence of *Escherichia coli* bacteriuria is not determined by bacterial adherence. Infect Immun 1991;59:2951–92.

18. Hedges S, Svanborg A. The mucosal cytokine response to urinary tract infections. Int J Antimicrob Ag 1994;4:89–93.

19. O'Grady F, Cattel WR. Kinetics of urinary tract infections: II. The bladder. Br J Urol 1966;38:156–62.

20. Chambers ST, Lever M. Betaines and urinary tract infections. Nephron 1996;74:1–10.

21. Pecha B, Low D, O'Hanley P. Gal-Gal pili vaccines prevent pyelonephritis by piliated *Escherichia coli*. J Clin Invest 1989;83:2102–8.

22. Stapleton A, Latham R, Johnson C, Stamm WE. Randomized, double blind, placebo-controlled trial post-coital antimicrobial prophylaxis for recurrent UTI. JAMA 1990;264:703–6.

23. Nicolle LE. Urinary tract infection in the elderly. J Antimicrob Chemother 1994;33(Suppl A):99–109.

24. Boscia JA, Kobasa WD, Abrutyn E, Levison ME, Kaplan AM, Kaye D. Lack of association between bacteriuria and symptoms in the elderly. Am J Med 1986;81:979–82.

25. Beer JH, Vogt A, Neftel K, Cottagnoud C. False positive results for leukocytes in urine dip stick test with common antibiotics. Br Med J 1996;313:25.

26. Kass EH. Bacteriuria and the diagnosis of infections of the urinary tract. Arch Intern Med 1957;100:709–14.

27. Stamm WE, Counts GW, Running KR, *et al.* Diagnosis of coliform infection in acutely dysuric women. N Eng J Med 1982;307:463–8.

28. Bailey RR. Cost-benefit considerations in the management of uncomplicated urinary tract infections in sexually active women. NZ Med J 1987;85:793–8.

29. Norrby SR. Short term treatment of uncomplicated lower UTI in women. Rev Infect Dis 1990;12:458–67.

30. Bailey RR. Management of lower urinary tract infections. Drugs 1993;45(Suppl 3):139–443.

31. Ronald AR, Boutros P, Mourtada H. Bacteriuria localisation and response to single dose therapy in women. JAMA 1976;235:1854–6.

32. Bailey RR. Quinolones in the treatment of uncomplicated urinary tract infections. Int J Antimicrob Ag 1992;2:19–28.

33. Kunin CM. The natural history of recurrent bacteriuria in school girls. N Engl J Med 1970;282:1443–8.

34. Wise R. Antibiotics. Br Med J 1987;294:42–6.

35. Lipsky BA. Urinary tract infections in men: epidemiology, pathophysiology, diagnosis, and treatment. Ann Intern Med 1989;110:138–50.

36. Nicolle LE, Bjornson J, Harding GKM, McDonnell JA. Bacteriuria in elderly institutionalized men. N Engl J Med 1983;309:1420–5.

37. Cafferky MT, Falkinen FR, Gillespie WA, Murphy DM. Antibiotics for the prevention of septicaemia in urology. J Antimicrob Chemother 1982;9:471–7.

38. Guglielmo BJ, Stoller ML, Jacobs RA. Management of candiduria. Int J Antimicrob Ag 1994;4:135–9.

39. Stamm WE, Running K, McKevitt M, Counts GW, Turck M, Holmes KK. Treatment of the acute urethral syndrome. N Engl J Med 1981;304:956–8.

Prostatitis, Epididymitis and Orchitis

Kurt G Naber & Wolfgang Weidner

PROSTATITIS

The diagnosis of prostatitis refers to a variety of inflammatory and noninflammatory conditions affecting the prostate. In 1978 a classification system was developed to differentiate inflammatory from noninflammatory entities (Fig. 58.1).[1] However, many aspects of chronic prostatic symptoms remain an enigma. A consensus conference at the National Institutes of Health categorized prostatitis into symptomatic and asymptomatic presentations:

- the symptomatic categories encompass both inflammatory and noninflammatory chronic prostatitis; and
- the asymptomatic entity identifies patients who are incidentally diagnosed from biopsies, evaluations for fertility disorders or routine examinations.

EPIDEMIOLOGY

DEFINITION AND NOMENCLATURE
Acute prostatitis is an acute febrile illness that may be characterized by intense pain in the perineum and rectum, fever, voiding difficulties, systemic symptoms of sepsis and a tender swollen prostate on rectal examination. The chronic prostatitis syndromes (bacterial, nonbacterial and prostatodynia) cause symptoms which cannot be differentiated from each other (see Fig. 58.2). Leukocytes are present in prostatic secretions of patients with true inflammation. Pathogens must be present in prostatic secretions for a conclusive diagnosis of bacterial prostatitis.[2] In prostatodynia, in contrast to 'true' prostatitis, no signs of inflammation are detectable (Fig. 58.1).

INCIDENCE AND PREVALENCE
Due to classification difficulties, few data are available to determine the incidence of prostatitis. Acute prostatitis is infrequent with a probable incidence of fewer than 1/1000 adult men. However, prostatic symptoms are common. In the USA approximately 30% of men between 20 and 50 years of age experience 'prostatitis-like' symptoms[3] and these symptoms are responsible for about 25% of physician office visits by men for genitourinary complaints.[3]

The term prostatitis implies inflammation, but only 5–10% of patients with this diagnosis actually have a proven bacterial infection.[3,4] The rest do not have 'significant' prostatic fluid bacterial counts. About 50% of these patients have nonbacterial prostatitis (NBP) with the prostatic fluid demonstrating an elevated leukocyte count.[2–9] The rest are categorized as having 'pelvic perineal' pain syndrome or prostadynia. This is a diagnosis of exclusion and in most cases it cannot be proved that the symptoms arise from the prostate.

RISK FACTORS
Urinary tract infections (UTIs) are the major underlying determinant of both acute and chronic bacterial prostatitis (CBP). Strains of *Escherichia coli* responsible for both acute and chronic prostatitis appears to have similar urovirulence determinants to the *E. coli* strains that cause pyelonephritis.[10] Prostatic calculi can account for recurrences of CBP.[2] Bacterial microcolonies enclosed within biofilms inside prostatic acini and ducts can be a foci for bacterial persistence.[7] In NBP it is hypothesized that intraprostatic reflux of urine causes inflammation, so triggering prostatic pain.[11] Other presumed and unproven causes of NBP are immunologic reactions, tissue response to spermatozoa and migration of sexually transmitted organisms from the urethra.

CLINICAL FEATURES

DIAGNOSIS
Acute bacterial prostatitis is diagnosed by its clinical presentation.[9] It presents as an acute febrile illness with irritative and obstructive voiding symptoms. Prostatic massage is contraindicated and the diagnosis depends upon:

- urine and blood cultures;
- a gentle examination of the prostate that demonstrates acute inflammation; and
- a urinalysis, which usually demonstrates pyuria.

Prostatic abscess may occur in patients with acute prostatitis. This diagnosis is made by clinical examination and transrectal ultrasonography. Focal hypoechoic zones with irregular internal echoes, septations and indirect borders with the surrounding parenchyma are typical patterns.

Fig. 58.1 Classification of chronic prostatitis.
EPS, expressed prostatic secretion. + = present; (+) = sometimes present; 0 = not present.

CLASSIFICATION OF CHRONIC PROSTATITIS					
	Evidence of inflammation in EPS (macrophages, neutrophils)	Positive culture		Etiologic organisms	Rectal examination (prostate)
		EPS	Bladder		
Chronic bacterial prostatitis	+	+	(+)	Enterobacteriaceae and *Enterococcus, Pseudomonas* and *Staphylococcus* spp.	Normal or enlarged with tenderness; may be nodular
'Nonbacterial' prostatitis	+	0	0	Unknown	Normal or enlarged
Prostatodynia	0	0	0	0	Normal

SYMPTOMS IN PATIENTS WITH THE CHRONIC PROSTATITIS SYNDROMES

Urethral symptoms	• Burning in the urethra during voiding • Discharge • Difficult urination • Stranguria • Frequency • Nocturia • Prostatorrhea • Leukocytospermia
Prostatic symptoms	• Pressure behind pubic bone • Perineal pressure tension in testes and epididymes • Inguinal pain • Anorectal dysesthesia • Diffuse anogenital syndromes • Lower abdominal discomfort
Sexual dysfunction	• Loss of libido • Erectile dysfunction • Ejaculatory dysfunction • Pain during or after orgasm
Other symptoms	• Myalgia • Headache • Fatigue

Fig. 58.2 Symptoms in patients with the chronic prostatitis syndromes.

The abscess may be distinct or more diffuse. Prostatic abscesses are usually due to the same uropathogens that are responsible for acute bacterial prostatitis, although a variety of anaerobes and fungi are implicated sporadically. Systemic mycoses, particularly *Cryptococcus neoformans, Blastomyces dermatitidis, Coccidioides immitis* or *Histoplasma capsulatum* can involve the prostate gland and produce prostatic abscesses. *Candida albicans* can also cause prostatic abscesses.

Chronic bacterial prostatitis is a less precise diagnosis (Fig. 58.2). Patients presenting with prostatic complaints should have a prostatic massage to localize the infection. The method of choice is the Meares and Stamey localization technique (Fig. 58.3).[12] Increased numbers of neutrophils and fat-laden macrophages are typical cytologic signs in the expressed prostatic secretion (EPS). Although increased numbers of leukocytes may be found in EPS, it is generally accepted that over 10 neutrophils/high-power field indicates prostatitis.[9,10] In patients for whom an EPS cannot be obtained increased numbers of neutrophils in the urine after prostatic massage (VB_3) is an indication of prostatitis if first voided urine (VB_1) and midstream urine (VB_2) do not contain these cells. In patients with CBP, bacterial pathogens will be present in the EPS or VB_3 in larger numbers, usually a 10-fold higher concentration than in the VB_1.[9,10] The exact technique for localizing infection with the Meares and Stamey technique is outlined in Figure 58.3 and should be followed carefully.[12]

The role of *Chlamydia trachomatis* and *Ureaplasma urealyticum* in bacterial prostatitis is uncertain and there are no widely accepted criteria

MEARES AND STAMEY LOCALIZATION TECHNIQUE

1. Approximately 30 minutes before taking the specimen, the patient should drink 400ml of liquid (two glasses). The test starts when the patient wants to void
2. The lids of four sterile specimen containers, which are marked VB_1, VB_2, EPS and VB_3, should be removed. Place the uncovered specimen containers on a flat surface and maintain sterility
3. Hands are washed
4. Expose the penis and retract the foreskin so that the glans is exposed. The foreskin should be retracted throughout
5. Cleanse the glans with a soap solution, remove the soap with sterile gauze or cotton and dry the glans
6. Urinate 10–15ml into the first container marked VB_1
7. Urinate 100–200ml into the toilet bowl or vessel and without interrupting the urine stream, urinate 10–15ml into the second container marked VB_2
8. The patient bends forward and holds the sterile specimen container (EPS) to catch the prostate secretion
9. The physician massages the prostate until several drops of prostate secretion (EPS) are obtained
10. If no EPS can be collected during massage, a drop may be present at the orifice of the urethra and this drop should be taken with a 10μl calibrated loop and cultured
11. Immediately after prostatic massage, the patient urinates 10–15ml of urine into the container marked VB_3.

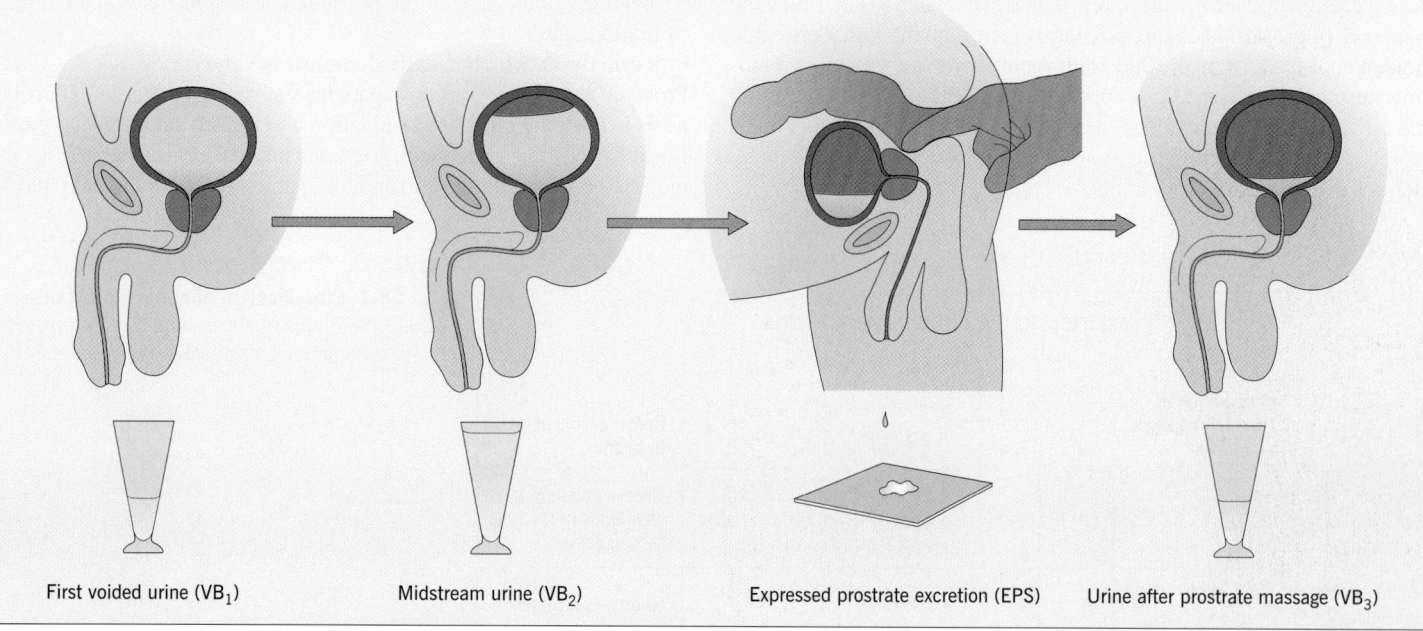

First voided urine (VB_1) Midstream urine (VB_2) Expressed prostrate excretion (EPS) Urine after prostrate massage (VB_3)

Fig. 58.3 Meares and Stamey[12] localization technique to diagnose chronic bacterial prostatitis. Prostate secretion can be more readily obtained if the patient has not ejaculated for approximately 3–5 days before the examination.

for defining prostatitis due to these or other infrequently isolated pathogens (Fig. 58.4).[13–15]

Ejaculate analysis is sometimes recommended in men with CBP to obtain further information, but studies of seminal fluid are mostly unhelpful. A proportion of men with CBP have bacteriospermia (>10³cfu/ml) and the organisms present are usually identical to those in the EPS.[16] Biochemical analysis of EPS has been used as an additional diagnostic criterion for CBP, but these observations have not been shown to be sufficiently sensitive or specific to add to the diagnosis (Fig. 58.5).[9,10] The pH is usually increased (>7.8) in the EPS from patients with CBP.

Biopsy under ultrasonographic guidance, particularly if nodules are present, is used for histology and culture.[2,5,17] Inflammatory findings in the prostate are usually nonspecific and the primary indication for biopsy is to exclude prostatic cancer.

Evaluation of bladder emptying by flow rate measurements and ultrasonography can be useful in patients with voiding disturbances.[17] On occasion this diagnostic work-up should include a voiding cysto-urethrogram. Urodynamic changes are present in about one-third of patients with CBP. In the presence of abnormal flow rate measurements, further studies should be performed to differentiate between functional and anatomic changes.

Urethrocystoscopy may reveal visible inflammatory changes in the posterior urethra. Prostatic sonography may demonstrate prostatic calculi (Fig. 58.6). Prostatic calculi may serve as nidi for pathogens and lead to CBP, but they are common and increase with age, and their role remains controversial. Figure 58.7 outlines the diagnostic investigation of patients who present with possible prostatitis.

Nonbacterial prostatitis is a less specific diagnosis. These patients have inflammatory cells in the EPS with negative cultures from both the

PROSTATITIS INFECTIONS BY UNCONVENTIONAL FASTIDIOUS PATHOGENS

Species	Clinical feature	Comment
Haemophilus influenzae		Single case reports
Neisseria gonorrhoeae	Associated with history of gonococcal urethritis	Decreasing due to effective antibiotic treatment
Mycobacterium tuberculosis	Urogenital manifestation	Associated with HIV infection
Anaerobes	Prostatic abscesses	
Candida spp.	In immunocompromised patients with indwelling urinary catheters	
Coccidioides immitis, Blastomyces dermatitidis, Histoplasma capsulatum	Disseminated disease	Associated with HIV infection
Trichomonas vaginalis	Chronic inflammation	May be associated with urethritis

Fig. 58.4 Prostatitis infections by unconventional fastidious pathogens.

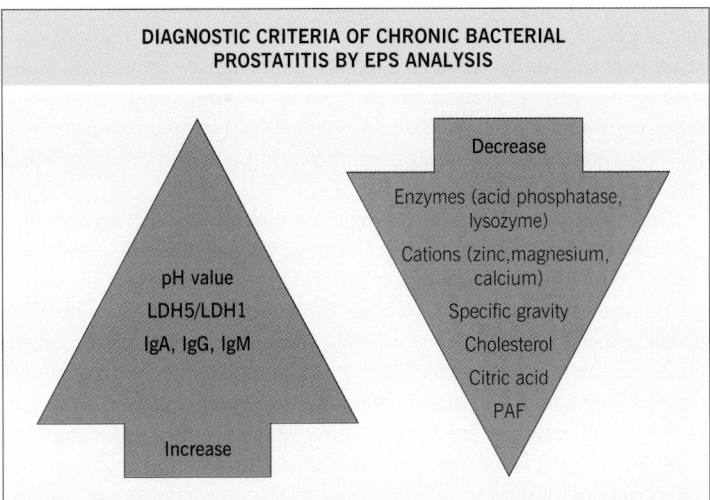

Fig. 58.5 Diagnostic criteria of chronic bacterial prostatitis by expressed prostatic secretion (EPS) analysis. LDH, lactate dehydrogenase; PAF, prostatic antibacterial factor.

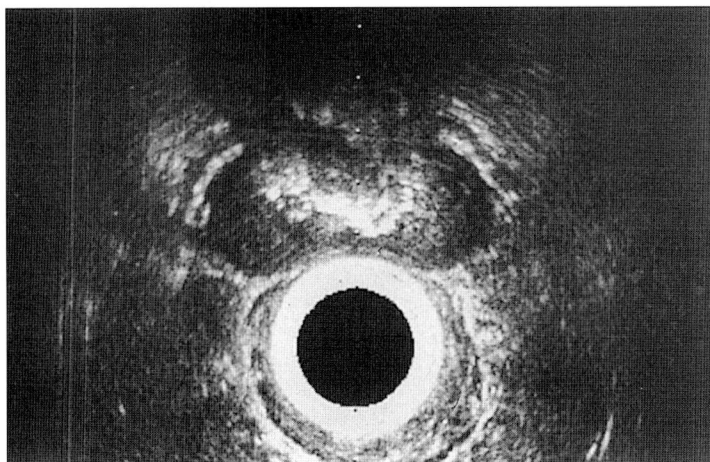

Fig. 58.6 Transrectal ultrasonography of the prostate with diffuse calcifications (prostatitis calcarea).

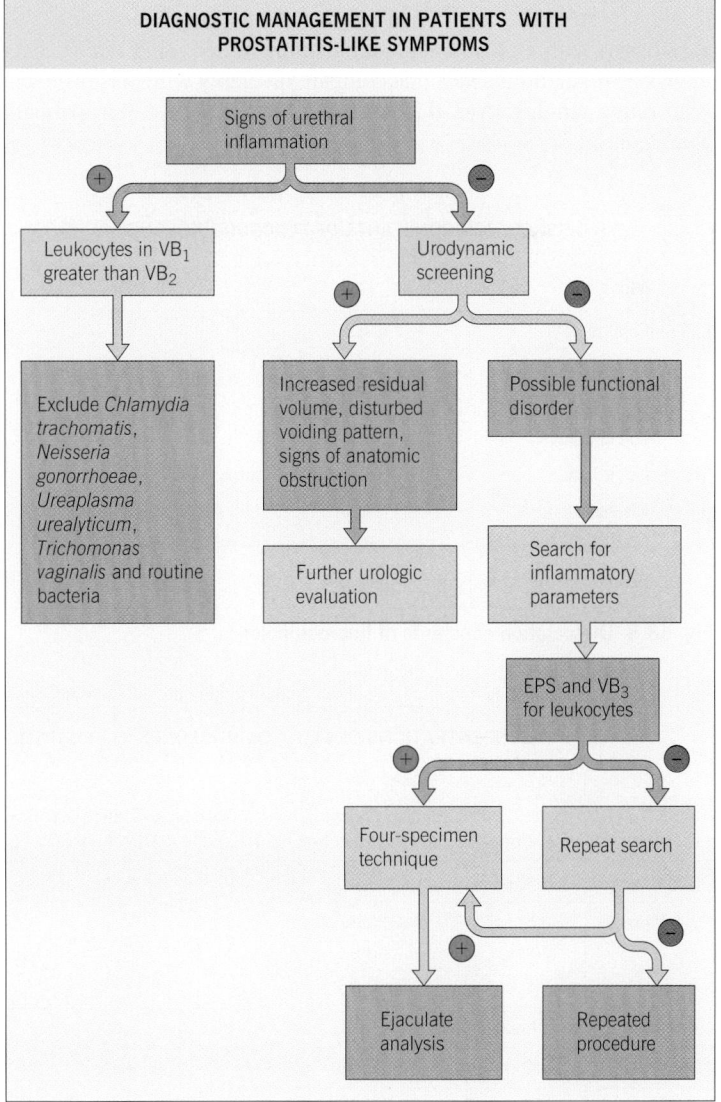

Fig. 58.7 Diagnostic management in patients with prostatitis-like symptoms. EPS, expressed prostatic secretion.

EPS and VB$_3$. Although numerous investigators have attempted to demonstrate that NBP is due to difficult-to-culture pathogens such as *C. trachomatis* or genital mycoplasma, there is no consensus that these organisms cause NBP.[13,18,19] As a result, this diagnosis is currently poorly defined and is presumed to be caused by unknown etiologic and pathogenetic processes. This entity is classified as inflammatory chronic pelvic pain syndrome (CPPS) according to the new definition of National Institute of Diabetes and Digestive and Kidney Disease (NIDDK).

MANAGEMENT

Treatment varies according to the severity of the patient's presenting symptoms and the probable etiologic agent. Antimicrobial treatment should be initiated immediately in patients with acute bacterial prostatitis after blood and urine cultures have been obtained. Prostatic massage is contraindicated. Parenteral treatment with trimethoprim–sulfamethoxazole (co-trimoxazole), a beta-lactam with an aminoglycoside, or a fluoroquinolone are all appropriate initial regimens. After initial improvement, a switch to an oral regimen is appropriate and should be prescribed for at least 6 weeks.

Patients with possible CBP require investigation for evidence of inflammation and an etiologic agent.

Selection of an appropriate antimicrobial agent that has optimal pharmacokinetics for prostatic tissue is important.[20] Antibacterial diffusion into prostate tissue depends upon the lipid solubility, molecular size and pKa of the agent.[20] For example, trimethoprim, a weak base with a pKa of 7.4, penetrates prostatic tissue well. However, because the pH of prostatic fluid in patients with CBP is often alkaline, tissue levels may be inadequate.[21,22] In contrast, the fluoroquinolones exist as zwitterions with a pKa in acid and alkaline milieus (Fig. 58.8). This allows prostatic fluid levels that compare favorably with plasma levels with ratios ranging from 0.12 to 0.48 (Fig. 58.9).[23,24,26] In patients

with CBP, the concentration of ciprofloxacin in alkaline seminal fluid may exceed that in plasma.[23,24,26] Other studies have examined fluoroquinolone concentrations in prostatic tissue obtained at transurethral resection and they appear to be consistently at or above corresponding plasma concentrations.[26] Macrolides also penetrate into prostatic and seminal fluids very well.[20,27]

Although it remains unproven, considerable evidence suggests that bacteria in prostatic tissue survive in a milieu protected by biofilms. Antimicrobial agents, particularly the fluoroquinolones and the macrolides, that penetrate through biofilm may be preferred drugs. Most studies in patients with CBP have not been well controlled and have been variably designed.[26,28] As a result, comparison is difficult. Duration of therapy has ranged from 14 to 150 days and follow-up investigation has not been standardized. An EPS should be obtained from all patients in therapeutic protocols 4–8 weeks after treatment to ensure that the pathogens have been eradicated. Overall, it appears that 60–80% of patients with *E. coli* and other Enterobacteriaceae can be cured with a 6-week course of therapy (Fig. 58.10).[3,29–35] However, prostatitis due to *Pseudomonas aeruginosa* and enterococci often fails to respond to treatment.

Chronic bacterial prostatitis can be a relapsing illness and recurrent episodes are best managed by either continuous low-dose suppressive therapy with an effective regimen such as fluoroquinolone, intermittent treatment whenever symptoms recur, or efforts to resect infected prostatic tissue, particularly prostatic calculi, in order to effect a surgical cure.[3] The latter is rarely successful and should only be carried out with very specific indications.

A prostatic abscess may require drainage in addition to antimicrobial treatment. Occasionally, anaerobes or mixed infections may be responsible for the abscess. Cultures should always be obtained, and if fungi are suspected the laboratory should be informed. Most treatment regimens should include an agent effective against anaerobes. Prostatic abscesses can be drained through the urethra, the perineum and occasionally through the rectum.

Nonbacterial prostatitis is managed empirically and no regimen has proved to be routinely successful. Occasionally patients appear to have a very specific response to antimicrobial therapy and whenever this occurs, a prolongation of therapy is indicated. However, most patients with NBP do not experience any change in symptoms with antibacterial therapy. Other treatment regimens include anti-inflammatory agents, α-adrenergic blocking agents, regular prostatic massage and weekly ejaculation. However, all regimens are empiric and treatment is often unsatisfactory.

Prostatodynia is an imprecise diagnosis for which therapy is controversial and unproven. Although the symptoms can mimic those of CBP, the absence of inflammation or any signs of infection are presumed to mean that no microbial agent is involved. This entity is classified as noninflammatory chronic pelvic pain syndrome (CPPS) according to the new definition of NIDDK. Treatment regimens similar to those used for NBP can be tried empirically.

DISSOCIATION CONSTANTS OF FLUOROQUINOLONES		
Quinolone	pK$_{a1}$	pK$_{a2}$
Ciprofloxacin	6.1	8.7
Enoxacin	6.3	8.7
Fleroxacin	5.5	8.1
Lomefloxacin	5.8	9.3
Norfloxacin	6.3	8.4
Ofloxacin	6.0	8.2
Pefloxacin	6.3	7.6
Sparfloxacin	6.2	8.6

Fig. 58.8 Dissociation constants of fluoroquinolones.

Fig. 58.9 Concentrations of fluoroquinolones in prostatic fluids of volunteers.[23,24,26]

CONCENTRATIONS OF FLUOROQUINOLONES IN PROSTATIC FLUIDS				
Quinolone	Dose (mg)	Median plasma concentration (mg/l)	Median prostatic fluid concentration (mg/l)	Median ratio of prostatic/plasma drug concentrations
Norfloxacin	800 po	1.40	0.14	0.12
Ciprofloxacin	200 iv	0.67	0.16	0.26
	200 iv	0.44	0.08	0.18
	750 po	0.88	0.23	0.23
Fleroxacin	400 po	3.71	1.00	0.28
Ofloxacin	400 po	2.00	0.66	0.33
Lomefloxacin	400 po	1.81	1.38	0.48

BACTERIOLOGIC CURE IN PATIENTS WITH CBP TREATED WITH FLUOROQUINOLONES

Quinolone	Dosage (mg q12h)	Duration of therapy (days)	Number of evaluable patients	% Bacteriologic cure	Duration of follow-up (months)	Year of study	References
Norfloxacin	400	28	14	64	6	1990	Schaeffer[29]
Norfloxacin	2–400	174	42	60	8	1991	Petrikkos[30]
Ofloxacin	200	14	21	67	12	1989	Pust et al.[31]
Ciprofloxacin	500	14	15	60	12	1987	Weidner et al.[32]
Ciprofloxacin	500	28	16	63	21–36	1991	Weidner et al.[33]
Ciprofloxacin	500	60–150	7	86	12	1991	Pfau[34,35]

Fig. 58.10 Eradication of pathogens (bacteriologic cure) in patients with chronic bacterial prostatitis (CBP) treated with fluoroquinolones. Only studies are listed in which the diagnosis was derived from application of the Meares and Stamey technique and a follow-up of at least 6 months was available.

CLASSIFICATION OF EPIDIDYMITIS AND ORCHITIS

Acute epididymitis or epididymo-orchitis	Granulomatous epididymitis or orchitis	Viral orchitis
Neisseria gonorrhoeae	Mycobacterium tuberculosis	Mumps
Chlamydia trachomatis	Treponema pallidum	Enteroviruses
Escherichia coli		
Streptococcus pneumoniae	Brucella spp.	
Klebsiella spp.	Sarcoid	
Salmonella spp.	Fungal	
Other urinary tract pathogens	Parasitic	
Idiopathic	Idiopathic	

Fig. 58.11 Classification of epididymitis and orchitis.

EPIDIDYMITIS AND ORCHITIS

Epididymitis is an acute painful swelling in the scrotum that is usually unilateral.[36] The testes may be involved in the inflammatory process as 'epididymo-orchitis'. Inflammatory processes of the testes, especially viral orchitis, less often involve the epididymis.

EPIDEMIOLOGY

Orchitis and epididymitis are classified as acute or chronic processes according to their cause (Fig. 58.11). Chronic inflammation with induration develops in about 15% of patients following an episode of acute epididymitis. Viral and bacterial inflammation of the testes can lead to testicular atrophy and destruction of spermatogenesis.[37]

Epididymitis is common among individuals who have high-risk sexual behaviors (frequent change of sexual partners) and is one of the leading causes of acute admission to hospital among military personnel. It occurs in 1–2% of patients with gonococcal and chlamydial urethritis, with an equal risk from each. It is usually unilateral and is due to an extension of the urethral infection via the vas deferens to the epididymis (see Chapter 2.63).

In middle-aged and older men, epididymitis is usually due to the same organisms as those that cause UTI and is presumably a direct extension from the urinary tract.

Epididymitis is more common in patients with indwelling catheters. Bladder outlet obstruction and urogenital abnormalities are also risk factors for acute and chronic epididymo-orchitis.

Mumps orchitis was common before widespread vaccination. It is now rare. It occurs in 20–30% of postpubertal men who have mumps. Other viral infections can also cause orchitis, particularly enteroviruses. The testes can also be involved as a continuation of epididymitis, particularly when suppurative UTI pathogens are involved. Granulomatous orchitis is a rare condition of uncertain etiology.[38]

Epididymo-orchitis can lead to abscess formation, testicular infarction, testicular atrophy, chronic epididymitis and infertility.[36]

CLINICAL FEATURES

Inflammation, pain and scrotal swelling characterize acute epididymitis.[36] Frequently the tail of the epididymis is involved first. The spermatic cord is usually tender and enlarged. The testes may be spared or may be involved to produce a contiguous large painful mass. Acute epididymitis always requires immediate evaluation by Doppler duplex scanning to differentiate between acute epididymitis and spermatic cord torsion. The latter requires urgent surgical intervention to prevent testicular infarction.

The microbiologic diagnosis of acute epididymitis and orchitis must be made as specifically as possible. A urethral Gram stain, urine culture and other studies for identification of Neisseria gonorrhoeae and C. trachomatis should be obtained for all patients. Blood cultures are valuable if the patient is febrile or has systemic signs of toxicity. Antibody and other specific serum investigations should be carried out to identify mumps, enteroviruses and other potential viral pathogens in patients with orchitis. Ejaculate analysis according to World Health Organization criteria including leukocyte analysis may be of value. A transient decreased sperm count or azoospermia is common. Infertility is a rare complication unless there is bilateral involvement.

MANAGEMENT

Antimicrobial agents should be chosen for initial empiric treatment based on the probability of the etiologic agent. In sexually active men who are at risk of C. trachomatis or N. gonorrhoeae a therapeutic regimen that covers both these pathogens is mandatory. Details of the treatment of these specific pathogens is provided in Chapter 2.63. Additional therapy includes bed rest and scrotal support. Abscesses may require surgical drainage. If urinary tract pathogens are considered to be the probable etiologic agent, the fluoroquinolones and trimethoprim–sulfamethoxazole are appropriate choices.

REFERENCES

1. Drach GW, Meares EM, Fair WR, Stamey TA. Classification of benign diseases associated with prostatic pain: prostatitis or prostatodynia. J Urol 1978;120:266.

2. Weidner W, Ludwig M. Diagnostic management in chronic prostatitis. In: Weidner W, Madsen PO, Schiefer HG, eds. Prostatitis. Berlin: Springer; 1994:49–65.

3. Lipsky BA. Urinary tract infections in men: epidemiology, pathophysiology, diagnosis, and treatment. Ann Intern Med 1989;110:138–48.

4. Weidner W, Schiefer HG, Krauss H, Jantos C, Friedrich HJ, Altmannsberger M. Chronic prostatitis: a thorough search for etiologically involved micro-organisms in 1461 patients. Infection 1991;19(Suppl 3):119–25.

5. de la Rosette JJMCH, Hubregtse MR, Meuleman EJH, Stolk-Engelaar MVM, Debruyne FMJ. Diagnosis and treatment of 409 patients with prostatitis syndromes. Urology 1993;41:301–7.

6. Weidner W, Schiefer HG. Inflammatory disease of the prostate: frequency and pathogenesis. In: Garraway M, ed. Epidemiology of prostate disease, Berlin: Springer; 1995:85–93.

7. Krieger J, Ross SO, Simonsen JM. Urinary tract infections in healthy university men. J Urol 1993;149:1046–8.

8. Schaeffer AJ. Diagnosis and treatment of prostatic infection. Urology 1990;36(Suppl 5):13–7.

9. Krieger JN, McGonagle LA. Diagnostic considerations and interpretation of microbiological findings for evaluation of chronic prostatitis. J Clin Microbiol 1989;27:2240–4.

10. Andrew A, Stapleton AE, Fennell C, et al. Urovirulence determinants in Escherichia coli strains causing prostatitis. J Infect Dis 1997:176;464–9.

11. Nickel JC, Olson ME, Barabas A, Benediktsson H, Dasgupta MK, Costerton JW. Pathogenesis of chronic bacterial prostatitis in an animal model. Br J Urol 1990;66:47–54.

12. Meares EM, Stamey TA. Bacteriologic localization patterns in bacterial prostatitis and urethritis. Invest Urol 1968;5:492–518.

13. Brunner H, Weidner W, Schiefer HG. Studies on the role of Ureaplasma urealyticum and Mycoplasma hominis in prostatitis. J Infect Dis 1983;147:807–13.

14. Shortliffe LMD, Sellers RG, Schachter J. The characterization of non-bacterial prostatitis: search for an etiology. J Urol 1992;148:1461–6.

15. Schiefer HG. Prostatic infection by unconventional, fastidious pathogens. In: Weidner W, Madsen PO, Schiefer HG, eds. Prostatitis. Berlin: Springer; 1990:229–44.

16. Weidner W, Jantos C, Schiefer HG, Haidl G, Friedrich HJ. Semen parameters in men with and without proven chronic prostatitis. Arch Androl 1991;26:173–83.

17. Meares EM. Prostatitis and related disorders. In: Walsh PC, Retik AB, Stamey TA, Vaughan ED, eds. Campbell's urology, 6th ed. Philadelphia: WB Saunders; 1992:807–22.

18. Doble A, Thomas BJ, Walker MM, Harris JRW, Witherow R, Taylor-Robinson C. The role of Chlamydia trachomatis in chronic abacterial prostatitis: a study using ultrasound guided biopsy. J Urol 1991;141–332.

19. Christansen E, Purvis K. Diagnosis of chronic abacterial prostato-vesiculitis by rectal ultrasonography in relation to symptoms and findings. Br J Urol 1991;67:173–6.

20. Stamey TA, Meares EM Jr, Winningham DG. Chronic bacterial prostatitis and the diffusion of drugs into prostatic fluid. J Urol 1970;103:187–94.

21. Stamey TA, Bushby SRM, Bragonje J. The concentration of trimethoprim in prostatic fluid: non-ionic diffusion or active transport? J Infect Dis 1973;129(Suppl):686–90.

22. Madsen PO, Kjaer TB, Baumeller A. Prostatic tissue and fluid concentrations of trimethoprim and sulfamethoxazole. Experimental and clinical studies. Urology 1976;8:129–32.

23. Naber KG, Kinzig M, Sörgel F, Weigel D. Penetration of ofloxacin into prostatic fluid, ejaculate and seminal fluid. Infection 1993;21:34–9.

24. Naber KG, Sorgel F, Kinzig M, Weigel DM. Penetration of ciprofloxacin into prostatic fluid in volunteers after an oral dose of 750 mg. J Urol 1993;150:1718–21.

25. Dalhoff A, Weidner W. Diffusion of ciprofloxacin into prostatitis fluid. Eur J Clin Microbiol 1984;3:360–6.

26. Naber KG. Role of quinolones in treatment of chronic bacterial prostatitis. In: Hooper DC, Wofson JS, eds. Quinolone antimicrobial agents, 2nd ed. Washington DC: American Society of Microbiology; 1993:285–97.

27. Sörgel F, Kinzig, Naber KG. Physiological disposition of macrolides. In: Bryskier AJ, Butzler J–P, Neu HC, Tulkens PM, eds. Macrolides. Chemistry, pharmacology and clinical uses. Paris: Arnette Blackwell; 1993:421–31.

28. Naber KG, Giamarellou H. Proposed study design in prostatitis. Infection 1994;22(Suppl 1):59–60.

29. Schaeffer AJ, Darras FS. The efficacy of norfloxacin in the treatment of chronic bacterial prostatitis refractory to trimethoprim-sulfamethoxazole and/or carbenicillin. J Urol 1990;144:690–3.

30. Petrikkos E, Peppas T, Giamarellou H, Peulios K, Zouboulis P, Sfikakis P. Four years experience with norfloxacin in the treatment of chronic bacterial prostatitis. Abstr. 1302; 17th International Congress of Chemotherapy, Berlin, Germany, June 23–28, 1991.

31. Pust RA, Ackenheil-Koeppe HR, Gilbert T, Weidner W. Clinical efficacy of ofloxacin in patients with chronic bacterial prostatitis. J Chemother 1989;(Suppl 4):869–71.

32. Weidner W, Schiefer HG, Dalhoff A. Treatment of chronic bacterial prostatitis with ciprofloxacin. Results of a one-year follow-up study. Am J Med 1987;82(Suppl 4A):280–3.

33. Weidner W, Schiefer HG, Brähler E. Refractory chronic bacterial prostatitis: a re-evaluation of ciprofloxacin treatment after a median follow-up of 30 months. J Urol 1991;146:350–2.

34. Pfau A. Therapie der unteren Harnwegsinfektionen beim Mann unter besonderer Berücksichtigung der chronischen bakteriellen Prostatitis. Aktuelle Urologie 1987;18:31–3.

35. Pfau A. The treatment of chronic bacterial prostatitis. Infection 1991;19(Suppl 3):160–4.

36. Weidner W, Schiefer HG, Garbe CH. Acute nongonococcal epididymitis: aetiological and therapeutic aspects. Drugs 1987;34(Suppl 1):111–7.

37. Nistal M, Paniagua R. Testicular and epididymal pathology. Stuttgart, New York: Thieme; 184.

38. Aitchison M, Mufti GR, Farrell J, Paterson PJ, Scott R. Granulomatous orchitis. Br J Urol 1990;66:312–4.

Pyelonephritis and Abscess of the Kidney

James R Johnson

Acute pyelonephritis, an acute infection (usually bacterial) of the kidney and renal pelvis, is one of the most common serious infectious diseases of otherwise healthy individuals, and is an even greater problem for compromised hosts. New approaches to the diagnosis and management of this disorder and its sequelae, including intrarenal and perinephric abscess, have resulted in improved outcomes for patients.

EPIDEMIOLOGY

Annually in the USA, approximately 100,000 adults are admitted to hospital for renal infection,[1,2] many others being managed as outpatients. In Manitoba, Canada, the annual adult risk of hospitalization for pyelonephritis is approximately 10/11,000 for women and 3/10,000 for men.[3]

COMPLICATED VERSUS UNCOMPLICATED PYELONEPHRITIS

Pyelonephritis can be stratified as 'complicated' or 'uncomplicated', depending on the presence of underlying urologic or medical conditions that predispose to kidney infection or that aggravate the severity or intransigence of such infections once they occur.[1,4] Uncomplicated and complicated pyelonephritis have distinctive host substrates, microbial flora, pathogenetic mechanisms, clinical presentations and requirements for and response to therapy.

RISK FACTORS

Although little is known about the specific risk factors for uncomplicated pyelonephritis, recognized risk factors for uncomplicated cystitis would be predicted to predispose to pyelonephritis also. Such associations include female gender and, among adult women, sexual intercourse, a history of previous urinary tract infections, use of spermicide–diaphragm contraception, the postmenopausal state and being a nonsecretor of blood group substances (see Chapter 2.56).[5,6] Among children, the P1 blood group phenotype is associated with an increased pyelonephritis risk.[7] Pyelonephritis in compromised hosts, which by definition is 'complicated', is promoted by almost any anatomic or functional abnormality of the urinary tract, urinary tract instrumentation, diabetes mellitus, immunosuppression, pregnancy (during which the risk of pyelonephritis is 1–2%) and conditions associated with sensory impairment (such as diabetic or alcoholic neuropathies and spinal cord injury).[1,4] Among the commonly implicated urologic conditions are posterior urethral valves (in infant boys), congenital vesico-ureteral reflux (in girls), indwelling or intermittent urinary catheterization, other instrumentation of the urinary tract, neurogenic bladder, urolithiasis, ureteral diversions, any obstruction to normal urinary flow and kidney transplantation.

Renal abscesses, which can be intrarenal, intrarenal with perirenal extension or entirely perirenal, typically develop as a consequence of acute pyelonephritis and are among the most serious local complications of this illness. They occur predominantly in compromised hosts, notably patients who have diabetes mellitus, or recent surgery or instrumentation of the urinary tract.[8–10] Urinary reflux and obstruction are prominent risk factors for renal abscesses. Rarely, renal abscesses may develop during a severe episode of otherwise uncomplicated pyelonephritis in an intact host.

PATHOGENESIS

ROUTE OF INFECTION

Irrespective of the presence of predisposing host conditions, in almost all patients acute pyelonephritis arises via an ascending route of infection.[1,4] The causative micro-organisms enter the urethra, colonize the bladder, then ascend the ureters to the renal pelvis and subsequently invade the renal parenchyma. In most cases, the pathogens arise from the host's own intestinal (and, in women, vaginal) flora,[11] although in patients who have indwelling catheters or nephrostomy tubes organisms may be transferred on the hands of health care workers and thus bypass the intestinal, vaginal and/or bladder colonization steps.

MICROBIAL FLORA

Organisms must have substantial intrinsic virulence to overcome the many defense mechanisms of a healthy urinary tract and cause pyelonephritis in an intact host. In contrast, organisms of lesser intrinsic virulence can infect the kidney in patients who have impaired urinary tract defenses. Paradoxically, the less virulent organisms associated with complicated pyelonephritis are more often resistant to antimicrobial agents than are the more virulent ones that cause uncomplicated pyelonephritis. This, together with the impaired defense mechanisms of compromised hosts, makes such infections more difficult to treat and cure than uncomplicated pyelonephritis.

In uncomplicated pyelonephritis the distribution of micro-organisms is similar to that in uncomplicated cystitis, with approximately 80% of isolates being *Escherichia coli* and the remainder other Gram-negative bacilli (predominantly *Klebsiella* and *Proteus* spp.), *Staphylococcus saprophyticus* (especially in young women), *Enterococcus* spp. (especially in older men) and occasionally group B or other streptococci.[1,4] The *E. coli* strains that cause uncomplicated pyelonephritis exhibit multiple virulence properties that contribute to their ability to invade the urinary tract and stimulate inflammation and tissue damage (Fig. 59.1).[12,13] Among the various adhesins expressed by these strains, the most prevalent and pathogenetically important are P fimbriae, which recognize Galα(1–4)Gal-containing receptors on host epithelial surfaces, including the mucosal lining of the colon, vagina and urinary tract. The P fimbrial adhesin molecule PapG is situated at the tip of the fimbrial stalk and mediates attachment to receptors on the host cell. PapG occurs in three known variants, of which the Class II variant is the most common among strains that cause pyelonephritis and bacteremic urinary tract infections (UTIs),[14,15] whereas the Class III variant predominates in cystitis.[15] Other important virulence factors of pyelonephritogenic *E. coli* include the cytotoxin α-hemolysin (which destroys or impairs the function of host epithelial cells, phagocytes and lymphocytes), the aerobactin iron sequestration system, polysaccharide capsules, lipopolysaccharide and serum resistance proteins (which protect the organism against phagocytosis and/or complement-mediated lysis).[12,13]

In complicated pyelonephritis, although *E. coli* still is the single most common pathogen, it is less prevalent than in uncomplicated pyelonephritis and is represented by less virulent strains. Other Gram-negative bacilli are more commonly encountered, including *Pseudomonas aeruginosa*, *Enterobacter* spp. and other Enterobacteriaceae.[1,4]

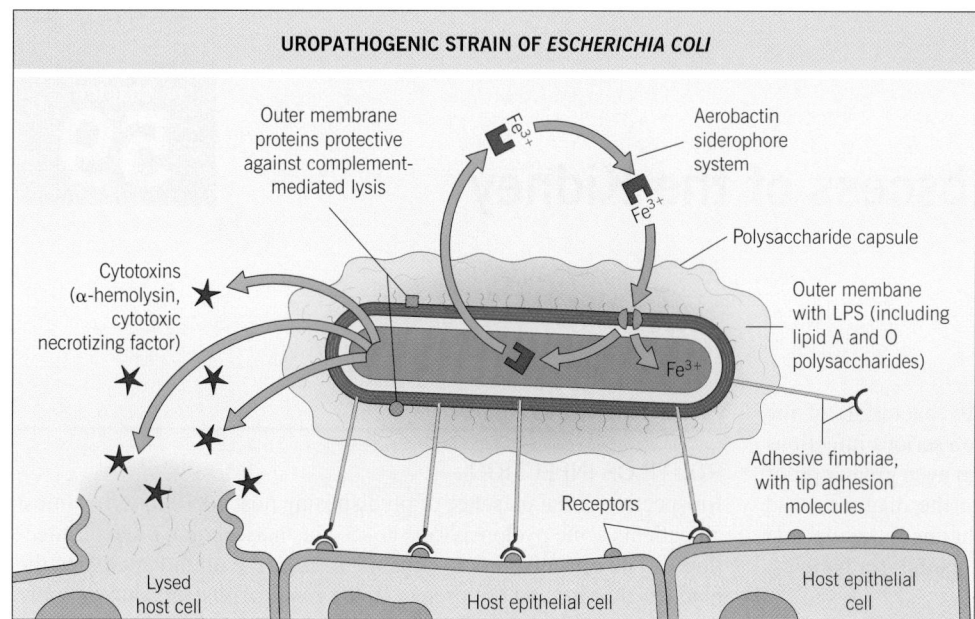

Fig. 59.1 Uropathogenic strain of *Escherichia coli*. Note the typical virulence properties, including adhesive fimbriae, cytotoxins, lipopolysaccharide (LPS), capsular polysaccharide, the aerobactin system, and outer membrane proteins important in serum resistance.

FACTORS PROMOTING ASCENDING INFECTION

Vaginal colonization with urovirulent organisms is promoted by sexual intercourse, particularly with the use of a spermicide, which kills normal lactobacillus-based vaginal flora and permits overgrowth with *E. coli* and other coliform bacteria.[11] Similar changes in the vaginal flora occur after the menopause as a result of estrogen depletion, and are induced by the use of certain antimicrobial agents, notably beta-lactams.

In women, sexual intercourse promotes the entry of periurethral bacteria into the bladder on a mechanical basis. In catheterized patients, bacteria can be introduced into the bladder at the time of catheter insertion, or can migrate into the bladder along the external or luminal surfaces of catheters.[16] With improper catheter care, infected urine from the collecting bag and drainage tubing can reflux into the bladder. Catheter-associated organisms persist within the urinary tract in part by cementing themselves to the catheter within glycocalyx matrices that protect them against natural host defense mechanisms and antimicrobial agents.

Ascent of pathogens from the bladder up the ureters is facilitated by vesico-ureteral reflux, which may be pre-existing or which in the intact host can result from a reversible ureteral aperistalsis induced by exposure of the ureteral wall to lipopolysaccharide from adherent bacteria.[17] Among several UTI-promoting physiologic alterations of pregnancy, ureteral hypotonia and some degree of ureteral obstruction may contribute to bacterial entry into the upper urinary tract in pregnant women and its persistence once there.[18] Once within the renal pelvis, microorganisms migrate up the collecting ducts into the tubules, a process promoted by intrarenal reflux (if present in the particular host) and by bacterial adhesins that recognize receptors along this epithelial surface or in subjacent tissues.[1,4,12,13,17]

PATHOLOGY

Within the urinary tract, pathogenic bacteria adhere to the mucosa and trigger a local cytokine network, with production of interleukin (IL)-1, IL-6, IL-8 and tumor necrosis factor-α and recruitment of polymorphonuclear leukocytes (PMNLs) and lymphocytes.[19] The influx of inflammatory cells leads to the generation of reactive oxygen species, leukotrienes, prostaglandins and other mediators of inflammation, which together with bacterial cytotoxins produce tissue damage, edema and, in the kidney, intense local vasoconstriction.[1,4] These phenomena are responsible for the characteristic signs and symptoms of pyelonephritis, including dysuria and suprapubic pain from bladder involvement, flank pain and costovertebral angle tenderness from kidney involvement, and fever and malaise from inflammatory cytokines that enter the systemic circulation.

Histologically, in acute pyelonephritis the mucosa and submucosa of the collecting system, the tubules and the interstitium are edematous and infiltrated with PMNLs (Fig. 59.2). Tubules may necrose. Microabscesses form within the mucosa and interstitium, and can coalesce to form macroscopic abscesses.[1,4]

Grossly, the kidneys are diffusely or focally swollen and edematous. On sectioning, streaks of yellowish inflammatory infiltrate extend from the papillae and medulla toward the cortex, sometimes reaching the capsule and rupturing it.[1,4] When macroscopic abscesses do form typically they localize at the corticomedullary junction, but they can be subcapsular or extend into the perirenal space.[8] In hyperglycemic diabetic patients, rapid fermentation of glucose by Gram-negative bacilli (or, rarely, yeasts) can produce gas within the renal parenchyma (emphysematous pyelonephritis) (Fig. 59.3), within an abscess (gas abscess) or within the renal pelvis and collecting system (emphysematous pyelitis).[20,21] Papillary necrosis, which occasionally complicates acute pyelonephritis among diabetic patients, may make the infection worse because of the obstruction caused by sloughed tissue (Fig. 59.4).[1,4]

Functionally, the intense interstitial inflammatory process leads to a reduction in urinary concentrating capacity. Decreased renal blood flow, functional tubular obstruction from inflammatory cells and necrotic debris, and inflammation-induced tubular dysfunction result in delayed excretion of radiographic contrast dye,[1,4] but only rarely manifest as clinically apparent renal dysfunction.[22]

Bacteremia develops in between 10 and 65% of patients who have acute pyelonephritis, depending on the severity of infection and increasing in proportion to the age of the host. Bacterial entry into the bloodstream may be promoted by P fimbriae[14] and by tissue destruction mediated by microbial cytotoxins.[23] Systemic complications of pyelonephritis, which are more common among patients who have Gram-negative bacteremia, include septic shock, disseminated intravascular coagulation and the acute respiratory distress syndrome (ARDS). Pregnant women with pyelonephritis are particularly prone to these complications, and also may develop premature labor as a result of the irritative effect of lipopolysaccharide on the uterus.[18]

HEMATOGENOUS RENAL ABSCESSES

Intrarenal abscesses can also be caused by certain hematogenously borne pathogens, most commonly *Staphylococcus aureus*, *Candida* spp. and *Mycobacterium tuberculosis*.[8] In contrast to abscesses that form during acute ascending pyelonephritis, hematogenously derived abscesses are usually cortical in location, are not prone to rupture into the perinephric space and are not associated with the characteristic clinical syndrome of pyelonephritis. Conversely, the typical pathogens of

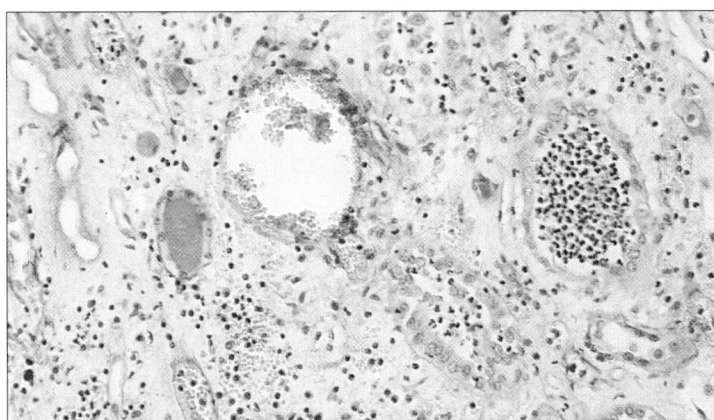

Fig. 59.2 Acute pyelonephritis. Note interstitial edema, tubules packed with polymorphonuclear leukocytes and a diffuse interstitial acute inflammatory infiltrate in this autopsy specimen from a diabetic with refractory *E. coli* urosepsis.

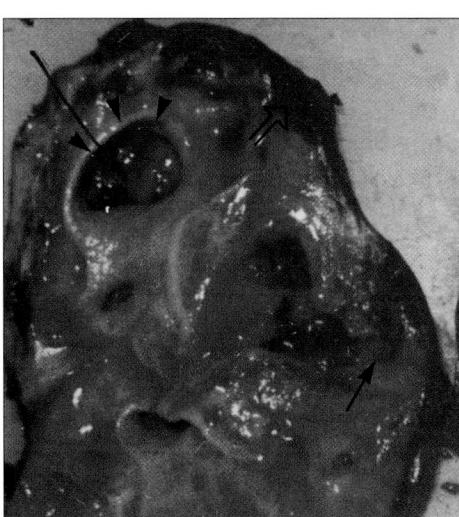

Fig. 59.3 Emphysematous pyelonephritis. Cortical necrosis (solid arrow), diffuse cortical hemorrhage (open arrow) and dilatation of the collecting system (arrowheads) in a nephrectomy specimen from a diabetic patient who received combined medical/surgical therapy and survived emphysematous pyelonephritis due to an unusual pathogen, *C. albicans*.

acute ascending pyelonephritis almost never cause renal abscesses in patients who have bacteremia arising from an extraurinary tract focus.[1,4]

PREVENTION

Little is known about the prevention of pyelonephritis or renal abscess. Presumably the same measures that can be recommended to noncompromised women who wish to reduce their risk of uncomplicated recurrent cystitis (e.g. avoiding spermicide–diaphragm contraception, use of chronic antimicrobial prophylaxis or early patient-initiated therapy for UTI symptoms) should decrease the risk of uncomplicated pyelonephritis.[24] Postmenopausal women can reduce their risk of bacteriuria with vaginal estrogen treatment;[12] this might also prevent pyelonephritis. Complicated pyelonephritis may be prevented by removing the precipitating factor. Urinary catheters should be avoided whenever possible, used according to current guidelines when unavoidable and removed as soon as no longer essential.[16] Correction of urologic abnormalities (whether surgically or medically) may reduce the associated infection risk, but treatment decisions must be carefully individualized based on the expected risks and benefits of the planned intervention(s). It is not known whether improved glycemic control among patients who have diabetes reduces their increased risk of pyelonephritis, but the other documented benefits of this therapy provide ample rationale for its use.

Prophylactic antimicrobial therapy can prevent UTIs in certain compromised hosts, for example renal transplant recipients in the early post-transplant period, but in many others is without clear benefit and often selects for resistant organisms and causes drug-related adverse effects.[24,25] At present there is no medically defined role for vaccines, cranberry juice, receptor analog therapy, lactobacillus preparations or yogurt in the prevention of UTI or pyelonephritis.[24]

CLINICAL FEATURES

The clinical manifestations of acute pyelonephritis vary considerably depending on characteristics of the host and pathogen. A typical history for the classic pyelonephritis syndrome, which is most commonly observed with kidney infections in otherwise healthy young women, includes several days of progressive flank pain, malaise, fever and chills, prostration and possibly nausea and vomiting, often preceded and/or accompanied by symptoms of acute cystitis.[1,4]

The physical examination characteristically shows an ill appearing, febrile, tachycardic patient, often with evidence of volume contraction. The pathognomonic physical finding of acute pyelonephritis is tenderness to palpation or percussion over one or both costovertebral angles. Mild to moderate abdominal and suprapubic tenderness are often also present.

Atypical presentations are common. Even otherwise healthy young

women with pyelonephritis may not have all of the classic symptoms or examination findings, and infants or young children, elderly or debilitated patients, and patients who have underlying systemic illnesses or neurologic impairment often have even less characteristic clinical pictures.[1,4] Abdominal pain, headache, nonspecific constitutional symptoms, diffuse back pain, pelvic pain or respiratory complaints may predominate, obscuring the diagnosis and suggesting other processes. A deceptively benign presentation, including sometimes even the complete absence of suggestive symptoms, can mask the presence of severe renal infections in immunocompromised or sensory-impaired hosts.[1,4,26] On the other hand, even in patients who have a classic presentation for acute pyelonephritis, other entities must be considered in the differential diagnosis, including (in the appropriate setting) pelvic inflammatory disease, acute appendicitis, urolithiasis, basal pneumonia and acute pancreatitis or biliary tract disease. The decision whether to perform a pelvic examination in a woman suspected of having pyelonephritis must be individualized, taking into consideration the patient's demographic characteristics, the specifics of the history (including the sexual history) and the findings on general physical examination.

In addition to the varied combinations of symptoms and physical findings encountered in patients who have acute pyelonephritis, a wide range of severity of illness is seen. At one extreme, patients who seem healthy and have what otherwise appears clinically to be acute cystitis may demonstrate a slight elevation of body temperature or report mild malaise, suggesting early renal involvement. At the other extreme, patients may present in full-blown septic shock, with multisystem organ failure. The severity of illness has a significant influence on subsequent management, as described below.

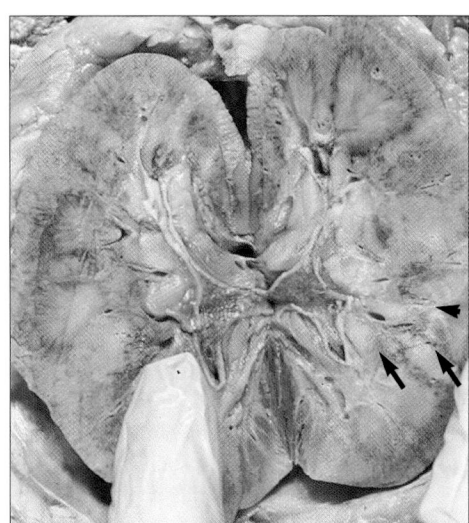

Fig. 59.4 Acute papillary necrosis (arrows) in an autopsy specimen from a diabetic patient who died from refractory *Escherichia coli* urosepsis. Necrotic papillae (arrows) failed to take up formalin, so appear pink, in contrast to the surrounding grayish-tan formalinized tissue.

ABSCESS

The initial history and physical examination usually provide few clues as to the presence of an intrarenal or perinephric abscess, although these entities should be kept in mind in high-risk patients. Presence of a palpable mass is suggestive of renal abscess, but is neither a sensitive nor specific finding.[10] Failure of a patient who is thought to have ordinary pyelonephritis to improve substantially after treatment for 48 hours increases the likelihood of abscess sufficiently to warrant further diagnostic studies.[1,4]

DIAGNOSIS

URINALYSIS AND URINE CULTURE

Acute pyelonephritis is a clinical diagnosis that is based on a combination of characteristic symptoms and signs together with supporting laboratory tests.[1,4] The minimal laboratory evaluation needed to make this diagnosis in the appropriate clinical setting is microscopic examination (whether by urinalysis or Gram stain) of a voided urine specimen to evaluate for the presence of pyuria, followed by quantitative urine culture. The Gram stain is also helpful by confirming the presence of bacteria in the urine (which are seen in unconcentrated urine specimens when the urine bacterial concentration is $>10^5$cfu/ml)[27] and by suggesting the likely bacterial type, although effective empiric treatment often can be selected without this information.[28]

In the absence of prior antimicrobial therapy, the urine culture almost always shows high concentrations ($>10^5$cfu/ml) of one or more bacterial species.[29,2] Pure growth of a single uropathogenic organism is typical of infections in noncompromised hosts, whereas polymicrobial infections are more common in compromised hosts. Lesser bacterial concentrations are occasionally encountered, and in the appropriate clinical context (e.g. a patient with typical symptoms and examination findings, plus pyuria) do not exclude the diagnosis of pyelonephritis. Antimicrobial susceptibility testing of urine isolates is essential, both to confirm that the empirically selected treatment regimen is appropriate, and for guiding selection of an effective oral agent for patients treated initially with a parenteral antimicrobial regimen.[24]

ANCILLARY TESTS

Other tests may be indicated depending on the severity of illness, the range of alternative diagnoses being considered and the presence of comorbid conditions. Pretherapy blood cultures are commonly collected, although interestingly, bacteremia (if present) predictably clears with appropriate therapy directed toward the urinary infection, and clinical outcomes are similar regardless of the presence or absence of bacteremia.[4] A pregnancy test is useful if the patient might be pregnant and treatment is being considered with an agent (such as an aminoglycoside or a fluoroquinolone) that might be toxic to the fetus.[18,24]

IMAGING STUDIES

Imaging studies are not routinely indicated for the diagnosis or management of acute pyelonephritis.[30] For patients in whom the initial diagnosis is unclear, those who fail to respond appropriately to therapy and those in whom abscess or obstruction are suspected for other reasons, CT can be used to clarify the anatomy and guide a mechanical intervention.[1,4,30–33] Of all urinary tract imaging modalities, contrast-enhanced CT provides the best anatomic definition of inflammatory processes in the urinary tract, including sensitive detection of abcesses and differentiation of abscesses (water density) from simple inflamed tissue (tissue density) (Figs 59.5–59.8).[30–33] Inflamed regions of the pyelonephritic kidney appear on enhanced CT as streaky or wedge-shaped hypodense areas that fail to concentrate contrast material normally in comparison with surrounding renal tissue. Focal bulges or diffuse swelling of the entire kidney are common, as is inflammatory stranding in the perinephric fat. Terms coined by radiologists in the 1980s for these changes, such as 'focal' (or 'lobar') nephronia and 'focal' (or 'diffuse') bacterial nephritis, were often confusing to the clinician and were applied inconsistently by dif-

ferent radiologists. The Society of Uroradiology has recently defined a new uniform terminology according to which all such changes are reported under the umbrella term 'acute pyelonephritis', with modifiers that describe the observed anatomic abnormalities.[31] The extent and severity of such CT findings at the time of presentation are predictive of the clinical course, including the likelihood of bacteremia, progression to abscess formation and death.[33]

Ultrasonography, although commonly used as an initial imaging test for patients who have a suspected focal infectious complication during pyelonephritis, is comparatively insensitive,[1,4,32,33] and is often followed by a CT scan irrespective of the ultrasound results. Consequently, it may be best to omit this test and proceed directly to CT. (However, serial directed sonographic examinations can be used subsequently to follow the response of abscesses or hydronephrosis to therapy, without the higher cost and exposure to radiation and contrast material of repeated CT scans.) Single photon emission CT using Technetium-99 dimercaptosuccinate (DMSA), the newest imaging modality for use in pyelonephritis, is slightly more sensitive than CT for identifying areas of inflammation within the kidney, which can be advantageous if the initial diagnosis is in question.[31] However, it cannot distinguish between frank abscesses and inflamed but viable tissue, so is of little help in evaluating the patient who fails to respond to the therapy. Excretory urography and MRI have little role in the management even of complicated pyelonephritis.[1,4] Nonenhanced spiral CT is more sensitive than excretory urography in detecting urinary calculi, and avoids exposing the patient to contrast material, so may be the modality of choice (when available) if urolithiasis is a concern (Talner LB, personal communication). Occasionally, antegrade or retrograde ureterography may be indicated, usually when stent placement or calculus removal is needed to relieve obstruction.[32]

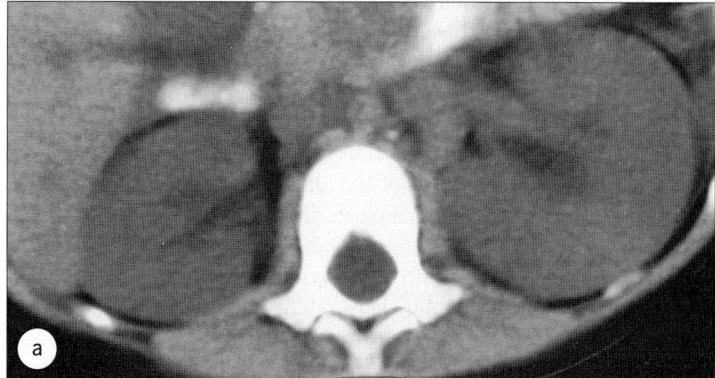

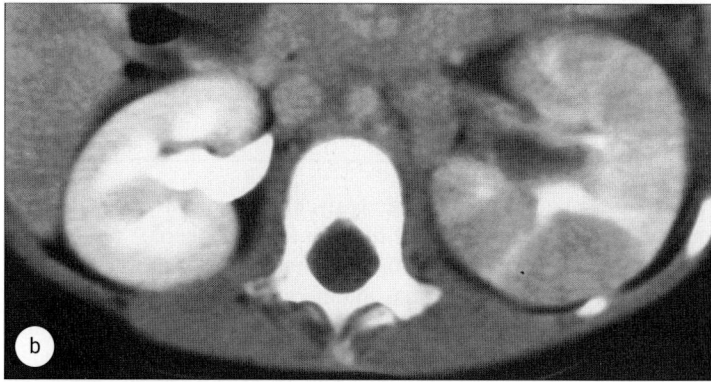

Fig. 59.5 Febrile urinary tract infection with white blood cell count of 36,000/ml (girl, 3 years). (a) Precontrast CT scan: left kidney is diffusely swollen; parenchymal attenuation is the same as that of the right kidney. (b) Postcontrast CT scan: wedge-shaped regions of hypoenhancing parenchyma in left kidney are most pronounced in the posterior portion. Inflamed parenchyma enhances from 32 to 93 Hounsfield unit (HU), whereas normal kidney enhances from 33 to 140 HU. Right kidney shows normal cortical enhancement and pronounced medullary blush. With permission from Talner.[31]

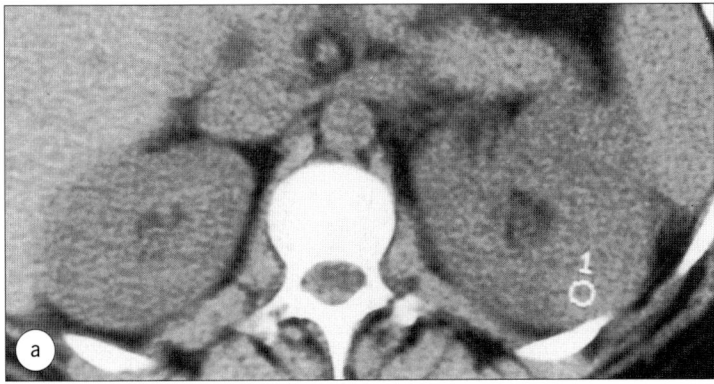

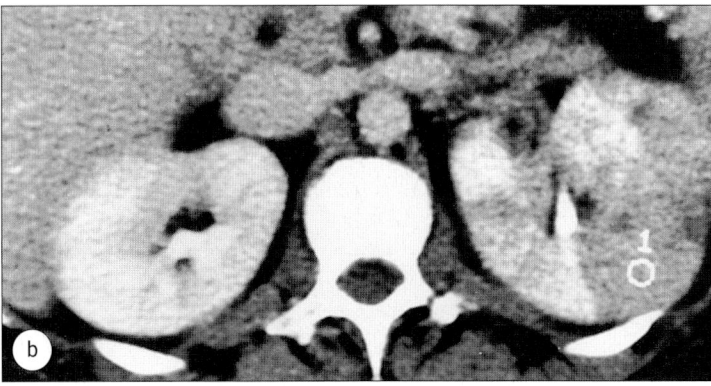

Fig. 59.6 Woman with clinical signs of acute pyelonephritis. (a) Precontrast CT scan: focal bulge present in anterolateral aspect of left kidney. Attenuation is the same as that of normal kidney parenchyma. (b) Postcontrast CT scan: rounded and streaky regions of hypoenhancing parenchyma in left kidney are most pronounced anterolaterally. Attenuation in the region of interest (cursor) was 22 HU on precontrast scans and increase to 93 HU on postcontrast scans. Normal parenchyma increased from 25 to 130 HU. With permission from Talner.[31]

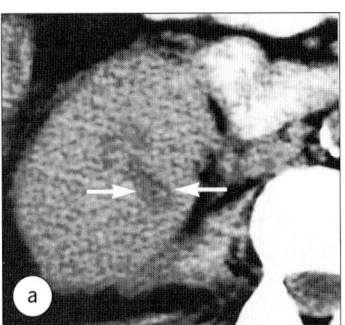

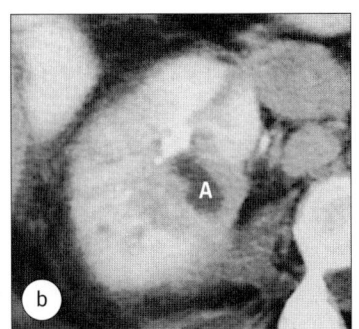

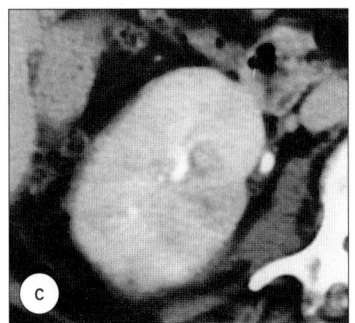

Fig. 59.7 Acute pyelonephritis with small intrarenal abscess. (a) Precontrast CT scan shows small region of low attenuation (arrows). (b) On the postcontrast CT scan, abscess A fails to enhance at all. Surrounding inflamed parenchyma bulges, and enhances less than adjacent normal parenchyma. (c) Follow-up CT scan obtained after prolonged antibiotic therapy. Abscess has resolved without drainage. Focal swelling is gone, but parenchyma still shows hypoenhancement. With permission from Talner.[31]

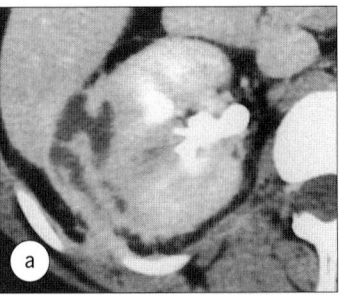

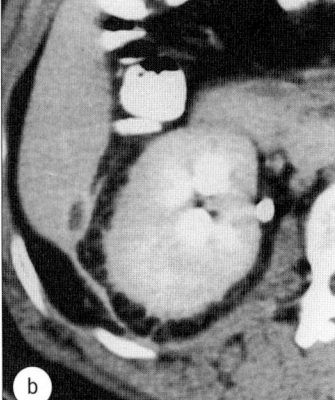

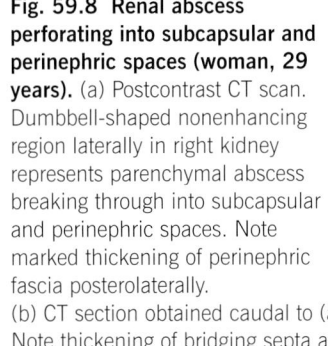

Fig. 59.8 Renal abscess perforating into subcapsular and perinephric spaces (woman, 29 years). (a) Postcontrast CT scan. Dumbbell-shaped nonenhancing region laterally in right kidney represents parenchymal abscess breaking through into subcapsular and perinephric spaces. Note marked thickening of perinephric fascia posterolaterally.
(b) CT section obtained caudal to (a). Note thickening of bridging septa as a manifestation of perinephric inflammation. At this level there is a small pararenal abscess pocket adjacent to the liver. With permission from Talner.[31]

MANAGEMENT

In comparison with the treatment of acute cystitis, which has been extensively studied, there have been relatively few large, high quality treatment trials for acute pyelonephritis on which to base therapeutic recommendations.[1,4,24,28] Much of the prevailing wisdom regarding the treatment of pyelonephritis comes from tradition, anecdotal experience, extrapolation from animal models or pharmacokinetic studies, small clinical trials involving heterogeneous patient populations and in-vitro susceptibility test results. Nonetheless, some guidelines can be suggested for key management issues.

INPATIENT VERSUS OUTPATIENT, AND PARENTERAL VERSUS ORAL THERAPY

Traditionally, most patients who have pyelonephritis have been hospitalized and given intravenous antimicrobial therapy, at least initially. However, evidence is accumulating that oral therapy on an ambulatory basis (with or without initial parenteral treatment and observation in the Emergency Department or short-stay unit) is acceptable for selected patients who have acute pyelonephritis.[34–36] Outcomes with oral therapy for otherwise healthy ambulatory patients who are clinically stable and can take medications by mouth have been similar to those obtained with sicker patients given traditional in-hospital parenteral therapy, at a considerable cost saving.[36] Oral therapy has even been used successfully with pregnant women,[37,38] in whom pyelonephritis has traditionally been considered to require in-hospital management.

Thus, there is no single right answer to the question of the optimal setting for treatment. The management plan must be individualized to the patient, taking into consideration the severity of illness (including the presence of nausea or vomiting), the patient's underlying host status and reliability level and the availability of a support system at home and a mechanism for medical follow-up (Fig. 59.9). Women with uncomplicated pyelonephritis who are only mildly ill can sometimes be treated successfully from the outset with oral therapy alone (Fig. 59.10). Moderately ill patients can be can be rehydrated with intravenous fluids (if needed) in the clinic or Emergency Department, given an initial parenteral dose of antibiotic and observed. If after several hours their condition has failed to improve sufficiently they can be admitted to the hospital for continued parenteral therapy, whereas if they are feeling better and are able to take fluids by mouth they can

INDICATIONS FOR HOSPITAL ADMISSION IN PATIENTS WITH ACUTE PYELONEPHRITIS	
Indication	**Rationale**
Severely ill, unstable (1)	Needs close monitoring, aggressive resuscitation
Moderate or severe host compromise	At risk of poor response to therapy, progression to 1
Suspected abscess, obstruction, stone	Needs diagnostic evaluation +/– intervention; at risk of progression to 1
Pregnant women*	At risk of progression to 1
Children*, men*	At risk of poor response to therapy, progression to 1
Persistent vomiting (despite antipyretic therapy and intravenous hydration)	Needs iv or im therapy†
No suitable oral therapy available	Needs iv or im therapy†
Unsuitable home situation, unreliable follow-up, or unreliable/noncompliant patient	At risk of progression to 1
*Selected patients with mild illness and suitable home situations may be treated orally as outpatients, with or without a first iv dose in the Emergency Department or clinic. †Home parental therapy acceptable (where available) for mildly or moderately ill patients.	

Fig. 59.9 Indications for hospital admission in patients with acute pyelonephritis.

be discharged to home with an appropriate oral antibiotic regimen (Fig. 59.10), with close follow-up arranged.

There is no published experience using oral therapy for pyelonephritis in men, children or women with complicating factors other than pregnancy. Clinical judgment may identify suitable cases even within these populations (for example, mildly ill patients who have only minor compromising conditions). However, most such patients should be admitted to the hospital initially for parenteral therapy, particularly if they are more than minimally ill.

ANTIMICROBIAL REGIMEN

Because urine culture and susceptibility testing takes several days to complete, the initial antimicrobial regimen for acute pyelonephritis is usually selected empirically (from among those agents that have suitable pharmacokinetic characteristics and a good 'track record' in pyelonephritis treatment trials) based on the predicted susceptibility patterns of the expected organism(s) (Fig. 59.10).[1,4,24,28] For all patients, activity against 'ordinary' Gram-negative bacilli is essential in the empiric regimen, and for patients who have complicated UTI or recent antimicrobial therapy, Gram-positive organisms and drug-resistant Gram-negative organisms must also be anticipated.

Suitable initial regimens are shown in Figure 59.10, which emphasizes aminoglycosides, fluoroquinolones, third-generation cephalosporins and beta-lactam–beta-lactamase inhibitor combination agents for parenteral use, and trimethoprim–sulfamethoxazole (co-trimoxazole; TMP–SMX), fluoroquinolones and amoxicillin–clavulanate for oral use. Because of the high prevalence among uropathogens of resistance to ampicillin, other penicillins and first- or second-generation cephalosporins, as well as these agents' adverse pharmacokinetic properties and inconsistent performance in clinical trials,[1,4,24,28] these drugs should be avoided as empiric monotherapy for even uncomplicated pyelonephritis. Whether oral third-generation cephalosporins should have a role in the empiric therapy of pyelonephritis in outpatients has not been adequately studied. The administration of intravenous antimicrobial agents can be simplified by using a single agent only (there being little rationale for combination therapy except in patients who are thought to have both Gram-positive and Gram-negative pathogens)[39] and by using twice-daily dosing with ciprofloxacin, ofloxacin and trimethoprim–sulfamethoxazole, and once-daily dosing with ceftriaxone and the aminoglycosides.

EMPIRIC TREATMENT FOR ACUTE PYELONEPHRITIS		
Uncomplicated pyelonephritis		
Modifying circumstances	**Treatment setting**	**Empiric treatment options**
Mild-to-moderate illness, no nausea or vomiting	Outpatient therapy acceptable	Oral* TMP–SMX, a fluoroquinolone (not in children) or amoxicillin–clavulanate for 10–14 days (Amoxicillin–clavulanate preferred if Gram-positive cocci are present)
Severe illness or possible urosepsis	Hospitalization required	Parenteral† TMP–SMX, 3rd-generation cephalosporin, fluoroquinolone (not in children), gentamicin or ampicillin–sulbactam until patient is better; then oral* agent (see above) to complete 14 days therapy (Initial regimen should include ampicillin if Gram-positive cocci are present)
Complicated pyelonephritis		
Modifying circumstances	**Treatment setting**	**Empiric treatment options**
Pregnancy, mild illness	Outpatient therapy acceptable	Oral* amoxicillin–clavulanate, cephalosporin or TMP–SMX‡, for 10–14 days (Amoxicillin–clavulanate preferred if Gram-positive cocci are present)
Pregnancy, with moderate-to-severe illness	Hospitalization required	Parenteral† third-generation cephalosporin, gentamicin caution‡, ampicillin–sulbactam or TMP–SMX caution‡ until patient is better; then oral* amoxicillin, amoxicillin–clavulanate, a cephalosporin, or TMP–SMX caution‡ for 14 days (Initial regimen should include ampicillin if pretherapy Gram stain shows Gram-positive cocci or no organisms, or is not done)
Not pregnant, mild illness, no nausea or vomiting	Outpatient therapy acceptable	Oral* fluoroquinolone (not in children) for 10–14 days
Not pregnant, with moderate-to-severe illness or possible urosepsis	Hospitalization required; imaging studies and urologic consultation often needed	Parenteral† gentamicin, fluoroquinolone, 3rd-generation cephalosporin, aztreonam, ticarcillin–clavulanate, piperacillin–tazobactam or imipenem–cilastatin until patient is better; then oral* agent (see above) for 14–21 days (Initial regimen should include a penicillin or imipenem–cilastatin if pretherapy Gram stain shows Gram-positive cocci or no organisms, or is not done)

*Oral regimens: TMP–SMX, 160mg + 800mg q12h; norfloxacin, 400mg q12h; ciprofloxacin, 500mg q12h; ofloxacin, 200–300mg q12h; lomefloxacin, 400mg daily; enoxacin, 400mg q12h; amoxicillin 500mg q8h; amoxicillin–clavulanate, 850mg q12h or 500mg q8h; cefpodoxime proxetil, 200mg q12h; and cefixime, 400mg daily

†Parenteral regimens: TMP–SMX, 160mg + 800mg q12h; ciprofloxacin, 200–400mg q12h; ofloxacin, 200–400mg q12h; gentamicin, 5mg per kg body weight daily; ceftriaxone, 1–2g daily; ampicillin, mezlocillin or piperacillin, 1g q6h; imipenem–cilastatin, 250–500mg q6h–q8h; ampicillin–sulbactam, 1.5g q6h; ticarcillin–clavulanate, 3.2g q6h–q8h; piperacillin–tazobactam, 3.375g q6h–q8h; and aztreonam, 1g q8h–q12h

‡Cautions: fluoroquinolones (norfloxacin, ciprofloxacin, ofloxacin, lomefloxacin and enoxacin) should not be used in pregnancy or in young children. TMP–SMX, although not approved for use in pregnancy, has been widely used. Gentamicin should be used with caution in pregnancy because of its possible toxicity to eighth-nerve development in the fetus. The fluoroquinolones norfloxacin, lomefloxacin, enoxacin can be administered orally only; ciprofloxacin and ofloxacin can be administered iv or orally

Fig. 59.10 Suggested empiric initial treatment regimens for acute pyelonephritis. 'Uncomplicated' is usually limited to noncompromised, non-pregnant adult women, but can include carefully selected men and children who lack compromising conditions and are only mildly ill. Adapted with permission from Stamm.[28]

CONVERSION TO ORAL THERAPY

Patients initially admitted to the hospital for intravenous therapy traditionally have been continued on parenteral therapy until susceptibility results are known. They are then placed on an oral agent selected on the basis of the susceptibility pattern of the urine organism, and are observed in the hospital for an additional 1 or 2 days to evaluate the success of oral therapy (Fig. 59.11). This approach leads to unnecessarily prolonged hospital stays in many patients. Conversion to oral therapy can be done safely as soon as the initial indications for parenteral therapy have resolved, as evidenced by the success of oral therapy for mildly ill ambulatory patients who have pyelonephritis. When the hospitalized patient is clinically ready for oral therapy before susceptibility results are available, an oral regimen can be selected empirically, much as is done in the Emergency Department for patients treated with an oral agent from the outset.[24,28,34] In the USA, the fluoroquinolones are predictably active against *E. coli*. Thus, despite their slightly higher cost than TMP–SMX (which might be the preferred agent for a known susceptible organism), these agents can yield a tremendous cost saving if they permit patients to be discharged sooner.

The practice of observing patients who have pyelonephritis in the hospital for 24 hours or longer on oral therapy before discharge is without empiric support. When examined retrospectively this approach was found to detect relapse in only 1% of patients, and intolerance of the new oral agent in only 4%.[2] Thus, patients can usually be safely discharged once they have demonstrated tolerance of the first dose of an appropriate oral agent, whether the drug is selected empirically or based on known susceptibility results.

EXPECTED CLINICAL COURSE

Nearly all patients who have pyelonephritis who ultimately will be cured by antimicrobial therapy alone experience substantial clinical improvement within the first 2 days of therapy, sometimes even after the first liter of intravenous rehydration fluid and before receiving any antimicrobial agent. Patients commonly continue to have fever and flank pain for several days on effective therapy, but these manifestations should begin to wane and there should be improvement in the patient's energy level, appetite and sense of wellbeing. If after 48 hours there is no improvement in any of these parameters, aggressive re-evaluation is needed.[1,4,24] Possibilities to be considered include a mistaken diagnosis, a mismatch between the urine organism and the selected antimicrobial regimen or an anatomic complication such as obstruction or abscess. A directed history and physical examination are indicated, as is repeated laboratory testing (including blood cultures and chemistries, urinalysis and urine culture plus Gram stain) and urinary tract imaging studies, beginning with enhanced abdominal CT. In some patients this evaluation will reveal a focal process in need of an invasive procedure, such as drainage of an abscess (Fig. 59.8) or an obstructed collecting system; in some patients, continued medical therapy (with or without adjustment) will suffice (Fig. 59.7). Consultation with an infectious diseases specialist and then subsequently with a urologic surgeon or interventional radiologist can be extremely helpful in problematic cases to ensure that all relevant options are considered and the appropriate procedures performed.

COMPLICATIONS

Supportive care for patients who develop septic shock, ARDS and multisystem organ failure during pyelonephritis, which is not specific to pyelonephritis, is discussed in Chapter 2.47. When infection is present, obstruction to urine flow (e.g. by a stone or tumor) must be relieved, either by removal of the obstruction or by provision of alternative drainage. When possible, removal of urinary calculi from patients who have pyelonephritis is probably best delayed until the bacterial load can be reduced and the patient stabilized with medical therapy. Gasforming UTIs have traditionally been managed surgically in most instances, often with nephrectomy in cases of emphysematous pyelonephritis (see Fig. 59.3).[20] However, reports of successful medical therapy of gas abscesses[21] and emphysematous pyelonephritis[40] indicate that even in these extreme situations therapy can be individualized.

Intrarenal (Fig. 59.7) and perinephric (Fig. 59.8) abscesses have also traditionally been managed with combined medical and surgical therapy.[9,11] Recent experience with closed (catheter-assisted) drainage or medical therapy alone suggests the possibility of alternative approaches in this setting as well.[9,41] Small abscesses, especially those occurring in otherwise intact hosts, are most likely to respond to medical therapy, whereas large collections, particularly in compromised hosts or in patients who have severe illness, are likely to require drainage. The cost and morbidity of a drainage procedure must be weighed against the cost and morbidity of the protracted antibiotic therapy that is usually required when abscesses are treated with antibiotics alone.[41] If an abscess is to be drained, the optimal method (open versus closed) depends in part on the anatomy, the host and local expertise. Perinephric abscesses (Fig. 59.8) have been described as requiring a more aggressive interventional approach than intrarenal abscesses,[8] but published experience suggests that drainage is not always needed even here.

DURATION OF THERAPY

The optimal duration of therapy for acute pyelonephritis, unlike that for acute cystitis, is largely undefined and remains a source of controversy.[39] As with other aspects of the management of pyelonephritis, because of the highly variable nature of the illness and the host substrate, it is probably best to tailor duration of therapy to the individual patient. Clinical trial data demonstrate that 14 days of a traditional sequential regimen that includes an intravenous aminoglycoside initially, followed by oral trimethoprim–sulfamethoxazole or ampicillin, eliminates the initial infection in 100% of women with moderate or severe uncomplicated pyelonephritis, with no relapses at the 6-week follow-up visit.[42] Thus, courses of therapy longer than 14 days should be unnecessary when similarly potent regimens are used in comparable hosts. In other trials, approximately 90% of patients who have uncomplicated pyelonephritis who were treated for only 5 days with aminoglycosides, third-generation cephalosporins or fluoroquinolones were cured,[39] although some of the 10% failure rate was attributable to relapses with the initial pathogen.[43] Whether there is a real or clinically meaningful difference in success rates between 5–7 days and 10–14 days of therapy for uncomplicated pyelonephritis is unknown. An ongoing treatment trial that compares 7 days of ciprofloxacin with 14 days of trimethoprim–sulfamethoxazole for ambulatory women with uncomplicated pyelonephritis of mild-to-moderate severity[44] should shed some light on this question, although its results will not necessarily be applicable to women with more severe uncomplicated infections or to patients who have complicated pyelonephritis.

It is generally recommended (but remains unproved) that patients who have complicated pyelonephritis should receive more extended courses of treatment. Duration of therapy for abscesses must be individualized, taking into consideration underlying host status, the nature of the abscess, adequacy of drainage (if undertaken) and response to therapy (both clinical and as revealed by serial imaging studies).

CRITERIA FOR CONVERSION TO ORAL THERAPY

Patient no longer severely ill or unstable

Patient taking fluids by mouth; no vomiting; adequate gut function

Suitable oral agent available:

- documented or predicted activity against causative organism(s)
- highly bioavailable
- good 'track record' in UTI therapy
- no contraindication to use, i.e. no history of previous adverse reaction, no drug–drug interactions, no fetal toxicity (pregnant women), no age-related toxicities (e.g. fluoroquinolones in children)

Fig. 59.11 Criteria for conversion to oral therapy.

FOLLOW-UP

Routine repeat urine cultures are commonly performed during therapy for pyelonephritis to confirm sterilization of the urine, but may add little beyond what is apparent from clinical evaluation and possibly from inspection of the urine for pyuria.[45] It is prudent to confirm at least by telephone that patients who are sent out from the Emergency Department with oral therapy are improving as expected. Whether routine post-therapy clinic visits, urine cultures and urinalyses contribute to favorable outcomes has not been studied. However, as it has been argued that in the setting of uncomplicated acute cystitis these measures are unnecessary,[24] it is possible that the same may be true with pyelonephritis, at least for uncomplicated cases in seemingly reliable and responsible patients. Post-therapy evaluations still are advisable in children, pregnant women,[18] and probably also in other compromised hosts.

UROLOGIC EVALUATION FOR PREDISPOSING CONDITIONS

In addition to the management of the acute pyelonephritis episode, in selected patients it is worth searching for an underlying urologic abnormality, as the surgical correction of such an abnormality might prevent future infections. The cost and morbidity of such a search must be weighed against the likelihood of finding a correctable abnormality, the morbidity of the possible corrective procedure itself and the infectious morbidity that can be averted by a successful procedure. In the absence of firm data, opinions differ as to the indications for imaging studies and corrective surgery after pyelonephritis.[24] One approach is to investigate all children and men who develop pyelonephritis, as they are the most likely to have an important correctable abnormality. Women probably should be studied if they have relapsing pyelonephritis with the same organism even after an extended course of appropriate antimicrobial therapy for a first relapse. Whether women who have multiple episodes of pyelonephritis caused by different organisms will benefit from urologic investigation is unknown.

SUMMARY

Acute pyelonephritis is a diverse entity that challenges the clinician to intervene sufficiently but not excessively, and for which the management approach must be tailored to the individual patient. New developments in the field, such as the use of at-home oral therapy, shorter treatment courses, single daily dose intravenous aminoglycoside or ceftriaxone therapy and early hospital discharge provide opportunities for cost savings and enhanced patient convenience. Alertness is required to anticipate and detect complications in high-risk patients or in those who fail to respond as expected to treatment. Intrarenal and perinephric abscesses, gas-forming renal infections and infections superimposed on urinary obstruction are potentially lethal processes that require aggressive therapy, often including mechanical interventions.

REFERENCES

1. Bergeron MG. Treatment of pyelonephritis in adults. Med Clin North Am 1995;79:619–49.
2. Caceres VM, Stange KC, Kikano GE, Zyzanski SJ. The clinical utility of a day of hospital observation after switching from intravenous to oral antibiotic therapy in the treatment of pyelonephritis. J Fam Pract 1994;39:337–9.
3. Nicolle LE, Friesen D, Harding GKM, Roos LL. Hospitalization for acute pyelonephritis in Manitoba, Canada, during the period from 1989 to 1992: impact of diabetes, pregnancy, aboriginal origin. Clin Infect Dis 1996;22:1051–6.
4. Meyrier A, Guibert J. Diagnosis and drug treatment of acute pyelonephritis. Drugs 1992;44:356–67.
5. Foxman B. Recurring urinary tract infection: incidence and risk factors. Am J Public Health 1990;80:331–3.
6. Hooton TM, Scholes D, Hughes JP, et al. A prospective study of risk factors for symptomatic urinary tract infection in young women N Engl J Med 1996;335:468–74.
7. Lomberg H, Svanborg Eden C. Influence of P blood group phenotype on susceptibility to urinary tract infection. FEMS Microbiol Immunol 1989;47:363–70.
8. Patterson JE, Andriole VT. Renal and perirenal abscesses. Inf Dis Clin Am 1987;1:907–26.
9. Lambiase RE, Deyoe L, Cronan JJ, Dorfman GS. Percutaneous drainage of 335 consecutive abscesses: results of primary drainage with 1-year follow-up. Radiology 1992;184:167–75.
10. Fowler JE, Perkins T. Presentation, diagnosis and treatment of renal abscesses: 1972–1988. J Urol 1994;151:847–51.
11. Hooton TM, Stamm WE. The vaginal flora and urinary tract infections. In: Warren JW, Mobley HLT, eds. Urinary tract infections: molecular pathogenesis and clinical management. Washington, DC: American Society of Microbiology Press; 1996:67–94.
12. Johnson JR. Virulence factors in E. coli urinary tract infection. Clin Micro Rev 1991;4:80–128.
13. Donnenberg MS, Welch RA. Virulence determinants of uropathogenic Escherichia coli. In: Urinary tract infections: molecular pathogenesis and clinical management. Washington, DC: American Society of Microbiology Press; 1996:135–74.
14. Otto G, Sandberg T, Marklund BI, Ullery P, Svanborg C. Virulence factors and pap genotype in Escherichia coli isolates from women with acute pyelonephritis, with or without bacteremia. Clin Infect Dis 1993;17:448–56.

15. Johanson I-M, Plos K, Marklund B-I, Svanborg C. Pap, papG and prsG DNA sequences in Escherichia coli from the fecal flora and the urinary tract. Microb Pathog 1993;15:121–9.
16. Warren JW. The catheter and urinary tract infection. Med Clin North Am 1991;75:481–93.
17. Roberts JA. Etiology and pathophysiology of pyelonephritis. Am J Kidney Dis 1991;17:1–9.
18. Plattner MS. Pyelonephritis in pregnancy. J Perinat Neonat Nursing 1994;8:20–7.
19. Svanborg C, Agace W, Hedges S, Linder H, Svensson M. Bacterial adherence and epithelial cell cytokine production. Zentralbl Bakteriol 1993;278:359–64.
20. Evanoff GV, Thompson CS, Foley R, Weinman EJ. Spectrum of gas within the kidney: emphysematous pyelonephritis and emphysematous pyelitis. Am J Med 1987;83:149–54.
21. Nickas ME, Reese JH, Anderson RU. Medical therapy alone for the treatment of gas forming intrarenal abscess. J Urol 1994;151:398–400.
22. Jones SR. Acute renal failure in adults with uncomplicated acute pyelonephritis: case reports and review. Clin Infect Dis 1992;14:243–6.
23. Mobley HLT, Green DM, Trifillis AL, et al. Pyelonephritogenic Escherichia coli and killing of cultured human renal proximal tubular epithelial cells: role of hemolysin in some strains. Infect Immunol 1990;58:1281–9.
24. Johnson JR. Treatment and prevention of urinary tract infections. In: Warren JW, Mobley HLT, eds. Urinary tract infections: molecular pathogenesis and clinical management. Washington, DC: American Society of Microbiology Press; 1995:95–118.
25. Nicolle LE. Urinary tract infection in the elderly. How to treat and when? Infection 1992;20:261–5.
26. Watson RA, Lennox K, Sridharan VC. Re: presentation, diagnosis and treatment of renal abscesses: 1972–1988. J Urol 1995;153:1239–40.
27. Jenkins RD, Fenn JP, Matsen JM. Review of urine microscopy for bacteriuria. JAMA 1986;255:3397–403.
28. Stamm WE, Hooton TM. Management of urinary tract infections in adults. N Engl J Med 1993;329:1328–34.
29. Ikäheimo R, Siitonen A, Heiskanen T, et al. Recurrence of urinary tract infection in a primary care setting: analysis of a 1-year follow-up of 179 patients. Clin Infect Dis 1996;22:91–9.
30. Rabushka LS, Fishman EK, Goldman SM. Pictorial review: computed tomography of renal inflammatory

disease. Urology 1994;44:473–80.
31. Talner LB, Davidson AJ, Lebowitz RL, Dalla Palma L, Goldman SM. Acute pyelonephritis: can we agree on terminology? Radiology 1994;192:297–305.
32. Merenich WM, Popky GL. Radiology of renal infection. Med Clin North Am 1991;75:425–69.
33. Huang J-J, Sung J-M, Chen K-W, et al. Acute bacterial nephritis: a clinicoradiologic correlation based on computed tomography. Am J Med 1992;93:289–98.
34. Pinson AG, Philbrick JT, Lindbeck GH, Schorling JB. Oral antibiotic therapy for acute pyelonephritis. J Gen Intern Med 1992;7:544–53.
35. Pinson AG, Philbrick JT, Lindbeck GH, Schorling JB. Management of acute pyelonephritis in women: a cohort study. Am J Emerg Med 1994;12:271–8.
36. Safrin S, Siegel D, Black D. Pyelonephritis in adult women: inpatient versus outpatient therapy. Am J Med 1988;85:793–8.
37. Angel JL, O'Brien WF, Finan MA, et al. Acute pyelonephritis in pregnancy: a prospective study of oral versus intravenous antibiotic therapy. Obstet Gynecol 1990;76:28–32.
38. Millar LK, Wing DA, Paul RH, Grimes DA. Outpatient treatment of pyelonephritis in pregnancy: a randomized controlled trial. Obstet Gynecol 1995;86:560–4.
39. Bailey RR. Duration of antimicrobial treatment and the use of drug combinations for the treatment of uncomplicated acute pyelonephritis. Infection 1994;22(Suppl 1):S50–2.
40. Nagappan R, Kletchko S. Case report: bilateral emphysematous pyelonephritis resolving to medical therapy. J Intern Med 1992;232:77–80.
41. Siegel JF, Smith A, Moldwin R. Minimally invasive treatment of renal abscess. J Urol 1996;155:52–5.
42. Johnson JR, Lyons MF II, Pearce W, et al. Therapy for women hospitalized with acute pyelonephritis: a randomized trial of ampicillin vs. trimethoprim sulfamethoxazole for 14 days. J Infect Dis 1991;163:325–30.
43. Bailey RR, Lynn KL, Robson RA, Peddie BA, Smith A. Comparison of ciprofloxacin with netilmicin for the treatment of acute pyelonephritis. NZ Med J 1992;105:102–3.
44. Talan DA. Infectious disease issues in the emergency department. Clin Infect Dis 1996;23:1–14.
45. Allen S, Alon V, Blowey D, et al. Follow-up urine cultures in patients with acute pyelonephritis. Pediatr Infect Dis J 1993;12:170–1.

Complicated Urinary Infection Including Postsurgical and Catheter-related Infections

Lindsay E Nicolle

The focus of this chapter is the group of urinary tract infections (UTIs) that is generally designated as 'complicated UTI'. This includes UTIs following urologic surgery. Infections associated with urinary catheterization, including intermittent catheterization and both short-term (<30 days) and long-term (>30 days) indwelling catheters, are also discussed.

EPIDEMIOLOGY

Urinary tract infection is the most common bacterial infection in adults. In the setting of structural or functional abnormalities of the genitourinary tract or after urologic interventions, its frequency may be exceptionally high (Fig. 60.1). For instance, for patients undergoing transurethral procedures with instrumentation or transurethral prostatectomy, the incidence of postintervention urinary infections is substantial for patients who do not receive antimicrobial prophylaxis.

Infection incidence on a population basis has not been reported. In a review of hospitalizations for acute pyelonephritis in Manitoba for 1989–1990, the total rate of admissions was 11/10,000 population for women and 3.3/10,000 for men. Of these, 34% of patients admitted to two tertiary care hospitals with pyelonephritis had complicating genitourinary factors. Of patients admitted to hospital for UTI other than pyelonephritis, 84% of subjects at one institution and 36% at a second had complicating factors.[7]

The urinary tract is also the most common source of infection in elderly individuals hospitalized with bacteremia and is responsible for 34% of such bacteremic episodes. Virtually all of these bacteremic elderly individuals had abnormalities of the urinary tract, primarily obstructing lesions and indwelling catheters.[8]

Urinary tract infection is the most frequent hospital-acquired infection and is almost always associated with indwelling catheters. It accounts for 40% of all nosocomial infections and occurs at a rate of approximately 2/100 patient discharges. The catheterized urinary tract is the most frequent source of nosocomial Gram-negative rod bacteremia.[5] With short-term catheterization, acquisition of infection approaches 5% of exposed subjects per day.

Approximately 5% of individuals resident in long-term care facilities in North America have a chronic indwelling catheter. The prevalence of bacteriuria in these subjects is 100%.

Intermittent catheterization is also associated with a high frequency of infection. For individuals with neurogenic bladders managed by intermittent catheterization the reported rates of infection are 4.06/100 patient days[6] or 17.2/patient years.[9]

Most catheter-associated infections are asymptomatic, but symptomatic infection, including bacteremia, sepsis syndrome and death, may occur. Although bacteremia occurs in only 2–4% of patients with catheter-acquired UTI, the high frequency of indwelling catheter use means that the absolute number of episodes of bacteremia secondary to catheter-acquired UTI is high.

PATHOGENESIS

RISK FACTORS

The normal genitourinary tract, apart from the distal urethra, is sterile. The usual colonizing flora of the distal urethra include *Staphylococcus epidermidis*, diphtheroids, streptococci and certain anaerobes. These organisms are rarely uropathogens. The sterility of the urine and genitourinary tract is primarily maintained through the flushing action of voiding of urine.

Obstruction to normal urine flow overwhelms all other factors in promoting infection. Other factors that may contribute to the development of UTI include the concentration and chemical composition of the urine, the bladder mucus layer and Tamm–Horsfall protein excreted from the kidneys. Therefore, in complicated UTI, including postsurgical infection and catheter-related infections, the major factor contributing to the initiation and persistence of bacteriuria is an impaired ability to flush organisms from the urinary tract. This may be due either:

- to obstruction to urine flow with a pool of urine remaining in the urinary tract after voiding; or
- to the presence of a protected environment, such as an infection stone or a bacterial biofilm on a catheter, from which organisms cannot be eradicated by usual antimicrobial therapy.

Many genitourinary abnormalities are associated with an increased incidence of UTI (Fig. 60.2). These are congenital or acquired functional, structural or metabolic abnormalities. The abnormality may be transient, for instance presence of a noninfected stone, a cystoscopy procedure or short-term catheterization. In this situation, the increased risk of UTI will resolve once the abnormality is corrected. If the abnormality cannot be corrected, as in a patient with an ileal conduit or with a neurogenic bladder maintained on intermittent catheterization, there is a continued risk for recurrent UTI.

Where UTI occurs in a patient with an indwelling urethral catheter, the organisms may have gained access to the bladder by two routes:

- ascending the mucous sheath from the periurethral area on the outside of the catheter; or
- intraluminally by ascension up the catheter.[10]

INFECTION RATES AFTER GENITOURINARY SURGERY, ESWL OR CATHETERIZATION	
Procedure	Proportion infected postprocedure
Genitourinary surgery	
Transurethral prostatectomy[1]	6–64%
Transurethral procedure with instrumentation for stone extraction[2]	25%
Extracorporeal shock wave lithotripsy (ESWL)[3]	
Negative urine culture before ESWL	1.5%
Positive urine culture before ESWL	21%
Sepsis	4.5%
Catheterization	
Urodynamic studies[4]	1.5–36%
Indwelling catheter[5]	5% per day
Intermittent catheterization[6]	4.06/100 patient days

Fig. 60.1 Infection rates after genitourinary surgery, extracorporeal shock wave lithotripsy (ESWL) or catheterization.

GENITOURINARY ABNORMALITIES ASSOCIATED WITH UTI

Type of lesion	Examples
Obstructing lesion	Tumor, stricture, urolithiasis, prostatic hypertrophy, diverticulum, pelvicalyceal junction obstruction, congenital abnormality, renal cysts
Foreign body	Indwelling catheter, ureteric stent, nephrostomy tube
Functional abnormality	Neurogenic bladder, vesicoureteral reflux
Metabolic illness	Diabetes mellitus, medullary sponge kidney, post-renal transplantation
Urinary instrumentation and urologic surgery	Prostatectomy, cystoscopy
Urinary diversion	Ileal conduit

Fig. 60.2 Genitourinary abnormalities associated with an increased frequency of urinary tract infection.

BACTERIA ISOLATED IN COMPLICATED UTI

Organism	Proportion of total organisms isolated (%)
Gram-negative organisms	
Escherichia coli	21–54
Klebsiella pneumoniae	1.9–17
Citrobacter spp.	4.7–6.1
Enterobacter spp.	1.9–10
Proteus mirabilis	0.9–10
Providencia spp.	1.9
Pseudomonas aeruginosa	2.0–19
Other Gram-negative organisms	6.1–23
Gram-positive organisms	
Enterococci	6.1–23
Coagulase-negative staphyloccoci	1.3–3.7
Staphylococcus aureus	0.9–2.0
Group B streptococci	1.2–3.5
Other Gram-positive organisms	1.9

Fig. 60.3 Frequency of isolation of different bacterial species in complicated urinary track infection.[14–17]

The intraluminal route appears to be more important in men than in women, in whom a shorter urethral length likely facilitates extraluminal ascension.

When infection occurs in the presence of a foreign body in the genitourinary tract, such as a ureteral stent, nephrostomy tube or indwelling catheter, a bacterial biofilm usually forms on the inert material.[11] A biofilm is an adherent colony of organisms with individual organisms encased in copious extracellular matrix. This biofilm provides a relatively protected environment for the bacteria by interfering with the diffusion of antibiotics and so contributing to relapsing infection.

Urinary tract infection may also be acquired in urologic practice as a result of organism transmission between patients on inappropriately cleaned diagnostic or therapeutic equipment.[12] In particular, contamination is a risk where instruments are not appropriately changed or cleaned between patients and where fluid is left standing for prolonged periods at room temperature. Multipatient use of urometers or urine collecting devices has also been repeatedly identified in the past as a cause of nosocomial outbreaks of infection.[13]

MICROBIOLOGY

The spectrum of micro-organisms isolated from individuals with complicated UTI is more varied than that observed in patients with uncomplicated UTI. Figure 60.3 summarizes the organisms isolated in a number of studies of complicated UTI. Although *Escherichia coli* remains an important infecting organism, the frequency with which it is isolated is substantially lower than that reported for acute uncomplicated UTI. *Escherichia coli* has unique virulence characteristics, which promote symptomatic infection in the person with a normal genitourinary tract (see Chapter 2.57). Where abnormalities of the genitourinary tract bypass the important nonspecific host resistance provided by complete voiding, organisms that do not possess unique virulence properties may also become important uropathogens. Therefore, there is a lower prevalence of genotypic or phenotypic expression of virulence factors by *E. coli* isolated from individuals with complicated genitourinary infection than by *E. coli* isolated from acute uncomplicated UTI.[18]

A wide variety of bacterial species other than *E. coli* is isolated in UTI. The distribution of organisms is determined by factors such as:
- whether organisms are isolated from initial or recurrent infection,
- whether acquisition is nosocomial- or community-acquired, and
- previous antimicrobial exposure.

Common organisms include Enterobacteriaceae such as *Klebsiella, Citrobacter, Serratia, Proteus* and *Providencia* spp., other Gram-negative organisms such as *Pseudomonas aeruginosa* and other nonfermenters, and Gram-positive organisms such as *Enterococcus faecalis* and group B streptococci. Coagulase-negative staphylococci are frequently isolated, although rarely the etiologic agent in symptomatic infection, and their pathogenicity is seldom clear. Yeast, primarily *Candida* spp., may be isolated, usually in individuals who have had prolonged or repeated courses of antimicrobial drugs. Anaerobic organisms are isolated rarely, and then in the setting of highly complicated urologic abnormalities and usually with abscess formation in the urinary tract.

The urease-producing organisms, principally *Proteus mirabilis, Providencia stuartii* and *Morganella morganii,* are important pathogens. Rarely, more unusual urease-producing organisms such as *Ureaplasma urealyticum* or *Corynebacterium* D2 may be isolated. These organisms maintain an alkaline environment, promoting persistence of infection and leading to the formation of struvite stones or catheter encrustation.

In addition to the much wider variety of infecting species in complicated UTI compared with uncomplicated UTI, there is also increased antimicrobial resistance among the infecting bacteria. Some of the infecting organisms, such as *P. aeruginosa*, are intrinsically more resistant to antimicrobials than *E. coli*. Two other factors also lead to increased resistance:
- repeated antimicrobial courses for previous UTI, and
- the high frequency of nosocomial infection.

PREVENTION

GENERAL MEASURES
Urinary tract infection in the abnormal genitourinary tract occurs because of the presence of an underlying abnormality or intervention that breaches normal defenses, and allows the introduction and persistence of micro-organisms. Therefore the most important interventions to prevent UTI are:
- to identify and, wherever possible, correct underlying abnormalities; and
- to avoid nonessential interventive procedures.

It is important to follow the appropriate aseptic technique for interventive procedures such as cystoscopy or urodynamic studies and for operative procedures. All fluids used in urologic procedures must be handled in a manner that ensures sterility. In particular, equipment must be disassembled after a procedure and reassembled using sterile components before the next procedure, and aseptic technique maintained.[12]

Institutions should establish and maintain appropriate infection surveillance programs to ensure endemic infection rates are known and early identification of and intervention in potential outbreaks.

CATHETER-ACQUIRED INFECTION

The frequency of catheter-associated UTI in institutional settings has led to extensive study of specific interventions to prevent catheter-acquired infection (Fig. 60.4).[5,10] The single most important practice in preventing infection in the catheterized patient is to maintain a closed urinary drainage system. In addition, use of an aseptic technique at insertion is important. Patients with indwelling catheters who receive antimicrobial therapy have a decreased incidence of infection acquisition during the initial 4 days of catheterization compared with that of patients who do not receive antimicrobials. After the first 4 days, the infection rates are similar, and patients receiving antimicrobials develop infections by more resistant organisms. Therefore antimicrobial therapy to prevent infection when an indwelling catheter *in situ* is currently not recommended.

Repeated evaluations of interventions using topical or local anti-infectives to prevent infection associated with indwelling catheters have consistently documented no benefit.[5] For instance, daily perineal cleansing with either soap or disinfectant does not decrease and may increase the rate of infection. Other measures that do not decrease the frequency of infection are the addition of disinfectants such as povidone–iodine or chlorhexidine to the drainage bag and the use of catheters impregnated with antimicrobial agents such as silver. It is in fact remarkable how consistently local anti-infective measures have failed to modify the occurrence of catheter-acquired infection.

The use of antimicrobials for preventing infection in patients with spinal cord injury who are maintained on intermittent catheterization has also been controversial. Clinical studies report prevention of both asymptomatic and symptomatic infection in the early postinjury months, but at the cost of increased antimicrobial resistance when infection occurs. Prophylactic therapy for the long term is likely not effective. Therefore, prophylactic antimicrobials are currently not recommended for such patients.[19]

POSTOPERATIVE INFECTION

The perioperative use of antimicrobials encompasses two issues:

- treatment of pre-existing bacteriuria to prevent the complications of invasive infection; and
- prophylaxis to prevent postoperative infection in individuals without positive preintervention urine cultures.

Treatment of bacteriuria preoperatively in individuals undergoing genitourinary interventions prevents postoperative bacteremia and sepsis and is indicated. It has been reported that postoperative sepsis was reduced from 6.2% to zero in patients with preoperative infected urine when appropriate antimicrobials were given 2–12 hours before operation.[20] The use of preoperative antimicrobials in this situation is most appropriately considered as therapy for UTI rather than prophylaxis, although it is prophylaxis for invasive infection. Antimicrobial therapy should be selected on the basis of the infecting organism and antimicrobial susceptibilities and initiated at least 1 hour before surgery.

There are some indications for the use of true prophylactic therapy in urologic surgery.[21] A summary of these indications is provided in Figure 60.5, with some reported rates of infection observed when selected prophylactic regimens are used. Most authorities[21,22] now suggest that antimicrobial prophylaxis is appropriate for transurethral prostatectomy even if the preprocedure urine culture is negative, although this recommendation has previously been controversial.[24]

There is no generally accepted 'standard' antimicrobial regimen for prophylaxis. Many different antimicrobials have been used. Generally, an aminoglycoside with or without a cephalosporin, or a fluoroquinolone is used. Studies have documented the efficacy of second- and third-generation cephalosporins, including cefotaxime, ceftriaxone, cefotetan, cefoxitin and ceftazidime, as well as fluoroquinolones. It is not clear, however, that these agents are superior to less costly alternatives such as aminoglycosides and trimethoprim–sulfamethoxazole (co-trimoxazole).

The recommended dosing regimen is one dose 1–2 hours preoperatively. The appropriate duration of antimicrobial therapy after therapy has not been defined. If an indwelling catheter remains *in situ* postoperatively some authors recommend continuation of antibiotics until the catheter is removed. However, recent studies suggest that, at least for some agents, a single dose is as effective as multidose therapy.[25,26] The shortest effective duration of therapy is preferred to limit cost, adverse effects and the emergence of antimicrobial-resistant organisms.

CLINICAL FEATURES

The clinical presentation of complicated UTI varies along a spectrum from asymptomatic bacteriuria without a measurable host response to septic shock and death.

INTERVENTIONS TO PREVENT CATHETER-ACQUIRED BACTERIURIA	
Proven effective	Avoid use of catheter Limit duration of catheterization Aseptic insertion Maintain closed drainage system Antibiotics first 4 days (not recommended)
Possibly effective	Antibiotics last 48h of catheterization Antimicrobial decontamination of gut
Proven not effective	Daily meatal care with soap or antiseptic Disinfectant (formaldehyde, chlorhexidine, hydrogen peroxide) in drainage bag Silver-coated catheters Continuous antibiotic or antiseptic irrigation

Fig. 60.4 Interventions to prevent catheter-acquired bacteriuria.[5,10]

Fig. 60.5 Prophylactic antimicrobial therapy in genitourinary surgery to prevent postoperative urinary tract infection.

PROPHYLACTIC ANTIMICROBIAL THERAPY IN GENITOURINARY SURGERY TO PREVENT POSTOPERATIVE UTI			
Procedure	Regimen	Infection rate with prophylaxis (%)	Infection rate without prophylaxis (%)
Transurethral instrumentation			
UTI with stone extraction[2]	Cefotaxime 1g iv, one dose	8.5	25
Sepsis[20]	Cefotaxime 1g iv, one dose	0	6.2
Prostatectomy			
Sterile urine preoperatively[22]	Various	3–22	6–70
Preoperative bacteriuria[22]	Various	35–41	65–92
Renal transplantation[23]	Trimethoprim–sulfamethoxazole 160mg–800mg daily for 4 months	8	35

In many clinical situations where chronic or recurring infection is anticipated, such as in the patient with a chronic indwelling catheter or the individual who has a neurogenic bladder and is maintained on intermittent catheterization, asymptomatic bacteriuria is the most common presentation. When symptomatic infection occurs the clinical features are those usually observed with a lower UTI such as frequency, suprapubic discomfort, dysuria and urgency.

With renal infection the characteristic presentation of upper UTI infection, including fever and costovertebral angle tenderness, is observed.

Obstruction and trauma to the genitourinary mucosa at any site predispose to bacteremia and more severe infection. Other contributing factors in determining the clinical presentation for a given infectious episode have not been well studied.

Infection may occasionally present as a high fever without any localizing findings, particularly in individuals who have indwelling catheters or neurologic impairment. Therefore the clinical presentation may suggest a urinary source of infection or be nonspecific. A diagnosis of UTI in the febrile patient who has a positive urine culture and no localizing findings must, however, be viewed critically. In populations with a high prevalence of asymptomatic bacteriuria the majority of such episodes are not due to UTI.[27]

Infection may be localized to the bladder or may involve the upper tract or kidney. In addition, in males, bladder infection may be secondary to or lead to prostatic infection. Presenting clinical symptoms are generally unhelpful in localizing the site of infection unless renal or prostatic tenderness can be demonstrated. Infection may manifest with lower UTI irritative symptoms alone despite the presence of upper tract or renal infection. In individuals with uncomplicated UTI, fever is a reliable localizing symptom for upper UTI. This is not the case for complicated and postsurgical infection or infection in the presence of an indwelling catheter. In these cases trauma to the bladder mucosa can lead to invasive infection and fever associated with lower UTI alone. In most cases, however, treatment decisions will not depend upon knowledge of the site of infection within the urinary tract.

PRESENTATION IN SELECTED PATIENT GROUPS

Selected patient groups may demonstrate some variation in presentation.

For spinal cord-injured patients who have a neurogenic bladder, the clinical presentation may differ from the usual irritative lower tract symptoms because of absent or altered sensation associated with the neurologic injury.[19] Signs and symptoms suggestive of UTI, in addition to fever, kidney pain or tenderness and bladder discomfort, may include an onset of or increase in urinary incontinence, autonomic hyperreflexia, increased sweating, increased spasticity, cloudy or odorous urine, and a general sense of being unwell.

In patients who have had renal transplantation, symptoms and signs may be absent or mild in the early post-transplant period, despite the presence of bacteremia. This lack of symptoms may be due to immunosuppressive therapy or uremia.

Occasionally, symptoms of the underlying genitourinary abnormality may be prominent. For instance, if UTI occurs in the setting of a ureteral stone, symptoms of renal colic may predominate, and the bacteriuric patient who has diabetes mellitus and papillary necrosis may have prominent symptoms of renal colic. A man with acute bacterial prostatitis may have prominent symptoms of urethral obstruction and even retention.

PRESENTATION WITH SPECIFIC INFECTING ORGANISMS

Infection by certain organisms may also produce a unique clinical presentation. *Corynebacterium* D2 infection is associated with the clinical syndrome of encrusted cystitis. This is encrustation of the bladder wall by struvite due to the urease production of the organism. Infections with Enterobacteriaceae, usually *E. coli* and *Klebsiella pneumoniae*, in patients who have diabetes mellitus and hyperglycemia and glycosuria may present as emphysematous cystitis or pyelonephritis. If a persistent fungal infection is identified, there may be a fungus ball of the bladder or kidney associated with obstruction.

RECURRENT INFECTION AFTER ANTIMICROBIAL THERAPY

Early recurrent infection after antimicrobial therapy is a characteristic clinical feature of individuals with persistent genitourinary abnormalities. It may be symptomatic or asymptomatic and may represent:
- relapse with recurrence of the pretherapy infecting organism after therapy; or
- re-infection with a new organism.

Selected reports that document this high frequency of recurrent infection are summarized in Figure 60.6.

Bacteriologic cure rates at 4–6 weeks (long-term follow up) are consistently less than 50% (i.e. recurrent infection is the expected outcome). If the underlying abnormality is transient or reversible, such as a single obstructing stone that is passed, permanent or long-term cure may, however, be achieved. If the underlying abnormality promoting infection cannot be resolved there will be recurrent infection by organisms with increasing antimicrobial resistance. Some patients may ultimately have infections for years with very resistant organisms such as *Pseudomonas* spp.

DIAGNOSIS

Clinical symptoms alone are not sufficient for a diagnosis of UTI. For definitive diagnosis an appropriately collected urine specimen must be obtained for bacterial culture. The large variety of potential infecting organisms and the high likelihood of antimicrobial resistance in infecting organisms mean that a urine culture is essential for appropriate antimicrobial management of patients with complicated UTI. The urine specimen must be collected before initiating antimicrobial therapy, using a urine collection method that limits contamination. A clean-catch voided specimen or, if a voided specimen cannot be obtained, a specimen obtained through in and out catheterization, is usually appropriate. For individuals with indwelling catheters, urine is collected by aseptic aspiration from the catheter port. Specimens may also be obtained by ureteric catheterization or percutaneous aspiration of the renal pelvis, but these invasive procedures are not recommended unless there is obstruction. There is no completely satisfactory way for collecting specimens for culture from people with ileal conduits. Specimens collected through the conduit will be contaminated with organisms colonizing the conduit.

Foreign material in the urinary tract, including indwelling urethral catheters, ureteric stents and nephrostomy tubes are rapidly coated with a bacterial biofilm after insertion. Organisms isolated from urine specimens for culture obtained through such devices may be more representative of the microbiology of the biofilm on the inner surface of

OUTCOME AFTER ANTIMICROBIAL THERAPY OF COMPLICATED UTI			
Regimen	Follow up after therapy	Cure (%)	Re-infection (%)
Complicated urinary infection			
Lomefloxacin[15]	5–9 days	59	5.9
	4–6 weeks	43	19
Trimethoprim–sulfamethoxazole[15]	5–9 days	33	1.5
	4–6 weeks	28	9.2
UTI secondary to spinal cord injury			
Norfloxacin 14 days[28]	5–7 days	53	14
	8–12 weeks	16	NS
Varied 7–14 days[29]	1 week	47	NS
Varied ≥28 days[29]	1 week	41	NS

Fig. 60.6 Outcome after antimicrobial therapy of complicated urinary tract infection. NS, not stated.

the catheter rather than of bladder urine. Therefore, it has been suggested that indwelling catheters should be changed before specimen collection and initiation of antimicrobial therapy.[10] The urine specimen is collected through the newly inserted catheter, which is free of biofilm, and is assumed to be representative of bladder bacteriuria and a more reliable identification of the bacterial species responsible for symptoms. However, no clinical study documenting that routine pretherapy catheter change for specimen collection leads to an improved clinical outcome has been published. Catheter replacement before therapy increases cost and may cause genitourinary trauma. Studies are therefore necessary to document its effectiveness before routine catheter change pretherapy can be promoted.

Urine specimens should be forwarded promptly to the laboratory for semiquantitative culture and appropriate susceptibility testing. Blood cultures should also be obtained from patients who have evidence of sepsis, including fever, rigors, hypothermia and confusion, and from early post-transplant patients who may be significantly immunosuppressed.

QUANTITATIVE BACTERIOLOGY

Current recommendations for quantitative bacteriology in the diagnosis of complicated UTI are provided in Figure 60.7. In the symptomatic patient, UTI may be diagnosed if the quantitative count of organisms in urine culture is $\geq 10^4$cfu/ml and there are symptoms consistent with genitourinary infection. For individuals who are asymptomatic, two specimens with a quantitative count of $\geq 10^5$cfu/ml and with the same organism(s) isolated on two consecutive occasions are necessary for diagnosis.[30]

Infections usually involve a single infecting organism, but there may be more than one bacterial species in the urine of patients with frequent recurrent infections. In the patient with a long-term indwelling catheter, isolation of 2–5 organisms is the norm.[5] In the presence of an indwelling catheter, small numbers of micro-organisms will usually increase to $\geq 10^5$cfu/ml in less than 24 hours and therefore any quantitative count may be significant.[31]

Rarely, less common organisms, such as yeast species, may not produce the usual quantitative counts. Unusual uropathogens such as *Mycoplasma hominis* or *Haemophilus influenzae*, which rarely cause infection, will not be isolated by routine laboratory methods for urine culture. Urine cultures may also be negative with symptomatic infection if the patient has had previous antimicrobial therapy or there is complete ureteric obstruction with infection localized proximal to the obstruction.

PYURIA

The presence of pyuria in a urine specimen may be useful in the diagnosis of UTI, but may be misleading. Pyuria reflects inflammation within the urinary tract, which is not necessarily caused by infection. Pyuria, by itself is not sufficient to diagnose a UTI in the absence of a positive urine culture. Although most UTIs have associated pyuria, underlying abnormalities associated with complicated UTI, inflammation following a surgical procedure, or a chronic indwelling catheter may be associated with pyuria in the absence of infection. Pyuria does not discriminate between symptomatic or asymptomatic infection. Therefore a dipstick test or urinalysis that shows evidence of pyuria is consistent with but not diagnostic of UTI.

MANAGEMENT

Essential elements in approaching the management of UTI in the setting of an abnormal genitourinary tract include:
- initial clinical evaluation and appropriate diagnostic specimen collection;
- initial antimicrobial therapy;
- appropriate supportive therapy;
- a review of urine bacteriology when available to ensure that the optimal antimicrobial regimen has been given; and

- an assessment of the need for genitourinary investigation and appropriate interventions to correct any abnormality.

ANTIMICROBIAL THERAPY

The empiric use of antimicrobials in this group of patients who have a high likelihood of recurrent infection will promote the emergence of organisms with increased antimicrobial resistance. Whenever possible, empiric therapy should be avoided and antimicrobial therapy should be specific for the infecting organism(s) identified in urine culture. This is frequently possible if the patient has mild symptoms. If the patient's symptoms are severe enough to warrant empiric therapy before the final culture results are available, a urine specimen for culture must be obtained before initiating therapy, and the antimicrobial therapy should be re-evaluated when the culture and susceptibility testing results are available, usually between 48 and 72 hours later.

The antimicrobial agents appropriate for therapy are similar to those used in the treatment of acute uncomplicated UTI or acute nonobstructive pyelonephritis (Figs 60.8 & 60.9). Initial parenteral therapy is preferred for individuals who have:
- hemodynamic instability,
- nausea and vomiting,
- questionable absorption of oral antimicrobials, or
- an infection by suspected resistant organisms for which oral therapy is not available.

In other situations, oral therapy can usually be initiated. The majority of patients can be managed without hospitalization or with a limited

QUANTITATIVE BACTERIOLOGY IN THE DIAGNOSIS OF COMPLICATED UTI	
Clinical situation	Bacteriologic count
Asymptomatic bacteriuria	$\geq 10^5$cfu/ml in two consecutive urine specimens
Symptomatic urinary infection	$\geq 10^4$cfu/ml in one specimen or $\geq 10^5$cfu/ml if collected by external catheter
Percutaneous aspiration in hydronephrosis	Any quantitative count
Diuresis, diuretic therapy, renal failure, selected infecting organisms (e.g. *Candida albicans*)	Lower quantitative counts ($<10^5$/ml) may occur in these situations

Fig. 60.7 Quantitative bacteriology in the diagnosis of complicated urinary tract infection.

ORAL THERAPEUTIC REGIMENS FOR THE TREATMENT OF COMPLICATED UTI	
Agent	Dose
Amoxicillin	500mg q8h
Amoxicillin–clavulanate	500mg q8h
Cephalexin	500mg q6h
Cefixime	500mg q24h
Nitrofurantoin	50 mg q6h
Nitrofurantoin macrocrystals	100mg q6h
Norfloxacin	400mg q12h
Ciprofloxacin	250–500mg q12h
Ofloxacin	400mg/day or 200mg q12h
Lomefloxacin	400mg/day
Enoxacin	200mg q12h
Fleroxacin	400mg/day
Trimethoprim	100mg q12h
Trimethoprim–sulfamethoxazole	160mg trimethoprim– 800mg sulfamethoxazole q12h

Fig. 60.8 Oral therapeutic regimens for the treatment of complicated urinary tract infection.

PARENTERAL REGIMENS FOR THE TREATMENT OF COMPLICATED UTI	
Agent	Dose
Ampicillin	1g q6h
Piperacillin	3g q6h
Ticarcillin–clavulanate	3.1g q6h
Piperacillin–tazobactam	4g pipericillin–500mg tazobactam q8h
Cefazolin	1–2g q8h
Cefotaxime	1g q8h
Ceftriaxone	1g q24h
Ceftazidime	1g q8–12h
Imipenem	500mg q6h
Gentamicin	5mg/kg/day q12h or q24h
Tobramycin	5mg/kg/day q12h or q24h
Amikacin	15mg/kg/day q12h or q24h
Trimethoprim–sulfamethoxazole	160mg trimethoprim–800mg sulfamethoxazole q12h
Ciprofloxacin	400mg q12h
Ofloxacin	400mg q12h
Fleroxacin	400mg/day

Fig. 60.9 Parenteral antimicrobial regimens for the treatment of complicated urinary tract infection.

(24–72h) admission to a short stay unit for initial parenteral therapy. Oral therapy is then started as soon as the patient is stable, often when pretherapy urine culture results are available to assist in selecting the appropriate medication.

The selection of a specific antimicrobial agent is based upon clinical presentation, the known or suspected infecting organism and its susceptibilities, patient tolerance, documented efficacy and, in some cases, cost. Comparative trials of different antimicrobials have not consistently reported that any one antimicrobial agent or class of antimicrobials is better than any other.[32] The selection of optimal antimicrobial therapy is further limited by a relative lack of relevant clinical trials. Although there are many published reports on the treatment of complicated UTI, few are useful in assisting with the selection of an antimicrobial in a specific clinical situation. One problem is the lack of an accepted 'standard' antimicrobial therapy with respect to agent, dose or duration to serve as a comparator for new agents.[30] In addition, studies have generally enrolled diverse and poorly characterized patient populations for whom different outcomes with therapy would be anticipated on the basis of underlying abnormalities. The severity of illness also varies, and subjects are enrolled into studies with clinical presentations ranging from an increase in incontinence or bladder spasms to a life-threatening illness with bacteremia.

In view of the very high frequency of relapse, therapeutic trials should provide both short-term (1 week post-therapy) and long-term (4–6 weeks post-therapy) outcomes.[30] Frequently, studies of therapy for complicated UTI have provided only short-term therapeutic outcomes. The many published studies therefore allow only a limited assessment of the comparative efficacy of different antimicrobials. They do, however, document the effectiveness of a wide variety of antimicrobial agents.

ORAL THERAPY

For oral therapy, the quinolone antimicrobials in particular have been widely studied and promoted. Benefits of fluoroquinolones include a wide antibacterial spectrum and good patient tolerance. Problems include increasing antimicrobial resistance with widespread use of quinoline antimicrobials and cost.

In studies of therapy for pyelonephritis, likely including some patients with complicated infection, cell-wall active agents such as amoxicillin or first-generation cephalosporins appear less effective than noncell-wall active agents such as trimethoprim–sulfamethoxazole or quinolones.[33] Appropriate comparative clinical trials have not shown whether these cell-wall active agents have a lower efficacy for

complicated UTI. For Gram-positive organisms such as group B streptococci and *Enterococcus* spp., amoxicillin or ampicillin would, of course, be the treatment of choice.

PARENTERAL THERAPY

For parenteral therapy, an aminoglycoside antimicrobial remains the treatment of choice because of the documented efficacy of this group of drugs over many years of use and the likelihood of effectiveness against more resistant organisms. The nephrotoxicity and ototoxicity of aminoglycosides are seldom a problem if the duration of therapy is limited, with a switch to oral therapy as soon as possible. If *Enterococcus* spp. may be present, ampicillin should be added. The increasing prevalence of ampicillin resistance in *Enterococcus faecium* and *Enterococcus faecalis* in many institutions means that vancomycin may be necessary to treat nosocomial enterococcal infection. Empiric use of vancomycin is, however, to be discouraged because widespread empiric use will promote the emergence of vancomycin-resistant organisms.

DURATION OF THERAPY

Few reported studies have directly addressed the question of the appropriate duration of therapy. The usual recommended duration is from 7 to 14 days.[30] There are selected clinical situations where alternative durations of therapy are appropriate:
- where relapsing infection is due to a prostate source, 6 or 12 weeks of antimicrobial therapy is appropriate;
- if symptomatic infection associated with an indwelling catheter is treated while the catheter remains *in situ*, it is recommended that the duration of therapy is as short as possible, usually 5–7 days, to limit the emergence of resistant organisms; and
- after successful extracorporeal shock wave lithotripsy for an infected struvite stone, antimicrobial therapy is continued for at least 4 weeks to prevent relapse and sterilize residual stone fragments.

SUPPORTIVE THERAPY

This should be given as appropriate. It may include hemodynamic monitoring, parenteral fluids, measurement of urine output and antiemetic medication. If any obstruction in the urinary tract is suspected, urgent ultrasound or CT scan should be obtained. Immediate drainage may be necessary if an obstruction is identified. If an indwelling catheter is obstructed or leaking, the catheter should be replaced.

RENAL FAILURE

Patients who have abnormalities of the genitourinary tract are more likely to have impaired renal function. Renal function should be determined, if not already known, for patients who present with possible complicated UTI. If there is renal impairment:
- appropriate modifications in antimicrobial dose are necessary, and
- nitrofurantoin and tetracyclines other than doxycycline should be avoided.

Some quinolones have been shown to lead to a reversible increase in serum creatinine in renal transplant recipients receiving cyclosporin. Quinolones should be avoided, if possible, in these patients.

In renal failure, renal perfusion is decreased and antimicrobials may not reach infected renal tissue or achieve high urine levels. The aminoglycosides, in particular, may be less effective.[32] The fluoroquinolone antimicrobials, trimethoprim–sulfamethoxazole, trimethoprim and extended spectrum beta-lactam antimicrobials appear, however, to be effective in treatment of UTI in the presence of significant renal failure. A more prolonged duration of antimicrobial therapy may also be necessary to cure UTI in patients who have renal failure.

An additional potential therapeutic problem is the patient who has normal measured renal function and satisfactory urinary antimicrobial levels, but disparate kidney function.[32] If the function of one kidney is severely impaired relative to the other, blood flow is preferentially increased in the functioning kidney and despite adequate urinary antibiotic levels, little antibiotic will be filtered by the

TREATMENT REGIMENS FOR FUNGAL UTI		
Agent	Dose	Cure rate (%)
Amphotericin B: parenteral	0.3mg/kg single dose or 6mg/kg body weight total dose	75
Amphotericin B: bladder irrigation	Continuous, 50mg/l for 5 days	72–88
Fluconazole	50–400mg/day for 7 days	70–80
5-Flucytosine	50–150mg/kg/day q6h	70

Fig. 60.10 Regimens for the treatment of fungal urinary tract infection.[34]

INDICATIONS FOR THE TREATMENT OF ASYMPTOMATIC BACTERIURIA	
Definite	Before an invasive genitourinary procedure[20] Pregnancy[38] Infection stone[37] Renal transplant[23]
Possible	Diabetes mellitus
Not indicated	In the elderly[39] For a schoolgirl[40] Intermittent catheterization[19] Indwelling urinary catheter[5]

Fig. 60.11 Indications for the treatment of asymptomatic bacteriuria.

poorly functioning kidney. Antimicrobial treatment may then not eradicate infection localized to the poorly functioning kidney. This has been documented with nitrofurantoin therapy, and nitrofurantoin should be avoided if there is a substantial difference in function between the two kidneys.

FUNGAL INFECTION

Optimal treatment and expected outcomes for fungal infection require further study.[34] The current treatment options and reported cure rates are listed in Figure 60.10. Currently recommended treatment for funguria is amphotericin B or fluconazole. Many nonalbicans *Candida* spp. have decreased susceptibility or are resistant to fluconazole. Comparative trials of fluconazole and amphotericin B and potentially other azoles are necessary to understand the relative roles for different agents. Previously, bladder irrigation with amphotericin B has been recommended. This approach, however, is costly and time consuming and is no longer consistent optimal therapy.[35]

Treatment of asymptomatic funguria remains controversial and requires further study. If there is an indwelling catheter, the catheter should be changed before treatment of funguria; if there is an asymptomatic infection persistence of funguria after catheter exchange should be documented before treatment. If there is symptomatic fungal infection the presence of a fungus ball in the bladder or kidneys should be excluded by ultrasound examination or other diagnostic imaging.

SUPPRESSIVE THERAPY

Suppressive therapy is long-term antimicrobial therapy given to prevent recurrent symptomatic infection in individuals with underlying abnormalities that cannot be corrected.[36] Long-term therapy, such as suppressive therapy, is infrequently indicated and should be used

selectively because of the potential for inducing the development of resistant organisms.

Suppressive therapy is recommended for the few individuals with a struvite (infection) stone that cannot be completely removed.[37] Prolonged suppressive therapy in this situation will usually prevent further stone enlargement and preserve renal function. When an abnormality leads to recurrent invasive infection in a patient for whom intervention cannot alleviate the problem, invasive episodes may be prevented by suppressive therapy. Another situation where suppressive therapy may be appropriate is in men who have frequent recurrent symptomatic episodes of cystitis from a prostatic source when prolonged antimicrobial therapy has failed to cure the infection.

ASYMPTOMATIC BACTERIURIA

Indications for the treatment of asymptomatic UTI remain controversial. Figure 60.11 summarizes current recommendations with respect to the treatment of asymptomatic bacteriuria in different patient populations. These recommendations for treatment or nontreatment are based on published studies. If treatment of asymptomatic bacteriuria is not indicated, therapy has not been shown to decrease morbidity, but is associated with a greater frequency of negative outcomes including the emergence of resistant organisms and adverse drug effects. Studies in children, in fact, suggest that the treatment of asymptomatic bacteriuria may increase the frequency of symptomatic infection. Asymptomatic bacteriuria should not be treated except where clinical studies have demonstrated a benefit. Following from this, screening for bacteriuria is not indicated except in those for whom treatment of asymptomatic bacteriuria is indicated.

INDICATIONS FOR INVESTIGATION

An important aspect of the management of UTIs is determining when to carry out urologic or imaging investigations to determine whether there are abnormalities in the genitourinary tract (see also Chapter 2.59). Single infections that are easily cured by antimicrobials are unlikely to be associated with significant underlying abnormalities. On many other occasions the abnormality may be obvious, such as the presence of an indwelling catheter. In selected other patients, genitourinary investigation should be considered. These clinical scenarios include:

- delayed or incomplete response to appropriate antimicrobial therapy; and
- early recurrence of infection after therapy.

Patients presenting with sepsis and hemodynamic instability may require urgent investigation to identify an abscess or obstruction requiring immediate intervention. Studies that define the relative efficacy of investigation in selected clinical scenarios are, however, necessary.

REFERENCES

1. Larsen EH, Gusser TC, Madsen PO. Antimicrobial prophylaxis in urologic surgery. Urol Clin N Am 1986;13:591–604.
2. Fourcade RO, the Cefotaxime Cooperative Group. Antibiotic prophylaxis with cefotaxime in endoscopic extraction of upper urinary tract stones: a randomized study. J Antimicrob Chemother 1990;26(Suppl A):77–83.
3. Charton M, Vallencien G, Veillon B, Prapotnich D, Mombet A, Brisset JM. Use of antibiotics in conjunction with extracorporeal lithotripsy. Eur Urol 1990;17:134–8.
4. Darouiche, RD, Smith MS, Markowski J. Antibiotic prophylaxis for urodynamic testing in patients with spinal cord injury: a preliminary study. J Hosp Infect 1994;28:57–61.
5. Warren JW. Catheter-associated urinary tract infections. Infect Dis Clin N Am 1987;1:823–54.
6. Mohler JL, Cower DL, Flanigan RC. Suppression and treatment of urinary tract infection in patients with an intermittently catheterized neurogenic bladder. J Urol 1987;138:336–40.
7. Nicolle LE, Friesen D, Harding GKM, Roos LL. Hospitalization for acute pyelonephritis in Manitoba, Canada, during the period from 1989 to 1991: impact of diabetes, pregnancy and aboriginal origin. Clin Infect Dis 1996;22:1051–6.
8. Esposito HL, Gleckman RA, Cram S, Crowley M, McCabe F, Drapkin MS. Community-acquired bacteremia in the elderly: analysis of one hundred consecutive episodes. J Am Geriatr Soc 1980;28:315–9.
9. Waites KB, Canupp KC, DeVivo MJ. Epidemiology and risk factors for urinary tract infection following spinal cord injury. Arch Phys Med Rehab 1993;74:691–5.
10. Stamm WE. Catheter-associated urinary tract infections: epidemiology, pathogenesis, and prevention. Am J Med 1991;91(Suppl 3B):65–71.
11. Nickel JC, Costerton JW, McLean RJC, Olson M. Bacterial biofilms: influence on the pathogenesis, diagnosis and treatment of urinary tract infections. J Antimicrob Chemother 1994;33(Suppl A):31–4.
12. Hamill RJ, Wright CE, Andres N, Koza MA. Urinary tract infection following instrumentation for urodynamic testing. Infect Control Hosp Epidemiol 1989;10:26–32.
13. Schaberg DR, Weinstein RA, Stamm WE. Epidemics of nosocomial urinary tract infections caused by multiply-resistant Gram-negative organisms – suggestions for control. J Infect Dis 1976;133:363–6.
14. Harding GKM, Nicolle LE, Ronald AR, et al. How long should catheter-acquired urinary tract infection in women be treated? Ann Intern Med 1991;116:713–9.
15. Nicolle LE, Louie TJ, Dubois J, Martel A, Harding GKM, Sinave C. Treatment of complicated urinary tract infections with lomefloxacin compared with trimethoprim–sulfamethoxazole. Antimicrob Agents Chemother 1994;38:1368–73.
16. Biering-Sorensen F, Hoiby N, Nordenbo A, Ravnborg M, Bruin B, Rahn V. Ciprofloxacin as prophylaxis for urinary tract infection. Prospective, randomized, cross-over, placebo controlled study in patients with spinal cord lesion. J Urol 1994;151:105–8.
17. Cox CE, Holloway WJ, Geckler RW. A multi-center comparative study of meropenem and imipenem/cilastatin in the treatment of complicated urinary tract infections in hospitalized patients. Clin Infect Dis 1995;21:86–92.
18. Johnson JR. Virulence factors in Escherichia coli urinary tract infection. Clin Microbiol Rev 1991;4:80–128.
19. Cardenas DD, Hooton TM. Urinary tract infection in persons with spinal cord injury. Arch Phys Med Rehab 1995;76:272–80.
20. Cafferkey MT, Falkiner FR, Gillespie WA, Murphy PM. Antibiotics for the prevention of septicaemia in urology. J Antimicrob Chemother 1982;9:471–7.
21. Del Rio G, Delet F, Chechile G. Antimicrobial prophylaxis in urologic surgery: does it give some benefit? Eur Urol 1993;24:305–12.
22. Grabe M. Antimicrobial agents in transurethral prostatic resection. J Urol 1987;138:245–57.
23. Tolkoff-Rubin NE, Cosimi AB, Russell PS, Rubin RH. A controlled study of trimethoprim–sulfamethoxazole prophylaxis of urinary tract infection in renal transplant receipients. Rev Infect Dis 1982;4:614–8.
24. Strickes PD, Grant ABF. Relative value of antibiotics and catheter care in the prevention of urinary tract infection after transurethral prostatic resection. Br J Urol 1988;61:494–7.
25. Hargreave TB, Botto H, Rikken GH, et al. European collaborative study of antibiotic prophylaxis for transurethral resection of the prostate. Eur Urol 1993;23:437–43.
26. Viitanen J, Talja M, Jussila E, et al. Randomized controlled study of chemoprophylaxis in transurethral prostatectomy. J Urol 1993;150:1715–7.
27. Orr P, Nicolle LE, Duckworth H, et al. Febrile urinary infection in the institutionalized elderly. Am J Med 1996;100:71–7.
28. Waites KB, Canupp KC, DeVivo MJ. Efficacy and tolerance of norfloxacin in treatment of complicated urinary tract infections in outpatients with neurogenic bladder secondary to spinal cord injury. Urology 1991;38:589–96.
29. Waites KB, Canupp KC, DeVivo MJ. Eradication of urinary tract infection following spinal cord injury. Paraplegia 1993;31:645–52.
30. Rubin RH, Shapiro ED, Andriole VT, Davis RJ, Stamm WE. Evaluation of new anti-infective drugs for the treatment of urinary tract infection. Clin Infect Dis 1992;15(Suppl 1):216–27.
31. Stark RP, Maki DG. Bacteriuria in the catheterized patient. What quantitative level of bacteriuria is relevant? N Engl J Med 1984;311:560–4.
32. Nicolle LE. A practical guide to the management of complicated urinary tract infection. Drugs 1997;53:583–92.
33. Pinson AG, Philbrick JT, Lindbeck GH, Schorling JB. Oral antibiotic therapy for acute pyelonephritis. J Gen Int Med 1992;7:544–53.
34. Fisher JF, Newman CL, Sobel JD. Yeast in the urine: solutions for a budding problem. Clin Infect Dis 1995;20:183–9.
35. Jacobs LG, Skidmore EA, Cardoso LA, Ziv F. Bladder irrigation with amphotericin B for treatment of fungal urinary tract infections. Clin Infect Dis 1994;18:313–8.
36. Sheehan GJ, Harding GKM, Haase DA, et al. Double-blind, randomized comparision of 24 weeks of norfloxacin and 12 weeks of placebo in the therapy of complicated urinary tract infection. Antimicrob Agents Chemother 1988;32:1292–3.
37. Chinn RH, Maskell R, Mead JA, Polak A. Renal stones and urinary infection: a study of antibiotic treatment. Br Med J 1976;2:1411–3.
38. Nicolle LE. Screening for asymptomatic bacteriuria in pregnancy. P100–107. The Canadian Guide to Clinical Preventive Health Care. Canadian Task Force on the Periodic Health Care Examination. Health Canada, Canada Communication Group, Ottawa, 1994.
39. Nicolle LE. Urinary tract infection in the elderly. J Antimicrob Chemother 1994;33(Suppl A):99–109.
40. Smith MBH. Screening for urinary tract infection in asymptomatic infants and children. P220–229. The Canadian Guide to Clinical Preventive Health Care. Canadian Task Force on the Periodic Health Examination, Health Canada. Canada Communication Group, Ottawa, 1994.

chapter
61

Tuberculosis of the Urogenital Tract

John David Hinze & Richard E Winn

The most common site for extrapulmonary tuberculosis (TB) next to lymphatic and pleural involvement is the genitourinary tract.

EPIDEMIOLOGY

The incidence and prevalence of genitourinary TB (GUTB) remains elusive. A large proportion of patients remain asymptomatic and symptoms that do arise are nonspecific and easily attributable to other causes. The incidence of GUTB has fallen over the past century, but at a slower rate than the decline of pulmonary TB. Extrapulmonary TB accounted for 22% of all TB cases in the USA in 1992.[1] When expressed as a proportion of extrapulmonary cases, GUTB accounts for 18%.[2] Genitourinary TB varies from an average of less than 1% in France[3] over a 10-year period to less than 2% of all TB cases in the USA[4] to over 20% in developing countries.[4–6]

Most cases occur in sexually active middle-aged adults aged 20–69 years. There is a male:female predominance of 2:1. The presence of TB at any site makes it mandatory to search for involvement at other sites.

PATHOGENESIS AND PATHOLOGY

Nearly all cases of GUTB are caused by *Mycobacterium tuberculosis*. Renal infection with *M. tuberculosis* begins from hematogenous seeding of the renal cortex from a pulmonary source. Either primary or reactivated pulmonary TB infection, that may or may not be clinically apparent, may seed the capillaries of the renal cortices. Other extrapulmonary sites should not, however, be excluded as potential sources. Given the high cardiac output delivery (20%) and therefore increased oxygen tension of the renal cortex, it is easy to understand the predilection of *M. tuberculosis* for the kidney among extrapulmonary sites. The vast majority of GUTB cases involve the kidney bilaterally, but progression of disease is almost uniformly unilateral.

Once important, *Mycobacterium bovis* from cattle was transmitted via ingestion of infected cows milk and caused gastrointestinal TB with the potential to spread to the genitourinary tract.

Mycobacterium kansasii and *Mycobacterium avium-intracellulare* have been cultured from the urine of immunocompromised persons (i.e. AIDS patients), but these cases are rare. *Mycobacterium avium-intracellulare* in the urine is of uncertain clinical significance.

Once infected, host immune status determines the extent of destruction. Macrophages, attracted to the site, halt the progression of the tubercle bacilli, leading to necrosis and eventual granuloma formation. In an immunocompetent individual, tubercle bacilli are isolated and contained and may ultimately be killed by cellular enzymes. However, a less vigorous response by the host's immune system may not kill all the bacilli and these microscopic foci may remain dormant for decades. Later, if the host's cellular immunity becomes compromised secondary to age, malnutrition, diabetes mellitus, malignancy, corticosteroid use, or chronic debilitating disease, reactivation TB may ensue. At this point, as infection spreads from the renal cortex, granuloma formation and subsequent necrosis advance with infection of the medulla and papilla (Fig. 61.1). As these foci coalesce, they form macroscopic

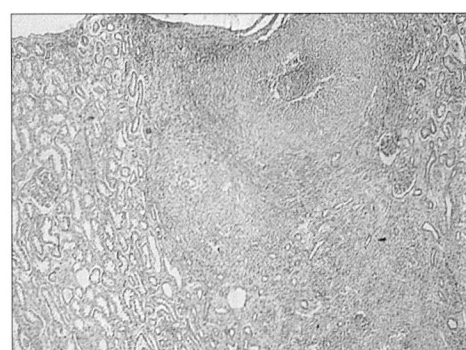

Fig. 61.1 **Granuloma formation in kidney biopsy.** Courtesy of Robert F. Peterson.

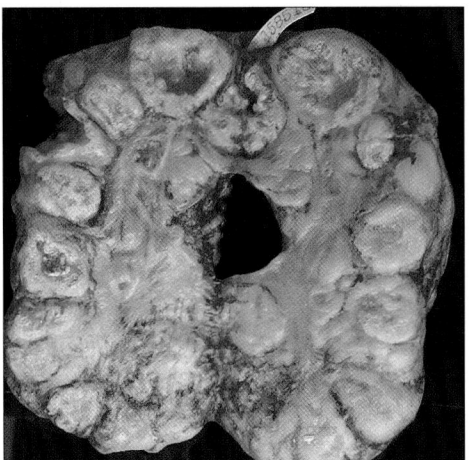

Fig. 61.2 **Chronic tuberculous nephritis with almost complete destruction of the kidney.** Courtesy of Robert F. Peterson.

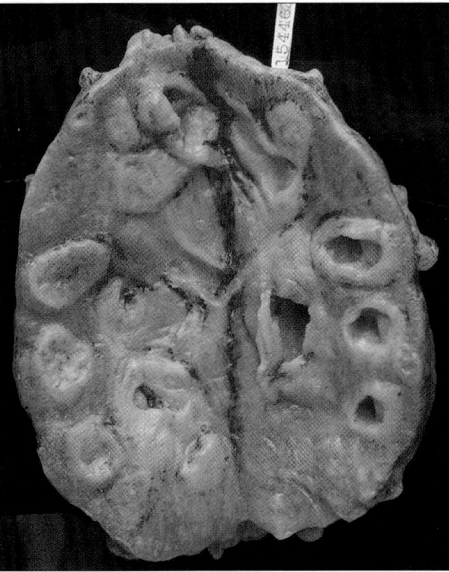

Fig. 61.3 **Diffuse acute tuberculous nephritis with abscess formation.** Courtesy of Robert F. Peterson.

cavitary lesions of caseation necrosis (Figs 61.2 & 61.3).[4,7] Infective debris can both infect and obstruct the calyces, ureters and bladder. Calyceal involvement by ulcerative and deforming lesions (Fig. 61.4) is responsible for many of the radiographic manifestations seen in

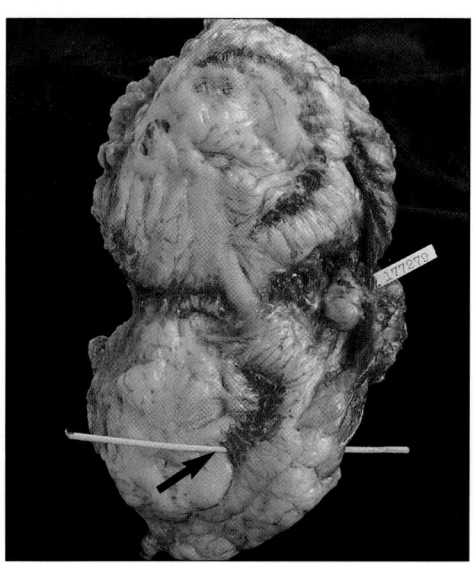

Fig. 61.4 Chronic tuberculous nephritis with destruction of all landmarks and pelvic calculus. The arrow shows a fistulous tract noted with the wooden probe. Courtesy of Robert F. Peterson.

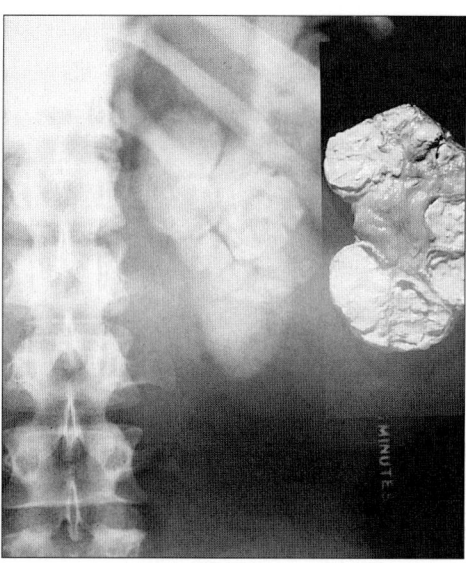

Fig. 61.5 Intravenous pyelogram of left kidney with bivalved surgical pathology specimen.

GUTB (Fig. 61.5).[4] If severe calyceal clubbing occurs with dilatation of the renal pelvis and ureter, then total destruction of the kidney ensues, termed 'autonephrectomy'.[8] Ureteral and bladder disease are secondary to renal involvement. During all stages of renal infection, tuberculous bacilluria is responsible for ureteral and bladder involvement, prostatitis and epididymitis.

In men, urologic spread of renal foci will infect, in descending order of frequency, the prostate, seminal vesicles, epididymis and testes.[9] However, genital TB without renal involvement does occur, suggesting bacillemic spread. In addition, TB of the prostate, epididymis and glans penis can occur with conjugal contact. Primary TB of the glans penis is extremely rare, with about 150 cases reported[10] and, although transmission may be secondary to hematogenous dissemination, local direct sexual contact is most probable.

In women, as in men, genital TB is almost always hematogenous in origin. Direct spread from an intra-abdominal or intraperitoneal source is possible, but GUTB may also be part of a miliary process. The fallopian tubes are involved in 90% of female cases[11] and chronic salpingitis is the most common manifestation. Fallopian TB is predominantly bilateral with a predilection for the ampullae.[12] From there the bacilli spread, in descending order, to the endometrium in 50–70% of cases, the ovaries 30% and cervix 5–15%; vulvar and vaginal disease are rare.[4,12,13]

In tuberculous endometritis, the typical lesion is the noncaseating granuloma formed by epithelial cells, lymphocytes and Langhans' giant cells.[12] Noncaseating granulomas are spread superficially and diffusely around the endometrium. Cases of vulvar or vaginal TB are usually secondary to hematogenous spread, but as in males, some may be sexually transmitted.

PREVENTION

The insidious nature of TB as well as the typical latency between onset of symptoms and medical therapy favor its communicability. Prevention of GUTB mirrors that of pulmonary TB with identification of infected sources and institution of appropriate antimicrobial therapy. In addition, prevention of primary venereal transmission of TB should follow safe sex guidelines, as the true incidence, although small, is unknown. The Advisory Council for the Elimination of Tuberculosis in the USA recommends a national standard centered on three prevention strategies:

- identifying and treating patients with active TB;
- screening contacts of active TB patients, determining whether they are infected, and if so, providing appropriate therapy; and
- screening high-risk populations and providing therapy to prevent progression to active TB.[14]

SYMPTOM FREQUENCY IN PATIENTS WHO HAVE GENITOURINARY TUBERCULOSIS				
	Study of 160 patients[3]	Study of 81 patients[6]	Study of 83 patients[15]	Study of 52 patients[5]
Dysuria (with urgency and frequency included) (%)	52	65	46	31
Gross hematuria (%)	30	36	43	31
Frank pain/ renal colic (%)	23	57	42	21
Fever (%)	12.5	35	23	ND
History of tuberculosis (%)	22.5	23.5	16	ND

Fig. 61.6 Symptom frequency in patients who have genitourinary tuberculosis. ND, no data.

Once at-risk contacts have been identified, the recommendations for chemoprophylaxis are the same as for pulmonary TB, especially for patients less than 35 years of age or in an 'at-risk' group.

CLINICAL FEATURES

Genitourinary TB is a relentless destructive process that may lie dormant or clinically inapparent for decades. Many people with pulmonary TB have coexistent asymptomatic GUTB.[14] The most common clinical symptoms of GUTB are:

- dysuria (including urinary frequency or urgency);
- recurrent urinary tract infections (UTIs); and
- pain (including back, flank, suprapubic and abdominal pain) (Fig. 61.6). Constitutional symptoms are generally uncommon, but may be more frequent in patients with advanced disease or those who are immunocompromised, and include fevers, chills, night sweats and weight loss. Hypertension is not generally a feature of tuberculous renal disease and is no more prevalent than in the general population, although case reports describe alleviation of hypertension after treatment of TB.[16]

In men, genital TB typically presents with a mildly tender or symptomless scrotal mass (epididymitis), and less commonly with prostatitis, orchitis, or scrotal fistulas.

For women with genital TB the most common presenting symptom is infertility[3,8,13] and it is estimated that 85% of patients have never been pregnant.[12] The next most common complaint is lower abdominal and pelvic pain, which occurs in 25–50% of the patients. As the disease progresses, so does the intensity of the pain, which may be exacerbated by activity or coitus. The clinical presentation might mimic that of pelvic inflammatory disease unresponsive to usual therapy. The third most frequent complaint is abnormal menstrual bleeding.

DIAGNOSIS

A healthy clinical suspicion is mandatory to diagnose GUTB early, given its insidious nature and the large proportion of patients who are asymptomatic. It should be considered in any patient with unexplained fever. An evaluation for GUTB is mandatory for any patient with a history of TB who develops dysuria or sterile pyuria from an unidentified cause. However, GUTB may exist despite negative urine cultures. Historic queries regarding past exposure to TB, evening pyrexia, weight loss, asthenia, fatigue and past medical history are helpful. Physical examination findings are nonspecific.

Over 50% of patients presenting with a UTI culture routine bacterial pathogens from the urine, obscuring the underlying GUTB. In men, a scrotal mass or nodular prostate may suggest TB. One study of 83 cases of GUTB from Turkey revealed tenderness of the costovertebral angle in 55% of patients.[15]

After an examination, initial laboratory work up should include:
- renal function tests;
- at least three first-morning urine specimens for acid-fast bacillus (AFB) stain and culture; and
- tuberculin skin testing.

Positive AFB stains of urine are usually due to *M. tuberculosis* (Richard Wallace, University of Texas Health Science Center at Tyler, personal communication). Of patients who have GUTB 77–92% will have positive urine cultures for *M. tuberculosis*,[4,5,13,15] and 90% of patients will have positive tuberculin skin tests.[17]

Early in the course of GUTB, radiologic manifestations are unremarkable. A chest radiograph should be obtained to assess for comorbid pulmonary TB. Simple abdominal radiography is generally nonspecific and commonly shows amorphous nephrocalcinosis or fine calcifications.

The 'gold standard' and most commonly used radiologic technique for evaluating the genitourinary system for *M. tuberculosis* remains the

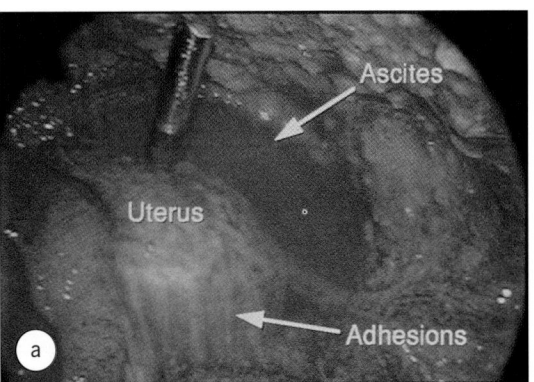

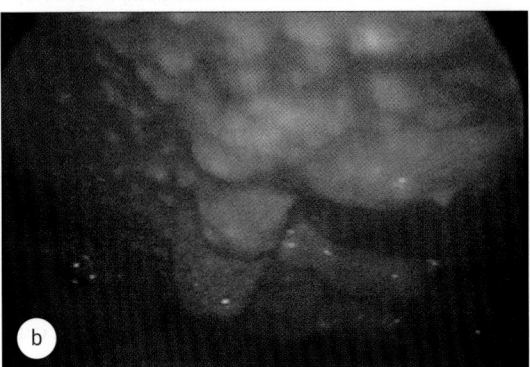

Fig. 61.7 Laparoscopic views in genitourinary tuberculosis. (a) Free and loculated ascites and fine fibrous adhesions. (b) Miliary nodular exudate in the anterior wall.

intravenous pyelogram (IVP) and excretory pyelogram.[18] The most valuable clue to renal TB is concurrent multiple abnormalities of both the upper and lower urinary tracts. Findings in progressive renal TB demonstrate abnormalities of the collecting system from the calyces to the bladder. Initially, an IVP may demonstrate irregular calyceal contours secondary to erosive inflammatory changes that later progress to delayed excretion, cavitation, 'moth eaten' calyces, or strictures with caliectasis. The characteristic finding of a 'phantom calyx' occurs when an IVP reveals an obstructed nonfunctioning calyx proximal to an infundibular stricture.[18] A 'hiked-up' renal pelvis is observed when the renal pelvis makes an acute angulation with the ureter and is highly suggestive of renal TB. Another highly suggestive lesion is the 'putty kidney' consisting of a heavily calcified caseous mass surrounded by a thin parenchymal shell.[18] Autonephrectomy is the end result. Ureteral TB may manifest as different combinations of strictures and obstructions, giving the appearance of 'beading,' 'corkscrewing', straight 'pipestems', focal calcification, or hydroureteronephrosis. Commonly, the bladder appears thickened and fibrotic with a small capacity.

In female genital TB, the hysterosalpingogram provides the most characteristic abnormalities, displaying a contracted deformed uterine cavity with associated intrauterine adhesions. The fallopian tubes may have ragged outlines and appear beaded or rigid.[12]

In the evaluation of GUTB, ultrasound, CT and MRI are not usually necessary, although sometimes have a role. A non-visualized kidney is best evaluated by ultrasound or CT,[18] and ultrasound has demonstrated small focal lesions in the kidneys in patients with renal TB.[18] In women, ultrasonography may reveal predominantly solid adnexal masses containing small scattered calcifications bilaterally. Abdominal and vaginal ultrasound may have a role in delineating the features of tuberculous peritonitis.[18] In men, testicular ultrasound is a rapid and easy way for assessing scrotal contents; however, it is nonspecific.[9] Transrectal ultrasound may also be helpful in delineating lower genitourinary tract pathology, but is also nonspecific. Sonography also has a use in providing a guide for fine-needle aspiration of genitourinary lesions.[13]

Computerized tomography is superior to IVP and serial examination at delineating anatomic detail and may prove to be beneficial in contributing to therapeutic decisions.[15] Typical CT findings in GUTB are caliectasis and focal cortical scarring (>80%).[18] Magnetic resonance imaging has also been used to describe tuberculous lesions due to enhanced contrast resolution and multiplanar capabilities. Tuberculous foci appear hypointense on T2-weighted images.[18]

Although a positive purified protein derivative skin test with classic radiologic findings may be suggestive of GUTB, diagnosis should only be made with positive bacteriologic or histologic evidence. If urine, menstrual blood, or seminal fluid cultures are negative, then ultrasound-guided or CT-guided fine-needle aspiration or diagnostic laparoscopy can be used to provide appropriate tissue for bacteriohistologic diagnosis.

The use of diagnostic laparoscopy in women with suspected genital TB may provide an earlier diagnosis (Fig. 61.7). The BACTEC system has sped culture time to roughly 1 week. In addition, rapid diagnostic DNA probes are being developed. The polymerase chain reaction (PCR) has been used to rapidly diagnose orificial TB and appears promising for speeding up the diagnosis of GUTB.

DIFFERENTIAL DIAGNOSIS

Differential diagnosis of GUTB should include amebiasis as well as those entities that mimic granulomatous disease such as sarcoid, other mycobacterial disease (including leprosy), actinomycosis, histoplasmosis, tularemia, berylliosis, silicosis, foreign body reactions and sexually transmitted diseases.[12] Other differential diagnoses include calyceal or diverticular stones, xanthogranulomatous pyelonephritis, obstructive pyonephrosis and congenital multicystic dysplastic kidney.[11] The salpingitis and infertility of genital TB in women needs to be differentiated from that due to pelvic inflammatory disease.

MANAGEMENT

Many authors believe that there is little difference between the treatment decisions for extrapulmonary and pulmonary TB. Genitourinary TB should be easier to treat than pulmonary TB for several reasons:
- the lower bacillary load;
- the kidneys' excellent blood supply;
- the high concentration of bactericidal medication in urine; and
- excellent drug penetration into closed cavities in lethal concentrations.[19]

Daily isoniazid, rifampin (rifampicin), and pyrazinamide (PZA) for 2–3 months, followed by isoniazid and rifampin for the remainder of the therapeutic course have been used successfully (Fig. 61.8). If the patient comes from an area where drug resistance is common then a fourth drug, usually ethambutol, is added until drug susceptibility tests for *M. tuberculosis* have been completed.[13]

A 4-month regimen for GUTB has been advocated, with excellent results.[20] However, a high incidence of surgical intervention was observed. A tailored regimen should be devised for each patient based on susceptibility. The recommended treatment of GUTB, if sensitive, is a 9-month course of INH and rifampin or, alternatively, a 6-month course with isoniazid, rifampin, pyrazinamide and ethambutol, as above. The mycobacterial burden is thought to be lower than in cavitary TB and the short course regimens are recommended for extrapulmonary disease in the same fashion.

A common problem in the management of GUTB is the progression of nephroureteric disease despite therapy with appropriate antimicrobials and negative sequential urine cultures. Obstructive fibrosis can occur anywhere along the urinary tract and is secondary to the healing process that begins after initiation of effective chemotherapy.[16] Corticosteroids, endoscopic balloon dilatation and placement of stents for ureteral strictures have been advocated and may obviate the need for reconstructive or ablative surgery.

Nephrectomy should be restricted to patients with intractable pain for longer than 1 year, uncontrollable or recalcitrant fever secondary to infection proximal to the stricture, life-threatening hematuria, uncontrollable hypertension secondary to renal TB and insurmountable drug resistance.[19] It has been suggested that surgical intervention for pelvic TB is indicated for:

Medication	Dose/day	Side effects
	MEDICATIONS COMMONLY USED FOR RENAL TUBERCULOSIS	
Isoniazid	5–10mg/kg–300mg (max)	Hepatitis, peripheral neuropathy (pyridoxine may decrease the incidence), systemic lupus erythematosus, Dupuytren's contracture
Rifampin	10mg/kg–600mg po, single dose on empty stomach	Gastrointestinal irritation, abnormal liver function tests, stains body secretions orange, flu-like syndrome, multiple drug interactions
Ethambutol	25mg/kg for 2 months then 15mg/kg po	Optic neuritis manifested as changes in visual acuity and red–green color blindness, gastrointestinal discomfort
Pyrazinamide	25mg/kg to a maximum of 2.5g po	arthralgia, hyperuricemia
Streptomycin	15 mg/kg im	Ototoxicity, nephrotoxicity
Capreomycin/ amikacin	0.75/1.0g for 2–3 months then 1.0g 2–3 times a week	Low potassium, low magnesium

Fig. 61.8 Medications commonly used for renal tuberculosis with dosages and common side effects.

- recalcitrant disease,
- persistent pain,
- abnormal bleeding, and
- nonhealing fistulas.[11]

Re-evaluation of GUTB should include urine cultures every 3 months and proof of cure must be documented by culture.[7] In addition, IVPs or ultrasounds should be considered every 6 months to rule out obstructive uropathy until the clinical regimen has been completed. In addition, renal function should be assessed every 6 months for 2 years after therapy. No other specific intervention is necessary unless the patient experiences a recurrence of symptoms.

REFERENCES

1. Cantwell MF, Snider DE Jr, Cauthen GM, Onorato IM. Epidemiology of tuberculosis in the United States, 1985 through 1992. JAMA 1994;272:535–9.
2. Extrapulmonary tuberculosis in the United States. United States Department of Health, Education and Welfare, Public Health Service. Center for Disease Control, HEW Pub. No. (CDC) 78–8360, 1978.
3. Poulios C, Malovrouvas D. Progress in the approach of tuberculosis of the genitourinary tract: remarks on a decade's experience over cases. Acta Urol Belg 1990;58:101–23.
4. Goldfarb DS, Saiman L. Tuberculosis of the genitourinary tract. In: Rom WN, Stuart MG, eds. *Tuberculosis.* New York: Little, Brown and Company, Inc.; 1996:609–22.
5. Allen FJ, de Kock ML. Genito-urinary tuberculosis – experience with 52 urology inpatients. S Afr Med J 1993;83:903–7.
6. Garcia-Rodriguez JA, Garcia Sanchez JE, Munoz Bellido JL. Genitourinary tuberculosis in Spain: a review of 81 cases. Clin Infect Dis 1994;18:557–61.
7. Rubin RH, Cotran RS, Tolkoff-Rubin NE. Urinary tract infection, pyelonephritis, and reflux nephropathy. In: Brenner BM, ed. The kidney, 5th ed. Philadelphia: WB Saunders Company; 1996:1597–1654.
8. Smith MHD, Weinstein AJ. Genitourinary tuberculosis. In: Schlossberg D, ed. Tuberculosis, 3rd ed. New York: Springer-Verlag; 1994:155–63.
9. Heaton ND, Hogan B, Michell M, Thompson P, Yates-Bell AJ. Tuberculous epididymo-orchitis: clinical and ultrasound observations. Br J Urol 1989;64:305–9.
10. Konohana A, Noda J, Shoji K, Hanyaku H. Primary tuberculosis of the glans penis. J Am Acad Dermatol 1992;26:1002–3.
11. Premkumar A, Lattimer J, Newhouse JH. CT and sonography of advanced urinary tract tuberculosis. Am J Radiol 1987;148:65–9.
12. Varma TR. Genital tuberculosis and subsequent fertility. Int J Gynaecol Obstet 1991;35:1–11.
13. Winn RE, Meier PA. Extrapulmonary tuberculosis. In: Hoeprich PD, Jordan MC, Ronald AR, eds. Infectious diseases: a treatise of infectious processes. Philadelphia: JB Lippincott Company; 1994:465–72.
14. Essential components of a tuberculosis prevention and control program, screening for tuberculosis and tuberculosis infection in high-risk populations. Atlanta, GA: Morbidity and Mortality Weekly Report. Recommendations of the Advisory Council for the Elimination of Tuberculosis; 1995 U.S. Centers for Disease Control No. RR-11.
15. Gokalp A, Gultekin EY, Ozdamar S. Genito-urinary tuberculosis: a review of 83 cases. Br J Clin Pract 1990;44:599–600.
16. Stockigt JR, Challis DR, Mirams JA. Hypertension due to renal tuberculosis: assessment by renal vein renin sampling. Aust N Z J Med 1976;6:229–33.
17. Alvarez S, McCabe WR. Extrapulmonary tuberculosis revisited: a review of experience at Boston City and other hospitals. Medicine 1984;63:25–55.
18. Neal DE Jr, Wasler E. Tuberculosis, fungal diseases, and parasitic diseases of the urinary tract. In: Resnick MI, Older RA, eds. Diagnosis of genitourinary disease, 2nd ed. New York: Thieme; 1997:285–302.
19. Weinberg AC, Boyd SD. Short-course chemotherapy and role of surgery in adult and pediatric genitourinary tuberculosis. Urology 1988;31:95–102.
20. Gow JG, Barbosa S. Genitourinary tuberculosis. A study of 1,117 cases over a period of 34 years. Br J Urol 1984;56:449–55.

Practice Points

Asymptomatic urinary infection in women with diabetes mellitus

Allan Ronald & George Zhanel

THE CLINICAL PROBLEM

A 40-year old white woman with a 26-year history of insulin-dependent diabetes mellitus consults you for moderate renal impairment [creatinine 290µmol/l (3.3mg/dl), urea 23.5mmol/l (66mg/dl)], proteinuria (3.5g in 24 hours), and pyuria (100 leukocytes per high-power field). The patient's diabetes has been stable on twice daily insulin and no other therapeutic agents. She denies any urinary tract symptoms except for nocturia three times each night. A first morning void urine culture obtained on two occasions showed $>10^5$ cfu/ml of *Escherichia coli*, which was susceptible to all antimicrobial agents tested. The patient has no previous history of urinary infection and has had no pregnancies.

BACKGROUND

Asymptomatic bacteriuria is common in women with diabetes, with a prevalence three times that of controls. Among patients with diabetes and asymptomatic bacteriuria, upper tract urinary infection is often present with 'localization studies' demonstrating renal infection in 50–70% of women. In this population, asymptomatic infection frequently progresses to acute pyelonephritis and acute renal infection is commonly complicated by bacteremia. Among women with diabetes, acute urinary tract infections (UTIs) are the second most frequent reason for hospital admissions. In a recent population-based study, the rate of hospitalization for acute pyelonephritis was 10 times greater among both men and women with diabetes than in the nondiabetic population. The determinants of asymptomatic bacteriuria and its complications among women with diabetes are mostly hypothetical and unsubstantiated. It is assumed that hyperglycemia and glycosuria with resulting impairment of leukocyte function and enhanced microbial metabolism, diabetic neuropathy with a neurogenic bladder, and renal microangiopathy each contribute to increased susceptibility to bacteriuria among women with diabetes. However, these hypotheses have not been tested in controlled studies. As a result, additional investigation is required to understand fully the factors that facilitate bacteriuria among women with diabetes.

No well-conducted prospective studies have shown that asymptomatic bacteriuria in diabetes contributes significantly to end-stage renal function; rather deterioration in renal function is almost always due to changes relating to progressive glomerulosclerosis.

Among patients with renal failure, regardless of the cause, asymptomatic bacteriuria is common. In most instances, these infections are presumably not due to the renal impairment but rather to multiple factors common in patients with renal failure including prior urologic investigation, failure to achieve adequate antibacterial concentrations in renal tissue or in the urine, and altered host defenses. Few large cross-sectional studies have been carried out in patients with asymptomatic bacteriuria and renal impairment and no definitive prospective studies are published. As a result, there is no information on the significance of asymptomatic bacteriuria in patients with renal failure, the importance of its treatment, or its contribution to further loss of renal function.

Diabetes is now the most common cause of renal failure, accounting for about one-third of patients in developed countries, and asymptomatic infection in patients with diabetes and impaired renal function is exceedingly common. As a result, the clinical scenario of a woman with either type 1 or type 2 diabetes, impaired renal function and asymptomatic bacteriuria is often encountered.

What are the appropriate recommendations for the management of this patient? Should the patient have been screened for bacteriuria? Does the presence of pyuria have any prognostic significance? Once she is discovered to have bacteriuria, should she have further investigation or treatment? Without more data, therapeutic regimens are empiric and unproven, and decisions must be based on anectodal experience and personal opinion.

SPECIFIC ISSUES
Diagnosis

The definitive diagnosis of asymptomatic UTI requires at least two urine cultures obtained as clean-voided midstream urine samples in order to have at least 95% assurance of bacteriuria. However, no studies have validated these criteria in patients with renal impairment. The presence of white blood cells provides credence to the diagnosis of asymptomatic bacteriuria. The microbial etiology of asymptomatic bacteriuria in diabetes is predominantly *E. coli* with more resistant organisms in patients who have had hospital admissions or instrumentation. Some pathogens, particularly *Proteus mirabilis*, may more often be associated with complications, and some physicians would treat these pathogens regardless of symptoms because of their propensity to cause struvite calculi. In some studies, they have also been associated with an increased occurance of acute pyelonephritis.

In patients with renal failure and complicated diabetes, clinical symptoms due to 'asymptomatic bacteriuria' can be difficult to exclude. Can asymptomatic infection cause nonspecific illness including fatigue, irritability, or malaise? Some patients after treatment of 'asymptomatic' infection relate improvement of symptoms that are not usually attributed to bacteriuria.

Imaging studies in these patients are also problematic. Ultrasound studies lack sensitivity and specificity. Intravenous pyelography is contraindicated by the presence of renal failure and diabetes. A helical computed tomography (CT) scan is the most effective means of excluding obstructing lesions, particularly calculi, evaluating renal size, and identifying other abnormalities. The net marginal cost of obtaining a noncontrast helical CT scan may be less than that of ultrasonography, and it should usually be the imaging procedure of choice. Contrast should not be used unless absolutely essential and, when it is necessary, the patient should be well hydrated and a low ionic formulation should be prescribed. Imaging, preferably with a helical

CT scan, is indicated in order to ensure that no remedial causes of renal impairment are present.

TREATMENT

In the presence of an intact urinary system and significant renal impairment presumed to be due to diabetes, how would we treat this asymptomatic infection? At present, no one can be dogmatic. We would choose treatment empirically in the hope that within several years clinical studies will have demonstrated the possible benefit of treatment or perhaps have identified a subset within this population in whom treatment is worthwhile. In treating such patients, we are hoping to prevent the complications of urinary infection that do occur with increased frequency in this population. However, there is no conclusive evidence that presumptive treatment prevents progression of renal impairment or acute complications, including acute pyelonephritis.

The choice of treatment is important. A therapeutic agent should be selected that will achieve reasonable levels in both renal tissue and urine despite impaired function. Renal tissue may be even further impaired regionally owing to altered perfusion with variable antimicrobial levels. Also, an agent should be selected that is not known to be toxic to the kidney. There is no urgency to treat asymptomatic infection, and susceptibility tests can identify one or more potential 'safe' agents. In this instance, we would choose a fluoroquinolone or trimethoprim alone. Sulfonamides, aminoglycsides and tetracyclines should not be prescribed. The fluoroquinolones, including ciprofloxacin, and the newer agents levofloxacin, trovofloxacin, gatifloxacin and others are well tolerated and diffuse widely in renal tissue. Nitrofurantoin should never be used in patients with impaired renal function because it does not achieve adequate urine or renal levels and metabolites rapidly accumulate and produce serious neurological toxicity.

We would prescribe the antibacterial agent for 14 days, obtain a urine culture on the last day of therapy to ensure temporary eradication of infection, and follow the patient. If the pathogen recurred within 2 weeks, after discussion with the patient we might prescribe a longer course of therapy with the intent that in this 'normal functioning' urinary tract, a cure of asymptomatic bacteriuria could be obtained and that this objective is worthwhile. However, if the patient continued to have recurrences, particularly with different organisms, and these remain asymptomatic, we would not pursue treatment or prescribe ongoing suppressive regimens or prophylaxis unless the patient appears to have clinical improvement in objective or subjective symptoms during the course of therapy.

In summary, this example illustrates our lack of knowledge in proper management strategies for patients with asymptomatic bacteriuria in the presence of diabetes or renal impairment. Careful clinical studies are necessary for a further understanding of the pathogenesis of UTIs in these patients and to enable bacteriuria to be managed on the basis of evidence rather than empiricism.

FURTHER READING

Kaplan DM, Rosenfield AT, Smith RC. Advances in the imaging of renal infection, helical CT and modern coordinated imaging. Infect Dis Clin North Am 1997;11:681–706.

Nicolle LE, Friesen D, Harding GKM, Roos LL. Hospitalization for acute pyelonephritis in Manitoba, Canada during the period from 1989 to 1992: impact of diabetes, pregnancy and aboriginal origin. Clin Infect Dis 1996;22:1051–6.

Stamm WE, McKevith M, Roberts DL, et al. Natural history of recurrent urinary tract infection in women. Rev Infect Dis 1991;13:77–84.

Zhanel GG, Harding GKM, Nicholle LE. Asymptomatic bacteriuria in patients with diabetes mellitus. Rev Infect Dis 1991;13:150–4.

Zhanel GG, Nicolle LE, Harding GKM and the Manitoba Diabetic Urinary Infection Study Group. Prevalence of asymptomatic bacteriuria and associated host factors in women with diabetes mellitus. Clin Infect Dis 1995;21:316–22.

Management of persistent symptoms of prostatitis _John N Krieger_

INTRODUCTION

'Prostatitis' is the diagnosis given to a large group of men who present with varied complaints referable to the lower urogenital tract and perineum. By one estimate, 50% of adult men experience symptoms of prostatitis at some time in their lives. Data from the National Health Center for Health Statistics indicate that there were 76 office visits per 1000 men per year for genitourinary problems, with prostatitis accounting for approximately 25% of these visits. Patients may experience symptoms for prolonged periods. Management of patients who experience persistent symptoms following repeated courses of treatment represents a clinical challenge.

PATHOGENESIS

Most prostate infections occur by ascending through the urethra. Therefore, mechanical factors such as urethral length, micturition, and ejaculation provide some protection, although the relative importance of such defenses is unclear. The oblique courses of the ejaculatory ducts and some prostatic ducts have also been proposed as mechanical defenses. Other host defenses include the antimicrobial activity in the prostatic secretions, particularly a zinc-containing polypeptide known as prostatic antibacterial factor. The prostate has higher concentrations of zinc than any other organ and prostatic secretions from normal men contain high zinc levels. Men with chronic bacterial prostatitis have low zinc concentrations in their prostatic fluid, but their serum zinc levels are normal and oral zinc supplements do not increase the zinc levels in the prostatic secretions. Local immunoglobulin production by the prostate also appears to be an important host defense. Many patients with prostatitis have increased leukocyte numbers in their prostatic secretions or semen, but the role of cellular immunity in resolving chronic prostatitis remains unresolved.

Hematogenous dissemination may result in prostatic infection in patients with systemic infections, such as tuberculosis or other granulomatous infections. This route is especially common in patients who are immunosuppressed or who have HIV infections. Rarely, patients develop prostatic infection or abscesses owing to involvement by infection of adjacent organs, for example with perforated appendicitis or diverticulitis.

MICROBIOLOGY
Uropathogenic bacteria

Bacteriuria is a hallmark of acute and chronic bacterial prostatitis. The agents are standard uropathogens associated with bacterial urinary tract infection (e.g. Enterobacteriaceae, pseudomonads, enterococci). Recurrent infections caused by the same organism are an indispensable criterion for the diagnosis of chronic bacterial prostatitis. Between episodes of bacteriuria these organisms may be 'localized' to the prostate as described below. Unfortunately, patients with well-documented acute and chronic bacterial prostatitis constitute a minority of patients presenting with prostatitis (less than 10% in our clinic).

CLASSIFICATION OF PROSTATITIS SYNDROMES				
Category		Characteristic clinical features	Bacteriuria	Inflammation
I	Acute bacterial prostatitis	Acute UTI	+	+
II	Chronic bacterial prostatitis	Recurrent UTI caused by the same organism	–	+
III	Chronic prostatitis/chronic pelvic pain syndrome	Primarily complaints of pain, but also of voiding problems and sexual dysfunction		
	A Inflammatory subtype (formerly 'nonbacterial prostatitis')		–	+
	B Non-inflammatory subtype (formerly 'prostatodynia')		–	–
IV	Asymptomatic	Diagnosed during evaluation of other genitourinary complaints	–	+

Fig. 62.1 **Classification of prostatitis syndromes.** This classification is produced by the National Institutes of Health. Inflammation refers to objective evidence of an inflammatory response in expressed prostatic secretions, postprostate massage urine or semen, or by histology.

Other genitourinary pathogens

Other genitourinary pathogens have been implicated as causes of prostatitis. The best evidence supports a role for sexually transmitted pathogens. In the preantibiotic era, *Neisseria gonorrhoeae* was a recognized cause of prostatitis and the most common cause of prostatic abscess. However, in current practice *N. gonorrhoeae* is seldom implicated. Some studies suggest a role for other sexually transmitted infections, particularly *Chlamydia trachomatis*, *Ureaplasma urealyticum*, and *Trichomonas vaginalis*. The role of each of these organisms remains controversial and the precise proportion of cases attributable to these pathogens is undefined.

Granulomatous infections

A few patients develop granulomatous prostatitis, an uncommon syndrome representing a characteristic histologic reaction of the prostate to a variety of insults. Granulomatous prostatitis may be classified as 'specific' when associated with particular granulomatous infections or as 'nonspecific' in other cases. Causes of nonspecific granulomatous prostatitis include:
• acute bacterial prostatitis,
• prostatic surgery, and
• rheumatoid diseases.
Specific causes of granulomatous prostatitis include:
• infection with *Mycobacterium tuberculosis*,
• infection with atypical mycobacteria,
• bacillus Calmette–Guérin vaccine after topical therapy for transitional cell carcinoma, and
• the deep mycoses (especially blastomycosis, coccidioidomycosis, and cryptococcosis).
The clinical point is that specific diagnostic studies are necessary to document sexually transmitted agents or granulomatous infections in patients who may be at risk. Accurate diagnosis is prerequisite for successful treatment, which may require antimicrobials seldom prescribed for standard uropathogens.

CLINICAL FEATURES

Prostatitis can be classified into four categories (Fig. 62.1):
• acute bacterial prostatitis,
• chronic bacterial prostatitis,
• chronic prostatitis/chronic pelvic pain syndrome, and
• asymptomatic prostatitis.

Acute bacterial prostatitis

The clinical features of acute bacterial prostatitis are readily apparent. Characteristic complaints include acute symptoms of urinary tract infection, such as:
• urgency,
• frequency,
• dysuria, and
• occasionally gross hematuria or acute urinary retention.
Patients may also have systemic symptoms of a 'flu-like' syndrome, with fever, chills, myalgias, or other symptoms associated with bacteremia. Patients may experience bladder outflow obstruction caused by acute edema of the prostate.

Physical examination may show a high temperature, lower abdominal or suprapubic discomfort owing to bladder infection, or urinary retention. The rectal examination is often impressive, with an exquisitely tender, tense prostate. Urinalysis reveals pyuria, and cultures will be positive for uropathogenic bacteria. Systemic leukocytosis is common, with increased numbers of segmented cells. Bacteremia may occur spontaneously or result from vigorous rectal examinations.

Chronic bacterial prostatitis

The characteristic clinical feature of chronic bacterial prostatitis is recurrent episodes of bacteriuria caused by the same organism. The patient may be totally asymptomatic or have only minimal symptoms between bouts of bacteriuria. The infected prostate remains a focus of organisms, causing relapsing infection in such patients. The prostate is usually normal on either rectal or endoscopic evaluation.

On occasion, chronic bacterial prostatitis presents as a systemic illness. Small numbers of bacteria in the prostate do not cause systemic illness. With acute exacerbations, bladder bacteriuria and secondary sepsis may result from the prostatic focus. This is especially true among older men, who may have the combination of prostatic obstruction and infection.

Chronic prostatitis

Chronic prostatitis/chronic pelvic pain syndrome is the new National Institutes of Health consensus term for the largest group of patients with prostatitis. Chronic pelvic pain is the most common presentation, especially perineal, lower abdominal, testicular, penile and ejaculatory pain. Other genitourinary tract complaints include sexual dysfunction and voiding complaints. Some patients have objective evidence of inflammation in their prostatic secretions, post-prostate massage urine, or semen (inflammatory subtype of chronic prostatitis/chronic pelvic pain syndrome, formerly termed 'nonbacterial prostatitis'), whereas others have no evidence of inflammation (noninflammatory subtype of chronic prostatitis/chronic pelvic pain syndrome, formerly called 'prostatodynia').

Asymptomatic prostatitis

Asymptomatic prostatitis may be diagnosed among men undergoing evaluation for other genitourinary tract problems. For example, some patients undergoing evaluation for infertility have increased concentrations of leukocytes in their seminal fluid. Chronic prostatitis is also the most common 'benign' diagnosis among men who undergo prostate biopsy for evaluation of elevated prostate specific antigen levels, suggesting the possibility of prostate cancer.

INVESTIGATIONS

The critical practice point is to distinguish patients with lower-urinary-tract complaints associated with bacteriuria from the larger number of men without bacteriuria. Careful review of the history, physical examination and previous laboratory studies is helpful in making this distinction. Patients with bacteriuria may have acute or chronic bacterial prostatitis, whereas these conditions are rare in patients with no history of bacteriuria.

Documentation of uropathogens

Urine culture and sensitivity testing is essential for men with acute lower urinary tract symptoms. Men with documented bacteriuria should have lower urinary tract localization studies (see Chapter 2.58). The purpose of this investigation is to document a prostatic focus of infection when the patient does not have an bacteriuria. Documenting persistent prostatic infection supports the need for continued antimicrobial therapy.

Unequivocal diagnosis of bacterial prostatitis requires that the colony count of a recognized uropathogen in post-massage urine [voided bladder (VB)$_3$] urine exceed the colony count in the first-void urine (VB$_1$) by at least a factor of 10. However, many men with chronic bacterial prostatitis harbor only small numbers of pathogenic bacteria in their prostates. Direct culture of the expressed prostatic secretions (EPS) is useful in this situation because colony counts in EPS are often 1 or 2 logs higher than comparable counts in the VB$_3$. The hallmark of chronic bacterial prostatitis is that the uropathogen present in VB$_3$ or EPS may be isolated on multiple occasions and is identical to the organism causing episodes of bacteriuria.

Documentation of other infectious agents

Patients with risk factors for sexually transmitted pathogens should have appropriate testing for *N. gonorrhoeae, C. trachomatis* and other agents (if possible). Serologic testing should be recommended for both syphilis and for HIV infection. Patients who have clinical findings suggesting granulomatous prostatitis should have appropriate studies for specific agents associated with this condition (often requiring histologic studies and cultures of prostate tissue).

Documentation of inflammation

Microscopic evaluation is important to identify EPS inflammation because this provides objective support for the diagnosis of chronic prostatitis. We prefer to define inflammation based on chamber counts with >1,000 leukocytes/mm^3. There appears to be little value in counting EPS leukocytes in patients with urethral inflammation, especially among men at risk for sexually transmitted diseases. Therefore, we examine a urethral smear before proceeding with the lower urinary tract localization study.

Other investigations

Our standard approach is to recommend noninvasive uroflow and post-void residual testing (by ultrasound). Patients with abnormal flow rates or significant postvoid residual urine have additional evaluation with a retrograde urethrogram to evaluate the possibility of urethral stricture, and video urodynamics are reserved for patients with abnormal uroflow findings and negative urethrograms. Cystoscopy is recommended if carcinoma *in situ* or interstitial cystitis are considered likely (e.g. in older patients, those with hematuria or a history of chemical exposure, or patients where painful voiding complaints are prominent). Urinary cytology is obtained if transitional cell carcinoma *in situ* is considered prominently in the differential diagnosis. For patients undergoing cystoscopy, we prefer general or regional anesthesia and recommend hydrodistension with appropriate bladder biopsies. Prostate specific antigen testing should be considered because occasional patients with carcinoma of the prostate present with persistent symptoms of prostatitis. However, such testing should not be recommended for patients with more acute symptoms, since temporary elevation of prostate specific antigen (and acid phosphatase) is common following acute episodes. Transrectal ultrasound evaluation may also be considered in selected patients to evaluate possible ejaculatory duct obstruction or complications such as prostatic abscess.

MANAGEMENT

Acute bacterial prostatitis

Appropriate therapy results in dramatic improvement. Many antimicrobials that do not penetrate the uninflamed prostate have proved effective. Thus, drugs appropriate for Enterobacteriaceae, pseudomonads or enterococci should be started once cultures are obtained. For men who require hospitalization, conventional therapy is the combination of an aminoglycoside plus a beta-lactam drug. The fluoroquinolones or third-generation cephalosporins are attractive alternatives for monotherapy.

For less severe infections the conventional choice for outpatient therapy is trimethoprim–sulfamethoxazole (TMP–SMX; co-trimoxazole). Beta-lactams or fluoroquinolones are also useful as oral therapy for patients with acute bacterial prostatitis who do not require hospitalization. We usually prescribe one of the newer quinolones for outpatient management.

Patients with acute urinary retention require bladder drainage. In this situation we prefer a suprapubic cystostomy tube, placed either using a percutaneous trocar or by open surgery. An indwelling transurethral catheter would pass through and obstruct drainage of the acutely infected prostate, increasing the risk for bacteremia and prostatic abscess. General measures are also indicated, including hydration, analgesics, and bed rest.

Chronic bacterial prostatitis

Trimethoprim–sulfamethoxazole is the 'gold standard.' Long-term therapy with trimethoprim (80mg) plus sulfamethoxazole (400mg) taken orally twice daily for 4–16 weeks is superior to shorter courses. Such therapy results in symptomatic and bacteriologic cure in approximately one-third of patients, symptomatic improvement during therapy in approximately one-third (who relapse after stopping treatment), and no improvement in the remaining patients.

During the past decade the fluoroquinolones have proved useful for treatment of chronic bacterial prostatitis. In contrast to the beta-lactams, concentrations of many fluoroquinolones are relatively high in prostatic fluid, prostatic tissue and seminal fluid compared to plasma levels. Good results were reported for men with bacterial prostatitis, including patients who failed therapy with TMP–SMX. Promising agents include norfloxacin, ciprofloxacin, ofloxacin and enoxacin. Currently our first choice for curative therapy for chronic bacterial prostatitis is usually an appropriate fluoroquinolone at full-dose for at least 3 months.

Patients who are not cured benefit from long-term suppressive treatment using low-dose antimicrobial agents. Because most patients are asymptomatic between episodes of bacteriuria, the goal of suppressive therapy is to prevent symptomatic of bacteriuria. Very low doses of drugs are remarkably effective. Available agents include penicillin G, tetracycline, nitrofurantoin, naladixic acid, cephalexin and TMP–SMX. Although effective, we seldom recommend fluoroquinolones for chronic suppression, because of cost and the potential for development of antimicrobial-resistant organisms.

Chronic prostatitis/chronic pelvic pain syndrome

Therapy is often unsatisfactory because the etiology of chronic prostatitis/chronic pelvic pain syndrome remains unclear. As outlined above, an etiologic role has been suggested for many infectious agents. Prostaglandins, autoimmunity, psychological abnormalities, neuromuscular dysfunction of the bladder neck or urogenital diaphragm, allergy to environmental agents, stress and other psychological factors have all been suggested as causes.

Antimicrobial drugs are often considered the first-line treatment. Patients with recognized uropathogens may respond to such empirical therapy. For men without evidence of infection by recognized pathogens, antimicrobial treatment often results in only temporary, if any, relief. Because long-term antimicrobial therapy offers limited benefit for patients with no evidence of urogenital infection, we recommend a thorough evaluation for infectious agents. We prescribe antimicrobials only for patients with documented infections rather than recommending repeated courses of empirical therapy.

Other recommended treatments include:
- prostate massage,
- anti-inflammatory drugs,
- anti-cholinergic drugs,
- allopurinol,
- muscle relaxants,
- transurethral resection of the prostate,
- other surgical procedures,
- sitz baths, diathermy, exercises, physiotherapy, and
- psychotherapy.

Some clinicians recommend increased frequency of ejaculation to relieve 'congestion.' Others recommend abstinence from ejaculation, alcohol, coffee, tea, spicy foods, etc. There is little objective evidence that any of these measures changes the natural history of chronic prostatitis/chronic pelvic pain syndrome.

CONCLUSIONS

Patients with documented bacteriuria may have acute or chronic bacterial prostatitis, while these conditions are rare in patients with no history of bacteriuria. Specific diagnostic studies are necessary to document uropathogens, sexually transmitted agents or granulomatous infections in patients with prostatitis. Other diagnoses should are possible in selected patients. Accurate diagnosis is prerequisite for successful treatment.

FURTHER READING

Kneger JN. Prostatitis syndromes. In: Holmes KK, Sparling PF, Mardh PA, *et al*, eds. Sexually transmitted diseases, 3rd ed. New York: McGraw-Hill; 1998.

Urinary tract infection in a 24-year-old woman with spinal cord injury and indwelling catheter

John Z Montgomerie & Kim Maeder

INTRODUCTION

Urinary tract infection (UTI) occurs in most patients with spinal cord injury (SCI) during initial hospitalization and rehabilitation and may be a recurrent problem throughout their lives. Until methods of urinary drainage were improved, infections were the dominant cause of bacteremia and renal failure. These complications, together with calculi and pyelonephritis, still occur more frequently in patients with indwelling urethral catheters. Indwelling catheters are used by more than 20% of patients with SCI in the USA.

PATHOGENESIS

The pathogenesis of UTI depends on the type of bladder drainage. Most patients immediately following SCI have an indwelling urethral catheter that is always associated with bacteriuria. In most SCI centers the catheter is removed within a few days and intermittent catheterization is the preferred method of urine drainage.

Changes in the bladder associated with the long-term use of indwelling catheters include squamous metaplasia, thickening and fibrosis of the bladder wall, bladder contraction, diverticuli, calculi, alkaline encrusting cystitis with urease-producing bacteria, and squamous cell carcinoma of the bladder. In male patients, penile and scrotal fistulae, abscesses and epididymitis are other complications.

MICROBIOLOGY

Studies of UTIs from different SCI centers have suggested a wide range of micro-organisms infect the urine with different bacteria predominating at different centers. *Escherichia coli*, *Pseudomonas* spp., *Kiebsiella* spp. and *Enterococcus* spp. have been the predominant micro-organisms causing UTIs in patients with SCI. Some centers have noted a high prevalence of *Proteus* spp.; this may relate to the more frequent use of indwelling catheters, which are also associated with multiple organisms. The presence of urease producers (*Proteus* spp., *Providencia* spp. and *Morganella* spp.) raises concerns about calculus formation.

Indwelling, urethral and suprapubic catheters are associated with calculi, multiple organisms and multiresistant Gram-negative bacilli. The patient's sex and level of spinal injury may affect the microbiology of bacteriuria and colonization. At our institution, male patients have had a high incidence of infection with *Klebsiella* spp. and *Pseudomonas* spp., which relates to the use of external condom catheters, the colonization of the perineum and urethra, and bowel flora and urine in the urine drainage bags. In female patients with SCI receiving intermittent catheterization, *E. coli* and *Enterococcus* spp. account for 71% of infections. It has not been possible to significantly alter the colonization of the perineal skin with increased bathing, the use of antiperspirants or antiseptics to clean the skin.

There are few studies of the modes of transmission of these micro-organisms. Although the patient's body sites and drainage bags are the immediate source of these infections, transmission on the hands of health care personnel is the most likely means of transmission among patients.

CLINICAL FEATURES

Because of loss of sensation, patients with SCI do not usually have the common symptoms of UTI such as frequency, urgency and dysuria. The clinical features of UTI may include fever, pyuria and 'soft' symptoms and signs such as discomfort over the back or abdomen during urination, onset of incontinence, increased spasticity, autonomic hyper-reflexia, malaise, lethargy or observation of cloudy urine with increased odor. The term 'soft' is used because increased spasticity (and other symptoms) may occur in patients without obvious cause. The presence of a catheter by itself may induce spasms. Identification of the infecting organism by urine culture is important. Blood cultures should be obtained if patients have a high fever. Calculus formation may occur with the infection and small stones (called 'gravel') may be present in the urine of patients with indwelling catheters.

INVESTIGATIONS

The exclusion of obstruction and other factors that might influence response to treatment is important. In those patients who void reflexly it is important to determine the residual volume. Ultrasound or intravenous pyelography may be important to confirm that there is no obstruction to urine flow and that there is adequate drainage from the kidneys and bladder. In patients with indwelling catheters it is important to change the catheter if there is any question of its being obstructed.

MANAGEMENT

We should be concerned that a woman with SCI has chosen to use an indwelling urethral catheter rather than intermittent catheterization. This, however, can be a rational choice for women because there are no reasonable external collection devices. As mentioned earlier, 20% of patients with SCI in the USA use indwelling catheters to drain the bladder. The choice is made if the patient is quadriplegic and she cannot use her hands and an assistant is not available. Others, particularly people with full-time jobs or people who travel, will make this decision because of the inconvenience of repeated catheterizations. They use the indwelling catheter to improve their quality of life despite the increased risks to their health. Unfortunately there are few studies of the optimal methods of care of the patient with a long-term indwelling catheter. The recommendations from our own institution and our own observations are listed in Figure 62.2. Urethral catheters need to be changed on a regular basis to prevent obstruction of the catheter that occurs with encrustation that includes struvite and apatite crystals and bacterial biofilm. Changes every 2–4 weeks are almost always adequate to prevent catheter obstruction. Occasional patients will need more frequent change of catheter. Silicone catheters have not been demonstrated to have sufficient advantage to be used routinely.

Studies of patients with long-term indwelling catheters indicate surprisingly few episodes of fever. Most episodes are of low-grade fever that last for less than 24 hours and resolve without antibiotics. Because patients with indwelling urethral catheters are colonized with three or more bacterial species and these change frequently, no useful purpose is served by routine culture. Culture and sensitivity tests should be reserved for patients who are starting on antimicrobial therapy. The laboratory should be notified that the urine was obtained from a patient with an indwelling catheter, otherwise the technicians may consider the multiple bacteria to be contaminants.

Because of a lack of evidence that treating asymptomatic bacteriuria reduces symptomatic bacteriuria or influences the long term function of the urinary tract or kidneys, bacteriuria in all patients with SCI should be treated when symptoms or signs are present. In the patient with SCI and indwelling catheter there are a combination of factors that make us even more reluctant to use antibiotics. Antimicrobial agents rarely eradicate micro-organisms in the presence of the catheter or other foreign bodies, and the bacteria in the urine may become resistant or may be replaced by resistant flora.

In considering the patient who is the topic of this discussion, bacteriuria and pyuria are usually present in the SCI patient with a long-term indwelling catheter. Occasional bladder spasms are also common, particularly with the physical presence of the catheter. By themselves these symptoms and signs do not constitute evidence of a need to treat with antibiotics. Fever is the main indication for treatment but the catheterized patient sometimes hase definite symptoms of UTI without fever. Patients who have had previous episodes of UTI with fever may recognize early symptoms, such as increased bladder spasms or sudden onset of cloudiness of the urine or change of odor. At the first evidence of infection patients should increase their fluid intake. A catheter change should be considered.

CARE OF LONG-TERM INDWELLING CATHETERS

Use the smallest catheter and balloon consistent with minimal leakage
Change catheters regularly each 2–4 weeks
Prevent trauma to the urethra
Maintain at least 2 liters fluid intake daily
Use nonrestrictive clothing
Ensure daily perineal care with soap and water
Urethral antisepsis and routine irrigations are not recommended

Fig. 62.2 Care of long-term indwelling catheters.

If the symptoms persist these patients will respond to oral antibiotics that are active *in vitro*. Appropriate duration of treatment has not been well studied in patients with indwelling catheters but they usually respond to relatively short courses of therapy (5–7 days). If there is evidence of renal infection, longer courses may be indicated. In symptomatic patients with high fever who may have bacteremia, broad coverage may be necessary until the results of the cultures are available because of the frequent presence of resistant bacteria colonizing these patients. Bacteremia in patients with SCI is usually the result of bacteriuria associated with catheterization or other bladder manipulation. In those episodes, enterococci, *E. coli* and *Pseudomonas aeruginosa* are the organisms most frequently isolated from the blood.

The formation of stones in the bladder is a not uncommon problem associated with urease-producing bacteria *(Proteus, Providencia* and *Morganella* spp.). Attempts to clear small stones (gravel) can be made by increasing fluid intake, acidifying the urine or by blocking urease production with acetohydroxamic acid. It is difficult to acidify urine by oral administration of methionine salts, especially in the presence of bacteriuria. Irrigation of the bladder with acid solutions such as Subys solution is sometimes used to dissolve stones, but the hazards of the procedure have not been adequately studied and these efforts should always be short term. Cystoscopy may be necessary to remove the stones.

There are a number of gaps in our understanding of the management of patients with indwelling catheters and further study of the optimal care of the catheter is needed.

FURTHER READING

Kamitsuka PF. The pathogenesis prevention and management of urinary tract infection in patients with spinal cord injury. Curr Clin Top infect Dis 1993;13:1–25.

National Institute on Disability and Rehabilitation Research (NIDRR) Consensus Statement. The prevention and management of urinary tract infections among people with spinal cord injuries. J Am Paraplegia Soc 1992;15:194–207.

Zejdlik CP. Maintaining urinary function. In: Zejdlik CP, ed. Management of spinal cord injury. Boston: Jones and Bartlett Publishers; 1991;353–95.

Gonococcal and Chlamydial Urethritis

Kimberley K Fox & Myron S Cohen

Neisseria gonorrhoeae and *Chlamydia trachomatis* are the two major pathogens responsible for urethritis, a syndrome characterized by urethral discharge and dysuria. Urethritis is defined by its pathognomonic laboratory finding: an increased number of polymorphonuclear leukocytes (PMNs) on the Gram stain of a urethral smear. Urethritis has generally been classified as gonococcal urethritis or nongonococcal urethritis (NGU). The causes of NGU have only recently been elucidated; in addition to *C. trachomatis*, these include *Ureaplasma urealyticum*, *Mycoplasma genitalium*, other infectious agents and a variety of chemical and physical irritants.

EPIDEMIOLOGY

Neisseria gonorrhoeae and *C. trachomatis*, along with most other agents of urethritis, are sexually transmitted pathogens. Both pathogens have a worldwide distribution, although prevalences vary tremendously from region to region. In the USA, the reported incidence of gonorrhea has declined steadily since 1975, but rates remain high in certain population groups. Two major trends characterize the changing epidemiology of gonorrhea in the USA. First, as rates have declined, the rate difference between whites and African-Americans has increased from 10-fold in 1981 to 35-fold in 1994.[1] Second, rates have declined less in those aged 15–19 years than in any other age group (Fig. 63.1). Consequently, the present overall rate of gonorrhea in the USA reflects very low rates in whites and individuals aged over 30 years, with an increasing concentration of the disease in minorities, adolescents and young adults.

Trends in chlamydial infection in the USA are less well documented because accurate tests for *C. trachomatis* have only recently become available and reporting of the infection is not yet required in all states. Chlamydial infection is probably several times more common than gonorrhea. However, currently reported rates of chlamydial infection (Fig. 63.2) reflect screening and reporting practices as much as they reflect the actual distribution of the disease. Specific testing for *C. trachomatis* has been especially limited in men, and reported rates of NGU, which are high and relatively stable, may better reflect the prevalence of this disease.[1]

In Europe, gonorrhea rates declined through the 1980s, reaching rates far lower than those in the USA. Chlamydial infection is still far more common than gonorrhea, as control programs were limited by the lack of diagnostic tests until recently.[2]

In the developing world, rates of gonococcal and chlamydial infection are less well known, but the public health burden of these diseases and their complications is clearly tremendous. In Africa, the prevalence of gonorrhea among pregnant women – the group for which rates are best known – ranges from 2 to 15%; rates of chlamydial infection range from 7 to 30%. Complications such as pelvic inflammatory disease and its sequelae in women, urethral stricture in men, and ophthalmia neonatorum in infants are common.[3]

Risk factors for urethritis are similar to those for other sexually transmitted diseases (STDs): multiple sexual partners, a recent new partner and other sexual behaviors which increase the likelihood of encountering a sexually transmitted pathogen. Young age, low socioeconomic

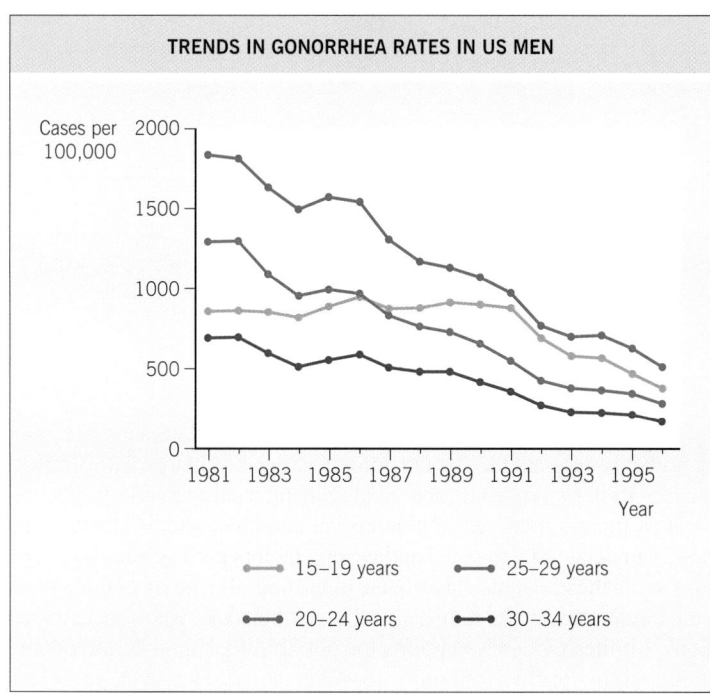

Fig. 63.1 Trends in gonorrhea rates among men aged 15–34 years in the USA, 1981–1996. Rates are cases per 100,000 population.

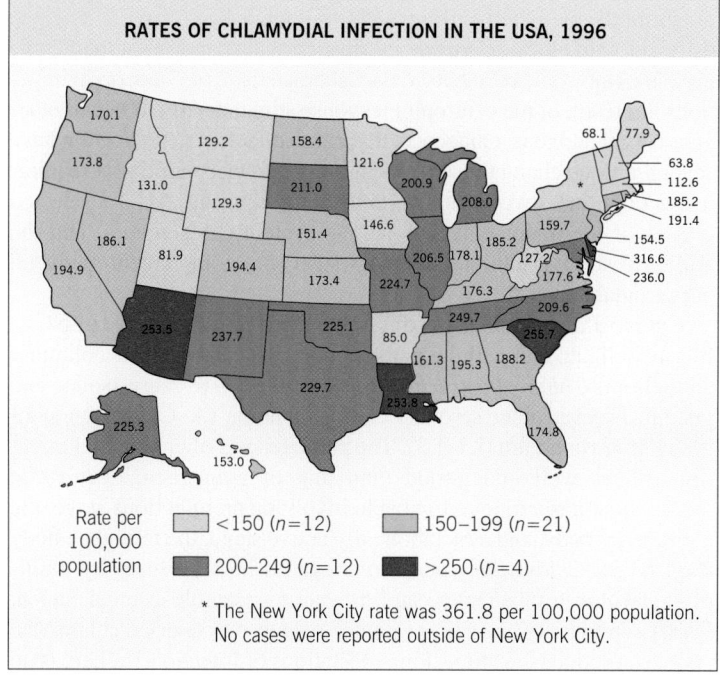

Fig. 63.2 Rates of chlamydial infection in the USA, 1996. Rates are cases per 100,000 population.

INFECTIOUS AND NONINFECTIOUS CAUSES OF URETHRAL DISCHARGE AND DYSURIA		
Major infectious causes	Minor infectious causes	Noninfectious causes
Neisseria gonorrhoeae	*Mycoplasma genitalium*	Chemical irritants (spermicides, bath products)
Chlamydia trachomatis	*Trichomonas vaginalis*	Tumor
Ureaplasma urealyticum	Herpes simplex virus	Foreign body
	Coliform bacteria	Stevens–Johnson syndrome
	Candida albicans	Wegener's granulomatosis
	Treponema pallidum	
	Human papillomavirus	

Fig. 63.3 Infectious and noninfectious causes of urethral discharge and dysuria.

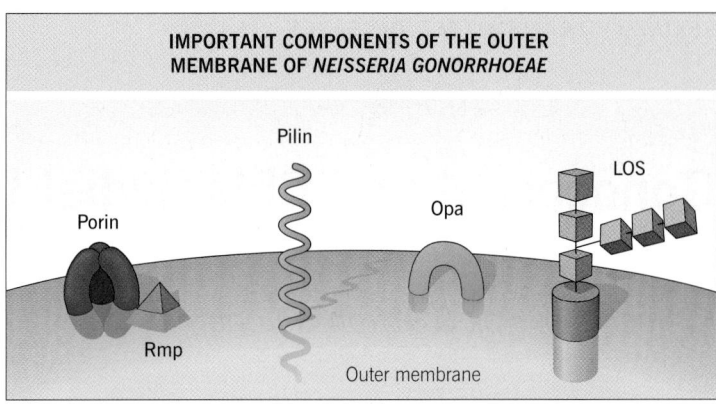

Fig. 63.4 Important components of the outer membrane of *Neisseria gonorrhoeae*. Porin is the major outer membrane protein. Reduction modifiable protein (Rmp) is the target of blocking antibodies that prevent bactericidal antibodies from binding to porin. Pilin and opacity protein (Opa) are important in adhesion. Lipo-oligosaccharide (LOS) stimulates PMN response and, when sialylated, blocks antibody-mediated killing.

status and minority race are recognized as risk markers for STDs. Men with NGU are more often white, better educated and of higher socio-economic status than men with gonorrhea, although there is substantial overlap and risk factors alone cannot be used to predict the cause of urethritis.[4,5] Heterosexual men have higher rates of NGU and chlamydial infection than homosexual men.[6] In addition, 10–30% of men with gonorrhea are co-infected with *C. trachomatis*.[7–9]

PATHOGENESIS AND PATHOLOGY

The large majority of urethritis cases are caused by sexually transmitted infectious agents, most commonly *N. gonorrhoeae* and *C. trachomatis* (Fig. 63.3). For both pathogens, humans are the only natural host. *Neisseria gonorrhoeae* is a Gram-negative diplococcus that is highly adapted for growth on the mucosal membranes, infecting primarily columnar and cuboidal epithelium. Urethral infection requires that the organism first attach to the epithelium and then evade host defenses well enough to survive and multiply. The gonococcus uses a set of complex mechanisms to accomplish these goals (Fig. 63.4).[10] At least two outer membrane proteins, pilin and Opa, are important in adherence. Mechanisms for evading ingestion by PMNs appear to include production of the antioxidant catalase, competition for molecular oxygen and DNA repair mechanisms. Other mechanisms important in the evasion of host defenses include production of an IgA protease, blocking of antibody-mediated killing with sialylated lipo-oligosaccharride (LOS) or with blocking antibodies directed against reduction modifiable protein (Rmp). The purulent exudate characteristic of gonococcal infections is a result of the neutrophil response stimulated by LOS and other gonococcal antigens. Gonococci that cause disseminated infection have several unique characteristics, including particular nutritional requirements (arginine-, hypoxanthine- and uracil-requiring; AHU⁻), selected classes of the major outer membrane protein (IA serovars) and the ability to survive humoral defenses such as a complement-mediated bactericidal attack.[11]

Chlamydia trachomatis is the single most common cause of NGU. It is an obligate intracellular pathogen that primarily infects columnar epithelium. *Chlamydia trachomatis* serovars D–K cause ocular and genital disease; other serovars cause trachoma (A–C) and lymphogranuloma venereum (L1–L3). The pathogenesis of chlamydial infection is less well understood than that of gonorrhea. *Chlamydia trachomatis* has a unique life cycle involving an infectious stage, the elementary body, and a metabolically active stage, the reticulate body (Fig. 63.5). *Chlamydia trachomatis* evades host defenses by multiplying within a phagosome and preventing phagolysosomal fusion. Direct cytotoxicity and a host immune response to selected chlamydial antigens produce the clinical manifestations of infection.[13] There is no evidence that *C. trachomatis* can persist in a truly latent state, but chronic, slowly replicating infection is probably common. Chronic

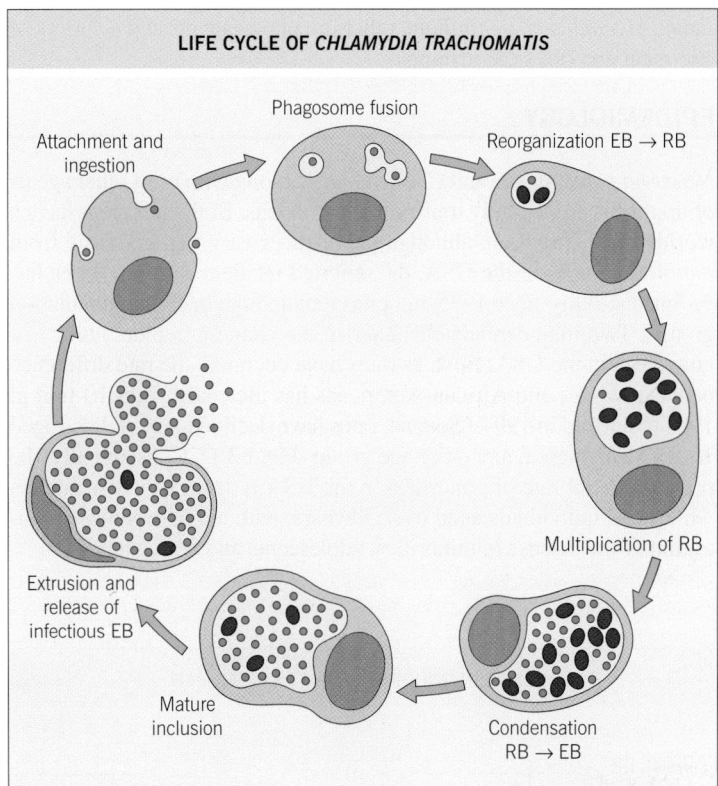

Fig. 63.5 The life cycle of *Chlamydia trachomatis*. The elementary body (EB) invades the host cell and then reorganizes into the metabolically active reticulate body (RB) while in a phagosome. The reticulate body multiplies, and the resultant reticulate bodies reorganize into elementary bodies, which are released by rupture of the host cell. Adapted from Jones, 1995.[12]

infection, with a long-lived humoral and cell-mediated immune response, is probably responsible for the complications of chlamydial infection such as Reiter's syndrome and tubal scarring leading to infertility.

Host factors involved in gonococcal and chlamydial infection are poorly understood. No racial and genetic factors predisposing to infection with these agents have been identified. Terminal complement deficiency predisposes to invasive, but not mucosal, gonococcal infections. Limited evidence supports the possibility of short-term, incomplete, strain-specific immunity to either agent. However, recurrent infections with these agents argue against a long-lived protective immune response after natural infection.

Nonchlamydial NGU is a group of syndromes caused by infectious and noninfectious agents. *Ureaplasma urealyticum* is the most common cause of nonchlamydial NGU, accounting for 10–40% of all NGU cases, although its role as a pathogen has been controversial.[14] *Ureaplasma urealyticum* clearly causes symptomatic infection that responds to specific therapy in some men, but has also been found to colonize as many as 60% of men attending STD clinics.[7,15] In the past decade, *Mycoplasma genitalium* has been recognized as a relatively frequent cause of nonchlamydial NGU.[14,16] *Mycoplasma hominis* is a frequent genital tract colonizer and was long suspected of causing urethritis, but studies have failed to confirm its role as a pathogen in men.

Of NGU cases 10–20% are caused by agents other than *C. trachomatis*, *U. urealyticum* and *M. genitalium*. Herpes simplex virus can cause urethritis, usually in primary infection and in conjunction with external ulcerative lesions.[17] *Trichomonas vaginalis* causes a variable proportion of NGU cases.[18] Coliform bacteria occasionally cause urethritis, especially if phimosis or urethral stricture are present or after urethral instrumentation. Distal urethritis may be caused by *Candida* spp. in association with yeast balanitis involving skin adjacent to the meatus. Urethral discharge without dysuria may be caused by an endourethral syphilitic chancre or by intraurethral condyloma acuminata. Limited evidence suggests that adenovirus, *Haemophilus influenzae*, *Clostridium difficile*, *Neisseria meningitidis* and anaerobic bacteria may occasionally cause urethritis.

A small percentage of NGU cases do not have infectious causes. Spermicides and some bath products can cause a chemical urethritis. An endourethral tumor or intraurethral foreign body can cause a mucoid or bloody discharge and may become secondarily infected with local skin flora. Repeated vigorous urethral stripping (see Physical examination) may eventually cause the production of a clear urethral discharge. Heavy crystalluria or calculous gravel in the urine can produce dysuria, and may have the appearance of a urethral discharge. Systemic illnesses such as Stevens–Johnson syndrome and Wegener's granulomatosis are occasionally associated with urethritis. Finally, the remnants of semen at the meatus or urinary incontinence may be misinterpreted by the patient as urethral discharge.

PREVENTION

The persistence of STDs such as gonococcal and chlamydial urethritis in a community requires the spread of disease from each infected person to, on average, at least one other susceptible person. This concept is expressed in the equation, $Ro = \beta cD$, where the number of secondary infections arising from each case, or reproductive rate (Ro), depends on the efficiency of transmission (β), the rate of sexual partner change (c) and the duration of infectiousness (D).[19] The value of each parameter varies by pathogen and by clinical and behavioural setting.

Gonococcal urethritis transmits infection with high efficiency, around 50–70% for a single act of vaginal intercourse.[20] Without treatment, gonococcal urethritis remains infectious for approximately 6 months, but most cases produce symptoms uncomfortable enough

that men rapidly seek treatment, shortening the infectious period to several days. Given these parameters, the maintenance of gonorrhea in a community in which treatment is readily available requires an average partner change rate of 13 partners per year.[21]

Chlamydial urethritis is transmitted with less efficiency than gonorrhea – approximately 20–50% for a single contact, or 70% for long-term partnerships.[22] Without treatment, chlamydial urethritis remains infectious for around 15 months, and because the majority of cases are asymptomatic, the infectious period remains long despite the ready availability of effective therapy. As a result of this long infectious period, the average partner change rate required to maintain chlamydial infection in a community is estimated at only four partners per year.[22] Most persons with gonococcal or chlamydial infection in fact have lower rates of partner change; however, a small group of people – the core group – with higher rates of partner change are critical in maintaining the spread of infection.[23] This core group for chlamydial infection encompasses a broader population than that for gonorrhea because of the lower number of partners required.

Preventive measures targeting one or more of these key parameters can result in lowered rates of STDs (Fig. 63.6). Treatment of STDs reduces the duration of infectiousness, thereby limiting secondary spread of disease. Highly effective single-dose therapies are recommended for gonorrhea, and single- or multiple-dose therapies for chlamydial infection (see Management). *Neisseria gonorrhoeae* is eliminated from the urethra within hours of oral or parenteral therapy;[24] elimination of *C. trachomatis* is slower. Treatment of the sexual partner is essential to prevent re-infection of the patient and spread to other individuals.

Screening, with prompt treatment of infected persons, is an important strategy to prevent secondary spread of asymptomatic or subclinical infections. Although the majority of gonococcal urethritis is symptomatic, men with asymptomatic infection contribute disproportionately to the spread of gonorrhea.[25] In addition, a large proportion of chlamydial urethritis is asymptomatic, so screening of persons with high-risk behaviors is especially important in limiting the spread of this disease. As chlamydial infection is highly prevalent in many areas now, clinicians should have a low threshold for screening any sexually active person.

Latex condoms are one of the most effective available tools for reducing the efficiency of transmission of gonorrhea and chlamydial infection.[26] The polyurethane female condom, marketed in the USA as Reality, has been demonstrated to reduce transmission of trichomoniasis,[27] and is being studied for effectiveness in preventing transmission of other bacterial STDs. However, this product has had limited user acceptance in the USA.

Vaginal microbicides such as nonoxynol-9 (marketed as a spermicide) have a limited, but perhaps important, role in reducing the transmission efficiency of gonorrhea and chlamydia. Nonoxynol-9 is a detergent, which acts by disrupting cell membranes and viral envelopes. Used intravaginally, without condoms or other barriers, nonoxynol-9 reduces the risk of acquiring gonorrhea by 10–70% and chlamydial infection by 25–40%.[28] The effect of nonoxynol-9 used alone on HIV transmission is unclear. Very frequent use of nonoxynol-9 can cause mucosal disruption and has been associated with an increased risk of HIV transmission. Therefore, the use of nonoxynol-9 alone for STD prevention can only be recommended in situations in which condom use is not feasible. However, there is some evidence that the use of nonoxynol-9 together with a condom is slightly more effective in preventing STDs than use of a condom alone.[29]

Finally, strategies to alter sexual behaviors to reduce the rate of partner change can decrease the spread of STDs. Changes in sexual behavior in the gay community were important in limiting the spread of HIV and other STDs in the 1980s.[30] At the same time, increasingly risky sexual behaviors among heterosexual adolescents have raised concern. The mean age at first intercourse has dropped, and an increasing proportion of adolescents are sexually active.[31]

PREVENTION OF GONOCOCCAL AND CHLAMYDIAL INFECTION	
Primary prevention	Secondary prevention
Male latex condoms	Screening of at-risk individuals
Male polyurethane condoms	Prompt treatment of infected individuals
Female polyurethane condoms	
Microbicides (nonoxynol-9)	
Sexual behavior change	

Fig. 63.6 Prevention of gonococcal and chlamydial infection. These preventive measures reduce the transmission efficiency, the duration of infectiousness, or the rate of sexual partner change.

CLINICAL FEATURES

Urethritis classically produces urethral discharge accompanied by dysuria. The discharge may be scant or copious, and may appear clear, white, yellow or green. Itching around the meatus is common. Frequency, urgency and hematuria are not generally part of this clinical syndrome and should lead to the consideration of alternative diagnoses.

The pattern of urethral symptoms and characteristics of the discharge can provide clues as to the etiologic diagnosis. In gonococcal urethritis, the incubation period is brief (2–6 days). The use of subcurative doses of antibiotics during this time can prolong the incubation period. Symptom onset is abrupt. Gonococcal urethritis usually produces copious, purulent, often yellow–green discharge along with marked dysuria.[4,8] Inguinal lymphadenopathy is absent, although small non-tender nodes, unrelated to the gonococcal infection, may be palpable in a majority of men. Up to 30% of men with gonorrhea are co-infected with *C. trachomatis*;[8,9]. The proportion of men with co-infection may be declining as dual treatment and, more recently, screening for *C. trachomatis* have become widely practiced.

Approximately 2–3% of men with urethral gonococcal infection are asymptomatic, especially those infected with strains that have selected serotypes and auxotypes.[32] These infections may play a disproportionate role in the spread of *N. gonorrhoeae*, as they are identified only through partner notification or by the screening of high-risk populations. Symptomatic gonococcal urethritis becomes asymptomatic if left untreated over a period of months.[33]

Gonococcal and nongonococcal urethritis can be accurately differentiated based on clinical grounds in three-quarters of patients.[4] Chlamydial urethritis has a longer incubation period (1–5 weeks) and produces more subtle symptoms than gonorrhea.[6,8] Onset of symptoms is subacute. The discharge is mucopurulent or mucoid and may be seen only after urethral stripping or in the morning before voiding. A small crust at the meatus may be the only visible discharge and may be associated with meatal itching. Dysuria is frequently present but may be less intense than in gonococcal infection. However, the presence of dysuria without urethral discharge is a very good (90%) predictor of NGU, including chlamydial infection.[4] As with gonorrhea, local lymphadenopathy is absent. One-quarter to one-half of men with chlamydial urethritis are asymptomatic.[6] The clinical manifestations of gonococcal and chlamydial urethritis appear to be similar in non-immunocompromised and immunocompromised patients, including those with HIV infection.

Urethritis caused by *U. urealyticum*, *M. genitalium* or *T. vaginalis* infection is clinically indistinguishable from chlamydial urethritis;[7] when available, laboratory testing for *T. vaginalis* may aid in diagnosis. Primary herpes simplex virus infection frequently results in urethritis accompanying external genital vesicles and ulcers.[17] Dysuria is severe and the mucoid discharge profuse; regional lymphadenopathy is common. Endourethral ulceration may result in localized tenderness along the urethra.

Several symptoms suggest diagnoses other than urethritis. Urinary frequency and urgency, with or without hematuria, suggest cystitis or upper urinary tract infection. Painless hematuria usually originates in the bladder or kidney from a variety of largely noninfectious causes. Hesitancy, dribbling and nocturia require evaluation for urologic and prostatic disorders. Prostate tenderness is not seen with simple urethritis, but may be found in the occasional case of prostatitis accompanying urethritis. Painful ejaculation without dysuria, blood in the ejaculate and pain radiating from the genitals to the pelvis or back are not seen in urethritis and mandate evaluation for other disorders.

COMPLICATIONS

Without treatment, gonococcal and chlamydial urethritis can lead to a variety of complications (Fig. 63.7). Epididymitis occurs in 1–2% of patients, with equal risk from *N. gonorrhoeae* and *C. trachomatis*.[6,34] In this setting, epididymitis is unilateral and is caused by extension of the urethral infection via the vas deferens to the epididymis. Most cases of epididymitis in adult men under the age of 35 years can be attributed to *N. gonorrhoeae* and *C. trachomatis*. Homosexual men who practice anal insertive intercourse may acquire urethritis and epididymitis caused by Gram-negative bacilli. Occasionally, epididymitis extends to the testis, producing epididymo-orchitis. Rapid differentiation of epididymitis and orchitis from testicular torsion is critical as the latter is a surgical emergency. Epididymitis and orchitis are discussed further in Chapter 2.58.

Conjunctivitis, following accidental self-inoculation, complicates as many as 1–2% of cases of gonococcal or chlamydial urethritis.[34] In the pre-antibiotic era, prostatitis and urethral stricture often resulted from prolonged untreated gonococcal urethritis. Periurethral abscess occasionally complicates urethritis caused by coliform bacteria, especially if phimosis or pre-existing urethral stricture are present.

A very small proportion of patients who have chlamydial urethritis develop Reiter's syndrome, with the triad of urethritis, conjunctivitis or uveitis, and arthritis.[35] Other clinical manifestations include painless erythema and ulceration of the glans (circinate balanitis), pustular or hyperkeratotic lesions of the soles of the feet (keratodermia blennorrhagica), nonarticular body pain and oral mucosal ulcerations. The majority of patients who have Reiter's syndrome have the HLA-B27 histocompatibility antigen. Pathogenesis is thought to involve an abnormal host response to antigens of *C. trachomatis*, which have been found in the synovium of affected joints. Reiter's syndrome also develops after infection with certain gastrointestinal pathogens (see Chapter 2.35).

Disseminated gonococcal infection (DGI) arises primarily from asymptomatic gonococcal urethritis caused by strains with particular serotypes (IA) and auxotypes (AHU⁻).[11] Strains associated with disseminated gonococcal infection are also resistant to killing by normal human serum, which presumably allows invasion of the bloodstream and dissemination to distant sites. Terminal complement deficiency predisposes to invasive gonococcal infections, but the majority of patients who have DGI have normal complement levels. Signs and symptoms of DGI include small numbers (usually fewer than 30) of papular, petechial or pustular skin lesions, usually on the hands, wrists and feet, tenosynovitis of the hands or feet or asymmetric polyarthritis involving few joints, and fever. Culture of joint fluid from a patient who has this dermatitis–arthritis syndrome is usually negative, although blood culture may be positive. A frank septic arthritis caused by *N. gonorrhoeae* may develop; in such cases, joint fluid culture is often positive and blood culture negative. Overall, around one-half of patients who have DGI have positive blood or joint fluid cultures. In those with negative sterile body site cultures, urethral, pharyngeal or rectal cultures frequently produce *N. gonorrhoeae* and thus support the diagnosis.

Increasingly, the importance of classic STDs in facilitating the sexual transmission of HIV infection has been recognized. The relationship between STDs and HIV is bidirectional; the presence of STDs in an HIV-negative person appears to increase the risk of acquiring HIV infection, whereas the presence of STDs in an HIV-positive individual appears to

COMPLICATIONS OF URETHRITIS CAUSED BY *NEISSERIA GONORRHOEAE* AND *CHLAMYDIA TRACHOMATIS*	
Neisseria gonorrhoeae	*N. gonorrhoeae* or *C. trachomatis*
Disseminated gonococcal infection (0.5–2%)	Epididymitis (1–2%)
Prostatitis (very rare)	Conjunctivitis (1–2%)
Chlamydia trachomatis	Urethral stricture (rare)
Reiter's syndrome (1–2%)	Enhanced transmission of HIV (risk increased 4- to 5-fold)

Fig. 63.7 Complications of urethritis caused by *Neisseria gonorrhoeae* and *Chlamydia trachomatis*. Approximate rates for each complication are provided in parentheses.

increase the potential for transmission of HIV. Gonococcal and chlamydial infection are associated with a four- to five-fold increased risk of acquiring HIV infection independent of sexual behaviors and other factors.[36] Community-wide treatment of STDs with effective therapies reduces the rate of new HIV infections.[37] Recent data provide biologic evidence supporting the concept of increased potential for HIV spread in persons dually infected with HIV and urethritis. HIV-infected men with gonococcal urethritis shed much larger quantities of HIV in their semen than those without gonorrhea; this shedding is reduced dramatically by treatment of the urethritis.[38]

PERSISTENT URETHRITIS

Persistent or recurrent urethritis develops in a small proportion of patients who have NGU. In many cases, this represents re-exposure to an untreated sexual partner, or infection with tetracycline-resistant *U. urealyticum* or with *T. vaginalis*. Repeat therapy, in the case of re-exposure, or empiric therapy directed at *U. urealyticum* and *T. vaginalis*, is appropriate; success of the therapy confirms the diagnosis. *Mycoplasma genitalium* has also been implicated in persistent urethritis and may respond to a 6-week course of erythromycin.[14] Accompanying prostatitis may be responsible for persistence or recurrence of urethritis until a long course of therapy (3–6 weeks) is provided.[39] Other less common agents, such as *Candida albicans*, genital warts and coliform bacteria, should be considered in cases of persistent or recurrent urethritis. Noninfectious causes may explain persistent symptoms despite antimicrobial therapy. Urologic evaluation, including urethroscopy to identify intraurethral lesions or foreign bodies, may be necessary.

URETHRITIS IN WOMEN

Urethral infection with *N. gonorrhoeae* and *C. trachomatis* occurs commonly in women; however, the clinical manifestations of concomitant cervicitis usually overshadow signs and symptoms related to urethral infection. In fact, DNA amplification techniques identify *C. trachomatis* in the first-voided portion of the urine from the vast majority of women with chlamydial cervicitis. In a small proportion of these women, careful examination may reveal urethral discharge.

The diagnosis of acute urethral syndrome is made in women with symptoms of cystitis and pyuria but fewer than 10^5 bacteria/ml urine. When low-level bacteriuria is present, the etiology is probably coliform organisms typical of cystitis; when bacteriuria is absent, *C. trachomatis* is often found and the symptoms respond to appropriate therapy.[40]

Dysuria in women is more commonly caused by cystitis and vulvovaginitis. Cystitis produces urgency, frequency and internal dysuria characterized by a deep burning sensation. Vulvovaginitis results in external dysuria caused by the irritant effect of urine contacting an inflamed perineum.

PHYSICAL EXAMINATION

Examination of the man with urethritis symptoms begins with assessment for urethral discharge. Ideally, the patient should not urinate for at least 2 hours before examination, as this washes discharge from the urethra. The examiner should look for evidence of spontaneous discharge, and note the color, quality and quantity of the discharge. The only evidence of mild discharge may be crusting at the meatus; meatal erythema should also be sought. If no discharge is found, the urethra should be stripped to bring discharge forward. Stripping is accomplished by applying pressure along the underside of the penis from the base to the meatus. In symptomatic men, stripping frequently produces a small amount of discharge. Urethral discharge should be collected on a swab and then rolled onto a glass slide for Gram staining (Fig. 63.8). If no discharge is produced, a urethral swab should be inserted 2–4cm into the urethra for collection of the specimen. Next the inguinal lymph nodes should be palpated; small, mobile, nontender lymph nodes are commonly felt, but enlarged or tender lymph nodes suggest a diagnosis other than gonococcal or chlamydial urethritis. The scrotal contents should be evaluated for

swelling, tenderness and warmth. Care should be taken to distinguish epididymitis and orchitis from testicular torsion, which requires prompt surgical attention (see Chapter 2.58).

Examination of the woman with urethritis symptoms should include a complete pelvic examination, with cervical specimens obtained for diagnostic testing (see Chapter 2.52). In the absence of apparent cervical infection, a urethral specimen may be useful; urethral stripping may be accomplished by compressing the urethra against the symphysis pubis using a forward motion. A urethral swab should only be inserted into the most superficial part of the female urethra. However, the recent availability of diagnostic tests applied to urine (see Diagnosis) may obviate the need for urethral and cervical specimens in some settings.

DIAGNOSIS

GRAM STAIN

Several laboratory studies are helpful in the diagnosis of urethritis. Once a specimen is obtained on a swab, the swab should be rolled on a slide for Gram staining (Fig. 63.8). The presence of more than four PMNs per oil-immersion field averaged over five fields in the maximally dense part of the slide is considered objective evidence of urethritis (Fig. 63.9). Because recent urination washes away urethral discharge, fewer PMNs may be seen in this setting. In addition, variation in specimen collection technique and intraobserver variability in reading the smear mean that some men infected with agents of urethritis have fewer PMNs. As many as one-third of men with urethral chlamydial infection may not exhibit abnormal numbers of PMNs on the urethral smear.[6] The presence of Gram-negative intracellular diplococci (Fig. 63.10) indicates gonococcal urethritis with 95% sensitivity and 98% specificity and is adequate justification for therapy.[4,20] Atypical intracellular or typical extracellular Gram-negative diplococci

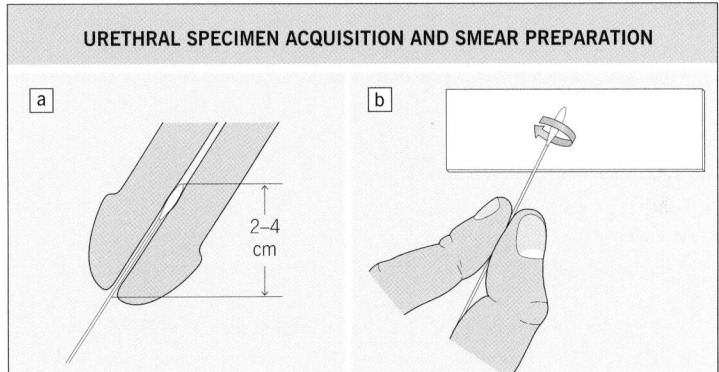

URETHRAL SPECIMEN ACQUISITION AND SMEAR PREPARATION

a

b

2–4 cm

Fig. 63.8 Procedure for obtaining a urethral specimen and preparing a smear for Gram stain. (a) If no discharge is present at the meatus, collect a specimen by inserting the urethral swab 2–4cm into the urethra and rotating for 5 seconds. (b) Roll the swab on a glass slide; rolling the swab preserves cell morphology.

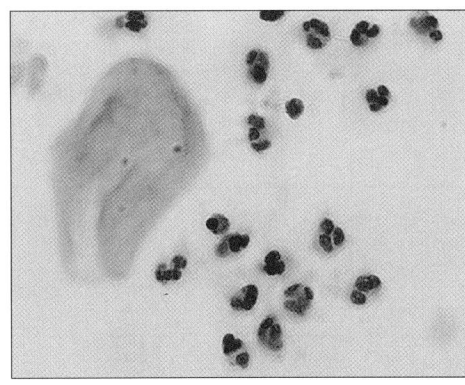

Fig. 63.9 Nongonococcal urethritis. Gram-stained smear of urethral discharge containing many PMNs but no visible bacteria.

may represent other micro-organisms; gonorrhea cultures are positive in 20–30% of these cases. Other Gram-positive and Gram-negative organisms usually reflect colonization of the first centimeter of the urethra and are a normal finding.

DIAGNOSTIC TESTS FOR GONORRHEA

Gonorrhea culture should be performed if the Gram-stained smear is negative or equivocal. *Neisseria gonorrhoeae* is a fastidious organism, requiring specialized media and conditions for growth. Modified Thayer–Martin, Martin–Lewis or other media designed specifically for culturing *N. gonorrhoeae* should be used. Optimally, the specimen should be plated at the bedside and placed into a carbon dioxide incubator or candle jar immediately. Transportable culture systems using carbon-dioxide-producing capsules have made culture possible in clinical settings when incubators are unavailable. Occasional strains sensitive to the concentrations of vancomycin used in the media result in false-negative cultures.

Culture has long been the gold standard for diagnosis of gonorrhea. However, the rigorous conditions necessary for successful culture have necessitated the development of new diagnostic methodologies (Fig. 63.11). The most important of these are the DNA probe and DNA amplification assays. The DNA probe test for gonorrhea has a sensitivity of 93–99% and specificity of 98–99.5%.[41] In situations in which optimal culture quality cannot be maintained, the DNA probe is more sensitive than culture. A DNA probe test is also available for *C. trachomatis*; a single swab can be submitted for both tests.

Two DNA amplification tests are available for the diagnosis of gonorrhea: ligase chain reaction (LCR) and polymerase chain reaction (PCR). These techniques appear to offer no advantage over culture in terms of sensitivity and specificity for detection of urethral infection.[42] However, unlike culture, DNA amplification tests can be applied to the first-voided portion of urine rather than urethral specimens with equivalent performance. All nonculture tests have the disadvantage of not producing an isolate that can be used for antimicrobial susceptibility testing; this may become important in the near future if fluoroquinolone resistance becomes more prevalent.

The diagnosis of DGI generally depends on the constellation of clinical findings rather than on specific laboratory tests. Patients suspected of having DGI should have genital, rectal and pharyngeal specimens cultured for *N. gonorrhoeae*. Joint fluid, if obtainable, should also be cultured. Blood cultures should be obtained for diagnosis and to exclude other infections associated with fever and petechial rash such as meningococcal sepsis. However, around 20% of patients who have DGI have no positive cultures. In the appropriate clinical setting, and with the exclusion of other bacterial infections of the joints or bloodstream, DGI is strongly suggested by the constellation of tenosynovitis, acral rash and fever.

DIAGNOSTIC TESTS FOR CHLAMYDIAL INFECTION

A wider variety of tests are available for the detection of *C. trachomatis* than for *N. gonorrhoeae* (Fig. 63.12). Although *C. trachomatis* can be cultured, the expense and complexity of this procedure have limited the clinical utility of culture as a diagnostic test. Several types of nonculture tests, including enzyme immunoassays (EIAs), direct fluorescent antibody tests (DFAs) and a DNA probe, have become the mainstay of chlamydial diagnostics. All of the nonculture tests can detect dead organisms, and accordingly should not be used within the 2–3 weeks after treatment of chlamydial infection. The EIAs and DFAs have sensitivities of 70–90% compared with culture, and specificities of 97–99% when a confirmatory test is used.[43] Sensitivity in asymptomatic men is lower than that found in symptomatic men, presumably because of a lower organism burden. The DNA probe generally performs a little better than the EIA or DFA, with a higher sensitivity (86–93%) and similar specificity.[44] The DNA probe test can be used to detect *N. gonorrhoeae* and *C. trachomatis* with the convenience of using a single swab. The performance of all of these tests is sensitive to the quality of specimen sampling, and to the presence or

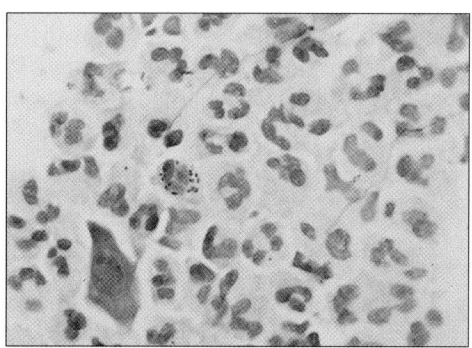

Fig. 63.10 Gonorrhea. Gram-stained smear of urethral discharge containing numerous PMNs and Gram-negative intracellular diplococci consistent with *Neisseria gonorrhoeae*.

DIAGNOSTIC TESTS FOR *NEISSERIA GONORRHOEAE*			
Test	Sensitivity (%)	Specificity (%)	Comment
Gram stain*	95 (symptomatic) 60 (asymptomatic)	98	Results available immediately
Culture†	90–97	98–99	Requires careful handling and proper facilities
DNA probe†	93–99	98–99.5	Can test for *C. trachomatis* with same swab
DNA amplification (LCR or PCR)†	98–99	>99	Can use first-voided portion of urine or urethral swab with equal performance, and *C. trachomatis* with same specimen

* Compared with culture

† Compared with enhanced reference standard comprising culture and DNA amplification or probe competition assay

Fig. 63.11 Diagnostic tests for *Neisseria gonorrhoeae*. Sensitivity and specificity are given for the diagnosis of urethritis in men, using urethral specimens unless otherwise stated.

DIAGNOSTIC TESTS FOR *CHLAMYDIA TRACHOMATIS*			
Test	Sensitivity (%)	Specificity (%)	Comment
EIA*	70–90	95–99	Readily done in high volume
DFA*	70–95	95–99	Depends on skill of microscopist; not amenable to high volume
Culture†	65–80	>99	Requires expert laboratory
DNA probe†	86–93	98–99.5	Can test for *N. gonorrhoeae* with same swab
DNA amplification (LCR or PCR)†	94–99	>99	Can use first-voided portion of urine or urethral swab with equal performance, and test for *N. gonorrhoeae* with same specimen

* Compared with culture

† Compared with enhanced reference standard comprising DNA amplification plus culture or DFA test

Fig. 63.12 Diagnostic tests for *Chlamydia trachomatis*. Sensitivity and specificity are given for the diagnosis of urethritis in men, using urethral specimens unless otherwise stated.

absence of symptoms, as this may reflect organism burden. Recently, rapid antigen detection tests have become available; these tests can detect *C. trachomatis* in less than 30 minutes and can be performed in the physician's office. However, until the sensitivity can be improved from the current 50% (compared with culture), such tests will have very limited utility.[45] A positive test for *C. trachomatis* using any of the above methodologies should be considered evidence of infection, although the clinician should recognize that even a highly specific test will yield some false-positive results, especially if the test is used to screen a low-prevalence population.

DNA amplification tests for *C. trachomatis* have recently become available and will revolutionize the diagnosis of urethritis. Comparisons of LCR and PCR with other tests for *C. trachomatis* suggest that the most sensitive test previously available, culture, detects only 65–80%

of infections.[46] In addition to having higher sensitivities (94–99% compared with a resolved gold standard) than any previously available test, LCR and PCR have extremely high specificities (>99%) and can be performed using the first-voided portion of urine or urethral swabs with equivalent performance.[46,47]

OTHER TESTS FOR URETHRITIS

Tests for causes of urethritis other than *N. gonorrhoeae* and *C. trachomatis* have limited utility and are often not available to the clinician. Although *U. urealyticum* is a major cause of urethritis, its role as a colonizer of the genital tract makes culture results difficult to interpret; culture is also not widely available. The same is also true for *M. genitalium*. *Trichomonas vaginalis* may rarely be seen in urethral Gram stains, but is better identified in a wet mount of the urethral specimen where motility can be appreciated (Fig. 63.13). However, most men infected with *T. vaginalis* have negative wet mounts. Culture and PCR for *T. vaginalis*, although not widely available, are much more sensitive than wet mount for urethral infection.[18] Despite use of all available diagnostic tests, 10–30% of NGU cases have no identified cause.

When the anatomic site of infection is in doubt, a urine sample can be used to distinguish urethritis from infection higher in the urinary tract. The presence of PMNs and mucous threads in the sediment of the first 10ml voided urine, while the remainder of the urine is clear, suggests urethritis;[48] equal numbers of PMNs in both parts suggests cystitis or pyelonephritis. The presence of at least 10 PMNs per

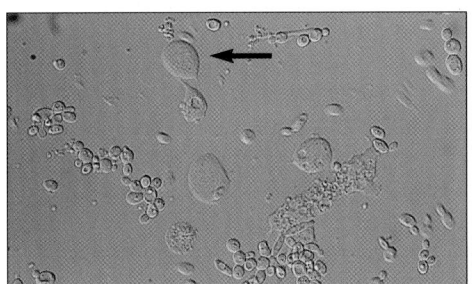

Fig. 63.13
Trichomonal infection.
Saline mount of *Trichomonas vaginalis* (arrow); characteristic ovoid shape and flagella can be seen.

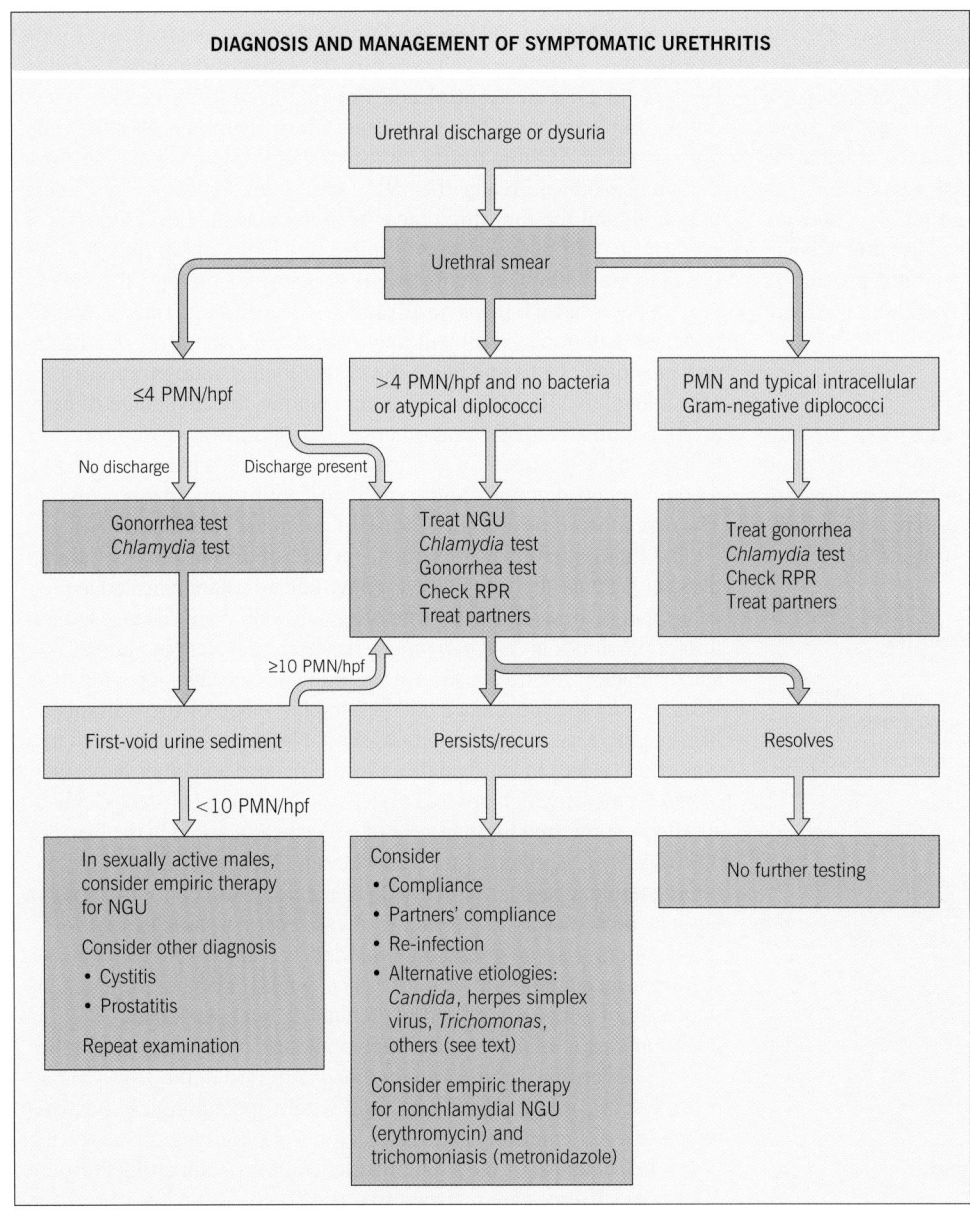

DIAGNOSIS AND MANAGEMENT OF SYMPTOMATIC URETHRITIS

Fig. 63.14 A simplified approach to the diagnosis and management of symptomatic urethritis. hpf, high-power field; RPR, rapid plasma reagin.

high-power field in the sediment of first-voided urine is considered objective evidence of urethritis.

DIAGNOSTIC APPROACH TO SYMPTOMATIC URETHRITIS

An algorithm for the diagnosis and management of symptomatic urethritis is outlined in Figure 63.14. The urethral smear classifies the patient as having gonococcal urethritis, NGU or no evidence of urethritis. The presence of typical intracellular Gram-negative diplococci is sufficient for the diagnosis of gonorrhea, requiring treatment for gonorrhea and possible co-infection with *C. trachomatis*. A test for *C. trachomatis* may be performed, as may a serologic test for syphilis, and partners should be treated.

A patient who has a urethral smear showing more than four PMNs per high-power field, but no bacteria or only atypical diplococci, is treated for NGU. A test for *C. trachomatis* allows an etiologic diagnosis, but treatment should not be delayed pending test results. Gonorrhea testing should always be performed on patients thought to have NGU, as the Gram stain is less than 100% sensitive. As with all STDs, partners should be treated and a serologic test for syphilis performed.

If NGU persists or recurs after therapy, several possibilities should be considered. First, if the patient was noncompliant with therapy or was re-exposed to an infected partner, repeat therapy should be effective. Otherwise, empiric therapy directed at tetracycline-resistant *U. urealyticum* (erythromycin) and at *T. vaginalis* (metronidazole) is most likely to resolve the urethritis. Less common causes of urethritis should also be considered at this time.

If four PMNs or fewer are seen per high-power field on the initial Gram stain, there is no objective evidence for urethritis. However, if a discharge is present, the patient should be managed as for NGU. Dysuria alone in a young sexually active man also suggests NGU; a single course of therapy directed at agents of NGU may be given before further evaluation. The presence of PMNs in first-voided urine supports the diagnosis of NGU. Whether or not treatment for NGU is given, testing for gonorrhea is necessary, and testing for *C. trachomatis* may be desirable. If no discharge is present, and there are no PMNs in first-voided urine, other diagnoses such as cystitis and prostatitis should be considered. Repeat examination after several hours without urination may also be helpful.

SCREENING FOR ASYMPTOMATIC URETHRITIS

A small percentage of men with gonorrhea and one-quarter to one-half of men infected with *C. trachomatis* are asymptomatic.[6] These men play a disproportionate role in spreading infection because they are unlikely to be identified and treated.[25] Attempts to improve identification of these men using leukocyte esterase testing of urine as a

preliminary test have been unsatisfactory owing to the poor sensitivity of this test. Newer DNA amplification tests simplify screening for *C. trachomatis* and *N. gonorrhoeae*. Urine-based LCR and PCR for these pathogens allows identification of asymptomatic infected men without the discomfort of a urethral swab and can be performed in settings in which clinicians or examination facilities are unavailable.

MANAGEMENT

Therapeutic regimens for the management of urethritis are outlined in Figure 63.15. Gonococcal urethritis is generally treated with single-dose therapy; a regimen active against *C. trachomatis* is added because of the high likelihood of co-infection. Nongonococcal urethritis or chlamydial urethritis is treated with a single-dose or multi-dose regimen. Recurrent or persistent urethritis may require more than one antibiotic or a long course of therapy. Sexual partners must also be treated, as the likelihood of infection is high. Abstinence is recommended until patient and partner have completed therapy.

The presence of an STD is a marker for high-risk sexual behavior. Therefore, all persons with an STD should have a serologic test for syphilis and should be counseled about STD and HIV prevention. Patients without immunity to hepatitis B should be vaccinated. Urethritis in HIV-infected persons is managed no differently from urethritis in persons not infected with HIV. The management of epididymitis complicating urethritis is discussed in Chapter 2.58.

MANAGEMENT OF GONOCOCCAL INFECTION

A variety of highly effective single-dose therapies are available for the management of gonococcal urethritis. Therapies recommended by the Centers for Disease Control and Prevention in 1998 include single doses of ceftriaxone 125mg intramuscularly, cefixime 400mg orally, ciprofloxacin 500mg orally or ofloxacin 400mg orally.[50] These therapies produce greater than 95% cure rates for genital and rectal infection, and the first three have been demonstrated to eliminate *N. gonorrhoeae* from the urethra within a few hours of administration.[24] Ceftriaxone 250mg, a mainstay of gonococcal therapy for several years, may be used but has no advantages over 125mg. The use of a 1% lidocaine solution as a diluent may reduce the discomfort of ceftriaxone injections. Cefixime has a lower therapeutic index (ratio of peak serum level to MIC) than ceftriaxone, but has the advantage of being orally administered. Several other cephalosporins have demonstrated efficacy in the treatment of gonorrhea, but have no advantages over the recommended therapies and experience with them is more limited. The cephalosporins are safe for use in pregnancy and in children.

The fluoroquinolones ciprofloxacin and ofloxacin provide alternatives for patients allergic to beta-lactams, but are contraindicated in pregnancy and in those under 18 years of age. In addition, resistance to these fluoroquinolones in *N. gonorrhoeae* has been prevalent in parts of Asia and the Pacific Islands for several years and has recently appeared in the USA.[51,52] As the prevalence and geographic range of these strains are likely to increase, fluoroquinolones should be used with caution to treat gonorrhea. Doses lower than those recommended and other fluoroquinolones, some of which are less effective, should not be used. Cephalosporins are preferred for treatment of gonorrhea acquired in the Far East, where rates of fluoroquinolone resistance are higher. If the prevalence of fluoroquinolone resistance in the USA increases, susceptibility monitoring may be necessary to ensure the effectiveness of these therapies.

An alternative to the recommended therapies for gonorrhea is spectinomycin 2g intramuscularly once, which can be used in patients intolerant of beta-lactams and in pregnancy, but is expensive, requires injection and is relatively ineffective against pharyngeal gonorrhea. Spectinomycin-resistant *N. gonorrhoeae* are rare in the USA, but are prevalent in some parts of the world where spectinomycin has been widely used. Penicillins and tetracyclines are no longer used to treat gonorrhea because of the high prevalence of resistant strains (around 30% of US isolates are resistant to one or both drugs).[52]

THERAPEUTIC REGIMENS FOR ACUTE URETHRITIS

Gonorrhea	Chlamydial infection	Nongonococcal urethritis (empiric therapy)
Ceftriaxone 125mg im once*†	Azithromycin 1g orally once‡	Azithromycin 1g orally once
Cefixime 400mg orally once*	Doxycycline 100mg orally q12h for 7 days	Doxycycline 100mg orally q12h for 7 days
Ciprofloxacin 500mg orally once†	Ofloxacin 300mg orally q12h for 7 days	Erythromycin 500mg orally q6h for 7 days
Ofloxacin 400mg orally once	Erythromycin 500mg orally q6h for 7 days*	Ofloxacin 300mg orally q12h for 7 days
Spectinomycin 2g im once*	Amoxicillin 500mg orally q8h for 7 days*	

* Considered safe for use in pregnancy

† Preferred for coexisting pharyngeal gonorrhea

‡ Safety in pregnancy not proved

Fig. 63.15 Therapeutic regimens for urethritis.[51] For treatment of recurrent or persistent urethritis, see discussion in text.

There are several additional considerations in managing the patient who has gonorrhea. First, any treatment for gonorrhea should be accompanied by a regimen effective for possible co-infection with *C. trachomatis* (see below). Second, all patients with an STD should be screened for syphilis with a serologic test such as the rapid plasma reagin, RPR. Patients who have incubating syphilis, however, have negative serologic tests and are accordingly difficult to identify; ideally, therefore, treatment for gonorrhea would also cure incubating syphilis. The cephalosporins, but not the quinolones or spectinomycin, have activity against *Treponema pallidum*. Azithromycin and doxycycline also have activity against *T. pallidum*, and azithromycin appeared to be effective in curing incubating syphilis in a small study.[53] Third, ceftriaxone and ciprofloxacin have been proved to be effective in the treatment of pharyngeal gonorrhea, with greater than 90% cure rates; data for other therapies are insufficient to recommend their use in pharyngeal gonorrhea. Follow-up is not necessary after treatment for uncomplicated gonorrhea because of the effectiveness of current therapies; however, all patients should be instructed to return if symptoms do not promptly resolve, and follow-up is advised for those who acquired infection overseas or in whom the diagnosis is unsure.

Disseminated gonococcal infection requires 7 days of antibiotic therapy, beginning with parenteral therapy and switching to oral therapy after 24–48 hours of improvement. Recommended parenteral therapies are ceftriaxone 1g intramuscularly or intravenously q24h, cefotaxime 1g intravenously q8h, or, for patients intolerant of cephalosporins, spectinomycin 2g intramuscularly q12h. For oral therapy, cefixime 400mg q12h or ciprofloxacin 500mg q12h may be used. Concurrent therapy active against *C. trachomatis* should be provided.

MANAGEMENT OF CHLAMYDIAL URETHRITIS
Chlamydial urethritis should be treated with a single-dose regimen of azithromycin 1g orally or with a multiple-dose regimen of doxycycline 100mg orally q12h for 7 days. Ofloxacin 300mg orally q12h for 7 days is also effective. Azithromycin has the advantage of a single-dose administration, but is more expensive than doxycycline. Azithromycin is approved for the treatment of respiratory infections in children over 2 years of age, so should also be safe for treatment of chlamydial infections in this age group; however, the appropriate dose for chlamydial infection in persons weighing <45kg has not been determined. The risks of azithromycin in pregnancy are assumed to be similar to those of erythromycin.[54] Doxycycline and ofloxacin are not recommended for use in pregnancy or in children. Ofloxacin is expensive and has no dosing advantages over doxycycline.

An alternative regimen for chlamydial infection is erythromycin 500mg orally q6h for 7 days. Erythromycin is inexpensive, but gastrointestinal upset may limit compliance. Amoxicillin 500mg orally q8h for 7 days is useful in pregnant women unable to tolerate erythromycin.[55]

Patients who have satisfactory resolution of symptoms generally do not require follow-up testing for *C. trachomatis*. However, if erythromycin or amoxicillin are used, post-treatment testing is advised. Testing should be delayed until at least 3 weeks after completion of therapy, as dead organisms may produce false-positive results on non-culture tests performed sooner.

MANAGEMENT OF NONGONOCOCCAL URETHRITIS
Treatment of NGU is directed at the likely etiologic agents, including *C. trachomatis, U. urealyticum* and *M. genitalium*. Symptoms resolve slowly, sometimes lasting for several days after the completion of therapy. Doxycycline 100mg orally q12h and azithromycin 1g orally once are equivalent in curing NGU. Erythromycin 500mg orally q6h for 7 days may be used as an alternative. For NGU that fails to respond to initial therapy, several alternatives may be considered. Repeat treatment with the same drug may be used if noncompliance or re-exposure to an untreated sexual partner is suspected. However, many doxycycline failures may be attributable to tetraycycline-resistant *U. urealyticum*, which may be successfully treated with a 7-day course of erythromycin, or to *T. vaginalis*, which may be cured with a single 2g oral dose of metronidazole. Some isolates of *U. urealyticum* are resistant to erythromycin but may respond to a 7-day course of ofloxacin 300mg orally q12h.[56] *Mycoplasma genitalium* has also been implicated in persistent NGU and may require a 6-week course of erythromycin for eradication.[14] Persistent NGU after two courses of therapy requires consideration of other diagnoses such as cystitis and prostatitis. Urologic evaluation may include urine flow measurements and urethroscopy or urethrography to assess the presence of foreign bodies, strictures and periurethral abscesses. If no cause can be found, a 3- to 6-week course of doxycycline or erythromycin can be tried,[39] although the long-term effectiveness of this is unknown.

REFERENCES

1. Division of STD Prevention. Sexually Transmitted Disease Surveillance, 1996. U.S. Department of Health and Human Services, Public Health Service. Atlanta: Centers for Disease Control and Prevention; 1997.
2. Piot P, Islam MQ. Sexually transmitted diseases in the 1990's: global epidemiology and challenges for control. Sex Transm Dis (suppl2) 1994;21:S7–13.
3. Buve A, Laga M, Piot P. Where are we now? sexually transmitted diseases. Health Policy Plann 1993;8:277–81.
4. Jacobs NF, Kraus SJ. Gonococcal and nongonococcal urethritis in men: clinical and laboratory differentiation. Ann Intern Med 1975;82:7–12.
5. Zimmerman HL, Potterat JJ, Dukes RL, et al. Epidemiologic differences between chlamydia and gonorrhea. Am J Public Health 1990;80:1338–42.
6. Stamm WE, Koutsky LA, Beneddeti JK, et al. Chlamydia trachomatis urethral infections in men prevalence, risk factors, and clinical manifestations. Ann Intern Med 1984;100:47–51.
7. Jacobs NS, Arum ES, Kraus SJ. Nongonococcal urethritis: the role of Chlamydia trachomatis. Ann Intern Med 1977;86:313–4.

8. Magder LS, Harrison R, Ehret JM, Anderson TS, Judson FN. Factors related to genital Chlamydia trachomatis and its diagnosis by culture in a sexually transmitted disease clinic. Am J Epidemiol 1988;128:298–308.
9. Bowie WR. Approach to men with urethritis and urologic complications of sexually transmitted disease. Med Clin North Am 1990;74:1543–57.
10. Cohen MS, Sparling PF. Mucosal infection with Neisseria gonorrhoeae: bacterial adaptation and mucosal defenses. J Clin Invest 1992;89:1699–705.
11. O'Brien JP, Goldenberg DL, Rice PA. Disseminated gonococcal infection: a prospective analysis of 49 patients and a review of pathophysiology and immune mechanisms. Medicine 1983;62:395–406.
12. Jones RB. Chlamydia trachomatis. In: Mandell GL, Bennett JE, Dolin R, eds. Principles and practice of infectious diseases, 4th ed. New York: Churchill Livingstone; 1995:1679–92.
13. Brunham RC, Peeling RW. Chlamydia trachomatis antigens: role in immunity and pathogenesis. Infect Agents Dis 1994;3:218–33.

14. Taylor-Robinson D. Infections due to species of Mycoplasma and Ureaplasma: an update. Clin Infect Dis 1996;23:671–84.
15. Taylor-Robinson D. The male reservoir of Ureaplasma urealyticum. Pediatr Infect Dis 1986;5(Suppl 6):S234–5.
16. Horner PJ, Gilroy CB, Thomas BJ, Naidoo ROM, Taylor-Robinson D. Association of Mycoplasm genitalium with acute non-gonococcal urethritis. Lancet 1993;342:582–5.
17. Corey L, Adams HG, Brown ZA, Holmes KK. Genital herpes simplex virus infections: clinical manifestations, course, and complications. Ann Intern Med 1983;98:958–72.
18. Krieger JN, Jenny C, Verdon M, et al. Clinical manifestations of trichomoniasis in men. Ann Intern Med 1983;118:844–9.
19. Anderson RM, May RM. Epidemiological parameters of HIV transmission. Nature 1988;333:514–9.
20. McCutchan JA. Epidemiology of venereal urethritis: comparison of gonorrhea and nongonococcal urethritis. Rev Infect Dis 1984;6:669–88.
21. Brunham RC. A general model of sexually transmitted disease epidemiology and its implications for control. Sex Transm Dis 1990;74:1339–52.

22. Quinn TC, Gaydos C, Shepherd M, *et al.* Epidemiologic and microbiologic correlates of *Chlamydia trachomatis* infection in sexual partnerships. JAMA 1996;276:1737–42.

23. Yorke JA, Hethcote HW, Nold A. Dynamics and control of the transmission of gonorrhea. Sex Transm Dis 1978;5:51–6.

24. Haizlip J, Isbey SF, Hamilton HA, *et al.* Time required for elimination of *Neisseria gonorrhoeae* from the urogenital tract in men with symptomatic urethritis: comparison of oral and intramuscular single-dose therapy. Sex Transm Dis 1995;22:145–8.

25. Potterat JJ, Dukes RL, Rothenberg RB. Disease transmission by heterosexual men with gonorrhea: an empiric estimate. Sex Transm Dis 1987;14:107–10.

26. Centers for Disease Control. Update: barrier protection against HIV infection and other sexually transmitted diseases. MMWR 1993;30:589–97.

27. Soper DE, Shoupe D, Shangold GA, *et al.* Prevention of vaginal trichomoniasis by compliant use of the female condom. Sex Transm Dis 1993;20:137–9.

28. Louv WC, Austin H, Alexander WJ, Stagno S, Cheeks J. A clinical trial of nonoxynol-9 for preventing gonococcal and chlamydial infections. J Infect Dis 1988;158:518–23.

29. Niruthisard S. Use of nonoxynol-9 and reduction in rate of gonococcal and chlamydial cervical infections. Lancet 1992;339:1371–5.

30. Martin JL, Garcia MA, Beatrice ST. Sexual behavior changes and HIV antibody in a cohort of New York City gay men. Am J Public Health 1989;79:501–3.

31. Centers for Disease Control. Premarital sexual experience among adolescent women–United States, 1970–1988. MMWR 1991;39:929–32.

32. Crawford F, Knapp JS, Hale J, Holmes KK. Asymptomatic gonorrhea in men caused by gonococci with unique nutritional requirements. Science 1977;196:1352–3.

33. Handsfield HH, Lipman TO, Narnisch JP, Tronca E, Holmes KK. Asymptomatic gonorrhea in men: diagnosis, natural course, prevalence and significance. N Engl J Med 1974;290:117–23.

34. Terho P. *Chlamydia trachomatis* in non-specific urethritis. Br J Venereal Dis 1978;54:251–6.

35. Svenungsson B. Reactive arthritis. Int J STD AIDS 1995;6:150–60.

36. Laga M, Manoka A, Kivuva M, *et al.* Non-ulcerative sexually transmitted diseases as risk factors for HIV-1 transmisssion in women: results from a cohort study. AIDS 1993;7:93–102.

37. Grosskurth H, Mosha F, Todd J, *et al.* Impact of improved treatment of sexually transmitted diseases on HIV infection in rural Tanzania: randomised controlled trial. Lancet 1995;346:530–6.

38. Cohen MS, Hoffman IF, Royce RA, *et al.* Reduction in concentration of HIV-1 in semen after treatment of urethritis: implications for prevention of sexual transmission of HIV-1. Lancet 1997;349:1868–73.

39. Wong ES, Hooton TM, Hill CC, McKevitt M, Stamm WE. Clinical and microbiological features of persistent or recurrent nongonococcal urethritis in men. J Infect Dis 1988;158:1098–101.

40. Stamm WE. Etiology and management of the acute urethral syndrome. Sex Transm Dis 1981;8:235–8.

41. Hale YM, Melton ME, Lewis JS, Willis DE. Evaluation of the PACE 2 *Neisseria gonorrhoeae* assay by three public health laboratories. J Clin Microbiol 1993;31:451–3.

42. Ching S, Lee H, Hook E, Jacobs MR, Zenilman J. Ligase chain reaction for detection of *Neisseria gonorrhoeae* in urogenital swabs. J Clin Microbiol 1995;33:3111–4.

43. Stamm WE. Diagnosis of *Chlamydia trachomatis* genitourinary infections. Ann Intern Med 1988;108:710–7.

44. Iwen PC, Walker RA, Warren KL, *et al.* Evaluation of nucleic acid-based test (PACE 2C) for simultaneous detection of *Chlamydia trachomatis* and *Neisseria gonorrhoeae* in endocervical specimens. J Clin Microbiol 1995;33:2587–91.

45. Hook EW, Spitters C, Reichart CA, Neumann TM, Quinn TC. Use of cell culture and a rapid diagnostic assay for 'Chlamydia trachomatis' screening. JAMA 1994;272:867–70.

46. Chernesky MA, Lee H, Schachter J, *et al.* Diagnosis of *Chlamydia trachomatis* urethral infection in symptomatic and asymptomatic men by testing first-void urine in a ligase chain reaction assay. J Infect Dis 1994;170:1308–11.

47. Bauwens JE Clark AM, Loeffelhholz MJ, Herman SA, Stamm WE. Diagnosis of *Chlamydia trachomatis* urethritis in men by polymerase chain reaction assay of first-catch urine. J Clin Microbiol 1993;31:3013–6.

48. Perera SA. Use of Kova-Slide II with grid and uncentrifuged segmented urine specimens in the diagnosis of nongonococcal urethritis: a quantitative technique. Sex Transm Dis 1985;12:14–8.

49. Fox KK, Isbey SF, Cohen MS, Carson CC. Urethritis, epididymitis, orchitis, and prostatitis. In: Root RK, Stamm W, Waldvogel F, Corey L, eds. Clinical infectious diseases: a practical approach. New York; Oxford University Press; in press.

50. Centers for Disease Control. 1998 Guidelines for treatment of sexually transmitted diseases. MMWR 1998;47(no. RR-1):1–111.

51. Centers for Disease Control. Fluoroquinolone resistance in *Neisseria gonorrhoeae* – Colorado and Washington, 1995. MMWR 1995;44:761–4.

52. Fox KK, Knapp JS, Holmes KK, *et al.* Antimicrobial resistance in Neisseria gonorrhoeae in the United States1988–1994: The emergence of resistance to the fluoroquinolones. J Infect Dis 1997;175:1396–403

53. Ennis DM, Stephens JG, Hook EW. A randomised comparative trial of azithromycin and benzathine penicillin G for prevention of syphilis in exposed patients [Abstract 307]. In: Proceedings of the Infectious Diseases Society of America 34th annual meeting (New Orleans). Infectious Diseases Society, Alexandria, VA 1996:93

54. Bush MR, Rosa CR. Azithromycin and erythromycin in the treatment of cervical chlamydial infection during pregnancy. Obstet Gynecol 1994;84:61–3.

55. Turrentine MA, Newton ER. Amoxicillin or erythromycin for the treatment of antenatal chlamydial infection: a meta-analysis. Obstet Gynecol 1995;86:1021–5

56. Waites KB, Cassell GH. Clinical applications of fluoroquinolones for genital *Mycoplasma* infections. Infect Med 1994;71–88.

chapter
64

Syphilis

George R Kinghorn

Syphilis is a chronic infectious disease caused by the spirochete *Treponema pallidum*, which is transmitted during sexual intercourse and other intimate contact; it may also be vertically transmitted by a pregnant woman to her fetus *in utero* or during birth.

The name of the disease was drawn from a poem *Syphilis sive morbus gallicus*, written by Fracastoro of Verona in 1530, in which the mythical swineherd Syphilis refused to make sacrifices to Apollo and was smitten as a result.[1]

EPIDEMIOLOGY

An epidemic of sexually transmitted syphilis spread across Europe at the end of the 15th century. There are conflicting views about the origin of syphilis in Europe – some believe that it was brought back from the New World by Columbus, and others believe that it had been endemic throughout the Middle Ages and became sexually acquired at the time of the epidemic. Syphilis had certainly become endemic in Europe by the 17th century, since when there have been several epidemic waves, notably during the Napoleonic wars and the period of industrialization in the 19th century, and during and after the two world wars of the 20th century.

In North America and the developed countries of northern Europe, syphilis had become predominately a disease of homosexual men by the 1970s. Although syphilis has continued to decline in northern Europe, there have been renewed outbreaks of heterosexual and congenital syphilis in North America during the late 1980s in the wake of the HIV epidemic.[2]

The global impact of AIDS in the 20th century has many similarities with the impact of syphilis in 16th-century Europe. The resurgence of syphilis has mainly been observed in commercial sex workers, in whom it is often associated with selling sex for drugs (especially crack cocaine), and in other persons of lower socioeconomic status. In 1994, there were 20,627 reported cases of primary and secondary syphilis in the USA (8.1 cases per 100,000 people, the rate being 60 times higher in non-Hispanic blacks than in Caucasians) compared with 304 cases in England (fewer than 0.6 cases per 100,000 people) (Fig. 64.1).[3] Although the North American trend has not yet been mirrored in western Europe, outbreaks of syphilis have been reported from eastern European countries during the 1990s, and neighboring Scandanavian countries have witnessed an increase in imported cases.[4]

The annual incidence of congenital syphilis in infants aged less than 1 year increased from 3.0 per 100,000 live births in 1980 to a peak of 107.3 per 100,000 live births in 1990. The very large increase in reported cases has been artificially elevated by the introduction of a new reporting system,[5–7] which takes account of epidemiologic factors, especially maternal treatment status, in addition to cases showing characteristic clinical stigmata (Fig. 64.2). The annual incidence has since declined to 30.4 per 100,000 live births in 1996.

The World Health Organization (WHO) estimates that the annual global incidence of syphilis is approximately 12 million cases, most of which occur in developing countries, where the disease has remained a prominent cause of genital ulcer disease in heterosexual men and

women, of stillbirth, and of neonatal morbidity and mortality.[8] The prevalence of pregnant seropositive women is 0.1–0.6% in developed countries, but it may exceed 10% in many developing countries. In some parts of South Africa, seroconversion during pregnancy has been reported to occur in more than 2% of women.[9]

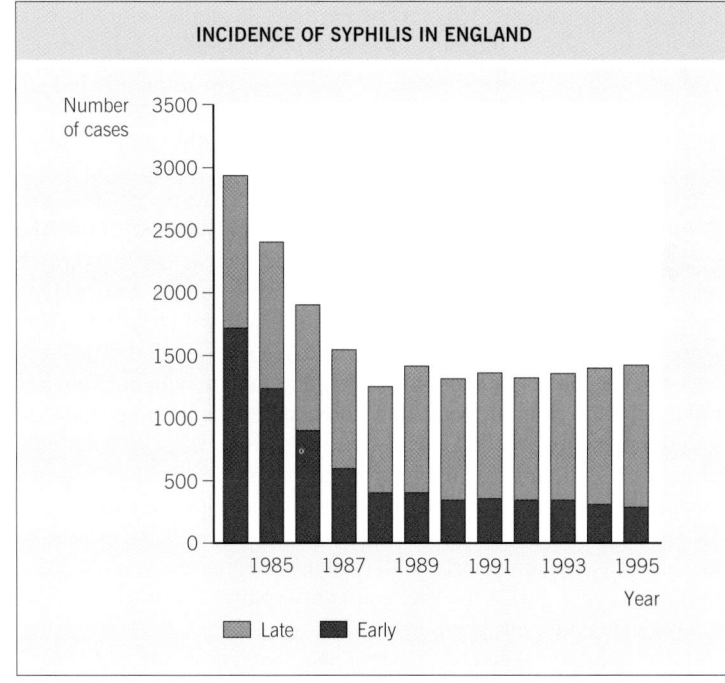

Fig. 64.1 Incidence of syphilis in England. Cases reported by genitourinary medicine clinics 1984–1995. Late is defined by latent syphilis of more than 2 years duration, cardiovascular syphilis, gummatous syphilis or neurosyphilis. Early is defined by primary syphilis, secondary syphilis or latent syphilis of less than 2 years duration.

DEFINITIONS OF CONGENITAL SYPHILIS	
Confirmed diagnosis	An infant in whom *Treponema pallidum* is identified by dark-field microscopy, fluorescent antibody, or other specific stains in specimens from lesions, placenta, umbilical cord, or autopsy material
Presumptive diagnosis	1. Any infant whose mother had untreated or inadequately treated syphilis at delivery, regardless of symptoms or signs in the infant 2. Any infant or child who has a reactive specific treponemal test for syphilis and one of the following: evidence of congenital syphilis on physical examination evidence of congenital syphilis on long-bone X-ray reactive CSF VDRL elevated CSF cell count or protein (without other cause) reactive test for FTA-ABS-IgM using fractionated serum

Fig. 64.2 Definitions of congenital syphilis.

TRANSMISSION

The organism is transmitted from the early mucocutaneous lesions, and enters the body through small breaches in epithelial surfaces of genital, anorectal, oropharyngeal and other cutaneous sites.

Prenatal transmission is greatest in cases of maternal infection of short duration, but it may also occur during the latent stages of syphilis. Disease manifestations are usual before 18 weeks *in utero*. Stillbirth caused by congenital syphilis has a maximum incidence at 6–8 months' gestation. Even when a previous pregnancy has resulted in an uninfected child, congenital syphilis may occur in subsequent offspring, and it may affect only one of twins. It is preventable with maternal treatment during pregnancy.

Syphilis is rarely transmitted during transfusion of blood or blood products, or through sharing needles by intravenous drug abusers.

PATHOGENESIS AND PATHOLOGY

The causative spirochete of syphilis, *Treponema pallidum* subsp. *pallidum*, is a facultative anaerobe that is 6–15μm long and 0.15μm wide. It can be identified in dark field microscopy by its characteristic morphology and movements, which typically include angling. It cannot be cultured on artificial media but it can be propagated in organ culture, such as rabbit testis. It has a slow growth rate with a doubling time of 30–36h. The organism is similar to and shares extensive DNA homology with three other pathogenic treponemes, which cause yaws, bejel and pinta (see Chapter 8.19).

Treponema pallidum initiates an inflammatory response at the site of inoculation and is disseminated during the primary infection. The organism has a surface-associated hyalouronidase enzyme, which may play a role in this process. Phagocytosis by cytokine-activated macrophages, as part of a predominant T-helper (Th1)-type early response, aids bacterial clearance and resolution of the primary lesion.[9] Virulent organisms promote adhesion of lymphocytes and monocytes to human vascular cells, and this is important in immunopathogenesis.[10] As with other organisms that cause chronic disease, *T. pallidum* has evolved mechanisms for evading immune responses. A Th1–Th2 switch occurs with macrophage suppression caused by prostaglandin E2 down-regulation; however the molecular mechanisms remain poorly understood.[11] Depressed cell-mediated responses occur during the later stages of syphilis, and lowered CD4+ lymphocyte count has been reported.[12]

It has been postulated that the immunoevasiveness of *T. pallidum* is the result of the organism's unusual molecular architecture. The outer membrane contains few poorly immunogenic transmembrane proteins; the highly immunogenic proteins are lipoproteins anchored predominately to the periplasmic leaflet of the cytoplasmic membrane.[13]

The dominant immunogen is a 47kDa membrane lipoprotein, which can induce synthesis of tumor necrosis factor-α. Immunoblotting has also shown IgG responses to an antigen of 65kDa that is shared with nonpathogenic treponemes, and antigens of 45, 17 and 15.5kDa that are specific for *T. pallidum*. The genome of the nonpathogenic Nichols strain has now been mapped and will provide new insight into the molecular biology of the organism; related techniques should permit the production of large quantities of treponemal proteins for use as antigens in serodiagnostic tests.

HISTOLOGIC APPEARANCES AND PATHOLOGY

Some manifestations of syphilis (e.g. neuropathy) are immune-complex mediated. In early lesions, perivascular infiltration by lymphocytes and plasma cells is accompanied by intimal proliferation in arteries and veins. This leads to ischemia and ulceration. Organisms are most numerous in the walls of capillaries and lymphatic vessels.

In late lesions, the characteristic lesion of mucocutanous surfaces is the syphilitic gumma. Granulation tissue forms with histiocytes, fibroblasts and epithelioid cells. Endarteritis obliterans and necrotic areas are pronounced. Gummas most often originate in subcutaneous tissues and spread in all directions. Spirochetes are not readily demonstrable in these lesions.

Heubner's arteritis occurs in cardiovascular and meningovascular syphilis. It is characterized by lymphocytic and plasma cell infiltration of the vasa vasorum and adventitia of large and medium-sized vessels. Occlusion of the vasa vasorum results in medial necrosis and fibroblast proliferation. There is associated subintimal proliferation, which leads to luminal occlusion and thrombosis.

PREVENTION

The risk factors for acquisition of syphilis mirror those of other sexually transmitted diseases (STDs) and primary prevention depends on similar methods, such as reducing the number of sexual partners and consistent use of condoms. Community outreach activities should target education at persons at high-risk.[14] There is no convincing evidence to support the use of chemoprophylactic agents, although administration of treponemicidal antibiotics to treat other STDs, such as gonorrhea and chancroid, may abort incubating concurrent syphilis. The inability to grow the organism on artificial media has inhibited the development of a vaccine against syphilis.

Secondary prevention by early diagnosis, treatment, partner notification, education and counseling remain the mainstay of prevention efforts. Access to prompt and appropriate services for infected persons is essential. In many developed countries, clinic-based specialist services have long been established. In developing countries, WHO has recommended that STD management be integrated into basic health care and reproductive health services.

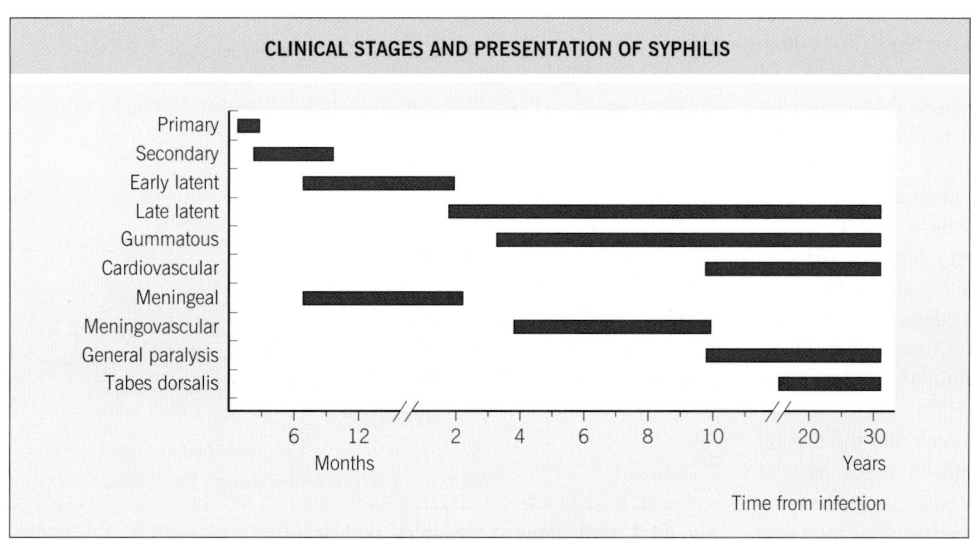

Fig. 64.3 Clinical stages and presentation of syphilis.

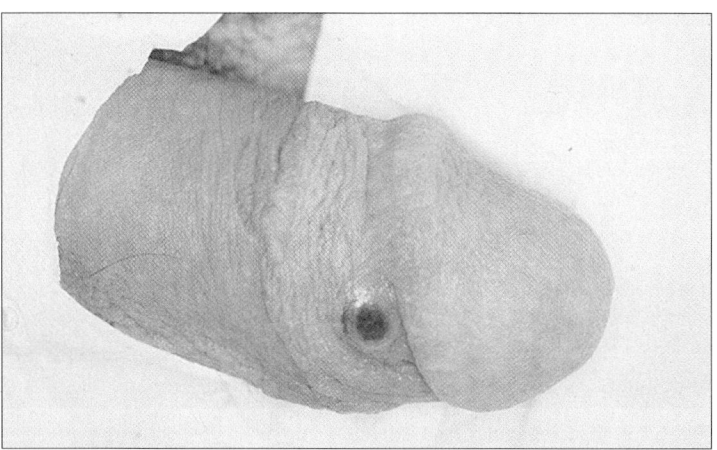

Fig. 64.4 Primary chancre in coronal sulcus in primary syphilis. A typical solitary lesion with raised everted edges, central ulceration and undermined base. With permission of The Medicine Group (Journals) Ltd.[37]

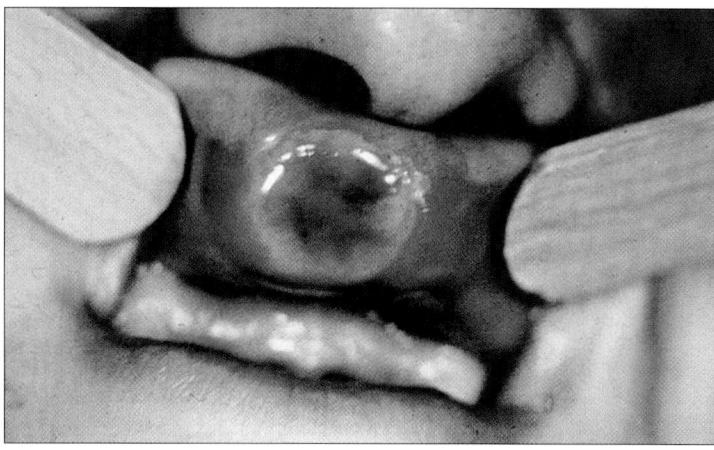

Fig. 64.5 Chancre of upper lip in primary syphilis. The chancre shows the characteristic features of a raised, rolled and everted edge; central ulceration; and a granular base. With permission of The Medicine Group (Journals) Ltd.[37]

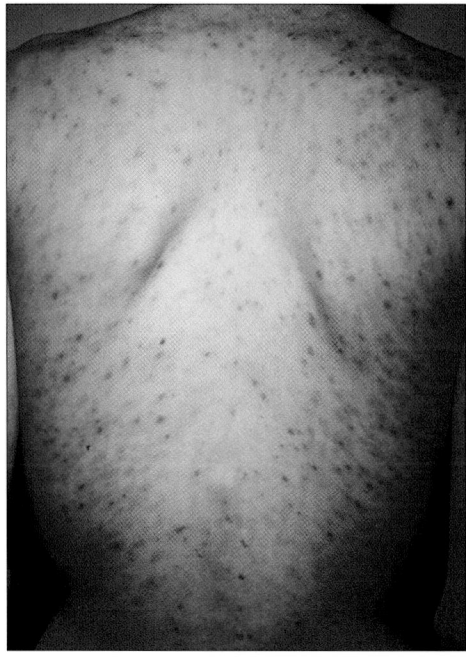

Fig. 64.6 Maculopapular rash on trunk in secondary syphilis. With permission of The Medicine Group (Journals) Ltd.[37]

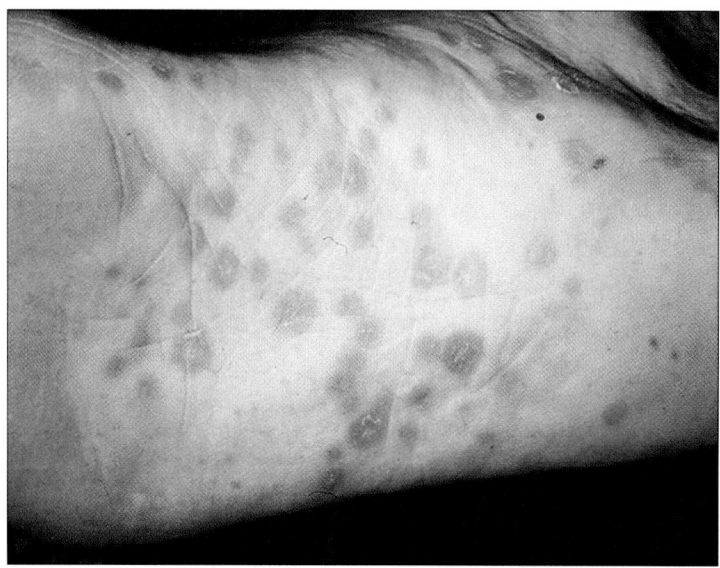

Fig. 64.7 Plantar syphilid in secondary syphilis. With permission of The Medicine Group (Journals) Ltd.[37]

Serologic screening for syphilis remains a cost-effective measure for control. Congenital syphilis may be prevented by maternal screening and treatment during early pregnancy. In Europe, screening remains a routine part of antenatal care, usually at about 12 weeks' gestation. In developing countries, where congenital syphilis is more common, the disease occurs when there has been no maternal screening, when no treatment has been administered in response to positive tests, or when primary infection occurs later in pregnancy. Repeat screening during the final trimester or at delivery is advocated in high prevalence regions.[15]

CLINICAL FEATURES

INCUBATION PERIOD

The time from transmission to the appearance of primary lesions averages 21 days with a range of 10–90 days; the incubation period varies inversely with the size of the spirochete inoculum.

The clinical presentation of syphilis is extremely diverse and may occur decades after initial infection. The time sequence of syphilis stages is shown in Figure 64.3.

PRIMARY SYPHILIS

The primary chancre appears at the site of initial treponemal invasion of the dermis. It may occur on any skin or mucous membrane surface and is usually situated on the external genitalia (Fig. 64.4). Initial lesions are papular but rapidly ulcerate. They are usually single, but 'kissing' lesions may occur on opposing mucocutaneous surfaces. Typically, the ulcers are nontender (unless there is co-existing infection) and indurated and have a clean base and raised edges (Fig. 64.5). There is often surrounding edema, especially with vulval lesions.[16] Chancres of the cervix, anorectum, or oropharynx are commonly silent. Nontender, nonsuppurative rubbery inguinal lymphadenopathy appears 1 week later and usually becomes bilateral after 2 weeks. The chancre usually heals spontaneously within 3–6 weeks but leaves a scar.

The differential diagnosis includes other sexually transmitted causes of genital ulcer disease (which may co-exist) such as chancroid, lymphogranuloma venereum, donovanosis, genital herpes, as well as traumatic ulceration, pyogenic lesions, aphthous ulceration and malignancy.[17]

SECONDARY SYPHILIS

The manifestations of generalized treponemal dissemination first appear about 8 weeks after infection. Constitutional symptoms consist

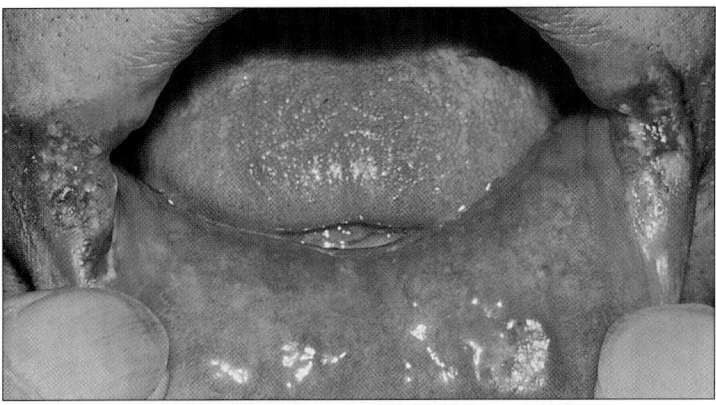

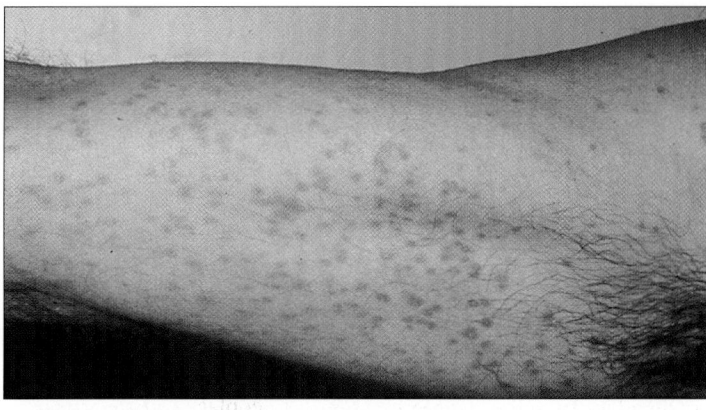

Fig. 64.8 Split papules at angle of mouth and mucous patch on lower lip in secondary syphilis. With permission of The Medicine Group (Journals) Ltd.[37]

Fig. 64.9 Maculopapular rash extending into axilla in secondary syphilis. With permission of The Medicine Group (Journals) Ltd.[37]

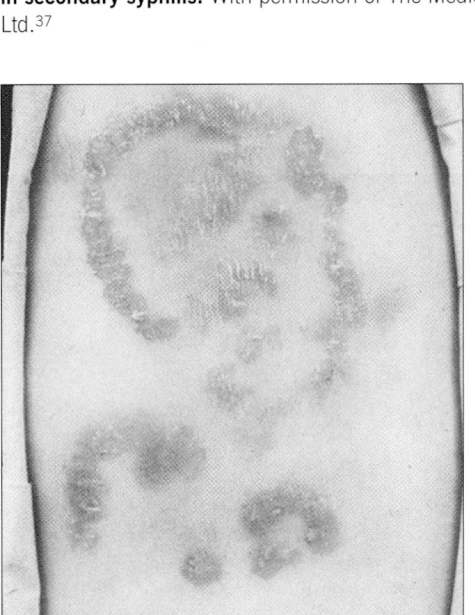

Fig. 64.10 Cutaneous nodular gummas of upper arm in tertiary gummatous syphilis. The lesions have a serpiginous outline. With permission of The Medicine Group (Journals) Ltd.[37]

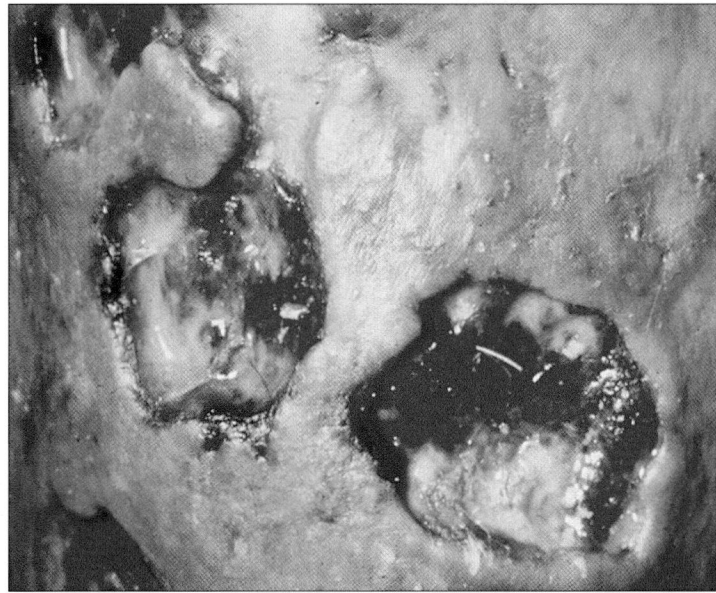

Fig. 64.11 Multiple gummatous ulcers of lower leg in tertiary gummatous syphilis. The lesions have a punched-out appearance with 'wash-leather' slough overlying a base of granulation tissue. They show a tendency for peripheral healing with thin tissue-paper scars. With permission of The Medicine Group (Journals) Ltd.[37]

of fever, headache, and bone and joint pains. There is wide diversity in physical features.

Skin rashes are the commonest feature. They are initially macular and become papular by 3 months. Lesions appear initially on the upper trunk (Fig. 64.6), the palms and soles (Fig. 64.7), and flexural surfaces of the extremities.[18] The later papulosquamous eruptions typically have a coppery color and often follow skin cleavage lines, as in pityriasis rosea. Facial lesions follow the hairline of the temporal and frontal scalp (the so-called corona veneris) and cause split papules at the angles of the mouth (Fig. 64.8). There may be hypopigmented lesions on the lateral neck (collaris veneris). Lesions in hairy areas cause moth-eaten alopecia of the scalp, beard, eye-brows and eye-lashes. Atypical facial plaques or ulcerated nodules (lues maligna) are more common with co-existing HIV infection.[19] Condylomata lata are moist flat-topped papules that appear in the moist intertriginous areas around the genitalia, anus, axillae (Fig. 64.9) and beneath the breasts about 6 months after infection. On mucous membranes, especially of the mouth, erythematous macules evolve into asymptomatic, slightly elevated flat-topped lesions covered by a hyperkeratotic grayish membrane. These mucous patches may coalesce to form 'snail-track' ulcers.

Generalized lymphadenopathy occurs in 50% of secondary syphilis

cases and has similar characteristics to the localized lymphadenopathy of primary infection. Other systemic features of secondary syphilis include panuveitis,[20] periostitis and joint effusions, glomerulonephritis, hepatitis, gastritis, myocarditis and aseptic meningitis.

The lesions of secondary syphilis resolve spontaneously in a variable time period and most patients enter the latency stage within the first year of infection. In some, especially the immunocompromised, primary or secondary lesions may recur.

The differential diagnosis is broad and includes exanthema associated with many infectious diseases, including primary HIV infection, dermatoses (e.g. pityriasis rosea and guttate psoriasis) and connective tissue disorders such as systemic lupus erythematosus. Condylomata lata must be differentiated from viral warts, scabies and lichen planus.

LATENT SYPHILIS

In latent syphilis there are no clinical stigmata of active disease, although disease remains detectable by positive serologic tests. In early latency, within 2 years of infection, vertical transmission of infection may still occur, but sexual transmission is less likely in the absence of mucocutaneous lesions. The late manifestations of syphilis subsequently arise, often decades later, in about 25% of those who have latent syphilis.

Genital Herpes

Diane Goade & Gregory Mertz

Genital herpes is one of the most common sexually transmitted diseases. Of these, the agents of genital herpes – herpes simplex virus (HSV) type 2, and less commonly, HSV type 1 – are among the most frequently encountered human pathogens.[1,2]

EPIDEMIOLOGY

Genital herpes infections are common, with estimates of 500,000–700,000 cases of symptomatic first episodes/year in the USA.[3–7] Humans are the natural reservoir for HSV, and virtually all cases of genital herpes are sporadic, acquired via person-to-person transmission. There are no reported epidemics of genital herpes.[2]

Herpes simplex virus infections have a worldwide distribution, with seroprevalence to either HSV-1 or HSV-2 approaching 90% in some age and sex groups.[3–7] Herpes simplex virus-1 infection is common early in life, with antibodies typically appearing in childhood and prevalence increasing with age; HSV-2 antibodies increase in prevalence with increasing age after the onset of sexual activity. Approximately 1 in every 3–4 adults in the USA is seropositive for HSV-2.[3–7] Herpes simplex virus-2 seroprevalence rates in the USA differ for some racial, sex and ethnic groups. Women acquire HSV-2 infections more readily than men, and overall have a higher seroprevalence rate.[8] Other risk factors for genital herpes include lower socioeconomic status, increased number of sexual partners, African-Caribbean race and Hispanic ethnicity.[4–7] The highest prevalence of HSV-2 antibodies is among commercial sex workers, and up to 70% of prostitutes in the USA have the infection. The lowest HSV-2 prevalence is in sexually abstinent groups, including nuns, where seroprevalence is 3% or lower.[4–7]

The incidence of seroconversion is approximately 5–10%/year when discordant couples are followed longitudinally. Among HSV-naive females with male partners who have the infection, seroconversion is as high as 15–30%/year. However, when the female partner has the infection first, less than 5% of male partners seroconvert/year.[8]

After infection with an HSV, antibodies to HSV-1 and HSV-2 type common antigens provide partial protection to infection with the counterpart virus. In prospective studies, women who have HSV-1 infection have a 5–20%/year lower rate of seroconversion to HSV-2 than women who do not have HSV infection.[8] Seroconversion to HSV-1 during childhood has decreased, particularly in upper and middle class socioeconomic groups in the Western developed countries, whereas symptomatic infection with HSV-2 during adulthood has increased.[4,5]

PATHOGENESIS

Herpes simplex viruses are large enveloped DNA viruses with a diameter of approximately 150nm, a dsDNA core, an icosahedral capsid composed of 162 capsomers, an amorphous tegument layer and a lipid envelope. There are 11 different glycoproteins projecting from the envelope that are crucial for virion–cell surface attachment and cell-to-cell spread (Fig. 65.1).[1,9]

Herpes simplex viruses are spread by direct contact, including contact with infected secretions:

- HSV-1 is typically spread through close contact with infected oral secretions, and genital herpes due to HSV-1 is usually due to oral-genital contact; and
- HSV-2 is primarily spread through intimate contact with infected genital secretions and tissues.

Intact skin is fairly resistant to virus infection, but abraded skin or mucous membranes are more susceptible.

The virus attaches to the cell surface and the viral envelope fuses with the cell membrane using a specific cellular receptor. Virion–cell surface attachment and virus intracellular penetration is mediated by viral surface glycoproteins. The viral nucleocapsid is released into the cytoplasm where it is transported to the nuclear pores of the cell. Following viral DNA replication and gene expression in the cell nucleus, the replicated nucleocapsid is assembled and buds through the nuclear membrane, acquiring an envelope. The enveloped nucleocapsid is translocated across the cytoplasm and cell membrane, acquiring surface glycoproteins at both the nuclear membrane and cell surface.[1,9]

Herpes simplex virus then infects and replicates in parabasal and intermediate skin cells. Replication results in lysis of the infected cell. Infection may spread locally by direct cell-to-cell invasion or to more distant sites via sensory nerve pathways. As virus replication spreads to involve the local autonomic and sensory nerve endings, retrograde transmission of virions (or possibly nucleocapsids) occurs with transport of virus particles to the regional sensory ganglia. Transient virus replication may occur in the ganglia at this point. From the sensory ganglia, antegrade virion migration along sensory nerves allows viral spread to other sites. By this method of spread, crops of herpetic lesions may arise at nonadjacent sites such as the thighs or buttocks. Virus replication is associated with cell lysis, cell destruction and local inflammation of all tissues except the sensory ganglia.[2,10,11]

Central nervous system disease may occur as an aseptic meningitis with primary HSV-2, or as a necrotic focal encephalitis with HSV-1 via spread through the cribriform plate to the temporal horns. Recurrent aseptic meningitis has been described, but is rare. Rarely, hematogenous dissemination may occur with visceral organ involvement.[2]

IMMUNE RESPONSE

Both cellular and humoral host immune responses appear to be elicited by genital herpes infection.[9–16] The lysis of infected epithelial cells results in local inflammation, macrophage recruitment and T-lymphocyte activation. In a murine model, there is induction of natural killer lymphocytes. Lymphocyte activation results in the appearance of antibodies, including virus-neutralizing antibodies and antibodies that provide passive protection against infection when given to animals who are then challenged with virus.[1,9] T-lymphocyte responses, including cytotoxic T-lymphocyte responses, appear to be crucial in limiting and clearing disease.[13] Murine models also indicate that the degree of macrophage function at the site of local invasion may contribute to limiting the spread of infection.[1]

Cytokine induction is less well described. In cell culture models, HSV-infected cells express the cytokines interleukin-2 , tumor necrosis factor-α and interferon-γ.[13] Peripheral blood mononuclear cells have been shown to produce interferon-α within hours of

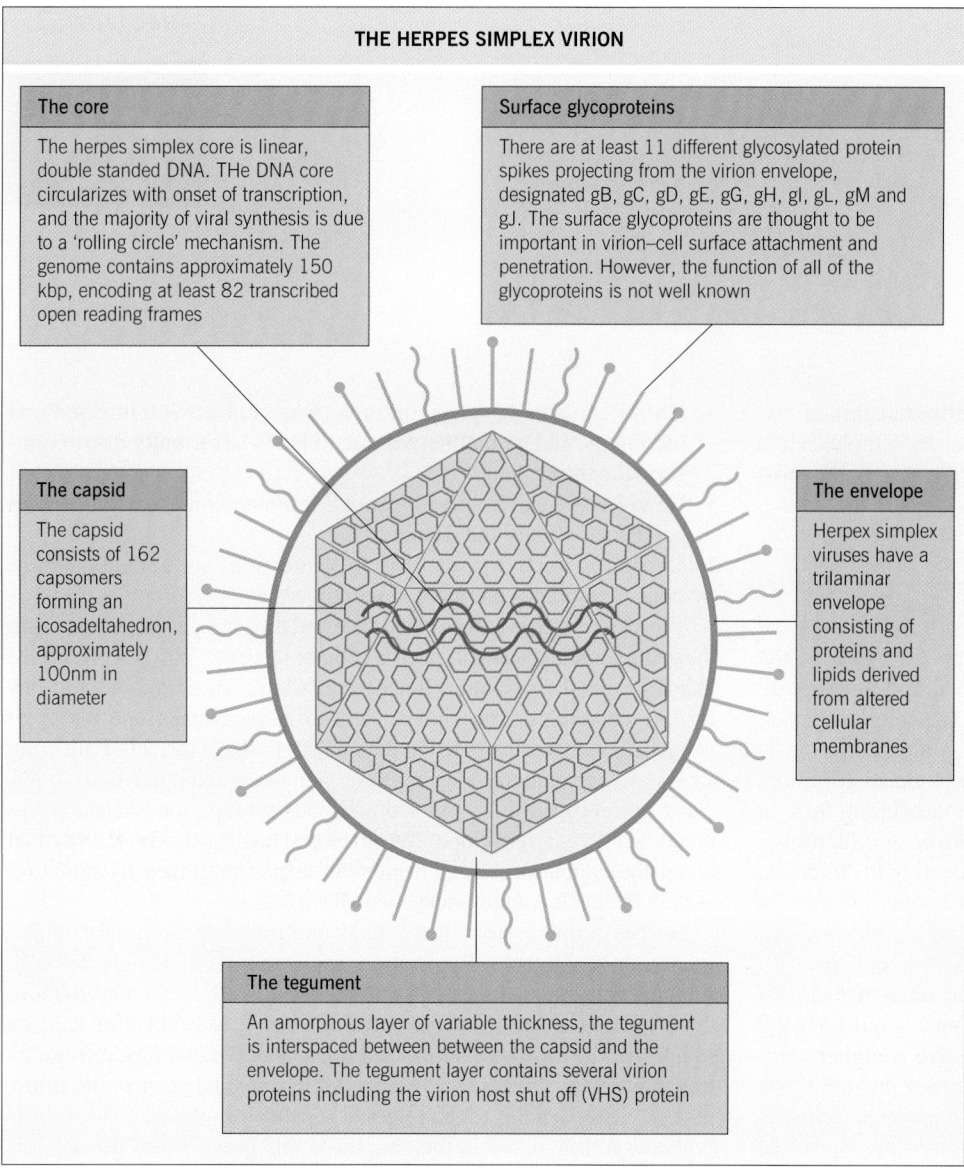

THE HERPES SIMPLEX VIRION

The core

The herpes simplex core is linear, double standed DNA. THe DNA core circularizes with onset of transcription, and the majority of viral synthesis is due to a 'rolling circle' mechanism. The genome contains approximately 150 kbp, encoding at least 82 transcribed open reading frames

Surface glycoproteins

There are at least 11 different glycosylated protein spikes projecting from the virion envelope, designated gB, gC, gD, gE, gG, gH, gI, gL, gM and gJ. The surface glycoproteins are thought to be important in virion–cell surface attachment and penetration. However, the function of all of the glycoproteins is not well known

The capsid

The capsid consists of 162 capsomers forming an icosadeltahedron, approximately 100nm in diameter

The envelope

Herpex simplex viruses have a trilaminar envelope consisting of proteins and lipids derived from altered cellular membranes

The tegument

An amorphous layer of variable thickness, the tegument is interspaced between between the capsid and the envelope. The tegument layer contains several virion proteins including the virion host shut off (VHS) protein

Fig. 65.1 The herpes simplex virion. The herpes simplex virion consists of a dsDNA core surrounded by a capsid, and amorphous tegument layer and a lipid envelope with numerous glycoprotein spikes. The overall diameter is 150–200nm. Virus replication takes place within the nucleus of the infected cell. The envelope is gained as the virion passes through the nuclear membrane. Replication of virus within the host cell results in cell lysis and destruction. Latent virus do not cause neural cell lysis within ganglia.

exposure to HSV virions.[11] Individuals with limited cellular immunity, including those at the extremes of life, patients with AIDS and bone marrow transplant recipients, tend to have prolonged severe disease with extensive tissue involvement and a higher rate of dissemination.[14]

Human humoral immune responses to HSV include the rapid generation of IgM antibodies following infection, with the appearance of detectable IgG and IgA antibodies approximately 10–14 days later. Antibodies appear first to certain structural proteins, and then sequentially to the various surface glycoproteins. Seroconversion to all virus antigenic determinants after infection may require months as measured by Western blot.[5,12,15] Lifelong virus neutralizing antibodies and antibody-dependent cellular cytotoxic antibodies are detectable approximately 1 month after infection. Lack of antibody-dependent cellular cytotoxic antibodies has been correlated with a poor clinical outcome and may be a factor in severe disease in the newborn.[1,16,17]

HISTOLOGY
The characteristic lesion of HSV infection is an erythematous macular or papular lesion, which progresses to a thin-walled vesicle on an erythematous base. Histologically, HSV infection is characterized by edema, multinucleate giant cells and Cowdry type A intranuclear inclusions. The inflammatory reaction present within HSV lesions consists of a mononuclear cell infiltrate of predominantly CD4+ T-lymphocytes (Fig. 65.2).[18]

LATENCY
Lifelong latency is a unique property of the herpesvirusesand is characterized by persistence of virus or viral DNA in an apparently quiescent or inactive state in sensory and autonomic ganglia.[1] Virus replication is limited or nonexistent during latency, and antiviral medications are unable to eradicate latent virus.[1,2,9]

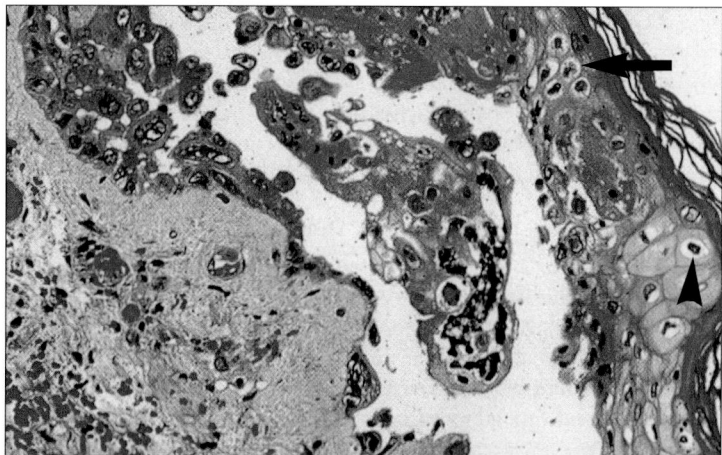

Fig. 65.2 Histology. Section of human skin showing typical HSV virus effects: multinucleated giant cells (arrowhead) and intranuclear inclusion (arrow).

Periodic recurrences of symptomatic disease are due to reactivation of latent virus. Latent virus begins to replicate and form active virus particles. The virus particles are transported by antegrade axonal flow from the ganglion to the epithelium in the genital tract. Following reactivation, fully infectious virus may be cultured from cutaneous lesions at the site of recurrence.

Reactivation of latent virus tends to be site- and virus-specific. HSV-2 reactivates much more readily from the sacral ganglia than HSV-1, and HSV-1 reactivates more readily from the trigeminal ganglia.[2,9,19] How the virus remains latent within the ganglia, and how reactivation occurs are not well understood. In the epithelial cell, actively replicating virus DNA exists in a circular form. During latency the viral DNA assumes a linear configuration, and latent viral DNA is not integrated into the host chromosome. Latency is not a wholly quiescent period, however, as some herpes simplex genes thought to be regulatory transcripts are expressed during this time.[1,2,9] Sequences within the herpes simplex genome specify 'latency-associated transcripts', which may be important in reactivation of virus replication. These sequences are highly divergent between HSV-1 and HSV-2 and may account for the preferential reactivation of virus type with its corresponding ganglion following latency.[2,9,19]

Virtually all recurrent genital herpes is due to reactivation of latent infection rather than from re-infection.[20] Several events may contribute to reactivation including trauma to the ganglia, immunosuppression and fever and possibly sexual activity.[2,19]

PREVENTION

The only proven prevention strategy in avoidance of skin-to-skin contact when HSV is present in the genital tract. This includes avoidance of close physical contact during clinically symptomatic outbreaks when virus is present in high concentrations. Most patients can recognize symptomatic clinical outbreaks even when their symptoms are 'atypical' or mild and can avoid intimate contact during this time.

Frequent, intermittent aymptomatic or subclinical shedding of low titers of virus from the genital tract occurs in both men and women[21] and accounts for most cases of the transmission of genital herpes.[21–23] There is no current method to predict when aymptomatic virus shedding is occurring. It has been demonstrated that use of suppressive aciclovir decreases both the number of days of virus shedding and the quantity of virus shed.[24] Studies are underway to address the question of whether decreased shedding decreases transmission risk.

VACCINES
Protective vaccines may become important preventative options. The increasing incidence of genital herpes, the large number of HSV-2-seropositive individuals who are unaware of their infection status and the risk of disease transmission from asymptomatic shedding underscore the need for an effective vaccine.[22,23]

In vaccine studies, various animal models, including a guinea pig vaginal HSV-2 model and a mouse footpad inoculation or scarification model, indicate that certain vaccine candidates provide protection from acquiring infection or ameliorate disease.[25,26] When studied in humans, these vaccine candidates have not been as effective as in the animal models. In a previous controlled trial in discordant couples, an inactivated HSV-2 glycoprotein vaccine failed to provide protection.[27] Recently, human trials have been completed or phase 3 trials are underway to evaluate recombinant surface glycoprotein vaccines.[28,29] No vaccine for HSV-2 is currently licensed.

BARRIER CONTRACEPTION
Barrier contraception such as latex condoms can reduce the risk of disease transmission by decreasing contact with the partner's infected skin or mucous membranes or infected secretions. Because herpesvirus may be present outside the portion of genital tract protected by barrier contraception, condom use is not infallible.

CLINICAL FEATURES

Genital herpes is a lifelong infection characterized by an initial infection followed by latency, and frequent recurrences. Infection may range from severe and symptomatic to asymptomatic. Herpes simplex virus disease is defined as:

- primary disease when a person lacking any antibodies to HSV acquires an infection with HSV-1 or HSV-2; and
- nonprimary first-episode disease when an individual with pre-existing antibodies to one serotype, typically HSV-1, acquires disease with the second type.

The presence of pre-existing type common antibodies and cell-mediated immune responses modifies the course of disease and so first episode nonprimary disease is typically less severe than primary disease.[2,9]

Genital herpes may recur from none to six or more times/year. Recurrent disease tends to be milder than symptomatic first episode disease, with fewer vesicles, less discomfort and a shortened duration of symptoms.[2,9]

Transmission of HSV-2 to a sexual partner or a neonate may be the first indication of the presence of genital herpes infection in an asymptomatic source partner.[23,30] The time and source of disease acquisition are often difficult to prove conclusively because:

- genital herpes can have a prolonged asymptomatic phase after acquisition and may be transmitted via asymptomatic shedding; and
- clinically silent or unrecognized disease is common.

PRIMARY FIRST-EPISODE GENITAL HERPES
Primary genital herpes is most often seen as a disease of sexually active teenagers and young adults. Following exposure, a clinically silent incubation period lasts for 2–7 days. Onset of clinically apparent disease may be heralded by fever, headache and local genital pain and burning. Patients may appear to be systemically ill. In general, females tend to have more severe disease than males, with estimates of urinary retention occurring in approximately 10% of females. Up to 25% of females manifest symptoms of aseptic meningitis.[2,9]

The characteristic painful lesions in the genital area initially present as erythematous macules, which then progress to vesicles on an erythematous base, pustules, ulcers and finally to crusts. Each crop of lesions takes an average of 8 days to heal completely, and successive crops of lesions may arise during the course of the disease. Untreated genital herpes may require weeks to resolve, averaging 3 weeks to cessation of lesions. Healing is usually complete, although particularly severe or large ulcers may result in scarring.[2]

In the male, lesions typically appear on the penis and glans penis. In females, lesions may be present throughout the genital tract including the perineum, vulva, labia, perianal regions and buttocks. The vesicles are typically distributed bilaterally in primary disease. Cervical involvement is usually present and may escape detection if limited external disease is present and a complete pelvic examination is not performed. A vaginal discharge may accompany cervical and, less commonly, vaginal herpes. In either sex, the perianal and rectal mucosa may be involved, especially if exposure was due to rectal intercourse. Tender bilateral inguinal adenopathy is generally present. Vesicles may also be present on the thighs.

If herpetic involvement of the urethra occurs, severe dysuria may result. Sacral radiculopathy may occur during the course of primary genital herpes, with urinary retention, neuralgias, dysesthesia and diminished rectal tone. Tenesmus and rectal pain may be present with rectal herpes.[2,9]

In HSV-naive individuals, primary genital disease due to either HSV-1 or HSV-2 is clinically indistinguishable, making identification of infection by genital cultures and virus typing important for diagnosis. Atypical symptoms are quite common, with up to 30% of genital herpes presenting as paresthesias or urinary retention rather than the classically described vesicular genital lesions.[2,9,31]

NONPRIMARY FIRST-EPISODE DISEASE

Nonprimary first-episode genital HSV-2 infection is typically intermediate in severity when compared with that of primary and recurrent genital herpes.[2] Untreated disease lasts for approximately 10–14 days, with fewer lesions and fewer crops of lesions than are typical for primary disease. Systemic symptoms, including fever, are less common than in primary genital herpes, and virus can be cultured less frequently from the cervix and genital tract.[2,9]

RECURRENT GENITAL HERPES

In approximately 50% of patients, a prodrome of symptoms heralds the onset of recurrent disease. Commonly reported prodromal symptoms include local burning and itching, tingling and dysesthesia. Patients may have their own recognizable cluster of symptoms. The prodromal symptoms may occur without the development of noticeable lesions or may be followed by the typical vesicular eruption lasting 6–10 days. In contrast to the widely distributed, bilateral lesions of primary genital herpes, the crop of vesicular lesions in recurrent disease tends to be localized and unilateral. Lesions are typically present on the vulva in women and the glans penis and penile shaft in men, although lesions may also present on the thigh or buttocks, in the rectum and at other sites. Paresthesia, dysesthesia, local edema, pain, regional adenopathy and local swelling may accompany recurrent cutaneous herpes.[2,9]

Recurrence rates vary widely from none to six or more episodes/year, with some individuals having one or more recurrences each month. Recurrences may be triggered by sexual activity, with high rates of recurrent disease in commercial sex workers. Immunocompromised patients may experience frequent, prolonged and severe recurrences.[32] Genital herpes due to infection with HSV-2 reactivates much more readily than genital herpes due to HSV-1. Recurrent genital herpes has been reported in over 80% of individuals following primary genital HSV-2, whereas recurrence in patients who had HSV-1 primary genital herpes was less than 50%.[2] Recurrence of genital herpes averages 0.33/month with HSV-2 disease, but only 0.02/month for HSV-1 genital disease.[19]

ASYMPTOMATIC SHEDDING

Landmark studies have demonstrated both by culture, and by polymerase chain reaction (PCR), that herpesvirus is frequently present in the genital tract when lesions are absent and skin is intact, or when small or unrecognized lesions are present (Fig. 65.3).[33,34] During periods of asymptomatic virus shedding, virus titers are typically lower than during a symptomatic acute outbreak. When detected by virus culture, asymptomatic shedding occurs on an average of 4% of days, whereas women with primary genital herpes may shed virus on up to 17% of days in the first few months following their primary outbreak.[21,22]

UNCOMMON SITES OF INFECTION

Although the majority of herpes virus infections occur in the genital and orolabial regions, cutaneous disease may occur in virtually any site, causing localized to widespread disease. Genital herpes may present as:
- rectal herpes, with symptoms of proctitis, including rectal discharge, anal pain and pain on defecation;
- sacral paresthesia with urine retention; and
- painful anal fissures.

Males with rectal herpes may also present with impotence as a manifestation of neurologic involvement with HSV.[2,9]

Neonatal herpes is a rare complication of genital herpes resulting from exposure of a newborn to HSV-2 from the maternal genital tract (see Chapter 2.54). Acquisition may occur during maternal primary genital disease via exposure to infectious virus in the birth canal during labor and delivery. Less commonly, the fetus acquires the infection during gestation. The incidence of neonatal herpes is approximately 1/3500 live births. An increased incidence is noted in preterm infants. Maternal acquisition of genital herpes during the third trimester of pregnancy increases the risk of neonatal transmission more than 10-fold

compared with the risk of transmission from longstanding maternal HSV infection.[30,35]

DISEASE IN THE IMMUNOCOMPROMISED HOST

Herpes simplex viruses may be significant pathogens in immunocompromised hosts (see Chapters 4.4 & 4.5). Patients who have AIDS may have both frequent and increased duration of recurrences of HSV mucocutaneous disease (see Chapter 5.11). Delayed healing and continued virus replication leads to local spread and large, painful ulcers extending through the cutaneous and subcutaneous layers. In patients with CD4+ lymphocyte count below 100/μl, treatment of genital herpes may be complicated by emergence of aciclovir-resistant HSV strains.[2,9,32,36]

DIAGNOSIS

Despite an overall increasing awareness of sexually transmitted diseases, recognition of genital herpes by both the patient and the health care provider is often limited, and the majority of infections are undiagnosed or unrecognized (Fig. 65.4).[4,5,31] Diagnosis of herpes simplex disease is important:
- to establish presence or absence of infection;
- to guide treatment considerations; and
- to allow the health care practitioner an opportunity to intervene in disease transmission.

Diagnosis may be accomplished by serologic and microbiologic methods.

VIRAL CULTURE

Viral culture and typing is the preferred method for identifying infection as it is the most accurate and most widely available diagnostic modality. It is recommended for all patients who have not had previous virologic confirmation of disease, including those with first-episode genital disease. Culture provides confirmation of the clinical diagnosis, and typing of virus predicts subsequent recurrence patterns. Culture of body fluids, vesicles and tissues from patients with symptomatic disease yields positive results in most cases when obtained early in the disease. Cervical cultures are positive in up to 90% of women with primary or first-episode genital herpes during the first week of symptoms, with decreasing rates of virus recovery during disease resolution. Virus may be recovered from mucocutaneous ulcers, cutaneous vesicles, CSF, rectum, urethra, urine and elsewhere in the genital tract.[2,40]

In recurrent disease, virus may not be present in readily detectable quantities. Culture of multiple sites such as urethra, rectum and genital tract improves the chance of virus recovery. Growth and typing of

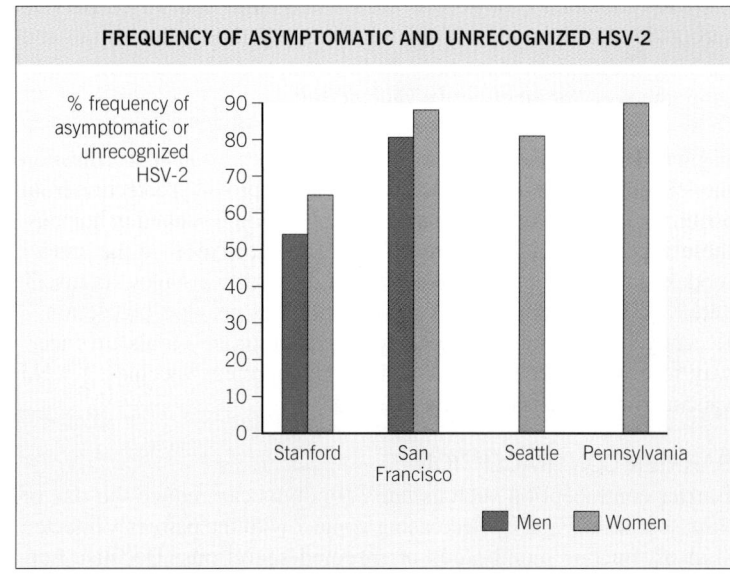

Fig. 65.3 Frequency of asymptomatic and unrecognized herpes simplex virus (HSV)-2 in four major US cities.[4,31,37–39]

virus requires less than 5 days, and modified culture techniques that detect herpes antigens (the shell-vial assays) yield preliminary results in 1–2 days.[33,40]

SEROLOGIC ASSAYS

Type-specific serologic diagnosis is important:
- for serosurveys to gauge prevalence rates;
- in situations where culture is not feasible or available; and
- for patient counseling in scenarios of sexually transmitted disease and other public health clinics.

Herpes simplex antibodies are readily detectable following infection, but it may take several months for complete antibody development to all antigenic determinants. Differentiating HSV-1 from HSV-2 antibodies is more problematic due to the antigenic similarity of the viruses.[1,9,15] Antibody responses in general are broadly cross-reactive between HSV-1 and HSV-2, and currently available commercial antibody detection-based assays do not differentiate between the two.[40] Antibodies to glycoprotein G are type-specific, and antibodies to portions of glycoprotein B are type specific.[41] Promising new tests such as sensitive and specific glycoprotein G-based serologic assays in enzyme-linked immunosorbent assay and immunodot forms are in development. Western blot analysis of antibodies to virus antigens including glycoprotein G is technically demanding, but is both sensitive and specific and has provided the basis for type-specific serosurveys.[41,42]

OTHER DIAGNOSTIC TECHNIQUES

The advent of the PCR allows amplification and detection of HSV gene segments even when present in virus copy numbers too low for detection by culture. Assays based on PCR are rapid and sensitive, but strict control measures are necessary to avoid false-positive results. Detection of HSV by PCR is most useful for herpes meningitis, encephalitis and other central nervous system infections that are not readily diagnosed by cerebrospinal fluid culture, or would otherwise require brain biopsy for diagnosis. Tthe sensitivity of HSV PCR approaches that of biopsy for the diagnosis of herpes encephalitis and that HSV-2 can be detected by PCR in a high proportion of people with recurrent aseptic meningitis.[1,9,43,44]

Use of the PCR to detect and quantify virus sequences on the skin and in the genital tract in the absence of lesions has provided important information about the duration and amount of asymptomatic virus shedding as the virus copy number is often below the threshold of detection by culture.[21] Neonatal herpes infection may also be diagnosed by PCR amplification of HSV gene segments in the serum and CSF.

DIFFERENTIAL DIAGNOSIS OF GENITAL HERPES	
Disease	Diagnostic clues
Syphilis	Lesions usually single and painless; positive darkfield microscopy
Chancroid	Nonindurated ulcers, positive bacterial cultures for *Haemophilus ducreyi*
Lymphogranuloma venereum	Constitutional symptoms follow onset of lesions; responds to doxycycline
Genital warts	Chronicity of lesions; no vesiculation; minimal pain
Fixed drug eruption	History; viral culture negative
Contact dermatitis	History; lack of systemic symptoms; no adenopathy
Trauma	History; lack of systemic symptoms; no adenopathy
Psoriasis	Chronicity of lesions; lesions elsewhere on body

Fig. 65.4 Differential diagnosis of genital herpes.

MANAGEMENT

Currently, the practitioner has a choice of effective, safe and well-tolerated medications (see Fig. 65.5). Antiviral therapy is effective:
- in the treatment of primary and first-episode genital herpes;
- for episodic treatment of recurrences; and
- for suppression of frequent recurrences.

Continuous antiviral therapy has also been shown to decrease viral shedding. Antiviral therapy has not yet been shown to affect latency, 'cure' genital herpes, or reduce the risk of transmission.

PHARMACOLOGIC AGENTS

Aciclovir is the acyclic analog of the nucleoside guanosine. In order to be active, it must first be phosphorylated by the virus-encoded enzyme, thymidine kinase, to aciclovir monophosphate. The monophosphorylated form is then further phosphorylated by cellular enzymes to the di- and triphosphate form. The active form, aciclovir triphosphate, inhibits the HSV-specific DNA polymerase and terminates the replicating DNA chain by competing with its analog deoxyguanosine triphosphate. Aciclovir lacks the 3´ hydroxyl group necessary for subsequent phosphodiester linkages, so that extension of the replicating DNA chain is no longer possible.[34]

ANTIVIRAL THERAPY			
Medication	Indication	Dose, route	Side effects
Aciclovir	Primary genital herpes	200mg po five times daily or 400mg po q8h for 10 days	Nausea
	Recurrent genital herpes	200mg po five times daily or 400mg q8h for 5 days	Nausea
	Suppression of frequent recurrences	400mg po q12h or 200mg po q8h	Nausea
	Severe or disseminated disease	5mg/kg slow iv q8h for 10 days	Reversible crystalline nephropathy, tremors
	Encephalitis	10mg/kg slow iv q8h for 10 days	Reversible crystalline nephropathy, tremors
Valaciclovir	Primary genital herpes	1g q12h for 10 days	Nausea
	Recurrent genital herpes	500mg q12h for 5 days	
	Suppression of frequent recurrences	500mg q12h or 1g daily	
Famciclovir	Primary genital herpes	250mg po q8h for 10 days	Nausea
	Recurrent genital herpes	125mg po q12h for 5 days	
	Suppression of frequent recurrences	250mg po q12h	
Foscarnet	Aciclovir-resistant herpes simplex virus	60mg/kg q8h, infuse over 2 hours for 10 days	Azotemia, seizures, hypo- or hyperkalemia and hypo- or hyperphosphatemia

Fig. 65.5 Antiviral therapy. Note that the topical aciclovir 5% ointment available in the USA is of little value in the treatment of genital herpes and is not recommended as effective therapy. Valaciclovir 1g daily and 500mg daily are both approved for chronic suppressive therapy, but the authors recommend 500mg q12h.

Aciclovir has proved to be a well-tolerated and effective medication with a wide margin of safety. Its safety and specificity results from the relative inability of cellular kinases to phosphorylate aciclovir to its active form and from the more potent inhibition of HSV DNA polymerase than human DNA polymerase by aciclovir triphosphate. Resistance to aciclovir occurs when HSV strains develop that lack thymidine kinase or less commonly by strains with an altered thymidine kinase or DNA polymerase.[34]

Aciclovir is currently available as an oral, topical and intravenous agent. Clearance is via the kidney, with approximately 90% of the drug excreted unchanged in the urine.[34] Side effects for the oral and topical forms are minimal. Topical aciclovir may cause burning and is not approved for use on mucous membranes.[45] Oral aciclovir may cause nausea, especially with high doses. These symptoms are generally mild and resolve over time with continued use of the drug.[46] Intravenous aciclovir may cause local pain and phlebitis if drug extravasates during administration.[34] The most common significant side effect of intravenous aciclovir is a reversible nephropathy secondary to crystallization of aciclovir in the renal tubules. Administration of intravenous doses slowly over 1 hour decreases the incidence of nephropathy. Aciclovir nephropathy is rarely seen in normal adults, but is more common in the elderly and in those with underlying renal dysfunction. Intravenous aciclovir may rarely cause neurologic complications, including lethargy, delirium and tremors.[34]

Other therapeutic agents

Antiviral medications that have recently become available include valaciclovir, penciclovir and famciclovir.

Valaciclovir. Oral bioavailability of aciclovir is limited, with only 15–20% of the oral dose absorbed. Valaciclovir, a prodrug of aciclovir, was developed to increase the oral bioavailability and is absorbed at levels 3–5 times greater than those for aciclovir. Following absorption, valaciclovir is then hydrolyzed to aciclovir. Oral administration of valaciclovir can lead to serum levels of aciclovir approaching those following intravenous administration of aciclovir.[47]

Penciclovir. Penciclovir is also an acyclic neucleoside analog. Like aciclovir, the drug must first be phosphorylated by the HSV-encoded thymidine kinase to penciclovir monophosphate. Cellular kinases then phosphorylate the compound to the di- and triphosphate forms. Like aciclovir triphosphate, penciclovir triphosphate is an inhibitor of HSV DNA polymerase. Although penciclovir is phosphorylated by thymidine kinase much more readily than aciclovir, this benefit is offset by reduced activity against the viral polymerase compared with that of aciclovir. DNA chain termination is not a significant property of penciclovir triphosphate. The intracellular half-life of penciclovir triphosphate is much longer than that of aciclovir triphosphate. It is unclear still whether these differences have an effect on the effectiveness or safety of penciclovir compared with those of aciclovir.[48,49]

Famciclovir. Famciclovir is an oral prodrug of penciclovir. Similar to valaciclovir, famciclovir was developed in an effort to increase oral bioavailability. Following ingestion, famciclovir is rapidly converted by deacetlyation to penciclovir. Approximately 60–70% of the dose is excreted in the urine as penciclovir.[50]

Foscarnet. Foscarnet is a pyrophosphate analog that inhibits viral DNA polymerase.[51] Because it does not require phosphorylation to become active, its efficacy is not dependent on the presence of HSV-specific thymidine kinases. As such, foscarnet is one of the few drugs available for the treatment of aciclovir-resistant herpes simplex due to thymidine kinase- or thymidine kinase-altered strains. Foscarnet is only available as an intravenous preparation. The most common side

DRUG COMPARISON TRIALS				
Medications	Indication	Authors	Results	Conclusions
Aciclovir 200mg po five times daily for 10 days versus placebo	First-episode genital herpes	Corey et al.[58]	With po or iv aciclovir, pain decreased by 4 days, viral shedding decreased by 7 days, time to healing reduced by 7 days, 60% fewer new lesions; topical aciclovir of limited value	Oral aciclovir significantly effective in treatment of first-episode genital herpes
Famciclovir various doses po q8h versus aciclovir 200mg po five times daily	First-episode genital herpes	Loveless et al.[60]	Famciclovir 125, 250 or 500mg q8h equal to aciclovir 200mg five times daily each given for 10 days; famciclovir 250, 500 or 750mg q8h equal to aciclovir 200mg five times daily each given for 5 days	Famciclovir equal in efficacy to standard dose aciclovir and required less frequent dosing interval
Valaciclovir 1g po q12h po versus aciclovir 200mg five times daily po	First-episode genital herpes	Fife et al.[73]	Valaciclovir q12h doses as effective as aciclovir five times daily	Valaciclovir as effective as aciclovir, but required less frequent dosing interval
Valciclovir 1g q12h po versus aciclovir 200mg five times daily po versus placebo	Recurrent genital herpes	Smiley et al.[65]	Time to healing equivalent for valaciclovir and aciclovir (115–116 hours) and shorter than with placebo (144 hours); duration of viral shedding also decreased in treated group	Treatment with valaciclovir or aciclovir significantly more effective than with placebo, and no difference between the two drug treatments (valaciclovir 500mg q12h now shown to be as effective as 1g q12h in a separate study)
Famciclovir 125, 250 or 500mg q12h po compared with placebo	Recurrent genital herpes	Sacks et al.[74]	Time to healing reduced by 1.1 days in treated group; significant reduction in shedding	Famciclovir effective in treatment of recurrent genital herpes
Aciclovir 400mg q12h po versus placebo	Suppression of frequent recurrences	Mertz et al.[69]	Mean number of recurrences 11.4/year for placebo group, 1.8/year for treated group; number free from recurrences for 1 year: 2% for placebo group, 44% for treated group	Aciclovir highly effective at suppressing frequent recurrences; minimal side effects, high patient compliance and satisfaction with treatment
Famciclovir various doses po versus placebo	Suppression of frequent recurrences	Mertz et al.[75]	Time to first recurrence 82 days for placebo, greater than 120 days for treatment; 250mg q12h most effective and 78% of patients with no recurrences at 120 days versus 42% of those treated with placebo	Famciclovir 250mg q12h effective for suppressing frequent recurrences
Aciclovir 400mg q12h po versus placebo	Suppression of asymptomatic viral shedding	Wald et al.[24]	Five of 34 treated shed virus during therapy compared with 25 of 34 in placebo group; days shed were 6.9% with placebo, 0.3% with aciclovir	Aciclovir dramatically decreases asymptomatic viral shedding

Fig. 65.6 Drug comparison trials.

effects include nephrotoxicity, electrolyte abnormalities, seizures and penile ulcers. Saline hydration decreases the renal toxicity and is recommended to diminish the risk of azotemia. Foscarnet-resistant HSV strains have occasionally developed in immunosuppressed hosts.[52]

Cidofovir or (S)-9-(3-hydroxy-2-phosphonylmethoxypropyl) cytosine. Cidofovir is an acyclic nucleoside phosphonate antiviral agent currently used in the treatment of cytomegalovirus retinitis. Cidofovir is active *in vitro* against HSV, and has activity against thymidine kinase negative and thymidine kinase-altered HSV strains. Trials of cidofovir in humans for the treatment of resistant genital herpes have not been completed. The primary toxicity of cidofovir at doses used to treat cytomegalovirus is nephrotoxicity. The doses of cidofovir necessary to treat aciclovir-resistant genital herpes have not been established.[53,54]

Ineffective therapies. These include BCG vaccination, topical betadine, topical vidarabine, topical idoxuridine and gammaglobulin. Topical therapy with foscarnet has been disappointing, with recent studies of treatment of recurrent genital herpes showing little to no benefit.[55] Lysine is a popular over the counter supplement purported to decrease the symptoms of genital herpes. Well-controlled clinical trials of lysine, including a double-blinded cross-over study, have failed to demonstrate efficacy.[56,57]

GENERAL TREATMENT GUIDELINES

Antiviral therapy decreases both the duration of symptoms and viral shedding in genital herpes. Maximum benefit occurs when antiviral therapy is initiated promptly, ideally with the first prodromal symptoms with recurrent genital herpes. With the wide margin of safety of the oral antiviral medications and the need to initiate therapy promptly, it is appropriate to begin medication before receiving culture results or other confirmatory test results.

Aciclovir, famciclovir or valaciclovir are all appropriate agents for the treatment of genital herpes. For some indications, valaciclovir and famciclovir offer more convenient dosing regimens. However, for many health care providers, generic aciclovir remains the drug of choice for the treatment of genital herpes due to the extensive clinical experience with the drug, its excellent safety and efficacy profiles, wide availability and lower cost (Fig. 65.6).

TREATMENT OF PRIMARY GENITAL HERPES

Antiviral therapy is clearly of benefit in the treatment of primary genital herpes. When compared with placebo it has been shown to reduce median:
- duration of viral shedding by 7 days;
- duration of pain by 4 days; and
- time to healing by 7 days.[58]

Antiviral therapy does not prevent the establishment of latency or affect the likelihood and frequency of recurrences when compared with placebo.[59] Higher than recommended doses of antiviral medications are no more effective in the treatment of genital herpes and may be associated with an increased risk of nausea.[46] Treatment for longer than 10 days in the normal host does not improve outcome when compared with the standard regimen.

Primary or first-episode genital herpes may be adequately treated with aciclovir at doses of 200mg five times daily or 400mg q8h for 10 days. Alternatively, valaciclovir 1g q12h for 7 days or famciclovir 250mg q8h for 7–10 days is also effective treatment for primary genital herpes.[57,60]

Individuals with severe disease or who are unable to take oral medications should be treated with intravenous aciclovir at doses of 5mg/kg administered over 1 hour q8h. Topical aciclovir is of little value in the treatment of primary disease.[58] The combination of oral and topical aciclovir offers no therapeutic advantage.[57,65]

Oral famciclovir and oral valaciclovir have been compared with oral aciclovir for the treatment of first-episode genital herpes in recent clinical studies. Oral famciclovir in doses of 125, 250 or 500mg q8h for 10 days has been shown to be as effective as aciclovir 200mg five times daily for

10 days.[57,62] Valaciclovir 1g q12h was also as effective as aciclovir 200mg five times daily in the treatment of first-episode genital herpes.[57,63] Neither famciclovir nor valaciclovir appear any more effective than aciclovir.

EPISODIC TREATMENT OF RECURRENT GENITAL HERPES

Recurrent genital herpes is generally milder and of shorter duration than primary disease, so the expected benefits of treating individual episodes with antiviral therapy are not as profound as those seen in primary disease. Episodic treatment of recurrent genital herpes with antiviral therapy results in only a modest decrease in disease severity, with a mean decrease in the duration of symptoms of 1 day or less.[62]

Aciclovir at a dose of 200mg five times daily or 400mg q8h for 5 days remains the recommended therapy.[64] Patient-initiated therapy at the time of onset of prodromal symptoms has been shown to be of significantly greater benefit than therapy delayed to initial lesion onset.[62]

Both valaciclovir and famciclovir have been evaluated for effectiveness in the treatment of recurrent genital herpes. Recent clinical trials comparing valaciclovir (1g q12h) with either aciclovir (200mg five times daily) or placebo showed the following in both treatment arms when compared with placebo:
- decreased time to lesion healing;
- decreased duration of pain; and
- reduced duration of viral shedding.[65]

Oral famciclovir at doses of 125, 250, or 500mg q12h reduced viral shedding and duration of symptoms and reduced time to healing when compared with placebo.[66] The lowest effective dose, 125mg q12h for 5 days, is the currently approved treatment dose. Neither famciclovir or valaciclovir appears to offer any therapeutic advantage over aciclovir.

The 5% topical aciclovir ointment available in the USA is not effective at reducing viral shedding, symptoms or time to healing, and is not licensed or recommended for treatment of recurrent genital herpes.[67] A different preparation available in Europe, a 5% topical aciclovir cream, has been shown to be effective and may be an appropriate alternative to oral therapy if available to the patient.[68]

SUPPRESSION OF FREQUENTLY RECURRING GENITAL HERPES

Chronic antiviral therapy has proven to be a safe and well-tolerated mechanism for suppressing symptomatic recurrences in patients with moderate to frequently (more than five episodes per year) recurring genital herpes.

Aciclovir

Aciclovir was the first antiviral agent evaluated for effectiveness in suppressing recurrent disease. In one study, patients with frequent recurrences had a reduction of recurrences from more than 12/year to an average of 1/year when treated with aciclovir 400mg q12h.[69]

Suppressive therapy is safe and well tolerated, with no long-term effects on sperm motility, no noted laboratory abnormalities and minimal side effects.[69,70]

Aciclovir has now been used for suppressive therapy for up to 10 years and has not been associated with development of tolerance or with any significant development of resistant strains in the normal host.[69,71,72] However, interruption of therapy at 1- or 2-year intervals is suggested to assess the frequency of episodes and need for suppressive therapy. It has recently been shown that suppressive therapy with aciclovir decreases the frequency of asymptomatic viral shedding in women.[24]

Famciclovir

Famciclovir is now licensed in the USA for suppressive therapy at a dose of 250mg q12h, the most effective dose tested in a dose-ranging study of famciclovir compared with placebo for suppression of frequently recurring genital herpes in women.[75] In this trial, once-daily dosing regimens were not as effective as the q12h dosing regimens at equal or higher cumulative daily doses. A subsequent 1-year trial in men and women also found that the 250mg q12h dosage was effective and well tolerated. At present, there are no results available of trials comparing the efficacy of suppressive therapy with famciclovir to therapy with valaciclovir or aciclovir.

Valaciclovir

Valaciclovir has also been used for suppression of genital herpes and has recently been licensed in the USA at a dose of 500mg or 1g orally daily for suppression of genital herpes in the normal host. The 500mg daily dose appears to be effective in persons with a history of 6–10 episodes/year. This regimen appears to be less effective than aciclovir 400mg orally q12h or valaciclovir 1g daily or 250mg q12h in patients with very frequent recurrences (ten or more episodes a year). Once-daily dosing with valaciclovir 1g appears to have acceptable efficacy in the normal host, but should not be used in the immunocompromised host because there is evidence of reduced efficacy in people who have HIV infection. Valaciclovir 1g daily or 250mg q12h and aciclovir 400mg q12h appeared equivalent in efficacy, even among people with frequent recurrences. For maximum efficacy, we prefer to use valaciclovir at a dose of 500mg q12h for suppression. This dose was found to be safe and was also significantly more effective than valaciclovir 1g orally daily in suppressing genital herpes in people who have HIV infection and a median CD4+ lymphocyte count of 320/μl.[76]

Summary

In summary, there are no data at present suggesting that suppressive therapy with either famciclovir or valaciclovir at the licensed doses is more effective than suppressive therapy with aciclovir 400mg q12h. In addition, cost comparisons favor the use of generic aciclovir rather than the newer agents.

CONCLUSION

Genital herpes is one of the most commonly encountered sexually transmitted diseases. Its management requires:
- recognition of disease,
- patient education about the unique features of the disease including latency and virus shedding, and
- judicious use of antiviral medications.

REFERENCES

1. Roizman B, Sears A. Herpes simplex viruses and their replication In: Fields BN, Knipe D, Howley PM, et al. eds. Fields virology, 3rd ed. Philadelphia: Raven Press; 1996:2231–95.
2. Corey L, Adams HG, Brown ZA, Holmes KK. Genital herpes simplex infections: clinical manifestations, course, and complications. Ann Intern Med 1983;98:958–72.
3. Genital herpes infection – United States, 1966–1984. MMWR Morb Mortal Wkly Rep 1986;35:402–4.
4. Breinig MK, Kingsley LA, Armstrong JA, et al. Epidemiology of genital herpes in Pittsburgh: serologic, sexual and racial correlates of apparent and inapparent herpes simplex infections. J Infect Dis 1990;162:299–305.

5. Nahmias AJ, Josey WE, Naib ZM, et al. Antibodies to herpes virus hominis types 1 and 2 in humans. I. Patients with genital herpetic infections. Am J Epidemiol 1970;91:539–46.
6. Johnson RE, Nahmias AJ, Magder LS, et al. A seroepidemiology survey of the prevalence of herpes simplex viruses type 2 infection in the United States. N Engl J Med 1989;321:7–12.
7. Gibson JJ, Hornung CA, Alexander GR, Lee FK, Potts WA, Nahmias AJ. A cross-sectional study of herpes simplex viruses types 1 and 2 in college students: occurrence and determinants of infection. J Infect Dis 1990;162:306–12.
8. Mertz GJ, Benedetti J, Ashley R, Selke S, Corey L. Risk factors for sexual transmission in genital herpes. Ann Intern Med 1992;116:197–202.

9. Whitley RJ. Herpes simplex viruses: In: Fields BN, Knipe D, Howley PM, et al., eds. Fields virology, 3rd ed. Philadelphia: Raven Press; 1996:2297–341.
10. Stanberry LR, Kern ER, Richards JT, Abbott TM, Overall JC Jr. Genital herpes in guinea pigs: pathogenesis of primary infection and description of recurrent disease. J Infect Dis 1982;146:397–404.
11. Capobianchi MR, Malavasi F, DiMarco P, Dianzani F. Differences in the mechanism of induction of interferon-alpha by herpes simplex virus and herpes simplex virus-infected cells. Arch Virol 1988;103:219–29.
12. Ashley R, Benedetti J, Corey L. Humoral immune response to HSV-1 and HSV-2 viral proteins in patients with primary genital herpes. J Med Virol 1985;17:153–66.

13. Whitton JL, Oldstone MB. Immune response to viruses. In: Fields BN, Knipe DM, Howley PM, eds. Fields virology, 3rd ed. Philadelphia: Raven Press; 1996:345–74.
14. Lopez C, Arvin AM, Ashley R. Immunity to herpes virus infections in humans. In: Roizman B, Whitley RJ, Lopez C, eds. The human herpes viruses. New York: Raven Press; 1993:397–425.
15. Ashley R, Koelle DM. Immune responses to genital herpes infection. Advances in host defense mechanisms. In: Quinn TC, ed. Sexually transmitted diseases. New York: Raven Press; 1992:201–38.
16. Oh SH, Douglas JM, Corey L, Kohl S. Kinetics of the humoral immune response measured by antibody-dependent cell-mediated cytotoxicity and neutralization assays in genital herpes virus infections. J Infect Dis 1989;159:328–30.
17. Whitley RJ, Nahmias AJ, Visintine AM, Fleming CL, Alford CA. The natural history of herpes simplex virus infection of mother and newborn. Pediatrics 1980;66:489–94.
18. Cunningham AL, Turner RR, Miller C, Para MF, Merigan TC. Evolution of recurrent herpes simplex lesions: an immunohistologic study. J Clin Invest 1985;75:225–33.
19. Lafferty WE, Coombs RW, Benedetti J, et al. Recurrences after oral and genital herpes simplex virus infection. Influence of site of infection and viral type. N Engl J Med 1987;316:1444–9.
20. Schmidt OW, Fife KH, Corey L. Reinfection is an uncommon occurrence in patients with symptomatic recurrent genital herpes. J Infect Dis 1984;149:645–6.
21. Wald A, Zeh J, Selke S, Ashley RL, Corey L. Virologic characteristics of subclinical and symptomatic genital herpes infections. N Engl J Med 1995;333:770–5.
22. Koelle DM, Benedetti J, Langenberg A, Corey L. Asymptomatic reactivation of herpes simplex virus in women after the first episode of genital herpes. Ann Intern Med 1992;116:433–7.
23. Mertz GJ, Schmidt O, Jourden JL, et al. Frequency of acquisition of first-episode genital infection with herpes simplex virus from symptomatic and asymptomatic source contacts. Sex Transm Dis 1985;12:33–9.
24. Wald A, Zeh J, Barnum G, et al. Suppression of subclinical shedding of herpes simplex virus type 2 with acyclovir. Ann Intern Med 1996;124:8–15.
25. Stanberry LR, Bernstein DI, Burke RL, Pachl C, Myers MG. Vaccination with recombinant herpes simplex virus glycoproteins: protection against initial and recurrent genital herpes. J Infect Dis 1987;155:914–20.
26. Burke RL. Contemporary approach to vaccination against herpes simplex virus. Curr Top Microbiol Immunol 1992;179:137–58.
27. Mertz GJ, Ashley R, Burke RL, et al. Double-blind, placebo-controlled trial of a herpes simplex virus type 2 glycoprotein vaccine in persons at high risk of herpes simplex infection. J Infect Dis 1990;161:653–60.
28. Straus SE, Savarese B, Tigges M, et al. Induction and enhancement of immune responses to herpes simplex type 2 in humans with a recombinant glycoprotein D vaccine. J Infect Dis 1993;167:1045–52.
29. Langenberg AGM, Burke RL, Adair SF, et al. A recombinant glycoprotein vaccine for herpes simplex type 2: safety and efficacy. Ann Intern Med 1995;122:889–98.
30. Brown ZA, Benedetti J, Ashley R, et al. Neonatal herpes simplex virus infection in relation to asymptomatic maternal infection at the time of labor. N Engl J Med 1991;324:1247–52.
31. Koutsky LA, Stevens CE, Holmes KK, et al. Underdiagnosis of genital herpes by current clinical and viral isolation procedures. N Engl J Med 1992;326:1533–9.
32. Quinnan GV Jr, Masur H, Rook AH, et al. Herpes virus infections in the acquired immune deficiency syndrome. JAMA 1984;252:72–7.

33. Mead PB. Proper methods of culturing herpes simplex virus. J Reprod Med 1986;31(Suppl 5):390–4.
34. Whitley RJ, Gnann JW. Acyclovir: a decade later. N Engl J Med 1992;327:782–9.
35. Whitley RJ. Perinatal herpes simplex infections. Rev Med Virol 1991;1:101–10.
36. Saral R. Management of mucocutaneous herpes simplex virus infections in immunocompromised patients. Am J Med 1988;85(Suppl 2a):57–60.
37. Siegel D, Golden E, Washington AE, et al. Prevalence and correlates of herpes simplex infections: the population-based AIDS in multiethnic neighborhoods study. JAMA 1992;268:1702–8.
38. Koutsky LA, Ashley RL, Holmes KK, et al. The frequency of unrecognized type 2 herpes simplex virus infection among women. Implications for the control of genital herpes. Sex Transm Dis 1990;17(2):90–4.
39. Kulhanjian JA, Soroush V, Au DS, et al. Identification of women at unsuspected risk of primary infection with herpes simplex virus type 2 during pregnancy. N Engl J Med 1992;326(14):916–20.
40. Ashley R. Laboratory techniques in the diagnosis of herpes simplex infection. Genitourin Med 1993;69:174–83.
41. Lentinen M, Koivisto V, Lentinen T, et al. Immunoblotting and enzyme-linked immunosorbent assay analysis of serological responses in patients infected with herpes simplex virus types 1 and 2. Intervirol 1985;24:18–25.
42. Ashley R, Militoni J, Lee F, Nahmias A, Corey L. Comparison of Western blot (immunoblot) and glycoprotein G-specific immunodot assay for detecting antibodies to herpes simplex virus types 1 and 2 in human sera. J Clin Microbiol 1988;26:662–7.
43. Lakeman FD, Whitley RJ. Diagnosis of herpes simplex encephalitis: application of polymerase chain reaction to cerebrospinal fluid from brain-biopsied patients and correlation with disease. National Institute of Allergy and Infectious Diseases Collaborative Antiviral Study Group. J Infect Dis 1995;171(4):857–63.
44. Domingues RB, Tsanaclis AM, Pannuti CS, Mayo MS, Lakeman FD. Evaluation of the range of clinical presentations of herpes simplex encephalitis by using polymerase chain reaction assay of cerebrospinal fluid samples. Clin Infect Dis 1997;25(1):86–91.
45. Corey L, Nahmias AJ, Guinan ME, Benedetti JK, Critchlow CW, Holmes KK. A trial of topical acyclovir in genital herpes simplex virus infections. N Engl J Med 1982;306:1313–9.
46. Wald A, Benedetti J, Davis G, et al. A randomized double-blind, comparative trial comparing high- and standard-dose oral acyclovir for first episode genital herpes infections. Antimicrob Agents Chemother 1994;38:174–6.
47. Beutner KR, Friedman DJ, Forszpaniak C, Andersen PL, Wood MJ. Valaciclovir compared with acyclovir for improved therapy for herpes zoster in immunocompetent adults. Antimicrob Agents Chemother 1995;39:1546–53.
48. Boyd MR, Safrin S, Kern ER. Penciclovir: a review of the spectrum of activity, selectivity, and cross-resistance pattern. Antiviral Chem Chemother 1993;4(Suppl):3–11.
49. Earnshaw DL, Bacon TH, Darlison SJ, et al. Mode of antiviral action of penciclovir in MRC-5 cells infected with herpes simplex virus type 1 (HSV-1), HSV-2, and varicella–zoster virus. Antimicrob Agents Chemother 1992;36:2747–57.
50. Pue M, Benet LZ. Pharmacokinetics of famciclovir in man. Antiviral Chem Chemother 1993;4(Suppl):47–55.
51. Obert B. Antiviral effects of phosphonoformate (PFA, foscarnet sodium). Pharmacol Ther 1989;40:213–85.

52. Chrisp P, Clissold SP. Foscarnet. A review of its antiviral activity, pharmacokinetic properties and therapeutic use in immunocompromised patients with cytomegalovirus retinitis. Drugs 1991;41:104–29.
53. Mills J. New drugs for cytomegalovirus infection. In: Mills J, Corey L, eds. New directions for clinical applications and research, vol. 3. New Jersey: Prentice–Hall; 1993:189–95.
54. Mendel DN, Barkhimer DB, Chen MS. Biochemical basis for the increased sensitivity to cidofovir of herpes simplex viruses with altered or deleted thymidine kinase [Abstract H10]. In: Abstracts of the 35th Interscience Conference on Antimicrobial Agents and Chemotherapy. San Francisco: American Society for Microbiology; 1995:181.
55. Sacks SL, Portnoy J, Lawee D, et al. Clinical course of recurrent genital herpes after treatment with foscarnet cream. Results of a Canadian multicenter trial. J Infect Dis 1987;155:178–86.
56. Milman N, Scheibel M, Jessen O. Lysine prophylaxis in recurrent herpes simplex labialis: a double-blind, controlled crossover study. Acta Dermatol Venereol 1980;60:85–7.
57. Drugs for non-HIV viral infections. Med Lett Drugs Ther 1997;39:69–76.
58. Corey L, Benedetti J, Critchlow C, et al. Treatment of primary first-episode genital herpes simplex virus infections with acyclovir: results of topical, intravenous and oral therapy. J Antimicrob Chemother 1983;12(Suppl B):79–88.
59. Mertz GJ, Benedetti J, Critchlow C, Corey L. Long-term recurrence rates of genital herpes infections after treatment of first-episode genital herpes with oral acyclovir. In: Kano R, ed. Herpes viruses and virus chemotherapy. Amsterdam: Elsevier; 1985:141–4.
60. Loveless M, Harris W, Sacks S. Treatment of first episode genital herpes with famciclovir [Abstract H12]. In: Abstracts of the 35th Interscience Conference on Antimicrobial Agents and Chemotherapy. San Francisco: American Society for Microbiology; 1995:181.
61. Kinghorn GR, Abeywickreme I, Jeavons M, et al. Efficacy of combined treatment with oral and topical acyclovir in first episode genital herpes. Genitourin Med 1986;62:186–8.
62. Reichman RC, Badger GJ, Mertz GJ, et al. Treatment of recurrent genital herpes simplex infections with oral acyclovir. A controlled trial. JAMA 1984;251:1203–7.
63. Fife KF, Barbarash RA, Rudolph T, Degregoria B, Roth R, the Valaciclovir International Herpes Simplex Virus Study Group. Valaciclovir versus acyclovir in the treatment of first-episode genital herpes infection: results of an international, multicenter, double-blind, randomized clinical trial. Sex Transm Dis 1997;24:481–6.
64. 1993 Sexually transmitted disease treatment guidelines. Centers for Disease Control and Prevention. MMWR Morb Mortal Wkly Rep 1993;42:1–102.
65. Smiley ML, The International Valaciclovir HSV Study Group. Valaciclovir and acyclovir for the treatment of recurrent genital herpes simplex virus infections [Abstract 1211]. In: Program of the 33rd Interscience Conference on Antimicrobial Agents and Chemotherapy. New Orleans: American Society for Microbiology; 1993.
66. Sacks SL, Aoki FY, Diaz-Mitoma F, et al. Patient-initiated treatment of recurrent genital herpes with oral famciclovir [abstract H4]. In: Abstracts of the 34th Interscience Conference on Antimicrobial Agents and Chemotherapy. Orlando: American Society for Microbiology; 1994:11.
67. Reichman RC, Badger GJ, Guinan ME, et al. Topically administered acyclovir in the treatment of recurrent herpes simplex genitalis: a controlled trial. J Infect Dis 1983;147:336–40.
68. Kinghorn GR. Topical acyclovir in the treatment of recurrent herpes simplex virus infections. Scand J Infect Dis 1985;47(Suppl):58–62.

69. Mertz GJ, Jones CC, Mills J, *et al.* Long-term acyclovir suppression of frequently recurring genital herpes simplex virus infection. A multicenter double-blind trial. JAMA 1988; 260:201–6.

70. Douglas JM, Davis LG, Remington ML, *et al.* A double-blind placebo-controlled trial of the effect of chronically administered oral acyclovir on sperm production in men with frequent recurrent genital herpes. J Infect Dis 1988;157:588–93.

71. Thin RN, Jeffries DJ, Taylor PK, *et al.* Recurrent genital herpes suppressed by oral acyclovir. A multicenter double-blind trial. J Antimicrob Chemother 1985;16:219–26.

72. Fife KH, Crumpacker CS, Mertz GJ, *et al.* Recurrence and resistance patterns of herpes simplex following cessation of ≥ 6 years of chronic acyclovir suppression. J Infect Dis 1994;169:1338–41.

73. Fife KH, Barbarash RA, Rudolph T, Degregorio B, Roth R. Valaciclovir versus acyclovir in the treatment of first-episode genital herpes infection. Results of an international, multicenter, double-blind, randomized clinical trial. The Valaciclovir International Herpes Simplex Virus Study Group. Sex Transm Dis 1997;24(8):481–6.

74. Sacks SL, Aoki FY, Diaz–Mitoma F, Sellors J, Shafran SD. Patient-initiated, twice-daily oral famciclovir for early recurrent genital herpes. A randomized, double-blind multicenter trial. Canadian Famciclovir Study Group. JAMA 1996;276(1):44–9.

75. Mertz GJ, Loveless MO, Levin MJ, *et al.* Oral famciclovir for suppression of recurrent genital herpes simplex virus infection in women. Arch Intern Med 1997;157:343–9.

76. Gold J, Bell A and the Valaciclovir International Study Group. Valaciclovir prevents herpes simplex virus recurrences in HIV-infected individual; a double-blind controlled trial [Abstract 4036]. International Congress of Chemotherapy. Sydney: 1997:118.

Papillomavirus Infections

Sten H Vermund, Sibylle Kristensen & Maria L Smith

INTRODUCTION

Human papillomavirus (HPV) is probably the most common sexually transmitted virus in humans. Infected persons are usually asymptomatic. Mild disease includes genital warts, verruga or cytologically evident dysplasia of the cervix or anus. Persistent anogenital infection is strongly associated with advanced cervical neoplastic disease and invasive carcinoma of the cervix. High-risk genotypes of HPV are likely to be responsible for a high proportion of squamous-origin carcinomas of the cervix, vagina, vulva, anus and penis worldwide.[1] Other types of HPV are associated with lower grade squamous lesions such as low-grade neoplasia and abnormal squamous cells of unknown significance.[2]

Nongenital types of HPV cause benign epithelial warts of the hands, feet and elsewhere, as well as a number of other dermatologic conditions not reviewed in this chapter (see Chapter 8.6). The significance of HPV infections in cancers of the oral cavity, the larynx and the esophagus is not known, but further research may elucidate the full role of this virus group in human carcinogenesis.[1] So-called 'low-risk types' such as HPV-11 can cause the severe non-neoplastic disease termed juvenile laryngeal papillomatosis characterized by laryngeal warts in children. This chapter reviews diagnostic, epidemiologic, molecular and therapeutic issues focusing on anogenital disease.

HUMAN PAPILLOMAVIRUSES

The HPVs are a family of DNA viruses with more than 142 related genetic types from which more than 80 have been fully sequenced (Fig. 66.1).[3] The genome consists of a circular double-stranded DNA about 7900bp long and is encapsidated in an icosahedral protein coat with no membrane envelope.[4] Most HPV genotypes have a similar organization consisting of:

- a transcription and replication control region;
- an early region encoding proteins for replication, regulation and modification of the host cytoplasm and nucleus; and
- a late region encoding capsid proteins.[3]

Human papillomaviruses are related to several papillomaviruses specific to many other vertebrates, including a wide variety of mammals, birds, amphibians and reptiles.[4]

EPIDEMIOLOGY, PATHOGENESIS AND PATHOLOGY

CERVICAL CANCER

Cervical HPV infection is the single most important risk factor for squamous intraepithelial lesions of the cervix.[5] The association between cervical cancer and a sexually transmitted etiologic agent was hypothesized long before identification of genital HPV infection. For several decades, cervical cancer risk has been recognized in association with early onset of sexual activity and multiple sexual partners. Although most women with cervical cancer are over 45 years of age when diagnosed, HPV infection and disease pathogenesis are known to begin at a much younger age. Early signs of cervical intraepithelial neoplasia (CIN) are detectable through cervical cytology screening programs that provide periodic Papanicolaou cervical smear testing (Pap smear). Nearly all cervical cancer cases occur in women receiving

HPV TYPES AND HPV-ASSOCIATED DISEASES	
HPV-associated diseases	HPV types
Skin warts	1,2,3,4,7,10,26,27,28,29,41,48,57, 60,63,65,75,76,77,78
Epidermodysplasia verruciformis benign lesions	3,5,8,9,12,14,15,17,19,20,21,22,23, 24,25,36,47,49,50
Epidermodysplasia verruciformis squamous cell carcinoma	5,8,14,17,20,47
Periungual squamous cell carcinoma	16,34,35
Laryngeal papillomas	6,11
Oral focal epithelial hyperplasia	13,32
Squamous cell carcinoma (tonsil)	16,33
Anogenital warts	6,11,40,42,43,44,54,55,74
Low-grade anogenital intraepithelial neoplasia	6,11,16,18,30,31,33,34,35,39,40,45,51,52, 56,57,58,59,61,64,66,67,68,70,71,72,73,74
High-grade anogenital intraepithelial neoplasia	16,18,31,33,34,35,39,45,51,52, 56,58,59,68
Squamous cell carcinoma (cervix mostly)	16,18,31,33,35,39,45,51,52,56, 58,59,68
Adenocarcinoma (cervix mostly)	16,18

Fig. 66.1 HPV types and HPV-associated diseases.[3,4]

suboptimal cervical screening regimens. Cervical cancer cases reflect failures in public health and preventive gynecology. Older women and women from ethnic minorities are more likely to be diagnosed with advanced stage disease.[6]

An estimated 500,000 new cervical cancer cases and 300,000 deaths occur worldwide each year and 75% of the deaths are in developing countries.[5] In many developing countries, cervical cancer is the most common cancer in women rivaled only by liver and gastric cancer.[5] In the absence of screening programs, 85% of the women with cervical cancer will die given the advanced stage of the disease at the time of diagnosis.[5]

Despite major progress in screening, cervical cancer is still the eighth most common cancer of women in the USA.[7] In 1996, there were about 15,700 cases and 4900 deaths from invasive cervical carcinoma in the USA and squamous carcinoma is the most common invasive malignancy of the cervix (77.1%). Cervical carcinoma *in situ* accounts for 78.5% of all cervical cancers when noninvasive malignancies are included in cancer statistics.[1] In 1995, the estimated cervical cancer prevalence in the USA was about 184,000, suggesting the long duration and under-recognition of most cervical cancers. In the USA, over 25% of invasive cervical cancers and 40–50% of deaths occur in women over 65 years of age.[8] Data from the Surveillance Epidemiology End Results program and from the 1992 National Health Interview Survey Cancer Control Supplement indicate an overall age-adjusted incidence rate for invasive cervical cancer in the USA of 8.5/100,000 women during 1988–1992. Among women under 45 years of age, the rates were similar for white and for black women (about 2.0/100,000). However, black women over 45 years of age were 66% more likely to develop invasive disease than white women over 45.[8] The lifetime risk for acquiring invasive cervical cancer in the USA is about 1%.[9] Cytologic screening in the USA involves the diagnosis and treatment of 750,000 or more women each year for cervical abnormalities thought by clinicians to represent precursor lesions.[9]

COFACTORS IN HUMAN PAPILLOMAVIRUS INFECTION AND CARCINOGENESIS

Molecular studies suggest that HPV has a direct mechanistic role in carcinogenesis.[10] Acute infections usually resolve spontaneously.[6] However, many patients continue to have detectable HPV DNA even after therapy for CIN or genital wart.[11] Immunosuppression facilitates the persistence of oncogenic HPV types and this may be important for carcinogenesis. Proteins of both HPV and endogenous origin influence deregulation of cell cycles and enable carcinogenesis to occur. Continued expression of HPV proteins has been demonstrated to be necessary for maintenance of the transformed state.[10] Metastases and recurrences from cervical cancer usually have the same viral types that were present in the primary tumor unless clonal diversity existed at the primary site.

Human papillomavirus infection with oncogenic viral types is ubiquitous in squamous cell tumors. A study of more than 1000 specimens from sequential patients with invasive cervical cancer from 32 hospitals in 22 countries, using polymerase chain reaction (PCR)-based assays capable of detecting more than 25 different HPV types confirmed HPV DNA in 93% of cervical tumors with no significant variation in HPV positivity rates among countries. Human papillomavirus-16 was present in 50%, HPV-18 in 14%, HPV-45 in 8% and HPV-31 in 5% of tumors. Human papillomavirus-16 was predominant everywhere except Indonesia, where HPV-18 was most prevalent. A clustering of HPV-45 was noted in western Africa, whereas HPV-39 and HPV-59 were largely found in Central and South America. In squamous cell tumors, HPV-16 was found in 51%, whereas HPV-18 predominated in adenocarcinomas (56%) and adenosquamous tumors (39%).[11] The more extensive the geographic and molecular reach in clinical studies, the more diversity and complexity is noted. The impact of ethnic and cultural factors is unknown.[12] Lower educational level and lack of preventive health care is associated with higher HPV and cervical disease rates presumably due, in part, to lower screening rates.

The etiology of risk may fall into several categories:
- viral pathogenicity;
- host immunogenetic factors;
- host immunosuppression;
- reinfection risk;
- acquired mucosal immunity;
- cofactor frequencies; and
- screening history.[9]

Viruses may differ substantially in their oncogenic potential.[11] Some people may have HLA profiles that are relatively unsupportive of viral colonization and replication. People infected with HIV, cancer chemotherapy recipients, renal transplant patients and other immunosuppressed persons have impaired ability to clear virus, permitting longer duration of infection and increased likelihood of oncogenic integration. Women who have HPV and are infected with more than one HPV type or have higher viral loads may be at higher risk for progression of HPV infection to high-grade CIN or cancer. Human papillomavirus persistence may be the major risk factor for carcinogenesis.[13]

Many infection cofactors have been implicated in disease pathogenesis. Herpes simplex virus type 2 has been suggested as a cancer cofactor.[14] Repetitive exposure to a variety of infectious antigens may accompany sexual encounters with many partners. Douching and bacterial vaginosis with amines, high vaginal pH and altered microbial

ecology may increase HPV risk.[13] Factors that affect the immunologic or physical integrity of the cervical epithelium like cervical trauma or pregnancy may increase the risk of carcinogenesis.[14]

Local inflammation from infectious or other causes may stimulate cytokine responses that impact on HPV expression.[14] Keratinocyte growth factor is a cytokine that downregulates HPV-16 expression and stimulates squamous epithelial growth. In contrast, a number of cytokines may have a dysfunctional role in upregulation of HPV expression as a consequence of nonspecific inflammation. When inflammatory cytokines are present in high concentration associated with other sexually transmitted infections, increased HPV expression may ensue. Local inflammation from infectious or other causes may stimulate cytokine responses such as intercellular adhesion molecule 1, vascular cellular adhesion molecule 1 and E-selectin that impact on HPV expression. These vascular adhesion molecules may enable local recruitment of immunocompetent cells.[15] Inflammatory cytokines from bacterial vaginosis or sexually transmitted infections may increase HPV expression.[14]

Human papillomavirus prevalence declines with age perhaps due to reduced risk behavior. Increased acquired immunity at the systemic and mucosal level over time may also contribute to lower HPV rates among older women. Women who do not clear their virus at these older ages may not have successfully developed an acquired immunity. Older women at highest risk are those in whom HPV is persistent.[6]

Male cofactor

A 'male factor' is apparent in the higher cervical cancer risk. Women married to men whose first wives had died of cervical cancer, monogamous women married to seafarers or traveling salesmen who were frequently away from home, and female sexual partners of men with penile cancer all have a higher than expected cervical cancer risk.[9] Lack of male circumcision has not been demonstrated as a risk factor for their sex partners.[9]

Risk for cervical cancer as a consequence of characteristics of a woman's sexual partner is consistent with an infectious etiology. Commercial sex workers have a high cervical cancer risk, but celibate nuns have a low risk. Multiple sexual partners, early age of first coitus, early age of first pregnancy and a history of sexually transmitted diseases have been associated with increased cervical cancer risk. The number of lifetime sex partners may be the best predictor of HPV risk. Unlike with other sexually transmitted pathogens, condom use is not associated clearly with HPV prevention, perhaps indicating higher infectiousness or the possibility of perineum–genital transmission. Sexual couples can be discordant in HPV infection status or type, demonstrating the transient nature of infection in many persons, its low level in at least one partner, or, theoretically, resistance to HPV by the uninfected partner perhaps through local immune or genetic factors.[13] Human papillomavirus-related genital cancers can cluster in families due to occult HPV transmission and reinfection.[12]

Transmission of human papillomavirus from mother to child

This can occur at delivery.[9] Conjunctival papillomas present during infancy may be caused by vertical HPV transmission during delivery. Mothers of infants with conjunctival papillomas should be examined for HPV disease.[16] Viral load in cervical and vaginal cells may be an important determinant for the risk of perinatal HPV transmission.[9] Whether acquisition of HPV during the perinatal period predisposes to an increased risk of CIN among female infants in later life is unknown, although evidence of persistent HPV infection throughout childhood is lacking.[16] Juvenile laryngeal papillomatosis can cause aphonia or severe respiratory obstruction; it is probable that vertical transmission results in laryngeal HPV infection that manifests in warts years later. Genital warts in children, in contrast, do not seem to occur from perinatal transmission and are nearly always the consequence of child sexual abuse when seen in immunocompetent children.

Smoking, diet and drugs

Smoking may be an independent risk factor for cervical cancer.[9] Cigarette smoke components can be found in high concentrations in cervical mucus. The carcinogenic impact of smoking could include formation of DNA adduct mutations in the host cells.[17]

Protection of mucosal immunologic integrity may depend upon nutritional factors. Implicated are retinoids like beta-carotene, antioxidants like vitamin C, and methylation agents like folic acid.[18] Chemicals and drugs may also affect cervical risk. Corticosteroids may increase risk, presumably through immunosuppression and facilitation of HPV persistence.[9] Oral contraceptives may increase the risk of cervical cancer in HPV-positive women, although this remains far from confirmed.[13]

Host genetics

A new research challenge is to investigate the role of host genetics in HPV acquisition, retention and disease pathogenesis. Theoretically, HLA type may affect the degree of host cell susceptibility, efficiency of viral replication, or nature of host immune responses.[2] Molecular techniques improve the precision and affordability of immunogenetic assessments within epidemiologic and clinical studies.[10] Impaired immunity increases susceptibility to many infections and malignancies. Immunosuppression from cancer, autoimmune infections and iatrogenic etiologies can trigger development or exacerbation of epithelial warts and facilitates persistence, pathogenicity and progression of HPV-induced neoplasia.[19]

Cervical and anal HPV infection and neoplastic changes are more common in HIV-infected persons than among persons with comparable behavioral risk who are HIV-seronegative.[19] In several studies, the magnitude of increased risk is proportionate to the severity of immunosuppression. Cervical intraepithelial neoplasia progresses more rapidly and recurs more often after primary therapy in HIV-infected women than in HIV-negative women. Human papillomavirus infection and HPV-associated disease can be multifocal in HIV-positive women and may include the vulva and the anus. Cervical cytology is an adequate screening tool for CIN in HIV-positive women, but the high recurrence rate and multifocal nature of this disease reinforces the need for regular screening at least once a year.[20]

OTHER GENITOURINARY CANCERS

Anal cancer in women and men is strongly associated with HPV. A high level of HPV infection may be important for development of squamous intraepithelial lesions (SILs).[21] Men and women who have anal sex have the highest anal cancer rates, but anal disease in women can occur without anal intercourse through perineal spread.[12] The HIV epidemic has been associated with a rise in anal cancer rates in the USA.[19]

Vulvar and vaginal neoplasia and invasive squamous carcinomas are not common. They are often associated with HPV infections of the same types as seen in cervical disease. Squamous carcinoma represents 74% of invasive vulvar malignancies and 71% of invasive vaginal malignancies.[7] Both HPV types 16 and 18 are associated with squamous cell carcinoma of the vulva,[22] although the prevalence of HPV-16 is lower than noted in cervical carcinoma.

Primary squamous cell carcinoma of the ovary is rare; most cases represent malignant transformation of ovarian teratomas and are not HPV related.[22] Oncogenic HPV types are associated strongly with carcinomas of the penis and urethra.[23] Human papillomavirus is much more often found in carcinoma tissue of the penis than in normal tissue from the same subjects. Other urologic malignancies (e.g. prostate, bladder) have not been convincingly demonstrated to reflect HPV etiology. It has been suggested but not demonstrated that HPV can act as an oncogenic agent in patients predisposed to bladder cancer.[23]

ONCOGENESIS

The integration of viral DNA is critical for malignant transformation. In benign warts and in preneoplastic lesions, the HPV genome is maintained in a nonintegrated form, whereas in cancers the circular viral DNA is usually integrated into the linear host cell genome.[24] The molecular mechanisms of HPV are currently the topic of intense investigation seeking the precise role of viral genes and proteins in carcinogenesis. The expression of some of the genes (E6/E7) of high-risk HPVs (16, 18 and others) seems to be an essential factor for malignant conversion of the cervical epithelium. The viral DNA usually integrates into the host DNA within the E1/E2 open reading frame of the viral genome.[25] Because the E2 region of the viral DNA normally represses the transcription of the E6 and E7 early viral genes, its division causes overexpression of the E6 and E7 proteins of HPV-16 and HPV-18.[25] Transformation occurs when the HPV E6 and E7 proteins bind the products of tumor suppressor genes p53 and *pRb*-1, respectively, modifying or inactivating their normal cell regulating functions. The *pRb*-1 and p53 genes normally regulate the transcription of genes involved in cell cycle control.[25] The E6/p53 and E7/*pRb*-1 interactions result in genomic instability, resulting in the accumulation of chromosomal abnormalities followed by clonal expansion of malignant cells.[3]

Gene mutations in the p53 region have been seen with high frequency in cervical and vulvar cancer specimens, although there is some controversy as to how central p53 is to the carcinogenic pathway.[3] The affinity of these transforming viral proteins for the products of the tumor suppressor genes differs depending upon the oncogenic potential of HPV. E6 and E7 proteins derived from high-risk HPVs bind to *pRb* and p53 with high affinity, whereas the E6 and E7 gene products of low-risk HPVs bind with low affinity.[24] The carcinogenic potential of the E6 and E7 genes of HPV has now focused attention on HPV as having the primary role as the carcinogenic initiator of cervical neoplasia. Additional cofactors and mutational events may be important through chromosomal rearrangements, proto-oncogene activation and other viruses acting as modulators.[25]

PREVENTION

Reduction of the incidence of cervical cancer has been achieved in industrialized nations through screening by cervical cytology (Pap smear). In countries where screening has been extensive, the mortality rate from cervical cancer has fallen markedly since the 1950s. Detection and treatment of precursors and identification of invasive cancer at an earlier more curable stage can save many lives. The rate of abnormal Pap smears and the number of women requiring medical intervention are orders of magnitude higher than the cervical cancer rate. Human papillomavirus detection methods are being evaluated to possibly complement cytologic detection of cervical disease. Use of HPV screening to help with the management of ambiguous Pap smears and for cytologic quality control is advisable. However, current HPV screening does not appear to add much to repetitive cytologic study alone.[26] Low-income women have the lowest Pap smear screening rates and the highest cervical cancer rates, resulting in even higher cervical cancer rates. More efforts and research are needed to increase overall screening among the indigent. Fiscal difficulties, challenges in health care organization, and women's health traditions that emphasize health of others (children and men) rather than themselves have inhibited effective Pap smear screening programs in most developing countries and in pockets of industrialized nations as well.[27]

A high public health priority is the development of vaccines targeted against HPV-16 and HPV-18.[12] Vaccines have been demonstrated to be feasible in several animal models. Safety and immunogenicity of a live recombinant vaccinia virus expressing the E6 and E7 proteins of HPV-16 and 18 (TA-HPV) has been evaluated in a phase I human clinical trial. Studies to investigate the use of TA-HPV for immunotherapy of cervical cancer are planned.[28] Vaccines proposed as immunomodulators or therapeutic adjuncts to radiation therapy are termed therapeutic vaccines. Among the most promising vaccine approaches for prevention of sustained HPV infection (preventive or prophylactic vaccines) is the use of recombinant virus-like particles. Virus-like particles are highly antigenic, protective in animal models and lack potentially carcinogenic viral DNA. Immunization with HPV peptides of tumor origin will be tested both for therapy and prophylaxis with a goal of tumor regression or prevention.[29]

CLINICAL FEATURES

Human papillomavirus infection may be asymptomatic or may be manifested in various benign or malignant lesions, most notably warts, on cutaneous and mucosal surfaces and anogenital neoplasia or carcinoma. Genital warts can be flat (condyloma lata) as is typical in the cervix or more papillary (condyloma acuminata) as is typical in the vulva, vagina or anus. Human papillomavirus is seen in all clinical circumstances: subclinical latent infection, clinically apparent warts, normal or abnormal genital cytology and squamous carcinoma.[30] Condylomata acuminata are often caused by low-risk HPV types 6, 11 or related types. Most tend to regress naturally and are very rarely associated with malignant progression. They are often multifocal, can be large and have a high rate of recurrence after treatment.[2]

Cervical intraepithelial neoplasia has been traditionally defined as a continuum of intraepithelial squamous abnormalities that exhibit nuclear atypia and possess some potential for progression to invasive carcinoma if not removed. The transformation zone of the cervix is particularly susceptible to neoplastic transformation following HPV infection. The usual cervical lesion is flat with warty colposcopic and cytopathic features and may be visualized when painted with 5%

acetic acid to reveal acetowhite thickening. Both CIN I and II may precede CIN III, and a small proportion progress to invasive carcinoma.[31] The majority of CIN I lesions regress to normal. Cervical intraepithelial neoplasia is considered within four sections by the Bethesda classification for Pap smear classification (Fig. 66.2): normal, low-grade SIL, high-grade SIL and invasive cancer. Low-grade SIL includes condylomatous atypia and CIN I. High-grade SIL includes CIN II (moderate dysplasia) and CIN III (severe dysplasia and carcinoma *in situ*).[2]

High-risk HPV types have been associated with all grades of CIN, whereas low-risk HPV types have segregated primarily in condylomata and CIN I. However, discrepancies between HPV type and morphology do exist, and cytology and histology provide variable, and at times conflicting, information.[31] Cells with inflammatory changes but no neoplastic characteristics are termed abnormal squamous cells of undetermined significance (ASCUS) or atypical cells (Fig. 66.3). A large multicenter clinical trial of ASCUS clinical management is currently sponsored by the National Institutes of Health (USA).

Human papillomavirus infections can be recognized by the characteristic raised appearance of the warts. Acetowhitening is helpful to clinicians examining the cervix, vagina and vulva under magnification (colposcopy) following an abnormal cytologic result in order to identify lesions requiring biopsy. It is not specific for HPV infection; however, a reliable reference standard for grading HPV-related anogenital pathology remains elusive, as clinical, microscopic and molecular diagnostic methods are all prone to misclassification (Figs 66.4–66.8).[2]

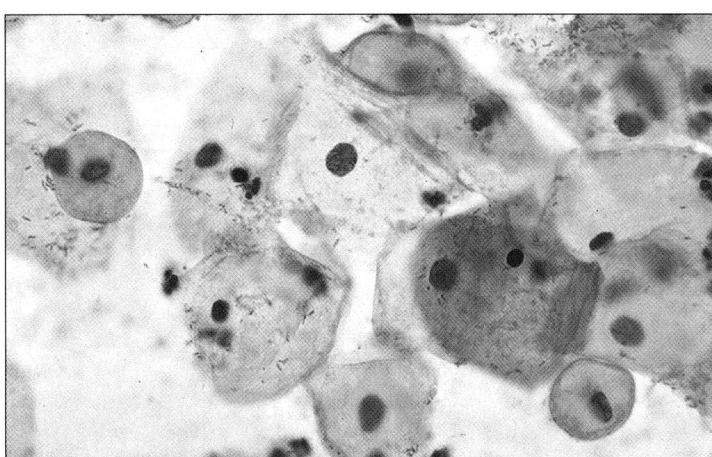

Fig. 66.2 Normal squamous cells and inflammatory cells. Courtesy of Dr William H Rogers. (Pap stain).

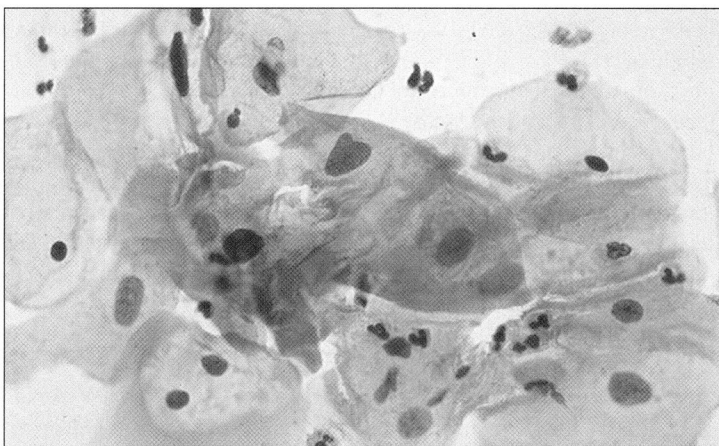

Fig. 66.3 Atypical squamous cells of undetermined significance. Here the cells are slightly enlarged and irregular relative to the cells in Figure 66.2 and contain perinuclear clear areas suggestive, but not diagnostic, of HPV infection. Courtesy of Dr William H Rogers. (Pap stain).

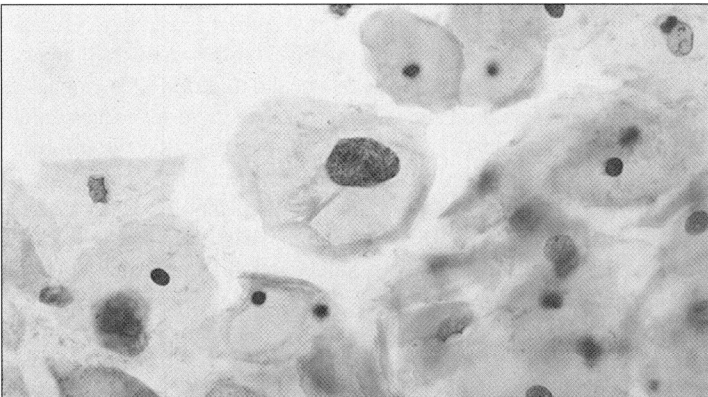

Fig. 66.4 Low-grade squamous intraepithelial lesion. In this case, the lesion would classically be called a mild dysplasia; the cell in the center of the photograph has a nucleus that is enlarged more than four times the size of the surrounding normal squamous cells; in addition, the nucleus has irregular nuclear outlines and hyperchromasia. Courtesy of Dr William H Rogers. (Pap stain).

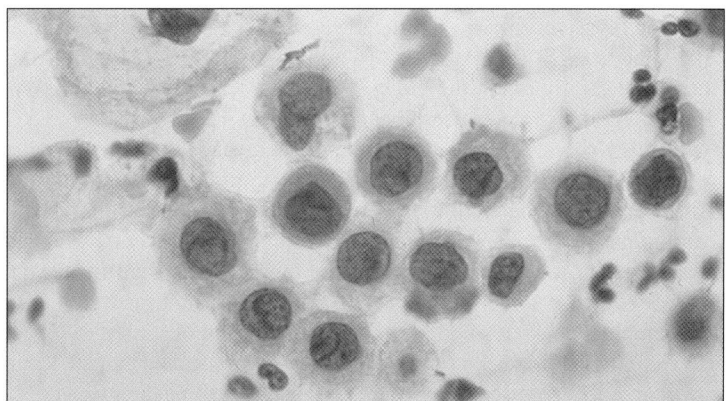

Fig. 66.5 High-grade squamous intraepithelial lesion. This contains small cells with an increased nuclear to cytoplasmic ratio and marked nuclear hyperchromasia; in the classic terminology, this would be considered a severe dysplasia or CIN III. Courtesy of Dr William H Rogers. (Pap stain).

On microscopic examination, the diagnosis is made by looking for dysplasia, which is termed koilocytotic if these cells pathognomonic for HPV infection are seen. Koilocytes are large cells with a clear enlarged cytoplasmic space. The nucleus is hyperchromatic, often irregular, and larger than normal. It may artefactually appear smaller than normal because the nucleus is within a larger-than-normal cell and cytoplasmic space.[2] A cytologic or pathologic description of koilocytotic atypia implies that no dysplasia is seen, but both low-grade dysplasia and koilocytic atypia are merged as low-grade SILs in the Bethesda classification system due to their similar prognosis.

DIAGNOSIS

The HPVs cannot be grown in culture. Using molecular techniques, more than 80 HPV genetic types have been sequenced and more are certain to be identified in the future. Oncogenic, high-risk HPV types are found in a large majority of squamous cell cervical cancers. Genital tract HPV types include 6, 11, 16, 18, 31, 33, 35, 39, 40, 42, 43, 44, 45, 51, 52, 53, 54, 55, 56, 57, 58, 59, 61, 66, 68, 70 and certainly others. High-risk types of major public health significance include 16, 18, 31, 33, 35, 39, 45, 51, 52, 54, 56, 58, 68, 70 and others.[3]

The PCR is so sensitive it can detect DNA in a very large proportion of sexually active women (typically 20–60%). Although it is the most sensitive technique for identifying HPV, a loss of specificity for predicting cervical disease means that the appropriate use of PCR in clinical screening remains to be determined. Older methods for molecular detection of HPV measure the presence of HPV DNA directly without PCR amplification, including Southern blot, in-situ hybridization, filter in-situ hybridization, and dot blot hybridization. These are hard to standardize across laboratories and some have unacceptably low sensitivity.[32] At the same time, Southern blot permits detailed characterization of nearly all viruses that may be present given the limits of its sensitivity.

Hybrid capture is a nonradioactive, rapid method of direct detection of HPV DNA. The technique allows semiquantitative estimation of one or many specific HPV types, and can be used with a variety of cervical specimen collection methods. A second-generation hybrid capture technology is now available using an enzyme-linked immunosorbent assay (ELISA)-type plate to enable lower cost and greater test volume without any loss in the sensitivity or high specificity of the test.[33] Hybrid capture is far more reproducible across laboratories than the PCR. Paradoxically, lower sensitivity of hybrid capture compared with PCR may be helpful in clinical screening by only detecting infections above a given quantitative threshold. It is probable that the 18 genotypes (including the 13 high risk) that the latest generation hybrid capture system can detect are associated with about 95% of HPV-related cancers.[34]

Cell sampling strategies include scrape, swab or brush technique, cervicovaginal lavage, home lavage performed by women at home, and even sampling from vaginal tampons. In many epidemiologic and

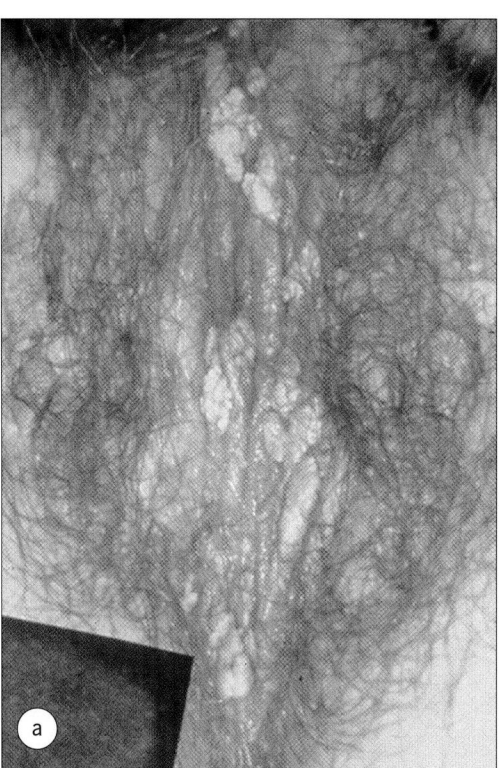

Fig. 66.8 Genital HPV infection. (a) Vaginal HPV infection. (b) Penile HPV infection.

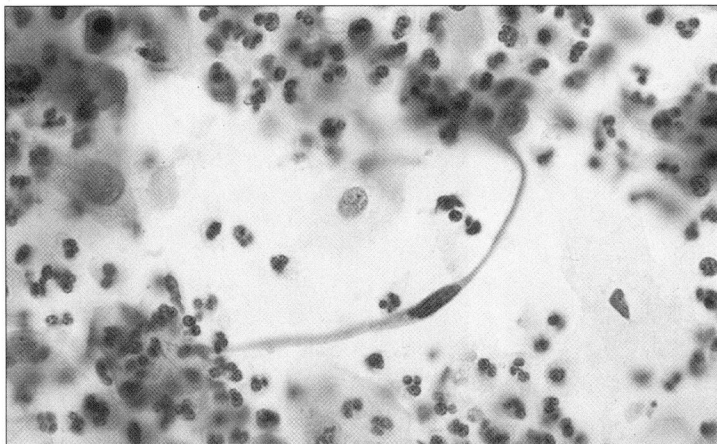

Fig. 66.6 Carcinoma *in situ*. The abnormal hyperchromatic cells have indistinct cell borders and form a pseudosyncytial arrangement. Courtesy of Dr William H Rogers. (Pap stain).

Fig. 66.7 Squamous cell carcinoma. This shows highly atypical, enlarged, abnormal keratinized cells. Courtesy of Dr William H Rogers. (Pap stain).

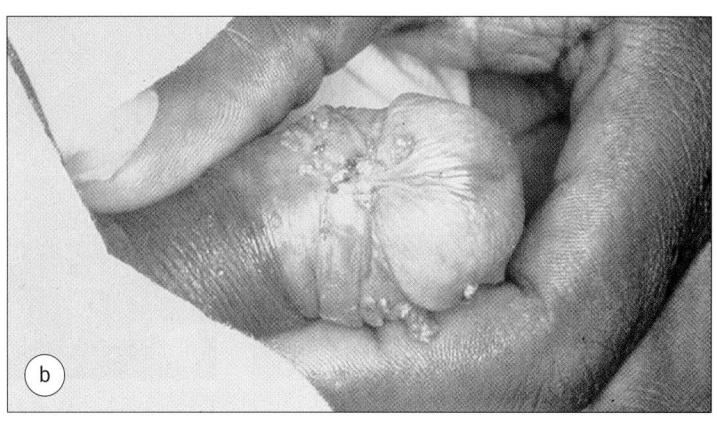

clinical investigations, high sensitivity of HPV assessment is desired to avoid false negative assessments. In such circumstances, the greater sensitivity of the cervicovaginal lavage method related directly to cell sample volume is desirable.[35] However, when only the squamo-columnar junction is to be sampled, the scrape–swab or scrape–brush techniques may be preferred to avoid oversampling desquamated cervical or vaginal cells obtained by lavage.

Current techniques incorporate serology in epidemiologic studies, risk assessment and in investigating possible correlates of protective immunity. Serology may become a tool to evaluate treatment successes, but it is not yet an adequate clinical diagnostic tool due to its suboptimal sensitivity and specificity and given the ubiquitous yet transient nature of HPV infection. Seroepidemiologic studies have emphasized antibody response to HPV-16 and HPV-18, and HPV-6 and HPV-11. A variety of test formats have been employed, including ELISA, Western blot, radioimmunoprecipitation assays and IgG and IgA levels in serum and in cervical secretions.[2]

Innovative diagnostic approaches are being developed, including infrared spectroscopy of cervicovaginal lavage fluid, automated PCR–ELISA-based techniques, laser-induced cervical fluorescence and semiquantitative techniques.[35] It is likely that some of these techniques will join the Pap smear, HPV testing, cervicography (high-resolution photography) (Fig. 66.9) and biopsy pathology as future screening and diagnostic tools.

MANAGEMENT

An accurate diagnosis and appropriate treatment plan can help eliminate the long-term sequelae of HPV disease. Primary prevention depends upon health care providers providing counseling to reduce sexual risk-taking.[36]

Current forms of treatment attempt to ablate the pathologic lesion and eliminate HPV. The first goal is realistic, whereas the second is elusive given multifocal infection and the ease of reinfection.

Ablation can be achieved by topical application of chemicals, cold (cryosurgery), heat (loop electrosurgery, laser), or surgery (cone biopsy, hysterectomy). Topically applied chemicals and medications include salicylic acid, cantharidin, podophyllin liquid, podophilox gel, trichloroacetic acid and topical 5-fluorouracil.[37] Cryosurgery applies liquid nitrogen with a swab, freezing superficial squamous epithelium.[38] Loop electrosurgical excision procedure is currently a popular option.[39] Recurrence rates associated with all modalities are high because these methods do not eradicate the subclinical or latent reservoir of HPV remaining in adjacent epithelial cells and mucous membranes.[30]

Warts of the vagina, urethral meatus, anus and oral mucosa may respond to cryotherapy with liquid nitrogen (a cryoprobe is not recommended for use in the vagina because of the risk of vaginal perforation and fistula formation). Podophyllin liquid with slightly different treatment regimens is available for warts of the vagina and urethral meatus unless the woman is pregnant. Trichloroacetic acid is used to treat vaginal and anal warts up to a maximum of six once-weekly treatments. Surgical removal may be indicated for severe anal warts, but recurrence rates are high.

Invasive and expensive treatment modalities such as carbon dioxide laser and surgery are usually reserved for patients with either extensive or refractory lesions.[40] Success in treating condylomata can be increased if the area is first soaked with 5% acetic acid to show the extent of the local infection more clearly. Both podofilox and podophyllin liquid are more efficacious when applied on warts occurring on moist mucosal surfaces than on lesions found on heavily keratinized epithelia.

During pregnancy, removal of visible warts is often advisable due to their propensity to proliferate and become friable. Similarly, high-grade CIN may need intervention. In contrast, treatment for subclinical genital HPV infection and low-grade CIN during pregnancy is not recommended as spontaneous improvement postpartum is common.

Immunologic therapy with interferons represents a promising new antiviral modality that can be directed against all sites of infection, including clinical, subclinical and latent disease. Interferons have been used successfully as monotherapy or in combination with traditional modalities to treat anogenital condyloma acuminatum.[30] They function as cytokines, which are intercellular signaling proteins that help regulate cell proliferation, differentiation and immune function. Interferons indirectly perform their diverse biologic activities by binding tightly to specific cellular receptors, resulting in transmembrane signaling and synthesis of effector proteins. Use of interferons in combination with other therapeutic modalities appears more efficacious than monotherapy.[30]

In the absence of HIV coinfection, currently available therapeutic methods (all modalities) are moderately successful (22–94%), with recurrence rates of 25% within 3 months. Exophytic genital warts may disappear without treatment. Follow-up is based on colposcopy and cytology.[40]

CHEMOPREVENTION

Chemoprevention is the use of agents to retard neoplastic progression. The desired effect for chemopreventive trials is complete regression or prevention of progression. However, spontaneous high regression rates, the subjective nature of CIN diagnosis and the impact of biopsy on regression complicate the evaluation.[41]

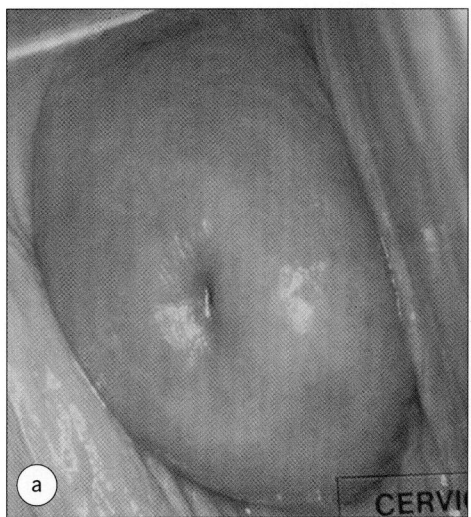
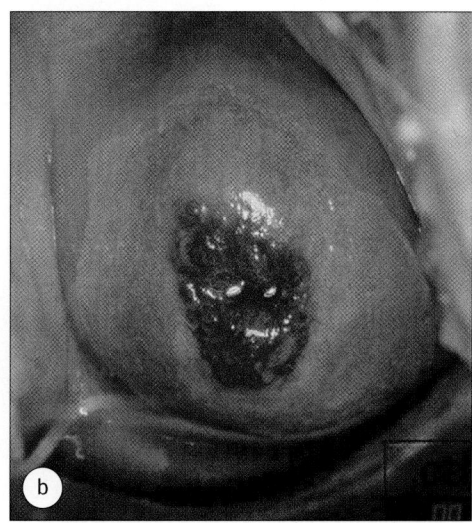
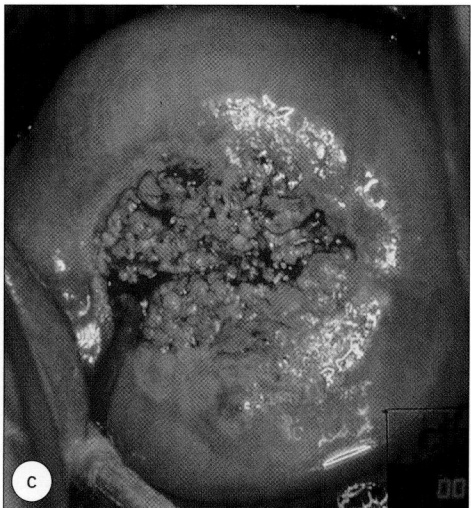

Fig. 66.9 Cervigrams. (a) Normal cervix. (b) Cervix with ectopy. (c) Cervix with microglandular hyperplasia.

Several processes in the HPV infection cycle are appropriate targets for the development of antiviral agents. The development of chemical compounds active against HPV could prevent the benign and malignant diseases associated with HPV infection.[42] Retinoids like dietary vitamin A (retinol) and carotenoids are being studied therapeutically early in the neoplastic process (either systemically or locally) to maintain normal cervical cell function and inhibit the disease progression. Retinoids do not necessarily act to inhibit proliferation of HPV-immortalized cervical cells via effects on HPV E6 and E7, but they may act to inhibit cervical proliferation by 'suppressing' the activity of the epidermal growth factor and insulin-like growth factor signaling pathways. This suggests that combined interferon–retinoid therapy could provide an enhanced beneficial effect to reduce cervical tumor size due to the fact that each agent inhibits cervical cell proliferation.[43]

The likelihood that a cervical precancerous lesion will progress increases with the severity of the atypia. However, even high-grade lesions may spontaneously regress.[44] For a low-grade SIL Pap smear, two options are suggested:

- serial Pap smear every 6 months for 2 years with a referral at the second abnormal Pap smear; and
- an immediate referral for colposcopy.

With high-grade SIL, immediate referral to a gynecologist for colposcopy, biopsy and appropriate therapy is indicated.[44]

In summary, HPV is a ubiquitous, often transient, infection that can cause squamous carcinoma when high-risk genotypes persist. Our understanding of viral pathogenesis has improved markedly in the past 2 decades. Diagnosis, therapy, and vaccine development are all evolving at a rapid pace. However, even more immediate progress in control of HPV-mediated genital tract cancers can result from expanded PAP smear screening and neoplasia treatment programs.

REFERENCES

1. Zur Hausen H. Papillomavirus infections – a major cause of human cancers. Biochim et Biophys Acta 1996;1288:F55–78.
2. Schiffman MH, Burk RD. Human papillomaviruses In: Evans AS, Kaslow RA, eds. Viral infections in humans, 4th ed. New York: Plenum Publishing Co; 1997.
3. Chow LT, Broker TR. *In vitro* experimental systems for HPV: epithelial raft cultures for investigations of viral reproduction and pathogenesis and for analyses of viral proteins and regulatory sequences. Clin Dermatol 1997;15:217–27.
4. Favre M, Ramoz N, Orth G. Human papillomaviruses: general features. Clin Dermatol 1997;15:181–98.
5. World Health Organization. Cervical cancer: experts confirmed virus a major cause, new detection technologies available. Press Release 47. Geneva: WHO; 1996.
6. Evander M, Edlund K, Gustafsson A, et al. Human papillomavirus infection is transient in young women: a population-based cohort study. J Infect Dis 1995;171:1026–30.
7. American Cancer Society, Inc. Cancer facts and figures 1996. 96–300M-No.5008.96. Atlanta: American Cancer Society; 1996.
8. National Cancer Institute. NCI cancer statistics fact book 1995. Bethesda: National Institutes of Health; 1996.
9. Herrero R. Epidemiology of cervical cancer. J Natl Cancer Inst Monographs 1996;21:1–6.
10. Munger K. The molecular biology of cervical cancer. J Cell Biochem 1995;23(Suppl):55–60.
11. Strickler HD, Dillner J, Schiffman MH, et al. A seroepidemiologic study of HPV infection and incident cervical squamous intraepithelial lesions. Viral Immunol 1994;7:169–77.

12. Bosch FX, Manos MM, Munoz N, et al. Prevalence of human papillomavirus in cervical cancer: a worldwide perspective. International biological study on cervical cancer (IBSCC) Study Group. J Natl Cancer Inst 1995;87:796–802.
13. Adimora AA, Quinlivan EB. Human papillomavirus infection: recent findings on progression to cervical cancer. Postgrad Med 1995;98:109–20.
14. Sikstrom B. Hellberg D. Nilsson S, et al. Gynecological symptoms and vaginal wet smear findings in women with cervical human papillomavirus infection. Gynecol Obstet Invest 1997;43:49–52.
15. Coleman N, Birley HD, Renton AM, et al. Immunological events in regressing genital warts. Am J Clin Pathol 1994;102:768–74.
16. Egbert JE, Kersten RC. Female genital tract papillomavirus in conjunctival papillomas of infancy. Am J Ophthalmol 1997;123:551–2.
17. Simons AM, Mugica van Herckenrode C, Rodriguez JA, et al. Demonstration of smoking-related DNA damage in cervical epithelium and correlation with human papillomavirus type 16, using exfoliated cervical cells. Br J Cancer 1995;71:246–49.
18. Romney SL, Palan PR, Basu J, et al. Nutrient antioxidants in the pathogenesis and prevention of cervical dysplasias and cancer. J Cell Biochem 1995;23(Suppl):96–103.
19. Vermund SH, Kelley KF, Klein RS, et al. High risk of human papillomavirus infection and cervical squamous intraepithelial lesions among women with symptomatic human immunodeficiency virus infection. Am J Obstet Gynecol 1991;165:392–400.
20. Shah KV, Solomon L, Daniel R, et al. Comparison of PCR and hybrid capture methods for detection of human papillomavirus in injection drug-using women at high risk of human immunodeficiency virus infection. J Clin Microbiol 1997;35:517–9.

21. Melbye M, Smith E, Wohlfahrt J, et al. Anal and cervical abnormality in women – prediction by human papillomavirus tests. Int J Cancer 1996;68:559–64.
22. Mai KT, Yazdi HM, Bertrand MA, et al. Bilateral primary ovarian squamous cell carcinoma associated with human papilloma virus infection and vulvar and cervical intraepithelial neoplasia. A case report with review of the literature. Am J Surg Pathol 1996;20:767–72.
23. Mvula M, Iwasaka T, Iguchi A, et al. Do human papillomaviruses have a role in the pathogenesis of bladder carcinoma? J Urol 1996;155:471–4.
24. Park TW, Fujiwara H, Wright TC. Molecular biology of cervical cancer and its precursors. Cancer 1995;76(Suppl):1902–13.
25. Tommasino M, Crawford L. Human papillomavirus E6 and E7: proteins which deregulate the cell cycle. Bioessays 1995;17:509–18
26. Hardy RE, Eckert C, Hargreaves MK, et al. Breast and cervical cancer screening among low-income women: impact of a simple centralized HMO intervention. J Natl Med Assoc 1996;88:381–4.
27. Borysiewicz LK, Fiander A, Nimako M, et al. A recombinant vaccinia virus encoding human papillomavirus types 16 and 18, E6 and E7 proteins as immunotherapy for cervical cancer. Lancet 1996;347:1523–7.
28. Hines JF, Ghim S, Schlegel R, et al. Prospects for a vaccine against human papillomavirus. Obstet Gynecol 1995;86:860–6.
29. Rockley PF, Tyring SK. Interferons alpha, beta and gamma therapy of anogenital human papillomavirus infections. Pharmacol Ther 1995;65:265–87.
30. Crum CP, McLachlin CM. Cervical intraepithelial neoplasia. J Cell Biochem 1995;23:71–9.
31. Miller KE. Women's health. Sexually transmitted diseases. Prim Care 1997;24:179–93.

32. Wideroff L, Schiffman MH, Nonnenmacher B, *et al.* Evaluation of seroreactivity to HPV type 16 virus-like particles in an incident case–control study of cervical neoplasia. J Infect Dis 1995;172:1425–30.

33. Hall S, Lorincz A, Shah F, *et al.* Human papillomavirus DNA detection in cervical specimens by hybrid capture: correlation with cytologic and histologic diagnoses of squamous intraepithelial lesions of the cervix. Gynecol Oncol 1996;62:353–9.

34. Vermund SH, Shiffman MH, Goldberg GL, *et al.* Molecular diagnosis of genital HPV infection: comparison of two methods used to collect exfoliated cervical cells. Am J Obstet Gynecol 1989;160:304–8.

35. Kaufman RH, Adam E, Icenogle J, *et al.* Relevance of human papillomavirus screening in management of cervical intraepithelial neoplasia. Am J Obstet Gynecol 1997;176:87–92.

36. Stone KM. Human papillomavirus infection and genital warts: update on epidemiology and treatment. Clin Infect Dis 1995;20(suppl 1):91–7.

37. Miller DM, Brodell RT. Human papillomavirus infection: treatment options for warts. Am Fam Physician 1996;53:135–43.

38. Mayeaux EJ, Harper MB, Barksdale W, Pope JB. Noncervical human papillomavirus genital infections. Am Fam Physician 1995;52:1137–46.

39. Vermund SH, Melnick SL. Human papillomavirus infection. In: Minkoff H, Dehovitz JA, Duerr A, eds. HIV infection in women. New York: Raven Press; 1995;11:189–227.

40. Ruffin MT, Ogaily MS, Johnston CM, *et al.* Surrogate endpoint biomarkers for cervical cancer chemopreventive trials. J Cell Biochem 1995;23:113–24.

41. Phelps WC, Alexander KA. Antiviral therapy for human papillomaviruses: rationale and prospects. Ann Intern Med 1995;123:368–82.

42. Eckert RL, Agarwal C, Hembree JR, *et al.* Human cervical cancer. Retinoids, interferon and human papillomavirus. Adv Exp Med Biol 1995;375:31–44.

43. Syrjanen KJ. Spontaneous evolution of intraepithelial lesions according to the grade and type of the implicated human papillomavirus (HPV). Eur J Obstet Gynecol Reprod Biol 1996;65:45–53.

44. Appleby J. Management of the abnormal Papanicolaou smear. Med Clin North Am 1995;79:345–60.

Lymphogranuloma Venerum, Chancroid and Granuloma Inguinale

Virginia R Roth & D William Cameron

LYMPHOGRANULOMA VENEREUM

Lymphogranuloma venereum (LGV) is a sexually transmitted disease caused by three serovars of *Chlamydia trachomatis*: L1, L2 and L3.

EPIDEMIOLOGY

Lymphogranuloma venereum is endemic in parts of Africa, India, Asia, South America and the Caribbean. It occurs sporadically in North America and Europe, usually in returning travelers or military personnel. Underdiagnosis and under-reporting of LGV is thought to be common. Men are six times more likely than women to have a clinically evident infection, and are only infectious until the primary ulcer heals. In contrast, women may harbor persistent asymptomatic cervical lesions that serve as reservoirs of infection.

PATHOGENESIS AND PATHOLOGY

Lymphogranuloma venereum is acquired sexually, but transmission through direct contact with infected tissues or fomites has been documented. Perinatal infection occurs as infants pass through an infected birth canal. After exposure, epithelial abrasions allow the organism to penetrate the mucosal barrier. Replication within the macrophages is followed by spread via the lymphatic system. The histopathologic changes on biopsy resemble those of other bacterial infections.[1]

CLINICAL FEATURES

Lymphogranuloma venereum begins in the genital region and spreads through the lymphatics. Clinical disease occurs in three stages. The transient primary lesion is a small, painless genital ulcer or papule. It appears 3–21 days after inoculation and generally goes unnoticed. It usually occurs on the coronal sulcus in men, and on the cervix, posterior vaginal wall or vulva in women. Urethral involvement may cause urethritis.

The second stage occurs days to weeks after the primary infection. It is characterized by painful regional lymphadenopathy and systemic symptoms. In men, the inguinal lymph nodes are affected, and node enlargement on either side of the inguinal ligament produces the characteristic 'groove sign'. In women, lymph drainage from the rectum and vagina results in pelvic lymphadenopathy. Involvement of these deep nodes causes lower abdominal and back pain. Initially, the lymph nodes are mobile and discrete, but with progressive inflammation they become fixed and suppurative with bubo formation. Buboes may spontaneously rupture or form chronically draining sinuses. Subsequent scarring and fibrosis results in lymphatic obstruction and genital edema (Fig. 67.1). Regional spread of LGV to the pelvis may cause salpingitis, pelvic adhesions and infertility. Hematogenous dissemination has been documented by the recovery of organisms from the blood and cerebrospinal fluid. Such patients experience nonspecific constitutional symptoms or, less commonly, present with meningoencephalitis, pneumonitis, arthritis or hepatitis. Skin lesions such as erythema nodosum classically follow surgical manipulation of infected tissue.

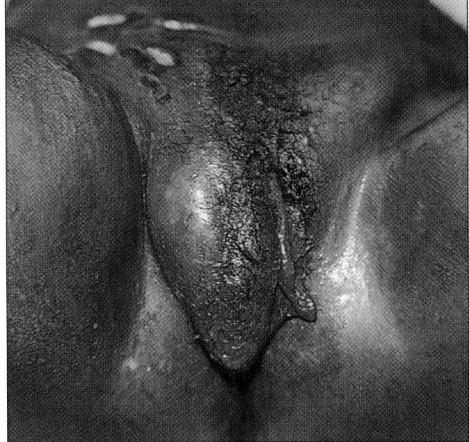

Fig. 67.1 Lymphogranuloma venereum causing unilateral vulvar lymphedema and inguinal buboes.

The tertiary or anorectal stage is predominantly seen in women and homosexual men. Rectal infection may result from anal intercourse, lymphatic spread or spread from vaginal secretions. Patients present with fever, rectal pain and mucopurulent or bloody discharge. The appearance on sigmoidoscopy resembles that of inflammatory bowel disease with mucosal ulceration and friable granulation tissue. Fibrosis can cause rectal strictures and bowel obstruction.

Conjunctival or oropharyngeal infection may be a result of autoinoculation or orogenital sex. The regional mandibular and cervical lymph nodes are involved, and subsequent spread to supraclavicular and mediastinal nodes has been reported to cause pericarditis.

DIAGNOSIS

When LGV is suspected clinically, other causes of genital ulcer disease should be excluded. Growth of the organism in cell culture is the most specific diagnostic test, but it is labor intensive with a recovery rate of only 50%.[2]

Serology has been the mainstay for the diagnosis of LGV. Complement fixation is currently the most sensitive and widely used test, and a titer of 1:64 or greater in the appropriate clinical setting is considered diagnostic. Other *Chlamydia* infections may result in a positive complement fixation test, but a titer of less than 1:16 essentially rules out acute LGV. Microimmunofluorescence is more specific but less sensitive than complement fixation. More recently, enzyme-linked immunosorbent assay (ELISA) and direct fluorescein-conjugated antibody tests have become available. Polymerase chain reaction (PCR) is highly sensitive and specific and will be a useful diagnostic tool in the future.

MANAGEMENT

Although LGV infections resolve spontaneously, this occurs over several weeks and may be complicated by fibrosis, stricture formation or superinfection. Antimicrobial therapy decreases the incidence of complications, but has not been shown to affect the rate of healing. The recommended therapy is doxycycline 100mg orally q12h for 3 weeks.

Alternative regimens are erythromycin 500mg orally q6h or trimethoprim–sulfamethoxazole (TMP–SMX; co-trimoxazole) q12h.[3] Asymptomatic sexual partners should also be treated. Patients should be followed to document clinical resolution. Repeated aspiration of buboes may be necessary to relieve pain and prevent rupture. Surgical intervention may be required for fistulae, strictures or genital elephantiasis.

CHANCROID

The etiologic agent of chancroid is *Haemophilus ducreyi*, a fastidious Gram-negative bacillus. It is a sexually transmitted cause of genital ulcer disease.

EPIDEMIOLOGY

Chancroid occurs worldwide. It is endemic in tropical climates and is the commonest cause of genital ulcer disease in many developing countries. It is much less frequent in North America and Europe where it occurs in sporadic outbreaks associated with prostitution, travel and returning military personnel. There have been sustained outbreaks in several cities in the USA associated with illicit drug use and prostitution. The prevalence is higher in men than women, and uncircumcised men are more susceptible to infection. A low clinical suspicion and a lack of readily available diagnostic tests have resulted in underreporting of the disease.

The spread of chancroid is related to the number of sexual partners of an infected person, and prostitution appears to be the main reservoir of infection. Because women are often asymptomatic, sexual activity continues despite active infection. Polymerase chain reaction testing of high-risk women without genital ulcers has confirmed that asymptomatic carriage of *H. ducreyi* does occur.[4]

Chancroid and other genital ulcer diseases are significantly associated with an increased rate of HIV transmission.[5,6] Conversely, the presence of HIV also increases the risk of chancroid. The significance of this codependency was emphasized in an epidemiologic study that estimated that genital ulcer disease increases the risk of HIV transmission per sexual exposure by 10–300 times.[7]

PATHOGENESIS AND PATHOLOGY

Haemophilus ducreyi is a bipolar-staining, pleomorphic Gram-negative coccobacillus. Three distinct histologic zones have been described on biopsy of the chancroid ulcer. The superficial zone, in which the organism is most readily seen, contains necrotic debris, fibrin and degenerated neutrophils. The middle zone is characterized by edematous inflammatory tissue with neovascularization, and the deep zone exhibits a dense cellular infiltrate. This infiltrate contains CD4+ lymphocytes and macrophages, which may contribute to the facilitation of HIV transmission.[8]

Chancroid is transmitted from person to person by direct contact. A break in the skin may allow the organism to penetrate, establish infection and evoke humoral and cellular immune responses. Despite the host immune response, re-infection and serial autoinfection can occur. Virulence factors have not been well defined. Pili have been demonstrated,[9] but their role in cellular adhesion is unknown. The production of lipo-oligosaccharides, heat-shock proteins and cytotoxin may contribute to tissue damage and ulceration. Evasion of host immune defense may be mediated in part through the lipo-oligosaccharides and outer membrane proteins.[10]

PREVENTION AND CONTROL

The role of chancroid in HIV transmission makes it a public health concern. Effective treatment of sexually transmitted diseases (STDs) decreases the population incidence of HIV.[11] Thus, treatment of infected persons and their sexual contacts, as well as the examination and treatment of prostitutes, are important measures. The future development of vaccines for genital ulcer diseases such as chancroid may also be highly effective in reducing the spread of HIV.

CLINICAL FEATURES

Patients who have chancroid generally present with painful genital ulcers within 4–7 days of exposure. An initial painless papule, usually unnoticed, develops into a pustule and progresses to form a painful ulcer about 1–2cm in size (Fig. 67.2). The ulcer margins are raised, irregular and sharply demarcated. Because the ulcer edge is not indurated, it is known as a 'soft chancre'. The friable, granular base is often covered with a necrotic exudate. Approximately one-third of patients develop multiple lesions, which may coalesce to form giant ulcers. Autoinoculation may result in 'kissing lesions' on opposing surfaces.

The clinical picture varies with gender, and men are more symptomatic then women. In men, the ulcer is usually located on the prepuce, coronal sulcus, penile shaft, glans or urethral meatus (Fig. 67.3). The scrotum and perineum are less frequently involved. In women, the clinical presentation may be atypical, with symptoms of dyspareunia or dysuria. Ulcers in women are more likely to be painless and are found on the forchette, labia, perineum, perianal region and the medial aspect of the thigh. Involvement of the vagina and cervix is rare. The ulcers may resemble those of syphilis, genital herpes or granuloma inguinale (GI). Co-infection with herpes simplex or syphilis commonly occurs.

Inguinal lymphadenitis is seen in about 50% of men and 35% of women, and may be bilateral. Lymph nodes progressively enlarge to become necrotic and fluctuant (buboes). Systemic symptoms are characteristically absent. Extragenital ulcers are rare, but have been described in the mouth, fingers and breasts. Co-infection with HIV may alter the clinical presentation, as these patients are more likely to have multiple genital lesions, to develop extragenital ulcerations and to experience a delayed or reduced response to treatment.[12,13] However, disseminated infection does not occur even in the immunocompromised. Although untreated ulcers usually heal spontaneously, they

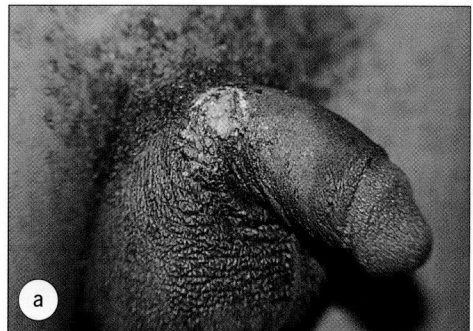
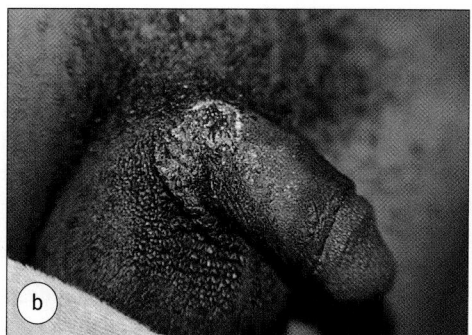
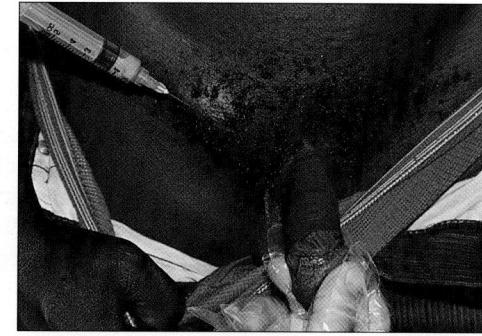

Fig. 67.2 Chancroid ulcer. (a) Before and (b) after the performance of a swab, demonstrating the friability of the ulcer base.

Fig. 67.3 Typical chancroid ulcer. Unilateral lymphadenitis and demonstration of the aspiration of a bubo.

can be complicated by secondary bacterial infection, tissue destruction, scarring, fistulae and stricture formation (Figs 67.4 & 67.5).

DIAGNOSIS

Laboratory methods for the identification of *H. ducreyi* have developed rapidly over recent years.[14] Because the accuracy of clinical diagnosis may be as low as 50%,[15] laboratory confirmation of infection should be obtained when possible. In addition, all patients who have suspected chancroid should be tested for HIV and for other, or coexisting, causes of genital ulcer disease.

Specimens are collected by swabbing the ulcer base. Bacterial contamination reduces the accuracy of the Gram stain, and its overall sensitivity and specificity are less than 50%. Culture of the organism is the preferred diagnostic test. A variety of culture media have been used (most commonly Mueller–Hinton or gonococcal agar base), and recovery rates can be improved by using more than one type of medium concurrently. Vancomycin is usually added as a selective agent. The sensitivity of a positive culture is 70–80% under ideal circumstances. Specimens should be inoculated onto culture plates within 1 hour of collection, or stored in an enriched medium and refrigerated for up to 1 week.[16] Culture plates are incubated at 33°C in maximal humidity and high CO_2. Growth is usually seen within 72 hours, but plates should be kept for 5 days before being reported negative. Colonies are raised; they are nonmucoid, yellow–gray in color and very cohesive. A positive culture may be confirmed by demonstrating the presence of nitrate reductase, cytochrome oxidase, alkaline phosphatase and the requirement for heme.

Antigen-detection techniques are of little clinical use. Serologic tests are available, but are primarily useful in epidemiologic studies. As a confirmatory test, PCR is useful due to its high sensitivity and specificity.

MANAGEMENT

The treatment of chancroid has been complicated by antimicrobial resistance and HIV co-infection. There are wide regional variations in antimicrobial susceptibilities, but increasing global resistance to tetracycline, aminoglycosides, sulfonamides and amoxicillin–clavulanic acid has been documented.

Current recommendations for treatment include azithromycin 1g orally in a single dose, ceftriaxone 250mg intramuscularly in a single dose or erythromycin base 500mg q6h for 7 days.[3,12] Single-dose ciprofloxacin 500mg orally or spectinomycin 2g intramuscularly are alternative regimens. The use of amoxicillin–clavulanic acid or TMP–SMX depends on local susceptibilities. Ease of administration and compliance makes single-dose therapies preferable. However, patients who have concurrent HIV infection experience higher failure rates after single-dose therapy, and therefore their treatment should be of longer duration.[12,13] Response to treatment is characterized by a decrease in pain within 48 hours; complete ulcer healing takes approximately 10 days. The development of fluctuant buboes may occur on treatment, and these should be drained by incision or needle aspiration.

GRANULOMA INGUINALE

Granuloma inguinale (or donovanosis) is caused by the Gram-negative bacterium *Calymmatobacterium granulomatis*. It is a fastidious organism that is difficult to culture and thus continues to evade taxonomic classification and definition of its biochemical characteristics.

EPIDEMIOLOGY

Granuloma inguinale is endemic in tropical and subtropical regions such as Papua New Guinea and India. It can also be found in Southeast Asia, parts of Africa, the Caribbean, central Australia and South America. In these regions the incidence varies from 0.3 to 7.6%. Granuloma inguinale is rare in North America and Europe. Underreporting probably occurs in nonendemic areas because of a low clinical suspicion and diagnostic difficulties.

The prevalence is highest among adults aged 20–40 years, although it does occur in children and in the elderly. The male to female ratio is about 2.5:1. Affected individuals are usually sexually active and may have a history of multiple sexual partners or contact with prostitutes. A significant association between granuloma inguinale and HIV seropositivity has been documented, particularly in men with genital ulcers of long duration.[17]

PATHOGENESIS AND PATHOLOGY

The exact mode of transmission is not known. It is widely believed to be sexually transmitted because of its predominance in sexually active persons, its predilection for the genital region, the high incidence of co-infection with other STDs and the association of anal lesions in men with receptive anal intercourse. However, occurrence in sexually inactive persons (including children) and the low rate of transmission between sexual partners suggests the possibility of nonsexual transmission.

On histopathology, large mononuclear cells containing inclusion bodies (Donovan bodies) are characteristic. The associated epithelial changes include ulceration, microabscesses, acanthosis, irregular elongation of the rete pegs and pseudoepitheliomatous hyperplasia. Untreated lesions may become hyperkeratotic. The dermal layer exhibits inflammatory changes, with a dense cellular infiltrate and varying degrees of fibrosis and edema.

PREVENTION

Serious morbidity is best prevented by early diagnosis and treatment. Sexual contacts should be examined, as the rate of infection in this group is as high as 50%. It has been suggested that annual screening may reduce the incidence of granuloma inguinale in endemic areas, and that condom use may decrease sexual transmission. As with other genital ulcer diseases, reducing the incidence of granuloma inguinale may be important in controlling the spread of HIV.[18]

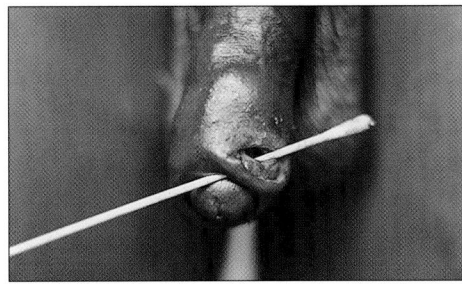

Fig. 67.4 Phagedenic chancroid with extensive tissue destruction.

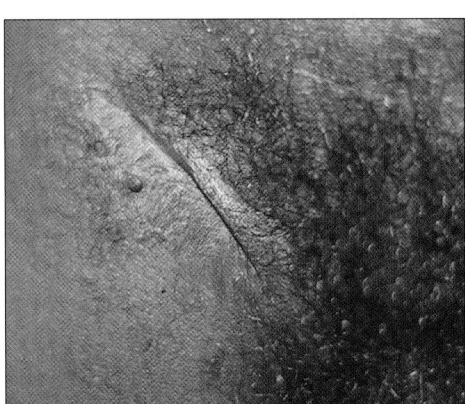

Fig. 67.5 Healed inguinal bubo with scar formation from previous chancroid infection.

CLINICAL FEATURES

Granuloma inguinale is a chronically progressive, ulcerative disease with no systemic symptoms. The incubation period appears to range between 3 and 30 days. Patients usually present with a nonsuppurative genital lesion. Less common presentations include vaginal bleeding or discharge, hematochezia, hematuria, pelvic inflammatory disease or a pelvic mass.

The initial lesion is a small firm papule at the site of infection, which erodes to form a painless ulcer (Fig. 67.6). The ulcer is granulomatous and 'beefy-red' with a nonpurulent base. Multiple lesions may develop on opposing surfaces or along skin folds. Lesions are usually found in the genital, perianal and inguinal regions. In women, cervical lesions may mimic dysplasia. Less frequently, extragenital sites such as the mouth, face or neck are involved. Abscess formation in the groin mimics lymphadenitis (pseudobuboes), but the lymph nodes themselves are rarely involved. This typical clinical picture may be altered if the genital lesions become superinfected, resulting in a purulent exudate and tender lymphadenopathy.

Without treatment, granuloma inguinale is slowly progressive, often resulting in soft tissue destruction and extensive scarring. Possible sequelae include genital adhesions, stenosis of the urethral, vaginal or anal orifices, rectovaginal fistulas and lymphatic obstruction with genital pseudoelephantiasis. Contiguous pelvic spread may result in a frozen pelvis or in hydronephrosis. Rarely, hematogenous spread to the bones or liver may occur. Even with treatment, there is a tendency for recurrence.

Granuloma inguinale may be confused with syphilis, ulcerated genital warts, squamous carcinoma, chancroid, LGV, genital herpes and traumatic ulceration. Co-infection with other STDs is common. Carcinoma of the penis and vulva may occur simultaneously with granuloma inguinale or in areas of previously healed ulcers. Causality has never been established, but it should be recognized that ulcers that do not respond to treatment or are recurrent may represent a malignancy. During pregnancy, granuloma inguinale is often more aggressive, with a higher rate of dissemination and a slower response to treatment. Perinatal infection is rare, but prophylactic antibiotics should be administered to the infant.

DIAGNOSIS

In nonendemic areas, a high index of suspicion is required to make a diagnosis of granuloma inguinale. Alternative or concomitant diagnoses must be ruled out. Clinical suspicion is confirmed by the demonstration of Donovan bodies on smear or biopsy. Reliable culture

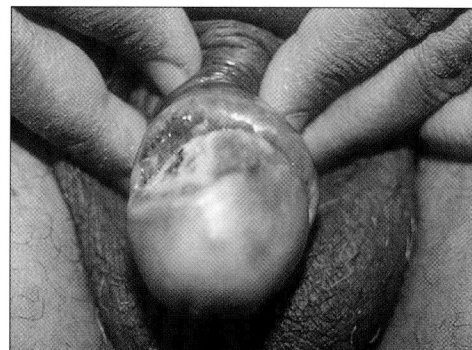

Fig. 67.6 Penile granuloma inguinale. Courtesy of Dr Don Low.

techniques and serologic tests are not available. To obtain a smear for diagnosis, the ulcer is scraped and the granulomatous tissue is spread directly onto a slide. The slide is air dried and stained with Wright or Giemsa stain. Donovan bodies are seen as darkly staining, ovoid organisms with or without a capsule. In the appropriate clinical setting, the 1-minute 'Quick test', in which the specimen is stained with eosin and thiazine dyes, is diagnostic.[19]

The smear is more likely to be negative if the lesion is early, sclerotic or superinfected. In such cases, a histologic diagnosis should be sought. The diagnosis may also be established using electron microscopy.

MANAGEMENT

Treatment regimens are empiric as in-vitro susceptibility testing is not available. One double-strength tablet of TMP–SMX q12h is favored because of the low recurrence rates associated with this treatment regimen and its lower toxicity.[3] Other commonly used regimens include doxycycline 100mg q12h, tetracycline or erythromycin 500mg q6h, chloramphenicol 500mg q8h and streptomycin 1g given intramuscularly q12h. Clindamycin, the fluoroquinolones and gentamicin are also effective. Clinical resistance to tetracycline, ampicillin and streptomycin have been reported. Combination therapy is used in more severe disease. Response to treatment is usually seen within 1 week but antibiotics should be continued until all the lesions have resolved, which may take months in advanced disease.

Relapses are common and may occur up to 2 years after apparently successful treatment, requiring an additional course of antibiotics. Complications such as strictures, sinus formation, extensive superinfection or disfiguration may require surgical intervention.

REFERENCES

1. Scieux C, Barnes R, Bianchi A, et al. Lymphogranuloma venereum: 27 cases in Paris. J Infect Dis 1989;160:662–8.
2. Joseph AK, Rosen T. Laboratory techniques used in the diagnosis of chancroid, granuloma inguinale, and lymphogranuloma venereum. Dermatol Clin 1994;12:1–8.
3. Centers for Disease Control and Prevention. 1998 Guidelines for treatment of sexually transmitted diseases. MMWR 1998;47:19–28.
4. Hawkes S, West B, Wilson S, et al. Asymptomatic carriage of Haemophilus ducreyi confirmed by the polymerase chain reaction. Genitourin Med 1995;71:224–7.
5. Cameron DW, Simonsen JN, D'Costa LJ, et al. Female to male transmission of human immunodeficiency virus type 1: risk factors for seroconversion in men. Lancet 1989;ii:403–7.
6. Wasserheit JN. Epidemiological synergy: interrelationships between HIV infection and other STDs. Sex Transm Dis 1992; 19:61–77.
7. Hayes RJ, Schulz KF, Plummer FA. The cofactor effect of genital ulcers on the per-exposure risk of

HIV transmission in sub-Saharan Africa. J Trop Med Hyg 1995;98:1–8.
8. King R, Gough J, Ronald A, et al. An immunohistochemical analysis of naturally occurring chancroid. J Infect Dis 1996;174:427–30.
9. Castellazzo A, Shero M, Apicella M, et al. Expression of pili by Haemophilus ducreyi. J Infect Dis 1992;165(suppl 1):S198–9.
10. Abeck D, Johnson AP. Pathophysiological concept of Haemophilus ducreyi infection chancroid. Int J STD AIDS. 1992;3:319–23.
11. Grosskurth H, Mosha F, Todd J, et al. Impact of improved treatment of sexually transmitted diseases on HIV infection in rural Tanzania: randomized control trial. Lancet 1995;346:530–6.
12. Schulte JM, Schmid GP. Recommendations for treatment of chancroid, 1993. Clin Infect Dis 1995;20(suppl 1):S39–46.
13. Tyndall MW, Agoki E, Plummer FA, et al. Single dose azithromycin for treatment of chancroid: a randomized comparison with erythromycin. Sex Transm Dis 1994;21:231–4.

14. Trees DL, Morse SA. Chancroid and Haemophilus ducreyi: an update. Clin Microbiol Rev 1995;8:357–75.
15. O'Farrell N, Hoosen AA, Coetzee KD, et al. Genital ulcer disease: accuracy of clinical diagnosis and strategies to improve control in Durban, South Africa. Genitourin Med 1994;70:7–11.
16. Dangor Y, Radebe F, Ballard RC. Transport media for Haemophilus ducreyi. Sex Transm Dis 1993;20:5–9.
17. O'Farrell N, Windsor I, Becker P. HIV-1 infection among heterosexual attenders at a sexually transmitted diseases clinic in Durban. S Afr Med J 1991;80:17–20.
18. O'Farrell NO. Global eradication of donovanosis: an opportunity for limiting the spread of HIV-1 infection. Genitourin Med 1995;71:27–31.
19. O'Farrell N, Hoosen AA, Coetzee KD, et al. A rapid stain for the diagnosis of granuloma inguinale. Genitourin Med 1990;66:200–1.

Practice Points

Persistent/recurrent vaginal discharge

Jonathan M Zenilman

INTRODUCTION

Vaginal discharge is one of the cardinal symptoms of lower tract gynecologic exudative infections. These disorders are classified by anatomic site of origin. For example, gonorrhea and chlamydial infections are cervical infections; bacterial vaginosis (BV), trichomoniasis and vaginal yeast infections are vaginal disorders. Herpes simplex and human papillomavirus can cause epithelial lesions on the external genitalia, but they can also cause cervicitis with discharge (see Chapter 2.52).

Initial steps

The first step in assessing a complaint of recurrent vaginal discharge is to differentiate between a normal physiologic discharge, a vaginal discharge, and cervical infections. Many women have a small amount of vaginal discharge (physiologic leukorrhea), which is clear or white, does not have an odor, and is composed predominantly of squamous epithelial cells; this may vary with the menstrual cycle.

Patients do not differentiate from cervical and vaginal disorders, but often report 'vaginal discharge', which may represent either cervical or vaginal pathology. Therefore, initial evaluation of a patient who has recurrent or persistent discharge should include assessment for cervical infection. 'Recurrent' chlamydial and gonococcal infection is most often due to either patient noncompliance with treatment regimens, re-exposure to an untreated sexual partner, or re-exposure (i.e. new-incident infection). New-incident gonococcal and chlamydial infection is particularly common among adolescents.

Assuming that gonococcal and chlamydial infection have been ruled out and that the problem has been localized to the vagina, the next step in managing recurrent vaginal discharge is to determine the specific etiology of the vaginitis. This involves taking a careful history, with attention to recent douching, antimicrobial use (including use of over-the-counter antifungal medications) and reproductive history, followed by a clinical examination, which should include microscopic evaluation of vaginal discharge and determination of vaginal pH. The differential algorithm proposed by Sobel is the standard in clinical assessment.

RECURRENT VAGINITIS DUE TO INFECTION

Recurrent trichomoniasis

Recurrent infection with *Trichomonas* spp. is most commonly due to re-infection from an untreated male partner or to re-exposure. Trichomoniasis in men is usually asymptomatic, and it is therefore imperative that all male partners of women who have trichomoniasis be treated with metronidazole, 2g orally, as a single dose.

Metronidazole-resistant trichomoniasis is rare (<1% of clinical isolates) and should be considered only after re-infection has been ruled out and the patient has failed two courses of therapy. In these patients, metronidazole resistance should be confirmed, and they will respond frequently to a prolonged course of metronidazole (2–4g daily for 10–14 days).

Recurrent candidal vaginitis

Candidal vaginitis is extremely common, and recurrences occur frequently, in up to 45–50% of cases in some studies. Local factors, such as frequent wearing of tight clothing, may occasionally be responsible. Recurrent candidiasis is found more frequently in women who are taking antimicrobial agents and in those who have uncontrolled diabetes mellitus. Immunosuppressed patients, such as persons who have advanced HIV disease, are also at higher risk of recurrent candidiasis as well as recurrent BV (see below).

After potential precipitating factors have been considered, there remains a subset of women who continue to get frequent recurrences. Careful microbiologic evaluation, with identification of the fungal species, may occasionally reveal a yeast that is resistant to the commonly used imidazole therapies, such as *Candida glabrata* or *Candida tropicalis*. These investigations are expensive and should be reserved for use only after the clinical and epidemiologic risks have been accounted for. Persons who have chronic, recurrent candidiasis that is known to be caused by *Candida albicans* often benefit from a course of long-term prophylaxis with fluconazole, 150mg weekly.

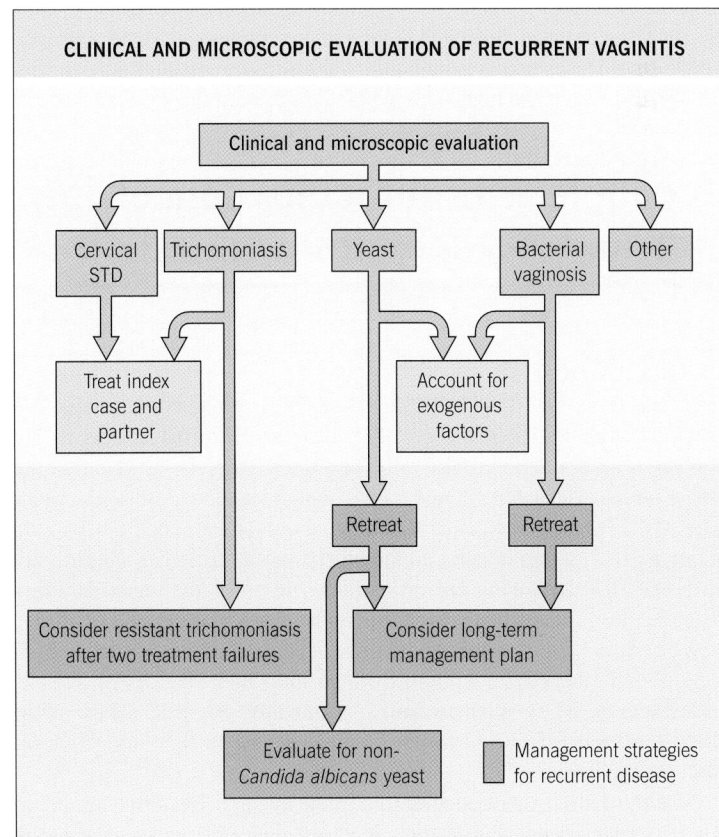

Fig. 68.1 Clinical and microscopic evaluation of recurrent vaginitis.

Recurrent bacterial vaginosis

Bacterial vaginosis is a disorder that occurs as a result of ecologic disturbances among the vaginal flora. Bacterial vaginosis is particularly prone to relapse. As above, the management of recurrent BV should account for the following:

- assurance that appropriate antimicrobial treatment was given initially. For example, many practitioners currently use a single dose regimen of metronidazole (2g orally), and this has a treatment failure rate of up to 20%. Persons who have suspected recurrence should be treated with a full multiday regimen, of metronidazole 500mg orally twice daily, or metronidazole vaginal gel (0.75%) 5g q12h for 5 days, or 2% clindamycin cream 5g q12h for 7 days.
- removal of exogenous factors that contribute to the pathogenesis of BV, including douching or long-term antimicrobials. Douching is particularly associated with the development of BV because of the disruption of the local mucosal surfaces and flora. Therefore, clinical recommendations include specific advice not to douche. Women who use spermicides are at higher risk for BV and must balance the risk and benefits of discontinuing spermicide use.
- ruling out the presence of cervical infection. Infections in the lower genital tract induce an inflammatory response, which in turn causes BV. For example, therefore, as above, ruling out cervical gonococcal and chlamydial infection is important early in the evaluation of persons who have recurrent BV.

There is a population of patients who have primary BV (i.e. BV without any identifiable cause). Primary BV resolves with treatment, but BV recurs frequently in these patients. The etiology in most cases is unknown. Recurrence rates are as high as 20–30% 1 month after treatment. In these cases, long-term treatment with metronidazole should be considered. In nonpregnant women, treatment should take into account the impact of symptoms on the patient's lifestyle. In pregnant women, because of the potential for perinatal complications, periodic evaluation and treatment for recurrences is recommended.

Other causes of recurrent vaginitis

Bacterial vaginosis and yeast vaginitis are the most common types of recurrent vagnitis. Uncommon causes include hypersensitivity vaginitis, especially to latex, which is managed by avoiding latex exposure. This is one situation in which natural membrane condoms may be appropriately used. Desquamative interstitial vaginitis is an uncommon disorder that is diagnosed by a high vaginal pH, a negative amine test, the absence of clue cells and the presence of polymorphonuclear leukocytes. These patients may respond to intravaginal 2% clindamycin cream, 5g q12h for 1 week; however, they are prone to frequent recurrence.

USE OF BIOLOGIC REMEDIES

Women who have frequently recurrent vaginitis will occasionally turn to biologic remedies obtained from health-food shops or over the Internet. These have included (among others) yoghurt douches, lactobacilli for vaginal instillation and prescriptions for eating large quantities of yoghurt. Controlled studies to date have failed to demonstrate any benefits of these remedies.

PATIENT COUNSELING

By the time they see a medical specialist, patients who have recurrent vaginal discharge have typically been seen by many medical care providers with limited results, and they are therefore often frustrated. Counseling on the etiology and pathogenesis of the disorder with frank explanation of the expected impact of therapy is a critical component of management. Issues of sexuality should also be explored, because patients may find intercourse either uncomfortable or embarrassing.

SUMMARY

Important points to remember are:

- take a complete history,
- account for exogenous factors,
- account for systemic diseases,
- rule out cervical sexually transmitted diseases,
- perform a complete evaluation including microscopy,
- consider episodic management and suppressive management, and
- counsel the patients intensively.

FURTHER READING

Amsel R, Totten PA, Spiegel CA, Chien KCS, Eschenbach D, Holmes KK. Nonspecific vagnitis. Diagnostic criteria and microbial and epidemiological associations. Am J Med 1983;74:14–21.

Eschenbach DA, Hillier S, Critchlow C, Stevens C, DeRouen T, Holmes KK. Diagnosis and clinical manifestations of bacterial vaginosis. Am J Obstet Gynecol 1988;158:819–28.

Spiegel CA. Bacterial vaginosis. Clin Microbiol Rev 1991;4:485–502.

Sobel JD. Epidemiology and pathogenesis of recurrent vulvovaginal candidiasis. Am J Obstet Gynecol 1985;152:924–35.

Sobel JD. Vaginitis. N Engl J Med 1997;337:1896–903.

A couple with difficulty conceiving: is it due to previous sexually transmitted diseases?

John W Sellors & John A Collins

INTRODUCTION

Pelvic infection and epididymo-orchitis are serious consequences of sexually transmitted disease (STD) that have known effects in the female on the function of the fallopian tubes (Chapter 2.53) and in the male on the ability to produce an adequate ejaculate. Although not all cases of STD have such clearly damaging outcomes, silent injury to the relevant tissues can occur, and the worry about fertility is a legitimate concern. The following case illustrates the problems raised and this Practice Point identifies reasonable approaches that may be helpful.

A couple have not conceived after 2 years of coitus during which they did not use contraception. Both partners had a history of STD as adolescents. They wish to know about any possible relationship between their infertility and STD and request further investigation and management.

Their question is not uncommon. In the average Western country, up to 10% of married couples are. In those under 30 years of age, the prevalences of *Chlamydia trachomatis* and *Neisseria gonorrhoeae* infections are approximately 7% and less than 1%, respectively, in asymptomatic women. The reported rates in men are less than one-sixth of these levels.

PATHOGENESIS

It has been estimated, from longitudinal studies among Swedish women, that about 8% of women develop laparoscopically proven salpingitis after infection caused by either *C. trachomatis* or *N. gonorrhoeae*. Less than 30% of cases of acute pelvic inflammatory disease have been proven to be due to *C. trachomatis* (by tubal specimens or serology), and a much smaller percentage has been linked to *N. gonorrhoeae*. The risk of tubal infertility in women is directly related to the number and severity of the episodes of pelvic inflammatory disease. Serologic studies in North American women have shown that at least half of the cases of tubal infertility and ectopic pregnancy are attributable to *C. trachomatis* infection.

Chlamydial and gonococcal infections frequently cause urethritis in young men. Spread into the upper genital tract can cause epididymo-orchitis, particularly in those who do not receive effective treatment. Although a link between epididymo-orchitis and infertility would be logical, a causal link has not yet been established. In epidemiologic studies, chlamydial serology was more often positive among infertile men but (with one exception – anti-chlamydial IgA in semen) the differences were not significant. A recent review found that studies linking prior STD infections and semen parameters among infertile men were methodologically flawed, and found a need for further research to demonstrate a link between STD and male infertility.

MICROBIOLOGY
The most accurate tests for *C. trachomatis* are amplified nucleic acid assays (based on the polymerase chain reaction or the ligase chain reaction). *Neisseria gonorrhoeae* is best isolated by routine culture. Cervical and urethral swab specimens are advisable to rule out infection in the woman and either urethral or first void urine specimens are acceptable in men. Cultures for *Mycoplasma* spp. have no proven clinical utility.

CLINICAL FEATURES
The most important clinical features of infertility are the duration of infertility, whether the partners have had a prior pregnancy together, and the female partner's age. The primary diagnoses (Fig. 68.2) occur in the following approximate order of frequency:
* ovulation defect 25%,
* seminal defect 25%,
* tubal defect 20%,
* endometriosis 5%, and
* unexplained infertility 25%.

Of the 20% with a tubal defect, tubal obstruction accounts for only one-quarter, and of the 25% with seminal defects, azoospermia accounts for only one-fifth. Although oligospermia may occur in men who have a history of STD, it also occurs among infertile men who do not have such a history, and among fertile men. A key concern for reproductive medicine specialists is the possibility that undetectable defects are the true cause of infertility in many couples.

More than 50% of women who have tubal infertility have no history of pelvic inflammatory disease. The characteristic findings are the same, however, with silent and manifest tubal disease. Visible changes include adhesions, loss of fimbria, tubal occlusion and hydrosalpinx. Microscopic changes range from minor impairment of the cilia to complete loss of epithelial function with evidence of chronic infection.

Although epididymo-orchitis is invariably accompanied by pain and obvious tenderness and swelling of the structures involved, urethritis and other infections in men may be asymptomatic and may not lead to overt clinical manifestations in the infertile male partner.

INVESTIGATIONS
Infertile couples should be managed together and both should undergo the testing that is deemed necessary in a given case. Testing includes general health screens, such as cervical cytology and rubella screening for the female partner. Investigation of infertility should include a semen analysis for the male partner and midluteal progesterone to confirm ovulation and a hysterosalpingogram in the female partner. A laparoscopy is indicated whenever there is a high risk of tubal disease or endometriosis or if the hysterosalpingogram is abnormal. Screening tests may also be included; these may include measurement of thyroid-stimulating hormone and prolactin levels and genital cultures. Specific further investigations are indicated if there is azoospermia or amenorrhea. Rare endocrine causes of azoospermia will respond to gonadotropin or gonadotropin-releasing factor stimulation of the testis and should not be overlooked. Chlamydial or gonococcal serologic studies are not helpful in the investigation of infertility in either sex. Testing for antibodies to HIV may sometimes be warranted but there is a duty to provide counseling to the couple both before and after HIV testing.

MANAGEMENT
Untreated couples with only 2 years of infertility have a 22% likelihood of having a conception within 12 months that will lead to live birth. The rate per month is just over 2% in the first 6 months.

In the majority of infertile male partners with a history of STD infection, the semen analysis will be within normal limits. There are no empiric treatments for the infertile male that have been demonstrated to be effective. Intrauterine insemination of prepared sperm is associated with a small, marginally significant improvement in pregnancy rate. With or without a history of STD, there may be male infertility manifested by azoospermia or oligospermia; in some cases this may be due to epididymo-orchitis or obstruction of the vas deferens. Donor insemination is the most common treatment in azoospermia. Typical couples experience pregnancy rates as high as 15% per cycle of insemination. In some obstructive causes of azoospermia, sperm may be retrieved from the vas, the epididymis or the testis for intracytoplasmic injection into oocytes. Severe oligospermia also can be treated by this means, and pregnancy rates in excess of 20% per cycle are frequently reported. Other treatments for oligospermia include intrauterine insemination of prepared sperm or, in the presence of a varicocele, surgical repair. Neither of these treatments is very effective.

Many infertile women who have a history of STD have no evidence of tubal disease. If tubal infertility is the sequel of STD in women, there may be bilateral or unilateral occlusion with or without adhesions. Bilateral tubal occlusion is optimally treated by means of in-vitro fertilization (IVF), although microsurgery is associated with pregnancy rates of 15–20%. Pregnancy rates with IVF are approximately 20% per cycle. With at least one open tube, however, there is uncertainty about the true cause of the infertility, and the treatments include IVF, surgery and various protocols of empiric therapy involving ovulation stimulation and intrauterine insemination.

Overall, less than 5% of infertile couples undergo the complete regimen of available treatments including IVF, and 40–50% are successful in having a child. To provide optimal advice it is crucial for the physician to understand the couple's values and to consider their preferences in the treatment choices. Optimal decisions blend evidence from medical care research with the patients' preferences along the following lines:
* medical care research guides the choice of treatments to achieve optimal effectiveness with minimal adverse effects at the lowest cost;
* the physician's experience and judgment serve to tailor the treatment options to the patient's circumstances; and
* the couple's preferences are the key to an appropriate overall treatment plan and the choices should be revisited as they progress through the plan.

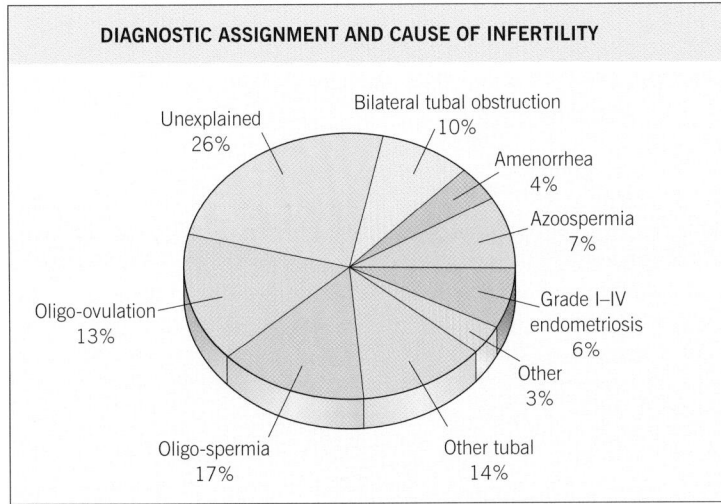

DIAGNOSTIC ASSIGNMENT AND CAUSE OF INFERTILITY

Unexplained 26%
Bilateral tubal obstruction 10%
Amenorrhea 4%
Azoospermia 7%
Grade I–IV endometriosis 6%
Other 3%
Other tubal 14%
Oligo-spermia 17%
Oligo-ovulation 13%

Fig. 68.2 Diagnostic assignment and cause of infertility.

FURTHER READING

Collins JA, Burrows EA, Willan AR. The prognosis for live birth among untreated infertile couples. Fertil Steril 1995;64:22–8.

de Mouzon J, Lancaster P. World collaborative report on in vitro fertilization preliminary data for 1995. J Assisted Reprod Genet 1997;14(suppl 5):251–26.

The ESHRE Capri Workshop. Guidelines to the prevalence, diagnosis, treatment and management of infertility, 1996. Hum Reprod 1996;11:1775–807.

Greenhall E, Vessey M. The prevalence of subfertility: a review of the current confusion and a report of two new studies. Fertil Steril 1990;54:978–83.

Mitchell AA. Intracytoplasmic sperm injection: offering hope for a term pregnancy and a healthy child? Br Med J 1997;315:1245–6.

Ness RB, Markovic N, Carlson C, Coughlin MT. Do men become infertile after having sexually transmitted urethritis? An epidemiologic examination. Fertil Steril 1997;68:205–13.

Schmidt L, Munster K, Helm P. Infertility and the seeking of infertility treatment in a representative population. Br J Obstet Gynaecol 1995;102:978–84.

Society for Assisted Reproductive Technology, The American Society for Reproductive Medicine. Assisted reproductive technology in the United States and Canada: 1994 results generated from the American society for Reproductive Medicine/Society for Assisted Reproductive Technology Registry. Fertil Steril 1996;66:697–705.

US Congress Office of Technology Assessment. Infertility: medical and social choices. Washington, DC: US Government Printing Office; 1988.

Westrom L, Joesoef R, Reynolds G, Hagdu A, Thompson SE. Pelvic inflammatory disease and fertility. Sex Transm Dis 1992;19:185–91.

World Health Organization Task Force on the Prevention and Management of Infertility. Tubal infertility: serologic relationship to past chlamydial and gonococcal infection. Sex Transm Dis 1995;22:71–7.

Special Problems in Infectious Disease Practice

Jonathan Cohen & Steven M Opal

3

Pathogenesis of Fever

Arif R Sarwari & Philip A Mackowiak

INTRODUCTION

Fever is best described as a complex physiologic response to disease, in which body temperature is elevated above the normal range as a result of the action of pyrogenic cytokines on the hypothalamic thermoregulatory center. In adult humans, body temperature, as reflected by oral readings, is normally tightly controlled between 96.0 and 99.9°F (35.6 and 37.7°C) and exhibits a circadian rhythm characterized by an evening peak and early morning trough. Such circadian rhythmicity is maintained during fever, and even during conditions such as bacterial endocarditis, in which circulating levels of exogenous pyrogens (e.g. bacterial products) are constant throughout the day.

NORMAL BODY TEMPERATURE

A survey published within the past 5 years of physicians' perceptions of body temperature suggests that there is widespread confusion over key features of the temperature of the human body during health and disease.[1] These perceptions, in all likelihood, originate from the writings of Carl Wunderlich who, in 1868, published a book on clinical thermometry that many regard, to this day, as the definitive work on the subject.[2,3] Unfortunately, several of Wunderlich's dicta on body temperature, like the perceptions of modern-day physicians, appear to be in error. In a recent descriptive analysis of 700 baseline oral temperature observations from 148 healthy men and women, a mean and median temperature of 98.2°F (36.8°C) was recorded.[4] Only 8% of the readings (Fig. 1.1) accounted for an oral temperature of 98.6°F (37°C). Mean temperature varied diurnally, with a 0600h nadir and a 0400–0600h zenith. Women had a statistically significantly higher average oral temperature than men – 98.4°F (36.9°C) versus 98.1°F (36.7°C) – but did not exhibit greater average diurnal temperature oscillations – 1.00°F (0.56°C) versus 0.97°F (0.54°C). This study suggested that 98.6°F (37°C) has no special significance vis-à-vis body temperature in healthy young adults when such temperature is measured orally using modern thermometers. Also, fever, as identified by a temperature above the 99th percentile, was defined as an early morning temperature of greater than 99.0°F (37.2°C) or a temperature of over 100°F (37.8°C) at any time during the day.

THERMOMETRY

In defining the febrile state, the quantitative effects of anatomic site and oral stimulation on estimates of body temperature must be considered.[5] In adults, mean rectal temperatures exceed concurrent oral readings by 0.8 ± 0.7°F (0.4 ± 0.4°C), which in turn exceed concurrent tympanic membrane readings by 0.7 ± 2.0°F (0.4 ± 1.1°C). Tympanic membrane readings show significantly more intra- and intersubject variability than rectal or oral readings, especially when cerumen is present in the external canal being examined. Mastication, smoking and exercise cause significant increases in oral temperature that may persist for periods of approximately 20 minutes.

HYPERTHERMIA

Hyperthermia (as distinguished from fever) is an unregulated elevation in body temperature, in which endogenous pyrogens do not appear to

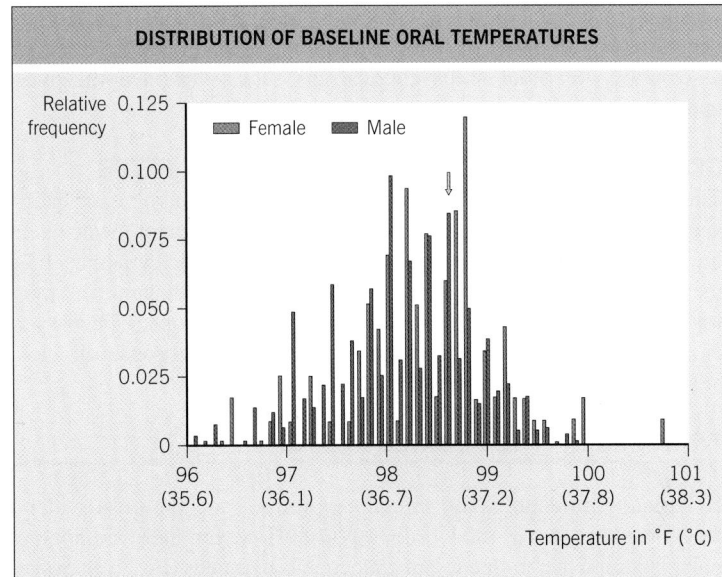

Fig. 1.1 Distribution of baseline oral temperatures in healthy men and women. Frequency distribution of 700 baseline oral temperatures obtained during 2 consecutive days of observation in 148 healthy young volunteers. Arrow indicates location of 98.6°F (37°C). With permission from Mackowiak *et al.*[4] Copyright 1992, American Medical Association.

CAUSES OF HYPERTHERMIA	
Increased heat production	Exercise-induced hyperthermia, thyrotoxicosis, pheochromocytoma, malignant hyperthermia, neuroleptic malignant syndrome
Decreased heat loss	Heat stroke, autonomic dysfunction, dehydration, drug-induced (e.g. atropine), occlusive dressings, severe anemia, congestive failure, absence of sweat glands
Hypothalamic disorders	Infection (e.g. granulomas), tumors, trauma, cerebrovascular accidents, drug-induced (e.g. phenothiazines)

Fig. 1.2 Causes of hyperthermia. These may be the result of increased heat production, decreased heat loss or hypothalamic disorders.

play a major role, and standard antipyretics are ineffective. It is the result of a failure of thermoregulatory homeostasis, in which there is either uncontrolled heat production, inadequate heat dissipation or failure of hypothalamic thermoregulation. Some causes of hyperthermia are listed in Figure 1.2.

Malignant hyperthermia is a rare hereditary disease transmitted by autosomal dominant inheritance with variable penetrance.[6] It is characterized by rapidly evolving hyperthermia, muscular rigidity and acidosis in patients undergoing general anesthesia. The disorder is related to excessive release of calcium from the sarcoplasmic reticulum in response to anesthetic agents. Although various inhalational anesthetic agents have been incriminated in the disorder, halothane – alone or in conjunction with succinylcholine (suxamethonium) – has been the most common offender. The condition is often presaged by sudden ventricular ectopic activity, tachypnea, circulatory instability and a sharp rise in body temperature. Metabolic acidosis and rhabdomyolysis are common and frequently severe. Mortality in acute cases varies between 28 and 70%.

Neuroleptic malignant syndrome, another form of hyperthermia, is characterized by an elevated body temperature, diffuse muscular rigidity, autonomic instability and altered consciousness. The syndrome is caused by dopaminergic receptor blockade in the corpus striatum, which leads to impaired hypothalamic thermoregulation and spasticity of skeletal muscles, with excess heat generation. It most often occurs as a side effect of haloperidol, but has also been reported in association with other antipsychotic drugs, such as the phenothiazines and thioxanthenes.[7]

GENERAL SCHEMA OF THE PATHOGENESIS OF FEVER

The preliminary steps in the pathogenesis of fever involve an interaction between various triggers and a host-derived effector mechanism mediated by endogenous pyrogens known as pyrogenic cytokines. It is the influence of these pyrogenic cytokines on the hypothalamic thermoregulatory center that culminates in a febrile response. The latter occurs in the context of an overall inflammatory response directed against pathogenic microbes and other disease states.

TRIGGERS OF THE FEBRILE RESPONSE

Historically, infections and infectious products are the most widely recognized triggers of the febrile response. However, these are not the only stimuli to the production of endogenous pyrogens (Fig. 1.3). Some endogenous molecules, such as antigen–antibody complexes, certain androgenic steroid metabolites, inflammatory bile acids, complement components and some lymphocyte products, also induce pyrogenic cytokines. The concept of cytokines inducing other cytokines is vital to understanding how noninfectious diseases produce fever. Vasculitis, acute exacerbations of rheumatoid arthritis, lupus, trauma, hemorrhage, thrombophlebitis, drug fever and cancer are examples in which fever is produced as a result of cytokines inducing other pyrogenic cytokines.[8]

EXOGENOUS PYROGENS

The term 'exogenous pyrogen' is most accurately applied to microbial exotoxins but is also frequently applied to microbial agents and their breakdown products. It is clear that exogenous pyrogens by themselves do not cause fever unless they elicit cytokine release. Gram-negative bacterial endotoxin [lipopolysaccharide (LPS)], for example, an otherwise potent exogenous pyrogen, induces few ill effects in murine strains that are unable to produce tumor necrosis factor (TNF-α).[9]

Gram-negative bacteria possess two pyrogens: LPS, which is a component of the bacterial outer membrane, and peptidoglycan, which forms a highly cross-linked lattice below the outer membrane. Lipopolysaccharide is a complex glycolipid consisting of lipid A, a core oligosaccharide, and peripheral O-antigenic chains composed of polysaccharides. The lipid A moiety is responsible for virtually all the biologic activity of LPS. Lipopolysaccharide is the most potent stimulus known for TNF-α production and release, and LPS is unquestionably a clinically important pyrogen.[10] Intravenous administration of 4ng/kg LPS to normal individuals results in a rapid rise in circulating TNF-α, followed by a fever that peaks in 3 hours. Pretreatment with the cyclo-oxygenase inhibitor, ibuprofen, prevents fever but not TNF-α release. Lipopolysaccharide also increases circulating levels of interleukin (IL)-1.

Peptidoglycan, although present in the cell walls of Gram-negative bacteria, is the major component of the Gram-positive bacterial cell wall. It is a complex polymer composed of alternating units of N-acetylglucosamine and its lactyl ether, N-acetylmuramic acid. Peptidoglycan is much less pyrogenic than LPS, with doses of 100mg being required to induce fever in rabbits. The basic subunit structure responsible for the pyrogenicity of peptidoglycans is muramyl dipeptide, a product of lysosomal degradation of Gram-positive bacteria. Like lipoteichoic acid and rhamnose glucose polymers, two other components of the Gram-positive bacterial cell wall, peptidoglycans cause fever by activating macrophages.

In addition to breakdown products, Gram-positive bacteria release exotoxins that can also cause fever. These pyrogenic exotoxins are structurally similar proteins belonging to a family of superantigenic exotoxins that includes the toxic shock syndrome toxin of *Staphylococcus aureus*, staphylococcal enterotoxin, streptococcal pyrogenic exotoxins and scarlet fever toxin.[11] Superantigens act by binding to major histocompatibility complex (MHC) class II molecules on antigen-presenting cells. The MHC–exotoxin complex is then able to bind to the Vβ domain of the T-lymphocyte receptor. As a result, not only is the antigen-presenting cell activated, but so are large numbers of T lymphocytes, causing the release of TNF-α and other cytokines (Fig. 1.4). *In vitro*, low concentrations (100ng/ml) of toxic shock syndrome toxin induce TNF-α and IL-1 secretion by monocytes.

TRIGGERS OF ENDOGENOUS PYROGENS	
Microbial agents	Viruses, bacteria, fungi, parasites
Microbial toxins	Endotoxin
	Exotoxins
	Enterotoxins, toxic shock syndrome toxin-1, streptococcal pyrogenic exotoxins, erythrogenic toxins
Microbial breakdown products	Peptidoglycans, muramyl peptides, lipoteichoic acid, rhamnose glucose polymers, lipoarabinomannan
Immune components and cytokines	Antigen–antibody complexes, complement components (C5a, C3a), lymphocyte products (IL-2, IFN), pyrogenic cytokines (IL-1, TNF-α)
Drugs	Etiocholanolone, bleomycin, penicillin (through lymphocyte products in sensitized individuals)
Tumors	Through production of pyrogenic cytokines

Fig. 1.3 Triggers of endogenous pyrogens. Substances that stimulate the production of endogenous pyrogens.

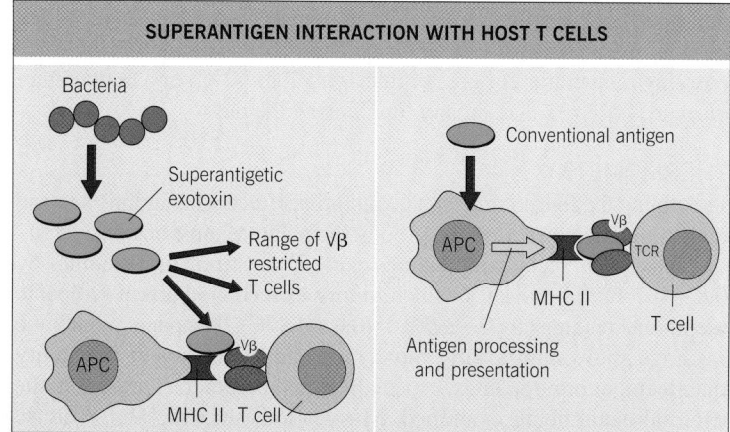

Fig. 1.4 Superantigen interaction with host T lymphocytes. Bacterial superantigens bind to the side of the class II HLA molecule (MHC II) of antigen presenting cells (APCs) and T-lymphocyte variable β chain (Vβ) to stimulate T-lymphocyte proliferation and cytokine production. Conventional antigen is processed and presented by APCs only to T cell receptors (TCRs) specific for that antigen.

Mycobacterial infections are notable for producing prolonged fevers. The lipid-rich cell wall of mycobacteria contains a unique phenolic glycolipid called lipoarabinomannan, which is a potent stimulus for TNF-α, IL-1 and IL-6 production by macrophages.[12]

EFFECTORS OF THE FEBRILE RESPONSE

Endogenous pyrogens are defined as endogenously produced molecules capable of evoking a febrile response by direct action on the hypothalamus. The concept that fever is mediated by endogenously produced molecules of leukocytic origin dates back to the 19th century. Initially, little was known about the chemical nature of such molecules. Subsequently, it was recognized that the endogenous pyrogens are distinct molecules that are synthesized *de novo* in response to appropriate stimuli. With the recognition of multiple distinct endogenous pyrogens came the realization that these same molecules have other distinctive nonpyrogenic biologic properties as important as their ability to evoke fever.[13] To date, the best characterized pyrogenic cytokines include IL-1, TNF-α and members of the glycoprotein (gp) 130 ligands. The latter include a family of cytokines that use the cell-signaling gp 130 apparatus such as IL-6, IL-11, oncostatin M, ciliary neurotrophic factor, cardiotropin-1 and leukemic inhibitory factor. Produced peripherally, these endogenous pyrogens reach the thermoregulatory center via the systemic circulation. They do not, however, appear to penetrate the blood–brain barrier or enter the brain tissue itself. Their effect is most likely exerted at the organum vasculosum laminae terminalis, also known as the circumventricular organ, where they stimulate endothelial cells to synthesize and release prostaglandin (PG) E_2.

INTERLEUKIN-1

Interleukin-1 is a prototypic endogenous pyrogen secreted by monocytes and macrophages.[14] Two different forms, IL-1α and IL-1β, are recognized, with only short segments of amino acid sequence homology. Both forms are translated as 31kDa precursor peptides that are processed enzymatically to the mature 17kDa form. The biologic activities of both forms are largely identical.

In activated cells, 10–50 times more IL-1β mRNA than IL-1α mRNA is usually found. Moreover, IL-1β is readily secreted from activated cells, whereas IL-1α remains primarily cell associated. Interleukin-1α is thus more likely relevant to local inflammation than systemic reactions.

TUMOR NECROSIS FACTOR-α

Tumor necrosis factor-α is a macrophage-derived product that is directly cytotoxic for certain tumor cells. Human TNF-α has been cloned and has the same amino acid sequence as a previously described effector molecule known as 'cachectin'. Tumor necrosis factor shares many biologic properties with IL-1.[15] For example, recombinant preparations of both molecules are involved in induction of hepatic acute-phase proteins, lymphocyte activation and the release of adrenocorticotropic hormones. The receptors for TNF-α, however, are distinct from those for IL-1.

Tumor necrosis factor is an endogenous inducer of IL-1. In large doses, TNF-α induces IL-1 *in vivo* in rabbits, and incubation of TNF-α with either human blood monocytes or cultured human endothelial cells induces IL-1 *in vitro*. Tumor necrosis factor has been implicated in the pathogenesis of endotoxin-induced fever and septic shock.[16]

INTERLEUKIN-6 AND OTHER GLYCOPROTEIN 130-TRANSDUCING CYTOKINES

Interleukin-6 is a polypeptide cytokine that was initially isolated from fibroblasts. Interleukin-6 produces typical endogenous pyrogen-mediated fever when injected into rabbits. In burn patients, a positive correlation has been observed between fever and IL-6 serum levels. Interleukin-6 production is influenced by many exogenous pyrogens and by IL-1 and TNF-α, which are potent stimulators of IL-6 gene expression and protein translation. Thus, IL-6 is often elevated in conditions in which IL-1 and TNF-α have been synthesized.[17]

Interleukin-6 belongs to the family of cytokines that triggers cells via the gp 130 signaling apparatus. This receptor is present on nearly all cells. Pyrogenic cytokines such as IL-11, oncostatin M, ciliary neurotrophic factor, cardiotropin-1 and leukemic inhibitory factor also use this receptor. Like IL-6, doses of ciliary neurotrophic factor required to induce fever are measured in mg/kg compared with ng/kg for IL-1 and TNF-α.

OTHER CYTOKINES

Interferons are also endogenous pyrogens. When injected into humans at doses of 0.1–1.0mg/kg, interferon (IFN)-α causes chills and fever.[18] Similar observations have been made with IL-2 and IL-12, but responses to the these interleukins appear to be mediated through IL-1 and TNF-α. The colony-stimulating factor, granulocyte–macrophage colony-stimulating factor might also manifest a febrile response that is mediated through TNF-α.

MODULATORS OF THE FEBRILE RESPONSE

Body temperature is regulated in the preoptic area of the anterior hypothalamus. Warm- and cold-sensitive neurons mediate activation of heat loss and heat production mechanisms, respectively. After systemic administration of exogenous or endogenous pyrogens, firing rates of warm-sensitive neurons generally decrease, whereas those of cold-sensitive neurons increase in a manner consistent with the decreased heat loss and increased heat production involved in the development of fever. However, approximately 60% of neurons are classified as temperature-insensitive, as they show little or no change in their firing rates when hypothalamic temperature is changed.

Initially, it was believed that cytokine-modulated fever involved direct central inhibition of warm-sensitive neurons and excitation of cold-sensitive neurons. However, because they are large hydrophilic peptides, pyrogenic cytokines are unable to traverse the blood–brain barrier. For this reason, it is currently believed that central signals of such molecules are transduced in areas of the brain in which the blood–brain barrier is imperfect, specifically in the organum vasculosum laminae terminalis, which lies in the midline of the preoptic area of the anterior hypothalamus, in the anteroventral wall of the third ventricle. Prostaglandin E_2 is believed to be a central transducer of pyrogenic cytokines.[19]

PROSTAGLANDIN E_2

Prostaglandin E_2 synthesis involves the cleavage of arachidonic acid released from membrane phospholipids into the prostaglandin endoperoxides, PGG_2 and PGH_2; PGH_2 is then quickly converted to PGE_2 by PGE_2 isomerase. The free arachidonic acid concentration is thus rate-limiting and, in the context of fever production, phospholipase A_2 is a key enzyme.[20] Its enhanced activation accounts for the release of arachidonic acid. The interaction between various pyrogenic cytokines and phospholipase A_2 activity has not yet been fully elucidated.

Ablation of the organum vasculosum laminae terminalis prevents fever caused by peripheral injection of endogenous pyrogens. Thus, it is likely that endothelial cells lining the organum vasculosum laminae terminalis either release or produce PGE_2 themselves on encountering endogenous pyrogens in the circulation. Prostaglandin E_2 may then act directly or through cyclic AMP to raise the thermal set-point by inhibiting warm-sensitive neurons. Another hypothesis proposes that PGE_2 is released by astrocytes in response to the binding of the endogenous pyrogens to the astrocytic terminals in the perivascular spaces of the organum vasculosum laminae terminalis. Astrocytes are, indeed, a potent source of PGE_2.

ENDOGENOUS ANTIPYRETICS

The upper limit of the febrile range has in the past received scant attention in the clinical literature.[21] In one of the earliest surveys concerned with this issue, only 4.3% of 1761 axillary and rectal temperature readings in patients with various febrile illnesses exceeded 106°F (41.1°C).

None were above 107.6°F (42°C), leading to the assumption that fever's upper limit lies between 106 and 107.6°F. Indeed, widespread organ dysfunction develops at body temperatures over 106–107.6°F.

Such evidence supporting an upper limit to the febrile range implies the existence of regulatory mechanisms involved in fever that prevent body temperature from rising above 106–107.6°F. These mechanisms are most likely complex and involve special properties of thermo-regulatory neurons themselves, circulating endogenous antipyretics and soluble receptors for the cytokine mediators of the febrile response. Among some of the proposed endogenous antipyretics are arginine vasopressin, α-melanocyte-stimulating hormone and somatostatin. Arginine vasopressin is present in the fibers and terminals of the ventral septal area and is released during fever. It appears to prevent or reduce fever through a receptor-mediated action that has no effect on normal body temperature. The neuropeptide, α-melanocyte-stimulating hormone, has not been identified in fibers projecting into the septum. The greatest increases in its central concentrations occur during the chill phase of fever, when the core temperature rises rapidly. The precise mechanisms by which endogenous antipyretic agents exert their effect on fever is unknown. A growing body of literature indicates that the release of pyrogenic cytokines such as IL-1 and TNF-α is followed by increased shedding of soluble receptors for such cytokines that function as endogenous inhibitors of the pyrogens. Although the specific biologic function of such cytokine inhibitors is not known, it is possible that they serve as a natural braking system for the febrile response.

THE FEBRILE RESPONSE

The culmination of the cascade of events triggered by endogenous pyrogens is a rise in core temperature in response to elevation of the hypothalamic temperature set-point. This thermal response should not be viewed as an isolated event but considered as part of a complex and highly co-ordinated response to disease that involves numerous other physiologic, immunologic and endocrinologic components. The major components of the febrile response are given in Figure 1.5.

THERMOREGULATION

Mammals utilize numerous thermogenic mechanisms to increase heat production during cold exposure and during the initiation of fever. Shivering is one such mechanism. Nonshivering thermogenesis, an important alternative mechanism in newborns, is most closely linked to brown adipose tissue. This specialized tissue is characterized by its brownish color, a profuse vascular system and an abundance of mito-chondria. Brown adipose tissue receives sympathetic adrenergic inner-vation and is located near the shoulder blades, neck, adrenals and deep blood vessels. Norepinephrine induces enzymatic hydrolysis of triglycerides in brown adipose tissue to glycerol and free fatty acids. These free fatty acids serve two roles in thermogenesis. First, they are the primary substrate oxidized by mitochondria to produce ATP and heat. Second, in brown fat cells, free fatty acids (or their derivatives) act as a signal to uncouple oxidative phosphorylation. This allows the mitochondria to bypass ATP synthesis and oxidize fatty acids rapidly, thus generating large amounts of heat.

Heat is distributed throughout the body via the circulatory system. Regulating cutaneous blood flow is important in determining heat loss from the skin surface by radiation, convection and conduction. When environmental temperatures approach body temperature, evaporation (e.g. sweating, panting) is the body's only means of heat loss. The bal-ance between heat production and heat loss, largely under control of the autonomic nervous system, helps maintain the hypothalamic temper-ature set-point around 98.2°F (36.8°C). This set-point temperature is believed to be determined by the 'functional overlap' of the activities of warm-sensitive and temperature-insensitive neurons. For each thermoregulatory effector neuron, the set-point occurs when the synap-tic output from warm-sensitive neurons is equal and opposite to the synaptic input from temperature-insensitive neurons. This synaptic

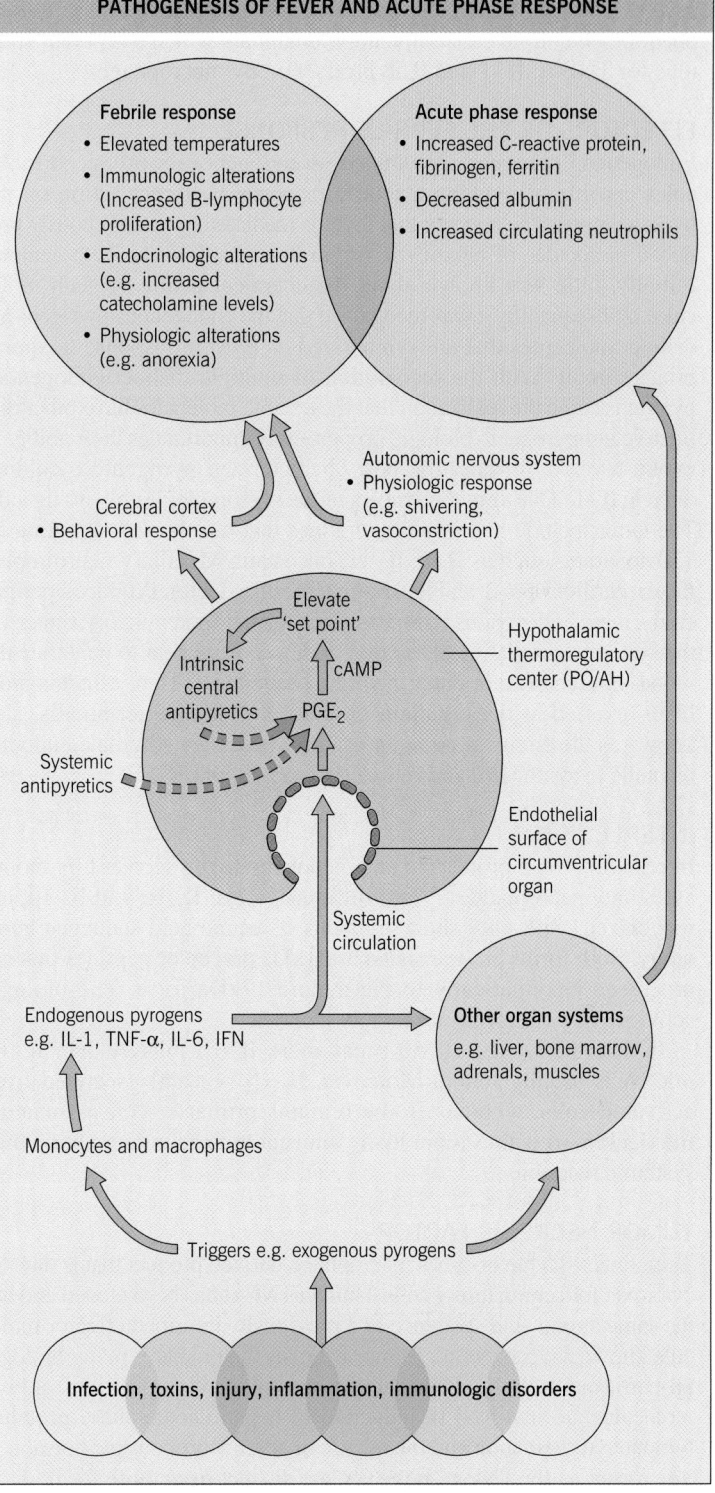

Fig 1.5 Pathogenesis of fever and acute phase response. Certain disease states, through the elaboration of exogenous pyrogens, stimulate monocytes and macrophages to produce endogenous pyrogens such as IL-1, TNF-α, IL-6 and IFN. These pyrogenic cytokines act at the endothelial surface of the circumventricular organ of the preoptic area of the anterior hypothalamus (PO/AH) to induce the production of PGE$_2$, which elevates the body's thermal set-point. Intrinsic central antipyretics and systemic antipyretics exert their effects by decreasing levels of PGE$_2$. Physiologic and behavioral responses may be invoked to raise body temperature to the new set-point. This febrile response needs to be considered in the context of an overlapping 'acute phase response' as a global nonspecific response to the original insult.

overlap normally occurs around 98.2°F (36.8°C). However, if the warm-sensitive neuronal activity is decreased by a pyrogen, the over-lap occurs at a higher temperature, such as 102.2°F (39°C) (Fig. 1.6). In response to the new temperature set-point, thermoregulatory

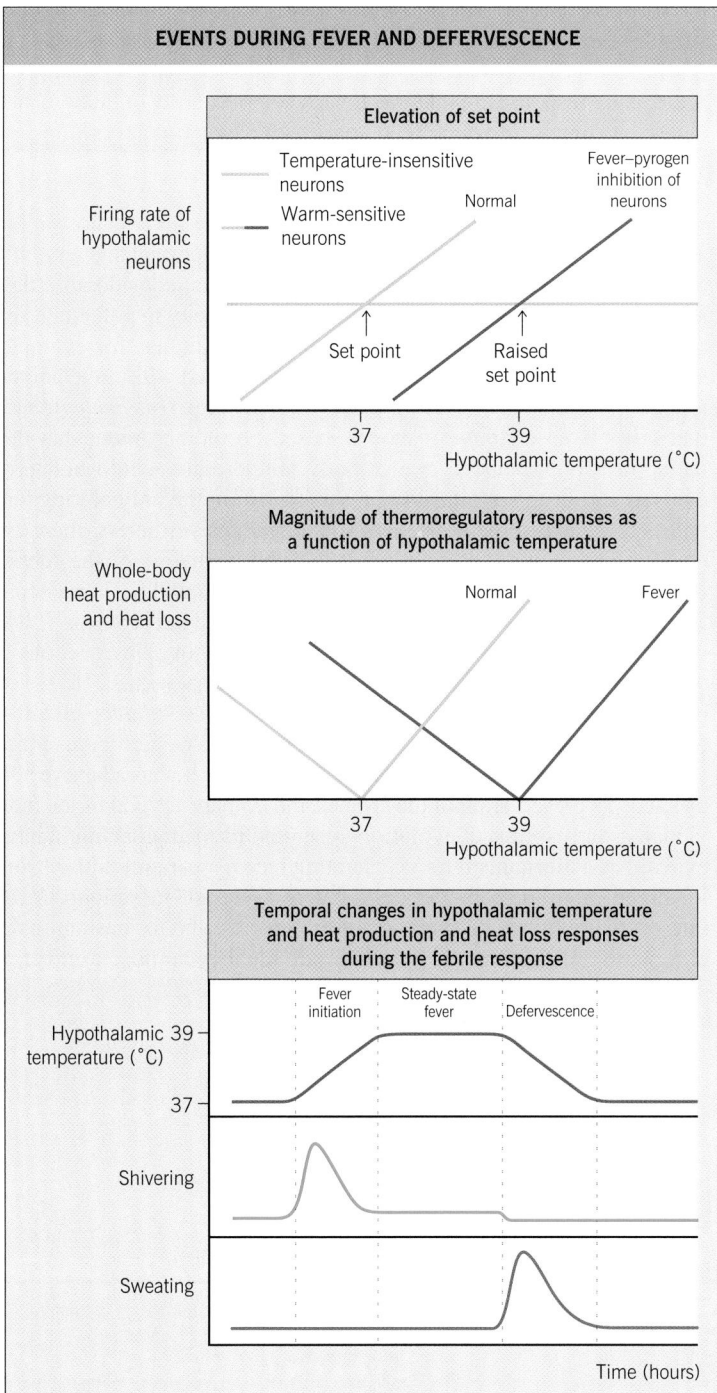

EVENTS DURING FEVER AND DEFERVESCENCE

Fig. 1.6 Events during fever and defervescence. When pyrogens are present in the pre-optic region, the whole-body and neuronal responses are as shown by the purple lines. Upper: normally the firing rates of warm-sensitive and temperature insensitive neurons functionally overlap at 37°C, the set-point of thermoregulatory neurons. During pyrogen inhibition of warm-sensitive neurons, this overlap occurs at the raised set point of 39°C. Center: during fever heat production is initially great, but as body temperature rises towards 39°C, heat production diminishes and should cease at 39°C. Lower: during fever initiation, shivering causes an increase in hypothalamic temperature and then ceases as the temperature reaches 39°C. During defervescence, the hypothalamus activates heat loss responses such as sweating. Adapted from Boulant, 1997.[22]

Pyrogenic cytokine	Biologic activity
IL-1	Acute phase response induction
	T-lymphocyte activation
	IL-2/ IL-2 receptor induction
	Fibroblast activation
	B-lymphocyte proliferation and differentiation
	Enhanced phagocyte microbial killing
	Accelerated wound healing
TNF-α	Septic shock
	Tumor necrosis
	Anorexia and cachexia
	Enhanced phagocyte microbial killing
	Osteoclast activation
	B-lymphocyte differentiation
IL-6	Acute phase response induction
	B-lymphocyte differentiation
	Myeloma proliferation
	Megakaryocyte maturation
	Weak antiviral activity
IFN	Macrophage priming
	Antiviral activity
	Enhanced TNF-α activity
	Enhanced natural killer cell activity
	B-lymphocyte differentiation

BIOACTIVITIES OF PYROGENIC CYTOKINES

Fig. 1.7 Bioactivities of pyrogenic cytokines. Examples of biologic activities of some of the currently recognized pyrogenic cytokines.

mechanisms are activated to increase the preoptic temperature to 102.2°F (39°C).[22]

This concept can be applied to the events that occur during fever and defervescence. As illustrated in Figure 1.6, the pyrogen-induced set-point temperature is 102.2°F (39°C). As body temperature is lower than the pyrogen-induced set-point, the hypothalamus employs heat

production responses such as shivering to warm the hypothalamus to the new 102.2°F (39°C) set-point. Initially, at 98.2°F (36.8°C), heat production is great, but as body temperature rises toward 102.2°F (39°C), heat production diminishes. When the temperature reaches 102.2°F (39°C), heat production should cease. This same response is also shown during fever initiation in the lower part of Figure 1.6; this is the rising phase of fever, when an initial, intense shivering is responsible for the increase in hypothalamic temperature. As temperature approaches and reaches 102.2°F (39°C), shivering diminishes and finally ceases. Although this example uses shivering to increase body temperature, depending on environmental conditions, a variety of thermoregulatory responses may be evoked (e.g. decrease in skin blood flow). These physiologic responses, however, cannot change the temperature by more than 3.6–5.4°F (2–3°C) and behavioral responses are often employed as well. In fact, behavioral thermoregulatory responses are often employed preferentially over autonomic responses to raise body temperature.

During the plateau or steady-state phase of fever the temperature is closely regulated at 102.2°F (39°C), often by skin blood flow and behavioral responses. Defervescence occurs when concentrations of preoptic pyrogenic substances decrease, either naturally or as a result of an antipyretic drug. Warm-sensitive neurons return to their original higher firing rates, resetting the temperature to around 98.2°F (36.8°C). To lower body temperature from the 102.2°F (39°C) level, the hypothalamus activates heat loss responses (e.g. sweating). The magnitude of the heat loss response can be determined from the solid line on the middle graph. Initially, at 102.2°F (39°C), heat loss is great, but as the body temperature decreases toward 98.2°F (36.8°C), heat loss diminishes. Defervescence is not confined to the sweating response. The hypothalamus controls a variety of autonomic and behavioral thermoregulatory responses and calls into action those most appropriate for given environmental conditions.

ACUTE PHASE RESPONSE

The acute phase response to disease consists of activation of new 'set-points' for homeostatic mechanisms that normally maintain a constant internal environment during health.[23] Fever is but one of the many changes in homeostatic settings that occurs during the acute phase response and is mediated by the same inflammatory cytokines that regulate other components of the acute phase response. Such cytokines have complex biologic activities (Fig. 1.7), and, in the broadest sense, each one is a component of the febrile response. Acute phase phenomena other than fever include somnolence, anorexia, changes in plasma protein synthesis and altered synthesis of numerous endocrine hormones such as corticotropin-releasing hormone, glucagon, insulin, adrenocorticotropic hormone, cortisol, adrenal catecholamines, growth hormone, thyroid-stimulating hormone, thyroxine, aldosterone and arginine vasopressin. The acute phase response is also characterized by inhibition of bone formation, negative nitrogen balance, gluconeogenesis and altered lipid metabolism. Serum zinc and iron levels typically fall, whereas copper levels rise. Leukocytosis and thrombocytosis occur in many patients. Decreased erythropoiesis resulting in 'anemia of chronic inflammation' is seen in patients with chronic inflammatory states.

Changes in concentrations of acute phase proteins reflect the reprogramming of the pattern of secretory protein gene expression by hepatocytes. Increases and decreases in the synthesis of hepatocyte secretory proteins occur. There are modest increases in the synthesis of ceruloplasmin, complement components C3 and C4, haptoglobin, α_1-acid glycoprotein, α_1-protease inhibitor, α_1-antichymotrypsin and fibrinogen. By contrast, C-reactive protein and serum amyloid A levels may increase by over 1000-fold. Albumin, transthyretin and transferrin levels characteristically diminish. The increased plasma concentrations of hepatic proteins, glycoproteins and globulins are responsible for the elevated erythrocyte sedimentation rate that characterizes the acute phase response.

The acute phase response involves complex interactions between the pyrogenic cytokines, other intercellular signaling molecules and intracellular events. The plasma protein response to inflammatory stimuli seen in hepatocytes is typical of the acute phase response in other organs. Changes in plasma protein synthesis occurring during the acute phase response are integrated via a complex array of humoral and paracrine signals, in which IL-6 appears to play a pivotal role.[24]

THE ADAPTIVE VALUE OF FEVER

The highly regulated nature of fever suggests that fever is not simply a by-product of infection but has evolved as an important and carefully orchestrated host defense response. Nevertheless, considerable data indicate that fever and its mediators have the capacity to potentiate and to impair resistance to infection. Phylogenetic studies, for example, have shown that the febrile response is widespread within the animal kingdom. Such data constitute some of the most persuasive evidence that fever is an adaptive response, based on the argument that this metabolically expensive rise in body temperature would not have evolved and been so faithfully preserved within the animal kingdom unless fever had some net benefit to the host. Nevertheless, there are equally convincing data to suggest that the mediators of the febrile response (i.e. pyrogenic cytokines such as TNF-α and IL-1) also contribute to the morbidity and mortality of Gram-negative sepsis.[25] It is difficult to reconcile these apparently contradictory observations if they are viewed solely from the standpoint of the individual. However, if viewed from the perspective of the species, the salutary effect of fever on mild to moderately severe infections and its pernicious influence on fulminating infections can both be interpreted as adaptive.[26] If one accepts preservation of the species, rather than survival of the individual, as the essence of evolution, fever and its mediators might have evolved as a mechanism for accelerating recovery of individuals from localized or mild to moderately severe systemic infections in the interest of continued propagation of the species, and for hastening the elimination of fulminantly infected individuals who pose a threat of epidemic disease to the species.

REFERENCES

1. Mackowiak PA, Wasserman SS. Physicians' perceptions regarding body temperature in health and disease. South Med J 1995;88:934–8.
2. Wunderlich C. Das Verhalten der Eiaenwasme in krankenheiten. Leipzig: Otto Wigard; 1868.
3. Wunderlich CA, Seguin E. Medical thermometry and human temperature. New York: William Wood & Co; 1871.
4. Mackowiak PA, Wasserman SS, Levine MM. A critical appraisal of 37°C (98.6°F), the upper limit of the normal body temperature, and other legacies of Carl Reinhold August Wunderlich. JAMA 1992;268:1578–80.
5. Rabinowitz RP, Cookson ST, Wasserman SS, Mackowiak PA. Effects of anatomic site, oral stimulation and body position on estimates of body temperature. Arch Intern Med 1996;156:777–80.
6. MacLennan DH, Duff, C, Zorzato, et al. Ryanodine receptor gene is a candidate for predisposition to malignant hyperthermia. Nature 1990;343:559–61.
7. Caroff SN, Mann SC. Neuroleptic malignant syndrome. Med Clin North Am 1993;77:185–202.
8. Mier JW, Souza LM, Allegretta M, et al. Dissimilarities between purified human interleukin-1 and recombinant human interleukin-2 in the induction of fever, brain prostaglandin and acute-phase protein synthesis. J Biol Response Med 1985;4:35–45.

9. Watson J, Kelly K, Largen M, Taylor BA. The genetic mapping of a defective LPS response gene in C3H/HeJ mice. J Immunol 1978;120:422–4.
10. Michie HR, Manogue KR, Spriggs DR, et al. Detection of circulating tumor necrosis factor after endotoxin administration. N Engl J Med 1988;318:1481–6.
11. Marck P, Kappler J. The staphylococcal enterotoxins and their relatives. Science 1990;248:705–11.
12. Barnes P, Chatterjee D, Abrams J, et al. Cytokine production induced by Mycobacterium tuberculosis lipoarabinomannan. J Immunol 1992;149:541–7.
13. Dinarello CA. Interleukin-1 and the pathogenesis of the acute phase response. N Engl J Med 1984;311:1413–8.
14. Dinarello CA. Biological basis for interleukin-1 in disease. Blood 1996;87:2095–147.
15. Dinarello CA. Interleukin-1 and its biologically related cytokines. Adv Immunol 1989;44:153–205.
16. Vassalli P. The pathophysiology of tumor necrosis factors. Annu Rev Immunol 1992;10:411–52.
17. Nijsten MW, de Groot ER, ten Duis HJ, et al. Serum levels of interleukin-6 and acute phase responses. Lancet 1987;2:921.
18. Horning SJ, Levine JF, Miller RA, Rosenberg SA, Merigan TC. Clinical and immunologic effects of recombinant leukocyte A interferon in eight patients with advanced cancer. JAMA 1982;247:1718–22.

19. Stitt JT. Prostaglandin E as the neural mediator of the febrile response. Yale J Biol Med 1986;59:137–49.
20. Smith JW, Urba WJ, Curti BD, et al. Phase II trial of interleukin-1 alpha in combination with indomethacin in melanoma patients. Proc Am Soc Clin Oncol 1991;10:293–9.
21. Mackowiak PA, Boulant JA. Fever's glass ceiling. Clin Infect Dis 1996;22:525–36.
22. Boulant JA. Thermoregulation. In: Mackowiak PA, ed. Fever: basic mechanisms and management, 2nd ed. Philadelphia: Lippincott-Raven; 1997:35–58.
23. Kushner I. The phenomenon of the acute phase response. Ann NY Acad Sci 1982;389:39–48.
24. Kushner I. Regulation of the acute phase response by cytokines. Perspect Biol Med 1993;36:611–22.
25. Casey LC, Balk RA, Bone RC. Plasma cytokine and endotoxin levels correlate with survival in patients with the sepsis syndrome. Ann Intern Med 1993;119:771–8.
26. Mackowiak PA. Fever: blessing or curse? A unifying hypothesis. Ann Intern Med 1994;120:1037–40.

Clinical Approach to the Acutely Febrile Patient

Harold Lambert

Fever is one of the most frequent symptoms that leads to consultation with a health professional. Vast numbers of febrile illnesses are of short duration and benign outlook, and few of these are diagnosed. However, in the midst of this mass of minor illness are patients whose illness is serious or likely to become so. Some of these serious illnesses also present a danger to others, and thus have a significance beyond that of the individual patient. This is the challenge of acute fever: to distinguish the threatening from the trivial in acute illnesses in which fever is a main feature.

In some cases, of course, the fever becomes prolonged and this topic of more long-lasting fever (fever of unknown origin; FUO) is discussed in Chapter 3.3. The distinction between fevers of short and those of longer duration is important in considering diagnostic possibilities. Many acute and short-lived fevers are of viral origin, and conversely viral fevers without particular diagnostic features rarely last longer than 1 or 2 weeks; thus, prolonged fever without distinguishing features is rarely caused by a virus, at least in immunologically normal patients.

HISTORY

As with any other medical problem, the history is the most productive component of the initial encounter. Hypotheses are generated from the patient's account and the physician's observations, and are successively pursued or rejected in the light of emerging data. In the case of acute fever, however, a few special features of the history stand out. One of these is the common difficulty in reaching agreement on the meaning of words and phrases used in this context. It is rare for the phrase 'I have a fever' to mean that the body temperature has been measured by a reliable method. More often, the phrase means that the patient has a subjective sensation of warmth, or a feeling of chilliness or undue sweating. 'Flu' is another word in common use and usually describes aching muscles, chills and shivering, but sometimes is used to denote upper respiratory symptoms such as a runny nose or scratchy throat, and sometimes to indicate a fever.

A second distinctive point when taking the history of a patient who has acute fever relates to the time-honored 'systems review'. This is usually employed, if at all, at the end of a history taking, but often has so little to contribute that it is discarded completely. In the case of acute fever, however, because the range of possibilities is so much wider than for many presenting symptoms, the systems enquiry is useful early in the history taking; it often reveals the only relevant localizing evidence, as patients may have forgotten or thought insignificant the symptoms that provide valuable clues. Among the apparently minor clues that may emerge on direct enquiry are minor respiratory, abdominal or urinary symptoms, a transient rash or previous episodes of illness of a similar nature. Apparent localizing features that are actually symptoms of the raised temperature may, however, give false leads. Thus, dark urine in a febrile patient may simply denote dehydration, and some patients, especially women, experience burning and discomfort passing urine when they are febrile. Muscle and joint pains are also hard to interpret during fever: severe pains suggest viral infections such as influenza or dengue, but

they are also a feature of some enteroviral infections (Bornholm disease) and of leptospirosis. Neurologic features are especially difficult. Some patients regularly experience headache when febrile, and many children and some older patients become delirious with a high fever; whether such clinical features indicate a specifically neurologic involvement obviously needs careful observation.

A history of medication may be important in acute febrile disease. A large number of drugs may themselves cause fever, often without a rash or other clear indicators. Among antimicrobial agents, penicillins, cephalosporins and sulfonamides are especially notable, but many others may be implicated. Anti-infective agents may suppress or modify infections, and so confound a diagnosis, and antipyretic agents may greatly modify the pattern of fever in an infection.

TRAVEL HISTORY

As rapid movements of vast numbers of people throughout the world have been made possible in the era of air travel, so have the possibilities of an infection developing in one country when it was acquired in another. A travel history must never be omitted in a patient who has fever and many tragic deaths from *Plasmodium falciparum* malaria testify to its importance. The history should be accurate as to time and place. The name of a country is not enough; a stay in a four-star hotel in a capital city presents different risks from those of a camping trek in rural areas of the same country. Timing is especially helpful, even though many infections have a wide range of recorded incubation periods. For example, an illness beginning more than about 10 days after return is unlikely to be one of the common acute respiratory infections, with the exception of *Mycoplasma pneumoniae* and perhaps Q fever; dengue, too, and other arbovirus infections would have developed by this time. An incubation period of more than 3 weeks excludes the hemorrhagic virus infections, such as Lassa fever, and almost excludes typhoid. On the other hand, longer periods still leave open the possibility of viral hepatitis, Katayama fever (acute schistosomiasis) and primary HIV infection. As to malaria, the incubation period of *P. falciparum* infection may be as little as 1 week, but after 6 or 8 weeks a first presentation of this form of malaria becomes uncommon. *Plasmodium vivax* and *Plasmodium malariae* infections may develop months or years after travel to a malarial area.

Other important aspects of the travel history are the immunization record and an account of medications, with special emphasis on antimalarial prophylaxis.

It is sometimes necessary to begin treatment before a definite diagnosis has been made, or when the causal organism but not its antibiotic susceptibility is known. The travel history is important here too, as the pattern of antibiotic resistance in many pathogens varies greatly from country to country, and will determine an appropriate choice of therapy. Notable examples are the differences in drug resistance in malaria in different countries, the spread of multi-resistant typhoid and shigellosis and the erratic distribution of pneumococcal resistance to penicillin. In each of these examples, the area in which infection was acquired may limit the options available for chemotherapy.

Every physician who sees a febrile traveler cannot be expected to have an up-to-date knowledge of the precise infective risks, let alone the antibiotic resistance patterns of possible pathogens, and therefore easy communication with a Tropical and Infectious Diseases Unit and with one of the specialized information services that deals with travel medicine, which are available in many countries, is essential.

What are the actual causes of acute fever in returning travelers? (As this chapter focuses on illnesses with a large element of fever, primarily diarrheal diseases, or sexually transmitted diseases with mainly local symptoms and signs, and many other health risks of travel are not discussed here, see Chapter 6.4). Contrary to popular myth, the 'classic' tropical diseases are rarely acquired by short-term travelers, with the vital exception of malaria. This ranks first among diagnoses of acute fever in returning travelers, followed by a large group of short-lived fevers for which no etiology is ever established. Other diagnoses obviously vary in their frequency with the pattern of travel to and from a particular country. As the traveler is exposed not only to exotic pathogens, but also to a changing ecologic background of widely distributed pathogens, it is not surprising that ordinary respiratory infections, ranging from colds to pneumonia, are common. So too are initially febrile presentations of diarrheal diseases and prodromes of hepatitis. Urinary infection, as one of the most common causes of fever in women not always accompanied by localizing symptoms, must also be remembered. Some diagnoses encountered with widely variable frequency in different units are listed in Figure 2.1.

FEVER IN RETURNING TRAVELERS
Common
Malaria
No diagnosis made
Respiratory infection
Diarrheal disease (fever before or accompanying gut symptoms)
Urinary tract infection
Viral hepatitis; febrile prodrome
Uncommon
Dengue
Typhoid
Tuberculosis
Acute HIV
Schistosomiasis
Rickettsial infections
Amebiasis

Fig. 2.1 Diagnoses made in travelers returning from tropical countries with fever as a principal symptom.

CONTACT HISTORY

Contact history may be relevant in travelers and in people staying at home. Information about local endemic or epidemic infections is to be sought. Most frequent of all, especially in the winter months, is a history of contact with acute respiratory infection, which is possibly relevant because so many respiratory infections begin with 1 or 2 days of indeterminate fever, but is impossible to interpret because of the very frequency of such infections. Even in places with high uptakes of routine immunization, measles is encountered, and tends then to be missed because of its low prevalence and because it may occur in older subjects in highly immunized populations. Measles is especially important when the patient, or a contact, is immunosuppressed. Rubella, a more difficult and uncertain clinical diagnosis, is clearly of the greatest import if the patient or a contact is pregnant. Known contact with meningococcal disease obviously demands immediate attention, although, owing to the vagaries of meningococcal carriage and immunity, very few patients who have this disease have a direct contact history. A story of 'food poisoning' or diarrheal disease in contacts may be relevant as shigellosis, salmonellosis and *Campylobacter jejuni* infections may all begin with a febrile phase, whereas ingestion of raw milk and some cheeses raises the possibilities of brucellosis and listerial infection. The long incubation periods of most forms of viral hepatitis should be remembered in exploring possible contact history.

OCCUPATIONAL HISTORY

Many occupational exposures are not particularly relevant to acute febrile presentations, but many of the points about contact history just discussed are especially applicable to health workers and to those involved in child care. Other specific risks arising from occupation that may present as an acute fever include leptospirosis in sewage workers and fish farmers, and the many infective risks in veterinary and abattoir work, including brucellosis and *Streptococcus suis* infection. Fever may be the first clinical manifestation of tuberculosis relevant to health professionals, especially those involved with the care of patients who have HIV, and to carers of the homeless.

Some fevers associated with occupation are not infective. Fever and chills may be caused by inhalation of metal fumes or breakdown products of polymers. Many occupational lung diseases manifest with primarily respiratory features, but in extrinsic allergic alveolitis fever and influenza-like symptoms may dominate the picture. These conditions are characterized by recurrent episodes related to the particular exposure.

PHYSICAL EXAMINATION

TEMPERATURE

Depending on the duration of the illness, few temperature measurements may be available for evaluation. Recorded temperatures of

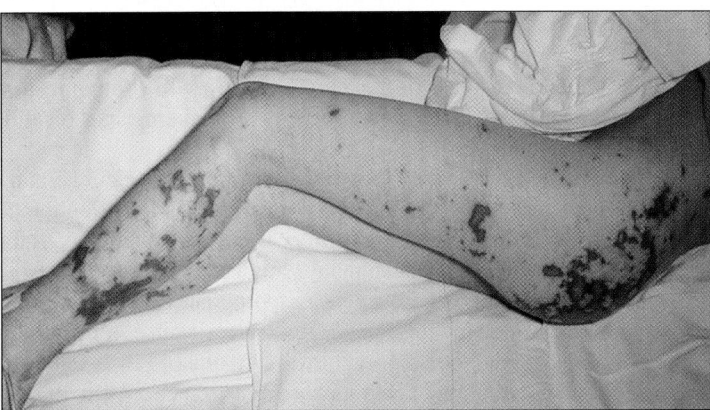

Fig. 2.2 Fully developed, almost pathognomonic hemorrhagic rash of meningococcal sepsis.

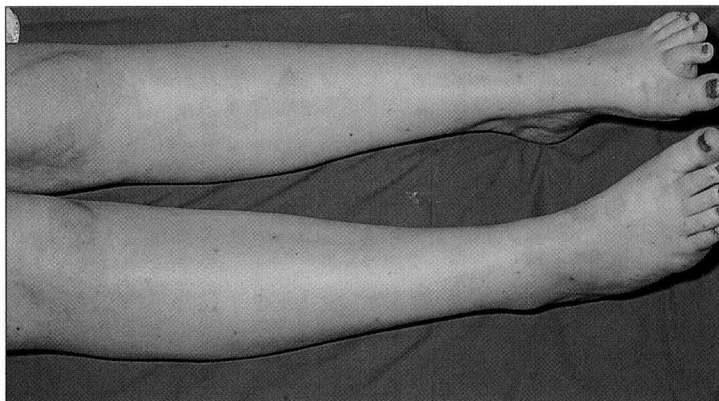

Fig. 2.3 Very early rash of meningococcal sepsis. A few petechiae only but meningococcal sepsis nonetheless. It can progress to the appearance in Figure 2.2 within minutes or hours. This is the window of opportunity for early treatment.

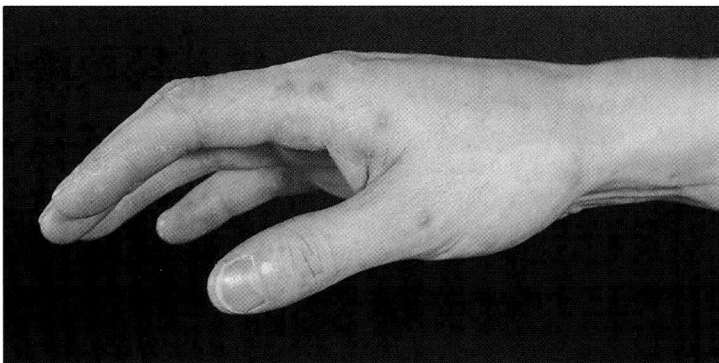

Fig. 2.4 Hand, foot and mouth disease. Shows scanty lax vesicles, found at these sites. There is often also a maculopapular rash, especially on the buttocks.

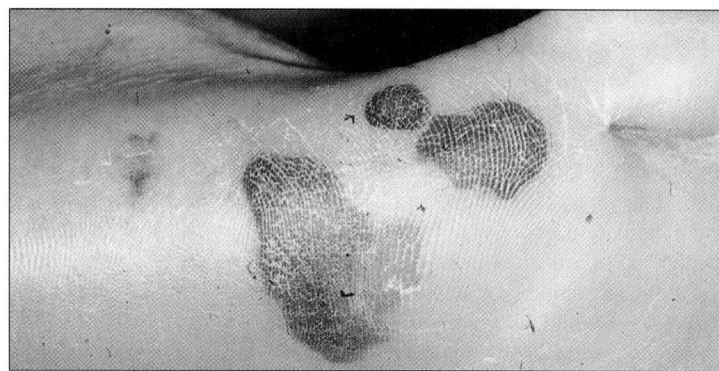

Fig. 2.5 Purpuric skin lesions in staphylococcal endocarditis.

RASHES ASSOCIATED WITH ACUTE VIRAL INFECTIONS		
Virus	Syndromes	Comment
Measles	Measles	Maculopapular followed by staining
Rubella	Rubella/German measles	Macular, often general facial flush
Herpesvirus 6	Roseola infantum	Macular or maculopapular after several days of fever
Parvovirus B19	Erythema infectiosum	Slapped cheeks, lacy on trunk and limbs, often rubelliform or hemorrhagic
Varicella-zoster	Chickenpox	Vesicular, rarely hemorrhagic
	Shingles	Neurological distribution, premonitary pain, erythema
Herpes simplex	Disseminated herpes Eczema herpeticum	
Epstein–Barr virus		Occasionally macular rash; severe rashes usually ampicillin-induced
Enteroviruses		Usually macular or maculopapular; sometimes hemorrhagic and/or vesicular (hand, foot and mouth disease; see Fig. 2.4)
Primary HIV	Mononucleosis-like illness	(Maculopapular rashes in chronic HIV; see Section 5)
Viral hemorrhagic fevers	See Section 6	Purpura, ecchymoses

Fig. 2.6 Rashes associated with acute viral infections.

RASHES ASSOCIATED WITH ACUTE BACTERIAL INFECTIONS		
Agent	Rashes	Comment
Neisseria meningitidis	Petechial/purpuric	Also nonhemorrhagic early rashes
Neisseria gonorrhoeae	Hemorrhagic vesicles, pustules	
Staphylococcus aureus	Pyogenic skin lesions Scalded skin syndrome Peripheral purpura Erythema	In staphylococcal endocarditis In toxic shock syndrome
Streptococcus pyogenes	Erysipelas Erythema	Local erythema, bullae In toxic shock syndrome
Salmonella typhi	Rose spots	
Pseudomonas aeruginosa	Ecthyma gangrenosum Cellulitis ± blebs	Also in *Aeromonas* and other Gram-negative bacillary infections
Haemophilus aegyptius	Brazilian haemorrhagic fever	

Fig. 2.7 Rashes associated with acute bacterial infections.

higher than 102.2°F (39.0°C) are more likely to be caused by a significant infection than are lesser degrees of fever, but very high fever must raise suspicion of a noninfectious cause such as heat stroke or substance abuse. The pattern of fever is much less valuable than is commonly supposed. This aspect is discussed more fully in Chapter 3.3, but a few points relevant to short-term fevers may be mentioned. A dramatic fever with wild swings between readings is suggestive of pyogenic infection and especially of abscess formation, and of acute pyelonephritis, but may also be seen in other conditions, including malaria and disseminated tuberculosis, also in Still's disease and occasionally in drug fever. Perhaps the most common reason for this kind of chart, however, is the use of antipyretics in a febrile patient, which often gives rise to this feature.

The most important caveats relate to malaria, and they cannot be emphasized enough. The temperature pattern in *P. falciparum* infections is often quite erratic, and this diagnosis must be considered in all febrile and some nonfebrile patients coming from a malarial area. Regular tertian or quartan (meaning every other day and every

third day, respectively) are not found in the early stages of malaria, and are a feature of relapse rather than initial infection. On the other hand, when present they are very characteristic of malaria.

RASHES

Many acute febrile illnesses are accompanied by a rash, which aids greatly in establishing a diagnosis. A few, notably those of meningococcal sepsis, are of vital importance in determining the need for urgent treatment or the protection of contacts (Figs 2.2 & 2.3). Some are pathognomonic, others only indicative (Figs 2.4 & 2.5), and the features of the rash must be placed in context with the other features of the illness. In hand, foot and mouth disease the distribution is pathognomonic. Figures 2.6–2.8 provide information about rashes associated with acute fevers, including those encountered in returning travelers, but a few specific points are worth emphasizing. In measles, easily forgotten in well immunized populations but by the same token important to remember in older age groups, fever precedes the Koplik spots and the exanthem by 2 or 3 days but sometimes by as much as 1 week, although respiratory features are prominent for most of this time. In rubella and in enteroviral infections, general symptoms only rarely precede the rash, and then only by 1 day or so. In dengue, the rash characteristically appears in the second phase of the biphasic illness. Conditions associated with pathognomonic or at least characteristic rashes may, however, also occur with nonspecific rashes; the early rash of meningococcal sepsis may be macular or maculopapular, and Lyme disease may exhibit nonspecific rashes in addition to erythema chronicum migrans.

Mouth

The mouth may show useful signs in a febrile patient (Figs 2.9 & 2.10). Especially in infancy and childhood, the tongue and mouth give some indication of dehydration, although mouth breathing and tachypnea often produce a similar appearance. The tongue is notably raw and red in scarlatina, in Kawasaki disease and in toxic shock syndrome. Vesicles are found, especially on the soft palate and anterior fauces, in some enteroviral infections (hand, foot and mouth disease). Palatal petechiae are fairly nonspecific, but are found in infectious mononucleosis and rubella in particular. Many important signs in HIV infection are to be found in the mouth and these are discussed in Section 5.

Eyes

Some degree of conjunctival suffusion is common in people with a high temperature. This is often prominent in measles, rubella, some adenovirus infections and in leptospirosis. In infections with a hemorrhagic rash, conjunctival hemorrhages may be present in addition to skin petechiae or purpura; this is especially helpful in patients who have dark skin, when petechiae are difficult to see. Other ocular signs that may be important in acute febrile illness are uveitis in acute sarcoid (although many patients who have acute sarcoid do not show ocular involvement) and in Still's disease. Choroiditis occurs in histoplasmosis and in toxoplasmosis. Although choroidoretinitis in toxoplasmosis is most frequently a late marker of congenital infection, it is now clear that a few patients who have acute acquired toxoplasmosis (and not HIV-infected) do have acute choroiditis. Miliary tuberculosis, with or without tuberculous meningitis, sometimes manifests as fever and general ill health; the diagnosis is immediately established if choroidal tubercles are seen.

Lymph nodes

Generalized node enlargement is relatively uncommon in acute febrile illness. Among the common infections of children and young adults, rubella, Epstein–Barr virus mononucleosis and cytomegalovirus infection are notable causes, to which must be added cat scratch disease and, in those at risk, secondary syphilis and primary HIV infection. These latter infections are especially important to remember in returning travelers. General node enlargement is also seen in some more specifically tropical diseases, of which dengue is the most likely to affect a short-term traveler. Acute histoplasmosis is another possibility after a first visit to an endemic area.

Focal nodes must direct a careful search of the relevant drainage area. For example, tender enlarged inguinal nodes may be more prominent than the source of infection, which may be insignificant-looking streptococcal lesions of the feet, perhaps superimposed on insect bites or fungal infection. Acquired toxoplasmosis in the immunocompetent host, although usually subclinical, manifests as a febrile illness with localized lymphadenopathy, most often in one or other cervical group but sometimes in nodes elsewhere. The persistent fallacy that toxoplasmosis is a cause of a 'glandular fever' syndrome must be firmly laid to rest. It is rare for the lymphadenopathy of acquired toxoplasmosis to be generalized, and atypical mononuclear leukocytes, if found at all on the blood film, are few in number.

Spleen

Acute and longer-term febrile illnesses make an interesting contrast here. Splenomegaly is found in so many of the infections and other conditions that can cause FUO that it is of little diagnostic value. By contrast, splenomegaly in a patient who has fever of a few days' duration certainly merits further attention. It may indicate a particular infection, such as infectious mononucleosis, rubella, a hepatitis prodrome, in which splenomegaly is especially common in children, or, in a returning traveler, malaria. Spenomegaly may be attributable to an

Fig. 2.8 Rashes associated with acute spirochetal and rickettsial infections.

RASHES ASSOCIATED WITH ACUTE SPIROCHETAL AND RICKETTSIAL INFECTIONS		
Agent	**Rashes**	**Comments**
Leptospirosis	Hemorrhages. Also other rashes	Weil's disease
Borrelia recurrentis (relapsing fever)	Petechiae	Often no rash; sometimes severe hemorrhages
Borrelia burgdorferi (Lyme disease)	Erythema chronicum migrans	Sometimes secondary annular or nonspecific rashes
Spirillum minus (rat-bite fever)	Blotchy macular, papular and urticarial rashes, beginning near the bite and spreading	Rashes also in the *Streptobacillus moniliformis* form of rat-bite fever
Rickettsial infections	Macular, papular petechial	Primary eschar (*tache noir*) in some syndromes

Fig. 2.8 Rashes associated with acute spirochetal and rickettsial infections.

ORAL SIGNS IN ACUTE FEVER	
Sign	**Diagnosis**
Dehydration	Any fever
Herpes simplex	Common in meningococcal and pneumococcal infection
Raw tongue	Scarlatina. Kawasaki disease. Toxic shock syndrome
Ulcers, vesicles	Varicella. Herpes simplex. Enteroviruses (herpangina, hand, foot and mouth disease). Aphthous stomatitis. Secondary syphilis. Erythema multiforme
Palatal petechiae	Nonspecific, but common in infectious mononucleosis and rubella

Fig. 2.9 Oral signs in acute fever.

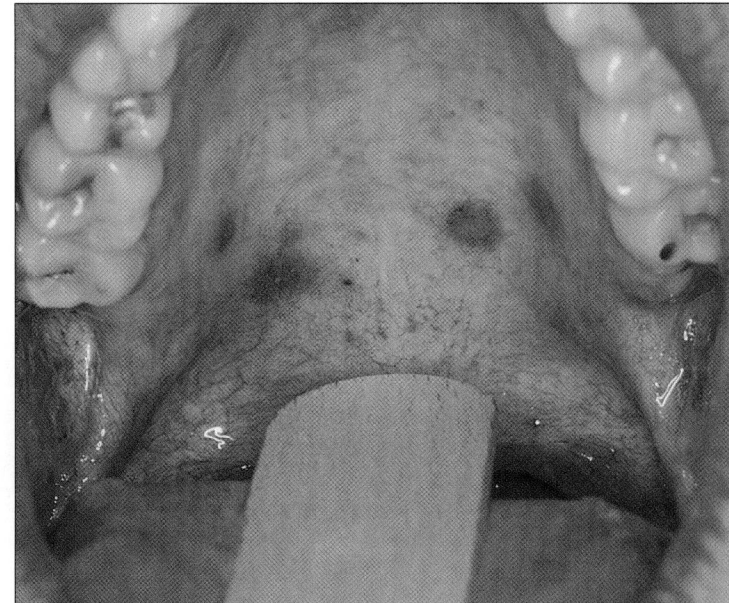

Fig. 2.10 Oral signs in hand, foot and mouth disease.

underlying hematologic condition, perhaps a hemolytic anemia or a lymphoma, itself the cause of the fever or a reason for increased susceptibility to infection.

MAKING A DECISION

Some specific factors in the history and examination suggest the need for a plan of management that goes beyond symptom relief. This may mean repeated observation, investigation or investigation combined with provisional treatment. The factors are:

- recent travel, especially to a malaria-risk country (see Chapter 6.26);
- chills and rigors;
- height of fever;
- fever and rash;
- extremes of age;
- any known or suspected immunosuppression;
- neurologic features;
- dehydration;
- parental or partner concern; and
- physician's impression.

Chills are common enough at the onset of respiratory infections, particularly at the onset of influenza. Nevertheless, the rapid rise in body temperature that they denote is also common in some more serious infections, and this caution applies with greater force if the patient has rigors. A temperature of more than 102.2°F (39°C) is common enough in the early stage of an ultimately minor infection, but higher temperatures sustained for more than a short time are more likely to be associated with serious infections.

The combination of fever and any kind of hemorrhagic rash (discussed fully in Chapters 2.5 & 3.3, see Figs 2.6–2.8), be it only a few petechiae, is especially important.

The elderly and babies are both subject to more rapid changes resulting from the metabolic stress of fever from whatever cause than are children and younger adults.

Many patients on immunosuppressive therapy are living and working normally in the community but are at increased risk of infection. In some conditions, notably asplenia from any cause, infection may take a fulminant course and any fever demands very prompt attention (see Chapters 4.7 & 4.9). In addition, some forms of immunosuppression may initially manifest with a febrile illness, and the possibility of a first presentation of HIV infection is especially to be borne in mind.

Depression of consciousness, meningism or localizing neurologic signs are clearly important. Children with high fever may exhibit mild confusion and experience hallucinations; this is seen less commonly at older ages. Whether such clinical features denote specific neurologic involvement needs careful assessment.

Children and the elderly are at greater risk of dehydration, but patients of any age with fever, especially in warm conditions and if anorexic or vomiting, may become fluid deficient.

Whatever the level of anxiety in patient or carer, someone close to the patient may well have an accurate notion of whether the illness is out of the ordinary, and their opinions should be carefully considered. The physician may form the impression that the illness is unusual, or serious, or likely to become serious. This is so common an issue as to merit more detailed discussion.

IS THE PATIENT ILL?

Even after the most meticulous history taking, physical examination and attention to the issues just discussed, there are large numbers of patients who have fever of short duration in whom no particular warning features are present. Fortunately, most patients who have fever of a few hours or a few days duration recover uneventfully within a few days without sequelae and without a diagnosis other than a meaningless attribution to ' viral infection'. How should one judge, in the home, in the health center or practice premises, or in the hospital Emergency Room, which of these patients should be further investigated, or investigated and given provisional empiric treatment? This must be one of the most frequent decisions that has to be made by clinicians all over the world and yet it is ignored in books on the subject of diagnosis. Decision theory is largely silent in this context because the elements of the decision involve multiple factors, usually heuristic in character, few of which can be assigned a numeric value.

It seems that the most common factor affecting the physician's decision is the impression that the patient has an infection with systemic and potentially hazardous features - for which the word 'toxic' is often used as shorthand – and this is the main determinant of further investigation and treatment in patients who have acute febrile illness. Few attempts have been made to analyze the basis of this impression and its value in management in adults, although some light was thrown on the problem in a hospital setting in a study of 473 patients in the Emergency Room of a large medical center in The Netherlands.[1] Blood cultures had been done for all the patients because of clinical suspicion of bacterial infection: 20% of them had positive cultures and 4% had septicemia, as defined by hemodynamic and hematologic criteria.

Attempts to analyze the physician's impression of illness have been more often pursued in children; this work had its origin in the increased use of blood culture in infants and children, most of whom did not look ill, taken to 'walk-in' clinics or hospital Emergency Rooms in the USA. Positive blood cultures were found in 2.8–8% of these infants. In most places the main organisms were *Streptococcus pneumoniae, Neisseria meningitidis* and, before general immunization against this organism, *Haemophilus influenzae*. A few of these children, perhaps 4–7%, went on to develop meningitis or other focal infections.[2] These findings spawned a vast amount of work on the early detection of potentially serious illness in febrile infants and on developing management plans for their care. Algorithms on this topic often begin with the question – Is the child toxic? – and efforts to define the basis of 'toxicity' have resulted in the Yale Acute Illness Observation Scale (AIOS), which assigns a three-point score to each of six aspects of the observations that precede physical examination.[3] The six aspects observed are:

- quality of cry,
- reaction of crying to parental comforting or holding,
- state variation (transition between sleeping and wakefulness),
- color,
- hydration, and
- response to social overtures.

This type of assessment, attempting to systematize what experienced physicians do without conscious thought, has confirmed the value of clinical judgment in predicting or excluding a high risk of serious disease in older infants and children. It is unsurprising that intermediate scores in the Yale AIOS assessment are common, and in these cases a total leukocyte count of greater than $15 \times 10^9/l$ is helpful in indicating an increased post-test probability of bacteremia. It is also sensible, if further investigations are decided upon, to include urine microscopy at this stage. The Yale system is of less value in infants younger than 3 months, in whom the detection of serious infection is notoriously difficult, and this problem is not addressed here.

A systematic approach to the diagnosis of acute febrile illness in older children and adults suitable for the education of students and junior staff needs to be developed and a useful contribution has been made in the particular case of suspected meningococcal disease in children and teenagers. A qualitative study of 83 cases seen in general practice in south Wales showed how clinical and contextual features helped to differentiate these patients from the many with acute self-limiting febrile illnesses.[4] The 'danger points' listed above are certainly important to note and act upon, but in the many febrile patients in whom none of these markers is present it seems impossible to dispense with the elusive but crucial clinical impression of illness, although even this may deceive in either direction. One reason for disasters associated

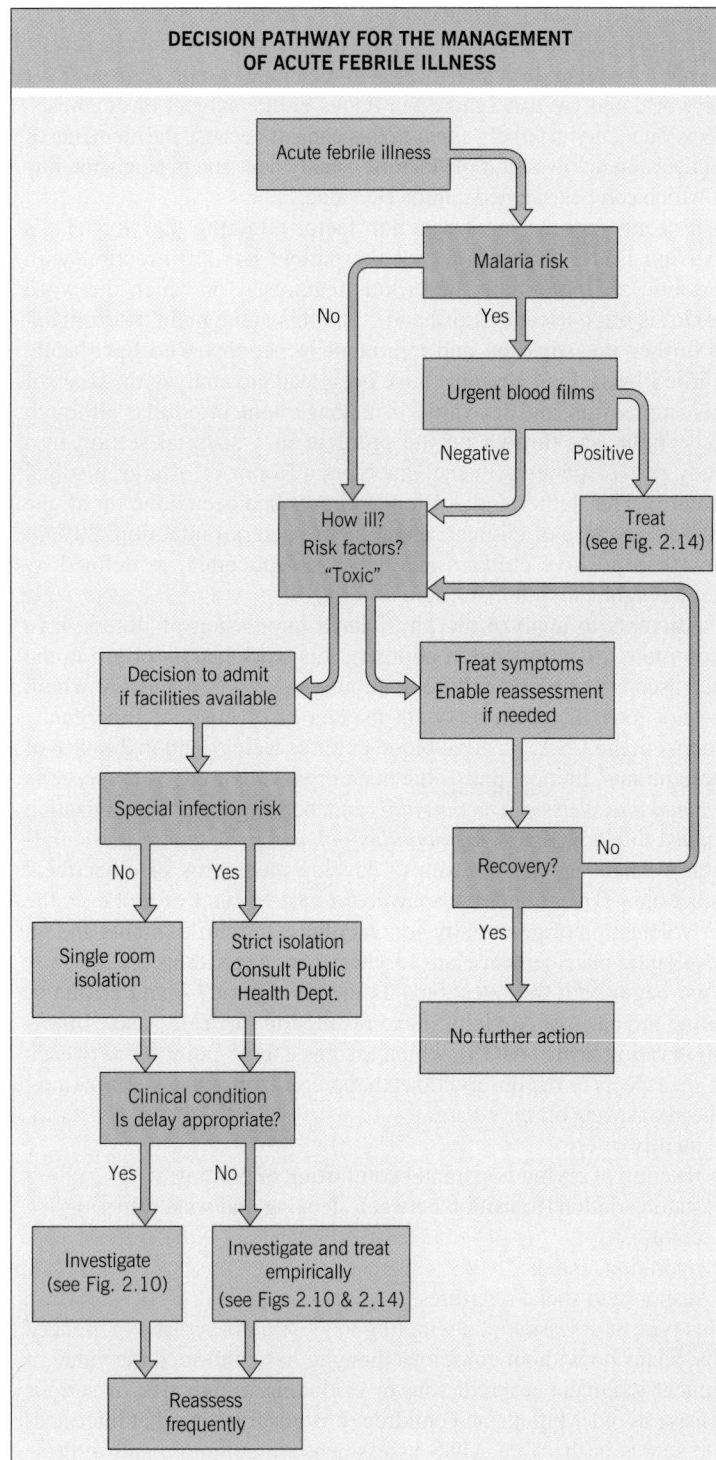

DECISION PATHWAY FOR THE MANAGEMENT OF ACUTE FEBRILE ILLNESS

Fig. 2.11 Decision pathway for the management of acute febrile illness.

BASIC INVESTIGATIONS IN ACUTE FEVER

- Routine blood count
- Stained blood film
- Urine microscopy and culture
- Chest radiograph
- Save serum

Fig. 2.12 Basic laboratory investigations in patients who have acute fever.

VALUE OF LEUKOCYTE COUNT IN ACUTE FEVER	
Neutrophilia	**Neutropenia**
Sepsis	Severe sepsis
Abscess	Malaria
Amebiasis (usually)	Typhoid
Leptospirosis (usually)	Brucellosis
Still's disease	Visceral leishmaniasis
Lymphoma (uncommon)	Rickettsial infections
Atypical mononuclear cells	**Eosinophilia**
Epstein–Barr virus	Schistosomiasis (Katayama fever)
Cytomegalovirus	Visceral larva migrans (toxocariasis etc.)

Fig. 2.13 Value of total and differential leukocyte count in acute fever. This table concerns acute illnesses in which fever is a principal feature; it does not include conditions such as tropical eosinophilia, in which respiratory features are dominant.

LABORATORY INVESTIGATIONS

With few exceptions, among them the classic infectious diseases such as measles and varicella, most acute and short-lived infections have no specific features that enable a clinical diagnosis to be made. Few of these illnesses are investigated. Facilities to do so are not available in most of the world and, when they are available, are unnecessary in patients who have mild and self-limiting illnesses. It follows that most of these infections remain undiagnosed, although a specific diagnosis can be assigned to a substantial number of them in research projects in which full virologic investigations are undertaken. This is the case especially in acute infections in children, who may experience a remarkably large number of viral infections in the course of a year.

Investigations are certainly indicated when any of the 'danger points' just described are present, and in any febrile patient whose general condition gives concern. The precise range of investigations chosen will obviously vary depending on the facilities available and on the vagaries of the clinical situation, but even a small and frequently accessible range of investigations (Fig. 2.12) greatly increases the possibility of establishing a diagnosis. When the features of the illness give no specific direction, the most useful investigations are a routine blood count together with careful examination of a stained blood film, blood culture, urine examination, and posteroanterior and lateral radiograph of the chest. When blood is taken, a serum specimen should be saved for later study.

Initial investigations are often, of course, much more extensive depending as they do on available resources and initial clinical clues. These will most commonly include liver function tests, stool microscopy and culture, antigen detection and serologic tests for particular pathogens, and relevant imaging especially abdominal ultrasound scanning and CT or MRI. The more extensive range of investigations is fully discussed in the context of FUO (see Chapter 3.3).

---

with *P. falciparum* malaria is the apparently good condition of the patient that may precede a rapid decline, whereas, conversely, patients may look much more ill than they are after an exhausting long journey or a lively party. Beyond the basic need for time and care in clinical assessment, a confident relationship between patient and physician and easy access for further consultation are perhaps the most important factors in ensuring that major illness is not missed.

A decision tree for the management of acute febrile illness is given in Figure 2.11.

THE TOTAL AND DIFFERENTIAL LEUKOCYTE COUNT

Modest degrees of neutrophilia, up to about $15 \times 10^9/l$ are of little help. More definite neutrophilia is principally found in pyogenic bacterial infections, but also in amebiasis, leptospirosis and in many non-infectious conditions such as thromboembolism, rheumatic fever, Still's disease, exacerbations of chronic liver damage and mechanical tissue damage (Fig. 2.13).

Neutropenia is common in many viral infections, including rubella and influenza, and, among infections of travelers, is often found in malaria, typhoid, brucellosis, rickettsial diseases and visceral leishmaniasis. Leukopenia is also a feature of severe and overwhelming sepsis, but the serious condition of patients who show this feature is usually only too evident. Thrombocytopenia is a very frequent feature of the blood film in malaria.

A substantial number of atypical mononuclear cells is found most commonly in acute Epstein–Barr virus and cytomegalovirus infections, whereas eosinophilia points to the tissue-invasive stage of many parasitic infections.

SPECIFIC DIAGNOSES FROM THE BLOOD FILM

Malaria is by far the most important finding from examination of the blood in those at risk, but other diagnoses that can sometimes be made in this way are listed in Figure 2.14. In addition to examination of the blood, a diagnosis may occasionally be aided by direct examination of material from a skin lesion, for example in meningococcal sepsis.

URINE EXAMINATION

Small degrees of proteinuria are of no significance in febrile patients. Dipsticks can be used to detect Gram-negative infections and pyuria, but should not be used alone in the diagnosis of fever because of the high false-negative rate of the nitrate test for bacteriuria. Urinary infection is best diagnosed by direct microscopy of a drop of urine with the finding of heavy pyuria, often some hematuria and visible organisms. The presence of organisms in association with pyuria in a freshly obtained specimen indicates significant bacteriuria ($> 1 \times 10/ml$) and a Gram stain can help in distinguishing positive cocci from negative bacilli. Urinary infection is one of the most common infections that sometimes manifests as a febrile illness with no localizing symptoms or signs.

CHEST RADIOGRAPH

The most important findings in a febrile but previously healthy patient are areas of consolidation in 'atypical' pneumonia, such as that associated with Q fever or *Mycoplasma pneumoniae* infection, in which general symptoms and fever may precede respiratory symptoms and signs by several days. The other crucial finding is that of pulmonary tuberculosis, in some communities to be suspected throughout the population, and in others more especially in the indigent and those infected with HIV. Other diagnoses may also be made, such as *Pneumocystis carinii* infection in HIV infection before respiratory features become evident, allergic pneumonias, visceral larva migrans and pulmonary emboli.

BLOOD CULTURE

The importance of blood culture in febrile patients thought ill enough to need investigation is evident but, important as it is, the information gained is necessarily delayed and thus irrelevant to the immediate management decisions.

SERUM

It is always sensible, if blood is drawn, to save a serum sample, especially for later comparative tests if the illness proves to be prolonged and remains undiagnosed.

ISOLATION

A few patients who have infections present a risk to other people. Because the diagnosis is often obscure at the time of admission to

---

DIAGNOSES FROM BLOOD FILM

- Malaria
- Babesiosis
- Trypanosomiasis
- Filariasis
- Leptospirosis (dark field)
- Relapsing fever (dark field or staining)
- Bartonellosis
- Ehrlichiosis
- Meningicoccemia
- Histoplasmosis

Fig. 2.14 Specific diagnoses from the blood film. Etiologies of acute fever sometimes established by examination of the stained blood film.

---

hospital of an acutely febrile patient, isolation is often advisable initially, if facilities are available. Sometimes, as for example in suspected Lassa fever, more elaborate measures involving the control-of-infection team in liaison with the public health authorities are indicated. These aspects of the management of infection are discussed in Chapter 3.10.

MANAGEMENT

SYMPTOMATIC TREATMENT

Drug therapy is unnecessary in many acute fevers, but discomfort can be alleviated by agents such as aspirin, paracetamol and non-steroidal anti-inflammatory agents, which act as cyclo-oxygenase inhibitors. There is little to choose between them as regards their effect on fever, but aspirin is avoided in infants because of its association with Reye's syndrome, and in many older patients because of its effects on the gastric mucosa.

The effectiveness of antipyretics in reducing fever does not seem to correlate with its cause. In a study of 1559 children with a temperature of more than 101°F (38.4°C) on arrival at the Emergency Room, reductions of temperature 1 and 2 hours after a single dose of paracetamol (acetaminophen) were slightly greater in patients who had a serious bacterial infection than in those who did not,[5] although it had been thought that fever with a serious cause might be less responsive to an antipyretic.

Sponging is still sometimes used as a method of reducing fever. It certainly does this, but it is often very uncomfortable, particularly if done with iced rather than tepid water. The vasoconstriction and shivering causing distress do not, however, produce a rise of core temperature. Combining paracetamol (acetaminophen) with sponging gives a slightly greater reduction of temperature than sponging alone.[6]

It is useful to know the timing of antipyretic action, especially if the aim is to reduce the likelihood of febrile convulsions. Both antipyretic drugs and sponging show an appreciable effect within about 30 minutes and have their maximal effects in 2–3 hours.

Corticosteroids are effective antipyretics but should be used only for specific indications in conjunction with appropriate anti-infective therapy for the known or presumed cause of the fever.

Maintaining hydration is important and not always easy in a warm climate as patients who have fever are often anorexic and sometimes suffer nausea or vomiting.

EMPIRIC TREATMENT

One of the most taxing and common decisions that has to be taken in acute febrile illness is whether to start empiric treatment based on one or more hypotheses about the diagnosis. On one side is the fear of rapid and perhaps irreversible deterioration, especially in *P. falciparum* malaria and in septic shock. On the other are the confounding effects of

DANGER POINTS IN ACUTE FEVER
• Petechial/purpuric rash
• Travel involving risk of malaria
• Chills and rigors
• Extremes of age
• Neurologic signs
• Asplenia
• Hypogammaglobulinemia
• Post bone marrow transplant

Fig. 2.15 Some dangerous features in patients who have acute fever.

EMPIRIC TREATMENT IN ACUTE FEVER		
Presumed diagnosis	Action	
Meningococcal sepsis	1.	Blood culture if possible
	2.	Benzyl penicillin
Septic shock in asplenia	1.	Blood culture if possible
	2.	Benzyl penicillin or cephalosporin*
Streptococcal sepsis	1.	Blood culture if possible
	2.	Local lesion, Gram stain and culture if possible
	3.	Benzyl penicillin +/- clindamycin
Staphylococcal sepsis	1.	Blood culture if possible
	2.	Local lesion, Gram stain and culture if possible
	3.	Flucloxacillin or similar agent*
Severe malaria	1.	Blood films
	2.	Quinine (or artemether or artesunate; see Section 6)
Lassa fever	1.	Strict isolation
	2.	Tribavirin (ribavirin)
	3.	Inform public health authorities

* Knowledge of local resistance patterns and antibiotic policy needed

Fig. 2.16 Suggested empiric regimens for use when urgent treatment is indicated in patients who have acute fever.

possibly inappropriate treatment, and the added problem of adverse drug reactions. If immediate treatment is given, it is nearly always possible to take blood before starting and this can be used for diagnostic tests.

Some indications for immediate treatment (Fig. 2.15) in acutely febrile patients can be firmly stated; others are indicative and depend on the precise details of the clinical and epidemiologic situation. The most urgent are the possibility of meningococcal sepsis and that of serious infection in asplenic subjects. Next in urgency are indications pointing toward streptococcal sepsis and, in returning travelers, the possibility of *P. falciparum* malaria with clinical deterioration. Immediate treatment should also be seriously considered if there is evidence of any immunologic disorder and, more generally, if other indicators of severe illness such as those already discussed (Fig. 2.15) are present. Figure 2.16 gives some recommendations for action in these circumstances. The antibiotic choice, as always, must take account of local susceptibility patterns, and for this reason, more than one option is given. For example, penicillin is no longer the agent of first choice in many places for serious pneumococcal infection, and the spread of meningococcal resistance to penicillin may make future changes necessary in the national policy in the UK for immediate treatment of suspected meningococcal sepsis.[7]

It has been written (by Garrison) that Wunderlich, the founder of clinical thermometry, 'found fever a disease and left it a symptom'. This chapter shows that fever remains an important and challenging symptom that demands meticulous analysis so as to achieve the best prospects for accurate diagnosis and treatment.

REFERENCES

1. van Deventer SJH, Buller HR, Ten Cate JW, Sturk A, Pauw W. Endotoxaemia: an early predictor of septicaemia in febrile patients. Lancet 1988;i:605–9.
2. Radetsky M. The febrile infant and assumption of risk. Curr Opin Infect Dis 1996;9:171–5.
3. McCarthy PL, Sharpe MR, Spiesel SZ, et al. Observation scales to identify serious illness in febrile children. Pediatrics 1982;70:802–9.
4. Granier S, Owen P, Pill R, Jacobson L. Recognising meningococcal disease in primary care: qualitative study of how general practitioners process clinical and contextual information. Br Med J 1988;316:276–9.
5. Baker MD, Fossarelli PD, Carpenter RO. Childhood fever: correlation of diagnosis with temperature response to acetaminophen. Pediatrics 1987;80:315–8.
6. Steele RW, Tanaka PT, Lara RP, Bass JW. Evaluation of sponging and oral antipyretic therapy to reduce fever. J Pediatr 1970;77:824–9.
7. PHLS Meningoccal Infections Working Group and Public Health Medicine Environmental Group. Control of meningococcal disease: guidance for Consultants in Communicable Disease Control. CDR Review 1995;5:R189–198.

Fever of Unknown Origin in the General Population and in HIV-infected Persons

Wendy Armstrong & Powel Kazanjian

INTRODUCTION

Fever of unknown origin (FUO) is one of the most challenging tests of the clinical acumen of the physician. The clinical characteristics of 1184 cumulative cases of FUO in the general population have been published in 15 separate reports that span 72 years, from 1930 to 1992 (Fig. 3.1).[1–15] Since the early case series from the USA on FUO were published,[1–7] important sociologic and technologic changes have occurred, for example, new microbiologic techniques[16] and radiographic diagnostic tools[17] have become routinely available, a growing number of people use intravenous drugs[18] or have implanted prostheses,[19] and patterns of immigration and travel destinations have expanded.[20] The incidence of newly described diseases such as AIDS[21] and Lyme disease[22] has risen. In developed countries, certain 'older' diseases such as rheumatic fever remain uncommon,[23] yet the frequency of tuberculosis has risen again after a decline during the 30 years preceding 1985.[24]

The Beeson and Petersdorf criteria for FUO, which standardized the definition of FUO in 1961,[8] are:

- A body temperature of more than 101°F (38.3°C) for at least 3 weeks.
- Failure to establish a diagnosis after 1 week investigation.

These criteria were designed to eliminate self-limiting diseases that may have been represented in the seven series on FUO reported before 1961.[1–7] Each of the seven subsequent published case series on FUO[9–15] used the classic Beeson and Petersdorf criteria. Some of the recent series[14,15] use a revised Petersdorf definition of FUO[25,26] that permits the investigation to take place in the ambulatory setting as well as in hospital, the originally specified setting. Furthermore, a subclassification of HIV-associated FUO has been added to the classification of FUO in the general population to account for the recognition of this new disease.[27] Fever of unknown origin associated with HIV infection has been reviewed in five series and in a total of 166 patients;[28–32] HIV-associated FUO has been defined as fever that lasts more than 4 weeks in outpatients or 3 days in hospitalized patients and that remains unexplained despite investigation. These series are reviewed later in this chapter.

CLASSIC FEVER OF UNKNOWN ORIGIN

DISEASE CATEGORIES

An etiology of FUO is identified in the majority of cases in each published series on FUO (average 73%, range 30–93% of cases). In early reports, the individual diseases causing FUO were limited to a small number of predominantly infectious diseases.[1–6] In contrast, recent series show that the diseases responsible for FUO are much more extensive, involving over 100 disorders.[13–15] Consequently, recent case series use disease categories rather than enumerating individual diseases to describe the clinical spectrum of FUO. The principal disease categories include infection, neoplasms and collagen diseases. For the sake of simplicity, the remaining diverse range of cases can be grouped together as 'miscellaneous' (Fig. 3.1).

		Number of patients with indicated diagnosis				
Study	Total no. of cases	Infection	Neoplasm	Collagen	Miscellaneous	Undiagnosed
Alt and Barker, 1930[1]	57	14	6	0	1	36
Hamman and Wainwright, 1936[2,3]	54	32	12	0	0	10
Keefer, 1939[4]	80	51	19	0	10	0
Wolf and Jacobs, 1947[5]	36	2	1	0	1	32
Bottinger, 1953[6]	68	16	11	4	4	33
Geraci et al., 1959[7]	70	15	21	0	20	14
Petersdorf and Beeson, 1961[8]	100	36	19	15	23	7
Petersson, 1962[9]	81	15	5	5	0	56
Sheon and Van Ommen, 1963[10]	60	12	11	8	6	23
Fransen and Bottinger, 1996[11]	60	8	19	2	4	27
Jacoby and Swartz, 1973[12]	128	51	26	19	22	10
Larson et al., 1982[13]	105	32	33	9	18	13
Knoeckaert et al., 1992[14]	199	45	14	42	47	51
Kazanjian, 1992[15]	86	28	21	18	11	8
Total	1184	357	218	122	167	320
Percentage		30%	19%	10%	14%	27%

DIAGNOSES IN CASES OF FEVER OF UNKNOWN ORIGIN REPORTED IN THE LITERATURE

Fig. 3.1 Diagnoses in cases of fever of unknown origin reported in the literature.

Certain changes in disease categories have occurred since the original description of FUO. Infections remain the most common cause of FUO in all but one series. Overall, 30% (range 6–70%) of cases of FUO are due to an infection. Neoplasms are responsible for 18% (range 7–34%) of cases, and the proportion of cases due to malignancy has remained constant. In contrast, there has been an increase in cases that are caused by collagen disorders. Although the overall percentage of cases in this category of diseases is 10% (range 0–22%), series published within the past 10 years indicate an increase in the number of cases caused by collagen diseases. Diseases falling under the category miscellaneous disorders are identified in 14% of cases (range 0–28%). The individual diseases represented within these disease categories are discussed below.

Infections

The major infections represented in older papers – tuberculosis, endocarditis and abdominal abscesses – continue to make up a significant proportion of FUO in recent series – 5%, 5%, and 10% respectively.[14,15] However, compared with earlier series, the type of infections causing FUO have become more diverse.[12–15] Recently described infections including HIV infection and Lyme disease, immunodeficiency-related infections such as *Pneumocystis carinii* pneumonia and atypical mycobacterial infection, and diseases such as typhoid fever and amebiasis in patients who have resided in developing countries, have been described for the first time in series reported within the past decade.[13–15] In addition, these reports describe infections that involve critically ill patients whose lives have been prolonged in an intensive care setting and who have developed superinfections with *Candida* spp. Other infections that make up a small percentage of FUOs include pyelonephritis, perinephric abscess, toxoplasmosis in the immunocompetent host and mononucleosis caused by Epstein–Barr virus (EBV) or cytomegalovirus (CMV).

There are several explanations why tuberculosis, abdominal abscesses, and infectious endocarditis make up the majority of the infectious causes of FUO. For example, tuberculosis continues to be prevalent in Africa and South East Asia, and tuberculosis afflicts intravenous drug users, the elderly, and HIV-infected persons.[20–22] Furthermore, the increase in prevalence among persons who have prosthetic valvular devices[19,23] has affected the number of cases of FUO caused by infectious endocarditis.[15] In addition, advances in microbiologic techniques permit the identification of fastidious organisms that cause valvular vegetations.[33] Finally, modern radiologic studies permit the detection of abdominal abscesses in cryptic locations such as the spleen.[34]

The first appearance of newly discovered diseases such as HIV infection[21] and Lyme disease[22] as causes of FUO reflects the increased recognition of these diseases. The increase in the number of immunocompromised persons reflects the increase in the incidence of opportunistic infections, such as *Pneumocystis carinii* pneumonia, *Mycobacterium avium* and disseminated candidiasis, as causes of FUO.[35]

Neoplasia

Hodgkin's and non-Hodgkin's lymphoma have remained the most common neoplastic diseases responsible for FUO, and lymphoma is the most common individual disease causing FUO.[13–15] Its ability to present in an insidious and protean fashion may explain why lymphoma continues to account for a sizable number of cases despite new diagnostic modalities.[36] For example, fever in some cases persists for months before a gland may become enlarged. In addition, it may be difficult to locate an involved lymph node on physical examination when the axilla is involved, and it is impossible when the retroperitoneal nodes or bone marrow are the only site of disease. Furthermore, a directed percutaneous needle biopsy of an involved gland or bone marrow may contain insufficient material to reveal diagnostic histopathology.[37] Thus, lymphoma may elude clinical detection for a long time. Malignant histiocytosis,[38] angioimmunoblastic lymphadenopathy with dysproteinemia[39] and Kikuchi's disease,[40] although uncommon, are causes of FUO with lymphadenopathy that were first recognized within the past 15 years.

Other neoplasms and solid tumors are less common causes of FUO than lymphoma.[13–15] The peripheral blood smear of certain leukemias and myelodysplastic syndromes may reveal no definitive findings (aleukemic leukemia); establishing the diagnosis requires bone marrow examination. Renal cell carcinoma may present with prolonged fevers and no other symptoms in a minority of cases.[41] Metastatic adenocarcinoma in the liver, regardless of the primary site, may also cause FUO.[41] In most situations, but not all, there is elevated hepatic alkaline phosphatase, hepatomegaly, or both. Other solid tumors that can cause FUO include leiomyosarcomas of the gastrointestinal tract, sarcomas, and atrial myxomas.[42]

Rheumatologic disorders

Adult Still's disease, for which there is no definitive laboratory test, remains the most common rheumatologic cause of FUO.[43] The typical clinical features are myalgias, leukocytosis, lymph node enlargement, splenomegaly and an evanescent rash that appears with febrile episodes; other causes of this clinical presentation must be excluded.

Temporal arteritis, with or without polymyalgia rheumatica,[44] should be considered in those aged over 50 years; the erythrocyte sedimentation rate (ESR) is nearly always elevated. The classic presentation of temporal arteritis, headache, jaw claudication, visual loss, or a palpable temporal artery, may be absent in one-third of patients with temporal arteritis.

Other less common rheumatologic causes of FUO include Wegener's granulomatosis and cryoglobulinemia; polyarteritis nodosa should be considered if there is mononeuritis multiplex, myalgias, skin lesions, abdominal pain (which is due to small intestinal ischemia) and azotemia.[45]

Miscellaneous

A diverse array of conditions, including granulomatous diseases, inflammatory illnesses and drug-related fevers, are classified as miscellaneous. Crohn's disease, sarcoidosis and granulomatous hepatitis are examples of granulomatous diseases.[46] Patients with granulomatous hepatitis require a biopsy of involved tissue and exclusion of other causes of this histologic pattern, such as infections with *Mycobacteria* spp., fungi, or bacteria (e.g. brucellosis, tularemia, cat scratch disease) and lymphoma.

Other conditions which need to be considered include alcoholic hepatitis,[47] pulmonary emboli,[48] subacute thyroiditis, Sweet's syndrome and familial Mediterranean fever.[49] Leukocytosis may occur with these conditions, but it is often especially prominent in alcoholic hepatitis and familial Mediterranean fever.[48] Fever most often resolves within a few days following anticoagulation in patients who have pulmonary emboli, but it may take longer in certain instances.[48] Familial Mediterranean fever causes recurrent fever, peritonitis and leukocytosis. Subacute thyroiditis may be difficult to diagnose because there are usually no systemic features of thyrotoxicosis and the thyroid function tests are usually normal. The thyroid gland may be nontender; however, it is commonly diffusely enlarged.[49] Schnitzler's syndrome (hyperostosis, lymph node enlargement and monoclonal IgM gammopathy) is a rare cause of FUO.[49]

Hematomas and drug fever may cause FUO.[50] Hematomas causing FUO may occur as a result of hemorrhages into the abdominal cavity or retroperitoneal space, but bleeding within the wall of an aneurysm or dissection of the thoracic or abdominal aorta has also been reported as being responsible.[50] In these cases, persistent fever and anemia typically follow an episode of chest, back, or abdominal pain that spontaneously resolves.[50] Trauma may predispose to the formation of hematomas that occur in extravascular spaces.

Drug fever can occur with virtually any medication, even those administered for long periods without previous problems (Fig. 3.2).[51]

DRUGS ASSOCIATED WITH FUO	
Common	Less common
Atropine	Allopurinol
Amphotericin	Hydralazine
Penicillins	Isoniazid
Cephalosporins	Rifampin (rifampicin)
Phenytoin	Macrolides
Procainamide	Clindamycin
Quinidine	Vancomycin
Sulfonamides	Aminoglycosides
Interleukin-2, interferon	

Fig. 3.2 Drugs associated with FUO.

DISEASES ASSOCIATED WITH DISTINCT PATTERNS OF FEVER		
Term	Description	Disease
Intermittent	Temperature elevation returns to normal at least once during most days	Abscesses, falciparum malaria, Still's disease
Remittent	Fevers do not return to normal each day	Tuberculosis, endocarditis, typhoid fever
Relapsing	Recurrent over days or weeks	Relapsing fever, brucellosis, malaria (tertian or quartan fever pattern), lymphoma (Pel-Ebstein fever pattern)
Biphasic	Recurs only once	Leptospirosis, dengue, Colorado tick fever, lymphocytic choriomeningitis
Continuous	Fever varies less than 1.8°F (1°C) over several days	Encephalitis, drug fever, salmonella, factitious fever

Fig. 3.3 Diseases associated with distinct patterns of fever.

There may be no eosinophilia.[51] There are no distinctive clinical features that are associated with drug fever that help to distinguish it from other causes of fever that have been mentioned above.

Other miscellaneous causes of FUO are rare. Endocrinologic causes of FUO include hyperthyroidism and adrenocortical insufficiency.[49] Factitious fever does not always follow a specific pattern of a characteristic patient population, although many have the features of Munchausen syndrome.[52] In order to provide objective evidence of fever, some patients may warm the thermometer when the health care worker is not in attendance. Others may subject themselves to mutilation through such maneuvers as injecting themselves with specimens that are contaminated with micro-organisms.

Undiagnosed fever of unknown origin

Between 7 and 30% of cases remain undiagnosed despite intensive evaluations.[1–15] The long-term follow-up, available in two FUO series, shows that fever resolves in the majority of these patients within a short time.[53] In one series, follow-up was available for 8 cases in whom no diagnosis was established.[15] Fever resolved within 3 weeks of the period of FUO in 87% of cases and within 4 months in all patients. The other series investigated the long-term follow up of 49 cases of undiagnosed FUOs taken from a larger cohort of 199 cases.[53] Fever resolved within a few weeks of discharge in 31 of the 49 cases (63%), and within 2 years of discharge in 83%. In the remaining 8 patients (17%), fever recurred and required repeated courses of nonsteroidal anti-inflammatory drugs (NSAIDs) and corticosteroids. Despite the lack of diagnosis in these patients, the mortality rate 5 years after discharge was small – only 3%. Thus, in most of these patients the fever abated without treatment, and rarely did a serious disorder emerge later.[15,53]

GENERAL APPROACH TO DIAGNOSIS

Although some disorders may be associated with a distinct pattern of fever (Fig. 3.3), the charted fever curve is rarely helpful in establishing an individual diagnosis. The following approaches should be pursued because most disorders that cause FUO do not have a specific fever pattern.

Routine noninvasive tests

Recent series have shown that a growing number of cases of FUO are being identified by a variety of noninvasive tests.[13–15] Several factors may explain this observation. The number of diseases diagnosed by microbiologic methods has risen, possibly because of advances in diagnostic capabilities.[16] For example, blood cultures utilizing the lysis–centrifugation technique may identify *Mycobacteria* spp. and obviate the need for a bone marrow aspiration.[54] The practice of incubating blood cultures in a carbon-dioxide-enhanced environment and subculturing broth even in the absence of turbidity has led to the detection of infectious endocarditis caused by fastidious organisms.[33] In other instances, the available serologic techniques have supplanted the need for pathologic analyses of surgically obtained tissue;[28] for example, elevated antibody titers to *Entamoeba histolytica* in patients with hepatic masses seen on CT scans supports the diagnosis of amebiasis and avoids the need for invasive procedures.[15] Advances in serologic testing are relevant for 'older' diseases as well; for example, systemic lupus erythematosus can now be detected in a person who is negative for antinuclear antibody.[15] Also, newly described diseases that have made their first appearance as causes of FUO, such as Lyme disease or HIV infection, can be diagnosed by serologic methods.

The number of cases of FUO diagnosed by noninvasive techniques is likely to increase in the future as noninvasive diagnostic testing improves. Blood culture with use of the lysis–centrifugation technique is a sensitive method of detecting common mycobacterial and fungal infections that cause prolonged fever in patients with AIDS.[54] The development of assays such as the polymerase chain reaction (PCR) for disseminated *Mycobacterium avium* infection, may further reduce the need for invasive procedures by identifying the organism far in advance of the time that is required to isolate it from blood cultures. The application of the PCR for diagnosis of other infections, such as acute HIV infection[55] or *Legionella* infection, could also avoid the need for an invasive procedure in selected circumstances. Finally, advances in obtaining expectorated sputum and analyzing it for the presence of *Pneumocystis carinii* will drastically reduce the need for bronchoscopy for the diagnosis of *P. carinii* pneumonia in persons with AIDS who have had prolonged fevers.

Testing guided by abnormal findings

In most instances of FUO, diagnostic testing is guided by notable findings on the physical examination or by abnormal values in a routine laboratory test.[56] The careful evaluation of patients that is necessary to reach a diagnosis cannot be replaced by the early use of new diagnostic tests such as transesophageal echocardiography and MRI in an effort to hasten a diagnosis.

A uniform diagnostic algorithm is not useful because studies are most helpful when performed in a guided fashion determined by each individual case. One study has identified the amount of time and resources required to establish the diagnosis.[15] This study showed that diagnosis required a mean time of 19 days (range 1 day to 8 months), including 11 days of hospitalization (range 3 days to 5 weeks), and four outpatient visits (range: 0–11). A substantial part of the evaluation should take place in an outpatient setting[57] if the patient's condition allows.

The approach to FUO is influenced by whether abnormal findings are present in the early or later stages of FUO. Several studies have reaffirmed the paramount importance of repeated evaluation of patients with FUO in whom no abnormal findings are present in the early stages of the illness.[1–15,56] Repeated histories and physical examinations are crucial for detecting new developments. If no group of findings occur early in the febrile course, then prolonged and meticulous observation is the most successful approach to discovering the cause of FUO. This approach yields crucial findings that do not become evident until a late stage of the illness. In one series, repetition of the physical examination, selected laboratory tests, or observation after specific therapeutic intervention led to a diagnosis in 28 of the 86 cases.[15]

This study has also shown that the late appearance of abnormalities on physical examination helps to direct further diagnostic testing.[15] In this report, excisional biopsy of a skin lesion that appeared late in the course of the fever in 2 patients showed polyarteritis nodosa and Sweet's syndrome in each of them, respectively. In addition, the visual appearance of keratoderma blenorrhagicum was diagnostic of a case of Reiter's syndrome. In other situations, neither the gross nor the microscopic appearance was specific, but the diagnosis of Still's disease, systemic lupus erythematosus, POEMS (polyneuropathy, organomegaly, endocrinopathy, M protein, skin changes) syndrome and essential mixed cryoglobulinemia was aided by the late appearance of a skin eruption. In some cases of lymphoma and in one case of angio-immunoblastic lymphadenopathy, fever persisted for months before a lymph gland became enlarged.

One case series has also demonstrated that the etiology of FUO may be established when diagnostic laboratory results first appear in the later stages.[15] Examples of cases diagnosed in this fashion include viral infections that were identified by a significant rise in serologic titers for CMV, EBV or HIV. Blood cultures facilitated a diagnosis of infectious endocarditis caused by *Actinobacillus actinomycetemcomitans* and *Enterococcus faecium* and of abdominal abscesses caused by *Listeria monocytogenes*. Eosinophilic pneumonia, bronchial adenoma, and cranial subdural empyema were diagnosed by evolution of findings on radiographic studies.

One series showed that abnormal findings may be present in the early stage of the febrile illness.[15] In these cases, the abnormal findings were discovered by the initial examining physician, who decided to initiate treatment for the most likely condition before testing for the presence of less likely diseases. When fever persisted, cessation of therapy and investigation for alternative explanations of the original clinical pattern proved to be an effective clinical approach. Examples of diagnoses established in this fashion included tuberculosis in a person who had pulmonary infiltrates that did not respond to empiric antibiotics. In another case, an open thoracotomy with pleural and lung biopsy was performed when fever persisted despite antimycobacterial therapy in a man who had a bloody lymphocytic exudate and a reactive tuberculin skin test. Histopathologic stains of tissue revealed lymphomatoid granulomatosis. In these cases, the true disease process was identified only when fever persisted despite initiation of therapy for the most likely cause of the condition. It is conceivable that diagnostic riddles solved by this approach may not be considered true FUOs in the future. Rapid diagnostic tests may become available and lead to a prompt identification of the illnesses considered in the differential diagnosis prior to the initiation of treatment.

The laborious process of investigating FUOs is difficult to accomplish in today's medical environment; carefully listening to and examining a patient, contemplating the problem in a quiet environment, and collaborating with others is an arduous task. Frustration, weariness and impatience intervene when a diagnosis is not promptly reached, and they render the physician vulnerable to overlooking the appearance of a valuable new finding. The physician must expect to devote a large amount of time to pacifying impatient relatives of the patient and justifying the length of stay to insurers and administrators who would prefer a quicker solution.

Blind testing in absence of abnormal findings

Although previous series and reviews have stressed the fact that tests that are not guided by abnormalities found on physical examination have a low diagnostic yield, one series showed that diagnoses were established by such tests in 10% of cases.[15] An example from this series is a biopsy of a temporal artery that revealed temporal arteritis in an elderly woman who had an elevated ESR but no localizing symptoms for that disorder. In addition, abdominal CT scanning led to a specific diagnosis in 6% of total cases; for example, one such CT scan showed extensive liver metastases in a man with stomach cancer who had no liver enlargement and normal liver function tests. In other cases, abdominal CT scans identified retroperitoneal lymphadenopathy despite the absence of abnormalities detected on physical examination; specific diagnoses were established by biopsies of the enlarged nodes.

Percutaneous CT-guided techniques are useful for obtaining diagnostic specimens in patients who have abnormalities identified by abdominal CT scan.[58] The quantity of the material obtained by these procedures may be inadequate to demonstrate characteristic histopathologic changes of neoplasms,[26] but it is often sufficient for microbiologic analysis to be able to establish the diagnosis of an infectious process. One series showed that the yield of these procedures is high for infection but low for tumor.[15] Exploratory laparotomy, now hardly ever required for diagnostic purposes,[59] continues to be a useful method for characterizing lesions that remain undiagnosed after percutaneous procedures or that were not amenable to this approach. Biopsies of tissue that are found to be abnormal by physical examination (e.g. lymph node) or diagnostic imaging techniques (e.g. lung) have been shown to have a higher yield (38%) than routine biopsies of bone marrow or liver (see below).

In contrast, 'blind' serologic and biopsy procedures are often fruitless at best and may actually prove misleading, thereby resulting in the pursuit of unnecessary diagnostic measures. For example, serologic testing for zoonotic infections such as tularemia, Lyme disease, or Rocky Mountain spotted fever should be performed only if the patient has been exposed to a relevant animal or tick; similarly, review of serial blood smears for malaria or serologic testing for conditions such as amebiasis or leishmaniasis should be undertaken only if the patient has been in an endemic region (Fig. 3.4).

The yield of routine bone marrow examination and liver biopsy has been mentioned in several case series.[13–15] The diagnostic yield of bone marrow examination varies but is low in most series, ranging from 0 to 14%.[13,15] Liver biopsy has been commented upon as being useful in several series,[60,61] but these series do not list the diagnostic yield. For example, Petersson's two series state that needle biopsy of the liver is of particular value in certain cases, even when hepatomegaly or jaundice are absent, because of the frequent involvement of this organ in systemic disease.[8,12] More recent series[13] report that the diagnostic yield of liver biopsy is 14%.

The previously useful diagnostic laparotomy has been supplanted by the abdominal CT scan,[15] and recent studies suggest that there is no longer an indication for routine exploratory laparotomy in the evaluation of FUO.[59]

The yield from biopsy of the temporal artery in elderly patients with an ESR above 40mm/h is not available in any case series. However, reports on temporal arteritis estimate that up to 30% of patients with this illness do not have the classic localizing symptoms. Moreover, several series comment that biopsy of the temporal artery should be performed early in the evaluation of an elderly patient with an ESR above 40mm/h, because giant cell arteritis is a common cause of FUO in this age group and also because early recognition and treatment of giant cell arteritis can prevent the sudden blindness that it sometimes causes. Figure 3.5 lists the distribution of conditions causing FUO in elderly patients.[62]

The usefulness of screening with radionuclide scans in patients with FUO remains unestablished.[63–65] Several reports suggest that the value of these scans in FUO has been over-rated and that the overall value of the test has been disappointing and potentially misleading. In one large series, approximately 14% of gallium-67 scans were helpful in providing a diagnosis but false-positive results that were potentially misleading and led to unnecessary testing occurred in 21% of patients.[13] This series was performed before the widespread use of abdominal CT scanning. Because abdominal CT scanning has proven to be of value in the evaluation of FUO, it may further reduce the value of gallium-67 scans in this setting. The diagnostic yield of indium-labeled leukocyte scanning,[64] technetium-labeled antigranulocyte antibody and indium-labeled polyclonal IgG[65] has not been systematically evaluated. Indium scans but may be even less useful than gallium scans because tumors may elude uptake of indium-labeled leukocyte scans. Because radionucleotide scans may give misleading results, they should not be part of the standard evaluation of FUO. Because of false-positive test results, physicians should be cautious in interpreting the findings and should not recommend invasive procedures based solely on positive radionucleotide scans.

Drug-related fevers

When a drug-related fever should be considered, necessary drugs can be changed to alternatives of a different class. After stopping the agent that is responsible for the fever, the fever will usually resolve within 3 days, although it may take as long as 2 weeks. Persistence of fever beyond this should direct the clinician to investigate an alternate source. If the fever remits, the clinician can definitively confirm the diagnosis by reinstituting the agent, which characteristically elicits fever again within a few hours. This procedure is safe unless drug-induced organ damage, such as interstitial nephritis or hepatitis, has occurred.

Therapeutic interventions

In most instances therapeutic trials should be discouraged in the early course of FUOs. The purpose of such trials is to establish a diagnosis by noticing an abatement of fever following the use of a therapeutic agent such as an antibiotic, a corticosteroid, or a NSAID. The empiric use of agents such as these may be misleading for several reasons:

- medical intervention makes it difficult to determine whether a new finding has resulted from the treatment of the underlying disease;
- fall of temperature may be fortuitous or it may result from the antipyretic effects of corticosteroids or NSAIDs; and
- improper use of antibiotics may lead to a false sense of therapeutic and diagnostic security and interfere with finding a diagnosis.

The spontaneous resolution of fever in stable patients is another reason against the empiric use of therapeutic trials. Employing empiric antibiotics except in the most urgent situations ultimately creates more frustration, confusion and despair for the physician and the patient.

Prolonged empiric therapy may have multiple deleterious consequences beyond unnecessary expense and inconvenience for the patient. When fever in a patient with a self-limiting illness coincidentally abates while receiving treatment for an unproven diagnosis (e.g. antibiotics for possible culture-negative endocarditis, antimycobacterial therapy for possible tuberculosis, or corticosteroid therapy for a collagen disorder) the patient may be exposed to unnecessary iatrogenic complications resulting from the treatment. In addition, complications resulting from unnecessary interventions may confuse further diagnostic strategies based on abnormalities on physical examination or laboratory findings. For these reasons, therapeutic interventions should be discouraged in stable patients. Nevertheless, these are occasional circumstances in which a patient has a rapidly progressive, potentially fatal illness in which empiric therapy becomes unavoidable. In such cases, for instance a pulminating vasculitis and even rarely, tuberculosis. high dose corticosteroid therapy can be lifesaving.

FEVER OF UNKNOWN ORIGIN IN HIV-INFECTED PERSONS

Fevers of unknown origin are not infrequent in the late stage of HIV infection[27] (see Chapters 5.8–5.21). One prospective study showed that fever occurred in 46% of patients with advanced HIV infection.[28] The number of FUO cases caused by AIDS-related diseases is likely to increase as HIV infection becomes more prevalent.

Several HIV-associated illnesses may present with fever before the onset of specific organ-related symptoms.[28–32,66–69] Examples include lymphoma, *Pneumocystis carinii* pneumonia, leishmaniasis and infections due to CMV, *Cryptococcus neoformans*, *Toxoplasma gondii* and *Mycobacterium tuberculosis*. Other illness, such as disseminated *Mycobacterium avium* infection and histoplasmosis, may present with constitutional symptoms alone in the absence of specific symptoms of organ involvement. To date, five series on FUO in HIV-infected persons have been published in the medical literature, with a total of 166 cumulative patients (Fig. 3.6). The mean CD4+ lymphocyte count, reported in three of the five series, were 160, 71 and 74 (range 71–180). Thus, in HIV-infected persons, FUO tends to occur in the late stage of HIV infection. A modified criteria for FUO was used in four of the five series: a fever in excess of 101°F (38.3°C) that persists for more than 4 weeks as an outpatient or 4 days as an in-patient and that has no obvious source.

EVALUATION OF FUO IN PATIENTS WITH RECENT TRAVEL, OCCUPATIONAL OR RECREATIONAL EXPOSURE

Exposure	Disease	Method of evaluation
Recent residence in or travel to an endemic region	Tuberculosis	Skin test, sputum smear
	Malaria	Blood smear
	Brucellosis	Serology, blood culture
	Hepatitis A, hepatitis E	Serology
	Typhoid fever	Blood culture
	Dengue	Serology
	Leptospirosis	Serology, urine culture
	Amebiasis	Serology, smears
Tick exposure	Relapsing fever	Blood smear
	Rocky Mountain spotted fever	Serology
	Lyme disease	Serology
	Tularemia	Serology, blood culture
Animal contact	Tularemia	Serology, blood culture
	Leptospirosis	Serology, blood culture
	Brucellosis	Serology, blood culture
	Q fever	Serology
	Psittacosis	Serology
	Murine typhus	Serology

Fig. 3.4 **Evaluation of FUO in patients with recent travel, occupational or recreational exposure.** All of the conditions that are endemic in a particular region have their own unique geographic distribution. All of the conditions associated with animal contact are caused by a unique pattern of animal exposure.

DISTRIBUTION OF CAUSES OF FUO IN THE ELDERLY

Cause of FUO	Percentage of cases of FUO
Infection (e.g. abdominal abscess, bacterial endocarditis, tuberculosis)	25–35
Connective tissue disorders (e.g. giant cell arteritis, polymyalgia rheumatica)	25–31
Neoplasia (e.g. lymphoma, carcinoma)	12–23
Unknown	9–16

Fig. 3.5 **Distribution of causes of FUO origin in the elderly.**

SUMMARY OF REPORTS OF FUO IN HIV-INFECTED PATIENTS

Report	Sepkowitz et al., 1993[28]	Bissuel et al., 1994[29]	Miralles et al., 1995[30]	Genne et al., 1992[31]	Prego et al., 1990[32]	Total no. cases	Percentage of total (%)
Total number of patients	25	57	50	22	12	166	
Mycobacterium tuberculosis	0	10	21	0	3	34	20
Mycobacterium avium	6	7	7	3	5	28	17
Other mycobacteria	0	6	0	0	0	6	3
Pneumocystis carinii pneumonia	4	3	1	3	0	11	6
Cytomegalovirus	0	5	1	1	1	8	5
HIV	1	1	0	6	0	8	5
Pyogenic infections	0	0	1	2	0	3	2
Lymphoma	4	4	2	1	0	11	6
Cryptococcosis	0	1	0	0	0	1	1
Leishmaniasis	0	4	7	1	0	12	7
Toxoplasmosis	1	2	1	0	0	4	2
Other diagnosis	5	6	3	2	0	16	10
Unknown	4	8	6	3	4	25	15
More than one causative disease	0	0	0	0	1	1	1

Fig. 3.6 Summary of reports of FUO in HIV-infected patients. In some cases, HIV itself as a cause of FUO was defined as a response to antiretroviral therapy. Included in the category of 'other diagnosis' are factitious fever, zidovudine toxicity, *Isospora belli* enteritis, *Candida* sepsis, aspergillosis, varicella-zoster encephalitis, drug fever, bleomycin pneumonitis, hepatitis B, malaria, disseminated histoplasmosis, pulmonary nocardiosis, and disseminated *Penicillium marneffei*.

Infections are the most common cause of FUO in HIV-infected persons, accounting for approximately 65% of cases (Fig. 3.6). Mycobacterial infections, both *M. tuberculosis* and *M. avium*, account for the majority of these cases. The remaining infections are due to pyogenic infections and to infections caused by *Toxoplasma gondii*, *Pneumocystis carinii*, *Cryptococcus neoformans* and *Leishmania* spp. Cytomegalovirus and HIV itself account for a small percentage of FUO, approximately 4% each. The cause of FUO was attributed to HIV alone when the diagnostic evaluation did not reveal a specific etiology and when the fever abated following antiretroviral therapy. Cases of infection with *Penicillium* spp. have been reported from South East Asia. Tumors, principally lymphomas, are responsible for 7% of cases. Miscellaneous causes, including drug fever, pelvic inflammatory disease and bleomycin lung toxicity, account for 10% of cases. The diagnosis remains unestablished in approximately 15% of cases. In 1% of cases, there was found to be more than one disease causing the unexplained fevers.

INDIVIDUAL DIAGNOSTIC TESTS

The utility of the available tests for FUO has not been determined from direct studies. Nevertheless, indirect information on their usefulness may be derived from studies that establish their sensitivity for the specific opportunistic infections that are responsible for causing FUO. The diagnostic modalities and the studies that establish their usefulness in the evaluation of HIV-associated FUO are discussed below.

Noninvasive tests

Blood cultures for bacteria, *Mycobacteria* spp., and fungi are valuable diagnostic tests in the evaluation of FUO. In one report, blood cultures had a sensitivity of 75% for disseminated *M. avium* infection; other reports suggest a sensitivity of 64–85% for *Mycobacteria* spp.[29] Available systems include Bactec, Dupont Isolator, and lysis–centrifugation systems; the comparative yield for each of these systems for FUO in HIV-infected persons is unknown. *Histoplasma capsulatum* has been grown from lysis–centrifugation system when it failed to grow in the routine biphasic blood culture system. In rare instances, other organisms may be recovered from isolator blood cultures, such as *Nocardia* spp. Buffy-coat culture for CMV infections has not been proved to be a useful test in establishing the diagnosis of disseminated CMV infection, both because patients may be viremic without having disease due to CMV infection, and because less than 50% of patients with documented CMV disease are viremic.[70]

Serum and urine antigen techniques are useful in identifying certain fungal and viral infections. The serum cryptococcal antigen is sensitive and specific for detecting dissemination with *Cryptococcus neoformans*; it is therefore a useful test for this purpose.[71] Recent reports suggest that serum antigen for CMV is sensitive for detecting dissemination due to CMV disease.[72] Antibodies for CMV are not helpful in establishing a diagnosis because 90% of HIV-positive patients have antibodies to CMV. Diagnosis of CMV esophagitis, colitis, gastritis or encephalitis requires pathologic evidence of the effects of the virus; retinitis may be diagnosed by funduscopic examination. *Histoplasma* antigen in urine or serum is a very sensitive and specific finding for the diagnosis of disseminated histoplasmosis;[73] serial antigen assessments has also been found useful in monitoring the response to therapy.

For the diagnosis of *Pneumocystis carinii* pneumonia, expectorated sputum is rarely diagnostic, because the cough is not productive in most cases. Nebulizer-induced sputum is a technique that is available in the ambulatory setting and is diagnostic in many cases because of the high number of organisms that are present in the alveoli. Published studies show that the sensitivity of the test for evaluating *P. carinii* pneumonia is 75–90%.[74,75] The technique involves centrifugation of liquefied sputum and staining the specimen with a direct fluorescent monoclonal antibody that reacts with the cyst wall. This test may establish the diagnosis of *P. carinii* pneumonia in a noninvasive fashion and avoid the need for bronchoscopy.

Invasive procedures

The introduction of sensitive noninvasive tests for diagnosing many conditions responsible for FUO in HIV-infected persons has reduced the need for invasive procedures. However, invasive procedures, such as biopsies of bone marrow, liver and abnormal lymph nodes, continue to have a role in evaluating FUO, especially when patients remain febrile despite a prolonged noninvasive evaluation.

The yield of bone marrow examination (BME) for FUO in HIV-infected persons has been investigated in several series and has ranged from 13 to 42%.[76–78] One series showed that in 86% of patients in whom a cause of the fever was identified by BME, the same diagnosis had been established by a noninvasive diagnostic modality.[78] This series also showed that in 53% of patients, the diagnosis was made by BME as rapidly as or sooner than it was by other modalities, and that in 16% of patients, the diagnosis was made exclusively by BME. The authors concluded that BME is indicated when a diagnosis is urgently sought or when an evaluation by other diagnostic modalities has been unsuccessful.[78]

The usefulness of liver and lymph node biopsy has been evaluated in several studies.[79–82] The yield from liver biopsy in evaluating FUO in HIV infected persons has varied between 40 and 58%. Biopsy of enlarged lymph nodes has been reported to have a high yield.[83–85] In a population at high risk for HIV, the yield of lymph node biopsy for tuberculosis was 57%. A fine-needle aspiration approach has also been reported to have a high diagnostic yield in one study.[85]

APPROACH TO THE DIAGNOSIS

An initial approach in the evaluation of FUO in HIV-infected persons should be to discontinue medications, especially antiviral agents and sulfonamides. The clinical features associated with opportunistic infections that cause prolonged fever often overlap with those associated with drug reactions (e.g. cytopenia and elevation of liver enzyme tests). If there is no response after 3 days, blood culture using the lysis–centrifugation technique is a sensitive method of identifying intracellular organisms that cause disseminated infections (e.g. *Histoplasma capsulatum, Cryptococcus neoformans, Mycobacterium avium*). However, because the mean time for cultures to turn positive is 18–25 days for *M. avium*,[69] other noninvasive tests should be performed simultaneously. Induced sputum for *P. carinii* and *M. tuberculosis* should be obtained because prolonged fevers may precede the onset of respiratory symptoms in both *P. carinii* pneumonia and tuberculosis. Tuberculin skin testing and antigen testing for *H. capsulatum* in serum and urine also should be performed. If the serum cryptococcal antigen is reactive at a titer of less than 1:16, a lumbar puncture should be performed, even if the patient does not complain of headache or demonstrate nuchal rigidity.[71] A dilated ophthalmologic examination should be performed to investigate retinitis due to CMV.

If the initial approach does not yield a specific diagnosis, the subsequent evaluation should include repeated physical examinations and routine laboratory work. Because abnormal findings of diagnostic importance (e.g. skin nodules, asymmetric and enlarging lymphadenopathy, and rapid and significant rise in serum alkaline phosphatase levels) may make their first appearance long after the onset of fever, abnormal organs should be biopsied and organisms looked for by special stains.

Other invasive procedures should not be performed while waiting for an organism to be isolated from lysis–centrifugation cultures if the patient remains stable, because cultures of material aspirated from bone marrow or lymph nodes or biopsied from the liver are no more sensitive than isolator blood cultures. If cultures of blood are still negative after 3 weeks, a bone marrow examination should be performed, even if the patient is stable, because the bone marrow examination has been shown to be the sole method of identifying an illness in approximately 5% of patients in whom all noninvasive tests have been unrevealing.[77,78]

In the evaluation of prolonged, unexplained fevers, the patient's previous exposures, stage of HIV infection and present epidemiologic setting often provide important clues. For example, tuberculosis should be suspected in anyone with HIV infection who has had an exposure to an infected person or who has resided in an endemic region. Similarly, histoplasmosis or coccidiomycosis may occur in persons who have been in an endemic region.[68] Leishmaniasis should be considered in people who have been in South America or the Mediterranean area. Infections caused by *Penicillium marneffei* should be considered in people who have lived in southern Asia. Extrapulmonary *Pneumocystis carinii* infections may be identified in patients in the late stages of HIV infection who have been receiving aerosolized pentamidine.[67] Infections due to *Bartonella henselae* should be considered in people who have had exposure to cats; the organism may be identified by serology or by isolator blood cultures. Finally, lymphoma should be considered in patients with no specific exposure history.

When the initial and subsequent evaluation for FUO has been unrevealing, abdominal CT scan occasionally proves to be a useful diagnostic tool. Occasionally, peritoneal masses or a group of enlarged retroperitoneal lymph nodes may be identified on the scan; a directed CT-guided biopsy of these abnormal areas on CT scan may reveal the cause of fevers. Gallium scans and indium-labeled leukocyte scans are frequently performed in the setting of prolonged unexplained fevers, but the tests are rarely of diagnostic value and are potentially misleading. Another test of uncertain significance is the buffy-coat culture of blood for CMV, because viremia may occur without symptoms and the test is insensitive for the detection of CMV disease.[72] A thorough evaluation of FUO as outlined above yields a diagnosis in approximately 85% of cases. Multiple causes for FUO will be identified in 2–10% of cases – the feature that distinguishes FUO in HIV-infected persons from those who are not infected with HIV.[32]

CONCLUSION

Since its original description in 1930, case series have shown that a careful, organized approach to the problem on the part of the physician remains of pre-eminent importance in identifying the cause of FUO. This remains true even though new diagnostic modalities that are useful in the evaluation of FUO have been introduced and the number of illnesses that are responsible for FUO has expanded. How to employ the available diagnostic tools must be individualized for each patient and remains a challenge for the physician. The role of exploratory laparotomy is limited to characterization of known lesions that remain undiagnosed after percutaneous procedures and of those that are not accessible by the percutaneous approach. Because blood culture with the use of the lysis–centrifugation technique is a sensitive method of detecting many of the infectious causes of HIV-associated FUO, invasive procedures may be avoided if the patient remains stable. Despite the introduction of new diagnostic modalities, the investigation of FUO in the general population or in HIV-infected persons remains one of the most challenging tasks for the clinician.

REFERENCES

1. Alt HL, Barker MH. Fever of unknown origin. JAMA 1930;94:1457–61.
2. Hamman L, Wainwright CW. The diagnosis of obscure fever. I. The diagnosis of unexplained, long-continuing, low-grade fever. Bull Johns Hopkins Hosp 1936;58:109–33.
3. Hamman L, Wainwright CW. The diagnosis of obscure fever. II. The diagnosis of unexplained high fever. Bull Johns Hopkins Hosp 1936;58:307–31.
4. Keefer CS. The diagnosis of the causes of obscure fever. Tex State J Med 1939;35:203–12.
5. Wolf HL, Jacobs S. Fever of undetermined origin. New Orleans Med Surg J 1947;99:441–47.
6. Bottiger LE. Fever of unknown origin with some remarks on the normal temperature in man. Acta Med Scand 1953;147:133–48.
7. Geraci JE, Weed LA, Nichols DR. Fever of obscure origin – the value of abdominal exploration in diagnosis: report of seventy cases. JAMA 1959;169:1306–15.
8. Petersdorf RG, Beeson PB. Fever of unexplained origin: report of 100 cases. Medicine (Baltimore) 1961;40:1–30.
9. Petersson T. Fever of obscure origin: a follow-up investigation of 88 cases. Acta Med Scand 1962;171:575–83.
10. Sheon RP, Van Ommen RA. Fever of obscure origin: diagnoses and treatment based on a series of 60 cases. Am J Med 1963;34:486–99.
11. Fransen H, Bottiger LE. Fever of more than two weeks duration. Acta Chem Scand 1966;179:147–55.
12. Jacoby GA, Swartz MN. Fever of undetermined origin. N Engl J Med 1973;289:1407–10.
13. Larson EB, Featherstone HJ, Petersdorf RG. Fever of undetermined origin: diagnosis and follow-up of 105 cases, 1970–1980. Medicine (Baltimore) 1982;61:269–93.
14. Knockaert DC, Vanneste LJ, Vanneste SB, Bobbers S. Fever of unknown origin in the 1980s: an update of the diagnostic spectrum. Arch Intern Med 1992;152:51–6.
15. Kazanjian PH. Fever of unknown origin: review of 86 patients treated in community hospitals. Clin Infect Dis 1992;15:968–73.
16. Washington JA, Ilstrup DM. Blood cultures: issues and controversies. Rev Infect Dis 1986;8:792–802.

17. Huang HK, Aberle DR, Luftkin R, Grant EG, Hanafee WN, Kangarloo H. Advances in medical imaging. Ann Intern Med 1990;112:203–20.

18. Centers for Disease Control. Urine testing for drug use among male arrestees – United States. MMWR Morbidity and Mortality Weekly Report 1989;38:780–3.

19. Sugarman B, Yound EJ. Infections associated with prosthetic devices: magnitude of the problem. Infect Dis Clin North Am 1989;3:187–98.

20. Hill DR. Tropical and travel-associated diseases: editorial overview. Curr Opin Infect Dis; 1991;4:261–4.

21. Centers for Disease Control. Current trends update: acquired immunodeficiency syndrome – United States, 1981–1989. MMWR Morb Mortal Wkly Rep 1989;38:229–36.

22. Steere AC. Lyme disease. N Engl J Med 1989;321:586–96.

23. Vyse T. Rheumatic fever: changes in its incidence and presentation. Br Med J 1991;302:518–20.

24. Snider DE, Roper WL. The new tuberculosis. N Engl J Med 1992;326:703–5.

25. Petersdorf RG. FUO: how it has changed in 20 years. Hosp Pract 1985;20:84I–84M, 84T–84V.

26. Petersdorf R. Fever of unknown origin: an old friend revisited. Arch Intern Med 1992;152:21–2.

27. Durack D, Street A. Fever of unknown origin: reexamined and redefined. In: Remington JS, Swartz MN, eds. Current clinical topics in infectious diseases, Vol. 11. Boston: Blackwell Scientific; 1991:35–51.

28. Sepkowitz KA, Telzak EE, Carrow M, Armstrong D. Fever among outpatients with advanced human immunodeficiency virus infection. Arch Intern Med 1993;153:1909–12.

29. Bissuel F, Leport C, Perronne C, Longuet P, Vilde JL. Fever of unknown origin in HIV-infected patients: a critical analysis of a retrospective series of 57 cases. J Intern Med 1994;236:529–35.

30. Miralles P, Moreno S, Perez-Tascon M, Cosin J, Diaz MD, Bouza E. Fever of uncertain origin in paitents infected with the human immunodeficiency virus. Clin Infect Dis 1995;20:872–5.

31. Genne D, Chave JP, Glaser MP. Fievre d'origine indterminee dans un collectif de patients HIV positifs. Schweiz Med Wochenschr 1992;122:1797–1802.

32. Prego V, Glatt AE, Roy V, Thelmo W, Dincsoy H, Raufman JP. Comparative yield of blood culture for fungi and mycobacteria, liver biopsy, and bone marrow biopsy in the diagnosis of fever of undetermined origin in human immunodeficiency virus-infected patients. Arch Intern Med 1990;150:333–6.

33. Koneman EW, Allen SD, Janda WM, et al. Miscellaneous and fastidious gram negative bacilli. In: Koneman EL, ed. Color diagnostic microbiology. Philadelphia: Lippincott; 1994:137–65.

34. Freund R, Pichl J, Heyder N, Rode W, Reimann JF. Splenic abscess – clinical symptoms and diagnostic possibilities. Am J Gastroenterol 1982;77:35–8.

35. Knockaert DC. Fever of unknown origin, a literature survey. Acta Clin Belg 1992;47:42–57.

36. Lobell M, Boggs DR, Wintrobe MM. The clinical significance of fever in Hodgkin's disease. Arch Intern Med 1966;117:335–42.

37. Tabbara SO, Frierson HH, Fechner RE. Diagnostic problems in tissues previously sampled by fine-needle aspiration. Am J Clin Pathol 1991;96:76–80.

38. Egeler RM, Schmitz L, Sonnevald P, Manniva IC, Nesbit ME. Malignant histiocytosis: a reassessment of cases formerly classified as histiocytic neoplasms and review of the literature. Med Pediatr Oncol 1995;25:1–7.

39. Freter CE, Cossman J. Angioimmunoblastic lymphadenopathy with dysproteinemia. Semin Oncol 1993;20:627–35.

40. Bailey EM, Klein NC, Cunha BA. Kikuchi's diseases with liver dysfunction presenting as fever of unknown origin. Lancet 1989;2:986.

41. Klastersky J, Weerts D, Hensgens C, Debusscher L. Fever of unexplained origin in patients with cancer. Eur J Cancer 1973;9:649–56.

42. Reynen K. Cardiac myxomas. N Engl J Med 1995;333:1610–7.

43. Pouchot J, Sampalis JS, Beaudet F, et al. Adult Still's disease: manifestations, disease course, and outcome in 62 patients. Medicine 1991;70:118–36.

44. Hunder GG. Giant cell (temporal) arteritis. Rheum Dis Clin North Am 1990;16:399–409.

45. Lhote F, Guillevin L. Polyarteritis nodosa, microscopic polyangiitis, and Churg–Strauss syndrome. Clinical aspects and treatment. Rheumatol Clin North Am 1995;21:911–45.

46. Zoutman DE, Ralph ED, Frei JV. Granulomatous hepatitis and fever of unknown origin. An 11-year experience of 23 cases with three years follow-up. J Clin Gastroenterol 1991;13:69–75.

47. Achord JL. Review of alcoholic hepatitis, and its treatment. Am J Gastroenterol 1993;88:1822–31.

48. Murray HW, Ellis GC, Blumenthal DS, Sos TA. Fever and pulmonary thromboembolism. Am J Med 1979;67:232–5.

49. Molavi A, Weinstein L. Persistent perplexing pyrexia: some comments on etiology and diagnosis. Med Clin North Am 1970;54:379–96.

50. Giladi M, Pines A, Averbuch M, Hershkoviz R, Sherez J, Levo Y. Aortic dissection manifested as fever of unknown origin. Cardiology 1991;78:78–80.

51. Mackowiak PA, LeMaistre CF. Drug fever: a critical appraisal of conventional concepts. An analysis of 51 episodes in two Dallas hospitals and 97 episodes reported in the English literature. Ann Intern Med 1987;106:728–33.

52. Aduan RP, Fauci AS, Dale DC, Herzberg JH, Wolff SM. Factitious fever and self-induced infection. A report of 32 cases and review of the literature. Ann Intern Med 1979;90:230–42.

53. Knockaert DC, Dujardin KS, Bobbaers HJ. Long-term follow-up of patients with undiagnosed fever of unknown origin. Arch Intern Med 1996;156:618–20.

54. Gill VJ, Park CH, Stock F, Gosey LL, Witebsky FG, Masur H. Use of lysis-centrifugation (Isolator) and radiometric (BACTEC) blood culture systems for the detection of mycobacteremia. J Clin Microbiol 1985;22:543–6.

55. Ou C-Y, Kwok S, Mitchell SW, et al. DNA amplification for direct detection of HIV-1 in DNA of peripheral blood mononuclear cells. Science 1988;239:295–7.

56. Brusch JL, Weinstein L. Fever of unknown origin. Med Clin North Am 1988;72:1247–61.

57. Jacobs C, Lamprey J. Diagnostic categories of review. In: Dahlgren R, Clark S, eds. The criteria for intensity of service, severity of illness and discharge screens – a review system with adult criteria. Westboro, Massachusetts: Interqual; 1988:28–32.

58. Gerzof S, Spira R, Robbins A. Percutaneous abscess drainage. Semin Roentgenol 1981;16:62–71.

59. Greenall MJ, Gough MH, Kettlewell MG. Laparotomy in the investigation of patients with pyrexia of unknown origin. Br J Surg 1983;70:356–7.

60. Mitchell DP, Hanes TE, Hoyumpa AM, Schenker S. Fever of unknown origin. Assessment of percutaneous liver biopsy. Arch Intern Med 1977;137:1001–4.

61. Holtz T, Moseley RH, Scheiman JM. Liver biopsy in fever of unknown origin. A reappraisal. J Clin Gastroenterol 1993;17:29–32.

62. Norman D, Yoshikawa T. Fever in the elderly. Infect Dis Clin North Am 1996;10:93–9.

63. Knockaert DC, Mortelmans LA, De Roo MC, Bobbaers HJ. Clinical value of gallium-67 scintigraphy in evaluation of fever of unknown origin. Clin Infect Dis 1994;18:601–5.

64. MacSweeney JE, Peters AM, Lavender JP. Indium labelled leukocyte scanning in pyrexia of unknown origin. Clin Radiol 1990;42:414–17.

65. Becker W, Dolkemeyer U, Gramatzki M, Schneider MU, Scheele J, Wolf F. Use of immunoscintigraphy in the diagnosis of fever of unknown origin. Eur J Nucl Med 1993;20:1078–83.

66. Katz MH, Hessol NA, Buchbinder SP, et al. Temporal trends of opportunistic infections and malignancies in homosexual men with AIDS. J Infect Dis 1994;170:198–202.

67. Cohen O, Stoeckle MY. Extrapulmonary Pneumocystis carinii infections in the acquired immunodeficiency syndrome. Arch Intern Med 1991;151:1205–14.

68. Wheat LJ, Connolly-Stringfield PA, Baker RL, et al. Disseminated histoplasmosis in the acquired immune deficiency syndrome: clinical findings, diagnosis, and treatment, and review of the literature. Medicine 1990;69:361–73.

69. Young LS. Mycobacterium avium complex infection. J Infect Dis 1988;157:863–7.

70. Zurlo JJ, O'Neill D, Polis MA, et al. Lack of clinical utility of cytomegalovirus blood and urine cultures in patients with HIV infection. Ann Intern Med 1993;118:12–7.

71. Powderly W, Clioud G, Dismukes W, et al. Measurement of cryptococcal antigen in serum and CSF: value in the management of AIDS-associated cryptococcal meningitis. Clin Infect Dis 1994;18:789–92.

72. Salzberger B, Franzen C, Fatkenheuer G, et al. CMV antigenemia in peripheral blood for the diagnosis of CMV disease in HIV-infected patients. J Acquir Immune Defic Syndr 1996;11:365–9.

73. Wheat LJ, Kohler RB, Tewari RP. Diagnosis of disseminated histoplasmosis by detection of Histoplasma capsulatum antigen in serum and urine specimens. N Engl J Med 1986;314:83–8.

74. Kovacs JA, Ng VL, Leong G, et al. Diagnosis of Pneumocystis pneumonia: Improved detection in sputum with use of monoclonal antibodies. N Engl J Med 1988;318:589.

75. Ng VL, Garner I, Weymouth LA, et al. The use of mucolysed induced sputum for the identification of pulmonary pathogens associated with HIV infection. Arch Pathol Lab Med 1989:113:488.

76. Nichols L, Florentine B, Lewis W, Sattler F, Rarick MU, Brynes RK. Bone marrow examination for the diagnosis of mycobacterial and fungal infections in the acquired immunodeficiency syndrome. Arch Pathol Lab Med 1991;115:1125–32.

77. Northfelt DW, Mayer A, Kaplan LD, et al. The usefulness of diagnostic bone marrow examination in patients with human immunodeficiency virus (HIV) infection. J Acquir Immune Defic Syndr 1991;4:659–66.

78. Engels E, Marks PW, Kazanjian P. Usefulness of bone marrow examination in the evaluation of unexplained fevers in patients infected with human immunodeficiency virus. Clin Infect Dis 1995;21:427–8.

79. Cavicchi M, Pialoux G, Carnot F, et al. Valve of liver biopsy for the rapid diagnosis of infection in human immunodeficiency virus-infected patients who have unexplained fever and elevated serum levels of alkaline phosphatase of γ-glutamyl transferase. Clin Infect Dis 1995;20:606–10.

80. Grinberg N, Martinez A, Cahn P, et al. Liver biopsy is a useful diagnostic tool in HIV disease. Inf Conf AIDS 8(2):B117 Abstract POB3183, Amsterdam, The Netherlands, 19–24 Jul 1992.

81. Oehler R, Loos U, Ferber J, Fischer HP. Diagnostic valve of liver biopsy in HIV patients with unexplained fever. Int Conf AIDS 8(2):B211 Abstract POB3722, Amsterdam, The Netherlands, 19–24 Jul 1992.

82. Rogeaux O, Priqueler L, Hoang C, et al. Diagnostic usefulness of liver biopsy for unexplained fever in HIV patients. Int Conf AIDS 9(1):446 Abstract PO-B19-1867, Berlin, Germany, 6–11 Jun 1993.

83. Brynes RK, Chan WC, Spira, et al. Value oflymph node biopsy in unexplained lymphadenopathy in homosexual men. JAMA 1983;250:1313–7.

84. Hewlett D, Duncanson FP, Jagadha V, et al. Lymphadenopathy in anninner city population consisting principally of intravenous drug users with AIDS. Am Rev Respir Dis 1988;137:1275–9.

85. Bottles K, McPhaul LW, Volberding P. Fine needle aspiration biopsy ofpatients with AIDS; experience in an outpatient clinic. Ann Intern Med 1988;108:42–5.

Chronic Fatigue

Nelson M Gantz

Fatigue is one of the most common complaints in ambulatory care and in one report in an adult primary care clinic, 24% of patients indicated that fatigue was a major problem.[1] Laboratory tests are not helpful in determining the cause of the fatigue in the majority of patients and at 1-year follow-up, about 75% of patients have persistent fatigue. Over the past decade there has been a worldwide increase in attention to patients reporting fatigue, cognitive difficulties, malaise, weakness, myalgias, arthralgias, headache and low-grade fever. This disorder has in recent years been called the chronic fatigue syndrome (CFS), myalgic encephalomyelitis and the postviral fatigue syndrome.[2–4] In the press, the disorder has been referred to as 'yuppie flu'.

The diagnosis of CFS continues to stir controversy. It is a waxing and waning illness, the fundamental nature of which remains uncertain. Some physicians deny its existence. Others specialize in the disorder, and evaluate patients who have a battery of viral serologies and various immunologic tests to confirm the diagnosis. Management strategies also evoke a diverse spectrum of responses. Some physicians use symptomatic treatment and others immediately prescribe a variety of exotic therapies, ranging from antiviral drugs to vitamins and herbal agents. Difficulty in identifying the cause of CFS has complicated the disorder's diagnostic definition, which, in turn, has introduced a measure of uncertainty when considering treatment options. The diagnosis is made by exclusion.

In my experience, about 20% of patients gradually improve and 80% have intermittent exacerbations. Unfortunately, some patients fail to respond to symptomatic therapy and must be considered disabled. Among those who fare poorly, some have a history of psychiatric illness, particularly depression. Unless an etiologic agent or unifying pathophysiology for CFS is identified, diagnosis will remain empiric and treatment largely supportive. It is important that clinicians recognize that CFS can be disabling, and provide support as the patient and family go through the difficult process of seeking disability benefits.

HISTORY

Chronic fatigue syndrome is not a new medical disorder. Patients who have a syndrome of fatigue, malaise and other somatic complaints have been recognized in the literature for more than 200 years (Fig. 4.1). In 1750, Sir Richard Manningham described febricula or little fever, an illness in which patients had weariness all over, pain, forgetfulness and low-grade fever.[5] In 1869, Beard coined the term neurasthenia to describe patients who lacked 'nerve strength', which he believed was the cause for the chronic fatigue.[6] Shortly after Beard's work was published, DaCosta described a syndrome of fatigue, breathlessness, palpitations, digestive problems, chest pain, sleep difficulties and dizziness in Civil War soldiers. DaCosta attributed the syndrome to an 'irritable heart'.[7] This syndrome was subsequently called the effort syndrome and the diagnosis continued to stir controversy in the 20th century, and it was supported on psychologic and physiologic grounds. In the 1940s, DaCosta's syndrome lost support as a distinct clinical entity.[15] Since then, numerous reports have appeared in the literature describing patients similar to those characterized by Beard with neurasthenia. Some of these outbreaks are listed in Figure 4.1.[8–14] In the British Commonwealth, because neurologic symptoms have

been prominent in some of the case clusters, the syndrome has been called benign myalgic encephalomyelitis.

Reports of patients who have fatiguing illnesses have also been attributed to various pathogens and to metabolic and environmental factors. In the 1930s, *Brucella* was erroneously linked as a cause of CFS.[16] Similarly, hypoglycemia, *Candida albicans* and the 'total allergy syndrome' have also been popular but unproved causes of this syndrome.[17,18] In the 1980s, chronic infection with Epstein–Barr virus (EBV) was thought to be associated with CFS.[19,20] However, when appropriate control populations were studied, EBV was not found to be a cause of CFS.[14] Other pathogens such as *Borrelia burgdorferi*, human herpesvirus-6 and human retroviruses have also been erroneously implicated as having a causative role in this disorder.[21–25]

Fibromyalgia, formerly called fibrosis, is a disorder that also has a long history and is seen commonly by rheumatologists.[26] The illness was described in the French literature in the 1850s and the clinical features overlap those seen in patients who have CFS.[27]

EPIDEMIOLOGY AND CASE DEFINITION

In 1987, the Centers for Disease Control and Prevention (CDC) convened a group of experts to develop a case definition for CFS for research and epidemiologic purposes. The definition required severe fatigue to be present for at least 6 months and no evidence of various illnesses that could produce chronic fatigue. In addition to these major criteria, the definition required the presence of eight criteria from the following symptoms or physical signs:
- the symptom criteria were fever and chills, sore throat, swollen neck or arm glands, muscle weakness, myalgias, post-exertional malaise, headaches, arthralgias, sleep disturbance, neuropsychiatric symptoms such as problems with memory, concentration and depression, and an acute onset;[2] and
- the physical sign criteria were low-grade fever, nonexudative pharyngitis and cervical or axillary lymphadenopathy.

SELECTED FATIGUING DISORDERS	
Condition	Year reported
Febricula[5]	1750
Neurasthenia[6]	1869
DaCosta's syndrome[7]	1871
Atypical poliomyelitis[8]	1934
Icelandic disease[9] (Akureyri disease)	1948
Epidemic of poliomyelitis-like illness[10] Adelaide, Australia	1949
Royal Free disease[11]	1955
Punta Gorda illness, Florida[12]	1956
Myalgic encephalomyelitis[13]	1956
Lake Tahoo illness[14]	1987

Fig. 4.1 Selected fatiguing disorders.

In 1991, a conference organized by the National Institutes of Health (NIH) proposed that certain patients be excluded: those who have chronic medical conditions, such as malignancy or autoimmune disease, psychotic depression, bipolar disorder or schizophrenia; those prone to substance abuse; and those who have postinfectious diseases, such as chronic active hepatitis B or C, untreated Lyme disease or HIV infection.[28] Patients who have a diagnosis of fibromyalgia, non-psychotic depression, somatoform disorders, or anxiety or panic disorders were to be included. The original case definition and the modifications proposed by the NIH conference were developed by consensus based on the anecdotal experience of the participants. Using this case definition, the CDC implemented a surveillance system in four US cities. The case records of 565 patients were reviewed and 23% were found to have fulfilled the case definition, 18% had unexplained chronic fatigue plus insufficient symptoms to meet the case definition, 42% had psychiatric disease before the onset of the fatiguing illness and 18% were found to have other medical disorders (unpublished CDC data). In this and another study, the physical examination criteria were found infrequently and did not contribute to the diagnosis.[29] The purpose of the definition was to select a homogeneous group of patients who have 'true CFS'. However, although the case definition did distinguish CFS cases from healthy controls and patients who have multiple sclerosis or depression, the criteria failed to separate CFS patients from other persons who have prolonged fatigue.[29]

At about the same time, a UK case definition and an Australian case definition were published.[30–32] The UK definition required the presence of severe fatigue and cognitive impairment. Patients who have medical conditions known to produce chronic fatigue and psychiatric disorders, such as schizophrenia, manic depressive illness, substance abuse, eating disorders, or organic brain disease, were excluded. Patients who have a fatiguing illness with a documented postinfectious onset should be identified.[30] The Australian case definition is similar to that of the UK;[31,32] three subtypes are recognized – a postinfectious type, a neuropsychologic type with depression and one associated with fibromyalgia.

In 1993, a meeting was held at the CDC to revise the original case definition published in 1988. The study group consisted of worldwide experts including persons involved in the earlier UK and Australian case definitions. The criteria for diagnosis are given in Figure 4.2.[33] Unexplained fatigue must be present for at least 6 months and CFS remains a diagnosis of exclusion. Four symptom criteria must be concurrently present for 6 months. Selected laboratory tests and mental status examination are performed to identify exclusionary disorders (Fig. 4.3). Patients who have severe fatigue for 6 months, the absence of other conditions to explain the fatigue, but less than four symptom criteria are designated as having idiopathic chronic fatigue. Patients who have anxiety and mild depression are not excluded. Fibromyalgia and depression are important overlapping disorders.

Chronic fatigue syndrome has been reported worldwide with most of the studies from the UK, Australia and the USA. The prevalence varies from study to study, reflecting differences in surveillance methods and in the case definition used. In a study from Australia, the prevalence rate was 37 cases per 100,000 persons.[32] A CDC study that collected data from four US cities found a prevalence rate of 2–7.3 cases per 100,000 persons using the 1988 case definition.[34] In a large community survey of fatigue in Washington state, USA, the prevalence rate of CFS ranged from 98 to 267 cases per 100,000 persons and the frequency of fatigue alone was much higher.[35] In a small study from Scotland, the prevalence of CFS was much higher with a rate of 560 per 100,000 persons.[36] Most studies show a female (75%) predominance with the average age ranging from 30 to 40 years. Disease also occurs in adolescents and the elderly.[37] All socioeconomic groups are affected. Cases occur sporadically and in outbreaks or clusters. No differences have been noted in sporadic cases compared with epidemic cases. Patients report three patterns of symptom onset: an acute onset of illness without precipitating cause, postinfectious onset or gradual onset of symptoms. Further studies are needed to compare

the type of onset with the course of the illness. Chronic fatigue syndrome does not appear to be contagious.

PATHOGENESIS AND PATHOLOGY

The etiology and pathogenesis of CFS is unknown. Patients who have CFS often cite an infectious illness such as a presumed viral respiratory tract infection as the inciting event. Much attention has focused on EBV as a possible cause of CFS in response to two reports in 1987.[19,20] However, other studies failed to demonstrate a difference in EBV antibody levels between cases and controls.[14,38] One UK report found

---

REVISED (1994) CFS CASE DEFINITION CRITERIA

1. Clinically evaluated, unexplained, persistent or relapsing fatigue for at least 6 months that:

- Is of new or definite onset
- Is not the result of ongoing exertion
- Is not substantially alleviated by rest
- Results in substantial reduction in previous levels of occupational, educational, social or personal activities

2. Four or more of the following concurrent symptoms on a persistent or recurrent basis during 6 or more consecutive months of illness, none of which may predate the fatigue:

- Self-reported impairment in short-term memory or concentration that is severe enough to cause substantial reduction in previous levels of occupational, educational, social or personal activities
- Sore throat
- Tender cervical or axillary lymph nodes
- Muscle pain
- Multijoint pain without joint swelling or redness
- Headaches of a new type, pattern or severity
- Unrefreshing sleep
- Post-exertional malaise lasting more than 24 hours

Both 1 and 2 are required conditions for a diagnosis of CFS.

Fig. 4.2 Revised (1994) CFS case definition criteria. With permission from Quadrant Healthcom.[68]

CONDITIONS THAT EXCLUDE THE DIAGNOSIS OF CFS

- Any active medical condition that may explain the presence of chronic fatigue, e.g. untreated hypothyroidism, sleep apnea, narcolepsy, adverse effects of medications, HIV disease

- Any previously diagnosed medical condition without resolution documented beyond reasonable clinical doubt, and for which continued activity may explain the chronic fatiguing illness, e.g. previously treated malignancies and unresolved cases of hepatitis B or hepatitis C virus infection

- Any past or current diagnosis of major depression with melancholic or psychotic features, bipolar affective disorder, schizophrenia of any subtype, delusional disorders of any subtype, dementias of any type, anorexia nervosa or bulimia

- Alcohol or other substance abuse within 2 years before the onset of the chronic fatigue and any time afterwards

- Severe obesity as defined by a body mass index (BMI)≥45:

$$BMI = \frac{weight\ in\ kg}{(height\ in\ m)^2}$$

- Any unexplained physical examination finding or laboratory or imaging test abnormality that strongly suggests the presence of an exclusionary condition

Fig. 4.3 Conditions that exclude the diagnosis of CFS. With permission from Quadrant Healthcom.[68]

higher levels of enterovirus in the stools of patients who have postviral fatigue syndrome than in those of control patients.[39] In another study, enteroviral RNA was identified in muscle biopsies from 20% of CFS patients compared with zero in control patients.[40] However, persistent enterovirus infection was not supported by a report from The Netherlands and another case–control study from the USA.[41,42] In one report, human T-cell leukemia/lymphoma virus (HTLV)-1 antibodies were detected in 50% of adults who had CFS and in none of the controls.[23] In the same study, HTLV-II gag sequences were found in the sera of 83% of adults who had CFS, 72% of children who had CFS and in none of the controls. These results were not confirmed by a study of 21 patients conducted by the CDC.[24] Other investigators have also failed to confirm the retrovirus finding and have not detected antibody to spumavirus in the blood, another CFS implicated retrovirus.[25] Antibody levels of other agents, including arboviruses, cytomegalovirus, human herpesvirus-6, varicella-zoster virus, respiratory viruses (adenovirus, parainfluenza virus types 1, 2 and 3, respiratory syncytial virus), hepatitis viruses, measles virus, *Rickettsia* spp., *Bartonella* spp., *B. burgdorferi*, *Chlamydia* spp. and *C. albicans,* were not found more frequently in CFS patients than in matched controls.[42] Although many different infectious agents have been suspected of having an etiologic role in CFS, none qualifies as the sole cause of the illness. It also appears that after certain acute infections, such as influenza, brucellosis or adequately treated Lyme disease, CFS can develop.[43–45] The mechanism that accounts for CFS in this setting after an acute infection is unknown.

Chronic fatigue syndrome may be a neuroendocrine rather than an infectious disorder. There is a clear association between stress, the immune system, the endocrine system and CFS. Symptoms of CFS such as fatigue, myalgias and sleep problems occur in patients who have adrenal insufficiency. Patients who have CFS have been reported as having reduced serum levels of basal evening glucocorticords and decreased 24-hour urinary free cortisol excretion compared with controls.[46] Plasma adrenocorticotropic hormone (ACTH) levels were not reduced and a decreased response of ACTH to ovine corticotropin-releasing hormone was noted. These results do not suggest either adrenal or pituitary insufficiency, but a possible hypothalmic problem. A controlled study that compared normal replacement doses of hydrocortisone with placebo doses in patients who have CFS showed no differences in symptoms (Straus S, personal communication). Plasma levels of 5-hydroxyindolacetic acid, a metabolite of serotonin, were noted to be increased in patients who have CFS.[47] In another study, prolactin levels were normal.[48] The interpretation of these various findings is unclear but future studies should clarify the meaning of such metabolic abnormalities.

In addition to fatigue, patients who have CFS often complain of lightheadedness and cognitive dysfunction. Reports have shown abnormal tilt table tests in patients who have CFS; 96% versus 29% for controls.[49] Therapy for this neurally mediated hypotension using increase in dietary salt intake, fludrocortisone, β-adrenergic blocking agents and disopyramide alone or in combination were associated with a reduction in symptoms in an uncontrolled study. A controlled trial using drugs to treat patients who have abnormal tilt table tests is needed.

A high frequency of atopy and positive immediate skin tests has been reported in patients who have CFS.[50,51] Further studies are needed to define the role of allergy in CFS.

Immunologic abnormalities similar to those reported with acute viral infections have frequently been noted in CFS patients.[52–54] Alpha-interferon and other cytokines such as interleukin (IL)-6 may be elevated in some patients who have CFS.[55] Flu-like symptoms have been associated with increased levels of various cytokines. The finding of persistent cytokine abnormalities in some studies along with an increase in CD8+ lymphocyte cell subsets showing activation markers is intriguing;[56] however, they do not provide a diagnostic test for CFS. It is important not to overinterpret the lymphocyte phenotyping data because the results have not been consistent, nor identified in the

majority of patients who have CFS. These abnormalities of increased cytokines and evidence of immune activation in many cases of CFS have led some to suggest that the illness be named 'chronic fatigue immune dysfunction syndrome'. This name or illness should not be confused with immune deficiency.

Possible factors in the pathogenesis of CFS are summarized in Figure 4.4. Likely predisposing factors include psychiatric illness, and genetic and environmental factors such as allergy. Delayed recovery from influenza virus infection was noted more frequently in patients who have pre-existing psychiatric illness.[44] Some studies have found a higher prevalence of psychiatric disorders such as depression in CFS patients before the onset of the illness compared with controls.[57–59] In contrast, another study reported the prior prevalence of major depression (12.5%) and of all psychiatric disorders (24.5%) in patients who have CFS to be no higher than in the general community.[60] Not surprisingly, depression and anxiety were common symptoms after the onset of the illness. A twin study is underway to evaluate the role of genetic factors in patients who have CFS. Infection or stress are often historically the precipitating or triggering factors. Possible perpetuating factors include physical deconditioning, concurrent psychiatric illness, misattribution of physical symptoms and increase in cytokines.

PREVENTION

There are no specific preventative measures because the etiology and mode of transmission are unknown, if there is one.

CLINICAL FEATURES

Fatigue is the hallmark of CFS and by definition should be present for at least 6 months (see Fig. 4.2). The fatigue refers to a state of severe mental and physical exhaustion that is not caused by activity or lack of rest. The fatigue is usually made markedly worse by activity and is not readily relieved by rest. This should not be confused with sleepiness, which indicates that the patient may have a sleep disorder such as sleep apnea, narcolepsy or depression. The fatigue is so severe that approximately 25% of patients report being often bedridden and unable to work.[61] Unfortunately, the precise measurement and definition of fatigue are difficult. The natural history of fatigue is poorly understood. Fatigue is usually measured using self-report instruments but these have limitations.

The majority of patients are female (about 70%) with a mean age of 35–40 years. Most patients (85%) report that the illness began suddenly, often with an initial 'flu-like' illness, although some report a gradual onset of symptoms with no triggering event. The disorder affects persons in all socioeconomic groups, but in most studies the patients are from the middle class.

In addition to the fatigue, patients note low-grade fevers, myalgias, sleep problems, impaired cognition, depression, headaches, sore throat, post-exertional malaise, arthralgias and dizziness.[61] The symptoms are present most of the time in the majority of patients and the illness typically waxes and wanes. As there is no diagnostic laboratory study, the clinical diagnosis rests upon the CFS case definition. Patients who have a diagnosis of fibromyalgia made by a rheumatologist often fit the case definition for CFS. Persons who

POSSIBLE PATHOGENESIS OF CFS		
Predisposing factors	Precipitating factors	Perpetuating factors
Psychiatric illness	Infection	Physical deconditioning
Genetic	Stress	Concurrent psychiatric illness
Environment, e.g. allergy, chemicals		Misattribution of physical symptoms
		Raised cytokines

Fig. 4.4 Possible pathogenesis of CFS.

have severe fatigue but fewer than four symptoms are classified as having idiopathic chronic fatigue.

The history is key in establishing the diagnosis. Epidemiologic clues related to travel, occupational and animal exposures, and substance abuse or alcohol misuse should be carefully sought. Patients should be questioned for HIV risk factors and, if positive, evaluated by testing.

A mental status examination is important to look for psychiatric disorders; if abnormalities are noted then a psychiatric or neurologic evaluation can be invaluable. Particular attention should be directed to depression, anxiety, suicide thoughts and a history of sexual abuse.

The diagnosis is based on self-reports and the physical examination is only helpful in identifying other causes of the patient's symptoms. The physical examination is usually normal and no pathognomonic physical findings have been reported. If a patient is found to have a temperature greater than 38.4°C (101°F), then another cause for the fever should be pursued. Similarly, generalized lymphadenopathy or a single large lymph node suggest another diagnosis.

The differential diagnosis of fatigue is extensive (Fig. 4.5). Psychologic disorders, particularly depression, are the most common causes of chronic fatigue. Other causes for fatigue such as multiple sclerosis, systemic lupus erythematosus or hypothyroidism should be considered.

MINIMUM RECOMMENDED TESTS TO EVALUATE SUSPECTED CFS	
Complete blood count	Calcium
Erythrocyte sedimentation rate	Phosphorus
Alanine aminotranferase	Electrolytes
Total protein	Glucose
Albumin	Blood urea nitrogen
Globulin	Urinalysis
Alkaline phosphatase	Other tests are based on history and results of physical examination
Creatinine	
Thyroid-stimulating hormone	

Fig. 4.6 Minimum recommended tests to evaluate suspected CFS.

MANAGING THE PATIENT WHO HAS CFS
1. Establish the diagnosis
2. Provide emotional support and refer patient to support groups
3. Prevent further disability by establishing a graded exercise program
4. Treat symptoms with appropriate medications, avoiding exotic untested remedies, and with cognitive behavior therapy
5. Follow up regularly and re-evaluate

Fig. 4.7 Managing the patient who has CFS.

DIAGNOSIS

No diagnostic tests are specific for CFS and the laboratory testing is to exclude possible causes for the fatigue and other symptoms. Laboratory studies should investigate the various diagnostic possibilities suggested by the history and physical examination. A minimum battery of recommended screening laboratory tests to evaluate a patient who has suspected CFS is given in Figure 4.6. The erythrocyte sedimentation rate is a key test, and results tend to be normal or low in patients who have CFS. Various immunologic tests can yield abnormal findings, but they are not indicated in clinical practice. Studies measuring cytokine levels and natural killer cell activity are best obtained in the research environment. There is no value in obtaining a battery of viral serologies, such as EBV titers, when chronic fatigue is suspected. MRI and single-photon emission CT studies of the heads of CFS patients are under investigation as diagnostic studies in such patients.

MANAGEMENT

Strategies for managing the patient who has CFS are outlined in Figure 4.7. The objectives of therapy are to help the patient develop realistic goals and expectations through education, to provide symptomatic relief and to preserve and improve the patient's ability to function. At the outset it is very important to acknowledge the sense of illness and debility expressed by these patients. Patient support groups can play an important role in helping the patient and their family cope with this frustrating chronic illness.

NONPHARMACOLOGIC THERAPIES

Chronic fatigue syndrome patients often avoid activity out of fear of exacerbating their symptoms. Complete bed rest should be avoided because of the problems associated with physical deconditioning. I believe that a balance between moderate levels of exercise and rest, dictated by common sense, is essential and that physical activity should be gradually increased as tolerated.

MOST COMMON DIFFERENTIAL DIAGNOSES OF CHRONIC FATIGUE			
Habit patterns	Caffeine habituation Alcoholism Other substance abuse	Occult malignancy	Lymphomas Gastrointestinal malignancy
Psychosocial	Depression Anxiety Stress reaction	Endocrine disorders	Hyperparathyroidism Hypothyroidism Apathetic 'hyperthyroidism' Adrenal insufficiency Cushing syndrome Hypopituitarism Diabetes mellitus
Medications	Corticosteroids Sedatives Chemotherapy		
Sleep disorders	Sleep apnea Narcolepsy	Hematologic problems	Anemia Myeloproliferative syndromes
Pregnancy	Anaemia Weight gain Fluid retention	Metabolic disorders	Hyponatremia Hypokalemia Hypercalcemia
Infectious diseases	Mononucleosis, cytomegalovirus, or EBV HIV infection Chronic hepatitis B or C virus infection Lyme disease Fungal disease Chronic parasitic infection Tuberculosis Brucellosis Subacute bacterial endocarditis Occult abscess	Cardiovascular disease	Low-output states Silent myocardial infarction
		Hepatic disease	Alcoholic hepatitis or cirrhosis
		Renal disease	Chronic renal failure
		Respiratory disorders	Chronic obstructive pulmonary disease
		Miscellaneous	Sarcoidosis Wegener's granulomatosis
Autoimmune disorders	Systemic lupus erythematosus Multiple sclerosis Thyroiditis Rheumatoid arthritis Myasthenia gravis		

Fig. 4.5 Most common differential diagnoses of chronic fatigue. This list is not meant to include every illness that can cause chronic fatigue. Rather, it is intended to highlight some of the illnesses that most commonly do so. Modified from Komaroff AL. Chronic fatigue. In: Branch WJ Jr ed. Philadelphia Office Practice and Medicine, 3E, Philadelphia: WB Saunders;1994.

Cognitive behavior therapy attempts to alter attitudes, perceptions and beliefs that can contribute to maladaptive behavior. Controlled trials using cognitive behavior therapy with a graded exercise program show reduced symptoms and increased activity in patients who have CFS and fibromyalgia, an illness that overlaps with CFS.[62] In some patients hypnotherapy and physical therapy are helpful for morning stiffness and muscle pain.

PHARMACOLOGIC THERAPY

Many therapeutic agents that have been used to treat CFS (Fig. 4.8). Information on the efficacy of most of these medications in treating CFS patients is limited to anecdotal reports, often in publications that are not peer-reviewed.[63]

Antiviral medications

Current data do not indicate the use of antiviral drugs. In a well designed placebo-controlled trial of 27 patients who have CFS, 46% of those given high-dose intravenous aciclovir and 41% given placebo responded favorably ($P > 0.05$).[64] In the aciclovir-treated group, most persons reported a return of symptoms soon after treatment was discontinued; immunologic tests and EBV serologic assays were unaffected and 12% developed reversible renal failure.

Amantadine, an agent used for the treatment of Parkinson's disease and influenza A virus, has been reported to decrease fatigue in patients who have multiple sclerosis. Only anecdotal information is available regarding its use in CFS patients, however.

Immunologically active medications

Immunoglobulin has been given to patients who have CFS based on the theory that CFS results from an immunoregulatory defect and because specific immunoglobulin subclass deficiencies have been found in some CFS patients. Two well designed controlled studies of high-dose intravenous immunoglobulin in CFS patients were conducted. In the USA, 28 adult CFS patients were given either placebo or 1g/kg intravenous immunoglobulin each month for 6 months; about 20% in each group improved symptomatically.[65] In Australia, 49 adult CFS patients were given either placebo or 2g/kg intravenous immunoglobulin each month for 3 months; 43% of those given immunoglobulin reportedly felt better compared with 12% of those given placebo.[66] Symptomatic improvement, however, was noted only at 3 months after the final infusion, and symptoms and disability returned 6 months after the end of therapy. Phlebitis occurred in 55% of patients and constitutional symptoms, such as headache, fatigue and diminished concentration, occurred in 82% of patients. Possible explanations for the different results between these studies include the smaller sample size and lower doses of immunoglobulin used in the US study, and differences in study populations and outcome assessments. There are no controlled studies on the value of immunoglobulin administered intramuscularly.

Transfer factor is a component of leukocytes that can transfer delayed-type hypersensitivity. In a double-blind trial, transfer factor given intramuscularly over a 4-week period was no more effective than placebo in improving immunologic parameters or the functional status of CFS patients.[56]

Poly(I)-poly($C_{12}U$) (Ampligen) consists of double-stranded RNA molecules with possible antiviral and immunomodulatory effects.[67] In a double-blind placebo-controlled study of 92 patients who have CFS, poly(I)-poly($C_{12}U$) given intravenously twice weekly for 6 months was associated with an enhanced capacity to perform activities of daily living and an improvement in memory.[67] Adverse effects included hepatic toxicity. This drug cannot be recommended until more data are available on its safety and efficacy.

Interferon-α given subcutaneously has been associated with improvement in some patients but the data are limited. Inosine pranobex, IL-2 and prednisolone in doses of 10–60mg/day have been attempted without beneficial effect.[68]

Antidepressant medications

Depression is common in CFS patients. In addition to their antidepressive effects, antidepressants may help improve sleep, fatigue and pain symptoms, and are a mainstay in the treatment of CFS (Fig. 4.9). Anecdotal reports suggest that antidepressant doses lower than normal may be effective; dosing can be increased gradually if there is no effect. The chosen agent should be used for 4–6 weeks before therapeutic failure is considered. The choice of agent depends, to a large extent, on expected side effects.

Although large controlled studies are lacking, tricyclic antidepressants and selective serotonin reuptake inhibitors (SSRIs) appear to be

SELECTED LIST OF AGENTS USED TO TREAT CFS PATIENTS			

Antidepressants	Tricyclic antidepressants
	  amitriptyline
	  desipramine
	  nortriptyline
	Monoamine inhibitors
	  phenelzine
		Calcium channel blockers	Nifedipine
			Nimodipine

		Stimulants	Amphetamines
		Vitamins and minerals	Cyanocobalamin Absorbic acid Zinc Magnesium

Selective serotonin reuptake inhibitors	Sertraline
	Paroxetine
	Venlafaxine
	Fluoxetine
	Nefazodone
		Psychoactive agents	Benzodiazepines
			  alprazolam
			  clonazepam
			Non-benzodiazepines
			  Carbamazepine
			  Buspirone

Immune modifiers	Transfer Factor Poly(I)-poly($C_{12}U$) Interferon-α Corticosteroids Cyclophosphamide IL-2 Isoprinosine Thymic extract		
		Antifungals	Ketoconazole Fluconazole Nystatin
		Antihistamines	H_2-receptor antagonists
Antibacterials	Ceftriaxone Ciprofloxacin Doxycycline Fusidic acid	Other agents	Germanium Kutapressin Primrose oil Vasopressin Herbs Pentoxifylline Essential fatty acids Hydrogen peroxide Galanthamine hydrobromide Quinacrine Fludrocortisone Atenolol Disopyramide
Antivirals	Acyclovir Amantadine Ganciclovir		

Anti-inflammatory agents	Hydroxychloroquine
	Nonsteroidal
	  anti-inflammatory
	  drugs
	Cyclobenzaprine		

Opium antagonists	Naltrexone		

Fig. 4.8 Selected list of agents used to treat CFS patients.

ANTIDEPRESSANTS USED TO TREAT CFS/FIBROMYALGIA	
Drug	Usual dose (mg/day)
Amitriptyline	100–150
Doxepin	100–150
Desipramine	150–200
Nortriptyline	75–100
Fluoxetine	20–40
Sertraline	50–150
Paroxetine	20
Bupropion	200–300
Venlafaxine	75–225
Nefazodone	200–500

Fig. 4.9 Antidepressants used to treat CFS/fibromyalgia.

beneficial. Tricyclic antidepressants are associated with sedative and anticholinergic effects. Anecdotally, patients who have difficulty sleeping sometimes respond well to agents such as amitriptyline or doxepin taken daily at bedtime.

In a study of patients who have fibromyalgia, 25mg amitriptyline at bedtime (rather than the usual dosages of 100–150mg) resulted in decreased fatigue and myalgias and improved sleep compared with placebo. Responses were usually seen in 3–4 weeks.[69] Desipramine is a less sedating tricyclic antidepressant. When sedation is not desirable, SSRIs, such as fluoxetine, sertraline or paroxetine, can be helpful. In a study of 79 CFS patients treated with 50mg sertraline daily for 6 months, 65% showed improvement in fatigue, myalgias, sleep disturbance and depression. Adverse effects, limited mainly to nausea and diarrhea, occurred in 8% of the patients.[70] Bupropion may be effective in patients who are unable to tolerate a tricyclic agent or SSRI.[71]

Anxiolytic medications

Panic disorders and anxiety occur frequently in patients who have CFS.[72] Although controlled studies in CFS patients are lacking, alprazolam plus ibuprofen were more effective than placebo in reducing pain and anxiety in patients who have fibromyalgia.[73]

Anecdotally, clonazepam, other benzodiazepines and buspirone also appear beneficial. Alprazolam may be particularly helpful in managing panic attacks; however, a dosage schedule of 3–4 times a day is required and the potential for habituation is substantial.

Pain medications

Acetaminophen, aspirin and other nonsteroidal anti-inflammatory drugs are often used to treat myalgias and arthralgias in CFS patients. In a study of patients who have fibromyalgia, naproxen (500mg q12h) plus amitriptyline were more effective than placebo in decreasing muscle aches.[69] In another randomized trial, amitriptyline (10–50mg at bedtime) was more effective than placebo in reducing myalgia in fibromyalgia patients.[74] Response was seen as early as 1–2 weeks after beginning therapy. In a placebo-controlled trial of the muscle relaxant cyclobenzaprine, a dosage of 10–40mg at bedtime for 12 weeks resulted in decreased pain and improved sleep in fibromyalgia patients.[75]

Sleep medications

Problems falling asleep and maintaining sleep, as well as awakening unrefreshed from sleep, are very common in CFS patients. Low doses of amitriptyline (25–50mg) or cyclobenzaprine (10–20mg) at bedtime may be beneficial. Other agents that have been anecdotally reported to be helpful are trazodone (25–50mg), doxepin (10–50mg) and clonazepam (0.5–1mg). In a controlled study, 10mg zolpidem in patients who have fibromyalgia improved sleep.[76]

Allergy medications

New allergies or exacerbation of old allergies are commonly reported by CFS patients. Food elimination diets, royal jelly, herbs and dietary supplements have not been shown to be helpful, however. Nonsedating antihistamines such as terfenadine, astemizole or loratadine can be tried, but in a small trial oral terfenadine versus placebo did not have a clinical benefit in alleviating CFS symptoms.[77] In one controlled study, nystatin did not reduce symptoms in patients who have the 'yeast connection'.[78] The yeast connection is a hypothesis that the *Candida* spp. present in the body produce products that cause symptoms of fatigue; however, there is no proof linking yeast with CFS.

Vitamins, minerals, and fatty acids

Liver extract, folic acid and vitamin B_{12} given intramuscularly were no better than placebo in adults who have CFS.[79] In a controlled trial intramuscular magnesium sulfate given weekly for 6 weeks was associated with increased energy, less pain and improved emotional state in patients who have CFS. In this study, red blood cell magnesium levels were lower in CFS patients than in healthy controls and became normal after treatment.[80] Other investigators have not found lower red blood cell magnesium levels in CFS patients.[81] I do not recommend magnesium therapy in CFS unless abnormally low red blood cell magnesium levels have been documented.

The treatment of CFS patients who have essential fatty acids has led to conflicting results. In one study, a combination of evening primrose oil and fish oil led to improvements in 85% of patients after 15 weeks, compared with 17% of those treated with placebo.[82] In another study, no difference was found between patients receiving essential fatty acids and those receiving placebo.[83]

TREATMENT OF NEURALLY MEDIATED HYPOTENSION

Patients who have CFS and a positive tilt table test should be tried on an increased dietary salt intake and fludrocortisone, 0.1–0.2mg/day, with the addition of a β-blocker or disopyramide if no response occurs with fludrocortisone. Approximately 40% of patients will respond to treatment but controlled studies are lacking.[49]

REFERENCES

1. Kroenke K, Wood DR, Mangelsdorff AD, Meier NJ, Powell JB. Chronic fatigue in primary care. JAMA 1988;260:929–34.

2. Holmes GP, Kaplan JE, Gantz NM, et al. Chronic fatigue syndrome: a working case definition. Ann Intern Med 1988;108:387–9.

3. Behan PO, Behan WMH, Bell EJ. The postviral fatigue syndrome – an analysis of the findings in 50 cases. J Infect 1985;10:211–22.

4. David A, Wessely S, Pelosi A. Myalgic encephalomyelitis or what? Lancet 1988;ii:100–1.

5. Manningham R. The symptoms, nature, causes and cure of the febricula or little fever: commonly called the nervous or hysteric fever; the fever on the spirits; vapours, hypo, or spleen, 2nd ed. London: J Robinson; 1750:52–3.

6. Beard G. Neurasthenia, or nervous exhaustion. Boston Med Surg J 1869;3:217–20.

7. DaCosta JM. On irritable heart: a clinical study of a form of functional cardiac disorder and its consequence. Am J Med Sci 1871;121:17–52.

8. Bigler M, Nielsen J: Poliomyelitis in Los Angeles in 1934: neurologic characteristics of the disease in adults. Bull Los Angeles Neurol Soc 1937;2:47.

9. Sigurdsson B, Sigurjonsson J, Sigurdsson JHJ, et al. A disease epidemic in Iceland simulating poliomyelitis. Am J Hyg 1950;52:222–38.

10. Pellew RAA. Clinical description of a disease resembling poliomyelitis. Med J Aust 1951;1:944–6.

11. The Medical Staff of the Royal Free Hospital. An outbreak of encephalomyelitis in the Royal Free Hospital group, London, 1955. Br Med J 1957;2:895–904.

12. Poskanzer DC, Henderson DA, Kunkle EC, et al. Epidemic neuromyasthenia. An outbreak in Punta Gorda, Florida. N Engl J Med 1957;257:356.

13. A new clinical entity? Lancet 1956;i:789–90.

14. Holmes GP, Kaplan JE, Stewart JA, et al. A cluster of patients with a chronic mononucleosis-like syndrome. Is Epstein–Barr virus the cause? JAMA 1987;260:2297–8.

15. Wood P. Aetiology of Da Costa's syndrome. Br Med J 1941;845–51.

16. Evans AC. Brucellosis in the United States. Am J Public Health 1947;37:139–51.

17. Stewart DE, Raskin J. Psychiatric assessment of patients with '20th-century disease' ('total allergy syndrome'). Can Med Assoc J 1985;133:1001–6.

18. Crook WG. The yeast connection: a medical breakthrough, 3rd ed. Jackson, TN: Professional Books; 1983.

19. Jones JF, Ray CG, Minnich LL, et al. Evidence for active Epstein–Barr virus infection in patients with persistent, unexplained illnesses: elevated anti-early antigen antibodies. Ann Intern Med 1985;102:1–7.

20. Straus SE, Tosato G, Armstrong G, et al. Persisting illness and fatigue in adults with evidence of Epstein–Barr virus infection. Ann Intern Med 1985;102:7–16.

21. Dale JK, Straus SE, Ablashi DV, et al. The Inoue-Melnicke virus, human herpes virus type 6, and the chronic fatigue syndrome. Ann Intern Med 1989;110:92–3.

22. Buchwald D, Cheney PR, Peterson DL, et al. A chronic illness characterized by fatigue, neurologic and immunologic disorders, and active human herpes virus type 6 infection. Ann Intern Med 1992;116:103–13.

23. DeFreitas E, Hilliard B, Cheney PR, et al. Retroviral sequence related to human T- lymphotropic virus Type II in patients with chronic fatigue immunodysfunction syndrome. Proc Natl Acad Sci USA 1991;88:2922–6.

24. Khan AS, Heneine WM, Chapman LE, et al. Assessment of a retroviral sequence and other possible risk factors for a chronic fatigue syndrome in adults. Ann Intern Med 1993;118:241–5.

25. Flugel RM, Mahnke C, Geiger A, et al. Absence of antibody to human spumaretrovirus in patients with chronic fatigue syndrome. Clin Infect Dis 1992;14:623–4.

26. Gowers WR. Lumbago: its lessons and analogues. Br Med J 1904;1:117–21.

27. Goldenberg DL, Simms RW, Geiger A, Komaroff AL. High frequency of fibromyalgia in patients with chronic fatigue seen in a primary care practice. Arthritis Rheum 1990;33:381.

28. Schluederberg A, Straus SE, Peterson P, et al. Chronic fatigue syndrome research: definition and medical outcome assessment. Ann Intern Med 1992;117:325–31.

29. Komaroff AL, Fagioli LR, Geiger AM, et al. An examination of the working case definition of chronic fatigue syndrome. Am J Med 1996;100:56–64.

30. Sharpe MC, Archard LC, Banatvala JE, et al. A report – chronic fatigue syndrome: guidelines for research. J Roy Soc Med 1991;84:118–21.

31. Lloyd AR, Wakefield D, Boughton C, Dwyer J. What is myalgic encephalomyelitis? Lancet 1988;i:1286–7.

32. Lloyd AR, Hickie I, Boughton CR, Spencer O, Wakefield D. Prevalence of chronic fatigue syndrome in an Australian population. Med J Aust 1990;153:522–8.

33. Fukuda K, Straus SE, Hickie I, et al. The chronic fatigue syndrome: a comprehensive approach to its definition and study. Ann Intern Med 1994;121:953–9.

34. Gunn WJ, Connell DB, Randall B. Epidemiology of chronic fatigue syndrome: the Centers for Disease Control study. In: Bock GR, Whelan J, eds. Chronic fatigue syndrome. Chichester, England: Wiley; 1993:83–93.

35. Buchwald D, Umali P, Umali J, Kith P, Pearlman T, Komaroff AL. Chronic fatigue and the chronic fatigue syndrome: prevalence in a pacific northwest health care system. Ann Intern Med 1995:123:81–8.

36. Lawrie SM, Pelosi AJ. Chronic fatigue syndrome in the community prevalence and associations. Br J Psychiatr 1995;166:793–7.

37. Carter BD, Edwards JF, Kronenberger WG, Michalczyk L, Marshall GS. Case control study of chronic fatigue in pediatric patients. Pediatrics 1995;2:179–86.

38. Buchwald D, Sullivan JL, Komaroff AL. Frequency of chronic active Epstein–Barr virus infection in a general medical practice. JAMA 1987;257:2303–7.

39. Yousef GE, Bell EJ, Maun GF, et al. Chronic enterovirus infection in patients with postviral fatigue syndrome. Lancet 1988;i:146–50.

40. Archard LC, Bowles NE, Behan PO, Bell EJ, Doyle D. Postviral fatigue syndrome: persistence of enterovirus RNA in muscle and elevated creatine kinase. J Roy Soc Med 1988;81:326–9.

41. Swanink CMA, Melchers WJG, Van Der Meer JWM, et al. Enteroviruses and the chronic fatigue syndrome. Clin Infect Dis 1994;19:860–4.

42. Mawle AC, Nisenbaum R, Dobbins JG, et al. Seroepidemiology of chronic fatigue syndrome: a case–control study. Clin Infect Dis 1995;21:1386–9.

43. Imboden JB, Canter A, Cluff LE, Trever RW. Brucellosis. III. Psychological aspects of delayed convalescence. Arch Intern Med 1959;103:406–14.

44. Imboden JB, Canter A, Cluff LE. Convalescence from influenza. A study of the psychological and clinical determinants. Arch Intern Med 1961;108:393–9.

45. Dinerman H, Steere AC. Lyme disease associated with fibromyalgia. Ann Intern Med 1992;11:281–5.

46. Demitrack MA, Dale JK, Straus SE, et al. Evidence for impaired activation of the hypothalamic-pituitary-adrenal axis in patients with chronic fatigue syndrome. J Clin Endocrinol Metab 1991;73:1224–34.

47. Demitrack MA, Gold PW, Dale JK, Krahn DD, Kling MA, Straus SE. Plasma and cerebrospinal monoamine metabolism in patients with chronic fatigue syndrome: preliminary findings. Biol Psychiatry 1992;32:1065–77.

48. Yatham LN, Morehouse RL, Chisholm T, et al. Neuroendocrine assessment of serotonin (5-HT) function in chronic fatigue syndrome. Can J Psychiatry 1995;40:93–6.

49. Bou-Holaigah I, Rowe PC, Kan J, Calkins H. The relationship between neurally mediated hypotension and the chronic fatigue syndrome. JAMA 1995;274:961–7.

50. Straus SE, Dale JK, Wright R, Metcalfe DD. Allergy and the chronic fatigue syndrome. J Allergy Clin Immunol 1988;81:791–5.

51. Steinberg P, McNutt BE, Marshall P, Schenck C, et al. Double-blind placebo-controlled study of the efficacy of oral terfenadine in the treatment of chronic fatigue syndrome.J Allergy Clin Immunol 1996;97:119–26.

52. Klimas NG, Salvato FR, Morgan R, Fletcher MA. Immunologic abnormalities in the chronic fatigue syndrome. J Clin Microbiol 1990;28:1403–10.

53. Lloyd AR, Hickie I, Brockman A, et al. Immunologic and psychologic therapy for patients with chronic fatigue syndrome: a double-blind, placebo-controlled trial. Am J Med 1993;94:197–203.

54. Straus SE, Dale JK, Peter JB, Dinarello CA. Circulating lymphokine levels in the chronic fatigue syndrome. J Infect Dis 1989;160:1085–6.

55. Linde A, Andersson B, Svenson SB, et al. Serum levels of lymphokines and soluble cellular receptors in primary Epstein–Barr virus infection and in patients with chronic fatigue syndrome. J Infect Dis 1992;165:994–1000.

56. Landay AL, Jessop C, Lennette ET, Levy JA. Chronic fatigue syndrome: clinical condition associated with immune activation. Lancet 1991:338:707–12.

57. Manu P, Matthews DA, Lane TJ. The mental health of patients with a chief complaint of chronic fatigue: a prospective evaluation and follow-up. Arch Intern Med 1988;148:2213–7.

58. Taerk GS, Thone BB, Sulit JE, et al. Depression in patients with neuromyasthenia (benign myalgic encephalomyelitis). Int J Psychiatry Med 1987;13:49–52.

59. Kruesi MJP, Dale J, Straus S. Psychiatric diagnoses in patients who have chronic fatigue. J Clin Psychiatry 1989;50:53–6.

60. Hickie I, Lloyd A, Wakefield D, Parker G. The psychiatric status of patients with the chronic fatigue syndrome. Br J Psychiatry 1990;156:534–40.

61. Komaroff AL, Buchwald D. Symptoms and signs of chronic fatigue syndrome. Rev Infect Dis 1991;13(Suppl 1):S8–11.

62. Sharpe M, Hawton K, Simkin S, et al. Cognitive behavior therapy for the chronic fatigue syndrome: a randomised controlled trial. Br Med J 1996:312:22–6.

63. Gantz NM, Holmes GP. Treatment of patients with chronic fatigue syndrome. Drugs 1989;38:855–62.

64. Straus SE, Dale JK, Tobi M, et al. Acyclovir treatment of the chronic fatigue syndrome: lack of efficacy in a placebo-controlled trial. N Engl J Med 1988;26:1692–8.

65. Peterson PK, Shepard J, Macres M, et al. A controlled trial of intravenous immunoglobulin G in chronic fatigue syndrome. Am J Med 1990;89:554–60.

66. Lloyd A, Hickie I, Wakefield D, et al. A double-blind, placebo-controlled trial of intravenous immunoglobulin therapy in patients with chronic fatigue syndrome. Am J Med 1990;89:561–8.

67. Strayer DR, Carter WA, Brodsky I, et al. A controlled clinical trial with a specifically configured RNA drug, Poly(I)-Poly (C12U), in chronic fatigue syndrome. Clin Infect Dis 1994;18(Suppl 1):S88–95.

68. Fukuda K, Gantz NM. Management strategies for chronic fatigue syndrome. Fed Pract 1995;12:12–27.

69. Goldenberg DL, Felsoon DT, Dinerman H. A randomized controlled trial of amitriptyline and naproxen in the treatment of patients with fibromyalgia. Arthritis Rheum 1986;29:1371–7.

70. Behan PO, Haniffah BAG, Doogan DP, Loudon M. A pilot study of sertraline for the treatment of chronic fatigue syndrome. Clin Infect Dis 1994;18(Suppl 1):S111–2.

71. Goodnick PJ, Sandoval R, Brickman A, Klimas NG. Bupropion treatment of fluoxetine-resistant chronic fatigue syndrome. Biol Psychiatry 1992;32:834–8.

72. Manu P, Matthews DA, Lane TJ. Panic disorder among patients with chronic fatigue. South Med J 1991;84:451–6.

73. Russell IJ, Fletcher EM, Michalek JE, et al. Treatment of primary fibrositis/fibromyalgia syndrome with ibuprogen and alprazolam: A double-blind, placebo-controlled study. Arthritis Rheum 1991;34:552–9.

74. Jaeschke R, Adachi J, Guyatt G, et al. Clinical usefulness of amitriptyline in fibromyalgia: The results of 23 N-of-1 randomized controlled trials. J Rheum 1991;18:447–51.

75. Bennett RM, Gatter RA, Campbell SM, et al. A comparison of cyclobenzaprine and placebo in the management of fibrositis: A double-blind controlled study. Arthritis Rheum 1988;31:1535–42.

76. Moldofsky H, Lue FA, Mously C, et al. The effect of zolpidem in patients with fibromyalgia: A dose ranging, double blind, placebo controlled, modified crossover study. J Rheum 1996;23:529–33.

77. Steinberg P, McNutt BE, Marshall P, et al. Double-blind placebo-controlled study of the efficacy of oral terfenadine in the treatment of chronic fatigue syndrome. J Allergy Clin Immunol 1966;97:119–26.

78. Dismukes WE, Wade JS, Lee JY, et al. A randomized, double-blind trial of nystatin therapy for the candidiasis hypersensitivity syndrome. N Engl J Med 1990;323:1717–23.

79. Kaslow JE, Rucker L, Onishi R. Liver extract-folic acid-cyanocobalamin versus placebo for chronic fatigue syndrome. Arch Intern Med 1989;149:2501–3.

80. Cox IM, Campbell MJ, Dowson D. Red-blood cell magnesium and chronic fatigue syndrome. Lancet 1991;337:757–60.

81. Gantz NM. Magnesium and chronic fatigue. Lancet 1991;338:66.

82. Behan PO, Behan WMH, Horrobin D. Effect of high doses of essential fatty acids on the postviral fatigue syndrome. Acta Neurol Scand 1990;82:209–16.

83. McBride SJ, McCluskey DR. Treatment of chronic fatigue syndrome. Br Med Bull 1991;47:895–907.

Infections from Pets

Donald Armstrong & Edward M Bernard

'The deviation of man from the state in which he was placed by nature seems to have proven to him a prolific source of diseases. From the love of splendor, from the indulgences of luxury, and from his fondness for amusement, he has familiarized himself with a great number of animals which may not, originally, have been intended for his associates. The wolf, disarmed of ferocity, is now pillowed in the lady's lap. The cat, the little tiger of our island, whose natural home is the forest, is equally domesticated and caressed' (Edward Jenner, London, 1796).[1]

Over 200 years ago, on 21 June 1778, Jenner introduced his treatise on using vaccination with cowpox to protect against smallpox with the above words. Would he have predicted the explosion in pet ownership that has occurred in the intervening two centuries? In the USA alone, estimates of the numbers of the most common pets are:

- dogs: 52.9 million;
- cats: 57 million;
- birds in cages: 12.6 million;
- reptiles: 3.5 million;
- rodents 4.8 million; and
- fish: 55.6 million.

In Australia, which has the highest incidence of pet ownership in the world, 66% of the 6 million households own pets. Thus, 12 million Australians are associated with pets.[2]

An early sign of a culture moving from the developing into the developed world is the appearance of pedigreed pets, most commonly cats, dogs and birds; such pets are usually expensive. These pets are usually kept in houses and live close to their human owners, sometimes sharing beds with them. This is in contrast to the working farm dog living in an outside doghouse or a cat living in the barn or other outbuildings. Thus, pets have increased as 'a prolific source of diseases'.[1]

A pet contact history should be a part of every infectious disease evaluation. The types of pets should be enumerated because some people do not consider birds or fish to be pets and therefore may not respond appropriately to the word 'pet'. Furthermore, although a person may not have a pet, he or she may have close contact with a neighbor's pet.

The organisms carried by each type of pet are listed under that animal in the tables that follow so that the reader can run through these when a positive animal contact history evolves. Excellent books, monographs and reviews have been written on zoonosis and infections contracted from pets, to which the reader is referred for more detailed descriptions.[3–10] All of the infections are covered in other chapters and the reader is referred to them for additional information on diagnosis, therapy and pathogenesis.

DOGS

Infectious organisms associated with dogs are listed in Figure 5.1.

BACTERIA

The most common adverse event from encounters with dogs is a bite (Fig. 5.2; see Chapter 6.15), but it is sufficient here to say that the first and most important part of the evaluation is to determine whether the dog could be rabid. If there is any question, then rabies immune

ORGANISMS CARRIED BY DOGS

Bacteria	Fungi	Parasites	Viruses
Mixed mouth flora	*Blastomyces dermatitidis*	*Giardia lamblia*	Rabies virus
Pasteurella multocida	*Microsporum* spp.	*Babesia* spp.	Lymphocytic choriomeningitis virus
Capnocytophaga canimorsis	*Trichophyton* spp.	*Toxocara canis*	Influenza virus
Streptococcus pyogenes		*Dipylidium caninum*	Mumps virus
Salmonella spp.		*Dirofilaria immitis**	
*Rickettsia rickettsii**		*Echinococcus*	
*Francisella tularensis**		*E. granulosus* and *E. multilocularis*	
Erhlichia spp.*		*Ancylostoma canium*	
Leptospira interrogans			
Burkholderi pseudomallei			
Brucella canis			
Mycobacteria spp.			
Yersinia enterocolitica			
Campylobacter jejuni			

*Transmitted by ticks or mosquitoes

Fig. 5.1 Organisms carried by dogs.

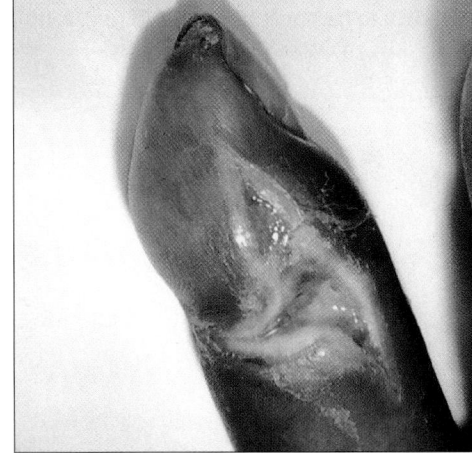

Fig. 5.2 Dog bite on finger after appropriate surgical drainage, but with poor clinical response.

globulin and vaccine should be administered (see Chapters 6.15 & 8.8). At the same time the wound should be well washed with whatever soap is available, preferably a disinfectant soap, and the wound should be drained if necessary. Anaerobic mouth flora along with *Pasteurella multocida* are the most common offenders in dog bites and are well treated by drainage and a beta-lactam antibiotic or a tetracycline, either of which would also kill or inhibit *Streptococcus pyogenes* (Fig. 5.3). Dogs may carry *S. pyogenes* in the throat or pass it in the feces, and they have been found to be responsible for repeated episodes of streptococcal pharyngitis in families.[11]

The duration of therapy depends on the extent and age of the wound; in older wounds that have not been treated and respond only slowly to appropriate therapy an underlying osteomyelitis should be considered (Figs 5.2–5.4).

Pasteurella multocida can spread from a wound via the bloodstream to the heart valves or the meninges; if it spreads to the liver an abscess results. Liver disease such as cirrhosis appears to predispose to dissemination of *P. multocida*.

Capnocytophaga spp., especially *Capnocytophaga canimorsis*, are carried in the mouths of dogs and can cause potentially lethal disease in the immunocompromised host (i.e. those who abuse alcohol or are neutropenic or who have been splenectomized).[12] Rarely, sepsis has been reported in an apparently normal host. A lick by a dog as well as a bite can introduce this fastidious facultative anaerobic Gram-negative rod into breaks in the skin, which may result in sepsis. The infection responds well to beta-lactam antibiotics and drainage when necessary.

Salmonella spp. and *Campylobacter* spp. are carried by dogs and may well be transmitted to humans by exposure to dog feces, but few cases have documented.

Mycobacterium genevense has been isolated from a dog, but its transmission to humans has not been observed.[13] It is a rare pathogen of the immunocompromised host (e.g. HIV-infected patients and homeless people, the latter presumably being malnourished). Infections that can be brought to humans by dogs carrying ticks include Rocky Mountain spotted fever, via the wood tick *Dermacentor andersoni* or the dog tick *Dermacentor variabilis*. How often dogs bring the deer tick *Ixodes dammini* to humans is uncertain, but that tick can carry:

- *Babesia microti*, the cause of babesiosis;
- *Borrelia burgdorferi*, the cause of Lyme disease; and
- *Ehrlichia* spp., the cause of ehrlichiosis.

FUNGI

Fungal diseases transmitted from dogs to humans are common only in the case of dermatophytes, *Microsporum* spp. and *Trichophyton* spp. They can cause annoying rashes but respond readily to treatment with topical or systemic azoles.

Blastomyces dermatitidis has been reported as causing pulmonary, skin and bone disease in dogs as well as in humans in the same household. In these cases both dogs and humans have been exposed to the same environment that is known to harbor *B. dermatitidis* (e.g. rotting wood and earth), and it is not certain that it passes from one animal to the other, or simply from environmental sources to both animals.

Dogs may carry many of the environmental fungi such as *Candida* spp. and *Aspergillus* spp. Their role in transmission of these organisms to immunocompromised hosts is uncertain.

PARASITES

Parasitic diseases may be transmitted from dog to humans, and geophagia or close contact among children and dogs may result in unusual, but sometimes complicated, infections. Children may become infected with *Toxocara canis*, which usually causes no disease, although rarely systemic infection does occur with a febrile illness with diffuse pulmonary infiltrates and eosinophilia.

Another potentially very disturbing consequence of infection with *T. canis* is that the eye lesion may be mistaken for a tumor; eye enucleation as a result has been reported. Most physicians caring for children and certainly pediatric ophthmalogists should be aware that this parasite can cause such lesions.

Giardia lamblia may infect dogs, but how often this parasite passes from dogs to humans is uncertain. One dog parasite that can be passed from infected dogs to humans by a mosquito is *Dirofilaria immitis*, the dog heartworm. In humans the organism causes few symptoms (e.g. mild cough and malaise) or no symptoms, but it results in a pulmonary lesion that can mimic a tumor. Because the parasite lodges in vessels, hemoptysis may occur. A serologic test exists for dogs, but the incidence of positive serologic tests in humans is uncertain so that most of these lesions are surgically removed. The infection can be controlled in dogs by prophylactic praziquantel during the mosquito season.

Echinococcosis, also referred to as hydatid disease, is due primarily to two organisms, *Echinococcus granulosus* and *Echinococcus multilocularis*, both tapeworms of dogs.[14] *Echinococcus granulosus* causes unilocular echinococcosis or cystic hydatid disease. The dog is the definitive host and grazing animals, such as sheep and cattle, along with humans are intermediate hosts. The organism is found worldwide, and camels, kangaroos or pigs may be part of the cycle. Humans contract the disease by swallowing eggs in dog feces. Signs and symptoms depend on the organs involved. Surgery may be necessary to remove cysts, and mebendazole or albendazole has been used in addition to surgery. Prevention is achieved through control of the disease in dogs and preventing dogs from eating intermediate hosts.

Echinococcus multilocularis causes multilocular or alveolar hydatid disease, usually involving the liver in humans. The tapeworms are found in dogs, foxes, wolves, coyotes and cats. Intermediate hosts include lemmings, voles, shrews and mice. The organism is found throughout the northern hemisphere. Diagnosis is usually by

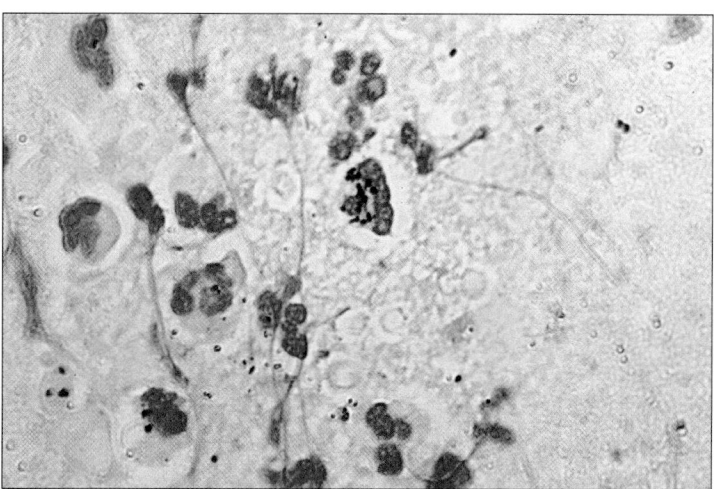

Fig. 5.3 Gram-stain of fluid after surgical drainage of a dog bite. The fluid grew anaerobic streptococci and *Pasteurella multocida*.

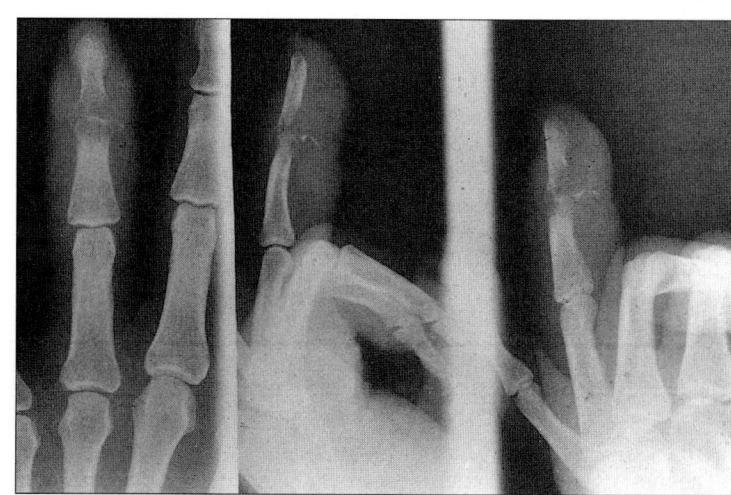

Fig. 5.4 Osteomyelitis of the medial and distal phalanx. X-ray of dog bite wound. The bone fragment yielded *Pasteurella multocida* on removal and culture, and the patient responded to penicillin.

histopathology, but a serologic test that appears reliable is under investigation. Surgery is usually necessary under cover of mebendazole or albendazole. Prevention strategies are similar to those for *E. granulosus*, and include the avoidance of contact with fecally contaminated soil or food and the control of the disease in dogs and cats.

Less commonly, infection with *Echinococcus vogeli* results in polycystic disease in liver, lungs and other organs.[10] Dogs are the definitive host. The paca, agouti and spring rat are intermediate hosts. Cases may occur in humans as accidental intermediate hosts in Columbia, Ecuador, Panama and Venezuela.[10]

Ancylostoma caninum and *Ancylostoma braziliense* are contracted through contact with dog or cat feces that contains larva. The larva are often found in sandy soil and after penetrating the skin cause serpiginous tracts, which can advance up to 2cm per day, accompanied by intense itching. The disease is self-limiting but relief can be hastened by freezing the area with ethyl chloride spray, ivermectin or albendazole therapy, or thiabendazole systemically or locally (see Chapter 7.17).

VIRUSES

The most dreaded virus infection transmitted from dogs to humans is rabies. This infection is discussed in detail in Chapter 8.8.

Influenza virus and lymphocytic choriomeningitis virus have been isolated from dogs, but transmission to humans has not been proven.

CATS

Infectious organisms associated with cats are listed in Figure 5.5.

BACTERIA

Cat bites result in the same sort of infections as dog bites, including infection with *P. multocida*. They should be treated in the same way. Cats may also carry *S. pyogenes*. A fastidious Gram-negative rod, formerly designated CDC-EF4, which is now regarded as a pasteurella-like bacterium has caused sepsis in immunocompromised patients, as have *Capnocytophaga* spp. Just as with *Capnocytophaga* spp. from dogs, the patients who suffer from sepsis from any of these organisms are almost all neutropenic, splenectomized or alcohol abusers. CDC-EF4 should respond to beta-lactam antibiotic therapy.

Bartonella henselae is a fastidious Gram-negative rod that has only recently been documented as the cause of cat scratch disease in the general population and of bacillary angiomatosis in HIV-infected patients. It is carried by cat fleas and is presumably spread to humans by contact with fleas. The incidence of this infection in cats, as detected by bacillemia, ranges from an amazing 41.5% in stray cats in San Francisco[15] to 6% in house (mostly apartment) cats in New York. Serologic studies showing a high incidence of antibody in both cats and humans suggest that most infection is asymptomatic. Even bacillemic cats may be without signs. Classic cat scratch disease in humans is manifest by regional lymphadenopathy with or without suppuration. The histopathology is a typical granuloma that is occasionally mistaken for Hodgkin's disease. The nodes usually subside on their own or do not recur after extirpation. Treatment with a macrolide or tetracycline antibiotic seems to hasten resolution of nodes. Rarely a more systemic illness is seen, including meningitis.

Bacillary angiomatosis, seen in HIV-infected patients, is manifest by red to purplish skin lesions, which sometimes resemble those of Kaposi's sarcoma, and biochemical evidence of hepatitis. Biopsy of skin lesions reveals involvement of vessels resembling that seen in bartonellosis. The presence of organisms in skin lesions are usually detected by DNA probes and seldom by isolation of the organism. To help to isolate the organisms, blood cultures should be incubated in liquid media for at least 3 weeks. Even in HIV-infected and immunocompromised patients, skin lesions and hepatitis should respond to antimicrobial therapy if the diagnosis is made early (see Chapter 5.14).

Afipia felis has also been described as a cause of classical cat scratch disease in children who are exposed to cats (often kittens). It has not

ORGANISMS CARRIED BY CATS			
Bacteria	**Fungi**	**Parasites**	**Viruses**
Mixed mouth flora	Dermatophytes	*Toxoplasma gondii*	Rabies
Pasturella multocida	*Cryptococcus neoformans*	*Echinococcus multilocularis*	Cowpox
Streptococcus pyogenes		*Ancyclostoma canium*	
Capnocytophaga spp.			
Pasteurella-like organism (EF4)			
Bartonella henselae*			
Coxiella burnetii			
Yersinia pestis*			
Francisella tularensis*			
Campytobacter jejuni			
Salmonella spp.			
Afipia felis			
*Transmitted through fleas or ticks			

Fig. 5.5 Organisms carried by cats.

been implicated in the more serious infections that occur in immunocompromised patients.

Cats, like dogs, may carry *Salmonella* spp. and *Campylobacter* spp. It is uncertain how often these organisms are transmitted to humans. An unusual infection of cats that can be transmitted to humans is Q fever. In one famous outbreak a parturient cat infected a group of poker players exposed in an enclosed basement.[16] However, transmission of Q fever seems to be rare. Cats may also transmit tularemia (*Francisella tularensis*) or the plague (*Yersinia pestis*) through saliva or scratching, but these are also rare occurrences.

FUNGI

Dermatophytes, some identical to dog dermatophytes, can be passed to humans from cats and the diagnosis and treatment are the same (see Chapter 2.6). Prevention requires diagnosis and therapy of the infections in cats.

Cryptococcus neoformans can infect cats and cause disease, including nasopharyngeal granulomas. Because these granulomas are filled with the organisms, they must be shed into the environment, but instances of spread to humans have not been documented.

PARASITES

Parasites that infect cats may transmit to humans include *Toxocara* spp. associated with visceral larva migrans. *Toxoplasma gondii* is the parasite spread from cats to humans that causes the greatest morbidity and, in the immunocompromised host, significant mortality. The trophozoites are passed in the stool of the cat into earth, sand or 'kitty litter' and from there are either ingested or inhaled by humans. The usual result is an asymptomatic infection or lymphadenopathy with or without a mild febrile illness. If the patient has a T-helper (T_H) lymphocyte defect, the infection may disseminate and cause pneumonia, myocarditis or encephalitis. The people most affected are those who have HIV infection, those who have undergone organ or bone marrow transplantation and those who have leukemia or lymphoma. In pregnant women the organism can infect the fetus and cause severe brain damage. It also tends to invade the eye and may result in blindness in the newborn.

The diagnosis of toxoplasmosis can be suspected by the characteristic histopathology of a lymph node biopsy supported by serology showing either high IgM titers or a four-fold rise in IgG titers. Immunocompromised hosts, such as AIDS patients, may not mount an antibody response and the clinical picture alone may warrant empiric therapy (see Chapter 5.13). Biopsy of lung or brain lesions often reveals the cysts or trophozoites both inside and outside host macrophages. Antigen or DNA (detected by polymerase chain reaction) of *T. gondii* may be found in the cerebrospinal fluid in infections of the central nervous system. In the newborn, IgM antibody is diagnostic; detection of the antigen or of DNA in the cerebrospinal fluid or other sterile body fluids can also be used for diagnosis.

Treatment is with sulfadiazine and pryrimethamine or clindamycin with pyrimethamine. Prevention is all-important, and pregnant women should be educated to avoid contact with cat feces (and to avoid the ingestion of rare beef, lamb or pork, which also results in infection); pregnant women who are cat owners should have themselves and the cat tested. Treatment with spinomycin and a combination of pyrimethamine and sulfadiazine during pregnancy and treatment of the child resulting from the pregnancy is beneficial (see Chapter 7.17).

Immunocompromised hosts such as AIDS patients, bone marrow transplant recipients and any patient who has a severe T_H lymphocyte defect should be educated to avoid infection and should be tested for *Toxoplasma* antibody because many of the infections are the result of reactivation; if antibody is present, prophylactic therapy or early presumptive therapy should be considered.

VIRUSES

Viruses contracted from contact with cats include rabies (although this is less common than infection from dogs). However, in general cats are less likely to bite than dogs, and an unprovoked bite should raise the question of rabies. In addition, cats may carry cowpox and transmit it to humans.[17] Cowpox is reappearing in the UK since the cessation of smallpox vaccination. Another reservoir for cowpox appears to be rodents. Cowpox is almost always a self-limiting disease in immunocompetent people, but infection in immunocompromised patients can be fatal.

BIRDS

Pet birds may vary from tiny finches to owls, hawks or peacocks. Contact may vary from kissing or feeding the bird from the owner's mouth to cleaning cages or allowing the bird free range of a home or a yard.

BACTERIA

The organisms carried by birds are listed in Figure 5.6. It is difficult to determine how often some of the organisms, such as *Campylobacter jejuni*, *P. multocida* or *Mycobacterium tuberculosis*, are passed to humans, but *Chlamydia psittaci* is regularly transmitted, as are *Salmonella* spp.

Chlamydia psittaci can be carried by any bird, pet or wild, not just psittacine birds such as parakeets or parrots, and all birds that carry the organism can pass it on to humans. (The disease is better called ornithosis rather than psittacosis.) Ducks and turkeys have been responsible for outbreaks of ornithosis in humans as well as birds kept in the home. Respiratory symptoms are the usual result of transmission from bird to humans, and there have been reports of human-to-human transmission, but apparently this is not common. Too little is known about the incidence of infection with *C. psittaci* because few studies have been done of different human populations using modern, accurate serologic techniques. If the respiratory symptoms are mild, the infection is often undiagnosed. Even in patients who have pneumonia, the diagnosis needs to be confirmed by showing a four-fold rise in acute and convalescent serum titers 2–4 weeks apart, but this is seldom pursued because:

- the diagnosis is not considered;
- an acute serum specimen is not obtained;
- most patients are better after 2 weeks and a convalescent serum is not obtained, even if an acute serum was;
- the serum usually has to be sent to a reference laboratory, and by the time the results are ready the patient has recovered; and

ORGANISMS TRANSMITTED FROM BIRDS TO HUMANS			
Bacteria	Fungi	Parasites	Viruses
Campylobacter jejuni	*Histoplasma capsulatum*	*Cryptosporidium* spp.	Influenza virus (from ducks)
Salmonella spp.	*Cryptococcus neoformans*	*Giardia lamblia*	Alphaviruses flaviviruses
Chlamydia psittaci			
Mycobacterium tuberculosis			
Pasteurella multocida			
Erysipelothrix rhusiopathiae			

Fig. 5.6 Organisms transmitted from birds to humans. All are transmitted by pet birds except alphavirses and flaviviruses, which are transmitted by wild birds.

- most reference laboratories only accept both acute and convalescent specimens (to be examined in the same test) and this is not easily arranged.

The diagnosis of acute disease is dependent on a high index of suspicion, and therapy must be empiric, because rapid diagnostic techniques are not available. A history of contact with a sick bird is highly suggestive, but well birds can carry the disease and a number of cases have been reported without a history of bird contact, although presumably there has been inapparent contact with bird excreta in the environment. Pigeon and other birds' feces abound in many urban environments, as does chicken or duck feces in rural environments.

The pneumonia in humans can be severe, and is often lobar accompanied by high fevers and chills. The sputum may be purulent with a lack of potential pathogens on smear, because *C. psittaci* does not take the Gram stain.

Once empiric therapy is decided upon, tetracycline is preferred, although erythromycin has been reported to be effective. A safe duration of therapy is 2 weeks, although a shorter period maybe adequate. Complications such as meningoencephalitis, arthritis or endocarditis may occur.

A specific diagnosis is important because epidemiologic factors may need to be investigated. A bird dealer may be importing carriers without appropriate quarantine and/or treatment and cases of human-to-human transmission may be uncovered including possible nosocomial spread. Control measures for *C. psittaci* infection of birds and humans are detailed in a recent report from the US Public Health Service.[15]

All of the organisms listed in Figure 5.6 have been isolated from birds; some, such as *Salmonella* spp. and *Giardia lamblia*, are clearly implicated in transmission to humans. Tuberculosis has been seen in patients in households where tuberculosis has been recognized in macaws. It is difficult to determine whether spread is from bird to humans or vice versa. Other psittacine birds may become infected with *M. tuberculosis*.[19]

FUNGI

Histoplasma capsulatum has been found in bird droppings, especially from chicken and blackbirds. *Histoplasma capsulatum* has been found throughout the world, but it is especially common in river valleys of the Americas and in the Caribbean and is thus considered a 'regional' fungus. Histoplasmosis is usually not due to exposures to pets, with the exception of exposure to chickens, which are sometimes kept and regarded as pets. The fungus grows in the feces of chickens, but does not infect them. Most human infections are asymptomatic but others may result in an influenza-like illness or rarely a progressive pneumonia (see Chapter 8.27). The majority of symptomatic infections are self-limiting; however, treatment when necessary (especially in the immunocompromised host) can be with amphotericin B initially followed by itraconazole or fluconazole for acute, progressive infections or itraconazole or fluconazole alone for more indolent disease. Prevention strategies should include advising immunocompromised people to avoid bird feces, especially from chickens.

Cryptococcus neoformans in found in soil throughout the world, but it appears to thrive in pigeon feces. Pigeon fanciers who keep flocks of pigeons for sport are exposed to *C. neoformans* more than the general population, as demonstrated by serologic testing; however, an increased incidence of disease has not been documented in these people. *Cryptococcosis* initially begins as a self-limiting respiratory infection. The fungus may disseminat widely to multiple organs including the central nervous system. It has a predilection for people who have T_H lymphocyte defects, and if untreated the meningitis it causes is associated with high mortality (up to 50%).[20] There may be significant morbidity and sequelae (e.g. internal hydrocephalus, blindness) (see Chapter 2.7).

The diagnosis is aided by the presence of cryptococcal polysaccharide antigens in the blood or cerebrospinal fluid, and a decrease in antigen titer is usually associated with a response to therapy in patients who do not have AIDS. In patients who have AIDS, high levels of antigen may persist indefinitely despite excellent clinical response to treatment. Amphotericin B with or without flucytosine is the treatment of the acute episode followed by fluconazole for more chronic therapy. Prevention should include advising immunocompromised people to avoid contact with pigeons.

PARASITES
Parasites that may spread to humans from birds include *G. lamblia* and *Cryptosporidia* spp, although direct spread from the latter is not as well documented as the former. Methods of diagnosis and treatment are covered in detail in Chapters 8.32 and 7.17.

VIRUSES
The alphaviruses and flaviviruses that pass from birds to humans are carried to humans by mosquitoes and ticks (see Chapter 8.11). The birds are almost always wild and not pets. Identical strains of influenza virus have been found in both humans and ducks where contact has been documented. The incidence of ducks or other birds serving as reservoirs for influenza is not certain.[22] In 1998, a large outbreak of influenza in Hong Kong was associated with chickens and caused several deaths. Thousands of birds were slaughtered in an attempt to control the infection.

SMALL MAMMAL PETS

Small mammal pets include mice, rats, hamsters, gerbils, guinea pigs and rabbits. People may also keep more exotic animals such as mink, ferrets and ocelots. These animals carry organisms similar to those carried by mice and rats; ocelots carry organisms similar to those carried by cats (Fig. 5.7).

ORGANSIMS CARRIED BY SMALL MAMMAL PETS			
Bacteria	Fungi	Parasites	Viruses
Campylobacter spp.	*Sporothrix schenckii*	*Cryptosporidium* spp.	Lymphocytic choriomeningitis virus
Spirillum minus	*Penicillium marneffei*		Hantavirus
Streptobacillus moniliformis			
Salmonella spp.			
Leptospira interrogans			
Francisella tularensis			
Yersinia pestis			
Listeria monocytogenes			
Pasteurella multocida			
Burkholderi pseudomallei			

Fig. 5.7 Organisms carried by small mammal pets.

BACTERIA
Most pets, regardless of type, can carry *Salmonella* spp. and *Campylobacter* spp. Many, including rabbits, carry *P. multocida* as part of their mouth flora. There are some that are more likely to carry certain organisms. Rats can carry *Spirillum minus* and *Streptobacillus moniliformis*. Rat bite fever or spirillary fever due to *S. minus* is seen worldwide but is most common in Asia. The fever is accompanied by a rash with reddish or purplish plaques. The healed bite wound may reactivate when fever develops. The diagnosis requires highly specialized laboratories for confirmation. Treatment consists of penicillin or a tetracycline.

Rate bite fever due to *S. moniliformis* (also called Haverhill fever) may be due to a rat bite or to exposure to contaminated milk or water during an outbreak. The fever is usually accompanied by maculopapular or petechial rash that is most pronounced on the extremities. Arthritis of large joints is common, as are relapses. Focal abscesses and endocarditis may occur. Diagnosis is confirmed by a specialized laboratory unless a sterile site is positive on culture. Treatment is with penicillin or a tetracycline.

FUNGI
Penicillium marneffei is endemic in South East Asia and southern China. It is carried by the bamboo rat and is found in water inhabited by these rodents. It is usually contracted in a natural setting and not through pets. In humans it causes a granulomatous disease resembling pulmonary tuberculosis except that skin lesions are common in penicilliosis. It is usually seen in immunocompromised hosts and, when diagnosed early, responds well to itraconazole or amphotericin B.

VIRUSES
Lymphocytic choriomeningitis virus is carried by mice and other rodents, including hamsters. It has been isolated from guinea pigs and dogs. Infection in humans results from exposure to the urine, feces or saliva of the rodent and may result in no symptoms, although a flu-like syndrome or meningitis may occur. The flu-like syndrome may be followed by recovery and then relapse with meningitis. Orchitis, parotitis and thrombocytopenia have also been observed. Diagnosis is made by isolation of the virus from a sterile site such as the cerebrospinal fluid or acute and convalescent serum specimens showing a four-fold rise in titer. There is no treatment. If a case occurs in one pet such as a hamster, the virus should be looked for in others in the hamster colony.

Hantavirus is spread from rodents to humans through urine and feces throughout the world (see Chapter 8.11). It is possible, but highly unlikely that pet rodents in cages in homes would be exposed.

MISCELLANEOUS PETS

Only the most common types of varied pets that people may try to tame and live with can be covered here.

MONKEYS
The most insidious and disastrous viral infection that a pet monkey can pass to a human is *Herpes simiae* (Herpes B virus). This latent infection of the monkey can be passed to humans by saliva or by a bite. It is almost always fatal in humans, in whom it causes a progressive encephalitis, which if it does not kill will leave severe sequelae in most cases (see Chapter 8.5 & 8.11). If diagnosed early, treatment with aciclovir may result in improvement and even recovery. Although attempts are made to screen pet monkeys, this does not always exclude carriers; unscrupulous dealers may not perform the test. Monkeys should not be pets.

REPTILES AND AMPHIBIANS
Any reptile or amphibian may carry *Salmonella* spp., which are excreted in the feces and may infect humans caring for the pet. This has been best exemplified by outbreaks in humans who have pet turtles.

FISH

Fish may also harbor *Salmonella* spp. and, in addition, *Mycobacterium marinum* has been found in fish tanks; this can cause granulomatous lesion of the hands in those cleaning the tanks and handling the fish. The diagnosis is made when the skin lesion is biopsied and cultured. Treatment with rifampin (rifampicin) and ethambutol, minocycline or trimethoprim–sulfamethoxazole (co-trimoxazole) have all been successful in eradicating this infection.

Erysipelothrix rhusiopathiae is an uncommon infection of food handlers, especially fishmongers. It causes erypiseloid, painful, indurated, irregular skin lesions, usually on the hands. It is very sensitive to penicillin. Penicillin-allergic patients can be treated with clindamycin.

REFERENCES

1. Jenner E. Vaccination against smallpox. Great Mind Series. New York: Prometheus Books; 1996:13.
2. Center for Information Management. US pet ownership and demographic source book. Schaumburg, IL: American Veterinary Medical Association; 1997.
3. Hubbert WT, McCulloch WF, Schnurrenberger PR (eds). Diseases transmitted from animals to man, 6th ed. Springfield, IL: Charles C Thomas; 1975.
4. Steele JH (ed). CRC handbook series in zoonoses (seven volumes). Boca Raton: CRC Press; 1979–1982. (Revised by Beran G, 1995.)
5. Acha PN, Szyfres B (eds). Zoonoses and communicable diseases common to man and animals. Washington, DC: Pan American Health Organization; 1987.
6. Bell, JC, Palmer SR, Panyne JM, eds. The zoonoses: infections transmitted from animals to man. London: Edward-Arnold; 1988.
7. Zoonosis updates from the Journal of the American Veterinary Medical Association. Schaumburg, IL: American Veterinary Medical Association; 1990.
8. Weinberg AN, Weber DJ, eds. Animal-associated human infections. Infect Dis Clin North Am 1991;5:1–177.
9. Goldstein EJ. Household pets and human infections. Infect Dis Clin North Am 1991;5:117–30.
10. Benenson AS, ed. Control of communiable disease in man, 16th ed. Washington DC: The American Public Health Association; 1995.
11. Cooperman SM. Cherchez le chien: household pets as reservoirs of persistent or recurrent streptococcal sore throats in children. N Y State J Med 1982;82:1685–7.
12. Kiehn TE, Hoefer H, Bottger EC, et al. Mycobacterium genavense infections in pet animals. J Clin Microbiol 1996;34:1840–2.
13. Hicklin H, Verghese A, Alvarez S. Dysgonic fermenter 2 septicemia. Rev Infect Dis 1987;5:884–90.
14. Bhatia G. Echiniococcus. Semin Respir Infect 1997;12:171–86.
15. Koehler, JE, Glaser CA, Tappero JW. Rochalimaea henselae infection. A new zoonosis with the domestic cat as reservoir. JAMA 1994;271:531–5.
16. Langley JM, Marrie TJ, Covert J, Waag DM, Williams JC. Poker players' pneumonia. An urban outbreak of Q fever following exposure to a parturient cat. N Engl J Med 1988;319:354–6.
17. Burton JL. Of mice and milkmaids, cats and cowpox. Lancet 1994;67:343.
18. Centers for Disease Control and Prevention. Compendium of measures to control Chlamydia psittaci infection among humans (psittacosis) and pet birds (avian chlamydiosis), 1998. MMWR Morb Mortal Wkly Rep 1998;47:1–14.
19. Washko RM, Hoefer H, Kiehn TE, Armstrong D, Dorsinville G, Frieden TR. Mycobacterium tuberculosis infection in a green-winged macaw (Ara chloroptera): report with public health implications. J Clin Microbiol 1998;36:1101–2.
20. White M, Armstrong D. Cryptococcosis. Infect Dis Clin North Am 1994;8:383–98.
21. Isolation of avian influenza A (HSN1) viruses from humans – Hong Kong May–December 1997. MMWR Morb Mortal Wkly Rep 1997;46:1204–7.

Infections from Non-domesticated Animals

James H Steele & Donald Armstrong

Zoonoses refer to infections transmitted from vertebrates to humans. Humans have contact with animals other than pets through a variety of activities. These include breeding and raising animals for commercial reasons, the care of animals in veterinary practices, handling of animals in zoos, and hunting or trapping or the handling of animals or their carcasses used for food. In addition, recreational activities such as hiking or boating may bring people into contact with various wild animals. There are so many opportunities for other animals to exchange micro-organisms with humans that only a brief overview can be given here.

There are numerous examples of zoonoses throughout this text and there are complete texts and manuals available on this subject.[1–4]

The physician can try to ascertain whether there is a history of contact with mammals, birds, reptiles, amphibians and fish through questions about travel, work and recreation and specific or general animal contact. A differential diagnosis and appropriate laboratory tests are needed to track down any potential infection. It may be difficult to carry out the laboratory tests because reference laboratories may be necessary and sending specimens may be complicated. Often the clinician must work through the local public health facilities to pursue the diagnosis. Serologic specimens are often necessary and must usually be stored in a refrigerator while awaiting a convalescent serum sample.

Because there is not sufficient space to cover each animal that can transmit a zoonosis, the organisms involved, the animals that can transmit them to humans and their geographic distribution are tabulated in Figure 6.1. More detailed descriptions can be obtained from other chapters in this book.

INFECTIONS FROM NON-DOMESTICATED ANIMALS				
Disease	Causative organism	Principal animals involved	Known distribution	Probable means of spread
Bacterial diseases (see Chapters 8.13, 8.14, 8.15, 8.19 & 8.22)				
Anthrax	*Bacillus anthracis*	Cattle, sheep goats, horses and wild herbivorous animals	Worldwide, common in Africa, Asia, South America and eastern Europe	Occupational skin exposure, food-borne in Africa, Russia and Asia; occasionally wounds or insect bites; rarely air-borne
Borreliosis	*Borrelia* spp.	Rodents	Worldwide	Soft ticks (*Ornithodoros* spp.)
Lyme disease	*Borrelia burgdorferi*	Deer, wild rodents	Worldwide	Hard ticks (*Ixodes* spp.)
Relapsing fever	*Borrelia recurrentis* (louse-borne or epidemic)	Transmitting lice have no animal reservoir	Epidemic	Crushing infected lice
	Borrelia hermsii (tick-borne or endemic)	Wild rodent ticks	Endemic	Tick bites
Brucellosis	*Brucella abortus*	Cattle, bison, elk and caribou	Worldwide, except North America	Occupational and recreational exposure
	Brucella melitensis	Goats and sheep	Worldwide	Milk, cheese and contact
	Brucella suis	Swine and caribou	Northern hemisphere	Air-borne
	Brucella canis	Dogs and coyotes	Rare	Genital secretion contact
Capnocytophaga infection	*Capnocytophaga canimorsus, Capnocytophaga cynodegmi*	Dogs and cats	USA	Bites and scratches
Campylobacter enteritis	*Campylobacter jejuni*	Domestic animals, dog, cats, poultry and wild birds	Worldwide; common	Mainly food-borne, milk, water-borne or occupational
	Campylobacter coli	Nonhuman primates and laboratory animals, domestic pigs	Common	
Cat-scratch disease	*Bartonella henselae, Bartonella quintana*	Cats	Worldwide	Scratches, bites and licks
Erysipeloid	*Erysipelothrix rhusiopathiae*	Swine, turkeys, pigeons, sea mammals and fish	Worldwide	Occupational and recreational exposure
Glanders	*Burkholderia mallei*	Equines	Rare except for some regions in Asia	Occupational exposure
Leptospirosis	*Leptospira interrogans* (200 serovars) in 23 serogroups	Domestic and wild animals; common in rodents and dogs	Worldwide	Occupational and recreational exposure, water- and food-borne

Fig. 6.1 Infections from non-domesticated animals. Adapted from Steele and Beran, 1995.[1]

INFECTIONS FROM NON-DOMESTICATED ANIMALS (continued)				
Disease	Causative organism	Principal animals involved	Known distribution	Probable means of spread
Parasitic diseases: trematode (fluke) diseases (continued)				
Schistosomiasis (bilharziasis) (continued	Schistosoma mattheei	Cattle	Southern Africa	
	Schistosoma mekongi	Dogs, monkeys	South East Asia	
	Schistosoma intercalatum	Cattle, sheep, antelopes and goats	Central Africa	
Swimmer's itch	Schistosome cercariae	Birds, mammals	Worldwide	Penetration of unbroken skin by cercariae from infected snails in fresh and salt water
Parasitic diseases: cestode (tapeworm) diseases (see Chapter 8.35)				
Dipylidiasis (dog tapeworm infection)	Dipylidium caninum	Dogs, cats and fleas	Worldwide	Accidental ingestion of tapeworm eggs in canine feces
Echinococcosis	Echinococcus granulosus	Dogs, sheep, cattle, swine, rodents, deer	Worldwide	Ingestion of tapeworm eggs
	Echinococcus multilocularis	Foxes, microtine rodents, coyotes, dogs, wolves, cats, voles, lemmings, shrews	Alaska, Canada, Asia, Europe	Ingestion of tapeworm eggs
	Echinococcus vogeli	Bush and hunting dogs, agouti, pacas and spiny rat	Central and South America	Ingestion of tapeworm eggs
Hymenolepiasis (dwarf tapeworm infection)	Hymenolepis nana	Humans, rodents	Worldwide	Accidental ingestion of tapeworm eggs or infected insects
Mouse or rat tapeworm	Hymenolepis nana, Hymenolepis diminuta	Rats, mice	Worldwide	Ingestion of cysticercoids in fleas and mealworms in food
Pork tapeworm disease	Taenia solium	Swine, humans	Worldwide where swine are reared; rare in USA, Canada, UK and Scandinavia	Ingestion of undercooked pork containing Cysticercus cellulosae; direct or autogenous transmission of T. solium ova in human may lead to cysticercosis
Asian taeniasis	Taenia saginata taiwanensis	Domestic and wild pigs, cattle and monkeys	East and south East Asia	Ingestion of undercooked meat
Sparganosis	Spirometra spp. (pseudophyllidean tapeworms, second larval stage)	Monkeys, cats, pigs, dogs, weasels, rats, chickens, snakes, frogs and mice	Worldwide; uncommon	Ingestion of infected Cyclops spp. or raw infected animal flesh
Taeniasis and cysticercosis, beef tapeworm disease	Taenia saginata	Cattle, water buffalo	Worldwide	Ingestion of undercooked meat containing Cysticercus bovis
Parasitic diseases: nematode (worm) diseases				
Anisakiasis (visceral larva migrans)	Larvae of Anisakis and Pseudoterranova spp.	Marine invertebrates, fish and mammals	Japan, Scandinavia, Western South America, Western Europe, USA	Ingestion of undercooked marine fish, squid or octopus
Filariasis: dirofilariasis	Dirofilaria immitis	Dogs, cats, raccoons, bears and mosquitoes	Worldwide	Bites of infected mosquitoes
Filariasis: Malayan filariasis	Brugia malayi	Cats, other carnivores, monkeys and mosquitoes	Asia; common	Bites of infected mosquitoes
Filariasis: tropical eosinophilia	Brugia pahangi			
Gnathostomiasis	Gnathostoma spinigererum	Dogs, cats and wild carnivores; copepods and freshwater fish.	East Asia, India and Australia	Ingestion of infected fish or poultry
Gongylonemiasis	Gongylonema pulchrum	Ruminants, domestic and wild swine and other mammals; beetles	Worldwide; rare	Ingestion of infected arthropods
Larva migrans, cutaneous (see also gnathostomiasis)	Ancylostoma braziliense, Ancylostoma caninum	Cats, dogs and wild carnivores	Worldwide in tropics and subtropics; common	Contact with infective larvae, which penetrate the skin
	Strongyloides stercoralis	Animals such as cats, dogs, sheep and swine	Worldwide in tropics and subtropics; rare to common	Contact with infective larvae, which penetrate the skin
Larva migrans, visceral (see also angiostrongyliasis and anisakiasis)	Toxocara canis, Toxocara cati	Dogs, cats	Worldwide	Ingestion of embryonated eggs shed in feces of dogs and cats
	Baylisascaris procyonis	Raccoons	North America, Europe	Accidental ingestion of embryonated eggs in soil
Oesophagostomiasis (ternidensiasis)	Oesophagostomum spp., Ternidens diminutus	Primates	Asia, Africa and South America	Accidental ingestion of infective larvae in soil
Strongyloidiasis	Strongyloides stercoralis, Strongyloides fuelleborni	Dogs, cats, foxes and primates	Worldwide; rare to common	Contact with infective larvae, which penetrate the skin

Fig. 6.1 Infections from non-domesticated animals continued.

		INFECTIONS FROM NON-DOMESTICATED ANIMALS (continued)		
Disease	Causative organism	Principal animals involved	Known distribution	Probable means of spread
		Parasitic diseases: nematode (worm) diseases (continued)		
Thelaziasis	*Thelazia* spp.	Dogs, cats, other domestic and wild animals, flies	East and South Asia; rare	Infected insects
Trichinosis	*Trichinella spiralis* and subspp.	Swine, rodents, bears, wild carnivores and marine mammals	Worldwide, especially sub-Arctic region	Ingestion of pork and flesh of wild animals containing viable cysts
Trichostrongyliasis	*Trichostrongylus* spp.	Cattle, sheep and wild ruminants	Worldwide	Ingestion of infective larvae on plant foods or in soil
Trichuriasis (whipworm infection)	*Trichuris trichiura,* other *Trichuris* spp.	Humans, other primates, domestic and wild canids and swine	Worldwide; common	Ingestion of embryonated eggs on plant foods or in soil
		Viral diseases (see Chapter 8.11)		
African hemorrhagic fever	Marburg and Ebola viruses	African green monkeys	Central and southern Africa	Contact with infected tissues
Filovirus infections	Ebola-related filoviruses	Cynomolgus monkeys	South East Asia	Person-to-person spread
Argentine hemorrhagic fever	Junin virus (arenavirus)	Rodents	Argentina	Rodent excretions and secretions
Bolivian hemorrhagic fever	Machupo virus (arenavirus)	Rodents	Bolivia	Rodent excretions
Brazilian hemorrhagic fever	Sabia virus (arenavirus)	Rodents are suspected	Brazil	Rodent excretions suspected; other aerosols
California group infections	California group of bunyaviruses			
La Cross encephalitis		Ground squirrels, other rodents	USA, Canada	Bites of mosquitoes (*Aedes* spp.)
Tahyna fever		Hares, rodents, other mammals	Europe, Africa	
Central European tick-borne encephalitis	CEE virus (flavivirus)	Rodents, hedgehogs, birds, goats and sheep	Europe	Bites of ticks of *Ixodes* spp. May be milk-borne
Colorado tick fever	CTF virus	Ground squirrels, chipmunks, porcupines and small rodents	Western USA; common	Bites of ticks (*Dermacentor andersoni*)
Contagious ecthyma (orf)	Orf virus (parapox)	Sheep, goats and wild ruminants	Worldwide; common	Occupational exposure
Cowpox	Cowpox virus	Cattle, rodents, cats and zoo cats	Worldwide; rare; no recent cases	Contact exposure
Crimean–Congo hemorrhagic fever	Crimean–Congo hemorrhagic fever virus (bunyavirus)	Cattle, rodents, sheep, goats, hares and birds	Southern Russia, Eastern Europe, Africa, Middle East, Asia	Bites of ticks (*Hyalomma* and *Boophilus* spp.)
Eastern equine encephalomyelitis	EEE virus (alphavirus)	Wild birds, domestic fowl, horses, mules and donkeys	Western hemisphere	Mosquitoes (*Culiseta melanura* and *Aedes* spp.)
Encephalomyocarditis	EMC virus (picornavirus)	Rats, mice, squirrels, swine and nonhuman primates	Worldwide	Environmental contamination
Far Eastern tick-borne encephalitis (Russian spring–summer encephalitis)	FE (RSSE) virus (flavivirus)	Birds, small mammals and sheep	Asia and Europe; rare	Bites of ticks (*Ixodes persulcatus* and *Ixodes ricinus*)
Foot-and-mouth disease	FMD virus (Aphthovirus spp. types A, O, C, SAT and Asia)	Cattle, swine and related cloven-hoofed animals	Europe, Asia, Africa and South America	Contact exposure; humans are quite resistant, but can be carriers
Hantaviral diseases	Hantaviruses (bunyavirus)	Rodents	Worldwide	Aerosols from rodent excretions and secretions
Hantaviral pulmonary syndrome	Sin Nombre virus, Black Creek Canal virus	*Peromyscus* spp., *Sigmodon hispidus*	USA, may be wider spread	
Hemorrhagic fever with renal syndrome (Korean hemorrhagic fever)	HFRS virus (Hantaan virus)	*Apodemus* spp.	China, Siberia, Korea, Manchuria, Japan	
Other hantaviral diseases	Dobrava virus	*Apodemus* spp.	Balkan countries	
	Pnumala virus	*Clethrionomys* spp.	Europe	
	Seoul virus	*Rattus* spp.	Worldwide	
Simian herpes B virus disease	Simian B virus	Old world monkeys; cell cultures	Worldwide; rare	Bites of monkeys, occupational exposures
Influenza including type A (swine and equine)	Influenzavirus (myxovirus)	Swine and ducks	Worldwide; common	Contact exposure; animals rarely a source

Fig. 6.1 Infections from non-domesticated animals continued.

INFECTIONS FROM NON-DOMESTICATED ANIMALS (continued)				
Disease	Causative organism	Principal animals involved	Known distribution	Probable means of spread
Viral diseases (continued)				
Japanese B encephalitis	JE virus (flavivirus)	Swine, wild birds and horses	Asia, Pacific islands from Japan to Philippines	Bites of mosquitoes (*Culex tritaeniorhyncus*, other *Culex* spp.)
Kyasanur Forest disease	KF virus (flavivirus)	Rodents and monkeys	India	Bites of ticks (*Haemaphysalis spinigera*)
Lassa fever	Lassa virus (arenavirus)	Wild rodents	Africa	Rodent excretions and secretions; contact in hospitals and laboratories
Louping ill	LI virus (flavivirus)	Sheep, goats, grouse and small rodents	UK; rare	Bites of ticks *Ixodes ricinus*
Lymphocytic choriomeningitis	LCM virus (arenavirus)	House mice, dogs, monkeys, guinea pigs and hamsters	Worldwide	Host excretions and secretions
Milker's nodules (pseudocowpox)	Pseudocowpox virus (parapoxvirus)	Cattle	Worldwide; common	Occupational exposure
Monkeypox	Monkeypox virus	Nonhuman primates	West Africa; very rare	Contact, aerosols
Murray Valley encephalitis	MVE virus (flavivirus)	Wild birds	Australia, New Guinea; rare	Bites of mosquitoes (*Culex annulirostris*)
Newcastle disease	ND virus (paramyxovirus)	Fowl and wild birds	Worldwide; common	Occupational exposure
Omsk hemorrhagic fever	OHF virus (flavivirus)	Rodents, muskrats	Omsk, Siberia; rare	Bites of ticks (*Dermacentor* spp.); direct contact (*Dermacentor marginatus*)
Rabies and rabies-related infections	Lyssaviruses, rabies virus, Duvenhage virus, Mokola virus, Ibadan shrew virus, Obodhiang virus	Wild and domestic dogs, skunks, raccoons, vampire and insectivorous bats	Worldwide, except Australia, New Zealand, UK, Ireland, Scandinavia, Japan and Taiwan; many smaller islands are free, including Hawaii	Bites of diseased animals; aerosols in closed environments
Rift Valley fever	RVF virus (phlebovirus)	Sheep, goats, cattle, camels	Africa; common to rare	Bites of mosquitoes (*Aedes* spp.); contact at autopsy or handling fresh meat
St Louis encephalitis	SLE virus (flavivirus)	Wild birds and domestic fowl	Western hemisphere	Bites of mosquitoes (*Culex tarsalis*, *Culex pipiensquinquefasciatus* complex, *Culex nigripalpus*)
Sindbis virus disease	Sindbis virus (alphavirus)	Birds	Eastern hemisphere; rare	Bites of mosquitoes (*Culex* spp.)
Ross River fever	Ross River virus (alphavirus)	Undetermined	Australia, South Pacific Islands	Bites of mosquitoes (*Culex annulirostris*, *Aedes* spp.)
Tanapox	Tanapox virus	Asian and African monkeys	Asia, Africa and in colonies of monkeys	Contact, aerosols
Venezuelan hemorrhagic fever	Gnanarito virus (arenavirus)	Rodents	Venezuela	Rodent excretions
Venezuelan equine encephalitis	VEE virus (alphavirus)	Rodents, equines	Western hemisphere; common	Bites of mosquitoes (*Mansonia*, *Aedes*, *Culex* spp.)
Vesicular stomatitis	VS virus (Indiana and New Jersey strains)	Swine, cattle, horses, bats, rodents; other wild mammals	North and South America	Contact exposure and insect bites including mosquitoes and biting flies (*Phlebotomus* spp.)
Wesselsbron fever	Wesselsbron virus (flavivirus)	Sheep	Southern Africa, South East Asia	Bites of mosquitoes (*Aedes*, *Mansonia*, *Culex* spp.)
West Nile fever	West Nile virus (flavivirus)	Wild birds, horses	Eastern hemisphere; common	Bites of mosquitoes (*Culex univittatus*, *Culex pipiens*, *Culex modestus*)
Western equine encephalomyelitis	WEE virus (alphavirus)	Wild birds, domestic fowl, horses, mules, donkeys, bats, reptiles and amphibians	Western and Central USA, Canada, South America	Mosquitoes (*Culex tarsalis* in USA; other *Culex* and *Aedes* spp. outside USA)
Yabapox	Yabapox virus	African monkeys	Africa; rare	Contact, aerosols
Yellow fever	YF virus (flavivirus)	Monkeys, baboons	Tropical South America, Africa; sporadic	Bites of mosquitoes (*Aedes aegypti* in urban cycles, *Haemagogus* spp. in jungle cycles in South America, *Aedes* spp. in jungle cycles in Africa)

CONCLUSION

The global zoonoses include a number of 'emerging' infectious diseases such as Ebola and Hantavirus infections. Understanding and control of these infections depend upon co-operation between human and veterinary physicians, researchers and epidemiologists. Public health support from the local community level through state and national governments to international organizations will be necessary for a co-ordinated response against these zoonotic infections.

REFERENCES

1. Steele JH, editor-in-chief. CRC handbook series in zoonoses, 7 volumes. Boca Rotan: CRC Press; 1979–1982. (Revised by Beran G., 1995.)
2. Acha PN, Szyfres B, eds. Zoonoses and communicable diseases common to man and animals. Washington: Pan American Health Organization; 1987.
3. Bell, JC, Palmer SR, Panyne JM, eds. The zoonoses: infections transmitted from animals to man. London: Edward Arnold; 1988.
4. Benenson AS, ed. Control of communicable disease in man, 16th ed. The American Public Health Association; 1995.

Food- and Water-borne Infections

Christopher P Conlon

INTRODUCTION

Food and water are essential for human existence. However, there is a constant risk of food and water becoming contaminated with potentially pathogenic organisms. Every human being risks exposure to disease when ingesting either food or water that may be vehicles of infection. A large number of such infections simply result in acute diarrhea and vomiting, a syndrome usually called 'food poisoning'. The term 'food-borne illness' is used whether the vehicle of infection is food or water. Also included in the definition of food poisoning are gastrointestinal illnesses caused by natural plant toxins, by heavy metals and by toxins such as scombroid that are associated with eating fish and other animals.

There are other food-borne and water-borne illnesses that are distinct from food poisoning. In these diseases, although food or water are the vehicles of infection and the gastrointestinal tract is the portal of entry, gastrointestinal symptoms are minimal and infection results in systemic symptoms or distant foci of disease.

Each year the average adult in a developed country drinks more than 500l of water and eats over 450kg of meat and vegetables, not to mention other foods. It is rare to find anyone who has not, at some time, been a victim of food poisoning. Many infections result from organisms derived from the gastrointestinal tract of other humans that have led to contamination of food or water, so-called fecal–oral transmission. Increasingly recognized, however, is the role of other species in food- and water-borne illness. Zoonoses such as brucellosis are well recognized, and more unusual problems, such as trichinella infection related to wild boar meat, are occasionally reported.[1] Much recent interest has focused on prions crossing species barriers, with good evidence that new variant Creutzfeld–Jacob disease is related to the consumption of beef from animals suffering from bovine spongiform encephalopathy (see Chapters 2.19 & 8.12).

This chapter outlines the problems related to infection caused by what we eat and drink.

EPIDEMIOLOGY

FOOD
The provision of food and water supplies has become increasingly complicated as society has become more urbanized and as the global economy has become more complex. In developed countries, the production and distribution of food has become highly sophisticated so that it is frequently consumed a long distance from its source and a long time after it has been produced. Often there are large, centralized facilities for food production with the risk that contamination early in the production process may lead to widespread infection in many different regions. In addition, there is an increasing tendency to eat food away from home and, in particular, there has been a huge increase in the consumption of convenience and 'take-away' foods. In contrast, in less developed countries food is usually consumed close to its source with much less centralization because refrigeration and other means of preservation are limited and food soon spoils if transported over any distance. Restaurants are less common and most food is prepared and

TYPES OF FOODS ASSOCIATED WITH VARIOUS PATHOGENS THAT CAUSE FOOD POISONING	
Pathogen	**Foods**
Staphylococcus aureus	Cream pastries, salads, meat products, cold foods
Bacillus cereus	Fried rice, vegetables, meat dishes, vanilla sauce
Clostridium perfringens	Cooked meats, gravies
Vibrio cholerae, Vibrio parahaemolyticus, Vibrio vulnificus	Shellfish, seafood
Campylobacter jejuni	Milk, poultry
Salmonella enteritidis	Eggs, poultry, other meats
Shigella spp.	Salads, milk, cold foods
Yersinia enterocolitica	Milk, pork products
Escherichia coli	Ground beef, milk, lettuce, unpasteurized cider
Listeria monocytogenes	Soft cheese, pâté, milk, coleslaw
Clostridium botulinum	Meats, home-canned fruit and vegetables
Hepatitis A and enteric viruses	Shellfish, various foods

Fig. 7.1 Types of foods associated with various pathogens that cause food poisoning.

consumed in the home. Thus, point source outbreaks of food poisoning, often on a massive scale, are relatively common in developed countries but rare in developing countries. In England and Wales between 1989 and 1991 there were 3012 reported outbreaks of food poisoning and in the USA there were 2423 outbreaks over a similar time period.[2,3] However, most cases of food-borne infection are sporadic (i.e. not part of an outbreak) whether they occur in the tropics or in temperate regions.

Almost every type of food has been associated with carrying infectious agents and some have been associated with noninfectious toxins (Fig. 7.1). There are numerous organisms that can cause food-borne infection, with some being recognized as very common causes of food poisoning. The data on the incidence and etiology vary geographically, largely because different countries have developed different surveillance systems. Most surveillance is passive, based on reports by clinicians and on laboratory reports of isolation of food-borne pathogens. In England and Wales, where food poisoning is notifiable and where laboratories report to the Public Health Laboratory Service, there were over 50,000 cases of food poisoning in 1991, giving a notification rate of 103 per 100,000 population. *Campylobacter* spp. was the most commonly reported cause of gastrointestinal illness, with *Salmonella* spp. infection second. The latter, however, was more commonly implicated in outbreaks. Similar figures are found in the USA. A program of active surveillance of food-borne diseases began in the USA in 1996; it involved five states and collected data on seven potentially food-borne infections (confirmed by culture).[4] This showed that

Campylobacter spp. were the most common with an incidence rate of 25 per 100,000 population, and *Salmonella* spp. were second with a rate of 16 per 100,000. There were regional and seasonal differences in the incidences of certain infections but the reasons for these were not clear. Information about food-borne illness in developing countries is scant because few developing countries have any surveillance systems in place because of resource limitations.

The morbidity of food poisoning is considerable but, in developed countries, the mortality is relatively low. Most deaths occur in debilitated people, often at the extremes of age. Studies in the USA and England show that salmonellosis is the most likely infection to lead to death, although listerial infections are more likely to lead to hospitalization than other causes of food poisoning. Statistics from the developing countries are not readily available but it is estimated that diarrheal disease (much of which is related to food-borne infection) is responsible for 3 million deaths a year in the tropics, mainly in children.[5]

WATER

Water becomes a vehicle for infection when contaminated by human or animal feces. The probability of becoming infected with an organism through this fecal–oral route depends on the availability of potable water. Thus, water-borne infection is relatively rare in developed countries where there are usually municipal supplies of treated drinking water and reliable sewage disposal systems to prevent contamination of the drinking water supply. However, failure of these sophisticated systems can result in large outbreaks of disease.[6] In recent years there have been outbreaks of illness caused by *Cryptosporidium* spp. from cattle feces contaminating reservoirs at times when water treatment procedures were inadequate. Sporadic water-borne infection may occur in developed countries as a result of poor hygiene but this is relatively uncommon. More common is the sporadic infection resulting from exposure to water inadvertently swallowed during leisure activities such as swimming, fishing, canoeing and surfing (see Chapter 3.12).[7] Some of these infections result from the dumping of raw sewage into rivers and into the sea (Fig. 7.2).

Water-borne infection is more common in developing countries, particularly in rural areas where basic sanitation may be rudimentary and access to clean water is limited. This can be a particular problem in times of drought. Contamination of drinking water is common and may even occur at the communal taps when piped water is supplied to a village. Firewood is usually scarce so drinking water is not boiled and water filters are usually too expensive. Constant exposure to unclean water not only leads to a large burden of acute and chronic diarrhea, but also increases the risk of parasitic disease (Fig. 7.3).

PATHOGENESIS AND PATHOPHYSIOLOGY

HOST FACTORS

The ability of the human gastrointestinal tract to withstand infection by contaminated food or water depends on a variety of host defenses, including human behavior. If food looks, smells or tastes bad because of contamination it may not be ingested. Most things we ingest are not sterile, even if they seem safe, but acid (pH<4) gastric secretions kill ingested bacteria relatively easily. Usually a large inoculum of organisms is required to overcome this acid barrier. However, relative achlorhydria, whether due to disease or to drugs (e.g. proton pump inhibitors or antacids), may allow bacteria to multiply within the stomach so that a relatively smaller initial inoculum is needed to cause disease.

Additional protection is provided by the normal bowel flora. In the human gut there are several hundred species of bacteria, almost all of which are anaerobes, and these organisms may physically prevent pathogenic bacteria from adhering to enterocytes, often a key prerequisite for causing disease.[8] This is sometimes termed colonization resistance. Normal gastrointestinal motility ensures a regular distribution of the bowel flora and may help eliminate potential pathogens.

The human gastrointestinal tract is also extremely active immunologically. Lymphocytes in the lamina propria, intraepithelial lymphocytes and lymphoid nodules, such as Peyer's patches in the small bowel, make up what is known as the gut-associated lymphoid tissue. Plasma cells in the lamina propria make specific antibody and most importantly produce secretory IgA, which can effectively block bacterial adhesion to enterocytes. Neonates receive immunoglobulin and lactoferrin in the colostrum of breast milk, which provides extra protection compared with formula feeds. Patients who are immunodeficient, such as those who have HIV infection or transplant recipients, are at greater risk of infection by enteric pathogens. Debilitated people, the very young and the very old are also at increased risk.

MICROBIAL FACTORS

Food- and water-borne organisms that cause disease must either cause damage to the intestinal mucosa or must be able to invade via the gastrointestinal tract to cause systemic or distant infection. The specific pathogenetic mechanisms for individual organisms will be

MICRO-ORGANISMS ASSOCIATED WITH WATER-BORNE INFECTIONS	
Bacteria	*Vibrio cholerae*
	Vibrio parahaemolyticus
	Campylobacter jejuni
	Shigella spp.
	Escherichia coli (especially enterotoxigenic *Escherichia coli*)
Viruses	Rotavirus
	Norwalk virus
	Small round-structured viruses
	Hepatitis A virus
	Hepatitis E virus
Protozoa	*Giardia lamblia*
	Entamoeba histolytica
	Cryptosporidium parvum
	Isospora belli
	Cyclospora cayetanensis
	Microsporidia spp.
	Dientamoeba fragilis
	Balantidium coli

Fig. 7.2 Micro-organisms associated with water-borne infections.

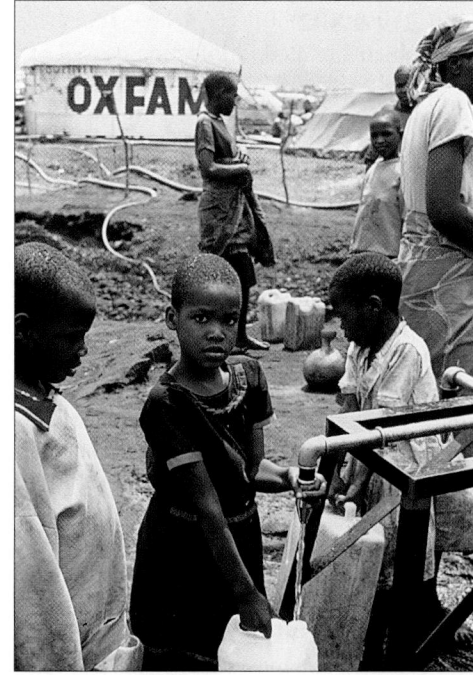

Fig. 7.3 Water source in a developing country at a refugee camp.

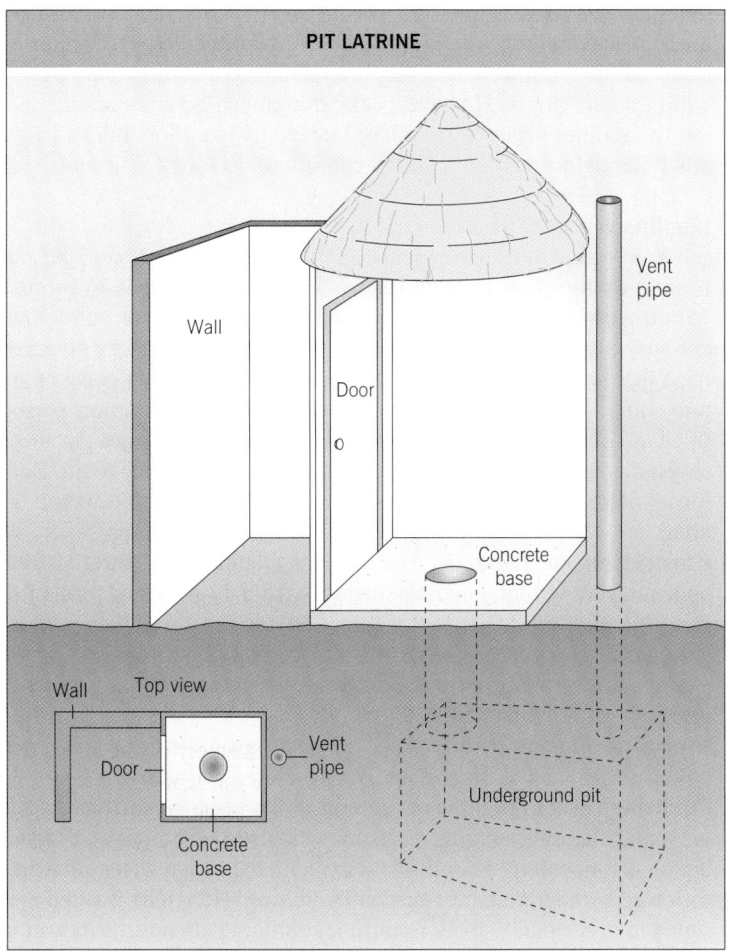

PIT LATRINE

Fig. 7.4 An example of a pit latrine.

found in detail in Chapters 2.35 and 2.37, but the general principles are outlined below.

Toxins

A large variety of toxins may be produced by enteric pathogens and these fall into three main categories:[9]

- enterotoxins,
- cytotoxins, and
- neurotoxins.

Enterotoxins. The best example of an enterotoxin is cholera toxin, which binds to the enterocyte by means of its 5 B-subunits, thus facilitating the entry of the A subunit into the cell, where it can activate adenyl cyclase; this in turn leads to net secretion of chloride ions and water into the gut lumen. This excess secretion overwhelms the normal resorptive capacity of the small and large bowel, leading to diarrhea. Most enterotoxins act in a similar manner, causing net secretion into the lumen but causing relatively little inflammation in the mucosa.

Cytotoxins. Cytotoxins, such as those produced by *Shigella* spp. or by enterohemorrhagic *Escherichia coli*, bind to enterocytes and lead to inflammation and usually to mucosal damage. Such cytotoxins are often associated with bloody diarrhea, or dysentery, because of the mucosal damage they cause.

Neurotoxins. Neurotoxins are less commonly implicated in food-borne illness. The most common example is staphylococcal food poisoning. The preformed toxin is ingested and causes profuse vomiting by stimulating the emetic center in the brain. Staphylococcal enterotoxins cause the coexisting diarrhea. Much more rare but more serious is botulism. The preformed toxin is extremely potent and once absorbed is widely disseminated, binding to nerve endings and inhibiting the release of acetylcholine, particularly in skeletal muscle. This leads to neuromuscular paralysis and, if not recognized and treated, death from respiratory failure.

Adherence

Most organisms cannot cause disease unless they can adhere to enterocytes. Some bacteria adhere using various adhesins, or fimbriae, which can be encoded by plasmids and are thus potentially transferrable to other species.[10] Some protozoa have specially adapted ways of sticking to the gut mucosa. *Giardia* spp. have suction plates on their ventral surface and microsporidia have a polar element that is inserted into the enterocyte. The helminth *Taenia solium* has a sucker and small hooklets that allow it to remain attached to the mucosa. Viruses, such as rotavirus, stick to the mucosa via ligands such as hemagglutinin protein.

Invasion

The ability of some organisms to invade mucosal cells and damage them may be associated with antigens in the bacterial cell wall. Virulence in *Shigella* spp. is related to the O antigen in the lipopolysaccharide cell wall, which may make it resistant to attack by complement. The production of some outer membrane proteins may enable the bacteria to survive intracellularly. Some of the genes controlling these attributes are chromosomal but others are on plasmids.

Other factors

The ability of bacteria to multiply quickly also provides an advantage against host defenses and this rapid multiplication allows for the exchange of genetic material, possibly with the acquisition of new virulence characteristics. Motility of enteric pathogens may be important in causing disease, either by aiding colonization of the mucosa or by evading phagocytes. Some viruses appear to cause selective damage to epithelial cells in the intestinal villi while leaving secretory cells in the crypts intact, thus favoring net secretion and the production of watery diarrhea.

PREVENTION

Food poisoning and other food-borne illnesses are often preventable through a combination of public health measures, personal hygiene and immunization and, sometimes, by chemoprophylaxis.

PUBLIC HEALTH

The provision of adequate housing and sanitation along with education about basic hygiene and food handling are major reasons why diarrheal illness has become much less common in developed countries than in underdeveloped ones. Modern sewage treatment plants and well-organized drinking water treatment and distribution dramatically reduce the risk of transmission of infection via the fecal–oral route. Good food production, refrigeration and distribution along with proper food handling in shops and restaurants is also important. For such systems to remain safe there need to be regular inspections, training of staff and registration of premises, all backed up by legislation. All of these methods are more likely to be found in developed countries but progress is also being made in less developed countries. Flush toilets are common in cities in the tropics and well-designed pit latrines, such as the Blair privy, are increasingly being built in urban townships and rural villages (Fig. 7.4).

These preventive efforts need to be strengthened by surveillance of food-borne illness based both on clinical cases and on laboratory reports. A system of compulsory notification of certain infections is essential. Such surveillance should lead to the prompt recognition of outbreaks, and the timely investigation of such outbreaks can often identify the source of the problem and lead to control measures aimed at preventing further infections.

PERSONAL MEASURES

The individual can play a major role in preventing food-borne illness. Attention to personal hygiene, especially hand washing, is an important way of reducing fecal–oral transmission. Proper food handling involving careful storage and preparation of both raw and cooked food is essential and, of course, easier to achieve in developed countries.

In countries with unreliable supplies of potable water, individuals may treat their personal drinking water in a variety of ways to minimize the risk of infection. Boiling and filtering water are time-honored methods of reducing contamination. Water can also be treated by chemicals such as chlorine or iodine to attempt to sterilize it. These methods are often used by travelers to less developed countries but can also be used by local residents if the methods are available and affordable. Travelers and others can reduce the chances of food-borne infection by careful eating, avoiding uncooked and unwashed fruit and vegetables, ice cubes and unpasteurized dairy produce. Chemoprophylaxis with drugs such as trimethoprim–sulphamethoxazole (co-trimoxazole), quinolones or doxycycline can reduce the risk of travelers' diarrhea (see Chapter 6.2).[11]

IMMUNIZATION

Polio vaccination is the most successful example of prevention of a food-borne illness, the disease having been virtually eliminated from many parts of the world. Hepatitis A virus infection, formerly prevented by repeated doses of gammaglobulin, is now easily preventable with the new vaccines, although the cost of these is prohibitive in most parts of the world where the virus is endemic. The risk of acquiring typhoid can also be reduced markedly by immunization, either with a polysaccharide parenteral immunization or a live, attenuated oral vaccine.

The old parenteral cholera vaccine offered less than 50% protection against infection and had serious side effects. However, new oral vaccines directed against cholera toxin have looked extremely promising in field trials.[12] Because the toxin is very similar to the toxin of enterotoxigenic *E. coli*, immunization may protect against disease caused by this organism as well.

CLINICAL FEATURES

The clinical consequences of food-borne infection depend, to some extent, on the infecting organism. However, with those organisms that cause food poisoning, with predominantly gastrointestinal symptoms, most patients develop diarrhea or vomiting or both, and the clinical features relate to whether the small or large intestine is affected. Invasive organisms can cause a variety of clinical features. In these diseases, gastrointestinal symptoms are mild or nonexistent but fever is often a feature.

BACTERIAL FOOD POISONING

Most patients who have food poisoning develop acute diarrhea, often with vomiting. Isolated vomiting may also occur but this is more unusual. Many infecting organisms, such as *Bacillus cereus*, elaborate enterotoxins that affect the small bowel, causing little mucosal inflammation and leading to a secretory diarrhea. Patients usually present with watery diarrhea without blood in the stool. There may be vomiting early on but this tends to settle before the diarrhea resolves. Other organisms such as *Shigella* spp. cause diarrhea via cytotoxins that cause inflammation of the intestinal mucosa and usually affect the distal small bowel and the large intestine. These patients may also have vomiting but diarrhea, often with blood (reflecting the mucosal inflammation), is the main feature and may last longer than with cases of secretory diarrhea. Generally, the incubation period from ingestion of the infected food or water until the onset of symptoms is longer with bacteria causing an inflammatory diarrhea. Some of the clinical features of individual infections are outlined below.

Infections with secretory diarrhea

Staphylococcal food poisoning. Often associated with cream-filled pastries and some tinned meats, staphylococci multiply in the food, producing various staphylococcal toxins. These preformed toxins are ingested and cause symptoms within a few hours. There is usually initial nausea followed quickly by severe vomiting. Diarrhea appears later and fever is rare. Most cases are self-limiting and recovery occurs within 24–48 hours. However, dehydration can be quite severe and, rarely, fatalities occur as a result of marked hypotension. In rare cases, other staphylococcal toxins may cause a toxic shock syndrome (see Chapter 8.13).

Bacillus cereus. There are really two syndromes associated with *B. cereus* infection, both toxin mediated.[13] In the first, ingestion of the preformed toxin, often in fried rice or vanilla sauce, leads to profuse vomiting within a few hours, accompanied by severe abdominal cramps. Diarrhea occurs in a minority of cases. The history of eating fried rice helps to differentiate this disease from staphylococcal food poisoning. The second syndrome has a longer incubation period (median 9 hours) and is characterized by watery diarrhea. In these cases, the bacteria multiply in the gut lumen and produce toxin. Both forms of *B. cereus* food poisoning are mild and resolve within 24 hours.

Clostridium perfringens. The clinical features of clostridial food poisoning are virtually indistinguishable from the diarrheal form of *B. cereus* infection. Most cases of infection due to *Clostridium perfringens* result from eating some form of cooked meat. The toxins are potent so there are often small outbreaks associated with a particular meal.

Vibrio parahaemolyticus. This organism grows best in a salt-rich environment and is thus usually associated with food poisoning following the consumption of seafood and, especially, shellfish.[14] The incubation period can range from a few hours to several days, depending on the inoculum. The illness starts with explosive watery diarrhea followed by abdominal cramps and vomiting. Headache is often present and occasionally there is sufficient inflammation of the bowel to cause fever and, rarely, some blood in the diarrhea. Most cases are self-limiting but may take several days to resolve.

Cholera. This disease, caused by *Vibrio cholerae*, is the classic example of a toxin-mediated secretory diarrhea.[15] Cholera usually follows the consumption of contaminated water but has been associated with eating shellfish. It is characterized by moderate to severe watery diarrhea without fever and with little vomiting. In severe cases, liters of fluid can be lost over 24 hours and severe prostration and even death may result from severe dehydration. In outbreaks, many infected people have few or no symptoms. With adequate fluid replacement, most cases are self-limiting. Almost all cases of cholera occur in the tropics and imported cases are rare, partly because of the short incubation period and the severity of symptoms and partly because the risk to travelers is small (Fig. 7.5).

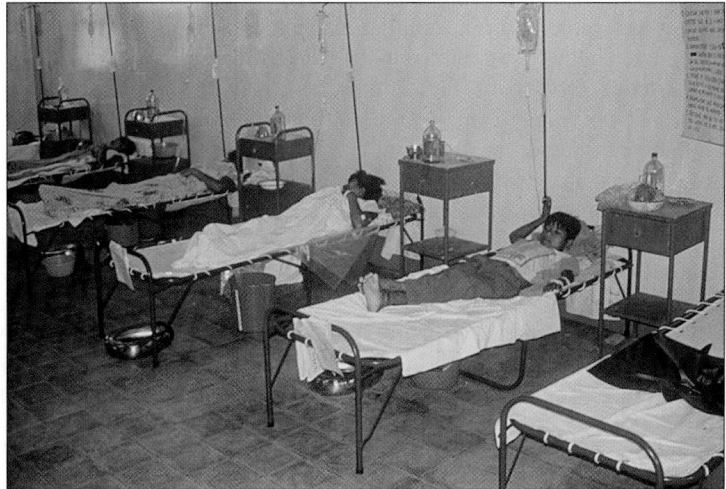

Fig. 7.5 A cholera ward in Peru. Courtesy of Dr J Vanchez.

Inflammatory diarrhea

Infections with Campylobacter *spp.*, Salmonella *spp.* and Shigella *spp.* *Campylobacter jejuni*, *Salmonella enteritidis* and other non-typhoidal salmonellae, *Shigella* spp. and enteroinvasive *E. coli* all produce an enterocolitis. *Campylobacter* spp. are sometimes associated with the consumption of milk or chicken and has also been associated with exposure to pets, such as puppies.[16] *Salmonella* spp. are particularly linked with poultry and eggs.[17] *Shigella* spp. have been found in association with a variety of foods and with contaminated water. The incubation period is often several days. Diarrhea is the principal symptom and there may be blood in the stool as a result of colonic inflammation. Vomiting is more common with *Salmonella* infection but can occur with any of these organisms. Abdominal pain is frequently severe and, particularly in campylobacter and *Salmonella* infections, may mimic an acute abdomen. Most cases are mild and resolve over the course of about a week. However, sometimes symptoms can be prolonged, raising the possibility of inflammatory bowel disease as a differential diagnosis. *Campylobacter* spp. and *Salmonella* spp. occasionally become invasive and cause an enteric fever syndrome with positive blood cultures. This is more likely in the elderly and the immunosuppressed. Both *Salmonella* and *Campylobacter* infections are associated with extraintestinal symptoms in the absence of bacteremia, such as arthritis. *Campylobacter* spp. are also strongly associated with Guillain–Barré syndrome (see Chapter 8.19).[18]

Yersinial infections. *Yersinia enterocolitica* can present in a number of ways. Most of the time it causes an entercolitis, presenting with acute diarrhea. Although it mainly affects young children, adults may sometimes be infected. The diarrheal illness may be severe and often resolves more slowly than that caused by other organisms. This organism may also cause a mesenteric adenitis and terminal ileitis in young children, which can mimic appendicitis. In such cases, diarrhea is rarely a feature. Sometimes infection with *Y. enterocolitica* is associated with extragastrointestinal features, such as arthritis, and rarely bacteremia occurs.

Escherichia coli *O157:H7*. Infection with *E. coli* O157:H7 causes an inflammatory colitis and is associated with hemolytic–uremic syndrome. It has become much more common in the past 2 decades and has been particularly associated with the consumption of hamburger meat.[19] Sporadic cases occur but major outbreaks have highlighted the seriousness of this infection. Most recently a large outbreak in Scotland caused 21 fatalities. The majority of cases present with diarrhea, which often contains frank blood and is frequently occult blood positive. Most of these infections are self-limiting. However, a proportion of infected patients develop hemolytic–uremic syndrome, which occurs 5–7 days after the onset of diarrhea and which carries a significant risk of death from renal failure, bleeding or cerebral infarction.

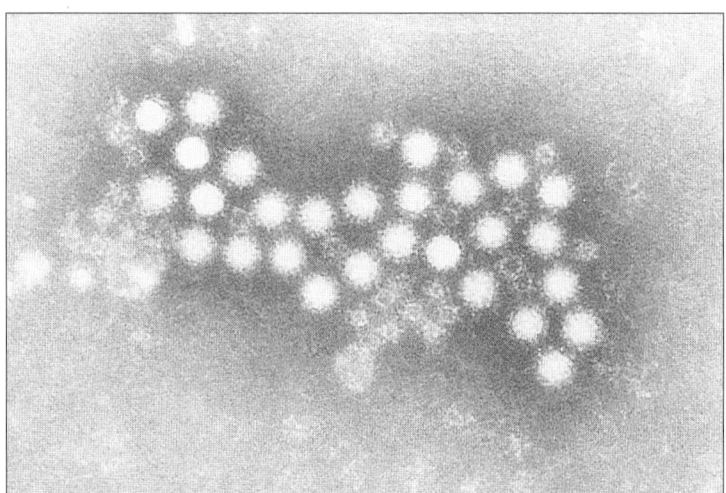

Fig. 7.6 Electron micrograph of small round-structured viruses.

Botulism. This disease is caused by food poisoning with a preformed neurotoxin produced by *Clostridium botulinum*. Many cases are related to home canning of produce but outbreaks related to commercially prepared food also occur from time to time.[20] The neurotoxin causes predominantly bulbar and ocular palsies, and therefore swallowing difficulties, double vision, blurred vision and ptosis are common. Limb weakness and respiratory difficulty are often present. The differential diagnosis thus includes myaesthenia gravis, Guillain–Barré syndrome and brain stem stroke.

VIRAL INFECTIONS
Gastrointestinal disease

Viral gastroenteritis is common and is usually mild and self-limiting.[21] Sporadic cases are most commonly due to rotavirus, which mainly affects infants and small children. There is usually an abrupt onset of fever and vomiting, followed later by watery diarrhea. Severe dehydration can result, particularly if the diarrhea is profuse or prolonged, but most cases resolve within a week. Adenoviruses and astroviruses cause similar, although usually milder, symptoms.

Norwalk virus and other small round-structured viruses affect adults and older children and may cause sporadic disease, but they are often associated with outbreaks (Fig. 7.6). Infection may occur from eating contaminated food or infected shellfish or from drinking water contaminated by sewage. These viruses may cause diarrhea or vomiting or both. There are often other symptoms such as mild fever, myalgia and headache. Although the symptoms tend to be quite debilitating they resolve quickly, usually within 24–48 hours. Symptomatic disease with any of these viruses leads to excretion of large numbers of viruses in the stool, so secondary cases are common.

PROTOZOAL INFECTIONS
Giardiasis

Giardia lamblia is the most common protozoal cause of diarrhea and is particularly common in travelers.[22] Affected people often develop nausea and abdominal bloating, frequently accompanied by foul-smelling flatulence and belches tasting of hydrogen sulfide. The parasite affects the proximal small bowel so watery diarrhea is the main symptom; the diarrhea is often explosive. Steatorrhea and even malabsorption can occur and, if untreated, symptoms may persist for up to 6 weeks. In some patients sufficient damage occurs to the villus brush border enzymes that a secondary lactose intolerance occurs, with prolongation of the diarrhea.

Amebiasis

Infection with *Entamoeba histolytica* occurs mainly in the tropics and, as with giardiasis, many people are asymptomatic carriers of the parasite.[23] Ingested cysts mature into trophozoites in the bowel lumen and symptoms usually occur between 2 and 6 weeks after exposure. Amebic trophozoites damage the large bowel mucosa, leading to dysentery (Fig. 7.7). Most patients have blood in their stools but some may not – some do not even have fecal occult blood. In adults, dehydration is uncommon and the systemic symptoms, such as fever, are mild. Bacillary dysentery and a first episode of ulcerative colitis need to be considered in the differential diagnosis. Infection with the large protozoan parasite *Balantidium coli* may also produce a syndrome resembling amebic dysentery. Children tend to get more severe diarrhea and fluid loss and often have severe abdominal pain. Sometimes colonic perforation occurs and rarely, usually in debilitated or immunocompromised patients, a fulminant colitis may occur; this is clinically indistinguishable from severe ulcerative colitis. An uncommon complication (occurring in less than 1% of cases) is the development of an ameboma, usually in the ileocecum, when there is marked inflammation and bowel thickening that may resemble a malignant tumor or even Crohn's disease.

Amebic trophozoites may also disseminate from the bowel and invade other tissues. Most commonly the parasite travels via the portal venous system to the liver, causing a mild hepatitis and, usually, an

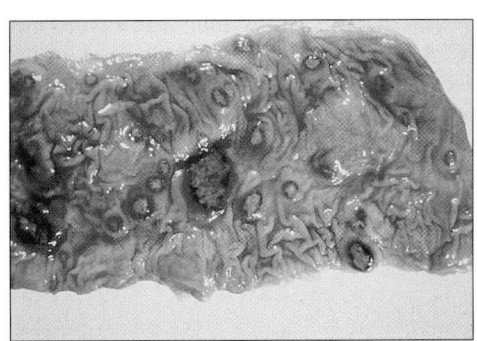

Fig. 7.7 Amebic dysentery. A post-mortem specimen. Note discrete flask-like ulcers with areas of hemorrhage.

amebic liver abscess. These patients usually complain of right upper quadrant pain, often with shoulder tip pain as well, and are frequently febrile. Less common sites of spread are the lungs and brain. More than half of the patients presenting with amebic abscess have no history of previous dysentery. Sometimes there is direct extension of the infection from the bowel to the overlying skin.

Cryptosporidiosis

The coccidian protozoan *Cryptosporidium parvum* causes a secretory diarrhea. Infection is almost always associated with drinking contaminated water and it is a not infrequent cause of travelers' diarrhea.[24] In addition to the diarrhea, nausea and anorexia are common. The incubation period ranges from a few days to a couple of weeks. Most people clear the parasite easily and symptoms abate within a few days. However, this can be a serious disease in people who have HIV infection and in children who have severe congenital immunodeficiency syndromes, in whom it results in severe, prolonged cholera-like diarrhea that is associated with malabsorption and profound weight loss. Some patients who have AIDS develop an ascending cholangitis with upper abdominal pain, abnormal liver function tests and, occasionally, frank jaundice. The inability of immunocompromised patients to clear this parasite is a particular problem because no effective treatment exists (see Chapter 5.13).

Cyclospora cayetanensis

This coccidian parasite has only relatively recently been discovered and described as a human pathogen.[25] Most cases are related to water consumption but outbreaks associated with imported, contaminated soft fruit have occurred in the USA. Symptoms initially include watery diarrhea and anorexia and often vomiting. These infections are usually self-limiting but some patients may take several weeks to recover and many of these suffer anorexia, profound fatigue and marked weight loss even after the diarrhea has resolved. Immunocompromised patients, such as those who have HIV infection, may develop chronic symptoms of diarrhea that are indistinguishable from those seen in cryptosporidiosis.

NATURAL TOXINS

Patients may present with gastrointestinal symptoms or neurologic symptoms as a result of eating or drinking naturally occurring toxins. Such illnesses often mimic food- or water-borne infection.

Plant toxins

There are various alkaloids and other plant toxins that may produce symptoms in humans who consume them. People who have glucose-6-phosphate dehydrogenase deficiency are unable to reduce oxidants contained in some legumes or beans. These toxins accumulate and lead to a mixture of symptoms known as favism. Early symptoms are headache and nausea and vomiting with a mild fever. The main problem, however, is marked hemolysis with hemoglobinuria and jaundice.

If casava is not prepared and cooked properly, its naturally occurring cyanide precursors remain and are ingested.[26] In heavy, acute exposure breathlessness, paralysis and coma ensue. More commonly,

chronic exposure leads to tropical spastic neuropathy. This is a particular risk for poor communities in times of severe drought.

Fish toxins

Neurotoxins associated with the consumption of shellfish lead to two distinct syndromes. Paralytic poisoning occurs within minutes to hours of ingestion and is characterized by breathlessness, muscle weakness and increasing respiratory difficulty.[27] Neurotoxic poisoning is milder, with some muscle weakness and paresthesiae but no respiratory problems.

Ciguatera poisoning follows the eating of fish that have consumed toxic microalgae. Such fish, like barracuda, have been feeding around coral reefs where the algae are most commonly found. Symptoms include acute diarrhea and vomiting and there is often a macular erythematous rash. Neurologic symptoms are common with circumoral paresthesiae and sometimes paralysis. Most cases are mild and fatalities are rare.[28]

Scombroid poisoning resembles acute histamine toxicity. Coarse feeding oily fish, like mackerel and tuna, are usually implicated.[29] The scombroid toxin is thought to be derived from the action of bacteria in the fish guts on histones in the flesh of the fish. The formation of the toxin is favored by heat, so the risk is highest in poorly cleaned fish that have been inadequately stored before cooking. Symptoms include headache, diarrhea, erythema and, usually, a marked urticarial rash.

Mushrooms

Some mushrooms, such as *Psylocybe* spp., cause hallucinations and may be eaten intentionally for this effect. Other mushrooms may be eaten in error with grave consequences.[30] *Amanita phalloides* contains a deadly toxin that initially causes abdominal cramps and diarrhea. These symptoms improve somewhat to be followed by inexorable liver and renal failure, which is often fatal.

Other mushrooms contain muscarine-like toxins leading to cholinergic symptoms such as excessive salivation, blurring of vision, sweating and diarrhea.

Heavy metals

Ingestion of either cadmium or thallium may cause acute diarrhea and vomiting, somewhat resembling staphylococcal food poisoning. The symptoms may be severe enough to cause acute dehydration and collapse. More chronic ingestion of cadmium results in nephropathy; chronic ingestion of thallium causes a peripheral neuropathy.

FOOD-BORNE INFECTIONS WITH SYSTEMIC RATHER THAN GASTROINTESTINAL SYMPTOMS

Some organisms, after ingestion, invade through the intestinal mucosa and cause little in the way of gastrointestinal upset; rather, they result in a myriad of systemic symptoms. Many of these infections have fever as a prominent symptom and usually have longer incubation periods than those associated with food poisoning, so it is more difficult to recognize food-borne outbreaks with these organisms.

Typhoid

Typhoid, or enteric fever, is the classic example of a food-borne infection leading to systemic disease. This condition is characterized by a chronic bacteremia, and fever is the main presenting complaint. Although older texts highlight relative constipation, diarrhea also occurs, although many patients have little in the way of bowel symptoms early in the course of the illness.[31] There is usually nonspecific malaise and headache, and a nonproductive cough is common. Also common is the so-called 'typhoid facies', a rather lethargic and apathetic facial expression. Most patients appear subacutely unwell; very few are acutely toxic or look as if they have a Gram-negative sepsis. When the bacilli re-invade the bowel, particularly the Peyer's patches, inflammation results and may lead to intestinal hemorrhage, which is sometimes torrential. Occasionally, severe ulceration results in small bowel perforation. Less common complications include myocarditis and meningitis.

Some cases are mild and self-limiting but most require specific antimicrobial therapy. Rarely, infected people become chronic carriers and excretors of *Salmonella typhi*. Carriage is particularly associated with the presence of gallstones.

Brucellosis

This disease is usually caused by *Brucella melitensis* acquired by eating unpasteurized cheese or milk. Most cases present with a fever without localizing symptoms or signs.[32] Associated symptoms such as headache, myalgia and chills are common. A less common presentation that has a more insidious onset is spondylitis; the main symptoms are back pain, related to the paraspinal inflammatory mass, and a milder fever. This may need to be differentiated from tuberculosis. Spinal cord compression is extremely rare in brucellar spondylitis. Rarely, both forms of brucellosis may have acute orchitis as a relatively early feature. Chronic brucellosis does not exist.

Listeriosis

Infection with *Listeria monocytogenes* most commonly presents with an acute meningoencephalitis, which may be associated with a bacteremia. Patients present with headache, confusion and, sometimes, vomiting. Most cases have neck stiffness and other signs of meningeal inflammation. In the more encephalitic presentations, differentiation from herpes simplex virus encephalitis is impossible clinically, especially as both conditions may have lymphocytes and red cells in the cerebrospinal fluid. Central nervous system infection is most common in the elderly and the immunocompromised.

Less commonly, patients are bacteremic and present with mild influenza-like symptoms, although occasionally there is shock and renal impairment. Some cases may have impaired liver function tests as a result of a granulomatous hepatitis. Pregnancy carries an increased risk of bacteremia if Listeria is ingested and infection in early pregnancy may lead to spontaneous miscarriage. Late in pregnancy infection can result in stillbirth or in severe neonatal septis or meningitis. Intrauterine infection is almost always fatal even when the illness in the mother has been mild.[33]

Mycobacteria

Mycobacterium bovis. Although the majority of intestinal tuberculosis results either from swallowed infected sputum or from bacteremic spread from a pulmonary focus of *Mycobacterium tuberculosis*, in some areas of the tropics cases still occur from consuming unpasteurized milk and dairy produce contaminated by *M. bovis*, a closely related species.[34] Intestinal tuberculosis may present in a variety of ways, ranging from malabsorption if the proximal small bowel is affected to intestinal obstruction due to inflammatory strictures. Diarrhea may occur, as may intestinal hemorrhage, but both are rare presenting features. Intestinal tuberculosis may mimic Crohn's disease.

Mycobacterium avium-intracellulare. *Mycobacterium avium-intracellulare* has become an important pathogen in the AIDS era. Late-stage HIV disease has been associated with an increased risk of disseminated *M. avium-intracellulare* infection, which commonly presents with fevers, accelerated weight loss, anemia and chronic diarrhea. The organism is ubiquitous in the environment.[35] Animal models of *M. avium-intracellulare* infection suggest that the gastrointestinal tract is the portal of entry (see Chapter 5.14).

Mycobacterium pseudotuberculosis. This organism is usually regarded as nonpathogenic. However, because of the similarities between intestinal tuberculosis and Crohn's disease, many researchers have sought a mycobacterial cause of Crohn's disease. Recently, molecular techniques have provided some evidence for the presence of *M. paratuberculosis* in the bowel of patients who have Crohn's disease, although this is controversial.[36] A causal link has yet to be proven.

Hepatitis viruses

Two of the hepatitis viruses, hepatitis A virus and hepatitis E virus, are acquired by the fecal–oral route. Hepatitis A virus is more common and is endemic in many countries, although its prevalence is highest in the tropics where it is a risk for nonimmune travelers. Hepatitis E virus is endemic in Asia, particularly in the Indian subcontinent, and is only rarely encountered as a disease of the returning traveler.[37,38] Hepatitis A has an incubation period of 2–6 weeks; the incubation period of hepatitis E is less certain. Both hepatitis A and hepatitis E present, like most cases of acute hepatitis, with a relatively acute onset of malaise, nausea, anorexia and mild fever followed soon after by jaundice. In the prodrome, many patients who normally smoke find they no longer feel like smoking. The jaundice usually only lasts about 2 weeks but some patients develop marked cholestasis with prolonged jaundice.

Hepatitis A virus infection is usually asymptomatic in children below the age of about 8 years. It always causes symptoms in adults, which are usually mild but characterized by marked fatigue. Death from hepatitis A is very rare unless there is pre-existing liver disease. Hepatitis E virus infection may cause a fatal fulminant hepatitis in pregnant women. Recovery from hepatitis A results in life-long immunity to re-infection and the same is probably true for hepatitis E (see Chapter 2.39).

Prions

In the past decade an epidemic of bovine spongiform encephalopathy in cattle was recognized in the UK and some other European countries, linked to the consumption by the cattle of feeds made up partly of protein derived from other cattle. Although control measures have been introduced and such feeds stopped, there is evidence that the prions causing bovine spongiform encephalopathy in cattle have entered the food chain and resulted in human disease. An unusual form of Creutzfeld–Jakob disease has occurred in young people and is believed to be linked to the consumption of beef from cattle infected with bovine spongiform encephalopathy. These cases differ from 'classic' Creutzfeld–Jakob disease epidemiologically, clinically and histologically, and have a distinct molecular configuration of the prion protein.[39] Such cases of new-variant Creutzfeld–Jakob disease have aroused widespread public concern, but it remains uncertain whether a major epidemic of new-variant Creutzfeld–Jakob disease will occur or whether prions from species other than cattle will infect humans (see Chapter 8.12 for detailed discussion).

Parasites

Protozoa. Most enteric protozoa, like *Giardia lamblia*, are associated with water or food contaminated with feces and are confined to the gut after ingestion. However, other protozoa with more complex lifecycles are parasites of other species and may cause disease in humans when the meat of the intermediate host species is eaten. The most common example is infection with *Toxoplasma gondii* when tissue cysts are ingested with undercooked meat.[40] Many infections are asymptomatic. Acute symptoms include a febrile illness with or without generalized lymphadenopathy. This is usually self-limiting. Infection in pregnancy carries a risk of vertical transmission and congenital toxoplasmosis. Patients who have HIV infection may reactivate dormant cysts in the brain, develop toxoplasmal abscesses and present with the features of a space-occupying lesion (see Chapter 5.13).

Helminths

Numerous helminths are ingested as infective ova, after which they undergo a complex lifecycle that includes larval migration around the human host and then re-entry into the gastrointestinal tract, where they develop into adult worms that may or may not cause symptoms (Fig. 7.8).[41]

Other worms are ingested as ova or larva but migrate out of the gut and cause problems unrelated to the gastrointestinal tract. Figure 7.9

FOOD-BORNE HELMINTHIC INFECTIONS THAT ARE CONFINED TO THE GUT
Ascaris lumbricoides Ancylostoma duodenale Trichuris trichiura Enterobius vermicularis Fasciolopis buski Taenia saginata Taenia solium Hymenolepis nana Diphyllobothrium latum

Fig. 7.8 Food-borne helminthic infections that are confined to the gut.

SYSTEMIC HELMINTHIC INFECTIONS THAT ARE TRANSMITTED BY FOOD OR WATER	
Helminth	Food vehicle
Dracunculis medinensis (guinea worm)	Crustacea in drinking water
Trichinella spiralis	Pork
Toxocara canis	Contaminated soil ingestion
Opisthorchis viverrini	Raw fish
Opisthorchis sinensis (Clonorchis sinensis)	Raw fish
Fasciola hepatica	Contaminated vegetables, watercress
Paragonimus westermani	Freshwater crabs, crayfish
Taenia solium (cysticercosis)	Pork
Echinococcus granulosis Echinococcus multilocularis	Contaminated food or water (with eggs in animal feces)

Fig. 7.9 Systemic helminthic infections that are transmitted by food or water.

outlines the main features of these infections, most of which are asymptomatic. Further details can be found Chapters 6.10 and 8.35.

DIAGNOSIS

FOOD POISONING
Microbiology
When a patient presents with symptoms suggesting food poisoning there may be clues about the infecting organism in the dietary history. A recent restaurant or take-away meal may highlight suspect foods whereas a story of recent tropical travel may raise the possibility of a protozoan parasite. Recent consumption of mayonnaise, soft-boiled eggs or barbecued chicken, for example, hint that *Salmonella* spp. may be the cause.

The microscopy and culture of a stool specimen is probably the most useful test and the diagnostic yield can be maximized by examining at least three specimens obtained at different times. Most causes of secretory diarrhea will produce negative stool tests as the diarrhea is usually caused by toxins and there is little inflammation in the intestinal mucosa. The presence of pus cells in the stool suggests infection and also indicates an inflammatory colitis. Red blood cells in the stool indicate colitis and may occur with any cause of inflammatory colitis. Infection with *E. coli* O157:H7 usually causes a hemorrhagic colitis so the presence of red cells in a stool specimen should alert the laboratory to the need to screen for this pathogen. If there is a history of tropical travel, blood in the stool may indicate shigellosis or amebic dysentery. Amebic trophozoites may be seen engulfing red cells but only if the stool is examined fresh or 'hot' because the trophozoites soon degrade *in vitro*.

Parasites, such as *Giardia* spp. and cryptosporidia, may be seen in stool specimens in heavy infections or in immunocompromised

patients. However, because they infect the small bowel and are shed intermittently in small numbers in the stool they may be missed on microscopy.[42] Microscopic examination of duodenal aspirates or the use of the entero-test, or string test, is more likely to yield results with these small bowel parasites; however, these investigations are more invasive. It should be noted that the nonpathogenic *Entamoeba dispar*, found in up to 50% of people in endemic areas, has cysts that are indistinguishable from those of *E. histolytica* so the finding of amebic cysts should be interpreted with caution in endemic areas or in patients returning from such areas (see Chapter 6.10).[43]

Electron microscopy has a role to play in the investigation of gastroenteritis caused by viruses. The characteristic appearances of rotavirus, astrovirus or small round-structured viruses such as the Norwalk virus clinches the diagnosis. Electron microscopy is particularly useful during outbreak investigations but it is not often routinely available for diagnosing individual cases.

Stool culture using a variety of selective media can identify the common bacterial causes of diarrhea unless the symptoms are due to preformed bacterial toxins in the food. The disadvantage is that the identification process can take several days. Culture methods may also be used to investigate water or food vehicles in suspected outbreaks.

There are now several commercially available latex and enzyme-linked immunosorbent assay (ELISA) kits for the identification of rotavirus in stool or vomit. These allow prompt diagnosis without the need for electron microscopy. Increasingly, reverse transcription polymerase chain reaction is being used to identify a variety of viruses in stool lysates.[44] Although not used in routine laboratories, ELISA can be used to identify bacterial toxins and are important when investigating outbreaks.

Serology has a minor role in the diagnosis of invasive amebiasis.[45] There are several tests available with variable predictive values. In endemic areas, up to one-quarter of the population may have positive tests because of previous asymptomatic infection. Other than for epidemiologic studies, the current IgG ELISA is most useful in patients from nonendemic areas but it is usually used, because of the turn-around time for the test, as a confirmatory test.

Hematology, biochemistry and immunology
Blood tests have little role in the specific diagnosis of food poisoning. The peripheral leukocyte count may be nonspecifically raised but it is commonly normal. Eosinophilia rarely occurs with invasive amebiasis; rather it is a feature of metaozoan (i.e. worm) infection, not protozoan infection. There may be mild anemia in hemorrhagic colitis. One key finding on the blood film is fragmented red cells, indicative of intravascular hemolysis in hemolytic–uremic syndrome in association with enterocolitis caused by *E. coli* O157:H7.

Biochemical tests are useful for gauging the extent of dehydration or renal impairment. Serum albumin may be low in more chronic diarrhea or if there is severe colonic inflammation or sepsis. The C-reactive protein may be significantly elevated in cases of inflammatory colitis due, for example, to *Campylobacter* spp. None of these tests is in any way specific.

Radiology
A plain abdominal radiograph is useful for assessing the severity of infective colitis. Infection with organisms causing inflammatory diarrhea may mimic ulcerative colitis and lead to large bowel dilatation and, sometimes, to a toxic megacolon. Plain radiographs may also show small bowel dilatation or fluid levels when there are inflammatory strictures in the ileocecum caused by infections with *Yersinia* spp. or amebae.

Barium enema examination can be used to demonstrate inflammation of the colon and may show ulceration in amebic dysentery, but this has largely been superceded by fiberoptic endoscopy. Computed tomography scans, MRI and labeled leukocyte scans have no role in the diagnosis of food poisoning.

Other investigations

Although stool culture and microscopy are the most important diagnostic tools, a useful adjunct is flexible sigmoidoscopy and large bowel biopsy. Endoscopy may show an active colitis, which can be macroscopically similar to that seen in ulcerative colitis, although the finding of frank pus points more towards infection. Amebic colitis causes inflamed mucosa around discrete ulcers with patches of normal mucosa in between, a useful feature that distinguishes it from ulcerative colitis. Rectal or colonic biopsy may show histologic features that differentiate between infection and inflammatory bowel disease (Fig. 7.10).

Microbiology

Many of the bacterial infections described above share the feature that, athough they enter via the gastrointestinal tract, they disseminate from there. Many of these spread via the bloodstream and hence, particularly early in the course of disease, blood cultures are essential. Typhoid is most easily diagnosed by blood culture, although bone marrow culture is even more sensitive.[46] Stool culture is less sensitive but is still valuable, particularly in areas where blood culture facilities are less readily available. Even a rectal swab can be used to diagnose typhoid with a sensitivity of about 30%. Brucellosis and listeriosis are also commonly diagnosed by positive blood culture. Brucellar spondylitis may result in a paravertebral mass, which may be positive on culture if aspirated or biopsied. Listeria may present with a meningoencephalitis, in which case the cerebrospinal fluid culture should be positive.

Mycobacterial infections affecting the gut are best diagnosed by tissue biopsy; specimens may show granuloma and, occasionally, acid fast-bacilli on histology, but they should always be sent for mycobacterial culture. In the setting of HIV infection, infection with *M. avium-intercellulare* is associated with large numbers of mycobacteria and very poorly formed granulomas. Patients may be bacteremic or have positive bone marrow cultures. Not infrequently, large numbers of acid-fast bacilli are seen in the stool, which will also be positive on culture. Intestinal biopsies will often show numerous acid-fast bacilli with little in the way of inflammatory reaction and certainly no caseation.

Serologic tests for brucellosis are useful in patients from nonendemic areas but even in endemic regions a rising titer can be diagnostic. The Widal test for typhoid is widely used in the tropics and is only partially useful in endemic areas if the test patterns in the population have been well-studied and validated. It cannot be relied upon to exclude typhoid in returning travelers or in patients in nonendemic areas. Previous typhoid immunization will lead to false-positive results.

Hepatitis due to enterically acquired viruses is diagnosed by appropriate serologic tests, usually in the form of an ELISA.

There are now a variety of commercial and research tests to detect pathogens by means of molecular biologic techniques.

Most diagnostic laboratories are not able to culture protozoa. Diagnosis of invasive protozoa like *T. gondii* rely on serologic tests such as an IgM seroconversion. In many cases there is detectable IgG to *Toxoplasma* spp., but this only defines previous exposure and does not prove that the current clinical problem is a disease caused by toxoplasmal infection.

Helminthic infections may be diagnosed by finding eggs in the stool or by the identification of adult worms passed in the stool (Fig. 7.11). Tapeworm infections may be diagnosed by finding segments, or proglottids, in the stool. Serologic tests may help identify invasive parasites causing problems such as cysticercosis or hydatid disease. However, these tests are best suited to returning travelers and are relatively unhelpful in endemic areas where large numbers of the population may be asymptomatically exposed.

Hematology and biochemistry

So-called routine blood tests are really of little value in the diagnosis of invasive food-borne infections and only serve an indirect purpose of assessing disease severity. Invasive helminths will commonly cause a peripheral blood eosinophilia. Viral hepatitis will result in raised levels of aminotransferase, such as aspartate aminotransferase, and in severe cases liver synthetic function is affected and hypoalbuminemia and abnormal clotting occur. Liver function tests may be abnormal in hydatid disease affecting the liver or if the biliary tree is obstructed by worms such as *Opisthorchis sinensis*.

Immunology

There are no specific immunologic tests that help in diagnosis. There are proponents of tuberculin testing to aid in the diagnosis of mycobacterial disease but in practice this is of limited use and is of no value in diagnosing atypical mycobacterial infections, such as *M. avium-intercellulare*.

Radiology

Plain radiographs are of little value in the diagnosis of these invasive diseases. Sometimes spondylitis caused by brucellosis may be seen on plain vertebral radiographs. Partially calcified hydatid cysts may be seen on plain radiographs but this usually represents inactive disease. Contrast radiology using, for example, a barium enema may find areas of disease, such as ileocecal abnormalities in intestinal tuberculosis, but will not yield a specific diagnosis.

Computed tomography scanning and MRI are particularly useful in delineating intracerebral lesions. In AIDS, cerebral toxoplasmosis appears as (usually multiple) ring-enhancing lesions or abscesses on

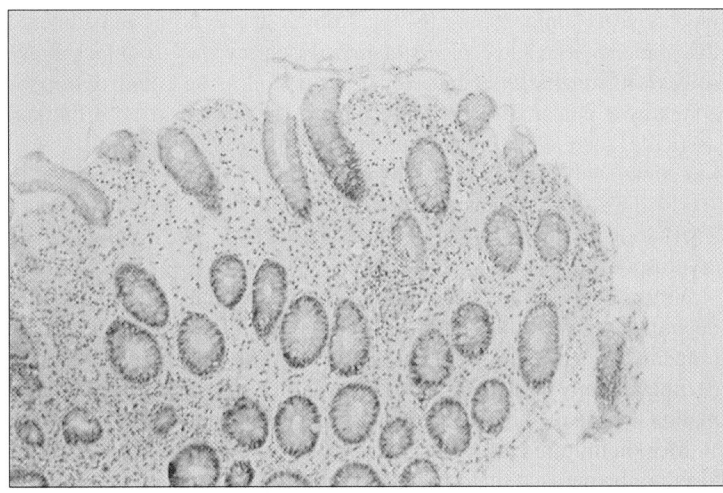

Fig. 7.10 Histology of infective colitis caused by *Campylobacter jejuni*.

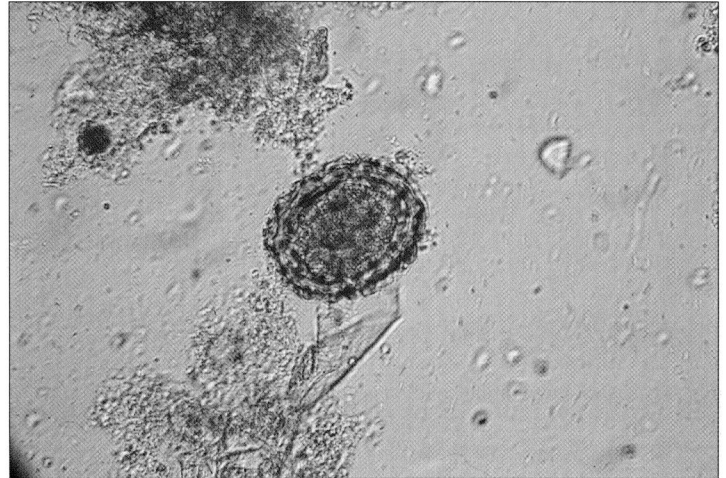

Fig. 7.11 Unfertilized egg of *Ascaris lumbricoides*.

CT scans or as multiple lesions on MRI. Neurocysticercosis presents with discrete, multiple lesions on these scans or with hydrocephalus if a cyst is blocking the fourth ventricle.

Histopathology
Tissue biopsy remains an important means of reaching a diagnosis in invasive disease. In addition to the histologic findings, specimens can be sent for culture (for *M. bovis*, for example). In-situ hybridization is increasingly used to demonstrate the infecting pathogen in tissue sections.

MANAGEMENT

FLUIDS
The mainstay of medical management for acute gastroenteritis is the administration of adequate fluid and electrolyte replacement to correct the intravascular volume and prevent cardiovascular collapse and renal impairment. For the vast majority of patients, oral rehydration is adequate but it should include electrolyte replacement as well as water.[47,48] A large number of commercial preparations of oral rehydration salts exist with flavorings to make them more palatable. They are based on the World Health Organization recommendations for oral rehydration therapy but those for use in developed countries tend to have a lower sodium content (Fig. 7.12) because fecal sodium losses are lower in temperate climates than in the tropics. The glucose content of these solutions is essential to allow active transport of water and electrolytes across the mucosa from the lumen.

Intravenous fluid replacement is required for those who are too frail and for those who are vomiting too much to tolerate oral therapy, as well as for those who have severe dehydration and near circulatory collapse. Crystalloid solutions are usually appropriate.

ANTIDIARRHEAL AGENTS
Drugs that inhibit intestinal motility have a small role to play in patients who have gastroenteritis. Loperamide, diphenoxylate and codeine phosphate all act in this way. Calmodulin, an antisecretory drug, may also have a role in reducing diarrhea. Only codeine is absorbed, with the advantage that it can act as an analgesic for those who have abdominal pain, but it carries the risk of side effects, such as nausea, and the danger of accumulation in patients who have renal impairment. Kaolin–pectin has no role in the management of diarrheal illness but some studies have shown a beneficial role of bismuth subsalicylate. Although one report suggested that the use of diphenoxylate–atropine is associated with an increased risk of bacterial invasion in acute shigellosis, no other studies have found this.[49] Equally, there is little evidence to suggest that these agents significantly prolong the carriage of infecting organsims or that they increase the risk of the development of toxic megacolon.[50]

ORAL REHYDRATION SOLUTION – WORLD HEALTH ORGANIZATION FORMULA

Sodium 90mmol/l

Potassium 20mmol/l

Chloride 80mmol/l

Citrate 10mmol/l

Glucose 110mmol/l

Total osmolality 310mmol/l

Fig. 7.12 Oral rehydration solution – World Health Organization formula. Note that commercial oral rehydration solutions for use in developed countries have a lower osmolality (240mmol/l) with a lower sodium content (60mmol/l) because fecal sodium losses are lower in developed countries than in the tropics.

OTHER SUPPORTIVE MEASURES
Patients who have severe shock from fluid loss may require intensive support, but this is very rarely needed with gastrointestinal infections. Some patients, particularly the elderly, may develop acute renal failure and require temporary renal support with hemofiltration or hemodialysis. This has been particularly true for those who have hemolytic–uremic syndrome following infection with *E. coli* O157:H7. There is also anecdotal evidence to suggest that patients who have hemolytic–uremic syndrome benefit from plasmapheresis.

Some food poisoning, such as botulism or paralytic shellfish poisoning, results in neurologic disease and impaired respiration. These cases often require respiratory support with artificial ventilation along with intensive physiotherapy.

ANTIMICROBIAL THERAPY
Most cases of food poisoning resolve spontaneously and do not require specific therapy. There is controversy about the role of antibiotics in community-acquired bacterial diarrhea.[51] Specific therapy may shorten the duration of illness and prevent complications but this is unproven in most cases. However, tetracycline treatment may reduce the duration of diarrhea in cholera and its use is important in epidemics. One problem is that therapy for most cases of diarrhea usually has to be empiric initially because it may take several days to isolate and identify a causative organism. Widespread use of empiric antibiotics for diarrhea may encourage the spread of resistant organisms, promote the development of diarrhea caused by *Clostridium difficile* and increase adverse reactions, such as rash. Studies have shown that the use of ampicillin for *Salmonella* enterocolitis may prolong excretion of the organism. There are also case–control study data to suggest that children who have hemolytic–uremic caused by *E. coli* O157:H7 who receive antibiotics may have a poorer outcome than those who do not.

Empiric antibiotics are appropriate for the elderly (aged over 70 years), those who have severe systemic symptoms, such as fever or joint inflammation, and the immunocompromised. In these cases, initial therapy is with a quinolone, such as ciprofloxacin (500mg q12h orally or 200mg q12h intravenously), because these drugs are well absorbed orally but are also available as intravenous preparations. They are effective against pathogens that can be invasive, such as *Salmonella* spp., *Campylobacter* spp. and *Yersinia* spp.; however, quinolone-resistant *Campylobacter* isolates are already well described.[52,53]

Most protozoa that cause food poisoning are treated with specific agents. Benzimidazoles, such as metronidazole or tinidazole, are effective against *Giardia* spp. (metronidazole 400–500mg q8h orally for 5 days) and amebae (metronidazole 750–800mg q8h orally for 5 days), although some strains of *Giardia* are relatively resistant to metronidazole. This resistance can be a problem because culture and sensitivity methods are not routinely available. In practice, those giardial infections that do not respond to metronidazole or tinidazole usually respond to mepacrine (100mg q8h orally for 7 days). It should be remembered that patients who have *E. histolytica* dysentery may re-infect themselves with amebic cysts carried in the gut. Following killing of trophozoites by a benzimidazole, these patients should be given a luminal cysticide, such as diloxanide furoate (500mg q8h orally for 10 days). Infections with *Isospora belli* and *Cyclospora cayetanensis* respond to 10–14 days of oral trimethoprim–sulfamethoxazole [960mg (160mg TMP/800mg SMX) q12h]. There is no specific treatment for cryptosporidiosis.

Viral infections are self-limiting. Rarely, patients who have acute hepatitis A virus infection may become deeply jaundiced with prolonged cholestasis. In such cases, a short course of oral prednisolone (0.5mg/kg daily reducing to nothing over 4 weeks) may reduce inflammation around the bile canaliculi and lead to resolution of the jaundice.

Most helminthic infections need specific therapy, which can be tailored to the parasite that is detected.

Most invasive food-borne infections, such as typhoid, need to be specifically treated, so it must be re-emphasized that every effort should be made to obtain samples for culture and sensitivity testing. This is increasingly important as antibacterial resistance of enteric organisms increases. The specific treatments for these conditions are described in Chapter 2.35.

SURGERY

Surgery has little role in the management of these infections. Infections caused by *Yersinia* spp., *Salmonella* spp. and other organisms may present in a manner resembling acute appendicitis, leading to laparoscopy or laparatomy. In severe, infective enterocolitis a toxic megacolon may arise. This sometimes leads to colectomy or to a decompressing colostomy. Surgery may also be required for the complications of typhoid, such as acute hemorrhage or intestinal perforation. Although surgical intervention may also be used to obtain tissue biopsies for histology and culture, such specimens are more often obtained by percutaneous biopsies guided with imaging techniques such as ultrasound or CT scanning.

PUBLIC HEALTH ISSUES

Hospitalized patients who have diarrhea or who are infected with an organism that can be spread by the fecal–oral route should be isolated in single rooms. Gloves and aprons should be worn when dealing with the patient's excreta to prevent nosocomial spread.

The diagnosis or suspicion of a food- or water-borne illness should be notified to the relevant public health officer. This is particularly important in suspected outbreaks, in institutions or when a food-handler is involved.

REFERENCES

1. Greenbloom SL, Martin-Smith P, Isaacs S, *et al*. Outbreak of trichinosis in Ontario secondary to the ingestion of wild boar meat. Can J Public Health 1997;88:52–6.
2. Sockett PN, Cowden JM, Le Baigue S, Ross D, Adak GK, Evans H. Foodborne disease surveillance in England and Wales: 1989–1991. Comm Dis Rep Rev 1993;3:R159–73.
3. Bean NH, Goulding JS, Lao C, Angulo FJ. Surveillance for foodborne-disease outbreaks – United States, 1988–1992. In: CDC Surveillance Summaries, 25 October 1996. Morb Mortal Wkly Rep 1996;45:1–13.
4. Centers for Disease Control and Prevention. Foodborne diseases active surveillance network, 1996. Morb Mortal Wkly Rep 1997;46:258–61.
5. Bern C, Martines J, de Zoysa I, Glass RI. The magnitude of the global problem of diarrheal disease: a ten year update. Bull World Health Organ 1992;70:705–14.
6. MacKenzie WR, Hoxie NJ, Proctor ME, *et al*. A massive outbreak in Milwaukee of *Cryptosporidium* infection transmitted through the public water supply. N Engl J Med 1994;331:161–7.
7. Keene WE, McAnulty JM, Hoesly FC, *et al*. A swimming-associated outbreak of hemorrhagic colitis caused by *Escherichia coli* O157:H7 and *Shigella sonnei*. N Engl J Med 1994;331:579–84.
8. Simon GL, Gorbach SL. Intestinal microflora. Med Clin North Am 1982;66:557–74.
9. Sears CL, Kaper JB. Enteric bacterial toxins: mechanisms of action and linkage to intestinal secretion. Microbiol Rev 1996;60:167–215.
10. Levine MM. *Escherichia coli* that cause diarrhea: Enterotoxigenic, enteropathogenic, enteroinvasive, enterohemorrhagic, and enteroadherent. J Infect Dis 1987;155:377–89.
11. DuPont HL, Ericsson CD. Prevention and treatment of traveler's diarrhea. N Engl J Med 1993;328:1821–7.
12. Cryz SJJ, Que JU, Levine MM, Wiedermann G, Kollaritsch H. Safety and immunogenicity of a live oral bivalent typhoid fever (*Salmonella typhi* Ty21a)–cholera (*Vibrio cholerae* CVD 103–HgR) vaccine in healthy adults. Infect Immun 1995;63:1336–9.
13. Lund BM. Foodborne disease due to *Bacillus cereus* and *Clostridium* species. Lancet 1990;336:982–6.
14. Hlady WG, Klontz KC. The epidemiology of *Vibrio* infections in Florida, 1981–1993. J Infect Dis 1996;173:1176–83.
15. Sanchez JL, Taylor DN. Cholera. Lancet 1997;349:1825–30.

16. Cowden J. *Campylobacter*: epidemiological paradoxes. Br Med J 1992;305:132–3.
17. Mishu B, Koehler J, Lee LA, *et al*. Outbreaks of *Salmonella enteritidis* infections in the United States, 1985–1991. J Infect Dis 1994;169:547–57.
18. Rees JH, Gregson NA, Hughes RAC. Anti-ganglioside GM_1 antibodies in Guillain–Barré syndrome and their relationship to *Campylobacter jejuni* infection. Ann Neurol 1995;38:809–16.
19. Bell BP, Goldoft M, Griffin PM, *et al*. A multistate outbreak of *Escherichia coli* O157:H7–associated bloody diarrhea and hemolytic uremic syndrome from hamburgers. JAMA 1994;272:1349–53.
20. Critchley EMR, Hayes P, Isaacs PET. Outbreak of botulism in Northwest England and Wales, June 1989. Lancet 1989;ii:849–53.
21. Blacklow NR, Greenberg HB. Viral gastroenteritis. N Engl J Med 1991;325:252–64.
22. Hill DR. Giardiasis. Issues in diagnosis and management. Infect Dis Clin North Am 1993;7:503–25.
23. Reed SL. Amebiasis: an update. Clin Infect Dis 1992;14:385–93.
24. Goodgame RW. Understanding intestinal spore-forming protozoa: cryptosporidia, microsporidia, isospora and cyclospora. Ann Intern Med 1996;124:429–41.
25. Ortega YR, Sterling CR, Gilman RH, Cama VA, Diaz F. Cyclospora species – a new protozoan pathogen of man. N Engl J Med 1993;328:1308–12.
26. Cliff J, NIcala D, Saute F, *et al*. Konzo associated with war in Mozambique. Trop Med Int Health 1997;2:1068–74.
27. Gessner BD, Middaugh JP. Paralytic shellfish poisoning in Alaska: a 20–year retrospective analysis. Am J Epidemiol 1995;141:766–70.
28. Lange WR, Snyder FR, Fudala PJ. Travel and ciguatera fish poisoning. Arch Intern Med 1992;152:2049–53.
29. CDSC. Scombrotoxic (histamine) fish poisoning. Commun Dis Rep Wkly 1993;3:163.
30. Cappell MS, Hassan T. Gastrointestinal and hepatic effects of *Amanita phalloides* ingestion. J Clin Gastroenterol 1992;15:225–8.
31. Wicks ACB, Homes GS, Davidson L. Endemic typhoid fever: a diagnostic pitfall. Q J Med 1971;40:341–54.
32. Ariza J. Brucellosis. Curr Opin Infect Dis 1996;9:126–31.
33. Schlech WF III. Lowbury lecture. Listeriosis: epidemiology, virulence and the significance of contaminated foodstuffs. J Hosp Infect 1991;19:211–24.

34. Cotter TP, Sheehan S, Cryan B, O'Shaughnessy E, Cummins H, Bredin CP. Tuberculosis due to *Mycobacterium bovis* in humans in the south-west of Ireland: is there a relationship with prevalence in cattle? Tubercle Lung Dis 1996;77:545–8.
35. von Reyn CF, Maslow JN, Barber TW, Falkinham JO 3rd, Arbeit RD. Persistent colonisation of potable water as a source of *Mycobacterium avium* infection in AIDS. Lancet 1994;343:1137–41.
36. Rowbotham DS, Mapstone NP, Trejdosiewicz LK, Howdle PD, Quirke P. *Mycobacterium paratuberculosis* DNA not detected in Crohn's disease tissue by fluorescent polymerase chain reaction. Gut 1995;37:660–7.
37. Koff RS. Hepatitis A. Lancet 1998;351:1643–9.
38. Rab MA, Bile MK, Mubarik MM, *et al*. Water-borne hepatitis E virus epidemic in Islamabad, Pakistan: a common source outbreak traced to the malfunction of a modern water treatment plant. Am J Trop Med Hyg 1997;57:151–7.
39. Will RG, Ironside JW, Zeidler M, *et al*. A new variant of Creutzfeld–Jakob disease in the UK. Lancet 1996;347:921–5.
40. Kapperud G, Jenum PA, Stray-Pedersen B, Melbye KK, Eskild A, Eng J. Risk factors for *Toxoplasma gondii* infection in pregnancy. Results of a prospective case–control study in Norway. Am J Epidemiol 1996;144:405–12.
41. Liu LX, Weller PF. Intestinal nematodes. In: Rustgi VK, ed. Gastrointestinal infections in the tropics. Basel: Karger; 1990:145–69.
42. Ignatius R, Eisenblatter M, REgnath T, *et al*. Efficacy of different methods for detection of low *Cryptosporidium parvum* oocyst numbers or antigen concentrations in stool specimens. Eur J Clin Microbiol Infect Dis 1997;16:732–6.
43. Jackson TF. *Entamoeba histolytica* and *Entamoeba dispar* are distinct species; clinical, epidemiological and serological evidence. Int J Parasitol 1998;28:181–6.
44. Gouvea V, Allen JR, Glass RI, *et al*. Detection of group B and C rotavirus by polymerase chain reaction. J Clin Microbiol 1991;28:2659–67.
45. Ravdin JI. Diagnosis of invasive amoebiasis-time to end the morphology era. In: Cook GC, ed. Gastroenterological problems from the tropics. London: BMJ Publishing Group; 1995:84–93.
46. Gilman RH, Terminel M, Levine MM, Hernandez-Mendoza P, Hornick RB. Relative efficacy of blood, urine, rectal swab, bone-marrow and rose-spot culture for recovery of *Salmonella typhi* in typhoid fever. Lancet 1975;1:1211–3.

47. Avery ME, Snyder JD. Oral therapy for acute diarrhea. The underused simple solution. N Engl J Med 1990;323:891–4.

48. Gore SM, Fontaine O, Pierce NF. Impact of rice based oral rehydration solution on stool output and duration of diarrhea: meta-analysis of 13 clinical trials. Br Med J 1992;304:287–91.

49. DuPont HL, Hornick RB. Adverse effects of Lomotil therapy in shigellosis. JAMA 1973;226:1525–8.

50. Bergstrom T, Alestig K, Thoren K, Trollfors B. Symptomatic treatment of acute infectious diarrheoa: loperamide versus placebo in a double-blind trial. J Infect 1986;12:35–8.

51. Farthing M, Feldman R, Finch R, *et al*. The management of infective gastroenteritis in adults. A consensus statement by an expert panel convened by the British Society for the Study of Infection. J Infect 1996;33:143–52.

52. Pilcher H, Diridl G, Wolf D. Ciprofloxacin in the treatment of acute bacterial diarrhea: a double-blind study. Eur J Clin Microbiol Infect Dis 1986;5:241–3.

53. Endtz HP, Mouton RP, van der Reyden T, Ruijs GJ, Biever M, van Klingeren B. Fluoroquinolone resistance in *Campylobacter* spp isolated from human stools and poultry products. Lancet 1990;335:787.

Infection in Burn Patients

David J Barillo & Albert T McManus

EPIDEMIOLOGY

Thermal burns are less common than other forms of trauma, but are unique in the production of the most severe physiologic stresses seen in any form of traumatic injury. It is estimated that 2 million people are burned annually in the USA, resulting in the need for 500,000 emergency department visits, 74,000 hospital admissions and 20,000 admissions to specialized burn treatment facilities.[1] Approximately 6500 people die each year from burns or exposure to fire in the USA.

Burn trauma is classified by depth of injury, extent of body surface area involvement and associated injuries.

- First-degree burns involve only the epidermal layer of skin, usually heal without medical intervention and normally do not become infected. First-degree burns are not included in estimations of burn size for the purposes of determining triage, need for fluid resuscitation or for survival estimates.
- Second-degree (partial thickness) burns involve varying layers of the dermis, and whether they heal without operative intervention depends upon depth of injury.
- Third-degree (full thickness) burns involve the full thickness of dermis and normally require operative debridement followed by split thickness skin grafting or other techniques to achieve wound closure.

The mortality of burn injury is proportional to the age of the patient and the size of the cutaneous second- and third-degree burn. Burn injury is poorly tolerated in the young, the elderly and in those with pre-existing chronic medical illness. For example, a burn sustained by an elderly diabetic while soaking a neuropathic foot in hot water may represent less than 3% total body surface area, but can easily evolve into a limb-threatening or life-threatening injury if treatment is inadequate or delayed.

Mortality from burn injury has decreased significantly over the past half century, primarily because of improved control of burn wound infection through the use of topical antimicrobial agents and aggressive surgical debridement. The LA_{50} (percentage body surface burned associated with a 50% mortality) now exceeds 80% in select age groups. (The combined effects of burn size and age on predicted mortality is demonstrated in Figure 8.1).

Infection remains the most frequent cause of morbidity and mortality in burn patients.[2] Although the incidence of invasive burn wound infection has significantly decreased, other infections, particularly pneumonia, remain a problem. Injury to the lungs from exposure to smoke is a significant comorbid factor, and predisposes the patient to nosocomial pneumonia.[3]

The American Burn Association has established criteria for the referral of patients who have thermal injury to specialized care facilities (Fig. 8.2). These criteria, endorsed by the Advanced Trauma Life Support and Advanced Burn Life Support programs[4,5] represent the standard of care in developed countries. The infectious disease specialist is often the first consultant to see the burn patient in a community hospital setting. Referral to a designated burn center may be the optimal approach in this situation.

PATHOGENESIS AND PATHOLOGY

Burn injury produces profound alterations in homeostasis, which are proportional to the size of the cutaneous injury. Virtually every organ system is affected, and changes in the cardiovascular and immunologic systems are particularly pertinent.

Thermal injury results in a significant and sustained hypermetabolic response. The causes of postburn hypermetabolism are poorly understood but may be related to a centrally mediated release of catecholamines, glucagon and cortisol.[2] Severe burn injury can result in resting metabolic rates that are twice normal levels, causing nutritional

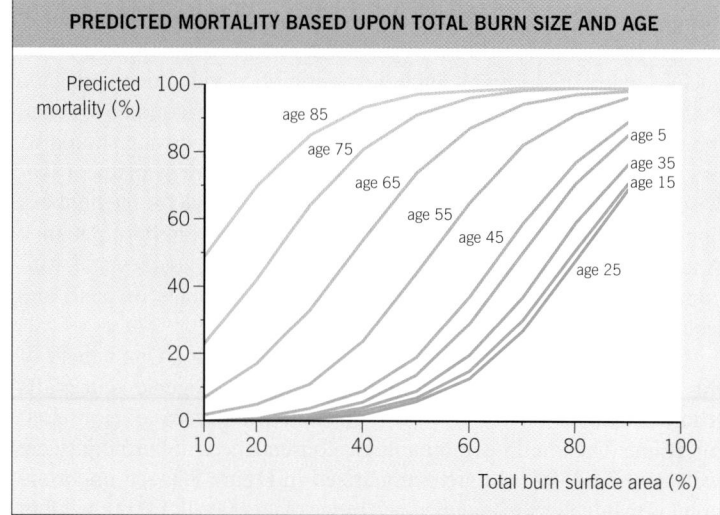

Fig. 8.1 Predicted mortality based upon total burn size and age.

AMERICAN BURN ASSOCIATION CRITERIA FOR REFERRAL TO A BURN CENTER

- Second- and third-degree burns >10% body surface area (BSA) in ages <10 or >50 years
- Second- and third-degree burns >20% BSA in other age groups
- Third-degree burns >5% BSA
- Second- and third-degree burns involving face, eyes, ears, hands, feet, genitalia, perineum or overlying major joints
- Electrical burns, including lightning injury
- Chemical burns
- Inhalation injury
- Burn injury in patients with pre-existing medical conditions that could complicate management, prolong recovery or affect mortality
- Burn injury with associated trauma
- Burn injury in patients with special social, emotional or rehabilitative needs, including suspected child abuse or neglect

Fig. 8.2 American Burn Association criteria for referral to a burn center.[4,5]

depletion if sufficient exogenous calories are not supplied. Burn hypermetabolism persists until the burn wounds are closed,[2] a process that may require several weeks.

The initial cardiovascular response to burn injury is a decrease in cardiac output along with an increase in systemic vascular resistance secondary to hypovolemia. With appropriate fluid resuscitation cardiac output returns to a normal level within 24 hours of injury. During the second 24 hours, the patient becomes hypermetabolic and cardiac output increases to supranormal (2–2.5 times predicted normal) levels. The elevation of cardiac output is accompanied by a reciprocal drop in systemic vascular resistance to 40–80% of normal levels.[6] Cardiac output remains elevated until the burn wounds are closed.[2] The stress on the cardiovascular system may precipitate myocardial infarction, particularly at the peak of the hypermetabolic response (1 week postburn).[2] It cannot be overemphasized that the pattern of elevated cardiac output and decreased systemic vascular resistance is a normal response to thermal injury, and is not indicative of sepsis.

The hypermetabolism of burn injury results in increased heat production, elevation of core temperature and a central upregulation of the thermoregulatory set point. Fever in the burn patient is thus often physiologic and not related to infection. Burn patients have poor temperature autoregulation while their wounds are still open. Loss of skin integrity results in high heat losses to the environment. Despite the hypermetabolic and thermogenic nature of burn injury, such patients may become hypothermic if the ambient temperature is not increased to compensate for these losses. The evaluation of hypothermia in the burn patient should start with consideration of an environmental cause. A final consequence of burn hypermetabolism is the increased clearance of many medications, including antibiotics and anticonvulsants. Patients on chronic medications pre-injury cannot be assumed to retain therapeutic levels on stable doses post-injury. Drug dosing should be based upon repeated serum measurements if these are available. Likewise, administration of antibiotics at dosages effective for the nonburn population will often result in subtherapeutic levels in burn patients. Antibiotic administration, particularly of aminoglycosides and vancomycin, must be guided by frequent measurements of peak and trough serum levels.

Thermal injury suppresses cell-mediated immunity. One benefit of this immunosuppression is the ability to utilize allogenic skin grafts (cadaver skin) as a temporary skin substitute without fear of early graft rejection.[2] The multiple immunologic consequences of burn injury are well described[2,7–11] and are summarized in Figure 8.3. An important point is that leukocyte counts in the range of 14,000–18,000 cells/ml or higher may be seen in burn patients in the absence of infection. The trend of white blood cell elevation rather than an isolated white blood cell elevation should alert the clinician to the possibility of infection.

A final immunologic consequence is the need for multiple transfusions of blood products. Transfusion is known to produce immunosuppression and may serve as a source of blood-borne pathogens. A study of 594 burn patients who have burn size over 10% body surface area surviving for more than 10 days showed an average transfusion rate of 19.7 units of packed red cells per patient.[12] A significant association exists between infectious morbidity and number of transfusions, independent of burn size or patient age.

In summary, a variety of metabolic events conspire to make the timely diagnosis of infection difficult in the burn patient. Hyperthermia, hypothermia, leukocytosis, tachypnea, tachycardia, disorientation, glucose intolerance and positive wound surface cultures are all seen in the absence or the presence of infectious processes, and are not sufficient to diagnose burn wound infection.[2]

PREVENTION

Several steps may be taken to reduce the risk of infectious complications in the burn population. As with any intensive care unit patient, infectious complications are reduced by the prompt extubation of the

respiratory, cardiovascular and genitourinary systems as clinical condition allows; the provision of adequate nutrition; and the timely mobilization of the patient to prevent pressure sores and atelectasis. The use of single-room isolation for burn patients delays the onset of colonization with *Pseudomonas aeruginosa* and reduces the incidence of wound infection, bacteremia and pneumonia associated with this pathogen.[13] Topical use of mafenide acetate in association with the avoidance of any pressure on the external ear reduces the incidence of suppurative chondritis.[14] The incidence of suppurative thrombophlebitis is decreased by the regular rotation of intravenous cannulation sites. At burn centers all indwelling venous lines should be replaced at the time of admission (if started outside of the burn center) and every 3 days thereafter by fresh venipuncture.[15] Line changes over guide wires are not performed. The incidence of nosocomial pneumonia is decreased by the use of high-frequency percussive ventilation, which facilitates the removal of endobronchial secretions and allows adequate ventilation at lower airway pressures than conventional techniques.[15,16] A bronchopneumonia incidence of 29.3% was reported in burn patients treated with high-frequency percussive ventilation compared with one of 52.3% in a matched cohort treated with volume-cycled ventilation.[16]

THE IMPACT OF THERMAL INJURY ON IMMUNE FUNCTION		
Circulating	IL-1	Initial increase in serum levels followed by decreased production Increased local production at sites of inflammation
	IL-2	Suppressed production
	TNF-α	Increased serum levels in severely infected burn patients
	IL-6	Increased serum levels in severely infected burn patients, increased local production at sites of inflammation
	Neopterin	Serum levels increased (nonspecific marker of macrophage stimulation)
	Immunoglobulins	Decreased serum levels in first week
	Prostaglandin E$_2$	Increased serum levels
	Thromboxane B$_2$	Increased serum levels
	Activation/depletion of alternative complement pathway	
	Secondary elevation of fibronectin levels	
	Reduction in serum opsonic activity	
Cellular	Initial leukopenia (margination) followed by leukocytosis	
	Generalized activation of circulating granulocytes by multiple pathways	
	Depression of neutrophil chemotaxis, phagocytosis and bacteriocidal activity	
	Depression of helper T cells	
	Generation of suppressor inducer T cells in animal studies	
	Increased production of suppressor effector T cells in animal studies	
	Suppression of IL-2 production by lymphocytes	
	Activation of macrophages	
Other	Loss of cutaneous skin barrier to infection	
	Smoke inhalation	increased risk of pneumonia (impaired mucociliary clearance mechanisms, defective alveolar macrophage function, distal airway obstruction, alveolar collapse, segmental atelectasis, increased requirements for airway intubation and mechanical ventilation)
	Requirement for long-term intubation of bladder and vascular system	
	Nutritional deficits	
	Impairment of reticuloendothelial system function	
	Multiple blood transfusions	

Fig. 8.3 **The impact of thermal injury on the immune system.**

Burn patients are prone to stress ulcers of the gastrointestinal system, and this process can be minimized by treatment with antacids and H₂-blocking agents. In one study nosocomial Gram-negative pneumonia occurred more frequently in patients requiring mechanical ventilation who received antacids and H₂-blocking agents than in a similar cohort receiving sucralfate.[17] Gram-negative colonization of the stomach secondary to elevation of gastric pH was a postulated mechanism. The study group was predominantly patients who have non-traumatic illness. Both regimens were compared in burn patients and no difference in rates of colonization of the respiratory or gastrointestinal tracts were observed, but a higher incidence of nosocomial pneumonia and upper gastrointestinal bleeding occurred in the sucralfate group.[18] An agent that prevents gastric ulceration and colonization would be ideal but is currently unavailable.

CLINICAL FEATURES

ORGANISMS CAUSING INFECTIONS

The history of burn wound infection has been largely influenced by therapeutic and environmental factors. Before the development of antimicrobial agents and the use of fluids to resuscitate the burn patient, essentially all those with serious burns died within a short period from the consequences of hypovolemic (burn) shock. Those patients who remained in hospital after the initial shock period were subject to streptococcal infection. It is this group of organisms that was targeted by Lister and others for topical protection for open burns with antiseptics. With the recognition of the requirement for resuscitation, patients who have severe burns began to survive the initial postburn period. This new patient population, with large wounds that remained open for months, led to the development of specialized burn centers, which were established at large hospitals and by the military. The traditional hospital open ward design was adapted for burn care and little could be done to prevent cross contamination. The situation of general ward care, large open wounds and the introduction of expanding generations of antimicrobial agents often resulted in wound infection by antimicrobial-resistant microbial pathogens. By the 1960s burn centers worldwide experienced infections from *P. aeruginosa* and other opportunists with intrinsic resistance to many antibiotics and with the capacity to acquire and propagate resistance mechanisms against newer generations of antimicrobials. Burn centers often gained notoriety for having a high incidence of infection and antimicrobial resistance.

With the recognition of the significance of cross contamination and the necessity to improve patient isolation, the design of most modern burn centers has changed to single rooms for the intensive phase of burn care. This change occurred at our burn center in 1983 and markedly changed the incidence, etiology and outcome of burn wound infections.[13,19]

In subsequent reviews the continued prevention of previously common infections with multiply resistant organisms and improved survival has been documented.[20] An example of such change is presented in Figure 8.4. These data document the incidence and outcome of *P. aeruginosa* bacteremia during the past 2 decades. In the first decade, the incidence of this infection was 9.4% and mortality in bacteremic patients was 73%. When this mortality is compared with that predicted for severity of injury alone, an excess attributable mortality of 61% is realized.[13] During the current decade, the incidence of this infection has dropped to 1.2% of admissions and the mortality noted is not different from that predicted based on severity alone.[20]

The review of infections and their causes in the past decade is presented in Figures 8.5 and 8.6. As can be seen, wound invasion, the hallmark of burn infections for many decades, has been reduced to 5% of infections.

Coincident with a decline in bacterial wound infection an increase in the incidence of fungal infection has been seen. A histopathologic review of all burn autopsy data at our institution between the years 1960 and 1969 showed a tenfold increase in the incidence of wound

infections caused by *Phycomycetes* and *Aspergillus* spp. coincident with the introduction of mafenide acetate burn cream in 1964.[21] Recent experience between the years 1979 and 1989 demonstrates a marked decrease in the incidence of bacterial wound infection, attributable to patient isolation, topical chemotherapy and surgical wound excision.[22] Interestingly, the incidence of fungal wound infection did not change

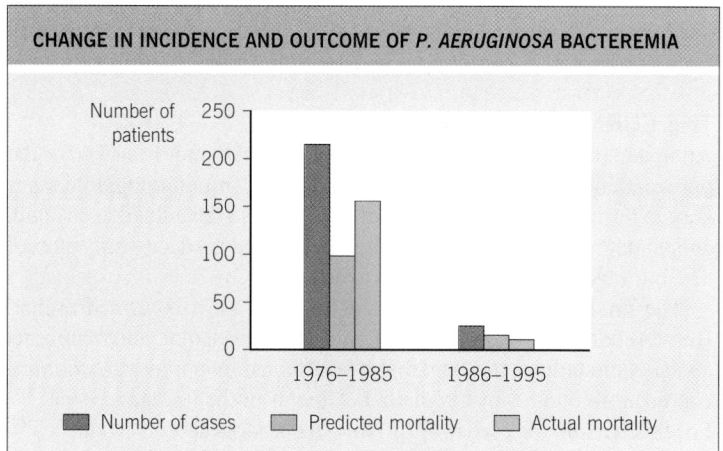

Fig. 8.4 Change in incidence and outcome of *Pseudomonas aeruginosa* bacteremia in burn patients over a 20-year period.

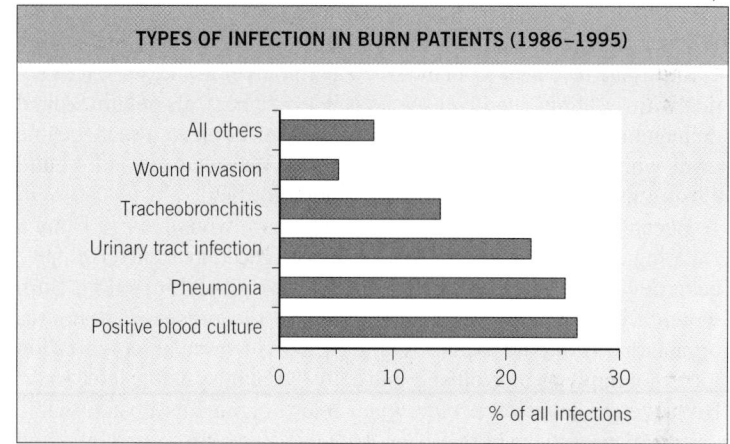

Fig. 8.5 Types of infections seen in burn patients over a 10-year period.

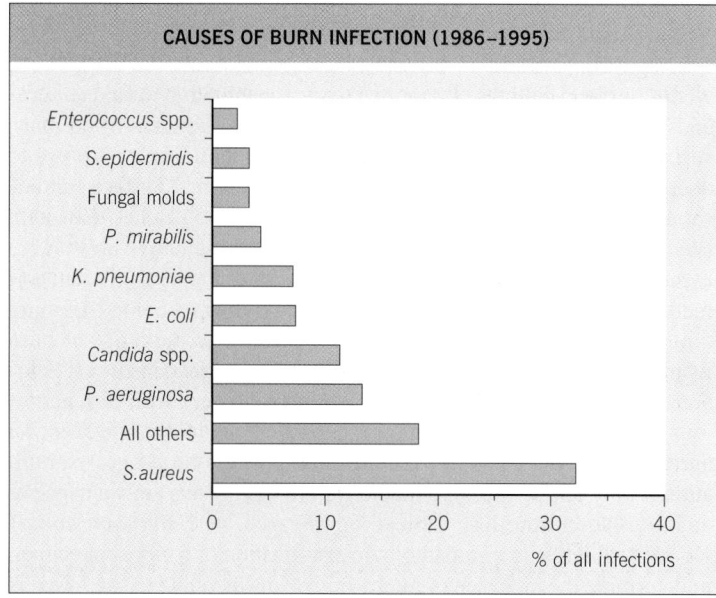

Fig. 8.6 Causes of infection in burn patients over a 10-year period. Each of the organisms in the 'All others' category account for <2% of burn infection.

during the same period. Bacterial and fungal wound infection were associated with large body surface area burns [mean 62.4% total body surface area (TBSA) burn for fungal infection and 54.4% TBSA for bacterial infection] and an increased incidence of smoke inhalation injury (74.5% of fungal patients versus 70.6% of bacterial patients). The immunosuppression of burn injury may predispose patients to fungal infection, which is difficult to prevent given the ubiquitous nature of fungi in the environment.[22] Indiscriminate use of systemic antibacterial agents in the absence of documented infection may suppress normal bacterial flora and result in fungal superinfection.

THE BURN WOUND

An understanding of the burn wound is key to an understanding of the burn patient. The physiologic, metabolic and immunologic changes seen in burn injury are proportional to the size of the cutaneous wound, and do not return to normal until the burn wound is successfully closed. The burn wound is the first site to examine when sepsis is suspected.

The thick leathery nonviable coating of a burn is termed eschar. Burn eschar is warm, protein rich, moist and avascular, and represents an excellent culture medium that is unaffected by parenterally administered antibiotics or by circulating elements of the immune system.[2,15] For this reason, the eschar of full thickness burns should be surgically excised as quickly as possible. Burn eschar normally becomes colonized with the patient's own flora (Gram-positive bacteria) within 3–5 days of injury.[9] This initial colonization is subsequently replaced by Gram-negative flora present in the hospital unit over a variable interval. The principal concern is eventual colonization of the subeschar space. When bacterial densities at the interface of eschar and underlying viable tissue reaches a level of 1×10^5 per gram of tissue, wound infection with systemic microbial spread is likely.[2] The goals of burn wound management are to contain microbial colonization to a manageable level with topical agents pending surgical debridement and wound closure with skin autografts or other modalities.[2]

Because the presence of bacteria in the burn wound *per se* is not a pathologic finding, a number of specialized procedures and terms have been developed to quantify the potential for wound infection. Burn wound colonization is the term given to the presence of micro-organisms within the eschar. As the eschar is avascular, colonization 'does not imply an unavoidable and active local or systemic infection'.[9] Burn wound invasion occurs when micro-organisms invade viable tissue adjacent to the burn eschar. True invasive burn wound infection is rarely seen in most burn centers when topical antimicrobial agents are properly and promptly employed. Invasion accompanied by a positive blood culture or by distant spread of micro-organisms or toxic products is termed burn wound septicemia.[9]

Diagnostic modalities include swab or plate cultures of the burn wound surface, cultures of debrided tissue, quantitative wound cultures and histologic examination of the burn wound. Cultures of the burn surface or of debrided tissue are useful for epidemiologic purposes to document resident flora in the event of true infection.[2,7] Surface cultures should be performed with contact plates (Fig. 8.7) rather than with swabs in order to sample a larger and more representative area and to avoid errors relating to prolonged incubation of the swab in transport media.[23] Quantitative wound cultures[24] or counts of colony-forming units per gram of tissue have limited diagnostic modality in burn wound care. A negative quantitative culture (bacterial density <10^5 cfu) correlates well (96.1% negative predictive power) with absence of invasive infection on histopathologic tissue evaluation; however, the agreement between positive cultures and positive histologic examination is only 35.7% (positive predictive power).[25] Thus, only a negative quantitative culture has clinical significance. The *sine qua non* of wound evaluation is histopathologic examination of a biopsy specimen to determine the presence of micro-organisms in viable tissue.[2] This is performed as a bedside procedure under local anesthesia. A 500mg sample of eschar (ellipse measuring 1–2cm) is excised to include the underlying viable tissue and submitted for microbial and pathologic

analysis.[2,23] Using a frozen section technique, results are available in 30 minutes.[26] The frozen section technique has a 3.6% false-negative rate, and should be confirmed by examination of permanent sections.[23,26] A rapid section technique that produces permanent sections in 4 hours has been described.[27] Results with either technique are communicated to the clinician using standardized nomenclature (Fig. 8.8).

The use of effective topical antimicrobial agents has decreased the incidence of true invasive wound infection. The percentages of infection-related deaths attributed to wound infection has decreased from 25.5% in 1979 to as low as 5.1% between 1987 and 1991.[15,28]

PNEUMONIA

As the incidence of wound infection decreases, pneumonia has emerged as the most frequent septic complication of burn injury.[15] With better microbial control of the burn wound, the route of pulmonary infection has changed from hematogenous to airborne, and the predominant radiographic pattern has changed from nodular infiltrates to bronchopneumonia.[15] Smoke inhalation injury results in mucociliary dysfunction, atelectasis, Ventilation/perfusion mismatch and impairment of polymorphonucleocyte function. These defects in pulmonary function increase the risk of pneumonia nearly five-fold.[2,7] The effects of inhalation injury and pneumonia on predicted mortality in burn injury are independent and additive: inhalation injury

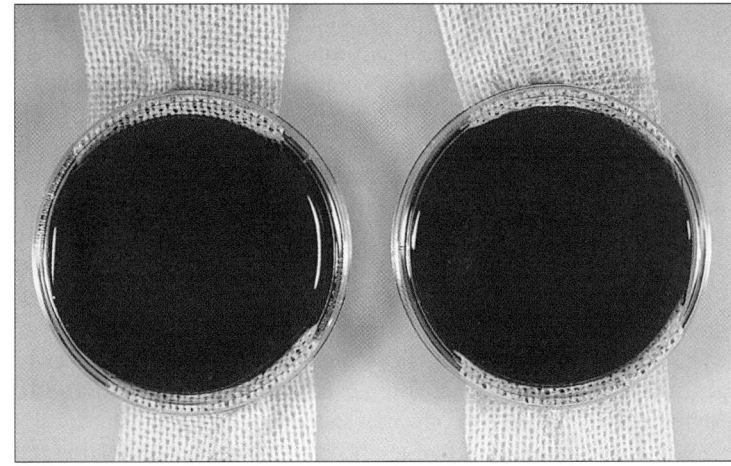

Fig. 8.7 Contact plate used for wound surveillance cultures. The culture media is lifted out of the Petri dish by the attached sterile gauze, placed in contact with the burn wound, then returned to the Petri dish for incubation.

HISTOLOGIC CLASSIFICATION OF BURN WOUND INFECTION		
Class 1 – Colonization	1A Superficial	Superficial bacterial colonization of the wound Micro-organisms present on wound surface
	1B Penetration	Penetration of the eschar by bacteria in variable thickness of eschar
	1C Proliferation	Multiplication of micro-organisms present in the subeschar space
Class 2 – Invasion	2A Microinvasion	Micro-organisms present in viable tissue immediately subjacent to subeschar space
	2B Generalized	Multifocal or widespread penetration of micro-organisms deep into viable tissue
	2C Microvascular	Involvement of small vessels and lymphatics

Fig. 8.8 Histologic classification of burn wound colonization and infection.

increases expected mortality by up to 20%; pneumonia increases mortality by up to 40%; and the combination of inhalation injury and pneumonia increases mortality by up to 60%.[3] For this reason, prevention of pneumonia has become a prime concern in patients who have smoke inhalation injury. As discussed earlier, the use of single-room isolation, volume diffusive ventilation techniques and certain stress-ulcer prophylaxis regimens may be associated with a lower risk of nosocomial pneumonia.

Criteria used at our burn center for the diagnosis of pneumonia in the burn patient are presented in Figure 8.9. Cases that meet criteria for diagnosis but lack radiographic evidence of an infiltrate are termed tracheobronchitis. Surveillance sputum cultures obtained three times per week provide an indication of the predominant organism when pneumonia or tracheobronchitis is diagnosed, allowing timely administration of an appropriate antibiotic. Pathogens commonly associated with bronchopneumonia in burn patients include *P. aeruginosa* and *Staphylococcus aureus*. The emergence of Gram-positive organisms as the predominant cause of bronchopneumonia has been a recent trend in many burn centers.[15] Staphylococcal pneumonia usually responds well to vancomycin. Our preference is to treat Gram-negative pneumonia with double antibiotic coverage, usually an aminoglycoside along with a broadspectrum beta-lactam antibiotic (see Chapter 2.28).

DIAGNOSTIC CRITERIA FOR PULMONARY INFECTION	
Pneumonia	1) Clinical findings consistent with pneumonia, i.e. pleuritic chest pain, fever, purulent sputum or other signs of sepsis
	2) More than 25 polymorphonuclear leukocytes on methylene blue stain of endotracheal secretions with less than 25 squamous epithelial cells per 100× field
	3) Roentographic findings consistent with pneumonia
	4) Positive sputum cultures (confirmatory but not essential for diagnosis)
Tracheobronchitis	As above without radiographic evidence of infiltrate

Fig. 8.9 Diagnostic criteria for pneumonia or tracheobronchitis in burn patients.

SUPPURATIVE CHONDRITIS

Burns to the ears may result in secondary infection of the cartilage. This process, termed suppurative chondritis, occurs in partial and full thickness burns, has a peak incidence between 3 and 5 weeks postburn, and may occur after skin healing is completed.[14] Before the widespread use of mafenide acetate, chondritis occurred in 20–25% of patients who have ear burns.[14,29] This incidence has decreased to 0–3.3% when burned ears are treated with this agent.[14] Silver sulfadiazine does not penetrate eschar well and is not as effective in the prevention of chondritis.

Suppurative chondritis has a rapid onset, manifesting as a throbbing ear pain poorly relieved by narcotics.[29] Over several hours the external ear becomes edematous with loss of the normal surface features of the antihelix and scapha (Fig. 8.10). Edema may create the appearance of the external ear being more prominent or anterior displaced compared with the contralateral side. The pathogens responsible may be polymicrobial with *Pseudomonas* spp. involved in 83–95% of cases, and *Staphylococcus* spp. involved in 55%.[14] Intravenous antibiotics are ineffective as the ear cartilage does not have an intrinsic blood supply and diffusion from the perichondrium is impaired by edema. Treatment of chondritis is surgical. Early cases may respond to local debridement, whereas established chondritis often requires a disfiguring bivalve incision with removal of a majority of the ear cartilage (Fig. 8.11). Wounds are packed open with fine mesh gauze soaked in an antimicrobial solution, then allowed to close by granulation.

SUPPURATIVE THROMBOPHLEBITIS

Suppurative thrombophlebitis occurs in up to 1.4–4.2% of burn patients.[30] Although the overall incidence is low, burn patients are at particular risk secondary to the need for long-term intravenous cannulation and to skin colonization with burn pathogens. The diagnosis is suggested by a positive blood culture in the absence of any obvious source. Clinical examination of current and previous intravenous cannulation sites is undertaken, although local signs of infection, including cellulitis, are present in only 35% of patients who have infected vessels. When the diagnosis is in doubt, surgical exploration is indicated. Infection is most frequently found at the vein site adjacent to the catheter tip; however, proximal migration and skip lesions are common, and the suspected vein should be excised proximally to the point at which the vessel becomes a tributary of the next larger order of veins (Fig. 8.12). In selected patients, resection may be terminated at a point at which the vein appears normal, has a lumen free of clot or

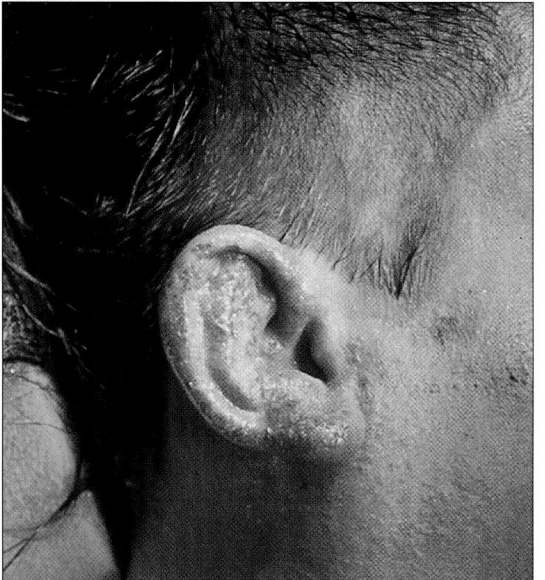

Fig. 8.10 Clinical appearance of suppurative chondritis.

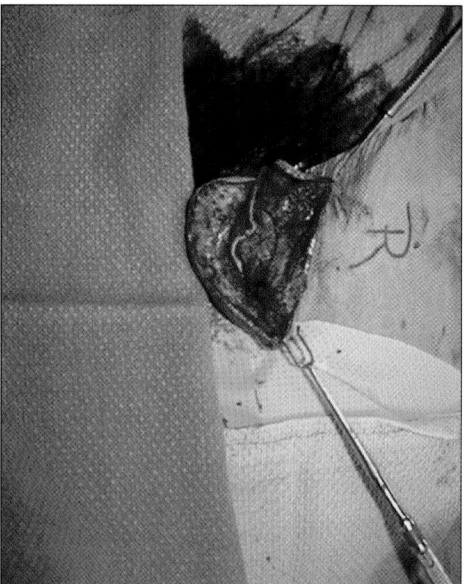

Fig. 8.11 Bivalve excision of infected cartilage.

intimal thickening and demonstrates brisk bleeding. The resected vessel should be sent for histologic and microbiologic analysis (Fig. 8.13). Failure to clear bacteremia after vein excision should prompt consideration of exploration of other vessels. Septic thrombophlebitis of central vessels is usually treated with systemic anticoagulation and intravenous antibiotics as surgical excision is impractical.

OTHER INFECTIONS

Sinusitis is a concern in burn patients because of the need for prolonged intubation of one or both nostrils. Nasotracheal intubation is the preferred airway access in burn patients for reasons of comfort and safety,[31] and nasojejunal tube feeding remains the method of choice for delivery of nutrients. The presence of sinusitis is suggested by headache, facial pain or purulent nasal discharge, although the diagnostic accuracy of clinical examination has been estimated to be only 60%. Plain film radiographs of the sinuses, particularly when taken with portable equipment, are difficult to interpret and add only 10% diagnostic accuracy to the clinical examination: for this reason the preferred diagnostic modality is CT scan of the sinuses. Treatment of sinusitis is removal of nasal tubes and administration of decongestants and culture-specific antibiotics. Antral puncture is infrequently required and should be reserved for patients who do not respond to conventional treatment (see Chapter 2.25 for further discussion on sinusitis).

Acute infective endocarditis is diagnosed in 1.3% of burn patients.[15] The right side of the heart is more commonly affected than the left; the offending organism is usually *S. aureus*. Heart murmurs are difficult to hear in burn patients, who are normally hyperdynamic, tachycardiac and frequently have the chest covered with dressings. The diagnosis is usually made with transesophageal echocardiography. Intravenous antibiotics are instituted and continued for 6 weeks after the last positive blood culture. The management of endocarditis is reviewed in detail in Chapter 2.50.

MANAGEMENT

Burn patients are prone to infection by virtue of loss of immune function and skin integrity. The daily care of burn patients requires meticulous infection control practices to avoid nosocomial infection. A microbial surveillance system is important to allow timely and exact diagnosis of infection and to guide antibiotic use. Because of the danger of superinfection from antibiotic-resistant organisms, the administration of antibiotics should strictly follow established protocols. The empiric administration of systemic antibiotics for fever, leukocytosis or nonspecific 'sepsis' in the absence of a known infectious source should be strongly discouraged.[15]

The nursing care of burn patients requires adherence to barrier precautions and reverse isolation techniques appropriate for the immunosuppressed. The use of an open dressing technique (application of topical antimicrobial to the burn without overlying dressings) allows earlier identification of potential wound infection and is the standard of practice at many burn centers. The use of open dressings, or the changing of closed dressings, requires all personnel entering the patient's room to wear gowns, head covers and gloves.[13] Barrier precautions have the added benefit of protecting the staff from occupational exposure to blood-borne pathogens. Medical supplies and equipment should not be moved from room to room, and stethoscopes are provided in each room to avoid cross contamination.

The use of single-bed isolation for burn patients is desirable. Compared with open ward housing, single-bed isolation significantly delays the onset of colonization with *P. aeruginosa* by 10 days and decreases the incidence of bacteremia, pneumonia and burn wound invasion.[13] A delay in colonization may decrease morbidity and mortality, as the patient may be more likely to resist infection later in their hospital stay as wound healing progresses.

Resistance isolation is utilized when a patient is identified as harboring a bacterial organism with multiple antibiotic resistance, or

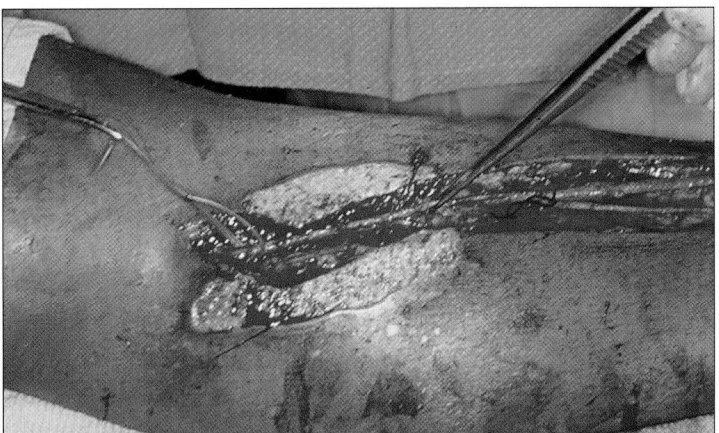

Fig. 8.12 Vein resection for suppurative thrombophlebitis.

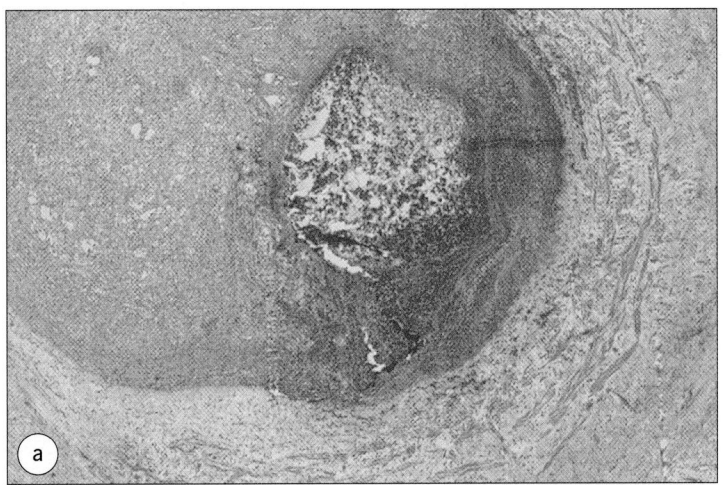
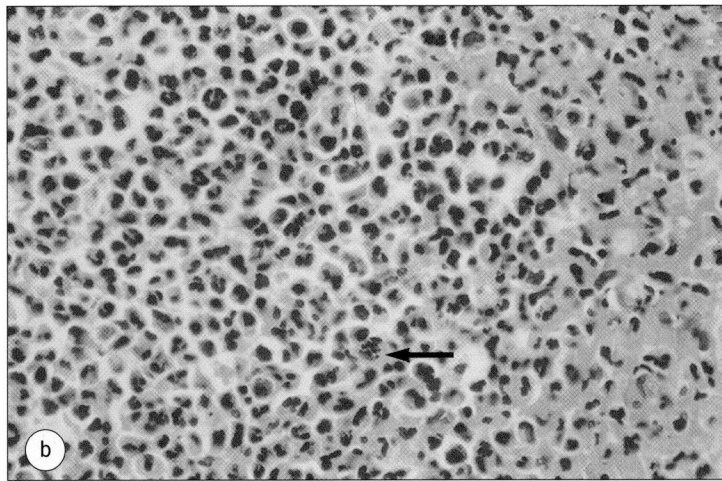

Fig. 8.13 Suppurative thrombophlebitis. (a) Histologic section of excised vein demonstrating thrombus. (b) Micro-organisms (Gram-positive cocci) present within thrombus (arrow).

when a patient is transferred after being an inpatient in another hospital for 7 days or more. Under resistance isolation, nursing staff are assigned to the same patient every day and normally do not enter the room of any other patient. Supplies are arranged to maximize patient care with minimal traffic in and out of the room, and physician care proceeds from nonisolated to resistance isolated areas as patient condition allows. Personnel providing resistance isolation care must change all garments, including scrub clothing, before entering other areas of the hospital. Under optimal conditions, nurses providing resistance isolation care are not reassigned to other patients until 48 hours after exposure to the isolated patient.

The microbial surveillance system in use at this and other burn center[9] consists of thrice weekly cultures of sputum, wound surfaces and urine of all patients. The surveillance system allows timely identification of patterns of antibiotic resistance, identifies nosocomial spread of flora and facilitates the rational choice of antibiotic when infection is identified. In general, the antibiotic sensitivities of flora seen in the burn center are different from similar species isolated from other nursing care units, and the regular hospital antibiogram should not be relied upon when choosing antibiotics. If a full burn surveillance system cannot be established, an alternative is to produce an antibiogram specific for isolates from the burn treatment unit.

Care of the burn wound centers on debridement of nonviable tissue and prevention of infection. Wounds are cleansed twice daily with chlorhexidine gluconate solution and then placed in 'alternating agents' consisting of mafenide acetate cream during the day and silver sulfadiazine cream at night. The combination of mafenide and silver sulfadiazine reduces the incidence of complications and drug resistance compared with that seen when either agent is used alone. Mafenide acetate provides the best penetration into nonviable eschar and may be employed as a single agent when the wound is obviously full thickness or when invasive infection is suspected. The advantages and disadvantages of this and other topical antimicrobial agents are summarized in Figure 8.14.

The entire wound surface must be inspected at least daily for signs of infection.[2] Wound care should be provided in the individual patient's room to avoid cross contamination between patients. Hydrotherapy or wound debridement in a Hubbard tank is no longer performed at most burn centers.

The ultimate goal of burn care is permanent wound closure. To this end, surgical excision of full thickness and deep partial thickness wounds commences 3–5 days after the burn injury and continues on a frequent basis until the entire burn is excised. Split thickness autografts harvested from unburned skin surfaces are used to cover the excised area. When donor sites are insufficient, temporary wound closure is performed with cadaver allograft. Donor sites may generally be re-harvested every 10–14 days, allowing eventual replacement of allograft with the patient's own skin.

TOPICAL ANTIMICROBIAL THERAPY OF THE BURN WOUND

Agent	Advantages	Disadvantages
Mafenide acetate 11.1% cream	Best eschar penetration, most widely studied agent; broad spectrum, bacteriostatic against Gram-positive and Gram-negative, especially effective against *Pseudomonas aeruginosa* and *Clostridia* spp.; no Gram-negative resistance	Painful to apply on partial thickness burns; metabolic acidosis from carbonic anhydrase inhibition; accentuates hyperventilation; minimal coverage of yeasts; poor coverage of *Providencia* spp.; most effective when utilized with open dressing technique
Mafenide acetate 5% aqueous solution	Good eschar penetration; useful in wet dressings to facilitate debridement; especially effective on wound bed after eschar removal; effective dressing for open granulating wounds or over meshed autografts	Requires wet dressings; may contribute to hypothermia; not Food and Drug Administration approved in USA
Silver sulfadiazine 1% cream	Painless on application; good Gram-negative and yeast coverage; infrequent hypersensitivity; may be used with open or closed dressings; may be combined with nystatin to increase yeast coverage	Poor eschar penetration; transient leukopenia; poor or no coverage of *Enterobacter*, *Klebsiella*, *Clostridia* and some *Pseudomonas* spp.; Plasmid-mediated resistance to this agent may extend to other antimicrobials
Silver nitrate 0.5% solution	Bacteriostatic against a broad spectrum of Gram-positive, Gram-negative and yeast-like organisms; effective for patients with toxic epidermal necrosis syndrome or burn patients allergic to sulfa drugs	Little to no eschar penetration; precipitates on tissue contact; works best on minimally colonized or debrided tissue; stains tissue, clothing and bedlinens; causes hyponatremia, hypokalemia and hypocalcemia; wet dressings may contribute to hypothermia; poor coverage of *Klebsiella* and *Providencia* spp.
Sodium hypochlorite 0.025% solution	Bacteriocidal against a broad spectrum of Gram-positive and Gram-negative organisms; inexpensive	Must be freshly compounded; requires wet dressings, which may contribute to hypothermia
Gentamicin sulfate 0.1% cream	Broad spectrum	Rapid emergence of resistant organisms; no longer in common use
Nitrofurazone 0.2% cream	Effective against *Staphylococcus* spp. [including methillin-resistant *Staphylococcus aureus* (MRSA)] and nonpseudomonad Gram-negative organisms	Poor coverage of *Pseudomonas* spp.
Mupirocin 2% cream	Effective against Gram-positive organisms, including MRSA; effective against some Gram-negative enteric organisms; useful for graft infection secondary to *Staphylococcus* spp.	Expensive; not a first line therapy
Nystatin 100,000 units/g	Effective against *Candida* spp. and most true fungi	No antibacterial coverage
Clotrimazole 1% cream	Broad-spectrum antifungal effective against *Candida*, *Trichophyton* and *Microsporum* spp.; minimal systemic absorption from topical use	No antibacterial coverage; poorly absorbed through normal skin; eschar penetration unknown

Fig. 8.14 Topical antimicrobial therapy of the burn wound.[2,7,9,22]

REFERENCES

1. Pruitt BA Jr, Mason AD, Goodwin CW. Epidemiology of burn injury and demography of burn care facilities. Probl Gen Surg 1990;7:235–51.

2. Pruitt BA Jr, Goodwin CW, Cioffi WG. Thermal injuries. In: Davis JH, Sheldon GF, Eds. Surgery – a problem solving approach. St Louis: Mosby-Year Book; 1995:643–719.

3. Shirani KZ, Pruitt BA Jr, Mason AD. The influence of inhalation injury and pneumonia on burn mortality. Ann Surg 1987;205:82–7.

4. Committee on Trauma, American College of Surgeons. Advanced trauma life support program for physicians. Chicago: American College of Surgeons; 1993.

5. Nebraska Burn Institute. Advanced burn life support. Lincoln: Nebraska Burn Institute; 1992.

6. Pruitt BA Jr, Mason AD, Moncrief JA. Hemodynamic changes in the early postburn patient: the influence of fluid administration and of a vasodilator (hydralazine). J Trauma 1971;11:36–46.

7. Shirani KZ, Vaughan GM, Mason AD, Pruitt BA Jr. Update on current therapeutic approaches in burns. Shock 1996;5:4–16.

8. Hinder F, Traber DL. Pathophysiology of the systemic inflammatory response syndrome. In: Herndon DN, ed. Total burn care. Philadelphia: WB Saunders; 1996:207–16.

9. Heggers J, Linares HA, Edgar P, Villarreal C, Herndon DN. Treatment of infections in burns. In: Herndon DN, ed. Total burn care. Philadelphia: WB Saunders; 1996:98–135.

10. Munster AM. The immunological response and strategies for intervention. In: Herndon DN, ed. Total burn care. Philadelphia: WB Saunders; 1996.

11. Demling RH. Physiologic changes in burn patients. In: Wilmore D, ed. American College of Surgeons care of the surgical patient. New York: Scientific American; 1990:1–8.

12. Graves TA, Cioffi WG, Mason AD, McManus WF, Pruitt BA Jr. Relationship of transfusion and infection in a burn population. J Trauma 1989;29:948–54.

13. McManus AT, Mason AD, McManus WF, Pruitt BA Jr. Control of *Pseudomonas aeruginosa* infections in burned patients. Surg Res Commun 1992;12:61–7.

14. Mills DC, Roberts LW, Mason AD, McManus WF, Pruitt BA Jr. Suppurative chondritis: its incidence, prevention and treatment in burn patients. Plast Reconstr Surg 1988;82:267–76.

15. Mozingo DW, Pruitt BA Jr. Infectious complications after burn injury. Curr Opin Surg Infect 1994;2:69–75.

16. Rue LW III, Cioffi WG, Mason AD, McManus WF, Pruitt BA Jr. Improved survival of burned patients with inhalation injury. Arch Surg 1993;128:772–80.

17. Driks MR, Craven DE, Celli BR, et al. Nosocomial pneumonia in intubated patients given sucralfate as compared with antacids or histamine type 2 blockers. N Engl J Med 1987;317:1376–82.

18. Cioffi WG, McManus AT, Rue LW III, et al. Comparison of acid neutralizing and non-acid neutralizing stress ulcer prophylaxis in thermally injured patients. J Trauma 1994;36:541–7.

19. Shirani KZ, McManus AT, Vaughan GM, et al. Effects of environment on infection in burn patients. Arch Surg 1986;121:31–6.

20. McManus AT, Mason AD, McManus WF, Pruitt BA Jr. A decade of reduced Gram-negative infections and mortality associated with improved isolation of burned patients. Arch Surg 1994;129:1306–9.

21. Nash G, Foley FD, Goodwin MN, et al. Fungal burn wound infection JAMA 1971;215:1664–6.

22. Becker WK, Cioffi WG, McManus AT et al. Fungal burn wound infection – a ten year experience Arch Surg 1991;126:44–8.

23. Pruitt BA Jr. The diagnosis and treatment of infection in the burn patient. Burns 1984;11:79–91.

24. Krizek TJ, Robson MC. Evolution of quantitative bacteriology in wound management. Am J Surg 1975;130:579–84.

25. McManus AT, Kim SH, McManus WF, Mason AD, Pruitt BA Jr. Comparison of quantitative microbiology and histopathology in divided burn-wound biopsy specimens. Arch Surg 1987;122:74–6.

26. Kim SH, Hubbard GB, McManus WF, Mason AD, Pruitt BA Jr. Frozen section technique to evaluate early burn wound biopsy: a comparison with the rapid section technique. J Trauma 1985;25:1134–7.

27. Kim SH, Hubbard GB, Worley BL, et al. A rapid section technique for burn wound biopsy. J Burn Care Rehab 1985;6:433–5.

28. Cioffi WG, Kim SH, Pruitt BA Jr. Cause of mortality in thermally injured patients. In: Lorenz S, Zellner PR, eds. Die Infektion beim Brandverletzten, Proceedings of the 'Infektionprophylaxe undv Infektions bekampfung beim Brandverletzten'. International Symposium. Darmstadt: Steinkopff Verlag; 1993:7–11.

29. Artz CP, Moncrief JA, Pruitt BA Jr. Burns – a team approach. Philadelphia: WB Saunders; 1979:317.

30. Pruitt BA Jr, McManus WF, Kim SH, Treat RC. Diagnosis and treatment of cannula-related intravenous sepsis in burn patients. Ann Surg 1980;191:546–54.

31. Bowers BL, Purdue GF, Hunt JL. Paranasal sinusitis in burn patients following nasotracheal intubation. Arch Surg 1991;126:1411–2.

Infective Complications After Trauma and Surgery

Jean Carlet, Maïté Garrouste-Orgeas, Jean-François Timsit & Pierre Moine

The two main complications after severe trauma and major surgery are infection and systemic inflammatory response syndrome (SIRS), an activation of the inflammatory cascade that is often, but not always, due to infection. Some patients develop the more severe complications multiple organ dysfunction syndrome (MODS) and multiple organ system failure (MOSF), which can both be fatal.[1] Infection is the most frequently identified cause of SIRS, MODS and MOSF.[2–5] The incidence of infectious complications is as high as 20–30%[6,7] following severe trauma, and up to 20% after surgery in very high-risk patients.[8,9] These events have a significant morbidity, mortality and cost.

SIRS AFTER TRAUMA AND SURGERY

SIRS AND MODS AFTER TRAUMA
Definition and natural history
Systemic inflammatory response syndrome is frequent during the early post-traumatic period, reflecting the consequences of the inflammation that occur after trauma. It may be either infective or non-infective in origin.

Systemic inflammatory response syndrome is the systemic inflammatory response to injury or other noninfectious insults to the host that results from activation of proinflammatory cytokines and other endogenous mediators. Systemic inflammatory response syndrome is characterized by two or more of the four clinical findings shown in Figure 9.1.

Sepsis is defined as the systemic inflammatory response associated with infection (Fig. 9.2).[1] Thus, sepsis has the same clinical manifestations as SIRS, along with microbial evidence that an infective process plays a direct part in the systemic inflammatory response. The term 'severe sepsis' is used when organ dysfunctions occur. The term septic shock is used when hemodynamic abnormalities are present. Multiple organ dysfunction syndrome and MOSF represent the presence of altered organ function in an acutely ill patient such that homeostasis cannot be maintained without intervention (see Chapter 2.47).

Pathogenesis
The pathogenesis of MODS and MOSF is a complex and inter-related mechanism. Trauma leads to activation of multiple humoral and cellular cascades and to activation of proinflammatory cytokine host defense mechanisms (see Fig. 9.3).[10] The importance of immune dysfunction[11,12,13] and gut barrier failure[14] has been stressed in this setting.

The acute physiologic response after injury is regarded as a natural healing phenomenon by means of an early, protective, inflammatory homeostatic response. It involves both a cellular and humoral immune response. The cytokine cascade plays an important role in modulating and amplifying the inflammatory response. The main cytokines involved in the modulation of this inflammatory response are tumor necrosis factor (TNF)-α, interleukin-1 (IL-1), IL-6, IL-8 and interferon-γ.[15,16] Interleukin-6 probably plays a pivotal role in modulating this acute phase response.[17]

Extensive injuries can sometimes lead to an uncontrolled, unregulated and prolonged hyperinflammatory response, characterized clinically by persistent fever, leukocytosis, tachypnea, tachycardia and increased metabolic rate. This clinical syndrome, SIRS,[1] is the first step

in a continuing clinical process that leads, in some circumstances, to major tissue injury, such as acute respiratory distress syndrome (ARDS), and to sepsis, severe sepsis, septic shock and MODS.[1]

Traumatic injuries are the leading cause of death among people younger than 40 years of age. In patients who do reach hospital, once hemorrhage has been controlled, the greatest risk to life is the development of late infection in and around the site of injury or at remote sites.[17,18]

The sources of infection in the trauma patient are primarily the wound if surgery is performed, and the site of injury itself. Secondary sources are contamination from the patient's own bacteria or from the team providing care, especially if there is prolonged use of foreign bodies in the intensive care setting. Experimental investigations into the nature of surgical infection have identified

---

SYMPTOMS OF THE SYSTEMIC INFLAMMATORY RESPONSE SYNDROME

Temperature greater than 100.4°F (38°C) or less than 96.8°F (36°C)

Heart rate greater than 90 beats per minute

Respiratory rate greater than 20 breaths per minute or arterial carbon dioxide tension less than 32torr

White blood cell count greater than 12,000/mm³ or less than 4000/mm³, or more than 10% band forms

Fig. 9.1 Symptoms of the systemic inflammatory response syndrome.

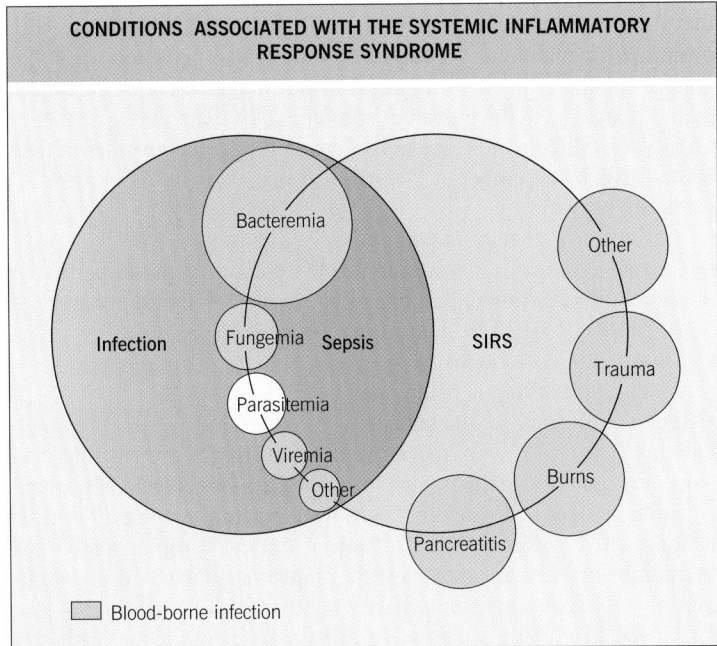

Fig. 9.2 Conditions associated with systemic inflammatory response syndrome. The complex and overlapping relationship between infection and inflammation.

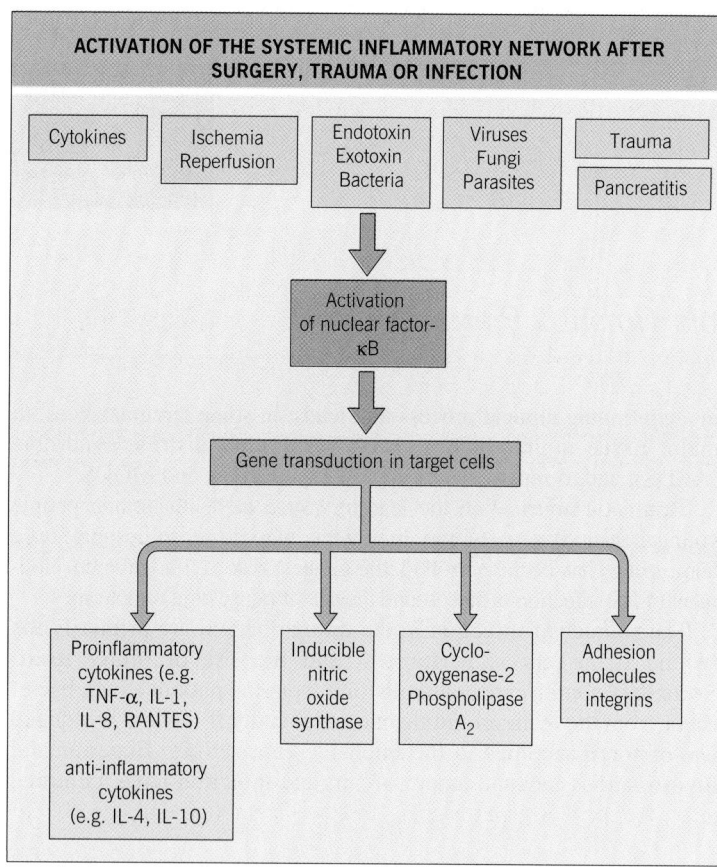

ACTIVATION OF THE SYSTEMIC INFLAMMATORY NETWORK AFTER SURGERY, TRAUMA OR INFECTION

Fig. 9.3 Activation of the systemic inflammatory network after surgery, trauma or infection.

conditions that are adjuvants for the invading bacteria. Among others, these include hypovolemic shock, vasoconstriction and immune suppression. Obviously, these factors are present in many severely injured patients.

Role of infection

The incidence of infective complications in trauma patients is estimated to be 20–30%, but it may be even higher in patients who require prolonged mechanical ventilation.[2,3,19,20] It has been reported that among trauma patients with stays in the intensive care unit longer than 30 days, 63% developed pneumonia, 69% bacteremia and 43% urinary tract infections.[21] The risk of developing infection after trauma is increased by a number of factors:[22]

- the severity of injury;
- the degree of contamination of the wounds;
- specific types of injury and injury to certain organs (in particular penetrating abdominal trauma, injury to the colon or other areas of the gastrointestinal tract, and open fractures);
- the amount of blood loss;
- the duration of hypotension; and
- the overall health of the patient.

Patients ($n = 457$), who had an Injury Severity Score over 15 and who were admitted to the trauma intensive care unit at Denver General Hospital in Denver, Colorado, USA, were recently reported. Of these patients, 30% suffered major infections and 16% minor infections. Major infections included pneumonia, empyema, lung abscess, abdominal or pelvic abscess, extensive wound infection, meningitis and urosepsis. Minor infections were urinary tract infections, catheter-related infections, wound infections not requiring debridement, sinusitis and conjunctivitis. Pneumonia was the most frequent infective complication, occurring in 30% of these patients. Bacteremia is also a

frequent complication in trauma patients, with a higher incidence than in general populations of intensive care patients.[23]

The role of infection in the pathophysiology of post-traumatic MODS and the exact timing of the events remains contentious. It has been suggested that MODS is the result of uncontrolled infection,[19] but there are no detectable differences between the response of patients with sepsis and those without.[24] It has become evident that patients can die of 'clinical sepsis' without an obvious focus of infection – although an infection may initiate MODS, a source of infection cannot be found in up to 50% of patients.[25] The type of micro-organism, if present, does not make a difference to the response. Two infectious models of MODS were proposed: in one, the insult causes ARDS and pulmonary sepsis, which leads to MODS; in the other, the insult causes sepsis, which leads to either ARDS or MODS or both.[26,27]

The role of infection has been considered as minimal by some authors,[28] whereas others have found that infection could be considered as a cause of multiple organ failure in up to 80% of patients with post-traumatic MODS.[29,30] Two different patterns have been described for the development of MODS (i.e. early MODS versus late MODS).[31] In 38% of the patients, multiple organ failure developed in the absence of infection and occurred rapidly, within 24–72 hours after trauma. In the group of delayed multiple organ failure, infection was present in 90% of the patients. Moreover, it has been shown that early post-traumatic multiple organ failure occurred in the great majority of the patients in the absence of infection.[32] The lack of infection in the early MODS patients could not be explained by the routine use of antibiotics, because most of the patients received only a single dose of antibiotics on the way to hospital. The potential impact of major infections on the clinical course of early MODS compared with late MODS has been studied.[33] Thirty-two major infections occurred in 23 of the 27 early MODS patients (85%). In contrast, 59 major infections occurred in 38 of the 43 late MODS patients (88%). Thus, early and late MODS patients experienced a similar high incidence of major infective complications. The majority of these occurred either early (and thus were unrelated to MODS) or late (and appeared to be symptoms of MODS). However, in the late MODS patients, major infections were classified because MODS triggers more often than in early MODS.

Collectively, these studies are consistent with the hypothesis that MODS occurs as a result of a dysfunctional inflammatory response.[33,34] It is speculated that severe trauma causes an early and short hyperinflammatory response. Following major trauma, patients are resuscitated into an early state of hyperinflammation (i.e. SIRS). The postinjury SIRS becomes activated as early as 6–12 hours after the injury.[35,36] Postinjury SIRS (see Fig. 9.3) is complex and involves multiple effector cells with overlapping mediator cascades. For example, hemorrhagic shock has been shown to affect nuclear factor κB regulatory mechanisms in the lung.[37] Mild to moderate SIRS is probably beneficial to the patient (i.e. it is the normal 'injury stress response'), whereas severe SIRS is potentially harmful. This can result in early MODS if the initial insult is massive (the 'one-hit' model) or if early secondary inflammatory insults occur (the 'two-hit' model).

SIRS AND MODS AFTER MAJOR SURGERY
Epidemiology

Most patients undergoing major and prolonged surgery develop (as in trauma patients) the symptoms of SIRS in the first few days after surgery. This represents a normal, adaptive, inflammatory response to the insult of surgical injury. Some patients will develop prolonged SIRS and MODS, which then become a life-threatening syndrome.

The exact incidence of SIRS and MODS after surgery is not known.[38] Factors that influence the development of these syndromes include the quality, the type and duration of the surgical procedure, the presence of an ischemic or reperfusion phenomenon, and the presence of an infection.

Pathophysiology

Cardiac surgery and vascular surgery with aortic cross-clamping are procedures that predispose to SIRS, MODS and ARDS, which is a frequent component of MODS. This could be due to the intensity of the ischemia and reperfusion, which is known to activate nuclear factor κB or other signaling pathways[37] and then induce the production of cytokines such as TNF-α, IL-1 and IL-8,[39,40] as well as oxygen radicals. Ischemia-paper fusion promotes the adhesion of leukocytes to the endothelium. Other mechanisms that may lead to MODS include bacterial translocation and the production of cytokines by the digestive tract.[41,42]

It has been demonstrated that cardiopulmonary bypass and aortic cross-clamping are able to induce the release of endotoxin.[41–43] However, antiendotoxin monoclonal antibodies are unable to prevent TNF-α production after aortic clamping in animals,[43] and this is an argument for a local production of cytokines, which has been suspected during human studies as well.[43] During cardiac surgery, although significant progress has been made on the quality of the cardiopulmonary bypass membranes, activation of the complement cascade and the inflammatory network is still possible.

The exact incidence of SIRS and MODS after other types of surgery (e.g. digestive, orthopedic, or urologic procedures) is not known. In these settings, infections are more often responsible for the activation of the inflammatory network. Peritonitis is an important cause of severe sepsis and represents up to 40% of the patients included in the trials designed to test new drugs such as anti-TNF antibodies during severe sepsis.[5,9]

BACTERIAL TRANSLOCATION

Bacterial translocation is a possible cause of activation of the inflammatory network after severe trauma and major surgery. Surgical and trauma patients are at high risk of bacterial translocation secondary to complications such as enteric overgrowth, intestinal ischemia, bowel stasis, or hemorrhagic shock. The importance of bacterial translocation, defined as the transmural passage of bacteria (dead or living) or endotoxins from the intestinal lumen to other sites (lymph nodes, liver, spleen and circulatory system),[44] is no longer debated in animal studies or in specific human populations such as neutropenic patients.[45] However, because its existence in humans is difficult to demonstrate, its clinical relevance is still very controversial.

In particular, the role of bacterial translocation as the initiating event in the development of multiple organ failure after trauma in the immediate postoperative period is not clear. A population of 20 patients requiring emergency laparotomy for abdominal injuries, which predisposed to multiple organ failure was studied.[46] Eight out of 212 (3.8%) portal blood samples were positive for bacteria; seven of these were presumed to be contaminated. In the first 48 hours, endotoxin was not detected, either in portal or in systemic samples, although 30% of the patients had multiple organ failure. Moreover, the role of bacterial or endotoxin translocation in the evolution and perpetuation of multiple organ failure in the later postoperative period remains obscure. No correlation was found between systemic endotoxin level and adverse outcome or multiple organ failure in patients with hemorrhagic shock caused by a ruptured abdominal aortic aneurysm.[47] A persistent increase in circulating cytokines has generally been associated with the development of multiple organ failure and death. In a recent report, plasma concentrations of TNF, IL-1β, IL-6 and IL-8 were prospectively examined in 251 consecutive unselected medical and surgical intensive care patients on admission and daily thereafter with respect to Acute Physiology and Chronic Health Evaluation (APACHE) III score and survival.[48] Plasma concentrations of these four cytokines fluctuated markedly on a day-to-day basis during critical illness and correlated poorly with concomitant physiologic derangements, APACHE III score, or outcome.

Although it is conceivable that bacterial or endotoxin translocation is a late event of multiple organ failure that occurs following disruption of the mucosal barrier induced by multiple insults in an immunocompromised host, no direct clinical evidence supports or refutes this hypothesis in the surgical or trauma population.[43]

IMMUNOSUPPRESSION AFTER TRAUMA AND MAJOR SURGERY

After the initial phase of injury, negative feedback systems downregulate early SIRS to limit potential autodestructive inflammation. The early hyperinflammatory response is followed by a long-lasting 'hypoinflammatory' state,[49] for which the name 'compensatory anti-inflammatory response syndrome' has been proposed (Fig. 9.4).[50]

The 'hypoinflammatory' state of injured patients may represent an autoprotective mechanism of the host to prevent the detrimental effects of overwhelming cytokinemia, which is thought to induce MODS. This results in delayed immunosuppression, which could be associated with major infectious complications. However, this has not yet been demonstrated clinically.

FOCAL INFECTIONS AFTER TRAUMA AND SURGERY

Bacterial infection remains a frequent event after trauma or major surgery. Infection is often endogenous in origin as improvements in the management of very ill patients results in prolonged stays in intensive care units, and predisposes to nosocomial infections (Fig. 9.5).

Mucosal resistance to colonization is reduced after trauma and surgery and in patients in intensive care units. Colonization is also increased in injured areas of the body (e.g. in the small bronchi during ARDS).[55] Broad-spectrum antibiotics play an important role in the selection of the more resistant strains (*Pseudomonas* spp., *Candida* spp.), which can then colonize many sites in the body, including the digestive tract.[56] Little is known about viral nosocomial

---

SEQUENTIAL EVENTS LEADING TO IMMUNE DEPRESSION AFTER MAJOR TRAUMA AND SURGERY

Release of endotoxin, bacterial products, free radicals

Activation of nuclear factor κB

Release of proinflammatory mediators (e.g. TNF-α, IL-1, IL-8)

Release of anti-inflammatory mediators (e.g. IL-4, IL-10)

Decrease in fibronectin and opsonic activity

Depressed neutrophil functions of chemotaxis, phagocytosis and intracellular killing

Shift from T-helper-1 lymphocytes to T-helper-2 lymphocytes[51]

Reduced monocyte and macrophage function[52,53]

Loss of skin reactivity

Decreased production of B lymphocytes and immunoglobulin

Fig. 9.4 Sequential events leading to immunodepression after major trauma and surgery.

TYPES OF INFECTION IN CRITICALLY ILL PATIENTS

Primary endogenous infection	Infections with normal endogenous flora (e.g. *Escherichia coli*, pneumococci, *Haemophilus* spp., methicillin-susceptible *Staphylococcus aureus*)
Secondary endogenous infections	Infections involving hospital strains, either selected in the initial flora, or transmitted from patient to patient [e.g. *Pseudomonas* spp., *Enterobacter* spp., methicillin-resistant *Staphylococcus aureus*, vancomycin-resistant enterococci (VRE)]
Exogenous infections	Transmitted from environment (e.g. methicillin-resistant *Staphylococcus aureus*, *Legionella* spp., *Aspergillus* spp.)

Fig. 9.5 Types of infection in critically ill patients. Adapted from Van Saene et al.[54]

infections and viral reactivation, which may more frequent than is usually thought.

The best data concerning nosocomial infections after surgery come from the network of hospitals prospectively followed for years by the Centers for Disease Control and Prevention (CDC) in the USA.[4,57] Some European data are available as well.[58–62] This chapter focuses on two main types of postsurgical infections: nosocomial pneumonias and infections of the surgical site.

NOSOCOMIAL PNEUMONIA

Nosocomial pneumonia is the second most common nosocomial infection (see Chapter 2.28). Nosocomial pneumonia developed at a rate of only 0.9 cases per 1000 patient-days in patients who did not require ventilatory assistance, compared with rates of 20.6 cases per 100 patient-days in patients who received mechanical ventilation.[63] Surgical patients in intensive care units were found to have consistently higher rate of nosocomial pneumonia than medical patients (relative risk 2.2).[64] Nosocomial pneumonia is particularly common after thoracoabdominal surgery[57] and trauma.[62–65]

Mortality

Nosocomial infections are associated with a high rate of mortality (30–70%).[66,67] However, it is difficult to evaluate this attributable mortality precisely because various well-designed case–control or cohort studies matched or adjusted on severity at admission have provided opposite results.[66–68] As the incidence of nosocomial pneumonia seems to be related to the severity of the underlying illness, the attributable mortality of nosocomial pneumonia might be largely overestimated.[66–68] However, nosocomial pneumonia induces a high morbidity because it increases severity scores and is probably associated with a 7 to 15-day increase in the duration of hospital stay.

Risk factors

Nosocomial pneumonia most commonly affects very young or very old patients with severe underlying disease, immunosuppression, depressed consciousness and cardiopulmonary disease.[69]

In trauma patients, emergency intubation, head injury, hypotension on admission, blunt trauma and a high Injury Severity Score have been found to be independently associated with nosocomial pneumonia.[70] Pulmonary contusion presumably presents a major risk factor for lower respiratory tract infections by increasing the degree of pulmonary edema and decreasing bacterial clearance by the lung.[71] Diminished mobility contributes to the increased likelihood of pneumonia in trauma victims by increasing stasis of secretions and atelectasis.[72] For example, early reduction of fractures, particularly those involving the femur, decreases the incidence of pulmonary complications, including nosocomial pneumonia, after trauma. Furthermore, in trauma patients, oscillating beds seem to decrease the incidence of lower respiratory tract infections. Other measures such as analgesia to reduce pain, particularly in the case of rib fractures, are useful in allowing adequate ventilation and physiotherapy.

In patients with burns, two major risk factors dramatically increase the risk of nosocomial infection: the major derangements of immune responsiveness that occur after burns and inhalation injuries (see Chapter 3.8).[73]

It should be stressed that most early-onset pneumonias that are considered to be nosocomial in origin are probably due to the early aspiration of gastric or oropharyngeal secretions, even before admission to hospital; they are thus similar to community-acquired pneumonias and should not be considered to be the result of poor quality of care.

Etiology

The cause of nosocomial pneumonia is highly dependent on the duration of stay in the intensive care unit, the duration of mechanical ventilation, antibiotic therapy given before the suspicion of pneumonia,[74] the specific ecology of the intensive care unit and the underlying illness. The main pathogens involved in early-onset pneumonias are methicillin-sensitive *Staphylococcus aureus*, *Streptococcus pneumoniae* and *Haemophilus influenzae*. In late-onset pneumonia, *Pseudomonas aeruginosa*, *Acinetobacter baumannii* and methicillin-resistant *S. aureus* are frequently recovered, especially from patients who have been treated with antibiotics.

After closed head injury, most cases of nosocomial pneumonia occur in the first 3 days of hospitalization.[75] In multiple trauma patients, *S. aureus* is the major causative agent, especially in comatose patients.[76]

Diagnosis

There is considerable controversy over how to diagnose nosocomial pneumonia in ventilated patients. The clinical definition of suspected nosocomial pneumonia is the association of new and persistent chest radiograph abnormalities with purulent tracheobronchial secretions, or fever, hypothermia or abnormality of blood leukocyte count, with a tracheal aspirate Gram stain showing more than 25 leukocytes and fewer than 10 squamous epithelial cells per low power field, with the recovery of a potential pathogen. Mechanically ventilated patients, however, frequently develop other conditions that either obscure these findings or give rise to a similar clinical picture. Nosocomial pneumonia is probably present in only 30–50% of patients in whom it is suspected.[77] Moreover, the accuracy of clinical judgment, even by a trained physician, in predicting pneumonia in patients suspected to have it is less than 70%.[77]

Clinical criteria, although sensitive, are probably insufficient to diagnose lung infection in ventilated patients with different forms of respiratory failure. This is especially true after trauma, because other kind of lung involvement (e.g. fat embolism) can occur (Fig. 9.6).

In order to increase the specificity of diagnosis of nosocomial pneumonia, many new approaches have been tested in the past 10 years.[78] Quantitative endotracheal aspirate has 80% sensitivity and specificity, but the method seems to recover a lot of contaminating micro-organisms. Various other procedures have been developed to obtain uncontaminated distal bacteriologic samples. The protected specimen brush has been widely tested, and if a threshold of 10^3 cfu/ml is used, it seems to have 60–100% sensitivity and 70–100% specificity. Other methods, such as the plugged telescoping catheter and bronchoalveolar lavage culture, appear to be more sensitive but less specific. As nosocomial pneumonia is patchy, distal samples might be obtained either blindly or in a directed way via a bronchoscope. However, bronchoscopy allowing airway visualization and distal sampling at the site of new progressive infiltrate may be preferred. The disadvantage of these techniques is that they provide a definite diagnosis only after 48 hours of culture.

The direct examination of bronchoalveolar lavage fluid accompanied by a calculation of the number of cells that contain bacteria has

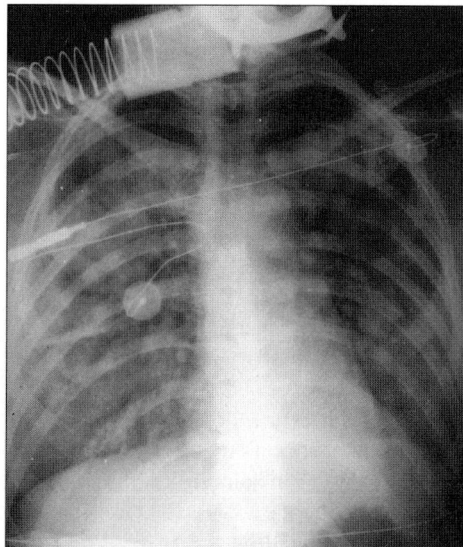

Fig. 9.6 Bilateral patchy consolidation during a fat embolism after multiple bone fractures.

been developed in the past few years. With a threshold of 2–5% of cells containing bacteria, this technique seems to provide good diagnostic accuracy only a few hours after the suspicion of pneumonia.

No definite prospective randomized study exists to confirm the cost effectiveness or superiority of invasive distal procedures. However, some preliminary data suggest that sampling that is directed via a bronchoscope is cost saving in trauma patients because it decreases unnecessary antibiotic treatment.[79]

Prevention

Preventive measures include staff education, infection surveillance, and interruption of transmission of micro-organisms by appropriate hand washing and adequate disinfection or sterilization of equipment.[69] Prevention of endogenous pneumonia by avoiding aspiration, which leads to contamination by gastric and oropharyngeal secretions, is probably the most important point. Measures such as removal of endotracheal, tracheostomy and enteral tubes as soon as possible are important. Other measures, such as avoidance of aspiration of subglottic secretions[80] and control of gastric acidity,[81] are much more debatable.

Some specific points must be mentioned. The duration of mechanical ventilation should be as short as possible, especially after chest trauma. Patients with flail chest injury and pulmonary contusion must be managed by avoiding mechanical ventilation except when it is mandated by other conditions (e.g. hypoxemia, head trauma, major surgery, shock, upper airway obstruction).

Appropriate management of pain with local or regional analgesia should be used to improve thoracic drainage, avoid hypoventilation and allow a rapid restoration of mobility. Other measures, such as physiotherapy with the use of an incentive spirometer or intermittent positive pressure, are still controversial.

SURGICAL SITE INFECTIONS

Surgical site infections (SSIs) are increasingly uncommon, but they still represent a challenge for surgical teams and can be considered as an accurate quality indicator of medical and surgical care in this setting. The risk of SSI is influenced by several factors, including the underlying condition of the patient, assessed, for example, by the American Society of Anesthesiologists score; the type of surgery, assessed by the Altemeier classification; and the duration of the procedure.[82]

The CDC have combined these risk factors to propose a risk index.[82] This seems to work very well for most surgical procedures, but not for all. This score is from 0 to 3 according to the combination of the three risk factors (Fig. 9.7).

The incidence of SSI ranges from a low level (often under 1%) in patients with a low risk (risk 0 in the CDC risk index) up to 20–25% in very high-risk patients (risk 3 in the CDC risk index; Fig. 9.8).

Infection can be classified as superficial (requiring only drainage) or deep (requiring antibiotic therapy and often reoperation). The most severe infective complication is gas gangrene (Fig. 9.9), which is now extremely unusual after scheduled surgery. Deep infections are often due to local complications such as leaks from digestive anastomoses. However, severe (although unusual) infections can occur after cardiac surgery (e.g. mediastinitis) or orthopedic surgery; these may cause significant mortality or morbidity (e.g. endocarditis, meningitis, mediastinitis) or greatly impair the functional status of the patient (e.g. infections after prosthetic joint replacement).

PREVENTION OF INFECTION AFTER TRAUMA AND SURGERY

GENERAL MEASURES

General hygienic measures are essential in reducing nosocomial infections after major trauma and surgery. They include hand washing, appropriate gloving, implementation of isolation procedures and standard precautions. Special emphasis must be put on the management of environmental factors, such as stethoscopes.

Antibiotic use policies are important in order to minimize the selective pressures that favor antibiotic-resistant bacterial organisms.[83] One method of preventing infection after trauma and surgery, which was first proposed several years ago, is selective digestive decontamination (SDD). This was initially suggested by Stoutenbeek et al.,[84] who used a combination of topical antibiotics (usually polymyxin E, tobramycin and amphotericin B) instilled in the oropharynx and the stomach q6h, plus a short course of systemic antibiotics (usually third-generation

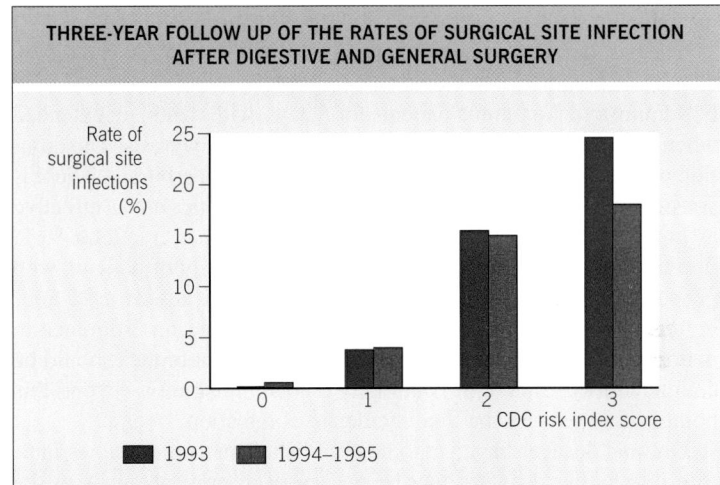

Fig. 9.8 Three-year follow up of the rates of surgical site infection after digestive and general surgery.

THE CDC RISK INDEX FOR SURGICAL SITE INFECTIONS

Contamination, according to the Altemeier classification	0 – clean or clean–contaminated 1 – contaminated or dirty
American Society of Anesthesiologists (ASA) score	0 – no underlying disease, or mild disease without any impairment of functional activity (ASA 1 and 2) 1 – ASA score 3, 4, or 5
Duration of the surgical procedure	0 – below 75th percentile of the distribution for the particular procedure 1 – above the 75th percentile of the distribution for the particular procedure
The total score is the sum of the three components to give a total of 0–3	

Fig. 9.7 The CDC risk index for surgical site infections. Adapted from Culver et al.[82]

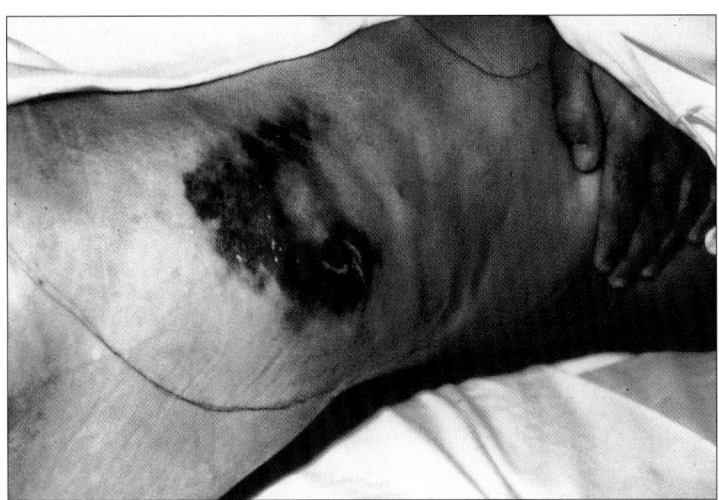

Fig. 9.9 Gas gangrene. Note the extensive local edema.

cephalosporins for 3–5 days). The intravenous component of SDD was supposed to prevent or treat early nosocomial pneumonia, and the topical component was supposed to prevent oropharyngeal and gastric colonization and thus the consequent secondary endogenous nosocomial infections.

Although a considerable amount of literature has been published in the past 10 years, including several meta-analyses,[85–88] the topic remains very controversial. The technique has been shown to be effective for preoperative prophylaxis in colon surgery, and more recently also in gastric surgery, where SDD was able to decrease not only SSI but also leakage from anastomoses.[89,90] Selective digestive decontamination is far more controversial in the intensive care setting. Although SDD is clearly able to reduce the incidence of nosocomial pneumonia in trauma and surgical intensive care patients, its effect on mortality and the risk of antibiotic resistance is less obvious.[91] However, a recent update of a meta-analysis published a few years ago[86] demonstrated a significant effect on mortality.

Additional measures aimed at enhancing host defenses seem helpful, but the data are not strong enough to recommend them at this stage. These measures include the administration of growth factors such as granulocyte colony stimulating factor,[92–96] interferon-γ[97,98] and immunoglobulins.[99,100]

SPECIFIC MEASURES
Prevention of infection in trauma patients
Clearly, antibiotic administration before injury is impossible for trauma patients. Nevertheless, there is evidence that administration of appropriate and safe systemic antibiotics as soon as possible after injury or before emergency surgery is associated with reduced wound infection rates.[35]

The best duration of initial therapy has not been studied in detail in the trauma situation. The traditional teaching is that antibiotics should be administered to trauma patients for 5 days, with treatment extended when a patient has an elevated temperature or leukocytosis. The duration of this early therapy (or prophylaxis) has been arbitrary. There is considerable evidence that short courses of antibiotics are as effective as longer ones for both penetrating trauma and open fractures.[101–104] Furthermore, a recent prospective randomized study of patients with penetrating abdominal trauma compared the efficacy of a 24-hour regimen with that of a 5-day regimen and reported no difference in major infection or death rate.[105] In our opinion, antibiotics should be continued for 24 hours. It is unlikely that administration beyond this point further reduces the final incidence of infection.

Optimal dosages have yet to be established, but some studies indicate that higher dosages may be necessary to prevent sepsis in the trauma victim.[102–106] There is concern that patients with major bleeding may lose a significant quantity of antibiotic in the shed blood and thus have only low levels of antibiotic in the serum and the wound. Significant fluid shifts and volume resuscitation may also contribute to low antibiotic levels. Furthermore, hemorrhagic shock has been shown to alter immune responses and to diminish the efficacy of antibiotics against both Gram-positive and Gram-negative organisms.[107,108] The decrease in antimicrobial efficacy reported in these experiments was postulated to be due to the failure of local host defenses to eliminate the residual bacteria remaining after administration of antibiotics. The

attainment of high levels (i.e. therapeutic concentrations) of antibiotic in serum and tissues during the early phase of treatment is probably more important than a long duration of administration.[104] In any case, the doses of antibiotics should be higher than those generally recommended (double the standard dosage), and subsequent doses should be administered frequently and at high levels if the volume of fluid resuscitation is great.[102,106]

The frequency of administration should also take into account the half-lives of the antibiotics.[102] One approach is to administer a second dose of antibiotic to any patient who, after the initial dose, has required replacement of one-half or more of the blood volume.[103,104]

One issue that is widely discussed is which drug and what antimicrobial spectrum is warranted. It is unlikely that all microbial forms can be destroyed. It seems advisable to use an agent or agents active against Gram-positive organisms including staphylococci, Gram-negative bacteria and anaerobic bacteria (clostridia, peptostreptococci and *Bacteroides fragilis*). Suitable regimens include flucloxacillin plus gentamicin plus metronidazole/amoxicillin–clavulanate.

Prevention of infection in surgical patients
Infection after surgery has decreased dramatically in the past few decades. Preventive measures include organizational and managerial improvements, skin preparation and antibiotic prophylaxis.[109] The literature demonstrating the effect of antibiotic prophylaxis on SSI is extensive, and precise guidelines are available is this setting.[110,111] Prophylaxis has to cover the surgical procedure and can be stopped either immediately after the procedure or a little later, but it must never extend for more than 36 hours. Topical antibiotics can be useful during digestive surgery,[89,90] including oesophageal, gastric and colon surgery. It is not known whether topical nasal mupirocin ointments can prevent postoperative staphylococcal infections in vascular, cardiac and orthopedic surgery.

Careful management of central temperature during and after surgical procedures is important, because hypothermia has been shown to increase the risk of SSI.[110]

During surgical procedures that are likely to cause significant ischemia and reperfusion, oxygen scavengers[111] or inotropes that are able to increase oxygen transport may be helpful, but this has not yet been confirmed. Finally, the role of nutritional support remains to be studied, because data are preliminary and controversial.[112–114]

CONCLUSION

Acute inflammation and infection are very frequent events after severe trauma and major surgery. These two events are closely linked, infection being both a trigger and a complication of inflammation, which is often followed by a period of immunodepression, which can predispose to infection. The balance is complex, and a better understanding of those events is necessary before we can modulate inflammation and prevent infection efficiently. In the meantime, very simple methods such as hygiene, adequate organization and management of the care teams, early detection of infection, proper antibiotic prophylaxis and curative antibiotic therapy still represent the most important measures in the prevention of postsurgical and post-traumatic infection.

REFERENCES

1. Members of the American College of Chest Physicians and the Society of Critical Care Medicine Consensus Conference Committee. Definitions for sepsis and organ failure and guidelines for the use of innovative therapies in sepsis. Crit Care Med 1992;20:864.

2. Brun-Buisson C, Doyon F, Carlet J, et al. Incidence, risk factors and outcome of severe sepsis and septic shock in adults. A multicenter prospective study in intensive care units. JAMA 1995;274:968–74.

3. Brun-Buisson C, Doyon F, Carlet J, et al. Bacteremia and severe sepsis in adults: a multicenter prospective survey in ICUs and wards of 24 hospitals. Am J Respir Crit Care Med 1996;154:617–24.

4. Vincent J, Bihari D, Suter P, et al. The prevalence of nosocomial infection in intensive care units in Europe: results of the European Prevalence of Infection in Intensive Care (EPIC) study. JAMA 1995;274:639–44.

5. Rangel-Frausto MS, Pittet D, Costigan M, Hwang T, Davis CS, Wenzel RP. The natural history of the systemic inflammatory response syndrome (SIRS). JAMA 1995;273:117–23.

6. Rodriguez JL, Gibbons KJ, Bitzer LG, Dechert RE, Steinberg SM, Flint LM. Pneumonia: incidence, risk factors, and outcome in injured patients. J Trauma 1991;31:907–12.

7. Waydhas C, Nast-Kolb D, Trupka A, et al. Posttraumatic inflammatory response, secondary operations, and late multiple organ failure. J Trauma 1996;40:624–30.

8. National Nosocomial Infections Surveillance (NNIS) System. National Nosocomial Infections Surveillance (NNIS) report: data summary from October 1986–April 1996. Am J Infect Control 1996;24:300–8.

9. Sands KE, Bates DW, Lanken PN, et al. Epidemiology of sepsis syndrome in 8 academic medical centers. JAMA 1997;278:234–40.

10. Deitch CA. Multiple organ failure: pathophysiology and potential future. therapy. Ann Surg 1992;216:117.

11. Faist E, Schinkel C, Zimmer S. Update on the mechanisms of immune. suppression of injury and immune modulation. World J Surg 1996;20:454–9.

12. Faist E, Wichmann M, Kim C. Immunosuppresion and immunomodulation in surgical patients. Curr Opin Crit Care 1997;3:293–8.

13. Lin E, Calvano SE, Lowry SF. The biologic control of systemic inflammatory response. Curr Opin Crit Care 1997;3:299–307.

14. Swank GM, Deitch EA. Role of the gut in multiple organ failure: bacterial translocation and permeability changes. World J Surg 1996;20:411–7.

15. Richard KS, Hoyt DB. Immunomodulation. Adv Trauma Crit Care 1994;9:135–67.

16. Casey LC, Balk RA, Bone RC. Plasma cytokine and endotoxin levels correlate with survival in patients with the sepsis syndrome. Ann Intern Med 1993;119:771–8.

17. Biffl WL, Moore EE, Moore FA, Peterson VM. Interleukin-6 in the injured patient. Marker of injury or mediator of inflammation? Ann Surg 1996;224:647–64.

18. Regel G, Lobenhoffer P, Grotz M, Pape HC, Lehmann U, Tscherne H. Treatment results of patients with multiple trauma: an analysis of 3406 cases treated between 1972 and 1991 at a German level I trauma center. J Trauma 1995;38:70–8.

19. Fry DE, Pearlstein L, Fulton RL, Polk HC. Multiple system organ. failure: the role of uncontrolled infection. Arch Surg 1980;115:136–40.

20. Thomason MH, Payseur ES, Hakenewerth AM, et al. Nosocomial pneumonia in ventilated trauma patients during stress ulcer prophylaxis with sucralfate, antacid and ranitidine. J Trauma 1996;41:503–8.

21. Goins WA, Reynolds HN, Nyanjom D, Dunham CM. Outcome following prolonged intensive care unit stay in multiple trauma patients. Crit Care Med 1991;19:339–45.

22. Regel G, Grotz M, Weltner T, Sturm JA, Tscherne H. Pattern of organ failure following severe trauma. World J Surg 1996;20:422–9.

23. Antonelli M, Moro ML, d'Errico RR, Conti G, Bufi M, Gasparetto A. Early and late onset bacteremia have different risk factors in trauma patients. Intensive Care Med 1996;22:735–41.

24. Goris RJA, te Boekhorst TPA, Nuytinck JKS, Gimbrere JSF. Multiple organ failure: generalized autodestructive inflammation? Arch Surg 1985;120:1109–15.

25. Carrico CJ, Meakins JL, Marshall JC, et al. Multiple organ failure syndrome. Arch Surg 1986;121:196–208.

26. Baue AE. Multiple progressive, or sequential systems failure. Arch Surg 1975;110:779.

27. Walker L, Eiseman B. The changing pattern of post-traumatic. respiratory distress syndrome. Ann Surg 1976;181:693.

28. Henao FJ, Daes JE, Dennis RJ. Risk factors for multiorgan failure: case control study. J Trauma 1991;31:74.

29. Lauwers LF, Rosseel P, Roelants A, et al. A retrospective study of 130 consecutive multiple trauma patients in an intensive care unit. Intensive Care Med 1986;12:296.

30. Waydhas C, Nast-Kolb D, Jochum M, et al. Inflammatory mediators, infection, sepsis and multiple organ failure after severe trauma. Arch Surg 1992;127:460.

31. Faist E, Baue AE, Dittmer H, et al. Multiple organ failure in polytrauma patients. J Trauma 1983;23:775.

32. Smail N, Messiah A, Edouard A, et al. Role of systemic inflammatory response syndrome and infection in the occurrence of early multiple organ dysfunction syndrome following severe trauma. Intensive Care Med 1995;21:813–6.

33. Moore FA, Sauaia A, Moore EE, Haenel JB, Burch JM, Lezotte DC. Postinjury multiple organ failure: a bimodal phenomenon. J Trauma 1996;40:501–12.

34. Biffl WL, Moore EE. Splanchnic ischaemia/reperfusion and multiple organ. failure. Br J Anaesth 1996;77:59–70.

35. Moore FA, Feliciano DV, Andrassy RJ, et al. Early enteral feeding, compred with parenteral, reduces postoperative septic complications. Ann Surg 1992;216:172.

36. Marshall JC, Christou NV, Meakins JL. The gastrointestinal tract: the undrained abscess of multiple organ failure. Ann Surg 1993;218:111.

37. Moine P, Shenkar R, Kaneko D, Le tulzo Y, Abraham E. Systemic blood less affects NF-κB regulatory mechanisms in the lungs. Am J Physiol 1997;273:L185–L192.

38. Cheadle WG, Polk HC. Prevention of sepsis and septic complications in surgical patients. Curr Opin Crit Care 1997;3:308–13.

39. Wan S, Leclerc JL, Vincent JL. Cytokine response to cardiopulmonary by pass: lessons learned from cardiac transplantation. Ann Thorac Surg 1997;63:269–76.

40. Wan S, Leclerc JL, Vincent JL. Inflammatory response to cardiopulmonary bypass: mechanisms involved and possible therapeutic strategies. Chest 1997;112:676–92.

41. Riddington DW, Venkatesh B, Boibin M, et al. Intestinal permeability, gastric intramucosal pH, and systemic endotoxemia in patients undergoing cardiopulmonary bypass. JAMA 1996;275:107–12.

42. Brinkmann A, Wolf CF, Berger D, et al. Perioperative endotoxemia and bacterial translocation during major abdominal surgery: evidence for the protective effect of endogenous prostacyclin. Crit Care Med 1996;24:1293–301.

43. Carlet J, Tamion F, Cabie A. Intestinal cytokines. In: Rombeau JL, Takala J, ed. Gut dysfunction in critical illness. Springer-Verlag, Berlin; 1996;177–88.

44. Van Leeuwen PAM, Boermeester MA, Houdijk APJ, et al. Clinical significance of translocation. Gut 1994;35(Suppl 1):S28–34.

45. Tancrede CH, Andremont AO. Bacterial translocation and Gram negative bacteremia in patients with hematological malignancies? J Infect Dis 1995;152:99–103.

46. Moore FA, Moore EE, Pogetti R, et al. Gut bacterial translocation via the portal vein: a clinical perpective with major torso trauma. J Trauma 1991;31:629–38.

47. Roumen RMH, Frieling JTM, Van Tits HWHJ, et al. Endotoxemia after major vascular operations. J Vasc Surg 1993;18:853–7.

48. Friedland JS, Porter JC, Daryanani S, et al. Plasma proinflammatory cytokine concentrations, Acute Physiology and Chronic Health Evaluation (APACHE) III scores and survival in patients in an intensive care unit. Crit Care Med 1996;24:1775–81.

49. Keel M, Schregenberger N, Steckholzer U, et al. Endotoxin tolerance after severe injury and its regulatory mechanisms. J Trauma 1996;41:430–7.

50. Bone RC. Sir Isaac Newton, sepsis, SIRS and CARS. Crit Care Med 1996;24(7):1125–8.

51. Decker D, Schonodorf M, Bidlingmaier F, Hirner A, Vonruecker AA. Surgical stress induces a shift in the type-1/type-2 T-helper cell balance, suggesting down-regulation of cell-mediated and up-regulation of antibody-mediated immunity commensurate to the trauma. Surgery 1996;119:316–25.

52. Munoz C, Carlet J, Fitting C, et al. Dysregulation of in vitro cytokine production by monocytes during sepsis. J Clin Invest 1991;88:1744–54.

53. Asadullah K, Woiciechowsky C, Döcke WD, et al. Very low monocytic HLA-DR expression indicates high risk of infection: immunomonitoring for patients after neurosurgery and patients during high dose steroid therapy. Eur J Emerg Med 1995;2:184–90.

54. Van Saene MKF, Danijanovic V, Murray AE, De la Cal M. How to classify infections in intensive care units: the carrier state, a criterium whose time has come? J Hosp Infect 1996;33:1–12.

55. De Bentzmann S, Plotkowski C, Puchelle E. Receptors in the Pseudomonas aeruginosa adherence to injured and repairing airway epithelium. Am J Respir Crit Care Med 1996;154:S155–62.

56. Bonten MJM, Bergmans DCJJ, Ambergen AW, et al. Risk factors for pneumonia, and colonization of respiratory tract and stomach in mechanically ventilated ICU patients. Am J Respir Crit Care Med 1996;154:1339–46.

57. Horan TC, Culver DH, Gaynes RP, et al. Nosocomial infections in surgical patients in the united states January 1986–June 1992. Infect Control Hosp Epidemiol 1993;14:73–80.

58. Jarlier V, Fosse T, Phillipon A and the ICU study group. Antibiotic susceptibility in aerobic gram-negative bacilli isolated in intensive care units in 39 French teaching hospitals (ICU study). Intensive Care Med 1996;22:1057–65.

59. Pittet J, Tarara D, Wenzel RP, et al. Nosocomial bloodstream infection in critical ill patients: excess of stay, extra costs, and attributable mortality. JAMA 1994;271:1598–601.

60. Moro M, Jepsen O, the EURONIS study group. Infection control practices in intensive care units of 14 European countries. Intensive Care Med 1996;22:872–9.

61. The Parisian Mediastinitis Study Group. Risk factors for deep sternal wound infections after stermotomy – a prospective multicenter study. J Thorac Cardiovasc Surg 1996;111:1200–7.

62. Chevret S, Hemmer M, Carlet J, Langer M, the European Cooperative Group on Nosocomial Pneumonia. Incidence and risk factors of pneumonia acquired in intensive care units. Intensive Care Med 1993;19:256–64.

63. George DL. Epidemiology of nosocomial pneumonia in intensive care unit patients. Clin Chest Med 1995;16:29–44.

64. Cunnion KM, Weber DJ, Broadhead WE, Hanson LC, Pieper CF, Rutala WA. Am J Respir Crit Care Med 1996;153:158–62.

65. Rello J, Ausina V, Castella J, Net A, Prats G. Nosocomial respiratory tract infections in multiple trauma patients. Chest 1992;102:525–9.

66. Timsit JF, Chevret S, Valcke J, et al. Does nosocomial pneumonia increase the risk of death in mechanically ventilated patients? Am Rev Respir Crit Care Med 1996;154:116–23.

67. Papazian L, Bregeon F, Thirion X, et al. Effect of ventilator-associated pneumonia on mortality and morbidity. Am J Respir Crit Care Med 1996;154:91–7.

68. Bjerke HS, Leyerle B, Shabot MM. Impact of ICU nosocomial infections on outcome from surgical care. Am Surg 1991:798–802.

69. Center for Disease Control and Prevention. Guideline for prevention of nosocomial pneumonia. Respir Care 1994;39:1191–236.

70. Rodriguez JL, Gibbons KJ, Bitzer LG, Dechert RE, Steinberg SM, Flint LM. Pneumonia: incidence, risk factors and outcome in injured patients. J Trauma 1991;31:531–7.

71. Richardson JD, Woods D, Johanson WG Jr, Trinkle JK. Lung bacterial clearance following pulmonary contusion. Surgery 1979;86:730–5.

72. Border JR, Hassett JM, Seibell R. Blunt multiple trauma (ISS 36), femur fracture and the pulmonary failure – septic state. Ann Surg 1987;206:427–48.

73. Shirany KZ, Pruitt BA, Mason AD Jr. The influence of inhalation injury and pneumonia on burn mortality. Ann Surg 1987;205:82–7.

74. Timsit JF, Misset B, Renaud B, Goldstein FW, Carlet J. Effect of previous antimicrobials on the accuracy of the main procedures used to diagnose nosocomial pneumonia in ventilated patients. Chest 1995;108:1036–40.

75. Hong Hao A, Bishop MJ, Kubilis PS, Newell DW, Pierson DJ. Pneumonia following closed head injury. Chest 1992;146:290–4.

76. Rello J, Ausina V, Castella J, Net A, Prats G. Nosocomial respiratory tract infections in multiple trauma patients. Chest 1992;102:525–9.

77. Fagon JY, Chastre J, Hance AJ, et al. Evaluation of clinical judgement in the identification and treatment of nosocomial pneumonia in ventilated patients. Chest 1993;103:547–53.

78. Griffin JG, Meduri GU. New approaches in the diagnosis of nosocomial pneumonia. Med Clin North Am 1994;78:1091–122.

79. Croce MA, Fabian TC, Shaw B, et al. Analysis of charges associated with diagnosis of nosocomial pneumonia: can routine bronchoscopy be justified? J Trauma 1994;34:721–7.

80. Valles J, Artigas A, Rello J, et al. Continuous aspiration of subglottic secretions in preventing ventilator associated pneumonia. Ann Intern Med 1995;122:179–86.

81. Bonten MJM, Gaillard CA, Van Der Geest S, et al. The role of intragastric acidity and stress ulcer prophylaxis on colonization and infection in mechanically ventilated patients: a stratified, randomized, double blind study of sulcralfate versus antacids. Am J Respir Crit Care Med 1995;152:1825–34.

82. Culver DH, Horan TC, Gaynes RP, et al. Surgical wound infection by wound class, operative procedure and patient risk index. Am J Med 1991;91:152S–7S.

83. Goldman DA, Weinstein RA, Wenzel RP, et al. Strategies to prevent and control the emergence and spead of antimicrobial resistant micro-organisms in hospitals. JAMA 1996;275:234–40.

84. Stoutenbeek CP, Van Saene HKF, Miranda DR, Zandstra DF. The effect of selective decontamination of the digestive tract on colonization and infection rate in multiple trauma patients. Intensive Care Med 1984;10:185–92.

85. Vanderbrouk-Grauls CM, Vanderbrouk-Grauls JP. Effect of selective decontamination of the digestive tract on respiratory tract infections and mortality in intensive care unit. Lancet 1991;338:859–62.

86. SDD Trialists' Collaborative Group. Meta-analysis of randomised controlled trials of selective decontamination of the digestive tract. Br Med J 1993;307:525–32.

87. Heyland DK, Cook DJ, Jaescher R, Griffith L, Lee HN, Guyatt GH. Selective decontamination of the digestive tract. An overview. Chest 1994;105:1221–9.

88. Kollef M. The role of selective digestive tract decontamination on mortality and respiratory tract infections. A meta-analysis. Chest 1994;105:1101–8.

89. Schardey H, Zimmer S, Strauss T, et al. Decontamination and cefotaxime prevent anastomatic leakage, septic complications and death following total gastrectomy. Interscience Conference on Antimicrobial Agents and Chemotherapy 1997; Abstract J 161:318.

90. Schardey HM, Joosten U, Finke U, et al. The prevention of anastomatic leakage after total gastrectomy with local decontamination: a prospective randomized, double-blind, placebo-controlled multicenter trial. Ann Surg 1997;225:172–80.

91. Verwaest C, Verhaegen J, Ferdinande P, et al. Randomized, controlled trial of selective digestive decontamination in 600 mechanically ventilated patients in a multidisciplinary intensive care unit. Crit Care Med 1997;25:63–71.

92. Gamelli RL, He LK, Liu H. Recombinant human granulocyte colony-stimulating factor treatment improves macrophage suppression of granulocyte and macrophage growth after brun and burn wound infection. J Trauma 1995;39:1141–7.

93. O'Reilly M, Silver GM, Greenhalgh DG, et al. Treatment of intra-abdominal infection with granulocyte colony-stimulating factor. J Trauma 1992;33:679–82.

94. Rao R, Prinz RA, Kazantsev GB, et al. Effects of granulocyte colony-stimulating factor in severe pancreatitis. Surgery 1996;119:657–63.

95. Weiss M, Gross-Weege W, Schneider M, et al. Enhancement of neutrophil function by in vivo Filgrastim treatment for prophylaxis of sepsis in surgical intensive care patients. J Crit Care 1995;10:21–6.

96. Wunderink RG, Leeper KV, Schein RMH, et al. Clinical response to Filgrastim (r-metHuG-CSF) in pneumonia with severe sepsis (abstract). Am J Respir Crit Care Med 1996;153S:A123.

97. Gennari R, Alexander JW, Eaves-Pyles T. IFN-gamma decreases translocation and improves survival following transfusion and thermal injury. J Surg Res 1994;56:530–6.

98. Dries DJ, Polk HC Jr. Interferon gamma related sepsis: result of two large multicenter studies. J Intensive Care 1994;20:123–6.

99. Gaar E, Naziri W, Cheadle WG, Pietsch JD, Johnson M, Polk HC Jr. Improved survival in simulated surgical infection with combined cytokine, antibiotic and immunostimulant therapy. Br J Surg 1994;81:1309–11.

100. Cheadle WG, Polk HC Jr. Prevention of sepsis and septic complications in surgical patients. Curr Opin Crit Care 1997;4:308–13.

101. Dellinger EP, Wertz MJ, LEnnard ES, Orescovich MR. Efficacy of short course antibiotic prophylaxis after penetrating intestinal injury: a prospective randomized trial. Arch Surg 1986;121:23–30.

102. Ericson CD, Fischer RP, Rowlands BJ, et al. Prophylactic antibiotics in trauma: the hazards of underdosing. J Trauma 1989;29:1356–61.

103. Dellinger EP, Caplan ES, Weaver LD, et al. Duration of preventive antibiotic administration for open extremity fractures. Arch Surg 1988;123:333–9.

104. Dellinger EP. Antibiotic prophylaxis in trauma: penetrating injury and open fractures. Rev Infect Dis 1991;13(Suppl 10):S847–57.

105. Fabian TC, Croce MA, Payne LW, et al. Duration of antibiotic therapy for penetrating abdominal trauma: a prospective trial. Surgery 1992;112:788–95.

106. Reed RL, Ericsson CD, Wu A, et al. The pharmacokinetics of prophylactic antibiotics in trauma. J Trauma 1992;32:21–7.

107. Livingston DH, Malangoni MA. An experimental study of susceptibility to infection after hemorrhagic shock. Surg Gynecol Obstet 1988;168:138–42.

108. Livingston DH, Malangoni MA. Increased antibiotic dosing decreases. polymicrobial infection following hemorrhagic shock. Surg Gynecol Obstet 1993;176:418–22.

109. Garner JS. CDC guidelines for prevention of surgical wound infections 1985. Infect Control 1986;7:194–200.

110. Kurz A, Sessler DI, Lenhardt R. Perioperative normothermia to reduce the incidence of surgical-wound infection and shorten hospitalization. N Engl J Med 1996;334:1209–15.

111. Kretzschmar M, Klein U, Palutke M, Schirmeister W. Reduction of ischemia–reperfusion syndrome after abdominal aortic aneurysmectomy by N-acetylcysteine but not mannitol. Acta Anaesthesiol Scand 1996;40:657–64.

112. Carr CS, Ling KDE, Boulos P, Singer M. Randomised trial of safety and efficacy of immediate postoperative enteral feeding in patients undergoing gastrointestinal resection. Br Med J 1996;312:869–71.

113. Hasse JM, Blue LS, Liepa GU, et al. Early enteral nutrition support in patients undergoing liver transplantation. J Parenter Enteral Nutr 1995;19:437–43.

114. Souba WW. Enteral nutrition after surgery – not routinely indicated in well nourished patient. Br Med J 1996;312:864.

Hospital Infection Control

Marc J Struelens

EPIDEMIOLOGY

DEFINITIONS OF HOSPITAL INFECTIONS

Hospital infection, also known as nosocomial infection, encompasses all types of infections acquired by patients while being cared for in an acute care institution, and those acquired by health care personnel and visitors. The rationale for categorizing these infections separately lies in our ability to prevent them through adequate organization of patient care in the hospital setting.

To study the epidemiology of hospital infection and to evaluate the efficacy of prevention strategies, hospital epidemiologists must use standardized definitions. An extensive set of criteria that are widely used internationally for the detection and classification of hospital infection has been published by the Centers for Disease Control and Prevention (CDC) (Fig. 10.1).[1,2] These definitions include a combination of clinical criteria and, when available, documentation by laboratory test results, pathologic findings and imaging data. Although these standard case definitions provide a useful basis for recording hospital infections, their application inevitably entails some degree of inter-observer bias and variability, because several criteria (e.g. visual detection of purulence) are based on subjective clinical judgment whereas others (microbiologic findings) rely on laboratory test usage and performance.

KEY POINTS IN CDC SURVEILLANCE DEFINITIONS OF MAJOR NOSOCOMIAL INFECTIONS IN ADULT PATIENTS	
Surgical site infection (SSI)	**Bloodstream infection (BSI)**
Infection affecting the surgical site and occurring within 30 days of the operative procedure, or within 1 year after implant surgery	Laboratory - confirmed BSI Infection was not present or incubating at time of admission and occurred during or after hospital stay, which meets one of the following:
Superficial incisional SSI At least one of the following: • Purulent drainage from the skin of subcutaneous tissue above fascia layer • Organism isolated from aseptically collected fluid or tissue from the superficial incision closed primarily • Surgeon deliberately opens the superficial incision, unless the culture is negative • Diagnosis by the surgeon or attending physician	• Recognized pathogen(s) isolated from blood culture and pathogen is not related to infection at another site or is related to an intravascular device (primary BSI) or related to nosocomial infection at another site (secondary BSI) • Fever, chills or hypotension and isolation of a common skin contaminant from two blood cultures or from a single blood culture in a patient with an intravascular device if physician institutes appropriate antibiotic therapy, or positive antigen test on blood
Deep incisional SSI At least one of the following: • Purulent discharge from the deep incision, i.e. fascia and muscle • Deep incision that spontaneously dehisces or is deliberately opened by the surgeon when the patient has fever and/or localized pain or tenderness, unless culture is negative • Abscess or other evidence of infection of deep incision seen on direct examination, during reoperation or by histopathologic or radiologic examination • Diagnosis by the surgeon or attending physician	**Urinary tract infection (UTI)**
	Symptomatic UTI Infection not present or incubating at the time of hospital admission which meets one of the following: • Fever, urgency, frequency, dysuria or suprapubic tenderness and urine culture with $\geq 10^5$ colonies /ml with no more than two organism species • Two of the preceding symptoms and pyuria, or positive leukocyte esterase or nitrate test, or positive Gram stain, or two urine cultures with repeated isolation of organism with $\geq 10^2$ colonies /ml, or one urine culture with $\leq 10^5$ colonies/ml if physician institutes appropriate antimicrobial therapy, or diagnosis or appropriate therapy by physician
Organ/Space SSI Infection of any organ/space located below the incision and opened or manipulated during the operative procedure, which meets at least one of the following: • Purulent drainage from a drain that is placed through a stab wound into the organ/space • Organism isolated from an aseptically obtained culture of fluid or tissue from organ/space • Abscess or other evidence of infection of the organ/space seen on direct examination, during reoperation or by histopathologic or radiologic examination • Diagnosis by the surgeon or attending physician	**Asymptomatic bacteriuria** One of the following: • Urine culture with $\geq 10^5$ colonies /ml with no more than two organism species in a patient with an indwelling catheter and no symptoms • Two urine cultures with $\geq 10^5$ colonies/ml of the same organism in a patient who had no indwelling catheter in previous 7 days and no symptoms
	Pneumonia
	Infection not present or incubating on admission, which meets one of the following: • Rales or dullness on chest percussion and new onset of purulent sputum, or pathogen isolated from blood, transtracheal specimen, bronchial brushing or biopsy • New lung infiltrate, consolidation, cavitation or pleural effusion on chest radiograph and one of above criteria, or positive direct or serologic diagnostic test for respiratory pathogen, or histopathologic diagnosis of pneumonia

Fig. 10.1 Keypoints in CDC Surveillance definitions of major nosocomial infections in adult patients. Adapted from Garner[1] and Horan[2].

INCIDENCE AND PUBLIC HEALTH IMPACT

Hospital infections are an important public health problem because of their frequency, attributable morbidity and mortality and cost. In the USA and in Europe, approximately 5–10% of hospitalized patients develop an infection during their hospital stay.[3–5] Higher incidence rates are reported in hospitals in developing countries.[6,7] The risk of infection varies by type of patient population and clinical area of care. For example, among critically ill patients the prevalence of hospital infection can reach 50% in intensive care units where patients stay for prolonged periods and undergo invasive therapeutic support, such as mechanical ventilation.[8] The most common types of hospital infection include, in order of decreasing frequency, urinary tract infection, surgical site infection, pneumonia and bacteremia. Record trends indicate that the incidence of hospital infection has increased over the past decades,[9,10] as illustrated by the rise of bacteremia incidence rates reported in hospitals of all sizes in the USA (Fig. 10.2).

Although the majority of hospital infections are minor, there is a wide range in the severity of clinical illnesses they cause; some have serious consequences, as in patients with infections of implanted prostheses who develop permanent disability or who need reoperation. The hospital length of stay is prolonged in infected patients, on average by 5–10 days.[11] The risk of death approximately doubles in patients who acquire hospital infection.[12] The mortality rates attributable to bloodstream infection and pneumonia are 25–50 and 7–27%, respectively, depending on the etiologic agent and underlying disease.[10–13] Estimates of direct and indirect costs associated with hospital infection vary widely according to differences in epidemiologic and econometric cost measures, patient population and health financing system. However, all studies consistently show that hospital-acquired infections are very expensive and contribute significantly to the escalating costs of health care.[11] It has been argued that, even if moderately effective, a hospital infection control program is one of the most cost-effective and cost-beneficial preventative medical interventions currently available.[14]

MODES OF ACQUISITION OF HOSPITAL INFECTIONS

A majority of hospital infections (approximately 80%) are acquired by the endogenous route through translocation of micro-organisms from the patient's mucocutaneous flora (Fig. 10.3). This auto-infection occurs as a result of predisposing host conditions (Fig. 10.4) and of exposure to invasive diagnostic and therapeutic procedures that lead to disruption of mucocutaneous barriers (Figs 10.5 & 10.6).[8] These factors interfere with the normal balance between host defenses and the invasive properties of the commensal microflora. Examples of endogenous translocation leading to common hospital infections include *Escherichia coli* urinary tract infection in a patient with indwelling bladder catheter and *Staphylococcus epidermidis* bacteremia in a patient who has a percutaneously inserted intravenous catheter. The micro-organisms will migrate from their mucosal or skin habitat along the external surface of the catheter and across the meatal or skin barrier to gain access to the site of infection. In addition, the commensal microflora changes during hospitalization because of mucosal modifications (pH, expression of

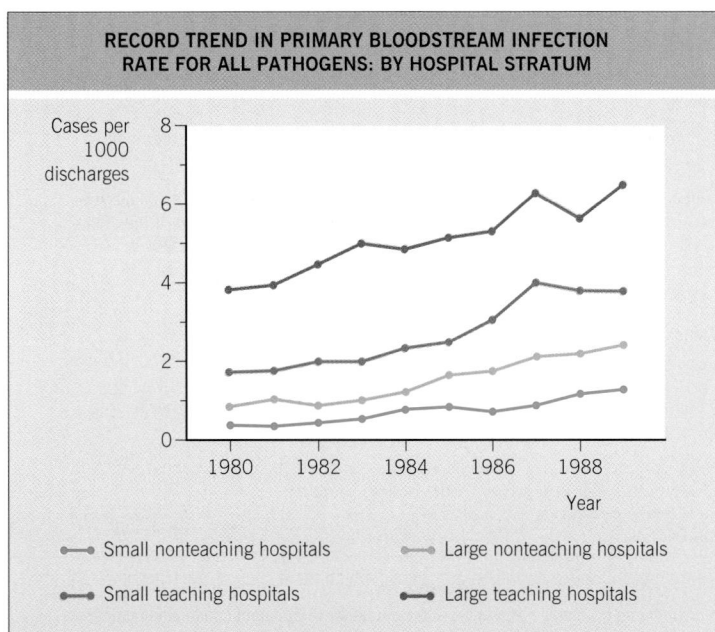

Fig. 10.2 Record trend in primary bloodstream infection rate for all pathogens. Record trend, 1980–1989, in primary bloodstream infection in US hospitals, National Nosocomial Infection Surveillance (NNIS) system, by hospital size. Data from Banerjee *et al.*[9]

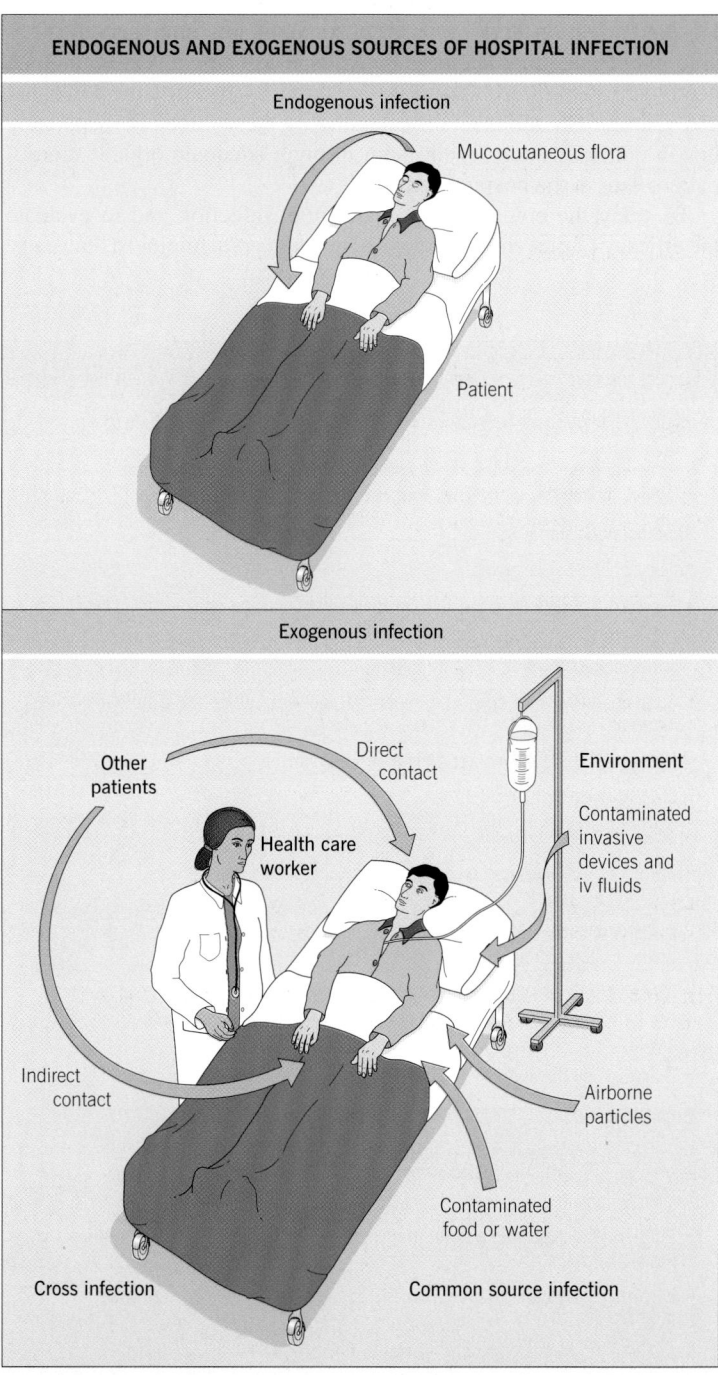

Fig. 10.3 Hospital infection can originate from an endogenous source or from an exogenous route. Endogenous infection by translocation of resident microflora secondary to a breach in host defense (top). Exogenous infection as a result of transmission from patient to patient or from health care worker to patient. It can also occur after exposure of a susceptible patient to a contaminated environmental source, such as inadequately disinfected medical devices (bottom).

surface receptors, etc.) and the selective pressure of antibiotics, favoring the multiplication of resistant organisms.

The second mechanism of acquisition of hospital infection is by the exogenous route, from a microbial reservoir in the hospital. This includes other patients, hospital staff or the inanimate environment.

The most common route is cross-infection or cross-colonization, for which the reservoir is the microbial flora of other patients. This flora is frequently transmitted by the hands of health care workers (Fig. 10.3). Cross-infection may account for approximately 10–20% of hospital infections. Contact spread is a mode of nosocomial transmission of environmentally sturdy and antibiotic-resistant bacteria that can be difficult to control.[15–17] Examples of pathogens spread by this route are given in Figure 10.7. In fact, most micro-organisms that cause endogenous hospital infection have been shown to contaminate transiently the hands of hospital staff and to be disseminated in this way.[15–17] Vehicles of cross-infection also include contaminated medical devices (such as inadaquately disinfected endoscopes, thermometers, electrodes or respirators), infected blood products or organ transplants (Fig. 10.7).

Person-to-person spread of pathogens can also follow the fecal–oral route, secretion droplet route and airborne route (Fig. 10.7). Pathogens transmitted from person to person in the hospital include community-acquired infectious agents, such as viruses [e.g. varicella-zoster virus, respiratory syncytial virus (RSV), influenza virus, herpes simplex virus, hepatitis A virus, rotavirus, adenovirus], bacteria (e.g. *Staphylococcus aureus, Neisseria meningitidis, Haemophilus influenzae, Mycobacterium tuberculosis*) and parasites (e.g. *Cryptosporidium* spp.). The risk of transmission of these pathogens in the hospital can vary depending upon the age and immune status of hospitalized patients, the staff-to-patient ratio, the number of patients sharing a room, the availability of handwashing facilities and geographic location of the health care facility. Seasonal and environmental changes may affect the prevalence of locally endemic infections in the community. Because many of these pathogens are virulent for normal, nonimmune hosts, these hospital outbreaks can involve infection of hospital personnel and visitors as well as patients.

Occasionally, healthy carriers or infected individuals among hospital personnel may be disseminators of pathogens and cause outbreaks of nosocomial infections (Fig. 10.7). Well documented examples include

HOST FACTORS PREDISPOSING TO HOSPITAL INFECTION

Factor	Example
Age	Neonates; elderly patients
Underlying disease	System or organ failure (e.g. liver cirrhosis, diabetes mellitus, chronic obstructive pulmonary disease, renal failure), cancer, neutropenia
Immunodeficiency	Congenital or acquired (e.g. AIDS, immunosuppressive therapy, malnutrition)
Specific immunity	Susceptibility to viral infections
Breach of mucocutaneous barriers	Trauma, burns, surgery, endoscopy, indwelling devices Mucosal and skin diseases
Anesthesia, sedation	Suppression of cough and peristalsis, hypoventilation
Antibiotics, antacids	Alterations of resident microflora and decrease of resistance to colonization by hospital flora Selection of antibiotic-resistant mutants and naturally resistant bacteria and yeasts
Colonizing flora	Carriage of opportunistic bacteria and fungi
Latent infection	Latent infection with intracellular pathogens reactivated by immunosuppression

Fig. 10.4 A variety of factors can alter host defenses and predispose hospitalized patients to infection.

INFECTIONS ASSOCIATED WITH INVASIVE DEVICES AND PROCEDURES

Device/procedure	Type of infection
Intravascular catheter	Bacteremia; catheter site infection
Bladder catheter	Urinary tract infection
Mechanical ventilation	Pneumonia; sinusitis
Stents	Pyelonephritis; cholangitis; meningitis
Surgery	Surgical site infection; pneumonia
Endoscopy	Bacteremia; pneumonia; gastroenteritis and cholangitis
Blood transfusion	Bacteremia and fungemia; viral infections

Fig. 10.5 Examples of important hospital infections that are directly related to the use of invasive diagnostic and therapeutic devices and procedures.

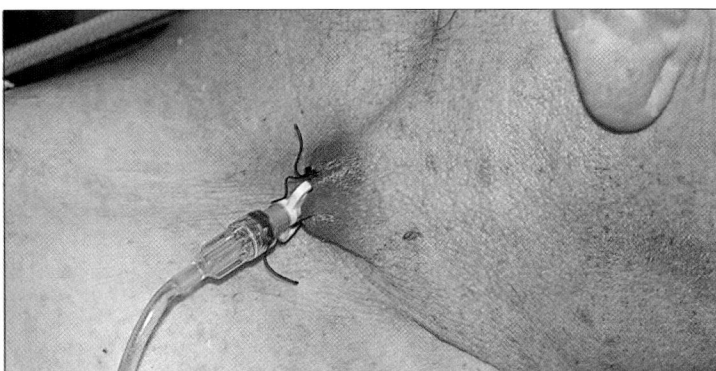

Fig. 10.6 Catheter exit site infection in a patient with central venous catheterization through the jugular vein. Courtesy of Dr JP Thys.

MODES OF TRANSMISSION OF NOSOCOMIAL PATHOGENS

Mode of transmission	Reservoir/source	Examples of pathogens
Contact	Patients/health care workers, fomites, medical devices	*Staphylococcus aureus* *Enterococcus* spp. Enterobacteriaceae *Clostridium difficile* Respiratory syncytial virus Rotavirus Adenovirus *Candida* spp.
Droplet spread	Health care workers, patients	*Staphylococcus aureus* Respiratory syncytial virus Influenza virus
Device-related	Water/respiratory equipment, endoscopes	*Pseudomonas aeruginosa* *Acinetobacter* spp. *Stenotrophomonas maltophilia*
Medication-related	Water/iv fluids, disinfectants	*Burkholderia cepacia* *Acinetobacter* spp. *Serratia marcescens*
Transfusion, needlestick	Patients/blood	Hepatitis B virus, hepatitis C virus, HIV, etc.
Transplantation	Patients/donor tissue	Cytomegalovirus *Toxoplasma gondii* Creutzfeld–Jacob agent
Airborne	Patients Hot water/showers Soil/dust	*Mycobacterium tuberculosis* *Legionella* spp. *Aspergillus* spp.
Foodborne	Animals/food products Water/enteral feeding	*Salmonella* spp. *Enterobacter* spp. *Pseudomonas aeruginosa*

Fig. 10.7 Modes of transmission and examples of sources of infection for selected nosocomial pathogens.

members of operating room personnel who are mucosal or skin carriers of *Streptococcus pyogenes*, *S. aureus* or *S. epidermidis* and become the source of epidemics of surgical site infection.[17–19] Certain

conditions, such as upper respiratory tract infection or dermatitis, appear to predispose individuals to become efficient airborne disseminators of these organisms.[20] Nosocomial outbreaks of adenovirus keratoconjunctivitis, of RSV and of influenza pneumonia have also been linked to infected health care workers.

Environmental acquisition is an uncommon route of hospital-acquired infection, accounting for less than 5% of cases. Common-source outbreaks can result from exposure of susceptible patients to air, water, food, medication, disinfectant or medical devices contaminated with micro-organisms originating from environmental reservoirs inside or outside the hospital (Figs 10.3 & 10.7). Airborne pathogens include *Legionella* spp.,[21] *Aspergillus* spp. and other filamentous fungi,[22] and *Nocardia* spp. These organisms represent a particular hazard to immunocompromised patients, especially those with cancer and transplant recipients. Waterborne outbreaks of infections in hospitals have been linked to patient bathing in hydrotherapy pools or enteral feeding with water contaminated with *Pseudomonas aeruginosa*, *Acinetobacter* spp. or *Legionella* spp. Foodborne outbreaks are most frequently caused by *Salmonella* spp. Enteric feeds contaminated with *Enterobacter* spp. can be a source of sepsis. Contamination of intravenous fluids, medications, antiseptics, blood products or medical devices with a variety of aquatic micro-organisms, such as *Serratia* spp., *Enterobacter* spp., *Acinetobacter* spp., *Pseudomonas* spp. and *Mycobacterium chelonae*, have caused hospital outbreaks of bacteremia, wound infection and pneumonia.[23,24] Extrinsic contamination occurs during hospital handling of medications and can lead to a local outbreak,[25] or, less commonly, intrinsic contamination takes place during manufacturing of the product, often triggering multi-hospital epidemics.[26] Outbreak investigations undertaken in US hospitals by the CDC over the past decade illustrate the wide spectrum of agents encountered (Fig. 10.8) and show a gradual increase in the proportion of outbreaks related to contaminated devices and products, or to invasive procedures.[23]

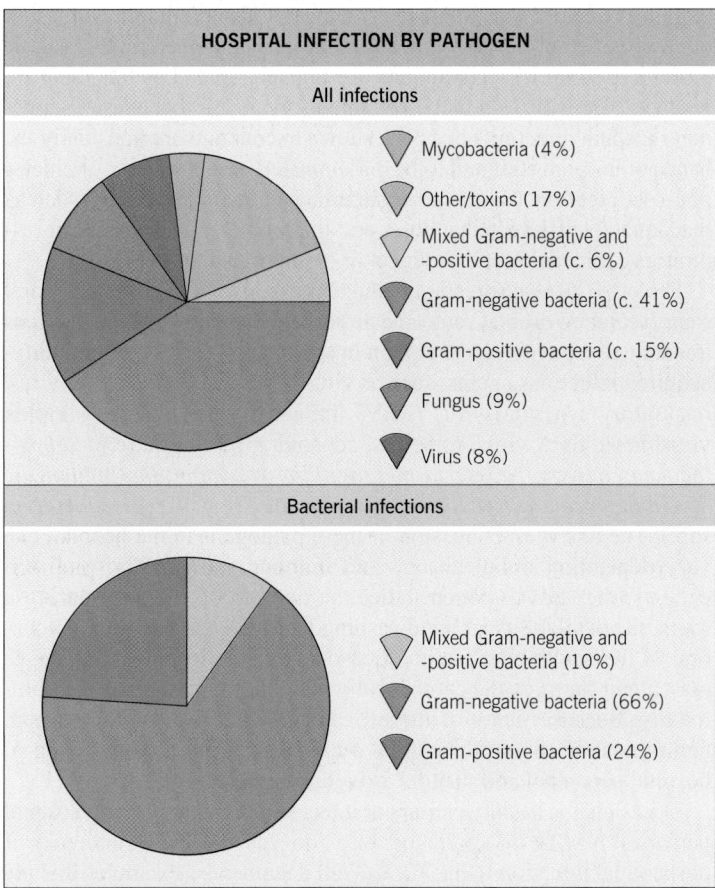

Fig. 10.8 Distribution of outbreaks of hospital infection investigated by the CDC, 1980–1990, by category of pathogen. Bacteria caused 62% of outbreaks, of which 66% were Gram-negative, 24% Gram-positive and 10% mixed bacterial pathogens. Data from Jarvis.[23]

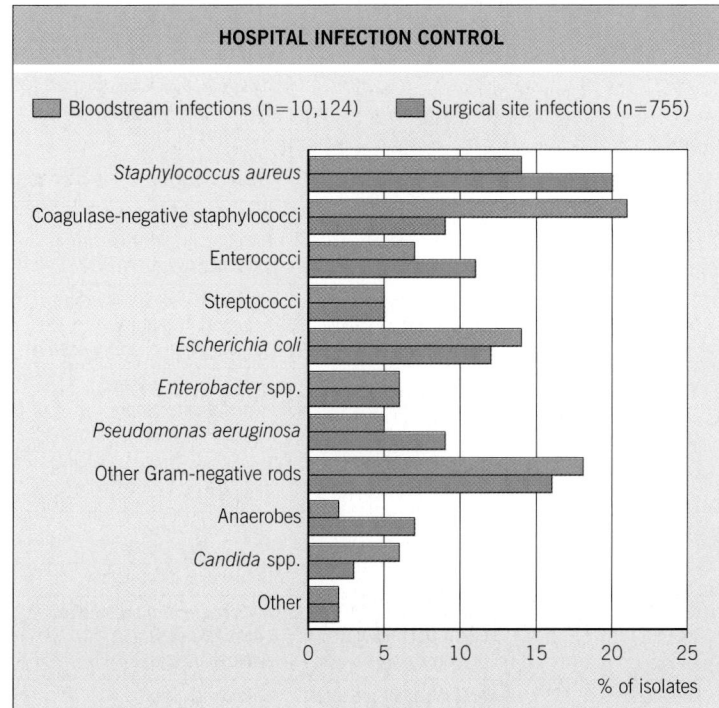

Fig. 10.9 Etiologic agents isolated from nosocomial bloodstream and surgical site infections in Belgian hospitals. National Program for the Surveillance of Infection in Hospitals, 1992–1995. Adapted from Mertens *et al.* (personal communication).

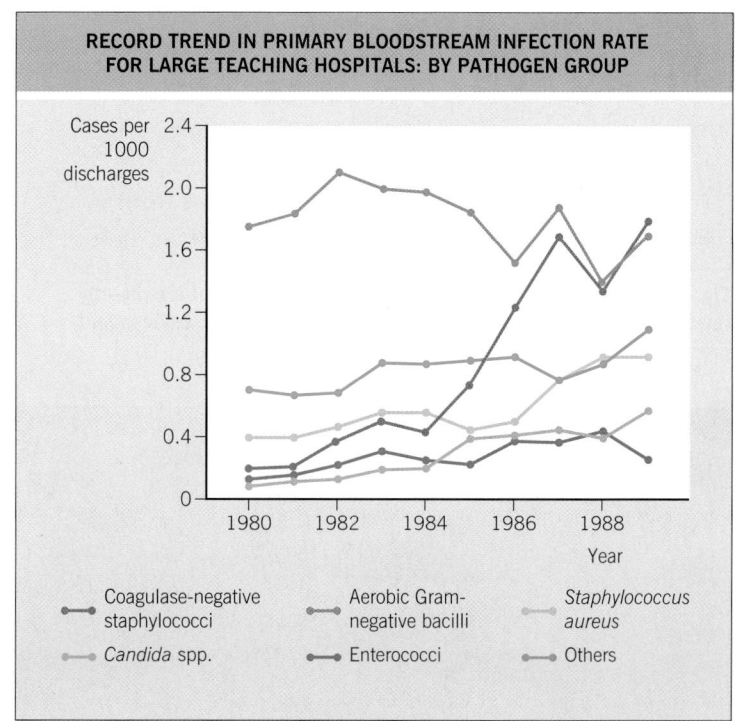

Fig. 10.10 Record trend in primary bloodstream infection rate for large teaching hospitals, by pathogen group, 1980–1989. NNIS system. Data from Banerjee *et al.*[9]

Pathogen	Resistance pattern	Selection of mutation	Gene spread	Clonal spread	Reservoir		Transmission	
					Human	Environment	Direct	Indirect
Staphylococcus aureus (MRSA)	Beta-lactam, multiple	+	+	+++	+++	+	+++	+
Enterococci	Glycopeptides, multiple	+	++	++	+++	+	+++	++
Klebsiella spp.	Extended spectrum beta-lactamase	+	++	+++	+++	−	+++	−
Enterobacter cloacae	Derepressed chromosomal beta-lactamase	+++	−	+	+++	−	+	−
Enterobacter aerogenes	Multiple	++	+	++	++	+	++	+
Acinetobacter baumannii	Multiple	++	+	+++	++	++	++	++
Pseudomonas aeruginosa	Multiple	+++	+	+	++	+	+	++

MECHANISMS OF INCREASED ANTIMICROBIAL RESISTANCE OF NOSOCOMIAL PATHOGENS

Fig. 10.11 Relative importance of mechanisms that contribute to the increasing frequency of antimicrobial resistance of selected nosocomial pathogens.

ETIOLOGIC AGENTS

A selection of important nosocomial pathogens and their major reservoirs and sources is presented in Figure 10.7. The majority of infections are caused by commensal bacteria, with *E. coli* and *S. aureus* being the most common.[7–10] Micro-organisms isolated from patients who have nosocomial bacteremia and surgical infection in Belgian hospitals are illustrated in Figure 10.9. The pattern of agents causing hospital infection can vary greatly according to the site of infection, the age and underlying conditions of the patients and their exposure to medical procedures, invasive devices and antimicrobials.

The spectrum of hospital pathogens has changed over the past decades, reflecting the evolution of medicine. In the pre-antibiotic era, most infections were caused by *S. pyogenes* and *S. aureus*. Gram-negative bacteria emerged as leading pathogens in the 1960s and 1970s in response to the increased use of anti-staphylococcal antibiotics. In the 1980s and 1990s, the massive use of broad-spectrum antimicrobials, the improved survival of critically ill patients, the growing population of compromised patients and the increased use of indwelling medical devices all contributed to the current emergence of multiple antimicrobial-resistant nosocomial pathogens. Well known examples are methicillin-resistant *S. aureus* (MRSA),[17] and *S. epidermidis*,[9] multiply resistant *Enterococcus faecium*[27] and *Enterobacter* spp.,[9] *Candida* spp.[9] and *Clostridium difficile*.[15] These changes are illustrated by the modification of organism-specific incidence rates of bloodstream infection in US hospitals (Fig. 10.10).[9] Another dramatic example of resurgence of a major pathogen is the multiply resistant *M. tuberculosis* outbreaks in hospitals caring for HIV-infected patients and in which adequate diagnostic and patient isolation facilities were not available.[28]

The increasing prevalence of antibiotic-resistant bacteria as agents of hospital infection has reached alarming proportions. Strains of organisms, such as *E. faecium* or *Acinetobacter baumannii*, that are resistant to all available antimicrobials with established clinical efficacy, leave no therapeutic option. To provide a sound basis for the control of this problem, research efforts have focused on improving the definition of the respective roles of selection by antibiotic treatment of naturally resistant micro-organisms from the endogenous flora, selection of resistant mutants and of mobile genetic determinants, such as transposons and plasmids, and dissemination of resistant clones between hospitalized patients.[29] A number of recent studies, performed in intensive care units in which antibiotic-resistant bacteria were frequent and clinically significant, showed that these various determinants generally interact in a multifactorial fashion.[30–36] Although variations are observed between different hospitals, general trends in the relative contributions of these mechanisms can be recognized as typical of each

resistant pathogen (Fig. 10.11). Clonal dissemination from patient to patient is a predominant mechanism of increased prevalence for the majority of resistant nosocomial pathogens. Among the common risk factors that predispose patients to develop colonization (which generally precedes infection) or infection with these resistant bacteria are the severity of underlying disease, the duration of stay in intensive care and in the hospital, and the intensity of exposure (number and duration) to broad-spectrum antimicrobial drugs and invasive devices such as intravascular and urinary catheters.[17,30–36]

CONTROL STRATEGIES

Before we examine the different components of an effective infection control program, it is worth considering exactly what the targets and objectives of the prevention strategies are, based on our understanding of the pathogenesis and epidemiology of hospital infection (Fig. 10.12). This classification is of course somewhat simplistic, as a single strategy may meet several objectives. For example, perioperative antibiotic prophylaxis reduces not only the bacterial inoculum released from the patient's own flora but also the bacteria released into the operative site from the surgical team's flora. However, this approach underlines the fact that further research into the mechanisms of acquisition of hospital infection is needed to design optimal prevention methods.

FUNCTIONS AND ORGANIZATION OF THE HOSPITAL INFECTION CONTROL PROGRAM

Major differences among countries in their health care resources and organization, and different medical cultures explain the diversity of approaches to the organization of hospital hygiene and infection control in hospitals around the world. The best known approach is the paradigm of hospital epidemiology developed over the past decades in the USA.[37,38] In the hospitals of industrialized countries today, the co-ordination of infection control typically operates on two levels: an executive body – the infection control team – and an advisory body to the hospital management – the infection control committee – which adopts the 'legislative' role of policy making. The functions of these bodies are to design, revise and foster good hygienic practices through continuing education of and interaction with health care personnel, to perform epidemiologic surveillance and outbreak management and to monitor and advise on the utilization of antimicrobial agents, sterilization, disinfection, waste management and housekeeping in the institution.

The infection control team should be organized to meet the needs of the hospital, which will vary greatly according to its size and the type of medical care it provides. In general, the team should include at least one or more physician and nurse specially trained in infectious diseases, microbiology, epidemiology and infection control. The hospital infection control physician is usually an infectious diseases specialist or less often a microbiologist. The landmark Study on the Efficacy of Nosocomial Infection Control, conducted in the 1970s in US hospitals, showed that the incidence of infection could be reduced by 32% in

A RATIONAL CLASSIFICATION OF HOSPITAL INFECTION PREVENTION STRATEGIES		
Target	**Objective**	**Example of strategy**
Endogenous infection	To prevent or neutralize the translocation of commensal flora	• Antibiotic prophylaxis in surgery • Skin antisepsis before surgery • Antiseptic-bound iv catheter • Intestinal decontamination of neutropenic patients • Pneumococcal immunization before splenectomy
Exogenous infection	To prevent cross-infection	• Hand hygiene for patient care procedures • Isolation and decolonization of carriers of transmissible pathogens • Sterilization or disinfection of invasive devices • Cleaning and disinfection of fomites • Outbreak detection and molecular epidemiologic studies to determine the mode and vehicles of spread
	To prevent common-source infection	• Ultra-clean air for prosthesis surgery or bone marrow transplant recipients • Disinfection of *Legionella* spp. in water systems • Environmental, water and food hygiene • Sterile parenteral drugs and implantable material • Outbreak detection and molecular epidemiologic studies to identify the source
Antimicrobial resistance	To prevent the emergence, and spread of resistance genes	• Restricted usage of broad-spectrum antimicrobial agents • Optimized anti-infectious therapy (agents, dosage and duration)
	To prevent the spread of resistant strains of micro-organisms	• Detection, monitoring and timely reporting of antimicrobial resistance • Isolation precautions and treatment of carriers of transmissible resistant strains • Molecular epidemiologic studies to distinguish between mutant selection, gene or clone dissemination

Fig. 10.12 A classification of strategies to prevent hospital infection and control antimicrobial resistance.

AIMS OF HOSPITAL INFECTION SURVEILLANCE
• To identify high-risk patients and procedures and assign infection control priorities • To monitor trends over time of incidence and patterns of infection • To detect outbreaks of hospital infection • To evaluate the efficacy of prevention and control interventions • To evaluate quality assurance programs • To educate and motivate heath care providers and decision makers

Fig. 10.13 A number of aims can be assigned to hospital epidemiologic surveillance systems.

hospitals with an adequately staffed infection control team (defined as one physician per 1000 beds and one nurse per 250 beds) and performing active surveillance activities compared with hospitals without such programs.[3] The infection control committee is typically composed of the physician hospital epidemiologist, hospital manager, hospital infection control practioners (often nurses), medical and nursing directors, leading medical and nursing representatives of clinical departments and representatives of other departments such as the microbiology laboratory, pharmacy, sterilization services, employee health clinic and safety committee.[37] This advisory body develops and regularly updates infection control policies and reviews the progress achieved toward the institution's objectives in this field. Policies are designed based on the published data documenting prevention strategies, guidelines and standards provided by national advisory committees and consensus conferences, and the local epidemiologic data and patient care resources. Extensive and detailed guidelines have been published by the CDC and the Hospital Infection Control Practice Advisory Committee (HICPAC). The latest version of these recommendations is available on the internet.[39] Each recommendation is categorized according to supporting scientific evidence, theoretical rationale and applicability. A method used for adaptation of some of these guidelines to settings with limited resources has been described.[40]

SURVEILLANCE

Epidemiologic surveillance is a systematic, ongoing process of data collection, analysis, interpretation and reporting, performed to monitor the temporal trends in disease frequency and associated risk factors in a population. The basic principle of its application to hospital infection surveillance is to measure the reduction of risk of infection as an outcome indicator of the effectiveness of the prevention efforts. Some of the objectives that can be assigned to surveillance activities are described in Figure 10.13. As a tool to evaluate the quality of care, outcome surveillance (i.e. monitoring the risk of hospital infection) can be coupled with the auditing of processes regulated by the infection control program, like compliance with standards of antimicrobial usage and hygienic care practice.

A key element to the usefulness of any surveillance system is to achieve a consensus with the patient care providers on what will be its objectives, indicators, and methods of case-finding and validation. Likewise, the involvement of clinical staff in data collection and interpretation of results is necessary for ensuring the credibility of the surveillance data as a guide to optimal care practices.

Because surveillance is a costly and time-consuming activity, each hospital must carefully tailor its system to its priorities and resources. Except in some US hospitals, staffing levels of infection control teams do not allow for comprehensive, hospital-wide surveillance of incidence rates of all infection types. Therefore, selective surveillance must be targeted to high-risk populations or procedures, particularly if specific control interventions are implemented. Haley provided a scheme to select surveillance objectives by site of infection based on the avoidable costs and morbidity associated with each infection type.[41]

Depending on the scope and objectives of the surveillance activities, different indicators and data collection methods can be used (Fig. 10.14). Outbreak warning can be largely accomplished by time-and-place cluster analysis of numerator laboratory data. This analysis will focus on patients colonized or infected by micro-organisms known to be transmissible by cross-infection or common-source acquisition, such as *C. difficile*, MRSA or *Legionella* spp. (alert organisms).

For the monitoring of overall risk of infection, repeated prevalence surveys are more cost-effective than continuous incidence surveillance and can be used successfully to evaluate the efficacy of control measures.[42,43] Data sources and collection methods used for the detection of patients who have hospital-acquired infection vary in their efficiency (i.e. the balance between accuracy and workload). A comparative evaluation of selective surveillance methods in a UK hospital reported a sensitivity of 76% for a time of 6.4 hours per 100 beds per week by using a laboratory-based and ward-liaison method.[44] This method consists of daily review of case records of patients who have a positive microbiology report and of patients reported by nursing staff to have an infection. The reference method,[44] based on exhaustive record review and staff interview, required 18.1 hours per 100 beds per week. In that study, laboratory-based detection had a sensitivity of 51% for a time requirement of only 3.1 hours per 100 beds per week. In US or Belgian hospitals this method achieved a sensitivity of 80–84%,[45,46] whereas it had only a 20% sensitivity in a Brazilian hospital. These discrepancies illustrate the fact that the efficiency of a surveillance method will depend on local factors, like the rate of utilization of microbiology tests. Other case detection methods based on review of temperature and drug prescription charts, or on patient risk factors also appear to be efficient.[44,47] Ideally, the sensitivity, specificity and inter-observer repeatability should be evaluated by comparison with an exhaustive case-finding reference method to validate the method used.[43,44]

The efficiency of hospital infection surveillance and quality assesment of antimicrobial prescription can be greatly enhanced by the development of computerized patient records and integrated hospital information systems that link clinical information, laboratory, radiology and pharmacy records into a single database.[48–50] Standardization of criteria for codification of risk factors, interventions and definitions of hospital infection is a first step toward inter-hospital comparison of rates.[50,51] National surveillance systems can provide baseline data for hospitals willing to compare the rate of infection in their institution with risk-adjusted rates in similar institutions.[51] However, methodologic issues remain unsettled on how best to adjust for confounding factors and to define similar institutions. National surveillance networks can also be set up to monitor the rate of nosocomial transmission of major pathogens, such as surveillance of incidence of MRSA acquisition in hospitals in which coordinated control policies have been implemented.[51]

When surveillance is used to assess the effectiveness of infection control interventions, a quantitative assessment of compliance with the recommended methods is a valuable component of the policy evaluation (Fig. 10.13). Direct methods of practice auditing (e.g. observation of patient care procedure such as glove use, hand disinfection or reprocessing of flexible endoscopes) are preferred for data collection but require significant staffing resources. Indirect methods, for example measuring the rate of material usage (e.g. gloves, disinfectant, isolation facilities), are more efficient but provide only partial and crude indicators of patient care practices.

OUTBREAK MANAGEMENT
An epidemic or outbreak can be defined as a significant temporal increase in the prevalence of infection above the expected baseline prevalence in a given population. The early detection and prompt management of outbreaks of hospital infection are important because of the frequent occurrence, clinical impact and preventable nature of epidemic infections.[52] The prevalence of outbreaks has been reported at approximately 1 per 10,000 admissions and the etiologic fraction can be estimated to account for 5–10% of all hospital-acquired infections.[52,53] In addition, even small clusters of infection that do not cross the threshold of statistical significance can be worth investigating, because identification of the mode of transmission can lead to effective prevention. The true magnitude of small-scale clustering caused by cross-infection remains to be defined. In a study employing molecular subtyping,[54] 13% of episodes of nosocomial infections detected in patients admitted to intensive care units were found to be possibly cross-transmitted.

The steps involved in the investigation and control of outbreaks have been well defined (Fig. 10.15).[52]

ROLE OF THE CLINICAL MICROBIOLOGY LABORATORY
The microbiology laboratory plays a key role in the detection, investigation and control of outbreaks of nosocomial infections (Fig. 10.16). This role includes accurate detection, species identification and susceptibility testing of micro-organisms causing hospital infection; archival and ongoing epidemiologic analysis of clinical test results; performing targeted microbiologic surveys of the hospital environment; and storage and epidemiologic typing of microbial isolates to support outbreak investigations.[53,55]

Rapid laboratory detection and reporting of 'alert' organisms that are known for their potential to cause outbreaks, for example *C. difficile*, MRSA or multidrug-resistant *M. tuberculosis* (Fig. 10.14), leads to the timely implementation of specific infection control precautions to reduce the risk of secondary spread.[53] The microbiology laboratory often provides the early warning that an outbreak is occurring. In the past decade, 63% of outbreaks were detected in our institution by prospective or retrospective reviews of laboratory data. Certain types of epidemics are difficult to identify, like those caused by organisms that are also common causes of endemic infections, or those caused by multiple strains. This type of epidemic can follow a break in disinfection technique, as

Scope	Objective, indicators and method of data collection	
SURVEILLANCE METHODS FOR THE EVALUATION OF INFECTION CONTROL PROGRAM OUTCOMES AND PROCESSES		
Outbreak warning	Objective	Detection and cluster analysis of transmissible organisms
	Indicators	Numerator: colonization or infection by specific micro-organism
	Case-finding	Laboratory-based
Prevalence of hospital infection	Objective	Periodic assessment of prevalence of infection: hospital-wide or selective
	Indicators	Numerator: infection by site, ward, procedure or device. Denominator: patient census on day of survey, procedures or devices
	Case-finding	Laboratory and/or ward liaison, chart review, computerized patient record
Incidence of hospital infection	Objective	Continuous monitoring of incidence of infection: hospital-wide or selective
	Indicators	Numerator: infection by site, ward, procedure or device. Denominator: patient admissions, hospital-days, procedures, device-days
	Case-finding	Laboratory and/or ward liaison, chart review, computerized patient record
Antibiotic usage	Objective	Continuous monitoring and quality assessment of antibiotic utilization patterns
	Indicators	Numerator: type of antimicrobial cures, doses and duration used for prophylaxis and treatment. Denominator: surgical interventions, documented infections (e.g. bacteremia), patient admissions
	Case-finding	Pharmacy records, operating room record, medical and nursing records, chart review, computerized patient record
Hygiene practices	Objective	Monitoring of compliance with, and quality assessment of, hygiene practices
	Indicators	Numerator: patient care procedures performed with appropriate hygiene precautions. Denominator: procedures requiring standard hygiene precaution, patient census, density of care index
	Case-finding	Ward observations, pharmacy and central supply records (gloves, disinfectants, etc.)

Fig. 10.14 **Surveillance methods can vary in scope and objectives.** The choice of indicators and case-finding methods will depend on the surveillance strategy selected.

observed in an outbreak of post-endoscopy biliary sepsis in which only molecular typing could distinguish multiple-strain cross-infection from endogenous infections.[24]

EPIDEMIOLOGIC TYPING

Epidemiologic typing is used for discrimination between unrelated isolates of the same microbial species and related isolates, derived by

STEPS IN THE INVESTIGATION AND CONTROL OF OUTBREAKS

1. Establish a case definition and define the population at risk

2. Confirm existence of a true outbreak
   - rule out pseudo-outbreaks (contamination of cultures during clinical sample collection or processing)
   - rule out surveillance artifacts (increase in laboratory utilization, or improved laboratory or surveillance methods)
   - determine space–time clustering and/or significant increase of incidence rate versus baseline period in exposed cohort

3. Determine clinical severity of infections and number of patients affected to define the degree of emergency; allocate time and resources for further investigation accordingly

4. Complete case-finding retrospectively and prospectively; ensure accurate microbiologic sampling and processing for optimal ascertainment of etiology; ensure storage and plan the typing of clinical isolates

5. Review the literature about risk factors and potential sources and compare with host and exposure factors revealed by reviewing the medical charts of infected patients

6. On the basis of descriptive epidemiology of epidemic cases in time, place, patient characteristics, and common exposure to devices, treatments and procedures, formulate tentative hypotheses about host factors, hospital exposure factors, reservoirs, source and mode(s) of transmission

7. Reinforce standard hygiene precautions and initiate temporary control measures based on hypotheses defined in step 6; follow-up impact on rate of transmission

8. If necessary, test hypotheses defined in step 6 by case–control, cohort and/or intervention studies and by epidemiologic typing of representative isolates

9. If necessary, initiate targeted culture surveys from potential reservoirs/sources (patients, personnel, environment, as appropriate); confirm the suspect epidemiologic link by comparative typing of isolates

10. Review results of the investigation with all concerned authorities and staff; report to the Infection Control Committee

11. Conduct follow-up surveillance to evaluate efficacy of control measures; update control measures if necessary; follow-up evaluation reports for the Infection Control Committee and all staff concerned

Fig. 10.15 Steps in the investigation and control of outbreaks. Adapted from Doebbeling.[52]

ROLE OF THE CLINICAL LABORATORY IN THE INVESTIGATION OF HOSPITAL INFECTION OUTBREAKS

Investigation step	Laboratory method	Aim
Outbreak detection	Identification and susceptibility testing of clinical isolates	Case finding, cluster detection
Outbreak confirmation and descriptive epidemiology	Epidemiologic typing of clinical isolates	Delineation of clonal spread
Identification of reservoirs and mode of transmission	Culture surveys of reservoirs and vehicles Typing of environmental isolates	Documentation of reservoir of epidemic clone(s) Test of transmission hypotheses
Follow-up of efficacy of control measures	Typing of clinical isolates, as part of post-outbreak surveillance	Test of interruption of transmission hypothesis

Fig. 10.16 The clinical microbiology laboratory has multiple roles in investigations of outbreaks of hospital infection. Adapted from Struelens.[53]

clonal descent from the same ancestor cell, as part of a common chain of transmission.[53–57] This can be achieved by scoring appropriate phenotypic or genotypic markers that exhibit sufficient intraspecies diversity. Typing systems can be used for different purposes, including to delineate the extent and patterns of dissemination of epidemic clone(s), to test hypotheses about the reservoirs, sources and vehicles of transmission, and to verify the interruption of transmission by application of control measures.[55–58]

A rapidly expanding number of laboratory techniques are available for the epidemiologic analysis of nosocomial pathogens. Figure 10.17 gives an overview of the underlying principles and performance of selected typing methods. For the evaluation of performance, several criteria are used,[56–58] including typeability, reproducibility, stability, discriminatory power and versatility:

- *typeability* refers to the proportion of isolates that can be assigned a type, ideally all isolates;
- *reproducibility* is the ability of the system to assign the same type on repeat testing of the same strain;
- *stability* is the probability that clonally derived isolates express the same type over time;
- *discriminatory power*, or the ability to distinguish epidemiologically unrelated isolates, is particularly important because it conditions the probability that isolates sharing the same type or clonal group of types are epidemiologically linked; and
- the *versatility* of a typing method, or its ability to type different pathogens, given minor technical modifications, is an important additional practical advantage for clinical laboratories involved in the study of nosocomial infections.

As yet there is no universally applicable, optimally discriminating, well standardized and easily interpretable system. It is recommended that a combination of typing systems be applied to assess microbial relatedness.

In contrast to most phenotypic typing systems, many methods based on the analysis of genomic DNA polymorphism have broad applicability. Similar reagents (e.g. restriction enzymes) and equipment (e.g. electrophoresis systems and pattern recognition software) can be used for typing different micro-organisms. The majority of these methods provide results within 1–3 days (i.e. rapidly enough to be useful in outbreak management). The methods, however, are readily available to very few hospitals. In general, molecular typing systems are more discriminating than phenotypic methods (Fig. 10.17), but the results produced, typically as an electrophoretic pattern of DNA fragments (Fig. 10.18), can be complex and difficult to interpret. Guidelines have been proposed for definitions of commonly used terms, such as strain and clone, and of criteria for epidemiologic relatedness, based on the results from some DNA typing systems, such as pulsed-field gel electrophoresis (PFGE) analysis.[58,59] Molecular typing systems have contributed greatly to our understanding of the mechanisms of acquisition of hospital infections. Difficult to type pathogens, like *Enterococcus faecalis* and *Candida albicans*, that were until recently believed to arise solely from an endogenous origin, have been shown by epidemiologic studies using genotyping to cause common-source or cross-infection outbreaks in hospitals.

Commonly used conventional and molecular methods are outlined below, and their advantages and limitations are briefly reviewed. It should be stressed that adequate comparative evaluations of these methods are not available for many of the newer methods or less well studied pathogens, making any comparative overview tentative and indicative only.

Phenotyping methods

Antibiogram. This conventional phenotypic method is still an important and routinely available first-line technique used to recognize outbreaks of hospital infection with resistant bacteria, including *S. aureus*[60] and *A. baumannii*.[61] However, as phenotypic characters that influence fitness undergo periodic selection, unrelated clones of nosocomial pathogens exposed to the selective pressure of

CONVENTIONAL AND MOLECULAR TYPING SYSTEMS FOR THE EPIDEMIOLOGIC ANALYSIS OF NOSOCOMIAL PATHOGENS						
Typing system	Principle	Versatility	Typeability	Discrimination	Reproducibility	Stability
Antibiogram	Susceptibility profile to a panel of antimicrobials	Broad	Excellent	Variable	Good	Variable
Biotype	Phenotypic characteristics, e.g. biochemical reaction profile	Narrow	Excellent	Variable	Good	Good
Serotype	Pattern of surface antigens, defined by a set of specific antibodies	Narrow	Good	Moderate	Good	Good
Phage type	Lysis susceptibilty pattern to a panel of specific bacteriophages	Narrow	Moderate	Good	Moderate	Moderate
Immunoblotting	Molecular weight patterns of protein antigens, separated by PAGE and identified with labeled antibodies	Narrow	Excellent	Good	Good	Moderate
Plasmid RFLP analysis	Pattern of restriction fragments of plasmid DNA by agarose electrophoresis	Moderate	Variable	Variable	Good	Moderate
Ribotyping	Pattern of restriction fragments of genomic DNA by Southern blot analysis with ribosomal RNA (or ribosomal DNA)-labeled probe	Broad	Excellent	Moderate	Excellent	Excellent
Southern blot RFLP analysis of genomic DNA	Pattern of genomic DNA restriction fragments by Southern blot analysis with specific DNA-labeled probe (e.g. Insertion sequence element, structural gene sequence)	Narrow	Excellent	Variable	Excellent	Excellent
PFGE of macrorestriction fragments of genomic DNA (PFGE analysis)	Pattern of large genomic DNA restriction fragments generated by rarely cleaving endonucleases and resolved by PFGE	Broad	Excellent	Excellent	Good	Good
PCR-mediated gene RFLP analysis	Pattern of restriction fragments of PCR-amplified polymorphic gene region (e.g. variable size tandem repeats)	Narrow	Excellent	Variable	Excellent	Excellent
AP-PCR and randomly amplified polymorphic DNA analysis	Pattern of low-stringency PCR-amplified genomic DNA segments lying between motifs partly homologous to short, arbitrary sequence primers	Broad	Excellent	Good	Moderate	Good
Inter-repetitive element spacer length polymorphism analysis (rep-PCR analysis)	Pattern of high-stringency PCR-amplified genomic DNA segments lying between repeat motifs (e.g. Insertion sequence elements, ERIC sequences) by using outwardly oriented primers	Variable	Variable	Good	Good	Excellent
AFLP analysis	Pattern of high-stringency PCR-amplified segments of adaptor-tagged genomic DNA restriction fragments	Broad	Excellent	Excellent	Excellent	Excellent
Nucleotide sequence analysis	Determination of DNA sequence of variable genomic regions	Universal	Excellent	Excellent	Excellent	Good

Fig. 10.17 An overview of conventional and molecular typing systems used for the epidemiologic analysis of nosocomial pathogens. A tentative assessment of the performance characteristics of the methods is proposed. Many methods are still under evaluation and their performance may vary according to the pathogen analyzed.

antimicrobials can display evolutionary convergence to the same advantageous resistance phenotype through mutations and multiple genetic exchanges. The level of discrimination of antibiogram varies according to the battery of test drugs used and the prevalence of acquired resistance traits in the study population.

Biotyping. This is based on diversity of colonial morphology, biochemical activity and other phenotypic characters, which tend to be unstable and poorly reproducible, unless highly specialized biotyping schemes are used.[53,58]

Serotyping. Surface antigens are characterized using a panel of species-specific polyclonal or monoclonal antibodies. It is a moderately discriminating tool used for strain delineation of several hospital pathogens, including *Legionella* spp., *P. aeruginosa* and *C. difficile*. For a number of reasons, surface antigens are not, however, reliable markers of population structure. Clonally related strains may show antigenic variation, as occurs, for example, among highly genomically related *Legionella pneumophila* strains isolated from an outbreak of legionellosis.[24]

Phage typing. This is based on susceptibility to cell lysis by a defined set of bacteriophages. Although very useful in past investigations and still used in some reference laboratories for typing important pathogens like *Salmonella* spp. and *S. aureus*, this highly specialized technique is limited by incomplete typeability, poor reproducibility and difficulties in pattern interpretation.[53]

Immunoblot analysis. Also known as Western blot analysis, this technique describes the separation of bacterial proteins using SDS polyacrylamide gel electrophoresis (SDS-PAGE), and their subsequent transfer onto a membrane and reaction with labeled, broad-spectrum antibodies. It has been applied successfully to the epidemiologic analysis of nosocomial infection with different bacterial pathogens, including *C. difficile*[15] and *A. baumannii*.[61–63] In comparison with genomic typing systems, immunoblotting shows good discrimination, but interpretation of pattern differences is not well defined.[62,63] Other phenotypic methods that can be valuable for epidemiologic typing, such as multilocus enzyme electrophoresis and pyrolysis mass spectrometry, are less widely used.[53,58]

Genotyping methods

Plasmid profile analysis. The first DNA-based typing method available for epidemiologic studies, this has now largely been replaced by methods that determine chromosomal DNA polymorphism because of the technical variability and biologic limitations of plasmid typing. Restriction endonuclease analysis of plasmid DNA improves reproducibility and discrimination and is useful for strain differentiation of important pathogens like *S. aureus*.[62,64] However, plasmids can be lost or acquired by conjugation, and can recombine internally or into the chromosome by transposition. The in-vivo instability of plasmids must be taken into account when interpreting typing results.[64] Plasmid analysis is essential for the epidemiologic analysis of hospital infections with multiple-antibiotic resistant organisms and for tracing dissemination of mobile antibiotic resistance genes[53].

DEMONSTRATION OF NOSOCOMICAL TRANSMISSION OF THREE CLONES OF *P. AERUGINOSA* VIA INADEQUATELY DISINFECTED ENDOSCOPES

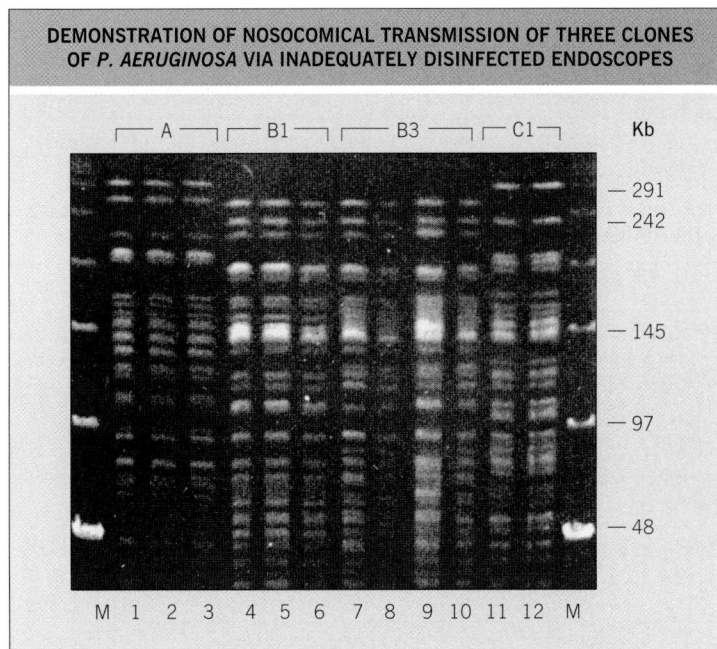

Fig. 10.18 Demonstration of nosocomial transmission of three clones of *Pseudomonas aeruginosa* via inadequately disinfected endoscopes. PFGE patterns of genomic DNA from *Pseudomonas aeruginosa* isolates restricted with the rarely cutting enzyme *XbaI*. Pattern A: bacteremic patients (lanes 1 and 2) and endoscope channel (lane 3); patterns B1and B3: bacteremic patients (lanes 4 and 5, and 7 and 8); endoscope channels (lanes 6 and 9); tap water (lane 10). Pattern C1: bacteremic patients (lanes 11 and 12). Lane M: molecular size markers, in kilobase pairs. Adapted from Struelens *et al.*[24]

RESTRICTION ANALYSIS OF BACTERIAL GENOME POLYMORPHISM

Fig. 10.19 Restriction endonuclease analysis of bacterial genome polymorphism. Chromosomal DNA is released after lysis of the bacterial cells. Restriction endonucleases that recognize commonly occurring sites will cut DNA in many small fragments. After conventional electrophoresis, these fragments are transferred onto a membrane and revealed by hybridization with labeled probes (Southern blot analysis). Alternatively, DNA can be restricted by endonucleases that recognize only rarely occurring sites. The few large, or macrorestriction, fragments are then separated by PFGE analysis.

Restriction fragment length polymorphism analysis. Genotyping can be performed by cleavage of chromosomal DNA with restriction endonucleases and electrophoretic separation of DNA fragments (Fig. 10.19). Restriction endonucleases that have frequent recognition sites produce complex fragment patterns by agarose or PAGE separation. The number and length of restriction fragments is affected by sequence variations that create or delete recognition sites, and by recombinational events that occur at or between restriction sites. To improve the resolution and facilitate the interpretation of genomic restriction fragment length polymorphism (RFLP) analysis two approaches are used:

- transfer of restriction fragments onto membranes, followed by Southern blot hybridization with DNA probes, and
- use of endonucleases that have infrequent (<30) recognition sites in the chromosome, followed by separation of these macrorestriction fragments by PFGE (Fig. 10.18).

Genome RFLP analysis by Southern blot hybridization. This can be applied by using different types of nucleic acid probes, including randomly cloned chromosomal fragments;[21] structural gene sequences;[65] insertion sequences and transposons[66] and ribosomal RNA or cloned ribosomal DNA sequences, also called ribotyping.[67] The performance of these systems depends on the organism and DNA probe. Probe sequence, restriction endonucleases, electrophoresis and hybridization conditions must be optimized for each species. In general, these RFLP typing techniques are less discriminating than other genotyping systems like PFGE and arbitrarily primed polymerase chain reaction (AP-PCR), described below.[53,62]

Ribotyping. This is the most versatile and the most widely used strategy. The evolutionary conservation of ribosomal RNA makes *E. coli* ribosomal RNA applicable as a universal bacterial probe. Most bacteria have more than five ribosomal operons per chromosome and produce ribotype patterns of 5–15 bands. An automated ribotyping system is commercially available. Ribotyping exhibits excellent reproducibility and stability, but only moderate discriminatory power.[53,67] In addition,

no consensus has been achieved on an optimal procedure and rules for pattern interpretation.

Genome macrorestriction analysis resolved by PFGE analysis. This has recently emerged as a gold standard for molecular typing of microbial pathogens.[53,57] Low-frequency cleaving enzymes cut the bacterial chromosome into fewer than 30 fragments, typically 10–700kb in size. Periodic change in the orientation of electric field during agarose electrophoresis, or PFGE, allows separation and size determination of these macrorestriction fragments (Fig. 10.19). It can be applied to any bacteria or yeasts, with minor technical modifications. In comparison with other typing methods, PFGE analysis shows equal or greater discriminatory power.[68] Consensus rules for interpretation of PFGE patterns are available.[58,59]

PCR-based strategies. They have been developed in recent years for strain typing of microbial pathogens.[69] In PCR-mediated gene RFLP typing, a polymorphic DNA target sequence is PCR-amplified at high stringency, cut with restriction endonucleases, separated by electrophoresis and isolates are compared by RFLP pattern. Careful identification of polymorphic gene sequences and selection of discriminant enzymes must be performed for each species. PCR-RFLP typing is a rapid, simple and reproducible technique, but it gives only moderate discrimination.[53,62]

AP-PCR typing and similar methods like random amplified polymorphic DNA analysis are based on low-stringency PCR amplification and use a single primer of arbitrary sequence. In the early cycles of the PCR, the primer anneals to multiple sequences with partial homology, and segments of DNA lying between closely spaced annealing sites are amplified to produce a strain-specific array of DNA fragments. This simple and rapid technique can be used for strain typing of bacteria, fungi and protozoans.[69] The discriminatory power varies according to the number and sequence of arbitrary primers and amplification conditions.[53,69] AP-PCR typing is, however, limited by problems in reproducibility and the lack of consensus rules for interpretation of pattern differences.[53,58] It is best used as a first-pass, efficient screening method to assess the genomic similarity of organisms during outbreak investigations.[2,32,53]

Repetitive element PCR (rep-PCR) typing consists of high-stringency PCR amplification of spacer fragments lying between repeat motifs of the genome by the use of two outwardly directed primers. Targets for rep-PCR analysis include the repetitive extragenic palindromes, the enterobacterial repetitive intergenic consensus (ERIC) sequences, insertion sequences and other species-specific repeat elements. rep-PCR typing shows moderate discriminatory power but a better reproducibility than AP-PCR analysis.

The amplified fragment length polymorphism (AFLP) analysis also has high resolution and excellent reproducibility. A restriction–ligation reaction produces restricted genomic DNA fragments tagged with specially designed adapters. Primers complementary to these adapters and adjacent nucleotides are used to amplify various parts of the tagged restriction fragments.

Determination of nucleotide sequence. This is the most accurate method for comparing strains based on localized genomic polymorphism. This method is important in the investigation of transmission of viruses, like the hepatitis C virus.[70] Progress in the efficiency of automated sequence analysis systems will enlarge the application of this approach.

Interpretation of typing results

Molecular typing systems are used to determine whether isolates are clonally derived and thus likely to belong to the same chain of transmission. The level of genomic similarity that can be used to define clonally or epidemiologically related organisms depends on the resolving power of the typing system used, the genomic plasticity of the organism and the time scale of the study.[56,58] Rules for interpretation of differences in PFGE patterns, as applied to outbreak investigations, correlate increase in the number of restriction fragment mismatches with increasing number of genetic differences and with decreasing probability of epidemiologic relatedness.[59] Restriction pattern similarity co-efficients are also useful for interpretation, particularly for large scale studies.[58] The nature of events giving rise to genomic polymorphisms scored by molecular typing systems requires additional study.

Implementing molecular typing systems

Given the diversity of nosocomial pathogens, broad-range typing systems are to be preferred. Confident assessment of clonality currently requires the use of two or three methods in combination. The methods used should be highly discriminatory and give reproducible results, at least within a single assay. Therefore, the methods currently best suited for hospital epidemiology are the antibiogram and, when appropriate, serotyping, followed by PCR-based methods for rapid clonal delineation. PFGE analysis can be used for confirmatory genotyping and more precise comparison of genomic relatedness. Whatever method is chosen, typing should always be undertaken with a clear purpose in mind. Specific hypotheses to be tested by typing will guide the selection of the appropriate method(s) and sample of isolates. Interpretation of results requires careful confrontation of clinical, epidemiologic and typing data.[56,58]

STERILIZATION AND DISINFECTION

To minimize the risk of transmission of micro-organisms during invasive procedures that involve effraction of mucosa or skin, complete or nearly complete removal of micro-organisms from invasive devices must be achieved by sterilization or disinfection. In addition, skin antisepsis is essential for reducing the risk of autoinfection in surgery and for preventing cross-colonization between patients via contaminated hands of health care personnel.

Sterilization is the process of removing or destroying all viable micro-organisms from an object. Disinfection consists of eliminating or killing the majority of potentially pathogenic micro-organisms from

a contaminated item.[71] These processes can be accomplished by using a variety of physical, chemical or physicochemical methods that denature proteins and nucleic acids (Fig. 10.20). Sterilization is most commonly performed by using steam heated under pressure (autoclaving), ethylene oxide gas or prolonged immersion in liquid sterilizing chemicals. Disinfection is usually achieved by using liquid chemicals for a shorter contact time. Different types of micro-organisms show varying levels of susceptibility to disinfectants. The most resistant forms are bacterial spores, followed by, in decreasing order of resistance, mycobacteria, non-lipid viruses, fungi, vegetative bacteria and lipid viruses.[72] Medical devices can be classified according to the level of invasiveness of their intended use, and are processed accordingly to ensure safe procedures. For example, critical devices that enter sterile tissues, such as surgical instruments or implants, require sterilization. Semicritical devices that come in contact with mucous membranes, such as endoscopes and rectal thermometers, must undergo high-level disinfection. This process should kill all micro-organisms, except for high levels of bacterial spores, and is achieved by using chemical or thermochemical methods (Fig. 10.20). Non-critical items and surfaces that come in contact with intact skin, such as stethoscopes, can be submitted to low-level disinfection procedures to kill the majority of pathogenic micro-organisms, with the exception of mycobacteria and bacterial spores.

Sterilization and disinfection must be preceded by meticulous cleaning to eliminate organic material from the device and to reduce the biologic burden. A number of technical factors are important to ensure adequate sterilization and disinfection of medical material: the type and load of contaminating micro-organisms, the nature and physical configuration of the object, the concentration of chemical agent used and the temperature and pH of the process.[72] To provide effective processing, it is preferable that high-level disinfection and sterilization are performed by specialized personnel in adequately centralized facilities. To monitor effectiveness, initial validation and regular quality control must be performed. Physical and chemical monitoring of each process cycle is necessary. Additional quality assurance can be achieved by periodically incorporating biologic indicators, generally a known inoculum of bacterial spores, and by testing their nonviability by culture after processing. Flexible fiberoptic endoscopes are especially difficult to clean internally and disinfect adequately, and specific reprocessing guidelines must be followed.[73]

	STERILIZATION AND DISINFECTION TECHNIQUES COMMONLY USED IN HOSPITAL PRACTICE		
Objective	Method	Principle of microbial inactivation	Example of use
Sterilization	Steam autoclaving	Thermal denaturation	Metallic surgical instruments
	Ethylene oxide	Thermochemical denaturation	Heat-labile surgical instruments
	Gamma-irradiation	Ionizing denaturation	Implantable medical devices (catheters, prostheses)
Disinfection	Chlorine	Chemical denaturation	Water disinfection
	Alcohols	Chemical denaturation	Skin antisepsis
	Iodophors	Chemical denaturation	Skin and mucosae antisepsis
	Glutaraldehyde	Chemical denaturation	Flexible endoscopes
	Peracetic acid	Chemical denaturation	Flexible endoscopes

Fig. 10.20 Techniques commonly used in hospitals for sterilization and disinfection of medical equipment and for skin antisepsis.

HAND HYGIENE AND ISOLATION PRECAUTIONS

To prevent transmission of potentially infectious micro-organisms from colonized or infected patients to other hospitalized patients, visitors or health care personnel, systematic hand hygiene precautions must be taken during patient care. In addition, patients who have certain conditions must be placed in special isolation to prevent transmission of pathogens by other routes. Isolation methods include special room requirements and the use of protective equipment, generally worn by patient care personnel.

Between 1970 and 1996, the CDC formalized a series of guidelines to implement isolation precautions. Category-specific precautions are based on the classification of infectious diseases into six categories according to their route of transmission: strict, contact, respiratory, tuberculosis, enteric and drainage–secretion precautions.[74] Disease-specific isolation is tailored according to the mechanism of transmission of each infectious disease. Although logical, these strategies are complex to implement. They tend to be difficult to apply to newly admitted patients who present with an undiagnosed, presumably infectious, syndrome.

In the face of the HIV pandemic, universal precautions were proposed to complement the disease-specific isolation precautions.[74] The goal was to protect health care workers from infection with bloodborne viruses such as HIV. Universal precautions[72] required the use of gloves and other barrier precautions to avoid contact with blood, internal body fluids and genital secretions. To reduce the risk of percutaneous exposure to blood and body fluids, minimal handling of needles and sharp instruments and their safe disposal was recommended.[71] At the same time, a simplified system, called the body substance isolation, was proposed as an attempt to merge the objectives of contact isolation and universal precautions.[75] This system is based on the premise that any contact with tissue, body fluids, wounds, mucous membranes and secretions is potentially contaminating and a source of transmission of infectious agents to health care workers and other patients. The systematic use of gloves, and other barrier precautions when necessary, was advocated for any contact described above with all patients. The latest CDC guidelines[76] incorporate this strategy with the additional need for handwashing after removing gloves, which was shown to recontaminate hands, as 'standard precautions' (Fig. 10.21). These systematic precautions are supplemented by patient-specific isolation precautions, grouped into three categories, for preventing the contact, droplet and airborne transmission of specific pathogens.[73] In addition to physical isolation in a private room and use of barriers such as gloves and gowns, cohort nursing can contribute to effective isolation, as shown for the prevention of nosocomial RSV infection.[77]

The growing importance of nosocomial transmission of multiple-antibiotic resistant pathogens has led national advisory bodies to issue specific guidelines for the early detection, isolation and decolonization of patients with infection or colonization with MRSA,[17,78,79] vancomycin-resistant enterococci,[80] and with vancomycin-resistant *S. aureus*.[81]

The optimal methods of hand hygiene in hospital practice remain under debate.[82] This relates to major problems with health care worker compliance and tolerance with traditional handwashing. The latter is generally practised only about 30–50% of the time it should be.[83] With the increasing use of gloves to prevent soiling of hands during contaminating procedures, greater emphasis is placed today on hand antisepsis, particularly in Europe. Handrub with alcohol-based disinfectants, such as 70% isopropyl-alcohol, is more effective, faster, easier to use and well tolerated compared with handwashing (Fig. 10.22).[82] Educational programs that include observation of health care workers' hand hygiene practices and regular feedback of compliance rates can improve these practices[83] and should be encouraged. Spread of infectious agents among patients in hospitals from health care workers' hands is a major and preventable cause of morbidity and mortality. It is mandatory to use whatever hand hygiene methods are available in a given hospital.

CONTROL OF ANTIBIOTIC RESISTANCE

In addition to the evaluation of isolation methods for preventing transmission of multiple resistant bacterial pathogens, strategies for the appropriate use of antimicrobials in the hospital are still in a state of empiric assesment.[84] Controlling the antimicrobial usage by restriction, such as methods based on antibiotic formularies, have been met with mixed success.[84,85] Studies linking intensive antibiotic control to an increase in micro-organism susceptibility are often difficult to interpret because of methodologic problems, including the failure to control for

OVERVIEW OF CDC/HICPAC ISOLATION PRECAUTIONS 1996				
Feature	Standard precautions	Contact precautions	Droplet precautions	Airborne precautions
Patient room	Standard	Private	Private	Private; door closed; well ventilated (minimum 6 air changes per hour; negative pressure)
Gloves	Contact with blood, body fluids, mucous membranes, secretions, excretions or broken skin	Before entering room	Standard	Standard
Handwashing	After glove removal; between patients	Standard; with antiseptic soap	Standard	Standard
Gown	Before procedure likely to generate projections of blood, body fluids, secretions or excretions	Contact with patient; if patient has diarrhea or open drainage of wounds or secretions	Standard	Standard
Mask	Before procedure likely to generate projections of blood, body fluids, secretions or excretions	Standard	If within 3 feet of patient	Before entering room
Examples of conditions	All patients	• Multidrug-resistant bacteria of special clinical and epidemiologic significance (e.g. MRSA, VRE) • Major abscess, cellulitis or decubiti • *Clostridium difficile* infection • Acute diarrhea, in an incontinent or diapered patient • RSV infections, bronchiolitis and croup in young infants	• Meningitis • Diphtheria • Pertussis • Influenza • Mumps • Rubella • Streptococcal pharyngitis, pneumonia or scarlet fever in young children	• Tuberculosis, or suspected tuberculosis • Measles • Varicella, disseminated zoster

Fig. 10.21 Key points in the 1996 CDC guideline for isolation precautions in hospitals. Adapted from Garner.[76] Refer to the original guideline for complete information.

HAND HYGIENE METHODS			
Feature	Handwashing	Hand alcohol antisepsis	Gloves
Advantages	• Removes soiling • Low cost	• High efficacy for removal of transient microflora (3–4 log) • Low cost • Fast and easy to use	• Prevents soiling • Protects health care worker
Disadvantages	• Low efficacy for removal of transient microflora (2 log) • Time consuming • Skin intolerance	• Efficacy decreased on soiled hands • Skin intolerance	• Contamination during removal • Skin intolerance • Cost

Fig. 10.22 The use of gloves to prevent hand soiling and to reduce hand contamination can be combined with alcohol antisepsis after glove removal. Frequent handwashing with plain soap and water, or with disinfectant – detergent and water – leads to considerable problems of skin intolerance.

confounding factors.[85] Studies have shown the impact of antibiotic restriction on decreased transmission of nosocomial pathogens, such as *C. difficile*, by molecular typing.[86] Computer-assisted support to medical decisions in prescribing antibiotics, based on locally defined consensus guidelines, can improve antibiotic use, reduce associated costs and stabilize the prevalence of antibiotic-resistant pathogens.[87] Further study of innovative strategies is needed to improve the control of antibiotic resistance of hospital pathogens.

REFERENCES

1. Garner JS, Jarvis WR, Emori TG, *et al.* CDC definitions for nosocomial infections, 1988. Am J Infect Control 1988;16:128–40.
2. Horan TC, Gaynes RP, Martone WJ, *et al.* CDC definitions of nosocomial surgical site infections, 1992: a modification of CDC definitions of surgical wound infections. Infect Control Hosp Epidemiol 1992;13:608–8.
3. Haley RW, Culver DH, White JW, *et al.* The efficacy of infection surveillance and control programs in US hospitals. Am J Epidemiol 1985; 121:182–205.
4. Haley RW, Culver DH, White JW, Morgan WM, Emori TG. The nationwide nosocomial infection rate: a new need for vital statistics. Am J Epidemiol 1985;121:159–67.
5. Emmerson AM. The impact of surveys on hospital infection. J Hosp Infect 1995;30(Suppl):421–40.
6. Western KA, St John R, Shearer LA. Hospital infection control – an international perspective. Infect Control 1982;3:453–5.
7. Ponce de Leon S. The needs of the developing countries and the resources required. J Hosp Infect 1991;18(Suppl A):376–81.
8. Vincent JL, Bihari DJ, Suter PM, *et al.* The prevalence of nosocomial infections in intensive care units in Europe. JAMA 1995;274:639–44.
9. Banerjee SN, Emori TG, Culver DH, *et al.* Secular trends in nosocomial primary bloodstream infections in the United States, 1980–89. Am J Med 1991;91(3B):86S–9S.
10. Pittet D, Wenzel RP. Nosocomial bloodstream infections. Secular trends in rates, mortality and contribution to total hospital deaths. Arch Intern Med 1995;155:1177–84.
11. Dixon RE. Costs of nosocomial infections and benefits of infection control programs. In: Wenzel RP, ed. Prevention and control of nosocomial infections. Baltimore: Williams & Wilkins; 1987:19–25.

12. Dinkel RH, Lebok U. A survey of nosocomial infections and their influence on hospital mortality rates. J Hosp Infect 1994;28:297–304.
13. Fagon JY, Novera A, Stepha F, Girou E, Safar M. Mortality attributable to nosocomial infections in the ICU. Infect Control Hosp Epidemiol 1994;15:428–34.
14. Wenzel RP. The economics of nosocomial infections. J Hosp Infect 1995;31:79–87.
15. McFarland LV, Mulligan ME, Kwok RYY, Stamm WE. Nosocomial acquisition of *Clostridium difficile* infection. N Engl J Med 1989;320:204–10.
16. Vaudry WL, Tierney AJ, Wenman WM. Investigation of a cluster of systemic *Candida albicans* infections in a neonatal intensive care unit. J Infect Dis 1988;158:1375–9.
17. Mulligan ME, Murray-Leisure KA, Standford HC, *et al.* Methicillin-resistant *Staphylococcus aureus*: a consensus review of the microbiology, pathogenesis, and epidemiology with implications for prevention and management. Am J Med 1993;94:313–28.
18. Boyce JM, Potter-Bynoe G, Opal SM, Dziobek L, Medeiros AA. A common source outbreak of *Staphylococcus epidermidis* infections among patients undergoing cardiac surgery. J Infect Dis 1990;161:493–9.
19. Mastro TD, Farley TA, Elliott JA, *et al.* An outbreak of surgical-wound infections due to group A streptococcus carried on the scalp. N Engl J Med 1990;323:968–72.
20. Sherertz RJ, Reagan DR, Hampton KD, *et al.* A cloud adult: the *Staphylococcus aureus* virus interaction revisited. Ann Intern Med 1996;124:539–47.
21. Struelens MJ, Maes N, Rost F, *et al.* Genotypic and phenotypic methods for the investigation of a nosocomial *Legionella pneumophila* outbreak and efficacy of control measures. J Infect Dis 1992;166:22–30.

22. Walsh TJ, Pizzo PA. Nosocomial fungal infections: a classification for hospital-acquired fungal infections and mycoses arising from endogenous flora or reactivation. Ann Rev Microbiol 1988;42:517–45.
23. Jarvis WR. Nosocomial outbreaks: the Centers for Disease Control's Hospital Infections Program Experience, 1980–1990. Am J Med 1991;91(3B):101S–6S.
24. Struelens MJ, Rost F, Deplano A, *et al. Pseudomonas aeruginosa* and Enterobacteriaceae bacteremia after biliary endoscopy: an outbreak investigation using DNA macrorestriction analysis. Am J Med 1993;95:489–98.
25. Bennett SN, McNeil MM, Bland LA, *et al.* Postoperative infections traced to contamination of an intravenous anesthetic, propofol. N Engl J Med 1995;333:147–54.
26. Chetoui H, Melin P, Struelens MJ, *et al.* Comparison of biotyping, ribotyping and pulsed-field gel electrophoresis for the investigation of a common-source outbreak of *Burkholderia pickettii* bacteremia. J Clin Microbiol;1997;35:1398–403.
27. Centers for Disease Control. Nosocomial enterococci resistant to vancomycin – United States, 1989–1993. Morb Mort Wkly Rep 1993;42:597–9.
28. Edlin BR, Tokars JI, Gieco MH, *et al.* An outbreak of multidrug-resistant tuberculosis among hospitalized patients with the acquired immunodeficiency syndrome. N Engl J Med 1992;326:1514–21.
29. Murray BE. Can antibiotic resistance be controlled? N Engl J Med 1994;330:1229–30.
30. Morris JG, Shay DK, Hebden JN, *et al.* Enterococci resistant to multiple antimicrobial agents, including vancomycin. Ann Intern Med 1995;123:250–9.
31. Chow JW, Fine MJ, Shlaes DM, *et al.* Enterobacter bacteremia: clinical features and emergence of antibiotic resistance during therapy. Ann Intern Med 1991;115:585–90.

32. De Gheldre Y, Maes N, Rost F, et al. Molecular epidemiology of an outbreak of multidrug-resistant Enterobacter aerogenes infections and in vivo emergence of imipenem resistance. J Clin Microbiol 1997;35:152–60.

33. Lucet JC, Chevret S, Decré D, et al. Outbreak of multiply resistant enterobacteriaceae in an intensive care unit: epidemiology and risk factors for acquisition. Clin Infect Dis 1996;22:430–6.

34. Lortholary O, Fagon JY, Buu Hoi A, et al. Nosocomial acquisition of multiresistant Acinetobacter baumannii: risk factors and prognosis. Clin Infect Dis 1995;20:790–6.

35. Go ES, Burns J, Kreiswirth B, et al. Clinical and molecular epidemiology of acinetobacter infections sensitive only to polymyxin B and sulbactam. Lancet 1994;344:1329–32.

36. Richard P, Le Floch R, Chamoux C, et al. Pseudomonas aeruginosa outbreak in a burn unit: role of antimicrobials in the emergence of multiply resistant strains. J Infect Dis 1994;170:377–83.

37. Wenzel RP, ed. Prevention and control of nosocomial infections, 2nd ed. Baltimore: William & Wilkins; 1993.

38. Wenzel RP. The evolving art and science of hospital epidemiology. J Infect Dis 1986;153:462–70.

39. Manangan LP. The infection control information system of the Hospital Infections Program, Centers for Diseases Control and Prevention. Am J Infect Control 1996;24:463–7.

40. Rhinehart E, Goldmann DA, O'Rourke EJ. Adaptation of the Centers for Disease Control guidelines for the prevention of nosocomial infection in a pediatric intensive care unit in Jakarta, Indonesia. Am J Med 1991;91(3B):213–20.

41. Haley RW. Surveillance by objective: a new priority-directed approach to the control of nosocomial infections. Am J Infect Control 1985;13:78–89.

42. French GL, Cheng AFB, Wong SL, Donnan S. Repeated prevalence surveys for monitoring effectiveness of hospital infection control. Lancet 1989;1021–3.

43. Dettenkofer M, Daschner FD. Cost-effectiveness of surveillance methods. In: Emmerson AM, Ayliffe GAJ, eds. Surveillance of nosocomial infections. Baillière's Clin Infect Dis 1996;3(2):289–382.

44. Glenister HM, Taylor LJ, Bartlett CLR, et al. An evaluation of surveillance methods for detecting infections in hospital inpatients. J Hosp Infect 1993;23:229–42.

45. Laxson LB, Blaser MJ, Parkhust SM. Surveillance for the detection of nosocomial infections and the potential of nosocomial outbreaks. Am J Infect Control 1984;12:318–24.

46. Struelens MJ. How can we integrate surveillance with prevention of nosocomial infection? 7th European Congress of Clinical Microbiology and Infectious Diseases. Abstracts Excerpta Medica Vienna, March 26–30, 1995:116.

47. Lima NL, Pereira CRB, Souza IC, et al. Selective surveillance for nosocomial infections in a Brazilian hospital. Infect Control Hosp Epidemiol 1993;14:197–202.

48. Broderick A, Mori M, Nettleman MD, et al. Nosocomial infections: validation of surveillance and computer modeling to identify patients at risk. Am J Epidemiol 1990;131:734–42.

49. Classen DC, Burke JP, Pestotnik SL, Evans RS, Stevens LE. Surveillance for quality assessment: IV. surveillance using a hospital information system. Infect Control Hosp Epidemiol 1991;12:239–44.

50. Mertens R, Ceusters W. Quality assurance, infection surveillance, and hospital information systems: avoiding the Bermuda Triangle. Infect Control Hosp Epidemiol 1994;15:203–9.

51. Struelens MJ, Ronveaux O, Jans B, Mertens R and the Groupement pour le Dépistage, l'Etude et la Prévention des Infections Hospitalières. Methicillin-resistant Staphylococcus aureus epidemiology and control in Belgian hospitals, 1991 to 1995. Infect Control Hosp Epidemiol 1996;17:503–8.

52. Doebbeling BN. Epidemics: identification and management. In: Wenzel RP, ed. Prevention and control of nosocomial infections, 2nd ed. Baltimore: William & Wilkins, 1993:177–206

53. Struelens MJ. Laboratory methods in the investigation of outbreaks of hospital-acquired infection. In: Emmerson AM, Ayliffe GAJ, eds. Surveillance of nosocomial infections. Baillière's Clin Infect Dis 1996;3(2):267–88.

54. Chetchotisak P, Phelps CL, Hartstein AI. Assessment of bacterial cross-transmission as a cause of infections in patients in intensive care units. Clin Infect Dis 1994;18:929–37.

55. McGowan JE, Metchock BG. Basic microbiologic support for hospital epidemiology. Infect Control Hosp Epidemiol 1996;17:298–303.

56. Arbeit RD. Laboratory procedures for the epidemiologic analysis of micro-organisms. In: Murray PR, ed. Manual of clinical microbiology, 6th ed. Washington DC: American Society for Microbiology Press, 1995:190–208.

57. Maslow JN, Mulligan ME, Arbeit RD. Molecular epidemiology: application of contemporary techniques to the typing of microorganisms. Clin Infect Dis 1993;17:153–64.58. Struelens MJ and the European Study Group on Epidemiological Markers. Consensus guidelines for appropriate use and evaluation of microbial epidemiologic typing systems. Clin Microbiol Infect 1996;2:1–11.

59. Tenover FC, Arbeit RD, Goering RV, et al. Interpreting chromosomal DNA restriction patterns produced by pulsed-field gel electrophoresis: criteria for bacterial strain typing. J Clin Microbiol 1995;33:2233–9.

60. Blanc DS, Lugeon C, Wenger A, et al. Quantitative antibiogram typing using inhibition zone diameters compared with ribotyping for epidemiological typing of methicillin-resistant Staphylococcus aureus. J Clin Microbiol 1994;32:2505–9.

61. Tankovic J, Legrand P, DeGatines G, et al. Characterization of a hospital outbreak of imipenem-resistant Acinetobacter baumannii by phenotypic and genotypic methods. J Clin Microbiol 1994;32:2677–81.

62. Tenover FC, Arbeit R, Archer G, et al. Comparison of traditional and molecular methods of typing isolates of Staphylococcus aureus. J Clin Microbiol 1994;32:407–15

63. Marcos MA, Jimenez De Anta MT, Vila J. Correlation of six methods for typing nosocomial isolates of Acinetobacter baumannii. J Med Microbiol 1995;42:328–35.

64. Hartstein AI, Phelps CL, Kwok RYY, Mulligan ME. In vivo stability and discriminatory power of methicillin-resistant Staphylococcus aureus typing by restriction endonuclease analysis of plasmid DNA compared with those of other molecular methods. J Clin Microbiol 1995;33:2022–6.

65. de Lancastre H, Couto I, Santos I, et al. Methicillin-resistant Staphylococcus aureus disease in a Portuguese hospital: characterization of clonal types by a combination of DNA typing methods. Eur J Clin Microbiol Infect Dis 1994;13:64–73.

66. Thorisdottir AS, Carias JL, Marshall, et al. IS6770, an enterococcal insertion-like sequence useful for determining the clonal relationship of clinical enterococcal isolates. J Infect Dis 1994;170:1539–48.

67. Bingen EH, Denamur E, Elion J. Use of ribotyping in epidemiological surveillance of nosocomial outbreaks. Clin Microbiol Rev 1994;7:311–27.

68. Grundmann H, Schneider C, Hartung D, et al. Discriminatory power of three DNA-based typing techniques for Pseudomonas aeruginosa. J Clin Microbiol 1995;33:528–34.

69. van Belkum A. DNA fingerprinting of medically important microorganisms by use of PCR. Clin Microbiol Rev 1994;7:174–84.

70. Allander T, Gruber A, Naghavi M, et al. Frequent patient-to-patient transmission of hepatitis C virus in a haematology ward. Lancet 1995;345:603–7.

71. Rutala WA. Disinfection, sterilization and waste disposal. In: Wenzel RP, ed. Prevention and control of nosocomial infections, 2nd ed. Baltimore: Williams & Wilkins; 1993:460–95.

72. Favero MS, Bond WW. Chemical disinfection of medical and surgical materials. In: Block SS, ed. Disinfection, sterilization and preservation, 4th ed. Philadelphia: Lea & Febiger; 1991:617–41.

73. Martin MA, Reichelderfer M. APIC Guideline for infection prevention and control in flexible endoscopy. Am J Infect Control 1994;22:19–38.

74. Edmond MB. Isolation. Infect Control Hosp Epidemiol 1997;18:58–64.

75. Lynch P, Cummings MJ, Roberts PL et al. Implementing and evaluating a system of generic infection precautions: body substance isolation. Am J Infect Control 1990;18:1–12.

76. Garner JS. Hospital Infection Control Practices Advisory Committee Guideline for isolation precautions in hospitals. Infect Control Hosp Epidemiol 1996;17:53–80.

77. Madge P, Paton JY, McColl JH, Mackie PLK. Prospective controlled study of four infection – control procedures to prevent nosocomial infection with respiratory syncytial virus. Lancet 1992;340:1079–93.

78. Duckworth G. Revised guidelines for the control of epidemic methicillin-resistant Staphylococcus aureus. J Hosp Infect 1990;16:351–77.

79. The Groupement pour le Dépistage, l'Etude et la Prévention des Infections Hospitalières – Groep ter Opsporing, Studie en Preventie van de Infecties in de Ziekenhuizen (GDEPIH-GOSPIZ). Guidelines for control and prevention of methicillin-resistant Staphylococcus aureus transmission in Belgian hospitals. Acta Clin Belgica 1994;49:108–13.

80. Hospital Infection Control Practices Advisory Committee (HICPAC). Recommendations for preventing the spread of vancomycin resistance. Am J Infect Control 1995;23:87–94.

81. Edmond MB, Wenzel RP, Pasculle AW. Vancomycin-resistant Staphylococcus aureus: prespectives on measures needed for control. Ann Intern Med 1996;124:329–34.

82. Larson EL. APIC guideline for handwashing and hand antisepsis in health care settings. Am J Infect Control 1995;23:251–69.

83. Larson E, Kretzer EK. Compliance with handwashing and barrier precautions. J Hosp Infect 1995;30:88–106.

84. Goldmann DA, Weinstein RA, Wenzel RP et al. Strategies to prevent and control the emergence and spread of antimicrobial-resistant microorganisms in hospitals. JAMA 1996;275:234–40.

85. McGowan JE. Do intensive hospital antibiotic control programs prevent the spread of antibiotic resistance? Infect Control Hosp Epidemiol 1994;15:478–83.

86. Pear SM, Williamson TH, Bettin KM, Gerding DN, Galgiani JN. Decrease in nosocomial Clostridium difficile-associated diarrhea by restricting clindamycin use. Ann Intern Med 1994;120:272–7.

87. Pestotnik SL, Classen DC, Scott Evans R, Burke JP. Implementing antibiotic practice guidelines through computer-assisted decision support: clinical and financial outcomes. Ann Intern Med 1996;124:884–90.

Employee Health Service

Kent A Sepkowitz

An active hospital employee health service (EHS), or occupational health service, is crucial to control of nosocomial infection. This is accomplished in several ways: identification and vaccination of workers susceptible to vaccine-preventable diseases; active surveillance for diseases such as tuberculosis (TB); and prompt diagnosis of transmissible illnesses such as respiratory syncytial virus (RSV) or hepatitis A virus infection in symptomatic workers. Recent articles have considered specific infectious disease problems frequently encountered by an EHS.[1-4]

ORGANIZATION OF EMPLOYEE HEALTH SERVICE

The organization of the EHS varies according to the size and administrative structure of a hospital. At larger hospitals, the EHS is staffed by full-time nurses and physicians, as well as by clerical staff. The model at smaller hospitals is characterized by fewer staff, limited hours and more limited capabilities (Fig. 11.1). The administrative reporting mechanisms for the EHS also vary considerably from hospital to hospital. The employee health service may be part of infection control, the Department of Nursing, or may report primarily to a senior hospital administrator.

Few studies have defined the scope of EHS activity.[5-7] In one analysis of 21,886 annual visits, 25% were for preventive services, such as vaccination and routine examinations; 25% were for occupationally related illnesses, including infectious diseases, stress and accidents; and 15% were for administrative procedures, such as prescription renewal, requests for letters and completion of forms.[5]

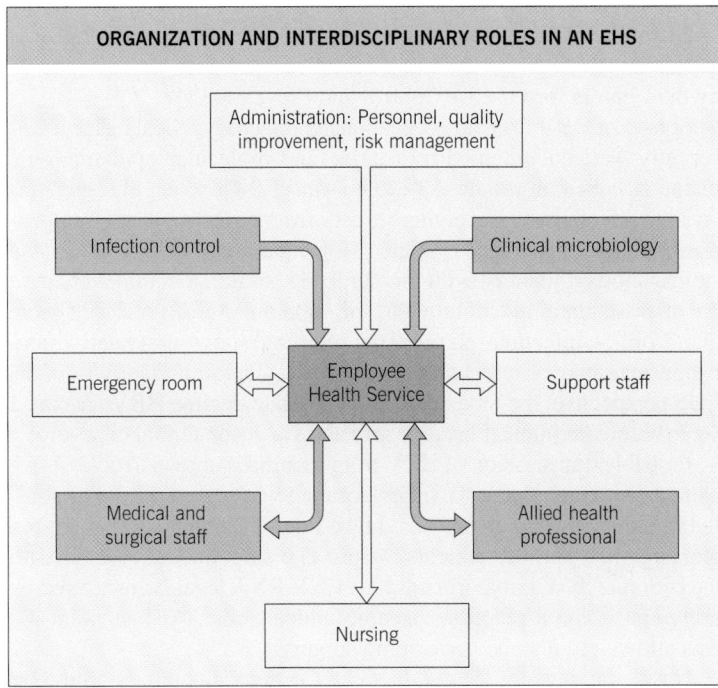

Fig. 11.1 Example of organization and interdisciplinary roles in an EHS.

Another study reviewing 3000 annual visits found 30% of visits to the EHS were for occupationally related illness or injury, and of these less than 3% were for fever.[6]

ROUTINE TESTS FOR NEW EMPLOYEES

The medical evaluation of new employees is a fundamental job for the EHS. In general, all new employees should have tests performed to evaluate for immunity to various potentially transmissible diseases (Fig. 11.2). These include serologic tests and a tuberculin skin test for TB. Routine chest radiography should be reserved only for those employees with known pulmonary problems, a previously abnormal chest radiograph, or a positive tuberculin skin test.

Serologic testing for numerous potential pathogens is essential, both for the safety of the health care worker and for patient safety. The Centers for Disease Control and Prevention has published recommendations on immunization of health care workers[8] and infection control in hospital personnel.[9]

Since 1992 the US Occupational Safety and Health Administration has required demonstration of seropositivity to hepatitis B virus (HBV) for all health care workers with occupational exposure to blood or body fluids.[10] Seronegative health care workers must either receive vaccine or formally decline the three-vaccine series, which is offered free of charge. The rates of vaccination have subsequently increased, but remain low, at about 50%.[10] The observed decrease in HBV-associated morbidity and mortality among health care workers is attributed to improved vaccine coverage.[11] Varicella-zoster virus (VZV) antibody status should also be determined. In some countries (e.g. the USA) vaccination of of susceptible employees is recommended.[12] Specific countries and regions may require evidence of immunity to other pathogens, such as measles, mumps and rubella.

Few hospitals track pneumococcal vaccine status of employees and none mandate or even suggest routine vaccination of health care workers. However, reports have appeared of outbreaks of pneumococcal disease,[13] including those caused by penicillin-resistant strains.[14] Although pneumococcus has not been firmly established as a nosocomial pathogen, additional reports of possible nosocomial spread may force a careful reconsideration of the issue. Finally, as new vaccines become available for such illnesses as RSV and cytomegalovirus, the EHS will be charged with assuring vaccine program implementation and delivery.

REGULAR FOLLOW-UP TESTING AND REVACCINATION

Routine surveillance to exclude infectious diseases is required for only a few illnesses, of which TB is a classic example. Tuberculosis control programs have waned in many developed nations, coincident with the national decrease in numbers of cases of TB. With the sudden rise in TB cases in many US cities in the late 1980s and with the recognition of several dramatic nosocomial outbreaks of the disease, hospitals have scrambled to implement effective TB control programs. These were plagued by poor or absent baseline data, nonspecific boosting as a result of frequent skin testing of employees, and concerns about the lack of effective prophylaxis against multidrug-resistant (MDR) TB.

IMMUNIZATIONS RECOMMENDED FOR HOSPITAL WORKERS			
Immunization against:	Indications	Vaccine dose and schedule	Contraindications
Hepatitis A virus	Employees working in high risk areas (e.g. food service, neonatal intensive care unit) without serologic evidence of previous hepatitis A virus infection	1.0ml im at 0 and 6–12 months	Known hypersensitivity to any component of the vaccine.
Hepatitis B virus	All employees at risk for occupational exposure to blood or body fluids	1.0ml im (deltoid) at 0, 1 and 6 months	Hypersensitivity to yeast
Influenza	All hospital employees	0.5ml im annually	History of anaphylactic reaction to eggs
Measles	Employees with no history of physician-diagnosed measles or no laboratory evidence of immunity	0.5ml subcutaneous of trivalent measles, mumps and rubella vaccine	Pregnancy, history of anaphylactic reaction to eggs or neomycin, severe febrile illness, immunosuppression, recent receipt of iv immunoglobulin
Mumps	Employees without a history of physician-diagnosed mumps, laboratory evidence of immunity, or proof of vaccination on or after their first birthday	As for measles (above)	As for measles (above)
Pneumococcus	Employees over 65 years of age or with underlying cardiac, pulmonary, liver, renal, or immunocompromising disease	0.5ml subcutaneous or im; booster dose every 6–10 years	Safety in pregnancy unknown
Rubella	Employees without verification of live vaccine delivery on or after their first birthday or proof of laboratory immunity	As for measles (above)	As for measles (above)
Tetanus-diphtheria	Employees who have not completed their initial series or who have not received a booster dose within 10 years	Initial series: 0.5ml im at 0, 1 and 6–12 months; booster dose for immunized employees: 0.5ml im every 10 years	History of neurologic or hypersensitivity reaction following a previous dose; first trimester of pregnancy
Varicella	Employees with patient contact who have no history of chickenpox and negative varicella titer	0.5ml at 0 and 4–8 weeks	Hypersensitivity to vaccine, gelatin, neomycin; immunosuppression or immunodeficiency; active tuberculosis; febrile illness; pregnancy

Fig. 11.2 Immunizations recommended for hospital workers. Data from Diekema and Doebbeling, 1995.[4]

The best approach is to maintain an effective ongoing TB control program, both during outbreaks and, as importantly, when no outbreaks are occurring. Such a program should test all tuberculin-negative employees every year, and every 6 months for those in high-risk jobs. Consideration should be given to 'two-step' testing of new employees, especially those who have received BCG vaccination or are older than 40–50 years. This minimizes the potential effect of the booster phenomenon, which is particularly seen in these groups (in serial skin tests the reaction may be 'boosted' in subsequent tests). Prophylaxis with isoniazid should then be offered according to standard guidelines.[15] Chemoprophylaxis for health care workers exposed to patients with isoniazid-resistant MDR-TB is complex and not standardized. This topic is discussed in detail in Chapter 2.30.

The EHS plays a central role in the annual drive to revaccinate against influenza. Despite demonstration of benefit both to health care workers and to patients, compliance rates for influenza vaccination remain poor, generally well below 50%.[16] Compliance rates for vaccinations given during identified outbreaks, such as of measles or pertussis, are much higher.

Recent measles outbreaks among previously vaccinated persons led to recognition of waning vaccine-induced immunity and gave rise to the new recommendation that an additional measles vaccine was necessary before or during teenage years.[17] Because of this observation, many have wondered about the durability of vaccine-induced immunity to infections such as varicella, pertussis and HBV. At present, there is no recommendation extant for routine follow-up surveillance to determine immunity to these vaccine-preventable diseases. However, if outbreaks of diseases continue to occur in well-vaccinated populations, as has been described with pertussis,[18] routine follow-up surveillance to demonstrate immunity may be advisable.[19] With measles programs, repeat serologic testing with targeted revaccination is significantly cheaper than simply vaccinating all workers.[20]

OUTBREAKS CAUSED BY HEALTH CARE WORKERS WHO ARE CARRIERS

Health care workers who are carriers are responsible for the spread of infections to other health care workers and to patients (Fig. 11.3).

Recent reports have documented the spread of HBV[21] and HCV[22] from health care workers to patients. This emphasizes the need for careful guidelines for the potentially infectious health care worker[23] that do not interfere with that person's individual rights.[24] These thorny issues surfaced in the USA in the early 1990s, when the possibility of mandatory testing for HIV of all health care workers was considered by the Centers for Disease Control and Prevention.[25]

Spread of HBV from an occupationally infected surgical resident was recently well-documented by routine and molecular epidemiologic methods.[21] In this report, 19 (13%) out of 144 susceptible persons became infected after receiving surgery from a surface- and e-antigen-positive thoracic surgery resident. Molecular analysis of 13 available strains showed identity with the surgeon's strain. A semiquantitative polymerase chain reaction test of the surgeon's serum revealed more than 1 billion infectious particles per milliliter, suggesting relative contagiousness may be a function of viral load. More importantly from the EHS perspective, the index case had chosen to decline HBV vaccine 2 years before he himself became infected via occupational exposure.

Probable transmission of HCV from a cardiac surgeon to at least five patients who underwent valve replacement was reported from Spain.[22] In this study, molecular analysis showed significant homology between the surgeon's and the patients' virus. The surgeon was treated with interferon-α2b and ribavirin until his HCV RNA level, as measured by polymerase chain reaction, became undetectable. At that point, he was allowed to resume performing surgery.

Nasal carriage of *Staphylococcus aureus*, which is found in 20–90% of health care workers, has been associated with outbreaks of infection, often in intensive care units. Poor handwashing by workers is frequently revealed as the cause. Chronic sinusitis may also contribute.[26] Recently, an additional means of transmission – the 'cloud adult' – has been described.[27] This refers to the occurrence of a viral upper respiratory infection in a patient with established nasal carriage of *S. aureus*. The associated sneezing results in aerosolization of the resistant bacteria, hence the term. In one study, a single 'cloud adult' surgeon was associated with spread of methicillin-resistant *S. aureus* to 8 out of 43 persons in an intensive care unit. The amount of bacteria aerosolized was significantly decreased when the surgeon wore a mask.[27] Nasal carriage can often be eradicated by local application of mupirocin ointment combined with oral ciprofloxacin and rifampin (rifampicin). Early recurrences are seen with this regimen, however, as has occurred with other regimens that have been used through the years. Selective screening of health care workers during nosocomial outbreaks of *S. aureus* infections is recommended.[28]

Outbreaks of group A streptococci traced to a health care worker have frequently been reported.[3] In many circumstances the health care worker is asymptomatic, but cultures of throat, vagina, rectum, or skin yields group A streptococci. When investigating a possible outbreak, it is essential to culture all potential sites routinely. The mode of spread may be by direct contact, via droplet transmission, or, in one report, through infected food.[29]

Dietary workers who are salmonella carriers have spread infection via the hospital kitchen, as may occur in restaurants.[30,31] In one study routine surveillance of all dietary staff failed to prevent a nosocomial outbreak, bringing into question the value of surveillance.[30] Interruption of another outbreak required treatment of all dietary staff with trimethoprim–sulfamethoxazole (co-trimoxazole).[31]

OUTBREAKS DUE TO HEALTH CARE WORKERS WHO ARE ILL

A significant problem is the ill health care worker who continues to work despite feeling ill and thus spreads disease to patients and other staff. Because of their younger age, medical students are particularly likely to be associated with outbreaks of vaccine-preventable infections, such as measles and rubella.[32] In one study, 12% of all health departments had reported that medical students or interns were probably the source case of a nosocomial outbreak of measles or rubella.[33]

Varicella may also be spread by health care workers. In one report, a susceptible pediatric resident failed to report an exposure and continued to work until he himself developed chickenpox.[34] This resulted in exposure of 250 patients or workers and a cost of about $US10,000. No secondary cases of varicella occurred. Recently, the Centers for Disease Control and Prevention and the Advisory Committee on Immunization Practices has recommended but not required varicella vaccination for health care workers.[12] Other methods of decreasing the likelihood of transmission of varicella from health care worker to patient, including wearing masks during the potentially infectious days and taking aciclovir pre-emptively, have also been suggested.[35]

Tuberculosis has been transmitted from staff to patients and to other staff.[36,37] In one report eight health care workers developed active TB, and tuberculin conversion rates ranged from 30% to 48% on wards housing patients with TB.[36] On one ward, transmission from health care worker to health care worker was strongly implicated by molecular fingerprint analysis. Distinction between community and occupational transmission may be difficult in health care workers who also socialize together.[37] Although older reports suggest that compliance with isoniazid prophylaxis in health care workers, particularly physicians, is poor, a recent report showed that more than half of eligible health care workers completed the recommended course of therapy.[38] Furthermore, rates of completion were higher among physicians (74%) than among nonphysicians (48%). The occurrence of several cases of TB among health care workers at this medical center might have resulted in higher compliance rates.

INFECTIONS SPREAD BY HEALTH CARE WORKERS TO PATIENTS OR OTHER HEALTH CARE WORKERS	
Infection	Comment
Hepatitis B virus[20]	e-Antigen positivity and high level of viremia associated with transmission
Hepatitis C virus[21]	Surgeon resumed work following medical control of his hepatitis C infection
Methicillin-resistant *Staphylococcus aureus*[22,23]	'Cloud adult' and chronic sinusits may facilitate spread
Group A streptococci[3]	Carriers may harbor the organism in throat, vagina, rectum, or skin
Salmonella[24,25]	Routine surveillance for dietary workers of unproven benefit
Tuberculosis[26]	Health care workers may spread disease through hospitals
Measles, rubella[27]	Unvaccinated medical students are source of many outbreaks

Fig. 11.3 Infections spread by health care workers to patients or other health care workers.

The well-publicized case of a Florida dentist who apparently spread HIV to at least four patients became the subject of a national debate regarding patients' right to know the health status of their physicians and dentists.[39] Numerous thorough 'look-back' studies of surgeons, other dentists and other practitioners, however, failed to demonstrate transmission.[25]

OCCUPATIONALLY ACQUIRED INFECTIONS IN HEALTH CARE WORKERS

Similar to many other occupations, health care workers are at risk for a wide variety of occupationally acquired illnesses (Fig. 11.4).[35,40] Three relatively simple interventions have been shown through the years to ensure the safety of workers. These include handwashing, vaccination and appropriate isolation of persons with known or suspected infectious diseases. More detailed consideration of this topic has recently been published.[35,40]

BLOOD-BORNE TRANSMISSION
Transmission of bloodborne infections has been the subject of intense scrutiny. Studies have demonstrated that HIV is transmitted in about 0.3% of exposures overall (Fig. 11.5).[41] To date, at least 54 health care workers have developed occupationally acquired HIV and another 132 have probably developed disease from an occupational exposure.[42] Five confirmed cases have been transmitted through mucocutaneous exposure, whereas the others have involved a percutaneous injury.

A recently published retrospective case-control study determined that zidovudine prophylaxis reduced transmission by about 80% compared with placebo (Fig. 11.6).[43] Factors associated with increased risk of transmission included a deep (intramuscular) injury (adjusted OR 15), visible blood on the sharp device (OR 6.2), injury from a needle that had been used to enter a blood vessel (OR 4.3) and a source patient who has terminal AIDS (OR 5.6). New US Public Health Service recommendations have suggested that therapy be tailored to the likelihood of transmission and that a one-, two-, or three-drug combination be selected and given for 1 month.[44] The recommended drugs include zidovudine, lamivudine and the protease inhibitor indinivir. This 14-pill per day regimen costs about $US1000 for medications and monitoring.[45]

The risks and rates of occupationally acquired HBV infection are even more disturbing. The Centers for Disease Control and Prevention estimates that 120–195 health care workers die each year in the USA as a result of occupationally acquired HBV.[46] The rate of transmission

INFECTIOUS DISEASES TRANSMITTED FROM PATIENT TO HEALTH CARE WORKER

Infection		Transmission rate	Comment
Blood-borne	HIV	0.3%	New recommendations include up to three-drug therapy for needlestick injuries
	Hepatitis B virus	e-Antigen negative: 3%	More than 100 health care workers die annually from hepatitis B virus complications
		e-Antigen positive: 30%	Vaccination rates improving
	Hepatitis C virus	3%	No known therapy or prophylaxis
	Cytomegalovirus	Very low	Studies do not demonstrate transmission risk to health care workers
	Ebola	Very high	Health care workers account for >30% of cases in recent outbreaks
Air-borne	Tuberculosis	20–50% in outbreaks	Several deaths from occupationally acquired multidrug-resistant tuberculosis and treatment
	Varicella	5–15%	New vaccine should decrease rates
	Measles	Very high	Physicians and nurses account for majority of occupational cases
	Rubella	13%	Affected health care workers have opted to terminate pregnancy
	Parvovirus B19	>25%	Spread is less dramatic than in schools
	Respiratory syncytial virus	>40%	Infection control interventions decreased spread to patients but not to health care workers
	Adenovirus	>20%	May be spread for efficiently if source case intubated
	Pertussis	43%	Spread in one outbreak to 87 health care workers (2% of all health care workers)
Enteric	Hepatitis A virus	20%	Vaccine now available
	Salmonella	5–20%	May spread to health care worker from food, excretions or from patient
	Helicobacter pylori	Unknown	Implications of higher seroprevalence among endoscopists unknown
	Norwalk virus	>50%	Extremely high rates of spread for nursing assistants
	Cryptosporidia	>30%	Animal handlers at particular risk
	Clostridium difficile	Unknown	One health care worker died of apparently occupationally acquired *Clostridium difficile* infection

Fig. 11.4 Infectious diseases transmitted from patient to health care worker. Data from Sepkowitz, 1996.[35,40]

is determined by the e-antigen status of the source case (about 3% for an e-antigen-negative and 30% for an e-antigen-positive source case).[47] A recent estimate has suggested that the annual number of deaths among health care workers may be decreasing, as a result of improved vaccine compliance.[11]

The morbidity and mortality of occupationally acquired HCV is not yet well defined. Transmission occurs in about 3% of percutaneous exposures.[40,48] The rate of progression of HCV to chronic liver disease, including cirrhosis, appears in excess of 80% for all patients.[49] The lack of an effective vaccine, therapy, or prophylaxis makes this disease of increasing concern for health care workers.[50]

Recent outbreaks of various viral hemorrhagic fevers, including Ebola virus, affected large numbers of health care workers in the treating hospitals.[40] Cytomegalovirus is a concern to pregnant health care workers, but recent studies have not demonstrated an increased rate of disease transmission to pediatric nurses or to other health care workers.[9,40]

AIR-BORNE TRANSMISSION

The risk of caring for patients with TB was demonstrated recently in the USA during several large hospital-based outbreaks of MDR-TB.[51] In these outbreaks at least 20 health care workers developed clinical MDR-TB,[52] whereas hundreds of others became latently infected and will remain at risk for re-activation disease during the decades ahead. At least one health care worker has died because of drug toxicity from a second-line regimen given for her MDR-TB[53] and several others have died of MDR-TB itself.[52] Recommendations for preventing transmission of TB in hospitals stress the need to place suspected cases into effective isolation.[9,15]

The introduction of the varicella vaccine should change the infection control strategy for containing VZV infection at many hospitals.[2,12] Transmission rates are poorly defined, but the incidence of new cases among susceptible individuals may exceed 10% per year if no

precautions are taken.[2,35] In addition, the problem of a potentially infectious health care worker is discussed above.

Measles virus may enter a hospital from the community or spread to the community from a hospital-based outbreak. Attack rates among susceptible individuals are high, vaccine failures occur, and physicians and nurses are at highest risk. Outbreaks of rubella[54] and parvovirus B19[55] are of particular concern to pregnant employees, because both infections may affect fetal development. Some health care workers in rubella outbreaks have opted to terminate pregnancies.[54] Transmission of RSV, adenovirus and pertussis to health care workers has been well-documented and probably occurs much more frequently than has been reported.[35]

FECAL–ORAL TRANSMISSION

Nosocomial outbreaks of hepatitis A virus with spread to health care workers have occasionally been reported, often from neonatal intensive care units. A recent report described an outbreak traced to a child with an immune defect that prevented a detectable antibody response to hepatitis A virus.[56] This delayed serodiagnosis resulted in spread to 15% of the staff, a rate similar to that in other outbreaks.

Salmonella may spread in hospitals in numerous ways: from a point source, such as contaminated food; from patient to health care worker; and from contact with contaminated excretions. As noted above, routine surveillance of hospital dietary employees may not be effective.[30,31] In addition to nurses, laundry workers appear at increased risk.[57]

Other common enteric infections such as Norwalk virus and cryptosporidiosis may spread to workers.[40] Norwalk virus, a small round structured virus, is particularly contagious, and may affect more than 90% of health care workers in close contact. A recent case of occupationally acquired *Clostridium difficile* diarrhea resulted in toxic megacolon and death in the health care worker concerned.[58] The clinical implications of elevated seroprevalence to *Helicobacter pylori* among persons who perform endoscopy are unknown.[40]

RISK CATEGORIES OF EXPOSURE TO POSSIBLE SOURCES OF HIV INFECTION

Exposure category	Definition
Highest risk – known HIV+ or highly suspect source	Device/needle/sharp from artery/vein/CSF/ pleural/pericardial/synovial fluids of source patient and penetrating injury to health care worker (blood evidence) and deep injury caused by hollow needle ≤21g or scalpel glass injury
High risk – known HIV+ or suspect source	Device/needle/sharp from artery/vein/CSF/ pleural/pericardial/synovial fluids of source patient and penetrating injury to health care worker (blood evidence)
Middle risk – known HIV+ or suspect source	Mucous membrane exposure to potentially infectious fluid or prolonged skin exposure (>5 minutes) to infectious fluid or skin exposure (with extensive skin-breaks) to infectious fluid or needle/sharp injury after subcutaneous injections from source patient
Low risk – known HIV+ or suspect source	Small volume of potentially infectious fluid, brief contact
No risk	Any type of exposure to urine, stool, vomit, tears, saliva or sweat

Fig. 11.5 Risk categories of exposure to possible sources of HIV infection.

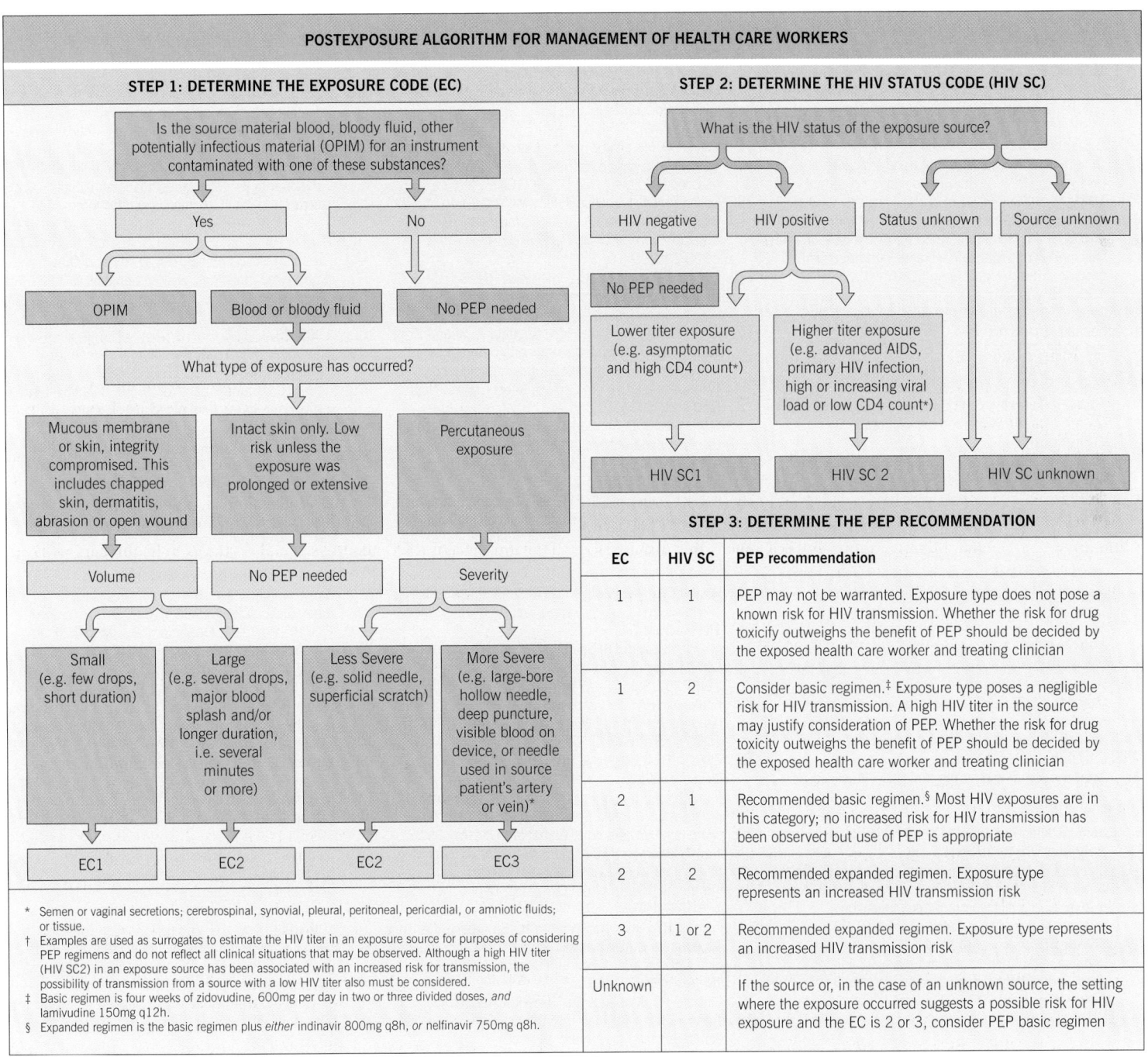

Fig. 11.6 Postexposure algorithm for management of health care workers who have been exposed to a known or suspected case of HIV. PEP, post-exposure prophylaxis; EC, exposure code, SC, status code.

REFERENCES

1. Weber DJ, Rutala WA. Management of healthcare workers exposed to pertussis. Infect Control Hosp Epidemiol 1994;15:411–5.

2. Weber DJ, Rutala WA, Hamilton H. Prevention and control of varicella-zoster infections in healthcare facilities. Infect Control Hosp Epidemiol 1996;17:694–705.

3. Weber DJ, Rutala WA, Denny FW. Management of healthcare workers with pharyngitis or suspected streptococcal infections. Infect Control Hosp Epidemiol 1996;17:753–61.

4. Diekema DJ, Doebbeling BN. Employee health and infection control. Infect Control Hosp Epidemiol 1995;16:292–301.

5. Lewy R. Visits to a hospital-based employee health service. J Occupat Med 1986;28:241–2.

6. Yannelli B, Gurevich I, Richardson J, Gianelli B, Cunha BA. Significance of fever in hospital employees. Am J Infect Control 1990;18:93–8.

7. Lewy R. Organization and conduct of a hospital occupational health service. Occupat Med 1987;2:617–49.

8. Centers for Disease Control and Prevention. Immunization of Health-Care Workers: recommendations of the Advisory Committee on Immunization Practices (ACIP) and the Hospital Infection Control Practices Advisory Committee (HICPAC). MMWR Morb Mortal Wkly Rep 1997;46(RR-18):1–42.

9. Bolyard EA, Tablan OC, Williams WW, et al. Guideline for infection control in health care personnel, 1998. Infect Control Hosp Epidemiol 1998;19:407–63.

10. Agerton TB, Mahoney FJ, Polish LB, Shapiro CN. Impact of the bloodborne pathogens standard on vaccination of healthcare workers with hepatitis B vaccine. Infect Control Hosp Epidemiol 1995;16:287–91.

11. Shapiro CN. Occupational risk of infection with hepatitis B and hepatitis C virus. Surg Clin North Am 1995;75:1047–56.

12. Advisory Committee on Immunization Practices. Prevention of varicella: recommendations of the Advisory Committee on Immunization Practices (ACIP). MMWR Morb Mortal Wkly Rep 1996;45(RR-11):13–5.

13. Hoge CW, Reichler MR, Dominguez EA, et al. An epidemic of pneumococcal disease in an overcrowded, inadequately ventilated jail. N Engl J Med 1992;331:643–8.

14. Nuorti JP, Butler JC, Crutcher JM, et al. An outbreak of multidrug-resistant pneumococcal pneumonia and bacteremia among unvaccinated nursing home residents. N Eng J Med 1998;338:1861–8.

15. Guidelines for preventing the transmission of Mycobacterium tuberculosis in health-care facilities, 1994. MMWR Morb Mortal Wkly Rep 1994;43(RR-13):1–132.

16. Heimberger T, Chang H-G, Shaikh M, Crotty L, Morse D, Birkhead G. Knowledge and attitudes of healthcare workers about influenza: why are they not getting vaccinated. Infect Control Hosp Epidemiol 1995;16:412–4.

17. Advisory Committee on Immunization Practices. General recommendations on immunization: recommendations of the Advisory Committee on Immunization Practices (ACIP). MMWR Morb Mortal Wkly Rep 1994;43(RR-1):1–38.

18. Christie CD, Marx ML, Marchant CD, Reising SF. The 1993 epidemic of pertussis in Cincinnati. Resurgence of disease in a highly immunized population of children. N Engl J Med 1994;331:16–21.

19. Christie CDC, Glover AM, Willke MJ, et al. Containment of pertussis in the regional pediatric hospital during the greater Cincinnati epidemic of 1993. Infect Control Hosp Epidemiol 1995;16:556–63.

20. Stover BH, Adams G, Kuebler CA, Cost KM, Rabalais GP. Measles–mumps–rubella immunization of susceptible hospital employees during a community measles outbreak: cost-effectiveness and protective efficacy. Infect Control Hosp Epidemiol 1994;15:18–21.

21. Harpaz R, von Seidlen L, Averhoff FM, et al. Transmission of hepatitis B virus to multiple patients from a surgeon without evidence of inadequate infection control. N Engl J Med 1996;334:549–54.

22. Esteban JI, Gomez J, Martell M, et al. Transmission of hepatitis C virus by a cardiac surgeon. N Engl J Med 1996; 334:555–60.

23. Recommendations for preventing transmission of human immunodeficiency virus and hepatitis B virus to patients during exposure-prone invasive procedures. MMWR Morb Mortal Wkly Rep 1991;40(RR-8):1–9.

24. Gerberding JL. The infected health care provider. N Engl J Med 1996;334:594–5.

25. Henderson DK. HIV screening for healthcare providers: can we provide sense and sensibility without pride or prejudice? Infect Control Hosp Epidemiol 1994;15:631–4.

26. Boyce JM, Opal SM, Potter-Bynoe G, Medeiros AA. Spread of methicillin-resistant Staphylococcus aureus in a hospital after exposure to a health care worker with chronic sinusitis. Clin Infect Dis 1993;17:496–504.

27. Sheretz RJ, Reagan DR, Hampton KD, et al. A cloud adult: the Staphylococcus aureus–virus interaction revisited. Ann Intern Med 1996;124:539–47.

28. Lessing MPA, Jordens JZ, Bowler ICJ. When should healthcare workers be screened for methicillin-resistant Staphylococcus aureus? J Hosp Infect 1996;34:205–10.

29. Decker MD, Lavely GB, Hutcheson RH, Schaffner W. Food-borne streptococcal pharyngitis in a hospital pediatrics clinic. JAMA 1985;253:679–81.

30. Khuri-Bulos NA, Khalaf MA, Shenabi A, Shami K. Foodhandler-associated salmonella outbreak in a university hospital despite routine surveillance cultures of kitchen employees. Infect Control Hosp Epidemiol 1994;15:311–4.

31. Linnemann CC, Cannon CG, Staneck JL, McNeely BL. Prolonged hospital epidemic of salmonellosis: use of trimethoprim–sulfamethoxazole for control. Infect Control 1985;6:221–5.

32. Kelley PW, Petruccelli BP, Stehr-Green P, Erickson RL, Mason CJ. The susceptibility of young adult Americans to vaccine-preventable infections: a national serosurvey of US Army recruits. JAMA 1991;266:2724–9.

33. Poland GA, Nichol KL. Medical students as sources of rubella and measles outbreaks. Arch Intern Med 1990;150:44–6

34. Miller PJ, Landry S, Searcy MA, Hunt E, Wenzel RP. Cost of varicella epidemic [letter]. Pediatrics 1985;75:989.

35. Sepkowitz KA. Occupationally-acquired infections in health care workers. Part I. Ann Intern Med 1996;125:826–34.

36. Zaza S, Blumberg HM, Beck-Sague C, et al. Nosocomial transmission of Mycobacterium tuberculosis: role of health care workers in outbreak propogation. J Infect Dis 1995;172:1542–9.

37. Blumberg HM, Moore P, Blanchard DK, Ray SM. Transmission of Mycobacterium tuberculosis among health care workers infected with human immunodeficiency virus. Clin Infect Dis 1996;22:597–8.

38. Camins BC, Bock N, Watkins DL, Blumberg HM. Acceptance of isoniazid preventive therapy by health care workers after tuberculin skin test conversion. JAMA 1996;275:1013–5.

39. Ciesielski C, Marianos D, Chin-Yih O, et al. Transmission of human immunodeficiency virus in a dental practice. Ann Intern Med 1992;116:798–805.

40. Sepkowitz KA. Occupationally-acquired infections in health care workers. Part II. Ann Intern Med 1996;125:917–28.

41. Marcus R and the CDC Cooperative Needlestick Surveillance Group. Surveillance of health care workers exposed to blood from patients infected with the human immunodeficiency virus. N Engl J Med 1988;319:1118–23.

42. Ippolito G, Puro V, De Carli G, and the Italian Study Group on Occupational Risk of HIV Infection. The risk of occupational human immunodeficiency virus infection in health care workers: Italian Multicenter Study. Arch Intern Med 1993;153:1451–8.

43. Case-control study of HIV seroconversion in health-care workers after percutaneous exposure to HIV-infected blood—France, United Kingdom, and United States, January 1988–August 1994. MMWR Morb Mortal Wkly Rep 1995;44:929–33.

44. Public Health Service. Update: provisional Public Health Service recommendations for chemoprophylaxis after occupational exposure to HIV. MMWR Morb Mortal Wkly Rep 1996;45:468–80.

45. Gerberding JL. Prophylaxis for occupational exposure to HIV. Ann Intern Med 1996;125:497–501.

46. Mast EE, Alter MJ. 'Prevention of hepatitis B virus infection among health-care workers.' In: Ellis RW, ed. Hepatitis B vaccines in clinical practice. New York: Marcel Dekker, Inc.; 1993:295–307.

47. Werner BG, Grady GF. Accidental hepatitis-B-surface-antigen-positive inoculations: use of e antigen to estimate infectivity. Ann Intern Med 1982;97:367–9.

48. Puro V, Petrosillo N, Ippolito G, and the Italian Study Group on Occupational Risk of HIV and Other Bloodborne Infections. Risk of hepatitis C seroconversion after occupational exposures in health care workers. Am J Infect Control 1995;23:273–7.

49. Sharara AI, Hunt CM, Hamilton JD. Hepatitis C. Ann Intern Med 1996;125:658–68.

50. Alter MJ. Occupational exposure to hepatitis C virus: a dilemma. Infect Control Hosp Epidemiol 1994;15:742–4.

51. Nosocomial transmission of multidrug-resistant tuberculosis among HIV-infected persons—Florida and New York. MMWR Morb Mortal Wkly Rep 1991;40:585–91.

52. Sepkowitz KA. AIDS, tuberculosis, and the health care worker. Clin Infect Dis 1995;20:232–42.

53. Weltman AC, DiFerdinando GT Jr, Washko R, Lipsky WM. A death associated with therapy for nosocomially acquired multidrug-resistant tuberculosis. Chest 1996;110:279–81.

54. Polk BF, White JA, DeGirolami PC, Modlin JF. An outbreak of rubella among hospital personnel. N Engl J Med 1980;303:541–5.

55. Bell LM, Naides SJ, Stoffman P, Hodinka RL, Plotkin SA. Human parvovirus B19 infection among hospital staff members after contact with infected patients. N Engl J Med 1989;321:485–91.

56. Burkholder BT, Coronado VG, Brown J, et al. Nosocomial transmission of hepatitis A in a pediatric hospital traced to an anti-hepatitis A virus-negative patient with immunodeficiency. Pediatr Infect Dis J 1995;14:261–6.

57. Standaert SM, Hutcheson RH, Schaffner W. Nosocomial transmission of salmonella gastroenteritis to laundry workers in a nursing home. Infect Control Hosp Epidemiol 1994;15:22–6.

58. Mathis S, Venkataraman L, Scheckman P, DeGirolami P, Samore M. Nosocomial outbreak of unusually severe C. difficile diarrhea with presumptive transmission to a health care worker [abstract S20]. Infect Control Hosp Epidemiol 1996;17:P32.

Recreational Infections

Alastair Miller

INTRODUCTION

It has been widely predicted that advancing technology will usher in an 'Age of Leisure', and people are spending their free time in increasingly varied and imaginative fashions. This chapter examines how these activities expose them to increased risks of infection and disease. As with many other factors that predispose to clinical infection, recreational behavior may either expose the host to infective organisms or modify the host's immune response, thereby increasing susceptibility to infection and disease. Recreational infection can be classified according to the activity that increases the risk of infection or according to the particular infections (or systems infected; Fig. 12.1) Inevitably there is considerable overlap with other sections of this book, such as Geographic and Travel Medicine (Section 6), Sexually Transmitted Diseases (Chapters 2.63–2.68) and Zoonotic Infections (Chapters 6.34 & 8.11).

TRAVEL

Travel is a common recreational activity either as an end in itself or in order to participate in other recreations. Travelers may be exposed to infection either during the journey or at their destination. During travel there may be exposure to gastrointestinal pathogens in mass-produced food or exposure to respiratory pathogens from air-conditioning units and fellow travelers. In addition the general fatigue of long-distance travel may perhaps lower resistance to infection in a nonspecific manner.

Outbreaks of food poisoning from airline food occur frequently and are well described,[1] and even cholera has been transmitted in this way.[2] On cruise ships, outbreaks of gastrointestinal illness have been caused by contaminated food and water,[3] and in addition there have been descriptions of more prolonged outbreaks of infection associated with the possibility of person-to-person transmission and environmental contamination. This type of outbreak is usually thought to be due to viral infection with organisms such as Norwalk agent or small round structured viruses.[4,5]

RECREATIONAL ACTIVITIES ASSOCIATED WITH RISKS OF INFECTION	
Activity	**Risk**
Travel	Infection during travel: gastrointestinal respiratory pathogens
	Geographic (tropical) infection
'Outdoor' recreation: hiking, backpacking, trekking, barbecues, etc.	Zoonoses: ingestion, inhalation, inoculation, arthropod spread
Water contact: jacuzzi, bathing, nonbathing water activity (wind surfing, canoeing, sailing, etc.)	Inhalation, inoculation, ingestion (see Fig. 12.2)
Contact sport: rugby, football, etc.	Skin infections, blood-borne pathogens
Strenuous exercise	Upper respiratory infection (possibly; see Fig. 12.3)

Fig. 12.1 Recreational activities associated with risks of infection.

Respiratory infection, including multidrug-resistant pulmonary tuberculosis, has also been transmitted during aircraft flight,[6,7] and there is a well-recognized association between outbreaks of *Legionella* infection and air-conditioning systems in holiday hotels.[8]

Western travelers are increasingly seeking more exotic destinations where, as a result of poverty and poor infrastructure in the local population, they may be at risk of infection with common pathogens (particularly of the gastrointestinal and respiratory tracts). They may also be at risk of more exotic infections that do not exist in their own country (e.g. malaria). By the nature of the travel, the patient with infection often may not have access to the level of diagnostic and therapeutic interventions that would be regarded as standard in the developed world, so empiric treatment of presumed infections is often required. These risks are discussed in detail in Chapter 6.2.

ZOONOSES

Zoonoses are infections of animals which can be transmitted to humans, who may act either as a dead-end host or may propagate the infection further. The resulting infection may or may not be clinically apparent. This topic is addressed in Chapters 6.24, 6.34, 8.8 and 8.11, but issues specifically related to recreation are discussed here. Many leisure activities increase the opportunity for contact between humans and animals, with consequent increased risk of infection.

Hiking and camping (particularly light-weight 'back packing') increase the risk of zoonoses. People may hike in a temperate climate or, increasingly, may choose to trek in a tropical or developing country. These activities increase the potential for contact with infected animals. Infection can then be transmitted by a number of possible routes such as:
- inhalation (e.g. 'Q' fever, anthrax);
- ingestion of contaminated food or water (e.g. *Salmonella*, *Brucella*);
- animal bites (e.g. rabies, skin infections);
- exposure of skin to contaminated water (e.g. leptospirosis, schistosomiasis); and
- via arthropod vectors (e.g. arboviruses, Lyme disease).

ZOONOTIC INFECTION ACQUIRED BY INHALATION
Inhaled zoonoses that can be acquired by the intrepid outdoor explorer include Q fever (caused by *Coxiella burnetii*) and brucellosis (more commonly acquired by ingestion). Rarer problems include plague, anthrax, tularemia and psittacosis.[9]

ZOONOTIC INFECTION ACQUIRED BY INGESTION
Many of the common 'food poisoning' organisms are zoonoses, and these are discussed in detail in Chapters 2.35, 6.3, 6.22, 6.24 and 6.25. However, there are certain recreational activities that particularly expose participants to increased risks of ingesting pathogenic organisms (which are often zoonotic, although they may be exclusively human parasites). Backpackers drinking inadequately boiled or purified water may become infected with *Cryptosporidium* spp., *Giardia* spp., hepatitis A, *Aeromonas* spp., and *Salmonella* spp. Barbecues are particularly notorious for leading to inadequately cooked meat (or fish) and consequent infection with *Salmonella* spp.,[10] *Campylobacter*

spp.,[11] and other more exotic organisms such as *Trichinella* spp. There have been well documented outbreaks of cryptosporidial infection in children having recreational visits to farm open days.[12,13]

ARTHROPOD-BORNE ZOONOSES

Viruses that must spend some of their lifecycle in a blood-sucking arthropod are known as arboviruses (see Chapter 8.11). Over 200 such viruses have been identified and over 70 have been reported as affecting humans. In 1994, 100 cases of presumed or confirmed arboviral disease were reported from 20 states of the USA.[14] These were all encephalitis viruses (mainly Californian and St Louis encephalitis), principally spread by mosquitoes. One case of tick-borne encephalitis (Powassan disease) was reported. Yellow fever is a life-threatening mosquito-borne, zoonotic viral infection and the illness remains a risk for travelers and residents during outdoor activites in endemic regions in Africa and south America In Europe, tick-borne encephalitis is regularly reported from Austria and southern Germany.[15] A major risk factor is outdoor recreation (in particular, walking through long grass while wearing short trousers). An inactivated vaccine is available.

Tick-borne rickettsiae (see Chapters 6.34Rickettsia & 8.24) are also potential pathogens among those who enjoy 'the great outdoors'.[16] They are mainly of the spotted fever group. In southern Europe, Africa and India, the disease is called tick typhus or boutonneuse fever and is caused by *Rickettsia conorii*. In the USA, it is Rocky Mountain spotted fever, caused by *Rickettsia rickettsii*. New rickettsioses identified during the past decade include Japanese spotted fever, Astrakhan fever, Flinders Island spotted fever, California flea typhus, African tick-site fever and *R. slovaca* infections in central France.

Scrub typhus may affect the trekker in eastern Asia. The infective organism is *R. tsutsugamushi*. The reservoir is rodents and the vector is the larva (chigger) of the trombiculid mite. Clinically the disease resembles other rickettsial infections, and prevention and treatment strategies are similar.

Lyme disease (see Chapter 2.45), caused by infection with *Borrelia burgdorferi*, is another condition that may be acquired by recreational exposure. The reservoir consists of mammals such as rodents and deer, with infection being spread by hard ticks (the *Ixodes ricinus* complex).

INFECTIONS CAUSED BY EXPOSURE TO WATER

A large number of infections can be caused by exposure to water (Fig. 12.2), and some of these have already been discussed in the section on zoonoses. Exposure to water can take place in a variety of recreational contexts. Trekkers and fishermen may wade through infected water, people may bathe in fresh water or sea water, and people may undertake other nonbathing recreational activities in water (e.g. water skiing, sailing, canoeing). There is also an increasing popularity of spa baths, whirlpool baths and jacuzzis.

As with arthropod-borne infections, infections related to water may be acquired by a number of routes, including ingestion, aspiration, inhalation of aerosols, and penetration of skin or mucous membranes by invasive organisms. A variety of clinical infections, including gastrointestinal infection, hepatitis, conjunctivitis, skin and soft tissue infection, pneumonia, may result, and numerous diverse organisms have been implicated.

Pathogenic organisms may enter the water from exogenous sources such as human contamination (sewage, etc.), animal and bird contamination, and farm effluent. Organisms may also come directly from aquatic animals or protozoa or be free living in the water supply.

INFECTION ASSOCIATED WITH WHIRLPOOLS

Jacuzzis, whirlpool baths, and spa baths, which are increasingly found in leisure resorts, are all based on the principle of being bathed in warm water through which jets of water and bubbles of air are blown in order to produce feelings of relaxation and pleasure. They therefore share the potential for the transmission of cutaneous, mucosal and respiratory infection. The main pathogens implicated in these infections are *Pseudomonas aeruginosa* and *Legionella pneumophila*. *Pseudomonas* infections of the skin were initially described in the early 1980s.[17] The first reports were of folliculitis, but infection of wounds, eyes, ears and urinary tract have now been described.[18] Fatal *Pseudomonas* pneumonia in an immunocompetent male has recently been associated with jacuzzi exposure.[19]

Legionella spp. (mainly *L. pneumophila*, but other species are also implicated) cause two distinct syndromes: legionnaires' disease (or legionnaires' pneumonia), which is usually a severe pneumonic illness requiring appropriate antibiotic treatment and Pontiac fever, which is generally a more benign self-limiting illness causing myalgia, fever and headache. The latter syndrome has frequently been associated with whirlpool use, although a prolonged outbreak of legionnaires' pneumonia among cruise ship passengers associated with exposure to a contaminated whirlpool spa has been described.[20]

INFECTION FROM BATHING

Numerous case reports and reviews have associated bathing in swimming pools, natural fresh water and the sea with gastrointestinal, respiratory and cutaneous infection. In swimming pools there have been reports of infection with *Shigella*, *Giardia* and *Cryptosporidium* spp., and various viruses including hepatitis A virus.[21]

The association of sea bathing and disease is a major political issue as millions of dollars are spent in the developed countries in an effort

INFECTIONS SPREAD BY RECREATIONAL CONTACT WITH WATER				
Mode of spread	Organisms			
	Bacteria	Viruses	Protozoa	Helminths
Fecal–oral spread (accidental ingestion)	*Vibrio* spp. *Salmonella* spp. *Campylobacter* spp. *Aeromonas* spp. *Escherichia coli* *Shigella* spp.	Enteroviruses (including polio) Hepatitis A Small round structured viruses	*Cryptosporidia* *Giardia*	
Spread by direct inoculation	*Pseudomonas* spp. *Aeromonas* spp. *Vibrio* spp. *Mycobacterium marinum* *Leptospira* spp.		*Acanthamoeba* *Naegleria*	*Schistosoma*
Spread by aerosol or aspiration	*Legionella* spp. *Pseudomonas* spp.	Adenoviruses		

Fig. 12.2 Infections spread by recreational contact with water.

to improve sewage disposal and enhance the 'quality' of bathing water. Microbiologic standards now exist for bathing water in Europe and North America. There is certainly a risk of infection from swimming in heavily contaminated water but the risk of minor symptomatic infection from swimming in less heavily polluted water remains contentious.[22] In the 1950s the UK Public Health Laboratory Service used a case-controlled method and showed no link between polio and sea bathing.[23] Cabelli's classic work under the aegis of the US Environmental Protection Agency in the 1970s suggested a dose–response relationship between the microbiologic contamination of bathing water and self-reporting of gastrointestinal symptoms.[24] These studies have been criticized for looking at self-reported symptoms in self-selected groups, with no control for other risk factors for gastrointestinal symptoms.

More recently, a large UK study attempted to address these criticisms by randomizing holiday makers to be 'swimmers' or 'nonswimmers'.[25] This study showed a significantly higher rate of gastroenteritis in the swimmers and demonstrated a dose–response relationship between occurrence of symptoms and concentrations of fecal streptococci (although only with the concentration measured at chest height). Currently, coliform counts are used to assess water quality and the authors of the above study could not demonstrate a correlation between symptoms and the coliform count.

In addition to gastroenteritis, an Australian study showed increased reporting of respiratory, eye and ear symptoms amongst swimming beach-goers as opposed to nonswimming ones. The incidence of the reported symptoms increased with increasing levels of pollution.[26] The authors of the UK study have now published their results of nonenteric illness acquired during bathing and their results are in broad agreement with those of the Australian study.[27]

INFECTION IN NONSWIMMING RECREATIONAL WATER ACTIVITIES

In addition to the hazards of bathing detailed above, many people are exposed to infection by recreational use of water where swimming is not the primary purpose. Such activities include angling, canoeing, water skiing, sailing and white water rafting.

Leptospirosis (see Chapters 6.34 Leptospirosis & 8.19) is traditionally regarded as a significant risk. It is estimated that on average in the UK there are 5 million recreational water users each year exclusive of bathers, and yet among this at-risk population there are only 2.5 cases of leptospirosis a year.[28] The annual total incidence of leptospirosis in England and Wales is more than 10 times that figure; it occurs principally among agricultural workers. Leptospirosis is a zoonotic infection that is mainly carried by rodents. It is estimated that about 25% of the rats in UK are infected. The risk of contracting infection relates less to the overall water quality than to the density of the local rodent population.

By the nature of the sport, canoeing involves high level exposure to water and, in addition to leptospirosis, other infections can be acquired. There is an increased incidence of gastrointestinal symptoms, and it has been shown that more than 50% of canoeists had experienced 'flu-like' symptoms shortly after canoeing.[29]

MISCELLANEOUS WATER-RELATED INFECTIONS

Naegleria and *Acanthamoeba* spp. are free-living amebae with no insect vector or human carrier state. They have been isolated on a worldwide basis from water and soil, and rarely they produce a severe amebic meningoencephalitis that is usually fatal (see Chapter 8.33). Schistosomiasis is dealt with in detail in Chapter 6.27. The cercaria of human schistosomes penetrate intact human skin and then migrate to their favored site to commence their maturation. Within 24 hours the penetration of the skin can produce a pruritic papular rash that is called 'swimmers itch'. Avian schistosomes are found in temperate climates, including in the Great Lakes of North America, and although they are unable to mature past the cercarial stage in a human host and therefore cannot give rise to later stage schistosomiasis, they can be responsible for producing a significant 'swimmers itch'.

Katayama fever occurs typically 4–8 weeks after infection and is associated with fever, chills, headache and cough. There is hepatosplenomegaly and lymphadenopathy, and usually a significant eosinophilia. It is caused both by *Schistosoma japonicum* and *S. mansoni*, the latter being particularly recognized in swimmers who have bathed in lake Malawi and the other rivers and lakes in East Africa.

INFECTION SPREAD BY DIRECT CONTACT

Many sports require close physical contact on the sports field and may also involve close contact in the changing rooms with shared towels, shaving equipment, etc. Tetanus is caused by contamination of a wound by the spores of *Clostridium tetani*. After contamination, the organism then elaborates a toxin that produces the clinical syndrome of tetanus. Although immunization against tetanus is widely practised there is still a risk to those playing contact sports (especially rugby and football), as well as to those pursuing more leisurely activities such as gardening.

The close contact in the scrum of rugby football may transmit herpes simplex virus and cause a condition called scrumpox or herpes gladiotorium. This is highly infectious and may spread rapidly between players. Acyclovir is effective treatment.

The moist atmosphere of changing rooms may promote the transmission of respiratory infections as well as a number of cutaneous infections such as verrucas, athletes foot (*Tinea pedis*) and Dhobie's itch (*Tinea cruris*). The spread of these tineal infections may be facilitated by sharing towels and washing equipment.

Gardening is usually considered a fairly safe past-time, but tetanus is a potential risk and sporotrichosis (see Chapter 8.28) can be acquired by scratches from rose thorns and similar injuries.

BLOOD-BORNE INFECTION TRANSMISSION IN CONTACT SPORT

The risk of transmission of blood-borne pathogens during contact sport is thought to be extremely low. There were large outbreaks of hepatitis amongst orienteers in Sweden from 1956 to 1966, and on the basis of the clinical and epidemiologic picture these were assumed to be due to hepatitis B virus (HBV), although a serologic test was not available.[30] As part of these outbreaks, five hundred and sixty-eight cases of hepatitis occurred between 1957 and 1963; several modes of transmission were postulated, including twigs contaminated with infected blood inoculating subsequent competitors, contaminated water in stagnant pools and transmission during washing after competition. It was established that 95% of orienteers received scratches or wounds during the competition. The outbreak was curtailed by the introduction of regulations that banned competitors who had hepatitis from competing for 15 months and that specified compulsory protective clothing. More cases were reported when these regulations were relaxed. There has also been a report of an outbreak of HBV infection among sumo wrestlers in Japan.[31] There is one report from Italy of an HIV-positive football player transmitting infection to another player during a collision when both players were bleeding profusely,[32] but the risks are generally considered to be negligible.

Numerous guidelines exist to limit the risk still further[31] – in rugby football, for example, a player with an open or bleeding wound must leave the field until the wound is covered and the bleeding controlled.

EFFECT OF EXERCISE ON THE IMMUNE SYSTEM

Although it is clear from the above that recreational activity can expose participants to numerous infective agents that they might not otherwise encounter, it is by no means so obvious whether recreation (in particular, vigorous exercise) has any clinically significant effect on immune function.[33] There is increasing evidence that physical exercise may bring benefit in terms of cardiovascular health. However, the evidence from the immunologic perspective is less obvious.

There are numerous anecdotal reports of increased incidence of upper respiratory infection in athletes and there have been attempts to examine this systematically. However, despite numerous reviews there is no consistent association between physical activity and incidence of clinical upper respiratory infection. Nor has any consistent immunologic abnormality been demonstrated in high-level athletes. This inconsistency has many parallels with the situation in chronic fatigue syndrome, and many top athletes who have recurrent infections develop a clinical condition indistinguishable from chronic fatigue syndrome.

The overall message from anecdotal reports, from case–controlled studies of symptoms, from animal studies and from laboratory test of immune function seems to be that moderate regular exercise enhances immunity whereas sudden unusual exertion or consistent, very high-grade training may have a deleterious effect. This is described as the 'J-shaped curve' correlating exercise and immunity.[33] Animal studies suggest that exercising before infection is beneficial, whereas exercising when infected is harmful. Some of the reported immunologic effects of exercise are listed in Figure 12.3.

It is generally advised that people who are suffering from acute infections do not participate in vigorous exercise. This seems common sense and most people would probably not feel like doing so, although definite evidence of harm remains contentious.

CONCLUSION

Recreational activities can expose participants to novel infectious agents that they are less likely to encounter in other contexts. In many of these the diagnosis may not be very obvious unless the condition is considered. Physicians need to add 'recreational history' to the already extensive list of travel, occupational and animal exposure details about which they need to enquire when evaluating a patient with a putative infection. Whether recreational activity can alter immune function remains more contentious, although there seems to be increasing consensus that regular physical exercise may be of benefit but that excessive exercise may increase risks of infection.

EFFECTS OF EXERCISE ON THE IMMUNE SYSTEM	
Symptoms/self-reported infections (anecdote and case–control)	Most studies suggest that moderate regular exercise reduces frequency and severity of upper respiratory tract infections but excessive training increases it
	Many studies are subjective and it may be that athletes are more aware of their symptoms than are controls
	Some increase in infection may be due to local factors such as mouth breathing rather than to any change in systemic immunity
Animal studies	Exhaustive exercise during experimental viral infection increases mortality and morbidity from that viral infection; the effect may be attenuated by exercise prior to infection Similar results have been shown in pneumococcal infection – exercise prior to infection protected against mortality but forced exercise after infection enhanced mortality
Immune function studies	Moderate exercise in HIV-positive people has been shown to produce some increase in CD4$^+$ lymphocyte count Excessive training in non-HIV-infected people has been shown to suppress CD4$^+$ lymphocyte counts
	Heavy exercise decreases lymphocyte proliferation and levels of IgA; the decreased levels of IgA may correlate with increased incidence of upper respiratory tract infections
	Regular moderate exercise will increase levels of natural killer lymphocytes
	Exercise generally increases the release of proinflammatory cytokines and acute phase proteins

Fig. 12.3 Effects of exercise on the immune system.

REFERENCES

1. Sockett P, Ries A, Wieneke AA. Food poisoning associated with in-flight meals. Commun Dis Rep CDR Rev 1993;3:103–420.
2. Eberhart-Phillips J, Besser RE, Tormey MP, et al. An outbreak of cholera from food served on an international aircraft. Epidemiol Infect 1996;116:9–13.
3. Mersom MH, Hughes JM, Wood BT, Yashik JC, Wells JG. Gasrointestinal illness on passanger cruise ships, 1986 through 1993. JAMA 1975;231:723–7.
4. McEvoy M, Blake W, Brown D, Green J, Cartwright R. An outbreak of viral gastroenteritis on a cruise ship. Commun Dis Rep CDR Rev 1996;6:188–92.
5. Gunn AG, Terranova WA, Greenberg HB, et al. Norwalk virus gastroenteritis aboard a cruise ship; outbreak on five consecutive cruises. Am J Epidemiol 1986;112:820–7.
6. Wenzel RP. Airline travel and infection. N Engl J Med 1996;345:981–2.
7. Kenyon TA, Valway SE, Ihle WW, Onorato IM, Castro KG. Transmission of multidrug-resistant Mycobacterium tuberculosis during a long airplane flight. N Engl J Med 1996;334:933–8.
8. Joseph CA, Hutchinson EJ, Dedman D, Birtles RJ, Watson JM, Bartlett CL. Legionnaires' disease surveillance: England and Wales 1994. Commun Dis Rep CDR Rev 1995;5:R180–3.
9. Weinberg AN. Respiratory infections transmitted from animals. Infect Dis Clin North Am 1991;5:649–61.
10. van de Giessen AW, Dufrenne JB, Ritmeester WS, Berkers PA, van Leeuwen WJ, Notermnas SH. The identification of Salmonella enteritidis-infected poultry flocks associated with an outbreak of human salmonellosis. Epidemiol Infect 1992;109:405–11.
11. Kapperud G, Skjerve E, Bean NH, Ostroff SM, Lassen J. Risk factors for sporadic Campylobacter infections: results of a case–control study in southeastern Norway. J Clin Microbiol 1992;30:3117–21.
12. Shield J, Baumer JH, Dawson JA, Wilkinson PJ. Cryptosporidiosis – an educational experience. J Infect 1990;21:297–301.
13. Sayers GM, Dillon MC, Connolly E, et al. Cryptosporidiosis in children who visited an open farm. Commun Dis Rep CDR Rev 1996;6:140–4.
14. Centres for Disease Control. Arboviral Disease – United States, 1994. MMWR Morb Mortal Wkly Rep 1995;44:641–4.
15. Christmann D, Staub-Schmidt T. Tick-borne encephalitis in Central and Eastern Europe. Presse Med 1996;25:420–3.
16. Weber DJ. Infections acquired in the great out-of-doors of North Carolina. North Carolina Med J 1993;54:537–42.
17. Brett J, Vivier A. Pseudomonas aeruginosa and whirlpools. Br Med J 1985;290:1024–5.
18. Hollyoak V, Allison D, Summers J. Pseudomonas aeruginosa wound infection associated with a nursing home's whirlpool bath. Commun Dis Rep CDR Rev 1995;5:100–4.
19. Parikh P, Nalitt B, Eisenberg ES. Case report: fatal Pseudomonas aeruginosa pneumonia and sepsis. N J Med 1995;92:165–6.
20. Jernigan DB, Hofmann J, Cetron MS, et al. Outbreak of Legionnaires' disease among cruise ship passengers exposed to a contaminated whirlpool spa. Lancet 1996;347:494–9.
21. Mahoney FJ, Farley TA, Kelso KY, Wilson SA, Horan JM, McFarland LM. An outbreak of hepatitis A associated with swimming in a public pool. J Infect Dis 1992;165:613–18.
22. Walker A. Swimming – the hazards of taking a dip. Br Med J 1992;304:242–5.
23. Public Health Laboratory Service. Sewage contamination of coastal bathing waters in England and Wales: a bacteriological and epidemiological study. J Hyg 1959;57:435–72.
24. Cabelli VJ, Dufour AP, McCabe LJ, Levin MA. Swimming-associated gastroenteritis and water quality. Am J Epidemiology 1982;115:606–16.
25. Kay D, Fleisher JM, Salmon, et al. Predicting liklihood of gastoenteritis from sea bathing: results from randomised exposure. Lancet 1994;334:905–9.
26. von Schirnding YE, Kfir R, Cabelli V, Franklin L. The health effects of swimming at Sydney beaches. The Sydney Beach Users Study Advisory Group. Am J Pub Health 1993;83:1701–6.
27. Fleisher JM, Kay D, Salmon RL, Jones F, Wyer MD, Godfree AF. Marine waters contaminated with domestic sewage: nonenteric illnesses associated with bather exposure in the United Kingdom. Am J Pub Health 1996;86:1228–34.
28. Philipp R. The public health response to increasing awareness about Weil's disease associated with recreational water exposure. Environ Health 1992;100:292–7.
29. Philipp R, King C, Hughes A. Understanding of Weil's disease among canoeists. Br J Sports Med 1992;26:223–7.
30. Ringertz O, Zetterberg B. Serum hepatitis among Swedish track finders. N Engl J Med 1967;308:1702–6.
31. Mast EE, Goodman RA, Bond WW, Favero MS, Drotman DP. Transmission of blood borne pathogens during sports: risk and prevention. Ann Intern Med 1995;122:283–5.
32. Torre D, Sampietro C, Ferraro G, Zeroli C, Speranza F. Transmission of HIV-1 infection via sports injury. Lancet 1990;335:1105.
33. Brenner IKM, Shek PN, Shephard, RJ. Infection in athletes. Sports Med 1994;17:86–107.

Occupational Infections

Rodrigo LC Romulo

Some individuals have an increased risk of acquiring infections as a result of their occupation. They include those whose occupations involve significant exposure to potentially infectious material such as:

- health care workers exposed to patients with communicable diseases;
- animal handlers;
- abattoir workers;
- raw animal product processors exposed to zoonotic infections; and
- workers exposed to sewage.

Biomedical laboratory workers are at risk of infection due to direct exposure to pathogenic micro-organisms in specimens being processed or isolated in culture. Forestry workers are more likely to contract arthropod-borne infections and certain mycoses than the general population. Irrigation workers and rice farmers in endemic areas are at risk of developing schistosomiasis.

Those whose livelihood requires travel and work in endemic areas have an increased risk of acquiring malaria, leishmaniasis, trypanosomiasis and diarrheal diseases. They include military personnel, missionaries, Peace Corp volunteers and disaster relief workers.

Military personnel living in barracks are exposed to outbreaks of air-borne infections such as pharyngoconjunctival fever and meningococcal disease. Individuals working in enclosed areas, such as factory workers, are susceptible to acquiring tuberculosis from infectious co-workers.

This chapter provides a quick reference for clinicians faced with patients for whom an occupational infection is suspected. The information is presented entirely in tabular form. Figures 13.1–13.5 offer possible diagnoses for specific clinical presentations considering the patient's occupation (e.g. possible anthrax in an animal handler with an enlarging pruritic papule that ulcerates, develops an eschar and becomes edematous). In the right column of each table the reader is referred to the appropriate chapter of this book for more detailed discussions of each infectious agent.

CUTANEOUS LESIONS AMONG ANIMAL HANDLERS				
Clinical presentation	Possible infectious agent	Possible animal sources	Comments	Chapter
Enlarging pruritic papule, which ulcerates, develops eschar and edema	*Bacillus anthracis* (anthrax)	Herbivores, particularly cattle, goats, donkeys, horses	Transmission via contact with animals sick with or who have died from anthrax or with contaminated raw animal materials[1]	2.2, 8.15
Papular or pustular lesions on arms or hands	*Listeria monocytogenes* (primary cutaneous listeriosis)	Domestic and wild mammals, birds, fish, ticks, crustaceans	Cases usually mild, resolve with treatment[2]	8.15
Localized painful cellulitis, slightly raised, violaceous, peripheral spread with central fading	*Erysipelothrix rhusiopathiae* (erysipeloid)	Wide range of vertebrates and invertebrates; mainly fish, swine, turkey, ducks, sheep	Greatest risk in fishermen, fish handlers, butchers, abattoir workers, veterinarians[3]	2.2, 8.15
Vesicular lesions resembling smallpox	Monkeypox virus	Monkeys from western and central Africa	Rare in humans, most cases in Zaire[4]	8.7
Vesicles progressing to pustules, which coalesce and scab	Parapoxvirus (orf)	Sheep and goats	Transmitted via direct contact with animal lesions; lesions mild, but can become painful and pruritic and may persist for weeks	8.7
	Parapoxvirus (pseudocowpox, paravaccinia, milker's nodule)[5]	Cattle		
	Parapoxvirus (sealpox)[6]	Gray seals		
Acute painful cellulitis following animal bite or scratch	*Pasteurella* spp.	Mostly cats and dogs; other wild and domestic mammals	Must consider if cellulitis develops within 24 hours of bite or scratch[7]	2.2, 6.15, 8.20
Mucocutaneous lesions, progressive encephalitis	Cercopithecine herpesvirus 1 (herpes B virus)	Macaque monkeys	Acquired from monkey bites or scratches or handling monkey tissues or cell cultures[8]	8.5
Necrotizing skin lesions, often hands or feet	*Vibrio vulnificus*	Fish and shellfish	Seen in fish 'farmers' or fishermen, often immunocompromised	2.3

Fig. 13.1 Cutaneous lesions among animal handlers. Animal handlers include animal farmers, fishermen, livestock handlers, veterinarians, zoo workers, animal laboratory workers, abattoir workers, butchers, meat inspectors and raw animal product processors.

ACUTE FEBRILE ILLNESS AMONG ANIMAL HANDLERS

Clinical presentation	Possible infectious agent	Possible animal sources	Comments	Chapter
Malaise, fatigue, fever, shaking chills, myalgias, arthralgias, dark urine	*Babesia bovis*, *Babesia divergens* (babesiosis)	Cattle (in Europe)	Thought to be transmitted to humans in Europe by cattle tick *Ixodes ricinus*	8.34
Fever, sweats, anorexia, headache, back pain	*Brucella abortus*	Mainly cattle; also buffalo, camels, yaks	Worldwide distribution, increased risk in veterinarians, livestock farmers, abattoir workers, meat inspectors	6.34
	Brucella melitensis	Goats, sheep, camels		
	Brucella suis biovars 1–3	Swine		
	Brucella suis biovar 4	Reindeer, caribou		
	Brucella canis	Dogs		
Fever, chills, headache, myalgias, abdominal pain, conjunctival suffusion, muscle tenderness, jaundice	*Leptospira* spp.	Wide range of mammals; rats most common source worldwide; also dogs, wild mammals, cats, pigs, other livestock	Worldwide distribution; cases usually result from contact with water or soil contaminated with infected urine	6.34
Acute onset fever, chills, headache, vomiting, migratory arthralgias	*Streptobacillus moniliformis* (USA), *Spirillum minus* (Asia) (rat-bite fever)	Rats, mice, squirrels; also cats, dogs, pigs, ferrets, weasels	Increased risk in animal laboratory workers[9]	6.15, 8.19
Fever, chills (endocarditis)	*Streptococcus suis*	Pigs	Rare in humans; mostly in pig farmers, others with close contact with pigs[10]	2.50, 8.14
	Streptococcus equinus	Horses	Case in UK farmer[11]	
Fever, headache, meningismus, declining sensorium (meningitis)	*Streptococcus suis*	Pigs	Close contact with pigs documented in most cases	8.14
Nonspecific febrile illness or atypical pneumonia	*Coxiella burnetti* (Q fever)	Most common reservoirs are cattle, sheep, goats	Worldwide distribution; usually affects those with direct contact with infected animals	2.27, 8.24
	Chlamydia psittaci (psittacosis)	Birds (poultry, parrot family, finches, pigeons, pheasants, egrets, seagulls, puffins); sheep[12]	Increased risk in poultry farmers, pet shop workers, abattoir and processing plant workers	2.27, 8.25
Fever, severe headache 3–5 days after flu-like illness	Lymphocytic choriomeningitis virus	Rodents	Increased risk in laboratory workers handling mice, hamsters	2.15, 8.11
Abrupt onset fever, chills, headache, malaise, anorexia, fatigue, tender lymphadenopathy, skin ulcer	*Francisella tularensis* (tularemia)	Voles, squirrels, rabbits, hares, muskrats, beavers, hamsters	Transmitted via insect bite, aerosol, contact with contaminated water or mud, animal bites; increased risk in farmers, animal laboratory workers, veterinarians, hunters, trappers, meat handlers	6.34
	Yersinia pestis (plague)	Rats most important reservoirs worldwide; also squirrels, prairie dogs and other urban and sylvatic rodents		6.34, 8.17
Fever, anorexia, nausea, vomiting, headache, pain or paresthesias at site of animal bite followed by hyperactivity, disorientation, bizarre behavior	Rabies virus	In developing countries mostly dogs; farm animals (e.g. cattle, horses, sheep), wild mammals (e.g. raccoons, skunks, foxes, coyotes, wolves, bats, cats)	Incubation period usually 20–90 days: bites on head 25–48 days; on extremity 46–78 days	6.15, 8.8
Hemorrhagic fever, hepatitis	Rift Valley fever virus	Sheep, cattle	Farmers and veterinarians handling animal carcasses in Africa[13]	6.34
Fever, chills, cough, chest pain, dyspnea, occasionally hemoptysis	*Burkholderia pseudomallei* (melioidosis)	Animals not reservoir for human disease	Farmers in Southeast Asia[14] and Northern Australia;[15] acquired by soil contamination of skin abrasions and possibly ingestion, inhalation or intranasal inoculation	6.34, 8.18

Fig. 13.2 Acute febrile illness among animal handlers.

DIARRHEAL ILLNESS AMONG ANIMAL HANDLERS				
Clinical presentation	Possible infectious agent	Possible animal sources	Comments	Chapter
Diarrhea or abdominal pain (pancreatitis)	*Cryptosporidium* spp.	Farm animals (cattle, sheep), laboratory animals (calves, rodents, rabbits)[16]	Transmission occurs animal to person, person-to-person, water-borne	6.25, 8.32
Acute diarrhea (watery or bloody), fever, abdominal pain	*Campylobacter jejuni*	Wild and domesticated cattle, sheep, goats, swine, dogs, cats, rodents, fowl	Worldwide distribution, transmission via ingestion of contaminated material, direct contact with infected animals	2.35, 8.19
	Campylobacter coli, C. hyointestinalis	Swine		
	Campylobacter upsaliensis	Dogs		
	Campylobacter fetus	Sheep, cattle, swine, poultry, reptiles		
	Shigella spp.	*Cynomolgus* macaque monkey	Outbreak of *S. flexneri* reported among workers in primate research unit[17]	2.35, 8.17
	Yersinia enterocolitica	Rodents, rabbits, sheep, pigs, horses, cattle, dogs, cats	Transmission mainly by ingestion of contaminated food or drink, less commonly direct contact with infected animals; Finnish butchers documented at higher risk[18]	2.35, 8.18
Chronic diarrhea	*Nanophyetus salmincola* (nanophyetiasis)	Coho salmon, other salminoid fish	Transmission usually by ingestion; also by handling infected fish[19]	6.28, 8.35

Fig. 13.3 Diarrheal illness among animal handlers.

INFECTIONS AMONG BIOMEDICAL LABORATORY WORKERS			
Clinical presentation	Possible infectious agent	Exposure	Chapter
Fever, sweats, sore throat, myalgias, maculopapular rash, headache, photophobia, meningismus	HIV	Percutaneous or mucous membrane exposure while processing infected blood or body fluid	3.10, 5.3
Fever, anorexia, malaise, then jaundice	Hepatitis viruses[20]		8.4
Fever, sweats, anorexia, headache, back pain	*Brucella* spp.[21]	Direct contact; air-borne spread among laboratory workers documented[22]	6.34
High fever, headache, myalgia, rash including palms and soles	*Rickettsia rickettsii* (Rocky Mountain spotted fever)	Transmitted in laboratory via infected aerosols or parenteral inoculation[23]	6.34, 8.24
Abrupt onset fever, chills, headache, malaise, anorexia, fatigue, tender lymphadenopathy, skin ulcer	*Francisella tularensis*	Direct contact with infected specimen or culture isolate	6.34
Gradually increasing fever, chills, headache, malaise	*Salmonella typhi*,[24] *S. paratyphi* A, B		6.24
Acute diarrhea	*Shigella* spp., nontyphoidal *Shigella* spp, nontyphoidal *Salmonella* spp., *Campylobacter* spp., *Vibrio cholerae*		6.22, 8.17, 8.19
Fever, purpuric/ecchymotic skin lesions, meningitis, shock	*Neisseria meningitidis*	Air-borne; 2 fatal cases described in laboratory workers[25]	2.15, 8.16
Hemorrhagic fever with renal syndrome	Hantavirus	Reported case probably due to contact with immunocytoma[26]	6.34
Chronic cough, fever, night sweats, anorexia, weight loss	*Mycobacterium tuberculosis*[19]	Inhalation of aerosolized droplet nuclei	2.30
Fever, chills, night sweats, productive cough, malaise, anorexia, arthralgias	*Coccidioides immitis*[27]	Inhalation of arthrospores from culture	2.7, 8.27
Cutaneous papules, pustules, nodules, ulcers or abscesses	*Coccidioides immitis*	Direct percutaneous inoculation of contaminated material	2.7, 8.27
Verrucous skin lesions with peripheral microabscesses or initial pustule that spreads into ulcer with red granulation tissue	*Blastomyces dermatitidis*[28]		2.7, 8.27

Fig. 13.4 Infections among biomedical laboratory workers.

OCCUPATIONAL INFECTIONS DUE TO ENVIRONMENTAL EXPOSURE

Clinical presentation: forestry workers	Possible infectious agent	Comments	Chapter
Red macule or papule with expanding borders and central clearing or migratory pain in joints, bursae, tendons, muscles; arthritis	*Borrelia burgdorferi*[29]	High seroprevalence in forestry workers, but asymptomatic infection more common	2.45
Abrupt fever, headache, photophobia, vomiting, meningismus, seizures, altered sensorium	Russian summer–spring encephalitis virus/ Central European encephalitis virus (tick-borne encephalitis virus, TBEV)	Higher antibody levels to TBEV found in Polish forestry workers[30]	2.16
Erythematous papulonodular lesion with several painless secondary nodules proximally along lymphatic channels	*Sporothrix schenckii* (sporotrichosis)	Outbreaks among forestry workers in USA associated with sphagnum moss[31,32]	2.7, 8.28
Hemorrhagic fever with renal syndrome	Puumala virus (nephropathia endemica)	Higher seroprevalence among forestry workers in Sweden,[33] but not in Netherlands[34]	6.34
Clinical presentation: sewer and irrigation workers			
Fever, malaise, anorexia, then jaundice	Hepatitis A	Sewer workers at higher risk than general population in developed countries[35]	8.4
Fever, chills, headache, myalgias, abdominal pain, conjunctival suffusion, muscle tenderness, jaundice	*Leptospira* spp. (leptospirosis)	Increased risk in sewer and public cleansing workers[36]	6.34
Intestinal parasitism	*Ascaris lumbricoides, Entamoeba histolytica, Enterobius vermicularis*	More common in Egyptian sewer workers than in controls[37]	6.25, 8.35
Fatigue, abdominal pain, intermittent diarrhea, hepatosplenomegaly	*Schistosoma japonicum, S. mansoni, S. mekongi* (schistosomiasis)	Rice farmers and freshwater fishermen in endemic areas	6.27, 8.35
Terminal hematuria, dysuria	*Schistosoma haematobium*		6.27

Fig. 13.5 Occupational infections due to environmental exposure: forestry, sewer and irrigation workers.

REFERENCES

1. Lew D. *Bacillus anthracis* (anthrax). In: Mandell GL, Bennett JE, Dolin R, eds. Principles and practice of infectious diseases. New York: Churchill Livingstone; 1995:1885–9.
2. McLaughlin J, Low JC. Primary cutaneous listeriosis in adults: an occupational disease of veterinarians and farmers. Vet Rec 1994;135:615–7.
3. Reboli AC, Farrar WE. *Erysipelothrix rhusiopathiae*: an occupational pathogen. Clin Microbiol Rev 1989;2:354–9.
4. Neff J. Variola (smallpox) and monkeypox viruses. In: Mandell GL, Bennett JE, Dolin R, eds. Principles and practice of infectious diseases. New York: Churchill Livingstone; 1995:1328–9.
5. Groves RW, Wilson-Jones E, MacDonald DM. Human orf and milker's nodule: a clinicopathologic study. J Am Acad Dermatol 1991;25:706–11.
6. Hicks BD, Worthy GA. Sealpox in captive grey seals (*Halichoerus grypus*) and their handlers. J Wildlf Dis 1987;23:1–6.
7. Boyce JM. *Pasteurella* species. In: Mandell GL, Bennett JE, Dolin R, eds. Principles and practice of infectious diseases. New York: Churchill Livingstone; 1995:2068–70.
8. Whitley RJ. Cercopithecine herpes virus 1 (B virus). In: Fields BN, Knipe DM, Chanock RM, et al., eds. Field's virology. New York: Raven Press; 1990:2063–74.
9. Anderson LC, Leary SL, Manning PJ. Rat-bite fever in animal research laboratory personnel. Lab Anim Sci 1983;33:292–4.
10. Ho AK, Woo KS, Tse KK, et al. Infective endocarditis caused by *Streptococcus suis* serotype 2. J Infect 1990;21:209–11.
11. Elliott PM, Williams H, Brooksby IA. A case of infective endocarditis in a farmer caused by *Streptococcus equinus*. Eur Heart J. 1993;14:1292–3.
12. Johnson FW, Matheson BA, Williams H, et al. Abortion due to infection with *Chlamydia psittaci* in a sheep farmer's wife. Br Med J 1985;290:592–4.

13. McIntosh BM, Russell D, dos Santos I, et al. Rift Valley fever in humans in South Africa. S Afr Med J 1980;1:77–83.
14. Suputtamongkol Y, Hall AJ, Dance DA, et. al. The epidemiology of melioidosis in Ubon Ratchani, Northeast Thailand. Int J Epidemiol 1994;23:1082–90.
15. Guard RW, Khafagi FA, Brigden MC, et al. Melioidosis in Far North Queensland: a clinical and epidemiological review of twenty cases. Am J Trop Med Hyg 1984;33:467–73.
16. Navin TR. Cryptosporidiosis in humans: review of recent epidemiologic studies. Eur J Epidemiol 1985;1:77–83.
17. Kennedy FM, Astbury J, Needham JR, et al. Shigellosis due to occupational contact with non-human primates. Epidemiol Infect 1993;110:247–51.
18. Merilahti-Palo R, Lahesmaa R, Granfors K, et al. Risk of yersinia infection among butchers. Scand J Infect Dis 1991;23:55–61.
19. Harrel LW, Deardorff TL. Human nanophyetiasis: transmission by handling naturally infected coho salmon (*Oncorhynchus kisutch*) J Infect Dis 1990;161:146–8.
20. Grist NR. Hepatitis and other infections in clinical laboratory staff, 1979. J Clin Pathol 1981;34:655–8.
21. Grist NR, Emslie JA. Infections in British clinical laboratories, 1988–1989. J Clin Pathol. 1991;44:667–9.
22. Gruner E, Bernasconi E, Galeazzi RL, et al. Brucellosis: an occupational hazard for medical laboratory personnel. Report of five cases. Infection 1994;22:33–6.
23. Johnson JE, Kadull PJ. Rocky mountain spotted fever acquired in a laboratory. N Engl J Med 1967;227:842–6.
24. Blaser MJ, Hickman FW, Farmer JJ, et al. *Salmonella typhi*: the laboratory as reservoir of infection. J Infect Dis 1980;142:934–8.
25. Laboratory-acquired meningococcemia – California and Massachusetts. MMWR Morb Mortal Wkly Rep 1991;40:46–7.

26. Lloyd G, Jones N. Infection of laboratory workers with hantavirus acquired from immunocytomas propagated in laboratory rats. J Infect 1986;12:117–25.
27. Johnson JE, Perry JE, Fekety FR, et al. Laboratory acquired coccidioidomycosis. A report of 210 cases. Ann Intern Med 1964;60:941.
28. Larson DM, Eckman MR, Alber RL, et al. Primary cutaneous blastomycosis: an occupational hazard to pathologists. Am J Clin Pathol 1983;79:253–5.
29. Kuiper H, de Jongh BM, Nauta AP, et al. Lyme borreliosis in Dutch forestry workers. J Infect 1991;23:279–86.
30. Prokopowicz D, Bobrowska M, Grzeszuck A. Prevalence of antibodies against tick-borne encephalitis among residents of north-eastern Poland. Scand J Infect Dis 1995;27:15–6.
31. Powell KE, Taylor A, Phillips BJ, et al. Cutaneous sporotrichosis in forestry workers. Epidemic due to contaminated sphagnum moss. JAMA 1978;240:232–5.
32. Coles FB, Schuchat A, Hibbs JR, et al. A multistate outbreak of sporotrichosis associated with sphagnum moss. Am J Epidemiol 1992;136:475–87.
33. Ahlm C, Linderholm M, Juto P, et al. Prevalence of serum IgG antibodies to Puumala virus (haemorrhagic fever with renal syndrome) in northern Sweden. Epidemiol Infect 1994;113:129–36.
34. Moll van Charante AW, Groen J, Osterhaus AD. Risk of infections transmitted by arthropods and rodents in forestry workers. Eur J Epidemiol 1994;10:349–51.
35. Heng BH, Goh KT, Doraisingham S, Quek GH. Prevalence of hepatitis A infection among sewage workers in Singapore. Epidemiol Infect 1994;113:121–8.
36. Chan OY, Chia SE, Nadarajah N, et al. Leptospirosis risk in public cleansing and sewer workers. Ann Acad Med Singapore 1987;16:586–90.
37. Hammouda NA, El-Gebali WM, Razek MK. Intestinal parasitic infection among sewage workers in Alexandria, Egypt. J Egypt Soc Parasitol 1992;22:299–303.

Practice Points

Management of candiduria in the intensive care unit   *Shiranee Sriskandan*

INTRODUCTION

Candiduria can be defined as the presence of greater than 10^5 fungal cfu/ml urine. The prevalence of candiduria varies between 6.5 and 20% among hospitalized patients, and it presents a dilemma to clinicians, who must decide whether such a finding represents colonization alone or is a feature of invasive fungal infection. Probably only 3–4% of cases of candiduria lead to candidemia, but 10% of all cases of candidemia are associated with a prior episode of candiduria. Indeed, studies based in the intensive care unit (ICU) have shown that candiduria can be associated with a rise in mortality from 19 to 50%.

PATHOGENESIS

Candiduria can arise in several ways: simple contamination of specimens at the time of procurement can account for many such cases, hence the need for a confirmatory second specimen. Colonization of the urinary tract may occur in the catheterized patient. Local infection of both the lower urinary tract (cystitis, urethritis) and upper tract (pyelonephritis) with *Candida* spp. is encouraged by urologic instrumentation, in particular catheterization. Other factors predisposing to such infections include ongoing broad-spectrum antibiotic therapy, diabetes mellitus, renal insufficiency and anatomic anomalies of the urinary tract. Finally, patients who have disseminated candidiasis may seed the urinary tract from blood stream spread (Fig. 14.1).

MICROBIOLOGY

The majority (50–70%) of candidal isolates from urine in the ICU are *Candida albicans,* which is sensitive to fluconazole. Indeed, provided that patients have not previously been exposed to fluconazole, it is reasonable to assume that any germ-tube-positive yeast will be sensitive to fluconazole. However, increasing numbers of yeasts other than *C. albicans* occur in the ICU setting and the prevalence varies between units. In particular, *Candida tropicalis* and *Candida glabrata* account for 10–20% of such isolates, the latter species being notable for its resistance to azole drugs (Chapters 7.16 & 8.26).

CLINICAL FEATURES

Candiduria alone does not cause symptoms; local infection can cause classical cystitis or urethritis, and pyelonephritis may lead to flank pain. Patients who have candiduria as a feature of disseminated candidiasis may have evidence of systemic candidal disease, which should be assiduously checked for; clinical features include sepsis, fever, lesions of the optic fundi, skin lesions and hepatosplenomegaly.

INVESTIGATIONS

From Figure 14.1, it is clear that a repeat fresh urine sample must be sent to the microbiology laboratory to confirm candiduria. Microscopy for the presence of white blood cells and casts may be useful in differentiating colonization from urinary tract infection. If the patient has not been catheterized or had urologic instrumentation recently, it is prudent to screen for diabetes mellitus and renal insufficiency by biochemical testing and for anatomic anomalies using ultrasound. Ultrasound of the renal tract can also demonstrate the presence of fungal balls in patients who have persistent candiduria. Simple tests to screen for the possibility of disseminated candidiasis would include a chest radiograph, abdominal ultrasound, C-reactive protein, cultures of other potentially infected sites (e.g. tracheal aspirate or bronchial lavage, bile, surgical drains, intravascular line tips) and blood cultures.

MANAGEMENT

The modern management of candiduria in the ICU setting is determined by the likely source of fungi (see Fig. 14. 2). It is clear that colonization can be treated by simply replacing the urinary catheter or, better, by removing it permanently. In all cases, rational reduction in the spectrum of antibacterial agents administered to patients will help eliminate fungal colonization and infection. These simple measures allow 40–60% of all patients who have candiduria to clear fungi from the urine. True infection of the urinary tract should be treated with a short, definitive course of an antifungal agent, usually fluconazole, in addition to catheter removal. Fluconazole can be administered intravenously or via the nasogastric tube in the oral formulation if the patient's gastrointestinal system is functioning. Infection with germ-tube-negative *Candida* spp. (other than *C. albicans*) may require intravenous amphotericin B. There is no case for local intermittent or continuous bladder irrigation with amphotericin B; the procedure necessitates instrumentation of the urinary tract, which might otherwise be unnecessary.

ETIOLOGY AND LABORATORY INVESTIGATION OF CANDIDURIA

Source of candiduria	Laboratory investigations
Inadvertent contamination	Repeat sample will be clear
Colonization of lower urinary tract	No leukocytes in urine; patient well
Infection of lower urinary tract	Leukocytes in urine; ultrasound if not instrumented; screen for diabetes mellitus and renal disease
Infection of upper urinary tract	Leukocytes and casts in urine; ultrasound; screen for diabetes mellitus and renal disease
Disseminated candidal infection	Blood cultures or cultures of other sterile site are positive for *Candida* spp.; chest radiograph; abdominal ultrasound; C-reactive protein levels high

Fig. 14.1 Etiology and laboratory investigation of candiduria.

MANAGEMENT OF CANDIDURIA IN THE INTENSIVE CARE UNIT		
Suspected cause of candiduria	Action	Additional considerations
Contamination	None	
Colonization	No antifungal medication necessary; remove or replace catheter; stop antibacterial agents if possible	If patient is at risk of infection or undergoing urologic procedure, fluconazole 400mg/day for 5 days
Lower urinary tract infection	Fluconazole 400mg/day for 5–10 days if due to Candida albicans	
Upper urinary tract infection	Fluconazole 400mg/day for 5–10 days if due to Candida albicans	
Disseminated infection	Fluconazole 800mg/day if Candida albicans or amphotericin B 0.6–1.0 mg/kg per day, depending on severity, for at least 2 weeks	If dissemination is confirmed, follow up for at least 3–6 months after discharge from intensive care unit in case of distant seeding

Fig. 14.2 Management of candiduria in the intensive care unit.

Furthermore, although local irrigation with amphotericin B can achieve prompt clearance of funguria, the effect is short-lived compared with clearance rates achieved by fluconazole.

Finally, the canduric patient who may have invasive fungal infection warrants more aggressive antifungal therapy. This must be based on careful assessment of combined clinical and laboratory findings. If *C. albicans* is isolated and the patient is stable, it is reasonable to treat with fluconazole for at least 2 weeks. However, if the same patient is clinically unstable, or if the isolate is not *C. albicans*, it would be prudent to treat with amphotericin B, as indicated in Figure 14.2. The appropriate duration of therapy in this setting is unclear and must be determined according to the individual clinical situation and response to therapy.

FURTHER READING

Ang BSP, Telenti A, King B, Steckelberg JM, Wilson WR. Candidemia from a urinary tract source: microbiological aspects and clinical significance. Clin Infect Dis 1993;17:662–6.

Edwards JE, Bodey GP, Bowden RA, et al. International conference for the development of a consensus on the management and prevention of severe candidal infections. Clin Infect Dis 1997;25:43–59.

Fisher JF, Newman CL, Sobel JD. Yeast in the urine: solutions for a budding problem. Clin Infect Dis 1995;20:183–9.

Hamory BH, Wenzel RP. Hospital-associated candiduria: predisposing factors and review of the literature. J Urol 1978;120:444–8.

Leu H-S, Huang CT. Clearance of funguria with short-course anti-fungal regimens: a prospective, randomized, controlled study. Clin Infect Dis 1995;20:1152–7.

Nassoura Z, Ivatury RR, Simon RJ, Jabbour N, Stahl WM. Candiduria as an early marker of disseminated infection in critically ill surgical patients: the role of fluconazole therapy. J Trauma 1993;35:290–5.

Management of the patient who has suspected viral hemorrhagic fever

Steven M Opal

INTRODUCTION

Continued expansion of human populations into tropical rain forests, economic pressures and changing ecologic conditions around equatorial regions of the world have increased the risk of exposure to a variety of tropical viral diseases. Global markets and expanded international trade in combination with improved access to remote areas by expanded international airline transportation makes it feasible that these viral illnesses could spread worldwide. Physicians in endemic areas need to be aware of the potential threat of viral hemorrhagic illnesses. Moreover, physicians in nonendemic regions need to recognize the potential risk of hemorrhagic viral illness in international travelers from tropical regions. Animal handlers in primate research laboratories throughout the world are also at risk.

It is important that physicians be aware of the potential risk of tropical viral hemorrhagic fevers for several reasons:
- to ensure appropriate diagnosis and management of index cases;
- to provide advice, counseling and possible prophylaxis to close contacts; and
- to minimize the risk of nosocomial transmission among health care workers (HCWs) caring for such patients.

Strict adherence to basic infection control techniques and some advance planning will minimize the risk to HCWs and allow rapid, compassionate and safe care of affected patients.

MICROBIOLOGY AND PATHOGENESIS

Hemorrhagic viruses in which person-to-person transmission has been documented include representatives of the arenavirus, bunyavirus and the filovirus groups. The most important examples are Lassa fever, Ebola virus and Marburg virus, and Crimean–Congo hemorrhagic fever, caused by a tick-transmitted bunyavirus, (see Chapter 8.11). Lassa, Ebola, Marburg and Crimean–Congo hemorrhagic fever viruses are particularly important to recognize because nosocomial transmission

to HCWs is a real possibility. Although the animal reservoir and mode of transmission to humans is reasonably well understood for Lassa and Crimean–Congo hemorrhagic fevers, the method of transmission of Ebola virus and Marburg virus remain an unsolved mystery.

These viral syndromes share many overlapping clinical features in humans. After an incubation period of between 3 and 21 days, patients develop the abrupt onset of fever, headache, myalgia, sore throat, respiratory symptoms, abdominal pain, nausea, vomiting, diarrhea and conjunctivitis with associated pharyngitis and cervical lymphadenitis. A macular skin eruption may occur in infections with Ebola and Marburg virus; this is less common in Lassa and Crimean–Congo hemorrhagic fever. Various degrees of mucosal and cutaneous hemorrhage occur associated with thrombocytopenia and disseminated intravascular coagulation. The geographic location or travel history of the patient is most useful in distinguishing between the different types of viral hemorrhagic fevers before virologic confirmation.

These viruses share rapid growth potential and the ability to invade a variety of cell types, resulting in high-grade viremia. The patient's blood and body fluids become potentially contagious to others who come in direct contact with them. Transmission may also occur through handling of bodies during burial rituals, as demonstrated in the most recent large Ebola outbreak in Kikwit, Congo. Although many other febrile illnesses, such as malaria, typhoid fever, meningococcemia, arboviral infections and leptospirosis, may present in a similar fashion, infection control measures need to be instituted to guard against potential transmission of viral hemorrhagic fevers until the diagnosis is established.

DIAGNOSIS AND MANAGEMENT

Recent improvements in the serologic diagnosis of viral hemorrhagic fevers now make it possible to make a specific diagnosis in the majority of acutely ill patients. An antigen-capture enzyme-linked immunosorbent assay has been developed for Ebola virus and may allow rapid diagnosis in acutely ill patients. Specific IgM and IgG capture enzyme-linked immunosorbent assay antibody studies are available for serologic diagnosis in convalescent samples. Unfortunately, diseases such as Ebola virus infection, in which mortality rates exceed 75%, do not often allow the opportunity to study convalescent samples. Virus isolation from the blood and body secretions of acutely ill patients is the definitive diagnostic method. This is, of course, a severe biohazard and it should only be attempted in biosafety level IV facilities. Reverse transcription and polymerase chain reaction for specific viral RNA is also a useful diagnostic method in patients who have viral hemorrhagic illnesses. Many of these methodologies are unavailable in regions of the world where these diseases are endemic. For this reason, the recent development of immunochemical staining method for skin biopsy samples is particularly valuable. This method allows for fixation of tissues at the site of diagnosis and eliminates the biohazard of transportation of infected human tissues.

Routine diagnostic methods to evaluate other common febrile illnesses should not be delayed because of suspected viral hemorrhagic fever. In particular, care must be taken to exclude falciparum malaria which may be fatal if unrecognized and left untreated. In practice, most cases of suspected VHF turn out to have malaria. Universal precautions when handling blood and body secretions should suffice to protect HCWs from hemorrhagic viruses (see Chapter 6.34).

INFECTION CONTROL METHODS

These viruses are transmitted through direct contact with the patient or the patient's secretions. There is a remote risk of air-borne transmission based upon studies with nonhuman primates, and one potential transmission by respiratory aerosol in a patient who had Lassa fever with extensive pulmonary involvement has been reported. Therefore, the primary infection control strategy is strict contact isolation, universal blood and body substance precautions, and enhanced preventive measures in the handling of blood and body fluids. Body substances are contagious during the acute febrile illness, but there is no evidence of transmission during the incubation phase of the illness. The guidelines listed in Figure 14.3 should be instituted in patients who have suspected viral hemorrhagic fevers.

POSTEXPOSURE PROPHYLAXIS

The arenavirus that causes Lassa fever is susceptible to ribavirin, and this antiviral agent may be of some value to HCWs exposed to blood or body fluids (e.g. by percutaneous needle stick accident). Passive immunotherapy with plasma from surviving patients with high-titer antibody has been shown to be of limited benefit in the prevention of viral hemorrhagic fevers.

REPORTING

It is essential that patients who have suspected viral hemorrhagic fever are reported to public health authorities as soon as possible. This allows a co-ordinated response to a potential epidemic situation and assures that diagnostic and therapeutic efforts will be handled appropriately. Expert international assistance may be necessary should a viral hemorrhagic fever occur in an international traveler.

INFECTION CONTROL METHODS FOR SUSPECTED VIRAL HEMORRHAGIC FEVERS

Isolation method	Comments
Isolation room	Negative-pressure room with an anteroom that has hand washing and isolation supplies; negative pressure with external venting should be verified on a daily basis
Personnel and visitors	Traffic flow into the patient's room should be restricted. A daily record of those who enter and leave the patient's room should be kept. Only essential personnel should be exposed to the patient and the patient's body fluids
Personal protection	Fluid-impervious gowns, gloves, face shields or surgical masks with eye protection (goggles); if cough, vomiting or extensive hemorrhage, respirators with filters (high-efficiency particulate air respirators) and leg and shoe coverings should be worn
Clinical samples	Clinical samples should be placed in plastic sealed bags and transported in a leak-proof container without contaminating the external surfaces. Samples should be handled in a biologic safety cabinet (biosafety level III). Serum should be pretreated with a polyethylene glycol phenolic for 1 hour before handling. Automated analyzers should be disinfected with 1:100 dilution of bleach after use. Fixation of blood smears and tissue samples will inactivate the virus and can be handled in a routine manner
Decontamination of the environment and of linen	Contaminated environmental surfaces should be disinfected using a registered hospital disinfectant or 1:100 dilution of bleach. Soiled linens can either be decontaminated by use of an autoclave or incineration. Hot cycle laundering with bleach may be acceptable
Human excrement and blood and body fluids	As an added precaution, human excreta, blood and body fluids should be decontaminated by 1:100 dilution of bleach for at least 5 minutes before disposal
Surgical procedures and autopsy	If a surgical procedure or autopsy is essential, extreme precautions must be used to avoid blood contamination. Double gloves, full face shields with high-efficiency particulate air filtration, water-impervious gowns and shoe covers should be worn. Every effort should be taken to avoid generation of an aerosol. Deceased persons should not be embalmed. The body should be placed in leak-proof, sealed material and cremated or buried in a sealed casket

Fig. 14.3 Infection control methods for suspected viral hemorrhagic fevers.

FURTHER READING

Centers for Disease Control and Prevention. Outbreak of Ebola viral hemorrhagic fever – Zaire, 1995. Morb Mortal Wkly Rep MMWR, 1995;44:381–2.

Centers for Disease Control and Prevention. Update: management of patients with suspected viral hemorrhagic fever – United States. Morb Mortal Wkly Rep MMWR, 1995;44:475–9.

Holmes GP, McCormick JB, Trock SC. Lassa fever in the United States – investigation of a case and new guidelines for management. N Eng J Med 1990;323:1120–3.

Peters CJ. Emerging infections – Ebola and other filo viruses. West J Med 1996;164:36–8.

Peters CJ, Sanchez A, Feldmann H, Rollin PE, Nichol S, Ksiaek TG. Filo viruses as emerging pathogens. Semin Virol 1994;5:147–54.

Treatment of dysentery in a pregnant woman
Sandra L Kweder

INTRODUCTION

Encountering dysentery or debilitating diarrhea in a pregnant woman sets the physician on a challenging path. Fetal health is inextricable from maternal health, making concerns about morbidity doubly important. Physiologic stresses of severe diarrhea may be well tolerated by a young woman but they may not be when she is pregnant.

Furthermore, her unborn child relies for its survival solely on maternal volume status by way of placental blood flow. The dysenteric pregnant woman should be hospitalized immediately if at all possible. The clinician must work quickly to ensure hydration, to establish a diagnosis and to select a rational management plan.

PATHOGENESIS

Etiologic considerations are the same for pregnant and nonpregnant patients, however, there are a few specific organisms to which a pregnant woman may be particularly predisposed. Noninfectious causes of dysentery should also be considered, particularly inflammatory bowel disease.

For example, physiologic changes of pregnancy may place the patient at risk for contracting or manifesting certain conditions. Cellular immunity is suppressed, predisposing the woman to intracellular pathogens, such as *Listeria* spp. The decreased gastrointestinal motility of pregnancy may allow for higher concentrations of enteric pathogens to accumulate in the bowel lumen, leading to more severe enteric illness.

The normal physiology of pregnancy can obscure diagnosis in the dysenteric patient. Leukocytosis is common. Uterine enlargement complicates the abdominal examination. Common symptoms of pregnancy can delay recognition of disease or lead to interventions that place the patient at risk of more significant dysenteric disease. For example, decreased bowel motility and laxity of the gastroesophageal sphincter, both caused by elevated estrogen levels, can cause severe gastroesophageal reflux and intestinal bloating and cramping. These symptoms may obscure the early recognition of enteric infections in pregnant women.

MICROBIOLOGY

The classic bacterial organisms associated with dysenteric disease are *Salmonella* spp. and *Shigella* spp., with the former more commonly associated with bacteremia and a carrier state. Enterohemorrhagic strains of *Escherichia coli* are an increasingly recognized cause of bloody diarrhea and may cause severe dysentery in pregnant women (Chapter 2.35).

Listeria monocytogenes infection typically causes a febrile diarrheal illness in pregnancy. Pregnancy is the most common independent risk factor for infection with *Listeria* spp., which are invasive, intracellular bacterial pathogens. Most reported cases of listeriosis in otherwise immunocompetent hosts are in pregnant women, particularly in the third trimester. Transplacental infection of the fetus and amnion, with severe outcomes, is well described even with mild maternal illness, making aggressive detection and treatment essential. The patient who has listeriosis may have additional signs and symptoms, including myalgia, pharyngitis or meningitis. She may, unfortunately, present with a mild febrile diarrheal illness and intrauterine fetal death, which should focus the clinician immediately on *Listeria* spp. (Chapter 2.53).

Campylobacter spp. are increasingly common agents of diarrheal illness that can afflict patients by multiple pathogenic mechanisms (Chapter 2.35). Symptoms are often suggestive of appendicitis, bowel perforation or inflammatory bowel disease. *Campylobacter* spp. have been described as a cause of abortion and perinatal sepsis, placing them alongside *Listeria* spp. as pathogens to be vigorously pursued in pregnant women who have diarrheal illness.

Parasitic infections deserve consideration in the pregnant patient who have diarrhea. *Entamoeba histolytica* may cause severe amebic colitis without typical symptoms of amebic dysentery in pregnant women. *Giardia lamblia*, although not a classic cause of dysentery, is problematic in pregnancy. Achlorhydria and any form of immunodeficiency each enhance risk of infection. Although pregnancy has never been identified as an independent risk factor for giardiasis, the disease may easily be missed in the pregnant patient who has intermittent bouts of gastrointestinal distress. Misdiagnosis can range from psychosomatic illness to hyperemesis gravidarum (Chapter 8.31).

CLINICAL FEATURES

What is most striking about pregnant women with any major illness is how quickly they can become severely ill, making early diagnosis and treatment essential. Pregnant women have at least a 20% greater plasma volume than nonpregnant women, with corresponding requirements for fluid intake. They tolerate fluid losses poorly, whether from diarrhea, fever or the decreased fluid intake that often accompanies enteric illness. Decreased peripheral vascular tone with vasodilatation contributes to a tendency for postural hypotension or presyncopal symptoms that may develop rapidly.

In the course of any significant infectious illness, particularly one with tissue invasion or associated Gram-negative bacteremia, the previously healthy pregnant woman is at substantial risk of developing pulmonary edema owing to the lowered colloid oncotic pressure of the gravid state. This is true even before rigorous hydration. A high index of suspicion for pulmonary edema is warranted in assessing and managing the pregnant patient with any infection. Her fetus will not tolerate hypoxemia as well as she does.

Many features of dysentery in pregnancy are no different from those in the nonpregnant patient; these include fever, abdominal cramping and bloody diarrhea. In *Shigella*, *Salmonella* and *Campylobacter* enteritis, the abdomen may be so tender that peritonitis is suspected. Peritoneal signs may be difficult to distinguish from chorioamnionitis in pregnancy. Vigilance and serial clinical examinations are essential to ensure prompt and proper diagnosis.

As with any infectious illness in a pregnant patient, infectious diarrhea or dysentery may present as preterm labor. In addition, the fetus may show signs of distress because of decreased uterine blood flow resulting from maternal volume depletion, hypoxemia or other physiologic alterations.

INVESTIGATIONS

When evaluating the pregnant woman who has a dysenteria-like illness, it is important to account for normal physiologic changes of pregnancy (Fig. 14.4).

Blood cultures may provide the definitive diagnosis in diarrhea

	NORMAL LABORATORY FINDINGS IN PREGNANCY			
Test	Increased	Unchanged	Decreased	Comment
Hemoglobin and hematocrit			√	Red cell indices unchanged Predominantly neutrophils
Leukocyte count	√			
Platelet count		√		
Blood urea nitrogen			√	
Serum creatinine			√	Usually less than 0.6mg/dl (<53µmol/L)
Sodium			√	
Potassium			√	
Chloride			√	
Bicarbonate			√	
Alanine aminotransferase		√		
Aspartate aminotransferase		√		
Bilirubin		√		
Alkaline phosphatase	√			
Albumin			√	
Creatinine clearance	√			1.5–2 times baseline

Fig. 14.4 Normal laboratory findings in pregnancy.

caused by *Salmonella* spp. or *Listeria* spp. If the patient is febrile, it is appropriate to culture all potentially infected body fluids, such as urine, stool and even amniotic fluid. Where there is a question of peritonitis or chorioamnionitis as well, amniocentesis is appropriate and is best performed by a qualified obstetrician.

A Gram stain of a stool specimen to look for evidence of mononuclear or polymorphonuclear white blood cells can quickly focus further investigations. Most importantly, bacterial isolates of enteric pathogens should undergo antibiotic susceptibility testing to avoid repeated trials of ineffective multiple antibiotics that lead to unnecessary and potentially injurious drug exposures in pregnant patients.

Ulcerative colitis or colonic Crohn's disease are often diagnosed by a flexible sigmoidoscope examination and biopsy, strategies with no excess risk in pregnancy. Occasionally, radiographic imaging of the abdomen is warranted. Fetal risks of radiation exposure must be weighed carefully against the risk of delayed or inaccurate diagnosis. However, fetal well-being depends on maternal well-being. A pregnant woman should not be denied a potentially life-saving diagnostic intervention, nor should it be delayed on account of her pregnancy.

MANAGEMENT

After an appropriate diagnostic evaluation (Fig. 14.5) empiric antimicrobial agents need to be considered. Further, if there is any suspicion of an infection that may be life-threatening to the mother or fetus, such as listeriosis, then empiric therapy should be instituted.

Numerous sources of information are available on the safety of antibiotics in pregnant women. Most readily available is the manufacturer's package insert, which usually includes a 'pregnancy category'. These categories are not always consistently applied. It is therefore wise to seek more detailed information from other sources, such as the on-line resources that are widely available in medical libraries and hospital pharmacies.

The number of commonly recommended antibiotics for diarrheal diseases is small. None of them are known teratogens. Ampicillin and other beta-lactam antibiotics (with the potential exception of ticarcillin) have a strong record of safety in pregnancy and are best administered in doses at the upper end of the therapeutic range for women in the second and third trimesters owing to altered pharmacokinetics.

Metronidazole is teratogenic in experimental animals and its use in pregnancy is controversial in some settings. Its use is probably warranted when the patient has a severe illness, such as symptomatic amebiasis. Fluoroquinolones are more controversial. As human data are scant, this class of agents is best avoided in pregnant women owing to the risk of arthropathy in the developing fetus, which has been well characterized in animal models. For all potential causes of dysenteric illness where fluoroquinolones are considered first-line

MANAGEMENT OF THE PREGNANT WOMAN WHO HAS DYSENTERY

1. Hospitalization
2. Fluid and electrolyte replacement
3. Oxygen monitoring
4. Fetal evaluation by an obstetrician
5. Begin diagnostic evaluation
6. Empiric therapy if indicated

Fig. 14.5 Management of the pregnant woman who has dysentery.

therapy, alternative agents exist that have better characterized safety risk profiles in pregnancy. Tetracyclines (which carry the risk of hepatotoxicity and staining of permanent teeth), chloramphenicol (which suppresses bone marrow), and prolonged courses of aminoglycosides (which are ototoxic) are best avoided in pregnancy if possible. Macrolides are generally safe, but even erythromycin has been occasionally associated with hypertrophic pyloric stenosis in infancy. Sulfa drugs should be avoided in the third trimester because of the potential increased risk of kernicterus. Trimethoprim–sulfamethoxazole (co-trimoxazole) has been associated in some studies with cleft palate when administered to rats at high doses, and it has the potential for interference with folate metabolism, raising concern about potential neural tube defects in the developing fetus. However, these have not been shown to be significant risks for humans.

The clinician unaccustomed to the uncertainties of prescribing in pregnancy may find little reassurance in such data. Absolute risk from a given agent in a given situation may be minimal, but the anxiety created by the unknown can be substantial. It must be remembered that delay of needed therapy may offer far more risk to the fetus than the therapy itself. Thus, as in the early stages of patient evaluation, the clinician must resist being paralyzed by indecision and the unknown regarding therapies. Rather, it is appropriate and wise to seek additional information. Most important, open and honest discussion of uncertainties with the patient and her obstetrician will serve all parties well.

FURTHER READING

Armon PJ. Amoebiasis in pregnancy and puerperium. Br J Obstet Gynecol 1978;85:264–9.

Burrow GN, Ferris TF. Medical complications during pregnancy. 4th ed. Philadelphia: WB Saunders; 1995.

Creasy RK, Resnik R. Maternal–fetal medicine: Principles and practice. 3rd ed. Philadelphia: WB Saunders; 1994.

Friedman JM, Polifka JE. The effects of drugs on the fetus and nursing infant: a handbook for health care professionals. Baltimore, London: The Johns Hopkins University Press; 1996.

Simor AE, Karmali MA, Jadavji T, Rosco M. Abortion and perinatal sepsis associated with *Campylobacter* infection. Rev Infect Dis 1986;8:397–402.

Tobak MA, Hart MD, Osborn LM. *Campylobacter* enteritis: prenatal and perinatal implications. Am J Obstet Gynecol 1983;147:845–6.

Management of fever that relapses and remits   *Nick Price*

INTRODUCTION

The patient who has recurrent febrile episodes commonly presents a particularly difficult diagnostic challenge. In addition to the classic criteria for fever of unknown origin (FUO) (Chapter 3.3), Knockaert *et al.* have defined 'recurrent' FUO as repeated febrile episodes with fever-free intervals of at least 2 weeks. The number of relapses or overall duration was not specified but, in practice, the clinical course is typically protracted. One limitation of this definition is that several important conditions that are typically associated with a recurrent fever pattern are excluded by the defining criteria (malaria is a notable example because of its periodic fever). However, a clear definition and strict adherence to defining criteria are helpful because they focus the diagnostic approach and are essential for meaningful comparative studies.

CAUSES

Infections, malignancy and multisystem inflammatory diseases are responsible for 60–70% of cases of classic FUO. If recurrent FUO is considered as a subset of classic FUO, these three causes account for only 20% of the cases; 50% go undiagnosed, and a collection of diverse 'miscellaneous' conditions forms the largest subgroup (Fig. 14.6).

Infectious causes

A silent focus of bacterial infection is the most common infectious cause that should be considered, rather than any of the limited number of specific infections listed (see Fig. 14.6). Other infections on the list of differential diagnoses that present with a relapsing and remitting fever pattern, which may not fulfill the stringent criteria for recurrent

CAUSES OF RECURRENT FEVER OF UNKNOWN ORIGIN

Infectious diseases

Focal bacterial infection (e.g. chronic prostatitis, subacute cholangitis)
Q fever endocarditis (*Coxiella burnetti*)
Rat-bite fever (*Spirillum minor, Streptobacillus moniliformis*)
Relapsing fever (*Borrelia recurrentis, Borrelia duttoni*)
Trypanosomiasis (*Trypanosoma gambiense, Trypanosoma rhodesiense*)
Whipple's disease (*Tropheryma whippelii*)
Yersiniosis (*Yersinia pseudotuberculosis, Yersinia enterocolitica*)

Multisystem diseases

Connective tissue diseases and vasculitides:
    Churg–Strauss disease
    Giant cell arteritis
    Polymyalgia rheumatica
    Mixed connective tissue disease
    Polyarteritis nodosa
    Systemic lupus erythematosus
    Wegener's granulomatosis

Rheumatologic diseases:
    Ankylosing spondylitis
    Relapsing polychondritis
    Rheumatoid disease
    Still's disease

Inflammatory diseases:
    Sarcoidosis

Neoplasia

Atrial myxoma
Colonic carcinoma
Lymphoma

Miscellaneous conditions

Castleman's disease
Cholesterol embolism
Crohn's disease
Cyclic neutropenia
Drug fever
Extrinsic allergic alveolitis
Factitious fever
Familial Mediterranean fever, familial Hibernian fever
Fume fever, hypersensitivity pneumonitis
Gaucher's disease, Fabry's disease
Hyper-IgD syndrome
Hypertriglyceridemia (type IV)
Mollaret's meningitis
Seizures ('thermal epilepsy')
Sweet's syndrome

Fig. 14.6 Causes of recurrent fever of unknown origin. The more common types are indicated in bold type. Adapted from Knockaert *et al.*, 1993.

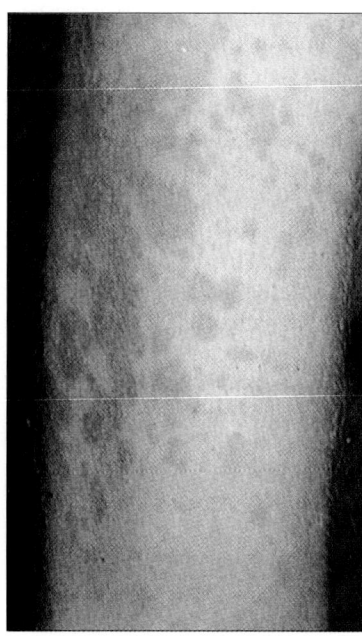

Fig. 14.7 Characteristic evanescent rash of Still's disease.

Miscellaneous causes

Crohn's disease is an important cause of recurrent FUO and may present with weight loss, fever and anemia without any gastrointestinal symptoms. Familial Mediterranean fever is characterized by recurrent polyserositis and can now be diagnosed by identification of the defective gene, which has recently been cloned (MEFV – the pyrin gene). It is unclear whether 'hyper-IgD syndrome' is a distinct clinical entity; patients typically have elevated IgD levels (>100U/ml), are usually European in origin and have similar clinical features to those individuals who suffer familial Mediterranean fever. Similarly, 'idiopathic granulomatosis' and 'granulomatous hepatitis' should not be readily accepted as final diagnoses because it is likely that they encompass a variety of different underlying conditions, which may be revealed during careful long-term follow up. Castleman's disease (or angiofollicular lymph node hyperplasia) may present with focal mediastinal or generalized lymphadenopathy. The localized type occurs in young adults and is curable by surgery. The generalized form affects older patients, has a less benign prognosis and may undergo malignant transformation. Sweet's syndrome is characterized by a painful neutrophilic dermatosis and is associated with joint pains and malignancy. Very rarely, epileptic seizures may produce periodic febrile confusion.

CLINICAL FEATURES

As for any FUO, a sharp clinical acumen is needed to make efficient use of the vast array of investigations. Associated clinical features are illustrated in Figure 14.8. In general, the pattern of the fever is seldom of diagnostic value. Cyclic neutropenia is a notable exception to this and causes a recurrent fever at a fixed interval of about 21 days.

It is vital to obtain a detailed travel history. In the tropical traveler, the risk of transmission from insect vectors should also be assessed by enquiring about visits to game parks, accommodation (camping, down-market hotels, log cabins) and protective measures such as bed nets. A tsetse fly (the vector in African trypanosomiasis) bite is often memorably painful and leaves an indurated lesion for days. In contrast, the bite in tick-borne relapsing fever is characteristically painless (Chapter 6.4). In addition, the patient's skin must be inspected closely for bites or chancres. Specific enquiry should also be made about consumption of unpasteurized milk (a cause of brucellosis), occupational exposure (e.g. fume fever), animal contact (e.g. rat-bite fever, Q fever, psittacosis), previous medical conditions (e.g. episodes of cholecystitis), drug treatment (especially if taken intermittently), and family history (e.g. Gaucher's disease and Fabry's disease).

FUO, include brucellosis, malaria, secondary syphilis, tuberculosis, trench fever (caused by *Bartonella quintana*), filariasis and visceral leishmaniasis.

Neoplastic causes

All common malignancies can cause FUO; however, those listed (see Fig. 14.6) have been specifically reported as causing recurrent FUO.

Multisystem diseases

All vasculitides or connective tissue diseases can flare up suddenly and remit spontaneously, producing a recurrent fever. Still's disease is a seronegative arthritis of unknown etiology; it is essentially a diagnosis of exclusion. The diagnosis should be strongly suspected in a young adult with the classic triad of high fever of >104°F (40°C), evanescent rash (Fig. 14.7) and arthritis (particularly if pharyngitis is also reported).

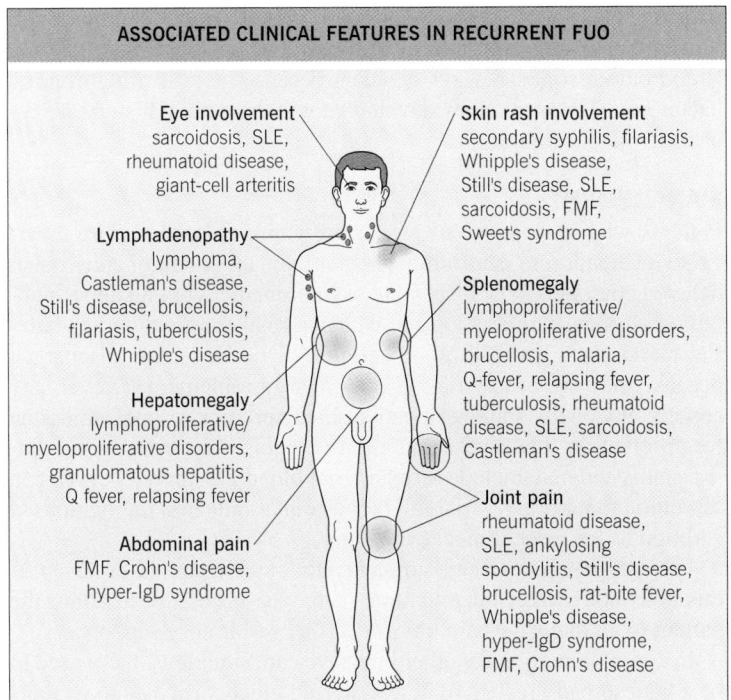

ASSOCIATED CLINICAL FEATURES IN RECURRENT FUO

Eye involvement
sarcoidosis, SLE,
rheumatoid disease,
giant-cell arteritis

Lymphadenopathy
lymphoma,
Castleman's disease,
Still's disease, brucellosis,
filariasis, tuberculosis,
Whipple's disease

Hepatomegaly
lymphoproliferative/
myeloproliferative disorders,
granulomatous hepatitis,
Q fever, relapsing fever

Abdominal pain
FMF, Crohn's disease,
hyper-IgD syndrome

Skin rash involvement
secondary syphilis, filariasis,
Whipple's disease,
Still's disease, SLE,
sarcoidosis, FMF,
Sweet's syndrome

Splenomegaly
lymphoproliferative/
myeloproliferative disorders,
brucellosis, malaria,
Q-fever, relapsing fever,
tuberculosis, rheumatoid
disease, SLE, sarcoidosis,
Castleman's disease

Joint pain
rheumatoid disease,
SLE, ankylosing
spondylitis, Still's disease,
brucellosis, rat-bite fever,
Whipple's disease,
hyper-IgD syndrome,
FMF, Crohn's disease

Fig. 14.8 Clinical features associated with recurrent fever of unknown origin. SLE, systemic lupus erythematosus; FMF, familial Mediterranean fever.

INVESTIGATIONS

The investigative work up is the same as for classic FUO (Chapter 3.3). Because the range of potential underling causes is so diverse, no comprehensive diagnostic algorithms exist.

Hematologic indices occasionally provide useful clues but are not always reliable (e.g. eosinophilia may indicate a parasitic infection, drug reaction, lymphoma or Churg–Strauss disease). In the tropical traveler, the causative organisms in relapsing fever and trypanosomiasis may be visualized on a thick blood film taken during a febrile episode. A moderately elevated acute phase response is not remarkable in itself, although it does exclude factitious fever. However, in some conditions, inflammatory indices are exceptionally high: an erythrocyte sedimentation rate >100mm/h is often seen in drug fever, malignancy,

giant-cell arteritis, Still's disease and hyper-IgD syndrome. In active Still's disease, a greatly raised serum ferritin level is also typical. Serologic and immunologic tests should be done as appropriate, but as in classic FUO they are often unrewarding.

Radioisotope-labeled white cell scanning is particularly useful at identifying occult foci of infection, but it may also yield positive results with diverse diseases such as sarcoidosis, colonic cancer, localized Castleman's disease and giant-cell arteritis. There should be a low threshold for investigating the gastrointestinal tract by endoscopy, small bowel transit study, colonoscopy or barium enema in order to look for inflammatory bowel disease and malignancy. In an elderly patient who has a very elevated erythrocyte sedimentation rate, temporal artery biopsy may be useful diagnostically where there is no prior localizing information.

GENERAL APPROACH

Because the cause of recurrent FUO is generally not life threatening, if no clues are provided by diagnostic tests, a 'watch-and-wait' strategy can be adopted. Periodic outpatient assessment is likely to reveal significant pathology in time. Most of the undiagnosed cases resolve spontaneously, but improved diagnostic techniques and the discovery of new pathogens (e.g. *Tropheryma whippelii*) will probably reduce the number of unidentified cases in the future.

Repeated attacks of fever may also represent a relapse of a pre-existing disease, particularly if treatment fails or is discontinued. Treatment compliance or antimicrobial resistance may therefore need to be addressed. In general, empiric trials of therapy are inadvisable. However, if empiric trials are felt to be absolutely necessary, a full course of treatment should be given so that complications arising from inadequate therapy are avoided.

FURTHER READING

Babior BM, Matzner Y. The familiar Mediterranean fever gene – cloned at last. N Engl J Med 1997;337:1548–9.

Knockaert DC, Vanneste LJ, Bobbaers HJ. Recurrent or episodic fever of unknown origin: review of 45 cases and survey of the literature. Medicine 1993;72:184–96.

Livneh A, Langevitz P, Zemer D, *et al.* The changing face of familial Mediterranean fever. Semin Arthritis Rheum 1996;26:612–27.

Van de Putte LB, Wouters JM. Adult-onset Still's disease. In: Sturrock RD, ed. Clinical rheumatology: rheumatic manifestations of haematological disease, vol V(2). London: Baillieres; 1991:263–75.

Infections associated with near drowning

Alastair Miller

INTRODUCTION

Drowning implies death due to cerebral hypoxia as a result of immersion in water. In the majority of cases water is aspirated into pulmonary air spaces. This produces a variety of pathologies depending on whether fresh or sea water is inhaled, but the end result is alveolar dysfunction causing venous blood to be shunted into the systemic circulation past underventilated alveoli to cause hypoxemia. In a minority of cases hypoxemia can result from apnea caused by several different mechanisms.

Drowning causes approximately 8000 deaths each year in the USA and it has been estimated that there are between two and 20 times more cases of near drowning. If the victim survives the initial hypoxic insult then a number of complications may ensue, including pulmonary edema, convulsions and infective problems such as pneumonia or sepsis.

PATHOGENESIS

The majority of people who have near drowning episodes have aspirated either sea water or fresh water. The resulting lung damage produces inflammation and edema, which damage alveolar defense mechanisms

and enhance the risk of infection. The relatively anaerobic conditions may also favor infection. Infecting organisms may include those already colonizing the lungs or upper airways that have been carried distally with the aspiration and have then taken advantage of improved conditions for growth. Alternatively, there may be organisms growing in the aspirated water and these may give rise to infective problems. Finally, an ill patient who has lung damage may be admitted to hospital (and to an intensive care unit) and therefore be exposed to all the risks of nosocomial pneumonia.

MICROBIOLOGY

The literature on the microbiology of near drowning consists mainly of reports of single cases rather than large-scale reviews, but some common themes do emerge. Organisms that have been implicated are shown in Figure 14.9, and these can be divided into those that are characteristically associated with pneumonia (either community-acquired or nosocomial) and those that are more specifically associated with immersion incidents. Gram-negative organisms predominate in the aquatic environment (both sea water and fresh water) but anaerobic organisms and

MICRO-ORGANISMS THAT HAVE BEEN IMPLICATED IN CAUSING PNEUMONIA OR SEPSIS AFTER NEAR DROWNING
Conventional respiratory pathogens (including atypical organisms and those associated with nosocomial pneumonias)
Staphylococcus aureus
Haemophilus influenzae
Streptococcus pneumoniae
Escherichia coli
Pseudomonas spp.
Moraxella spp.
Klebsiella spp.
Legionella spp.
Pathogens specifically related to immersion
Aeromonas spp.
Pseudomonas putrefaciens
Francisella philomiragia
Chromobacterium violaceum
Burkholderia pseudomallei
Vibrio spp.
Pseudallescheria boydii
Aspergillus spp.

Fig. 14.9 Micro-organisms that have been implicated in causing pneumonia or sepsis after near drowning.

Staphylococcus spp. can also be found. There may be some organisms that are more likely depending on whether immersion took place in sea water or fresh water and depending on whether the water was clean or contaminated. It may also be that certain organisms are more common in particular geographic areas. For example, one might anticipate exposure to *Burkholderia pseudomallei* following a near-drowning episode in the paddy fields of South East Asia (Chapter 6.34).

Several cases of infection with *Aeromonas* spp. exist in the literature and these are associated with a high proportion of positive blood cultures and a high mortality. Fungal infections can also cause problems and there are reports of *Aspergillus* pneumonia and disseminated aspergillosis after immersion incidents. Infection is commonly polymicrobial.

CLINICAL FEATURES

The clinical features of infection after near drowning are similar to those seen when the particular infection arises from more conventional causes and depend on the site of infection. The main complication is pneumonia (as might be predicted from the portal of entry) but there is often an associated bacteremia, which may produce clinical features of sepsis. There have also been case reports of meningitis after near drowning.

Noninfective pulmonary edema is a common complication of near drowning and can progress to full adult respiratory distress syndrome. Pulmonary edema can be difficult to distinguish clinically and radiographically from pneumonia. In one series of 125 near drowning episodes, the incidence of pulmonary edema was 43% whereas the incidence of pneumonia was 14.7%. These figures are sensitive to changes in case definition, and clearly many patients who initially have pulmonary edema may subsequently go on to develop pneumonia, which tends to be a later complication.

Most patients who have pneumonia have fever (although recognition of this may be confounded if there is any residual hypothermia from the immersion). They may have clinical features of pulmonary consolidation or edema, or both.

INVESTIGATIONS

Near-drowning victims should have a chest radiograph on admission and this may well be clear or show nonspecific shadowing. They should also have a full blood count and arterial blood gas analysis. It is unlikely that an asymptomatic patient who has normal arterial blood gases and chest radiograph will develop any pulmonary complications. Leukocytosis is usual in patients who have pneumonia but is not specific for infection.

Pulmonary secretions must be examined microbiologically; these may include expectorated sputum or tracheal aspirates in intubated patients. There may be pus cells in the samples and it is common to find infecting micro-organisms by stain and by subsequent culture. Blood cultures must always be taken because there is a high rate of bacteremia. Empyema may develop later in the natural history, necessitating pleural aspiration.

MANAGEMENT

Patients who have survived a near drowning episode require emergency evaluation to determine whether they are at risk of subsequent delayed complications. If they are asymptomatic, with no abnormalities on physical examination and with a normal chest radiograph, arterial blood gases and full blood count, they can be safely discharged because they are at low risk of pulmonary problems. However, any abnormality on this initial evaluation should prompt hospital admission for observation. The level of monitoring required depends on the clinical status and may include serial arterial blood gas analysis or oxygen saturation monitoring, serial full blood counts and chest radiographs in addition to frequent clinical evaluation.

If hypoxemia is present, supplemental oxygen should be given. If this does not correct the situation, it may be necessary to admit the patient to an intensive care unit for further respiratory support.

In common with many other intensive care situations, there used to be a widespread practice of administering glucocorticoids to patients who had undergone aspiration. There has never been evidence of benefit in near-drowning incidents and this practice is not recommended.

ANTIBIOTICS

Prophylactic antibiotics have been shown of no benefit in at least one study and their use is not recommended. However, there should be a low threshold for instituting antimicrobial therapy if there is any suspicion of developing pneumonia or sepsis (Fig. 14.10). Features giving rise to concern include deteriorating arterial blood gases, new infiltrates on chest radiograph, hemodynamic disturbance or the development of fever or leukocytosis. It is likely that antibiotics will have to commence before any microbiologic information is available from the laboratory (although initial Gram stains may be helpful). Therefore, broad-spectrum empiric cover with good pulmonary penetration is indicated.

Numerous antibiotics have been used, including aminoglycosides, monobactams, carbapenems, cephalosporins and extended spectrum penicillins (with and without beta-lactamase inhibitors). There are no large-scale trials to guide rational therapy. I suggest the use of clindamycin, which has good penetration and will provide good Gram-positive cover as well as treating anaerobic infection. This should be combined with ciprofloxacin to cover the Gram-negative organisms and also provide some cover against *Legionella* spp. Other reasonable combinations would be ticarcillin–clavulanate with gentamicin and ceftazidime with metronidazole, although neither of these two regimens offers cover against *Legionella* spp. Clearly the initial regimen may need to be modified in the light of subsequent information from the microbiology laboratory, but it is important to remember that polymicrobial infection is common. If there is no adequate response, it may be necessary to consider the use of antifungal treatment.

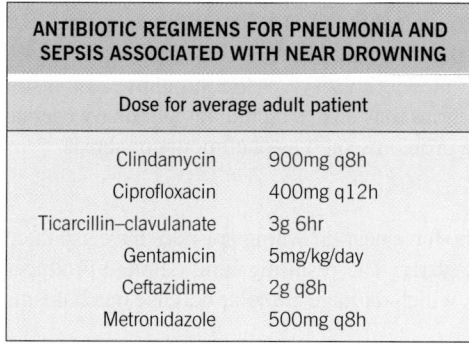

ANTIBIOTIC REGIMENS FOR PNEUMONIA AND SEPSIS ASSOCIATED WITH NEAR DROWNING	
Dose for average adult patient	
Clindamycin	900mg q8h
Ciprofloxacin	400mg q12h
Ticarcillin–clavulanate	3g 6hr
Gentamicin	5mg/kg/day
Ceftazidime	2g q8h
Metronidazole	500mg q8h

Fig. 14.10 Antibiotic regimens for pneumonia and sepsis associated with near drowning. All these antibiotics are administered intravenously.

FURTHER READING

Dworzack DL. New causes of pneumonia, meningitis and disseminated infections associated with immersion. Infect Dis Clin North Am 1987;1:615–33.

Ender PT, Dolan MJ. Pneumonia associated with near drowning. Clin Infect Dis 1997;27:896–907.

Ender PT, Dolan MJ, Dolan D, Farmer JS, Melcher GP. Near-drowning-associated *Aeromonas* pneumonia. J Emerg Med 1996;14:737–41.

Modell JH. Current concepts: drowning. N Engl J Med 1993;328:253–6.

Stewart RD. Submersion incidents: drowning and near drowning. In: Auerbach PS, Geehr EC, eds. Management of wilderness and environmental emergencies, 2nd ed. St Louis: Mosby 1989;908–32.

van Berkel M, Bierens JJ, Lie RL, Kool LJ, van de Welde EA, Meinders AE. Pulmonary oedema, pneumonia and mortality in submersion victims; a retrospective study in 125 patients. Intensive Care Med 1996;22:101–7.

Diagnostic work up of the potentially septic burn patient

David J Barillo & Albert T McManus

The presence of fever, leukocytosis, elevated cardiac output, low systemic vascular resistance and positive wound surface cultures all represent 'normal' physiology in the burns patient. These clinical features may exist in the absence of sepsis and are not of themselves diagnostic of infection. Nevertheless, given the fact that infection remains the major source of morbidity and mortality in burns patients, careful and repeated examination for septic foci is indicated in this population (Chapter 3.8).

Acute infection may be suggested by the presence of any of the above findings, or more commonly by a change in hemodynamic status, body temperature or clinical condition. Increased need for ventilatory support or the new onset of ileus, glycosuria or glucose intolerance also indicate the need for a septic work up. We do not consider acute burn patients to be febrile until core (rectal or pulmonary artery catheter thermistor) temperature exceeds 102.5°F (39.2°C) and do not perform 'fever work ups' below this level. An exception is the patient who has nearly closed burn wounds who has previously returned to a 'normal' body temperature [98.6°F (37°C)]; such patients are considered febrile by the usual criteria.

A septic work up starts with a complete physical examination. In addition to the usual examination of the ears, oropharynx, sinuses, lungs and abdomen, specific attention should be directed at the burn wound (see below) and to any current or previous site of intravenous cannulation. Rectal examination should be performed to rule out prostatitis in males and perirectal disease in both sexes. Cultures of blood, sputum and urine are obtained, along with a chest radiograph. A time frame of initial presentation of infection by site is presented in Figure 14.11.

Intra-abdominal processes producing sepsis include acalculous cholecystitis, bowel ischemia or necrosis, pancreatitis and, rarely, perforation of a gastric or duodenal ulcer. Pancreatitis or cholecystitis is

evaluated by abdominal ultrasound. Triple-contrast (nasogastric/rectal and intravenous) CT scans of the abdomen may be useful. We have found diagnostic peritoneal lavage, as normally performed for acute abdominal trauma, to have a sensitivity of 86%, a specificity of 100% and an overall accuracy of 94% in the diagnosis of intraperitoneal infection in burn patients, and this technique remains our primary diagnostic modality for the abdomen.

Children may develop idiopathic fevers in the 103°F (39.5°C) range early in the course of burn care. The fever usually resolves without a source being identified; however, all febrile burned children should be carefully examined with particular attention to the middle ears, oropharynx and urinary system. Asymptomatic colonization of the pediatric oropharynx with Lancefield group A β-hemolytic streptococci is a theoretic concern, because spread of streptococci to the burn wound can result in a rapidly spreading cellulitis or loss of previously placed autograft (Chapter 6.17). Some advocate the prophylactic administration of penicillin to pediatric burn patients or to all burn patients. Given the low incidence of β-hemolytic streptococcal infection in burn patients, such routine prophylaxis is probably unjustified. A middle course is to obtain pediatric throat cultures at the time of admission, and to administer penicillin only to those children from whom streptococci are isolated.

Electrical injury is a special category of burns trauma in which extensive muscle necrosis may occur along the route of the passage of the electric current. Because the external position of the skin allows rapid heat dissipation, it is common to encounter necrotic muscle covered by skin that is entirely normal in appearance. The work up of fever or sepsis in the electrical injury patient should include prompt surgical exploration of body regions known or suspected to be involved if another septic source is not immediately apparent.

Positive blood cultures in the absence of wound infection should prompt examination of intravenous cannulation sites and consideration of endocarditis. When a single positive blood culture is inconsistent with the clinical picture, treatment may be deferred pending repeat culture results. Two blood cultures that are positive for the same organism and that are uncontaminated by passage through the burn wound should be treated with systemic antibiotics even in the absence of systemic signs. Gram-negative bacteremia (but not Gram-positive bacteremia) in burns patients is associated with a significantly increased mortality. The association of fungemia with increased mortality is equivocal.

Radionucleotide studies such as indium or tagged leukocyte scans are, in general, of little use in the burns patient. Areas of open burn wound or skin donor sites frequently concentrate isotope, making interpretation difficult.

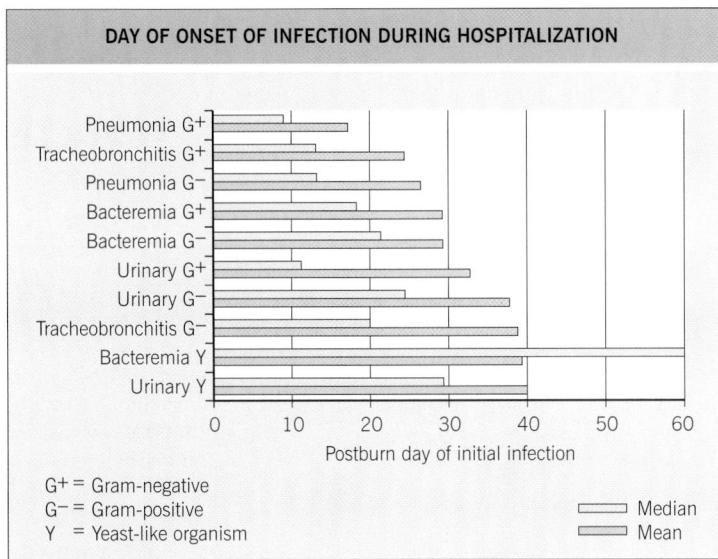

DAY OF ONSET OF INFECTION DURING HOSPITALIZATION

Postburn day of initial infection

G+ = Gram-negative
G− = Gram-positive
Y = Yeast-like organism

Median
Mean

Fig. 14.11 Time of onset of infection in burns patients during hospitalization.

EVALUATION AND TREATMENT OF THE BURN WOUND AS A POSSIBLE SOURCE OF SEPSIS

The burn wound should be examined on at least a daily basis, and at the first sign of systemic infection. Cellulitis is diagnosed by the presence of expanding erythema at the margins of the burn wound. Erythema surrounding second- or third-degree burn injury that does not increase in size may also represent areas of first-degree burn. Burn wound cellulitis usually responds well to a penicillin.

True burn wound infection is suspected on the basis of signs such as:

- early eschar separation,
- conversion of partial-thickness to full-thickness injury,
- subeschar hemorrhage,
- degeneration of granulation tissue,
- dark red, brown or black discoloration of eschar (Fig. 14.12),
- violaceous discoloration of unburned skin at the wound margins and
- ecthyma gangrenosum (green discoloration of subcutaneous fat as a result of infection with *Pseudomonas* spp.)

Diagnosis of invasive wound infection is confirmed by wound biopsy and histologic examination. When invasive bacterial infection (stage 2A, 2B or 2C) (see Chapter 3.8) is diagnosed, the wound should be continuously covered with mafenide acetate cream and all other agents discontinued. Systemic antibiotics are then instituted on the basis of the predominant organism in the biopsy specimen or of surveillance cultures; Gram-negative organisms are most frequently implicated. The wound should be surgically excised as soon as possible. Subeschar injection of systemic antibiotics (clysis) is a useful adjunct and should be performed immediately on diagnosis and repeated 6 hours before

surgical excision. One half of the daily dose of a semisynthetic penicillin (piperacillin or carbenicillin) may be mixed in sufficient diluent (1 liter of normal saline) for injection through a 20 gauge spinal needle. Clysis may be repeated twice a day for patients who are too unstable to tolerate surgical excision.

Fungal infection of the burn wound is most commonly caused by *Aspergillus* spp., *Candida* spp., *Mucor* spp. or *Rhizopus* spp. Wound colonization involving *Candida* spp. is commonly treated with topical nystatin or clotrimazole, although few studies have addressed the effectiveness of these agents in burn care. *Aspergillus* spp. characteristically produce superficial colonization or infection that is amenable to local surgical excision. *Mucor* spp. may produce a rapidly spreading fascial infection with early microvascular involvement. Radical surgical debridement or amputation may be required to control this type of infection.

We reserve the use of systemic antifungal therapy (amphotericin B) for cases where disseminated or systemic fungal infection is known or suspected, or when wound biopsies are positive at a stage 2C level. We do not use other systemic antifungal agents such as fluconazole at present.

FURTHER READING

Artz CP, Moncrief JA, Pruitt BA Jr. Burns – a team approach. Philadelphia: WB Saunders; 1979.

Becker WK, Cioffi WG, McManus AT, *et al.* Fungal burn wound infection: a ten year experience. Arch Surg 1991;126:44–8.

Behrman RE, Kleigman RM, Nelson WE, Vaughan VC III, eds. Nelson's textbook of pediatrics, 14th ed. Philadelphia: WB Saunders; 1992.

Heggers J, Linares HA, Edgar P, *et al.* Treatment of infections in burns. In: Herndon DN, ed. Total burn care. Philadelphia: WB Saunders: 1996.

Hinder F, Traber DL. Pathophysiology of the systemic inflammatory response syndrome. In: Herndon DN, ed. Total burn care. Philadelphia: WB Saunders; 1996.

McManus AT, McManus WF, Mason AD, Pruitt BA Jr. Beta-hemolytic streptococcal burn wound infections are too infrequent to justify penicillin prophylaxis [letter]. Plast Reconstr Surg 1994;93:650.

McManus WF, Goodwin CW, Pruitt BA Jr. Subeschar treatment of burn wound infection. Arch Surg 1983;118:291–4.

Mason AD, McManus AT, Pruitt BA Jr. Association of burn mortality and bacteremia. Arch Surg 1986;121:1027–31.

Mozingo DW, Cioffi WG, McManus WF, Pruitt BA Jr. Peritoneal lavage in the diagnosis of acute surgical abdomen following surgical injury. J Trauma 1995;38:5–7.

Pruitt BA Jr, Goodwin CW, Cioffi WG. Thermal injuries. In: Davis JH, Sheldon GF, eds. Surgery – a problem solving approach. St Louis: Mosby-Year Book; 1995.

Robson MC, Burns BF, Smith DJ. Acute management of the burned patient. Plast Reconstr Surg 1992;89:1155–68.

Shirani KZ, Vaughan GM, Mason AD, Pruitt BA Jr. Update on current therapeutic approaches in burns. Shock 1996;5:4–16.

Timmons MJ. Acute management of the burned patient [letter]. Plast Reconstr Surg 1993;91:1175.

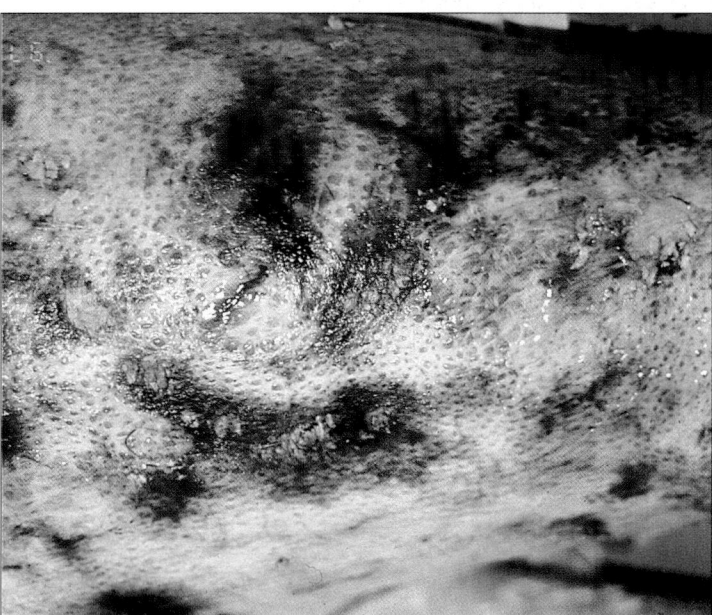

Fig. 14.12 Invasive pseudomonal burn wound infection, stage 2C.

Infections in the Immunocompromised Host

Paul G Quie & Claus O Solberg

4

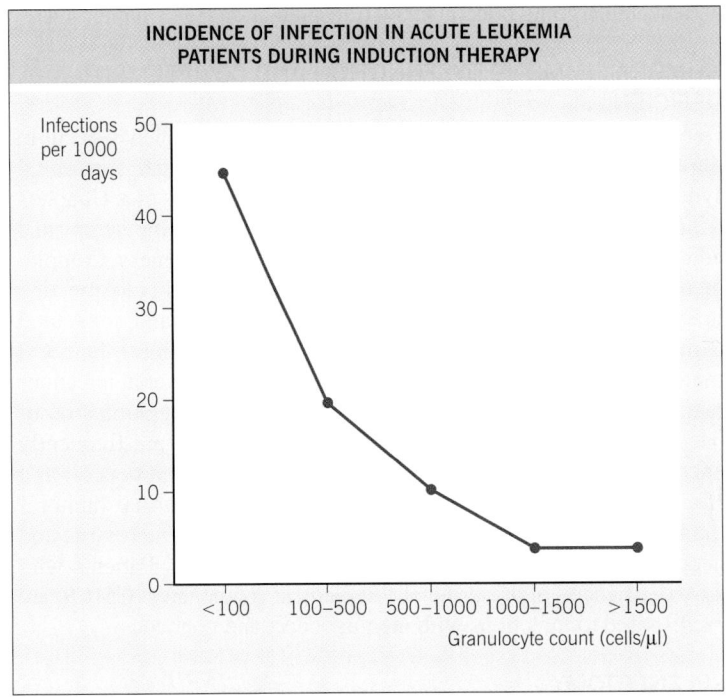 at top right corner:

Introduction

Claus O Solberg & Paul G Quie

The term immunocompromised host describes individuals with defects of nonspecific (skin, mucosa, phagocytes, complement or cytokines) and/or specific (humoral or cellular) immunity to infection. These individuals are at increased risk of infection with a variety of micro-organisms, including micro-organisms with no pathogenicity for healthy individuals (i.e. opportunistic agents). This chapter gives a brief overview of infections in the immunocompromised host. The following chapters in this section present comprehensive reviews of infectious disease problems specific to the circumstances of immunocompromise.

EPIDEMIOLOGY

During the past three decades, major advances have been made in cancer chemotherapy, transplantation, and treatment of a variety of immunologically mediated diseases. This success has resulted in a steadily increasing population of immunocompromised patients, such as patients who have severe malignancy (e.g. leukemia, lymphoma, multiple myeloma and cancer metastases), solid organ and bone marrow transplants, collagenoses and advanced diabetes mellitus, and patients receiving immunosuppressive or cytotoxic drug therapy.[1,2] Infection is a common feature in these individuals, and during the past 20–30 years, infection in the immunocompromised host has evolved from an esoteric subject of interest mainly in academic centers to one that involves physicians in nearly all fields of medicine. Furthermore, the advent of the catastrophic AIDS epidemic has markedly stimulated the interest in individuals with acquired immunocompromise and has captured the attention of the general public to a greater extent than any other disease in modern time.

PATHOGENESIS

A useful approach to infections in the immunocompromised host is the recognition of the major predisposing factors, because each is associated with infections caused by an array of pathogens that usually do not overlap.[1,3] Knowledge of the major immunocompromising factors contributes to appropriate diagnosis and management of infection in specific patients. The most important predisposing factors are:
• granulocytopenia and qualitative phagocyte defects,
• cellular immune dysfunction,
• humoral immune dysfunction and complement deficiency and
• splenectomy.

Various medical procedures and several disease conditions also contribute to immunocompromise and increased susceptibility to infection.

GRANULOCYTOPENIA AND QUALITATIVE PHAGOCYTE DEFECTS

The most common and serious abnormality is granulocytopenia (i.e. neutropenia). The risk of infection increases very little until the granulocyte count drops below 500 cells/μl and rises rapidly as the count approaches zero (Fig. 1.1).[4] However, the risk of infection is much more pronounced in patients who have a rapidly falling granulocyte count than in patients who have prolonged stationary granulocytopenia as in aplastic anemia. Also the duration of the granulocytopenic phase

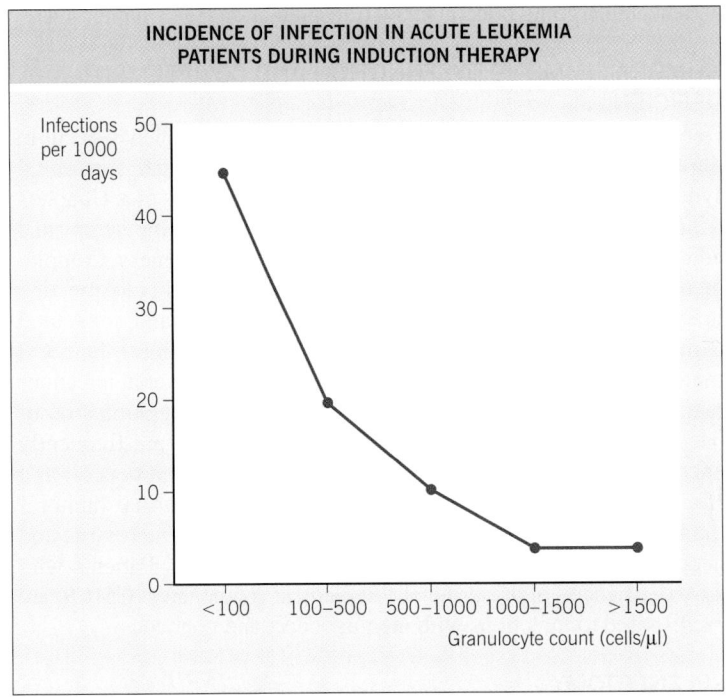

INCIDENCE OF INFECTION IN ACUTE LEUKEMIA PATIENTS DURING INDUCTION THERAPY

Fig. 1.1 Incidence of infection during induction therapy of 52 patients who have acute leukemia. The incidence of infection rises as the granulocyte count is reduced. Data from Bodey *et al.*[4]

correlates with infection. This is clearly illustrated in bone marrow transplant patients with 20–25 days of granulocytopenia, who have a much higher infection rate than do patients who have shorter granulocytopenic periods (e.g. patients receiving intensive chemotherapy for lung or testicular carcinoma).

The most common sites of infection in granulocytopenic patients include the oropharynx, perianal area, skin, lung and colon. Local infections spread easily and invasion of the blood stream is frequent. The most prevalent bacteria causing infection include *Escherichia coli, Klebsiella pneumoniae, Pseudomonas aeruginosa*, coagulase-negative staphylococci, α-hemolytic streptococci and *Staphylococcus aureus* (Fig. 1.2). Most fungal infections are caused by *Candida albicans, Candida tropicalis, Aspergillus fumigatus*. and *Aspergillus flavus*. Generally, the infections are caused by micro-organisms that have colonized the site at which the infection develops; more than 50% are hospital-acquired pathogens.

The risk of infection is also increased in patients who have qualitative abnormalities in phagocyte function (e.g. defects in chemotaxis, phagocytosis or ingestion, or metabolic factors involved in the killing of micro-organisms). The abnormalities may be congenital (see Chapter 4.2) or secondary to various underlying diseases such as leukemia and lymphoma. Radiotherapy, corticosteroids, certain antibiotics and antineoplastic agents may also contribute to phagocytic dysfunction (see Chapter 4.5).

CELLULAR IMMUNE DYSFUNCTION

Impaired cellular immune responses occur with HIV infection, Hodgkin's disease, non-Hodgkin's lymphoma, bone marrow transplantation, sarcoidosis, advanced cancer, use of cytotoxic or immunosuppressive drugs, cytomegalovirus infection, uremia and congenital syndromes associated with abnormal T-lymphocyte function. These conditions predispose patients to infections with a wide variety of micro-organisms, including many opportunistic agents (Fig. 1.2). Most of these organisms are intracellular pathogens, and many of the infections represent reactivation of a latent agent (e.g. infections with varicella-zoster virus, herpes simplex virus, *Toxoplasma gondii* and *Pneumocystis carinii*). The prevalence and severity of infections are most pronounced in patients who have AIDS (see Section 5) and in patients undergoing bone marrow transplantation (see Chapter 4.4).

HUMORAL IMMUNE DYSFUNCTION AND COMPLEMENT DEFICIENCY

Defects in humoral immunity caused by antibody deficiency occur in multiple myeloma, chronic lymphocytic leukemia and congenital syndromes associated with low immunoglobulin levels (see Chapters 4.2 & 4.5). In addition, radiation therapy, anticancer chemotherapy and adrenocorticosteroids may depress immune responsiveness. Complement deficiency may contribute to increased susceptibility to infection in systemic lupus erythematosus, sickle cell anemia and congenital complement deficiency syndromes. Patients who have humoral immune dysfunction have an increased incidence of bacterial infections mainly because of deficient opsonization, lysis and agglutination of bacteria. Respiratory tract infections and bacteremia are frequently encountered. Encapsulated bacteria such as pneumococci and *Haemophilus influenzae* are common pathogens. Normal humoral immune function is also essential for the control of enterovirus and hepatitis virus infections in the acute viremic phase. Patients who have deficiencies of the terminal complement components (C5–C9) are predisposed to infections with meningococci and gonococci.

SPLENECTOMY

The spleen filters out opsonin-coated and nonopsonized micro-organisms from the circulation and is the principal organ for the production of antibody to polysaccharide antigens (see Chapter 4.7). Splenectomized patients have decreased levels of IgM and properidin and may be deficient in other phagocytosis-promoting peptides. They are at increased risk of fulminant septicemia due to encapsulated bacteria, particularly pneumococci, but also *H. influenzae*, meningococci and some other pathogens, such as Capnocytophaga canimorsus (DF-2) and *Babesia* spp. (see Chapter 4.7). Splenectomized children, especially those aged under 2 years, are more susceptible to overwhelming bacterial sepsis than are adults.

VARIOUS MEDICAL PROCEDURES AND DISEASE CONDITIONS

Granulocytopenia and cellular and humoral immune deficiencies are often associated with other less specific factors that act in concert with neutropenia or the immune deficiency and predispose patients to infection. Cancer chemotherapy is often associated with damage to the mucosa of the alimentary and respiratory tract. These mucosal lesions frequently serve as portals of entry for micro-organisms that colonize the mucosal surface. In the absence of granulocytes or an adequate immune response, these micro-organisms may easily cause local infections or gain access to the vascular system, causing severe septicemia. Intravenous cannulae, tracheostomas and catheters in various body orifices designed to maintain vital functions are notorious points of entry for bacteria and fungi, and are particularly dangerous in patients who have granulocytopenia or other impaired immune responses. Patients who have leukemia or lymphoma frequently have breaks in skin and mucosal surfaces, allowing micro-organisms to invade and multiply. Tumors that obstruct a bronchus or a segment of the urinary tract impede normal drainage and, together with granulocytopenia or impaired immunity, encourage pulmonary or urinary tract infection. Central nervous system dysfunction as a result of cerebral hemorrhage, tumor or infection may lead to impairment of the gag reflex and an increased risk of aspiration pneumonia. Nutritional deficiencies common in patients with malignancy or who have AIDS may further depress immune function and enhance susceptibility to infection.

SHIFT IN ENDOGENOUS MICROBIAL FLORA

Immunocompromised patients frequently develop infections with hospital-acquired organisms that have colonized the site at which the infection develops.[5–7] In neutropenic patients, more than 80% of microbiologically documented infections are caused by organisms that are part of the endogenous flora, and approximately 50% of the causative agents are acquired by the patient subsequent to hospital admission.[5,7] Three factors appear to be of major importance for the shift in the endogenous flora:
• the underlying disease,
• the use of antibiotics and
• invasive techniques.
In healthy individuals, the skin and mucous membranes are colonized by relatively innocuous normal flora, primarily aerobic Gram-positive bacteria and a variety of anaerobic organisms. As disease and general debilitation occur, a shift toward Gram-negative bacilli occurs, and in the more severely ill patients Gram-negative bacilli and fungi, often from the hospital environment, become the predominant endogenous flora.[8] This shift seems partly mediated by changes in the receptors for micro-organisms on epithelial cell surfaces.

Antimicrobial agents notoriously produce a shift in microbial flora.

INFECTIONS IN IMMUNOCOMPROMISED PATIENTS: PREDISPOSING FACTORS AND PREDOMINATING PATHOGENS

Granulocytopenia	Cellular immune dysfunction		Humoral immune dysfunction
Escherichia coli	*Listeria monocytogenes*	Herpes simplex virus	*Haemophilus influenzae*
Klebsiella pneumoniae	*Legionella pneumophila*	Varicella-zoster virus	*Streptococcus pneumoniae*
Pseudomonas aeruginosa	*Mycobacterium avium* or	*Cryptosporidium*	Enteroviruses
Staphylococcus aureus	*M. intracellulare*	*Pneumocystis carinii*	Hepatitis viruses
Staphylococcus epidermidis	*M. tuberculosis*	*Toxoplasma gondii*	
α-hemolytic streptococci	*Salmonella* spp.	*Strongyloides stercoralis*	
Aspergillus flavus and *A. fumigatus*	*Cryptococcus neoformans*	HHV6 parvovirus	
Candida albicans and *C. tropicalis*	*Coccidioides immitis*	Measles virus	
	Histoplasma capsulatum	Respiratory syncytial virus	
	Cytomegalovirus	*Microsporidia*	
	Epstein–Barr virus		

Fig. 1.2 Infections in immunocompromised patients: predisposing factors and predominating pathogens.

Broad-spectrum antibiotics will suppress the beneficial normal flora that provides protection against colonization and infection by more pathogenic micro-organisms. In animal experiments, it has been demonstrated that the anaerobic flora of the gastrointestinal tract prevents colonization with new organisms, the so-called colonization resistance phenomenon.[9] Several antibiotics excreted partly via the hepatobiliary tract (e.g. cefoperazone, ciprofloxacin and piperacillin) will suppress the anaerobic flora of the gastrointestinal tract and predispose the patients to colonization with antibiotic resistant bacteria or fungi from the hospital environment. Concurrently, if the mucosa is damaged, the organisms may produce local infections.

Invasive procedures often lead to shifts in flora. The pharynx and larynx of patients who have tracheostomies become colonized with Gram-negative bacilli within a few days of the tracheotomy, and pneumonia developing in these patients is often caused by these organisms. Histamine type-2 blockers (cimetidine, ranitidine) also increase the colonization of the hypopharynx by Gram-negative bacilli in addition to anaerobic bacteria and fungi, and predispose the patients to infection with these micro-organisms.[10] Intravenous cannulae and urinary catheters also create pathways for bacteria and fungi.

Because colonization precedes infection, surveillance cultures may sometimes be helpful in the care of high-risk immunocompromised patients.[6,10] Information about the colonization with special organisms such as antibiotic resistant Gram-negative bacilli, *Candida* spp. or *Corynebacterium* spp. in the throat or rectum and *Aspergillus* spp. in the nares may be helpful when empiric antibiotic treatment is needed for a febrile patient.

PREVENTION

Several measures have been tried to prevent infection in immunocompromised patients by reducing the endogenous flora and/or the acquisition of exogenous pathogens (Fig. 1.3). Granulocytopenic patients in particular have been studied. Because the gastrointestinal tract is the source of many of the pathogens causing infections in these patients, oral nonabsorbable antibiotics have been used to suppress the endogenous gastrointestinal flora. Lack of patient compliance because of poor tolerance, malabsorption, high cost and development of antibiotic resistance have markedly limited indications for this regimen, and prophylaxis with oral nonabsorbable antibiotics is usually not recommended except in patients nursed in ultraclean environments (e.g. laminar airflow rooms).

Selective decontamination is a modified antimicrobial regimen for suppressing the potentially pathogenic aerobic flora while preserving the anaerobic flora, thus reducing subsequent colonization with new

organisms.[11] The most commonly used agents are trimethoprim–sulfamethoxazole (co-trimoxazole) or fluoroquinolones, and initial studies in neutropenic patients demonstrated reduction in most infections. However, drug toxicity, prolonged periods of granulocytopenia and antibiotic resistance development have been reported in subsequent studies with prolonged trimethoprim–sulfamethoxazole (co-trimoxazole) prophylaxis. Fluoroquinolone prophylaxis has been associated with increased prevalence of infections with Gram-positive bacteria, particularly viridans streptococci and coagulase-negative staphylococci, and also with resistance development. The potential advantages of prophylaxis with trimethoprim–sulfamethoxazole (co-trimoxazole) or fluoroquinolones in neutropenic patients are minimized by the serious disadvantages (see Chapters 1.4, 4.4 & 4.5).

The marked prevalence of invasive mycosis in profoundly immunocompromised patients (e.g. patients who have acute leukemia, those who have AIDS, or those undergoing bone marrow transplantation) has prompted extensive prophylactic use of antifungal drugs (polyenes, imidazoles and triazoles). Decrease in colonization and superficial infections with fungi may be achieved and indeed the incidence of invasive mycosis was reduced in one study.[12] However, overgrowth and invasion by resistant fungi, especially *Aspergillus* spp. and *Candida krusei*, have also been reported.[13] So far, significant benefit from antifungal prophylaxis in profoundly immunocompromised patients seems not to have been proven except in allogeneic bone marrow transplant patients, and widespread antifungal chemoprophylaxis is not recommended (see Chapters 1.4, 4.4, 4.5 & 5.9)

Viral infections are common in some immunocompromised patients, and antiviral chemoprophylaxis is indicated in certain situations (see Chapters 1.4, 4.4, 4.5 & 5.9).[1,2,14] Immunization (see Chapters 4.5, 4.7 & 4.8) and cytokine therapy to accelerate granulocyte recovery (see Chapters 4.4 & 4.5) are also important prophylactic measures in these patients.[1,2]

Bone marrow transplant patients have been given oral nonabsorbable antibiotics together with skin antiseptics and antibiotic ointments to suppress intestinal and body flora, and have been nursed in ultraclean rooms with constant positive pressure airflow, that is, laminar airflow rooms or plastic isolators (Fig. 1.4).[7,15] The ultraclean environment was maintained by sterilization of all objects that entered the room, including food. The combined use of these measures does reduce the number and severity of infections in profoundly immunocompromised patients. However, strict isolation of patients in laminar airflow rooms for prolonged periods of time is psychologically disturbing and the oral nonabsorbable antibiotics add to the problem of patient compliance because of their gastrointestinal side effects. Furthermore, these measures are expensive, and the survival of patients undergoing marrow transplantation

Fig. 1.3 Methods for preventing infection in immunocompromised patients.

METHODS FOR PREVENTING INFECTION IN IMMUNOCOMPROMISED PATIENTS		
Suppress endogenous microbial flora and/or prevent acquisition of environmental micro-organisms		**Stimulate host defense**
Prophylactic antibacterial agents	Isolation rooms	Immunization
Oral nonabsorbable antibiotics	Ultraclean (e.g. laminar airflow)	Viral and bacterial vaccines
Fluoroquinolones or trimethoprim–sulfamethoxazole ('selective decontamination')	Reverse isolation	Pooled or specific immunoglobulins
Prophylactic antifungal agents	Total protected isolation	Increase granulocyte recovery
Imidazoles	Laminar airflow room and prophylactic antimicrobial agents	Granulocyte colony-stimulating factor and granulocyte-macrophage colony-stimulating factor
Polyenes		
Triazoles		Granulocyte transfusions
Prophylactic antiviral agents		
Aclclovir		
Amantadine		
Ganciclovir		

has not been substantially improved. However, if a laminar airflow room with appropriate support is available, it seems reasonable to use it for bone marrow transplant patients and other patients who have profound neutropenia (see Chapters 4.4 & 4.5). If ultraclean facilities are not available, the combined use of positive pressure isolation facilities and the wearing of surgical gowns and masks by all visitors is recommended by some. Positive pressure rooms present a potential problem if the patients develop respiratory illnesses such as tuberculosis which could pass to other patients in nearby rooms. The most important anti-infective measure is careful handwashing practices by all personnel.

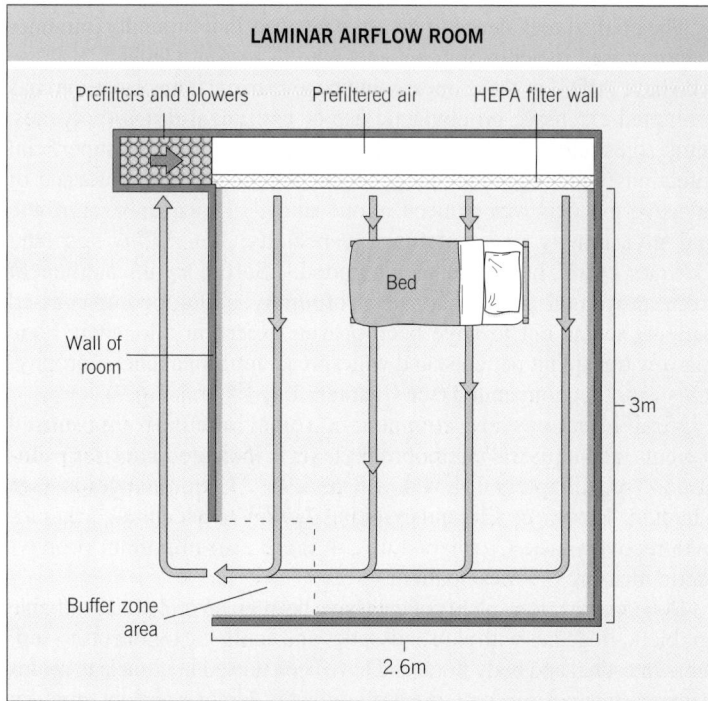

Fig. 1.4 Laminar airflow room. One entire wall is made up of high-efficiency particulate air-filters (HEPA) capable of removing 99.99% of all particles larger than 0.3μm in diameter. Virtually all bacteria, fungi and protozoa are filtered out at this standard of efficiency, and virus particles that may exist as individual particles smaller than 0.3μm in diameter are also removed by virtue of Brownian movement. The bed is oriented perpendicular to the airflow at the filter wall of the room so that all activities take place downstream from the patient, and any infective particle that might originate from the personnel is carried away from the patient by the airflow. To prevent infection by contact, all personnel entering the room dress in sterile uniforms in the buffer zone area and all materials are presterilized.

CAUSES OF PERSISTENT FEVER IN IMMUNOCOMPROMISED PATIENTS WHO HAVE NEGATIVE BACTERIAL AND FUNGAL CULTURES

- Cytomegalovirus infection
- Epstein–Barr virus infection
- Hepatitis A, B, C and E, anicteric stage
- Cryptic abscess
- Tuberculosis or other granulomatous infections
- Drug fever
- Pulmonary emboli
- Allergic reactions
- Graft-versus-host disease
- Splenic infarcts
- Underlying disease

Fig. 1.5 Causes of persistent fever in immunocompromised patients who have negative bacterial and fungal cultures.

CLINICAL FEATURES

The initial evaluation of the patient should always include a careful history and physical examination supported by Gram's stain of wound drainage, cutaneous lesions, transtracheal aspirate, urine, etc. In severely immunocompromised patients, bacterial sepsis, widespread wound infection or pneumonia are often fulminant, and the physical examination should be carried out as expeditiously as possible. It must always be borne in mind that severely immunocompromised patients, particularly granulocytopenic patients, usually fail to develop an adequate inflammatory response, and characteristic local signs of infection may not be present. Instead of abscess formation with pus and fluctuation, only cutaneous cellulitis may be present, and cough, purulent expectoration, and even stethoscopic and radiographic findings may be absent despite widespread bacterial invasion in patients who have pneumonia. Empyema and abscess rarely occur. Patients who have urinary tract infection may not have significant symptoms and may not develop pyuria. The characteristic sign of nuchal rigidity may be absent in patients who have meningitis. However, headache and mental changes are usually present.

Once it is recognized that the patient is immunocompromised, the following factors or conditions should be carefully analyzed: predisposing factors, organ defining symptoms, possible sources of infection and previous infections.

PREDISPOSING FACTORS

Generally, each major predisposing factor is associated with infections caused by a spectrum of pathogens, and these often do not overlap (Fig. 1.2). Thus, knowledge of the major compromising factors may give a clue to the diagnosis and management of infection in the specific patient. Patients who have rapidly dropping neutrophil counts, for example, are those at the highest risk of infection with Gram-negative bacilli and opportunistic fungal infections. Splenectomized patients and patients who have multiple myeloma are most likely to have infections with encapsulated bacteria. Knowledge about radiotherapy, drug treatment or diseases associated with cellular immune dysfunction is of great importance in the evaluation of pulmonary infiltrates (see Chapter 4.5).

ORGAN DEFINING SYMPTOMS

Specific symptoms that suggest the underlying pathology, such as sore throat, cough, dysuria or vaginal discharge, should be carefully evaluated to localize the source of infection and tailor antibiotic therapy. In neutropenic patients, local pain or tenderness and erythema are often present and represent major clues for defining the site of infection.[16] Information about illness in the patient's family or community, recent travel and exposure to pets or to any unusual material that has been injected or smoked may be helpful in diagnosis.

POSSIBLE SOURCES OF INFECTION

A common problem in immunocompromised patients is fever for which a source of infection cannot be found despite a thorough clinical evaluation, including inspection of intravenous catheter sites, the oral cavity, the skin and the perirectal area. In such situations, various viral infections, tuberculosis, cryptic abscesses and not least noninfectious causes of fever must be considered (Fig. 1.5). Cytotoxic drugs, allergic reactions, pulmonary emboli, graft-versus-host disease, splenic infarcts and reaction to blood products are all potential sources of fever. The underlying disease itself may also be the source of fever. However, this diagnosis should only be made after careful reevaluation to detect an infectious cause of the fever.

PREVIOUS INFECTIONS

Infections in immunocompromised patients may persist or recur even after appropriate therapy. If the patient has experienced a microbiologic and clinical cure of a documented infection, reappearance of fever often signals the onset of a new infection, and a careful search for the etiology of the new infection must be undertaken. Knowledge about previous antibiotic treatment is important because recurrent infections tend to be caused by organisms resistant to recently used antimicrobial agents.

DIAGNOSIS

It is of fundamental importance to obtain cultures of blood and any body fluid or site suspected of being infected. Initially, two peripheral blood cultures from separate venipuncture sites should be obtained and three blood cultures are usually enough to diagnose bacteremia. Blood culture bottles should be incubated aerobically and anaerobically at 37°C for 7 days. Most aerobic bacteria show detectable growth after 3 days of incubation, and more than 90% of bacteremias will be diagnosed by incubation of three sets of blood cultures for 3 days. If, however, the patient has received antibiotics, growth may be suppressed for longer. The significance of blood cultures obtained through intravenous catheters is often difficult to interpret. Positive cultures may reflect catheter-associated infection rather than true bacteremia and fungemia. Fungal cultures generally require prolonged periods of incubation, sometimes several weeks or even months. For some unknown reason, blood cultures obtained from patients who have widespread disseminated mycotic disease often fail to grow fungi. Thus, if disseminated mycotic disease is strongly suspected, antifungal therapy should be instituted empirically.

Intravenous catheters should be carefully examined and cultured. Skin lesions should be aspirated, cultured and biopsied. Occasionally, morphology alone can establish the etiologic diagnosis. Cultures of transtracheal aspirates and material from any abscess are indicated.

Serologic tests may be helpful in the diagnosis of infection, particularly in hepatitis A–E, cryptococcosis, coccidioidomycosis and toxoplasmosis. Results of serologic tests are less reliable for aspergillosis, histoplasmosis and systemic candidiasis.

Standard laboratory tests (i.e. white blood cell count, erythrocyte sedimentation rate, C-reactive protein measurement and urinalysis) and noninvasive diagnostic procedures (i.e. radiographs, radionuclide scanning, ultrasonography, CT and MRI) are at least as important in the diagnosis of infection in the immunocompromised host as in other patients. However, it should be borne in mind that neutropenic patients usually fail to develop a neutrophilic response even in the presence of extensive bacterial infection. A routine chest radiograph provides an important baseline for comparison with later films and should be obtained in all febrile neutropenic patients, even in the absence of pulmonary symptoms.

MANAGEMENT

Characteristic for infection in the immunocompromised patient, particularly neutropenic patient, is the sudden onset of symptoms and the often fulminant course of the disease. Therefore, antimicrobial therapy has to be instituted as early as possible, usually before microbiological results are available. The early institution of empiric antimicrobial therapy has remained a major advance in the management of infection in the immunocompromised patient. Before this strategy was introduced, nearly 80% of patients who had serious infections caused by Gram-negative bacilli died[17] compared with 20–40% once early empiric therapy was administered.

Bacterial infections predominate in the immunocompromised host, and 85–90% of pathogens associated with new episodes of fever are bacteria.[18,19] Because of the wide spectrum of bacteria that causes infection, any empiric regimen must have a broad antibacterial spectrum. The most common regimens have been combinations of an extended spectrum beta-lactam antibiotic and an aminoglycoside, which produce response rates up to 80–85%. Recently, good results (often equal to the results obtained with the combined beta-lactam–aminoglycoside regimen) have been obtained with a combination of two beta-lactam agents or monotherapy with ceftazidime or imipenem–cilastatin (see Chapter 4.5).

Today, such a large armamentarium of highly effective antibiotics is available that it is difficult to recommend a specific antibiotic or combination of antibiotics for the initial treatment of the febrile immunocompromised host.[20,21] The physician should modify therapy according to prevalent bacterial species and their current susceptibility to antibiotics, as these factors differ markedly between institutions and from country to country. However, a combination of an aminoglycoside and an extended spectrum beta-lactam antibiotic (e.g. azlocillin, piperacillin, ceftazidime or cefoperazone) is usually recommended for empiric therapy (Fig. 1.6). If the patient has eighth cranial nerve damage or impaired kidney function or is receiving concomitant treatment with nephrotoxic drugs (e.g. cisplatinum, amphotericin B or cyclosporin), nephrotoxic and ototoxic antibiotics such as aminoglycosides should be avoided and beta-lactam agents may be used. If infection with S. aureus or coagulase-negative staphylococci is suspected, an isoxazolylpenicillin or vancomycin should be added. In institutions in which methicillin-resistant staphylococci or enterococci are infrequent, vancomycin should not be included. If infection with Pseudomonas spp. is suspected, a combination of tobramycin and a beta-lactam antibiotic with antipseudomonal activity (e.g. azlocillin or ceftazidime) should be used. Antibiotic therapy should also be modified if the site of infection is known because this is the single most important factor indicating the etiology of infection (see Chapter 4.5).

If a pathogenic agent has been identified and antibiotic susceptibility determined, the antibiotic regimen should be changed to provide optimal treatment. Treatment should be continued until the causative agent is eradicated, all sites of infection have been resolved, the patient has no symptoms or signs of infection, and, in neutropenic patients, the neutrophil count is rising (preferably to the level of 500 cells/µl). Profoundly neutropenic patients are at greatest risk of recurrence and more prolonged antibiotic therapy may be required.

If fever persists after 3–4 days of antibacterial therapy in neutropenic patients and reassessment has not identified a cause, antifungal therapy should be instituted. It has been demonstrated that up to 33% of febrile neutropenic patients who do not respond to antibiotic therapy for a week have systemic fungal infection, caused in most cases by Candida or Aspergillus spp. Less frequently infection is caused by a virus, a protozoa or even a helminth. Usually, good therapeutic agents are available in these situations (see Chapters 4.2, 4.4 & 4.5).

GUIDELINES FOR INITIAL TREATMENT OF THE FEBRILE (≥38.3°C) IMMUNOCOMPROMISED PATIENT	
Neutrophil count/specific situations	Therapy
Neutrophil count <500 cells/µl	Aminoglycoside + beta-lactam (ureidopenicillin, ceftazidime, cefapime or cefoperazone)
	If resistant staphylococci suspected add isoxazolylpenicillin or vancomycin
Neutrophil count <500 cells/µl and eighth cranial nerve damage, renal impairment, and/or nephrotoxic drugs	Two beta-lactam drugs (e.g. ceftazidime + ureidopenicillin)
	If staphylococci suspected add isoxazolylpenicillin or vancomycin
Neutrophil count >500 cells/µl	Aminoglycoside + first generation cephalosporin, or ceftazidime or imipenem–cilastatin alone
Additional therapy in specific situations	Pulmonary infiltrates: trimethoprim–sulfamethoxazole or erythromycin (Legionella pneumophila)
	Abdominal symptoms: metronidazole or tinidazole

Fig. 1.6 Guidelines for the initial treatment of the febrile (≥ 38.3°C) immunocompromised patient.

REFERENCES

1. Wade JC. Epidemiology and prevention of infection in the compromised host. In: Rubin RH, Young LS, eds. Clinical approach to infection in the compromised host. New York: Plenum;1994:5–31.
2. Freifeld AG, Hathorn JW, Pizzo PA. Infectious complications in the pediatric cancer patient. In: Pizzo PA, Poplack DG, eds. Principles and practice of pediatric oncology. Philadelphia: JB Lippincott;1993:987–1019.
3. Schimpff SC. Infections in the cancer patient – diagnosis, prevention, and treatment. In: Mandell GL, Bennett JE, Dolin L, eds. Principles and practice of infectious diseases. New York: Churchill Livingstone;1995:2666–75.
4. Bodey GP, Buckley M, Sathe YS, Freireich EJ. Quantitative relationships between circulating leukocytes and infection in patients with acute leukemia. Ann Intern Med 1966;64:328–40.
5. Schimpff SC, Young VM, Greene WH, Vermeulen GD, Moody MR, Wiernik PH. Origin of infection in acute nonlymphocytic leukemia: significance of hospital acquisition of potential pathogens. Ann Intern Med 1972;77:707–14.
6. Cohen ML, Murphy MT, Counts GW, Buckner CD, Clift RA, Meyers JD. Prediction by surveillance cultures of bacteremia among neutropenic patients treated in a protective enviroment. J Infect Dis 1983;147:789–93.
7. Solberg CO, Meuwissen HJ, Needham RN, Good RA, Matsen JM. Infectious complications in bone marrow transplantation. Br Med J 1971;1:18–23.
8. Johanson WG, Pierce AK, Sanford JP. Changing pharyngeal bacterial flora of hospitalized patients. Emergence of Gram-negative bacilli. N Engl J Med 1969;281:1137–40.
9. van der Waaij DD, Berghuis J, Lekkerkerk JEC. Colonization resistance of the digestive tract of mice during systemic antibiotic treatment. J Hyg (Camb) 1972;70:605–10.
10. Wells CL, Ferrieri P, Weisdorf DJ, Rhame FS. The importance of surveillance stool cultures during periods of severe neutropenia. Infect Control 1987;8:317–9.
11. Dekker AW, Rozenberg-Arska M, Verhoef J. Infection prophylaxis in acute leukemia: a comparison of ciprofloxacin with trimethoprim–sulfamethoxazole and colistin. Ann Intern Med 1987;106:7–11.
12. Goodman JL, Winston DJ, Greenfield RA, et al. A controlled trial of fluconazole to prevent fungal infections in patients undergoing bone marrow transplantation. N Engl J Med 1992;326:845–51.
13. Wingard JR, Merz WG, Rinaldi MG, Johnson TR, Karp JE, Saral R. Increase in Candida krusei infection among patients with bone marrow transplantation and neutropenia treated prophylactically with fluconazole. N Engl J Med 1991;325:1274–7.
14. Merigan TC, Renlund DG, Keay S, et al. A controlled trial of ganciclovir to prevent cytomegalovirus disease after heart transplantation. N Engl J Med 1992;326:1182–6.
15. Levine AS, Siegel SE, Schreiber AD, et al. Protected environments and prophylactic antibiotics: a prospective controlled study of their utility in the therapy of acute leukemia. N Engl J Med 1973;288:477–83.
16. Sickles EA, Greene WH, Wiernik PH. Clinical presentation of infection in granulocytopenic patients. Arch Intern Med 1975;135:715–9.
17. McCabe WR, Jackson GG. Gram-negative bacteremia. II. Clinical, laboratory, and therapeutic observations. Arch Intern Med 1962;110:856–64.
18. Schimpff SC. Overview of empiric antibiotic therapy for the febrile neutropenic patient. Rev Infect Dis 1985;7(suppl 4):5734–40.
19. Pizzo PA, Robichaud KJ, Wesley R, Commers JA. Fever in the pediatric and young adult patient with cancer: a prospective study of 1001 episodes. Medicine (Baltimore) 1982;61:153–65.
20. Infectious Diseases Society of America. Guidelines for the use of antimicrobial agents in neutropenic patients with unexplained fever. J Infect Dis 1990;161:381–96.
21. Immunocompromised Host Society. The design, analysis, and reporting of clinical trials on the empirical antibiotic management of the neutropenic patient: report of a consensus panel. J Infect Dis 1990;161:397–401.

Primary Immunodeficiency Syndromes

John C Christenson & Harry R Hill

It is essential that a diagnosis of a congenital immunodeficiency disease is made as soon as possible. Survival and quality of life have improved for almost all conditions for which the basic underlying pathophysiology of the immune defect has been elucidated. The genetics of many primary immunodeficiencies have been clearly defined, making prenatal and early neonatal diagnosis feasible for many of these conditions.[1] Early use of immunotherapy and prophylactic antimicrobial therapy can prevent many serious infections in these patients. In some instances, bone marrow or stem cell transplantation has proved curative. The prospect of gene therapy must also be considered.

In this chapter we provide an overview of the most important primary immunodeficiencies and their associated infections. We emphasize the preventive and therapeutic management of these complex patients.

EPIDEMIOLOGY

An underlying immunodeficiency should be suspected in individuals with recurrent, chronic or unusually severe infections. The causative organisms and the age at which these infections occur provide important clues to the presence and type of disorder. Although such disorders are rare, early diagnosis can prevent a number of serious infections and their consequences, including the development of chronic lung disease, local suppurative infections and overwhelming sepsis.

The incidence of primary immunodeficiencies is approximately 1/10,000 live births with the exception of asymptomatic selective IgA deficiency, which occurs with an incidence of 20/10,000 live births.[2-4] Although geographic differences have been noted, antibody deficiencies have comprised approximately 50% of all recognized cases of immunodeficiency. Combined antibody and cellular immunodeficiency make up approximately 20% of the total, whereas phagocytic disorders comprise 20%, cellular-mediated disorders 8%, and complement deficiencies 2% of the total (Fig. 2.1).

Nearly 75% of immunodeficiency disorders are diagnosed in the first 5 years of life. Approximately 50% of these are diagnosed in the first year. Only about 5–10% of cases are diagnosed in adulthood. The

INCIDENCE OF PRIMARY IMMUNODEFICIENCY DISORDERS	
Immunodeficiency disorder	Number of cases/number of live births
IgA deficiency, asymptomatic	20/10,000
X-Linked agammaglobulinemia	1/103,000
DiGeorge syndrome	1/66,000
Severe combined immunodeficiency	1/66,000
Combined variable immunodeficiency	1/83,000
Chronic mucocutaneous candidiasis	1/103,000
Chronic granulomatous disease	1/181,000

Fig. 2.1 Incidence of primary immunodeficiency disorders. Relationship between the number of patients with primary immunodeficiency disorders and the number of live births.

majority of immunodeficiencies occur in males, reflecting the fact that the majority are X-linked.[4] A family history of an immune disorder may help in making a diagnosis of immunodeficiency. This is usually present in 25% of cases.

With the exception of respiratory viral infections, no clear evidence of seasonality can be observed in patients with primary immunodeficiencies. Viral and bacterial infections of the upper respiratory tract are especially common during the winter season. The clinician should be attentive during this time of the year and initiate prompt specific therapy to prevent further progression of infection. Although not sufficiently emphasized at times, contact with clinically ill individuals should be limited to minimize the likelihood of infection.

PATHOGENESIS AND PATHOLOGY

This section reviews the major congenital immunodeficiency syndromes and discusses their major host defense abnormalities. A summary of the most serious and most common causative agents of infections in these patients is given in Figure 2.2.

COMBINED B- AND T-LYMPHOCYTE DEFECTS
Severe combined immunodeficiency disease
This disease occurs as an X-linked form and as an autosomal recessive form. It is characterized by:
- lymphopenia,
- a marked decrease in T- and B-lymphocyte numbers,
- low serum immunoglobulins,
- a lack of antibody response following immunization,
- negative skin test reactions, and
- severe and recurrent infections.

In X-linked severe combined immunodeficiency disease (SCID), the gene at the Xq13.1–13.3 locus is abnormal. This gene is responsible for the interleukin (IL)-2 receptor γ chain, which serves as the receptor for several cytokines including IL-2, IL-4 and IL-7, which promote growth and development of T and B lymphocytes.[1] Autosomal recessive SCIDs may be due to deficiency of ZAP-70, a protein kinase that maps to chromosome 2q12 and is important in T-lymphocyte receptor signal transduction.

Purine pathway enzyme deficiencies
Patients with autosomal recessive SCIDs may have defects in their purine metabolic pathways. Their infections are similar to those of the X-linked form except there may be a later onset and they are often less severe as patients may have some immune function.[5,6]

The immunodeficiency in these patients probably results from the accumulation of substances that are toxic to the developing immune system because of a enzyme deficiency. Adenosine deaminase (ADA) and purine nucleoside phosphorylase (PNP) deficiencies have both been associated with combined B- and T-lymphocyte abnormalities. Generally, some immune functions remain, so initial symptoms of infection may not appear until 6–12 months of age.

Examination of the patient's erythrocytes for ADA or PNP levels is diagnostic because these are extremely low in affected patients. Serum or urine uric acid concentrations are also quite low because of the

MOST COMMON ASSOCIATED INFECTIONS IN PRIMARY IMMUNODEFICIENCY DISORDERS	
Immunodeficiency	Infections
T-lymphocyte defects (severe combined immunodeficiency, purine pathway enzyme deficiency, Wiskott–Aldrich syndrome, ataxia–telangiectasia, DiGeorge syndrome, chronic mucocutaneous candidiasis)	*Pneumocystis carinii* pneumonia Listeriosis Candidiasis Salmonellosis Aspergillosis Severe, persistent or recurrent viral infections (RSV, parainfluenza, CMV, poliovirus, enterovirus, HSV, EBV) Disseminated or pulmonary mycobacterial infection
B-lymphocyte disorders (transient or X-linked hypogammaglobulinemia, hypogammaglobulinemia with increased IgM, selective IgM or IgA deficiency, common variable hypogammaglobulinemia), ataxia–telangiectasia	Bacterial sepsis/meningitis (*Streptococcus pneumoniae, Haemophilus influenzae, Pseudomonas aeruginosa*) Recurrent otitis media Recurrent sinopulmonary infections Chronic enteroviral infections Recurrent or chronic gastrointestinal infections (*Giardia lamblia*, rotavirus, *Cryptosporidium* spp.) Arthritis due to *Ureaplasma urealyticum*
Complement disorders	Severe or recurrent infections with encapsulated bacteria (*Neisseria meningitidis, Neisseria gonorrhoeae, Haemophilus influenzae, Streptococcus pneumoniae*)
Phagocytic/chemotactic disorders	Pyogenic infections due to *Staphylococcus aureus*, opportunistic Gram-negative bacteria, *Nocardia* spp., fungi (aspergillus, *Candida* spp.)

Fig. 2.2 Most common infections in patients who have primary immunodeficiency disorders. CMV, cytomegalovirus; EBV, Epstein–Barr virus; HSV, herpes simplex virus; RSV, respiratory syncytial virus.

purine metabolic block and may be used as a screening test for the disorder. The gene for ADA deficiency has been mapped to chromosome 20q13, whereas that for PNP deficiency maps to chromosome 14q13.1.[1]

Wiskott–Aldrich syndrome

The major host defense abnormality in these patients is an inability to make antibody directed at polysaccharide (and to a lesser degree protein) antigens. The basic defect is unknown, but many believe it results from abnormal macrophage processing of antigen.[7] Later, these patients seem to lose T-lymphocyte function, making this a combined B- and T-lymphocyte abnormality. Along with eczema, thrombocytopenia (50,000–100,000/mm[3] or lower) often suggests the diagnosis. Infections are seldom a problem until maternal immunoglobulin disappears in the infant 4–6 months after delivery. Recently, a novel gene termed *WASP*, which encodes a Wiskott–Aldrich syndrome protein, has been found to have point mutations or single base deletions in patients with the disorder.[1]

Ataxia–telangiectasia

These patients develop cerebellar ataxia, telangiectasia (most prominent on the bulbar conjunctiva, nose, ears and antecubital fossae) and recurrent sinopulmonary infections. Many have depressed skin test reactivity and lymphocyte responses, and may have absent IgA and IgE as well as depressed IgG_2 and/or IgG_4. A single ataxia telangiectasia gene has been located on chromosome 11q22.23 by positional cloning.[1]

CONGENITAL PURE T-LYMPHOCYTE IMMUNODEFICIENCIES

Cellular immunodeficiency with immunoglobulins

Cellular immunodeficiency with immunoglobulins is primarily a T-lymphocyte defect, although immunoglobulin synthesis abnormalities are also observed. These are thought to be secondary to the primary defect in T lymphocytes. In addition, these patients may fail to produce adequate antibodies against T lymphocyte-dependent antigens. The disease may be inherited in an autosomal recessive pattern or may be sporadic, and is characterized by failure to develop a thymus. The time of onset of infections varies, but is usually at 6–12 months of age. Recent evidence suggests that a number of these patients have PNP deficiency. The deficiency of PNP maps to chromosome 14q13.1.[1]

DiGeorge syndrome

This syndrome, which results from abnormal embryologic development of the third and fourth pharyngeal pouches, often results in total or partial absence of the thymus and a marked deficiency in the T-lymphocyte system. Abnormalities of the aortic arch, the parathyroid glands and occasionally the thyroid gland may also occur, along with characteristic dysmorphic facial features. Monosomy of chromosome 22 can be demonstrated by fluorescent in-situ hybridization in most of the patients.[1] Although immunoglobulins are usually normal, there may be some problems in making specific antibodies to T lymphocyte-dependent antigens.

Chronic mucocutaneous candidiasis

Chronic mucocutaneous candidiasis probably represents a spectrum of diseases; defective function has been observed at different sites in the immune system in different patients. An autosomal recessive pattern has been detected as well as sporadic disease. The disease may also occur in association with multiple endocrine abnormalities including hypoparathyroidism, diabetes mellitus and Addison's disease. Abnormal immune parameters may include:
- decreased skin test and in-vitro lymphocyte mitogenic responses to *Candida,* and other antigens; and
- a specific defect in skin test and in-vitro mitogenic responses to *Candida,* but absent production of migration inhibition factor (MIF) by lymphocytes challenged with candida antigen.

B-LYMPHOCYTE IMMUNODEFICIENCY

Congenital abnormalities of the B-lymphocyte system are associated with severe and recurrent infections and may be classified as follows.

Transient hypogammaglobulinemia of infancy

A small number of infants have a lag in antibody production that may or may not be associated with increased infections. This condition is usually overdiagnosed and is often used as the pretext for inappropriate use of immunoglobulin. One study[8] suggested that most such patients do not have serious bacterial infections and most can make specific antibodies when immunized.

Sex-linked hypogammaglobulinemia

This disease, which is X-linked, occurs exclusively in males and is associated with:
- extremely low levels (<100mg/dl) of IgG, IgM and IgA;
- low numbers of (or absent) mature B lymphocytes;
- absent germinal centers in lymph nodes; and
- a marked decrease in plasma cells.

The disorder is caused by the absence of 'Bruton's tyrosine kinase (Btk)', which is encoded on the X chromosome and is apparently critical for B lymphocyte maturation to pass the pre-B lymphocyte stage.[9] Infections usually begin at 4–6 months of age when maternal antibody disappears from the infant.

Hypogammaglobulinemia associated with hyperimmunoglobulinemia M

This is a sex-linked disorder characterized by:

- normal-to-increased levels of IgM and IgM-producing B and plasma cells; and
- low levels of IgG and IgA.

The disorder is due to a primary dysfunction of isotype switching.[10] In the majority of cases, which occur in a sex-linked pattern, the disorder results from the absence on T lymphocytes of the ligand for CD40 on B lymphocytes. Binding of the ligand to CD40 on the B lymphocytes is essential for isotype switching. A minority of cases have an autosomal recessive pattern of inheritance and are due to improper signaling through CD40 on the B lymphocyte. The patients may also have neutropenia, thrombocytopenia and hemolytic anemia, and develop lymphomas. Antibodies directed against polysaccharide antigens such as isohemagglutinins or opsonins for *Streptococcus pneumoniae* and *Haemophilus influenzae* are present in the serum and are of the IgM variety. Antibody levels of IgG and IgA are low to absent in tissue fluids and respiratory and gastrointestinal secretions, however. These patients therefore have respiratory, soft tissue and gastrointestinal infections, but do not often suffer overwhelming episodes of sepsis.

Selective IgM deficiency

This disease is probably of genetic origin, but the exact inheritance pattern is unclear. It is characterized by extremely low levels (<20mg/dl) of IgM without other detectable abnormalities. These patients lack production of IgM antibodies directed against the polysaccharide capsules of many pyogenic bacteria, so they tend to have severe systemic infections caused by *Strep. pneumoniae*, *H. influenzae* and *Escherichia coli* as well as other encapsulated pathogens.

Selective IgA deficiency

This immunodeficiency is one of the most prevalent abnormalities in the host defense mechanism. These individuals usually have an absence of serum and secretory IgA, but the number of IgA-bearing B lymphocytes are normal or only slightly decreased. There appears to be a terminal block in B lymphocyte differentiation into plasma cells and subsequently a block in actual IgA synthesis. Other individuals lack secretory piece and have undetectable IgA in external secretions, but normal serum levels of IgA.[11] Absence of IgA has been found in a number of normal individuals who have no increased incidence of infection.[12] Such individuals may, however, have an increased incidence of cutaneous, respiratory and gastrointestinal allergies, indicating that secretory IgA has a major role in preventing absorption of allergens. Autoimmune diseases such as rheumatoid arthritis and systemic lupus erythematous are also more common in these patients. Recently, a common susceptibility gene located in the MHC class III region on chromosome 6 has been implicated in both IgA deficiency and common variable immunodeficiency.[13]

Common variable hypogammaglobulinemia

This immunodeficiency is usually classified as acquired; however, studies have indicated a possible genetic basis, perhaps related to IgA deficiency mentioned above.[13] This is the most common form of serious antibody deficiency. It has its onset several years to several decades after birth and is characterized by a variable incidence of immunoglobulin deficiency. Concentration of IgG is usually low, with or without low concentrations of IgM and IgA. Approximately 35% of patients have defective T-lymphocyte function, and 25% of them eventually develop malignancies, including thymomas and lymphoreticular tumors. The exact pathogenesis of this disorder is not known, although deficiency of production of T-lymphocyte cytokines such as IL-2 has been implicated in some patients.[1,13]

COMPLEMENT COMPONENT DEFICIENCIES

The complement system represents an important aspect of the humoral portion of the host defense mechanism. Individual components play a major role in:

- bacterial and yeast opsonization (C3b, iC3b and C5b);
- viral neutralization (C4b);
- phagocyte chemotaxis (C5a); and
- lysis of some micro-organisms (C5, C6, C7, C8 and C9).

Total or partial deficiency of individual components is genetically determined by autosomal codominant inheritance with the exception of properdin deficiency, which is sex-linked. The homozygous state generally results in serious disease and complete absence of the component, whereas heterozygous deficiency leads to minor or no symptoms.[14–20]

Infections in patients with complement deficiencies vary significantly according to the nature of the missing component. The classic complement pathway involving C1, 4, 2, 3, 5, 6, 7, 8 and 9 is triggered predominantly by antigen–antibody complexes. In the absence of antibody, the alternative pathway, which involves properdin, factor A or C3b, and factor B or C3 proactivator, is triggered and acts directly on C3 to activate the terminal part of the system. In general, therefore, the classic pathway, which is more efficient, is important in the immune host, whereas the alternative pathway functions in individuals lacking antibodies to certain bacteria. Two of the most important functions of the complement system are:

- to generate chemotactic factors and inflammatory mediators (C3a and C5a); and
- to opsonize micro-organisms (C3b and iC3b).

Early classic pathway component deficiencies

Deficiencies of Clq, r, s, C2 and C4 do not usually result in an increased incidence of infection, probably because the alternative complement pathway is intact, but individuals with these deficiencies may, have disorders resembling collagen vascular disorders.[21–23] Nephritis is particularly common and may be associated with rashes, Raynaud's phenomenon and arthritis. Severe infections occasionally occur and are usually due to polysaccharide-coated bacteria such as *Strep. pneumoniae*. The gene for C2 is located within the MHC on the short arm of chromosome 6. Inheritance of C2 deficiency is autosomal recessive, as is inheritance of the components of the C1 complex (C1q, r, s) and C4.

C3 and C5 deficiency

C3 and C5 breakdown products play a major role in the host defense mechanism, assisting in immune adherence, opsonization and chemotaxis, and being important as inflammatory mediators. Absence of C3 leads to infections that are similar to and may be even more severe than those in patients with hypogammaglobulinemia.

C6, C7 and C8 deficiency

Absence of the sixth, seventh and eighth components of complement often results in infections.[16–18] In one study 13 out of 24 patients with an absence of one of these components had at least one and usually several episodes of disseminated *Neisseria meningitidis* or *Neisseria gonorrhoea* infection.[19]

Alternative pathway defects

Absence or deficiency of alternative pathway components may be congenital, developmental or acquired. Newborn infants have low levels of factor B and impaired nonspecific serum opsonic activity. This is apparently developmental because the levels subsequently become normal. Patients with the nephrotic syndrome apparently lose factor B in their urine and therefore also have defective nonspecific opsonic activity. Congenital deficiency of factor B has also been described in association with C2 deficiency.[24]

An absence of properdin associated with recurrent infections has been reported as a sex-linked disorder.[25]

People with defects in the alternative complement pathway have an unusually high incidence of severe and often overwhelming infections.

MANNOSE-BINDING PROTEIN DEFICIENCY

Mannose-binding protein (MBP) belongs to a group of calcium-dependent lectins, which are known as collectins.[26] These recognize mannose and *N*-acetylglucosamine on the surface of micro-organisms and promote their killing by acting as an opsonin or by activating complement.[26,27] Three mutations have been detected in exon 1 of the MBP gene.[28] Low levels of MBP have been associated with recurrent infections in children and adults including skin infections, abscesses, diarrhea, pneumonia, meningitis and recurrent herpes simplex infections.

PHAGOCYTE ABNORMALITIES

The importance of phagocytes, including polymorphonuclear leukocytes (PMNLs), macrophages and other fixed tissue histiocytes, is illustrated best in the individual who has a marked deficiency of these cells. Profound neutropenia from a variety of causes including congenital, autoimmune or toxic causes, or those associated with malignancy, usually results in severe infections and often death (see Chapter 4.5). In addition, the infections that occur in patients who have phagocyte abnormalities are not commonly observed in individuals with adequate numbers and function of phagocytes and include:
- severe sepsis with Gram-negative and Gram-positive bacteria;
- severe pneumonia (Fig. 2.3);
- perirectal and abdominal abscesses;
- cutaneous and systemic candidiasis; and
- aspergillus infection (Fig. 2.4).

Many of these patients have normal antibody and complement levels as well as adequate T-lymphocyte function, but still contract these serious infections, indicating the critical role that phagocytes play in the host defense mechanism against a number of bacterial, fungal, and even viral pathogens.

Congenital neutropenias

Several forms of congenital neutropenia occur that may result in serious infection. Recent published articles provide an excellent review of all these clinical disorders of neutropenia and enumerates their work up and therapy.[29,30] The disorders are briefly discussed below.

Infantile lethal agranulocytosis. This is an autosomal recessive disease associated with profound neutropenia, eosinophilia and monocytosis. The bone marrow reveals a striking absence of neutrophilic precursors. Corticosteroids, splenectomy and other maneuvers have little effect, and the patients suffer severe infections with staphylococci, *E. coli*, *Proteus mirabilis*, *Pseudomonas aeruginosa*, streptococci and *Candida* spp. Despite antibiotic prophylaxis and prompt therapy of individual infections, patients usually die early in life. These patients were first described in several Swedish families,[31] but similar cases have been described elsewhere. Recently, therapy with colony stimulating factors has proven lifesaving.

Chronic benign neutropenia. This is usually a sporadic disease, but autosomal recessive inheritance has been reported. Unlike the fatal neutropenia described above, this condition has a much milder course. Patients also have eosinophilia and often a marked monocytosis, which may help to explain their ability to overcome infections. Bone marrow examination reveals arrest at the myelocyte or metamyelocyte stage. During acute infection, some of these patients appear to be able to mount an adequate neutrophil response.

Neutropenia with hypogammaglobulinemia and increased IgM. As mentioned under B-lymphocyte immunodeficiency (above), patients with this sex-linked disease have profound neutropenia, which contributes to their infectious complications, including pneumonias, episodes of sepsis, and occasional cervical adenitis and abscesses. The neutropenia in this disease may be cyclic or constant in nature.

Chemotactic defects

A number of individuals have severe and repeated infections secondary to phagocyte chemotactic defects. Animal studies have shown that a critical 2- to 4-hour period exists during which phagocytes must arrive at the site of microbial invasion if infection is to be suppressed or contained. Individuals with chemotactic defects develop a variety of infections, which are usually confined to the skin, lymph nodes, mucous membranes and respiratory tract.

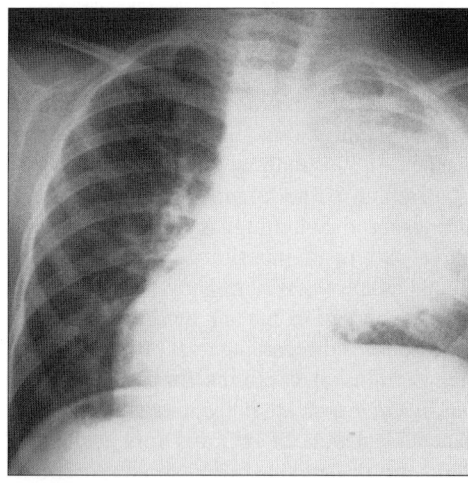

Fig. 2.3 Severe *Nocardia* pneumonia in a patient with chronic granulomatous disease.

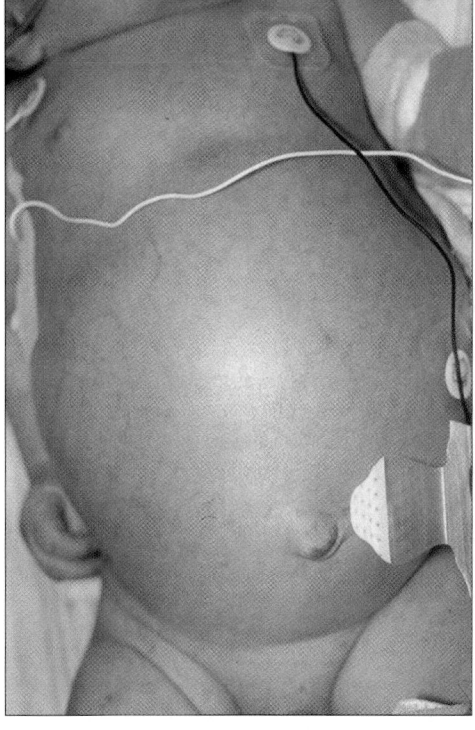

Fig. 2.4 Aspergillus abdominal infection in a patient with chronic granulomatous disease.

The 'lazy-leukocyte' syndrome. Two children were described in 1971 who had gingivitis, recurrent otitis media, rhinitis and stomatitis.[32] Each had marked neutropenia, but in addition, PMNL random migration and chemotactic function were markedly abnormal. Both patients grew normally, and severe life-threatening infections were not reported.

Congenital ichthyosis. Two kindreds with congenital ichthyosis were described[33] who had chronic recurrent *Trichophyton rubrum* infections as well as otitis media, recurrent upper respiratory infections, deep abscesses and generalized impetigo. Peripheral neutrophil counts were normal, as was the random motility of their PMNLs, but chemotaxis was markedly depressed.

Hyperimmunoglobulinemia E, defective chemotaxis and recurrent infection. Over 100 patients with a syndrome of hyperimmunoglobulinemia E, allergic manifestations, recurrent infection and defective PMNL and monocyte chemotaxis have been described.[34–37] These patients have characteristic facies with doughy skin, a broad nasal bridge and nasal alae and a prominent lower lip (Fig. 2.5).

Several aspects of the syndrome, including its association with bone disease, have been reviewed.[38] There appears to be a familial pattern in the inheritance.[39] Those with the syndrome have usually had severe eczema,[34,36,37] although urticaria[40] and allergic rhinitis have also been reported. The infections vary from multiple superficial cutaneous

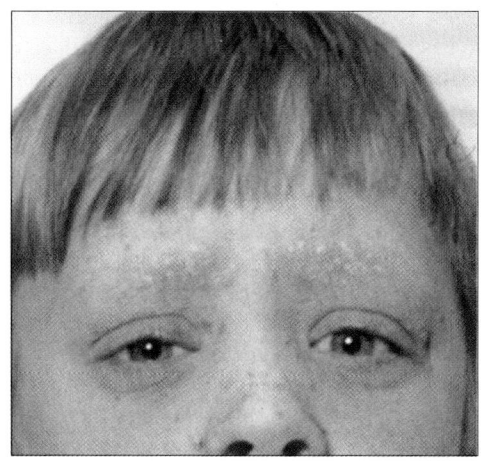

Fig. 2.5 Patient with the characteristic facial features of Job's syndrome.

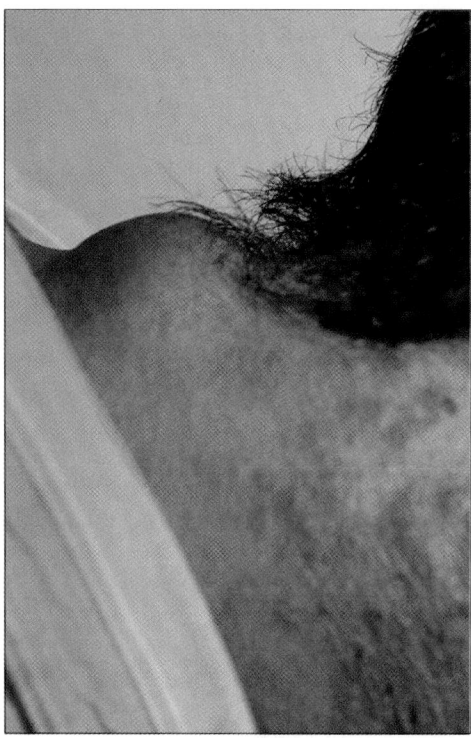

Fig. 2.6 Cervical staphylococcal abscess in a patient with Job's syndrome.

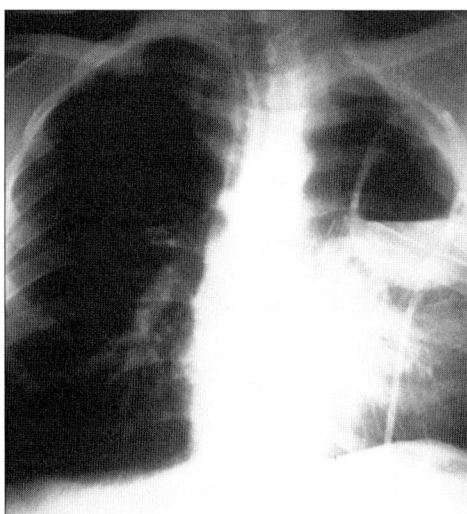

Fig. 2.7 Pneumonia with pneumatocele and abscess formation in a patient with Job's syndrome.

abscesses to deep-seated abscesses in the buttocks, scalp or other tissues (Fig. 2.6).[34,36,37,40] Chronic rhinitis, bronchitis and otitis media also occur. Serious systemic infections such as sepsis and pneumonia (Fig. 2.7) have been reported.[40] These are almost always caused by staphylococci, but infections with streptococci, *P. aeruginosa* and *Aspergillus*

spp. have also been recognized. Chronic cutaneous candidiasis may also be a problem.[35,36]

These patients may be related to those described by Buckley and co-workers[38] and their condition is certainly a variant of Job's syndrome, which was originally described by Davis *et al*.[42] In fact, we studied the original Job's syndrome patients, who were red-haired females with severe eczema, hyperimmunoglobulinemia E and recurrent staphylococcal abscesses, and found them to have a profound defect in chemotactic function.[43] The chemotactic defect in Job's syndrome patients is not always present and may be related to the release of allergic mediators that can depress PMNL chemotaxis.[34,40]

Of interest are findings suggesting that allergen-induced reactions can depress chemotactic function and several of these patients had high levels of IgE antibody directed against staphylococci and *Candida*, their most prominent pathogens.[44] Thus, staphylococci may evoke a strong IgE response in individuals with appropriate genetic factors that on subsequent challenge leads to an allergic release of mediators, thereby depressing the phagocyte system.

Lymphocytes of patients with the hyperimmunoglobulinemia E syndrome have an imbalance in interferon (IFN)-γ production in relation to IL-4 production. This would increase serum IgE concentrations and possibly result in poor activation of PMNLs and macrophages because IFN-γ is a major activator of these cells.[45]

Actin dysfunction. An infant with blepharitis, vesicular skin lesions, abscesses and sepsis with organisms including *Staphylococcus aureus*, *Candida albicans*, *Enterococcus faecalis* and *E. coli* has been described.[43] This patient had a profound defect in PMNL chemotaxis and phagocytosis and had actin that polymerized poorly after treatment with potassium chloride and eventually received a bone marrow transplant. More recent evidence suggests that patients with actin dysfunction may actually have a form of leukocyte adhesion deficiency.

Monocyte chemotactic deficiency. Defective monocyte chemotactic responsiveness has occasionally been observed in the patients with hyperimmunoglobulinemia E. In addition, patients with chronic mucocutaneous candidiasis with defective monocyte chemotaxis have been reported.[47]

Microbicidal defects
Microbicidal defects in phagocytes also result in serious infections and may lead to marked sequelae. The major microbicidal mechanism of the PMNLs involves the production of toxic oxygen products or radicals including hydrogen peroxide, superoxide and perhaps singlet oxygen (Fig. 2.8). Additional important factors in microbicidal activity include the lysosomal enzyme myeloperoxidase, and a halide. There are several possible defects in this system and these result in the intracellular survival or even multiplication of bacteria. The most common syndromes associated with microbicidal defects are described below.

Chronic granulomatous disease. Chronic granulomatous disease (CGD) was the first granulocyte defect to be described and have its mechanism elucidated.[48] Of individuals with this disease, 60% have a sex-linked form, but CGD also occurs in an autosomal recessive form or in association with severe glucose-6-phosphate dehydrogenase (G6PD) deficiency. Following phagocytosis, the cells of these patients:
- fail to undergo the respiratory burst;
- do not activate their hexose monophosphate shunt; and
- do not produce the toxic oxygen products necessary for microbicidal activity.

The phagocytes also fail to reduce the histochemical dye nitroblue tetrazolium (NBT) to a blue–black deposit after stimulation with endotoxin or phorbol myristate acetate, unlike normal phagocytes (Fig. 2.9). These patients fail to heal normally after surgical drainage of infection (Fig. 2.10). In the sex-linked form of the disease, this was thought to be caused by the absence of a nicotinamide–adenine dinucleotide phosphate (NADP) or the reduced form of NADP (NADPH) oxidase required to activate the cell. However, evidence indicates that the abnormality is due to the absence of the 91kDa heavy chain of cytochrome *b* 558, which is responsible for electron transfer in the initial stages of the respiratory burst (Fig. 2.11). Glutathione peroxidase deficiency was once believed to be behind the autosomal-recessive form of the disease. It appears that these autosomal-recessive forms are due, however, to the absence of a 47kDa or 67kDa cytosolic protein necessary for activity of the oxidase or to the absence of the 22kDa light chain of the cytochrome (Fig. 2.11). The gene for the 91kDa cytochrome *b* 558 heavy chain is located at Xp21.1 (gp 91 phox), whereas that for the 22kDa light chain is at 16q24 (gp 22 phox).[1] The gene for the 47kDa cytosolic factor is at 7q11.23, but that for the 67kDa factor is at 1q25 (gp 67 phox).[1]

Myeloperoxidase deficiency. Hereditary deficiency of the lysosomal enzyme myeloperoxidase has been described in association with candidal infections.[49] In addition, patients with Chédiak–Higashi syndrome who have recurrent infections, oculocutaneous albinism and giant PMNL lysosomal granules also have a relative deficiency of myeloperoxidase because their granules do not readily discharge myeloperoxidase into phagocytic vacuoles (Fig. 2.12). The gene for this autosomal recessive disorder is on chromosome 1. Absence or deficiency of myeloperoxidase results in delayed killing of bacteria and may play a major role in killing yeasts such as *C. albicans*. Infections include those caused by *Candida* spp., which may be cutaneous or systemic, and also abscesses caused by *Staph. aureus*.

Down syndrome. Patients who have Down syndrome may have defective PMNL bactericidal activity against *Staph. aureus*, which may result in recurrent infections.[50] The PMNLs of these patients cause less reduction of NBT dye than those of controls, but other metabolic parameters have not been systematically examined. Patients who have Down syndrome probably have an increased incidence of abscesses and pneumonia due to *Staph. aureus*.

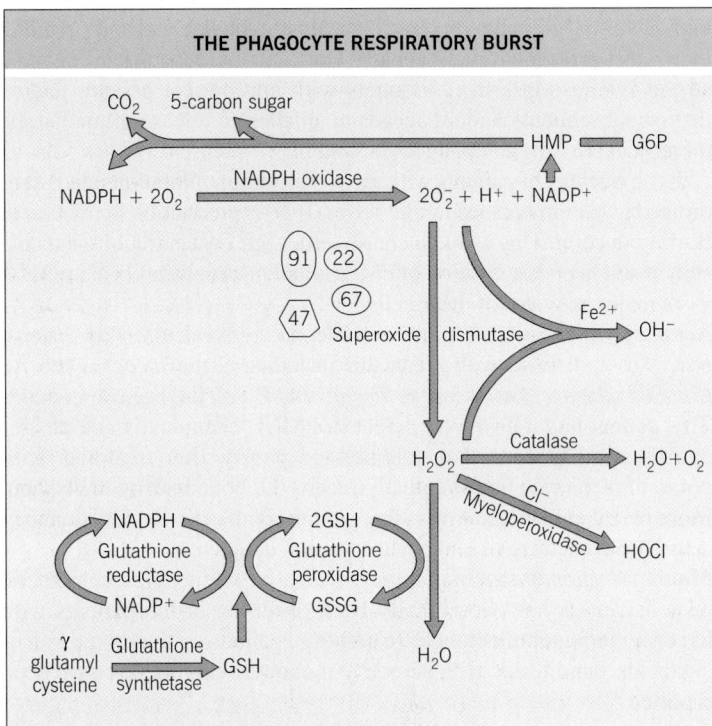

THE PHAGOCYTE RESPIRATORY BURST

Fig. 2.8 The phagocyte respiratory burst. G6P, glucose-6-phosphate; GSH, reduced glutathione; GSSG, oxidized glutathione; HOCl, hypochloric acid; HMP, hexose monophosphate shunt; NADP, nicotinamide–adenine dinucleotide phosphate; NADP+, the oxidized form of NADP; NADPH, the reduced form of NADP; 91kDa, cytochrome *b* 558 heavy chain; 22kDa, light chain; 47 and 67kDa, cytosolic components.

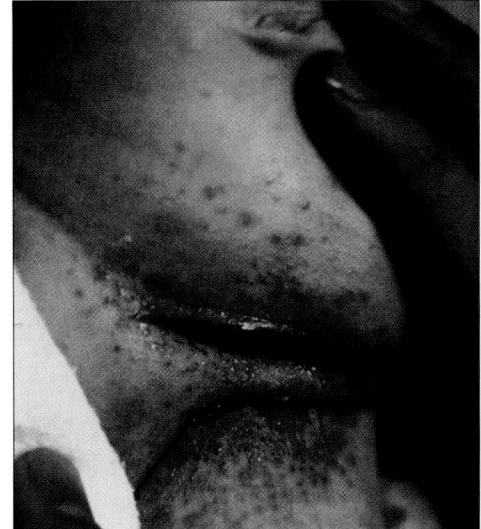

Fig. 2.10 Poor wound healing in a patient who has chronic granulomatous disease after incision and drainage of an inguinal lymphadenitis.

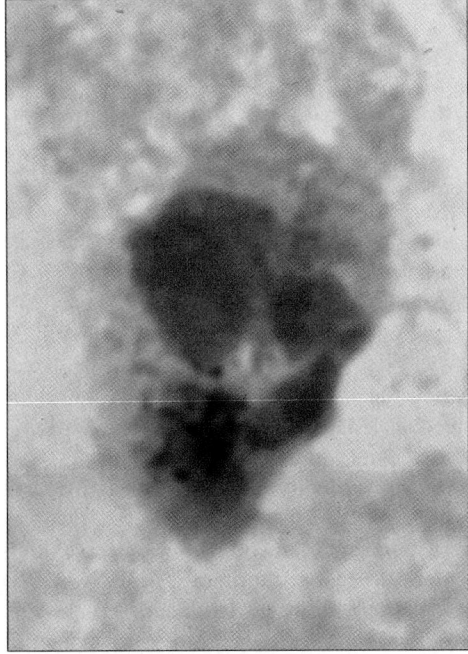

Fig. 2.9 Reduced nitroblue tetrazolium dye in normal polymorphonuclear leukocytes.

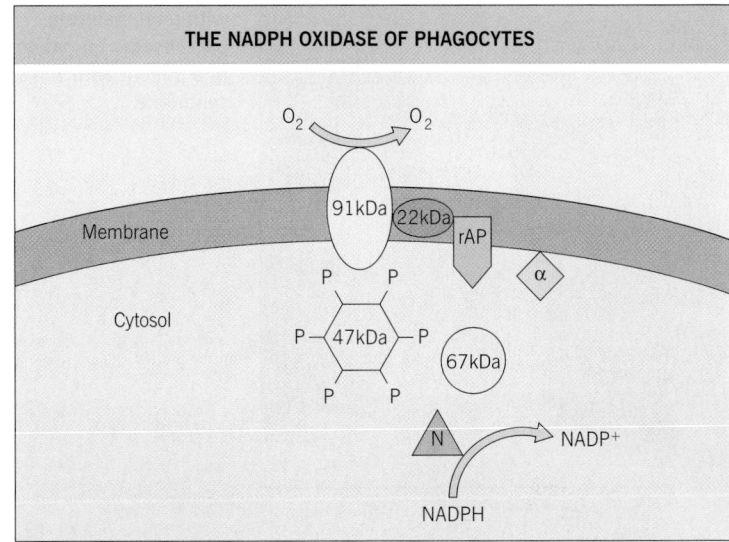

THE NADPH OXIDASE OF PHAGOCYTES

Fig. 2.11 Components of the reduced form of nicotinamide–adenine dinucleotide phosphate (NADPH) oxidase of phagocytes. NADP+, the oxidized form of NADP. N, NADPH binding subunit; rAP, regression-associated protein; α, alpha unit. Adapted with permission from Yang KD and Hill HR. J Pediatr 1991;119:343–54.

Leukocyte adhesion deficiency

The deficiency of CD11/CD18 – leukocyte adhesion deficiency (LAD) type I – complex is transmitted as an autosomal recessive trait. The gene encoding for CD18 has been mapped to chromosome 21 at 21q22.3.[1] This deficiency is characterized by abnormal neutrophil mobilization, which is frequently associated with:

- marked leukocytosis; and
- frequent infections such as gingivitis, perirectal abscesses, otitis media, sinusitis, sepsis and pneumonia.

The infections are commonly caused by *Staph. aureus*, group A streptococci, *Proteus mirabilis*, *P. aeruginosa* and *E. coli*. A history of delayed umbilical cord separation may be obtained, along with markedly elevated peripheral leukocyte counts. This syndrome is associated with absent or deficient expression of the plasma membrane glycoprotein leukocyte function antigen (LFA)-1 (CD11a/CD18), macrophage antigen (Mac)-1 (CD11b/CD18) and p150/95 (CD11c/CD18) due to defective production of the common CD18 component. The function of these surface glycoproteins is to promote a series of leukocyte adhesion-dependent interactions including binding to iC3b, aggregation, adhesion to endothelial cell surfaces, chemotaxis, phagocytosis and particle-induced respiratory burst activity of phagocytes, lymphoproliferative response of lymphocytes and cytotoxicity mediated by T lymphocytes.[51]

There appear to be two variants of this disease:

- a severe form with a complete absence of CD11/CD18 expression; and
- a moderate form with 5–20% of normal expression.

The severity of the patient's clinical manifestations is closely related to the variant of the disease. Patients who have severe deficiency are likely to die in the first year of life, whereas those with mild-to-moderate disease may live into adulthood.

In the second form of the disease LAD type II, sialyl-Lewis X, the ligand on neutrophils for E-selectin is missing.[52,53] The cells from these patients are unable to roll along the endothelium due to the lack of interaction with the endothelial cell selectins. The clinical manifestations are similar to those of LAD type I.

PREVENTION

GENERAL MEASURES

Figure 2.13 provides a summary of general preventive measures against infections for patients who have primary immunodeficiency. The most important objective is to prevent the long-term sequelae of infections.

Acute, recurrent and chronic infections often lead to the development of serious sequelae. Death of patients with antibody-deficiency syndromes, for instance, is often the result of respiratory failure secondary to bronchiectasis and recurrent pneumonias. Similar respiratory problems may occur in ataxia telangiectasia and even in diseases associated with phagocyte disorders such as CGD and Job's syndrome. On occasion, recurrent staphylococcal pneumonias with abscess and pneumatocele formation and chronic pulmonary fibrosis have resulted in lobectomy (Fig. 2.14) and other interventions. When infection becomes manifested in other lobes, the patient with a history of lobectomy is even more compromised. For this reason, such procedures are approached cautiously in most centers. Postural drainage and physiotherapy cannot be overstressed in the management of these patients because adequate removal of plugs, inflammatory cells and bacterial debris contributes greatly to the prevention of long-term pulmonary complications. Patients with pulmonary disease should have at least once-yearly chest radiography and pulmonary function studies. We use antibiotics when clinical or radiographic findings point to an increasingly purulent bronchitis or pneumonia.

The patient who has chronic sinusitis may benefit from drainage procedures such as the Caldwell–Luc procedure, whereas patients who have recurrent otitis media may benefit from adenoidectomy, or more importantly from insertion of tympanic membrane drainage tubes.

Patients who have recurrent skin abscesses, especially those caused by staphylococci, may respond to skin decontamination with vigorous washing with an agent containing povidone–iodine or chlorhexidine. These preparations tend to dry out the skin, however, and may actually increase breaks in the skin barrier and result in abscess formation. In some individuals with severe, essentially incapacitating abscess formation, we have had to resort to chronic long-term antimicrobial prophylaxis. We do not advocate the indiscriminate use of antibiotic prophylaxis, but in a few instances it can be useful. In general, the choice of such therapy should be limited to situations in which:

- one etiologic agent predominates;
- the therapy is not associated with significant toxicities; and
- resistance is not likely to develop readily.

In general, we have tended to use full therapeutic doses rather than the low-dose therapy commonly associated with prophylaxis. We believe that low-dose therapy might favor the selection of resistant organisms.

The combination of trimethoprim–sulfamethoxazole (co-trimoxazole) may have several uses in the therapy or prevention of infection in immunodeficient patients with recurrent infections. The preparation has been used in children with recurrent episodes of otitis media and recurrent urinary tract infections with success. Also, sulfonamides have a beneficial effect in patients who have CGD. A review[54]

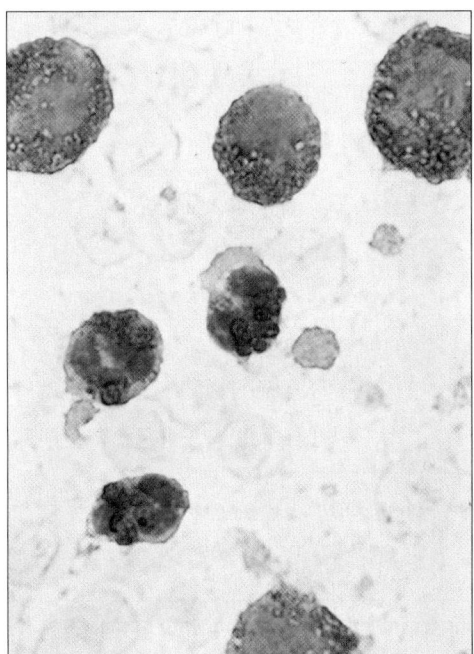

Fig. 2.12 Myeloperoxidase stain of the giant neutrophil granules of a patient with Chédiak–Higashi syndrome.

GENERAL MEASURES FOR PREVENTION OF INFECTION IN PRIMARY IMMUNODEFICIENCIES

- Avoid contact with individuals with respiratory infections
- Postural drainage and chest physiotherapy for patients with pneumonia or pulmonary disease
- Avoid live viral and bacterial vaccines; oral poliovirus vaccine should not be given to close contacts or household members
- Immunize normal close contacts against vaccine-preventable diseases (i.e. chickenpox, measles, influenza)
- Irradiate all blood products (3000–5000rad) before administration to avoid graft-versus-host disease
- Use red blood cells for transfusion from cytomegalovirus-seronegative donors or leukocyte filtered red blood cells
- Avoid splenectomy if possible
- Treat all minor infections with appropriate antimicrobial therapy to avoid severe infections and complications

Fig. 2.13 General measures for prevention of infection in patients with primary immunodeficiencies.

summarizes the advantages and disadvantages of antimicrobial prophylaxis in patients who have CGD.

Drugs that concentrate within the PMNL such as rifampin (rifampicin) and clindamycin are also attractive agents for patients with phagocytic disorders. The potential for the emergence of resistance and side effects needs to be considered when making the decision to institute a prophylactic agent, however. In addition, periodic rotation of the antibiotics being used every 10–14 days may help prevent the development of resistance.

IMMUNOTHERAPY

Figure 2.15 provides the recommended preventive options for patients with specific primary immunodeficiencies.

Antibody deficiency

In antibody-deficient patients, prevention of chronic infections and sequelae is aided significantly by the use of immunoglobulin. Intramuscular immunoglobulin (65mg/ml) is administered prophylactically in a dose of approximately 0.6ml/kg every 3 weeks after an initial loading dose of 1.2ml/kg. In larger individuals, this dose can result in a substantial injection volume. For this reason, many such patients prefer weekly doses amounting to approximately one-third of the dose: 10ml/week usually offers reasonable protection against pyogenic infections in most patients. We do not routinely check immunoglobulin levels following injection because the level seldom correlates specifically with protection against infection. An attempt is made, however, to adjust the dose according to the patient's symptoms.

Approximately 10% of patients develop reactions following immunoglobulin administration. Most are caused by inadvertent injection into small veins in the muscle. The aggregates contained within the intramuscular preparation may result in complement activation and an anaphylaxis-like picture. Patients may also develop IgE or IgG antibodies directed against various proteins in the immunoglobulin preparations. Patients with a total absence of IgA are likely to develop such antibodies to this immunoglobulin. This may result in anaphylactoid reactions after intramuscular or intravenous administration. These patients may be skin tested for such reactivity using low concentrations of the preparation. Both types of reactions, and especially those caused by aggregates, may be managed subsequently through the use of intravenous gammaglobulin, or in the IgA-deficient patient, by an IgA-depleted intravenous immunoglobulin (IVIG). This must be administered carefully and emergency equipment must be readily available in case the patient has a reaction.

Intravenous immunoglobulin preparations appear to represent a significant advance in the therapy of patients with antibody-deficiency disease.[55,56] The use of intravenous gammaglobulin as a prophylactic agent has clearly resulted in a reduction of morbidity in patients who have:
- X-linked agammaglobulinemia,
- hypogammaglobulinemia with IgM, and
- common variable hypogammaglobulinemia.

Intravenous gammaglobulin has significant advantages over plasma

PREVENTION OF INFECTIONS IN IMMUNODEFICIENCY	
Immunodeficiency	Preventive measures
Antibody deficiency	Intravenous immunoglobulin
	Prevention of vaccine-associated infections (no live virus or bacterial vaccines; IPV for household contacts)
Severe combined immunodeficiency and combined variable immunodeficiency	Intravenous immunoglobulin
	Prevention of vaccine-associated infections (no live virus or bacterial vaccines; IPV for household contacts)
	Trimethoprim–sulfamethoxazole (co-trimoxazole) prophylaxis for pneumocystis pneumonia
	Bone marrow transplantation
Ataxia–telangiectasia	Breast cancer screening
	Plasma therapy
	IgA-depleted intravenous immunoglobulin
Wiskott–Aldrich syndrome	Intravenous immunoglobulin
	Prevention of vaccine-associated infections (no live virus or bacterial vaccines; IPV for household contacts)
	Trimethoprim–sulfamethoxazole prophylaxis for *Pneumocystis* pneumonia
	Platelet transfusions
	Bone marrow transplantation
	Oral nystatin, ketoconazole or fluconazole
DiGeorge syndrome	Trimethoprim–sulfamethoxazole for *Pneumocystis* pneumonia
	Intravenous immunoglobulin
	Prevention of vaccine-associated infections
	Fetal thymus transplantation
	Bone marrow transplantation
Complement deficiencies	Meningococcal, pneumococcal and *Haemophilus influenzae* type b conjugate vaccines
Severe neutropenia	Granulocyte colony-stimulating factor
Chronic granulomatous disease	Recombinant interferon-γ
	Trimethoprim–sulfamethoxazole
Leukocyte adherence defect	Trimethoprim–sulfamethoxazole
	Bone marrow transplantation
Hyperimmunoglobulinemia E	Trimethoprim–sulfamethoxazole or dicloxacillin
	Fluconazole or ketoconazole
	Interferon-γ may be tried
	Immunomodulator therapy

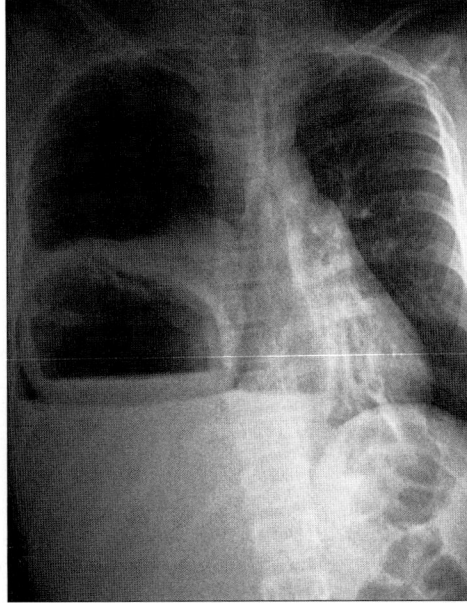

Fig. 2.14 Pulmonary abscess in a patient with Job's syndrome that required right lower lobectomy.

Fig. 2.15 Prevention options for infections in patients with primary immunodeficiencies. IPV, inactivated poliovirus vaccine.

therapy and intramuscular gammaglobulin therapy. Multiple studies have demonstrated the efficacy of IVIG as a therapeutic and prophylactic agent.[55–58]

Long-term immunoglobulin replacement therapy in people with selective IgM or IgA deficiency is not indicated because commercial preparations contain low levels of these immunoglobulins, and the half-life of both is quite short between 5–7 days.

Hyperimmune respiratory syncytial virus (RSV) immunoglobulin (RSVIG) has recently been shown to be effective in reducing the incidence and morbidity of RSV infection in infants with chronic pulmonary disease. Although studies are lacking, anecdotal experience points to a beneficial effect in selected immunocompromised hosts, so the use of this preparation should be considered for immunodeficient infants during the RSV season.[59] In fact, all immunodeficient children under 2–3 years of age should receive RSVIG rather than conventional IVIG.

Anti-allergic therapy for rhinitis or asthma may also benefit certain individuals with IgA deficiency. Plasma therapy has occasionally had a beneficial effect despite the fact that little infused IgA can be demonstrated in external secretions. Both IgG_2 and IgG_4 deficiency may accompany IgA deficiency in up to 20% of patients who have IgA deficiency who suffer recurrent infections. If such patients have an increased incidence of infections, IVIG administration may be beneficial. Because of the possibility of allergic reactions to infused IgA in IgA-deficient patients, only IVIG depleted of IgA should be used.

Severe combined immunodeficiency disease
Permanent reconstitution in SCID is generally attempted after acute infections have been controlled and is best carried out with an HLA-matched sibling bone marrow transplant. Marrow from a parent that has been treated to remove mature T lymphocytes may also be used. More recently peripheral stem cell or cord blood stem cell transplant has been employed. Alternative procedures include fetal liver transplantation with or without fetal thymus transplant.

Purine pathway enzyme deficiency
Therapy for patients with purine pathway enzyme deficiencies is similar to that given above for SCID. In addition, these patients may respond with partial immunologic reconstitution to the administration of glycerol-frozen packed erythrocytes containing high levels of the missing enzymes. Polyethylene glycol (PEG) ADA is also used to treat these patients. Immunoglobulin therapy should be included when there is evidence of defective antibody production.

Disorders treated with transfer factor and thymosin
A number of substances derived from human or animal sources or synthesized chemically have been used in attempts to enhance the host defense mechanism of immunodeficient patients.

Transfer factor, a low molecular weight (<10,000), nonimmunogenic protein derived from human leukocyte lysates, has been used with some success to prevent infections in patients with Wiskott–Aldrich syndrome or chronic mucocutaneous candidiasis.[60,61] However, results have been variable, and use of this agent has been associated with renal toxicity and the development of hemolytic anemia in a few patients.[60]

Thymosin, a partially purified extract of beef thymic tissue, was reported to increase T-lymphocyte numbers in a variety of congenital and acquired immunodeficiency syndromes.[62] Conversion to positive mitogenic responses and mixed leukocyte reactions has followed in-vitro incubation with the agent, whereas in-vivo therapy has resulted in clinical improvement in patients who have:
- Nezelof syndrome of cellular immunodeficiency with immunoglobulins,
- ataxia–telangiectasia,
- DiGeorge syndrome, and
- Wiskott–Aldrich syndrome.
The beneficial clinical effects, however, have not been permanent. In addition, allergic reactions and hepatitis have occurred during the use of this agent.

Neither transfer factor nor thymosin are available in a standardized form and they are not currently being used in the treatment of immunodeficiency to our knowledge. Both transfer factor and thymosin have been reported to cause at least a temporary improvement in some patients with chronic mucocutaneous candidiasis, but are not standard therapy at this time.

Disorders treated with bone marrow, fetal thymus and fetal liver transplants
Bone marrow, fetal thymus and fetal liver transplants have been used in the management of a variety of immunodeficiency diseases. Marrow transplantation between HLA-matched siblings (especially HLA-D matched, mixed lymphocyte culture nonreactive pairs) has been successful in a number of patients who have SCID and in patients who have Wiskott–Aldrich syndrome.[63] Excellent results have been obtained when HLA-matched donors have been available. Almost all patients who receive marrow from an individual not matched at the D locus have died of severe graft-versus-host disease and overwhelming infection within the first 1–2 months after transplantation. Recent attempts at transplanting mismatched marrow have employed lectin or monoclonal antibody removal of mature T lymphocytes from donor marrow.

Fetal thymic and hepatic tissue obtained before immunocompetence has been established have been used for patients who have SCID and for whom no HLA-D-matched marrow donor has been available. Reconstitution has been successful in several instances, but has not usually been longlasting.

Transplantation of fetal thymus or thymic epithelial cells maintained in vitro has been attempted in a variety of immunodeficiency disorders including DiGeorge syndrome, Nezelof syndrome and ataxia--telangiectasia. Transient improvements in skin test reactions and in-vitro lymphocyte responses and a decrease in the incidence or severity of infectious complications have been reported following such therapy, but permanent reconstitution has been rare. Transplantation of cord blood or peripheral stem cells from HLA-matched siblings or even unrelated donors has now been acomplished in several immunodeficiency disorders and appears to be a major hope for future therapy of these disorders.

Disorders treated with immune-potentiating agents
Patients with congenital agranulocytosis are given recombinant human granulocyte colony-stimulating factor (G-CSF), which will increase their absolute neutrophil counts. This results in a decreased morbidity and reduced need for antimicrobial therapy.

A number of substances with possible immune-potentiating effects have been investigated in patients with congenital immunodeficiencies.
- We and others[64] have shown that neutrophil chemotaxis and lysosomal enzyme release are modulated, in part, by cyclic 3´,5´-guanosine monophosphate (cGMP) and cyclic 3´,5´-adenosine monophosphate (cAMP). In addition, microtubular polymerization and function appeared to be dependent on the intracellular levels of these cyclic nucleotides.
- Patients who have Chédiak–Higashi syndrome, who have PMNLs filled with large lysosomal granules and chemotactic and bactericidal defects, have disordered microtubular function that can be corrected in vitro with cGMP or acetylcholine.[65] A patient with Chédiak–Higashi syndrome was subsequently treated with ascorbic acid (an agent that has been shown to alter cGMP and cAMP and leukocyte function),[66] and following such treatment, the patient improved clinically and had partial reversal of his in-vitro leukocyte function abnormalities.
- More recently, we have used moderately high doses of ascorbic acid in several patients with hyperimmunoglobulinemia E, recurrent infections and defective PMNL chemotaxis, and in several such patients we have observed a decrease in infections after in-vivo therapy with 1000–2000mg/day ascorbic acid, although no effect has been observed in others.

- It was recently reported that ascorbic acid improved leukocyte function and decreased infectious episodes in a group of patients with altered chemotactic function.[67]

As in the other congenital immunodeficiency syndromes that have a variable course, it is difficult to evaluate such therapy.

Interferon-γ and other agents

A dramatic improvement in the health of patients with CGD has been achieved with the use of IFN-γ. A reduction in serious infections in recipients of IFN-γ was observed in a recent study published by a large collaborative study group.[68] It has also recently been shown that recombinant human IFN-γ significantly improves the chemotactic responsiveness of neutrophils of patients with hyperimmunoglobulinemia E.[69] It was subsequently reported that IFN-γ administered subcutaneously three times weekly in a dose similar to that used in the CGD study improved neutrophil chemotaxis in Job's syndrome and probably benefitted 3 out of 4 patients.[70] Granulocyte colony-stimulating factor has also been reported to be of some benefit to these patients.

Levamisole is capable of enhancing chemotactic function both *in vitro*[71] and *in vivo*.[72] A controlled study with this agent in people who have Job's syndrome failed to show any decrease in the number of serious infections, even though chemotactic function was increased.[73]

Following in-vitro studies that indicated that histamine H_2-blocking agents might improve chemotaxis in patients with hyperimmunoglubinemia E,[40] such a patient was treated with 200mg of cimetidine q6h.[74] The chemotaxis remained normal throughout the treatment period.

Patients who have common variable hypogammaglobulinemia who failed to make IL-2 have been treated with this cytokine and have shown clinical and immunologic improvement.[75]

CLINICAL FEATURES

Patients who have primary immunodeficiency diseases are seldom entirely free from pyogenic infections. The antibody-deficient patient therefore often has recurrent or chronic episodes of sinusitis, otitis media, mastoiditis or bronchitis. Patients with an absence of C3 or C5 have similar problems, whereas those with phagocyte movement or killing defects have recurrent abscesses, adenitis, episodes of cellulitis and pneumonias. These recurrent acute infections impair the patient's quality of life and may evolve into either severe life-threatening or chronic indolent infections. Every attempt should be made to control these infections by using both antimicrobial therapy and immunologic regimens. In many cases, the etiologic agents may differ from those seen in normal hosts and may have unusual antibiotic sensitivity patterns, in part because of the chronic use of antimicrobial agents. The acute processes may be divided into respiratory, gastrointestinal and cutaneous infections.

RESPIRATORY INFECTIONS
Acute sinusitis and otitis media

Acute sinusitis is common in patients who have a deficiency of antibodies, C3 or C5, or phagocyte dysfunction. The infection is characterized by low-grade fever, congestion and postnasal drip, and pressure and tenderness over the involved sinus. Such infection may be associated with recurrent otitis media. The organisms involved are often similar to those in the normal host and include *H. influenzae, Strep. pneumoniae*, and occasionally *Streptococcus pyogenes* or *Neisseria* spp. Anaerobic bacteria may also be involved. In contrast to nonimmunodeficient patients, organisms such as *Staph. aureus* or Gram-negative bacilli such as *P. aeruginosa* may be isolated from the middle ear of immunodeficient hosts in association with symptoms of otitis media or tympanic membrane perforation and otorrhea. Antimicrobial agents should be administered for clinically apparent disease.

Acute bronchitis and pneumonia
Acute bronchitis and pneumonia are also common in patients with primary immunodeficiency. Low-grade fever, cough and sputum production with bronchitis are common in patients with antibody deficiencies and may also be seen in patients with T-lymphocyte and phagocyte abnormalities. Typeable and nontypeable *H. influenzae* are often isolated from sputum specimens. A host of other organisms may also be involved. A Gram stain of expectorated sputum combined with culture results should be the guide to therapy. It is important to remember that bronchitis-like illnesses in older children may be caused by *Mycoplasma pneumoniae* or *Chlamydia pneumoniae*.

Recurrent pneumonia is one of the most common problems faced by physicians caring for immunodeficient patients. Pyogenic infections caused by *H. influenzae* and *Strep. pneumoniae* as well as a variety of other pathogens occur in patients with antibody deficiencies. In patients with phagocyte dysfunction, *Staph. aureus* is more prevalent as an etiologic agent. Sputum or transtracheal cultures should be obtained as well as blood, urine and pleural fluid when possible for culture and examination. If the patient appears toxic and if empyema or pneumatocele are present, the patient should be hospitalized and treated with parenteral antibiotics. For the less ill patient, we have been successful with oral therapy combined with chest physiotherapy and postural drainage and close follow-up evaluation.

Respiratory viruses such as parainfluenza virus, adenovirus and RSV have long been recognized as significant causes of morbidity and mortality in patients with compromised immune systems.[76–78]

GASTROINTESTINAL INFECTIONS

The gastrointestinal tract is one of the prime sites for microbial challenge in both nonimmunodeficient and immunodeficient patients. Therefore, it is not unusual that this should be a major focus of infection in the compromised individual. Most patients with combined T- and B-lymphocyte defects have some diarrhea and malabsorption.[79]

Patients with isolated IgA deficiency or IgA deficiency associated with other immunoglobulin abnormalities often have chronic diarrhea due to *Giardia lamblia, Cryptosporidium parvum* or rotavirus infection. These agents are probably the leading cause of infectious diarrhea in immunodeficient patients. Patients with giardiasis may have symptoms of cramping abdominal pain, nausea and diarrhea, and occasionally low-grade fever. The disease may last for weeks or months in the immunodeficient individual. The diagnosis may be established by examining multiple stool specimens for cysts and trophozoites. The diagnosis can also be made by examining fresh duodenal or jejunal aspirates or biopsies. Because of the lack of sensitivity of stool examination and the difficulty examining aspirates, detection of giardiasis can be achieved by performing antigen detection assays on stools using either an enzyme-linked immunosorbent assay (ELISA) or direct fluorescent antibody (DFA) assay. A DFA assay can also be used to detect the presence of *C. parvum*. Both assays are highly sensitive and specific. A sensitive ELISA to detect the presence of rotavirus can also be used.

CUTANEOUS INFECTIONS

Recurrent cutaneous infections are the hallmark of patients with phagocyte defects. Abscess formation is common in patients with neutrophil and macrophage chemotactic, phagocytic and killing defects. These may consist of small 'pimples', larger boils or huge abscesses. Interestingly, the patients with the largest abscesses often have phagocyte motility defects leading to their recurrent infections. The large abscesses in patients with chemotactic defects probably result from delayed accumulation of the first wave of phagocytes. This allows further bacterial multiplication with subsequent production of an increased quantity of inflammatory mediators via the complement system and other pathways. This added stimulus continues to call in additional cells and results in the large abscesses observed.

Chronic granulomatous disease
Patients with CGD usually have an early onset of:

- recurrent abscesses, especially around the nose and mouth,
- cervical lymphadenitis,
- hepatic abscesses,
- pneumonias, and
- osteomyelitis.

The organisms involved are either catalase positive or do not make hydrogen peroxide. *Streptococcus pneumoniae*, group A streptococci, enterococci and viridans group streptococci are killed normally by these patients' cells. In contrast, *Staph. aureus*, *Staphylococcus epidermidis*, *E. coli*, *Serratia marcescens*, and *C. albicans* are not killed by the PMNLs of these patients. *Aspergillus* spp. as well as disseminated BCG infection have also been reported in these individuals.[80] Fungal infections are common in patients who have CGD.

In addition to these infections, many of these patients have gastrointestinal symptoms including diarrhea and stomach outlet obstruction secondary to granuloma formation. Granulomas also form in the abdomen and urinary tract and can lead to obstruction and additional infectious complications. Infection is usually caused by staphylococci, with *Klebsiella* spp., *E. coli*, *S. marcescens*, *C. albicans*, *Pseudomonas*, *Aspergillus*, *Proteus* and *Salmonella* spp. also being involved on occasion. A multiply-resistant pathogen, *Burkholderia cepacia* (formerly *Pseudomonas cepacia*), has been recognized as an emerging pathogen in patients with CGD, causing necrotizing pneumonia and lymphadenitis.[81] Sepsis is rare in these patients.

The microbicidal defects such as those of CGD allow:
- intracellular growth of bacteria;
- lysis of PMNLs and other cells; and
- release of important inflammatory mediators that result in accumulations of bacteria, phagocytes and debris.

Needle aspiration or open drainage usually yields an etiologic agent on which susceptibility testing can be performed.

Many patients who have CGD have serious problems in wound healing, so recently we have not recommended incision and drainage except where absolutely necessary. When possible, aspiration with a large-bore needle has been successful in relieving pressure and obtaining an etiologic diagnosis. Therapy is then instituted with an appropriate bactericidal agent and continued for an extended period of time. Such medical management of what used to be considered surgical cases has resulted in far less overall morbidity in CGD patients. At times, however, drainage procedures are required.

Cutaneous and mucocutaneous candidiasis have been observed in patients with phagocyte abnormalities. Some also have T-lymphocyte disorders, so the exact role of each abnormality in the overall clinical picture is unknown.

Cellulitis caused by streptococci, staphylococci and other agents has occasionally been a problem in patients with phagocyte disorders.[34] This generally requires a rapid diagnosis based on blood cultures or local needle aspirates of the infected area and is treated initially with parenteral bactericidal antimicrobial agents followed by oral agents.

DIAGNOSIS

A critical factor in the detection of immunodeficient patients is to maintain a high degree of suspicion in order to discover such individuals as early as possible. In one study of patients with acquired common variable hypogammaglobulinemia, a period of approximately 10 years lapsed between the onset of recurrent infections and a diagnosis of the antibody deficiency. This is unacceptable today because simple tests are available in most laboratories to screen for hypogammaglobulinemia. There are several excellent reviews on detecting the patient with a primary immunodeficiency,[4,82–84] and we shall briefly review those aspects that should alert the clinician to the possibility of a defect and then list the readily available tests that are useful in screening suspected patients. Figure 2.16 provides a summary of clinical features that should suggest a diagnosis of an immunodeficiency.

Deciding which patients have a host defense abnormality and which

require further investigation is difficult in many instances. A careful history detailing the number, type and severity of infections is critical. Particular attention should be addressed to determining whether the infection and its etiology are documented by culture results, radiographs, scans and serologic antigen detection or DNA-based tests, or other means. This is essential because often a diagnosis of pneumonia or 'bloodstream infection' is mentioned by the patient or parent without any documentation being available. A complete family history, concentrating on recurrent infections, early deaths, malignancies and consanguinity, may also yield valuable data. A thorough physical examination and appropriate laboratory tests should be performed to rule out physical or anatomic defects that might lead to recurrent infections. Recurrent meningitis because of a dermal sinus or basilar skull fracture and recurrent urinary tract infections secondary to ureteral problems are prime examples of such anatomic abnormalities. Figure 2.17 provides a summary of clinical conditions that do not suggest an immunodeficiency.

In addition, one must exclude those patients who are normal, but who are exposed to a number of respiratory illnesses in their environment and are therefore often ill. It has been shown that preschool and school-aged children have 6–12 respiratory infections per year. An adult probably averages 2–4 respiratory infections/year. These figures are very useful in explaining recurrent infections to the individual who turns out on testing to have a normal immune system.

After determining that a patient's recurrent infections are not the result of anatomic defects or epidemiologic exposure, it is important to divide the host defense mechanism into its major components and consider the type of infection generally seen with defects in each system.

CLINICAL FEATURES SUGGESTIVE OF IMMUNODEFICIENCY	
Immunodeficiency	Clinical features
Severe combined immunodeficiency	Eczema, chronic diarrhea, failure to thrive, chronic interstitial pneumonitis
	Persistent mucocutaneous candidiasis
	Pneumocystis carinii pneumonia
	Hepatosplenomegaly
Antibody-deficiency disorders	Recurrent sinusitis
	Recurrent episodes of pneumonia, sepsis or meninigitis
Ataxia–telangiectasia	Chronic sinopulmonary infections
Complement deficiencies	Recurrent *Neisseria meningitidis* infections
	Sepsis with encapsulated bacteria
	Recurrent sinusitis
	Lupus-like syndrome and Raynaud's phenomenon
	Ankylosing spondylitis
Congential neutropenia, chemotaxis defects	Perirectal abscesses
	Mouth ulcerations, gingivitis
Chronic granulomatous disorders	Recurrent cutaneous abscesses
	Cervical lymphadenitis
	Fungal infections with *Aspergillus* spp.
	Necrotizing pneumonia due to *Burkholderia cepacia*
DiGeorge syndrome	Neonatal hypocalcemia and seizures
	Right-sided congenital heart defects

Fig. 2.16 Clinical features suggestive of primary immunodeficiency.

CELL-MEDIATED DEFICINECY

Patients with abnormalities in cell-mediated immunity tend to have severe or recurrent viral infections caused by varicella-zoster virus, RSV, rotavirus, herpes simplex virus or cytomegalovirus, or fungal infections such as those caused by *C. albicans*. A variety of intracellular bacterial and *Pneumocystis carinii* infections also occur. Abnormalities in T-lymphocyte numbers and function can be screened for fairly simply employing skin tests for delayed hypersensitivity, lymphocyte mitogen and antigen responses, and enumeration of T lymphocytes and T-lymphocyte subsets (Fig. 2.18). More recently, analysis of the production of specific cytokines has also been used.

The diagnosis of DiGeorge syndrome should be suspected in the presence of seizures resulting from hypocalcemia, and cardiac anomalies in a newborn. Radiographic studies may reveal an absence of thymic tissue, and T-lymphocyte quantitation will be low. Cardiac and parathyroid gland complications may therefore alert the clinician to the diagnosis before infections occur. Later, chronic mucocutaneous candidiasis, chronic rhinitis and recurrent pneumonias develop. *Pneumocystis carinii* pulmonary infection is not uncommon. Diarrhea and failure to thrive may also occur.

ANTIBODY-DEFICIENCY SYNDROMES

One of the major functions of antibody in the host defense mechanism is to opsonize or coat bacteria so that phagocytic cells can ingest and kill them. Antibody-deficiency syndromes are often characterized, therefore, by severe and recurrent pyogenic bacterial infections. Almost all such patients have recurrent respiratory infections which include draining otitis media, mastoiditis, sinusitis, bronchitis and multiple episodes of pneumonia. This often leads to the development of bronchiectasis and chronic respiratory problems. These patients also often have chronic diarrhea and may have systemic infections such as sepsis, meningitis or osteomyelitis.

A diagnosis of hypogammaglobulinemia is supported by:
- a history of severe or recurrent bacterial infections;
- low immunoglobulin levels; and
- the inability to make specific antibodies (Fig. 2.8).

Hypogammaglobulinemia is best documented by determining quantitative IgG, IgM and IgA levels. Recurrent sinopulmonary infections strongly suggest an immunoglobulin deficiency. In patients with normal IgG concentrations, a selective deficiency in an IgG subclass is also a possibility.[85]

The ability of an individual to make specific antibody to an antigen can also be assessed using common serologic techniques (Fig. 2.18). Anti-blood group A and B titers or isohemagglutinins can be determined wherever blood typing is performed. These are predominantly IgM antibodies directed against cross-reacting polysaccharide antigens on bacteria normally present in the gastrointestinal flora. By 6 months of age, a child should have a titer of 1:8 or greater against A or B substance unless the blood type is AB. Other serologic tests that can be used to assess specific antibody production include:

- the antistreptolysin O or anti-DNAase B if a patient has had a past streptococcal infection; and
- rubella titer if the patient has received this vaccine.

Alternatively, one can measure influenza, diphtheria or tetanus antibody titers following immunization with influenza or diphtheria–tetanus toxoid vaccines. In addition, specific antibody responses to polysaccharides can be measured after immunization with *H. influenzae* type b conjugate and meningococcal and pneumococcal vaccines. The assessment of an immune response to polysaccharides is important for detecting those patients with normal immunoglobulin levels who have an impaired response to these antigens.[86] Finally, one can enumerate the number of peripheral blood lymphocytes that have immunoglobulin on their surface or surface markers for B lymphocytes.

CONGENITAL COMPLEMENT DEFICIENCIES

Congenital deficiencies in the complement system are often associated with infections similar to those observed in hypogammaglobulinemia, and include respiratory infections, sepsis and meningitis.[14–20] Complement activity and factors should be measured in patients who have recurring respiratory infections, sepsis and meningitis (Fig. 2.18).

PHAGOCYTE ABNORMALITIES

Infections in patients with phagocyte abnormalities often manifest as abscesses or episodes of cellulitis. Staphylococci predominate as the etiologic agents; this is probably because the organisms are the most numerous among the skin flora. Infections with streptococci and Gram-negative bacteria as well as *C. albicans* also occur. The metabolic activity of phagocytes, which relates to their ability to activate the hexose monophosphate shunt and generate toxic oxygen radicals essential to microbicidal activity, can be assessed with the NBT dye reduction test (Fig. 2.9),[87] a procedure employing the detection of chemiluminescence,[88] or more recently, dihydrorhodamine fluorescence (Fig. 2.18).[89,90] Myeloperoxidase deficiency may also be detected using the chemiluminescence assay as well as by using a histochemical stain for this enzyme (Fig. 2.12). All suspected defects in microbicidal activity should be confirmed by more classic phagocytosis and killing assays[48] as well as identification of the missing cytochrome chain or phagocyte oxidase (Fig. 2.11).

The measurement of the serum level of IgE, may be of value in the diagnosis of a number of patients who have hyperimmunoglobulinemia E, recurrent infections and defective PMNL chemotaxis.[34] Extremely high levels of IgE are usually present in subsets of these patients,[8,15] including those who have the Hill–Quie syndrome[34] and Buckley syndrome,[41] as well those who have the closely related or identical syndrome of Job.[43] Neutrophil chemotaxis is usually abnormal in these patients as measured in the Boyden chamber filter or in an under agarose assay (Fig. 2.19).

SEVERE LIFE-THREATENING INFECTIONS

Patients with congenital immunodeficiency are especially prone to develop sudden overwhelming and often fatal infections. In such cases, it is absolutely essential that the clinician has an understanding of the basic underlying defect in the host defense mechanism, the most likely etiologic agents and the available therapeutic modalities.

Early diagnosis of infection and correct identification of the etiologic agent are most important in managing severe life-threatening infections in immunodeficient hosts. A high degree of suspicion must be maintained for infection in these patients. A variety of diagnostic tests lend additional support in suggesting the presence of infection. These include:
- routine and more specialized cultures of transtracheal aspirates, lung aspirates, bronchoalveolar lavage, or open biopsies in diagnosing pneumonias;
- examination of cerebrospinal fluid (CSF) or even brain biopsies for central nervous system (CNS) infections; and
- a variety of scans that have proven useful in defining infections in these patients, including technetium-99m bone scans, indium-111 white blood cell scans, CT and MRI.

CLINICAL FEATURES NOT SUGGESTIVE OF AN IMMUNODEFICIENCY

- Uncomplicated isolated episodes of tonsillitis and pharyngitis
- Recurrent episodes of urinary tract infection
- Uncomplicated common colds
- Isolated recurrent episodes of otitis media
- Infections related only to indwelling devices
- Recurrent episodes of infections at the same site (e.g. osteomyelitis, septic arthritis)
- Infections associated with anatomic defects (e.g. dermal sinus)

Fig. 2.17 Clinical features that do not suggest an immunodeficiency.

IMMUNOLOGIC SCREENING TESTS	
Part of the immune system to be tested	Tests
Cell-mediated	Total lymphocyte count (complete blood count, differential)
	Delayed hypersensitivity skin tests (*Candida albicans*, tetanus, diphtheria, *Trichophyton* spp.)
	Total T lymphocytes, T-lymphocyte subsets
	Mitogen and antigen proliferation responses
	HIV antibody test
Antibody-mediated	Serum quantitative immunoglobulin levels (IgA, IgG, IgM)
	Serum IgG subclass levels
	IgG response to vaccine proteins (diphtheria, tetanus) and polysaccharides (pneumococcus, meningococcus)
	Isohemagglutinin titers (anti-A, anti-B)
Complement	Total hemolytic complement activity (CH50)
	Quantitation of serum complement components (C2, C3, C4, C6, factor B or other individual components)
Phagocytic function	Complete white blood cell count, differential count
	Quantitative nitroblue tetrazolium test, chemiluminescence assay or dihydrorhodamine fluorescence for respiratory burst activity
	Serum IgE level
	Chemotaxis assay
	Flow cytometric analysis of CD11/18

Fig. 2.18 Immunologic screening tests. For use in patients with suspected primary immunodeficiency syndromes.

Although a positive result with these techniques may be helpful, a negative result does not rule out the presence of infection in an immunocompromised host.

Sinus or middle ear fluid cultures should be taken in the immunodeficient patient, and antimicrobial susceptibility patterns determined on significant isolates. This is in contrast to the usual practice in the normal host with acute otitis or sinusitis where such cultures are usually not indicated and are not cost-effective.

Failure to evaluate infections in the immunodeficient host with appropriate cultures and antimicrobial susceptibility determinations often results in a significant delay in the initiation of appropriate therapy. In addition, if the infection disseminates and becomes life-threatening, the initial culture and susceptibility results can be of great benefit in selecting appropriate therapy.

There are excellent reviews of the proper use of diagnostic microbiology laboratory tests that provide guidance for clinicians in diagnosing bacterial and viral infections.[91,92]

MANAGEMENT

The initial evaluation of the febrile patient with primary immunodeficiency should always include a careful history and physical examination supported by Gram stain and culture of material obtained from cutaneous lesions, expectorate, wound drainage, etc. Selecting an appropriate antimicrobial regimen for the severely ill immunocompromised host may be a difficult task. Initial therapeutic regimens should be designed to stem the progression of infection quickly and pre-

vent a fatal outcome. The antimicrobial agents should be chosen based on the patient's host defense defect and the most likely pathogen involved (Figs 2.2 & 2.20). In addition, an attempt should be made to select bactericidal rather than bacteriostatic antibiotics when possible because the host's immune system may not be capable of microbial killing. Intravenous therapy is indicated for all serious infections.

Initial antimicrobial therapy for deep-seated bone or tissue infections should always include a penicillinase-resistant penicillin such as nafcillin. It may be combined with an aminoglycoside for synergism or to cover enteric Gram-negative bacilli. Several investigators have used agents such as rifampin, clindamycin or chloramphenicol, which appear to penetrate leukocytes more efficiently. Such agents have been shown to have better activity *in vitro* in the presence of PMNLs. Therapy must be continued for long periods. After an initial 2 to 3-week period, oral antimicrobial agents may be substituted for parenteral therapy.

For patients with antibody deficiencies, less than 6 hours may elapse between the onset of symptoms and death. It is critical that clinicians managing such patients are aware of this and that they inform the patients or the parents of the possible consequences of severe infection. Immediately upon evaluating a patient with fever, we recommend that blood, urine and CSF cultures are obtained, followed within minutes by the administration of high intravenous doses of a third-generation cephalosporin such as cefotaxime or ceftriaxone. *Streptococcus pneumoniae* and *H. influenzae* are by far the most likely pathogens and these agents should cover both pathogens. Critically ill patients should receive intravenous gammaglobulin. Patients with the Wiskott–Aldrich syndrome are particularly susceptible to the development of serious overwhelming infections with *Strep. pneumoniae, H. influenzae* and other encapsulated bacteria because they fail to make adequately-functioning antibodies to polysaccharide antigens.[7] A number of individuals with this syndrome have died of such infections.

The use of extensive surgical procedures in patients with CGD should be limited because these individuals heal very poorly. In addition, the use of pulmonary lobectomy should be discouraged because the patients often go on to develop disease in other lobes and are then even more compromised. Limited incision and drainage of abscesses are often required for patients with hyperimmunglobulinemia E, and large volumes of purulent material will often be obtained. Healing from surgical procedures is usually satisfactory in contrast to that of patients with CGD.

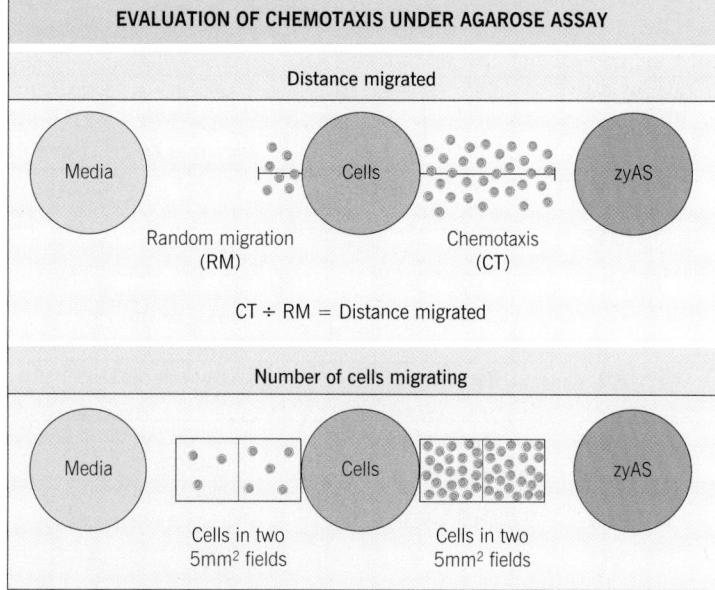

Fig. 2.19 Chemotaxis of leukocytes or monocytes assessed in the under agarose assay. Cells, leukocytes or monocytes; ZyAS, zymosan-activated serum.

INITIAL ANTIMICROBIAL THERAPY IN PATIENTS WITH PRIMARY IMMUNODEFICIENCY

Immunodeficiency	Type of infection	Suggested therapy
Severe combined immunodeficiency (SCID)	Bacterial pneumonia or sepsis	Cefotaxime, ceftriaxone
	If *Staphylococcus aureus* suspected	Add nafcillin or oxacillin
	If *Pseudomonas aeruginosa* suspected	Ceftazidime plus aminoglycoside or extended-spectrum penicillin plus aminoglycoside
	If methicillin-resistant *Staphylococcus aureus* or drug-resistant *Streptococcus pneumoniae*	Use vancomycin as Gram-positive coverage
	Herpes simplex virus or varicella-zoster virus infections	Aciclovir
	Cytomegalovirus infection	Ganciclovir, foscarnet
	Mucocutaneous candidiasis	Fluconazole
Purine pathway enzyme deficiencies	Similar to SCID	Similar to SCID
Wiskott–Aldrich syndrome	Bacterial pneumonia or sepsis	Cefotaxime or ceftriaxone
	If methicillin-resistant *Staphylococcus aureus* or drug-resistant *Streptococcus pneumoniae*	Add vancomycin
Ataxia–telangiectasia	Chronic sinopulmonary infections, mild-to-moderate	Amoxicillin–clavulanate, cefuroxime*
	Severe	Cefotaxime or ceftriaxone
Mucocutaneous candidiasis	Mild-to-moderate fungal disease	Fluconazole, ketoconazole, nystatin, topical amphotericin B
	Systemic fungal disease	Amphotericin B
Antibody-deficiency disorders, common variable hypogamma-globulinemia	Pneumonia or sepsis†	Third-generation cephalosporin or piperacillin–tazobactam plus aminoglycoside or imipenem–cilastatin plus aminoglycoside
	Otitis media, sinusitis	Amoxicillin–clavulanate, cefuroxime*
	Chronic enteroviral meningoencephalitis	Intravenous immunoglobulin
Selective IgA deficiency	Upper respiratory tract infections	Amoxicillin–clavulanate or cefuroxime
	Giardiasis	Metronidazole or quinacrine
Complement disorders	Pneumonia, sepsis or meningitis	Ceftriaxone or cefotaxime†
Neutropenia disorders	Perirectal abscesses	Amoxicillin–clavulanate or piperacillin–tazobactam or imipenem–cilastatin or clindamycin plus aminoglycoside
Chemotactic disorders	Pneumonia	Clindamycin or dicloxacillin
Hyperimmuno-globulinemia E	Cutaneous infections	Nafcillin or oxacillin plus aminoglycoside
Chronic granulomatous disease	Musculoskeletal or soft tissue infections	Clindamycin plus aminoglycoside or nafcillin or oxacillin plus aminoglycoside

*If drug-resistant *Streptococcus pneumoniae* is suspected, add clindamycin.
†If drug-resistant *Streptococcus pneumoniae* is suspected, add vancomycin.

Fig. 2.20 Suggested initial antimicrobial therapy for specific infections in patients with primary immunodeficiency disorders.

Because giardiasis is so common in IgA- and combined immunoglobulin-deficient patients, initiating therapy with metronidazole is considered acceptable before a specific diagnosis has been made after stool specimens have been collected for examination. Therapy is continued usually for 1 week. Relapses may occur, requiring retreatment and longer courses of therapy. The symptomatic patient may be treated with an alternative antimicrobial agent if no response is observed following initial therapy. A suspension of furazolidone can be used for young children who are unable to swallow tablets.

Bacterial overgrowth in the small intestine has also been suspected as a cause of diarrhea in immunodeficient patients. Reliable data are not available correlating bacterial counts in the small bowel content and symptomatology. On occasion, an immunodeficient patient with marked diarrhea and no specific identified pathogen will respond to antimicrobial therapy. A nonabsorbable drug such as neomycin may be employed, or sometimes an absorbable drug such as tetracycline will be of benefit to the older patient. Although data on such therapy are practically nonexistent, a trial may be indicated for the patient with marked diarrhea after specific pathogens have been ruled out as the etiology. Other investigators have suggested the use of oral immunoglobulin in these patients.[93]

Other important gastrointestinal pathogens commonly reported to cause disease in the immunodeficient host are rotavirus and *Cryptosporidium* spp. Both are well-recognized causative agents of chronic diarrhea in this population. Although various agents such as spiramycin, azithromycin and paromomycin have been used, there is still no recognized effective therapy for cryptosporidiosis. Clinical trials are in progress to evaluate the efficacy of clarithromycin, bovine immunoglobulin concentrate and nitazoxanide in the treatment of cryptosporidiosis in AIDS patients (see Chapter 5.13). Enteral immunoglobulins have been used with favorable results in some patients with chronic diarrhea caused by rotavirus.[95] Because of the frequent exposure to antimicrobial agents, the immunodeficient patient is also susceptible to infection by *Clostridium difficile*.

Plasma infusions or IVIG often decrease the severity and frequency of diarrhea in the immunodeficient patient.[93] The reason for this is unclear because the IgA in plasma does not appear to cross into the gastrointestinal tract. Perhaps the plasma contains other factors such as lymphocyte products that are helpful in enhancing local secretory immunity. One or two units of plasma may be given on a biweekly basis to such patients, and this is often followed by dramatic improvement. Because of the risks associated with plasma infusions, even from close relatives, IVIG is now used much more often than plasma.

Recurrent episodes of perirectal abscesses in a young child should suggest a possible immunodeficiency. Commonly patients with leukocyte adherence defects may present with perirectal abscesses requiring broad-spectrum antibiotics and surgical drainage.

Patients who have CGD often develop severe pneumonias and other infections caused by staphylococci because their leukocytes fail to kill these organisms following ingestion. A CGD patient who has severe pneumonia should be treated initially with antimicrobial agents directed against staphylococci, and especially agents that penetrate into cells.

Patients who have congenital defects of their terminal complement components (C6, C7, C8) often have repeated disseminated infections with *Neisseria meningitidis* or *Neisseria gonorrhoeae*.[16–19] An acutely toxic patient known to have such a defect should receive appropriate intravenous antimicrobial therapy for these organisms. Anecdotal experience suggests that IVIG, including hyperimmune RSVIG, used prophylactically and therapeutically may be beneficial in high-risk immunocompromised patients. Although the use of aerosolized ribavirin is questionable in immunocompetent individuals, anecdotal experience with and without IVIG, suggests it may be effective in the treatment of the immunocompromised host who has RSV, adenovirus or parainfluenza pneumonia.[95–97] Due to the scarcity of patients with immunodeficiencies who have RSV infection or an infection by other viral pathogens in any given medical center, controlled trials are unlikely in the near future.

FUNGAL INFECTIONS

Candidiasis in immunodeficient patients is usually difficult to treat and may require prolonged topical therapy; systemic therapy may be needed for a brief period of time. Nystatin has generally been used in topical therapy, with agents such as amphotericin B and 5-flucytosine being used occasionally for severely affected patients. Ketoconazole is quite effective against superficial infections, but is less successful when used against deep infections such as those in bones and joints.

Newer antifungal agents such as fluconazole and itraconazole are promising agents in the treatment of fungal infections in the immuno-compromised host. The latter agent has in-vitro activity against aspergillus infection, which is a major problem in many of these patients.

THERAPIES TO ENHANCE HOST DEFENSES

After appropriate cultures and laboratory tests have been obtained and antimicrobial therapy has been instituted in the critically ill congenitally immunodeficient patient, the clinician must consider therapies that may enhance host defenses.

Granulocyte transfusion therapy has been used on occasion for severe infection in patients with CGD, but a marked improvement has not been observed. Today a number of older individuals have CGD, and it appears that infections become less severe with age. Granulocyte transfusions have also been given to patients with marked neutropenia. Good results have been reported in patients treated with daily infusions of 3–4 units of granulocytes. However, the use of granulocyte transfusions has decreased in the past few years because of the availability of G-CSF.[98,99]

Attempts to correct T-lymphocyte abnormalities in acutely ill patients have not met with much success and are best carried out after the infection has been controlled. Efforts at transplantation during such episodes have not often resulted in survival.

In the antibody-deficient patient, an effort should be directed towards supplying the missing antibodies.[100] In the acutely ill individual, IVIG 400–750mg/kg infused over 2–4 hours should be administered. It ameliorates the severity of the illness and improves survival.[51–53] Such IVIG preparations are superior to intramuscular globulin preparations in reducing specific acute illnesses and reducing the number of days that hypogammaglobulinemic individuals require antibiotics.[96] Furthermore, they are effective in preventing symptomatic cytomegalovirus infection following transplantation; in treating chronic ECHO-virus encephalitis; and for treatment and prophylaxis of infections caused by rotavirus and RSV.[56,59,94] Intravenous immunoglobulin has also been used with some success in patients who have Wiskott–Aldrich syndrome, ataxia–telangiectasia and complement component deficiencies.

REFERENCES

1. Shyur S-D, Hill HR. Recent advances in the genetics of primary immunodeficiency syndromes. J Pediatr 1996;129:8–24.
2. Hayakawa H, Inata T, Yata J, Kobayashi N. Primary immunodeficiency in Japan. I. Overview of a nationwide survey on primary immunodeficiency syndrome. J Clin Immunol 1981;1:31–9.
3. Robertson DM, Shelton MJ, Hosking CS. Incidence of primary immunodeficiency disorders in childhood (abstract). Fifth International Congress of Immunology, 1983.
4. Stiehm ER. Immunodeficiency disorders: general considerations. In: Stiehm ER, ed. Immunologic disorders in infants and children, 4th ed. Philadelphia: WB Saunders; 1996:201–52.
5. Parkman R, Gelfand EW, Rosen FS, et al. Severe combined immunodeficiency and adenosine deaminase deficiency. N Engl J Med 1975;292:714–9.
6. Stoop JW, Zegers BJM, Hendricks GFM, et al. Purine nucleoside phosphorylase deficiency associated with selective cellular immunodeficiency. N Engl J Med 1977;96:651–5.
7. Blaese RM, Strober W, Waldmann TA. Immunodeficiency in Wiskott–Aldrich syndrome. Birth Defects 1975;11:250–4.
8. Tiller TL Jr, Buckley RN. Transient hypogammaglobulinemia of infancy: review of the literature, clinical and immunologic features of 11 new cases, and long-term followup. J Pediatr 1978;92:347–53.
9. Tsukada S, Saffran DC, Rawlings DJ, et al. Deficient expression of a B cell cytoplasmic tyrosine kinase in human X-linked agammaglobulinemia. Cell 1993;72:279–90.
10. Levitt D, Haber P, Rich K, et al. Hyper IgM immunodeficiency. J Clin Invest 1983;72:1650–7.
11. Strober W, Krakauer R, Klaeveman HL, et al. Secretory component deficiency: a disorder of the IgA immune system. N Engl J Med 1976;294:351–6.
12. Ammann AJ, Hong R. Selective IgA deficiency: presentation of 30 cases and a review of the literature. Medicine (Baltimore) 1971;50:223–6.

13. Sneller MC, Strober W, Eisenstein E, Jaffe JS, Cunningham-Rundles C. New insights into common variable immunodeficiency. Ann Intern Med 1993;118:720–30.
14. Alper CA, Colten HR, Gear JSS, et al. Homozygous human C3 deficiency. J Clin Invest 1976;57:222–9.
15. Ballow M, Shira JE, Harden L, et al. Complete absence of the third component of complement in man. J Clin Invest 1975;56:703–10.
16. Boyer JT, Gall EP, Norman ME, et al. Hereditary deficiency of the seventh component of complement. J Clin Invest 1975;56:905–13.
17. Leddy JP, Frank MM, Gaitner I, et al. Hereditary deficiency of the sixth component of complement in man. J Clin Invest 1974;53:544–53.
18. Petersen BH, Graham JA, Brooks GF. Human deficiency of the eighth component of complement. J Clin Invest 1976;57:283–90.
19. Petersen BH, Lee TJ, Snyderman RJ, et al. Neisseria meningitidis and Neisseria gonorrhoeae bacteremia associated with C6, C7, or C8 deficiency. Ann Intern Med 1979;90:917–20.
20. Rosenfeld SI, Baum J, Steigbigel RT, et al. Hereditary deficiency of the fifth component of complement in man. J Clin Invest 1976;57:1635–43.
21. Day NK, Geiger H, Stroud R, et al. C1r deficiency: an inborn error associated with cutaneous and renal disease. J Clin Invest 1972;51:1102–8.
22. Klemperer MR, Woodworth HC, Rosen FS, et al. Hereditary deficiency of the second component of complement (C'2) in man. J Clin Invest 1966;45:880–90.
23. Gilliland BC, Schaller JG, Leddy JP, et al. Lupus syndrome in a C4-deficient child. Arthritis Rheum 1975;18:401.
24. Newman SL, Vogler LB, Feigin RD, et al. Recurrent septicemia associated with congenital deficiency of C2 and partial deficiency of factor B and the alternative complement. N Engl J Med 1978;299:290–2.
25. Neu RL, Stockman JA III, Spitzer RE, et al. 46,XY/46,XY,21q-mosaicism in an infant with neutropenia and properdin deficiency. J Med Genet 1976;13:332–4.

26. Sumiya M, Summerfield JA. The role of collectins in host defense. Semin Liver Dis 1997;17:311–8.
27. Snowden N, Stanworth S, Donn R, Davies E, Ollier B. Mannose-binding protein genotypes and recurrent infection. Lancet 1995;346:1629–31.
28. Summerfield JA, Ryder S, Sumiya M, et al. Mannose binding protein gene mutations associated with unusual and severe infections in adults. Lancet 1995;345:886–9.
29. Boxer LA, Blackwood RA. Leukocyte disorders: quantitative and qualitative disorders of the neutrophil, Part 1. Pediatr Rev 1996;17:19–28.
30. Boxer LA, Blackwood RA. Leukocyte disorders: quantitative and qualitative disorders of the neutrophil, Part 2. Pediatr Rev 1996;17:47–50.
31. Kostmann R. Infantile genetic agranulocytosis. Acta Paediatr 1956;45:1–78.
32. Miller ME, Oski FA, Harris MB. Lazy-leukocyte syndrome. Lancet 1971;1:665–9.
33. Miller ME, Norman ME, Koblenzer PJ, et al. A new familial defect of neutrophil movement. J Lab Clin Med 1973;82:1–8.
34. Hill HR, Quie PG. Raised serum-IgE levels and defective neutrophil chemotaxis in three children with eczema and recurrent bacterial infections. Lancet 1974;1:183–7.
35. Clark RA, Root RK, Kimball HR, et al. Defective neutrophil chemotaxis and cellular immunity in a child with recurrent infections. Ann Intern Med 1973;78:515–9.
36. Van Scoy RE, Hill HR, Ritts RE Jr, et al. Familial neutrophil chemotaxis defect, recurrent bacterial infections, mucocutaneous candidiasis and hyperimmunoglobulinemia E. Ann Intern Med 1975;82:766–71.
37. Jacobs JC, Norman ME. A familial defect of neutrophil chemotaxis with asthma, eczema, and recurrent skin infections. Pediatr Res 1977;11:732–6.
38. Hill HR. The syndrome of hyperimmunoglobulinemia E and recurrent infections. Am J Dis Child 1982;136:767–71.
39. Hill HR, Augustine NH, Alexander G, et al. Familial occurrence of Job's syndrome of hyper-IgE and recurrent infections. J Allergy Clin Immunol 1977;99:S395.

40. Hill HR, Estensen RD, Hogan NA, et al. Severe staphylococcal disease associated with allergic manifestations, hyperimmunoglobulinemia E, and defective neutrophil chemotaxis. J Lab Clin Med 1976;88:796–806.

41. Buckley RH, Wray BB, Belmaker EZ. Extreme hyperimmunoglobulinemia E and undue susceptibility to infection. Pediatrics 1972;49:59–69.

42. Davis SD, Schaller J, Wedgwood RJ. Job's syndrome: recurrent 'cold' staphylococcal abscesses. Lancet 1966;1:1013–7.

43. Hill HR, Quie PG, Pabst HF, et al. Defect in neutrophil granulocyte chemotaxis in Job's syndrome or recurrent 'cold' staphylococcal abscesses. Lancet 1974;2:617–9.

44. Schopfer K, Baerlocher K, Price P, et al. Staphylococcal IgE antibodies, hyperimmunoglobulinemia E and Staphylococcus aureus infections. N Engl J Med 1979;300:835–8.

45. Del Prete G, Tiri A, Maggi E, et al. Defective in-vitro production of gamma interferon and tumor necrosis factor-alpha by circulating T cells from patients with hyper-immunoglobulinemia syndrome. J Clin Invest 1989;84:1830–5.

46. Boxer LA, Hedley-Whyte ET, Stossel TP. Neutrophil actin dysfunction and abnormal neutrophil behavior. N Engl J Med 1974;291:1093–9.

47. Snyderman R, Altman LC, Frankel A, et al. Defective mononuclear leukocyte chemotaxis: a previously unrecognized immune dysfunction. Ann Intern Med 1973;78:509–13.

48. Quie PG, White JG, Holmes B, et al. In vitro bactericidal capacity of human polymorphonuclear leukocytes: diminished activity in chronic granulomatous disease of childhood. J Clin Invest 1967;46:668–79.

49. Salmon SE, Cline MJ, Schultz J, et al. Myeloperoxidase deficiency. N Engl J Med 1970;282:250–3.

50. Rosner F, Kozinn PJ, Jervis GA. Leukocyte function and serum immunoglobulins in Down's syndrome. NY State J Med 1973;73:672–5.

51. Anderson DC, Schmalsteig FC, Finegold MJ, et al. The severe and moderate phenotypes of heritable Mac-1, LFA-1 deficiency: their quantitative definition and relation to leukocyte dysfunction and clinical features. J Infect Dis 1985;152:668–89.

52. Etzioni A, Harlan JM, Pollack S, Phillips LM, Gershoni-Baruch R, Paulson JC. Leukocyte adhesion deficiency (LAD) II: a new adhesion defect due to absence of sialyl Lewis X, the ligand for selectins. Immunodeficiency 1993;4:307–8.

53. Phillips ML, Schwartz BR, Etzioni A, et al. Neutrophil adhesion in leukocyte adhesion deficiency syndrome type 2. J Clin Invest 1995;96:2898–2906.

54. Gonzalez LA, Hill HR. Advantages and disadvantages of antimicrobial prophylaxis in chronic granulomatous disease of childhood. Pediatr Infect Dis J 1988;7:83–5.

55. Stiehm ER. New pediatric indications for IVIG. Contemp Pediatr 1991;8:29.

56. Stiehm ER. Human intravenous immunoglobulin in primary and secondary antibody deficiencies. Pediatr Infect Dis J 1997;16:696.

57. NIH Consensus Conference. Intravenous immunoglobulin. Prevention and treatment of disease. JAMA 1990;264:3189–93.

58. Roifman CM, Gelfand EW. Replacement therapy with high dose intravenous gamma-globulin improves chronic sinopulmonary disease in patients with hypogammaglobulinemia. Pediatr Infect Dis J 1988;5:S92–6.

59. Meissner HC, Welliver RC, Chartrand SA, Fulton DR, Rodriguez WJA, Groothuis JR. Prevention of respiratory syncytial virus infection in high risk infants: consensus opinion on the role of immunoprophylaxis with respiratory syncytial virus hyperimmune globulin. Pediatr Infect Dis J 1996;15:1059–68.

60. Ballow M, Dupont B, Good RA. Autoimmune hemolytic anemia in Wiskott–Aldrich syndrome during treatment with transfer factor. J Pediatr 1973;83:772–80.

61. Wybran J, Levin AS, Spitter LE, et al. Rosette-forming cells, immunologic deficiency diseases and transfer factor. N Engl J Med 1973;288:710–3.

62. Wara DW, Ammann AJ. Activation of T-cell rosettes in immunodeficient patients by thymosin. Ann NY Acad Sci 1975;249:308–14.

63. Ozsahin H, Le Deist F, Benkerrov M, et al. Bone marrow transplantation in 26 patients with Wiskott–Aldrich syndrome from a single center. J Pediatr 1996;129:238–44.

64. Hill HR, Estensen RD, Quie PG, et al. Modulation of human neutrophil chemotactic responses by cyclic 3'5'-guanosine monophosphate and cyclic 3'5'-adenosine monophosphate. Metabolism 1975;24:447–56.

65. Oliver JM, Zurier RB. Correction of characteristic abnormalities of microtubule function and granule morphology in Chédiak–Higashi syndrome with cholinergic agonists. J Clin Invest 1976;57:1239–47.

66. Boxer LA, Watanabe AM, Rister M, et al. Correction of leukocyte function in Chédiak–Higashi syndrome by ascorbate. N Engl J Med 1976;295:1041–5.

67. Levy R, Shriker O, Porath A, Riesenberg K, Schlaeffer F. Vitamin C for the treatment of recurrent furunculosis in patients with impaired neutrophil functions. J Infect Dis 1996;173:1502–5.

68. The International Chronic Granulomatous Disease Cooperative Study Group. A controlled trial of interferon gamma to prevent infection in chronic granulomatous disease. N Engl J Med 1991;324:509–16.

69. Jeppson JD, Jaffe HS, Hill HR. Use of recombinant human interferon gamma to enhance neutrophil chemotactic responses in Job syndrome of hyperimmunoglobulinemia E and recurrent infections. J Pediatr 1991;118:383–7.

70. Petrak BA, Augustine NH, Hill HR. Recombinant human interferon-gamma treatment of patients with Job's syndrome of hyperimmunoglobulinemia E and recurrent infections. Clin Res 1994;42:1A.

71. Hogan NA, Hill HR. Levamisole enhances PMN chemotaxis and elevates cellular cyclic GMP. J Infect Dis 1978;138:437–44.

72. Wright DG, Kirkpatrick CH, Gallin JI. Effects of levamisole on normal and abnormal leukocyte locomotion. J Clin Invest 1977;59:941–50.

73. Donabedian H, Alling DW, Vallin JI. Levamisole is inferior to placebo in the hyperimmunoglobulin E recurrent infection (Job's) syndrome. N Engl J Med 1982;307:290–2.

74. Mawhinney H, Killen M, Fleming WA, et al. The hyperimmunoglobulinemia E syndrome – a neutrophil chemotactic defect reversible by histamine H_2 receptor blockade? Clin Immunol Immunopathol 1980;17:483–91.

75. Cunningham-Rundles C, Kazbay K, Hassett J, Zhou Z, Mayer L. Brief report: enhanced humoral immunity in common variable immunodeficiency after long-term treatment with polyethylene glycol-conjugated interleukin-2. N Engl J Med 1994;331:918–21.

76. Hall CB, Powell KR, MacDonald NE, et al. Respiratory syncytial viral infection in children with compromised immune function. N Engl J Med 1986;315:77–81.

77. Wendt CH, Weisdorf DJ, Jordan MC, Balfour HH, Hertz MI. Parainfluenza virus respiratory infection after bone marrow transplantation. N Engl J Med 1992;326:921–6.

78. Lewis VA, Champlin R, Englund J, et al. Respiratory disease due to parainfluenza virus in adult bone marrow transplant recipients. Clin Infect Dis 1996;23:1033–7.

79. Ament ME. Immunodeficiency syndromes and gastrointestinal disease. Pediatr Clin North Am 1975;22:807–25.

80. Raubitschak AA, Levin AS, Stites DP, et al. Normal granulocyte infusion therapy for aspergillosis in chronic granulomatous disease. Pediatrics 1973;51:230–3.

81. O'Neil KM, Herman JH, Modlin JF, Moxon ER, Chir B, Winkelstein JA. Pseudomonas cepacia: an emerging pathogen in chronic granulomatous disease. J Pediatr 1986;108:940–2.

82. Albano EA, Pizzo PA. The evolving population of immunocompromised children. Pediatr Infect Dis J 1988;7:S79–86.

83. Shyur S-D, Hill HR. Immunodeficiency in the 1990s. Pediatr Infect Dis J 1991;10:595–611

84. Rosen FS, Cooper MD, Wedgwood RJP. The primary immunodeficiencies. N Engl J Med 1995;333:431–40.

85. Heiner DC. Recognition and management of IgG subclass deficiencies. Pediatr Infect Dis J 1987;6:235–8.

86. Gigliotti F, Herrod HG, Kalwinsky DK, et al. Immunodeficiency associated with recurrent infections and an isolated in vivo inability to respond to bacterial polysaccharides. Pediatr Infect Dis J 1988;7:417–20.

87. Baehner RL, Nathan DG. Quantitative nitroblue tetrazolium test in chronic granulomatous disease. N Engl J Med 1968;278:971–80.

88. Cheson BD, Christensen RL, Sperling R, et al. The origin of the chemiluminescence of phagocytizing granulocytes. J Clin Invest 1976;58:789–96.

89. Vowells SJ, Sekhsaria S, Malech HL, Shalit M, Fleisher TA. Flow cytometric analysis of the granulocyte respiratory burst: a comparison study of fluorescent probes. J Immunol Meth 1995;178:89–97.

90. Vowells SJ, Fleisher TA, Sekhsaria S, Alling DW, Maguire TE, Malech HL. Genotype-dependent variability in flow cytometric evaluation of reduced nicotinamide adenine dinucleotide phosphate oxidase function in patients with chronic granulomatous disease. J Pediatr 1996;128:104–7.

91. Christenson JC. Laboratory diagnosis of infection due to bacteria, fungi, parasites, and rickettsiae. In: Long SS, Pickering LK, Prober CG, eds. Principles and practice of pediatric infectious diseases. New York: Churchill Livingstone; 1996:1516–32.

92. Overall JC. Laboratory diagnosis of infection due to viruses, chlamydia, and mycoplasma. In: Long SS, Pickering LK, Prober CG, eds. Principles and practice of pediatric infectious diseases. New York: Churchill Livingstone; 1996:1532–53.

93. Melamed I, Griffiths AM, Roifman CM. Benefit of oral immune globulin therapy in patients with immunodeficiency and chronic diarrhea. J Pediatr 1991;119:486–9.

94. Guarino A, Guandalini S, Albano F, Mascia A, De Ritis G, Rubino A. Enteral immunoglobulin for treatment of protracted rotaviral diarrhea. Pediatr Infect Dis J 1991;10:612–4.

95. Whimbey E, Champlin RE, Englund JA, et al. Combination therapy with aerosolized ribavirin and intravenous immunoglobulin for respiratory syncytial virus disease in adult bone marrow transplant recipients. Bone Marrow Transplant 1995;16:393–9.

96. Johnson DW, Lum G, Nimmo G, Hawley CM. Parainfluenza virus respiratory infection after heart tranplantation: successful treatment with ribavirin. Clin Infect Dis 1995;21:1040–1.

97. McCarthy AJ, Bergin M, De Silva LM, Stevens M. Intravenous ribavirin therapy for disseminated adenovirus infection. Pediatr Infect Dis J 1995;14:1003–4.

98. Welte K, Zeidler C, Reiter A, et al. Differential effects of granulocyte-macrophage colony-stimulating factor and granulocyte colony-stimulating factor in children with severe congenital neutropenia. Blood 1990;75:1056–63.

99. Hammond WP, Price TH, Souza LM, Dale DC. Treatment of cyclic neutropenia with granulocyte colony-stimulating factor. N Engl J Med 1989;320:1306–11.

100. Cunningham-Rundles C, Siegel FP, Smithwick EM, et al. Efficacy of intravenous immunoglobulin in primary humoral immunodeficiency disease. Ann Intern Med 1984;101:435–9.

Solid Organ Transplantation

David L Dunn & Robert D Acton

INTRODUCTION

Solid organ transplantation is becoming a common therapy for a variety of disease processes, and more than 20,000 solid organ transplants are performed each year in the USA.[1] Although renal transplant procedures predominate, liver, pancreas, heart, lung, bowel and multivisceral transplants are increasingly being performed. Surgical and medical advances have led to improved results as measured by patient and allograft survival.

Even though remarkable advances have been made in the diagnosis, prevention and treatment of infections, solid organ transplant patients continue to be highly susceptible to serious infectious diseases. Infection is associated with significant morbidity and mortality in this patient population. Therefore, knowledge of the epidemiology, etiology, pathogenesis, pathology and principles of diagnosis and treatment is essential for physicians who care for these patients.

Approximately 80% of solid organ transplant recipients suffer at least one significant episode of infection during the first year after transplant.[2] Successful allogeneic solid organ transplantation requires exogenous immunosuppression, and all immunosuppressive agents diminish immune responsiveness in a relatively nonselective fashion. For example, corticosteroids, azathioprine, cyclosporin, FK-506, mycophenolate mofetil, deoxyspergualin, antithymocyte globulin and OKT3 have different mechanisms of action but they all suppress T-lymphocyte function and, concurrently, other components of antimicrobial host defense.

Several immunosuppressive agents are usually given in balanced combination so as to avoid the side effects that occur with high doses of individual agents. However, recipient–allograft interaction is not static, and intermittent episodes of acute rejection or underlying indolent chronic rejection (or both) are the rule rather than the exception. The transplant clinician attempts to achieve a balance between sufficient immunosuppression to prevent and treat rejection, thereby aiming at acceptance of the allograft by the recipient, and excessive immunosuppression, which may contribute to sequelae of infection and malignancy. Higher doses of immunosuppressive agents are usually administered during the first months after transplant; these doses are gradually reduced if allograft function is stable. Clinical and pathologic evidence of allograft rejection requires doses of immunosuppressive agents similar to those given immediately after transplantation in order to restore recipient–allograft homeostasis.

Unfortunately, patients requiring exogenous immunosuppression to preserve allograft function exhibit a higher rate of infection and malignancy.[3,4] Infection in patients requiring repeated high-dose immunosuppressive therapy is frequently viral or fungal in etiology, which is evidence of compromise of the cell-mediated immune function in these patients. A goal of experimental and clinical investigation is the development of immunosuppressive agents that specifically block foreign antigen recognition but that do not affect components of the immune system critical to host defense against infection. This goal has yet to be achieved.

EPIDEMIOLOGY

Solid organ transplant patients are at risk of infection not only from microbial pathogens that infect the normal host; they are also, as a consequence of immunosuppression, susceptible to the organisms generally categorized as 'atypical' or 'opportunistic.' Micro-organisms considered to be contaminants, commensals or saprophytes when cultured from patients with an intact immune system must be considered as potential pathogens when cultured from one or more body sites of a solid organ transplant recipient. Furthermore, microbes associated with either mild or self-limiting infection in normal hosts may cause significant disease in transplant patients. Similarly, microbial pathogens associated with serious but readily treatable infections in normal hosts are capable of disseminating quickly and producing a rapidly fatal illness in transplant recipients. The usual signs and symptoms of common infections are often masked by immunosuppressive therapy, further challenging the clinician's diagnostic skills.

Transplant recipients are at highest risk of infection during the first year after transplant and after treatment of rejection. These infections tend to fall into predictable patterns depending on the organ transplanted, the time since the transplant and the extent of current and composite exogenous immunosuppression.[5,6] Infections during the first 30 days after transplant are typically postoperative infections associated with the operative site or with organisms harbored by either the recipient or the transplanted organ. Common postoperative infections include wound infections, pneumonia, urinary tract infections (UTIs), line sepsis and intra-abdominal infections secondary to anastomotic complications.[2,3,7]

Many postoperative infections appear to localize at the site of allograft implantation, which may be related to operative trauma. In addition, the inflammatory response may be either acute and vigorous or chronic and minimal, with the consequence of reduced host defense. Interestingly, renal transplant recipients typically develop UTIs; hepatic, small bowel and pancreas transplant recipients develop intra-abdominal abscesses; and cardiac and lung transplant recipients develop mediastinitis, bronchitis or pneumonia.

Infections that occur 1–6 months after transplant are often caused by viral and fungal pathogens: viruses transmitted from the donor organ, reactivation of latent viruses in the recipient or newly acquired opportunistic organisms.[6,8] The period from 6 months to 1 year after transplant is associated with infection from more routine bacterial and viral agents. The epidemiology of infection during the postoperative period is less well characterized epidemiologically because recipients routinely reside at home, often at a distance from their transplant center.[8] It must be remembered that post-transplant patients exhibit increased susceptibility to a wide variety of infectious agents and even minor signs or symptoms of local or generalized illness may be a manifestation of serious infection.

RISK FACTORS FOR INFECTION

Within the entire group of solid organ transplant patients, specific factors can be identified that increase the risk of serious infections. The patient's underlying disease process that caused organ failure is a major risk factor. For example, patients with diabetes or hepatitis have great susceptibility to various types of infection after transplantation. Patients who receive a cadaver allograft require more immunosuppression than recipients of organs donated from close relatives (e.g. HLA-identical siblings), and they are highly susceptible to infection. In particular, patients who require multiple courses of antirejection therapy for several months at a time or who suffer recurrent or refractory rejection episodes that necessitate the use of potent antilymphocyte antibody preparations are at highest risk. Patients who have undergone splenectomy or who develop leukopenia from their immunosuppressive drugs and those who remain uremic or jaundiced after transplant suffer the most frequent and severe infectious problems and exhibit high rates of allograft loss and mortality.[4]

PREOPERATIVE EVALUATION

EVALUATION OF RECIPIENTS

Prospective transplant recipients are at increased risk of infection because of organ failure, and this risk is compounded by immunosuppressive medications. Thorough evaluation for possible infection that could be treated before transplantation is essential (Fig. 3.1). The

history will reveal evidence of exposure to *Mycobacterium* spp. and sexually transmitted agents and any unusual susceptibility to skin and wound infection. A chest radiograph is needed to exclude indolent infection or malignancy.

A history of sinusitis, duodenal or gastric ulcer disease or cholecystitis warrants investigation and possibly, elective pretransplant intervention. Liver transplant recipients require perioperative or preoperative selective bowel decontamination (often at the time they are placed on the waiting list) and recipients with cystic fibrosis undergoing a lung transplant receive perioperative antibiotics targeted at those organisms identified as colonizing the tracheobronchial tree.

The vaccination history of all potential transplant recipients is especially important and all routine vaccines should be brought up to date. Recipients should not be given live attenuated vaccines [measles, mumps, rubella, oral polio virus, varicella-zoster virus (VZV), yellow fever or oral typhoid] because of immunodeficiency associated with organ failure and post-transplant immunosuppression. Inactivated vaccines or toxoid preparations (diphtheria, pertussis, tetanus, influenza, parental typhoid; inactivated polio, pneumococcal polysaccharide, *Haemophilus influenzae* type b, meningococcal, recombinant hepatitis B, inactivated hepatitis A and influenza) can be administered. Response to vaccines may be subnormal after transplant and some

PRETRANSPLANT EVALUATION OF POTENTIAL SOURCES OF INFECTION IN PROSPECTIVE SOLID ORGAN TRANSPLANT RECIPIENTS			
Potential site of infection		**Evaluation**	**Treatment**
Oropharynx and esophagus	Dental abscess	Dental examination	Dental extraction
	Oropharyngeal candidiasis	Oral examination	Oral nystatin
	Esophageal candidiasis	Endoscopy	Oral nystatin plus either iv amphotericin B or fluconazole if refractory
Gastrointestinal tract	Duodenal ulceration	Upper gastrointestinal series or endoscopy	Elective antiulcer procedure
	Colonic diverticulosis	Barium enema	Elective colonic resection
	Perirectal fistulae or abscess	Proctosigmoidoscopy	Internal sphincterotomy, drainage
	Cholelithiasis	Abdominal ultrasound	Cholecystectomy
	Strongyloidiasis	Stool microscopy	Eradicative therapy
Lungs and pleural cavity	Pulmonary infiltrates	Chest radiograph, bronchoscopy	Antibiotics if infection is present
	Pulmonary nodule	Obtain previous chest radiograph	If stable, observe
	Enlarging pulmonary nodule or cavity	Chest radiograph, chest CT, bronchoscopy with biopsy or transthoracic biopsy	Resection
	Pulmonary effusion	Aspiration	Drainage and antibiotic therapy if infected
Skin and soft tissues	Access sites	Site culture	Remove
	Superficial skin abscess	Site culture	Incision and drainage
	Fungal skin lesions	Site culture	Topical antifungal therapy
	Extremity ulcers	Site culture, transcutaneous oxygen measurement; consider arteriography	Antibiotic therapy, debridement, arterial dilatation or bypass if stenosis identified
Genitourinary system	Kidneys, ureter and bladder	Urine analysis and culture, intravenous pyelogram, voiding cystourethrogram, cystoscopy	Antibiotic therapy, bilateral nephrectomy if reflux and persistent infection are present
	Genitalia	Examination	Antibiotic therapy if infection is present
Serum	Cytomegalovirus	Cytomegalovirus IgM, IgG, rapid antigen determination	Increased risk of primary infection if cytomegalovirus-negative recipient receives a cytomegalovirus-positive donor organ. Active disease represents contraindication until treated
	Epstein–Barr virus	Epstein–Barr virus IgM, IgG	Possible increased risk for Epstein–Barr virus and post-transplant lymphoproliferative disorders if Epstein–Barr virus positive donor organ. Active disease represents contraindication until treated
	Varicella-zoster virus	Varicella-zoster virus IgG	Immunize pretransplant in selected cases
	Herpes simplex virus	None, unless active mucocutaneous disease present	Observe for reactivation after transplant. Active disease represents contraindication until treated
	Human immunodeficiency virus	HIV antigen and antibody	Contraindication for transplantation
	Hepatitis A, B, C and D viruses	Hepatitis A, B, C and D virus antibody	Immunize if hepatitis B virus negative
	Toxoplasmosis	Toxoplasma immunofluorescence assay	Baseline for reference

Fig. 3.1 Pretransplant evaluation of potential sources of infection in prospective solid organ transplant recipients.

recipients require an additional immunizing booster 4–6 months after completing their initial immunization.[8]

EVALUATION OF DONORS

Organ donors are evaluated with the goal of minimizing the risk of transmitting microbes from donor to recipient.[2] The risk of transmission of viral agents via donor organs is greatest for cytomegalovirus (CMV) and Epstein–Barr virus (EBV). Although rates of positive bacterial culture in kidney preservation fluid and duodenal cuff cultures (associated with whole organ donor pancreas) range from 2 to 25%, positive findings are not invariably associated with infection in the recipient of the contaminated organ because knowledge of a positive culture from the organ preservation fluid prompts administration of appropriate antibiotics to the recipient.[9,10]

ORGAN SYSTEMS INVOLVED

The urinary tract, lungs, intra-abdominal cavity and skin are the primary sites of infection in patients receiving solid organ transplants.

URINARY TRACT INFECTIONS
Epidemiology

Most UTIs occur during the first few months after transplant and are related to the surgical procedure itself and the high levels of immunosuppression during this period. Bacteriuria is reported in up to 83% of renal transplant recipients. During the immediate post-transplant period, UTIs are associated with an increased incidence of wound infection and systemic sepsis. The most frequent organisms involved are common Gram-negative aerobic bacteria, with a high incidence of *Candida* spp. as well.[3,11] Contributing factors include:

- long duration of preoperative hemodialysis,
- bladder catheterization,
- decreased renal function, and
- prolonged (>48 hours) perioperative antibiotic prophylaxis.[12]

The renal allograft is also susceptible to pyelonephritis in the first 3–6 months post-transplant, especially in recipients with small contracted bladders who develop reflux into the allograft renal pelvis. However, this entity is quite rare.

Solid organ transplant recipients other than those receiving bladder-drained pancreas transplants (i.e. liver, heart, lung and small bowel recipients) do not appear to be at increased risk of developing a UTI. They do not routinely have their urinary tracts manipulated except for the brief perioperative period of bladder catheterization. Their incidence of UTIs is between 8 and 30% in the immediate postoperative period, which is a similar rate to that of other seriously ill patients undergoing extensive operations.

Prevention

Perioperative prophylaxis with intravenous broad-spectrum antibacterial agents, usually a cephalosporin combined with instillation of a topical solution of an antimicrobial agent into the urinary bladder at the inception of the renal transplant procedure, and early catheter removal help to reduce the incidence of UTIs.[3,13] Recipients with recurrent UTIs may require prolonged courses of intravenous antibiotics.[5] Transplant recipients with urinary tract dysfunction and an inability to void spontaneously can perform intermittent self-catheterization. This form of manipulation is associated with a slightly higher incidence of UTIs and urosepsis than urinary diversion is; however, intermittent catheterization is often preferred by recipients because of ease of care and social acceptability.[14] Young children with renal failure secondary to posterior urethral valves are at increased risk of UTIs if vesicoureteral reflux persists.[15]

Routine use of internal or internal–external ureteral stents to protect the ureteroneocystostomy or uteropyelostomy remains controversial because their use is associated with an increased incidence of UTIs. In one study, a UTI rate of 35% was reported and one-third of these UTIs cleared only after stent removal. Transplant surgeons generally do not employ stents for routine renal transplant procedures, using them for technically difficult anastomoses and for short periods of time. Consideration should be given to administering an oral antimicrobial agent such as trimethoprim–sulfamethoxazole (TMP–SMX; co-trimoxazole) while the stent remains *in situ*.[16]

Clinical features and management

As with most post-transplant infections, many recipients may not complain of classic symptoms of dysuria, frequency and burning and irritation with voiding. The only symptoms may be a fever, or signs such as hematuria or an elevation in white blood cell count with or without fever.[3] Therefore, a high index of concern and a very low threshold for obtaining a urinalysis and urine culture is required. Empiric use of antimicrobial agents may be necessary before culture results are available. In the early postoperative period (the first 90 days after transplant), intravenous antimicrobial agents may be necessary if clinical signs suggest a systemic infection.

If the UTI is diagnosed 6 months or more after transplantation or after recent treatment of acute rejection, treatment as an outpatient with an oral antimicrobial agent may be appropriate.[2] Indeed, UTIs occurring 6 months or more after transplant are less frequently associated with systemic sepsis and mortality and generally respond to an appropriate oral antimicrobial agent.[17] Although several studies have demonstrated that these late infections do not adversely affect either allograft or patient survival in renal transplant recipients, we recommend that oral TMP–SMX should be given immediately after transplant and continued on a lifelong, daily basis. In our experience, few patients receiving this drug regimen have developed infection from TMP–SMX-sensitive opportunistic pathogens (e.g. *Pneumocystis carinii, Nocardia asteroides, Listeria monocytogenes, Legionella pneumophila, Toxoplasma gondii*).[18–20]

Bladder-drained pancreas transplants. Bladder-drained pancreas transplant recipients often require prolonged urinary catheterization postoperatively and are at increased risk of UTIs. The bladder anastomosis must heal and bladder function normalize to prevent urine leak and associated intra-abdominal sepsis (Fig. 3.2).[21] Recipients of bladder-drained pancreatic transplants are severely diabetic and may harbor severe peripheral vascular disease associated with nonhealing extremity wounds. In addition, a renal allograft may be transplanted concurrently, and these patients are highly immunosuppressed. Recurrent UTIs do not appear to effect long-term allograft survival; however, we routinely administer lifelong TMP–SMX to these patients. One final issue in relation to this group of patients bears mention: the pancreas transplant patient with discomfort and pain with voiding, frequency and urgency does not invariably harbor a UTI. Cystitis and urethritis secondary to pancreatic exocrine secretions may occur within the urinary bladder and cause symptoms identical to those of a UTI. Persistent symptoms not controlled with routine conservative management may require conversion of the pancreas to enteric drainage.

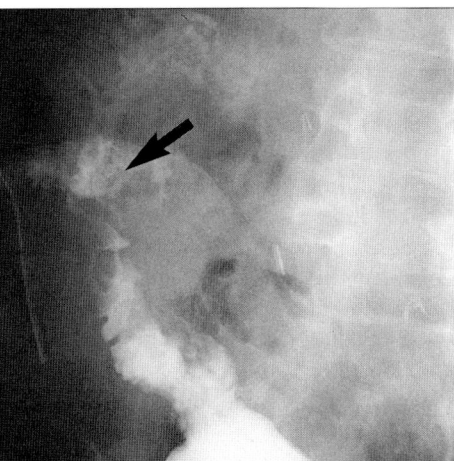

Fig. 3.2 Cystogram demonstrating a bladder leak (arrow) in a patient who has undergone combined kidney and pancreas transplantation.

WOUND AND PERIALLOGRAFT INFECTIONS

Wound and periallograft infection is a frequent and serious complication of solid organ transplantation. It is associated with increased morbidity, allograft loss and mortality. Periallograft infections present difficult surgical management problems, often requiring repeated operative intervention and an extended period of time for wound healing by secondary intention. There are three categories of wound infection:

- superficial infections, consisting of infections above the fascia;
- deep infections, occurring below the fascial closure and within the body cavity in which the transplant operation was performed; and
- combined infections (i.e. infections with communication between both superficial and deep wound compartments).[3]

The rates of superficial and deep wound infections vary by transplant type, and the different categories of wound infection have different causes and require different treatment. The total incidence of superficial, deep and combined wound infections ranges from 1 to 2% in renal transplant recipients up to 25–30% in pancreas and small bowel transplant recipients.[3,21,22] Wound infections are typically apparent within 2–4 weeks of the transplantation, although some manifest as late as 6–8 weeks postoperatively.

The incidence of wound infection has been quantified precisely in renal transplant recipients, historically the largest and most carefully studied group of solid organ transplant patients. Renal transplantation is classified as a 'clean contaminated (class 2)' type of surgical procedure with regard to the potential for wound infection, because the urinary bladder is entered. Not surprisingly, the etiologic agents are usually common urinary tract pathogens: Gram-negative aerobic bacteria, Gram-positive skin microflora and occasionally *Candida* spp. When deep wound infections occur, transplant nephrectomy is often necessary; this is associated with increased morbidity and occasional mortality. The reduced incidence of wound infection in this patient population has been accomplished through improvements in surgical technique and the use of prophylactic antimicrobial agents.[23]

The incidence of wound infection in heart transplant recipients ranges from 0 to 8% and approaches that of nonimmunosuppressed recipients undergoing heart surgery.[24–26] As expected, primary pathogens are skin microflora (i.e. *Staphylococcus aureus* and *Staphylococcus epidermidis*). However, fungal and other unusual pathogens are often found. Lung and heart–lung transplant recipients exhibit a higher rate of wound infection (4–8%).[27–29] In addition, these patients suffer a very high rate of pneumonia and pulmonary infections with associated anastomotic disruption, bronchopleural fistulae, hemorrhage, mediastinitis and empyema.[30] An infected surgical field precludes retransplantation; therefore, open wound care, prolonged courses of antimicrobial agents and reduction in immunosuppression are required.

Liver transplant procedures are also associated with higher rates of wound infection than renal transplants: 6–8% of patients develop superficial wound infections and 15–19% develop deep wound infections (including intra-abdominal abscesses). The most common sites of infection include intra-abdominal abscesses (associated with biliary leaks), and subdiaphragmatic, subhepatic and intrahepatic abscesses.[31–33] These infections are typically caused by enteric Gram-negative aerobic and anaerobic bacteria, although fungi are not uncommon. Deep wound infections in liver transplant recipients may lead to life-threatening disruption of both bowel and arterial anastomoses. Liver transplant recipients are also at risk of developing cholangitis and biliary tract stricture, which requires stenting or operative repair. Cholangitis after liver transplant is associated with 33% mortality.[31]

Pancreas allografts present a variety of problems, and technical failure in the immediate perioperative period accounts for approximately 20% of allograft losses.[21] Additional problems include wound and intra-abdominal infection, allograft thrombosis, allograft pancreatitis and anastomotic disruption at the site of exocrine drainage.[34,35] Pancreas transplant recipients develop wound infections with high frequency (superficial infections at a rate of 10–40%, deep infections at a rate of 15–22% and combined infections at a rate of 8%). A mor-

tality rate of 27% has been observed.[22,34] Microbial agents in abdominal infection are either low-virulence organisms (e.g. *Enterococcus faecalis*, *E. faecium*, *S. epidermidis*, *Candida albicans*) or virulent Gram-negative aerobic microbes (e.g. *Pseudomonas aeruginosa*). Multi-agent antimicrobial therapy is necessary; recommendations include 10–14 days of either a carbapenam or a penicillin plus a β-lastamase inhibitor (ampicillin–sulbactam, ticarcillin–clavulanate) piperacillin–tazobactam plus vancomycin. Amphotericin B may also be necessary in one-third of cases.

Severe infection around the allograft predisposes recipients to pseudoaneurysm formation, often involving the allograft anastomosis itself. Rupture is both limb- and life-threatening, and requires immediate allograft removal and vascular reconstruction.[21,33,35] When periallograft infections develop several months after the initial procedure, a well-defined intra-abdominal fluid collection is usually identified, which may be managed by percutaneous drainage.

Small bowel transplant recipients are highly susceptible to infections (they have an infection rate of 25–45%).[36] Causes of infection relate to contamination at the time of transplant, anastomotic leak, rejection, bacterial translocation and perforation. Not surprisingly, organisms isolated from infected periallograft fluid collections are characteristic of bowel flora and include both Gram-negative and Gram-positive aerobic (e.g. *Escherichia coli*, *Enterococcus faecalis*, *E. faecium*, *S. epidermidis*), and anaerobic bacteria (e.g. *Bacteroides fragilis* and other species) and *Candida albicans*. Cytomegalovirus appears to play a significant role as a pathogen in this group of recipients, and it may be the antecedent cause of perforation and infection in some cases.[36–38] Antibiotic therapy is similar to that described for pancreas transplant patients with periallograft infection.

Multiple factors predispose solid organ transplant recipients to wound infection (Fig. 3.3). High degrees of global immunosuppression, whether due to underlying disease (e.g. diabetes mellitus, hepatitis C) or to receiving a cadaver donor organ, are clearly associated epidemiologically with an increased incidence of wound infection.[3,39,40] Other factors that predispose transplant recipients to wound infections include:[12,21,31]

- re-exploration via the same incision;
- periallograft hematoma formation;
- infection involving the allograft (e.g. donor UTI before renal donation, prolonged intubation in lung donation);
- contamination of the allograft, leakage from the drainage site of the organ (e.g. ureteric and bladder leaks in renal or bladder-drained pancreas recipients, biliary tract leaks in liver recipients, bowel anastomotic leaks in bowel-drained pancreas or small bowel transplant recipients); and
- concomitant infection at distant sites and the use of wound drains.

Pancreatic transplant patients are especially vulnerable because pancreatic exocrine enzymes contribute to the creation of an excellent culture medium in the space surrounding the allograft.[22] After pancreas transplantation, the incidence of concordance is high (74%) between the organisms that cause wound infections and those cultured from the donor duodenum at the time of procurement but by no means absolute.[22]

FACTORS PREDISPOSING TO WOUND INFECTIONS AFTER TRANSPLANTATION

Immunosuppression
Cadaver donor organ
Re-exploration
Infected allograft
Anastomotic leakage
Wound drains
Allograft contamination

Fig. 3.3 Factors predisposing to wound infections after transplantation.

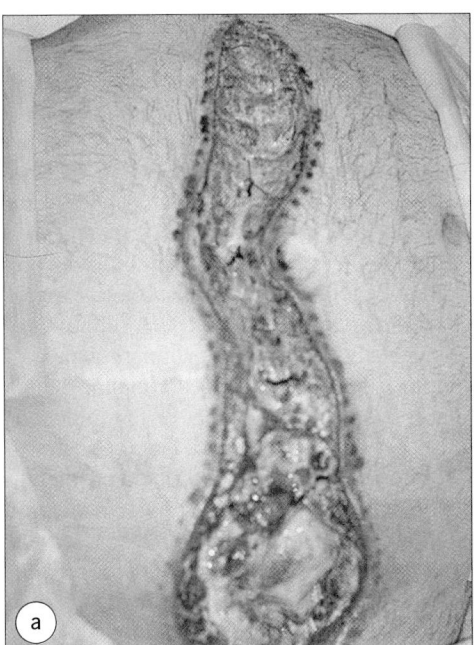
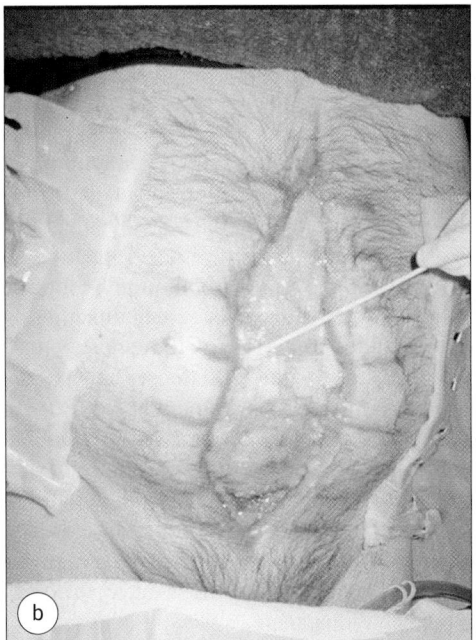
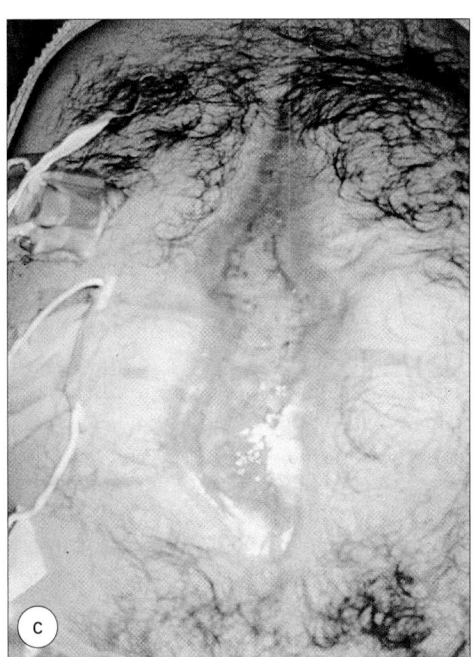

Fig. 3.4 Abdominal wound healing by secondary intention subsequent to severe intra-abdominal sepsis.
(a) At diagnosis, (b) 1 month later and (c) 10 months later.

Renal allograft contamination may also contribute to severe wound infection and mycotic aneurysm formation after transplantation. *Pseudomonas* spp. in particular appear to predispose to this type of infection. Colonization of donor lungs or the recipient's remaining lung in single-lung transplant recipients after prolonged intubation is also of great concern.[41] Recipients with cystic fibrosis may be at risk of pneumonia caused by *Pseudomonas* spp. However, correlation with wound infections remains problematic.[42] Prevention is difficult because it is not always possible to avoid use of contaminated donor organs. Cadaver organ preservation time is especially critical in pulmonary, cardiac, hepatic, small bowel and pancreatic transplants, and culture results from donor organs may not be available before the transplant. When positive cultures from the donor organ are obtained, a course of appropriate antimicrobial agents to which the organism is sensitive is recommended.

Diagnosis

Diagnosing a wound infection in transplant recipients is difficult because the usual, common symptoms and signs of infection may not be present. Wound swelling and serous drainage without fever or local symptoms are common and often the white blood cell count may be elevated without significant signs of infection. Purulent drainage may not occur, especially in the immediate postoperative period, which is when recipients are most heavily immunosuppressed and do not mount a leukocyte response to infection. A small elevation in temperature or white blood cell count in the immediate postoperative period should prompt investigation of a possible wound infection. Cultures of any wound drainage and searches for fluid collections by ultrasound or CT scans of the wound and surrounding region are helpful for diagnosing wound infections. When microbes are identified by Gram stain or culture of wound drainage, the superficial wound should be opened, debrided, packed and then either closed later (by delayed primary closure) or allowed to heal by secondary intention. A diligent search should also be made for evidence of a concurrent deep wound infection, intra-abdominal infection (in renal, pancreas, hepatic and small bowel transplant recipients) or mediastinal or pleural infection (in heart and lung transplant recipients).[3] Evidence of a significant fluid collection on ultrasound or CT, even without evidence of microbes in Gram stains or cultures, should not deter the surgeon from opening the wound or from considering re-exploration of the wound and periallograft region if there is evidence of ongoing infection.

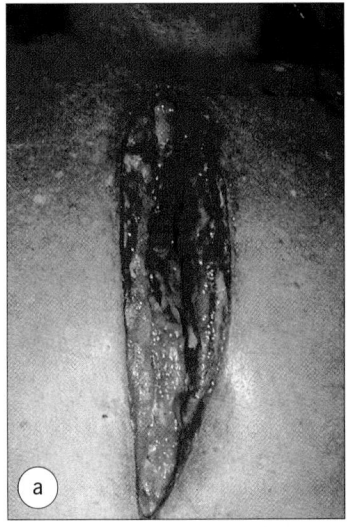
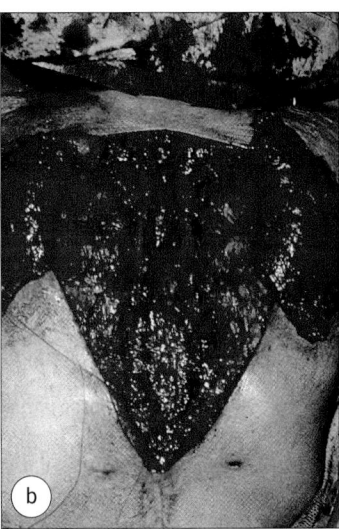

Fig. 3.5 Sternal wound infection demonstrating defect at the time of debridement and closure. (a) Open wound, (b) pectoralis pedicle flaps.

Management

Wound infections in transplant patients have significant sequelae, and even in the case of superficial infections the wound should be opened, debrided, packed and allowed to heal by secondary intention, an extremely slow process in immunosuppressed patients. The high doses of systemic corticosteroids in the immediate postoperative period and the greatly reduced inflammatory response contribute to delayed wound healing. An infected wound in an otherwise healthy surgical patient usually heals within 4–6 weeks; however, 4–6 months may be required in a transplant recipient (Fig. 3.4). Such wound infections are often associated with a large fascial defect and a ventral hernia in abdominal transplant patients and with an open sternal or chest wound in thoracic transplant patients. Sternal wound infections in cardiac transplant recipients often require aggressive sternal debridement and creation of pedicle flaps (from pectoralis muscle or omentum) to achieve adequate soft tissue coverage of the sternal defect (Fig. 3.5).[24,25]

Delay in diagnosis of superficial wound infections in this patient population may contribute to necrosis of soft tissue near the wound site. Although rare, this process usually is diagnosed at the time of re-exploration and requires extensive debridement of the surrounding muscle and fascia. Deep wound infections in renal, pancreas, hepatic or small bowel recipients (in the last three groups presenting as intra-abdominal infections) are extremely serious events that are frequently associated with systemic sepsis or pseudoaneurysm formation at the site of vascular anastomosis, or both. For kidney or pancreas recipients this process can be limb-threatening because the iliac arteriovenous system is used for transplantation.[3,20] Allograft removal and vascular reconstruction may both be necessary.

Prevention

All transplant patients should undergo skin scrubs and showers with a bactericidal soap and receive an intravenous dose of an antimicrobial agent before incision. If the procedure lasts for more than 4 hours, the same drug should be administered again to patients with normal renal function. In general, a single dose is sufficient for patients undergoing renal transplantation. Heart transplant recipients should receive a first-generation cephalosporin, and a second- or third-generation cephalosporin active against both Gram-negative and Gram-positive pathogens is appropriate for renal transplant recipients. Patients undergoing a hepatic, pancreas, small bowel or pulmonary transplantation should receive broad-spectrum antimicrobial agents that are active against both Gram-negative and Gram-positive aerobic and anaerobic pathogens because of the possibility of enteric, biliary, or tracheo-bronchial contamination during organ procurement and the transplant procedure. A single broad-spectrum agent such as a carbapenem or a penicillin plus a β-lactamase inhibitor or a second- or third-generation cephalosporin plus an antianaerobic agent are generally chosen.

Additional doses of prophylactic antimicrobial agents are administered postoperatively in those patients at high risk of wound infection. Pancreas and small bowel transplant recipients generally receive a treatment course of 3–7 days. These patients are especially susceptible to fungal pathogens, and they may receive a triazole drug such as fluconazole as well. Such therapy is administered in an attempt to reduce the morbidity and mortality associated with wound infections in these particular subgroups of transplant patients; however, efficacy has not been established.

INTRA-ABDOMINAL COMPLICATIONS

Post-transplant gastrointestinal complications are frequent, occurring in 2–4% of patients, and may involve the upper or lower gastrointestinal tract. Intra-abdominal infection may result from peptic ulcer disease with perforation of a gastric or duodenal ulcer or from diverticulitis and colon perforation.[43–46]

Perforation of a viscus in a post-transplant patient is difficult to diagnose because corticosteroid administration masks many of the usual signs and symptoms. Rapid institution of appropriate therapy is necessary to prevent secondary bacterial peritonitis, a serious event in any group of immunosuppressed patients.[45,46] In transplant recipients mortality rates of 50 and 77% have been reported.[44,47]

Cytomegalovirus infection may also play an important role in the development of gastroduodenal and colonic ulceration in post-transplant patients. Cytomegalovirus-induced ulceration may occur in both the upper and lower gastrointestinal tract and may be associated with perforation. Corticosteroid therapy is a major factor causing inhibition of mucosal cell replication, fibroblast function, lymphoid aggregation and tissue repair within the bowel wall.[48]

Immunosuppression may contribute to inhibition of peritoneal host defenses against intra-abdominal infection. Reduced lymphocyte and granulocyte recruitment leads to poor containment of the infectious process and minimal clinical signs and symptoms. Therefore, aggressive diagnostic evaluation is necessary in transplant patients with minimal abdominal discomfort. Imaging procedures should include an upright chest radiograph, upright and supine abdominal radiographs and upper and lower gastrointestinal series with a water-soluble contrast agent to look for evidence of a perforated viscus. Computed tomography scans or ultrasound examination of the abdomen may be extremely helpful (Fig. 3.6).

Management

Evidence of a perforated viscus (e.g. free intraperitoneal air) mandates an emergency laparotomy. Simultaneously, an empiric broad-spectrum antimicrobial agent (e.g. imipenem–cilistatin, ticarcillin–clavulanate or piperacillin-tazobactam with or without vancomycin) should be administered. Antibiotics with nephrotoxic properties are avoided because transplant patients often receive nephrotoxic agents (e.g. cyclosporin) as part of their immunosuppressive drug regimen.

At the time of operation, we routinely lavage the abdominal cavity with 6–8 liters of a first-generation cephalosporin and 1–2 liters of an amphotericin B-containing solution. Perforation of the stomach or duodenum is usually managed by closing the open site with either a Graham patch of omentum or the serosal surface of a loop of small bowel. Recipients who develop small gastric perforations may be treated by limited, local gastric resection with primary closure. Patients with a history of peptic ulcer disease and large perforations may require pyloroplasty or highly selective vagotomy.

Perforation of the small bowel can usually be managed via resection and primary anastomosis; however, in extremely ill patients, both proximal and distal ends of the bowel should be exteriorized. Colonic perforation should be managed by resection of the involved region of the bowel and exteriorizing the proximal colonic segment. All feculent and infected material must be removed and the abdomen copiously irrigated. Resection and primary anastomosis of the colon should not be performed during the initial operation because it is associated with an anastomotic leak rate of about 50% and high mortality.[43,48] The skin edges of the wound should not be closed after an operation in a heavily contaminated field; in general, the wound should be packed and allowed to heal by secondary intention. Occasional patients recover expeditiously and benefit from delayed primary closure.

Antimicrobial therapy should be continued postoperatively for 7–10 days, although no precise standards for duration of therapy in this patient population exist. Most clinicians initiate antifungal therapy (e.g. amphotericin B, fluconazole) if *Candida* spp. are cultured; however, if patients are recovering rapidly, the initial antibiotic regimen should not be altered. Patients who exhibit deteriorating after surgery should undergo diagnostic imaging and not merely a change in the antibiotic regimen. If no ongoing source of peritoneal contamination is present (e.g. perforated viscus, leaking anastomosis) and the patient has sequestered the infection as an intra-abdominal abscess, treatment with percutaneous drainage is usually possible (Fig. 3.7).

If diagnostic tests are unrevealing and no extra-abdominal sources of infection are identified, the patient should be returned to the

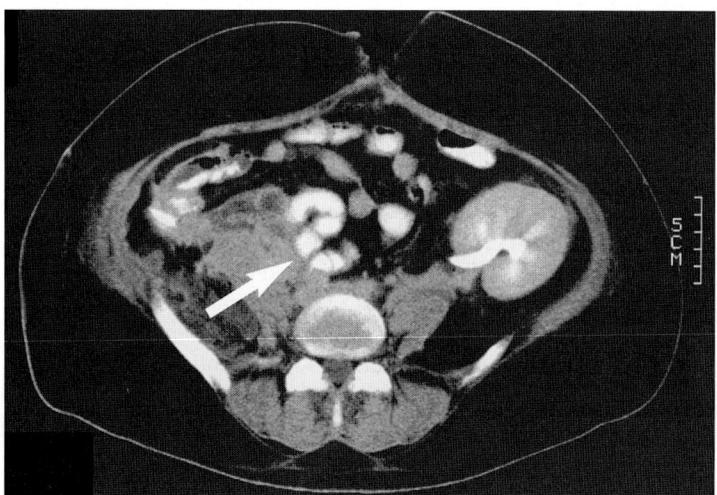

Fig. 3.6 Abdominal CT scan revealing the presence of pancreatic periallograft fluid collection that proved to be an intra-abdominal abscess (arrow).

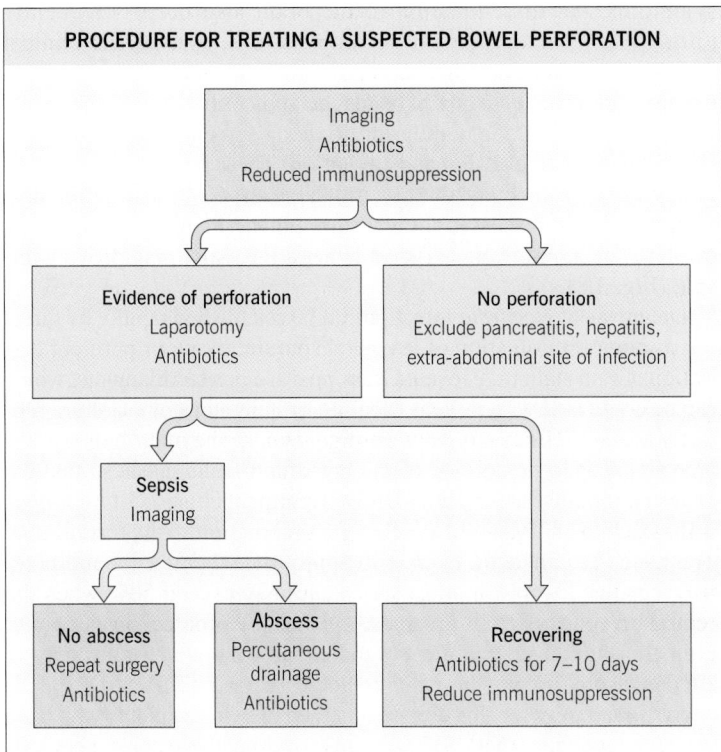

PROCEDURE FOR TREATING A SUSPECTED BOWEL PERFORATION

Imaging
Antibiotics
Reduced immunosuppression

Evidence of perforation
Laparotomy
Antibiotics

No perforation
Exclude pancreatitis, hepatitis,
extra-abdominal site of infection

Sepsis
Imaging

No abscess
Repeat surgery
Antibiotics

Abscess
Percutaneous
drainage
Antibiotics

Recovering
Antibiotics for 7–10 days
Reduce immunosuppression

Fig. 3.7 Procedure for treating a suspected bowel perforation.

operating room for re-exploration if the clinical condition continues to deteriorate postoperatively. Evidence of poorly contained, ongoing intra-abdominal infection (also termed tertiary microbial peritonitis) may require repeated re-exploration with peritoneal debridement and copious irritation. This disease process is associated with the appearance of low-virulence or resistant pathogens (*Enterococcus* spp., *S. epidermidis*, *Candida* spp. and *P. aeruginosa*) within the peritoneum, and there is a high mortality rate (>50%). Perhaps not surprisingly, this appears to be the same group of pathogens that are cultured from pancreas transplant patients who develop periallograft infection. Immunosuppressive therapy may be gradually increased during recovery. Removing the allograft is not necessary in renal transplant recipients who have intra-abdominal sepsis because the allograft is not infected. In contrast, patients who have deep wound infections, which, in most cases, involve the allograft, require removal of the allograft.[4] However, intra-abdominal sepsis does not mandate removal of a hepatic allograft, which, by definition, the patient requires for survival. These recipients will recover if surgical care is meticulous and if the focus of infection is separate from the allograft.

BACTERIAL PNEUMONIA

Approximately 4% of solid organ transplant patients develop postoperative pneumonia, an event that typically occurs within the first few months after transplantation. The incidence varies by organ type: renal transplant recipients demonstrate the lowest incidence of pneumonia (1–2%) and lung transplant recipients exhibit the highest incidence (22%). Heart, pancreas and liver transplant recipients fall midway between these extremes, with incidences of between 5 and 17%.[49] The overall mortality from these infections is significant (20–60%), and this disease process represents an important cause of death in the early post-transplant period.[49,50]

The most common causative organisms during the first 3 months after transplant are aerobic Gram-negative bacteria (e.g. *Klebsiella* spp., *Enterobacter* spp. and *P. aeruginosa*), *S. aureus* and *Legionella* spp. During the early post-transplant period, pulmonary infections are most commonly polymicrobial. Cytomegalovirus or *Candida* spp. are commonly cultured in concert with bacteria, making diagnosis and treatment more difficult. A concurrent CMV infection is an independent risk factor for development of bacterial pneumonia, increasing the risk by between three and eight times.[49,51,52] After 3 months, usual pathogens include *Streptococcus pneumoniae*, *H. influenzae*, *Chlamydia trachomatis*, *Listeria* spp., *Nocardia* spp., *Pneumocystis carinii* and *Mycobacterium tuberculosis*.

Several factors contribute to the increased risk of pneumonia in transplant patients. Organ failure requires frequent pretransplant hospitalizations and may require mechanical ventilation.[53] Heart failure and pulmonary edema contribute to increased pulmonary colonization with bacteria,[49] although post-transplant pneumonia is not always caused by the microbial agents that colonized the patient before the transplant.[42] Surgical procedures involving upper abdominal or thoracic incisions are associated with atelectasis and pneumonia, and finally, treatment of acute rejection in the immediate post-transplant period places recipients at increased risk.[49]

Lung allograft recipients are at 1.5–10 times greater risk for pneumonia than other solid organ transplant recipients, for the following reasons:[28]
• the lung is the only transplanted organ directly exposed to the environment;
• the transplanted lung is a denervated organ with impaired mucociliary function and cough reflex; and
• patients receiving lung transplants typically require higher levels of immunosuppression to prevent rejection.

Moreover, an increasing number of recipients are being transplanted for end-stage disease secondary to cystic fibrosis. These patients are universally colonized or infected with highly resistant strains , including *Burkholderia cepacia* (*Pseudomonas cepacia*). Aggressive care, including sinus drainage, surveillance cultures, and early bronchoscopy, is necessary. Recipients with cystic fibrosis warrant extremely close observation in the first 6 months after transplant.[42,54–56] Evaluation of the transplanted lung should consist of early bronchoscopy for biopsy and culture to differentiate acute rejection from infection, as both have similar clinical features of cough, dyspnea and infiltrate on chest radiograph.[55,57,58]

Fever, malaise and cough are common symptoms of any type of pulmonary infection, although they may be minimal or absent in immunosuppressed patients. Generally, patients develop an infiltrate on chest radiograph that may be associated with a pleural effusion. As with most other types of infection, bacterial pneumonia occurs more frequently in cadaver allograft recipients and often occurs after antirejection therapy. Unfortunately, sputum samples are often difficult to obtain or are not diagnostic, particularly in critically ill recipients maintained by ventilator support.[49,57,58] More commonly, bronchoscopy plus bronchoalveolar lavage is used to obtain a specimen for culture.

In lung transplant recipients, a transbronchial biopsy is necessary to rule out rejection. Bronchoalveolar lavage or biopsy often reveal the diagnosis when more standard tests fail. If cultures remain negative and the patient continues to deteriorate, an open or thoracoscopic lung biopsy should be considered to establish the etiology of the pulmonary process.[49] If a pulmonary effusion also exists, it should be percutaneously sampled and drained and the specimen evaluated by microbiologic and cytologic techniques. Empiric antimicrobial therapy based on the initial microbiologic results (Gram, potassium hydroxide, Giemsa, methenamine-silver and Ziehl–Neelsen stains) is recommended. Gram-positive organisms such as staphylococci and streptococci, as well as Gram-negative aerobic pathogens, are frequently cultured. Because of the high incidence of infections with *Pseudomonas* spp. in lung transplant recipients, empiric therapy must include agents effective against strains that are prevalent at the particular institution. Progression of pneumonia to empyema and lung abscess is associated with extremely high mortality (50%). Aggressive therapy with immediate drainage of the infected collection is necessary.

Legionella pneumophila and *L. micdadei* can cause pulmonary infection in solid organ transplant recipients and, in many cases, a water source within the hospital environment is identified. Most infections with these organisms occur within the first few months after transplant or after a recently treated rejection episode. Patients usually complain initially of 'flu-like' symptoms and have a patchy lobular or diffuse interstitial infiltrate on chest radiograph. The exact incidence of *Legionella* pneumonia in the transplant population is hard to estimate, but between 6 and 15% of all cases of pneumonia requiring hospitalization in the general population are caused by *Legionella* spp.[59] Extrapulmonary *Legionella* infections also occur but are extremely rare.[60]

Both *L. pneumophila* and *L. micdadei* are obligate aerobic microbes and are difficult to isolate. Cultures and direct immunofluorescent studies may substantiate the presence of these pathogens; however, at endemic sites, patients suspected of *Legionella*-related pneumonia should be treated empirically with erythromycin and rifampin (rifampicin). Erythromycin and TMP–SMX are also useful as prophylactic agents for *Legionella* pneumonia.[59,61]

BACTEREMIA

The majority of episodes of bacteremia occur in the early post-transplant period, with a wide range of incidence figures (10–41%) being reported.[3,4] Most episodes are caused by infection at a specific site, although translocation of bacteria across the bowel may occur during acute rejection in small bowel recipients or during profound leukopenia (absolute neutrophil count <500 cells/mm^3).[38] Specific infections in transplant recipients that are associated with systemic bacteremia include UTIs, infected central venous catheters, pneumonia and infected wounds. Receiving a cadaveric organ, antirejection treatment and leukopenia are important risk factors. The cause of bacterial sepsis in transplant patients is usually a Gram-negative pathogen, with *E. coli*, *Klebsiella* spp., *Enterobacter* spp. and *Serratia* spp. heading the list.[22,27]

Mortality from bacterial sepsis and shock in recipients of solid organ transplants is extremely high (>50%). Therefore, if bacteremia is suspected, empiric antimicrobial therapy with an extended-spectrum β-lactam in combination with a fluoroquinolone or aminoglycoside is advised. If intra-abdominal sepsis is suspected as the source, agents active against anaerobic bacteria should be added. Several large clinical trials to determine the efficacy of new forms of therapy, including antiendotoxin and anticytokine agents, have unfortunately not demonstrated efficacy in septic patients.[62]

Splenectomy used to be performed before renal transplantation or at the same time because splenectomized recipients were noted to tolerate larger doses of azathioprine without severe leukopenia. However, splenectomy increases susceptibility to bacterial sepsis, often caused by encapsulated organisms such as *Streptococcus pneumoniae* or *H. influenzae*.[3] For this reason, most centers have abandoned routine pretransplant splenectomy, reserving it for recipients of ABO-mismatched organs. Pneumococcal, meningococcal, and *H. influenzae* type b vaccination should be given before splenectomy and prophylactic antibiotics should be administered daily after splenectomy. We currently vaccinate all patients pretransplant.

UNUSUAL BACTERIAL ORGANISMS

Listeria monocytogenes can be the etiologic agent of meningitis or cerebritis, as well as of bacteremia and pneumonia in transplant recipients. An overall mortality rate of 26% was reported after *Listeria* infection in renal transplant patients.[63] Therefore, patients who present with even vague neurologic symptoms should undergo a complete evaluation, including lumbar puncture, and be given empiric antimicrobial therapy such as ampicillin with an aminoglycoside.[64] Infection of the nervous system occurs infrequently in our institution, presumably because our transplant recipients are given long-term TMP–SMX prophylaxis.

Nocardia asteroides may be a cause of brain abscess as well as of pulmonary, dermal, eye, joint and disseminated infections. The incidence of *Nocardia* infection varies among transplant centers (range 0–20%, mean 3%). Most patients (80–90%) have pulmonary symptoms, but dissemination to the brain also occurs frequently (30–40%).[65,66] Patients with nocardiosis have nonspecific clinical findings (e.g. fever, cough, sputum production, anorexia, hemoptysis, dyspnea, pleuritic chest pain, headache and confusion). Chest radiograph findings include nodular infiltrates, segmental and multilobar infiltrates, pleural effusion and cavitation. These findings may mimic tuberculosis with lung abscess, invasive mycosis or malignancy. *Nocardia* brain abscesses show a ring-enhancing lesion on CT scan or MRI.[65–67] Even if the CT scan is negative, MRI may prove valuable (Fig. 3.8).

Diagnosis of *Nocardia* infection can be established rapidly by direct microscopic examination of involved sputum, tissue or purulent collection. Gram stain may reveal Gram-positive beaded filaments, which can be confirmed with a Ziehl–Neelsen or Kinyoun stain. Culture routinely takes 5–21 days to grow the organism, so the microbiology laboratory needs to be notified of the presumptive diagnosis so that the plates are not discarded prematurely. Treatment consists of high-dose sulfisoxazole or TMP–SMX, often in combination with an additional agent such as amikacin. Even with appropriate therapy, the mortality rate remains 25–50% in most series and may exceed 50% when the central nervous system is involved.[65–67] Relapse of infection can occur, even after prolonged treatment of more than 4 months; for this reason, after invasive disease the patient should receive TMP–SMX indefinitely.[68] We rarely see this disease and then only in recipients who have not been receiving TMP–SMX because of drug allergy or noncompliance. Other infecting *Nocardia* spp. include *N. brasiliensis*, *N. otitidiscaviarum*, *N. transvalensis* and *N. farcinica*, none of which is particularly common as a pathogen.[65]

MYCOBACTERIAL INFECTIONS

In transplant recipients, mycobacterial infections can assume a wide variety of forms. They occur with an incidence of 1–2% in this patient group, making it 50–100 times more common than it is in the general population in the USA. They are associated with a mortality rate that approaches 30%. As with the other opportunistic infections, the majority of mycobacterial infections arise within the first year after transplant and are often temporally associated with a rejection episode.[69] Between 60 and 75% of these infections are caused by *M. tuberculosis*; atypical mycobacteria cause the remainder. Isolated pulmonary disease is the most common presentation, but dissemination is frequent, occurring in 40% of cases; resultant conditions include locally invasive pleuropulmonary disease, granulomatous hepatitis, gastrointestinal disease, bone and monoarticular joint disease, brain abscesses and miliary disease.[69–71]

It is difficult to establish the exact route of infection in the majority of post-transplant mycobacterial infections. It appears that

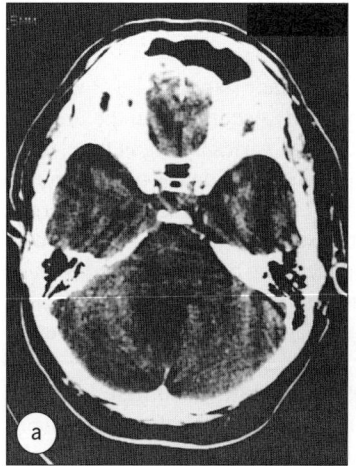
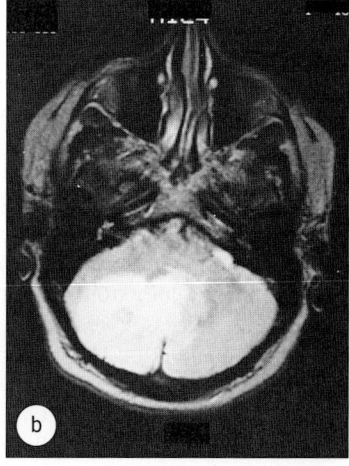

Fig. 3.8 Cerebral nocardiosis occurring after renal transplantation. (a) The CT scan of the head was unrevealing. (b) The MRI scan of the head revealed ring-enhancing lesions, in particular in the posterior fossa.

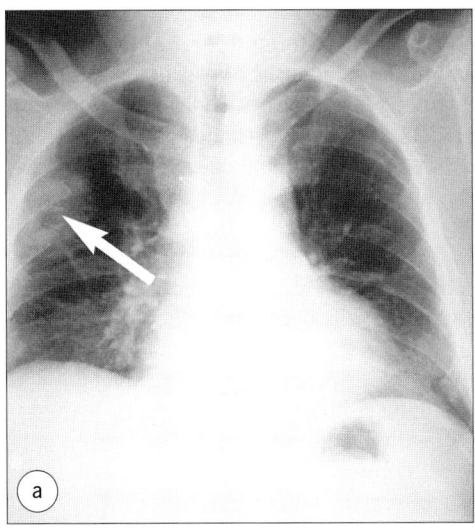

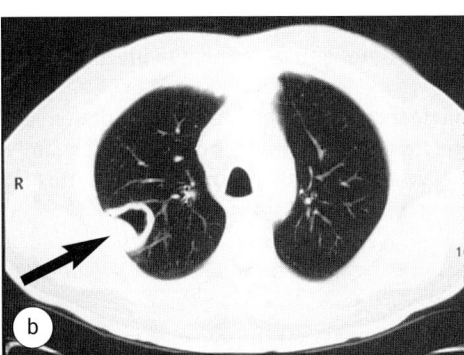

Fig. 3.9 Chest radiograph (a) and CT scan (b) demonstrating the presence of a pulmonary cavity caused by aspergillosis (arrows).

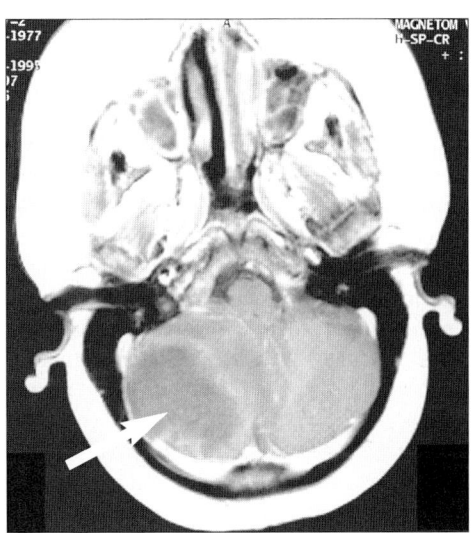

Fig. 3.10 Computed tomography of the head demonstrating cerebral aspergillosis (arrow).

approximately 40% are due to reactivation and the remainder are due to primary infection or, very rarely, transmission of disease via the donor organ.[72,73] Nosocomial transmission of *M. tuberculosis* has also been documented in transplant units.[74] Diagnosis is more difficult in solid organ transplant patients because 70% or more are anergic owing to immunosuppression or their preoperative uremic condition, and tuberculin skin tests are rarely revealing.[75]

Mycobacterium tuberculosis infection must be part of the differential diagnosis in any transplant patient presenting with an infiltrate or cavitation on chest radiograph. Bronchoscopy, or in some patients, transbronchial biopsy is useful and the latter provides tissue for culture. Treatment requires multiple drugs including isoniazid, rifampin plus ethambutol.[69,76] The use of tuberculosis prophylaxis in high-risk ethnic groups, such as native Americans or Asians, or in recipients who provide a previous history of significant exposure or a history of a positive tuberculin skin test and inadequate treatment or prophylaxis is a controversial issue; however, we recommend this approach.

FUNGAL INFECTIONS
Fungal infections are common after solid organ transplantation, accounting for 30% of serious post-transplant infections. The incidence ranges from a low of approximately 5% in kidney allograft recipients to a high of approximately 40% in liver and pancreas transplant recipients; there is a high rate of mortality due to invasive infection (30–50%).[77] The majority of fungal infections occur within the first 3 months after transplant and vary from colonization and overgrowth at mucosal surfaces to cavitary pneumonia, abdominal abscesses and cerebral abscesses. Commonly encountered infections are caused by opportunistic fungi belonging to the genera *Aspergillus*, *Candida*, *Coccidioides*, *Cryptococcus*, *Histoplasma*, *Mucor*, *Rhizopus*, *Tinea* and *Torulopsis*. Soil fungi such as *Fusarium* spp. and *Pseudallescheria boydii* may also cause infections in these patients. When high-dose immunosuppression is required, fungal infections occur in concert with other microbial infections; fungi are more frequently sole agents of infection during maintenance immunosuppression.[2,77,78]

Aspergillus spp.
Infection with *Aspergillus* spp. occurs in 1–4% of organ transplant recipients. Disseminated disease occurs in 50% of these patients and is almost invariably fatal.[78–80] *Aspergillus* spp. infections account for 20–27% of all fungal infections in solid organ transplant recipients, and in heart transplant recipients these pathogens account for 68% of all fungal infections.[77]

Recipients infected with *Aspergillus* spp. most commonly develop a fever and cough. Diffuse pneumonia with patchy infiltrates is observed on chest radiograph, although consolidation (with or without cavitation) of a pulmonary lobe or segment may resemble the radiographic appearance of bacterial pneumonia (Fig. 3.9). If pulmonary disease is unresponsive to antibacterial agent, a fungal etiology should be considered.[78]

Dissemination frequently involves the central nervous system and few patients survive (Fig. 3.10).[80–82] *Aspergillus* spp. may also infect the upper respiratory tract, oropharynx, ears, eyes, sinuses, skin and bone marrow. Endocarditis, blood vessel invasion leading to pulmonary infarction, embolization with widespread dissemination of fungal elements, and disseminated intravascular coagulation are also complications of infections with *Aspergillus* spp.

Diagnosis of pulmonary aspergillosis is established by stains and cultures from a transbronchial biopsy. However, empiric therapy with amphotericin B is often necessary. Liposomal amphotericin B preparations or itraconazole are also used in selected patients, particularly those with renal dysfunction or highly drug resistant organisms. Patients with cavitary disease should receive initial antifungal therapy followed by resection of the involved pulmonary segment. Cerebral abscesses are treated with long-term administration of antifungal agents and eventual resection; however, only a few survivors of cerebral infection have been reported.[50,78,81–83]

Candida spp.
Candida spp. are the most frequently isolated fungus in transplant recipients, accounting for 40% of all fungal infections in these patients.[78,84] In heavily immunosuppressed patients, especially those with indwelling catheters, aggressive local and systemic infection can develop, with a resultant mortality of more than 50%. *Candida* spp. are frequently copathogens with Gram-negative bacteria during intra-abdominal sepsis and deep and superficial wound infection.[22,84] Pancreas, liver and small bowel transplant recipients are highly susceptible, perhaps owing to the presence of *Candida* spp. in the duodenum and biliary tract. In renal transplant recipients, *Candida* spp. are most frequently identified in the urine and are frequent causes of UTIs. Although often identified in sputum, *Candida* spp. rarely cause invasive pneumonia.[85] Predisposing factors in transplant recipients include:[77]

- high-doses immunosuppressive therapy,
- persisting neutropenia,
- diabetes, and
- prolonged broad-spectrum antimicrobial treatment.

The diagnosis of invasive candidal disease is confirmed by culture evidence of bloodstream invasion, positive cultures from a normally sterile tissue, evidence of chorioretinitis and positive cultures from several body sites, and candidal hyphae in biopsy specimens. Fluconazole is acceptable as first-line therapy for candidal UTIs. However, persistent fever requires re-evaluation and systemic antifungal therapy. Amphotericin B is the 'gold standard' treatment of candidemia and aggressive candidal infections. Fluconazole is often effective, although *Candida krusei* is resistant to it.

Cryptococcus neoformans

Cryptococcus neoformans may be a cause of pneumonia with subtle clinical findings (i.e. low-grade fever, malaise and a nonproductive cough). Chest radiograph findings are quite variable but circumscribed pulmonary nodules are the most common finding.[86] The central nervous system is frequently involved in patients with cryptococcal pulmonary disease. Therefore, cerebrospinal fluid (CSF) should be examined in all patients with cryptococcal disease. High protein, low glucose and a mild lymphocytic leukocytosis are typical findings in CSF. India ink preparations may demonstrate the organism in CSF. Serum and CSF antigen determinations are useful in diagnosis. Treatment with amphotericin B for 2–3 weeks followed by fluconazole is standard treatment for cryptococcal disease.[86,87]

Coccidioides immitis

Infection with *Coccidioides immitis* is a risk for transplant recipients living in or visiting an endemic area (e.g. southwestern USA or northern Mexico). The incidence is 7–9% for recipients living in these areas. Mortality is approximately 25% for pulmonary disease, and it may be as high as 72% in disseminated disease. The brain, genitourinary tract, spleen, liver, joints and skin may be involved. Diagnosis is confirmed by culture, antigen detection or visualization of spherules in tissue. Long-term administration of amphotericin B is used for treatment.[78,88]

Histoplasma capsulatum and Blastomyces dermatitidis

Histoplasma capsulatum and *Blastomyces dermatitidis* are endemic in the Mississippi and Ohio River valleys in the USA, with an incidence of infection of 0.5–2% in solid organ transplant recipients. Reactivation may be a cause of disease for recipients residing in nonendemic areas. Transplant patients living in endemic areas acquire *H. capsulatum* and *B. dermatitidis* by inhalation of conidial spores. The organisms rapidly disseminate via the bloodstream and the lymphatic vessels and are concentrated in the reticuloendothelial system.[78,89] Skin lesions resemble erythema nodosum, and recognition of these lesions is key to the diagnosis. Diagnosis is confirmed by culture or histopathologic identification of the fungus from lesions or bone marrow. Bone marrow samples usually grow before material obtained from the skin, and a periodic acid–Schiff or methenamine silver stain is useful for diagnosis. Amphotericin B is used for treatment. Intraconazole may be an alternative (see Chapter 2.7).[78,89]

Mucormycosis

Mucormycosis is caused by several fungi found in soil, bread and fruit, including *Mucor* spp., *Rhizopus* spp. and *Absidia* spp. These organisms are inhaled as spores and produce locally destructive rhinocerebral infections in highly immunosuppressed patients. Aggressive surgical debridement and reduction in exogenous immunosuppression are required. These fungi may be resistant to most antifungal agents, including amphotericin B.[78] Treatment with amphotericin B (often a liposomal formulation) is prolonged and additional agents such as itraconazole, 5-fluorocytosine or rifampin are added.[77,78,87]

VIRAL INFECTIONS

Viral infections assume a wide variety of forms that range from asymptomatic infection that is diagnosed solely on the basis of a progressive increase in antibody titer to fulminant, tissue invasive disease with high mortality. Viral infections may be caused by latent viruses, by viral agents transmitted via donor organs or by viral agents in the environment to which the immunosuppressed host is exposed.[2]

Herpesviruses

Infection caused by herpesviruses is frequent after all solid organ transplants, and occurs most commonly during the periods of maximal immunosuppression immediately after transplant and during anti-rejection therapy.

Cytomegalovirus

Cytomegalovirus is the most common viral pathogen in solid organ transplant patients, exerting a significant detrimental effect on both allograft and patient survival. Some authors have reported an extremely high incidence (90%) of post-transplant CMV, diagnosed by evidence of seroconversion or viral shedding with or without overt manifestations of disease.

In our experience, the incidence of asymptomatic and symptomatic CMV infection after solid organ transplantation is approximately 50–75%; CMV infections that cause disease occur in 10–35% of solid

MANIFESTATIONS OF CYTOMEGALOVIRUS INFECTION AND DISEASE IN SOLID ORGAN TRANSPLANT RECIPIENTS	
Severity of infection	Findings
Asymptomatic CMV infection	**No clinical syndrome**
	>fourfold rise in anti-CMV antibody titer
	or
	positive CMV rapid antigen or antigenemia test
	or
	positive CMV culture obtained from blood, urine, bronchoalveolar lavage or tissue site
CMV disease	**Viral syndrome**
	Mild Fever Leukopenia (white cell count <2500 cells/mm³) Malaise, myalgias, lethargy
	Moderate Pulmonary symptoms (e.g. cough, dyspnea) with interstitial pneumonitis on chest radiograph Gastrointestinal symptoms (e.g. abdominal pain, nausea, vomiting, diarrhea) plus evidence of gastritis, duodenitis or colitis on endoscopy Retinitis
	Severe Respiratory failure Severe hypotension Massive gastrointestinal hemorrhage or perforation Hepatitis Pancreatitis
	Evidence of CMV as the primary pathogen
	The above plus Rapid antigen/antigenemia detection test *or* CMV inclusion bodies obtained from sample of bronchoalveolar lavage or tissue site

Fig. 3.11 Manifestations of cytomegalovirus infection and disease in solid organ transplant recipients. CMV, cytomegalovirus.

organ transplant patients, with higher rates in recipients of liver, heart and lung allografts. Primary infection, reactivation and superinfection can occur. Cytomegalovirus-naive recipients who receive a blood transfusion or an organ from a donor in whom a CMV titer is present (in most cases indicative of a latent CMV infection in the donor) are at highest risk for development of primary CMV disease.[89–92] The presumed source of CMV is leukocytes, as they are the target cells for the virus itself during both active and latent infection.[93] Disease can occur because of reactivation of a strain of CMV that caused an initial infection or by exposure to a second strain of CMV. However, primary infection causes the most severe type of disease and accounts for the majority of patient deaths and allograft losses. Cytomegalovirus disease due to superinfection is less severe, and reactivation disease most frequently is mild.[94] Concurrent herpes simplex virus (HSV) and CMV infection has a higher mortality and rate of allograft loss than CMV infection alone.[94,95]

A direct correlation is noted between CMV infection, disease and the amount of immunosuppressive therapy. Patients who receive a cadaveric organ, those who are treated for rejection with additional immunosuppressive medication and those who are treated with extremely potent immunosuppressive agents such as antilymphocyte antibody are more likely to develop CMV disease. Even after clinical remission and seroconversion, permanent cure cannot be assured; there is a relatively high rate (about 25%) of recurrence, and many asymptomatic recipients will continue to excrete CMV for many years.[96]

Cytomegalovirus infection may become manifest in several different ways (see Fig. 3.11):
- asymptomatic infection diagnosed by an increase in serum anti-CMV antibody titer or shedding (intermittent or chronic) of CMV from one or more sites (e.g. urine, sputum, saliva);
- symptomatic infection in which CMV is the sole causative agent and the patient manifests a specific syndrome related to the site of infection or disseminated disease with systemic manifestations; and
- symptomatic infection that occurs in conjunction with other infectious agents.

We have attempted to define significant CMV disease as that which causes a clinical syndrome and is clearly invading tissue and involving a specific organ site such as the lung or that which is associated with viremia.[90–98]

Typical mild clinical manifestations of CMV infection include fever, leukopenia, malaise and myalgias; more severe manifestations include pneumonitis and pneumonia, upper and lower gastrointestinal hemorrhage (which is sometimes massive) owing to CMV ulceration (Fig. 3.12), pancreatitis, hepatitis and retinitis. A very severe, lethal form of the disease, with hypoxemia, hypotension and multiple system organ failure, can also occur.[90]

Anti-CMV antibody (IgG and IgM) can be quantified by enzyme-linked immunosorbent assay, immunofluorescent detection, latex agglutination and complement fixation assays. A four-fold increase in the anti-CMV titer supports the diagnosis. Tissue can be examined for presence of characteristic CMV inclusion bodies, but often these are not observed (Fig. 3.13). Samples of urine, blood, sputum or tissue for viral culture provide more definitive information but take up to 3 weeks to evaluate.[94] The former tests have become outmoded, and more rapid diagnosis can be accomplished by use of the 'shell vial' culture technique, in which the culture specimen is cultured with fibroblasts for 18–36 hours, centrifuged, stained with an immunofluorescent-labeled anti-CMV-specific murine monoclonal antibody and examined using immunofluorescent microscopic techniques. This assay is as sensitive as routine cultures and provides data in a relatively short period of time. An antigenemia assay for CMV involves staining of patient leukocytes for CMV antigen with specific, high-affinity antibody. However, this test may produce false negative results in recipients with neutropenia (<500–1000 cells/mm^3) and should be repeated once the white blood cell count has returned to the normal range.[99] Finally, the presence of viral DNA can be detected using polymerase chain reaction techniques that are extremely sensitive; this approach is being used increasingly for diagnosis and to guide therapy.

Prophylactic measures to prevent the occurrence of CMV disease after transplantation include:
- donor–recipient matching for CMV status, which avoids transplantation of an organ from a CMV-positive donor into a CMV-seronegative recipient;
- vaccination with attenuated CMV virus (Towne strain);
- use of anti-CMV immunoglobulin preparations;
- aciclovir administration; and
- ganciclovir administration.

Donor–recipient matching often precludes patient access to scarce donor organs and does not prevent reactivation CMV disease. Vaccination has not provided consistent benefit and is not available for general clinical use, although clinical trials have been re-instituted. Administration of anti-CMV antibody to recipients of bone marrow, liver and renal allografts, both immediately after surgery and for several months after transplant, has led to a reduction in the incidence and severity of CMV infection and disease, although the currently available polyclonal antibody preparations are

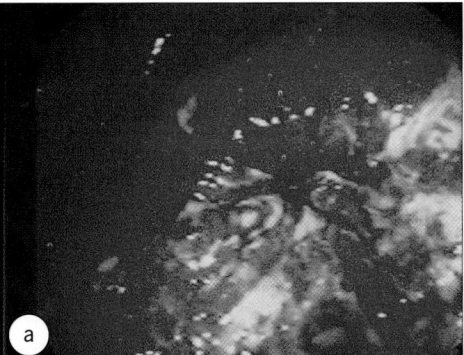
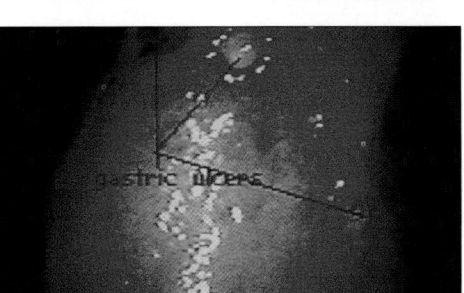

Fig. 3.12 Gastric CMV infection. (a) CMV gastritis with focal areas of inflammation. (b) Severe infection due to CMV with gastric ulceration.

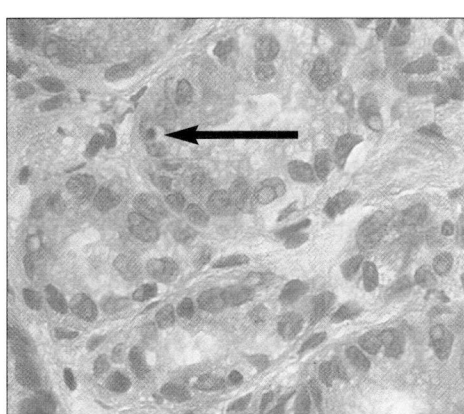

Fig. 3.13 Gastric biopsy demonstrating the presence of CMV inclusion bodies (arrow).

expensive. Aciclovir therapy has not been successful in the treatment of CMV disease, but administration of aciclovir intravenously after bone marrow transplantation and orally after cadaveric renal transplantation has led to a reduction in the incidence of CMV disease, particularly in those CMV-seronegative recipients receiving organs from CMV-positive donors. Intravenous ganciclovir administered postoperatively in heart and liver transplant recipients has been effective in reducing the incidence of subsequent CMV disease in seropositive recipients but less so in seronegative recipients. Prophylactic ganciclovir therapy has also been studied in several types of solid organ transplant recipients and during antirejection therapy in kidney transplant recipients. This form of intervention appears to lead to a reduction in the incidence and severity of disease in renal transplant and delays disease in lung transplant recipients.[98,100–108]

Ganciclovir has become the mainstay of treatment for CMV. Although its efficacy has not been tested in a randomized fashion, ganciclovir is more effective against CMV and less nephrotoxic than aciclovir.[90] Ganciclovir therapy can be limited, however, because of bone marrow suppression.[90,98] Recently, an oral formulation has become available.

Foscarnet (trisodium phosphonoformate), another agent that possesses activity against CMV, has been used to treat CMV disease in a limited number of transplant recipients. The antiviral activity of this drug is distinct from either aciclovir or ganciclovir, and it is a suitable agent if ganciclovir resistance is identified.[3,94]

Herpes simplex virus

In solid organ transplant patients, HSV-1 (and less commonly HSV-2) can cause severe oropharyngeal ulceration as well as disseminated epidermal infection, gastrointestinal tract disease, fulminant hepatitis, pneumonia and encephalitis. The majority of cases are secondary to reactivation of latent virus.[109,110] Herpes simplex virus pneumonia is reported to occur with an incidence of 0.8–10%, the highest-risk group being heart and lung transplant recipients. However, a detrimental effect of HSV alone on either patient or allograft survival has not been documented.[95]

Diagnosis of HSV is established by identifying the virus in lesions on Tzank smear, culture, immunofluorescent monoclonal antibody staining for antigen or histopathologic changes. A four-fold rise in antibody titer and seroconversion provide indirect evidence of infection. Treatment with aciclovir applied topically to cutaneous lesions or administered orally or intravenously is generally effective in controlling HSV infection. Some solid organ transplant recipients with frequent recurring HSV may require long-term prophylaxis with oral aciclovir. If fulminant disseminated HSV is suspected the patient requires immediate high-dose intravenous aciclovir and suspension of immunosuppression, with the exception of low doses of corticosteroids.

Epstein–Barr virus

Epstein–Barr virus infection can be identified in a large proportion (25–82%) of transplant recipients.[111] The diagnosis of EBV infection can be established if a fourfold rise in anti-EBV titer to viral capsid and nuclear antigens occurs; the virus may also be identified by immunohistologic staining and histopathologic changes in tissue specimens. Epstein–Barr virus may cause a lymphocytic interstitial pneumonitis; recipients present complaining of fever, cough, fatigue and dyspnea. Severe EBV infections can involve the liver, causing significant elevations in hepatic enzymes but only vague symptomatology.[111]

The danger of this ubiquitous virus is its ability to cause post-transplant lymphoproliferative disorders (PTLDs), which encompass a spectrum of conditions from benign, self-limiting infections resembling mononucleosis to aggressive malignant disease in the form of polyclonal and monoclonal B-cell lymphomas.[111–116] Post-transplant lymphoproliferative disorder occurs in only 1% of renal transplant recipients but it has been reported to occur in approximately 9% of heart–lung transplant recipients and in 30% of small bowel recipients.[33,112,115,116] Disseminated PTLD may mimic sepsis syndrome and multiple system organ failure.[117]

The diagnosis of PTLD is made by abdominal, chest and head CT studies, bone marrow biopsy and lumbar puncture to locate foci of lymphoma. If pulmonary or gastrointestinal involvement is suspected, upper and lower gastrointestinal endoscopy should be performed. Treatment of EBV infections that resemble mononucleosis or isolated EBV hepatitis or pneumonitis entails administration of aciclovir or ganciclovir (the latter if concurrent CMV is suspected or identified). Severe disease requires a reduction in exogenous immunosuppression as well.[116,117] Epstein–Barr virus is rarely fatal unless PTLD develops; PTLD carries a mortality rate of over 50%.[116] Investigational regimens for PTLD include interferon-α-2b, standard lymphoma chemotherapy and interleukin-2-activated natural killer cell infusion (often with a concurrent reduction in immunosuppression).

Varicella-zoster virus

Varicella-zoster virus (VZV) typically causes pain along a specific dermatome with or without skin eruptions. Between 5 and 26% of transplant recipients develop shingles.[118] Nonimmune adults and immunosuppressed patients may develop complications related to dissemination, such as pneumonitis or encephalitis. Pediatric transplant recipients without immunity to VZV are at high risk of disseminated VZV infection.[119] Approximately 5% of recipients without immunity develop chickenpox, which has a mortality of 11% in these patients. Diagnosis of VZV infection may be based on identification of typical VZV skin lesions, and cultures of skin lesions or respiratory secretions may be positive for VZV.

Aciclovir is the drug of choice for the treatment of active VZV infection. Varicella-zoster immune globulin may prevent disease if it is administered soon after exposure, but is generally not thought to be helpful in the treatment of severe disease,[119] for which suspension of exogenous immunosuppression and intravenous aciclovir is necessary.[109] Mild VZV infection typically responds rapidly to aciclovir therapy and a complete response is achieved without a reduction in immunosuppression. Recently, an attenuated viral vaccine has become available. This should not be administered to immunosuppressed transplant patients.

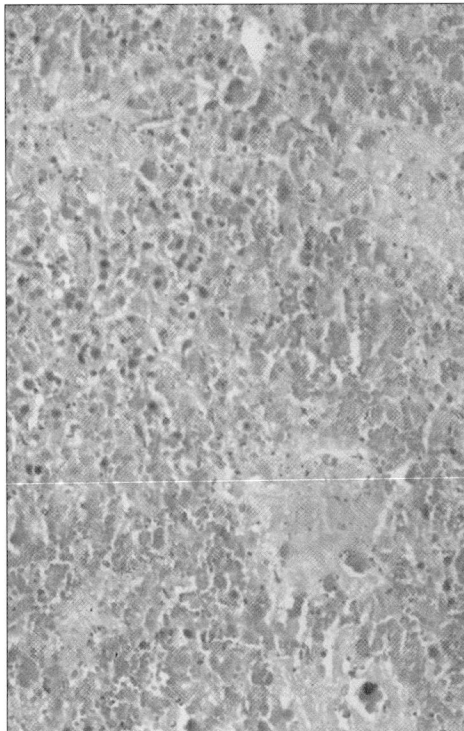

Fig. 3.14 Fulminant hepatic necrosis secondary to adenovirus hepatitis occurring after liver transplantation.

Viral hepatitis

Viral hepatitis may be diagnosed by:

- alterations in liver enzymes;
- the identification of viral antigens in the bloodstream; and
- an antibody response to hepatitis virus antigens.

Exposure to various hepatitis viruses carries the risk of hepatitis, ranging in severity from mild disease to fulminant hepatitis with hepatic coma and death, as well as the potential sequelae of chronic hepatitis with eventual hepatic failure and the risk of hepatic carcinoma.[120] Hepatitis B virus and hepatitis C virus are common causative agents, although hepatitis D virus, hepatitis E virus and other hepatitis viruses have also been identified in transplant recipients. Patients may acquire hepatitis viruses while patients are being treated with hemodialysis due to transfusion of blood products while awaiting transplantation. Progressive liver dysfunction in recipients with chronic antigenemia after transplantation is associated with an increased susceptibility to superinfection with nonviral pathogens.[121] Adenovirus, HSV, CMV, EBV and VZV have also been implicated in the etiology of progressive liver disease after transplantation. Herpes simplex virus and adenovirus hepatitis may be associated with fulminant acute hepatitis (Fig. 3.14).

Limiting the exposure of recipients to blood products before and during transplantation is often difficult, although more widespread use of erythropoietin therapy may reduce transfusion requirements in uremic patients. The presence of hepatitis B virus or hepatitis C virus is associated with considerable morbidity, and danger of transmission precludes organ donation from patients with a history of viral hepatitis.[121,122] However, some patients who are hepatitis C positive have received organs from hepatitis-C-positive donors, but these patients suffer a variety of long-term sequelae, including liver failure and infection. Hepatitis B immune globulin is available (pooled from human sources) for use in conjunction with hepatitis B vaccine and should be administered to nonimmunized transplant recipients as soon as possible after exposure. It is not clear at present whether this form of passive immunotherapy invariably prevents the disease, reduces the severity of disease, or merely prolongs the incubation period.[123–126] As previously mentioned, vaccination of all transplant candidates should be undertaken using recombinant hepatitis B vaccine.

Other viruses

Papilloma viruses occur much more frequently in immunosuppressed transplant recipients and have been implicated in the development of malignancy, multifocal leukoencephalopathy, ureteral stricture, renal allograft dysfunction and pancreatitis.[3]

Adenoviruses can cause severe disease in transplant recipients, such as diffuse interstitial pneumonia or fulminant hepatitis, either of which may be lethal.[109,127]

Respiratory syncytial virus (RSV) is a highly contagious virus that may cause pneumonia in adult transplant recipients, although the disease is usually self-limiting. Pediatric transplant recipients are at greater risk for severe RSV disease. Diagnosis is made by culture identification of RSV antigens in nasopharyngeal washes, sputum or bronchoalveolar lavage fluid. Treatment with ribavirin appears to be beneficial in some pediatric and severe adult cases.[109,128]

Human immunodeficiency virus has been transmitted via organs obtained from donors who have been identified to be HIV positive. Recipients develop an acute viral syndrome with splenomegaly and leukopenia and deteriorate clinically after renal transplantation. HIV-positive serology is a contraindication for solid organ transplantation.[129,130] Transplant patients who become HIV positive typically require reduction in exogenous immunosuppression.

Human herpesvirus 6 has been recently described and is capable of causing fever, malaise and other mild systemic symptoms in transplant patients.[131]

PROTOZOAL AND PARASITIC PATHOGENS

Pneumocystis carinii is a frequent cause of pulmonary disease in immunosuppressed transplant recipients. Cough, tachypnea and mild fever with unexpectedly severe hypoxia are typical presenting signs. Bilateral diffuse alveolar and interstitial pneumonia is commonly observed on the chest radiograph (Fig. 3.15).[132] The diagnosis must be established rapidly via bronchoscopy and, in some cases, open lung biopsy because of the high attendant mortality of untreated disease. Empiric treatment with parenteral TMP–SMX or pentamidine is instituted when a diagnosis of *P. carinii* pneumonia is suspected. Dapsone plus TMP represents an alternative therapy for patients who are allergic to sulfa drugs. Patients diagnosed with pneumocystic disease should receive lifelong suppressive therapy with TMP–SMX or pentamidine nebulizers.[133] Because all patients receiving exogenous immunosuppression at our institution receive TMP–SMX we rarely encounter this disease.

Toxoplasma gondii infections are associated with severe neurologic symptoms and death in immunosuppressed solid organ transplant recipients.[134] Transmission from the donor organs has been noted most frequently in cardiac allograft recipients, presumably because heart tissue contains more cysts than other organs. Histologic evidence obtained from lymph node or by endothelial biopsy in cardiac allograft recipients mandates therapy with pyrimethamine and sulfadiazine.

Parasitic infections are more common in allograft recipients in tropical environments, with *Strongyloides stercoralis* the most common. Pulmonary and visceral manifestations may be fatal. Schistosomiasis, malaria, cryptosporidiosis, amebiasis, *Taenia* spp., *Enterobius* spp. and other parasitic infections have also been reported in renal transplant recipients.[135]

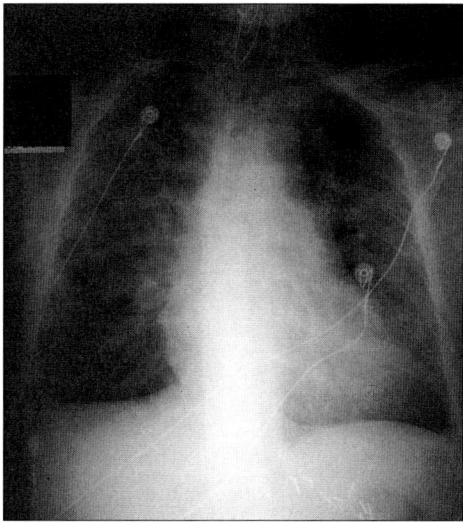

Fig. 3.15 Diffuse interstitial infiltrates secondary to *Pneumocystis carinii* infection. This chest radiograph is from a renal transplant patient who was not receiving TMP–SMX.

REFERENCES

1. United Network for Organ Sharing, Scientific Registry data, 1998. See website: www.unos.org.
2. Nicholson V, Johnson PC. Infectious complications in solid organ transplant recipients. Surg Clin North Am 1994;74:1223–45.
3. Dunn DL. Problems related to immunosuppression: infection and malignancy occurring after solid organ transplantation. Crit Care Clin 1990;6:955–77.
4. Brayman KL, Stephanian, E, Matas J, et al. Analysis of infectious complications occurring after solid organ transplantation. Arch Surg 1992;127:38–48.
5. Rubin RH, Wolfson JS, Cosimi AB, Tolkoff–Rubin NE. Infection in the renal transplant recipient. Am J Med 1981;70:405–11.
6. George DL, Arnow PM, Fox A, et al. Patterns of infection after pediatric liver transplantation. Am J Dis Child 1992;146:924–9.
7. Colonna JO II, Winston DJ, Brill JE, et al. Infectious complications in liver transplantation. Arch Surg 1988;123:360–4.
8. Green M, Michaels MG. Infectious complications of solid-organ transplantation in children. Adv Pediatr Infect Dis 1992;7:181–204.
9. Gottesdiener KM. Transplanted infections: donor-to-host transmission with the allograft. Ann Intern Med 1989;110:1001–16.
10. Spees EK, Light JA, Oakes DD, Reinmuth B. Experiences with cadaver renal allograft contamination before transplantation. Br J Surg 1982;69:482–5.
11. Prat V, Horciekova M, Matousovic M, Liska M. Urinary tract infection in renal transplant patients. Infection 1985;13:207–10.
12. Lapchik MS, Castelo-Filho A, Pestana JO, Silva-Filho AP, Wey SB. Risk factors for nosocomial urinary tract and postoperative wound infections in renal transplant patients: a matched-pair case–control study. J Urol 1992;147:994–8.
13. Hoy WE, Kissel SM, Freeman RB, Sterling WA. Altered patterns of posttransplant urinary tract infections associated with perioperative antibiotics and curtailed catheterization. Am J Kidney Dis 1985;5:212–6.
14. Gill IS, Hayes JM, Hodge EE, Novick AC. Clean intermittent catheterization and urinary diversion in the management of renal transplant recipients with lower urinary tract dysfunction. J Urol 1992;148:1397–400.
15. Mochon, M, Kaiser BA, Dunn S, et al. Urinary tract infections in children with posterior urethral valves after kidney transplantation. J Urol 1992;6:1874–6.
16. Nicol DL, P'Ng K, Hardie DR, et al. Routine use of indwelling ureteral stents in renal transplantation. J Urol 1993;150:1375–9.
17. Tolkoff-Rubin NE, Cosimi AB, Russell PS, Rubin RH. A controlled study of trimethoprim–sulfamethoxazole prophylaxis of urinary tract infection in renal transplant recipients. Rev Infect Dis 1982;4:614–8.
18. Simmons RL, Migliori RJ. Infection prophylaxis after successful organ transplantation. Transplant Proc 1988;20(Suppl 8):7–11.
19. Fox BC, Sollinger HW, Belzer FO, Maki DG. A prospective, randomized, double-blind study of trimethoprim–sulfamethoxazole for prophylaxis of infection in renal transplantation: clinical efficacy, absorption of trimethoprim–sulfamethoxazole, effects on the microflora, and the cost-benefit of prophylaxis. Am J Surg 1990;89:255–74.
20. Sollinger HW, Ploeg RJ, Eckhoff DE, et al. Two hundred consecutive simultaneous pancreas–kidney transplants with bladder drainage. Surgery 1993;114:736–44.
21. Douzdjian V, Abecassis MM, Cooper JL, Smith JL, Corry RJ. Incidence, management and significance of surgical complications after pancreatic transplantation. Surg Gynecol Obstet 1993;177:451–6.

22. Everett JE, Wahoff DC, Statz C, et al. Characterization and impact of wound infection after pancreas transplantation. Arch Surg 1994;129:1310–7.
23. Judson RT. Wound infection following renal transplantation. Aust N Z J Surg 1984;54:223–4.
24. Wornom IL III, Maragh H, Pozez A, Guerraty AJ. Use of the omentum in the management of sternal wound infection after cardiac transplantation. Plast Reconstr Surg 1995;95:697–702.
25. Ascherman JA, Hugo NE, Sultan MR, Patsis MC, Smith CR, Rose EA. Single-stage treatment of sternal wound complications in heart transplant recipients in whom pectoralis major myocutaneous advancement flaps were used. J Thorac Cardiovasc Surg 1995;110:1030–6.
26. Rabito FJ, Pankey GA. Infections in orthotopic heart transplant patients at the Ochsner Medical Institutions. Med Clin North Am 1992;76:1125–34.
27. Kramer MR, Marshall SE, Starnes VA, Gamberg P, Amitai Z, Theodore J. Infectious complications in heart-lung transplantation analysis of 200 episodes. Arch Intern Med 1993;153:2010–6.
28. Mauer JR, Tullis DE, Grossman RF, et al. Infectious complications following isolated lung transplantation. Chest 1992;101:1056–9.
29. Herridge MS, deHoyos AL, Chaparro C, Winton TL, Kesten S, Maurer JR. Pleural complications in lung transplant recipients. J Thorac Cardiovasc Surg 1995;110:22–6.
30. Sielaff TD, Everett JE, Shumway SJ, Wahoff DC, Bolman RM III, Dunn DL. Mycoplasma hominis infections occurring in cardiovascular surgical patients. Ann Thorac Surg 1996;61:99–103.
31. Kusne S, Dummer JS, Singh N, et al. Infections after liver transplantation, an analysis of 101 consecutive cases. Medicine 1988;67:132–43.
32. Keating MR, Wilhel MP. Management of infectious complications following liver transplantation. Curr Clin Top Infect Dis 1993;13:226–49.
33. Ozaki CF, Katz SM, Monsour HP, et al. Surgical complications of liver transplantation. Surg Clin North Am 1994;74:1155–67.
34. Hesse UJ, Sutherland DER, Simmons RL, Najarian JS. Intra-abdominal infections in pancreas transplant recipients. Ann Surg 1986;203:153–62.
35. Sutherland DER, Dunn DL, Goetz FC, et al. A ten year experience with 290 pancreas transplants at a single institution. Ann Surg 1989;210:274–88.
36. Todo S, Reyes J, Furukawa H, et al. Outcome analysis of 71 clinical intestinal transplantations. Ann Surg 1995;222:270–82.
37. Asfar S, Zhong R, Grant D. Small bowel transplantation. Surg Clin North Am 1994;74:1197–210.
38. Todo S, Tzakis A, Abu–Elmagd K, et al. Abdominal multivisceral. Transplantation 1995;59:234–40.
39. Trail KC, Stratta RJ, Larsen JL, et al. Results of liver transplantation in diabetic patients. Surg 1993;114:650–8.
40. Singh N, Gayowski T, Wagener M, et al. Increased infections in liver transplant recipients with recurrent hepatitis C virus hepatitis. Transplantation 1996;61:402–6.
41. Low DE, Kaiser LR. The donor lung: infectious and pathologic factors affecting outcome in lung transplantation. J Thorac Cardiovasc Surg 1993;106:614–21.
42. Flume PA, Egan TM, Paradowski LJ, Detterbeck FC, Thompson JT, Yankaskas JR. Infectious complications of lung transplantation. Impact of cystic fibrosis. Am J Respir Crit Care Med 1994;149:1601–7.
43. Church JM, Fazio VW, Braun WE, Novick AC, Steinmuller DR. Perforation of the colon in renal homograft recipients. Ann Surg 1986;203:69–76.
44. Pollak R, Hau T, Mozes MF. The spectrum of peritonitis in renal transplant recipients. Am Surg 1985;51:617–20.

45. Alexander P, Schuman E, Vetto RM. Perforation of the colon in the immunocompromised patient. Am J Surg 1986;151:557–61.
46. Pirenne J, Lledo-Garcia E, Benedetti E, et al. Colon perforation after renal transplantation: a single-institution review. Clin Transplant 1997;11:94–7.
47. Hau T, Van Hook EJ, Simmons RL, et al. Prognostic factors of peritoneal infections in transplant patients. Surgery 1978;84:403–8.
48. Dunn DL, Najarian JS. Abdominal catastrophes in the immuno-suppressed patient. In: Najarian JS, Delaney JP, eds. Trauma and critical care surgery. Chicago: Year Book Medical Publishers; 1987:271–9.
49. Mermel LA, Maki DG. Bacterial pneumonia in solid organ transplantation. Semin Respir Infect 1990;5:10–29.
50. Dunn DL, Najarian JS. Infectious complications in transplant surgery. In: Shires GT, Davis J, eds. Principles and management of surgical infection. Philadelphia: JB Lippincott; 1990:425–64.
51. Deusch E, End A, Grimm M, et al. Early bacterial infections in lung transplant recipients. Chest 1993;104:1412–6.
52. Keating MR, Wilhelm MP, Walker RC. Strategies for prevention of infection after cardiac transplantation. Mayo Clin Proc 1992;67:676–84.
53. Horvath J, Dummer S, Loyd J, Walker B, Merrill WH, Frist WH. Infection in the transplanted and native lung after single lung transplantation. Chest 1993;104:681–5.
54. Snell GI, deHoyos A, Krajden M, Winton T, Maurer JR. Pseudomonas cepacia in lung transplant recipients with cystic fibrosis. Chest 1993;103:466–71.
55. Steinbach S, Sun L, Jiang RZ, et al. Transmissibility of Pseudomonas cepacia infection in clinic patients and lung-transplant recipients with cystic fibrosis. N Engl J Med 1994;331:981–7.
56. Egan TM, Detterbeck FC, Mill, MR, et al. Improved results of lung transplantation for patients with cystic fibrosis. J Thorac Cardiovasc Surg 1995;109:224–235.
57. Johnson PC, Hogg KM, Sarosi GA. The rapid diagnosis of pulmonary infections in solid organ transplant recipients. Semin Respir Infect 1990;5:2–9.
58. Cazzadori A, Di Perri G, Todeschini G, et al. Transbronchial biopsy in the diagnosis of pulmonary infiltrates in immunocompromised patients. Chest 1995;101:101–6.
59. Ampple NM, Wing EJ. Legionella infection in transplant recipients. Semin Respir Infect 1990;5:30–7.
60. Tokunaga Y, Concepcion W, Berquist WE, et al. Graft involvement by Legionella in a liver transplant recipient. Arch Surg 1992;127:475–7.
61. Weeratna R, Marrie TJ, Logan SM, et al. Legionnaires' disease in cardiac transplant patients: a cell-mediated immune response develops despite cyclosporine therapy. J Infect Dis 1993;168:521–2.
62. Suffredini AF. Current prospects for the treatment of clinical sepsis. Crit Care Med 1994;22(Suppl 7):S12–7.
63. Stamm AM, Dismukes WE, Simmons BP, et al. Listeriosis in renal transplant recipients: Report of an outbreak and review of 102 cases. Rev Infect Dis 1982;4:665–82.
64. Tolkoff-Rubin NE, Rubin RH. Opportunistic fungal and bacterial infection in the renal transplant recipient. J Am Soc Neph 1992;2(Suppl 12):S264–9.
65. Chapman SW, Wilson JP. Nocardiosis in transplant recipients. Semin Respir Infect 1990;5:74–9.
66. Wilson JP, Turner HR, Kirchner KA, Chapman SW. Nocardial infections in renal transplant recipients. Medicine 1989;68:38–57.
67. Aduino RC, Johnson PC, Miranda AG. Nocardiosis in renal transplant recipients undergoing immunosuppression with cyclosporin. Clin Infect Dis 1993;16:505–12.

68. King CT, Chapman SW, Butkus DE. Recurrent nocardiosis in a renal transplant recipient. South Med J 1993;86:225–8.

69. Sinnott JT, Emmanuel, PJ. Mycobacterial infections in the transplant patient. Semin Respir Infect 1990;5:65–73.

70. Hall, CM, Willcox PA, Swanepoel CR, Kahn D, Van Zyl Smit R. Mycobacterial infection in renal transplant recipients. Chest 1994;106:435–9.

71. Higgins RSD, Kusne S, Reyes J, et al. Mycobacterium tuberculosis after liver transplantation: management and guidelines for prevention. Clin Transplant 1992;6:81–90.

72. Ridgeway AL, Warner GS, Phillips P, et al. Transmission of Mycobacterium tuberculosis to recipients of single lung transplants from the same donor. Am J Respir Crit Care Med 1996;153:1166–8.

73. Peters TG, Reiter, CG, Boswell RL. Transmission of tuberculosis by kidney transplant recipients. Transplantation 1984;38:514–6.

74. Jereb J, Burwen DR, Dooley SW, et al. Nosocomial outbreak of tuberculosis in a renal transplant unit: application of a new technique for restriction fragment length polymorphism analysis of Mycobacterium tuberculosis isolates. J Infect Dis 1993;168:1219–24.

75. Delaney V, Sumrani KN, Hong JH, Sommer B. Mycobacterial infections in renal allograft recipients. Transplant Proc 1993;25:2288–9.

76. Miller RA, Lanza LA, Kline JN, Geist LJ. Mycobacterium tuberculosis in lung transplant recipients. Am J Respir Crit Care Med 1995;152:374–6.

77. Paya CV. Fungal infections in solid-organ transplantation. Clin Infect Dis 1993;16:677–88.

78. Zeluff BJ. Fungal pneumonia in transplant recipients. Semin Respir Infect 1990;5:80–9.

79. Keating MR, Guerrero MA, Daly RC, Walker RC, Davies SF. Transmission of invasive aspergillosis from a subclinically infected donor to three different organ transplant recipients. Chest 1996;109:1119–24.

80. Kusne S, Torre-Cisneros J, Manez R, et al. Factors associated with invasive lung aspergillosis and the significance of positive Aspergillus culture after liver transplantation. J Infect Dis 1992;166:1379–83.

81. Polo JM, Fabrega E, Casafont F, et al. Treatment of cerebral aspergillosis after liver transplantion. Neurology 1992;42:1817–9.

82. Denning DW, Stevens DA. Antifungal and surgical treatment of invasive aspergillosis: review of 2,121 published cases. Rev Infect Dis 1990;12:1147–201.

83. Denning DW, Lee JY, Hostetler JS, et al. NIAID mycoses study group multicenter trial of oral itraconazole therapy for invasive aspergillosis. Am J Med 1994;97:135–44.

84. Nieto-Rodriguez JA, Kusne S, Manez R, et al. Factors associated with the development of candidemia and candidemia-related death among liver transplant recipients. Ann Surg 1996;223:70–6.

85. Chugh KS, Sakhuja V, Jain S, et al. Fungal infections in renal allograft recipients. Transplant Proc 1992;24:1940–2.

86. Watson AJ, Russell RP, Cabreja RF, Braverman R, Whelton A. Cure of cryptococcal infection during continued immunosuppressive therapy. Q J Med 1985;55:169–72.

87. Denning DW, Tucker RM, Hanson LH, Stevens DA. Itraconazole in opportunistic mycoses: crytococcosis and aspergillosis. J Am Acad Dermatol 1990;23:602–7.

88. Cohen KM, Galgiani JN, Potter D, Ogden DA. Coccidioidomycosis in renal replacement therapy. Arch Intern Med 1982;142:489–94.

89. Davies SF, Sarosi GA, Peterson PK, et al. Disseminated histoplasmosis in renal transplant recipients. Am J Surg 1979;137:686–91.

90. Dunn DL, Mayoral JL, Gillingham KJ, et al. Treatment of invasive cytomegalovirus disease in solid organ transplant patients with ganciclovir. Transplantation 1991;51:98–106.

91. Boivin G, Erice A, Crane D, Dunn DL, Balfour HH. Ganciclovir susceptibilities of cytomegalovirus (CMV) isolates from solid organ transplant recipients with CMV viremia after antiviral prophylaxis. J Infect Dis 1993;168:332–5.

92. Ettinger NA, Bailey TC, Trulock EP, et al. Cytomegalovirus infection and pneumonitis, impact after isolated lung transplantation. Am Rev Respir Dis 1993;147:1017–23.

93. Gerna G, Zipeto D, Percivalle, et al. Human cytomegalovirus infection of the major leukocyte subpopulations and evidence for viral replication in polymorphonuclear leukocytes from viremic patients. J Infect Dis 1992;166:1236–44.

94. Dunn DL, Najarian JS. New approaches to the diagnoses, prevention, and treatment of cytomegalovirus infection after transplantation. Am J Surg 1991;161:250–5.

95. Dunn DL, Matas AJ, Fryd DS, Simmons RL, Najarian JS. Association of concurrent herpes simplex virus and cytomegalovirus with detrimental effects after renal transplantation. Arch Surg 1984;119:812–7.

96. Sawyer MD, Mayoral JL, Gillingham KJ, Kramer MA, Dunn DL. Treatment of recurrent cytomegalovirus disease in patients receiving solid organ transplants. Arch Surg 1993;128:165–70.

97. Arabia FA, Rosado LJ, Huston CL, Sethi GK, Copeland JG III. Incidence and recurrence of gastrointestinal cytomegalovirus infection in heart transplantation. Ann Thorac Surg 1993;55:8–11.

98. Dunn DL, Gillingham KJ, Kramer MA, et al. A prospective randomized study of aciclovir versus ganciclovir plus human immune globulin prophylaxis of cytomegalovirus infection after solid organ transplantation. Transplantation 1994;57:876–84.

99. Erice A, Holm MA, Gill PC, et al. Cytomegalovirus (CMV) antigenemia assay is more sensitive than shell vial cultures for rapid detection of CMV in polymorphonuclear blood lukocytes. J Clin Microbiol 1992;30:2822–5.

100. Metselaar HJ, Rothbarth PH, Brouwer RML, Wenting GJ, Jeekel J, Weimar W. Prevention of cytomegalovirus-related death by passive immunization. Transplantation 1989;48:264–6.

101. Snydman DR, Werner BG, Dougherty NN, et al. Cytomegalovirus immune globulin prophyalxis in liver transplantion a randomized, double-blind, placebo-controlled trial. Ann Intern Med 1993;119:984–91.

102. Balfour HH, Chase BA, Stapleton JT, Simmons RL, Fryd DS. A randomized, placebo-controlled trial of oral acyclovir for the prevention of cytomegalovirus disease in recipients of renal allografts. N Engl J Med 1989;320:1381–7.

103. Freise CE, Pons V, Lake J, Burke E, Ascher NL, Robert JP. Comparison of three regimens for cytomegalovirus prophylaxis in 147 liver transplant recipients. Transplant Proc 1991;23:1498–500.

104. Merigan TC, Renlund DG, Keay S, et al. A controlled trial of ganciclovir to prevent cytomegalovirus disease after heart transplantation. N Engl J Med 1992;326:1182–6.

105. Hibberd PL, Tolkoff-Rubin NE, Conti D, et al. Preemptive ganciclovir therapy to prevent cytomegalovirus disease in cytomegalovirus antibody-positive renal transplant recipients. Ann Intern Med 1995;123:18–26.

106. Bailey TC, Trulock EP, Ettinger NA, Storch GA, Cooper JD, Powderly WG. Failure of prophylactic ganciclovir to prevent cytomegalovirus disease in recipients of lung transplants. J Infect Dis 1992;165:548–52.

107. Brayman KL, Dafoe DC, Smythe WR, et al. Prophylaxis of serious cytomegalovirus infection in renal transplant candidates using live human cytomegalovirus vaccine. Arch Surg 1988;123:1502–8.

108. Plotkin SA, Friedman HM, Fleisher GR, et al. Towne-vaccine-induced prevention of cytomegalovirus disease after renal transplants. Lancet 1984;1:528–30.

109. Anderson DJ, Jordan MC. Viral pneumonia in recipients of solid organ transplants. Semin Respir Infect 1990;5:38–49.

110. Carrier M, Pelletier GB, Cartier R, Leclerc Y, Pelletier LC. Prevention of herpes simplex virus infection by oral acyclovir after cardiac transplantation. Can J Surg 1992;35:513–6.

111. Langnas AN, Castaldo P, Markin RS, Stratta RJ, Wood RP, Shaw BW. The spectrum of Epstein–Barr virus infection with hepatitis following liver transplantation. Transplant Proc 1991;23:1513–4.

112. Hanto DW, Frizzera G, Gajl-Peczalska KJ, et al. Epstein–Barr virus-induced B-cell lymphoma after renal transplantation. N Engl J Med 1982;306:913–8.

113. Cockfield SM, Preiksaitis JK, Jewell LD, Parfrey NA. Post-transplant lymphoproliferative disorder in renal allograft recipients. Transplantation 1993;56:88–96.

114. Rostaing L, Icart J, Durand D, et al. Clinical outcome of Epstein–Barr viremia in transplant patients. Transplant Proc 1993;25:2286–7.

115. Swinnen LJ, Costanzo-Nordin MR, Fisher SG, et al. Increased incidence of lymphoproliferative disorder after immunosuppression with the monoclonal antibody OKT3 in cardiac-transplant recipients. N Engl J Med 1990;323:1723–8.

116. Stephanian E, Gruber SA, Dunn DL, Matas AJ. Posttransplant lymphoproliferative disorders. Transplant Rev 1991;5:120–9.

117. Stephanian E, Brayman KL, Manivel JC, Sutherland DER, Dunn DL. Fulminant post-transplant lymphoproliferative disorder presenting as multisystem organ failure. Clin Transplant 1992;6:361–8.

118. Straus SE, Ostrove JM, Inchauspe G, et al. Varicella–zoster infections biology, natural history, treatment, and prevention. Ann Intern Med 1988;108:221–37.

119. Lynfield R, Herrin JT, Rubin RH. Varicella in pediatric renal transplant recipients. Pediatrics 1992;90:216–20.

120. Fagiuoli S, Shah G, Wright HI, Van Thiel DH. Types, causes, and therapies of hepatitis ocurring in liver transplant recipients. Dig Dis Sci 1993;38:449–56.

121. Dusheiko G, Song E, Bowyer S, et al. Natural history of hepatitis B virus infection in renal transplant recipients-a fifteen-year follow-up. Hepatology 1983;3:330–6.

122. Valeri M, Pisani F, De Paolis P, et al. Hepatitis C virus infection in kidney transplant recipients. Transplant Proc 1993;25:2284–5.

123. Samuel D, Muller R, Alexander G, et al. Liver transplantation in European patients with the hepatitis B surface antigen. N Engl J Med 1993;329:1842–7.

124. Rimoldi P, Belli LS, Rondinara GF, et al. Recurrent HBV/HDV infections under different immunoprophylaxis protocols. Transplant Proc 1993;25:2675–6.

125. Mion F, Boillot O, Gille D, Chevallier P, Paliard P. Liver transplantation for posthepatitic B-Delta cirrhosis: prevention of recurrence with high-dose anti-HBs immunoglobulins. Transplant Proc 1993;25:2638–9.

126. Berner J, Kadian M, Post J, et al. prophylactic recombinant hepatitis B vaccine in patients undergoing orthotopic liver transplantation. Transplant Proc 1993;25:1751–2.

127. Michaels MG, Green M, Wald ER, Starzl TE. Adenovirus infection in pediatric liver transplant recipients. J Infect Dis 1992;165:170–4.

128. Pohl C, Green M, Wald ER, Ledesma-Medina J. Respiratory syncytial virus infections in pediatric liver transplant recipients. J Infect Dis 1992;165:166–9.

129. Oliveira DBG, Winearls CG, Cohen J, Ind PW, Williams G. Severe immunosuppression in a renal transplant recipient with HTLV-III antibodies. Transplantation 1986;1:260–2.

130. L'age-Stehr J, Schwarz A, Offermann G, *et al*. HTLV-III infection in kidney transplant recipients. Lancet 1985;2:1361–2.

131. Gudnason T, Dunn DL, Brown NA, Balfour HH Jr. Human herpes virus 6 infections in hospitalized renal transplant recipients. Clin Transplantation 1991;5:359–64.

132. Dummer JS. *Pneumocystis carinii* Infections in transplant recipients. Semin Respir Infect 1990;5:50–7.

133. Saukkonen K, Garland R, Koziel H. Aerosolized pentamidine as alternative primary prophylaxis against *Pneumocystis carinii* pneumonia in adult hepatic and renal transplant recipients. Chest 1996;109:1250–5.

134. Luft BJ, Naot Y, Araujo FG, Stinson EB, Remington JS. Primary and reactivated toxoplasma infection in patients with cardiac transplants. Ann Intern Med 1983;99:27–31.

135. Date A, Vaska K, Vaska PH, Pandey AP, Kirubakaran MG, Shastry JCM. Terminal infections in renal transplant patients in a tropical environment. Nephron 1982;32:253–7.

Blood and Marrow Transplantation

Raleigh A Bowden

INTRODUCTION

Infection continues to be a leading cause of morbidity and mortality after blood and marrow transplantation (BMT). However, advances that have been made in the past decade have had an important impact on the relative importance and timing of infections. First, effective prophylaxis for cytomegalovirus (CMV) and invasive candidiasis is now available, and so the attention and focus of clinical research has shifted to other pathogens such as *Aspergillus* spp. and respiratory viruses. Second, we are learning that effective prophylaxis during the early post-BMT period results, in some cases, in an increase in the occurrence of infection once prophylaxis is discontinued. Third, increasing cost pressures are changing the way in which patients are managed, with less emphasis on routine laboratory screening and more focus on management outside hospital. Specifically, cost considerations are having a major impact on the approach to protecting patients from infection. For example, the use of laminar air flow protection is becoming increasingly difficult to justify from the point of view of cost as more patients receive most of their care as outpatients.

Recent advances have also occurred in the delivery of hematopoietic stem cells. Historically, all stem cells came from bone marrow, but advances in technology have allowed the use of peripheral blood as a source of stem cells following myeloablative therapy.[1] Thus, the term 'marrow transplantation' is increasingly being replaced by 'peripheral blood stem cell (PBSC) transplantation'. Further, additional sources of stem cells, including umbilical cord blood, are currently being investigated to increase the availability of this potentially life-saving procedure; this may add a new dimension to the profile of post-BMT infectious complications in the future. Therefore, to acknowledge this changing technology, the term 'blood and marrow transplantation' (BMT) will replace the use of the traditional term 'bone marrow transplantation' throughout this chapter to reflect this changing clinical practice.

Stem cell products that are obtained from peripheral blood differ somewhat from those obtained from marrow, in that PBSC products deliver up to 10 times more T lymphocytes than marrow does. Peripheral blood stem cell transplantation facilitates earlier engraftment; however, it may be associated with an increased incidence of graft-versus-host disease (GVHD). Infectious complications may be similar to those that occur after marrow transplantation if the advantages of early engraftment are offset by the increased incidence of GVHD. Data presented in this chapter will mainly reflect the timing and spectrum of infections that follow traditional marrow transplantation. When available, differences in the characteristics of infectious complications between marrow and PBSC transplantation will be noted.

Despite changes in technology and the effects that anti-infective prophylaxis have had on the timing of infectious complications, our approach to the management of infectious complications has not changed appreciably over the past several decades. In general, prevention of infections of all types is clearly more effective than treatment after infections are well established. This is particularly true for viral and fungal disease after BMT, where the mortality rate for patients with established infections continues to be high despite available therapy. Furthermore, it is now apparent that re-exposure to antigens may be

critical to the reconstitution of normal immunity after transplant for some types of infections. This is particularly true for the herpesviruses. For example, when effective antiviral suppression is instituted to prevent infection with CMV in the early post-BMT period, there is a shift in the timing of the onset of CMV infection to the late period (after day 100 post-transplant).[2] Advances in our ability to facilitate immune reconstitution may assist in the control of infections in the future by manipulation of the immune system rather than simply by suppression of infection with anti-infective drugs. An example is the use of adaptive immunotherapy for CMV.[3] Such an approach offers the potential of facilitating long-lasting immunity and reducing the risk of delaying infections such as CMV from the early to the late period post-transplant.

As improvement in the prevention of CMV during the first 100 days after transplant becomes the standard of care, invasive fungal infection, and specifically aspergillosis, may become the leading infectious cause of death during the first 100 days after transplant.[4,5] Late infections are also becoming increasingly important as patients tend to survive longer and as prophylaxis delays infection until the late post-transplant period.

This chapter reviews the major causes of infectious complications following BMT and highlights changes in epidemiology with the introduction of recent prevention measures. Specific details are provided for current diagnostic, preventative and treatment approaches to the common and less common infections, with emphasis on approaches that are unique to the BMT setting.

EPIDEMIOLOGY

The risk for various types of infectious complications after stem cell transplantation depends, in large part, on both the specific immune deficiency and timing of recovery following myeloablative conditioning. Therefore, epidemiology and morbidity of the various infectious diseases following BMT are closely linked. In general, taking all types of BMT patients into consideration, the two most powerful determinants of infectious risks and outcomes are:

- whether the transplanted marrow is from an allogeneic or an autologous stem cell donor source; and
- the time after transplant that the infection occurs.

This holds true with all types of infection: bacterial, viral, fungal and parasitic. The critical distinguishing factor in determining infectious risk between allogeneic and autologous grafts is the associated risk of immunosuppression from GVHD itself or from therapy for it.

TIMING OF INFECTIOUS COMPLICATIONS

The organisms that cause the majority of serious infectious complications after BMT come either from endogenous flora or from latent viral infections with the DNA viruses. Important exceptions to this include *Aspergillus* spp., community-acquired respiratory virus infections and nosocomially transmitted bacterial infections (e.g. vancomycin-resistant *Enterococcus* spp. and *Clostridium difficile*). Aspergillosis results from inhalation of spores from the environment and may occur with higher frequency during the dry and warmer (and thus the dustier) months.[6] Respiratory virus infections following BMT classically occur during the winter months; the specific virus depends on what is epidemic in the community.[7] The exception is parainfluenza virus, which may occur throughout the year and nosocomial outbreaks of respiratory syncytial virus (RSV), which may cause infection outside the observed season in the community.[7] Knowledge of the source and timing of specific infections provide the basis for much of our infection prevention strategies.

The risk for all types of infection following stem cell transplantation can also be predicted from a knowledge of the immunologic deficiencies that remain after myeloablative conditioning therapy. Historically, the risk periods were divided into the neutropenic period, the early postengraftment period (engraftment until day 100) and the late period (after day 100). This historic division reflects a time when the majority of transplants were performed with matched allogeneic donors.[8] Figure 4.1 shows the major risk periods for bacterial, viral and fungal infections when no routine prophylaxis was given and relates the risk of infection to the major host defense defects, including neutropenia and GVHD. Although the first several weeks after transplant are characterized by both neutropenia and lymphopenia, most of the infections that occur during this period are related to neutropenia. Neutropenia remains the overriding risk for serious bacterial infections, particularly Gram-negative bacterial infections,

during the early post-transplant period. However, the risk for the most common cause of bacteremia, coagulase-negative *Staphylococcus* spp., is related to the length of time that the indwelling intravenous catheter remains in place; coagulase-negative *Staphylococcus* spp. infection occurs with equal frequency both before and after engraftment until the central line is removed (Fig. 4.2).[9]

After engraftment, the continued need for indwelling catheters and the disruption of the gastrointestinal mucosa (due either to chemotherapy or to GVHD) both add to the risk for bacterial infection. The risk for all types of infection is increased by defects in neutrophil function in patients with acute GVHD; corticosteroids used in the treatment of GVHD can also compound this effect. As T-lymphocyte function recovers during the first 100 days in patients who do not develop GVHD, the risk for viral infection diminishes and host defense recovers, usually becoming normal by about 18 months after transplant.[10] In patients with continuing GVHD, especially those receiving corticosteroids, the risk of bacterial, viral and fungal infection continues.[11,12]

With recent advances in strategies for the prevention of infection, the risk periods for certain types of infections is changing. These changes, some of which may affect the time of onset of infection, include:

- shortening of the duration of neutropenia by the use of growth factors and PBSC infusions as a source of stem cells; and
- the increasing shift of viral (and specifically CMV) and fungal infection to the late period (after day 100) as effective early prevention strategies have been developed.

As new prophylactic measures become the standard of care, the thinking about how best to divide the remaining risk periods following transplant is changing.

Figure 4.3 shows the same risk factors as outlined in Figure 4.1 but with standard prophylaxis and with serologically screened or filtered blood for prevention of primary CMV, ganciclovir prophylaxis for prevention of reactivation of CMV in the seropositive recipient, fluconazole prophylaxis for prevention of candidiasis and trimethoprim–sulfamethoxazole (co-trimoxazole) prophylaxis for *Pneumocystis carinii* infection. The initial risk period begins with the onset of myeloablative conditioning therapy and ends at engraftment. The risk periods for bacterial infections for patients receiving autologous and allogeneic grafts are quite similar. In contrast to what is shown in Figure 4.1, herpes simplex virus (HSV) infection in the setting of routine aciclovir prophylaxis has been for the most part eliminated during the first month, but it now occurs with a relatively increased frequency, although less frequently than before prophylaxis during the second period after aciclovir has been discontinued (Fig. 4.4). Ganciclovir is highly effective for prophylaxis of CMV (Fig. 4.5). *Pneumocystis carinii* disease has also been significantly reduced with routine use of trimethoprim–sulfamethoxazole.

The second risk period, from engraftment until day 100, remains a high-risk period for the allogeneic patient, particularly those with acute GVHD. A new, late post-transplant risk period for the allogeneic patient with continuing GVHD begins at approximately day 100 and ends when the patient regains normal immunity, generally by 18 months after transplant in patients who are not being treated with immunosuppressive medication and who remain free from GVHD. *Aspergillus* spp. infection is a major risk during the late post-transplant risk period, with CMV, varicella-zoster virus (VZV) and encapsulated bacteria added to the continuing risk of infection in these patients. In a review of late infections in 386 patients, the most common infections were sinusitis (241 episodes), pneumonia (235 episodes) and otitis media (124 episodes).[11] For patients with life-long GVHD, a late risk period persists for as long as therapy for chronic GVHD is required. In addition, it has recently been appreciated that CMV disease is becoming a leading cause of death in the late post-transplant period.[2] It is likely that aspergillosis will also play a significant role in infection-related mortality during the late risk period, but the frequency of aspergillosis has not yet been defined.

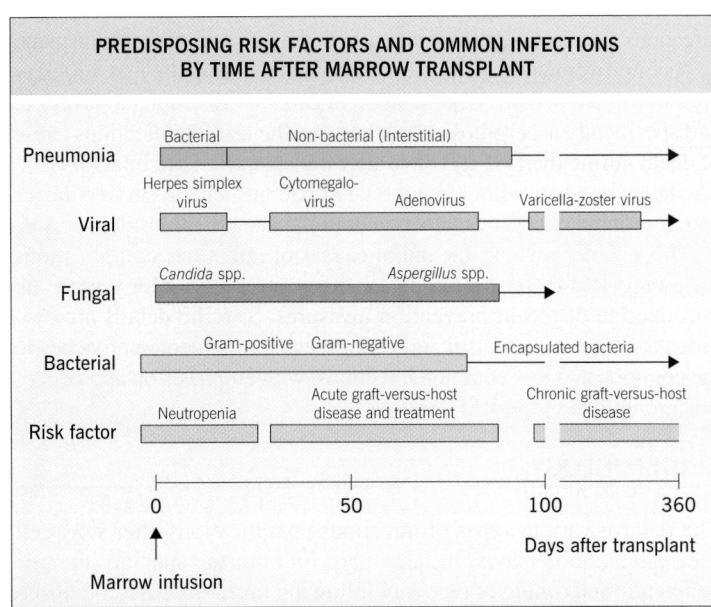

PREDISPOSING RISK FACTORS AND COMMON INFECTIONS BY TIME AFTER MARROW TRANSPLANT

Fig. 4.1 **Predisposing risk factors and common infections by time after marrow transplant, when no routine antimicrobial prophylaxis is given.**

OCCURRENCE OF GRAM-POSITIVE BACTEREMIA BY DAY AFTER TRANSPLANT

First day of positive culture	Number of patients	Number of positive blood cultures (Gram-positive isolates only)
0–10	33	56
11–20	11	44
21–30	13	25
31–40	17	40
41–50	16	60
51–60	22	33
61–70	9	20
71–80	9	27
81–90	13	21
91–100	5	12

Fig. 4.2 **Occurrence of Gram-positive bacteremia by day after transplant.** Data from Walter and Bowden.[9]

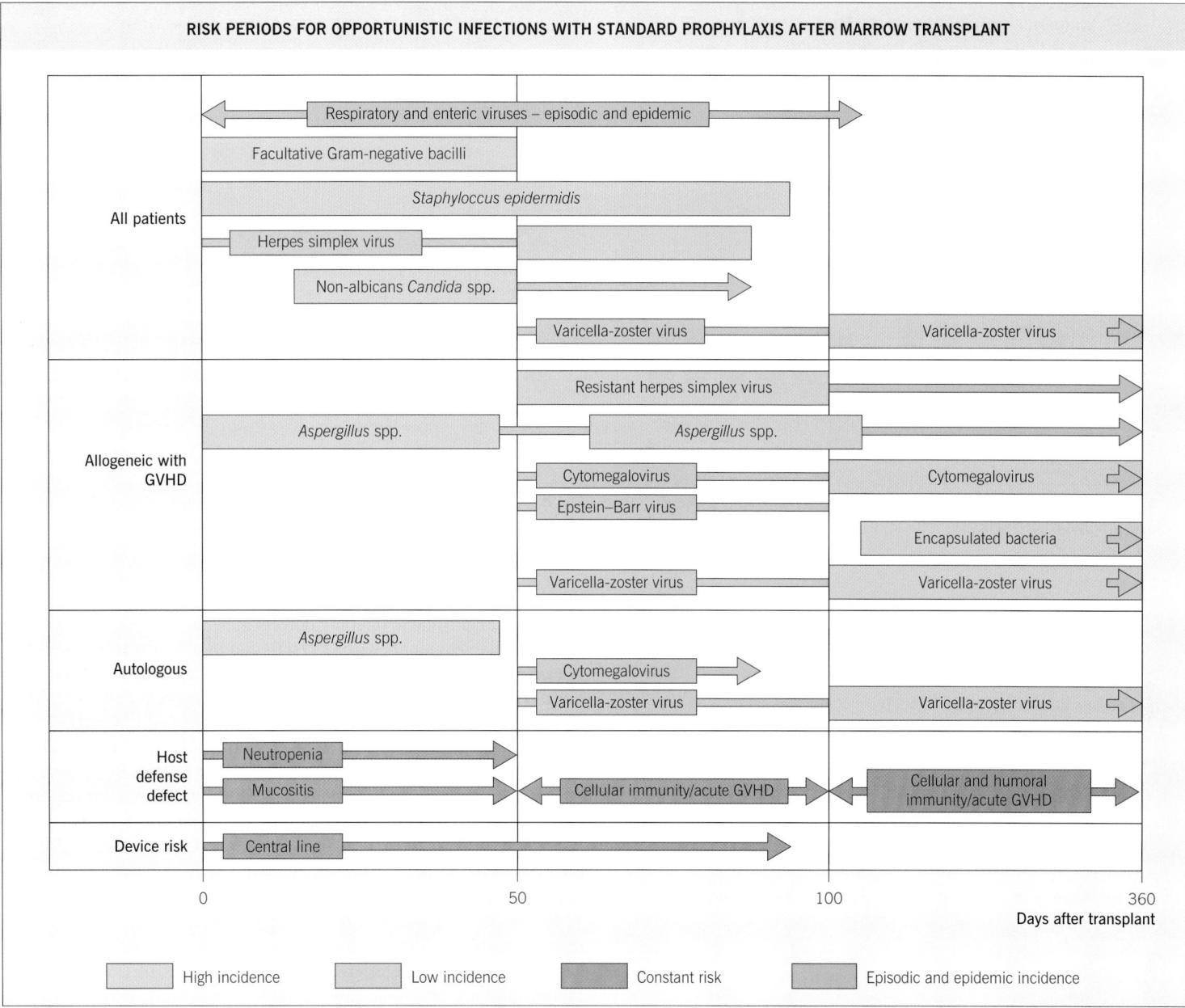

Fig. 4.3 Risk periods for opportunistic infections with standard prophylaxis after marrow transplant. Standard prophylaxis includes trimethoprim–sulfamethoxazole for *Pneumocystis carinii* pneumonia, screened or filtered blood and ganciclovir for cytomegalovirus, empiric antibiotics for febrile neutropenia, fluconazole for *Candida albicans*, and aciclovir for herpes simplex virus. GVHD, graft-versus-host disease.

PATHOGENESIS AND PATHOLOGY

Blood and marrow transplant results in a unique profile of infectious complications predictable by time after transplant. A major factor that determines the incidence, timing and severity of infection is the degree of HLA matching between the patient and the stem cell donor. In general, the risk for infectious complications is the lowest and has the shortest duration when the patient and the donor match exactly (i.e. in syngeneic transplant and autologous transplant settings). At the other end of the risk spectrum is the HLA-mismatched allogeneic family or unrelated donor–patient transplant setting, in which maximal immunosuppression may continue for an extended period of time and result in the highest risk for serious infection with the poorest outcome. Intermediate risk for infection exists for the patient with a matched family member stem cell donor. Despite advances in HLA-matching techniques and improved supportive care, the delayed and dysregulated immune reconstitution following transplant remains the main reason that infections continue to be the major cause of early

and late post-transplant morbidity and mortality. Both autologous transplantation and allogeneic transplantation from unrelated donors are being used increasingly for a variety of malignant and non-malignant conditions.

Whether transplantation is performed using stem cells from marrow or peripheral blood, and whether the stem cells come from the patient (autologous) or from a family member or an unrelated donor (allogeneic), all patients have two major defects in host defense function in the early post-transplant period. First, all patients have neutropenia of varying duration following conditioning chemotherapy or irradiation, although the period of neutropenia is relatively short in the autologous setting. Second, after recovery of peripheral blood cells, there is a period of abnormal T-lymphocyte function. In the allogeneic setting, the T-lymphocyte dysfunction is most apparent during the first 100 days after transplantation in patients without significant GVHD. Approximately one-third of patients experience chronic GVHD and in these patients T-lymphocyte dysfunction may be more severe and prolonged. Finally, other abnormalities in host defense, including

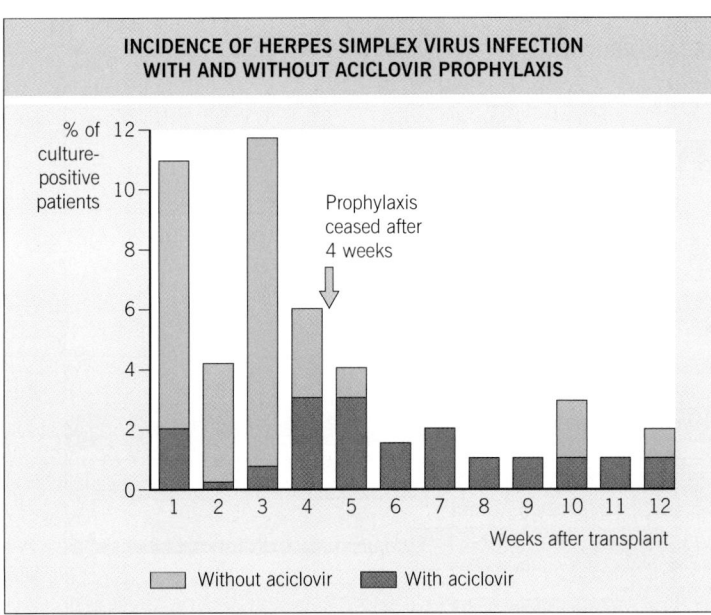

Fig. 4.4 **Incidence of herpes simplex virus infection with and without aciclovir prophylaxis.** The figures refer to the first positive culture after marrow transplant.

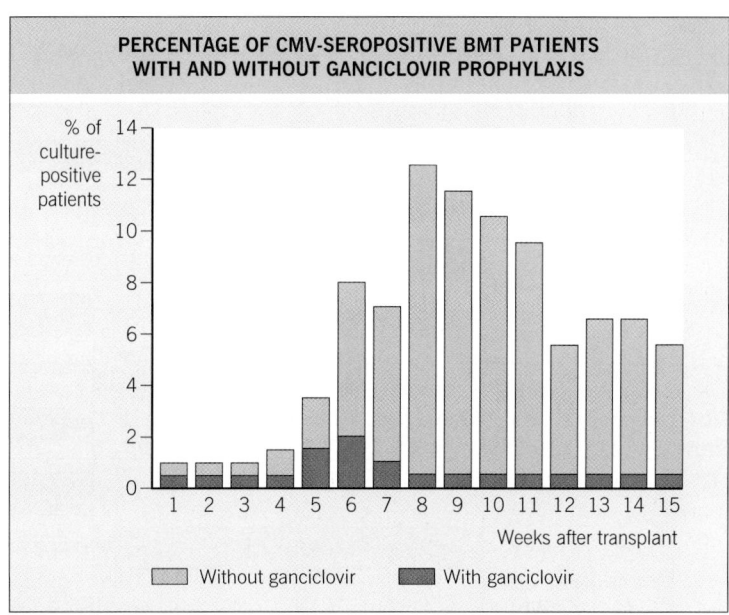

Fig. 4.5 **Percentage of cytomegalovirus-seropositive bone marrow transplant patients with and without ganciclovir prophylaxis.** The figures refer to positive blood culture by week after transplant.

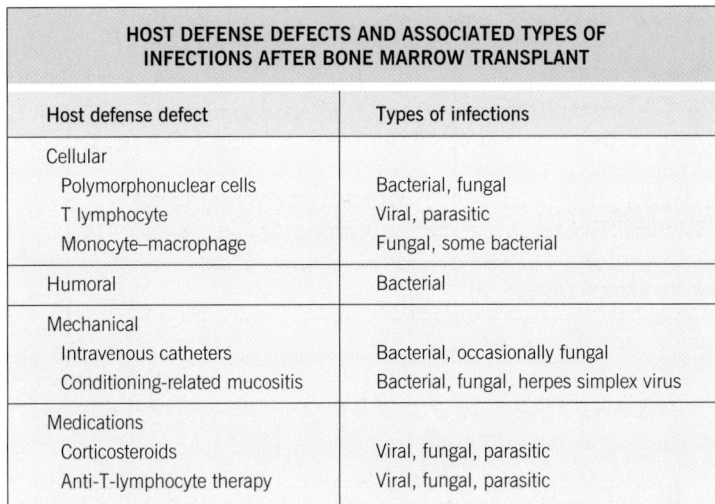

HOST DEFENSE DEFECTS AND ASSOCIATED TYPES OF INFECTIONS AFTER BONE MARROW TRANSPLANT	
Host defense defect	Types of infections
Cellular	
Polymorphonuclear cells	Bacterial, fungal
T lymphocyte	Viral, parasitic
Monocyte–macrophage	Fungal, some bacterial
Humoral	Bacterial
Mechanical	
Intravenous catheters	Bacterial, occasionally fungal
Conditioning-related mucositis	Bacterial, fungal, herpes simplex virus
Medications	
Corticosteroids	Viral, fungal, parasitic
Anti-T-lymphocyte therapy	Viral, fungal, parasitic

Fig. 4.6 **Host defense defects and associated types of infections after bone marrow transplant.**

dysfunction of humoral immunity and macrophage dysfunction, are most apparent in the late post-transplant period.

HOST DEFENSE DEFECTS ASSOCIATED WITH RISK FOR INFECTION

Specific host defense defects and associated infections can be divided into cellular, humoral, mechanical and medication-related defects (Fig. 4.6). All these defects are associated with increased risk for infection. In the early post-transplant period mechanical defects, including those caused by mucositis and central venous catheters, provide increased access for normal skin organisms and gastrointestinal mucosal flora to otherwise sterile body sites. The disruption in membrane barriers is further complicated by the common use of broad-spectrum antibiotics, which shifts the normal gastrointestinal flora, allowing overgrowth of potentially pathogenic organisms.

The continued importance of neutrophils for host defense against bacterial infection has been outlined above, and neutropenia is the single most important risk factor for bacterial infection, especially with Gram-negative organisms. Neutrophils are also critical for host defense against fungal infection in the early post-transplant period.

Following engraftment, ongoing defects in neutrophil phagocytic function continue in patients with GVHD[13] and in patients who are receiving corticosteroids, whether these have been used to ameliorate the toxic effects of the conditioning regimen or to prevent or treat GVHD. Graft versus host disease itself results in decreased chemotaxis and phagocytosis, whereas the use of corticosteroids for prevention or treatment of GVHD compounds the defects of GVHD by its interference with normal chemotaxis and phagocytosis. The risk for infection with encapsulated bacteria, including *Pseudomonas* spp., pneumococci and *Haemophilus influenzae* in patients with chronic GVHD after day 100 is also increased because phagocytic cell dysfunction persists in these patients.

Reconstituted T lymphocytes have abnormal function for a variety of reasons, including a requirement for re-exposure to specific viral antigens, which may be interfered with by the affects of GVHD and its treatment (corticosteroids, anti-T-lymphocyte therapy) and ganciclovir therapy for CMV.[14] T lymphocytes are critically important for the prevention of viral infection and for recovery from it, particularly herpes virus infection. Without ganciclovir prophylaxis, CMV continues to be a major problem in patients with GVHD. Recent studies that have documented the role of both CD4+ T helper lymphocytes and CD8+ cytotoxic T lymphocytes (CTLs) have now clearly demonstrated that defective CTL activity is associated with serious CMV infection and disease.[15] Ganciclovir therapy appears to delay recovery of function of CTLs, either by a direct effect on lymphocytes[16] or by limiting the amount of antigen exposure to lymphocytes.[14] This immunodeficiency can be reversed when CTLs are given adoptively.[3,17] From this work, it is apparent that adaptively transferred cells can be given safely and retain viral specificity that lasts for several months at least. Until this technology becomes routinely available, patients will need antiviral protection during the first 100 days after transplant. Following day 100, patients without GVHD and patients without normal CMV-specific T lymphocyte function may need ongoing prophylaxis.

The major defect in humoral immunity in the early period is the absence of specific antibody production. Patients receiving a matched sibling BMT show a transient drop in IgG levels below normal 3–4 months after transplant.[10] After several months, recovery to normal levels is seen in most patients. Patients undergoing autologous transplant may have a similar pattern but with faster recovery. Severe hypogammaglobulinemia, defined as IgG levels of less than 400mg/dl, may occur in patients with chronic GVHD and is associated with recurrent pneumococcal infections and obstructive lung disease.[18] Administration of intravenous immunoglobulin (IVIG) during the first 100 days (even to patients who are not hypogammaglobulinemic) reduces the number of bacterial infections between engraftment and day 100, evidence that humoral immunity is important for protection against bacterial infection during this period.[18]

The major defects in humoral immunity in the late risk period occur in patients with GVHD and include a reduction in the production of opsonizing antibody and a low level of production of all classes of IgG and IgA antibodies.[10] This immunodeficiency is further complicated by poor splenic function. These defects translate into an increased risk of encapsulated bacterial infection and an increased risk of infections in the sinuses and lungs, as mentioned above. For example, as many as 20–25% of patients who have received a transplant from an unrelated stem cell donor may be hypogammaglobulinemic, and this is associated with an increased risk of encapsulated bacterial infections, particularly sinopulmonary infection and otitis media.[18] This risk can be minimized by regular IVIG replacement. Intravenous immunoglobulin does not appear to be of benefit to patients with normal levels of IgG and IgA during the late period.

CHILDREN
Because pediatric patients are at lower risk for GVHD, they are probably also at somewhat lower risk for a variety of infectious complications. However, this reduced risk has not been well defined for a majority of infectious complications after transplant and the approach for children therefore remains similar to that for adults. One important difference, however, is that dosing regimens for many antibiotics in children differ from those in adults.

RECENT ADVANCES IN IMMUNE RECONSTITUTION
Most advances in the control of infection after BMT have resulted from careful studies of the application of anti-infective agents rather than by earlier or more effective immune reconstitution. One exception is the successful reconstitution of CMV-specific T lymphocytes that can be achieved through the use of adoptive immunotherapy associated with protection from CMV disease.[3] Such an approach is potentially very exciting and holds great promise for the future if it can be used in routine clinical practice. Furthermore, it has the potential of improving protection against other life-threatening infections. The use of growth factors, although shortening the duration of neutropenia, has not been associated with a reduction in the risk of serious infection or with an improvement in the outcome from serious infections. Major changes in host defenses in the post-transplant setting are related to the source of stem cells; however, the impact of these changes on incidence, timing and severity of infections is not clear at this time.

PREVENTION

One of the basic principles of infection control in the BMT setting is the prevention of infections. Treatment that is initiated once infection is well established is not as effective as prevention. Prevention of exposure to infectious agents is perhaps the most effective way of managing the infectious complications of transplantation, but this approach is not possible for all infections that occur after BMT. Prevention of exposure is particularly important for infections for which there is no effective treatment and for those where the currently available treatment has little impact on outcome (e.g. aspergillosis and community-acquired respiratory virus infections). Management of subclinical infection to prevent disease (pre-emptive therapy) is part of a continuum that includes prevention.

There are currently several infections for which prevention of exposure has been demonstrated to be clearly effective. One of the best examples is the use of CMV-safe blood products (serologically screened seronegative blood products[19] or filtered blood products[20]) to prevent transmission of CMV from blood by ensuring that CMV-seronegative

patients receive CMV-seronegative stem cells. Prevention of exposure reduces the risk of some other infections but does not completely eliminate it, so other means of prevention or treatment are needed. An example of this strategy is the use of antiviral suppressive therapy.

There are four approaches to the prevention of infection in the BMT setting:
- prevention of exposure;
- prevention of infection by the enhancement of host immune reconstitution, including the use of immunoglobulin, vaccination and growth factors;
- complete suppression of infection during the high-risk period with anti-infective chemotherapy; and
- pre-emptive therapy in subclinically infected patients who are identified as being at high risk of developing serious disease.

This last-mentioned, pre-emptive approach involves prevention of clinical disease rather than true prevention of infection. This section will deal specifically with those infections for which prevention of infection is the primary approach to management. The pre-emptive approach will be discussed in the section on treatment. Similarly, prevention of life-threatening bacterial infection during neutropenia includes both prophylaxis and early empiric therapy. Prophylaxis will be discussed here and empiric therapy will be discussed in the section on management.

PREVENTION OF BACTERIAL INFECTION
Because of the high mortality associated with bacterial infection during the neutropenic period, there are currently two approaches to the management of bacterial infection. The first involves the use of prophylactic systemic antibiotics, which are administered when the neutrophil count drops below 500/mm^3 regardless of fever. Antibiotics are continued until the neutrophil count recovers.[21] The other common approach is the use of empiric therapy, or therapy initiated with a first fever of 100.4°F (38°C) or more during neutropenia. Gastrointestinal decontamination, a popular means of prophylaxis in the past, is controversial and is no longer used in most centers.

PREVENTION OF VIRAL INFECTION
Herpes simplex virus
Because HSV infection occurs in 80% of seropositive recipients, prophylaxis with aciclovir (250mg/m^2 q12h intravenously[22] or 400mg q8h orally[23]) has become standard practice. Prophylaxis is initiated at the time of conditioning and continues until mucositis has diminished. Oral therapy is preferred for cost reasons whenever possible. Newer agents, including valaciclovir, may provide effective alternatives for prophylaxis but they have not been studied specifically in the BMT setting.

Varicella-zoster virus
Approximately 95% of VZV infection is a result of reactivation in the seropositive patient. Several studies have shown that infection can be effectively prevented with aciclovir. Six months of aciclovir has been shown to be too short for this purpose because it results in rebound infection between 6 months and 1 year, resulting in an infection rate by the end of the first year that is similar to that in patients who are given no prophylaxis.[24] If prophylaxis is continued for 1 year, such rebound infection is not observed, because by this time VZV-specific immunity has recovered despite antiviral therapy.[25] Controversy remains whether all patients should be given prophylaxis because only 40% of patients reactivate the virus during the first year and the majority of infections are localized and can be successfully managed once infection is identified.

Cytomegalovirus
There are now several successful strategies for preventing primary CMV infection in the seronegative autologous or allogeneic transplant patient. These strategies include the use of either screened blood[19] or filtered blood.[20] Both strategies have effectively reduced the incidence of CMV infection to 1–3% compared with an historic incidence of 40%, a rate that

will persist until more sensitive serologic screening methods are available to identify the seronegative recipient and for screening donor blood.

Respiratory viruses

The key to management of respiratory viruses in this setting is prevention. Strict attention to handwashing and careful isolation of patients is the best approach during the respiratory virus season. Special attention should be given to keeping family members and health care workers with upper respiratory infections away from patients. Vaccination of family members against influenza may help control exposure of the transplant recipient to this infection. Immunoglobulin prophylaxis with RSV-specific globulin has not been studied in the BMT setting. Amantidine or rimantidine prophylaxis may be useful during significant outbreaks; however, routine use should be avoided without further study because of side effects associated with therapy and the risk of rapid development of resistance.

PREVENTION OF INVASIVE FUNGAL INFECTIONS
Candidiasis and aspergillosis

The standard approach to the prevention of invasive fungal infections includes both prophylaxis and the use of empiric therapy for persistent febrile neutropenia in patients already on broad-spectrum antibiotics. The only effective preventative therapy that has been demonstrated by definitive studies is fluconazole prophylaxis for invasive candidiasis, particularly when caused by *Candida albicans*.[26,27] It is given from the time of conditioning until either engraftment[27] or until day 75;[26] the latter strategy has been associated with improved survival. Fluconazole does not protect against *Candida krusei*, which is innately resistant to fluconazole and breakthrough infections with *C. glabrata* and *C. parapsilosis* occur.

Fluconazole prophylaxis has now been well established as being of benefit in prevention of invasive fungal infection after allogeneic transplant. It is less clear whether it should be used after autologous transplantation because of the lower risk of invasive fungal infection as well as the relatively shorter period of risk. However, autologous patients undergoing conditioning regimens that are associated with significant mucositis may benefit from fluconazole prophylaxis during the neutropenic period.

There are currently no proven effective means of preventing invasive aspergillosis. There is a clear need for prospectively controlled studies to help determine the most effective strategies for prevention and treatment of aspergillosis in the BMT setting. Much of the data that guide therapy in this area come from historically controlled studies that are difficult to interpret because the incidence of aspergillosis varies from year to year and from institution to institution.

The use of low-dose amphotericin B for prevention of candidiasis and aspergillosis has been reported but none of the studies is prospectively controlled in the higher-risk allogeneic setting.[28,29] Furthermore, these studies have not clearly demonstrated that low-dose amphotericin B is necessarily associated with fewer infusion-related problems or nephrotoxicity. Other strategies for the prevention of aspergillosis, including the use of nasal spray and aerosolized amphotericin B, are descriptive only and concurrently controlled studies have not been done.

Pneumocystis carinii

The incidence of *P. carinii* infection has been reduced since the availability of effective prophylaxis with trimethoprim–sulfamethoxazole. This drug is generally administered as one double-strength tablet q12h, 2 days a week. Most patients with a history of sulfa allergies can be safely given trimethoprim (160mg), sulfamethoxazole (800mg) prophylaxis after desensitization.[30] An alternative for patients with refractory allergies is dapsone.

VACCINATION AND IMMUNOGLOBULIN REPLACEMENT
Vaccination

Patients undergoing BMT eventually lose immunity to the common childhood diseases and should be re-immunized between the first and second year after transplant, when their recovering immune system can respond to such vaccination. Data support the reimmunization of allogeneic transplant patients to polio at 1 year, using inactivated intramuscular vaccine,[31] and vaccination to mumps, measles and rubella at 2 years in patients without GVHD or in patients who have discontinued all GVHD therapy.[32]

In general, although autologous transplant patients are less immunosuppressed than allogeneic transplant patients, the differences in the ability to maintain sufficient immune responses are minimal between the two groups,[33,34] and thus a rationale could be made for treating them on a similar immunization schedule. The recommendations for bacterial vaccination are less clear, because patients who need protection (i.e. patients with chronic GVHD) are the least likely to respond. However, it has become standard practice to administer pneumococcal[35] and *H. influenzae* type b conjugate vaccine[36] to such patients at 1 year and again at 2 years after transplant. Vaccination with the live-attenuated VZV vaccine is contraindicated without careful study to demonstrate safety in the BMT setting. Susceptible family members, however, should receive VZV vaccine.

Replacement immunoglobulin

Patients undergoing allogeneic transplantation, particularly those undergoing unrelated donor transplantation or those with chronic GVHD who develop severe hypogammaglobulinemia, are at particularly high risk for bacterial infection after transplant.[10] Replacement intravenous immunoglobulin (IVIG) (200–500mg/kg every 1–2 weeks) is recommended for allogeneic transplant recipients with low immunoglobulin levels, which is defined as serum IgG levels less than 400mg/dl at day 90. Intravenous immunoglobulin has been studied for prevention of both early infections before day 90[37] as well as late infections occurring between day 90 and the end of the first year after BMT;[38] a difference in reduced rates of sepsis and localized infection when IVIG replacement is given was only observed in the early period after transplant.[37]

The role of hyperimmune globulin in the prevention of specific infections is less clear. The most thoroughly studied has been the use of high-titer CMV immunoglobulin for prevention of CMV infection and disease. The results of multiple controlled studies in the 1980s gave inconsistent results, although meta-analyses performed subsequently have suggested that it does have a role in the prevention of both CMV infection and CMV disease. The more recent availability of effective antiviral drugs have been shown to provide more complete protection against CMV disease. Better protection afforded by antiviral drugs as well as cost considerations have led to a decrease in the use of CMV immunoglobulin in many BMT centers. Hyperimmune RSV immunoglobulin is now available but has not yet been studied in the BMT setting for treatment or prevention. Virus-specific monoclonal antibodies as preventative therapy for both RSV and CMV are currently under investigation in the BMT setting.

SUMMARY OF PROGRESS IN THE PAST DECADE

Major progress has been made in the prevention of early CMV disease. Unfortunately, this has led to a shift in CMV disease to the later post-transplant period, which is a particular problem for patients with ongoing immunodeficiency from GVHD or its therapy. Better means of prevention are urgently needed for late-onset CMV disease, respiratory virus infections and aspergillosis, which continue to be major causes of morbidity and mortality in transplant patients.

CLINICAL FEATURES

BACTEREMIA

Bacteremia is the single most common cause of documented bacterial infection after transplant. Approximately 60% of episodes of febrile neutropenia in the early period following BMT are associated with documented infection, one-third of those being bacteremias.[39,40] A patient with bacteremia typically presents with fever but often without other focal signs of infection. However, patients receiving corticosteroids for prevention or treatment of treatment-related toxicity or GVHD may develop bacteremia yet remain afebrile. Risk factors for bacterial infection in this setting include the type of underlying malignancy or marrow dysplasia, the intensity of chemotherapy, the degree of neutropenia, a prior history of bacterial infection, the presence of colonizing organisms or intravenous catheters and the use of prophylactic antibiotics. A shift in the spectrum of organisms has occurred in the past decade. In the 1970s, bacteremia in the marrow transplant and neutropenic cancer patients was most frequently caused by Gram-negative organisms.[41,42] Gram-positive organisms now account for approximately 60% of documented cases of bacteremia infections in these clinical settings.[41,43]

Possible reasons for this shift include the use of indwelling catheters, mucositis associated with intensive conditioning therapy and the use of prophylactic antibiotics, especially the newer generation cephalosporins and quinolones. Although the skin flora is traditionally thought to be the primary source of these organisms, recent data suggest that the gastrointestinal tract may also be a significant reservoir. *Staphylococcus epidermidis* remains the most common species identified from blood. However, streptococcal species, including *Streptococcus pyogenes* and *S. mitis*, as well as *Enterococcus* spp., have emerged as important causes of bacteremia in some centers.[44] The incidence of *Pseudomonas* spp. has decreased substantially in many centers in recent years, presumably because of more effective antibiotics used for empiric therapy. However, other Gram-negative organisms continue to be frequent causes of bacteremia.

Although bacteremia has historically occurred during the neutropenic period, a substantial number of bacteremias, particularly with coagulase-negative staphylococci, occur following engraftment and continue to occur as long as central intravenous catheters remain in place. Figure 4.2 shows the incidence of Gram-positive blood cultures by day after transplant from a review of all positive blood cultures between 1991 and 1993.[9] More than 60% of all infections occurred after engraftment. The risk of bacteremia decreases during the first 2 months after transplant, except in patients with continuing immunosuppression due to GVHD or its therapy, or in patients who develop recurrent neutropenia secondary to graft failure or drug-related marrow suppression (e.g. induced by ganciclovir).

In patients who have chronic GVHD, the risk of infection with encapsulated organisms persists. Recent studies of late infection after marrow transplant have shown that patients with unrelated matched sibling donors have twice the incidence of bacteremia or sepsis than HLA-matched donors do.[11] A similar increase in late infections was found in patients with unrelated donors compared with patients whose donors were family members.[12] Patients with unrelated donors are at increased risk of late infections, even in the absence of GVHD.[12]

SINUSITIS

Sinusitis is the most common localized infection more than 100 days after transplantation; it accounts for nearly 50% of all late infections.[18] A diagnosis of sinusitis before day 100 is quite common, although the exact incidence, etiology and natural history have not been well described. This is due in part to the fact that sinus abnormalities, particularly sinus thickening, on radiographic examination are quite common and often occur with or without typical clinical symptoms and may be temporally related to the occurrence of mucositis at other sites related to the conditioning regimen. Furthermore, because evaluation of the sinuses often involves an invasive procedure, the sinuses are often not specifically cultured and thus the true incidence of infectious sinusitis is likely to be under-appreciated. Interpretation of cultures from sinus aspirates is also difficult.

PNEUMONIA

Pneumonia continues to be a common problem after marrow transplant.[45] Most patients who develop pneumonia have typical associated signs and symptoms (i.e. cough, shortness of breath) associated with diffuse or focal findings on chest X-ray. Most viral pneumonias, including CMV and respiratory viruses, cause diffuse interstitial changes; however, focal changes early in the course of infection are also seen. The unreliability of radiographic characteristics for predicting the cause of pneumonia cannot be overemphasized (Fig. 4.7).

In the 1970s and 1980s, 40–60% of patients undergoing marrow transplant experienced pneumonia during the first 100 days after transplant.[46] The most common types of pneumonia included idiopathic interstitial pneumonia, more recently renamed idiopathic pneumonia syndrome[47] and CMV pneumonia. Less frequent types of pneumonias included *P. carinii* pneumonia, bacterial pneumonia, community-acquired respiratory virus pneumonia and fungal pneumonia. In general, the spectrum of pneumonia has not changed appreciably with the introduction of peripheral blood as a stem cell source. The most common types of pneumonia seen today are bacterial or fungal pneumonia, and in some centers, respiratory viral pneumonia. CMV pneumonia now occurs in less than 5% of patients during the first three months after transplant.

Idiopathic pneumonia syndrome is a noninfectious syndrome that is characterized clinically by diffuse interstitial infiltrates and varying degrees of respiratory failure. It is thought to be related to the chemotherapy or total body irradiation used as part of the conditioning regimen.[48] Idiopathic pneumonia syndrome occurs in 12–17% of patients,[49,50] has an equal frequency after autologous and allogeneic

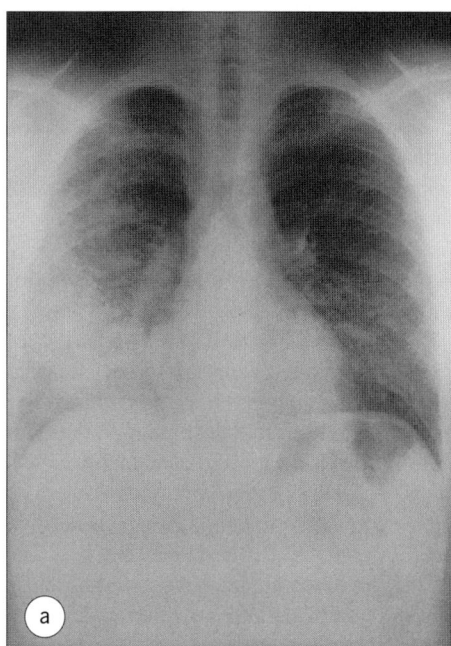

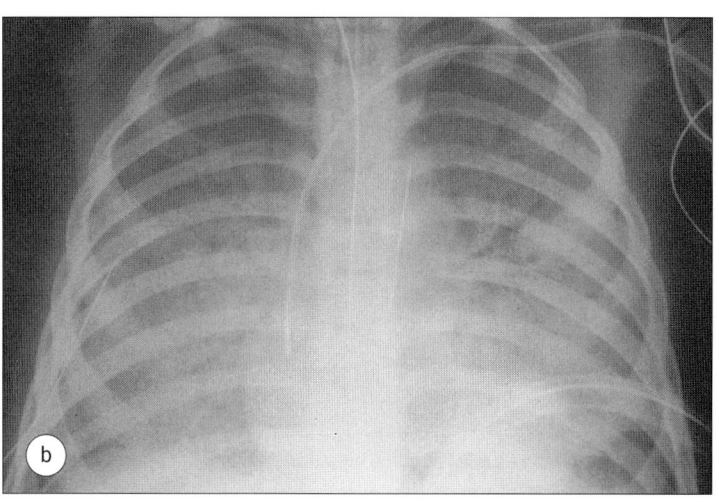

Fig. 4.7 Pneumonia after marrow transplant. (a) Radiograph from a patient at 12 hours after the onset of shortness of breath, fever and cough. The pneumonia appears to be lobar in nature, which is suggestive of a bacterial process. (b) A repeat radiograph 24 hours after the onset of symptoms and shortly before the patient required intubation revealed the diffuse interstitial changes typically associated with CMV pneumonia. Bronchoalveolar lavage confirmed the diagnosis of CMV in this case.

transplantation and is associated with a mortality rate of 60–80%. Idiopathic pneumonia syndrome occurs classically in two peaks, one early (in the first few weeks after transplant) and one late (in the second and third month after transplant).[49]

Pulmonary complications during the first month after transplant include bacterial pneumonia and noninfectious causes such as pulmonary edema, hemorrhage, adult respiratory distress syndrome and idiopathic pneumonia syndrome. Cytomegalovirus pneumonia is distinctly unusual before engraftment.[51] Community-acquired respiratory viral pneumonia can occur with increased frequency pre-engraftment during the respiratory virus season. Following engraftment, bacterial pneumonia is seen less commonly. Viral pneumonia, notably caused by CMV and fungi, particularly *Aspergillus* spp., are major problems during the early postengraftment period.

Bacteria remain a common cause of pneumonia in the late post-transplant period in allogeneic transplant patients who have chronic GVHD. Patients who have chronic GVHD have a 59% risk of pulmonary infection in the late risk period compared with a 3% risk in patients receiving autologous PBSC.[11] Pneumonia is often associated with chronic obstructive pulmonary disease in which lung histopathology shows obliterative bronchitis.[52] The etiology and pathogenesis of obliterative bronchitis is not well understood. Approximately 50% of late pneumonias are due to noninfectious interstitial pneumonitis.[49,50]

Respiratory viruses are increasingly becoming recognized as a cause of pneumonia. They are associated with high morbidity and mortality.[7,53] Before 1988, little had been described about the incidence and role of respiratory viruses following marrow transplantation. It is now known that up to 15% of patients may become infected during the winter months.[54,55] The most common causes of respiratory viruses by frequency include RSV, parainfluenza virus, rhinovirus and influenza virus;[54] RSV[56] and parainfluenza[57] virus are associated with the highest incidence of progression to pneumonia among infected patients and the highest mortality after BMT.

Patients with respiratory virus infection typically present first with upper respiratory infection symptoms, fever or both. Respiratory syncytial virus infection progresses to pneumonia in approximately 50% of patients with upper respiratory tract infection, whereas parainfluenza virus causes pneumonia in approximately 22% (Fig. 4.8). The role of rhinovirus has not been well described. In a recent review of more than 30 consecutive isolates, only one with rhinovirus was from a bronchoalveolar specimen from the lower respiratory tract.[54] The mortality with RSV infection remains 80% despite therapy with aerosolized ribavirin;[56] the mortality for parainfluenza pneumonia is 32%.[57] Influenza, of which the incidence of type A far exceeds that of type B, infrequently progresses to pneumonia,[7] although little data

exist as to the exact progression rate. Patients who develop respiratory virus pneumonia before engraftment have poorer outcomes.[7,53]

Another infrequent cause of pneumonia following BMT is *P. carinii*. Prophylactic trimethoprim–sulfamethoxazole or alternative agents are successful in preventing *P. carinii* pneumonia in most cases. The role of other community-acquired agents such as *Chlamydia* or *Mycoplasma* spp. in the etiology of pneumonia has not been defined in the BMT setting.

ACUTE ABDOMINAL PAIN AND GASTROINTESTINAL INFECTION

Diarrhea and abdominal pain are frequent complaints in the early post-transplant setting. However, they are rarely caused by infection. In a recent review, diarrheal specimens were cultured for a variety of infectious agents but an infectious agent was identified in only 10% of samples.[58] In this study, the most common infectious agents identified were *C. difficile*, adenovirus and CMV. *Clostridium difficile* is becoming an increasing problem because of its high rate of nosocomial transmission: up to 20% of hospitalized patients may be colonized with *C. difficile*.[59] It is not clear what the pattern of transmission is in the BMT setting, because no prospective studies have been reported in this patient population.

Clostridium difficile is being seen with increasing frequency; presumably this is associated with prolonged parenteral antibiotic therapy. The epidemiology of *C. difficile* infection following BMT has not been well defined and most of the available data describe the incidence only in toxin-positive patients, rather than culture-positive patients. Recent data suggest that the culture-positive rate, including asymptomatic carriage, may be as high as 60% in nontransplant patients in a hospital setting.[59] Outbreaks of diarrhea have also been associated with a variety of agents, including *Cryptosporidium*[60] and enterovirus spp.,[61] but overall these agents are rare causes of gastrointestinal infection following transplant. Diarrhea is most commonly associated with noninfectious causes, including GVHD, in which the diarrhea is usually bloody and associated with crampy abdominal pain, and treatment-related toxicity; diarrhea is especially common with busulfan conditioning therapy. Rotavirus is an extremely uncommon cause of diarrhea in this setting, accounting for less than 1% of all thoroughly investigated cases of diarrhea.[58]

Another less common cause of acute abdominal pain associated with infection is abdominal VZV. The diagnosis of this presentation of VZV is often delayed until the infection is quite advanced because the abdominal pain, which is often associated with hepatitis, may precede the appearance of skin lesions by several days.[62] The typical presentation of abdominal VZV occurs in patients with GVHD on corticosteroids several months after transplant and is characterized by severe acute abdominal pain with few other symptoms. The mortality rate is quite high, often related to a delayed diagnosis. A high index of suspicion and early institution of aciclovir may be lifesaving.

Hepatitis is a frequent complication following marrow transplant, but viral hepatitis is relatively uncommon, except in patients with a known history of or exposure to hepatitis B or C viruses (see Chapter 2.39). Infectious hepatitis must be distinguished from several common noninfectious causes, including veno-occlusive disease related to the conditioning regimen, GVHD and chemical hepatitis related either to drugs or to hyperalimentation.

SKIN INFECTION

Although skin rashes following BMT are common, skin infections as a cause of rashes are uncommon. One common cause of skin rash includes the skin changes associated with conditioning therapy (i.e. sudden onset of marked erythema over large areas of the body, often associated with blistering on the hands and feet). Other common noninfectious causes of skin rashes include skin GVHD and drug eruptions associated with antibiotics or other drugs used in this setting. A skin biopsy can be invaluable in distinguishing infectious from noninfectious causes of skin changes.

The most frequent infections that involve the skin include:

Virus	Total number of cases	Upper respiratory tract (nose, pharynx, trachea) (%)	Sputum (%)	Lower respiratory tract (bronchoalveolar lavage) (%)
Respiratory syncytial	47	24 (51)		23 (49)
Parainfluenza				
Type 1	18	6 (33)	8 (45)	4 (22)
Type 2	3	2 (66)		1 (33)
Type 3	51	40 (78)		11 (22)
Influenza				
Type A	17	16 (94)	1 (6)	
Type B	4	3 (75)	1 (25)	
Rhinovirus	29	28 (97)	1 (3)	

SITE OF COMMUNITY-ACQUIRED RESPIRATORY VIRUS ISOLATION AFTER MARROW TRANSPLANT

Fig. 4.8 Site of community-acquired respiratory virus isolation after marrow transplant.

- VZV,
- catheter-related exit site or tunnel infections,
- superficial dermatophyte infections, which are particularly common in the perineal area, and
- skin involvement with disseminated bacterial or fungal infections.

Focal areas of bacterial cellulitis are distinctly uncommon.

CATHETER-RELATED EXIT SITE AND TUNNEL INFECTIONS

Infections of the bloodstream associated with intravenous catheters are common and occur in up to 50% of patients during the first 100 days after transplant. The most common causative organisms are Gram-positive bacteria, followed in frequency by Gram-negative bacteria and atypical *Mycobacteria* spp.

In the absence of bacteremia, most exit site infections can be managed with local skin care unless the erythema extends for more than 1–2 cm up the catheter from the exit site. The most common cause of exit site and line tunnel infections are Gram-positive cocci. Other causes include Gram-negative infections and, less commonly, atypical mycobacterial infection. Atypical mycobacterial tunnel infections, although infrequent, are particularly important because their diagnosis requires a strong index of suspicion. An acid-fast stain as part of the initial microbiologic evaluation is needed for their diagnosis. The usual causes of mycobacterial tunnel infections are the rapid growing atypical mycobacterial organisms of which *Mycobacterium chelonei* and *M. fortuitum* are among the most common.[63] Management of atypical mycobacterial tunnel infection always involves removal of the line and surgical excision of the tunnel tract. This aggressive approach is generally not required with infections caused by other organisms when the patient responds to initial antibiotic management.

VIRAL INFECTIONS

Cytomegalovirus

Dramatic progress has been made in the past decade in the control of CMV infection with prophylactic and pre-emptive ganciclovir therapy. Knowledge of the risk for CMV provides the rationale for providing antiviral protection during the early post-BMT period. In the absence of antiviral prophylaxis, CMV reactivation and infection will occur in 80% of patients who were CMV seropositive prior to transplant and in 40% of seronegative patients, either because of the use of unscreened blood products or seropositive stem cells.[8,9] In the absence of antiviral prophylaxis, the median time of onset is approximately day 62 after BMT. Cytomegalovirus disease prior to engraftment is rare.[51] Cytomegalovirus disease, of which CMV pneumonitis or gastroenteritis are the most common manifestations, occurs in 35% of patients who develop CMV infection during the first 100 days after transplant.[64] Cytomegalovirus gastroenteritis is characterized by anorexia and nausea and sometimes by diarrhea. It is often associated with GVHD of the gastrointestinal tract. The diagnosis is made by endoscopy.

Until the 1990s, CMV pneumonia was the leading cause of death from infection in the first 100 days after transplant, occurring in up to 35% of CMV-seropositive allogeneic patients[64] and in 2–7% of autologous patients.[65,66] Some autologous patients, such as those undergoing autologous transplant for breast cancer, may be at substantially lower risk for CMV pneumonia[67] such that ganciclovir prophylaxis cannot be justified. Cytomegalovirus pneumonia now occurs in less than 5% of CMV-seropositive allogeneic patients who receive ganciclovir prophylaxis during the first 100 days.[66] Recently, however, a shift in the onset of CMV pneumonia to the later post-transplant period has become apparent in patients who receive early ganciclovir prophylaxis or pre-emptive therapy[68,69] (see Fig. 4.3). Currently, late CMV disease accounts for 75% of all CMV disease during the first year after allogeneic transplantation.

Progress has been made since 1986 in the reduction of CMV disease by the introduction of ganciclovir prophylaxis during the first 100 days (see Fig. 4.5), but this reduction has been accompanied by the emergence of late CMV disease (Fig. 4.9). Despite an initial apparent improvement in survival in reports where ganciclovir was combined

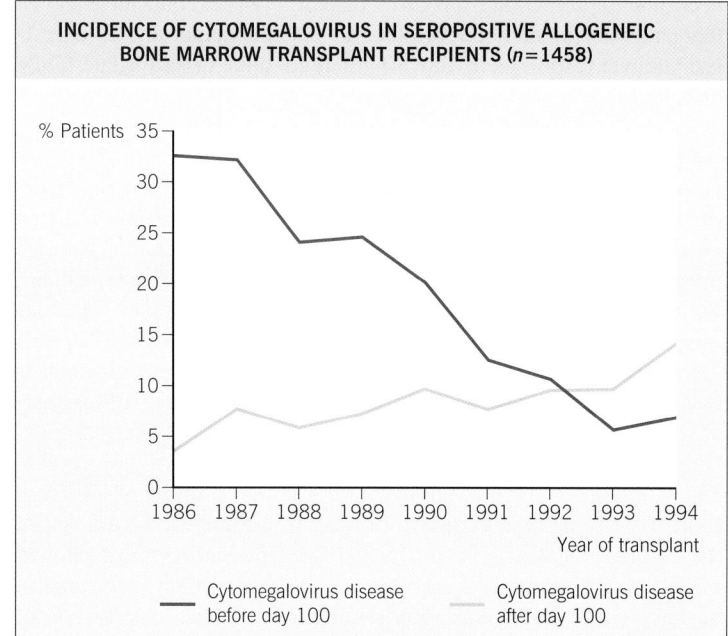

Fig. 4.9 **Incidence of cytomegalovirus disease in seropositive allogeneic bone marrow transplant recipients.** The data are from the Fred Hutchinson Cancer Research Center by year of transplant.

Manifestation	Total number (%) of patients
CLINICAL MANIFESTATIONS OF LATE CYTOMEGALOVIRUS DISEASE	
Pneumonia	122 (62.9)
Pneumonia only	110
Pneumonia associated with disseminated disease	12
Gastrointestinal disease	50 (25.8)
Retinitis	10 (5.2)
Retinitis only	8
Retinitis associated with disseminated disease	2
Graft failure	5 (2.6)
Hepatitis	4 (2.1)
Sinusitis	3 (1.5)
Total	194

Fig. 4.10 **Clinical manifestations of late cytomegalovirus disease.**

with IVIG for treatment,[70,71] outcome remains poor for patients with CMV pneumonia. Approximately 70% have a fatal outcome despite combined therapy with ganciclovir and IVIG and regardless of whether CMV pneumonia occurs before or after day 100.[2]

Once the leading cause of death from infection after allogeneic transplant, pre-emptive and prophylactic strategies with ganciclovir have reduced the incidence of CMV disease in seropositive allogeneic patients from 35%[64] to approximately 5% in the first 100 days after transplant.[69] Figure 4.5 compares the timing of first positive culture in patients receiving routine surveillance before ganciclovir prophylaxis was routine and since its use has become standard.

The decrease in early CMV disease that has accompanied the use of ganciclovir prophylaxis has been accompanied by a shift of CMV disease to the late post-transplant period[2] (Fig. 4.10). As with the other herpesviruses, development of a CMV-specific immune response is critical to protection from CMV disease.[17] Recent data have shown that patients who do not develop CMV-specific helper or cytotoxic T-lymphocyte responses by day 80 are at continued risk for late CMV disease.[2]

Herpes simplex virus

Herpes simplex virus infection is a common problem in HSV-seropositive patients if they do not receive aciclovir prophylaxis. Of seropositive patients 80% are at risk for HSV infection. The large majority of infections occur during the first 50 days after transplant, with a peak incidence between 2–3 weeks after transplant.[72] In contrast, less than 1% of HSV-seronegative patients excrete HSV following transplant, suggesting that HSV infection after transplant is due almost exclusively to reactivation of latent virus.[72] Before aciclovir was available, mouth lesions caused by HSV were common (Fig. 4.11), but this clinical presentation is now totally preventable and is no longer seen in centers where aciclovir prophylaxis is given routinely for the first 30 days following transplant. In the era before the availability of aciclovir, only 10% of patients who developed infection did so more than 6 weeks after transplant, presumably because earlier HSV infection stimulated immune reconstitution. The use of aciclovir prophylaxis delays the reconstitution of T-lymphocyte immunity[73] and this knowledge has resulted in the clinical practice of allowing patients to tolerate a mild reactivation after day 30 without treatment.

With aciclovir prophylaxis, the overall incidence and morbidity of HSV mucositis has been substantially reduced (see Fig. 4.4). A recent unpublished review of data in over 1500 consecutive HSV-seropositive marrow transplant patients at the Fred Hutchinson Cancer Research Center showed 370 infections (25%) in the first 100 days after transplant. The median time of onset of first excretion was 52 days (range 0–90 days). The majority of infections were confined to the oropharynx, although occasionally the infection extended directly to the esophagus or lungs, or by autoinoculation to adjacent skin areas of the face. Rarely, the infection disseminates to involve distal skin areas, the central nervous system (CNS), or visceral organs.

Varicella-zoster virus

Infection with VZV occurs in approximately 30–50% of adults and 25% of children who receive no antiviral prophylaxis during the first year after transplant.[74–77] The majority of VZV infections occur after the first 100 days after transplant, with only 15% of infections in the early post-transplant period. The median time of onset is 5 months after transplant.[75] Risk factors for VZV infection are similar to those for other herpesviruses; they include GVHD, allogeneic transplantation and transplantation for treatment of hematologic malignancies other than chronic myelogenous leukemia.[74,75]

Varicella-zoster virus infections present as localized, dermatomal zoster in 85% of patients. Although VZV can present with the typical dermatomal vesicles where bedside diagnosis is easy, it can often present atypically such that laboratory confirmation is essential. Approximately 16% of patients present with dissemination, sometimes referred to as varicelliform zoster, which involves visceral organs in 40–50% of these patients.[75,76] Graft-versus-host-disease is a strong predictor of VZV dissemination.[75] The fatality rate for untreated VZV infection is 35% during the first year after transplant.[75] The patients for whom VZV infection is most likely to be fatal are those who present with disseminated zoster or abdominal zoster,[62] or those who have GVHD and are started on suboptimal doses of aciclovir or in whom therapy is initiated relatively late.

The risk of acquiring a second primary VZV infection in patients who are already VZV-seropositive is unknown; this is undoubtedly very rare, although it has been reported. Therefore, the major risk of primary VZV is in patients who have never had VZV infection before transplant.

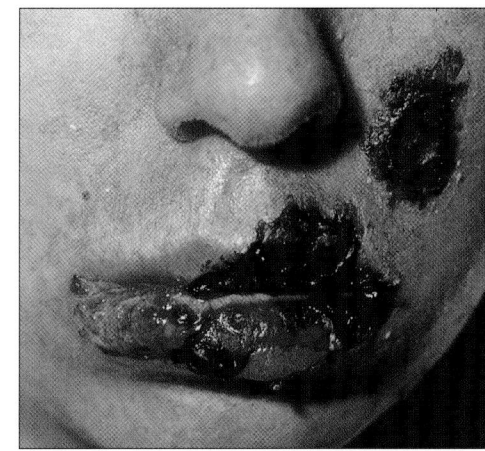

Fig. 4.11 Oral and facial lesions caused by herpes simplex virus. These lesions occurred 14 days after allogeneic transplant and are typical of those that used to occur in the era before aciclovir was available. This clinical presentation is now totally preventable.

Adenovirus

Adenovirus infection occurs in approximately 5% of patients in the allogeneic transplant setting.[78] Because adenovirus becomes latent and because chronic shedding in the absence of clinical disease can occur in the normal host, it is likely that many of the infections observed in the post-BMT period result from reactivation. However, adenovirus can also be acquired from respiratory droplet transmission and the role of this route of infection compared with reactivation of latent virus is not known.[78,79]

Support for reactivation as the major source of infection comes from the lack of observed seasonality and the timing of infection, which is similar to that of CMV in the BMT setting. Infection with adenovirus occurs a mean of 44 days after transplant (range 13–199 days).[78] These figures have not changed with the recent introduction of antiviral agents that are effective against the herpesviruses. Graft-versus-host disease is an important risk factor for adenovirus infection after BMT.[78] Adenovirus is also known to be associated with hemorrhagic cystitis.[80] Systemic infection occurs in less than 20% of patients infected with adenovirus, but when it does occur the most common sites of infection are the lung, liver and kidney.[78,80,81] Infections have been reported to occur in as many as 18% of children.[81]

Other viral infections

There are several other viral infections that are either less frequent or whose role in the post-BMT setting remains ill-defined. Epstein–Barr virus (EBV) is a ubiquitous DNA virus that belongs to the herpesvirus group; it is known to cause a lymphoproliferative disorder associated with the ongoing use of anti-T lymphocyte immunosuppressive therapy following BMT as well as solid organ transplantation. The role of EBV in hepatitis and fever following BMT has not been defined. Human herpesvirus type 6 (HHV-6) is another ubiquitous DNA virus first associated with marrow failure[82] and possibly pneumonitis.[83] Human herpesvirus type 6 appears to reactivate commonly in the early post-BMT setting; reactivation can be demonstrated in 46% of patients by culture and in 27% by seroconversion.[84] As many as 100% patients will be positive for HHV-6 when tested for increased levels of HHV-6 DNA by polymerase chain reaction (PCR) in the blood.[83] Most strains of HHV-6 identified in blood and urine after BMT appear to be the B variant, but a mixture of A and B have been reported in the lung.[83] The correlation of symptoms with HHV-6 infection remains ill-defined in the BMT setting.

Parvovirus B19 is a rare diagnostic consideration following BMT, as are BK virus and JC virus (both polyoma viruses). Parvovirus B19 is commonly associated with aplastic crises outside the marrow transplant setting and is the causative agent of erythema infectiosum in nontransplanted children. Only case reports of infection exist in the BMT setting.[85] BK virus causes mild respiratory infection in children. It has been detected in the urine following BMT and has been reported to occur in up to 44% of patients without obvious associated clinical symptoms.[86] It has been associated with hepatic dysfunction.[87] JC virus, a cause of multifocal leukoencephalopathy, has been found in the urine of patients following BMT.[88] There are currently no specific therapies other than supportive care for any of these more unusual viruses.

FUNGAL INFECTIONS

Invasive fungal infections are increasingly realized to be a significant cause of morbidity and mortality as better prevention of life-threatening CMV disease has been developed. The major causes of invasive fungal disease include *Candida* spp., *Aspergillus* spp. and (less frequently) molds other than *Aspergillus*.

Candidiasis

Risk factors for invasive candidiasis include neutropenia,[89] mucositis, and the use of broad spectrum antibiotics[90] and corticosteroids.[91] The dust from building works and the drier months of the year are particular risks for aspergillosis.[6] Patients undergoing allogeneic transplantation are 10 times as likely to have an invasive fungal infection as patients receiving an autologous graft.[88]

Candidiasis generally occurs in the early post-transplant period, with a median onset of 3 weeks after transplant.[92] Recently, with more widespread use of fluconazole prophylaxis, there has been a shift in the types of *Candida* spp. causing invasive fungal disease. Before fluconazole was available, *C. albicans* and *C. tropicalis* predominated as the causes of candidiasis;[93] now, however, invasive fungal disease due to *C. krusei*, *C. glabrata* and *C. parapsilosis* is increasing.[94] This shift may not be entirely due to fluconazole, because it is also being observed in centers where fluconazole is not being used.[94]

Candidiasis is acquired from species colonizing the gastrointestinal tract, the risk of which is increased by a combination of neutropenia, breakdown of the normal mucosal barrier due to conditioning therapy, and overgrowth of *Candida* spp. associated with the use of broad-spectrum antibiotics. The most common manifestations of candidiasis include fungemia and visceral candidiasis. Because the primary site of entry of *Candida* spp. from the gastrointestinal tract is through the portal circulation, it is no surprise that the liver, spleen and kidney are the most commonly involved visceral organs. Disease above the diaphragm, including pneumonia and CNS infection, is uncommon. When candidal pneumonia does develop, it is usually in the setting of fungemia and presents as a diffuse miliary pattern on chest radiograph. *Candida* spp. are second in frequency to *Aspergillus* spp. as the cause of CNS infection following BMT.[95]

Aspergillosis

Aspergillosis has become the leading cause of death from infection during the first 100 days after transplant.[4,5] Aspergillosis occurs in a bimodal pattern, with the first peak at a median of 16 days after transplant and a second peak occurring a median of 96 days after BMT[6] (see Fig. 4.3). In autologous patients, virtually all of aspergillosis is temporally associated with neutropenia.[6] *Aspergillus* is acquired as spores from the environment, inhaled into the upper respiratory tract. Therefore, the most common sites of infection include the lung and sinuses. Direct extension of infection to the brain, either from the sinuses or via the blood, is next. Invasive disease below the diaphragm is uncommon and occurs late in the course of infection.

Infection with molds other than *Aspergillus*

The third most common cause of invasive fungal infection is that caused by molds other than *Aspergillus*. The genus and species of molds responsible vary in frequency from institution to institution. The clinical presentation of these infections is typically similar to that of aspergillosis, with sinus and lung disease predominating. Fungal infections caused by the dimorphic fungi, including coccidioidomycosis, histoplasmosis and blastomycosis, are quite unusual despite the high endemic rate of these infections in certain parts of the world. Similarly, infection with *Cryptococcus* spp. is quite unusual, in contrast to its frequent occurrence in patients infected with HIV.

OTHER INFECTIONS

Pneumocystis carinii pneumonia is extremely rare now with routine prophylaxis with trimethoprim–sulfamethoxazole or alternative agents such as quinolones. It sometimes occurs after autologous transplantation, including PBSC transplantation, although the frequency appears to be low. The use of prophylaxis in this setting has not been clearly defined and may need to be re-evaluated as more autologous transplants using peripheral blood as the stem cell source are performed. Before the routine use of prophylaxis, *P. carinii* pneumonia in allogeneic transplant patients had an incidence of approximately 7% and a median time of onset of 41–80 days after transplant and it was associated with a 5% risk of death.[30] Patients typically present with dyspnea, cough and fever; 58% of patients have bilateral infiltrates, whereas 15% of patients have either minimal radiographic changes or none.[96]

Toxoplasmosis is rare after transplant and unfortunately the majority of cases are diagnosed *post mortem*.[97] It appears to result from reactivation of prior infection; this supposition is supported by the observation that all cases reported to date have occurred in seropositive recipients. The incidence probably varies with the endemic infection rate. For example, in France, where the seroprevalence rate is 70%, the reported incidence is 2–3%;[98] on the other hand, at the Fred Hutchinson Cancer Research Center, where the seroprevalence before transplant is 40%, the reported incidence is 0.3%.[97] Risk factors include pre-transplant seropositive *Toxoplasma* serology and GVHD.[97] Because diagnosis is difficult, it is most often fatal before treatment is considered.

Clinical presentations of toxoplasmosis include focal cerebral lesions and disseminated infection in blood, lungs and other organs.[97,98] Blood cultures taken for viral isolation have unexpectedly demonstrated toxoplasmosis, but this usually occurs weeks after the sample was drawn and often after the patient has died.[99]

SUMMARY OF CHANGES IN THE PAST DECADE

One of the major changes in the clinical presentation of infections in the BMT setting is the shift of infections such as CMV to the later post-transplant period as more effective antiviral prevention has been developed. There has also been an increased recognition of the seriousness of respiratory virus infections in this setting. Finally, fungal infections have become the leading cause of death from infections as better prevention of CMV disease has been achieved.

DIAGNOSIS

GENERAL APPROACH TO DIAGNOSIS

Diagnostic approaches in the evaluation of infection after BMT are guided by knowledge of which organisms are likely during any specific risk period, the type of transplant (autologous or allogeneic) and the time post-transplant at which the signs and symptoms of infection occur. An accurate diagnosis also depends on a thorough physical examination focusing on sites that are likely to involve infection in the BMT patient. A BMT-specific examination should focus on:

- the sinuses, looking for tenderness or symptoms of postnasal drainage;
- the oropharynx and perirectal area, looking for tenderness, ulceration, or black, necrotic areas;
- the catheter exit sites; and
- all skin surfaces.

A careful physical examination may identify skin lesions that are critical to the diagnosis of fungal infection in patients whose blood cultures are otherwise negative. It cannot be over-emphasized that all suspicious lesions should be cultured or biopsied immediately.

In general, the clinical signs and symptoms of infection following BMT are similar to those in other settings. Fever remains the most common presenting symptom; however, it may be absent in patients receiving large doses of corticosteroids for GVHD. Subtle behavioral changes may be the only symptom of an evolving CNS abscess.

DIAGNOSIS OF BACTERIAL INFECTION

Blood cultures should be taken daily in all patients with a fever of 100.4°F (38°C) or more. The blood culture system should be sensitive enough to identify yeast, either by using one of the newer automated blood culture systems or the isolator blood culture system. In some centers, blood cultures are routinely obtained once or twice a week in patients receiving high dose corticosteroids. Patients who develop fever during neutropenia should be evaluated aggressively, even in the absence of localizing signs and symptoms. An evaluation should include a chest X-ray, and, if fever persists despite broad-spectrum antibiotics, a sinus X-ray should also be considered. Although urinary tract infections are uncommon in this setting, a urinalysis and urine culture may be helpful in the evaluation, especially in women with a history of urinary tract infections. Evaluation of the cerebrospinal fluid is rarely helpful in febrile patients; bacterial meningitis is rare in this setting because broad-spectrum antibiotics that have CNS penetration, such as cephalosporins, are used for empiric antibiotic therapy. During the respiratory virus season, all patients with respiratory symptoms should have a sample from the nasopharynx cultured for respiratory viruses.

The diagnosis of bacterial infection is made primarily by culturing blood or areas of localized inflammation (e.g. the tunnel tract of an infected intravascular catheter). A high index of suspicion should guide the use of special cultures or stains; for example, all material from an infected tunnel tract should be examined for the presence of acid-fast bacilli (indicating an atypical mycobacterial infection). In general, bacterial surveillance cultures are not cost-effective on a routine basis.

Invasive procedures to obtain material for diagnosis should be performed early in the course of infection if blood cultures are not revealing. Such procedures may include bronchoalveolar lavage, to evaluate the cause of pulmonary disease, and a sinus aspirate, to obtain material for culture and Gram stain. Determining the etiology of newly evolving symptoms and distinguishing them from noninfectious causes may be greatly enhanced by Gram-staining aspirated material. Skin biopsies should be routine in the evaluation of newly appearing skin lesions in a sick patient. Careful thought and communication with the diagnostic laboratory will facilitate consideration of more unusual pathogens depending on the patients symptomatology.

Evaluation of the patient before transplant should include serologic evaluation of herpesvirus status (CMV, HSV and possibly VZV) to assist in providing appropriate antiviral prophylaxis following transplant. In certain areas of the world, *Toxoplasma* serology may be helpful in defining patients at higher risk of developing toxoplasmosis in the post-transplant period. Routine bacterial, fungal and viral surveillance cultures, either before or after transplant, are of limited value and are no longer considered cost-effective.

DIAGNOSIS OF VIRAL INFECTION

Viral infections are diagnosed either by culture or with the aid of type-specific monoclonal antibodies. Herpes simplex virus grows rapidly in viral culture and can be identified in 24–48 hours. In contrast, VZV is best diagnosed by scraping the base of a vesicle and examining the cells with VZV-specific monoclonal antibodies, because VZV is a fastidious virus and often does not withstand the time required to transport the specimen to the diagnostic laboratory. Tissue from biopsy of lung, gastrointestinal tract, or other visceral organs can be examined by histology, immunohistochemical techniques or culture.

Techniques to identify the patient who is infected with CMV have changed dramatically in the past 20 years. There is a continuum of techniques that have been used to identify patients with latent infection (seropositive only), early reaction and overtly culture-positive infection (Fig. 4.12). With the rapid development of a variety of early diagnostic approaches to CMV, there is no longer a major role for standard tube

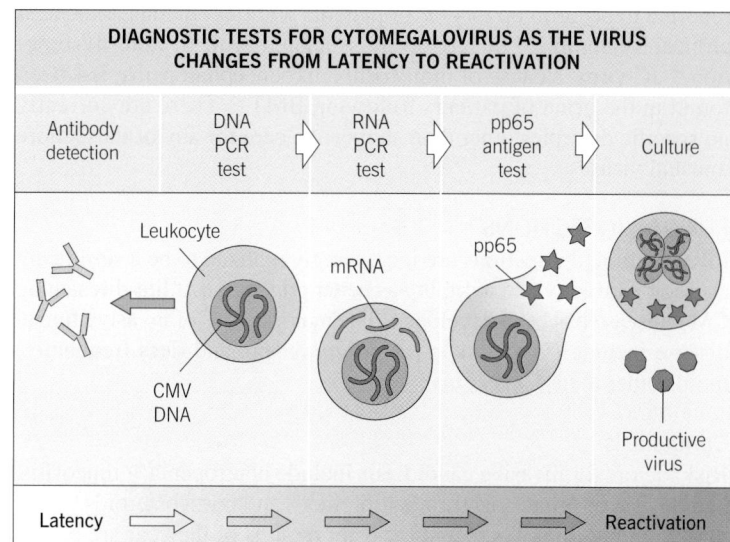

Fig. 4.12 Diagnostic tests for cytomegalovirus as the virus changes from latency to reactivation.

cultures specifically for CMV. Shell-vial technology has replaced tube cultures in many laboratories[100] and is useful for rapid identification of CMV from clinical specimens, especially material from bronchoalveolar lavage and biopsy. More recently, with the availability of effective antiviral therapy for CMV, CMV antigen testing[101] and PCR[102] have replaced routine viral shell-vial screening for CMV in many centers.

Antigen testing identifies pp65, which is a late structural protein of CMV that can readily be detected in the leukocytes of infected patients.[101] It is highly sensitive and specific, it is more sensitive at identifying patients before the onset of CMV disease than viral blood cultures, and results are available in 24–48 hours. Commercial kits are now available to assist the clinical diagnostic laboratory in performing the assay. The disadvantage of antigen testing is that patients must have detectable circulating neutrophils in order for the test to become positive, so it is not helpful in identifying infection in patients before engraftment. Fortunately, the incidence of CMV before engraftment is very low.[51]

Currently, both CMV antigen testing and PCR are considered excellent methods for early CMV detection. Antigen testing reliably identifies CMV infection before the onset of CMV disease[101] and can be used to guide pre-emptive therapy with ganciclovir.[103] Some laboratories prefer PCR,[102] and some use two consecutive same tests[104] to identify patients who might benefit most from pre-emptive ganciclovir therapy. Polymerase chain reaction is more sensitive than antigen testing, and it therefore becomes positive earlier and remains positive longer after ganciclovir therapy is initiated (Fig. 4.13). It may require more effort at standardization than the commercially available CMV antigen testing kits. Weekly screening allows identification of patients who might benefit most from pre-emptive therapy with ganciclovir.

DIAGNOSIS OF RESPIRATORY VIRUSES

Cultures, both standard and shell-vial, viral antigen testing and direct fluorescent antibody staining of nasal secretions are alternative investigations for the diagnosis of respiratory infections in BMT patients who develop respiratory symptoms.[105] In the past, community-acquired upper respiratory viral infections were not thought to result in significant clinical disease, and many centers therefore do not routinely evaluate patients for such infections during the respiratory virus season. However, as recent outbreaks are being reported[56] and high mortality is being appreciated in the marrow transplant setting,[7,53] routine screening of all patients with upper respiratory symptoms during the winter months should be considered. Such cultures may not only identify patients for whom early antiviral intervention might be appropriate but may also assist in maintaining appropriate infection-control procedures.

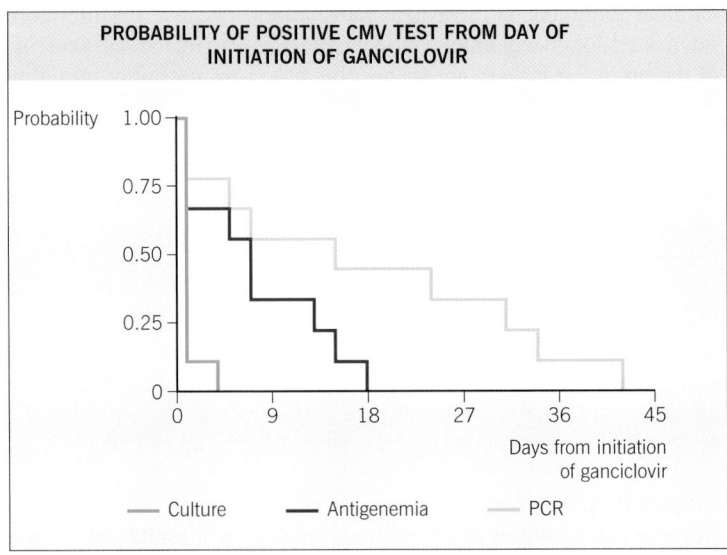

Fig. 4.13 Probability of a positive test for cytomegalovirus from the day of initiation of ganciclovir therapy.

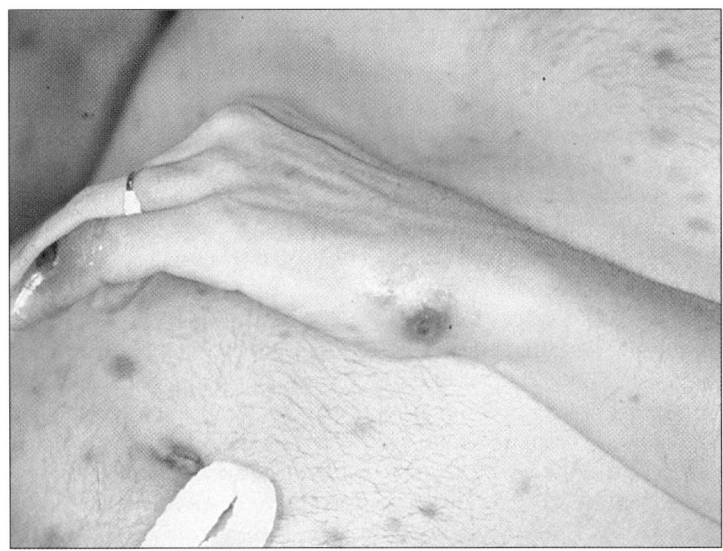

Fig. 4.14 Skin lesions of a patient with disseminated fusariosis.

DIAGNOSIS OF UNUSUAL VIRAL INFECTIONS

There are a number of viral infections for which there is currently no effective therapy. Thus, early diagnosis may be of limited therapeutic value, although it may be important to establish the diagnosis so a search for other causes of fever or other symptoms can be stopped. Examples of such infections include adenovirus, HHV-6, JC virus, BK virus and parvovirus.

Adenovirus is diagnosed by direct tissue culture of blood, urine, stool or tissue or by immunofluorescence.[106] Human herpesvirus 6 can be identified by coculture techniques with lymphocytes[84] or by PCR.[83] JC virus can be identified by culture techniques,[88] and BK virus is detected by antigen detection methods, enzyme-linked immunosorbent assay or DNA hybridization.[87] Parvovirus is detected by antibody detection or PCR.

DIAGNOSIS OF FUNGAL INFECTIONS

The availability of accurate early diagnostic tests for invasive fungal infections lags behind that for other types of infections. This presents particular difficulty in the BMT setting because invasive fungal infections have become the leading cause of death from infection. Culture remains the gold standard, although blood cultures for *Candida* spp. are often negative in the face of disseminated infection that is identified later, including *post mortem*.[93,107] Blood cultures for molds are rarely positive,[108] except in the case of *Fusarium* spp. Therefore, culture and histologic evaluation of tissue may be the only way of adequately diagnosing an invasive infection. The skin is particularly accessible when disseminated skin lesions are present (Fig. 4.14). A disadvantage of culture is that, in some cases, fungal organisms are identified by Gram stain or histology but do not grow in the laboratory. In a recent large series of documented cases of infections with *Aspergillus* spp., approximately 10% were diagnosed by histology without confirmation by positive culture.[6] Even when septate hyphal elements typical of *Aspergillus* spp. are present, one cannot be sure that this does not represent one of the other molds. Especially in tissue section, the distinction between yeasts and molds based on histology alone can be difficult.

The diagnostic dilemma presented by invasive fungal infection is further complicated in a situation in which a patient develops, for example, typical nodular lesions on CT scans that are consistent with invasive aspergillosis, but the patient is either too ill to undergo a bronchoalveolar lavage or is too thrombocytopenic for an open biopsy (Fig. 4.15). In such cases, the patient must often be managed empirically with antifungal therapy, always leaving some doubt as to the exact etiology of the infection. *Nocardia* spp., for example, can also

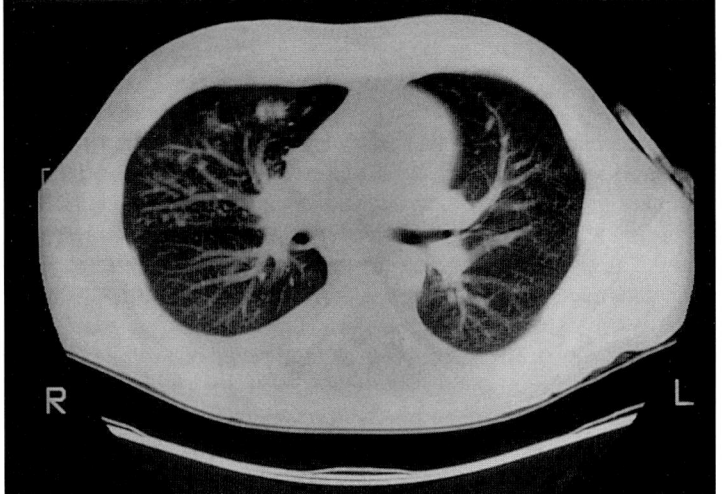

Fig. 4.15 Computed tomography scan of the chest in a patient with aspergillosis, demonstrating typical nodular lesions on the right.

present as a nodular appearance on chest CT scan. Whenever possible, the diagnosis should be confirmed by biopsy, culture, or both, because this will help guide the use of potentially toxic or costly therapy. Without such confirmation, the decision to continue therapy is always more difficult to justify.

A variety of diagnostic tests have been evaluated for early diagnosis of invasive fungal infection. Serologic evaluation of fungal infections is unreliable.[109] Antigen detection has been studied for both *Candida*[110] and *Aspergillus* spp.[111] but has not been routinely adopted in the clinical laboratory. Polymerase chain reaction appears to hold promise[112] but remains investigational at present because the sensitivity and specificity of this method have not been tested in large numbers of clinical samples from BMT patients or patients who are immunocompromised for other reasons.

SUMMARY OF DIAGNOSTIC CHALLENGES OF INFECTION IN THE BONE AND MARROW TRANSPLANTATION SETTING

Early diagnosis continues to be critical to successful outcome of infection after BMT. Significant progress has been made in the past decade in using early diagnostic testing to guide pre-emptive ganciclovir therapy. A major challenge for the next decade is the development of more sensitive and specific tests for the diagnosis of invasive fungal infections.

MANAGEMENT

With a few exceptions, infections in the BMT setting cannot be completely prevented. Therefore, aggressive management of established infection remains an important of post-transplant supportive care. Treatment remains difficult for many infections in the BMT setting, in part because of the inability to diagnose some types of infections early. This is particularly important because immunocompromise during the early post-transplant period and severe GVHD contribute to rapid progression of infection.

In general, a successful treatment of patients who develop infections in the BMT setting depends on rapid identification of the causative organism. Blood cultures, biopsies of suspicious skin lesions, mucous membranes or visceral organs and bronchoalveolar lavage early in the course of suspected pulmonary infection should result in the early institution of life-saving therapy. Duration of therapy as well as associated side effects may also be reduced by early specific treatment.

BACTERIAL INFECTIONS

Several bacterial infection syndromes that are specific to the BMT setting are discussed here because their management is sometimes unique to this setting. Please refer to other sections in this book for treatment of specific organisms.

Empiric antibiotic therapy

Management of febrile neutropenia includes empiric antibiotics and the majority of patients receive this therapy in the early post-BMT period. Persistent febrile neutropenia in the face of broad-spectrum antibiotics continues to be a major clinical challenge because the differential diagnosis includes a variety of noninfectious causes of fever, i.e. GVHD, tissue trauma resulting from the conditioning regimen and drug-related fever. The choice of antibiotic coverage is determined by the types of bacterial organisms occurring in a particular center, cost and whether inpatient or outpatient therapy is being considered. For example, it has been well established that coagulase-negative staphylococci rarely cause significant mortality, thus justifying the exclusion of empiric Gram-positive coverage for febrile neutropenic episodes in many centers.[113] In contrast, the virulent streptococcal species cause substantial morbidity and mortality, thus justifying initial institution of antibiotics for these organisms in centers with a high incidence of these infections. Persistent fever while receiving broad-spectrum antibiotics is frequently due to fungal infection, and thus the addition of antifungal coverage after 5–7 days of persistent fever is part of our standard of care (see Chapter 4.5).[114]

The long-standing tradition of initiating antibiotic therapy and continuing until recovery of the neutrophil count and resolution of the fever continues to be the standard of care in the febrile neutropenic patient.[113] In high-risk settings, such as neutropenia or severe GVHD in which a definite diagnosis of infection has not been made, the presumed cause of infection should be treated with a full course of antibiotic. Obviously, the risk of continuing expensive, toxic therapy when the specific cause of infection has not been proved must be considered.

Catheter-related infections

Most of the serious catheter-associated infections are bacterial in etiology. In terms of clinical management, a catheter exit site infection can be defined as an infection that does not extend more than 1cm from the exit site. Such infections are often associated with minimal tenderness and some drainage. They can often be managed with good local care and without systemic antibiotics, even in neutropenic patients. Once the infection progresses more than 1cm from the exit site or it becomes associated with tenderness or erythema along the tunnel tract, fever, or a positive blood culture, more aggressive management with systemic antibiotics and possibly removal of the line should be considered. Many catheter-associated bacteremias can be successfully managed without removing the line (see Chapter 4.5).

Clinical judgment is critical in these cases, because the literature often does not give definitive guidance for specific infections. One rule of thumb is that if there are no positive blood cultures after initiation of appropriate antibiotic therapy and a satisfactory clinical response, the catheter can often be left in place for 2 weeks' antibiotic therapy. One absolute indication for removal of the catheter is infection due to atypical mycobacterial infection. Because the catheter tunnel tract may be involved, surgical debridement is often necessary in addition to line removal for complete eradication of infection.

VIRAL INFECTIONS

As with many infections in the BMT setting, treatment of established viral disease is much more difficult than prevention. In general, prophylaxis is considered, particularly for the latent herpesviruses, when the incidence of reactivation and associated morbidity and mortality is high.

Herpes simplex virus

Because reconstitution of HSV immunity is critical for the prevention of reactivation and because aciclovir may reduce the ability to develop an HSV-specific T-lymphocyte response,[73] aciclovir treatment of milder HSV infections which occur after prophylaxis is discontinued is generally avoided. In general, treatment should be reserved for patients who develop HSV infection that interferes with adequate oral intake or that is associated with severe pain. Valaciclovir may be an acceptable alternative, depending on cost, and it is particularly attractive because it can be given orally at a less frequent dosing schedule than aciclovir.

One of the current problems in the management of HSV infection in the later post-transplant period includes the development of resistant HSV. Although the precise incidence is not known, HSV resistance typically develops following repetitive courses of oral aciclovir for recurrent infection, particularly when absorption is unpredictable. Thus, low-dose or repeated therapy should be avoided when possible. Infections with resistant HSV, although initially thought not to result in progressive serious HSV disease, have now been reported to cause HSV pneumonia in marrow transplant patients.[115] Resistant HSV infection can be treated with foscarnet.[116] Cidofovir is a potential alternative for treatment of resistant HSV infection, but associated nephrotoxicity may make administration difficult in the marrow transplant setting (see Chapter 7.15).

Varicella-zoster virus

High dose aciclovir (500mg/m^2 intravenously q8h) has been the treatment of choice for VZV infection,[117] although valaciclovir may become the treatment of choice, particularly for uncomplicated VZV infection, because it gives predictably higher drug levels than aciclovir and can be administered orally. Aggressive early therapy has been recommended in all patients in the first 9 months after transplant because this has been shown to be the highest period of risk.[75,118] Deaths continue to occur from VZV infection when treatment is given orally at suboptimal doses or initiated late in disseminated infection; this includes abdominal presentations of VZV where the skin lesions appear late in the course of infection.

Cytomegalovirus

For the CMV-seronegative allograft recipient of CMV-seropositive stem cells as well as for the seropositive BMT patient, there are currently no effective ways of totally eliminating the risk of CMV infection and disease. Seronegative patients with seropositive stem cell donors continue to have an infection rate of approximately 17%, of which half will result in CMV disease, even when CMV-safe blood products are used.[119]

Cytomegalovirus-seropositive allogeneic transplant recipients continue to be at highest risk of serious CMV disease. The first antiviral study that has shown significantly reduced incidence of CMV infection and disease in CMV-seropositive allogeneic patients was published by Meyers *et al.*, who used high-dose intravenous aciclovir from conditioning until day 30 after BMT.[64] The patients who received aciclovir had a 50% reduction in both infection and biopsy-proven disease compared with placebo patients. Both this study in the USA and a subsequent study in Europe have demonstrated an improvement in survival in patients receiving aciclovir, although the reason is not clear in the later study because the incidence of CMV disease was not statistically different between the groups.[120] Although high-dose aciclovir continues to be used for CMV prophylaxis in Europe, most USA centers have discontinued this strategy now that ganciclovir has become available.

More recently, a series of studies has demonstrated that ganciclovir can significantly reduce CMV disease during the first 100 days after allogeneic transplantation. Although it is clear that one can 'prevent' CMV disease in the early post-transplant seropositive patient using ganciclovir prophylaxis at the time of engraftment,[121,122] this strategy results in significantly longer neutropenia with an increased risk of secondary bacterial infection.[68]

Therefore, an alternative approach to the prevention of CMV is ganciclovir treatment at the first sign of reactivation of infection using a pre-emptive antiviral strategy.[68,69,102] Such pre-emptive ganciclovir strategies have included those guided by bronchoalveolar lavage,[70] first positive culture,[121] CMV antigen detection[69] and PCR[102] (see Fig. 4.12).

In addition to the fact that true prophylaxis at engraftment for all CMV-seropositive patients is associated with the lowest CMV disease rate, it also results in more patients being treated who would never have developed CMV disease and a higher incidence of late CMV disease.[68] With pre-emptive therapy, once CMV is identified by an early detection method, patients are treated with 5–7 days of induction ganciclovir therapy, followed by maintenance therapy until the CMV test becomes negative[102] or until day 100.[69] Data presented in more recent studies indicate that early CMV antigen testing or PCR are clearly superior to cultures, including viral blood cultures, and these are the preferred method of guiding ganciclovir therapy in most centers. Although ganciclovir can be safely discontinued in some settings when the CMV test becomes negative,[102] in higher-risk settings where GVHD is a problem, discontinuation of therapy before day 100 is associated with a higher CMV disease rate.[69] This may depend, in part, on the number of patients undergoing unrelated BMT, the use of T-lymphocyte depletion, or the incidence of GVHD at a particular center. Both strategies are associated with an increase in late CMV disease.

Oral ganciclovir is not an effective alternative to intravenous therapy in the BMT setting. Foscarnet prophylaxis has been studied after autologous transplantation but is associated with significant nephrotoxicity.[123] Forscarnet toxicity did not limit drug administration in a recent study.[124]

With the availability of ganciclovir, which has better antiviral activity than aciclovir, the use of aciclovir with or without ganciclovir is controversial. A recent study concluded that aciclovir in combination with ganciclovir prophylaxis does not provide additional benefit.[125]

Cytomegalovirus-seropositive autologous transplant patients can be effectively managed with a pre-emptive ganciclovir strategy of 7 days of induction followed by 3 weeks of maintenance using CMV antigen detection to guide therapy.[103] Seronegative patients can be given CMV-safe blood products as an alternative to ganciclovir, and in patients receiving minimal immunosuppression (e.g. for breast transplantation) consideration can be given to not using prophylaxis because the incidence of CMV disease is less than 1%.

The more difficult patient management situation with regard to CMV prevention is the CMV-seronegative allogeneic patient receiving a CMV-seropositive graft. Because the ratio of CMV disease to infection is higher in this transplant setting than in any other allogeneic CMV graft combination,[119] the most rational approach in the absence of specific studies is the use of CMV-safe blood products and pre-emptive ganciclovir therapy once CMV is identified by rapid antigen detection or PCR.

Treatment of established CMV disease continues to be difficult. The most frequent manifestation of CMV disease following BMT is CMV pneumonia, which is currently treated with a combination of ganciclovir (5mg/kg intravenously q12h for 10–21 days) plus IVIG (500mg/kg every second day for 14–21 days).[71] There are, to date, no controlled studies that have evaluated strategies for the treatment of CMV pneumonia. There are also no data to show that CMV-specific immunoglobulin improves outcome, and thus standard IVIG at high doses is generally used, depending on cost.

Treatment of CMV enteritis also remains difficult, and the one controlled study demonstrated no clinical improvement after 2 weeks of intravenous ganciclovir.[126] In the absence of further data, treatment of patients with protracted CMV enteritis includes ganciclovir and immunoglobulin or an induction course of ganciclovir alone followed by several weeks of ganciclovir maintenance therapy to facilitate gastrointestinal healing.

Respiratory viruses
There are no controlled studies evaluating the treatment of RSV or other respiratory viral infection in the BMT setting. The treatment of established RSV pneumonia is associated with high mortality. Both aerosolized ribavirin and a combination of ribavirin and IVIG have been used, and survival appears to be higher when treatment is initiated before significant hypoxia develops.[56,127] In patients with positive nasopharyngeal cultures for RSV, pre-emptive therapy with aerosolized ribavirin appears promising.[7,53]

Other viral infections
To date, no treatments for adenovirus, EBV, HHV-6, or other unusual viruses such as rotavirus, parvovirus, BK virus or JC virus have been demonstrated to be effective. Hepatitis B and C is difficult to treat following BMT (see Chapter 2.39).

FUNGAL INFECTIONS
Options for management of invasive fungal infection remain relatively limited compared with treatment options for other opportunistic infections in the BMT setting. Treatment of most invasive fungal infections remains empiric because there have been no prospectively controlled studies demonstrating optimal therapy or duration of therapy in this setting. It is recommended that treatment of candidemia or visceral candidiasis during the neutropenic period should include a total dose of 1–2g amphotericin B (given intravenously at a dose of 0.5mg/kg per day). Careful hydration can often avoid nephrotoxicity, and pre-medication with diphenhydramine and domperidol is often required to control infusion-related side-effects. An alternative treatment for visceral candidiasis in the engrafted patient includes the use of fluconazole (400mg/day).[128] A randomized controlled study that compared lipid-complexed amphotericin B with standard amphotericin B in the treatment of invasive candidiasis in cancer patients showed that lipid-complexed amphotericin B has significantly less nephrotoxicity, although no improvement in infusion-related side effects or outcome was noted.[129]

Treatment of invasive aspergillosis remains difficult despite the recommended treatment with a total dose of 2–3g amphotericin B. Two studies have shown that lipid-complexed amphotericin B and amphotericin B colloidal dispersion are both associated with less nephrotoxicity than standard amphotericin B.[130] The improvement in survival noted in both these studies is difficult to interpret, because neither was a randomized controlled study and both used historic controls as the comparator group.

Itraconazole offers a potential alternative to amphotericin B in the treatment of invasive aspergillosis.[131] However, the capsule formulation of itraconazole is relatively poorly absorbed and the administration of the drug is complicated by multiple drug–drug interactions in the BMT setting. Furthermore, it takes several weeks to achieve therapeutic drug levels, owing to the large volume of distribution of the drug. A newer formulation, itraconazole solution, has improved oral bioavailability and potentially overcomes some of the absorption problems of the capsule. Itraconazole should not be used to treat aspergillosis in the marrow transplant setting without obtaining blood drug levels to ensure adequate absorption of standard doses of drug. Newer drugs that are safe and effective and that have good oral bioavailability are clearly needed.

The treatment of choice for *Pneumocystis carinii* infection is trimethoprim–sulfamethoxazole. Pentamidine is used in patients who are allergic to trimethoprim–sulfmethoxazole or who cannot tolerate it.

PROTOZOAN INFECTIONS

Toxoplasmosis occurs so infrequently in many centers, particularly in the USA, that prophylaxis is not routinely justified. In some European communities, however, where the seropositivity rate is higher, pyrimethamine–sulfadoxine may be appropriate.[132] The treatment for established infection is pyrimethamine. For treatment of other parasitic infections, see Section 6.

CONCLUSIONS

Infection remains an important post-BMT complication. Progress in the development of strategies to prevent invasive candidiasis and CMV disease has had an important impact on improving survival during the first 3 months after transplant. Challenges remain, however, in developing ways of preventing the occurrence of late CMV disease and of improving the diagnosis and treatment of invasive fungal disease and, most importantly, invasive aspergillosis, which has become a leading infectious cause of death after transplant. Increasing emphasis is being placed on prevention in general and cost-effective strategies that allow delivery of such therapy in the outpatient setting.

REFERENCES

1. Meropol N, Overmoyer B, Stadtmauer E. High-dose chemotherapy with autologous stem cell support for breast cancer [published erratum appears in Oncology 1993;7:105]. Oncology 1992;6:53–60, 63 [discussion 63–4, 69].
2. Boeckh M, Riddell S, Cunningham T, et al. Increased incidence of late CMV disease in allogeneic marrow transplant recipients after ganciclovir prophylaxis is due to a lack of CMV-specific T cell responses. 38th Annual Meeting of the American Society of Hematology. Blood 1996;88:302a.
3. Riddell S, Watanabe K, Goodrich J, Li C, Agha M, Greenberg P. Restoration of viral immunity in immunodeficient humans by the adoptive transfer of T cell clones. Science 1992;257:238–42.
4. Pannuti C, Gingrich R, Pfaller M, Kao C, Wenzel R. Nosocomial pneumonia in patients having bone marrow transplant: attributable mortality and risk factors. Cancer 1992;69:2653–62.
5. Peterson P, McGlave P, Ramsay N, et al. A prospective study of infectious diseases following bone marrow transplantation: emergence of aspergillus and cytomegalovirus as the major causes of mortality. Infect Control 1983;4:81–9.
6. Wald A, Leisenring W, van Burik J, Bowden R. Natural history of aspergillus infections in a large cohort of patients undergoing bone marrow transplantation. J Infect Dis 1997:175;1459–66.
7. Bowden R. Respiratory virus infections after marrow transplant: The Fred Hutchinson Cancer Research Center experience. In: Whimbey E, Englund JA, Ljungman P, eds. Community respiratory viral infections in the immunocompromised host 1997;(Suppl) 102:27–30.
8. Meyers J. Infection in recipients of marrow transplants. In: Remington JS, Swartz MN, eds. Current clinical topics in infectious diseases. New York: McGraw-Hill; 1985:261–92.
9. Walter E, Bowden R. Infections in the bone marrow transplant recipient. Infect Dis Clin North Am 1995;9:823–47.
10. Witherspoon R, Storb R, Ochs H, et al. Recovery of antibody production in human allogeneic marrow graft recipients: influence of time posttransplantation, the presence or absence of chronic graft-versus-host disease, and antithymocyte globulin treatment. Blood 1981;58:360–8.
11. Sullivan K, Nims J, Leisenring W, et al. Determinants of late infection following marrow transplantation for aplastic anemia and myelodysplastic syndrome. Blood 1995;86:213a.
12. Ochs L, Shu X, Miller J, et al. Late infections after allogeneic bone marrow transplantations: comparison of incidence in related and unrelated donor transplant recipients. Blood 1995;86:3979–86.
13. Rinehart J, Balcerzak S, Sagone A, LoBuglio A. Effects of corticosteroids on human monocyte function. J Clin Invest 1974;54:1337–43.
14. Li C, Greenberg P, Gilbert M, Goodrich J, Riddell S. Recovery of HLA-restricted cytomegalovirus (CMV)-specific T-cell responses after allogeneic bone marrow transplant: correlation with CMV disease and effect of ganciclovir prophylaxis. Blood 1971;83:1971–9.
15. Reusser P, Riddell S, Meyers J, Greenberg P. Cytotoxic T-lymphocyte response to cytomegalovirus after human allogeneic bone marrow transplantation: pattern of recovery and correlation with cytomegalovirus infection and disease. Blood 1991;78:1373–80.
16. Bowden R, Digel J, Reed E, Meyers J. Immuno-suppressive effects of ganciclovir on in vitro lymphocyte responses. J Infect Dis 1987;156:899–903.
17. Walter E, Greenberg P, Gilbert M, et al. Reconstitution of cellular immunity against cytomegalovirus in recipients of allogeneic bone marrow by transfer of T-cell clones from the donor. N Engl J Med 1995;333:1038–44.
18. Sullivan K, Mori M, Sanders J, et al. Late complications of allogeneic and autologous marrow transplantation. Bone Marrow Transplant 1992;10:267.
19. Bowden R, Sayers M, Flournoy N, et al. Cytomegalovirus immune globulin and seronegative blood products to prevent primary cytomegalovirus infection after marrow transplantation. N Engl J Med 1986;314:1006–10.
20. Bowden R, Slichter S, Sayers M, et al. A comparison of filtered leukocyte-reduced and cytomegalovirus (CMV) seronegative blood products for the prevention of transfusion-associated CMV infection after marrow transplant. Blood 1995;86:3598–603.
21. Petersen F, Buckner C, Clift R, et al. Infectious complications in patients undergoing marrow transplantation: a prospective randomized study of the additional effect of decontamination and laminar air flow isolation among patients receiving prophylactic systemic antibiotics. Scand J Infect Dis 1987;19:559–67.
22. Wade J, Newton B, McLaren C, Flournoy N, Keeney R, Meyers J. Intravenous aciclovir to treat mucocutaneous herpes simplex virus infection after marrow transplantation. Ann Intern Med 1982;96:149–52.
23. Wade J, Newton B, Flournoy N, Meyers J. Oral aciclovir for prevention of herpes simplex virus reactivation after marrow transplant. Ann Intern Med 1984;100:823–8.
24. Ljungman P, Lonnqvist B, Gahrton G, Ringden O, Sundqvist V, Wahren B. Clinical and subclinical reactivations of varicella-zoster virus in immunocompromised patients. J Infect Dis 1986;153:840–7.
25. Bowden R, Meyers J, Digel J, Keller C. Successful immunologic reconstitution to varicella zoster virus (VZV) infection in asymptomatic marrow transplant patients given long-term oral aciclovir (ACV): Ablation of rebound VZV. The 32nd Interscience Conference on Antimicrobial Agents and Chemotherapy. Blood 1992:168.

26. Slavin M, Osborne B, Adams R, *et al*. Efficacy and safety of fluconazole for fungal infections after marrow transplant: a prospective, randomized, double-blind study. J Infect Dis 1995;171:1545–52.

27. Goodman J, Winston D, Greenfield R, *et al*. A controlled trial of fluconazole to prevent fungal infections in patients undergoing bone marrow transplantation. N Engl J Med 1992;326:845–51.

28. Rousey S, Russler S, Gottlieb M, Ash R. Low-dose amphotericin B prophylaxis against invasive aspergillus infections in allogeneic marrow transplantation. Am J Med 1991;91:484–92.

29. O'Donnell M, Schmidt G, Tegtmeier B, *et al*. Prediction of systemic fungal infection in allogeneic marrow recipients: impact of amphotericin prophylaxis in high-risk patients. J Clin Oncol 1994;12:827–34.

30. Walter E, Chauncey T, Boeckh M, Hackman B, Kennedy M, Bowden R. PCP prophylaxis after marrow transplantation: efficacy of trimethoprim sulfamethoxazole (TS), role of TS desensitization and IV pentamidine. Interscience Conference on Antimicrobial Agent and Chemotherapy 1993:125 .

31. Ljungman P, Duraj V, Magnius L. Response to immunization against polio after allogeneic marrow transplantation. Bone Marrow Transplant 1991;14:225–7.

32. Ljungman P, Fridell E, Lonnqvist B, *et al*. Efficacy and safety of vaccination of marrow transplant recipients with a live attenuated measles, mumps, and rubella vaccine. J Infect Dis 1989;159:610–15.

33. Pauksen K, Daraj V, Ljungman P, *et al*. Immunity to and immunization against measles, rubella and mumps in patients after autologous bone marrow transplantation. Bone Marrow Transplant 1992;9:427–32.

34. Pauksen K, Hammerstrom V, Ljungman P, *et al*. Immunity to poliovirus and immunization with inactivated poliovirus vaccine after autologous bone marrow transplantation. Clin Infect Dis 1994;18:547–52.

35. Giebink G, Warkentin P, Ramsay N, *et al*. Titers of antibody to pneumococci in allogeneic bone marrow transplant recipients before and after vaccination with pneumococcal vaccine. J Infect Dis 1986;154:590–6.

36. Barra A, Cordonnier C, Preziosi MP, *et al*. Immunogenicity of *Haemophilus influenzae* type b conjugate vaccine in allogeneic bone marrrow recipients. J Infect Dis 1992;166:1021–8.

37. Sullivan K, Kopecky K, Jocom J, *et al*. Immunomodulatory and antimicrobial efficacy of intravenous immunoglobulin in bone marrow transplantation. N Engl J Med 1990;323:705–12.

38. Sullivan K, Storek J, Kopecky K, *et al*. A controlled trial of long-term administration of intravenous immunoglobulin to prevent late infection and chronic graft-versus-host disease following marrow transplantation: clinical outcome and effect on subsequent immune recovery. Biol Blood Marrow Transplant 1996;2:44–53.

39. Schimpff S. Empiric antibiotic therapy for granulocytopenic cancer patients. Am J Med 1986;80:13.

40. Bodey G, Buckley M, Sathe Y, Freireich E. Quantitative relationships between circulating leukocytes and infection in patients with acute leukemia. Ann Intern Med 1966;64:328.

41. Zinner S. New pathogens in the immunocompromised host. Recent results in cancer research. Berlin, Heidelberg: Springer-Verlag; 1993:238.

42. Winston D, Chandrasekar P, Lazarus H. *et al*. Fluconazole prophylaxis of fungal infections in patients with acute leukemia: results of a randomized placebo-controlled, double-blind, multicenter trial. Ann Intern Med 1993;118:495–503.

43. Winston D. Prophylaxis and treatment of infection in the bone marrow transplant recipient. Curr Clin Top Infect Dis 1993;13:293.

44. From the EORTC and National Cancer Institute of Canada. Vancomycin added to empirical combination antibiotic therapy for fever in granulocytopenic cancer patients. J Infect Dis 1991;163:951.

45. Gentile G, Micozzi A, Girmenia, C *et al*. Pneumonia in allogenic and autologous bone marrow recipients – a retrospective study. Chest 1993;104:371–5.

46. Krowka M, Rosenow E, Hoagland H. Pulmonary complications of bone marrow transplantation. Chest 1985;87:237–46.

47. Crawford S. Idiopathic pneumonia syndrome and respiratory failure after marrow transplantation. Semin Respir Crit Care Med 1996;17:401–7.

48. Crawford S. Supportive care in bone marrow transplantation: pulmonary complications. In: Winter JN, ed. Blood stem cell transplantation. Kluwer Academic Publishers, The Netherlands; 1997:231–54.

49. Meyers J, Flournoy N, Thomas E. Nonbacterial pneumonia after allogeneic marrow transplantation: a review of ten years' experience. Rev Infect Dis 1982;4:1119–32.

50. Wingard J, Mellits E, Sostrin M, *et al*. Interstitial pneumonia after allogeneic marrow transplantation. Medicine (Baltimore) 1988;67:175–86.

51. Limaye A, Bowden R, Myerson D, Boeckh M. CMV disease before engraftment in marrow transplant patients. Clin Infect Dis 1997;24:830–5.

52. Chan C, Hyland R, Hutchen M, *et al*. Small-airways disease in recipients of allogeneic bone marrow transplants. Medicine 1987;66:327–40.

53. Whimbey E, Englund J, Couch R. Community respiratory virus infections in immunocompromised patients with cancer. In: Whimbey E, Englund J, Ljungman P, eds. Community respiratory viral infections in the immunocompromised host 1997;102:10–8.

54. Bowden R. Other viruses after marrow transplantation. In: Forman S, Blume K, Thomas E, eds. Bone marrow transplantation. Boston: Blackwell Scientific Publications; 1994:443–53.

55. Ljungman P, Gleaves C, Meyers J. Respiratory virus infection in immunocompromised patients. Bone Marrow Transplant 1989;4:35–40.

56. Harrington R, Hooton T, Hackman R, *et al*. An outbreak of respiratory syncytial virus in a bone marrow transplant center. J Infect Dis 1992;165:987–93.

57. Wendt C, Weisdorf D, Jordan M, Balflour H, Hertz M. Parainfluenza virus respiratory infection after bone marrow transplantation. N Engl J Med 1992;326:921–6.

58. Cox G, Matsui S, Lo R, *et al*. Etiology and outcome of diarrhea after marrow transplantation: a prospective study. Gastroenterology 1994;107:1398–407.

59. McFarland L, Mulligan M, Kwok R, Stamm W. Nosocomial acquisition of *Clostridium difficile* infection. N Engl J Med 1989;320:204–10.

60. Collier A, Miller R, Meyers J. Cryptosporidiosis after marrow transplant: Person-to person transmission and treatment with spiramycin. Ann Intern Med 1984;101:205–6.

61. Yolken R, Bishop C, Townsend T, *et al*. Infectious gastroenteritis in bone-marrow-transplant recipients. N Engl J Med 1982;306:1010–12.

62. Schiller G, Nimer S, Gajewski J, Golde D. Abdominal presentation of varicella-zoster infection in recipients of allogeneic bone marrow transplantation. Bone Marrow Transplant 1991;7:489–91.

63. Wallace R. Spectrum of disease due to rapidly growing mycobacteria. Rev Infect Dis 1983;5:657–79.

64. Meyers J, Flournoy N, Thomas E. Risk factors for cytomegalovirus infection after human marrow transplantation. J Infect Dis 1986;153:478–88.

65. Reusser P, Fisher L, Buckner C, Thomas E, Meyers J. Cytomegalovirus infection after autologous bone marrow transplantation: occurrence of cytomegalovirus disease and effect on engraftment. Blood 1990;75:1888–94.

66. Wingard J, Sostrin M, Vriesendorp H, *et al*. Interstitial pneumonitis following autologous bone marrow transplantation. Transplantation 1988;46:61.

67. Holland H, Dix S, Geller R, *et al*. Minimal toxicity and mortality in high-risk breast cancer patients receiving high-dose cyclophosphamide, thiotepa, and carboplatin plus autologous marrow/stem-cell transplantation and comprehensive supportive care. J Clin Oncol 1996;14:1156–64.

68. Goodrich J, Bowden R, Fisher L, Keller C, Schoch G, Meyers J. Ganciclovir prophylaxis to prevent cytomegalovirus disease after allogeneic transplant. Ann Intern Med 1993;118:173–8.

69. Boeckh M, Gooley T, Myerson D, Cunningham T, Schoch G, Bowden R. CMV pp65 antigenemia-guided early treatment with ganciclovir versus ganciclovir at engraftment after allogeneic marrow transplant – a randomized double-blind study. Blood 1996;88:4063–71.

70. Schmidt G, Kovacs A, Zaia J, *et al*. Ganciclovir/immunoglobulin combination therapy for the treatment of human cytomegalovirus-associated interstitial pneumonia in bone marrow allograft recipients. Transplantation 1988;46:905–7.

71. Reed E, Bowden R, Dandliker P, Lilleby K, Meyers J. Treatment of cytomegalovirus pneumonia with ganciclovir and intravenous cytomegalovirus immunoglobulin in patients with bone marrow transplants. Ann Intern Med 1988;109:783.

72. Meyers J, Flournoy N, Thomas E. Infection with herpes simplex virus and cell-mediated immunity after marrow transplant. J Infect Dis 1980;142:338–46.

73. Wade J, Day L, Crowley J, Meyers J. Recurrent infection with herpes simplex virus after marrow transplant: role of specific immune response and aciclovir treatment. J Infect Dis 1984;149:750–6.

74. Atkinson K, Meyers J, Storb R, Prentice R, Thomas E. Varicella-zoster virus infection after marrow transplantation for aplastic anemia or leukemia. Transplantation 1980;29:47.

75. Locksley R, Flournoy N, Sullivan K, Meyers J. Infection with varicella-zoster virus infection after marrow transplantation. J Infect Dis 1985;152:1172.

76. Schuchter L, Wingard J, Piantadosi S, Burns W, Santos G, Saral R. Herpes zoster infection after autologous bone marrow transplantation. Blood 1989;74:1424–7.

77. Wacker P, Hartmann O, Benhamou *et al*. Varicella-zoster virus infections after autologous bone marrow transplantation in children. Bone Marrow Transplant 1989;4:191.

78. Shields A, Hackman R, Fife K, Corey L, Meyers J. Adenovirus infections in patients undergoing bone marrow transplantation. N Engl J Med 1985;312:529–33.

79. Miyamura K, Minami S, Matsuyama T, *et al*. Adenovirus-induced late onset hemorrhagic cystitis following allogeneic bone marrow transplantation. Bone Marrow Transplant 1987;2:109–15.

80. Ambinder R, Burns W, Forman M, *et al*. Hemorrhagic cystitis associated with adenovirus infection in bone marrow transplantation. Arch Intern Med 1986;146:1400–1.

81. Wasserman R, August C, Plotkin S. Viral infections in pediatric bone marrow transplant patients. Pediatr Infect Dis J 1988;7:109–15.

82. Drobyski W, Dunne W, Burd E, *et al*. Human herpesvirus-6 (HHV-6) infection in allogeneic bone marrow transplant recipients: evidence of a marrow-suppressive role for HHV-6 in vivo. J Infect Dis 1993;167:735–9.

83. Cone R, Hackman R, Huang M, *et al*. Human herpesvirus 6 in lung tissue from patients with pneumonitis after bone marrow transplantation. N Engl J Med 1993;329:156–61.

84. Kadakia M, Rybka W, Stewart J, *et al*. Human herpesvirus 6: infection and disease following autologous and allogeneic bone marrow transplantation. Blood 1996;87:5341–54.

85. Niitsu H, Miura A, Nobuo Y, Sugamura K. Pure red cell aplasia induced by B19 parvovirus during allogeneic bone marrow transplantation. Clin Transplant 1989:315.

86. Drummond J, Shah K, Saral R, Santos G, Donnenberg A. BK virus specific humoral and cell mediated immunity in allogeneic bone marrow transplant (BMT) recipients. J Med Virol 1987;23:331–44.

87. O'Reilly R, Lee F, Grossbard E, et al. Papovirus excretion following marrow transplantation: incidence and association with hepatic dysfunction. Transplant Proc 1981;13:362–6.

88. Myers C, Frisque R, Arthur R. Direct isolation and characterization of JC virus from urine samples of renal and bone marrow transplant patients. J Virol 1989;63:4445–9.

89. Gerson S, Talbot G, Hurwitz S, Strom B, Lusk E, Cassileth P. Prolonged granulocytopenia: the major risk factor for invasive pulmonary aspergillosis in patients with acute leukemia. Ann Intern Med 1984;100:345–51.

90. Wade J. Chapter 5: Epidemiology of candida infections. In: Bodey G, ed. Candidiasis: pathogenesis, diagnosis and treatment. New York: Raven Press; 1993:85–107.

91. Stuck A, Minder C, Frey F. Risk of infectious complications in patients taking glucocorticosteroids. Rev Infect Dis 1989;11:954.

92. Goodrich J, Reed E, Mori M, et al. Clinical features and analysis of risk factors for invasive candidal infection after marrow transplantation. J Infect Dis 1991;164:731–40.

93. Meyers J. Fungal infections in bone marrow transplant patients. Semin Oncol 1990;17:10–13.

94. Wingard J. Importance of candida species other than C. albicans as pathogens in oncology patients. Clin Infect Dis 1995;20:115–25.

95. Hagensee M, Bauwens J, Kjos B, Bowden R. Brain abscess following marrow transplantation: The Fred Hutchinson Cancer Research Center experience 1984–1992. Clin Infect Dis 1994;19:402–8.

96. Tuan I, Dennison D, Weisdorf D. Pneumocystis carinii pneumonitis following bone marrow transplantation. Bone Marrow Transplant 1992;10:267.

97. Slavin M, Meyers J, Remington J, Hackman R. Toxoplasma gondii infection in marrow transplant recipients: a 20-year experience. Bone Marrow Transplant 1994;13:549.

98. Derouin F, Devergie A, Auber P, et al. Toxoplasmosis in bone marrow-transplant recipients: report of seven cases and review. Clin Infect Dis 1992;15:267.

99. Shepp D, Hackman R, Conley F, Anderson J, Meyers J. Toxoplasma gondii reactivation by detection of parasitemia in tissue culture. Ann Intern Med 1985;103:218–21.

100. Gleaves C, Smith T, Shuster E, Pearson G. Rapid detection of cytomegalovirus in MRC-5 cells inoculated with urine specimens by using low-speed centrifugation and monoclonal antibody to an early antigen. J Clin Microbiol 1984;19:917–19.

101. Boeckh M, Bowden R, Goodrich J, Pettinger M, Meyers J. Cytomegalovirus antigen detection in peripheral blood leukocytes after allogeneic bone marrow transplantation. Blood 1992;80:1358–64.

102. Einsele H, Ehninger G, Hebart H, et al. Polymerase chain reaction monitoring reduces the incidence of cytomegalovirus disease and the duration and side effects of antiviral therapy after bone marrow transplantation. Blood 1995;86:2815–20.

103. Boeckh M, Stevens-Ayers T, Bowden R. Cytomegalovirus pp65 antigenemia after autologous marrow and peripheral blood stem cell transplant. J Infect Dis 1996;174:907–12.

104. Ljungman P, Lore K, Aschan J, et al. Use of a semi-quantitative PCR for cytomegalovirus DNA as a basis for pre-emptive antiviral therapy in allogeneic bone marrow transplant patients. Bone Marrow Transplant 1996;17:583–7.

105. Englund J, Piedra P, Jewell A, et al. Rapid diagnosis of respiratory syncytial virus infections in immunocompromised adults. J Clin Microbiol 1996;34:1649–53.

106. Mahafzah A, Landry M. Evaluation of immunofluorescent reagents, centrifugation, and conventional cultures for the diagnosis of adenovirus infection. Diagn Microbiol Infect Dis 1989;12:407–11.

107. Thaler M, Pastakia B, Shawker TH, O'Leary T, Pizzo PA. Hepatic candidiasis in cancer patients: the evolving picture of the syndrome. Ann Intern Med 1988;108:88–100.

108. Duthie R, Denning D. Aspergillus fungemia: report of two cases and review. Clin Infect Dis 1995;20:598–605.

109. Young R, Bennett J. Invasive aspergillosis: absence of detectable antibody response. Am Rev Resp Dis 1971;104:710–16.

110. Morrison C, Hurst S, Bragg S, Pruit W, Gorelkin L, Reiss E. Aspartyl proteinase (AP): An antigenic marker in the diagnosis os systemic candidiasis by enzyme immunoassay (EIA). ICAAC 1992:287.

111. Patterson T, Miniter P, Patterson J, Rappeport J, Andriole V. Aspergillus antigen detection in the diagnosis of invasive aspergillosis. J Infect Dis 1995;171:1553–8.

112. van Deventer A, Goessens W, van Belkum H, van Vliet E, Verbrugh H. Improved detection of Candida albicans by PCR in blood of neutropenic mice with systemic candidiasis. J Clin Microbiol 1995;32:2962–7.

113. Hughes W, Armstrong D, Bodey, GP, et al. Guidelines for the use of antimicrobial agents in neutropenic patients with unexplained fever. J Infect Dis 1990;161:381–96.

114. Pizzo P, Robichaud K, Gill F, Witebsky F. Empiric antibiotic and antifungal therapy for cancer patients with prolonged fever and granulocytopenia. Am J Med 1982;72:101–11.

115. Ljungman P, Ellis M, Hackman R, Shepp D, Meyers J. Aciclovir-resistant herpes simplex virus causing pneumonia after marrow transplantation. J Infect Dis 1990;162:244–8.

116. Safrin S, Crumpacker C, Chatis P, et al. A controlled trial comparing foscarnet with vidarabine for aciclovir-resistant mucocutaneous herpes simplex in the acquired immunodeficiency syndrome. The AIDS Clinical Trials Group. N Engl J Med 1991;325:551–5.

117. Shepp D, Dandliker P, Meyers J. Treatment of varicella-zoster virus infection in severely immunocompromised patients. N Engl J Med 1986;314:208–12.

118. Han C, Miller W, Haake R, Weisdorf D. Varicella zoster infection after bone marrow transplantation: incidence, risk factors and complications. Bone Marrow Transplant 1994;13:277–83.

119. Bowden R, Fisher L, Rogers K, Cays M, Meyers J. Cytomegalovirus (CMV)-specific intravenous immunoglobulin for the prevention of primary CMV infection and disease after marrow transplant. J Infect Dis 1991;164:483–7.

120. Prentice H, Gluckman E, Powles R, et al. Impact of long-term aciclovir on cytomegalovirus infection and survival after allogeneic bone marrow transplantation. European Aciclovir for CMV Prophylaxis Study Group. Lancet 1994;343:749–53.

121. Goodrich J, Boeckh M, Bowden R. Strategies for the prevention of cytomegalovirus disease after marrow transplantation. Clin Infect Dis 1994;19:287–98.

122. Winston D, Ho W, Bartoni K, et al. Ganciclovir prophylaxis of cytomegalovirus infection and disease in allogeneic bone marrow transplant recipients. Results of a placebo-controlled, double-blind trial. Ann Intern Med 1993;118:179–84.

123. Reusser P, Gambertoglio J, Lilleby K, Meyers J. Phase I-II trial of foscarnet for prevention of cytomegalovirus infection in autologous and allogeneic marrow tranplant recipients. J Infect Dis 1992;166:473–479.

124. Ljungman P, Oberg G, Aschan J, et al. Foscarnet for pre-emptive therapy of CMV infection detected by a leukocyte-based nested PCR in allogeneic bone marrow transplant patients. Bone Marrow Transplant 1996;18:565–8.

125. Boeckh M, Gooley T, Reusser P, Buckner C, Bowden R. Failure of high dose aciclovir to prevent cytomegalovirus disease after autologous marrow transplantation. J Infect Dis 1995;172:939–43.

126. Shepp D, Dandliker P, de Miranda P, et al. Activity of 9-[2-hydroxy-1-(hydroxymethyl)ethoxymethyl]guanine (BW B759U) in the treatment of cytomegalovirus pneumonia. Ann Intern Med 1985;103:368–83.

127. Whimbey E, Couch R, Englund J, et al. Respiratory syncytial virus pneumonia in hospitalized adult patients with leukemia. Clin Infect Dis 1995;21:376–9.

128. Torres-Valdivieso M, Lopez J, Melero C, et al. Hepatosplenic candidosis in an immunosuppressed patient responding to fluconazole. Mycoses 1994;37:443–6.

129. Anaissie E, White M, Uzun O, et al. Amphotericin B lipid complex vs. amphotericin B for treatment of invasive candidiasis: a prospective, randomized, multicenter trial. 35th Interscience Conference on Antimicrobial Agents and Chemotherapy 1995:330.

130. Hiemenz J, Walsh T. Lipid formulations of amphotericin B: recent progress and future directions. Clin Infect Dis 1996;22(suppl 2):133–44.

131. Denning D, Lee J, Hostetler J, et al. NIAID mycoses study group multicenter trial of oral itraconazole therapy for invasive aspergillosis. Am J Med 1994;97:135–44.

132. Foot A, Garin Y, Ribaud P, Devergie A, Derouin F, Gluckman E. Prophylaxis of toxoplasmosis infection with pyrimethamine/sulfadoxine (Fansidar) in bone marrow transplant recipients. Bone Marrow Transplant 1994;14:241–5.

Hematologic Malignancy

Robert Bjerknes, Øystein Bruserud & Claus O Solberg

Infection remains a major problem in the management of patients who have hematologic malignancy. This is particularly true for adult patients who have acute leukemia and individuals with therapy-resistant lymphoma receiving intensive cytotoxic drug treatment. Characteristic features of infection in these patients are the sudden onset of symptoms, the rapid progression of the disease, the difficult diagnosis and the high mortality. However, during the past two to three decades, the outcome of patients who have hematologic malignancy has steadily improved as a result of more aggressive radiation and chemotherapy, bone marrow transplantation, advances in supportive care, improved management of infection and better knowledge of host defense mechanisms against infection.

Malignant hematologic diseases originate from lymphoid or myeloid cells, and on the basis of their origin the diseases are classified into myeloproliferative and lymphoproliferative disorders (Fig. 5.1).[1] Patients who have these diseases frequently have defects of host defense mechanisms, including defects of nonspecific (skin, mucosa, phagocytes or complement) and specific (humoral or cellular) immunity. However, the single most important cause of impaired host defense is neutropenia (<500 cells/mm^3), which is followed by humoral immune deficiency in advanced disease.

CLASSIFICATION OF MALIGNANT HEMATOLOGIC DISEASES

Category	Subclassification	
Myeloproliferative disorders	Preleukemic myelodysplastic syndromes	Primary myelodysplasia
		Secondary myelodysplasia after irradiation or cytotoxic drug therapy
	Acute myelogenous leukemia	Primary (*de novo*) leukemia
		Secondary leukemia after myelodysplasia, irradiation or cytotoxic drug therapy
	Chronic myeloproliferative disorders (subclassified by affected pathway of differentiation)	Chronic myelogenous leukemia
		Polycythemia vera
		Essential thrombocytosis
		Chronic myelofibrosis
Lymphoproliferative disorders	Leukemia	Acute lymphoblastic leukemia (highly malignant)
		Chronic lymphocytic leukemia (slowly progressive)
	Lymphoma	Hodgkin's disease
		Non-Hodgkin's lymphoma
	Plasma cell dyscrasia	Multiple myeloma
		Waldenström's macroglobinemia

Fig. 5.1 Classification of malignant hematologic diseases. On the basis of their origin from myeloid or lymphoid cells the diseases are classified into two major categories: the myeloproliferative and the lymphoproliferative disorders. The less common prolymphocyte leukemia and hairy cell leukemia (not included in the figure) are related to chronic lymphocytic leukemia.

EPIDEMIOLOGY

INCIDENCE OF INFECTION

Infection is a common complication in patients who have hematologic malignancy and is most frequent in patients who have acute leukemia or lymphoma undergoing intensive (i.e. potentially curative) chemotherapy. Severe and prolonged neutropenia nearly always occurs in these patients. Intensive induction chemotherapy to achieve hematologic remission in acute leukemia patients is usually followed by 16–20 days of severe neutropenia, and 60–80% of patients develop microbiologically or clinically documented infections during this period.[2–4] The less intensive chemotherapy to maintain hematologic remission (i.e. consolidation therapy) is most often followed by 8–12 days of neutropenia, and 35–50% of patients develop infections.[2] Neutropenia is less frequent in patients who have Hodgkin's disease or non-Hodgkin's lymphoma given less intensive but potentially curative therapy.[5,6] Infections occur in 30–50% of these patients, most often in patients who have advanced disease.[6]

Infection is also prevalent in patients who have other forms of hematologic malignancy, including patients given palliative chemotherapy for low-grade malignant lymphoproliferative disorders (e.g. chronic lymphocytic leukemia), multiple myeloma or chronic myeloproliferative disorders. The overall incidence of infection in patients who have chronic lymphocytic leukemia is 0.25–0.50 episode per patient-year and increases up to 1.8 episodes per year in patients who have advanced disease.[7] Similar incidences are recorded in patients who have chronic myeloproliferative disorders or in individuals given palliative chemotherapy for low-grade malignant non-Hodgkin's lymphoma.

Intravenous catheters which are frequently used for administration of therapeutic agents in patients who have hematologic malignancy are notorious points of entry for bacteria and fungi, particularly in patients who have neutropenia. The frequency of catheter-related infections varies between 0.5 and 2.5 per 1000 catheter-days, including local and systemic infections.[8] Neutropenia and intensive chemotherapy are associated with a high frequency of infection.

MORTALITY

Infection is a major cause of mortality in patients who have hematologic malignancy, particularly adult patients who have acute leukemia and individuals with therapy-resistant lymphoma receiving intensive cytotoxic drug treatment. Infection alone accounts for almost 70% of deaths in patients who have acute leukemia, and hemorrhage and infection together for another 10%.[9] Hence, some 75% of deaths in patients who have acute leukemia are attributable to infection.

Age above 50 years is an important risk factor for the development of fatal infections in patients who have hematologic malignancies, and with few exceptions the incidence of these diseases increases with increasing age (Fig. 5.2).[10–12] Chemotherapy-induced neutropenia is also more severe in elderly patients, particularly those aged over 50–60 years, and fatal infections during induction therapy for acute leukemia are significantly more common in elderly patients.[3] Less than 5% of patients who have acute leukemia develop fatal infections during the consolidation period.[2–4]

Infection is also the most important cause of death in patients who have chronic hematologic diseases who do not receive intensive chemotherapy. In patients given palliative chemotherapy for low-grade malignant lymphoproliferative disorders, 70–80% of deaths are attributable to infection, even in the absence of neutropenia.[7] Infection is also a frequent cause of death in patients who have myelodysplastic syndromes.[10]

PATHOGENESIS AND PATHOLOGY

There are several reasons for the impaired host defense against infection in patients who have hematologic malignancy, including the malignant disease itself, the chemotherapy, the old age of many patients, and the local damage to skin and mucous membranes. A useful approach to the diagnosis and management of infections in these patients is recognition of the major predisposing factors, because each factor is associated with infections caused by a spectrum of pathogens and these usually do not overlap.[13,14] The most important predisposing factors are:

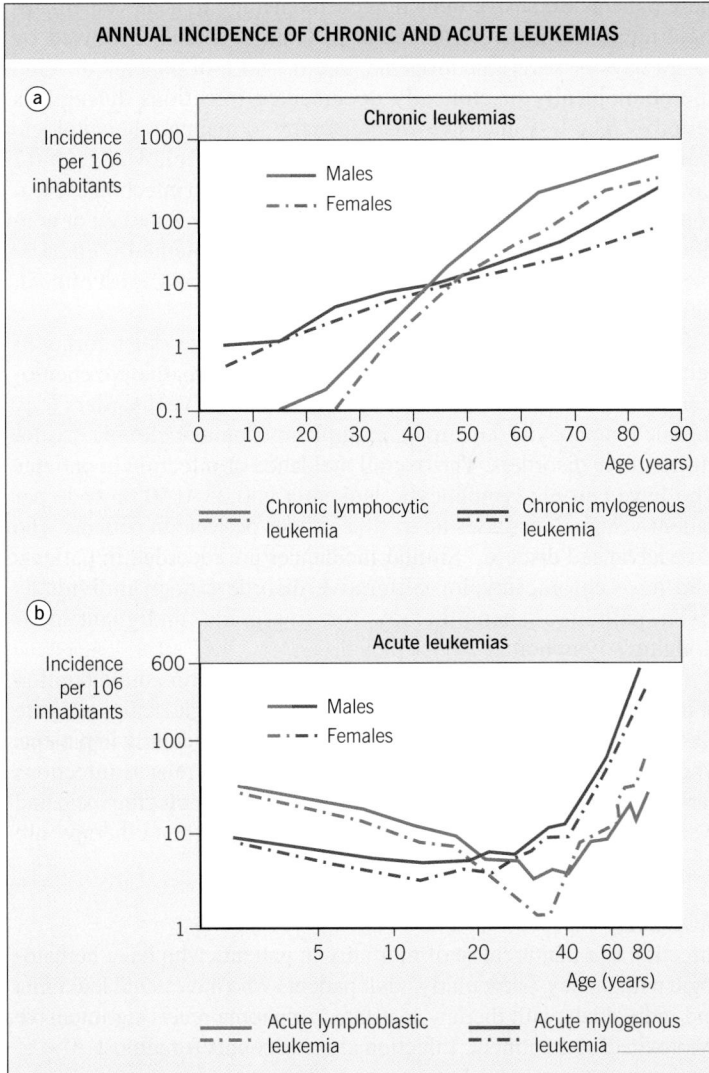

Fig. 5.2 Annual incidence of chronic and acute leukemias. (a) The incidence of chronic myelogenous and chronic lymphocytic leukemia increases with age; a markedly increased incidence is observed above the age of 50 years. A similar increase in incidence is observed at age 40–50 years for myelodysplastic syndromes, acute myelogenous leukemia, lymphomas and plasma cell dyscrasias. (b) The incidence of acute myelogenous leukemia also increases with age. The incidence of acute lymphoblastic leukemia peaks in children, decreases to a minimum by the age of 30 years and then rises after the age of 50 years. The incidence curve for Hodgkin's disease is also bimodal, with an initial peak between 15 and 25 years of age and an increasing incidence after the age of 50 years. Adapted from Finch[11] and Stevens.[12]

• neutropenia and qualitative phagocyte defects,
• humoral immune dysfunction,
• cellular immune dysfunction,
• deficiency of the complement and cytokine systems,
• splenectomy,
• shift in endogenous microbial flora and
• various medical procedures and disease conditions (Fig. 5.3).

In most patients complex interactions between these factors exist.

NEUTROPENIA AND QUALITATIVE PHAGOCYTE DEFECTS

Neutrophil granulocytes ingest and kill micro-organisms, and normal levels of circulating cells are essential for proper host defense against infections. Mature neutrophils lack the ability to replicate by cell division. They remain in the circulation for only a few days before they die, and normal levels of circulating cells depend on a continuous renewal from the bone marrow.

The risk of infection increases very little until the neutrophil count drops below 500 cells/mm³ and rises rapidly as the count approaches zero.[15] However, the risk of infection is much more pronounced in patients who have a rapidly falling neutrophil count after intensive chemotherapy than in patients who have prolonged stationary neutropenia as occurs in myelodysplastic syndromes. Also the duration of the neutropenic phase correlates with infection. This is clearly illustrated by the much higher infection rate in acute leukemia patients who have 16–20 days of neutropenia after intensive chemotherapy than in patients who have shorter neutropenic periods (e.g. patients receiving palliative chemotherapy for chronic lymphocytic leukemia, multiple myeloma or chronic myeloproliferative disorders).

The main reasons for neutropenia in patients who have hematologic malignancy include intensive chemotherapy, displacement of normal bone marrow by malignant cell infiltration and bone marrow failure as occurs in patients who have myelodysplastic syndromes. Intensive chemotherapy is nearly always followed by severe neutropenia that usually lasts for 16–20 days. In palliative chemotherapy, neutropenia is usually avoided by careful dose estimations. However, neutropenia sometimes occurs, particularly in patients who have advanced disease or in those given several chemotherapy courses. It usually appears 10–14 days after treatment and lasts for only a few days. Radiation therapy also causes leukopenia and may further aggravate chemotherapy-induced neutropenia. Treatment with interferon-α (e.g. in chronic myelogenous leukemia, essential thrombocytosis or hairy cell leukemia) may cause chronic, dose-dependent granulocytopenia.

In patients who have highly malignant hematologic diseases (e.g. acute leukemia or lymphoblastic lymphoma), bone marrow infiltration with blast cells very soon leads to impaired hematopoiesis with neutropenia, thrombocytopenia and anemia. However, during the early course of several malignant hematologic diseases or in low-grade malignancy, bone marrow infiltration is scarce and general marrow failure is absent. This is particularly true for patients who have chronic lymphocytic leukemia, low-grade malignant non-Hodgkin's lymphoma or early multiple myeloma. In these patients, peripheral blood cell counts may remain normal for a considerable time, even for years in some patients.

Patients who have myelodysplastic syndromes and marrow failure nearly always have anemia, whereas neutropenia and thrombocytopenia usually develop in advanced disease.[10,16] Patients who have chronic myeloproliferative disorders most often have normal or elevated peripheral neutrophil counts, and neutropenia is common only in patients who have chronic myelofibrosis.

Common sites of infections in patients who have neutropenia are the oropharynx, periodontium, perianal area, colon, skin, lung and distal esophagus. Rapid progression of local infection with bloodstream invasion and septicemia is frequent. Bacterial infections are caused by *Escherichia coli*, *Klebsiella pneumoniae*, *Pseudomonas aeruginosa*, *Staphylococcus epidermidis*, α-hemolytic streptococci and *Staphylococcus aureus* (Fig. 5.4). The etiologic agents of most fungal infections are *Candida albicans*, *Candida tropicalis*, *Aspergillus flavus* and

INFECTIONS IN HEMATOLOGIC MALIGNANCY: PREDISPOSING FACTORS

Predisposing factors	Hematologic malignancy	Treatment
Neutropenia	Acute leukemia, chronic lymphocytic leukemia, myelodysplasia	Intensive chemotherapy of acute leukemia and lymphoma
Qualitative phagocyte defects	Acute leukemia, chronic myelogenous leukemia, myelodysplasia	Radiation and chemotherapy, corticosteroid treatment
Humoral immune dysfunction	Multiple myeloma, chronic lymphocytic leukemia, myelodysplasia	Intensive chemotherapy of acute leukemia and Hodgkin's disease
Cellular immune dysfunction	Chronic lymphocytic leukemia, Hodgkin's disease, non-Hodgkin's lymphoma, myelodysplasia	Cytotoxic and immunosuppressive drug therapy
Complement deficiency	Acute leukemia, lymphoma, multiple myeloma, chronic lymphocytic leukemia	Uncertain
Splenectomy	Chronic lymphocytic leukemia	Surgical
Shift in endogenous microbial flora, damage to skin and mucous membranes	Most diseases, particularly severe forms	Intensive chemotherapy

Fig. 5.3 Factors predisposing to infections in patients who have hematologic malignancy.

Aspergillus fumigatus. The infections are frequently caused by micro-organisms that have colonized the site at which the infection develops, and more than 50% are hospital-acquired pathogens.

Patients who have hematologic malignancy are also at increased risk of infection as a result of qualitative abnormalities in phagocyte function (e.g. defects in chemotaxis, phagocytosis or ingestion, or metabolic factors involved in the killing of micro-organisms). Infection caused by defects in phagocytosis and intracellular killing of micro-organisms is particularly demonstrated in patients who have immature phagocytes (e.g. patients who have myelogenous leukemias) or undergoing intensive chemotherapy.[17,18] In myelodysplasia, defects in neutrophil chemotaxis or phagocytosis also occur, even in the absence of neutropenia. The defects are most pronounced in patients who have advanced disease. Moreover, patients who have chronic myeloproliferative disorders have impaired neutrophil chemotaxis.[18] Radiotherapy, corticosteroids, certain antibiotics and antineoplastic agents also contribute to phagocyte dysfunction.

HUMORAL IMMUNE DYSFUNCTION

Defects in humoral immunity caused by decreased serum antibody levels are common in patients who have hematologic malignancy, particularly in patients who have chronic lymphocytic leukemia and multiple myeloma (Fig. 5.3). About 60–80% of patients who have chronic lymphocytic leukemia have deficiencies in at least one immunoglobulin isotype, and one-third has panhypogammaglobulinemia.[19] The latter is most prevalent in long-term survivors and patients who have advanced disease. Correction is not possible by the present mode of chemotherapy.

The majority of patients who have multiple myeloma have decreased serum levels of immunoglobulins, often less than 20% of normal.[20] Most often the deficiencies are combined IgG, IgM and IgA defects. Usually they persist throughout life and may even be accentuated by standard chemotherapy with alkylating agents and corticosteroids. Characteristic findings include a prolonged induction time for IgM responses and a decreased peak antibody titer followed by a rapid decline in antibody levels.[21] Primary antibody responses are more severely affected than secondary responses.

NEUTROPENIA WITH HEMATOLOGIC MALIGNANCY: PREDOMINATING PATHOGENS AND SITES OF INFECTION

Predominating pathogens		Sites of infection
Bacteria	Fungi	
Escherichia coli	*Aspergillus fumigatus*	Oropharynx
Klebsiella pneumoniae	*Aspergillus flavus*	Periodontium
Pseudomonas aeruginosa	*Candida albicans*	Perianal area
Staphylococcus aureus	*Candida tropicalis*	Colon
Coagulase-negative staphylococcus	*Candida* spp.	Skin
α-hemolytic streptococci	*Trichosporon* spp.	Lung
	Fusarium spp.	Esophagus

Fig. 5.4 Predominating pathogens and sites of infection in neutropenic patients who have hematologic malignancy.

INFECTION IN HEMATOLOGIC MALIGNANCY: PREDISPOSING IMMUNE DYSFUNCTIONS AND PREDOMINATING PATHOGENS

Humoral immune dysfunction	Cellular immune dysfunction	
Haemophilus influenzae	*Listeria monocytogenes*	Cytomegalovirus
Streptococcus pneumoniae	*Legionella pneumophila*	Epstein–Barr virus
Neisseria meningitidis	*Mycobacterium avium/intracellulare*	Herpes simplex virus
Other streptococci		Varicella-zoster virus
Enteroviruses	*Mycobacterium tuberculosis*	Measles virus
Hepatitis viruses	*Mycobacterium* spp.	HHV6 parvovirus
	Salmonella spp.	Respiratory syncytial virus
	Pneumocystis carinii	
	Cryptococcus neoformans	*Cryptosporidium*
		Microsporidium
	Coccidioides immitis	*Toxoplasma gondii*
	Histoplasma capsulatum	*Strongyloides stercoralis*

Fig. 5.5 Infections in patients who have hematologic malignancy: predisposing immune dysfunctions and predominating pathogens.

Hypogammaglobulinemia occurs in about 20% of patients who have myelodysplastic syndromes.[16] The intensive chemotherapy in acute leukemia may also result in decreased immunoglobulin levels, particularly IgG$_2$ levels, and impaired host defense against bacterial infections.[17] The defect may persist after chemotherapy is discontinued. Additionally, in Hodgkin's disease intensive chemotherapy together with radiation therapy may result in humoral immune dysfunction.

Patients who have humoral immune dysfunction have an increased incidence of bacterial infections, mainly because of deficient opsonization, lysis and agglutination of bacteria. Respiratory tract infections and bacteremia are frequently encountered in patients who have IgG and IgM deficiencies. Encapsulated bacteria such as pneumococci and *Haemophilus influenzae* are common pathogens (Fig. 5.5). Normal humoral immune function is also essential for the control of enterovirus and hepatitis virus infections in the acute viremic phase. The clinical picture in patients who have IgA deficiency is variable; they may be asymptomatic or experience recurrent sinopulmonary infections with viruses or bacteria.

CELLULAR IMMUNE DYSFUNCTION

Impaired cellular immune responses occur with chronic lymphocytic leukemia, non-Hodgkin's lymphoma, Hodgkin's disease, myelodysplastic syndromes and the use of cytotoxic or immunosuppressive drugs. The defects are often present in the absence of lymphopenia. In patients who have chronic lymphocytic leukemia, the defects occur particularly in those who also have hypogammaglobulinemia.[7] Cytotoxic drugs (e.g. fludarabine) or high doses of corticosteroids (e.g. treatment of multiple myeloma) cause CD4+ lymphopenia.[22] The corticosteroid-induced lymphopenia is rapidly reversible whereas lymphopenia after cytotoxic drug therapy may persist for several months. Acquired cellular immunity to *C. albicans* may prevent progression of mucosal colonization to symptomatic infection in immunocompetent individuals. This seems to be the result of an interdependence between cellular immunity and granulocyte functions, and the combination of defects in these systems may be important in the increased susceptibility to fungal infections in neutropenic patients who have hematologic malignancy.

Patients who have cellular immune dysfunction frequently develop infections with a wide variety of micro-organisms, including many opportunistic agents (Fig. 5.5). Most of these organisms are intracellular pathogens, and many of the infections represent reactivation of a latent agent (e.g. infections with varicella-zoster virus, herpes simplex virus, *Toxoplasma gondii* or *Pneumocystis carinii*).

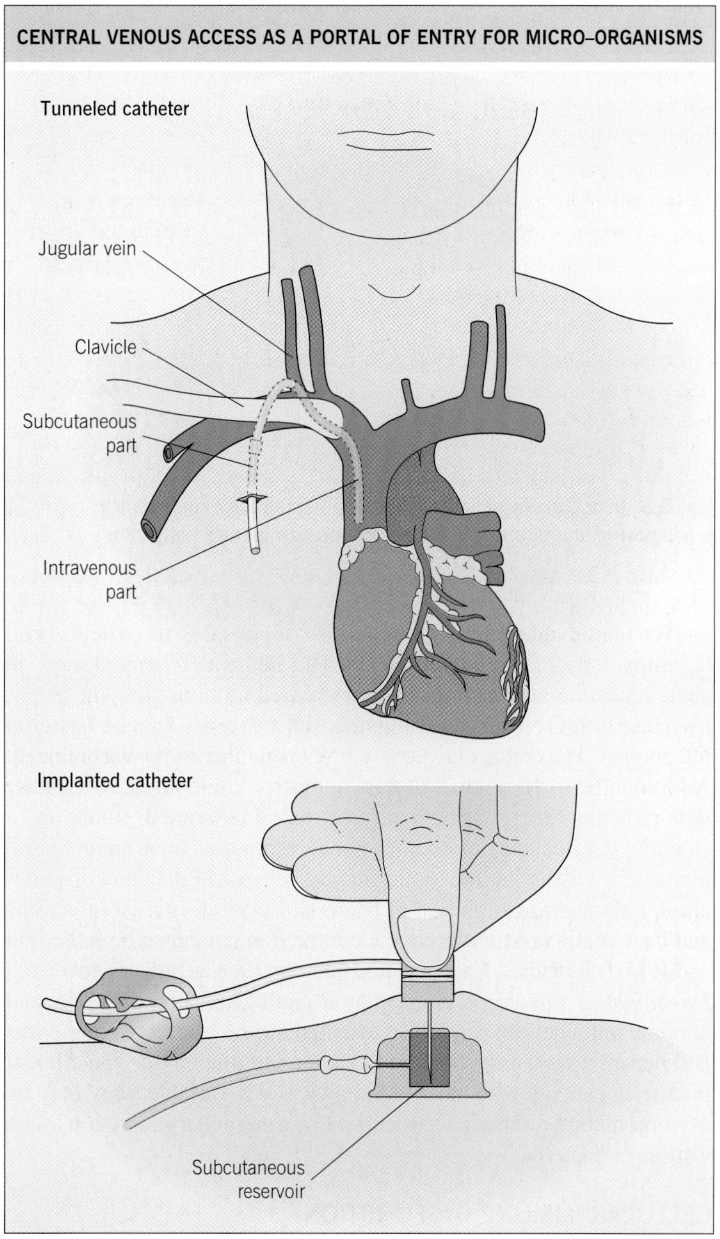

DEFICIENCY OF THE COMPLEMENT AND CYTOKINE SYSTEMS

Deficiencies of the complement system sometimes occur in patients who have acute leukemia, lymphoma, multiple myeloma or chronic lymphocytic leukemia. Patients who have chronic lymphocytic leukemia may have decreased serum levels of isolated complement factors or combinations of several factors.[7,23] The defects are most frequent in patients who have advanced disease. The complement system is of major importance for opsonization and killing of micro-organisms, and phagocyte chemotaxis. Defects predispose to infection with encapsulated bacteria (*Neisseria* spp., *Streptococcus pneumoniae* and *H. influenzae*) and *C. albicans*.

Decreased cytokine levels are often encountered in patients who have hematologic malignancy, but even neutropenic patients respond with increased cytokine production during infection.[24] The membrane forms of adhesion molecules are important for the migration and effector function of many immunocompetent cells. These molecules also exist in biologically active soluble forms. In neutropenic patients, the serum levels of the soluble molecules are modulated by complicating infections.[24] However, the specific role of these soluble molecules in the pathogenesis of infection in immunocompromised patients is not defined.

SPLENECTOMY

The indications for splenectomy in patients who have hematologic malignancy are limited and include mainly chronic lymphocytic leukemia complicated with hypersplenism or autoimmune thrombocytopenia or hemolysis. The procedure is also indicated in selected patients who have chronic myeloproliferative disorders. In patients who cannot undergo splenectomy, splenic irradiation is an alternative. Splenectomized patients are at increased risk of fulminant septicemia with encapsulated bacteria, particularly pneumococci, but also *H. influenzae*, meningococci and some other bacteria (see Chapter 4.7). Splenectomy further reduces impaired host defense in patients who have hematologic malignancy.

SHIFT IN ENDOGENOUS MICROBIAL FLORA

In healthy individuals, the skin and mucous membranes are colonized by relatively innocuous normal flora, mainly aerobic Gram-positive bacteria and a variety of anaerobic organisms. As disease and general debilitation occur, a shift toward Gram-negative bacilli occurs (see Chapter 4.1). In the more severely ill patients, such as many patients who have hematologic malignancy, Gram-negative bacilli and fungi, often from the hospital environment, become the predominant endogenous flora and the cause of infection. In neutropenic patients, more than 80% of microbiologically documented infections are caused by organisms that are part of the endogenous flora, and about one-half of the etiologic agents are acquired by the patient subsequent to hospital admission.[25]

Antimicrobial agents are frequently used in patients who have hematologic malignancy. They suppress the beneficial normal flora of the skin that provides protection against colonization and infection with more pathogenic agents. Several antibiotics excreted partly via the hepatobiliary tract (e.g. cefoperazone, ciprofloxacin or piperacillin) will suppress the anaerobic flora of the gastrointestinal tract and facilitate colonization with antibiotic-resistant Gram-negative bacilli and fungi from the hospital environment. If the mucosa becomes damaged (e.g. by intensive chemotherapy) the organisms may easily cause local infection and gain access to the circulation. Because colonization precedes infection, surveillance cultures may sometimes be helpful in the care of high-risk patients who have hematologic malignancy.

VARIOUS MEDICAL PROCEDURES AND DISEASE CONDITIONS

In patients who have hematologic malignancy, neutropenia and immune deficiencies are often associated with other less specific factors that act in concert with neutropenia and immune deficiency and predispose the patients to infection. Intravenous cannulae and catheters

Fig. 5.6 Central venous access as a portal of entry for micro-organisms. A tunneled catheter is inserted through a subcutaneous tunnel into the vein; the exit site causes damage to the skin. An implanted catheter system is connected with a subcutaneous reservoir and is inserted into a central vein. For infusion the skin and the reservoir are punctured with a needle; the skin remains intact when the system is not in use.

CENTRAL VENOUS ACCESS AS A PORTAL OF ENTRY FOR MICRO–ORGANISMS

Tunneled catheter / Jugular vein / Clavicle / Subcutaneous part / Intravenous part / Implanted catheter / Subcutaneous reservoir designed to maintain vital functions and therapeutic measures are notorious points of entry for bacteria and fungi and are particularly dangerous in patients who have neutropenia or an impaired immune response (Fig. 5.6). Patients who have leukemia and lymphoma and bleed easily frequently have breaks in skin and mucosa, which allows micro-organisms to invade and multiply. Corticosteroid therapy causes

skin atrophy and breaks and these become infected easily. Intensive chemotherapy in acute leukemia or lymphoma is often associated with damage to the mucosa of the gastrointestinal (e.g. methotrexate) and respiratory tracts. These mucosal lesions frequently serve as portals of entry for micro-organisms that colonize the mucosal surface. In the absence of granulocytes or an adequate immune response, these organisms may easily cause local infections or invade the vascular system causing severe septicemia. Some patients who have untreated acute leukemia or lymphoma have malignant cell infiltrates in their gastrointestinal tract. During initial chemotherapy, the infiltrates will regress leaving a damaged mucosa, which may serve as a portal of entry for micro-organisms colonizing the site.

PREVENTION

Methods to prevent infection in patients who have hematologic malignancy include reducing the acquisition of new micro-organisms, suppressing or eliminating endogenous microbial flora and improving host defenses (Fig. 5.7). A number of measures have been introduced; each has advantages and problems (Fig. 5.8). However, the most important anti-infective measure remains the simplest: careful handwashing practices by all personnel and visitors who come into contact with the patient.

PREVENTING THE ACQUISITION OF NEW MICRO-ORGANISMS

Patients who have hematologic malignancy frequently develop infections with hospital-acquired micro-organisms that have colonized the site at which the infection develops.[13,25] In neutropenic patients, more than 80% of microbiologically documented infections are caused by organisms that are part of the endogenous flora and approximately 50% of the causative agents are acquired by the patients subsequent to hospital admission (see Chapter 4.1). Thus, it is important to minimize the acquisition of hospital organisms. Upon hospital admission, patients whose neutrophil counts are expected to drop below 500 cells/mm^3 should be placed in a single room, preferably with positive air pressure to prevent airborne bacteria and spores from entering the room from more contaminated adjacent areas. If the patient is not placed in a protected environment (e.g. single room with positive air pressure) until after their neutrophil count has dropped to below 500 cells/mm^3, they may already have become colonized with hospital organisms liable to cause infection when the neutrophil count drops. The number of visitors should be kept to a minimum. Although practices vary, we require staff members to wear surgical gowns and masks to prevent the transfer of micro-organisms from staff to patient. Visitors are also required to wear a nonsterile-type mask upon entering the room, to prevent upper respiratory tract infections in particular because these infections are often communicable before symptoms appear. To have

PREVENTING INFECTIONS IN PATIENTS WITH HEMATOLOGIC MALIGNANCY

Prevent acquisition of environmental micro-organisms and suppress endogenous flora	Isolation rooms
	Single, positive air pressure
	Ultraclean (e.g. laminar airflow and prophylactic antimicrobial agents)
	Prophylactic antibacterial agents
	Oral nonabsorbable antibiotics
	Trimethoprim–sulfamethoxazole ('selective decontamination')
	Isoniazid
	Prophylactic antifungal agents
	Nystatin
	Imidazoles
	Triazoles
	Prophylactic antiviral agents
	Aciclovir
	Ganciclovir
	Foscarnet (?)
	Prophylactic agents against *Pneumocystis carinii*
	Trimethoprim–sulfamethoxazole
	Aerosolized pentamidine
	Dapsone
Improve host defenses	Immunizations
	Viral and bacterial vaccines
	Specific or pooled immunoglobulins
	Increase granulocyte recovery
	Granulocyte colony-stimulating factor
	Granulocyte–macrophage colony-stimulating factor
	Monocyte colony stimulating factor
	Granulocyte transfusions

Fig. 5.7 Methods for preventing infections in patients who have hematologic malignancy.

PREVENTING INFECTIONS IN PATIENTS WITH ACUTE LEUKEMIA UNDERGOING REMISSION-INDUCTION CHEMOTHERAPY: EFFICACY AND DISADVANTAGES

Parameter	Ultraclean environment	Nonabsorbable antibiotics	Trimethoprim–sulfamethoxazole	Fluoroquinolones
Reduced infection	Yes	No	Possibly	Possibly
Decreased fever	Yes	No	No	No
Reduced need for antibacterial and antifungal agents	No	No	Possibly	Possibly
Increased survival	No	No	No	No
Good compliance	No	No	Fairly	Yes
Bone marrow suppression	No	No	Yes	No
Emergence of resistant bacteria	Yes	Yes	Yes	Yes
Increased cost	Yes	Yes	Moderately	Yes

Fig. 5.8 Methods for preventing infections in patients who have acute leukemia undergoing remission-induction chemotherapy: efficacy and disadvantages. Ultraclean environment includes laminar airflow room, oral nonabsorbable antibiotics and sterilization of all objects entering the room.

visitors and staff wear a mask upon entering the room may also have an important effect in reminding them to wash their hands before touching the patient. Positive pressure rooms can be responsible for the spread of respiratory pathogens, e.g. tuberculosis in other patients.

Foods are naturally contaminated with bacteria, particularly Gram-negative bacilli such as *E. coli*, *K. pneumoniae* and *P. aeruginosa*. To reduce the acquisition of new micro-organisms, all foods should be cooked, placed on sterile dishes and covered before being served to the patient. Fresh fruit and vegetables should be excluded from the diet unless they are properly decontaminated or peeled. Sterile water or bottled water should be used for drinking purposes. Flowers should not be brought into the patient's room. Housekeeping procedures that tend to redisperse micro-organisms into the air (e.g. dry mopping) should be avoided.

Ultraclean rooms with constant positive pressure airflow (i.e. laminar airflow rooms or plastic isolators) have been adapted for care of patients who have a high risk of infection (see Chapters 4.1 & 4.4). The ultra-clean environment is maintained by sterilization of all objects that enter the room, including food. Patients nursed in these rooms are given oral nonabsorbable antibiotics together with skin antiseptics and antibiotic ointments to suppress intestinal and body flora. The combined use of these measures does reduce the number and severity of infections in neutropenic patients,[13,26] and cases of airborne infections (e.g. aspergillosis and mucormycosis) have been exceedingly rare. However, strict isolation of patients in laminar airflow rooms for prolonged periods of time is psychologically disturbing and expensive. Furthermore, the patient survival has not been substantially improved because the treatment of established infections has improved in recent years. Laminar airflow rooms are not necessary for the treatment of patients who have hematologic malignancy but they may be of value to patients who are likely to experience prolonged periods (>2–3 weeks) of profound neutropenia or patients undergoing bone marrow transplantation.

SUPPRESSION OF ENDOGENOUS MICRO-ORGANISMS
Because the gastrointestinal tract is the source of many of the pathogens that cause infections in patients who have hematologic malignancy, particularly during neutropenic periods, oral non-absorbable antimicrobial agents have been used to suppress the endogenous gastrointestinal flora. These regimens have usually included an aminoglycoside, colistin, nystatin, polymyxin B or vancomycin. Several of these agents are distasteful and cause nausea and vomiting, making compliance a significant problem, particularly in patients receiving endogenic chemotherapy. Development of anti-biotic resistance has also been a problem, especially when an amino-glycoside was included in the regimen. Lack of patient compliance as a result of poor tolerance, development of antibiotic resistance, malabsorption and high cost have markedly limited the indications for these regimens, and prophylaxis with oral nonabsorbable antibiotics is not recommended except in patients nursed in ultraclean environments (e.g. laminar airflow rooms).

Selective decontamination is a modified antimicrobial technique for suppressing the potentially pathogenic aerobic flora of the gastro-intestinal tract while preserving the anaerobic flora that provides resistance against colonization by new aerobic bacteria and fungi.[27] The most commonly used agents are trimethoprim–sulfamethoxazole (co-trimoxazole) or fluoroquinolones.[28,29] Initial studies with these agents in neutropenic patients demonstrated reduction in most infections. However, follow-up studies have given conflicting results.[29] Drug toxicity, prolonged periods of neutropenia caused by myelo-suppression and the development of antibiotic resistance have been reported during prolonged trimethoprim–sulfamethoxazole prophy-laxis. Fluoroquinolone prophylaxis has been associated with an increased prevalence of infections with Gram-positive bacteria, partic-ularly viridans streptococci and coagulase-negative staphylococci, and also with resistance development. The potential advantages of pro-phylaxis with trimethoprim–sulfamethoxazole or fluoroquinolones in

neutropenic patients are minimized by the serious disadvantages (see Chapters 4.1 & 4.4).

A patient who has not previously been treated for tuberculosis but has a positive skin test or a Ghon complex on chest radiograph should receive isoniazid, 300mg/day, if they are receiving prolonged and/or high dose steroid therapy. A negative skin test does not preclude the need for isoniazid because of the frequent anergy to such tests.

The increasing incidence of invasive fungal infections in patients who have hematologic malignancy, particularly neutropenic patients who have acute leukemia, has stimulated extensive prophylactic use of antifungal drugs (nystatin, imidazoles, triazoles). Such use has dec-reased colonization and superficial infections with fungi. However, this has not resulted in a decreased incidence of invasive disease except in one study of fluconazole prophylaxis in bone marrow transplant patients.[30] In contrast, antifungal prophylaxis in patients who have acute leukemia has resulted in overgrowth and invasion by resistant fungi, particularly *Aspergillus* spp. and *Candida krusei*,[31] and increased patient survival has not been demonstrated. Significant benefit from antifungal prophylaxis in patients who have hematologic malignancy seems not to have been proved, and widespread antifungal chemo-prophylaxis is not recommended.

Patients undergoing induction therapy for leukemia or lymphoma often experience reactivation of herpes simplex virus infection with extensive mucocutaneous lesions. At least 50% of patients who have acute leukemia will experience reactivation within 2–3 weeks of initiation of induction therapy, and antiviral therapy seems warranted in about 90% of these patients.[13,32] Reactivation may be prevented by either intravenous or oral administration of aciclovir during the first 2–3 weeks after initiation of induction chemotherapy.

Cytomegalovirus is frequently isolated from patients who have disorders of cell-mediated immunity, and can cause a variety of serious infections, including esophagitis, enterocolitis, pneumonitis, chorio-retinitis and encephalitis (see Chapter 8.5). Prevention of cytomegalo-virus infection among seronegative patients is achieved by use of seronegative or leukocyte-depleted blood products. The role of specific immunoglobulin prophylaxis remains unclear. Prevention of cyto-megalovirus infection among seropositive patients may be achieved with the use of ganciclovir[33] or high-dose aciclovir. Foscarnet has a good therapeutic effect against cytomegalovirus infection, and may also become an effective prophylactic agent.

Children undergoing remission-induction therapy for acute lympho-blastic leukemia or lymphoma are at particular risk of developing *P. carinii* pneumonia. Most of these infections occur during remission. Effective prophylaxis is achieved by administration of trimethoprim–-sulfamethoxazole. Alternative agents include aerosolized pentamidine or dapsone. However, not all children require prophylaxis. The intensity of immunosuppressive or cytotoxic therapy and the pre-valence of pneumocystosis should be considered when deciding whether prophylaxis should be given.

IMPROVEMENT OF HOST DEFENSES
Improvement of host defenses may be achieved by active and passive immunization and stimulation of bone marrow by hematopoietic growth factors.

Live virus vaccines are generally contraindicated in immuno-compromised patients who have hematologic malignancy because of the risk of serious adverse effect. An exception appears to be the judicious use of live varicella vaccine in children with acute lympho-blastic leukemia in remission, in whom the risk of natural varicella out-weighs the risk from the attenuated vaccine virus.[34] Inactivated polio vaccine should be routinely used for the patient and for siblings and other household contacts because live attenuated vaccine strains are transmissible to the immunocompromised individual. However, siblings and household contacts can receive live measles, rubella and mumps vaccines because transmission of these vaccine viruses does not occur. Patients who have leukemia in remission and whose chemotherapy has been terminated for at least 3 months may receive live virus vaccines for infections to which they are still susceptible.

Patients who have Hodgkin's disease are at increased risk of pneumococcal infection and possibly also of *H. influenzae* type b infection and should be immunized against these micro-organisms. Patients undergoing splenectomy for hematologic malignancy should receive pneumococcal and *H. influenzae* type b vaccine, and children should also receive meningococcal vaccine (see Chapter 4.7). To optimize antibody response, the vaccines should be administered in periods of no chemotherapy and at least 2 weeks before splenectomy. The humoral antibody response to pneumococcal immunization in patients who have multiple myeloma has been disappointing.

Passive immunization with varicella-zoster immune globulin reduces the incidence of severe infection and the mortality rate in immunocompromised patients who have primary varicella infection. Varicella-zoster immune globulin should be given within 72 hours of exposure to immunocompromised patients who are seronegative. A single dose is protective for approximately 1 month.

Deficient antibody production could contribute to the enhanced susceptibility to infection in patients who have hematologic malignancy, and intravenous immunoglobulins have reduced the frequency of respiratory tract infections in patients who have multiple myeloma or chronic lymphocytic leukemia.[35] However, the incidence of fever or infection has not been reduced in neutropenic patients given intravenous immunoglobulins. This is an exceptionally expensive intervention that has not improved the survival of the patients.[36] Its role in the prevention of bacterial infections in patients who have hematologic malignancy has not been defined.

Granulocyte colony-stimulating factor (G-CSF) and granulocyte-macrophage colony-stimulating factor (GM-CSF) stimulate the proliferation and maturation of bone marrow progenitor cells and increase the number of circulating blood cells. When given prophylactically to patients receiving chemotherapy for hematologic malignancy or solid tumors, the duration and severity of neutropenia and the incidence of fever are reduced, as is the use of systemic antibiotics.[37] However, these growth factors may also stimulate the proliferation of malignant myeloid cells. They are expensive and a beneficial effect has not been demonstrated on survival of patients who have hematologic malignancy. Thus, for patients who have neutropenia of short duration (i.e. <10 days) and a low risk of infection, these agents seem unnecessary. However, for patients who have prolonged neutropenia and a high risk of infection the use of G-CSF or GM-CSF seems indicated. The prophylactic and therapeutic use of transfused leukocytes has been abandoned, mainly because of the use of colony-stimulating factors, but also because of serious questions about clinical efficacy, safety and cost-effectiveness.

CLINICAL FEATURES

FEVER

The most common clinical manifestation of infection in patients who have hematologic malignancy is fever; in neutropenic patients especially, fever may be the first and only sign of infection. However, fever can also develop as a manifestation of the neoplastic disease itself. In addition, other noninfectious causes of fever must be considered, including drugs, transfusion reactions, emboli, splenic infarcts, thrombophlebitis, radiation injury and allergic reactions (Fig. 5.9).

The evaluation of the febrile patient who has hematologic malignancy should include a careful history and a prompt and thorough physical examination (Fig. 5.10). The history should reveal organ-defining symptoms (e.g. sore throat, cough, diarrhea, perianal pain and dysuria), as these are indispensable for the localization and specific treatment of the infection. The mode of onset and the rate of progression of the febrile reaction may also give useful clues as to the diagnosis. Information on other illnesses (e.g. diabetes mellitus) and previous and current therapy that may have influenced the host defense or the microbial colonization (e.g. high-dose corticosteroids, cytotoxic

treatment, radiation and antimicrobial medication) must be obtained. Knowledge about neutropenia or lymphopenia is vital for the correct evaluation and management of the patient. The duration of the immunosuppressed state should also be defined, because this is an important indicator of the etiology of the infection. Hence, a patient

CAUSES OF FEVER IN PATIENTS WHO HAVE HEMATOLOGIC MALIGNANCY
• Infection (viruses, bacteria, fungi, protozoa)
• Underlying malignant disease
• Pyrogenic medications (e.g. cytotoxic drugs)
• Radiation injury
• Transfusion reactions
• Emboli (e.g. pulmonary emboli)
• Infarcts (e.g. splenic infarcts)
• Thrombophlebitis
• Hematomas
• Allergic reactions
• Pulmonary edema

Fig. 5.9 Causes of fever in patients who have hematologic malignancy.

CLINICAL EVALUATION OF PATIENTS WHO HAVE HEMATOLOGIC MALIGNANCY AND FEVER	
History	Examples
Obtain information about: The febrile reaction	Mode of onset and rate of progression
Organ-defining symptoms	Sore throat, cough, diarrhea, abdominal or perianal pain, dysuria and headache
Complicating diseases	Diabetes mellitus
Previous infections	Tuberculosis and hepatic candidiasis
Previous and current therapy	High-dose corticosteriods, cytotoxic treatment, radiation, splenectomy and antimicrobial medication
Predisposing factors	Intravenous catheters, endotracheal tubes and urinary catheters
Recent invasive procedures	Bone marrow aspiration, lumbar puncture and biopsy
The nature of the underlying malignancy	
Microbial colonization	
Neutropenia	Severity and duration
Physical examination	Examples
Perform a complete and thorough examination without delay. In neutropenic patients give special attention to: Skin	Redness tenderness
Lungs	Cough, tachypnea
Perioral area	Blisters
Perianal area	Pain, fissures
Colon	Tenderness, resistance
Wounds	Wounds
Sites of procedure	Venipuncture, bone marrow aspiration and central venous catheter insertion
Foreign bodies	Indwelling venous catheters, endotracheal tubes and urinary catheters

Fig. 5.10 Clinical evaluation of patients who have hematologic malignancy and fever.

who has acute leukemia presenting for the first time with cough and tachypnea most probably has a bacterial infection, whereas the same patient who has fever and pneumonia after 3 weeks of chemotherapy and broad antibacterial treatment is at high risk of having an invasive fungal infection. The history should also include information about previous infections (e.g. tuberculosis or hepatic candidiasis) and predisposing factors like splenectomy or the presence of indwelling catheters or other foreign material. Furthermore, the nature of the underlying malignancy has to be taken into consideration. Hence, patients who have lymphoma often have abnormalities of the cellular immune system that heighten their risk of infections with viruses (e.g. herpes simplex and varicella-zoster) and fungi (e.g. *Cryptococcus* spp.). Moreover, the fever in Hodgkin's disease is sometimes of a characteristic type and a manifestation of the disease itself. However, the fever curve alone is usually of limited predictive value for the determination of the cause of fever in the individual patient. Information on microbial colonization may sometimes be helpful. At least 80% of documented infections that occur in patients who have neutropenia are caused by organisms that are part of the endogenous microflora, usually at sites near the source of infection.[25,38] However, multiple potential pathogens are often isolated from a single site, making it difficult to predict the exact micro-organism causing the infection.[39]

The spectrum of infectious complications in neutropenic patients who have hematologic malignancy and fever is different from that of non-neutropenic patients. Thus, in febrile neutropenic patients special attention should be given to the sites that are most commonly the source of infection, i.e. the skin, the lungs and the perioral and perianal areas (Fig. 5.10). Any wound or site of previous procedure (e.g. venipuncture, bone marrow aspiration, lumbar puncture or central venous catheter insertion) should be carefully examined. Signs of herpetic blisters and ulcers and of mucositis should be sought. Cough, expectoration, tachypnea and cyanosis should be registered, and careful abdominal palpation should reveal tenderness or resistance. Although examination of the perirectal area should always be performed, digital rectal examination should only be carried out when the findings are suggestive of a localized inflammatory site (e.g. distinctive pain or fluctuation). In patients who have neutropenia, symptoms and signs indicating infection (i.e. pain, swelling, erythema or pus formation) may be blunted or even lacking because of an inadequate inflammatory response.[40] In these patients even subtle indications of inflammation must be considered as presumptive signs of invasive infection. Mild perirectal erythema and tenderness may be caused by a perianal cellulitis, and even slight erythema and secretion at the exit site of a Hickman catheter indicate a tunnel infection. It should, however, be borne in mind that the initial evaluation of febrile neutropenic patients reveals a defined site of infection in less than 50% of cases,[41] and that failure to determine the cause of the febrile response must not lead to delayed institution of proper therapy (see also below).

In the absence of neutropenia, the infections are often related to defects of cell-mediated or humoral immunity, secondary to either the underlying disease or side effects of treatment (e.g. high-dose corticosteroids or cytotoxic drugs). In these patients, it is important to recognize the association of specific infectious syndromes with specific defects. Consistently, children with leukemia in remission receiving maintenance chemotherapy are at increased risk of *P. carinii* pneumonia or *H. influenzae* sepsis,[42] whereas patients who have lymphoma are particularly susceptible to infections with viruses, fungi or facultative intracellular micro-organisms (see Pathogenesis and pathology).[43,44]

Specific therapeutic procedures may also be associated with specific infections. Febrile patients who have an indwelling venous catheter, for example, are at increased risk of bloodstream infections with staphylococci,[45] whereas splenectomized patients are at increased risk of serious bacterial infections caused primarily by pneumococci or *H. influenzae*.[46] The initial presentation of even overwhelming infection may be misleadingly subtle in asplenic patients, with fever being the only sign. Thus, splenectomized

patients who have hematologic malignancy and fever should be treated initially as being potentially septic.

PATIENTS WHO HAVE DOCUMENTED INFECTION
Bacteremia, fungemia and sepsis

The recovery of bacteria or fungi from blood cultures may be a transient phenomenon not associated with bloodstream infection or the serious extension of an invasive infectious disease. Transient bacteremia is frequent after instrumentation of the gastrointestinal and the genitourinary tracts, and after surgery.[47] In addition, pseudobacteremia may be associated with contaminated disinfectants, heparinized flushes, intravenous infusates or contaminated equipment. On the other hand, bacteremia and fungemia may precede or coincide with local foci of infection such as cellulitis or endocarditis. Patients who have hematologic malignancy are at increased risk of developing persistent bacteremia and metastatic infection.

For most episodes of bacteremia, the etiologic agent and the site of origin are difficult to predict at the onset of fever. However, indwelling central venous catheters and totally implanted venous access systems represent significant sources of bacteremia and fungemia.[45] Among immunocompromised patients who have no such devices, the respiratory tract is the most commonly identified site of origin (25%), followed by the perianal and perioral areas (10%) and the gastrointestinal (10%) and the genitourinary tracts (10%).[41] This contrasts with the situation in the general hospital population in whom the genitourinary tract is the most common site of origin for bacteremias.

Bacteria are most frequently isolated from blood cultures and, up to 1980, Gram-negative aerobic organisms (e.g. *E. coli*, *P. aeruginosa* and *K. pneumoniae*) were the most frequently isolated pathogens in neutropenic patients.[9,48] During the past decade the pattern of infection has shifted, and Gram-positive micro-organisms (most commonly *S. aureus*, *S. epidermidis* and *Streptococcus* spp.) are now isolated more often than Gram-negative bacteria at most cancer centers.[9,48–50]

In recent years, the relative proportion of disseminated fungal infections has increased.[9,48,51] *Candida* spp. dominate, but other fungi are not infrequent. Patients who have hematologic malignancy at special risk of developing fungal infection include those with neutropenia lasting more than 1 week, those who have experienced a fungal infection earlier and those who have received broad-spectrum antibiotics or corticosteroids in combination with cytotoxic drugs (Fig. 5.11). Special attention must be given to patients who continue to be febrile while on broad-spectrum antibacterial treatment.

Sepsis is defined as clinical evidence of infection (e.g. positive blood cultures) combined with signs of a systemic inflammatory response (fever, tachycardia, hyperventilation or hypoventilation, and leukocytosis or leukopenia).[52] The onset is usually characterized by

INVASIVE FUNGAL INFECTIONS IN PATIENTS WHO HAVE HEMATOLOGIC MALIGNANCY
Predisposing factors
Neutropenia >7 days
High-dose corticosteroid therapy in combination with cytotoxic drugs or antibiotics
Previous fungal infection
Chemotherapy-induced mucositis
Clinical signs
Fever >5–7 days despite broad-spectrum antibiotic therapy
Progressive debilitation during antibiotic therapy
Diffuse pulmonary infiltrates not respecting natural anatomic borders
Progressive unexplained liver or renal failure

Fig. 5.11 **Predisposing factors and clinical signs of invasive fungal infections in patients who have hematologic malignancy.**

nonspecific symptoms, including chills, sweats, nausea, vomiting, breathlessness and headache. Sometimes cough, dysuria or other symptoms suggestive of the underlying process occur. On examination, the patient is febrile, tachypneic and tachycardic. Progression of the systemic inflammatory response may lead to shock and multiorgan failure, with hypotension, cardiac arrhythmias, oliguria, coagulopathy, ileus and signs of encephalopathy (see Chapter 2.47).

Signs of sepsis in patients who have hematologic malignancy call for immediate and thorough evaluation. Information about the origin of infection and the nature of the infecting micro-organism has implications for therapy and is important for the estimation of prognosis. However, sepsis in patients who have hematologic malignancy is often associated with a rapid progression and a high mortality, and a full assessment may have to be postponed until resuscitation and empiric antimicrobial treatment have been instituted.

In small children, in the elderly and in neutropenic patients, the symptoms and signs of sepsis may be altered or even lacking. Hence, severe sepsis may manifest with hypothermia in infants, and sepsis originating from a perirectal cellulitis in neutropenic patients may almost completely lack local signs of inflammation. Thus, in these patients sepsis should be considered as a possible differential diagnosis of any unexplained illness.

Intravascular catheters
Indwelling venous (e.g. Hickman catheters) or arterial catheters and totally implanted venous access devices represent major sources of infection in patients who have hematologic malignancy. The infectious complications are commonly categorized:
• bacteremia and septic infections,
• tunnel infections and
• exit site infections.

Exit site infections are local infections of the tissue at the point at which the catheter exits, whereas tunnel infections are local infections of the subcutaneous track from the skin to the site of entry into the central blood vessel (see Fig. 5.6).

Catheter-associated bacteremia may be completely symptom free, whereas in the case of dissemination, the patient may develop all common symptoms of sepsis. Erythema, swelling, tenderness or discharge at the catheter exit site are suggestive of a tunnel or exit site infection. However, in neutropenic patients most of these signs may be absent because of the blunted inflammatory response.

Whatever the underlying disease, Gram-positive cocci, especially coagulase-negative staphylococci and *S. aureus*, account for the majority (60–65%) of septic catheter-associated infections.[45,53] Gram-negative bacilli constitute 25–30% of the isolates, whereas fungi (mostly *Candida* spp.) are less common (about 2–6%).[45,53]

Although indwelling central venous catheters may become infected secondary to a bacteremia arising from a distant focus, especially in the presence of a catheter thrombus,[54] the majority of catheter infections arise through external contamination.[45] Totally implanted venous access systems eliminate the chronic catheter exit site wound, and the use of such devices seems to be associated with fewer infections and thrombotic complications than are other long-term catheters.

Upper respiratory tract infections
Children with hematologic malignancy, like healthy children, often develop acute otitis media after a viral respiratory illness, and the symptoms range from the typical complaints of fever, pain, irritability and drainage to nearly no complaints. The most common micro-organisms isolated are *S. pneumoniae*, *H. influenzae* and *Moraxella catarrhalis*. Neutropenic patients are also susceptible to other Gram-positive and Gram-negative bacteria that may have colonized the oropharynx and nasopharynx during hospitalization.

Patients who have obstruction of the sinuses by a tumor (e.g. Burkitt's lymphoma) are especially at risk of developing sinusitis. Characteristic findings in patients who have acute sinusitis include facial pain, local tenderness and purulent nasal drainage. If, however, the outlet to the nasal cavity is obstructed or the patient is severely neutropenic, only minimal drainage may be observed. When the ethmoid sinuses are involved, edema of the eyelids may develop. Fever in sinusitis is of variable occurrence and is generally inversely related to age and the duration of the illness. In immunosuppressed patients, the classic symptoms and signs of infection may be absent. Thus, any sinus tenderness in a neutropenic patient warrants further examination.

In the non-neutropenic patient, *S. pneumoniae*, *H. influenzae* and *M. catarrhalis* are the most common pathogens causing sinusitis. Fungi (e.g. *Aspergillus* spp., *C. albicans* and *Mucor* spp.), particularly, cause complicated forms of sinusitis in patients with prolonged neutropenia.[55]

Pulmonary infections
Lower respiratory tract infections are among the most common complications in patients who have hematologic malignancy. The lungs are involved in about 75% of immunocompromised patients who develop fever, and at autopsy evidence of pulmonary infection is present in more than 90% of patients.[56,57] In addition, patients who have lung injury from noninfectious processes have a high risk of secondary infection, which is often the immediate cause of death.

The risk of developing invasive pulmonary infection in patients who have hematologic malignancy depends on the immunosuppression caused by the underlying disease process and the therapeutic regimen, as well as a variety of local factors, including mucosal ulceration, obstructing tumor masses and foreign bodies (e.g. endotracheal tubes). Furthermore, the shift in the pattern of colonization of the upper respiratory tract from predominantly Gram-positive to Gram-negative flora provides a new source of pathogens in direct proximity to the lower respiratory tract.[58] Once oropharyngeal colonization with Gram-negative bacteria has occurred, it tends to persist either alone or in combination with *Candida* spp. or other fungi.

Even though bloodborne or inhaled micro-organisms represent a significant microbiologic challenge to the lungs, the large majority of pneumonias in immunocompromised patients results from the transportation of virulent micro-organisms to the lower respiratory tract by aspiration of oropharyngeal or gastric content. The elevation of gastric pH after the use of antacids or histamine type-2 blockers and after enteral feeding favors gastric colonization with Gram-negative bacteria. This overgrowth promotes duodenal–gastric reflux, which further elevates the gastric pH and increases the bacterial growth. Aspiration of oropharyngeal or gastric contents is facilitated during sleep, in situations of decreased consciousness and depressed gag and cough reflexes, and by endotracheal or nasogastric tubes.

The general signs of lower respiratory tract infection include chills, high fever, cough, expectoration, tachypnea and grunting and distressed respiration. Auscultation may reveal diminished breath sounds and fine crackling rales in the affected area. Irritation of the pleura is accompanied by chest pain, and a friction rub may be present over the involved region. The development of pleural effusion or empyema usually leads to increased dyspnea and reduced pleural pain, dullness on percussion and reduction of breath sounds on auscultation.

The symptoms and signs of pneumonia vary with the pathogen, the age of the patient and the severity of the immunosuppression. Some micro-organisms are associated with a specific pattern of disease, such as the lobar pneumonia of pneumococci and the empyema, abscess, and pneumatocele formation of *S. aureus*. In young infants, the symptoms may be nonspecific and the findings on physical examination scarce. In neutropenic patients, the clinical presentation may be subtle because of the reduced inflammatory response, and cough, purulent expectoration and pleural symptoms may be nearly nonexistent.[41] Because the survival of neutropenic patients who have pulmonary infection depends mainly on the speed with which the diagnosis is made and effective therapy is instituted, even subtle clinical findings must be promptly and carefully evaluated.

A variety of micro-organisms may cause lung infections in patients

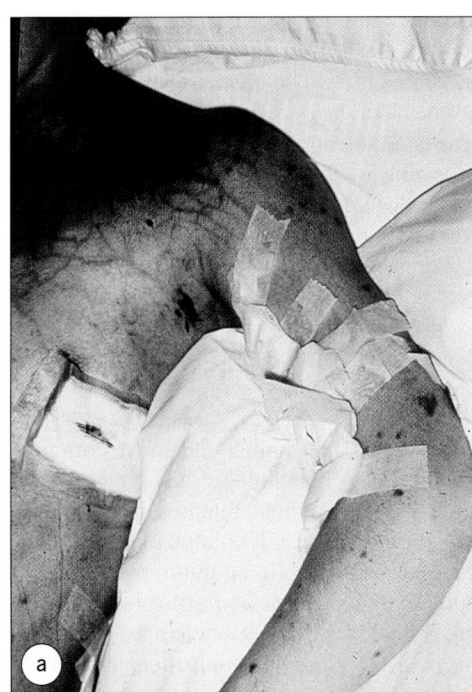

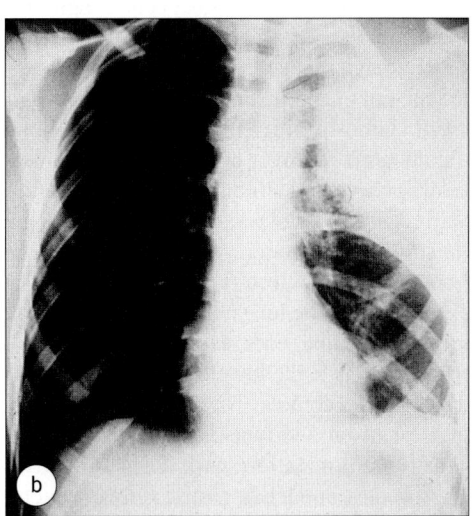

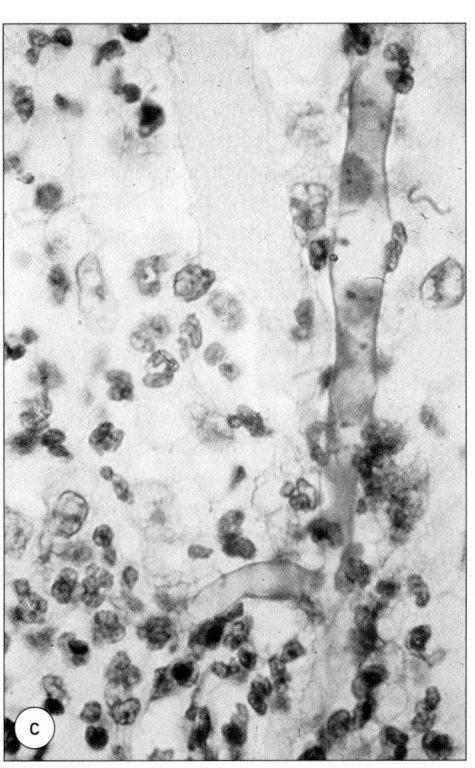

Fig. 5.12 Patient with acute myelogenous leukemia with disseminated phycomycosis. (a) Left shoulder and arm of a young female with acute myelogenous leukemia and disseminated phycomycosis involving the left lung, pleura and shoulder, the left side of the neck, the left thigh, the kidneys and the brain. The marked edema and varicose veins are caused by vascular invasion by the fungus and secondary thrombosis. (b) Chest radiograph of the patient who has a density (10 x 14cm) in the upper lateral area of the left lung. (c) Biopsy from the pulmonary lesion with broad nonseptate hyphae with right angle branching characteristic of the phycomycetes. The patient responded to prolonged treatment with amphotericin B and surgery, but died suddenly 5 months after debut of symptoms from subarachnoid hemorrhage caused by fungal invasion of the basilar artery.

who have hematologic malignancy, including *S. pneumoniae*, *H. influenzae*, opportunistic Gram-negative bacteria, *Nocardia* spp., mycobacteria, fungi, protozoa and viruses. However, a variety of noninfectious causes of pulmonary infiltrates must also be considered,[59] including the underlying malignancy, radiation pneumonitis, drug reactions, emboli, pulmonary edema, leukoagglutinin-transfusion reactions and hemorrhage secondary to severe thrombocytopenia (Fig. 5.9). In addition, secondary infections of noninfectious pulmonary processes are common and should not be overlooked.

Even though patients who have hematologic malignancy often experience infections with opportunistic micro-organisms, pneumonia caused by common bacteria (i.e. pneumococci and *H. influenzae*) or *Mycoplasma* spp. occurs most frequently.[59] Patients receiving immunosuppressive therapy (e.g. high-dose corticosteroids) are at particular risk of tuberculosis and atypical mycobacterial disease,[60] and nocardiosis. Pneumonia caused by *Legionella* spp. is also common.[61] Even though legionellosis is a multiorgan infection, the lung is the primary target organ. The initial symptoms are usually nonspecific, with fever, malaise, anorexia, lethargy and headache. Most patients develop dyspnea and a nonproductive cough, and in some patients chest pain may be significant. Diarrhea may precede or follow the respiratory symptoms. Neurologic symptoms affect up to one-third of the patients and range from headache and disorientation to seizures and encephalopathy.

Neutropenic patients who have hematologic malignancy and have received broad-spectrum antibacterial therapy are especially susceptible to invasive fungal disease, most commonly caused by *Candida* and *Aspergillus* spp. However, other fungi (i.e. *Phycomycetes*, *Histoplasma* and *Coccidioides* spp. and cryptococci) may also cause lung infection in immunocompromised patients (Fig. 5.12). The incidence of pulmonary infections caused by *Aspergillus* spp. has increased in recent years.[59,62] As *Aspergillus* spp. have a tendency to invade blood vessels, a necrotizing pneumonia is typical, sometimes with life-threatening hemoptysis. A common symptom is chest pain, which may develop before the appearance of pulmonary infiltrates. *Aspergillus* spp. may also cause saprophytic colonization of lung cavities in immunocompromised and in immunocompetent patients, producing aspergillomas. The most common symptom is hemoptysis, which may range from intermittent bloodstained sputum to massive hemoptysis. *Aspergillus* spp. may also cause allergic phenomena like extrinsic allergic alveolitis.

Patients who have lymphoma or those who are on consolidation therapy for acute lymphoblastic leukemia are at high risk of *P. carinii* pneumonia.[48,63] The clinical presentation is highly variable and depends primarily on the host defense in the individual patient. The onset may be insidious with clinical progression over 3 or more weeks, or it may be fulminant with rapid progression over 2–3 days. The patients usually present with variable fever, nonproductive cough, tachypnea and dyspnea. Tachypnea, nasal flaring and intercostal, sub-costal or supracostal retractions are common, whereas wheeze or rales are usually not detected until later in the course as resolution occurs.

Herpesviruses (e.g. herpes simplex virus, varicella-zoster virus and cytomegalovirus) are the most common cause of viral lung infection in patients who have hematologic malignancy. Respiratory syncytial virus, adenovirus, measles virus, enterovirus and rhinovirus are less common. Primary varicella-zoster virus infection is associated with significant mortality in patients who have hematologic malignancy.[64] The lung is the major site of dissemination, and is usually involved 3–7 days after the onset of skin lesions. Visceral dissemination with lung involvement is less common in zoster than after primary varicella-zoster virus infection.

Cytomegalovirus can cause serious interstitial pneumonia in patients who have hematologic malignancy, manifesting with fever and dry, nonproductive cough followed by 1 or 2 weeks' progression to dyspnea, wheezing and retractions, a situation often necessitating ventilatory support. Reactivation of latent virus or acquisition of virus from blood products are the most important causes of infection.[65]

Disseminated cytomegalovirus disease is often accompanied by abdominal pain and hemorrhagic diarrhea.

The clinical presentation of pneumonia varies with etiologic agents, and the mode of onset and the rate of progression of the disease process may give important clues as to the diagnosis. Moreover, the spectrum of pulmonary infections is highly modified by the neutrophil count and by the duration of neutropenia. Bacteria dominate as causative pathogens for pneumonia in patients who have neutropenia lasting less than 14 days. Patients who have longer periods of low neutrophil counts are more susceptible to viral (e.g. cytomegalovirus, varicella-zoster and herpes simplex) or fungal (e.g. *Candida* or *Aspergillus* spp.) infections.

When a patient who has hematologic malignancy and possible pulmonary infection is evaluated, the mode of clinical presentation should always be combined with the information on neutropenia and results of a chest radiograph. Such an approach will restrict the etiologic possibilities and make the problem more manageable for the clinician (see Diagnosis).

Skin and soft tissue infections

The skin may be infected primarily or in association with bacteremia, fungemia or viremia. Skin lesions may be pathognomonic for certain infections and permit early diagnosis of infection in a patient who has hematologic malignancy. A thorough examination of the skin should therefore always be performed when a patient who has hematologic malignancy and fever is evaluated. Signs to aid diagnosis include the vesicular lesions of herpes simplex virus infection (Fig. 5.13), the disseminated vesicles of primary varicella-zoster virus infection (Fig.

5.14), the crops of vesicles and pustules distributed along a dermatome in zoster, peripheral emboli in endocarditis and ecthyma gangrenosum in patients who have neutropenia and *P. aeruginosa* bacteremia. Lesions similar to ecthyma gangrenosum have also been reported in disseminated candidiasis and infections due to molds.

Herpes simplex virus may cause significant morbidity in patients who have hematologic malignancy. In children, herpes simplex virus infection is more common in those with myeloid leukemia than in those with lymphocytic leukemia, and the risk increases with neutropenia and chemotherapy.[66] The infections tend to remain localized, and the most common sites of infection are in and around the mouth (Fig. 5.13), the nares and the esophagus. Patients who have a history of genital or perianal herpes may also experience reactivation. Dissemination to distant areas of the skin, viscera (e.g. lungs, liver and adrenals) and the central nervous system (CNS) occurs. The lesions begin as papules and blisters that progress to bullae. In immunocompromised patients, further progression includes large, coalescing, hemorrhagic or ulcerated lesions, eroding into the subcutaneous tissue. Pain is a prominent symptom. The lesions must be differentiated from bacterial, fungal and other viral infections, and pyoderma gangrenosum and chemotherapy-induced ulcers. Secondary infections of cutaneous and mucosal lesions represent portals of entry for bacteria into the bloodstream.

In patients who have leukemia and lymphoma, primary varicella-zoster virus infection is usually severe and progressive (Fig. 5.14). The fever is higher than in otherwise healthy individuals, and the cutaneous lesions can sometimes develop atypically with more deep-seated and umbilicated lesions. Visceral involvement first of all includes the lungs, but dissemination to the CNS and the liver is also common.[64,67] Dyspnea,

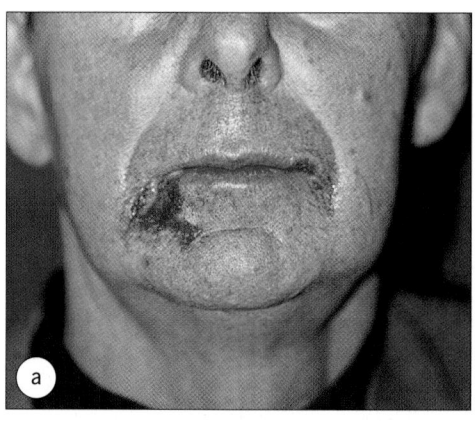
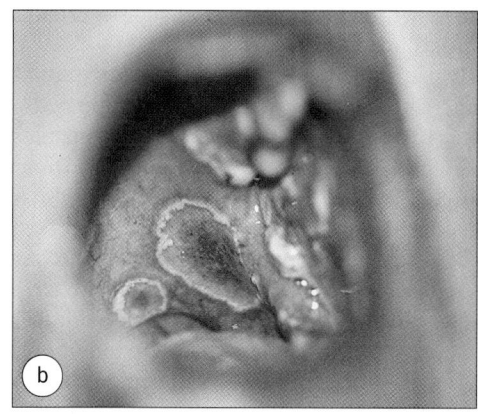

Fig. 5.13 Herpes simplex virus infection in a patient who has lymphoma. (a) Cutaneous lesions. (b) Mucosal lesions in the mouth of the same patient. Herpes simplex virus was demonstrated in fluid from oral blisters.

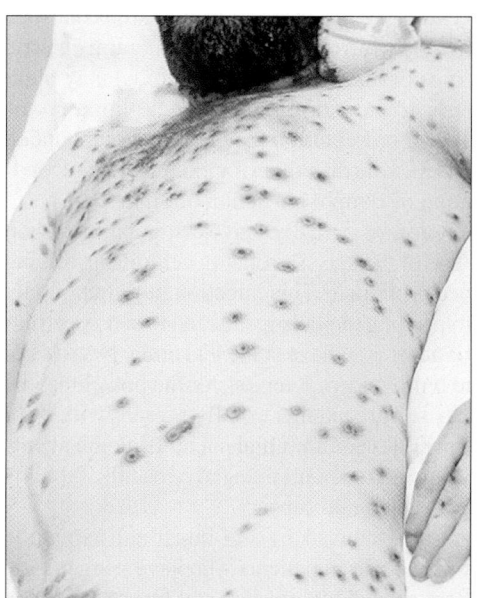
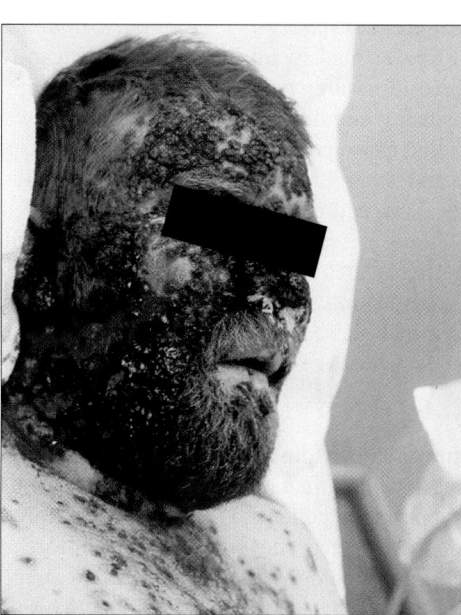

Fig. 5.14 Primary varicella-zoster virus infection in a patient who has marked lymphopenia and neutropenia after chemotherapy for Hodgkin's disease. The lesions are deep-seated, hemorrhagic and umbilicated. The patient also had pneumonia most likely caused by varicella-zoster virus. He recovered from his infection and the lymphoma went into remission.

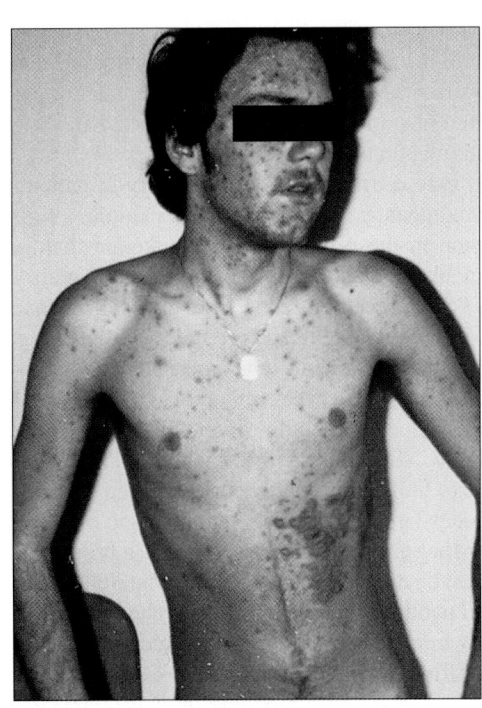

Fig. 5.15 Generalized herpes zoster in a patient who has lymphoma.

severe headache, abdominal pain, back pain and inappropriate secretion of antidiuretic hormone may indicate multisystem involvement.

Zoster represents reactivation of latent varicella-zoster virus disease and is frequent in patients who have hematologic malignancy (Fig. 5.15). Patients who have Hodgkin's disease, followed by those with non-Hodgkin's lymphoma, are at highest risk of developing zoster. Furthermore, the infection is common in patients receiving intensive immunosuppressive therapy and in those with advanced neoplastic disease. Zoster manifests with painful grouped vesicles surrounded by an erythematous base and typically distributed along the dermatomes of one to three sensory nerves. The lesions are usually unilateral and most prevalent in the thoracic region, although any dermatome may be involved.

In neutropenic patients, cutaneous punctures (e.g. needle sticks, venipunctures and bone marrow aspiration punctures) and minor abrasions may result in severe infections caused by staphylococci, *Corynebacterium jeikeium* and by colonizing *Enterobacteriaceae* or *P. aeruginosa*. In these patients, minor trauma should always be considered a potential source of bacteremia.

Perianal infections mainly represent a clinical problem in neutropenic patients,[48,68] especially in those with long-lasting and profound neutropenia. Predisposing factors include perianal mucositis caused by chemotherapy or radiotherapy, hemorrhoids, constipation and any type of rectal manipulation (e.g. repetitive manual rectal examinations, rectoscopy or barium enema). Mucosal fissures may serve as portals of entry for micro-organisms, causing cellulitis or abscess formation. The most common pathogens that cause perianal cellulitis include aerobic Gram-negative bacteria and anaerobic bacteria. The patients may complain of painful defecation, and usually they present with erythematous tender lesions without abscess formation. Although a thorough examination of the perirectal area should always be performed, unnecessary digital rectal examination should be avoided as this may induce bacteremia, sepsis, or metastatic infections, particularly in neutropenic patients.

Oropharyngeal infections
Oral mucositis is a common complication of treatment with cytotoxic drugs, and offers a potential site for microbial invasion and infection (Fig. 5.16). Gingivitis and periodontitis are very common in patients who have hematologic malignancy, and cultures of infected sites usually reveal mixed aerobic and anaerobic flora. Necrotizing gingivitis characterized by erythematous periapical gingiva is caused by anaer-

obic bacteria. In some situations, the infectious gingivitis may be clinically indistinguishable from gingival leukemic infiltrates.

The most common mucosal infection in patients who have hematologic malignancy is thrush, a superficial oral infection caused by *Candida* spp. (Fig. 5.17). The patients present with creamy white patches with slightly indurated borders. The lesions bleed easily when scraped. Oropharyngeal candidiasis may compromise food intake and serve as a nidus for systemic dissemination.

Herpes simplex is the most common viral pathogen isolated from oromucosal lesions. Clinically, the lesions usually appear as blisters and ulcera. However, the lesions may be atypical and be confused with the mucositis usually attributed to radiation or chemotherapy. Herpes simplex virus stomatitis contributes to poor nutrition. The mucosal disruption may also be infected with bacteria or fungi.

Sinus infections
Bacteria, especially *P. aeruginosa*, as well as mouth flora may cause sinusitis in the neutropenic patient. Fungi to anticipate causing sinusitis include Zygomycetes, *Aspergillus* spp. and *Fusarium* spp.

Esophagitis
Patients who have esophagitis often present with subacute onset of retrosternal or epigastric burning pain that usually is aggravated by swallowing. In non-neutropenic patients, infectious esophagitis is rare and esophagitis is most commonly caused by chemical irritation from refluxed gastric contents (e.g. occurring in association with the emesis of intensive chemotherapy).

Fungi (especially *Candida* spp.), viruses (e.g. herpes simplex virus and cytomegalovirus) and bacteria can cause esophagitis, and perforation may even occur (Fig. 5.18). Extension of oral thrush to the esophagus is common. However, absence of oral thrush does not rule out candidal esophagitis.

Gastrointestinal infections
Normally, the gastrointestinal mucosa acts as a barrier, but in patients who have hematologic malignancy it can be disrupted by tumor invasion or damage from chemotherapy or radiotherapy. The normal microbial balance is also altered by reduced bowel motility and antimicrobial therapy, further contributing to altered colonization and infection.

Patients who have abdominal infections and present with distinct abdominal or back pain, nausea, vomiting, fever and diarrhea must be evaluated without delay, and careful abdominal and pulmonary examination should be performed, including in this case a rectal examination. Several factors modulate the symptoms and clinical findings in patients who have hematologic malignancy, fever and abdominal complaints. The clinical presentation of peritonitis and even common abdominal processes like appendicitis or infectious diarrhea may be significantly altered by neutropenia. Moreover, antineoplastic therapy (e.g. cytotoxic drugs or high-dose corticosteroids) may blunt the inflammatory response to infection and induce symptoms of reduced intensity. The clinical presentation may also be compounded by the malignant disease itself. Diarrhea may, for example, be secondary to bowel wall infiltration of lymphoma and not to infection.

Some abdominal infections are virtually only seen in patients who have malignant disease. One of these is necrotizing cellulitis involving the cecum and often termed typhlitis.[69] This infection most commonly occurs in association with prolonged neutropenia and broad-spectrum antimicrobial therapy in patients who have acute leukemia. Necrosis of leukemic infiltrates of the lymphoid-rich regions of the bowel may be involved in the pathogenesis. The patients usually present with right lower quadrant pain, diarrhea, fever and fatigue. The etiologic agents include anaerobic bacteria and aerobic Gram-negative bacilli. Typhlitis can lead to perforation, peritonitis and sepsis.

A hyperinfection syndrome caused by the intestinal nematode *Strongyloides stercoralis* may occur in patients who have hematologic malignancy. This disorder is caused by invasion and ulceration of the gastrointestinal mucosa by filariform larvae and may be followed by polymicrobial sepsis. The patients usually present with fever, nausea, vomiting, diarrhea and abdominal pain.

Pseudomembranous colitis particularly associated with clindamycin and broad-spectrum beta-lactam antibiotic treatment is caused by colonization of the gut with *Clostridium difficile*. Colonization is followed by bacterial overgrowth, toxin production and mucosal lesions. In patients who have hematologic malignancy, a locally-invasive condition, called neutropenic enterocolitis, may develop which is usually associated with *C. septicum*. The patients typically present with abdominal pain and distention, and watery or mucoid diarrhea, and often go on to develop shock.

Hepatic infections

Hepatitis may be caused by a variety of infectious agents, including those that infect the liver primarily (e.g. hepatitis A, B, C and the delta agent) and secondarily (e.g. herpes simplex virus, cytomegalovirus, varicella-zoster virus, Epstein–Barr virus, coxsackie B virus, *T. gondii* and *C. albicans*).

Cytomegalovirus hepatitis in patients who have hematologic malignancy is usually mild, with little jaundice and moderate hepatomegaly.[66] Epstein–Barr virus infection in immunocompromised patients usually runs a course similar to that in immunocompetent individuals, whereas hepatitis caused by herpes simplex virus is associated with more severe disseminated disease.

Focal hepatic candidiasis has mainly been reported in patients who have leukemia and chronic neutropenia.[70,71] These patients usually present with upper right quadrant abdominal pain, nausea and fever refractory to broad-spectrum antibiotics and the disease persists even after the recovery of the neutrophil counts. The patients may also have nonspecific gastrointestinal symptoms such as diarrhea. Jaundice, abdominal pain and hepatomegaly may be present.

Genitourinary tract infections

The genitourinary tract is a less common source of infection in immunocompromised patients who have malignant hematologic disease. However, local obstruction, neurologic dysfunction and therapeutic procedures (e.g. bladder catheterization) predispose these patients to genitourinary infection. Gram-negative aerobic bacteria (e.g. *E. coli*, *Klebsiella* spp., *Proteus* spp. and *P. aeruginosa*) and enterococci are the most common causative agents. The typical symptoms of urinary tract infection (i.e. dysuria, urgency, frequency and fever) may be absent in neutropenic patients.

Colonization of the urinary tract with fungi (usually *Candida* spp.) also occurs, especially in patients who have indwelling catheters or those receiving broad-spectrum antibiotic therapy. Invasive fungal infection is usually insidious with few, if any, symptoms. However, fever and sometimes flank pain may be present.

Infections of the central nervous system

Infections of the CNS are infrequent in patients who have hematologic malignancy. Nonetheless, symptoms suggestive of CNS dysfunction should lead to immediate clinical evaluation of the patient.

Patients who have hematologic malignancy experience encephalitis with herpesviruses (e.g. Epstein–Barr virus, cytomegalovirus, varicella-zoster virus and herpes simplex virus) more frequently than do healthy individuals, and those with altered cell-mediated immunity are also more susceptible to encephalitis with measles virus and adenovirus.[64] Symptoms include fever, signs of meningeal irritation and evidence of altered mental state. Confusion may progress to coma. Seizures and focal neurologic signs are relatively common. Progressive multifocal leukoencephalopathy (PML) is a rare, rapidly progressive neurodegenerative condition which usually occurs in patients with lymphoma or chronic lymphocytic leukemia. It is caused by JC virus, a polymavirus.

Bacterial or fungal meningitis is most frequently encountered in patients who have impaired cell-mediated immunity (e.g. lymphoma or high-dose corticosteroids). Prevalent micro-organisms include *Listeria monocytogenes*, *Mycobacterium tuberculosis*, *Candida* spp. and *Cryptococcus neoformans*. Cryptococcal meningoencephalitis is usually insidious in onset with low-grade fever, headache, dizziness, nausea and altered mental state.[72] Cranial nerve involvement may result in a variety of ocular symptoms (e.g. diplopia, blurred vision and nystagmus). Meningeal signs like nuchal rigidity may be absent.

Brain abscess represents an important differential diagnosis to meningeal and cerebral infiltration with malignant cells. Predisposing factors include adjacent infected sites (e.g. otitis media, sinusitis or dental abscesses), a history of penetrating cranial trauma, congenital heart disease, endocarditis, intrathecal injections and pulmonary infections. Aerobic and anaerobic bacteria, fungi and *Nocardia* spp. are common in immunosuppressed patients who have brain abscesses. Abscesses caused by fungi or *Nocardia* spp. are usually associated with

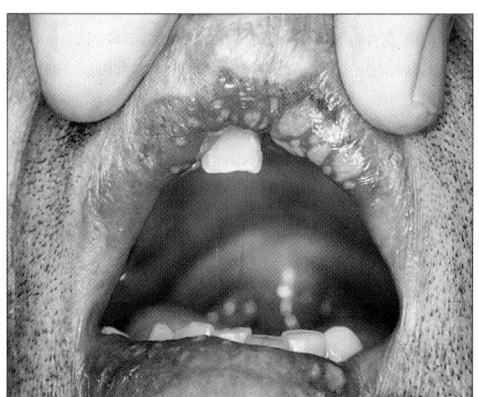

Fig. 5.16 Oral mucositis complicating cytotoxic drug treatment in a patient who has acute leukemia. The ulcerated lesions are painful and easily become infected.

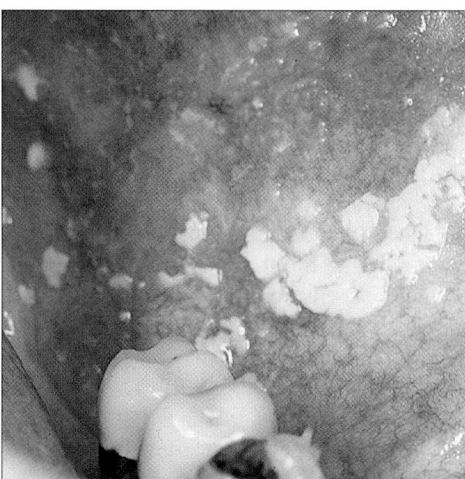

Fig. 5.17 Oral thrush in a patient who has acute leukemia. The white patches usually have indurated borders and bleed easily when scraped.

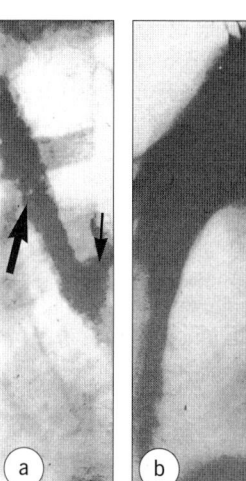
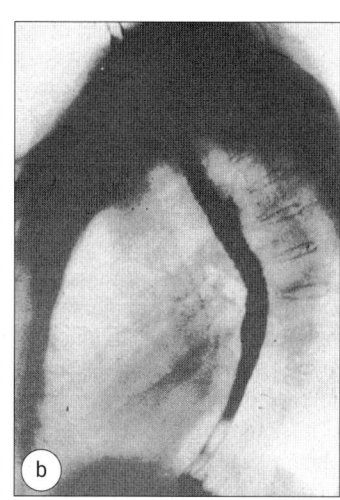

Fig. 5.18 Esophagus perforation: (a) contrast in esophagus (large arrow) and mediastinum (small arrow) in a neutropenic patient who has acute leukemia and esophagitis caused by *C. albicans* and bacterial superinfection. (b) Conservative treatment with amphotericin B and broad-spectrum antibiotics was successful, i.e. contrast only in esophagus.

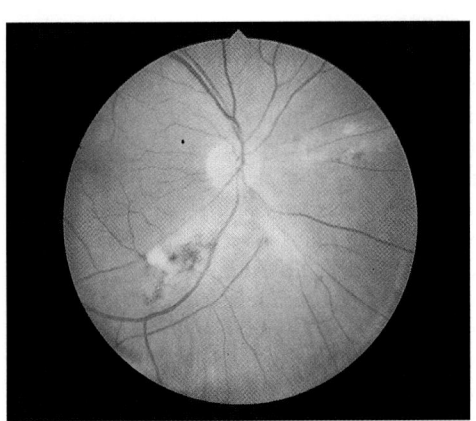

Fig. 5.19 Cytomegalovirus retinitis in a patient who has lymphoma. The patchy lesions are typically white, granular and associated with hemorrhage.

LIMITED VALIDITY OF SPUTUM EXAMINATIONS IN PATIENTS WHO HAVE HEMATOLOGIC MALIGNANCY AND PULMONARY INFILTRATES

- Patients who have neutropenia fail to produce adequate sputum
- Sputum specimens are frequently contaminated by potential pathogens from the upper respiratory tract
- Common pathogens (e.g. mold) shed insufficient numbers of micro-organisms into the sputum to permit diagnosis by microscopy and culture
- Sputum examination will not detect noninfectious causes of pulmonary infiltrates

Fig. 5.20 Reasons for the limited diagnostic value of sputum examinations in patients who have hematologic malignancy and pulmonary infiltrates.

pulmonary infiltrates. *Toxoplasma gondii* infection may also manifest as single or multiple abscesses.

Eye infections
In patients who have hematologic malignancy, conjunctivitis may be caused by viruses, bacteria or *Chlamydia* spp. It may also be secondary to chemotherapy.[73] Keratitis may be caused by herpes simplex virus and varicella-zoster virus and is usually related to reactivation with eruptions along the territory of a particular nerve. If the herpes simplex virus infection involves the ophthalmic distribution of the trigeminal nerve, blisters develop on the eyelid, and the patients complain of pain and foreign body sensation. Redness, photophobia and visual disturbances are common. The herpes simplex virus keratitis may be accompanied by scarring, blepharitis and conjunctivitis. Zoster ophthalmicus can involve any part of the eye, but in the majority of cases the cornea is involved.[73] The patients present with pain, paresthesias, lacrimation and a vesicular and ulcerating eruption that may progress to crustating and scarring. Conjunctivitis, uveitis and optic neuritis may also occur.

Retinitis is the most common manifestation of systemic cytomegalovirus disease (Fig. 5.19). The patients may be asymptomatic or present with progressive loss of vision. Ophthalmoscopy shows patchy, white, granular lesions associated with hemorrhage. The retinitis leads to scarring and may be associated with retinal detachment.

In systemic candidiasis, up to 50% of patients have ocular manifestations.[73] The eye involvement usually manifests with multiple, white, cotton-like lesions often associated with vitreous infiltrates. Progression results in retinitis, retinal detachment and endophthalmitis.

Infections of the cardiovascular system
In spite of the increasing use of indwelling venous catheters, cardiovascular infections are relatively uncommon among patients who have hematologic malignancy. Although Gram-positive bacteria (e.g. staphylococci, enterococci and streptococci) most commonly cause endovascular infections, aerobic Gram-negative bacteria and fungi may cause disease. The clinical manifestations of endocarditis in immunosuppressed patients are similar to those in immunocompetent individuals, that is, nonspecific complaints of fever, chills, malaise, fatigue, night sweats and weight loss.

Osteomyelitis and arthritis
Osteomyelitis and arthritis occur from time to time in patients who have hematologic malignancy. Micro-organisms can be introduced into the bone or joint by direct inoculation, by local invasion from a contiguous infection or by hematogenous implantation secondary to bacteremia. The primary etiologic agent in immunocompetent patients is *S. aureus*, followed by streptococci, Gram-negative bacilli and *H. influenzae*. In immunocompromised patients, fungi and mycobacteria may also cause osteomyelitis and arthritis. The symptoms depend on the site of infection, but low-grade fever, localization-defining pain and redness and swelling of affected joints are usually present.

DIAGNOSIS

When infection is suspected in a patient who has hematologic malignancy, a thorough and expeditious clinical examination should always be performed (see Fig. 5.10). Cultures of blood and any body fluid suspected of being infected should be obtained without delay. In neutropenia, even subtle signs of inflammation should be considered as possible signs of infection, and accessible sites aspirated for Gram staining and culture. The initial evaluation should also include a chest radiograph and standard hematologic and biochemical tests (see below).

MICROBIOLOGY
Specimens for microbiologic examination should always be obtained before institution of antibiotic therapy. The results from these tests may be important for later therapeutic strategies, particularly if the initial empiric treatment fails. The microbiologic examination should include blood cultures, analysis of urine and cultures from all wounds and venous access sites. Depending on the clinical picture, samples from sputum, stools, pleural effusions, joint fluid or cerebrospinal fluid should also be obtained. A tuberculin skin test is often of limited value and should only be performed in patients who have suspected tuberculosis.

The risk of hemorrhage after invasive diagnostic procedures must always be considered in patients who have hematologic malignancies. Many of these patients have thrombocytopenia. Moreover, because of impaired platelet function, many patients experience bleeding even with normal or increased platelet counts (e.g. patients who have myelodysplasia or chronic myeloproliferative disorders).[74] A careful history and a complete physical examination together with platelet counts are therefore essential for the evaluation of the risk of hemorrhage in these patients.

Bacterial, fungal and protozoan infections
Blood cultures. Two separate sets of blood cultures (a total of 40ml blood) should be obtained from patients who have suspected infections. If the patient has an indwelling venous catheter, at least one set should be drawn from each catheter lumen. The blood should be cultured aerobically and anaerobically for at least 7 days.

Sputum and bronchoalveolar lavage fluid. Expectorated sputum should always be examined by microscopy and culture. Gram staining should be performed, and Ziehl–Nielsen staining if a mycobacterial infection is suspected.[75] The sputum should be cultured for aerobic and anaerobic micro-organisms, including mycobacteria and fungi. The validity of a sputum examination should only be trusted if microscopy verifies <10 squamous cells per low-power field together with an excess of neutrophils (>25 cells per low-power field). Even with these criteria the validity of sputum examinations may be questioned in patients who have hematologic malignancies (Fig. 5.20). The reason for this is that many patients who have such disorders, particularly those with marked neutropenia, fail to produce sufficient amounts of sputum. Furthermore, the expectorated sputum may become contaminated by potentially pathogenic micro-organisms (particularly Gram-negative bacilli and fungi) that colonize the upper respiratory tract, and differentiation between micro-organisms truly invading the lung and those colonizing the pharynx is difficult. Also, certain pathogens (e.g. mold) usually shed insufficient numbers of organisms into the sputum to permit diagnosis by culture or microscopy.

Induced sputum is better suited for examination than spontaneously expectorated specimens, particularly when pneumocystis pneumonia is suspected. However, the sensitivity of sputum examination in pneumocystosis is low in patients who have leukemia or lymphoma compared with other immunocompromised patients because of the low burden of infecting organisms in patients who have hematologic malignancies. Transtracheal aspirates may be difficult to obtain in patients who have hematologic malignancies because of the risk of complicating hemorrhage or infections.

Bronchoalveolar lavage is particularly useful in diagnosing *P. carinii* infection. The lavage fluid should be examined by microscopy and culture. The diagnosis of *P. carinii* infection is confirmed by the detection of cysts or trophozoites in material stained with toluene blue or silver nitrate (Fig. 5.21), or by immunofluoresence using monoclonal antibodies against *Pneumocystis* antigens.[76] Bronchoalveolar lavage fluid can also be used for the diagnosis of bacterial and fungal infections.[77,78] However, the results from lavage fluid investigations must be interpreted with caution, as it may be very difficult to differentiate between colonization and true infection. In neutropenia, bronchoalveolar lavage

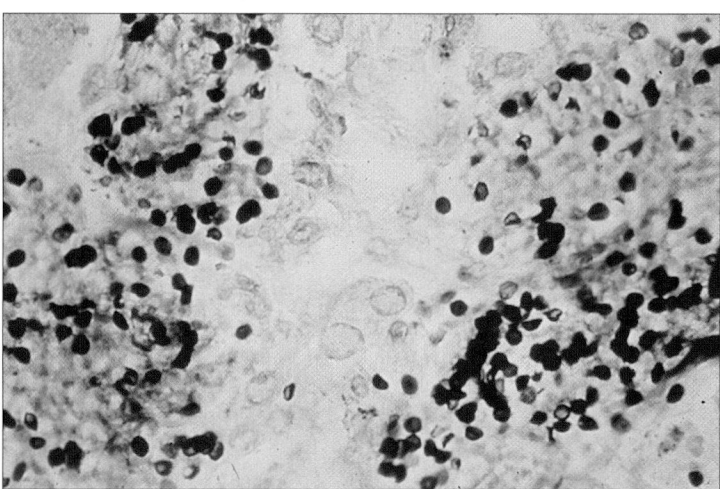

Fig. 5.21 *Pneumocystis carinii* (silver nitrate staining) in induced sputum from a patient who has non-Hodgkin's lymphoma and pneumonia. The pneumonia developed after intensive chemotherapy. Treatment with trimethoprim–sulfamethoxazole was successful.

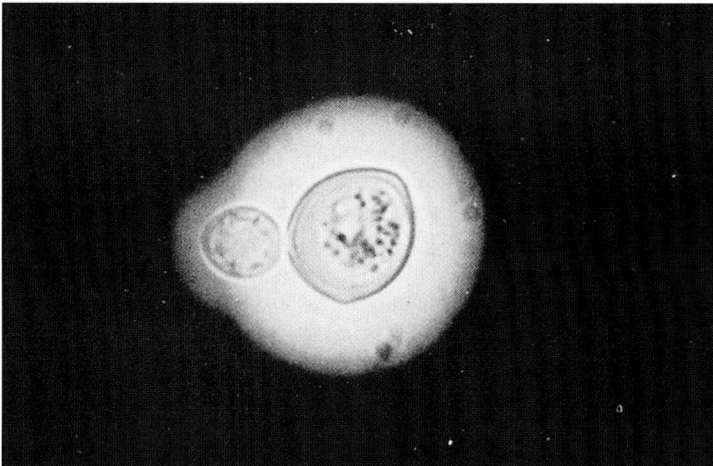

Fig. 5.22 *Cryptococcus neoformans* in cerebrospinal fluid from a patient who has non-Hodgkin's lymphoma and meningitis. Indian ink staining.

is of limited value in the diagnosis of pulmonary infection, particularly fungal infection. This is because of a high rate of false-positive bacterial isolates caused by contamination from the upper airway and a low yield in diagnosing invasive fungal infections. In neutropenia, there is also a significant risk of complicating bacteremia or pneumonia after the bronchoscopic procedure (see below).

Urine. A urine culture should always be performed in patients who have hematologic malignancy and fever. In cases with silent hematuria or unexplained pyuria, a tuberculous infection should be suspected. In such cases tuberculosis may be reactivated as a result of the immunosuppression caused by the disease itself or by the chemotherapy.

Cerebrospinal fluid. If the patient has symptoms of a CNS infection, a lumbar puncture should be performed, preferably after an MRI shows no evidence of increased intracranial pressure, and the cerebrospinal fluid examined.[79] A lumbar puncture should only be carried out in patients who have platelet counts exceeding 30,000/mm³. In thrombocytopenic patients, the puncture should be performed during an ongoing platelet transfusion. The cerebrospinal fluid should be examined by direct microscopy and culture for bacterial and fungal pathogens, and glucose and protein concentrations should be measured. Latex agglutination tests may be of significant help in the rapid diagnosis of bacterial or fungal infections. In mycobacterial and fungal infections, the number of infecting organisms in the cerebrospinal fluid is low, and at least 2ml cerebrospinal fluid should be collected for microbiologic examination. In such situations, increased sensitivity may be obtained using antigen detection methods and in some cases PCR.

Characteristic cerebrospinal fluid findings in bacterial meningitis include increased cell counts with a predominance of neutrophils, increased protein content and markedly decreased glucose levels. Splenectomized patients and patients who have hypogammaglobulinemia are especially susceptible to infections with *S. pneumoniae*, *H. influenzae* and *Neisseria meningitidis*, whereas patients who have cellular immune defects particularly experience infections with *L. monocytogenes* and *C. neoformans* (Fig. 5.22).[80] Characteristic cerebrospinal fluid findings in *Listeria* and cryptococcal meningitis include slightly increased leukocyte counts and moderately elevated protein levels. In cryptococcal infections, lymphocytes predominate. In *Listeria meningitis*, the leukocyte count may range from 5 to 10,000 cells/mm³, and both mononuclear and polymorphonuclear cells may predominate. Tuberculous meningitis must also be considered in patients who have increased lymphocyte counts and low glucose levels.

In patients who have hematologic malignancy and neurologic symptoms, CNS infiltration with malignant cells has to be considered.[81] Malignant cell infiltration of the CNS is rather uncommon, but occurs particularly in patients who have acute lymphoblastic leukemia, non-Hodgkin's lymphoma or the myelomonocytic variants of acute myelogenous leukemia. Common findings include increased cerebrospinal fluid protein concentrations and decreased levels of glucose. The diagnosis depends on careful cytologic examination of the cerebrospinal fluid, and immunologic techniques may be helpful to distinguish between leukemia blast cells and reactive mononuclear cells. Intrathecal chemotherapy may also cause a slight cerebrospinal fluid pleocytosis.[81]

Stools. In patients who have hematologic malignancy and diarrhea or abdominal pain, stools must be examined by microscopy and culture. Strongyloidiasis is diagnosed by microscopic demonstration of larvae in fresh stool specimens or duodenal contents. *C. difficile* as a cause of antibiotic-associated colitis is demonstrated in stool cultures, and the toxins A and B are detected by latex agglutination tests or polymerase chain reaction (PCR)-based techniques. The micro-organism is frequently harbored by asymptomatic carriers, and the demonstration of the organism or the toxins in stool specimens should always be taken together with the clinical symptoms. In neutropenic patients who have hematologic malignancy, endoscopic examinations to establish the diagnosis of antibiotic-associated colitis should not be performed, because of the risk of mucosal damage and invasive infection.

Viral infections

Even though the diagnosis of a viral infection can sometimes be made from the clinical picture alone (e.g. the typical skin lesions of herpes simplex virus or varicella-zoster virus), additional information to establish a diagnosis is often needed from immunofluorescence analyses, viral cultures, histopathologic examinations, electron microscopy, in-situ nucleic acid hybridization assays, PCR-based techniques or serologic tests (see Chapter 1.3).[64,66,82,83] Suitable specimens include mouth and throat washings, expectorate (Fig. 5.23), swabs or scrapings of skin or mucosal lesions, blister fluid, stools, buffy coat, bronchoalveolar lavage fluid, cerebrospinal fluid and biopsies.

In patients who have hematologic malignancy, viral cultures may be helpful in the discrimination between mucosal herpes simplex virus infections, chemotherapy-induced mucositis and ulcerations caused by bacteria, fungi or local irritation (e.g. peptic esophagitis). The cytopathic effects of herpes simplex virus can usually be demonstrated within 24–48 hours. For a more rapid diagnosis, herpes simplex antigens may be demonstrated in scrapings from suspected lesions by immunohistochemical methods or in-situ DNA hybridization. The cerebrospinal fluid findings in viral meningitis are characterized by a mild lymphocytic pleocytosis, slightly elevated protein levels and normal or slightly decreased glucose values. Viruses can be detected either by culture or by demonstration of viral antigens.

SEROLOGY

Serologic tests are of limited value in the early diagnosis of infection in patients who have hematologic malignancy and fever because therapy has to be instituted before seroconversion or increased antibody titers are demonstrated. An exception is infection with *Mycoplasma pneumoniae* in which specific IgM antibodies, highly predictive of an acute infection, may be demonstrated during the first week of the infection.[84] Serologic tests are also helpful in the diagnosis of toxoplasmosis, cryptococcosis, coccidioidomycosis and some viral infections (e.g. hepatitis A–E and Epstein–Barr virus infection). Results of serologic tests are less reliable for aspergillosis, histoplasmosis and systemic candidiasis.

HISTOLOGY AND CYTOLOGY

Aspirates or biopsies may be necessary for the documentation of invasive infection or disseminated infectious disease (see below). Demonstration of bacteria, fungi, virus components or protozoa in tissue specimens, together with an inflammatory reaction (e.g. leukocyte infiltration, microabscesses, fibrosis, granuloma formation or necrosis) establishes the diagnosis.

HEMATOLOGY AND BIOCHEMISTRY

Hemoglobin concentration, total and differential leukocyte counts and platelet count should be obtained in all patients who have hematologic malignancy and fever. Neutrophilia (i.e. >10,000 neutrophils/mm³ or >5000 nonsegmented neutrophils/mm³) suggests infection. It is most important to document leukopenia, and especially neutropenia (i.e. <500 neutrophils/mm³), because this finding has direct consequences for the strategy of therapy. A low hemoglobin concentration and thrombocytopenia indicate the need for transfusion, whereas low platelet counts together with coagulopathy suggest disseminated intravascular coagulation.

Analysis of arterial blood gases is a very useful test of pulmonary function. Hypoxemia usually indicates severe or disseminated pulmonary infection (e.g. *P. carinii* pneumonia). However, other causes of hypoxemia (e.g. pulmonary emboli or pneumothorax) should be considered. In serious infections (e.g. sepsis), respiratory alkalosis is an early finding, whereas metabolic acidosis develops late.

Results of liver and kidney function tests, blood glucose, serum electrolyte, albumin, amylase and creatinine kinase analyses, and results of tests for coagulation and fibrinolysis may all be useful in the demonstration of the origin of infection and in the diagnosis and follow-up of complications.

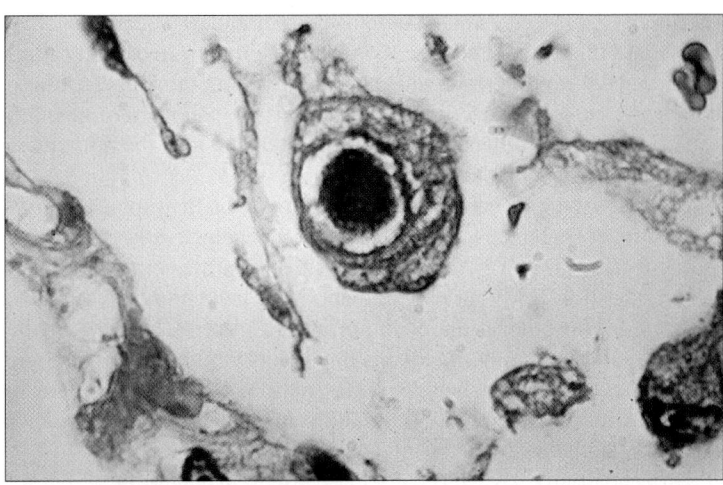

Fig. 5.23 Inclusion body ('owl's eye') in sputum from a patient who has Hodgkin's disease and cytomegalovirus pneumonia. The pneumonia developed after intensive chemotherapy. Treatment with ganciclovir was successful. The inclusion body is pathognomonic for cytomegalovirus infection.

MICRO-ORGANISMS CAUSING LOCALIZED INFILTRATES IN PATIENTS WITH HEMATOLOGIC MALIGNANCY AND PULMONARY INFECTION		
	Non-neutropenic patients	Neutropenic patients
Acute infection (develops in <24h)	*Streptococcus pneumoniae* *Haemophilus influenzae* *Legionella* spp. *Chlamydia* spp.	Any Gram-positive and Gram-negative bacterium
Subacute/chronic infection (develops in days–weeks)	Respiratory syncytial virus, adenovirus *Mycoplasma pneumoniae* Mycobacteria *Cryptococcus* spp. *Histoplasma*	Herpes simplex virus, varicella-zoster virus Mycobacteria *Nocardia* spp. *Aspergillus* spp., *Candida* spp., *Cryptococcus* spp., *Histoplasma* spp.

Fig. 5.24 Micro-organisms causing localized infiltrates in patients who have hematologic malignancy and pulmonary infection. (Listed according to the neutrophil count and the rate of progression of symptoms.)

RADIOLOGY

Radiographic examinations are most helpful in the diagnosis of infectious complications in patients who have hematologic malignancy. Infections of the respiratory tract are most frequent and a chest radiograph should be obtained, particularly in neutropenic patients. In addition, radiographs of sinuses, CT examinations of the chest, abdomen, pelvis and brain, ultrasound examinations of abdominal organs and the heart and various MRI techniques may be indispensable for the localization of an infection. Their use should be guided by organ-defining symptoms (e.g. pulmonary wheeze or rales, hepatomegaly or peritoneal irritation) and biochemical parameters (e.g. hypoxemia or elevated liver enzymes).

Chest radiography

Anteroposterior and lateral view films should be obtained, upright and at full inspiration. A decubitus film should be included if pleural fluid is suspected. Although no particular chest radiographic pattern is specific for a given pathologic process or infection, certain patterns are more characteristic for some processes than others. Hence, the recognition of such patterns may narrow the differential diagnostic possibilities significantly.

Radiographic characteristics that are useful for establishing a correct diagnosis include the time of appearance and progression of abnormalities, and their distribution and localization (focal, diffuse, central or peripheral). Other findings that should be looked for include lung opacities (consolidations with air bronchograms, peribronchovascular infiltrates or noduli), atelectases, pleural fluid, cavitation and lymphadenopathy (for examples see below).

The clinical presentation and rate of progression of clinical symptoms should always be taken into consideration when evaluating the febrile patient who has pulmonary infiltrates. In addition to infection, the hematologic malignancy itself and the noninfectious causes of pulmonary infiltrates (e.g. cytotoxic drugs, radiation therapy or pulmonary emboli) should be considered. The impaired inflammatory response in neutropenia or high-dose glucocorticosteroid treatment may greatly modify and delay the appearance of pulmonary infiltrates. Hence, in severe neutropenia, an atelectasis may be the only radiologic sign of pneumonia. Moreover, radiologic evidence of fungal infection, which is normally associated with a weaker inflammatory response than occurs in bacterial infection, will develop very slowly in neutropenia. A chest radiograph can serve as a valuable baseline in patients who have neutropenia, even in the absence of pulmonary symptoms,

and it is recommended that this test be included in the work-up of most patients who have hematologic malignancy and fever.

When evaluating febrile patients who have hematologic malignancy and pulmonary infiltrates, a useful approach is to categorize the patients according to the rate of clinical progression, the anatomic distribution of the infiltrate (i.e. localized or diffuse) and the neutrophil count (i.e. absence or presence of neutropenia) (Figs 5.24 & 5.25).[48,59] This classification is a useful tool in the identification of etiology and the evaluation of appropriate therapy.

Typically, an acute onset over less than 24 hours suggests a common bacterial infection. A subacute onset over days suggests an infection with a virus, *Mycoplasma* spp., *Chlamydia* spp. or *P. carinii*, whereas a more chronic progression over weeks typically suggests nocardial, fungal or tuberculous infection.

A localized infectious pulmonary infiltrate in a non-neutropenic patient who has hematologic malignancy is usually caused by micro-organisms identical to those that cause pneumonia in the immunocompetent host (Fig. 5.24). Hence, viruses, *H. influenzae* and pneumococci dominate (Fig. 5.26). Non-neutropenic patients who receive immunosuppressive therapy are at increased risk of tuberculosis or pulmonary infections with other mycobacteria or fungi. The most relevant differential diagnoses include an atelectatic segment of the lung, a pulmonary embolus or a localized reaction to a cytotoxic drug (particularly methotrexate, cyclophosphamide or bleomycin). However, drug reactions are more commonly manifested as diffuse infiltrates.

A localized infectious pulmonary infiltrate in a neutropenic patient may be caused by pathogens identical to those in the non-neutropenic patient, but in addition, a variety of opportunistic micro-organisms must be considered (Figs 5.24 & 5.27). However, bacterial pathogens dominate if the neutropenia has lasted for less than 2 weeks. Patients who have longer periods of low neutrophil counts are more likely to develop fungal (e.g. *Candida* spp., *Aspergillus* spp. *Trichosporon* spp. or *Phycomycetes* spp.) or viral (e.g. cytomegalovirus, herpes simplex virus or varicella-zoster virus) infections. Fungi are the most common cause of a localized pulmonary infiltrate in the patient who has hematologic malignancy and protracted neutropenia. *Candida* pneumonia usually manifests as a progressive pulmonary infiltrate in a patient who has persistent fever and neutropenia. It tends to suggest hematogenous spread of the yeast, however, the diagnosis is difficult and there is no definite radiographic pattern pathognomonic for this

MICRO–ORGANISMS CAUSING DIFFUSE OR MULTIPLE INFILTRATES IN PATIENTS WITH HEMATOLOGIC MALIGNANCY AND PULMONARY INFECTION		
	Non-neutropenic patients	Neutropenic patients
Acute infection (develops in <24h)	Respiratory syncytial virus, herpes simplex virus, varicella-zoster virus, cytomegalovirus *Pneumocystis carinii*	Any Gram-positive and Gram-negative bacterium Herpes simplex virus, varicella-zoster virus, cytomegalovirus, adenovirus, respiratory syncytial virus *Pneumocystis carinii* *Phycomycetes* spp., *Strongyloides*
Subacute/chronic infection (develops in days–weeks)	*Chlamydia* spp. *Mycoplasma* spp. *Legionella* spp. Mycobacteria *Nocardia* spp. *Cryptococcus* spp., *Histoplasma*	Any Gram-positive and Gram-negative bacterium, mycobacteria, *Legionella* spp. *Nocardia* spp. *Aspergillus* spp., *Candida* spp., *Histoplasma* spp., *Cryptococcus* spp.

Fig. 5.25 Micro-organisms causing diffuse or multiple infiltrates in patients who have hematologic malignancy and pulmonary infection. (Listed according to the neutrophil count and the rate of progression of symptoms.)

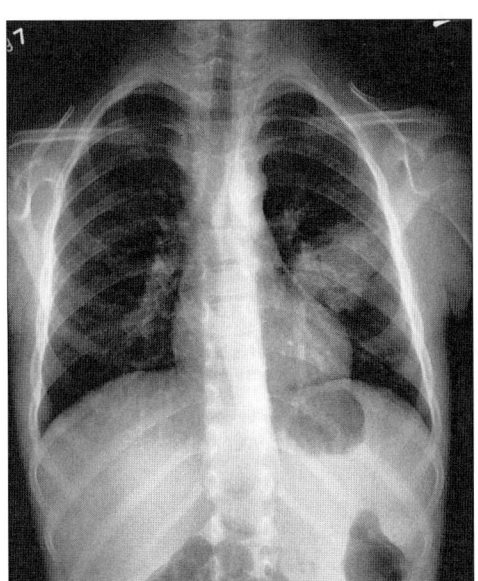

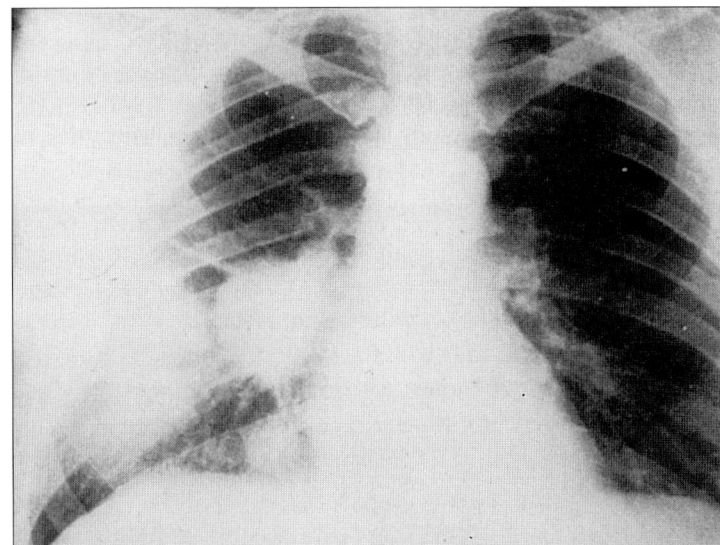

Fig. 5.26 Pneumococcal pneumonia in a child with acute lymphocytic leukemia. A consolidation is seen in the left lung. *Streptococcus pneumoniae* was demonstrated in blood cultures and the patient recovered on penicillin treatment.

Fig. 5.27 Pulmonary cryptococcosis in a neutropenic young male with acute myelogenous leukemia. Extensive infiltrates in the right lower and middle lobe and perihilar infiltrates in the left lung. *Cryptococcus neoformans* was demonstrated in aspiration-needle biopsy from the right lung. The patient suddenly developed *Staphylococcus aureus* septicemia and died. At autopsy, *Cryptococcus neoformans* and *Staphylococcus aureus* were demonstrated in both lungs and in liver and kidney abscesses.

infection. The findings range from a normal appearing radiograph to a localized perihilar infiltrate or a miliary pattern. *Aspergillus* spp. produce aspergillomas by colonization of lung cavities in immuno-competent patients or by invasive infection in neutropenic patients. An aspergilloma represents a ball of mycelia growing in a poorly drained lung space that communicates with the bronchial tree. The characteristic radiologic finding is an apical, pulmonary meniscus sign (i.e. crescent-shaped air adjacent to an intracavitary body with surrounding fibrocavitary changes). Cavitation also suggests other necrotizing infections (e.g. infections caused by other fungi, *Nocardia* spp., *Klebsiella* spp., *Pseudomonas* spp. or *S. aureus*). *Legionella* spp. should also be considered in the neutropenic patient who has hematologic malignancy. The radiologic abnormality is a patchy, alveolar infiltrate involving a single lobe. However, translobar consolidation may occur.

Diffuse infectious pulmonary infiltrates in non-neutropenic patients who have hematologic malignancy are most commonly caused by *P. carinii* (Fig. 5.25).[85] The radiographic findings are characteristic with bilateral fluffy alveolar infiltrates, often originating from the hili and extending peripherally. Several viruses, including cytomegalovirus, measles, herpes simplex virus and varicella-zoster virus, also cause diffuse pulmonary infiltrates. *Mycobacteria* spp., *Mycoplasma* spp. and *Chlamydia* spp. should also be considered. The most common differential diagnoses include radiation pneumonitis, drug reactions or a leukoagglutinin reaction.[59] The leukoagglutinin reaction is an uncommon cause of fever, respiratory distress and patchy multifocal pulmonary infiltrates. The reaction develops within the first few hours after a blood transfusion and is caused by interaction between preformed agglutinating antibodies and antigens on leukocyte surfaces.

Diffuse infectious pulmonary infiltrates in patients who have hematologic malignancy and neutropenia can be caused by any Gram-positive or Gram-negative bacterium, several fungi and viruses, and *P. carinii* (Fig. 5.25). Although rare, *T. gondii* and *Strongyloides* should also be considered.

CT of the chest

Although conventional chest radiography remains the first procedure when evaluating a febrile patient who has hematologic malignancy and pulmonary symptoms, the high sensitivity and precise localization possible with CT scanning may lead to earlier diagnosis and treatment. The recently developed high-resolution CT allows detection of subtle pneumonias sooner than do other techniques. In addition, spiral CT allows multiplanar reconstructions by which an infiltrate can be distinguished from tumor masses or vascular structures.[86] Modern CT techniques may reveal specific patterns of pulmonary pathology that, in conjunction with the clinical findings, may suggest the etiology of the infection. Hence, lobar and lobular bacterial pneumonias appear as increased lung density because of air-space filling. Alveolar edema may give rise to the 'ground-glass' pattern, usually seen in viral or pneumocystis pneumonia and aspergillosis is said to produce a characteristic 'halo' sign. A focal lung mass with a thickened wall and an air-fluid level indicates a lung abscess (Fig. 5.28), whereas cavitation suggests a necrotizing infection. CT examination is also most helpful in the demonstration of other pathologic processes that may manifest as possible infection (i.e. radiation pneumonitis or drug-induced pneumonitis).[59] Radiation pneumonitis in its early phase appears on CT scans as homogenously increased attenuation that progresses to patchy and later more dense consolidation.

CT and ultrasonography of abdomen and pelvis

Abdominal or pelvic CT examinations are especially helpful if an abscess is suspected. In hepatic candidiasis, the granulomatous lesions consist of an inner core of necrosis surrounded by a ring of inflammatory tissue and an outer ring of fibrosis. With ultrasound, the typical 'bull's eye' lesion of hepatic candidiasis can be observed.[87] These imaged lesions change over time, and with therapy they calcify. Small abscesses may remain undetected by ultrasound and CT, and in such cases MRI of the liver is more sensitive.[88]

Other radiologic evaluations

Echocardiography should be performed if endocarditis is suspected. A radiograph of the sinuses will demonstrate signs of sinusitis and a CT scan of the brain will reveal an abscess. Because of the possible induction of bacteremia or fungemia, invasive radiologic procedures (e.g. barium enema) should be avoided in severely neutropenic patients.

SCINTIGRAPHY

In selected patients, nuclear medicine assays can be useful, especially for the detection of focal infections in the lungs, bones, joints, soft tissues or the abdomen. Leukocyte scintigraphy using the patient's own leukocytes labeled with indium-111 is laborious,[89] but human IgG labeled with indium-111 represents an alternative that can be used even in neutropenia.[90]

INVASIVE DIAGNOSTIC PROCEDURES

Although ultrasonography, CT scans or MRI can demonstrate evidence of localized infections (e.g. pulmonary infiltrates or hepatosplenic abscesses), a definitive diagnosis can only be reached by microbiologic methods, cytology or histology (see above). The choice of invasive procedure depends on the degree of illness, the rate of disease progression and the type of radiographic findings. Percutaneous sampling and drainage procedures (e.g. puncture of superficial or deep abscesses or thoracocentesis), preferably performed with guidance by ultrasound or CT, provide material for cytologic, histologic and microbiologic examination. Liver biopsy is, for example, most helpful in establishing the diagnosis of hepatic candidiasis. Invasive diagnostic procedures are also particularly useful in patients who have hematologic malignancy and lung infection, and percutaneous needle aspiration is well suited for diagnosing focal peripheral lung infiltrates caused by fungi, *Nocardia* spp. or mycobacteria.[91] In contrast, if the patient has diffuse lung infiltrates, bronchoscopic approaches (e.g. bronchoalveolar lavage or transbronchial biopsy) are preferred.[92] Open lung biopsy should be considered if the pulmonary infiltrates are diffuse or multifocal and spreading rapidly.[59,93] The definite diagnostic procedure in patients who have hematologic malignancy with signs of peritonitis may be exploratory laparotomy. Brain biopsy may also be informative in selected cases. However, these procedures, like open lung biopsy, should only be considered if the infection is progressing rapidly, and the prognosis for the underlying disease is hopeful (see Management).

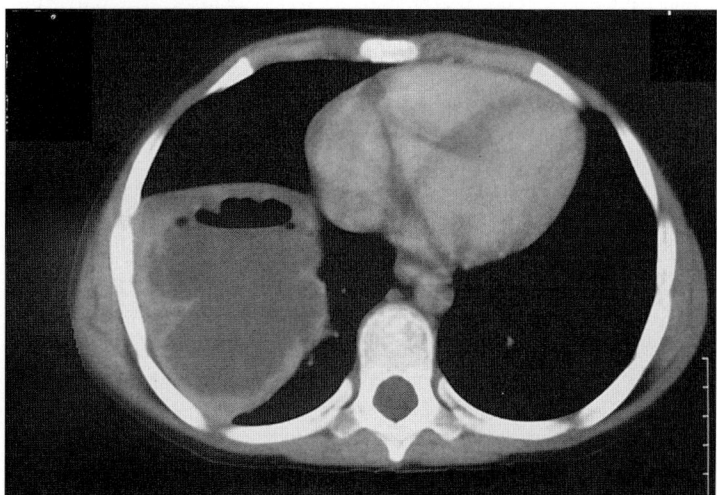

Fig. 5.28 CT scan of an abscess in the right lung of a child who has lymphoma.

MANAGEMENT

The single most important advance in the management of the febrile patient who has hematologic malignancy and neutropenia has remained the early institution of empiric antimicrobial therapy. Before this strategy was adopted, the mortality of patients who have infections caused by Gram-negative bacilli was close to 80%[94] compared with 20–40% after the introduction of early empiric antibiotic treatment.[9,48]

The initial evaluation of the febrile patient should always include a careful history and physical examination supported by Gram's stain and culture of cutaneous lesions, wound drainage, intravenous catheter infections, transtracheal aspirate, urine, etc. (Fig. 5.29). In neutropenic patients, bacterial sepsis, widespread wound infection, or pneumonia are often fulminant, and the physical examination should be carried out as expeditiously as possible. A clinically or microbiologically documented site of infection is demonstrated in only 50% of febrile neutropenic patients. Usually these patients fail to develop an adequate inflammatory response and characteristic local signs of infection may not be present. Instead of abscess formation with pus and fluctuation, only a slight cutaneous cellulitis may be present, and cough, purulent expectoration and even stethoscopic and radiographic findings may be absent, despite widespread bacterial invasion in patients who have pneumonia. Accordingly, subtle signs of inflammation such as slight erythema and pain should be considered as possible signs of infection, and, if accessible, any clinically suspicious site of infection should be aspirated for culture and Gram staining. It is also of fundamental importance to obtain cultures of blood and any body fluid suspected of being infected. Initially, two peripheral blood cultures from separate venipuncture sites should be obtained. Patients who have diarrhea should have their stools cultured. A routine chest radiograph provides an important baseline for comparison with later films and should be obtained in febrile neutropenic patients. As soon as the evaluation is accomplished, febrile neutropenic patients should receive empiric broad-spectrum antibiotic therapy (see below). In febrile non-neutropenic patients, empiric antimicrobial therapy is not recommended except when patients have serious infections and the etiologic agent is not established (e.g. sepsis, severe pneumonia or extensive wound infections).

NEUTROPENIC PATIENTS WHO HAVE UNEXPLAINED FEVER

A common problem in neutropenic patients who have hematologic malignancy is fever for which a source of infection cannot be found despite a thorough clinical evaluation. In some of these patients, cytotoxic drugs, allergic reactions, splenic infarcts, reaction to blood products or even the underlying hematologic disease itself may be the source of fever. However, the majority of the patients seem to have occult infections that remain undefined because of the poor inflammatory reaction and the early institution of empiric antibiotic therapy.

Empiric antibiotic therapy

Bacterial infections predominate in neutropenic patients who have hematologic malignancy, and 85–90% of pathogens associated with new episodes of fever are bacteria.[41,95] Because of the wide range of bacteria that causes infection, any empiric regimen must cover a broad antibacterial spectrum and provide high bactericidal serum levels of the drugs. The most common regimens have been combinations of an extended spectrum beta-lactam antibiotic and an aminoglycoside that cover a broad spectrum of bacteria and produce response rates up to 80–85%.[96–98] Two antibiotics may also have synergistic activity and decrease antibiotic resistance development.

Recently, good results have been obtained with a combination of two beta-lactam antibiotics or monotherapy with ceftazidime, meropenem or imipenem–cilastatin.[96,99,100] The major disadvantages of using two beta-lactams are the occasional selection of resistant microorganisms, the high cost and the possibility of antagonism with some combinations.[101] The major concern over ceftazidime monotherapy has remained the poor activity against Gram-positive cocci, particularly coagulase-negative staphylococci and enterococci; the latter are virtually resistant. Furthermore, ceftazidime has variable activity against *Enterobacter* spp. and *Pseudomonas* spp. other than *P. aeruginosa*, and increased antibiotic resistance may become a problem in hospitals where large amounts of third-generation cephalosporins are used. Imipenem–cilastatin and meropenem have a broader antibacterial spectrum than ceftazidime, but some bacterial species that are not infrequent causes of infection in patients who have hematologic malignancy may be resistant to these agents, including methicillin-resistant staphylococci, *Enterococcus faecium*, *Stenotrophomonas maltophilia*, and some strains of *Listeria* spp., *Corynebacterium* spp. and *Bacteroides* spp. However, good results – often equal to the results obtained with the combined beta-lactam–aminoglycoside regimen – have been obtained with monotherapy provided the patient is closely monitored and therapy modified if single-agent treatment is failing.

Today, such a large armamentarium of highly effective antibiotics is available that it is difficult to recommend a specific antibiotic or combination of antibiotics for the initial treatment of the febrile neutropenic patient who has hematologic malignancy.[96,97] The decision about an appropriate regimen should be individualized at each institution according to prevalent bacterial species and their current antimicrobial susceptibility, because these factors differ markedly between institutions and from country to country. However, a combination of an aminoglycoside

---

INITIAL MANAGEMENT OF NEUTROPENIC PATIENTS WHO HAVE HEMATOLOGIC MALIGNANCY AND UNEXPLAINED FEVER

- Admit patient to a single room, preferably with positive air pressure (see Prevention)
- Carry out physical examination expeditiously (<0.5h)
- Aspirate any suspicious site of infection for culture and Gram staining
- Obtain cultures of blood and any body fluid suspected of being infected
- Obtain a chest radiograph
- Initiate prompt empiric broad-spectrum antibiotic therapy according to the flora prevalent at the institution

Fig. 5.29 General principles for initial management of neutropenic patients who have hematologic malignancy and unexplained fever.

EMPIRIC ANTIBIOTIC TREATMENT IN NEUTROPENIC PATIENTS WHO HAVE HEMATOLOGIC MALIGNANCY AND UNEXPLAINED FEVER

Antibiotics	Comments
Aminoglycoside and extended spectrum beta-lactam (e.g. azlocillin, piperacillin, ceftazidime or cefoperazone)	Broad antibacterial spectrum, potential synergistic effect. Nephrotoxic and ototoxic. Should be replaced by ceftazidime or imipenem–cilastatin if the patient has eighth cranial nerve damage, impaired kidney function or receives nephrotoxic drugs (e.g. cisplatinum, amphotericin B or cyclosporin)
Ceftazidime	Poor activity against Gram-positive cocci (enterococci are resistant), variable activity against *Enterobacter* spp. and some *Pseudomonas* spp.
Imipenem–cilastatin	Broad antibacterial spectrum. Methicillin-resistant staphylococci, *Enterococcus faecium*, *Stenotrophomonas maltophila*, and strains of *Listeria*, *Corynebacterium* and *Bacteroides* spp. are resistant
Cefapime	Broad antibacterial spectrum including Gram-positive cocci *Enterbacter* spp. and *Klebsiella* spp.

Fig. 5.30 Empiric antibiotics in neutropenic patients who have hematologic malignancy and unexplained fever.

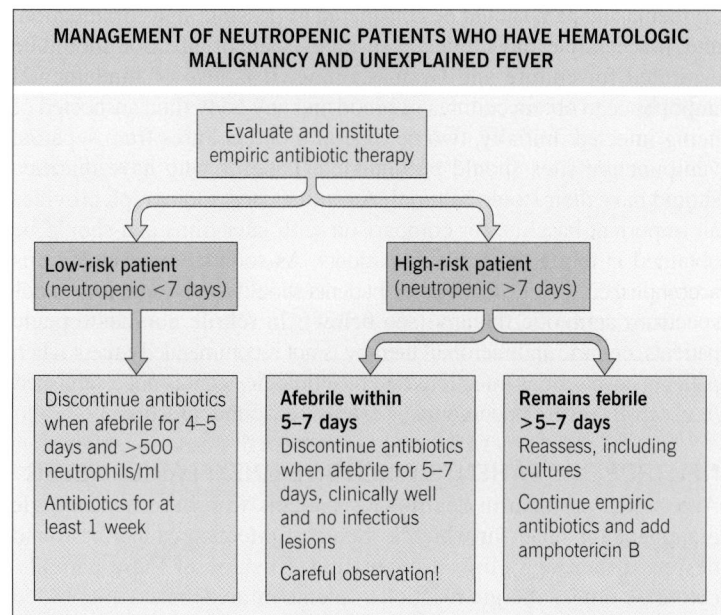

Fig. 5.31 Management of neutropenic patients who have hematologic malignancy and unexplained fever.

and an extended spectrum beta-lactam antibiotic (e.g. azlocillin, piperacillin, ceftazidime or cefoperazone) is usually recommended for initial therapy (Fig. 5.30). If the patient has eighth cranial nerve damage or impaired kidney function or is receiving concomitant treatment with nephrotoxic drugs (e.g. cisplatinum, amphotericin B or cyclosporin), nephrotoxic and ototoxic antibiotics such as aminoglycosides should be avoided and beta-lactam agents may be used. If infection with *S. aureus* or coagulase-negative staphylococci is suspected (e.g. in patients who have vascular access devices), an isoxazolyl-penicillin or vancomycin should be added. In institutions in which methicillin-resistant staphylococci or enterococci are infrequent, vancomycin should not be included. If infection with *Pseudomonas* spp. is suspected, a combination of tobramycin and a beta-lactam antibiotic with antipseudomonal activity (e.g. azlocillin or ceftazidime) should be used.

Changes and duration of antibiotic therapy

If a pathogenic agent is identified, the initial antibiotic regimen should be changed to provide optimal treatment. However, broad-spectrum coverage to prevent breakthrough infections should be maintained in patients who have prolonged neutropenia (>7 days). If no etiologic agent is isolated, the initial antibiotic regimen should be continued.

Little is known about the optimal duration of antimicrobial therapy in neutropenic patients who have unexplained fever. However, the single most important factor is the neutrophil count. When the neutrophil count exceeds 500 cells/mm^3, the likelihood of persistence or recurrence of infection is markedly reduced. Patients whose neutrophil counts rise to 500 cells/mm^3 within a week of initiation of antibiotic therapy usually have an uneventful recovery and antibiotic treatment may be discontinued when they are clinically well and have been afebrile for 4–5 days (Fig. 5.31). However, all febrile neutropenic patients will require at least 1 week of antibiotic therapy. If antibiotic treatment is discontinued at an earlier stage, reappearance of fever is frequent.

If neutropenia lasts for more than 1 week and there is no evidence of bone marrow recovery, the patient is at high risk of serious infections and the proper antibiotic course is less well defined. However, it seems reasonable to discontinue antibiotic treatment when the patient has been afebrile for 5–7 days, appears well clinically and has no discernible infectious lesion (e.g. no mucositis, ulcerations or bleeding sites) and no radiographic or laboratory evidence of infection. This approach should only be taken if the patient can be carefully observed, and no invasive procedures or intensive chemotherapy are impending.

On recurrence of fever, intravenous antibiotic therapy should be re-instituted immediately. Antibiotic therapy throughout the neutropenic period should be considered in patients who have profound neutropenia (<100 cells/mm^3), mucous membrane lesions of the mouth or gastrointestinal tract, and who are clinically unstable. Patients who have myelodysplasia or myelofibrosis, in whom it is unlikely that the neutrophil count will ever reach 500 cells/mm^3, should receive antibiotic treatment until they are afebrile and clinically stable, and treatment should be discontinued under close observation.

Empiric antifungal therapy

If neutropenia and fever persist after 5–7 days of broad-spectrum antibiotic therapy, and a cause of fever is not identified despite careful reassessment of the patient, including reculture of blood and specific sites of infection and diagnostic imaging of any organ suspected of localized infection, empiric antifungal therapy should be added to the empiric antibacterial regimen. Up to 33% of febrile neutropenic patients not responding to broad-spectrum antibiotic therapy for 4–7 days will have systemic fungal infection, caused in most cases by *Candida* spp. or *Aspergillus* spp.[102] Institution of empiric antifungal therapy is also supported by the observation that ante-mortem diagnosis of even disseminated fungal infection is difficult in an immunocompromised host. Furthermore, the outcome of these infections in immunocompromised patients is improved by early antifungal therapy.[103]

Amphotericin B remains the most reliable antifungal agent for empiric therapy and for the treatment of invasive disease. The potential value of liposomal amphotericin B, fluconazole and itraconazole remains to be established by prospective, randomized clinical trials. Little is known about the optimal duration of empiric antifungal therapy, and a common approach is to continue treatment until the resolution of neutropenia. If no fungal agent is identified, but the patient's fever abates, treatment should be continued for at least 1 week after the patient has become afebrile. Persisting fever in spite of empiric antibacterial and antifungal therapy calls for a thorough re-evaluation of the patient to document other causes of fever, including infections with viruses, resistant bacteria or less susceptible fungi (e.g. *Aspergillus* spp., *Fusarium* spp., *Mucor* spp., *Pseudallescheria boydii* and *Trichosporon* spp.), allergic reactions and reactions to blood products or therapeutic agents. Patients who have documented fungal infections should be treated according to established guidelines (see Chapter 2.7).

Empiric antiviral therapy is not recommended for febrile neutropenic patients who have no evidence of viral disease. However, if skin or mucous membrane lesions caused by herpes simplex or varicella-zoster viruses are present, aciclovir therapy is usually indicated.

PATIENTS WHO HAVE DOCUMENTED INFECTIONS

During neutropenic periods, patients who have hematologic malignancy are at risk of multiple episodes of infection and may require prolonged empiric antimicrobial therapy. However, therapy has to be modified when the site of infection is known, because this is the single most important factor indicating the etiology.

Bacteremia and fungemia

About 20% of febrile patients who have hematologic malignancy and neutropenia have bacteremia. Gram-positive bacteria are more frequently isolated than Gram-negative. The prevalence of *P. aeruginosa* has decreased in recent years. The mortality from bacteremia is high, particularly in neutropenic patients, and empiric broad-spectrum antibacterial therapy as indicated for unexplained fever has to be instituted as early as possible after the patient has been examined and appropriate cultures obtained. When the pathogenic agent is identified, the initial antibiotic regimen should be changed according to the antibiotic sensitivity pattern of the isolate to provide optimal treatment and to avoid unnecessary use of antibiotics and resistance development. In patients who have prolonged neutropenia (i.e. >7 days), however, narrowing of the spectrum of the initial antibiotic regimen allows proliferation of resistant bacteria, which may result in breakthrough infections. Accordingly, if the empiric antibacterial spectrum is narrowed, patients who have prolonged neutropenia should be carefully monitored and the antibacterial coverage broadened if the condition deteriorates. The minimal duration of therapy is 10–14 days in non-neutropenic patients and patients neutropenic for less than 1 week. Patients who have prolonged neutropenia require longer therapy (see Neutropenic patients who have unexplained fever).

Fungemia is prevalent in patients who have acute leukemia and prolonged neutropenia. Treatment follows established guidelines (see Chapter 7.16).

Catheter-associated infections

Infections of indwelling vascular access devices (e.g. Hickman–Broviac catheter) are frequent causes of bacteremia. Most of these infections are caused by staphylococci. Usually they respond to parenteral antibiotic therapy without removal of the catheter unless a subcutaneous tunnel or pocket infection has become established. In double- or triple-lumen catheters, the antibiotic infusions should be rotated among each of the catheter lumens. However, catheter-associated bacteremia caused by *Bacillus* spp. or *C. jeikeium* or fungemia (usually *Candida* spp.) responds poorly to antimicrobial therapy, and removal of the catheter is usually necessary (Fig. 5.32). Also, if blood cultures remain positive despite 2–3 days of antimicrobial therapy, the catheter should be removed. Patients who have catheter-associated infection should be treated for at least 10 days.

Upper respiratory tract infections

Non-neutropenic patients who have hematologic malignancy usually experience the same infectious disease problems as immunocompetent patients. The most likely pathogens in otitis media are *S. pneumoniae* and *H. influenzae*. An acute ear infection in a non-neutropenic patient is managed with amoxicillin, amoxicillin plus clavulanic acid, or trimethoprim–sulfamethoxazole. Neutropenic patients also develop ear infections with bacteria that have colonized the nasopharynx, and a broad-spectrum antibiotic regimen is necessary unless a specific pathogen has been identified. Patients should be treated for 10–14 days.

Sinusitis in non-neutropenic patients is caused by *S. pneumoniae*, *H. influenzae*, *M. catarrhalis* and not infrequently by anaerobic bacteria. Patients who have acute leukemia and other conditions associated with neutropenia are also susceptible to fungal pathogens (e.g. *Aspergillus* spp., *C. albicans* and *Mucor* spp.). Acute sinusitis in non-neutropenic patients is managed with amoxicillin plus clavulanic acid or trimethoprim–sulfamethoxazole. In neutropenic patients, broad-spectrum antibiotic treatment is necessary. If a neutropenic patient does not improve within 72 hours, aspiration or biopsy of the sinus should be performed and antimicrobial therapy tailored to the etiologic agent. The diagnosis of fungal sinusitis requires histopathologic documentation of tissue invasion. Early institution of amphotericin B is a must. Surgical debridement of involved tissue is often required. A successful outcome depends on recovery of bone marrow function.

Pulmonary infections

The management of patients who have hematologic malignancy and pulmonary infections represents a great challenge to the clinician (Fig. 5.33). A major problem is the large number of pathogens that must be considered, ranging from common viruses and bacteria to exotic fungal and protozoan agents. Furthermore, a clinical picture similar to that produced by infection may be caused by a number of noninfectious causes of inflammation, including drug reactions, radiation lung injury, the underlying hematologic disease itself, pulmonary hemorrhage, leukoagglutinin transfusion reactions and pulmonary emboli. These noninfectious lung injuries have a high rate of secondary infection, which is often the immediate cause of death. In many patients, particularly neutropenic patients, the clinician's task is further complicated by the subtlety of the clinical presentation as a result of the impaired inflammatory response, the rapid progress of the infection and the difficulties in obtaining an etiologic agent because of serious disease conditions or bleeding disorders (e.g. thrombocytopenia). Of all host defense defects, neutropenia has the most profound effect on the course of pulmonary infection and treatment result. Careful attention has to be given to all these elements to arrive at the appropriate treatment.

Patient evaluation. The initial evaluation of the patient who has suspected pulmonary infection includes a chest radiograph, standard laboratory tests (i.e. white blood cell count with differential count, erythrocyte sedimentation rate, CRP measurement and urinalysis), two peripheral blood cultures from separate venipuncture sites, analysis of arterial blood gases, examination of sputum and, in patients who have suspected tuberculosis, a skin test for this disease (Fig. 5.34). In patients who have less obvious clinical pictures an acute-phase serum specimen should be stored for serologic testing or viral examinations.

INDICATIONS FOR REMOVAL OF INTRAVENOUS CATHETER TO CONTROL INFECTION

- Subcutaneous tunnel or pocket infection
- Bacteremia caused by *Bacillus* spp. or *Corynebacterium jeikeium*
- Fungemia (usually *Candida* spp.)
- Positive blood cultures despite 2–3 days antimicrobial therapy

Fig. 5.32 Indications for removal of intravenous catheter to control infection.

MAJOR CHALLENGES IN THE MANAGEMENT OF PATIENTS WITH HEMATOLOGIC MALIGNANCY AND PULMONARY INFECTIONS

- A large number of etiologic agents has to be considered (viruses, bacteria, fungi and protozoa)
- Noninfectious causes of pulmonary inflammation must be ruled out (drug reactions, radiation lung injury, underlying hematologic disease, pulmonary hemorrhage, leukoagglutinin transfusion reactions and pulmonary emboli)
- Secondary infections of noninfectious pulmonary injuries are frequent and must not be overlooked
- Because of serious disease conditions or bleeding disorders (e.g. thrombocytopenia) an etiologic agent is often difficult to obtain
- Disease progression is often rapid and necessitates prompt institution of antibiotic therapy

Fig. 5.33 Major challenges in the management of patients who have hematologic malignancy and pulmonary infections.

INITIAL EVALUATION OF PATIENTS WITH HEMATOLOGIC MALIGNANCY AND SUSPECTED PULMONARY INFECTION

- Chest radiograph
- Standard laboratory tests (i.e. white blood cell count with differential count, erythrocyte sedimentation rate, CRP measurement and urinalysis)
- Two peripheral blood cultures
- Analysis of arterial blood gases
- Sputum examination
- Skin test for tuberculosis (in suspected patients)
- An acute phase serum specimen (to be stored for serologic testing or viral examinations)

Fig. 5.34 Initial evaluation of patients who have hematologic malignancy and suspected pulmonary infection.

Appropriate therapy of patients who have hematologic malignancy and pulmonary infection requires a rapid and precise diagnosis. The sooner the etiologic diagnosis is made, the better the outcome. The diagnostic evaluation should always be initiated by examination of Gram's stain and culture of expectorated sputum specimens. However, sputum examinations are often of limited diagnostic value in immuno-compromised patients, and particularly patients who have hematologic malignancy. The reason for this is that many of these patients, particularly those with marked neutropenia, fail to produce sputum and expectorated sputum specimens are frequently contaminated by potential pathogens that colonize the upper respiratory tract of these patients. In addition, certain micro-organisms that are common causes of pneumonia in this population, particularly fungi, usually shed insufficient numbers of micro-organisms into the sputum to permit diagnosis by microscopy and culture. Finally, examination of sputum specimens will not detect the noninfectious causes of pulmonary infiltrates. Accordingly, more invasive diagnostic procedures are frequently required, including bronchoscopic techniques, percutaneous needle biopsy and the gold standard of open lung biopsy.[59] However, it should be borne in mind that

patients who have hematologic malignancy and pneumonia on first presentation almost always have infections with common pathogens, mostly bacteria, rather than opportunistic agents, and almost never require an invasive diagnostic procedure before initiating effective antimicrobial therapy. In contrast, these same patients after 2–3 weeks of chemotherapy-induced neutropenia and broad-spectrum antibacterial therapy are at high risk of opportunistic infections, and invasive diagnostic procedures may then be required to tailor antimicrobial therapy.

The choice of invasive procedure depends on the degree of illness, the rate of disease progression and the type of chest radiograph finding (Fig. 5.35). Open lung biopsy should be considered if the pulmonary infiltrates are diffuse or multifocal and spreading rapidly, the arterial hypoxia is intensifying and the life expectancy from the underlying disease is good, that is, can be measured in years (e.g. Hodgkin's disease, but not relapsing acute myelogenous leukemia).[59,93] A specific diagnosis is reached in about 80% of patients undergoing open lung biopsy. If the pulmonary process and hypoxia are progressing more slowly, and the disease is more of a diagnostic problem than a therapeutic emergency, less invasive techniques should be used, and the open lung biopsy should be kept in reserve should these techniques fail.

Bronchoalveolar lavage is particularly useful in diagnosing *P. carinii* infection and pulmonary hemorrhage, but is of little value in the diagnosis of pulmonary infiltrates in neutropenic leukemia patients.[59,104] The procedure can be safely performed in patients who have platelet counts as low as 30,000/mm^3. Transbronchial biopsy is most useful in the diagnosis of leukemic infiltrates, interstitial pneumonia and radiation or drug-induced pulmonary changes.[59,92] The procedure should not be performed in patients who have platelet counts less than 50,000/mm^3. In neutropenic patients, any bronchoscopic procedure may cause serious bacteremia and pneumonia. To avoid these complications, intravenous broad-spectrum antibiotics should be given as soon as adequate specimens are obtained.

Aspiration-needle biopsy is the diagnostic procedure of choice for focal lung disease, particularly peripheral lung infections such as *Nocardia* spp., and fungal infections and tuberculosis.[91] The sensitivity is greater than 80% for infection and 90% for malignancy. The diagnostic yield is particularly high if cavitation is present. The incidence of hemoptysis is less than 1% provided 22-gauge thin-wall needles are used and the patient's platelet count is more than 75,000/mm^3.[59]

In certain situations, empiric antimicrobial therapy should be considered without burdening the patient with an invasive diagnostic procedure. The most common situations are relapsing acute myelogenous leukemia and other advanced malignancies with limited life expectancy because of the severity of the underlying disease, serious bleeding disorders or marked impairment of pulmonary function that do not allow invasive techniques, and patient refusal. In such situations, the choice of empiric antimicrobial therapy is based on epidemiologic and clinical features, the nature of the underlying process, the progress of the pulmonary disease and results of laboratory investigations, including chest radiographs.

Infections in non-neutropenic patients. The causes of pulmonary infection in non-neutropenic patients who have hematologic malignancy are similar to those in immunocompetent patients. Common bacteria, mycoplasmas and viruses are most frequent (see Figs 5.24 & 5.25), and antimicrobial therapy is similar to that for immunocompetent patients (see Chapter 2.27). However, non-neutropenic patients who receive immunosuppressive therapy are at increased risk of tuberculosis, atypical mycobacterial disease, *P. carinii* infection and viral pneumonia. Patients who have tuberculosis infection should receive treatment with at least two effective antituberculous agents (e.g. isoniazid and rifampin) for 9 months. Treatment of atypical mycobacterial infection is more complex and should be individualized (see Chapter 2.30). *Pneumocystis carinii* causes bilateral diffuse pulmonary infiltrates. Trimethoprim–sulfamethoxazole is the treatment of choice for pneumocystis pneumonia (see Chapter 5.10), and improvement in alveolar air exchange and clinical condition usually occurs within 3–4 days. On the

INVASIVE PROCEDURES IN THE DIAGNOSIS OF PULMONARY INFILTRATES IN PATIENTS WITH HEMATOLOGIC MALIGNANCY

Procedure	Indications
Bronchoalveolar lavage	*Pneumocystis carinii* infection or pulmonary hemorrhage
Transbronchial biopsy	Leukemic infiltrates, interstitial pneumonia, or radiation or drug-induced injuries
Aspiration-needle biopsy	Focal lung disease, particularly peripheral lung infections (e.g. *Nocardia* or fungal infections or tuberculosis)
Open lung biopsy	Rapidly spreading diffuse or multifocal infiltrates with intensifying arterial hypoxia. Life expectancy from underlying disease should be good (i.e. measured in years)

Fig. 5.35 Invasive procedures in the diagnosis of pulmonary infiltrates in patients who have hematologic malignancy. Patients who have serious bleeding disorders, marked impairment of pulmonary function or advanced malignancies with limited life expectancy (e.g. relapsing acute myelogenous leukemia) should not be burdened with an invasive diagnostic procedure, but should be given empiric antimicrobial therapy.

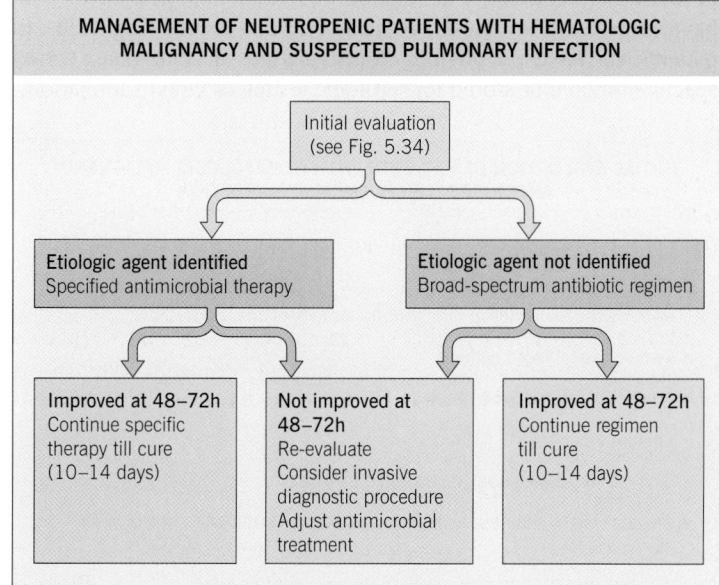

Fig. 5.36 Management of neutropenic patients who have hematologic malignancy and suspected pulmonary infection.

basis of studies in AIDS patients who have pneumocystosis a 21-day course of prednisone is given to patients who have moderate to severe pneumocystis pneumonia.[105] If trimethoprim–sufamethoxazole cannot be used, pentamidine, dapsone plus trimethoprim, or atovaquone alone should be considered (see Chapter 5.10).

The exact cause of viral pneumonia is difficult to establish, and specific therapy for most viral infections is lacking. However, infections with cytomegalovirus can be detected in a matter of days, and combined therapy with ganciclovir and intravenous immunoglobulin (pooled or cytomegalovirus hyperimmune) has markedly improved survival in allogeneic bone marrow transplant patients who have cytomegalovirus pneumonitis.[106] These results have led to the acceptance of ganciclovir and immunoglobulin as standard treatment for patients who have cytomegalovirus pneumonitis. Pneumonia caused by respiratory syncytial virus may be diagnosed within a few hours. Ribavirin seems to have a beneficial effect in children with severe respiratory disease caused by respiratory syncytial virus.[107] Although few studies are reported on the effect of ribavirin in immunocompromised patients who have respiratory syncytial virus pneumonia, it seems reasonable to recommend ribavirin in serious pulmonary infection caused by this agent.

Infections in neutropenic patients. In addition to the pathogens isolated from pulmonary infections in non-neutropenic patients, a large number of opportunistic pathogens may cause pneumonia in neutropenic patients, including a wide variety of Gram-positive or Gram-negative bacteria and several viruses, fungi and protozoa (see Figs 5.24 & 5.25). Bacteria predominate in patients who have neutropenia of less than 14 days' duration. Patients who have more prolonged neutropenia are at greater risk of fungal or viral infections. Unless the clinical picture or the results of sputum examination indicate specific antimicrobial therapy, a 48- to 72-hour trial of a broad-spectrum antibiotic regimen (see above) should be instituted before attempting to arrive at a specific diagnosis by invasive procedures (Fig. 5.36). If the patient has improved or stabilized by 72 hours, treatment should be continued until the patient is cured, which usually takes 10–14 days. If the patient has not improved or stabilized, bronchoalveolar lavage or another invasive diagnostic procedure should be performed and antimicrobial treatment adjusted according to test results.

Fungi are frequent causes of pulmonary infection in patients who have prolonged neutropenia, particularly in patients already receiving broad-spectrum antibacterial agents.[59,108–110] *Aspergillus* spp. are most prevalent followed by *Candida* spp. and *Phycomycetes* spp. Typically, these fungi cause a localized pulmonary infiltrate. *Coccidioides immitis, C. neoformans* and *Histoplasma capsulatum* more commonly cause diffuse or nodular pulmonary infiltrates. The clinical and radiographic features of pulmonary fungal infections are indistinguishable from those of other pulmonary processes, and a definitive diagnosis requires microbiologic or histopathologic confirmation in specimens obtained by transbronchial or open lung biopsy.[59] Optimal therapy is provided by amphotericin B. In *Aspergillus* pneumonia, doses of 1–1.5mg/kg/day should be given. The addition of 5-fluorocytosine (100–150mg/kg/day in three divided doses) may be helpful although there is disagreement on this which lacks controled trials. Blood levels of 5-fluorocytosine should be kept in the range of 40–60mg/L to prevent side effects. The potential value of liposomal amphotericin B remains to be established in prospective randomized clinical trials. Therapy of pulmonary infections caused by phycomycetes, especially *Mucor* spp. and *Rhizopus* spp., consists of amphotericin B (1mg/kg/day) and extensive surgical debridement. Treatment results are poor unless bone marrow recovery occurs.

Patients who have prolonged neutropenia are also at increased risk of pulmonary infections with *Legionella pneumophila, Nocardia asteroides* and *Nocardia brasiliensis*. Erythromycin (40–50mg/kg/day; maximum 4g/day) in four divided doses per day for 3 weeks is the treatment of choice for *Legionella* pneumonia. In seriously ill patients, rifampin (20mg/kg/day in two doses) may be given in addition to erythromycin. Usually, improvement occurs within 24–48 hours. Doxycycline is an alternative to erythromycin. Azithromycin, clarithromycin and ciprofloxacin may represent therapeutic improvements. Sulfadiazine (100mg/kg/day for 6 months) is the drug of choice for the treatment of *Nocardia* pneumonia. Patients who have disseminated *Nocardia* infection have a high mortality, approximately 30%.

Skin and soft tissue infections

Skin infections may represent a primary focus of infection or may occur as a result of bacteremia, fungemia or viremia. Examination of aspirate or biopsy from skin lesions suggesting disseminated disease may allow early diagnosis and institution of appropriate antimicrobial therapy.

Perianal cellulitis is a common lesion in patients who have acute leukemia, particularly those with prolonged (>7 days) and profound neutropenia (<100 cells/mm³). The most common pathogens are aerobic Gram-negative bacilli and anaerobic bacteria. In neutropenic patients, broad-spectrum antibiotic therapy, including antianaerobic agents, should be instituted at the first complaints of tenderness. Supportive measures include stool softeners, sitz baths and low-bulk diet. Unnecessary rectal examinations should be avoided.

Life-threatening varicella-zoster virus infection leading to visceral dissemination is a well known complication in immunocompromised patients, particularly in children with leukemia. Treatment with aciclovir should be instituted promptly. If a seronegative patient who has leukemia or lymphoma is exposed to varicella, varicella-zoster immune globulin should be administered promptly, but not more than 96 hours after exposure. Varicella vaccine is now available and provides a high degree of protection. Extension of genital herpetic lesions to the thighs and perianal area is common in patients who have hematologic malignancy. Treatment is with aciclovir.

Oropharyngeal infections

Gingivitis and periodontitis are frequent in patients who have acute leukemia, and hygienic measures are important. Necrotizing gingivitis is caused by anaerobic bacteria and should be managed with antianaerobic antibiotics.[111] Oropharyngeal candidiasis is the most common mucosal lesion in patients who have hematologic malignancy and is usually controlled by topical antifungal agents (e.g. clotrimazole troches). Oral fluconazole 50–100mg/day is highly effective. Herpes simplex stomatitis is more extensive and protracted in neutropenic patients than in immunocompetent hosts and may serve as a nidus for bacterial and fungal invasion. Aciclovir (750mg/m² per day in three divided doses) is the treatment of choice. Patients who have acute leukemia and are seropositive should receive prophylactic aciclovir when undergoing bone marrow transplantation or induction regimens.

Esophagitis

Infectious esophagitis most commonly occurs in neutropenic patients on antibiotic therapy. Infections with *Candida* spp. or herpes simplex virus are most prevalent, followed by bacterial infections.[112] Therapy should be based on findings at esophagoscopy. However, if the etiology has not been established, oral fluconazole plus parenteral broad-spectrum antibacterial therapy should be instituted. If the patient does not respond to this regimen within 48–72 hours, fluconazole should be replaced by intravenous amphotericin B. If symptoms persist for another 48–72 hours, *Candida* spp. are unlikely to be the etiologic agents and a trial of aciclovir is recommended on account of the high prevalence of herpes simplex virus esophagitis. In difficult therapeutic situations, microbiologic and histologic examinations of specimens obtained by esophagoscopy may be of significant aid in establishing a definitive diagnosis.

Gastrointestinal infections

Necrotizing enterocolitis (typhlitis) most often occurs in patients who have acute leukemia, particularly during periods of neutropenia and antibiotic therapy.[69] Etiologic agents include Gram-negative bacilli and anaerobic bacteria, especially *Clostridium* spp. Management involves broad-spectrum antibacterial therapy, fluid replacement and surgery to resect necrotic bowel. The mortality rate is high, 30–40%.

Clostridium spp. also cause severe peritonitis and bacteremia in patients who have acute leukemia, particularly during prolonged periods of neutropenia and antibiotic therapy. Management involves antibiotic therapy and supportive care. Partly because of the frequent use of antibiotics in neutropenic patients, *C. difficile* associated colitis is prevalent. Treatment with oral vancomycin or metronidazole is as for immunocompetent patients. Relapse is not unusual and may follow cancer chemotherapy. Patients who have hyperinfection syndrome caused by *S. stercoralis* are treated with thiabendazole. Immunocompromised patients should be treated for 2–3 weeks.

Hepatic candidiasis
Focal hepatic candidiasis has mainly been reported in patients who have leukemia and resolving neutropenia. The disease represents a therapeutic challenge, and eradication of microabscesses is difficult to achieve. Prolonged therapy with amphotericin B is necessary and a total amount of 4–5g may be needed. Experimental studies suggest that the combination of amphotericin B and 5-fluorocytosine is preferable. Good results have also been obtained with fluconazole or amphothericin B incorporated in liposomes.[113] Resolution of infection is confirmed by biopsy.

Urinary tract infections
Urinary tract infections constitute 5–10% of documented infections in neutropenic patients. Gram-negative aerobic bacilli and enterococci are the most common etiologic agents. Antibiotic treatment should be tailored to the sensitivity of the causative agent. Febrile neutropenic patients who have urinary tract infection should receive broad-spectrum antibiotic therapy.

Fungal invasion of the urinary tract is usually insidious even in neutropenic patients who have acute leukemia. Superficial bladder infections are effectively treated with oral fluconazole or instillation of amphotericin B into the bladder. However, isolation of a particular fungal species (usually *Candida* spp.) in two or more urine cultures in the presence of fever and deteriorating kidney function should prompt the institution of systemic amphotericin B.

Infections of the central nervous system
Splenectomized patients are at increased risk of meningitis with encapsulated bacteria, particularly *S. pneumoniae*, and patients who have other hematologic malignancies undergoing heavy immunosuppressive therapy are prone to develop meningitis with *C. neoformans* and *L. monocytogenes*. Management of these infections follows the same guidelines as for immunocompetent patients (see Chapters 2.15, 2.16 & 2.17).

Eye infections
The management of conjunctivitis or keratitis in patients who have hematologic malignancy usually follows the same guidelines as for immunocompetent patients (see Chapter 2.11). Bacterial conjunctivitis is treated with topical antibiotics. Herpes simplex virus may cause conjunctivitis, blepharitis and stromal keratitis. Treatment includes local debridement and topical antiviral agents (i.e. aciclovir, vidarabine or trifluorothymidine). Varicella-zoster ophthalmitis in immunocompromised patients should be treated with intravenous aciclovir because of the relatively poor bioavailability of the oral compound. Cytomegalovirus retinitis is managed with ganciclovir, and invasive fungal eye infection requires intravenous amphotericin B.

Infections of the cardiovascular system
Cardiovascular infections are less common among patients who have hematologic malignancy. In endocarditis, Gram-positive cocci (i.e. *S. aureus*, viridans streptococci and enterococci) are the most common etiologic agents followed by Gram-negative bacilli and fungi (i.e. *Candida* spp. and *Aspergillus* spp.). Therapy should be directed at the specific agents (see Chapter 2.49). Valve replacement is most often required in fungal endocarditis.

REFERENCES

1. Sullivan AK. Classification, pathogenesis, and etiology of neoplastic diseases of the hematopoietic system. In: Lee GR, Bithell TC, Foerster J, Athens JW, Lukens JN, eds. Wintrobe's Clinical Hematology, 9th ed. Philadelphia: Lea & Febiger;1993;1725–91.

2. Bishop JF, Matthews JP, Young GA, *et al.* A randomized study of high-dose cytarabine in induction in acute myeloid leukemia. Blood 1996;87:1710–7.

3. Mayer RJ, Davis RB, Schiffer CA, *et al.* Intensive postremission chemotherapy in adults with acute myeloid leukemia. N Engl J Med 1994;331:896–903.

4. Larson RA, Dodge RK, Burns CP, *et al.* A five-drug remission induction regimen with intensive consolidation for adults with acute lymphoblastic leukemia: Cancer and leukemia group B study 8811. Blood 1995;85:2025–37.

5. Feld R, Bodey GP. Infections in patients with malignant lymphoma treated with combination chemotherapy. Cancer 1977;39:1018–25.

6. Notter DT, Grossman PL, Rosenberg SA, Remington JS. Infections in patients with Hodgkin's disease: a clinical study of 300 consecutive adult patients. Rev Infect Dis 1980;2:761–800.

7. Molica S. Infections in chronic lymphocytic leukemia: risk factors, and impact on survival, and treatment. Leukemia and Lymphoma 1994;13:203–14.

8. Severien C, Nelson JD. Frequency of infections associated with implanted systems vs cuffed, tunneled silastic venous catheters in patients with acute leukemia. Am J Dis Child 1991;145:1433–8.

9. Young LS. Management of infections in leukemia and lymphoma. In: Rubin RH, Young LS, eds. Clinical approach to infection in the compromised host, 3rd ed. New York: Plenum;1994:551–79.

10. Hamblin T. Clinical features of MDS. Leukemia Res 1992;16:89–93.

11. Finch SC, Linet MS. Chronic leukaemias. Baillière's Clin Haematol 1992;5:27–56

12. Stevens RG. Age and risk of acute leukemia. J Natl Cancer Inst 1986;76:845–8.

13. Wade JC. Epidemiology and prevention of infection in the compromised host. In: Rubin RH, Young LS, eds. Clinical approach to infection in the compromised host, 3rd ed. New York: Plenum;1994:5–31.

14. Schimpff SC. Infections in the cancer patient – diagnosis, prevention, and treatment. In: Mandell GL, Bennett JE, Dolin R, eds. Principles and practice of infectious diseases. New York: Churchill Livingstone;1995:2666–75.

15. Bodey GP, Buckley M, Sathe YS, Freireich EJ. Quantitative relationships between circulating leukocytes and infections in patients with acute leukemia. Ann Intern Med 1966;64:328–40.

16. Hamblin T. Immunologic abnormalities in myelodysplastic syndromes. Hematol Oncol Clin North Am 1992;6:571–86.

17. de Boer AW, de Vaan, GAM, Weemaes CMR, Bakkeren JAJM. Iatrogenic IgG$_2$ deficiency in a leukaemic child. A case report. Eur J Pediatr 1992;151:271–3.

18. Bogomolski-Yahalom V, Matzner Y. Disorders of neutrophil function. Blood Rev 1995;9:183–90.

19. Gamm H, Huber C, Chapel H, *et al.* Intravenous immune globulin in chronic lymphocytic leukaemia. Clin Exp Immunol 1994;97(suppl 1):17–20.

20. Pilarski LM, Mant MJ, Ruether BA. Analysis of immunodeficiency in multiple myeloma: observations and hypothesis. J Clin Lab Anal 1987;1:214–28.

21. Hargreaves RM, Lea JR, Griffiths H, *et al.* Immunological factors and risk of infection in plateau phase myeloma. J Clin Pathol 1995;48:260–6.

22. Heredia A, Hewlett IK, Soriano V, Epstein JS. Idiopathic CD4+ T lymphocytopenia: a review and current perspective. Transfusion Med Rev 1994;8:223–31.

23. Schlesinger M, Broman I, Lugassy G. The complement system is defective in chronic lymphatic leukemia patients and in their healthy relatives. Leukemia 1996;10:1509–13.

24. Bruserud Ø, Halstensen A, Peen E, Solberg CO. Serum levels of adhesion molecules and cytokines in patients with acute leukaemia. Leukemia and Lymphoma 1996;23:423–30.

25. Schimpff SC, Young VM, Greene WH, *et al.* Origin of infection in acute nonlymphocytic leukemia: significance of hospital acquisition of potential pathogens. Ann Intern Med 1972;77:707–14.

26. Levine AS, Siegel SE, Schreiber AD, *et al.* Protected environments and prophylactic antibiotics: a prospective controlled study of their utility in the therapy of acute leukemia. N Engl J Med 1973;288:477–83.

27. van der Waaij DD, Berghuis J, Lekkerkerk JEC. Colonization resistance of the digestive tract of mice during systemic antibiotic treatment. J Hyg (Camb) 1972;70:605–10.

28. Dekker AW, Rozenberg-Arska M, Verhoef J. Infection prophylaxis in acute leukemia: a comparison of ciprofloxacin with trimethoprim–sulfamethoxazole and colistin. Ann Intern Med 1987;106:7–12.

29. Bow EJ, Ronald AR. Editorial: antimicrobial chemoprophylaxis in neutropenic patients – where do we go from here? Clin Infect Dis 1993;17:333–7.

30. Goodman JL, Winston DJ, Greenfield RA, et al. A controlled trial of fluconazole to prevent fungal infections in patients undergoing bone marrow transplantation. N Engl J Med 1992;326:845–51.

31. Wingard JR, Merz WG, Rinaldi MG, et al. Increase in Candida krusei infection among patients with bone marrow transplantation and neutropenia treated prophylactically with fluconazole. N Engl J Med 1991;325:1274–7.

32. Bustamente CI, Wade JC. Herpes simplex virus infection in the immunocompromised cancer patient. J Clin Oncol 1991;9:1903–15.

33. Schmidt GM, Horak DA, Niland JC, et al. A randomized, controlled trial of prophylactic ganciclovir for cytomegalovirus pulmonary infection in recipients of allogeneic bone marrow transplants. N Engl J Med 1991;324:1005–11.

34. Gershon AA, Steinberg SP, and the National Institute of Allergy and Infectious Diseases Varicella Vaccine Collaborative Study Group. Live attenuated varicella vaccine: protection in healthy adults compared with leukemic children. J Infect Dis 1990;161:661–6.

35. Cooperative Group for the Study of Immunglobulin in Chronic Lymphocytic Leukemia. Intravenous immunoglobulin for the prevention of infection in chronic lymphocytic leukemia: a randomized, controlled clinical trial. N Engl J Med 1988;319:902–7.

36. Weeks JC, Tierney MR, Weinstein MC. Cost effectiveness of prophylactic intravenous immune globulin in chronic lymphocytic leukemia. N Engl J Med 1991;325:81–6.

37. Roilides E, Pizzo PA. Modulation of host defenses by cytokines: evolving adjuncts in prevention and treatment of serious infections in immunocompromised hosts. Clin Infect Dis 1992;15:508–24.

38. Solberg CO, Meuwissen HJ, Needham RN, Good RA, Matsen JM. Infectious complications in bone marrow transplantation. Br Med J 1971;1:18–23.

39. Kramer BS, Pizzo PA, Robichaud KJ, Witesbsky F, Wesley R. Role of serial microbiologic surveillance and clinical evaluation in the management of cancer patients with fever and granulocytopenia. Am J Med 1982;72:561–8.

40. Sickles EA, Greene WH, Wiernik PH. Clinical presentation of infection in granulocytopenic patients. Arch Intern Med 1975;135:715–9.

41. Pizzo PA, Robichaud KJ, Wesley R, Commers JR. Fever in the pediatric and young adult patient with cancer: a prospective study of 1001 episodes. Medicine (Baltimore) 1982;61:153–65.

42. Bartlett AV, Zusman J, Daum RS. Unusual presentations of Haemophilus influenzae infections in immunocompromised patients. J Pediatr 1983;102:55–8.

43. Sinkovics JG, Smith JP. Septicemia with Bacteroides in patients with malignant disease. Cancer 1970;25:663–71.

44. Fisher RI, DeVita VT, Bostick F, et al. Persistent immunologic abnormalities in long-term survivors of advanced Hodgkin's disease. Ann Intern Med 1980;92:595–9.

45. Decker MD, Edwards KM. Central venous catheter infections. Pediatr Clin North Am 1988;35:579–612.

46. Green DM, Stutzman L, Blumenson LE, et al. The incidence of post-splenectomy sepsis and herpes zoster in children and adolescents with Hodgkin disease. Med Pediatr Oncol 1979;7:285–97.

47. Vindenes H, Bjerknes R. The frequency of bacteremia and fungemia following wound cleaning and excision in patients with large burns. J Trauma 1993;35:742–9.

48. Freifeld AG, Hathorn JW, Pizzo PA. Infectious complications in the pediatric cancer patient. In: Pizzo PA, Poplack DG, eds. Principles and practice of pediatric oncology, 2nd ed. Philadelphia: JB Lippincott;1993:987–1019.

49. Koll BS, Brown AE. The changing epidemiology of infections at cancer hospitals. Clin Infect Dis 1993;17(suppl 2):S322–8.

50. Rubio M, Palau L, Vivas JR, et al. Predominance of Gram-positive micro-organisms as a cause of septicemia in patients with hematologic malignancies. Infect Control Hosp Epidemiol 1994;15:101–4.

51. Horn R, Wong B, Kiehn TE, Armstrong D. Fungemia in a cancer hospital: changing frequency, earlier onset, and results of therapy. Rev Infect Dis 1985;7:646–55.

52. Bone RC, Balk RA, Cerra FB, et al. Definitions for sepsis and organ failure and guidelines for the use of innovative therapies in sepsis. Chest 1992;101:1644–55.

53. Hiemenz J, Skelton J, Pizzo PA. Perspective on the management of catheter-related infections in cancer patients. Pediatr Infect Dis 1986;5:6–11.

54. Raad II, Luna M, Khalil S-AM, et al. The relationship between the thrombotic and infectious complications of central venous catheters. JAMA 1994;271:1014–6.

55. McGill TJ, Simpson G, Healvy GB. Fulminant aspergillosis of the nose and the paranasal sinuses: a new clinical entity. Laryngoscope 1980;90:748–54.

56. Rosenow EC III, Wilson WR, Cockerill FR III. Pulmonary disease in the immunocompromised host. 1.Mayo Clin Proc 1985;60:473–87.

57. Wilson WR, Cockerill FR III, Rosenow EC III. Pulmonary disease in the immunocompromised host. 2. Mayo Clin Proc 1985;60:610–31.

58. Johanson WG, Pierce AK, Sanford JP. Changing pharyngeal bacterial flora of hospitalized patients. N Engl J Med 1969;281:1137–40.

59. Rubin RH, Greene R. Clinical approach to the compromised host with fever and pulmonary infiltrates. In: Rubin RH, Young LS, eds. Clinical approach to infection in the compromised host, 3rd ed. New York: Plenum;1994:121–61.

60. Kaplan MH, Armstrong D, Rosen P. Tuberculosis complicating neoplastic disease. A review of 201 cases. Cancer 1974;33:850–8.

61. Edelstein PH. Legionnaires' disease, pontiac fever, and related illnesses. In: Feigin RD, Cherry JD, eds. Textbook of pediatric infectious diseases, 3rd ed. Philadelphia: WB Saunders;1992:1141–8.

62. Levitz SM. Aspergillosis. Infect Dis Clin North Am 1989;3:1–18.

63. Hughes WT, Feldman S, Aur RJA, et al. Intensity of immunosuppressive therapy and the incidence of Pneumocystis carinii pneumonitis. Cancer 1975;36:2004–9.

64. Whitley RJ. Varicella-zoster virus. In: Mandell GL, Douglas RG Jr, Bennett JE, eds. Principles and practice of infectious diseases. New York: Churchill Livingstone;1989:1153–9.

65. Adler SP. Transfusion-associated cytomegalovirus infections. Rev Infect Dis 1983;5:977–93.

66. Hirsch MS. Herpes group virus infections in the compromised host. In: Rubin RH, Young LS, eds. Clinical approach to infection in the compromised host, 3rd ed. New York: Plenum;1994:379–96.

67. Straus SE. Varicella-zoster virus infections. Biology, natural history, treatment, and prevention. Ann Intern Med 1988;108:221–37.

68. Glenn J, Cotton D, Wesley R, Pizzo PA. Anorectal infections in patients with malignant disease. Rev Infect Dis 1988;10:42–52.

69. Skibber JM, Matter GJ, Pizzo PA, Lotze MT. Right lower quadrant pain in young patients with leukemia: a surgical perspective. Ann Surg 1987;206:711–6.

70. Haron E, Feld R, Tuffnell P, et al. Hepatic candidiasis: an increasing problem in immunocompromised patients. Am J Med 1987;83:17–26.

71. Bodey GP. Hematogenous and major organ candidiasis. In: Bodey GP, ed. Candidiasis: pathogenesis, diagnosis, and treatment, 2nd ed. New York: Raven;1993:279–329.

72. Perfect JR. Cryptococcosis. Infect Dis Clin North Am 1989;3:77–102.

73. Rothenhaus TC, Polis MA. Ocular manifestations of systemic disease. Emerg Med Clin North Am 1995;13:607–30.

74. Schafer AI. Bleeding and thrombosis in the myeloproliferative disorders. Blood 1984;64:1–12.

75. Murray PR, Washington JA II. Microscopic and bacteriologic analysis of expectorated sputum. Mayo Clin Proc 1975;50:339–44.

76. Kovacs JA, Ng VL, Masur H, et al. Diagnosis of Pneumocystis carinii pneumonia: improved detection in sputum with use of monoclonal antibodies. N Engl J Med 1988;318:589–93.

77. Saito H, Anaissie EJ, Morice RC, Dekmezian R, Bodey GP. Bronchoalveolar lavage in the diagnosis of pulmonary infiltrates in patients with acute leukemia. Chest 1988;94:745–9.

78. Kovalski R, Hansen-Flaschen J, Lodato RF, Pietra GG. Localized leukemic pulmonary infiltrates: diagnosis by bronchoscopy and resolution with therapy. Chest 1990;97:674–8.

79. Armstrong D, Polsky B. Central nervous system infections in the compromised host. In: Rubin RG, Young LS, eds. Clinical approach to infection in the compromised host, 2nd ed. New York: Plenum;1988:163–91.

80. Chernik NL, Armstrong D, Posner JB. Central nervous system infections in patients with cancer. Changing patterns. Cancer 1977;40:268–74.

81. Chessells JM. Central nervous system directed therapy in acute lymphoblastic leukaemia. Baillière's Clin Haematol 1994;7:349–63.

82. Drew WL. Nonpulmonary manifestations of cytomegalovirus infection in immunocompromised patients. Clin Microbiol Rev 1992;5:204–10.

83. Kellogg JA. Culture vs. direct antigen assays for detection of microbial pathogens from lower respiratory tract specimens suspected of containing the respiratory syncytial virus. Arch Pathol Lab Med 1991;115:451–8.

84. Uldum SA, Jensen JS, Søndergaard-Andersen J, Lind K. Enzyme immunoassay for detection of immunoglobulin M (IgM) and IgG antibodies to Mycoplasma pneumoniae. J Clin Microbiol 1992;30:1198–204.

85. Sepkowitz KA, Brown AE, Telzak EE, Gottlieb S, Armstrong D. Pneumocystis carinii pneumonia among patients without AIDS at a cancer hospital. JAMA 1992;267:832–7.

86. Wheeler JH, Fishman EK. Computed tomography in the management of chest infections: current status. Clin Infect Dis 1996;23:232–40.

87. Thaler M, Pastakia B, Shawker TH, O'Leary T, Pizzo PA. Hepatic candidiasis in cancer patients: the evolving picture of the syndrome. Ann Intern Med 1988;108:88–100.

88. Lamminen AE, Anttila V-JA, Bondestam S, Ruutu T, Ruutu PJ. Infectious liver foci in leukemia: comparison of short-inversion-time inversion-recovery, T1-weighted spin-echo, and dynamic gadolinium-enhanced MR imaging. Radiology 1994;191:539–43.

89. Dutcher JP, Schiffer CA, Johnston GS. Rapid migration of [111]indium-labeled granulocytes to sites of infection. N Engl J Med 1981;304:586–9.

90. Oyen WJG, Claessens RAMJ, Raemaekers JMM, et al. Diagnosing infection in febrile granulocytopenic patients with Indium-111-labeled human immunoglobulin G. J Clin Oncol 1992;10:61–8.

91. Perlmutt LM, Johnston WW, Dunnick NR. Percutaneous transthoracic needle aspiration: a review. Am J Roentgenol 1989;152:451–5.

92. Rosenow EC III. Diffuse pulmonary infiltrates in the immunocompromised host. Clin Chest Med 1990;11:55–64.

93. Catterall JR, McCabe RE, Brooks RG, Remington JS. Open lung biopsy in patients with Hodgkin's disease and pulmonary infiltrates. Am Rev Respir Dis 1989;139;1274–9.

94. McCabe WR, Jackson GG. Gram-negative bacteremia. II: clinical, laboratory, and therapeutic observations. Arch Intern Med 1962;110:856–64.

95. Schimpf SC. Overview of empiric antibiotic therapy for the febrile neutropenic patient. Rev Infect Dis 1985;7(suppl 4):S734–40.

96. Infectious Diseases Society of America. Guidelines for the use of antimicrobial agents in neutropenic patients with unexplained fever. J Infect Dis 1990;161:381–96.

97. Immunocompromised Host Society. The design, analysis, and reporting of clinical trials on the empirical antibiotic management of the neutropenic patient: report of a consensus panel. J Infect Dis 1990;161:397–401.

98. EORTC International Antimicrobial Therapy Cooperative Group. Ceftazidime combined with a short or long course of amikacin for empirical therapy of Gram-negative bacteremia in cancer patients with granulocytopenia. N Engl J Med 1987;314:1692–8.

99. Winston DJ, Ho WG, Bruckner DA, Gale RP, Champlin RE. Controlled trials of double beta-lactam therapy with cefoperazone plus piperacillin in febrile granulocytopenic patients. Am J Med 1988;85(suppl 1A):21–30.

100. Pizzo PA, Hathorn JW, Hiemenz JW, et al. A randomized trial comparing ceftazidime alone with combination antibiotic therapy in cancer patients with fever and neutropenia. N Engl J Med 1986;315:552–8.

101. Gutmann L, Williamson R, Kitzie MD, Acar JF. Synergism and antagonism in double beta-lactam antibiotic combinations. Am J Med 1986;80(suppl 5C):21–9.

102. Pizzo PA, Robichaud KJ, Gill FA, Witebsky FG. Empiric antibiotic and antifungal therapy for cancer patients with prolonged fever and granulocytopenia. Am J Med 1982;72:101–11.

103. EORTC International Antimicrobial Therapy Cooperative Group. Empiric antifungal therapy in febrile granulocytopenic patients, part I. Am J Med 1989;86:668–72.

104. Kahn FW, Jones JM. Diagnosing bacterial respiratory infection by bronchoalveolar lavage. J Infect Dis 1987;155:862–9.

105. Gagnon S, Boota AM, Fischl MA, et al. Corticosteroids as adjunctive therapy for severe Pneumocystis carinii pneumonia in the acquired immunodeficiency syndrome. N Engl J Med 1990;323:1444–50.

106. Emanuel D, Cunningham I, Jules-Elysee K, et al. Cytomegalovirus pneumonia after bone marrow transplantation successfully treated with a combination of ganciclovir and high-dose intravenous immune globulin. Ann Intern Med 1988;109:777–82.

107. Smith DW, Frankel LR, Mathers LH, et al. A controlled trial of aerosolized ribavirin in infants receiving mechanical ventilation for severe respiratory syncytial virus infections. N Engl J Med 1991;325:24–9.

108. Edwards JE, Lehrer RI, Stiehm ER, Fischer TJ, Young LS. Severe candidal infections: clinical perspective, immune defense mechanisms, and current concepts of therapy. Ann Intern Med 1978;89:91–106.

109. Krick JA, Remington JS. Opportunistic invasive fungal infections in patients with leukemia and lymphoma. Clin Haematol 1976;5:249–310.

110. Rinaldi MG. Invasive aspergillosis. Rev Infect Dis 1983;5:1061–77.

111. Peterson D, Minah GE, Overholser CD. Microbiology of acute periodontal infection in myelosuppressed cancer patients. J Clin Oncol 1987;5:1461–8.

112. Walsh TJ, Belitsos N, Hamilton SR. Bacterial esophagitis in immunocompromised patients. Arch Intern Med 1986;146:1345–8.

113. Anaissie E, Bodey GP, Kantarjian H, et al. Fluconazole therapy for chronic disseminated candidiasis in patients with leukemia and prior amphotericin B therapy. Am J Med 1991;91:142–50.

Immunologically Mediated Diseases

Jonathan Cohen

This chapter is concerned with a diverse group of conditions that have in common the fact that their cause is thought to be related to disordered immune processes, and their treatment involves high-dose immunosuppressive therapy. In the past these diseases have been called 'autoimmune', 'autoallergic', 'collagen-vascular' or 'vasculitis', but I think they are better referred to as simply immunologically mediated diseases (IMD; Fig. 6.1).

EPIDEMIOLOGY

The importance of IMD to the infectious diseases practitioner lies in the fact that these patients frequently have severe multisystem disease and require high-dose immunosuppressive therapy, so the risk of opportunistic infection is high. Furthermore, they differ from other types of immunosuppressed patients in that they often receive several different modalities of immunosuppression (Fig. 6.2), and the duration of their treatment is much longer than that for a patient who has leukemia or cancer, for instance, in whom the neutropenic period is nowadays often not much more than 1 week in duration.

Infection is a major cause of morbidity and mortality in patients who have IMD,[1] but the incidence of infection in these patients varies considerably depending on the stage of the disease and the intensity of the immunosuppression. In a study of 75 heavily immunosuppressed patients who had a variety of IMD, we found a rate of 0.74 infections/patient/week.[2] More recently, an overall rate of just 0.008 infections/patient/week was reported for a series of 102 patients who have systemic lupus erythematosus (SLE) followed for several years.[3] Notably though, the incidence of major infection was 20 times greater during the month after a course of methylprednisolone.

PATHOGENESIS AND PATHOLOGY

Whereas organ or bone marrow transplant recipients are a homogeneous population, patients who have IMD can represent a very complex challenge to the infectious diseases physician. Factors that need to be taken into account in assessing the patient include the nature of the underlying disease and the particular type of immunosuppression used, its duration and its dose. Although specific diseases are not generally complicated by particular infections, there are some associations of note; salmonellosis frequently occurs as a complication of SLE, for instance, although the mechanism is not at all clear.[4] In some cases, there may be an etiologic association between an infection and the disease itself. A good example of this is the role of the hepatitis viruses in the pathogenesis of cryoglobulinemia, polyarteritis nodosa and other types of systemic vasculitis.[5,6] Recently, there have been intriguing reports suggesting that Wegener's granulomatosis may be caused by an abnormal response to an unknown infection, and that relapses of Wegener's granulomatosis can be prevented by chronic administration of trimethoprim–sulfamethoxazole (co-trimoxazole).[7]

Although certain types of treatment are associated with particular defects in immune function,[8] patients who have IMD commonly receive combinations of drugs, and this makes predictions very difficult. Certainly, high-dose corticosteroid therapy is complicated by

IMMUNOLOGICALLY MEDIATED DISEASES

Systemic lupus erythematosus	Mixed connective tissue disease
Polyarteritis nodosa	Progressive systemic sclerosis
Wegener's granulomatosis lymphomatoid granulomatosis bronchocentric granulomatosis	Polymyositis/dermatomyositis
	Relapsing polychondritis
Antiglomerular basement membrane disease (Goodpasture's syndrome)	Behçet's syndrome
	Sjögren's syndrome
Mixed essential cryoglobulinemia	Churg–Strauss syndrome
Rheumatoid arthritis Still's disease Felty's syndrome	Henoch–Schönlein purpura
	Hemolytic uremic syndrome/thrombotic thrombocytopenic purpura

Fig. 6.1 Immunologically mediated diseases. A list of IMD in which high-dose immunosuppression is often used and major opportunistic infection is a common problem. The list excludes generally less severe diseases such as asthma; although such patients may occasionally need high-dose immunosuppression, it is much less common.

IMMUNOSUPPRESSIVE AGENTS AND PROCEDURES

Corticosteroids	Cyclosporin and related drugs FK506 (tacrolimus) Rapamycin
Thiopurines 6-Mercaptopurine Azathioprine	
	Total lymphoid irradiation
Alkylating agents	Antilymphocyte globulin
Cyclophosphamide	Plasma exchange

Fig. 6.2 Immunosuppressive agents and procedures. Types of immunosuppression typically used in patients who have IMD. It is common for several of these agents to be used in combination.

infections such as *Listeria*, herpesviruses and fungi, whereas patients who develop neutropenia as a consequence of cyclophosphamide, for instance, are susceptible to the same kinds of infections as neutropenic bone marrow transplant recipients. Plasma exchange is a form of immunosuppression used particularly in these patients, and this has its own complications.[9,10] It is generally true that the differential diagnosis of infection in patients who have IMD is considerably wider than in other kinds of immunosuppressed patients (see Clinical features and management).

It is not just the longer list of possible infections that makes assessment more difficult in these patients. It is frequently very hard to be sure whether the patient has infection or simply a relapse of the underlying disease. An acute flare-up of SLE involving the central nervous system can be indistinguishable from infective meningitis or encephalitis as a consequence of the immunosuppressive therapy. This leaves the clinician on the horns of an unpleasant dilemma; should the immunosuppression be reduced in order to allow antimicrobial therapy to be more effective, or should it be increased to bring the underlying disease back under control? It is helpful to ask whether the clinical features at this presentation are the same as on previous occasions when it was known to be disease activity. Individual patients tend to be consistent in the form of disease they get when it is active.

A further complication is the phenomenon of 'infection provoked relapse'; in patients who have IMD an intercurrent infection can precipitate a relapse of the underlying disease.[11] The infection and the vasculitis need to be treated simultaneously.

PREVENTION

Patients who have IMD, as with all immunosuppressed patients, are constantly at risk of a very wide range of infections but it is neither practicable nor desirable to try and prevent all of them. Some approaches that can be used and the possible indications are given in Figure 6.3. Tuberculosis is a particular problem because its presentation may be atypical and extrapulmonary disease is common. Patients who are receiving more than 15mg/day prednisolone for prolonged periods and who have a clinical history or radiologic evidence of past tuberculosis should be given prophylaxis with isoniazid 300mg/day plus pyridoxine 10mg/day. If the risk is less clear, the complications of isoniazid need to be considered (see Chapter 7.13), although my practice is to err on the side of advising prophylaxis. In my opinion, the routine use of trimethoprim–sulfamethoxazole to prevent *Pneumocystis carinii* pneumonia is not warranted in this population, even if they are receiving corticosteroids, because of the low incidence of the infection. In marked contrast to patients who have AIDS, relapse of pneumocystis pneumonia is most uncommon in this population and secondary prophylaxis is not indicated.

CLINICAL FEATURES AND MANAGEMENT

FEVER AND PULMONARY INFILTRATES

The development of fever and new pulmonary infiltrates is one of the most common and most difficult clinical syndromes that occurs in patients who have IMD. The differential diagnosis is extraordinarily wide (Fig. 6.4), and includes infective and noninfective conditions. Details of specific infections may be found elsewhere in this book; here I consider some general principles that apply to the initial assessment and management of patients who have IMD who develop fever and pneumonia.

- There may be very rapid deterioration, from low-grade fever and cough to severe hypoxia needing mechanical ventilation within 12 hours, particularly if the patient is liable to develop pulmonary hemorrhage.
- Radiologic appearances are very nonspecific. It is rare to be able to 'guess' the diagnosis just on the basis of the X-ray, with the possible exception of pneumocystis pneumonia.
- Multiple infections are common. Even if the physician correctly recognizes the clinical and radiologic features of pneumocystis pneumonia, the patient may be co-infected with an additional, equally treatable pathogen such as cytomegalovirus (CMV).
- Sputum microbiology can be confusing. The presence of *Candida* spp., for instance, may indicate nothing more than colonization of the nasopharynx, whereas important pathogens such as *Aspergillus* spp. or *Pneumocystis* spp. often do not appear in the sputum.

Consideration of the nature of the underlying disease and the immunosuppression and epidemiologic features in the history is helpful in guiding therapy. The single most important factor is gauging the speed of progression of the condition. It cannot be overemphasized that in IMD patients a seemingly trivial community acquired chest infection can proceed to life-threatening pneumonia and/or pulmonary hemorrhage within a frighteningly short period. Urgent evaluation and investigation is essential. All patients should have simple, basic laboratory investigations performed, including a full blood count, sputum and blood cultures, measurement of blood gas concentrations and a chest radiograph. Much has been written about the radiologic features of certain infections. It is perfectly true, for instance, that pneumocystis pneumonia classically

produces a bilateral 'ground glass' appearance, but so too does CMV infection and acute pulmonary hemorrhage in a patient who has pulmonary vasculitis. Combining the clinical and radiologic data results in a 'short list' of likely diagnoses, but too great a reliance on this is very hazardous. The main value of the chest X-ray is in indicating the extent and rate of progression of the process, not in guessing the pathogen.

Empiric antibacterial therapy is usually indicated when the risk of a major opportunistic pathogen is judged to be low. Factors pointing toward this conclusion are:

INFECTION PREVENTION		
Intervention		Indication
Immunizations	*Streptococcus pneumoniae* (Pneumovax)	Splenic dysfunction, or splenectomy
	Haemophilus influenzae (Hib vaccine)	
	Influenza	Any chronic lung disease in an immunosuppressed patient
Chemoprophylaxis	Oral quinolone antibiotics	Neutropenia*
	Fluconazole	
	Itraconazole	Previous confirmed invasive aspergillosis plus continued immunosuppression
	Isoniazid	Significant corticosteroid use

* The same considerations govern the use of prophylactic agents as in other types of neutropenic patients (see Chapter 4.5)

Fig. 6.3 Infection prevention. Some approaches to the prevention of infection in patients who have IMD.

CAUSES OF FEVER AND PULMONARY INFILTRATES		
Infective	Bacteria	Conventional respiratory pathogens* Mycobacteria *Nocardia*[12] 'Atypical' bacteria (*Mycoplasma* spp., *Coxiella* spp.) *Legionella* spp.
	Fungi	*Aspergillus* spp.[13]* *Candida* spp. Mucor Primary systemic fungi (*Histoplasma* spp., *Blastomyces* spp., etc.) Other systemic fungi (rarely) (e.g. *Sporothrix schenckii*) *Pneumocystis* spp.*
	Parasites	*Strongyloides stercoralis* *Toxoplasma* spp.
	Viruses	Cytomegalovirus* Herpes simplex Varicella-zoster Respiratory synctial virus Adenovirus
Noninfective		Edema* Hemorrhage[14]* Infarction Emboli Tumor Radiation Chemotherapy Vasculitis Leukoagglutinin reaction

* Most common causes

Fig. 6.4 Causes of fever and pulmonary infiltrates in patients who have IMD. The list is long but incomplete and, in practice, any organism isolated in pure or predominant culture from a bronchoalveolar lavage or open lung biopsy should be regarded as a pathogen until proved otherwise. Further details about some of the conditions are provided in the references, where indicated.

- slow onset/development,
- modest immunosuppression (e.g. <10mg prednisolone daily),
- absence of hypoxia and
- clinical, epidemiologic or microbiologic evidence of a conventional pathogen (e.g. *Streptococcus pneumoniae*).

Pneumocystis pneumonia is said to often have a very characteristic presentation, and some advocate empiric therapy (see Chapter 8.30). However, this strategy is unwise in patients who have IMD because of the wide differential diagnosis and the possibility of co-infection with other pathogens.

In the majority of patients further specific investigations should be performed. The most useful is a bronchoscopy with a bronchoalveolar lavage. Close liaison with the laboratory is essential to ensure a rapid response and the maximum diagnostic yield. Two other tests deserve mention. CT scans will undoubtedly give additional and sometimes useful information but in my experience are rarely diagnostic. In contrast, pulmonary function tests can be very valuable in this group of patients, in particular measurement of carbon monoxide uptake (the K_{CO}) to detect intrapulmonary hemorrhage.[15]

What if the patient fails to respond to the initial treatment regimen? Infection with more than one organism is not uncommon; for example, in two recent studies of pneumocystis pneumonia in non-AIDS patients, additional pathogens were found in 35 and 58% of cases.[16,17] A repeat diagnostic procedure should be considered; the choice usually lies between a second bronchoscopy or an open lung biopsy. There are no published studies that adequately address this question. Comparisons between diagnostic procedures have been made, usually in the setting of solid tumors or hematologic malignancy, but these are not readily extrapolated to second procedures in a different patient population. Although open lung biopsy is more invasive and has a significant morbidity, it should be carefully considered. In a patient who is not responding to first-line therapy, the second procedure will usually be the last chance to make a diagnosis.

When a specific organism is identified the treatment follows conventional guidelines. 'Blind' empiric therapy is rarely advisable because of the wide differential diagnosis.

ACUTE NEUROLOGIC PROBLEMS

A wide differential diagnosis also exists for neurologic problems, and prompt evaluation, investigation and treatment are essential.[18] Knowledge of the nature of the immune deficit can narrow down the list of possibilities. This information can be linked to the clinical presentation to provide useful clues; thus, a patient who has a defect in cellular immunity as a result of high-dose steroid therapy who develops a subacute meningitis is likely to have *Listeria*, cryptococcal or tuberculous meningitis, whereas in a neutropenic patient *Aspergillus* or a pyogenic bacterial infection are more common.[19] These mental exercises are intellectually challenging, but in reality the clinician is faced with a patient in whom even the 'short list' of likely causes all demand quite different treatment. Clearly, it is most important to make the diagnosis as quickly as possible.

The initial assessment should include a detailed clinical and epidemiologic history and a careful neurologic examination. Key areas are:

- exposure to family members or others as a potential source,
- relevant foreign travel (not forgetting malaria),
- previous episodes of neurologic manifestations associated with relapse of underlying disease and
- speed of progression of the disease.

Immediate investigations include a blood film and full blood count, blood and urine cultures and a chest X-ray. If there are new skin lesions they should be biopsied for immediate smear and culture. If a CT scan is available it is invaluable, and a lumbar puncture should be performed provided there are no contraindications.

Meningitis

Meningitis (Fig. 6.5) can be caused by common bacteria (*Streptococcus pneumoniae*, *Neisseria meningitidis*), but in immunosuppressed patients

Listeria monocytogenes is particularly important. Despite the name, the cerebrospinal fluid (CSF) usually contains neutrophils, not mononuclear cells. Polymicrobial meningitis (particularly with aerobic Gram-negative bacteria) can be a clue to the presence of hyperinfection with strongyloidiasis, a complication of corticosteroid therapy, and also infection with human T-cell leukemia/lymphoma virus type. Enteroviruses are common causes of meningitis in normal hosts; rather curiously, they also occur in patients who have hypogammaglobulinemia.[20] Tuberculosis, cryptococcosis (and much more rarely, *Nocardia*) all manifest with a subacute picture and are recognized causes of meningitis in patients who have IMD. The serum cryptococcal antigen test cannot be used as a surrogate for CSF examination, unlike in AIDS patients in whom the burden of infection is often very high. Meningitis is rarely caused by relapse of the underlying disease, but it can occasionally be caused by drugs used in its treatment, notably non-steroidal anti-inflammatory drugs (NSAIDs).[21]

Abscesses

In IMD patients, abscesses are usually nonbacterial (Fig. 6.5). The commonest causes of focal neurologic lesions are fungi (especially *Aspergillus* spp.) and toxoplasma. *Nocardia* spp. infections classically cause multiple focal abnormalities but occur less often. Tuberculoma and cryptococcoma are more common in textbooks than in patients. The diagnosis of single or multiple space-occupying lesions in IMD patients is particularly difficult. Neither the radiologic features nor the CSF findings are pathognomonic; it is rare for the causative organism to be identified from the CSF and, with the exception of the cryptococcal latex agglutination test, serologic tests are unhelpful. Particular care is needed in making a presumptive diagnosis of toxoplasmosis. Whereas in other groups of immunosuppressed patients the appearance of multiple enhancing lesions on the CT scan will often be sufficient grounds to commence empiric therapy, in patients who have IMD the differential diagnosis is much wider and if at all possible a tissue diagnosis should be obtained. Noninfective causes should not be forgotten. Cerebral vasculitis can certainly cause focal neurologic signs but here the CT appearances will be helpful in excluding mass lesions.

Encephalitis

Encephalitis can be caused by infective and noninfective processes (Fig. 6.5). Listeriosis and toxoplasmosis can manifest with an encephalitic picture, as can measles. Cerebral vasculitis (typically in SLE) is a particularly important consideration. It can cause a florid and life-threatening illness that can be extremely difficult to distinguish from an opportunist infection. Evaluation is complicated by the fact that high-dose corticosteroid therapy can itself cause neuropsychiatric manifestations. It is helpful if the patient is known to have past history of cerebral vasculitis, but sometimes the only course of action is to treat with immunosuppression and antimicrobial agents until the picture becomes clearer. Two infections merit comment because of their rarity:

NEUROLOGIC PROBLEMS IN IMMUNOSUPPRESSED PATIENTS		
Meningitis	**Abscesses**	**Encephalitis**
Common pyogenic bacteria	Toxoplasmosis	Toxoplasmosis
Mycobacterium tuberculosis	*Aspergillus* spp.	*Listeria* spp.
	Mucor spp.	Measles
Listeria monocytogenes	*Nocardia* spp.	Progressive multifocal leukoencephalopathy
Nocardia spp.	Tuberculoma	
Cryptococcus spp.	Cryptococcoma	Varicella-zoster virus
Candida spp.	Pyogenic bacteria and anaerobic bacteria	Herpes simpex virus
Echoviruses		Cytomegalovirus
Drugs (e.g. NSAIDs)	Cerebral lymphoma	Cerebral vasculitis
		Steroid-induced disease

Fig. 6.5 Causes of neurologic syndromes in patients who have IMD.

herpes simplex encephalitis seems to be uncommon, despite the fact that local cutaneous reactivation often occurs, and likewise CMV encephalitis is very unusual in this population.

GASTROINTESTINAL PROBLEMS

Although immunosuppressed patients are susceptible to a wide range of bacterial, fungal, viral and protozoal infections of the gut,[22] it is largely those that are a feature of high-dose corticosteroid therapy that occur in patients who have IMD. The clinical features of common infections are often modified: herpetic stomatitis can be very severe, for instance (Fig. 6.6). Three infections merit comment. Extrapulmonary tuberculosis is more common in immunosuppressed patients and even if suspected (e.g. because a patient comes from the Indian subcontinent) can sometimes be hard to prove. The use of polymerase chain reaction to detect mycobacterial DNA in ascitic fluid is just becoming available and will be invaluable; meanwhile peritoneal biopsy is often the only diagnostic procedure of use. Not infrequently the only option is empiric therapy. Cytomegalovirus enteritis is perhaps underdiagnosed. It can affect any part of the gut, but particularly the colon. Ganciclovir has been very effective.[23] *Strongyloides stercoralis* can be present for many years without causing symptoms, but after corticosteroid therapy can cause subacute

obstruction, pulmonary infiltrates and polymicrobial bacteremia or meningitis. Thiabendazole or mebendazole is effective, but it must be given in larger doses and for a longer period than in nonimmunosuppressed patients. Vasculitis (especially in SLE) can cause symptoms and signs indistinguishable from acute infection, including diarrhea, obstruction and perforation. Again, there are no diagnostic tests and management must depend on clinical evaluation and, if necessary, a therapeutic trial.

SKIN, SOFT TISSUE AND JOINTS

Many organisms cause skin disease in immunosuppressed patients and the clinical manifestations are protean (Figs 6.7 & 6.8).[24] In patients receiving plasma exchange, infections of the vascular access sites can be troublesome. Many noninfective causes of skin rash need to be remembered, including cutaneous vasculitis and drug eruptions. Soft tissue infections are unusual except that patients who have hypogammaglobulinemia are susceptible to enterovirus polymyositis,[25] although myositis is much more likely to be caused by the underlying disease (dermatomyositis, polymyositis or polyarteritis nodosa). Acute arthritis is always an indication for aspiration to exclude infection: *Staphylococcus aureus* is the most common isolate. Once again, relapse of the underlying disease is an important part of the differential diagnosis.

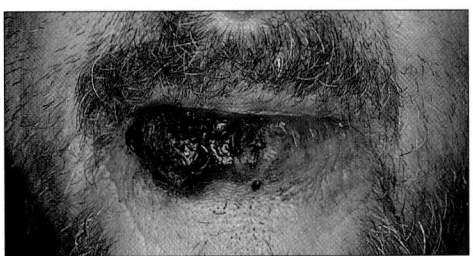

Fig. 6.6 A large necrotizing lesion caused by herpes simplex type-1 in a patient who has a teratoma. Herpetic stomatitis is common in immunosuppressed patients and is often atypical; any ulcerating lesion in the perioral region should be considered to be herpetic until proved otherwise.

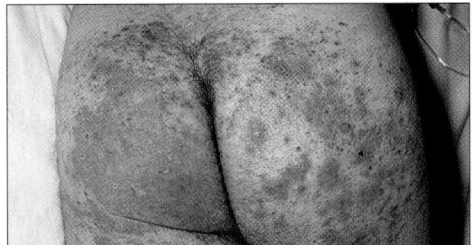

Fig. 6.7 Extensive dermatophyte infection in a bone marrow transplant recipient. Many other infections (and graft-versus-host disease) can give a similar appearance but the diagnosis is quickly established by biopsy and microscopy. This condition is limited to the skin but nevertheless requires systemic antifungal therapy.

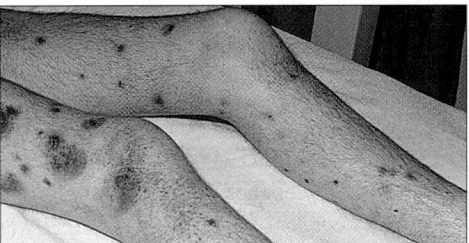

Fig. 6.8 Extensive skin lesions caused by *Mycobacterium cheloneae* in a patient who has polyarteritis nodosa. They were palpable but not especially painful.

REFERENCES

1. Payan DG. Evaluation and management of patients with collagen vascular disease. In: Rubin RH, Young LS, eds. Clinical approach to infection in the compromised host. New York: Plenum; 1994:581–600.
2. Cohen J, Pinching AJ, Rees AJ, et al. Infection and immunosuppression. A study of the infective complications of 75 patients with immunologically-mediated disease. Q J Med 1982;51:1–15.
3. Paton NI, Cheong IK, Kong NC, et al. Risk factors for infection in Malaysian patients with systemic lupus erythematosus. Q J Med 1996;89:531–8.
4. Pablos JL, Aragon A, Gomez-Reino JJ, et al. Salmonellosis and systemic lupus erythematosus. Report of ten cases. Br J Rheumatol 1994;33:129–32.
5. Guillevin L, Lhote F, Cohen P, et al. Polyarteritis nodosa related to hepatitis B virus. A prospective study with long-term observation of 41 patients. Medicine Baltimore 1995;74:238–53.
6. Somer T, Finegold SM. Vasculitides associated with infections, immunization, and antimicrobial drugs. Clin Infect Dis 1995;20:1010–36.
7. Stegeman CA, Tervaert JW, De Jong PE, et al. Trimethoprim–sulfamethoxazole (co-trimoxazole) for the prevention of relapses of Wegener's granulomatosis. N Engl J Med 1996;335:16–20.
8. Rees AJ, Lockwood CM. Immunosuppressive drugs in clinical practice. In: Lachmann PJ, Peters DK, Rosen FS, Walport MA. Clinical aspects of immunology. Cambridge, MA: Blackwell; 1993:929–72.

9. Singer DR, Roberts B, Cohen J. Infective complications of plasma exchange. A prospective study. Arthritis Rheum 1987;30:443–7.
10. Wing EJ, Bruns FJ, Fraley DS, et al. Infectious complications with plasmapheresis in rapidly progressive glomerulonephritis. JAMA 1980;244:2423–6.
11. Pinching AJ, Rees AJ, Pussell BA, et al. Relapses in Wegener's granulomatosis. the role of infection. Br Med J 1980;281:836–8.
12. Lerner PI. Nocardiosis. Clin Infect Dis 1996;22:891–905.
13. Verhaeghe W, Noppen M, Meysman M, et al. Invasive pulmonary aspergillosis. unusual diagnosis after corticosteroid treatment for obstructive pulmonary disease. Eur J Intern Med 1996;7:57–60.
14. Bowley NB, Hughes JM, Steiner RE. The chest X-ray in pulmonary capillary haemorrhage. correlation with carbon monoxide uptake. Clin Radiol 1979;30:413–7.
15. Ewan PW, Jones HA, Rhodes CG, et al. Detection of intrapulmonary hemorrhage with carbon monoxide uptake. Application in Goodpasture's syndrome. N Engl J Med 1976;295:1391–6.
16. Yalle SH, Limper AH. *Pneumocystis carinii* pneumonia in patients without acquired immunodeficiency syndrome: associated illnesses and prior corticosteroid therapy. Mayo Clin Proc 1996;71:5–13.
17. Arend SM, Kroon FP, van't Wout JW. *Pneumocystis carinii* pneumonia in patients without AIDS, 1980 through 1993. An analysis of 78 cases. Arch Intern Med 1995;155:2436–41.

18. Hooper DC, Pruitt AA, Rubin RH. Central nervous system infection in the chronically immunosuppressed. Medicine 1982;61:166–87.
19. Armstrong D, Wong B. Central nervous system infections in immunocompromised hosts. Ann Rev Med 1982;33:293–308.
20. Wilfert CM, Buckley RH, Mohanakumar T, et al. Persistent and fatal central-nervous-system ECHO virus infections in patients with agammaglobulinemia. N Engl J Med 1977;296:1485–9.
21. Hoppmann RA, Peden JG, Ober SK. Central nervous system side effects of nonsteroidal anti-inflammatory drugs. Aseptic meningitis, psychosis, and cognitive dysfunction. Arch Intern Med 1991;151:1309–13.
22. Boyd Jr WP, Bachman BA. Gastrointestinal infections in the compromised host. Med Clin N Am 1982;66:743–53.
23. Ross CN, Beynon HL, Savill JS, et al. Ganciclovir treatment for cytomegalovirus infection in immunocompromised patients with renal disease. Q J Med 1991;81:929–36.
24. Kaye ET, Johnson RA, Wolfson JS, et al. Dermatologic manifestations of infection in the compromised host. In: Rubin RH, Young LS, eds. Clinical approach to infection in the compromised host. New York: Plenum; 1994:105–15.
25. Crennan JM, Van Scoy RE, McKenna CH, et al. Echovirus polymyositis in patients with hypogammaglobulinemia. Failure of high-dose intravenous gammaglobulin therapy and review of the literature. Am J Med 1986;81:35–42.

Splenectomy and Splenic Dysfunction

Steven M Opal

The spleen in postnatal life functions primarily as a specialized lymphatic organ. It clears particulate elements from the circulation and promotes a co-ordinated immune response to systemic antigens. The rapidly progressive and highly lethal syndrome of overwhelming postsplenectomy infection (OPSI) attests the critical importance of the spleen to host defense against disseminated infections in the systemic circulation.

EPIDEMIOLOGY

The incidence of fatal postsplenectomy sepsis has been estimated at approximately 1 per 300 patient-years in children and 1 per 800 patient-years in adults.[1] Serious infectious complications may also occur in patients who have splenic hypofunction found in a broad array of systemic disorders (Fig. 7.1).[2–6] Functional asplenia is suggested by the presence of Howell–Jolly bodies (nuclear remnants within erythrocytes) and target cells in the peripheral blood smear, and a decreased uptake of radioactivity by spleen scan. The most common cause of functional asplenia is sickle-cell disease, which leads to repeated infarction of splenic tissue over the first few years of life. Infants born with congenital asplenia are at particularly high risk of death from systemic infection within the first 12 months of life.[7]

PATHOGENESIS AND PATHOLOGY

STRUCTURE–FUNCTION RELATIONSHIPS IN THE SPLEEN

The spleen is organized to provide an optimal environment for particulate antigen clearance and immunologic surveillance within the systemic circulation. Although the spleen is a small structure that accounts for only 0.25% of body weight, it receives 5% of cardiac output and contains up to 25% of the total lymphocyte population within the body.[8] Blood enters the spleen through central arteries, which branch into penicilary arterioles (Fig. 7.2). These vessels are cuffed with T lymphocytes, forming a periarterial lymphocytic sheath. The white pulp of the spleen surrounds arterioles and consists of large populations of T lymphocytes with lesser numbers of B lymphocytes

and natural killer cells. The marginal zone surrounds the white pulp and principally consists of large concentrations of B lymphocytes with lesser numbers of T lymphocytes and antigen-presenting cells. Memory cells of the B-lymphocyte lineage are found primarily within the marginal zones of the spleen. The white pulp and marginal zone bring antigen-presenting cells, particulate antigens, T lymphocytes and B lymphocytes in close proximity. This microenvironment promotes a co-ordinated immune response to systemic antigens.[1–9]

The majority of the spleen consists of red pulp and venous sinuses. Before formed elements within the blood can reach the venous sinuses of the spleen, they must negotiate the red pulp with its tightly compact network of endothelial cells and macrophages (the cords of Billroth). This slow filtration process allows for careful immunologic surveillance and removal of damaged cellular elements and foreign particulate matter.

IMMUNOLOGIC DEFECTS AND FACTORS PREDISPOSING FOR POSTSPLENECTOMY SEPSIS

A number of immunologic defects have been described in the postsplenectomy state (Fig. 7.3).[1,9–11] The principal immunologic defect associated with the postsplenectomy state is an impairment in clearance of poorly opsonized particulate antigens.[12] Invasive, encapsulated bacteria possess an outer surface polysaccharide capsule that impedes opsonization by immunoglobulin or complement upon entry to the systemic circulation. The spleen is much more efficient than the liver in removing poorly opsonized bacterial pathogens. After splenectomy, decreased clearance of these encapsulated organisms results in disseminated intravascular infection and the OPSI syndrome.

Multiple host factors determine the cumulative risk of OPSI. A number of the most important host determinants of infection after surgical or functional asplenia are listed in Figure 7.4. The principal determinant of risk of postsplenectomy sepsis is the age and immunologic experience of the patient before splenectomy.[12,13] In a recent

CONDITIONS ASSOCIATED WITH FUNCTIONAL ASPLENIA	
Atrophic spleen	Normal-sized or enlarged spleen
Ulcerative colitis	Other hemoglobinopathies
Celiac disease	Sarcoidosis
Graft-versus-host disease after bone marrow transplantation	Amyloidosis
Splenic irradiation	Systemic lupus erythematosus, rheumatoid arthritis
Thyrotoxicosis	Epstein–Barr virus infection
Dermatitis herpetiformis	Vasculitis with antineutrophil cytoplasmic antibodies
Idiopathic thrombocytopenia	Liver disease – portal hypertension
Sickle-cell disease	AIDS, immunosuppressive agents

Fig. 7.1 Conditions associated with functional asplenia.

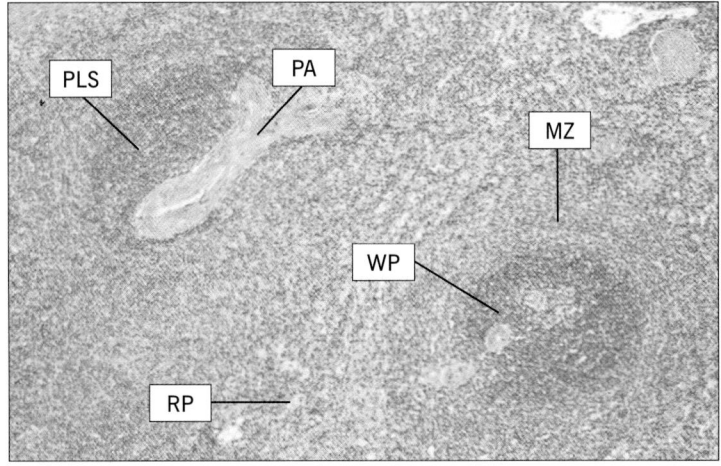

Fig. 7.2 Normal splenic architecture in the adult human. PLS, periarterial lymphatic sheath; PA, penicillary arteriole; MZ, marginal zone (B lymphocytes predominate); WP, white pulp (T lymphocytes predominate); RP, red pulp (vascular cords and venous sinuses). H & E stain.

review of over 12,000 patients who had undergone splenectomy, the incidence of serious postsplenectomy infections was found to be 15.7% in infants, 10.7% in children under the age of 5 years, 4.0% in children under 16 years and 0.9% in adults.[11]

The spleen is particularly important in the primary immunologic response to polysaccharide antigens. This is a largely T-cell-independent B-cell response that requires the spleen for an optimal immune response and occurs in the marginal zone of the spleen where B cells are abundant for immunologic surveillance in the systemic circulation. This immune response is attenuated after splenectomy. T-cell-dependent B-cell responses to protein antigens and cellular immune responses are reasonably well preserved after splenectomy.[14–16] Consequently, carbohydrate neoantigens are not recognized and processed efficiently in the postsplenectomy state. This results in delayed clearance of pathogens as they first enter the systemic circulation.

If the growth rate of the pathogen exceeds the clearance rate of the host, overwhelming intravascular infection occurs with potentially lethal consequences. In experimental studies, macrophage synthesis of tumor necrosis factor (TNF)-α is upregulated after splenectomy. Enhanced TNF synthesis may increase the risk of systemic activation of the proinflammatory cytokines, thus contributing to postsplenectomy sepsis.[17] Patients who have HIV infection tolerate splenectomy reasonably well;[18] nonetheless, severe pneumococcal infections have occurred in splenectomized HIV-positive patients.

PREVENTION OF BABESIOSIS

Individuals living in areas where babesia is endemic should be advised to avoid areas where ticks are common or, if unavoidable, to check daily for the presence of ticks in endemic areas. If the tick is removed within 24 hours it appears to protect against transmission of *Babesia* spp. Babesiosis can be morbidly persistent in splenectomized adults as well as children and in some cases has required exchange transfusion as well as treatment with clindamycin and quinine. This infection needs to be prevented in splenectomized people. Chills, fever, anemia, leukopenia and thrombocytopenia can all accompany babesiosis. The diagnosis is usually evident if suspected and sought for on the blood smear. Babesiosis can be confused with *Plasmodium falciparum* malaria.

PREVENTION

SPLENIC SALVAGE METHOD

The well recognized risk of OPSI indicates a need to prevent these infections if at all possible. The most direct approach is to minimize the frequency with which splenectomy is performed.[19] Elective splenectomy for congenital hemolytic disorders should be delayed until after the first 5 years of life if possible (Fig. 7.5). Surgical repair of splenic hematomas, conservative management of splenic trauma without splenectomy, percutaneous drainage of splenic abscesses and a decreased use of splenic irradiation have led to fewer patients at risk of postsplenectomy infectious syndromes.[20,21]

Partial splenectomy and surgical repair of splenic injury have been utilized along with autotransplantation of splenic tissue in an attempt to limit the risk of OPSI.[22,23] Enthusiasm for these splenic salvage maneuvers is tempered by the finding that these methods do not uniformly protect against sepsis in animal models of splenectomy,[24] and case reports exist of overwhelming infections despite these maneuvers.[25] Preservation of residual splenic tissue, if possible, may be preferable to total splenectomy in selected patients. One comparative study found two episodes in 18 children with splenectomy and no episodes in 16 children who had undergone partial splenectomy.[26] The overall clinical applicability and practical value of splenic salvage techniques remain to be demonstrated in a large patient series.

IMMUNIZATIONS TO PREVENT POSTSPLENECTOMY SEPSIS

Immunization with the pneumococcal vaccine is safe and offers significant protection in children with sickle-cell disease.[27] The efficacy of the pneumococcal vaccine is also suggested in other patient groups after splenectomy.[9,16,28,29] To optimize antibody response against T-cell-independent immunogens, it is recommended that the pneumococcal

IMMUNOLOGIC DEFECTS AFTER SPLENECTOMY

Defects	Comments
Decreased clearance of particulate antigens	Hepatic Kupffer cells will partially correct this defect
Diminished clearance of poorly opsonized bacterial antigens	The spleen is the most efficient organ for this purpose
Diminished primary humoral immune response to neoantigens	IgM levels and T-cell-independent antibody responses decrease
Diminished antibody response to polysaccharide antigens	Increased risk of infections with encapsulated bacteria
Decreased tuftsin and fibronectin levels	Diminished levels of this tetrapeptide and serum protein reduce nonspecific attachment and phagocytosis
Quantitative and qualitative defects in the alternative complement pathway	Functional defects in the alternative complement pathway interfere with opsonization

Fig 7.3 Immunologic defects after splenectomy.

RISK FACTORS FOR POSTSPLENECTOMY SEPSIS

Risk factors	Comments
Patient age	Immunologic experience (vaccines and naturally acquired infections) before splenectomy decreases subsequent risk
Absence of spleen at birth	Congenital asplenia results in serious bacterial infections in over 50% of patients in the first year of life
Time interval after splenectomy	Greatest risk of infection is within the first few years after splenectomy
Traumatic versus other indications for splenectomy	Splenosis (splenic implants within the peritoneum) after trauma offers some protection against infection
Immunocompromised states	Patients with hematologic malignancies and continuing need for immunosuppressive medications are at increased risk of postsplenectomy sepsis

Fig 7.4 Risk factors for postsplenectomy sepsis.

MEASURES TO PREVENT POSTSPLENECTOMY INFECTION

Method	Comments
Salvage splenic tissue (splenorrhaphy, autotransplants)	Reasonable but unproved benefit
Delay elective splenectomy past childhood	Greatest risk of OPSI is in childhood, provide immunizations before splenectomy
Immunizations	Pneumococcal, meningococcal and *Haemophilus influenzae* vaccines provide partial protection before splenectomy when possible
Antimicrobial prophylaxis	Indicated in childhood and immunocompromised, efficacy in adults uncertain
Early empiric therapy	Unproved yet rational approach to rapidly progressive disease
Medical alert bracelet	Reminder for patient and health care workers

Fig 7.5 Measures to prevent postsplenectomy infection.

vaccine be administered at least 2 weeks before an elective splenectomy.[12] Nonetheless, adequate antibody responses have been measured after splenectomy in nonimmunocompromised patients.[14] Current recommendations of the Adult Immunization Practices Task Force include repeat pneumococcal immunization every 6 years from the initial immunization.[30] The role of experimental polysaccharide–protein conjugate pneumococcal vaccine awaits further clinical trials in the asplenic population.[5]

Haemophilus influenzae type b conjugate vaccine is indicated in all children, including those who have functional or surgical asplenia.[30] It is unclear whether the *H. influenzae* type b vaccine is useful in adults who have not been vaccinated before splenectomy. The risk–benefit ratio would argue in favor of immunizing children and adults who have undergone splenectomy if they have not been previously immunized.[31] The same rationale is used to recommend meningococcal vaccine in children and young adults who undergo splenectomy.[13,14,31,32] The duration of protection and vaccine efficacy against *H. influenzae* type b and meningococci in the asplenic patient is speculative. Vaccination is limited by variable antibody responses of uncertain duration and incomplete coverage of important serogroups within *Streptococcus pneumoniae* and *Neisseria meningitidis* (i.e. serogroup B). Vaccine failures are well known in splenectomized patients and therefore additional preventative measures are needed.

ANTIBIOTIC PROPHYLAXIS

The efficacy of long-term penicillin prophylaxis to prevent pneumococcal infection has been studied in children. Sufficient clinical evidence now exists to support the recommendation for penicillin prophylaxis in the first 5 years of life in asplenic children.[33,34] Some authors suggest that prophylaxis be continued indefinitely in immunocompromised patients.[3,12,16,31] Amoxicillin may be preferable to penicillin V in that it is better tolerated and has activity against most strains of *H. influenzae*.[31]

The value of penicillin prophylaxis in adults is more controversial. The uncertain benefits of penicillin prophylaxis in the adult must be weighed against the potential risk of acquisition of penicillin-resistant strains of *S. pneumoniae* and infections by other organisms not susceptible to penicillin.[1,9,12,14] Some authorities recommend penicillin prophylaxis for 2 years after splenectomy in adult patients at high

risk of OPSI (hematologic malignancies, severe liver disease, immunocompromised states) other recommend prophylaxis indefinitely. Expectant early empiric therapy for symptoms suggestive of OPSI is recommended for nonimmunocompromised, asplenic adults.

An alternative strategy to continuous prophylaxis is to educate the patient to administer an initial dose of oral amoxicillin at the onset of symptoms compatible with systemic infection. Ideally, patients should have blood cultures taken before empiric antimicrobial therapy; however, this may not be feasible in all patients and treatment should not be delayed if symptoms compatible with OPSI exist.

A medical alert bracelet should be provided to patients after splenectomy. This bracelet serves to remind the patient as well as health care workers that the patient is at risk of OPSI and that urgent management for this potentially devastating syndrome may be life saving. Patients have developed severe infections up to 4 decades after splenectomy.[9] The alert bracelet should provide continued awareness of the risk of infection long after surgical removal of the spleen.

CLINICAL FEATURES OF OPSI

A large variety of bacterial, fungal, parasitic and viral pathogens have been reported to cause serious infection in patient who have splenic hypofunction or asplenia (Fig. 7.6).[1,3,9,13,35] *Streptococcus pneumoniae* continues to account for the majority of bacterial infection associated with OPSI. *Haemophilus influenzae* and *N. meningitidis* contribute approximately 25% of bacterial infections in the postsplenectomy state.

The syndrome of overwhelming pneumococcal sepsis after splenectomy is one of the most dramatic and rapidly fatal infections in clinical medicine. Symptoms often begin with a vague sense of general malaise, sore throat, myalgia and gastrointestinal symptoms. Fever and true shaking chills are often seen during the prodromal phase of OPSI. Although some patients note lower respiratory tract symptoms or symptoms of meningitis, the primary source of the bacteremic infection is not localized in the majority of patients.

Within 24–48 hours of onset of symptoms patients rapidly deteriorate with progressive hypotension, diffuse intravascular coagulation, purpuric lesions in the extremities, acute respiratory insufficiency, metabolic acidosis and coma. The rapidly progressive nature of the illness is suggestive of primary meningococcemia. The patient may develop refractory hypotension and die within hours of the onset of symptoms.[1,10,12] Long-term sequelae in survivors include gangrene of the extremities, bilateral adrenal hemorrhage, osteomyelitis from vascular insufficiency, endocarditis, meningitis and neurosensory hearing loss.[9] The polysaccharide capsular serotypes 12, 22 and 23 account for the majority of cases of OPSI from *S. pneumoniae*.[12] All three serotypes are found in the current 23 valent pneumococcal polysaccharide vaccine.[30]

DIAGNOSIS OF OPSI

The diagnosis of OPSI is often readily apparent upon clinical examination. It is important to remember that even a remote history of previous splenectomy should raise suspicion of possible OPSI. Supporting laboratory findings are compatible with a consumptive coagulopathy, lactic acidosis, hypoxemia and acute renal failure. Children are more likely to have concomitant bacterial pneumonia or meningitis than adults.[1,9] As a consequence of high-grade bacteremia, micro-organisms can often be identified in the peripheral blood smear (Fig. 7.7). The blood smear should be reviewed for evidence of parasitemia from *Plasmodium* or *Babesia* spp. A Gram stain of the buffy coat may readily reveal organisms as the level of bacteremia may exceed 1 million cfu/ml.

Patients who have concomitant bacterial meningitis may have large numbers of organisms in the cerebrospinal fluid (CSF) with minimal pleocytosis (Fig. 7.8). Blood cultures, bacterial cultures and results of antigen detection measures in the spinal fluid, sputum and urine will confirm the diagnosis.

MICRO-ORGANISMS ASSOCIATED WITH SYSTEMIC POSTSPLENECTOMY INFECTION	
Micro-organisms	Comments
Streptococcus pneumoniae	Most common, highly lethal, characteristic presentation
Haemophilus influenzae	Increased risk, especially in childhood
Neisseria meningitidis	Possibly increased risk, typical features of primary meningococcemia
Salmonella spp.	Increased risk, especially sickle-cell disease
Other streptococci, enterococci	Possibly increased risk of infection
Capnocytophaga canimorsus	Gram-negative rod may cause infection after dog bites
Babesia microti	Tick-associated or blood transfusion-associated protozoa may cause severe infection in asplenic patients
Plasmodium spp.	Sporadic reports of activation of latent malaria and fulminant course in non-falciparum malaria
Anaerobic bacteria, Gram-negative bacteria, *Pseudomonas* spp., fungi, protozoa and viruses	Case reports, true association is unclear

Fig 7.6 Micro-organisms associated with systemic postsplenectomy infection.

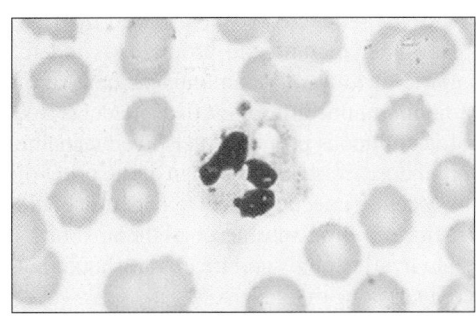

Fig. 7.7 Peripheral blood smear of an asplenic patient who has pneumococcal sepsis and meningitis. Note polymorphonuclear leukocyte with several bacterial diplococci in the cytoplasm (Wright stain).

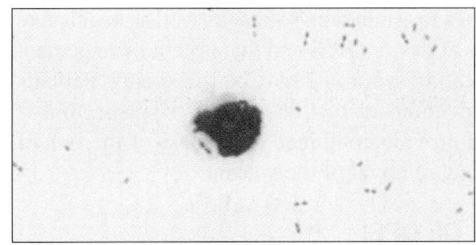

Fig. 7.8 Gram stain of CSF of an asplenic patient who has pneumococcal meningitis. Note numerous Gram-positive cocci in pairs and a single lymphocyte.

MANAGEMENT OF OPSI

This disease is a true medical emergency requiring immediate administration of antimicrobial agents and intensive care support.

High-dose intravenous benzylpenicillin has been the standard treatment for postsplenectomy pneumococcal sepsis. Vancomycin and ceftriaxone should be used in areas in which penicillin-resistant *S. pneumoniae* is prevalent. Moreover, broad-spectrum bactericidal antibiotics such as an extended spectrum cephalosporin or a carbapenem should be used along with an aminoglycoside when the suspected micro-organism cannot be identified on Gram strain of the buffy coat or CSF.

Passive immunotherapy with intravenous immunoglobulin is of benefit in experimental models of postsplenectomy sepsis.[36] The therapeutic efficacy of passive immunotherapy in human OPSI is worthy of further clinical investigation. Fluid resuscitation, vasopressor agents, fresh-frozen plasma, ventilatory support and expert acid–base and electrolyte management are essential to survival in these critically ill patients (see Chapter 2.47).

The mortality rate for OPSI caused by *S. pneumoniae* has been reported to be between 50 and 70%.[1,2,9–12] With early recognition and treatment combined with skilled supportive care the mortality rate has decreased to as low as 10% in recent series.[16,37]

During the convalescent period, it may be necessary to excise necrotic tissues that have been irreparably damaged by the prolonged hypotension and intravascular coagulation that often accompanies this syndrome. Late complications such as adrenal insufficiency, osteomyelitis and endocarditis should be sought in patient who have persistent fever after an episode of OPSI. Patient education, vaccination and a medical alert bracelet should be offered to survivors to prevent recurrences.

REFERENCES

1. Stryrt B. Infection associated with asplenia: risks, mechanisms, and prevention. Am J Med 1990;88:35–42.
2. Eichner ER. Splenic function: normal, too much and too little. Am J Med 1979;66:311–9.
3. Zarrabi MH, Rosner F. Serious infections in adults following splenectomy for trauma. Arch Intern Med 1984;144:1421–4.
4. Sunder-Plassman G, Geissler K, Penner E. Functional asplenia and vasculitis associated with antineutrophil cytoplasmic antibodies. N Engl J Med 1992;327:437–8.
5. Loite F, Engle J, Gilmore N, Osterland CK. Asplenism and systemic lupus erythematosus. Clin Rheumatol 1995;14:220–3.
6. Kalhs P, Panzer S, Kletter K, et al. Functional asplenia after bone marrow transplantation, a late complication related to extensive chronic graft-versus-host disease. Ann Intern Med 1989;109:461–4.
7. Phoon CK, Neill CA. Asplenia syndrome – risk factors for early unfavorable outcome. Am J Cardiol 1994;673:1235–7.
8. Brown AR. Immunological functions of splenic B-lymphocytes. Crit Rev Immunol 1992;11:395–403.
9. Brigden ML. Overwhelming post-splenectomy infection: still a problem. West J Med 1992;157:440–3.
10. Cullingford GL, Watkins DN, Watts AD, Mallon DF. Severe late post-splenectomy infection. Br J Surg 1991;78:716–21.
11. Holdsworth RJ, Irving AD, Cuschieri A. Post-splenectomy sepsis and its mortality rate: actual versus perceived risks. Br J Surg 1991;78:1031–8.
12. Hosea SW, Brown EJ, Hamburger MI, Frank MM. Opsonic requirements for intravascular clearance after splenectomy. N Engl J Med 1981;304:245–50.
13. Loggie BW, Hinchey EJ. Does splenectomy predispose to meningococcal sepsis? An experimental study and clinical review. J Pediatr Surg 1989;21:326–30.
14. Siber GP, Gorham C, Martin P, et al. Antibody response to pretreatment immunization and post-treatment boosting with bacterial polysaccharide vaccines in patients with Hodgkin's disease. Ann Intern Med 1986;104:467–75.
15. Cohn DA, Schiffman G. Immunoregulatory role of the spleen in antibody responses to pneumococcal polysaccharide antigens. Infect Immunol 1987;55:1375–80.
16. Jockhovich M, Mendenhall NP, Sonbeck MD, et al. Long-term complications of laparotomy in Hodgkin's disease. Ann Surg 1994;219:615–21.
17. McCarthy JE, Redmon PH, Duggan SM, et al. Characterization of the defects in murine peritoneal macrophage function in the early post-splenectomy period. J Immunol 1995;155:387–96.
18. Genet P, Lionnet F, Pulik M, et al. Severe pneumococcal infections in splenectomized HIV-positive individuals. AIDS 1994;8:850–1.
19. Carroll A, Thomas P. Decision-making in surgery: splenectomy. Br J Hosp Med 1995;54:147–9.
20. Lucas CE. Splenic trauma. Choice of management. Ann Surg 1991;213:98–112.
21. Vallalba MR, Howells GA, Lucas RJ, et al. Nonoperative management of the adult ruptured spleen. Arch Surg 1990;125:836–9.
22. Timens W, Leemans R. Splenic autotransplantation and the immune system. Adequate tesing required for evaluation of effect. Ann Surg 1992;215:256–60.
23. Alvarez SR, Fernandez-Excalante C, Rituerto C, et al. Assessment of post-splenectomy residual splenic function – splenic autotransplants. Int Surg 1987;72:149–53.
24. Horton J, Ogden MF, William S, Coln D. The importance of splenic blood flow in clearing pneumococcal organisms. Ann Surg 1982;195:172–6.
25. Moore GE, Stevens RE, Moore EE, Aragon GE. Failure of splenic implants to protect against fatal pneumococcal infection. Am J Surg 1983;146:413–4.
26. Greene JB, Shackford SR, Sise MJ, Powell RW. Post-splenectomy sepsis in pediatric patients for trauma: a proposal for a multi-institutional study. J Pediatr Surg 1986:19:269–72.
27. Ammann AJ, Adiego J, Wara DW, et al. Polyvalent pneumococcal-polysaccharide immunization of patients with sickle-cell anemia in patients with splenectomy. N Engl J Med 1977;297:897–900.
28. Rutherford EJ, Livengood J, Higginbotham M, et al. Efficacy and safety of pneumococcal revaccination after splenectomy for trauma. J Trauma 1995;39:448–52.
29. Chahopadhyay B. Splenectomy, pneumococcal vaccination and antibiotic prophylaxis. Br J Hosp Med 1989;41:172–4.
30. Task force on adult immunization and infectious diseases society of America. American College of Physicians Guide for Adult Immunization/ACP, 3rd ed. Philadelphia, PA: American College of Physicians; 1994.
31. Waghorn DJ. Prevention of postsplenectomy sepsis. Lancet 1993;341:248–9.
32. Ruben FL, Hankins WA, Zeigler Z, et al. Antibody responses to meningococcal polysaccharide vaccine in adults without a spleen. N Engl J Med 1984;76:115–21.
33. Buchanan GR, Smith SJ. Pneumococcal septicemia despite pneumococcal vaccine and prescription of penicillin prophylaxis in children with sickle cell anemia. Am J Dis Child 1986;140:428–32.
34. Gaston MH, Verter JI, Woods G, et al. Prophylaxis with oral penicillin in children with sickle cell anemia. N Engl J Med 1986;314:1593–5.
35. Fish HR, Gschia JK, Shakir KM. Post-splenectomy sepsis caused by Group A streptococcus in an adult diabetes millitus. Diabetes Care 1985;8:608–9.
36. Camel JE, Kim KS, Tchejeyan GH, Mahour GH. Efficacy of passive immunotherapy in experimental post-splenectomy sepsis due to *Haemophilus influenzae* type B. J Pediatr Surg 1993;28:1441–4.
37. Green JB, Shackford SR, Sise MJ, Fridlund P. Late septic complications in adults following splenectomy for trauma: a prospective analysis in 144 patients. J Trauma 1986;26:999–1004.

Special Populations

Jos WM van der Meer & Bart-Jan Kullberg

In daily practice, many patients are encountered with impaired host defense mechanisms as a consequence of age, nutrition, lifestyle, disease or medication. The defects in host defense may range between subtle and severe. The types of infection in such patients may indicate the nature of the specific host defense mechanism affected and, conversely, knowing the host defense defect one may be able to predict the type of infection. The host defense system with its defects and consequent infections are listed in Figure 8.1.

The integument comprises the skin, respiratory tract, alimentary tract, and the genitourinary tract, and provides the first line of defense against microbial invasion. The intact skin and mucosa are capable of resisting colonization with exogenous microflora (Fig. 8.1), and a variety of mechanisms co-operates to clear invading organisms, including desquamation, ciliary motion, ventilation, coughing and frequent voiding. Unless the continuous layer of the skin and mucosal surfaces is damaged, the first line of defense forms an extremely important barrier against invading micro-organisms. The second line of defense is made up of humoral and cellular defense mechanisms (Fig. 8.1) that act in close co-operation. Thus, the division between humoral and cellular defense mechanisms is a somewhat artificial approach.

This chapter describes a variety of conditions in which host defense is impaired in specific populations. The relevant host defense defects are summarized schematically in Figure 8.2.

PATHOGENESIS AND PATHOLOGY

NEONATES

The neonatal period is the part of life during which a healthy individual is most susceptible to infection. The causative agents of neonatal infection are markedly different from those in other age groups. Approximately 60–70% of infections are caused by *E. coli*, group B streptococci, or *Listeria monocytogenes*. The bacteria are usually acquired from the mother during the intrapartum period. Neonatal sepsis is one of the most prevalent manifestations in this patient group. The infection may spread to the meninges in a substantial proportion of patients. The vulnerable state of the neonate is multifactorial: the umbilicus is an important portal of entry for micro-organisms; the barrier between the bloodstream and the meninges is still imperfect, and most host defense mechanisms are still immature. The neonate has no resident flora providing 'colonization resistance' against pathogens newly encountered on the skin or in the gut.

Many effector systems of host defense mechanisms function suboptimally during the neonatal period.[1] Humoral defense mechanisms have been thoroughly studied; complement factors, especially those of the alternative pathway, are present in low concentrations.[2] During the neonatal period, the alternative pathway of complement may be particularly important, as antibodies are not yet available. As a consequence, opsonization for phagocytosis of micro-organisms such as *Escherichia coli* is poor.[3] Initially, IgM and IgA are absent, and the antibody response to the so-called T-lymphocyte-independent polysaccharide antigens, such as the capsular polysaccharides of

HOST DEFENSE DEFECT AND CAUSE OF INFECTION		
Defect	**Infectious agent**	
Damaged skin or mucosa	Colonizing (endogenous) microflora Exogenous microflora	
Humoral defects Complement deficiency Early factors C6–C9	*Haemophilus influenzae* *Streptococcus pneumoniae* *Staphylococcus aureus* *Neisseria meningitidis* *Neisseria gonorrhoeae*	
Immunoglobulin deficiency	*Haemophilus influenzae* *Streptococcus pneumoniae* *Campylobacter jejuni* *Salmonella* spp.	*Mycoplasma hominis* *Ureaplasma* spp. Enterovirus *Giardia lamblia*
Phagocyte defects	Gram-positive cocci Aerobic Gram-negative rods Fungi	Herpes simplex virus Epstein–Barr virus Human herpes virus type 6
Defective cellular immunity	Varicella-zoster virus Cytomegalovirus *Chlamydia trachomatis* *Listeria monocytogenes* *Salmonella* spp. *Legionella* spp. *Mycobacterium* spp. *Nocardia* spp. *Cryptococcus neoformans* *Pneumocystis carinii* *Toxoplasma gondii* *Leishmania* spp.	*Strongyloides stercoralis* Measles *C. pneumoniae* *Histoplasma capsulatum* *Coccidioides immitis* *Rhodococcus equi* *Cryptosporidia* spp. *Microsporidia* spp. *Cyclosporidia cayetanensis*

Fig. 8.1 Host defense defect and cause of infection.

Streptococcus pneumoniae and *Haemophilus influenzae*, is weak. The production of cytokines, especially interferon (IFN)-γ, is also substantially impaired.[4]

Although the numbers of neutrophils in the circulation are high in the neonate, bone marrow production of neutrophils may be insufficient, especially in cases of infection.[1] The chemotactic activity of granulocytes and monocytes in neonates is low.[5,6] Phagocytic function of granulocytes and monocytes is generally normal, although it has been reported that phagocytosis of group B streptococci by monocytes is impaired.[3] Although difference of opinion exists on the microbicidal function of phagocytic cells in the newborn, monocytes particularly seem to be defective in the killing of Gram-positive micro-organisms such as staphylococci and streptococci.[7]

CLINICALLY RELEVANT HOST DEFENSE DEFECTS IN SPECIFIC POPULATIONS									
	Surface and mucosal barriers	Complement	Antibodies	B lymphocytes	Polymorpho-nuclear neutrophils	Macrophages	Cytokines	T lymphocytes	Natural killer cells
Neonates	●	●	●	●	●	●	●		
The elderly	●		●	●	●		●	●	
Malnutrition	●	●			●		●	●	●
Alcoholism	●	●	●	●	●	●		●	●
Cirrhosis		●						●	
Drug abuse	●				●	●		●	
Diabetes	●	●			●	●			
Renal failure					●	●		●	
Hemodialysis	●	●	●	●					
Chronic ambulatory peritoneal dialysis	●	●	●						
Corticosteroids	●				●	●	●	●	

Fig. 8.2 Clinically relevant host defense defects in specific populations. The icons represent the relevant host defense defects in each of the specified populations.

Antigen presentation by monocytes is abnormal in the neonate, and the same is true for the function of natural killer cells.[8,9] The benefit of human breast milk for the host defense should be stressed. Human breast milk provides not only immunoglobulins, in particular IgA, but also cytokines and growth factors, which may accelerate the development of the neonate's mucosal barrier. Moreover, Gram-positive lactobacilli and the iron-sequestering lactoferrin provided by breastfeeding may encourage the development of a protective intestinal flora.[10]

THE ELDERLY

The proportion of the population that is elderly continues to rise. In the 1990s, it is estimated that patients over age the of 65 years use one-third of the acute care hospital beds and 90% of all long-term care facilities in developed countries. It is estimated that after the turn of the century, at least 50% of the costs of health care will be spent on the elderly.

In nursing homes, infection is a significant cause of morbidity and mortality. Prevalence rates range from 2 to 18%. Urinary tract infection and lower respiratory tract infection are the most frequent types of infection encountered. In hospitalized patients, the rate of nosocomial infection increases markedly in patients older than 50 years, reaching a peak in those aged over 70 years (Fig. 8.3). Although underlying diseases strongly influence the risk of nosocomial infections, several studies have identified an age greater than 60 or 70 years as an independent risk factor for acquiring a nosocomial infection.[11]

The increasing prevalence of urinary tract infections in the elderly is well established. The rate is about 1% in randomly selected ambulatory young women and rises to about 20% at the age of 70 years. Urinary tract infections are rarely seen in men under the age of 50 years and occur in about 4% of men aged 70 years. Among nursing home residents and hospitalized patients, the incidence of bacteriuria is significantly higher than among age-matched ambulatory persons. Although a small group of elderly patients who have persistent bacteriuria exists, about 95% of individuals have intermittent or transient bacteriuria that responds well to antimicrobial therapy.

Older people are also at significant risk of lower respiratory tract infection. In the early 1990s, pneumonia and influenza constituted the fifth largest cause of death in the USA. Although few studies have addressed the age-related incidence of pneumonia in nonhospitalized patients, it has been well established that the incidence increases with age. Moreover, age has been shown to be an independent risk factor for a complicated course of pneumonia, requiring hospital admission (Fig. 8.3).

For bacteremia among hospitalized patients, the incidence is limited during the first 5 decades of life, but steadily increases thereafter. In a Dutch study, the mortality rate from bacteremia was 27% in patients over 40 years of age compared with 12% among the younger group. Likewise, both the incidence and attributable mortality of bacterial endocarditis have been shown to increase significantly with increasing age.[12]

The question that regularly arises in relation to the increased frequency of infection in the elderly is that of causation. It is tempting to assume that specific host defense mechanisms become less effective, but it is also reasonable to assume that infections in the elderly are facilitated by functional and anatomic defects, underlying disease and drug use, which are inevitably linked to aging. Although few data exist on the relative contributions of these divergent factors to the increased incidence to infection in the elderly, the effects of aging on host defense mechanisms is discussed in this chapter.

The major infections in the aged are most probably a consequence of the decline in the quality of the first line of defense. Atrophy and dryness of skin and mucous membranes, together with impairment of repair processes, increase the chance of invasion by pathogens. Impaired ciliary movement, decreased cough, microaspiration and immobilization may affect the incidence of respiratory infection. Gastric atrophy and impaired gut motility may lead to gastrointestinal infection, whereas reduced fluid intake, decreased voiding frequency and anatomic changes affect the defense against urinary tract infections.

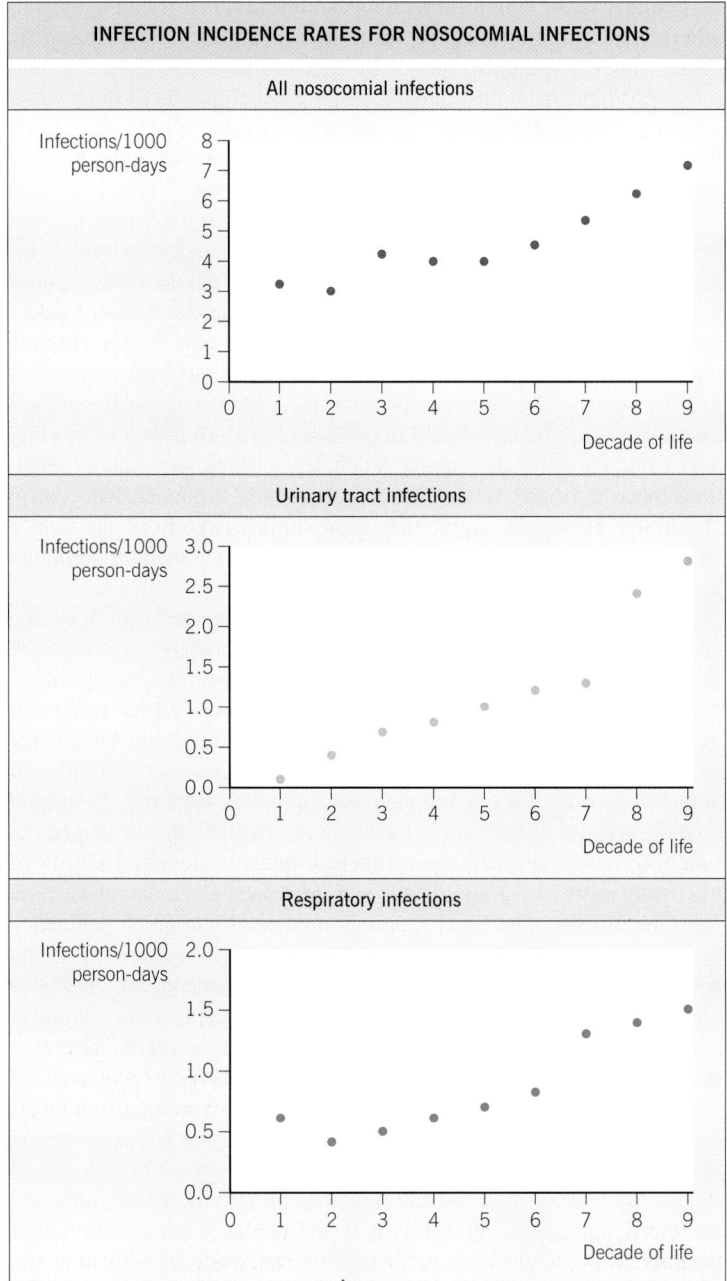

INFECTION INCIDENCE RATES FOR NOSOCOMIAL INFECTIONS

All nosocomial infections

Infections/1000 person-days

Decade of life

Urinary tract infections

Infections/1000 person-days

Decade of life

Respiratory infections

Infections/1000 person-days

Decade of life

Fig. 8.3 Infection incidence rates for nosocomial infections per decade of life. Adapted from Saviteer *et al.,* 1988.[11]

MEDICATION THAT INTERFERES WITH HOST DEFENSE

Drug	Effect on host defense
Antacids, H₂-blockers, H⁺ pump inhibitors	Increased gastrointestinal colonization and infection
Parasympaticolytic drugs	Interference with secretory host defense barrier, gastrointestinal motility and urine voiding
Morphinomimetic drugs	Inhibition of ventilation, cough and gastrointestinal motility; phagocyte and lymphocyte dysfunction
Psychotropic drugs	Inhibition of ventilation, cough
Glucocorticosteroids	Atrophy of skin, decreased repair, impaired cytokine response, impaired phagocyte influx, impaired T-lymphocyte function

Fig. 8.4 Medication that interferes with host defense.

The consequences of this phenomenon for host defense against infection are not yet clear.

It is assumed that aging has no significant effect on the numbers and functions of granulocytes, monocytes or macrophages. Studies addressing granulocyte adherence, chemotaxis and granulocyte degranulation have revealed no abnormalities, although others have demonstrated a reduced migration and adherence of granulocytes obtained from elderly subjects. There is also evidence that oxidative metabolism of granulocytes is reduced in elderly persons. This deficit, which is of uncertain clinical significance, can be improved by the administration of growth hormone.[14]

It has long been recognized that a high proportion of the elderly show a negative delayed-type hypersensitivity response to skin tests. This phenomenon has not only been found with the tuberculin test, but also with other antigens to which the patient has had previous exposure, although complete anergy to all antigens tested is rare. This phenomenon may at least in part be attributable to the effect of aging on the numbers of circulating T lymphocytes, leading to a decline that may be as large as 20–30%.[15] In addition, T-lymphocyte functions are impaired, as has been demonstrated by reduced T-lymphocyte responses upon stimulation with mitogens and an impaired production of T-lymphocyte-derived cytokines such as IL-2. It has been suggested that the reduced capacity of aged lymphocytes to produce IL-2 upon stimulation by macrophage-derived cytokines is a pivotal factor in the reduced immune response in the elderly,[16] but other factors must also be taken into account.[17] Herpes zoster and the occasional reactivation of tuberculosis that occurs in elderly individuals may be consequences of this impaired T-lymphocyte function. Although no major defect has been demonstrated for B lymphocytes, primary and secondary specific humoral immune responses are apparently suboptimal in the elderly. In particular the level of IgM gradually falls, and a reduced antibody response to specific antigens has been well documented, including a reduced humoral response to a variety of vaccines.[18] The degree of functional ability is a major determinant for the magnitude of the antibody response to influenza.[19] Whether the deficits in antibody responses in the elderly are such that they account for increased susceptibility to infection is questionable.

The effects of nutrition on the mechanisms of host defense are discussed in the next paragraph. Especially in the elderly, however, slight signs of protein-energy, mineral or vitamin deficiency may be present. The chronic illnesses and multiple pathologies in elderly individuals may cause anorexia and interfere with their ability to purchase and prepare food. This sequence often leads to combined effects on host defense mechanisms that are caused by aging, deficiencies and the underlying illness itself.

Reduced mobility and increased risk of trauma may also contribute to an increased susceptibility to infection. In addition, underlying diseases in the elderly and the medication prescribed (Fig. 8.4) may interfere with various types of host defense mechanisms.

The production of most cytokines, including interleukin (IL)-1, IL-2, interferon (IFN)-γ is decreased in the elderly, and the production of the hematopoietic growth factors granulocyte-colony stimulating factor (G-CSF) and granulocyte-monocyte (GM)-CSF is also reduced. The decreased response of these colony-stimulating factors may explain the relatively blunted neutrophil response in the elderly. Likewise, the inability of a subgroup of elderly patients to develop fever during acute infections may be the result of decreased pyrogenic cytokine production. Other mechanisms, such as a hypothalamic dysfunction or a decreased capacity to conserve warmth by vasoconstriction, may also explain the differences in fever between elderly and younger patients. Interestingly, the production of tumor necrosis factor (TNF)-α is upregulated in elderly patients and in infection models in senescent mice.[13] It has been hypothesized that a defect in the glucocorticoid-directed downregulation of TNF-α is responsible for the elevated circulating TNF-α concentrations.

MALNUTRITION

At the global level, malnutrition is probably the major cause of defective host defense against infection. Although a severe problem in poor areas of the world, a deficient nutritional status also occurs in developed countries, for example in the elderly or in hospitalized patients who have severe underlying illness. Protein-energy malnutrition is thought to contribute to the development of a variety of infections in hospitalized or seriously ill patients, including tuberculosis, bacterial diarrhea, bacterial and viral respiratory tract infection, aspergillosis, candidiasis and pneumocystosis.[20]

In the developing countries, protein-energy malnutrition exists in two major forms, which often go together: marasmus and kwashiorkor. Nutritional marasmus, resulting from deficient intake of bulk nutrients, is characterized by wasting of muscle and fat tissue, leading to extreme weight reduction. In marasmus there is little dysfunction of organs and homeostasis mechanisms, and the prognosis on refeeding is good, whereas the treatment of kwashiorkor is difficult. Children with kwashiorkor are clinically characterized by failure to thrive, weight reduction, edema, hepatomegaly, loss or depigmentation of hair, and skin desquamation. Diarrhea, purpura and ecchymoses are often encountered. Kwashiorkor children are at higher risk of infection than children with marasmus. The major manifestations of infection include bacterial skin infections, which are often necrotizing, and fungal infections of the mucous membranes (stomatitis, vulvitis, balanitis). Herpes simplex infections and measles occur frequently, the latter often leading to measles pneumonia with a poor outcome. Anecdotal reports have suggested that the febrile response to infection may be reduced during protein-energy malnutrition. In contrast to the increased susceptibility to many types of infections, certain infections, such as malaria, show a less severe course in patients who have protein-energy malnutrition. In spite of similar rates of infection, malnourished children show a lower incidence of cerebral malaria and lower degrees of parasitemia than well nourished children.

Different aspects of host defense are affected by protein-energy malnutrition. First, the epithelial barrier function of skin and mucous membranes may become impaired as a result of thinning of the mucosa and a decreased production of lysozyme and secretory IgA.[21] Humoral defense mechanisms are relatively well conserved. It is remarkable that the immunoglobulin concentrations and the specific antibody responses to foreign proteins are normal in protein-energy malnourished individuals, with the exception of the above-mentioned decrease in secretory IgA. Malnutrition does affect the complement system: both the classic and the alternative pathway become impaired affecting, in particular, the opsonization of micro-organisms. Neutrophils of patients who have protein-energy malnutrition show a reduced chemotactic response, probably because of the defects in the complement system. Phagocytosis is normal or only slightly decreased, whereas the intracellular killing of bacteria and *Candida* spp. by the neutrophils of malnourished patients is impaired. It is unclear whether these phagocyte defects are clinically relevant. Natural killer cell function is also depressed in malnourished children, but whether this leads to clinically apparent susceptibility to viral infection is uncertain.[22] Malnutrition reportedly gives rise to impaired cell-mediated immunity, probably caused by deficient T-helper lymphocyte function and disturbances in thymic morphology and function.[23]

Little is known about the effect of protein-energy malnutrition on the network of cytokines and other inflammatory mediators. The production of proinflammatory cytokines, such as TNF-α and IL-1β, appears to be reduced in patients and in experimental animals with protein-energy malnutrition. This phenomenon may contribute to the observation that fever and signs of inflammation may be reduced in infected patients who have malnutrition, as well as to the increased signs or severity of infection on refeeding, as has been shown for malaria.[24] In malnourished children, the capacity of stimulated blood cells to produce IL-1, TNF-α and IL-6 is reduced, whereas the concentrations of circulating soluble TNF-receptors are increased,

particularly in the subgroup with kwashiorkor. It is difficult to discern whether such findings are the result of an immune defect caused by protein-energy malnutrition, or by concomitant infections. In fact, infections have been postulated to trigger development of the kwashiorkor variant of protein-energy malnutrition, and it has been hypothesized that these ongoing infections lead to a secondary down-regulation of proinflammatory cytokine production.[25]

Deficiency of micronutrients also has an important impact on host defense against infection. In particular the role of vitamin A in susceptibility to infection has been well described.[22] In the 1980s, several controlled double-blind studies in developing countries demonstrated a reduction of mortality attributable to all causes of up to 30% in children receiving vitamin A supplements.[26,27] Certain infections, such as measles, greatly increase the demand for vitamin A, so that supplementation dramatically improves survival in areas with vitamin A deficiency (Fig. 8.5). Children with mild vitamin A deficiency develop respiratory infections twice and diarrhea three times as frequently as nondeficient control children.[22] However, supplementation studies have not consistently shown a beneficial effect on diarrhea or respiratory infections, although the severity of these infections has been reduced by vitamin A.

As is suggested by the increased susceptibility to respiratory and gastrointestinal infection, vitamin A affects the integrity of the mucosa. In vitamin A deficiency, the numbers of mucus-producing epithelial cells in the respiratory, genitourinary and gastrointestinal tracts are decreased, and the concentration of secretory IgA is reduced. Deficiency of vitamin A leads to impaired humoral immunity, in particular to antigens that require a T-lymphocyte-dependent response. In animal models, vitamin A deficiency impairs natural killer cell and phagocytic function; defective phagocytic function leads to impaired killing of micro-organisms by granulocytes and decreased clearance of bacteria from the bloodstream. Finally, animal models of vitamin A deficiency have demonstrated increased production of cytokines, such as TNF-α and IL-1β, upon infection. To what extent these mechanisms are present in humans and contribute to the increased morbidity is presently unknown.

Deficiency of zinc, which in experimental animals increases susceptibility to *Listeria* and *Salmonella* spp., gives rise to defects of the immune response. Zinc deficiency impairs cell-mediated immunity, including the number of CD4+ helper T lymphocytes and suppression of lymphocyte proliferative responses to mitogens and antigens.[28] Interleukin-2 production and natural killer cell activity are also impaired in zinc deficiency. Neutrophils and monocytes from zinc-deficient patients show decreased chemotactic migration, reduced activation and

EFFECT OF VITAMIN A SUPPLEMENTS ON MORTALITY OF CHILDREN IN DEVELOPING COUNTRIES

Country	Number enrolled	Interval between doses (months)[‡]	Outcome*	P-value
Indonesia (N.Sumatra)	25,200	6	0.73	0.024
Nepal (Lowland)	28,630	4	0.70	0.003
Nepal (Highland)	7197	Once only	0.74	0.058
India (Tamil Nadu)	15,419	0.25	0.46	0.01
India (Andhra Pradesh)	15,775	6	0.94	0.82
Ghana	21,906	4	0.81	0.03
Sudan[†]	28,492	6	1.06	0.76

* Ratio of treated to control mortality rates. A ratio <1 indicates a positive effect of supplements

[†] This study found a highly significant correlation between dietary vitamin A deficiency and risk of mortality in the same community

[‡] In most studies, a dose of 200,000 IU was given at baseline and repeated once. In the Tamil Nadu study, each dose contained 8333 IU

Fig. 8.5 Effect of vitamin A supplements on mortality of children in developing countries. Adapted from Bates, 1995.[26]

decreased microbicidal activity. Deficient phagocytic activity in zinc deficiency affects intracellular killing of bacteria, fungi and parasites.[28]

In patients, zinc deficiency is correlated with impaired delayed-type hypersensitivity to common antigens, and zinc supplementation has reportedly corrected the anergy. Zinc deficiency probably contributes to the host defense defects encountered in protein-energy malnutrition. Zinc deficiency may result from dietary deficiency, malabsorption or increased zinc loss. In hospital, zinc deficiency occurs in patients treated with total parenteral nutrition and in those with sickle-cell disease.

Likewise, deficiency of phosphate, which may also occur during parenteral hyperalimentation, leads to impaired granulocyte function and thereby to increased susceptibility to bacterial and fungal infections.[29] Apart from its effects on zinc and phosphate concentrations, parenteral nutrition itself may affect host defense mechanisms. For example, infusion of lipid emulsions leads to saturation of macrophage endocytosis and impairs the oxidative killing of micro-organisms by granulocytes. Moreover, administration of lipids alters the expression of receptors for cytokines and other mediators on phagocytic cells, and may interact with circulating serum microbicidal factors.[30] In contrast, the capacity of infused lipids to bind and neutralize bacterial lipopolysaccharides may contribute to a decreased susceptibility to Gram-negative sepsis.[31] Likewise, it has been suggested that severe hypolipoproteinemia may result in a decreased lipopolysaccharide clearance, but the impact of this observation on the susceptibility to infections in clinical practice is unknown.

Whether iron deficiency leads to a significantly increased susceptibility to infection in humans is uncertain.[32] However, the killing of micro-organisms by neutrophils and the function of T-lymphocytes are abnormal in patients who have iron deficiency. In contrast, iron repletion and iron overload predispose to infection, probably by making iron available to micro-organisms as a nutrient. Iron is an essential growth factor for most bacteria. The organisms obtain iron by producing chelators called siderophores, which bind iron for uptake into the bacteria. Several micro-organisms, for example *Yersinia enterocolitica*, are thought to be of low virulence because they lack siderophores. During iron overload, listeriosis and severe yersiniosis have been reported, as has the rare but severe infection with the fungi of the class of Zygomycetes, zygomycosis or mucormycosis.[33,34] These infections are particularly seen in patients treated with deferoxamine , as this agent can be utilized by micro-organisms as an exogenous siderophore, leading to increased iron uptake and enhanced outgrowth.

ALCOHOLISM, CIRRHOSIS AND DRUG ABUSE
Alcohol
Most people drink alcohol, and excessive alcohol intake or alcoholism probably is one of the most common forms of exogenous offence to the host defense system. Only a minority of alcoholics are among the stereotypical homeless or slum inhabitants, in whom the risk of infection is increased because of the combined effects of lifestyle, poor hygiene, trauma and alcohol abuse. In these groups, the most common problems are skin infections, and tuberculosis and other pneumonias. Bacterial pneumonia in these patients is most commonly caused by pneumococci, mixed anaerobic and aerobic flora and *Legionella* spp. The majority of those with excessive alcohol consumption, however, are 'average' patients who have a relatively normal lifestyle. For these patient groups, very few data exist on the relative contribution of alcoholism to the incidence of infection.

Alcohol clearly affects the first line of defense. Oral and gastric contents may be aspirated, aspiration being facilitated by reduced consciousness, a depressed cough reflex and reduced glottal closure. Consequently, patients are at greater risk of bacterial pneumonias. The second line of defense is also affected by alcoholism. Although a final proof of a causal relationship is difficult to obtain, the infections commonly seen in alcoholism seem to correlate quite well with the defects in host defense mechanisms that are caused by alcohol *in vitro*.[35,36] There have been reports of subtle defects in the complement cascade, with

consequences for chemotactic responses of granulocytes. Although the secondary antibody response seems to be normal, the response to new antigens is clearly impaired in alcoholics. Adherence of neutrophils is impaired after exposure to alcohol, and this finding may explain the leukopenia and the blunted leukocyte response during bacterial infection that may be observed in alcoholics.[36] The function of the neutrophils, including phagocytosis and intracellular killing, is otherwise normal. In contrast, macrophages are significantly affected by alcoholism; clearance of particles from the bloodstream is impaired and an abnormal response to cytokines has been noted. In addition, cell-mediated immunity is depressed in severe alcoholism.[36] T lymphocytes may be fewer in number and a reduced response to mitogens has been found. Likewise, impaired natural killer cell function has been described.[37]

A variety of additional risk factors may be present in patients who have presumed alcoholism-related infection, including hepatic damage, cirrhosis and poor nutrition. Alcohol consumption yields large amounts of carbohydrates without proteins, vitamins and minerals. Most vitamins absorbed from the intestine may be deficient in alcoholism, including vitamin A, which has important effects on host defenses. Likewise, zinc deficiency may occur as a result of dietary deficiency, contributing to impaired wound healing and reduced delayed-type hypersensitivity.

Cirrhosis
A variety of infections are reportedly related to cirrhosis and end-stage liver disease. In most patients, cirrhosis, whether attributable to chronic alcoholism or to other causes, is insidious in onset, and in some patients the diagnosis is only made after occurrence of accompanying infectious sequelae or at autopsy. In patients who have cirrhosis, prominent infections are aspiration pneumonia, sepsis and spontaneous bacterial peritonitis. These infections are also frequently seen in patients who have end-stage liver disease awaiting transplantation. In those who are hospitalized, intravascular line-related sepsis can be added to the list. Apart from the specific defects in host defense mechanisms described below, the risk of aspiration pneumonia may be caused by hepatic encephalopathy, leading to a reduced glottal closure, microaspiration and a decreased cough reflex. Aerobic and anaerobic oral flora, and Gram-negative organisms in hospitalized patients, are frequent in such individuals.

Spontaneous bacterial peritonitis is a constant risk in patients who have liver disease accompanied by ascites.[38] *Enterobacteriaceae*, mostly *E. coli* and *Klebsiella pneumoniae*, and *S. pneumoniae*, other streptococci and enterococci are the most frequently recovered pathogens. The route of infection in spontaneous bacterial peritonitis has not been completely elucidated. It is assumed that enteric micro-organisms pass directly to the peritoneal cavity through the intact intestinal wall. This phenomenon of translocation occurs in experimental animal models of cirrhosis and ascites. A hematogenous route of infection has also been postulated. Clearance of particles from the bloodstream is impaired, and this can probably be at least partly explained by changes in hepatic blood flow.[39] Reduced clearance of bacteria from the portal circulation may allow micro-organisms to cause metastatic infection in the peritoneal fluid. Together with the other host defense defects in cirrhotic patients, this phenomenon may also explain the increased incidence of sepsis and Gram-negative endocarditis in this patient group. Especially in patients who have very advanced liver disease, the ascitic fluid has low concentrations of albumin, complement and other proteins that have opsonic activity and provide protection against bacteria. The risk of developing spontaneous bacterial peritonitis inversely correlates with the concentration of complement factor C3 in ascites fluid.[40]

In patients who have cirrhosis, a variety of other host defense abnormalities has been found, but their relative importance in the increased susceptibility to infection is unclear. Serum from cirrhotic patients shows a poorer chemotaxis for neutrophils compared with normal serum, probably because of a specific inhibitor.[41] Complement activity and opsonization are usually normal in patients who have alcoholic cirrhosis, but occasional abnormalities have been reported. Phagocytosis and intracellular killing by granulocytes and monocytes are normal. Depressed T-lymphocyte reactivity in cirrhosis has been identified.

Drug abuse

Infection is the leading cause of death in intravenous drug abusers. Infections of the skin and soft tissues are the most common, including cellulitis, cutaneous abscesses, thrombophlebitis and necrotizing fasciitis. Injections without a sterile technique frequently lead to bacterial contamination of the site of administration, with subsequent infection. In addition, the illicit substance injected itself, diluents or impurities may cause inflammation, vasospasm, tissue necrosis and ulceration. Spread of local infections resulting in mediastinitis or cervical abscesses with erosion of the carotid arteries has been reported. *Staphylococcus aureus* has been the most frequent pathogen, followed by *Streptococcus* spp. Certain techniques may lead to contamination of the drugs or injection paraphernalia with oral flora and infections with *Streptococcus milleri*, pneumococci and anaerobic bacteria may occur. Necrotizing fasciitis is relatively frequent in intravenous drug users, requiring aggressive combined surgical and antibiotic treatment. Hematogenous infections of the bones and joints are frequent, usually as a result of spread from a skin or soft tissue infection. Infective endocarditis is the best known infection attributed to intravenous drug use, although skin and soft tissue infections are far more frequent than endocarditis. In cases of infective endocarditis, *S. aureus* and *Streptococcus* spp. are the most common organisms. Gram-negative bacteria such as *Pseudomonas aeruginosa*, *Serratia marsescens* and *Candida* spp. have also been reported frequently. Unlike native valve endocarditis in other patients, the valves of intravenous drug users with endocarditis have almost always been normal until development of the disease. Mycotic aneurysms, caused by either hematogenous seed during endocarditis or direct trauma at the site of injection, are common in intravenous drug users. Respiratory symptoms may represent septic pulmonary emboli, which may evolve to abscesses in right-sided (tricuspid) endocarditis (Fig. 8.6). Initially, these manifestations may be difficult to differentiate from pneumonias caused by common respiratory pathogens, which are also frequent in drug users. Furthermore, pulmonary tuberculosis is encountered, especially in the homeless and HIV-infected population. Other opportunistic infections secondary to HIV infection and hepatitis B, C and D are common in these individuals.

Not all of the infections are strictly related to intravenous drug use. For example, smoking of cocaine used in its alkaloid form (crack) is associated with tuberculosis as well as with a series of noninfectious pulmonary complications (infarction, pulmonary edema, atelectasis and hemorrhage), which may become secondarily infected. Smoking of marijuana contaminated with *Aspergillus* spp. may lead to pulmonary aspergillosis, especially in HIV-infected patients.[42]

Drug addiction may predispose to infection in various ways.[43] Most of the bacterial infections relate to lifestyle, poor hygiene, needle sharing and unsterile injection practices, all of which compromise primarily the first line of defense. Increased rates of skin colonization with *S. aureus* have been reported. Specific organisms causing infection in HIV-negative intravenous drug users (e.g. *Candida* spp., *Serratia* spp.) seem to be related to contamination of injected drugs or certain practices, rather than to host defense defects (Fig. 8.7). Whether injection of insoluble additives (such as starch, talc and other particulate matter) temporarily leads to blockade of the phagocytic capacity of the mononuclear phagocyte system has not been established. In contrast, recurrent immunologic stimulation by these foreign materials has been associated with the increased concentrations of immunoglobulins found in intravenous drug users, and no evidence exists of impaired humoral immunity in these patients.

Other effects of narcotic drugs may contribute to increase susceptibility to infection. Opiates interfere with pulmonary defense mechanisms through depression of respiration and the cough reflex. In addition, opiates alter a variety of immune responses through their indirect and direct effects on immune cells. First, the effects of morphine on the central nervous system include activation of the hypothalamic–pituitary–adrenal axis, with secondary effects on the immune system mediated through induction of glucocorticoids.[44] Second, a variety of immune cells express a specific opiate receptor that can be inhibited by naloxone. Through binding to this receptor, morphine inhibits phagocytosis of micro-organisms by neutrophils and macrophages, their ability to produce oxygen radicals (respiratory burst) required for intracellular killing of pathogens and the capacity of macrophages to produce TNF-α and IFN-γ.[44] The chemotaxis of neutrophils is inhibited by opiates, as is the expression of adhesion molecules on these cells. In addition, opiates impair lymphocyte responsiveness and natural killer cell function.[45] In animal models, morphine treatment not only leads to increased outgrowth of bacteria during disseminated infection through its suppressive effects on neutrophil function, but also to increased sensitivity to bacterial endotoxin.[46] Delayed-type hypersensitivity skin reactions are frequently absent in intravenous drug users, as is in-vitro lymphocyte proliferation in response to antigens and mitogens. Moreover, natural killer cell function is significantly reduced after administration of morphine. From these data, it is clear that opiates influence the host defense system at many levels, particularly affecting cellular immunity, and granulocyte and macrophage function, including influx at the site of infection, phagocytosis and killing of micro-organisms. To what extent these mechanisms contribute to an increased susceptibility to sepsis in intravenous drug users, or likewise in postoperative patients, remains to be established.

DIABETES MELLITUS

Diabetes mellitus is the most common endocrine disease. It is estimated that 6–11% of the population have diabetes mellitus or impaired glucose

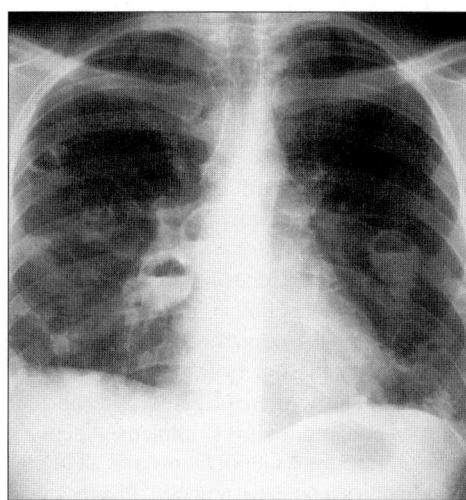

Fig. 8.6 Lung abscesses caused by septic pulmonary embolism in right-sided *Staphylococcus aureus* endocarditis in a 22-year-old male intravenous drug user.

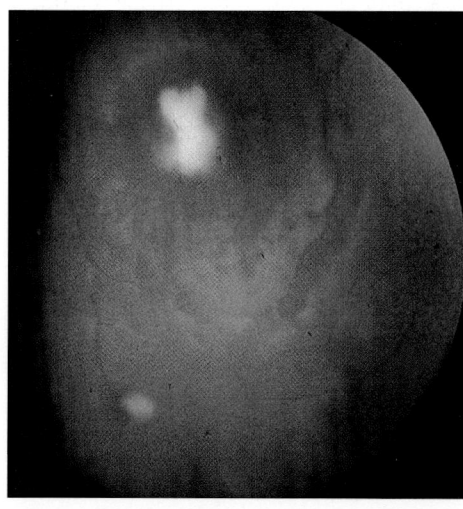

Fig. 8.7 *Candida albicans* endophthalmitis in a 29-year-old male intravenous drug user.

tolerance, depending on the diagnostic criteria. Among the many sequelae of long-standing diabetes mellitus, some types of infection may occur more frequently than in normal individuals, whereas other infections tend to have a more severe course. Although formal evidence is difficult to provide, it is generally believed that diabetes mellitus is associated with impaired host defense. Breaches in the first line of defense as a result of injections, diabetic vascular disease and neuropathy are important causes of infections. The prominent infections in diabetic patients are those of skin and underlying soft tissues and bones. These infections are mainly caused by *S. aureus*, hemolytic streptococci and *Candida* spp. The development of foot ulcers is a special problem in the diabetic patient (Fig. 8.8). Diabetic neuropathy, leading to abnormal pressure distribution and reduced recognition of pain in cases of minor trauma or pressure, is the initial step in the pathogenesis of diabetic foot ulcers. Vascular disease contributes to the development of the lesion, and secondary bacterial infection is common. *Staphylococcus aureus* is the most common pathogen. In more severe cases, the infection is commonly polymicrobial. *Staphylococcus aureus*, enteric Gram-negative bacteria, and *Streptococcus* spp. are the major pathogens in these cases, together with enterococci, anaerobic streptococci and *Bacteroides* spp. Patients who have diabetes mellitus and inject insulin, like other regular users of needles, have a high incidence (35%) of *S. aureus* skin carriage.[47] However, diabetic persons who are not insulin-dependent also carry *S. aureus* more frequently than normal individuals.

Furthermore, urinary tract infections caused by enteric Gram-negative rods, enterococci and *Candida* spp. are often encountered in patients who have diabetes mellitus. High concentrations of glucose in urine and secretions may promote colonization by *Candida* spp. and other micro-organisms. It is less easy to explain the association of diabetes mellitus with mucormycosis and with malignant external otitis. The latter is an invasive, necrotizing infection that spreads from the ear canal into the soft tissue, cartilage and mastoid. Further spread to the jugular bulb, meninges and brain may cause life-threatening disease. Malignant external otitis is usually caused by *P. aeruginosa* and occurs almost exclusively in elderly patients who have diabetes mellitus.[48]

Rare but rather specific for the diabetic patient is rhinocerebral zygomycosis, which manifests particularly during diabetic ketoacidosis (see Chapter 4.9, Approach to the patient with zygomycosis). Zygomycosis (also called mucormycosis) is caused by fungi belonging to the class Zygomycetes and the order Mucorales.[49] These organisms are strongly dependent on iron supply, and compete with serum apotransferrin for the uptake of iron. It has been demonstrated that the change of pH during diabetic ketoacidosis reduces the affinity of serum transferrin to bind iron, thus during acidosis, increased amounts of iron may be available to the micro-organism, leading to enhanced outgrowth.[50]

In diabetes, a number of abnormalities of the second line of defense have been found. Nonenzymatic glycosylation of the complement factor C3 has been reported, an abnormality that may lead to impaired opsonization of bacteria and *Candida* spp.[51] The antibody responses are generally considered normal. The inflammatory response at the site of infection in diabetic experimental animals is impaired. In this respect, the finding that chemotactic activity of granulocytes is impaired in individuals with diabetes mellitus is relevant.[52] This phenomenon is not related to ketoacidosis. Defective chemotaxis has also been found in monocytes, possibly as a consequence of auto-oxidative cell damage.

Many studies have addressed the function of phagocytic cells in diabetes mellitus.[53] Adherence of leukocytes and phagocytosis tend to be reduced at high glucose concentrations, high osmolarity and low pH. Phagocytic function of mononuclear phagocytes as assessed by the capacity to clear aggregated albumin from the bloodstream appears to be normal. Abnormalities of the bactericidal function of granulocytes have also been described; the impaired glucose metabolism of the phagocytes could well be the basis of these observed abnormalities.[54] Myeloperoxidase deficiency, a disorder of the oxidative killing mechanisms of granulocytes and mononuclear phagocytes, occurs in 1 out of 2000–4000 healthy individuals and does not seem to have a

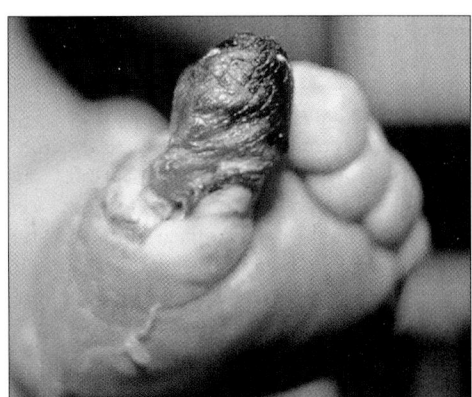

Fig. 8.8 Diabetic foot ulcer in a 53-year-old male patient with diabetes mellitus.

significant impact on the host defense to infection in these subjects. However, when present in patients who have diabetes mellitus, myeloperoxidase deficiency seems to predispose to serious infections, and invasive fungal infections have been described in these patients. Therefore, the occurrence of a deep-seated fungal infection in a patient who has diabetes mellitus suggests that the myeloperoxidase activity in their leukocytes should be determined.

T-lymphocyte function is normal in most patients who have diabetes mellitus, although patients who have poorly controlled glucose concentrations have depressed T-lymphocyte function. Animal experiments have provided some evidence for altered cell-mediated immunity, but the consequences for host defense in diabetic patients are unclear.

CHRONIC RENAL FAILURE

Although many clinicians believe that uremia predisposes to infection, it is hard to find evidence to support this notion. Humoral defense mechanisms are not affected by chronic renal failure *per se*. In contrast, specific abnormalities of the cellular defense mechanisms have been reported in patients who have renal failure. The marrow pool reserve of granulocytes is decreased in uremic patients and, in addition, impaired neutrophil accumulation *in vivo* and impaired neutrophil chemotaxis *in vitro* have been observed. Impaired generation of chemotactic factors in uremic serum may be responsible for these findings. This anomaly can be partially corrected by peritoneal dialysis, but not by hemodialysis.[55] The impaired granulocyte response upon infection seems to be fully explained by this impairment of chemotaxis, as opsonization, together with adherence, phagocytosis and intracellular killing by granulocytes, reportedly is normal in patients who have chronic renal failure. In contrast, phagocytosis of micro-organisms by mononuclear phagocytes has been reported to be abnormal *in vitro* and *in vivo*.[56,57] Delayed-type hypersensitivity skin reactions to assess cell-mediated immunity are reduced in chronic renal failure and do not improve with hemodialysis. This effect is probably caused by lymphocytopenia, which may be present in uremia, and by impaired lymphocyte function, as suppression of lymphocyte proliferation has been demonstrated in the presence of uremic serum.[58] It is controversial whether the proliferative responses of lymphocytes to mitogens and antigens are abnormal in uremic patients.

The susceptibility to infection may increase with hemodialysis. In patients on hemodialysis, the first line of defense becomes compromised by multiple punctures, which may lead to intravascular infection, especially when prosthetic shunts are present. In addition, these patients have an unexplained but clearly increased incidence of nasal carriage of *S. aureus* and infections caused by this organism.

The use of certain dialysis membranes causes hemodialysis to activate complement, leading to adherence of granulocytes and subsequent margination and sequestration in the pulmonary circulation. On the basis of trials of hepatitis B vaccination, it has become clear that the antibody response is abnormal in patients on hemodialysis. In view of the finding in these patients that cell-mediated immunity is impaired, several investigators have tried to restore the vaccine response by concomitant administration of cytokines such as IL-2 and IFN-γ; however, the results of these efforts are inconsistent.

Iron overload in hemodialysis patients increases the risk of bacteremia.[34,59] *Listeria monocytogenes* and *Y. enterocolitica* have been reported as the cause of bacteremia in such patients. Three mechanisms may be responsible for the increased susceptibility to these pathogens in iron-overloaded hemodialysis patients. First, iron overload impairs phagocytosis and the killing of micro-organisms by neutrophils.[33] Second, iron is a growth factor for certain strains of bacteria and, *in vitro*, their virulence is directly correlated with the iron content of the medium (see Malnutrition). Third, attempts to chelate aluminium or iron with deferoxamine have been shown to be associated with an increased risk of acquiring infections, in particular yersiniosis and zygomycosis, the latter a rare but often fatal invasive fungal infection (see Chapter 4.9, Approach to the patient with zygomycosis). An international registry of zygomycosis in hemodialysis patients has revealed a considerable number of patients who were overloaded with either iron or aluminium and approximately 80% were receiving deferoxamine at the time of the infection. Zygomycetes depend on iron as a growth factor and require a siderophore to facilitate its uptake. For one of the common causative agents of zygomycosis, *Rhizopus microsporus*, rhizoferrin has been isolated as the endogenous fungal siderophore.[60] During deferoxamine therapy, deferoxamine is used by the fungus as an exogenous siderophore in place of its endogenous rhizoferrin, leading to increased iron uptake and enhanced outgrowth (Fig. 8.9). An important proportion of the iron bound to rhizoferrin is taken up by serum apotransferrin. Thereby, this protein makes iron unavailable to *R. microsporus*, contributing to the fungistatic properties of human serum. In contrast, the iron within deferoxamine is not trapped by serum apotransferrin and it is easily utilized by *R. microsporus*.[60] Patients who have normal renal function and are treated with deferoxamine only occasionally develop zygomycosis. This contrast is explained by the pharmacokinetic changes in uremia. Hemodialysis patients have reduced clearance of deferoxamine, with levels of the iron–deferoxamine complexes that are continuously sufficient to reverse the fungistatic properties of serum and to promote the growth of the fungus.

Similarly, deferoxamine enhances in-vitro growth of various other micro-organisms, such as *Klebsiella* spp., *Salmonella typhimurium* and some serotypes of *Y. enterocolitica*. Indeed, hemodialysis patients have been reported to develop bacteremia caused by *Y. enterocolitica* strains that lack an endogenous siderophore. These strains depend on the availability of exogenous siderophores, and are able to take up iron from the iron–deferoxamine complex.[34]

Patients on chronic ambulatory peritoneal dialysis (CAPD) are at risk of infectious peritonitis, most often caused by Gram-positive micro-organisms, in particular *Staphylococcus epidermidis* and *S. aureus*. A series of factors predispose to such infection: exogenous contamination of the catheter, the transcutaneous path of the intraperitoneal catheter and infection of the peritoneal contents through intestinal disease, for example diverticulitis. Peritoneal macrophages of patients on CAPD exhibit normal phagocytic and microbicidal functions. However, a serious deficiency of opsonins (IgG and C3) in the peritoneal dialysis effluent has been demonstrated.[61,62] The reduced opsonic activity correlates well with the incidence of *S. epidermidis* peritonitis in these patients. It is remarkable that CAPD patients who have diabetes mellitus do not seem to be at increased risk of peritonitis compared with nondiabetic patients on CAPD, and remarkably the peritoneal effluent of diabetic patients exhibits high opsonic activity.[62]

GLUCOCORTICOSTEROIDS
Since the early days of the therapeutic use of glucocorticosteroids, it has been clear that these drugs predispose users to infection by interference with host defense mechanisms. The infections associated with glucocorticosteroid treatment mainly point to defective phagocyte function, such as infections caused by *S. aureus*, enteric Gram-negative bacteria, *Candida* spp. and *Aspergillus* spp., and to defective cellular immunity, as demonstrated through infections caused by varicella-zoster virus, *L. monocytogenes*, *Salmonella* spp., mycobacteria, and *Pneumocystis carinii*.

The risk of infection is related to duration of treatment and dose, as was demonstrated in a meta-analysis of controlled trials (Fig. 8.10).[63] According to this analysis, infectious complications occur particularly in patients who have been given the equivalent of more than a cumulative dose of 700mg prednisone. These data suggest that either short-term administration of high doses (e.g. 7 days of 100mg) or prolonged administration of lower doses (e.g. 70 days of 10mg) have a similar effect on host defense whenever a cumulative dose of approximately 700mg has been exceeded. Doses of less than 10mg/day do not appear to be associated with increased risk of infection. Conversion to a single dose of glucocorticosteroid given on alternate days reduces the chance of infectious complications in patients needing prolonged treatment with these drugs.

Glucocorticosteroids potentially affect all lines of host defense. Characteristic damage to the first line of defense includes atrophy, bruising and delayed healing, and these effects may contribute to the acquisition of infections.

Humoral defense mechanisms are less affected. Immunoglobulin concentrations may decrease during glucocorticosteroid treatment, but rarely to levels that lead to infectious complications. The complement system seems to function normally. Glucocorticosteroids inhibit the production of proinflammatory cytokines, such as IL-1 and TNF-α, and this has an impact on the activation of T-lymphocytes, granulocytes and mononuclear phagocytes, and on the development of fever and other aspects of the acute phase response.[64]

Cellular defense mechanisms are a main target for glucocorticosteroids. Granulocytopoiesis is enhanced and the bone marrow reserve is poured into the circulation, leading to peripheral blood granulocytosis. However, the negative effects of glucocorticosteroids on granulocyte function seem to outweigh these apparently positive effects.[65] The influx of granulocytes at inflammatory sites is reduced after glucocorticosteroid treatment. Impaired margination and chemotactic responsiveness seem to be the mechanisms behind the impaired accumulation of white cells. Other functions of granulocytes, such as phagocytosis and intracellular killing, are not affected unless phagocytes are exposed to very high glucocorticosteroid concentrations, and these impairments may not be clinically relevant.

The cells of the mononuclear phagocyte lineage are also affected by glucocorticosteroid treatment. Monocytopenia and impaired monocyte

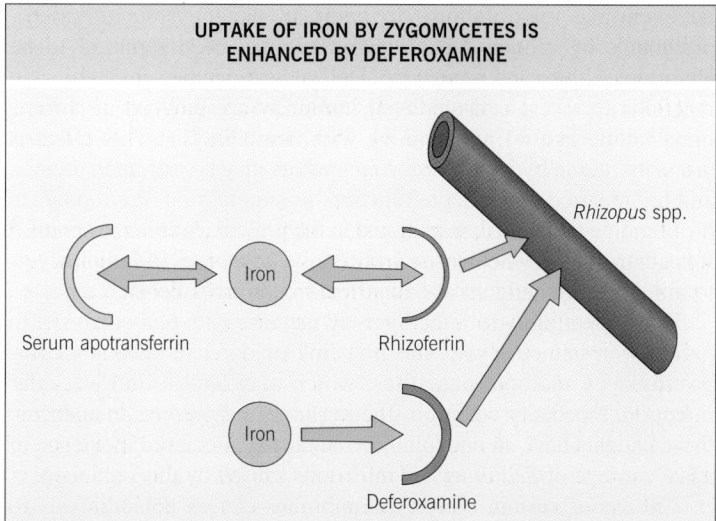

UPTAKE OF IRON BY ZYGOMYCETES IS ENHANCED BY DEFEROXAMINE

Rhizopus spp.

Iron

Serum apotransferrin

Rhizoferrin

Iron

Deferoxamine

Fig. 8.9 Uptake of iron by zygomycetes is enhanced by deferoxamine. The endogenous siderophore of the fungus, rhizoferrin, competes with serum apotransferrin for the uptake of iron. By limiting the fungal uptake of iron, apotransferrin acts as a fungistatic serum factor. Apotransferrin does not compete with the iron–deferoxamine complex, and fungal iron uptake in the presence of deferoxamine is markedly enhanced.

chemotaxis are prominent. Impaired killing of micro-organisms by mononuclear phagocytes does not seem to occur unless very high dosages are being applied.[66] The clearance of particles from the bloodstream is reduced. Moreover, activation of macrophages for enhanced killing of intracellular pathogens is impaired after glucocorticosteroid treatment as a result of the decreased production of proinflammatory cytokines. *In vitro*, the impaired killing of bacteria or fungi by granulocytes and monocytes exposed to glucocorticosteroids can be reversed by the addition of IFN-γ, and addition of G-CSF has a similar effect on the granulocyte defect. The clinical impact of these findings is unclear.

The primary effect of glucocorticosteroid administration on lymphocytes is the induction of a profound lymphocytopenia within hours of administration. Mainly, circulating T lymphocytes are reduced, but there is also some effect on B lymphocytes. In humans, redistribution of lymphocytes is the main mechanism responsible for this effect, in contrast to the lymphocytolysis that has been reported in rodents after glucocorticosteroid treatment.[59] The redistribution of lymphocytes and the reduced production of proinflammatory cytokines appear to be the major explanations for the impairment of cellular immunity during glucocorticosteroid treatment.

PREVENTION AND MANAGEMENT

Advances in medical and surgical treatment frequently interfere with the quality of host defense mechanisms of patients. Knowledge of the defenses of the host is a necessary first step in the prevention of infections that are caused by such interference.

In the patient who has impaired host defense mechanisms, prevention of infection is a primary goal. Measures to avoid damage to the first line of defense are of great importance. In compromised hosts, punctures of skin and mucous membranes should be avoided as much as possible, as should be the introduction of indwelling catheters and other devices. Each breach of the first line of defense should be viewed as a serious threat that may lead to subsequent infection.

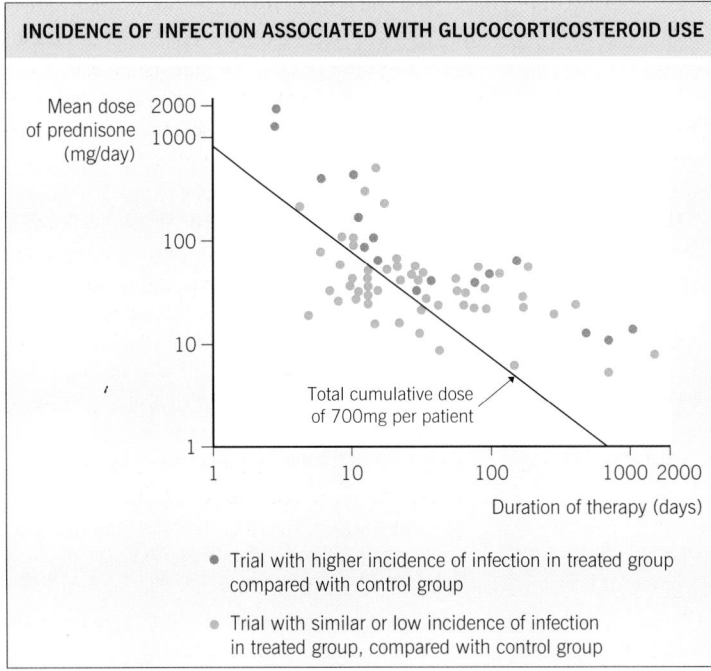

INCIDENCE OF INFECTION ASSOCIATED WITH GLUCOCORTICOSTEROID USE

Mean dose of prednisone (mg/day) — y-axis: 2000, 1000, 100, 10, 1

Duration of therapy (days) — x-axis: 1, 10, 100, 1000 2000

Total cumulative dose of 700mg per patient

● Trial with higher incidence of infection in treated group compared with control group

● Trial with similar or low incidence of infection in treated group, compared with control group

Fig. 8.10 Incidence of infection associated with glucocorticosteroid use.
In this meta-analysis of 71 placebo-controlled trials of prednisone, all trials in which there was a higher incidence of infection in the treated group (compared with the controls) were located above the isodose line of 700mg. This indicates that, independent of the regimen used in the trial, patients who had a cumulative dose of less than 700mg did not have an increased risk of infectious complications. With permission from Stuck *et al.*[63]

Likewise, pharmaceuticals that affect host defense, such as H₂-blockers of parasympathicolytics, should be avoided (see The elderly). Adequate nursing, physical therapy and maintenance of a good nutritional state are measures that are relatively easy to accomplish.

More sophisticated methods to improve the first line of defense are still in their infancy, for example increasing the integrity of epithelial layers with cytokines such as IL-13, or acceleration of wound healing using epidermal growth factors and other cytokines. Depending on the risk of colonization of skin or mucous membranes with certain potentially pathogenic micro-organisms (e.g. *S. aureus*, *Salmonella* spp.), prophylactic antimicrobial strategies may be initiated to eradicate such a carrier state.

Options to improve the second line of defense are manifold as well. Complement factors may be replenished by administration of fresh plasma. Because the complement system is a strong proinflammatory cascade system, such substitution should be done cautiously, as it may induce inflammation and tissue damage. Although many data exist on the intravenous administration of cryoprecipitates rich in fibronectin during sepsis, with the aim of improving opsonization, such treatment has not been shown to be successful.

In compromised hosts a variety of vaccines may be of benefit, provided that vaccination can mount an immune response in this patient group. The most important vaccines currently are hepatitis B vaccine, pneumococcal polysaccharide vaccine, *H. influenzae* type b conjugate vaccine and varicella vaccine. Potentially important vaccines that are on the horizon are the new meningococcal vaccines. As patients who have defective host defense mechanisms may exhibit poor antibody responses and poor cellular immune responses to vaccines, there is a great need for improved vaccine adjuvants. Bacterial products (monophosphoryl lipid A, trehalose dimycolate) and proinflammatory cytokines (IL-1, IL-2, IL-6, IFN-γ) are currently being studied for this purpose.

The recombinant proinflammatory cytokines, in particular IL-1, IL-2, IFN-γ, IL-12 and TNF-α, may be applied to enhance cellular effector mechanisms, although strategies to circumvent toxicity need to be developed. Several of these cytokines, including TNF-α, are strong activators of neutrophil function and are essential in host defense against fungal infection. Moreover, cytokines like TNF-α, IL-12 and IFN-γ are essential in the granulomatous response to infection and the containment and killing of intracellular pathogens. The medical community will have to learn how to use these substances for therapeutic purposes in immunocompromised patients.

The recombinant hematopoietic growth factors (G-CSF, GM-CSF, M-CSF) are another area of great therapeutic interest. So far, these substances have mainly been used in patients who have neutropenia. Although the benefit of these growth factors in patients who have chemotherapy-induced neutropenia has not been well established, recombinant G-CSF has been shown to be cost-effective in patients who have congenital neutropenia. Whether these factors will benefit patients who have infection and malfunctioning or even normal granulocytes is currently under study.

Immunoglobulin preparations mainly have their place in the treatment of patients who have antibody-deficiency syndromes, but are now also being considered for severe staphylococcal and streptococcal toxic shock syndrome. Patients who have these diseases may suffer from a selective deficiency of neutralizing antibodies against the relevant bacterial toxins, which act as superantigens (see Chapter 1.2). Restoration of these antibodies by infusion of immunoglobulin from pooled donors may be beneficial, although trials to substantiate this hypothesis are still in progress. Immunoglobulins are also being employed to combat neonatal infections, such as those caused by *S. epidermidis*.

Immunoglobulin preparations with high titers against cytomegalovirus are being used in conjunction with antiviral drugs, especially ganciclovir, in severely immunocompromised patients who have cytomegalovirus pneumonitis. Likewise, antirespiratory syncytical virus (RSV) globulin is under study along with vibovirin for the treatment of RSV pneumonia.

REFERENCES

1. Quie PG. Antimicrobial defenses in the neonate. Sem Perinatol 1990;14:2–9.
2. Adamkin D, Stitzel A, Urmson J, et al. Activity of the alternative pathway of complement in the newborn infant. J Pediatr 1978;93:604–8.
3. Maródi L, Leijh PCJ, Braat A, et al. Opsonic activity of cord blood sera against various species of microorganisms. Pediatr Res 1985;19:433–6.
4. Wilson CB, Lewis DB. Basis and implications of selectively diminished cytokine production in neonatal susceptibility to infection. Rev Infect Dis 1990;12(Suppl 4):410–20.
5. Maródi L, Jzerniczky J, Csorba S, et al. Chemotactic and random movement of cord blood granulocytes. Experientia 1984;40:1407–10.
6. Maródi L, Csorba S, Nagy B. Chemotactic and random movement of human newborn monocytes. Eur J Pediatr 1980;135:73–85.
7. Maródi L, Leijh PCJ, Van Furth R. Characterization and functional capacities of human cord blood granulocytes and monocytes. Pediatr Res 1984;18:1127–31.
8. Van Tol MJD, Zijlstra J, Thomas CMG, et al. Distinct role of neonatal and adult monocytes in the regulation of the in vitro antigen-induced plaque-forming cell response in man. J Immunol 1902;133:1902–8.
9. Kohl S, Frazier JJ, Greenberg SB, et al. Interferon induction of natural killer cytotoxicity in human neonates. J Pediatr 1981;98:379–84.
10. Xanthou M, Bines J, Walker WA. Human milk and intestinal defense in newborns. An update. Adv Pediatr 1995;42:171–208.
11. Saviteer SM, Samsa GP, Rutala WA. Nosocomial infections in the elderly. Increased risk per hospital day. Am J Med 1988;84:661–6.
12. Van der Meer JTM, Thompson J, Valkenburg HA, Michel MF. Epidemiology of bacterial endocarditis in the Netherlands. I. Patient characteristics. Arch Intern Med 1992;152:1863–8.
13. Peterson PK. Ageing, cytokines, and infectious diseases. In: Van der Meer JWM, Michel MF, Verbrugh HA, eds. Infections in the elderly. Proceedings of the 6th SB Kurhaus workshop on antibiotics. Rijswijk: Smithkline Beecham; 1994:23–32.
14. Wiedermann CJ, Niedermühlbichler M, Beimpold H, et al. In vitro activation of neutrophils of the aged by recombinant growth hormone. J Infect Dis 1991;164:1017–20.
15. Saltzman RL, Peterson PK. Immunodeficiency of the elderly. Rev Infect Dis 1987;9:1127–39.
16. Nagel JE, Chopra RK, Chrest FJ et al. Decreased proliferation, interleukin-2 production and interleukin-2 receptor expression are accompanied by decreased mRNA expression in phytohemagglutinin stimulated cells from elderly donors. J Clin Invest 1988;81:1096–102.
17. Miller RA. The aging immune system. Primer and prospectus. Science 1996;273:70–3.
18. Phair J, Kauffman CA, Bjornson A. Failure to respond to influenza vaccine in the aged. Correlation with B cell number or function. J Lab Clin Med 1978;92:822–8.
19. Remarque EJ, Cools HJM, Boere TJ, et al. Functional disability and antibody response to influenza vaccine in elderly patients in a Dutch nursing home. Br Med J 1996;312:1015.
20. Chandra RK. Nutrition and the immune system. Proc Nutr Soc 1993;52:77–83.
21. Keusch GT, Wilson CS, Waksal SD. Nutrition, host defenses and the lymphoid system. In: Gallin JI, Fauci AS, eds. Advances in host defense mechanisms, vol II. New York: Raven Press; 1983:275–359.
22. West CE, Rombout JHW, Van der Zijp AJ, et al. Vitamin A and immune function. Proc Nutr Soc 1991;50:251–62.

23. Salimonu LS, Ojo Amaize E, Williams AIO, et al. Depressed natural killer cell activity in children with protein calory malnutrition. Clin Immunol Immunopathol 1982;24:1–7.
24. Sauerwein RW, Mulder JA, Mulder L, et al. Inflammatory mediators in children with protein-energy malnutrition. Am J Clin Nutr 1997;65:1543–9.
25. Keuter M, Dharmana E, Gasem MH, et al. Patterns of proinflammatory cytokines and inhibitors during typhoid fever. J Infect Dis 1994;169:1306–11.
26. Bates CJ. Vitamin A. Lancet 1995;345:31–5.
27. Rhamatullah L, Underwood BA, Thulasiraj RD, et al. Reduced mortality among children in southern India receiving a small weekly dose of vitamin A. N Engl J Med 1990;323:929–35.
28. Chandra RK, McBean LD. Zinc and immunity. Nutrition 1994;10:79–80.
29. Craddock PR, Yawata Y, Van Santen L. Acquired phagocyte dysfunction. A complication of the hypophosphatemia of parenteral hyperalimentation. N Engl J Med 1974;290:1403–7.
30. Netea MG, Demacker PNM, De Bont N, et al. Hyperlipoproteinemia enhances susceptibility to acute disseminated Candida albicans infection in low-density-lipoprotein-receptor-deficient mice. Infect Immun 1997;65:2663–7.
31. Read TE, Grunfeld C, Kumwenda ZL, et al. Triglyceride-rich lipoproteins prevent septic death in rats. J Exp Med 1995;182:267–72.
32. Bullen JJ, Griffiths E, eds. Iron and infection. Chichester: Wiley; 1987.
33. Van Asbeck BS, Verbrugh HA, Van Oost BA, et al. Listeria monocytogenes meningitis and decreased phagocytosis associated with iron overload. Br Med J 1982;284:542–4.
34. Boelaert JR, Van Landuyt HW, Valcke YJ, et al. The role of iron overload in Yersinia enterocolitica and Yersinia pseudotuberculosis bacteremia in hemodialysis patients. J Infect Dis 1987;156:384–7.
35. Gluckman SJ, Dvorak VC, MacGregor RR. Host defenses during prolonged alcohol consumption in a controlled environment. Arch Intern Med 1977;137:1539–43.
36. MacGregor RR. Alcohol and immune defense. JAMA 1986;256:1474–9.
37. Saxena QB, Mezey E, Adler WH. Regulation of natural killer activity in vivo. The effect of alcohol on human peripheral blood natural killer activity. Int J Cancer 1980;26:413–7.
38. Wilcox CM, Dismukes WE. Spontaneous bacterial peritonitis. A review of pathogenesis, diagnosis and treatment. Medicine 1987;66:447–56.
39. Rimola A, Soto R. Reticuloendothelial system phagocytic activity in cirrhosis and its relation to bacterial infection and prognosis. Hepatology 1984;4:53–8.
40. Runyon BA. Patients with deficient ascites fluid opsonic activity are predisposed to spontaneous bacterial peritonitis. Hepatology 1988;8:632–5.
41. Blussé van Oud Alblas A, Janssens AR, Leijh PCJ, et al. Functions of granulocytes and monocytes in primary biliary and alcoholic cirrhosis. Clin Exp Immunol 1985;62:724–31.
42. Denning DW, Follansbee SE, Scolaro M, et al. Pulmonary aspergillosis in the acquired immunodeficiency syndrome. N Engl J Med 1991;324:654–62.
43. Cherubin CE, Sapira JD. The medical complications of drug addiction and the medical assessment of the intravenous drug user: 25 years later. Ann Intern Med 1993;119:1017–28.
44. Peterson PK, Molitor TW, Chao CC. Mechanisms of morphine-induced immunomodulation. Biochem Pharmacol 1993;46:343–8.
45. Tubaro E, Borelli G, Croce C, Cavallo G, Santiangeli C. Effects of morphine on resistance to infection. J Infect Dis 1983;148:656–66.

46. Hillburger ME, Adler MW, Truant AL, et al. Morphine induces sepsis in mice. J Infect Dis 1997;176:183–8.
47. Sheagren JN. Staphylococcus aureus the persistent pathogen (first of two parts). N Engl J Med 1984;310:1368–73.
48. Rubin J, Yu VL. Malignant external otitis: insights into pathogenesis, clinical manifestations, diagnosis and therapy. Am J Med 1988;85:391–8.
49. Meyers BR, Wormser G, Hirschman SZ, et al. Rhinocerebral mucormycosis. Premortem diagnosis and therapy. Arch Intern Med 1979;139:557–63.
50. Artis WM, Fountain JA, Delacher HK, Jones HE. A mechanism of susceptibility to mucormycosis in diabetic ketoacidosis: transferrin and iron availability. Diabetes 1982;31:1109–14.
51. Hostetter MK. Effects of hyperglycemia on C3 and Candida albicans. Diabetes 1990;39:271–5.
52. Mowat AG, Baum J. Chemotaxis of polymorphonuclear leucocytes from patients with diabetes mellitus. N Engl J Med 1971;284:621–7.
53. McMahon MM, Bistrian BR. Host defenses and susceptibility to infection in patients with diabetes mellitus. Infect Dis Clin North Am 1995;9:1–9.
54. Nolan CM, Beaty HN, Bagdade JD. Further characterization of the impaired bactericidal function of granulocytes in patients with poorly controlled diabetes. Diabetes 1978;27:889–94.
55. Salant DF, Glover AM, Anderson R, et al. Depressed neutrophil chemotaxis in patients with chronic renal failure and after renal transplantation. J Lab Clin Med 1976;88:536–45.
56. Urbanitz D, Sieberth HG. Impaired phagocytic activity of human monocytes in respect to reduced antibacterial resistance in uremia. Clin Nephrol 1975;4:13–7.
57. Ruiz P, Gomez F, Schreiber AD. Impaired function of macrophage Fcg receptors in end-stage renal disease. N Engl J Med 1990;322:717–22.
58. Newsberry WM, Sanford JP. Defective cellular immunity in renal failure. Depression of reactivity of lymphocytes to phytohemagglutinin by renal failure serum. J Clin Invest 1971;50:1262–71.
59. Boelaert JR, Daneels RF, Schurgers ML, et al. Iron overload in haemodialysis patients increases the risk of bacteraemia: a prospective study. Nephrol Dial Transplant 1990;5:130–4.
60. De Locht M, Boelaert JR, Schneider YJ. Iron uptake from ferrioxamine and from ferrirhizoferrin by germinating spores of Rhizopus microsporus. Biochem Pharmacol 1994;47:1843–50.
61. Verbrugh HA, Keane WF, Hoidal JR, et al. Peritoneal macrophages and opsonins. Antibacterial defense in patients on chronic peritoneal dialysis. J Infect Dis 1983;147:1018–29.
62. Holmes CJ. Peritoneal host defense mechanisms in peritoneal dialysis. Kidney Int 1994;48:58–70.
63. Stuck AE, Minder CE, Frey FJ. Risk of infectious complications in patients taking glucocorticosteroids. Rev Infect Dis 1989;11:954–63.
64. Knudsen PJ, Dinarello CA, Strom TB. Glucocorticosteroids inhibit transcriptional and posttranscriptional expression of interleukin-1 in U937 cells. J Immunol 1987;139:4129–35.
65. Dale DC, Fauci AS, Wolff SM. Alternate-day prednisone. Leukocyte kinetics and susceptibility to infections. N Engl J Med 1974;291:1154–8.
66. Rinehart JJ, Sagone AL, Balcerzak SP, et al. Effects of corticosteroid therapy on human monocyte function. N Engl J Med 1975;292:236–41.

Practice Points

Intravenous immunoglobulin therapy in immunodeficiency disease

Harry R Hill &
John C Christenson

INTRODUCTION

In dealing with the immunocompromised host, the clinician has no more powerful tool than immunoglobulin therapy. Immune serum therapy was used to treat infections before the development of antimicrobial therapy. There is currently a resurgence of interest in such therapy in the immunocompromised host as well as in the 'normal' host because of the lack of efficacy of current regimens in certain infections and because of the emergence of resistant pathogens. In the various forms of combined immunodeficiency disease as well as in the classic antibody deficiency states, immunoglobulin prophylaxis and treatment of infections is life saving. More recently, a number of patients have been discovered who may have normal concentrations of immunoglobulins and immunoglobulin subclasses but who fail to make antibody to specific antigens and therefore suffer from significant recurrent sinopulmonary infections. Immunoglobulin therapy may also prove beneficial in these patients, as well as in immunocompetent patients who become infected with a pathogen to which they have no antibody.

PATHOGENESIS

The pathogenesis of disorders amenable to immunoglobulin therapy or prophylaxis fall into three categories:
• genetic disorders,
• acquired disorders, and
• infectious or epidemiologic disorders.

The vast majority of the classic immunodeficiency diseases, for which immunoglobulin therapy is useful, are genetically determined (see Chapter 4.2). This includes most forms of severe combined immunodeficiency, Bruton's agammaglobulinemia, hypogammaglobulinemia with increased IgM, Wiskott–Aldrich syndrome and ataxia telangiectasia (Fig. 9.1). In others, such as common variable immunodeficiency and IgA deficiency, the susceptibility to acquire the disease is inherited. Acquired disorders may result from infections, malignancies, radiation or as yet undetermined environmental exposures. Infections such as those with HIV may lead to poor antibody production and recurrent pyogenic infections, and these may benefit from immunoglobulin therapy. Lastly, there is a large group of 'normal' patients who are deficient in specific protective antibodies because of lack of epidemiologic exposure to certain pathogens, and they may thus be susceptible to overwhelming infection with these pathogens.

MICROBIOLOGY

The pathogens that usually infect antibody-deficient hosts are encapsulated pyogenic bacteria, such as *Streptococcus pneumoniae, Haemophilus influenzae, Neisseria meningitidis, Klebsiella pneumoniae* and *Escherichia coli,* as well as the enteroviruses, including poliovirus, echovirus and the Coxsackie viruses. Respiratory viruses, such as respiratory syncytial virus (RSV) and adenovirus may also present problems in antibody-deficient hosts.

CLINICAL FEATURES

Patients who have antibody deficiency syndromes suffer infections at the sites where exposure to most bacteria and viruses occurs: the sinopulmonary and gastrointestinal tracts. Essentially all of these patients suffer from sinopulmonary infections such as sinusitis, otitis, bronchitis and pneumonia, and 60% or more have chronic diarrhea. Poliomyelitis resulting from the attenuated oral vaccine may also occur. In addition, chronic central nervous system infections caused by enteroviruses may develop. In IgG subclass deficiencies or specific antibody deficiency, infections may be limited to the sinopulmonary tract. Occasionally abscesses may result from a deficiency of serum opsonins in disorders such as IgM or IgG_3 deficiency.

IMMUNODEFICIENCY DISEASES IN WHICH INTRAVENOUS IMMUNOGLOBULIN MAY BE OF BENEFIT	
Combined immunodeficiency	Severe combined immunodeficiency
	Wiskott–Aldrich syndrome
	Ataxia-telangiectasia
	X-linked lymphoproliferative syndrome
Primary antibody deficiency	Bruton's X-linked agammaglobulinemia
	Hypogammaglobulinemia with hyperimmunoglobulinemia M
	IgG subclass deficiency
	Common variable immunodeficiency
	Transient hypogammaglobulinemia of infancy
	Specific antibody deficiency
Secondary antibody deficiency	HIV infection
	Post-transplantation (bone marrow)
	Protein loosing enteropathy
	Monoclonal gammopathies

Fig. 9.1 Immunodeficiency diseases in which intravenous immunoglobulin may be of benefit.

INVESTIGATIONS

Patients suspected of having an antibody deficiency syndrome should have serum concentrations of IgM, IgG, IgA and IgE measured by nephelometry or radial immunodiffusion. The values should always be compared with those of age-matched controls performed by the same methods. In selected patients who have low or borderline low IgG concentrations and a clinical history strongly suggesting an antibody deficiency disease, results of IgG subclass measurements may be of value. Measurements of IgG subclass should also be performed in any patient who has low or absent IgA, because an IgG subclass deficiency may often be present. In patients who have hypogammaglobulinemia who are over 20 or 30 years of age, it is essential that an immuno-fixation electrophoresis of the serum (and perhaps urine) be performed to rule out a monoclonal gammopathy, because either a myeloma or a monoclonal gammopathy of unknown significance may lead to suppression of other immunoglobulins, hypogammaglobulinemia and recurrent infections. Unless the IgG concentration is in the range 200–300mg/dl (2–3g/l) range, we do not start immunoglobulin therapy until we have proven that the patient also cannot make antibody. We generally immunize all patients suspected of antibody deficiency with the pneumococcal, diphtheria, tetanus and influenza vaccines. One month after vaccination, pre- and postvaccine-specific antibody concentrations are measured, allowing the assessment of the patient's ability to respond to polysaccharide, protein and viral antigens.

MANAGEMENT

We consider immunoglobulin therapy only in patients who have significant recurrent infections along with a significantly lowered serum IgG or IgG subclass level or a documented inability to respond to vaccination (Fig. 9.2). Moreover, in patients who have subclass deficiencies or specific antibody deficiency, it is appropriate to attempt to control infections with antibiotic prophylaxis for 3–6 months before initiating immunoglobulin therapy. In nonallergic patients, we generally employ trimethoprim–sulfamethoxazole (co-trimoxazole), or a rotating weekly schedule of amoxicillin, a cephalosporin and clarithromycin.

If the patient meets the criteria outlined above for the use of immunoglobulin prophylaxis, it is important to first advise him or her of the various hazards of immunoglobulin therapy (Fig. 9.3). All human gammaglobulin is made from multiple plasma donors, with from 3000 to as high as 100,000 individual donors contributing to some preparations. It should always be stressed that immunoglobulin is a biologic product that has a number of inherent risks, including the possibility of severe and even fatal complications. The most serious reactions occur in patients who have no IgA and recognize the IgA as foreign. To some degree IgA is present in all intramuscular and intravenous immunoglobulin preparations. These patients may make IgE or IgG$_4$ skin-sensitizing antibody to IgA. After several injections this can lead to the development of anaphylactic reactions, which can be very severe and require appropriate resuscitative measures. It is essential that a person trained in the management of such emergencies and the appropriate medications [such as epinephrine (adrenaline), an antihistamine and corticosteroids] should be available during any immunoglobulin administration.

Preparations of immunoglobulin are treated to prevent the formation of aggregates and to allow intravenous infusion. The processes employed vary significantly and include alkylation and reduction, pepsin treatment, lowering the pH, treatment with polyethylene glycol and other processes. These processes are effective, and reactions due to aggregates are rare with the currently available intravenous immunoglobulin (IVIG) preparations. However, other impurities may be present in different preparations resulting in various minor reactions. Administration of aspirin (15mg/kg) or acetaminophen (paracetamol) (15mg/kg), diphenhydramine (1mg/kg) or hydrocortisone (6mg/kg) 30–60 minutes before the IVIG infusion may prevent many of these reactions.

A variety of rate-related reactions may be associated with IVIG administration, including headache, backache and flushing. These can generally be prevented or aborted by slowing the infusion rate when the patient first has symptoms. We initially infuse the dose of IVIG over 2–3 hours; later the patients may tolerate standard doses over as little as 30 minutes.

Another serious complication which may result from IVIG administration is infection. In the fractionation process, most immunoglobulin is treated with approximately 25% alcohol, which, it was previously thought, would inactivate most viral pathogens. Only more recently have there been documented cases of hepatitis C virus (HCV) infection transmitted by licensed IVIG preparations; this has probably occurred since generalized screening and elimination of HCV-antibody positive samples from donor pools was mandated. Most commercially available preparations have now added an additional solvent detergent step or even pasteurization in order to inactivate HCV and similar viruses. Human immunodeficiency virus and even the slow-virus-induced Creutzfeldt–Jakob disease must also be considered as potential risk factors in IVIG therapy, even though no cases have ever been documented as a result of such therapy.

Rare patients may develop an aseptic meningitis with cerebrospinal fluid pleocytosis after IVIG therapy. This is self limiting and no pathogens have been isolated. Reasonably frequently, in our experience, severely hypogammaglobulinemic patients who have chronic infections of the lungs or sinuses may have reactions several hours after initial infusions of IVIG. These include chills, fever, malaise and other symptoms of acute infection. We believe this results from the provision of opsonins and the ingestion of infecting bacteria by macrophages and other antigen-presenting cells in the body. This results in the release of cytokines, which probably cause the observed response. In general, acetaminophen or nonsteroidal anti-inflammatory agents may prevent or ameliorate these symptoms; they seldom recur on second infusion. However, the patient should be warned of them.

INDICATIONS FOR IMMUNOGLOBULIN THERAPY IN IMMUNODEFICIENCY
• Significant recurrent infections
• Depressed IgG or IgG subclass concentrations
• Inability to form specific antibody when vaccinated

Fig. 9.2 Indications for immunoglobulin therapy in immunodeficiency.

POTENTIAL SIDE EFFECTS OF INTRAVENOUS IMMUNOGLOBULIN THERAPY	
Side effect	Incidence
Headache	Common
Backache	Common
Fever	Common
Rash	Common
Hypertension or hypotension	Common
Malaise	Common
Aseptic meningitis	Rare
Hepatitis C	Rare
Anaphylaxis	Very rare
Thrombosis	Very rare
Arthritis	Very rare
Noninfectious hepatitis	Very rare
Creutzfeldt–Jakob disease	Potential only
HIV infection	Potential only

Fig. 9.3 Potential side effects of intravenous immunoglobulin therapy.

The usual starting dose for IVIG in an immunodeficient patient is 400mg/kg given every 3–4 weeks. In severely hypogammaglobulinemic, symptomatic patients, a second dose given within the first week following the initial dose is sometimes indicated so as to give more rapid adjustment of the baseline concentrations to a higher level in order to supply all tissues throughout the body with adequate immunoglobulin. Each person metabolizes IVIG differently and therefore may require different doses or dosing schedules. Some patients, especially those who have refractory sinusitis or lung infections may require doses up to and above 750–1000mg/ kg. It is unwise, in our opinion, to exceed a dose of 1200mg/kg, because evidence appears in animal models and in humans of antagonism of the IVIG with the effects of antibiotics on infection. Some patients may need therapy as often as every 2 weeks. We attempt to maintain an IgG trough concentration, taken just before the next dose of IVIG, of 500mg/dl (5g/l) or higher. However, it is very important to listen to the patients and decide whether they are suffering an increase in infections, respiratory secretions or even increasing fatigue in the days just before the next dose. This may indicate a need to adjust the dose upwards or to decrease the interval between doses. For medicolegal purposes we like to check the patient for HCV by polymerase chain reaction before initiation of therapy, and to follow liver enzyme levels, renal function tests and complete blood counts every 6 months while the patient is on therapy. Infants less than 3 years of age, maybe older, should be given RSV-hyperimmune IVIG during the RSV season to help prevent this serious complication in immunodeficient patients.

FURTHER READING

Ballow M. Mechanisms of action of intravenous immune serum globulin therapy. Pediatr Infect Dis J 1994;13:806–11.
NIH Conference. New insights into common variable immunodeficiency. Ann Intern Med 1993;118:720–30.
Pfeffer KD, Hill HR. Pulmonary infections in patients with primary immune defects. In: Fishman JA, ed. Pulmonary diseases and disorders, 3rd ed. New York: McGraw-Hill; 1998:2165–78.
Shyur SD, Hill HR. Recent advances in the genetics of primary immunodeficiency syndromes. J Pediatr 1996;129:8–24.
Shyur SD, Hill HR. Immunodeficiency in the 1990s. Pediatr Infect Dis J 1991;10:595–611.
Stiehm ER. Human intravenous immunoglobulin in primary and secondary antibody deficiencies. Pediatr Infect Dis J 1997;16:696–707.

Antimicrobial prophylaxis in primary immunodeficiency disorders

John C Christenson & Harry R Hill

INTRODUCTION

Infections are a major cause of morbidity and mortality in patients who have immunologic disorders. Although advances in the diagnosis and therapy of immunologic disorders have evolved, opportunistic infections continue to be a threat to the well being and survival of these patients (Fig. 9.4). The risk and type of these infections depends on the type and severity of the underlying immunologic disorder. At times, infections may be a consequence of the therapies used to treat the underlying immune disorder. This chapter summarizes the important aspects of prophylaxis using antimicrobial agents in patients who have immunologic disorders.

MANAGEMENT

Despite a better understanding of the epidemiology of infections in immunodeficient hosts, the use of prophylactic antimicrobial therapy is still controversial. Much of our experience with this issue is derived from anecdotal data from individual clinicians providing care to a small number of patients. The limited number of patients who have specific immune disorders has made it difficult to develop large clinical trials to allow us to answer issues of efficacy and potential side effects. To understand better the need for microbial prophylaxis, the clinician must have a good understanding of the pathogenesis of the underlying immune disorder. In addition, certain therapies predispose for certain types of infections. These topics are discussed in detail in Chapter 4.2.

Antimicrobial prophylaxis is intended to prevent infection, but no regimen can prevent all infections. Regimens need to be targeted toward specific pathogens that are more likely to cause the greatest morbidity and mortality in patients who have a particular immunodeficiency disorder. In addition, the prophylaxis against certain micro-organisms may have the undesired effect of selecting for colonization with other micro-organisms. An example of this phenomenon has been observed with the use of fluconazole as a prophylactic and therapeutic agent in bone marrow transplant patients. This agent is effective in treating infections caused by *Candida albicans,* but an increase in the colonization of treated patients with fluconazole-resistant isolates of *Candida krusei* and *Candida glabrata* has been observed. Bone marrow transplant recipients receiving fluoroquinolones such as norfloxacin and ciprofloxacin have an increased number of infections caused by α-hemolytic streptococci. It appears that the use of the antimicrobial agents may significantly alter the microbial flora of immunocompromised patients. Because of this the benefits of using prophylatic regimens should always outweigh the potential risks of the agents being used.

Agents that achieve high intracellular concentrations are more likely to be efficacious in the immunocompromised host, especially in patients who have phagocytic disorders. The experience with agents producing lower intracellular concentrations, such as beta-lactams, suggests that they are less efficacious and may alter the microbial flora of the host more. Rather than using lower doses of antimicrobial agents, which may achieve subinhibitory concentrations in blood or other potential sites of infection, full doses are usually recommended to minimize the selection of resistant organisms. Agents that have a very broad spectrum of activity can be counter-productive and select for highly resistant organisms.

Newer prophylactic regimens are also being developed to broaden coverage against pathogens such as *Aspergillus* spp. (e.g. itraconazole, low-dose amphotericin B), and to diminish potential side effects of

RECOMMENDED ANTIMICROBIAL PROPHYLAXIS FOR IMMUNODEFICIENCY DISORDERS		
Immunologic disorders	Common pathogens	Antimicrobial prophylaxis
Neutrophil disorders (chronic granulomatous disease, Job's syndrome/hyper-immunoglobulinemia E, Chediak– Higashi syndrome)	*Staphylococcus aureus* Gram-negative bacilli	Trimethoprim–sulfamethoxazole (co-trimoxazole)
T-lymphocyte disorders	*Pneumocystis carinii*	Trimethoprim–sulfamethoxazole
Splenic deficiency (congenital asplenia, splenectomized patients)	Encapsulated organisms (e.g. *Streptococcus pneumoniae, Haemophilus influenzae*)	Amoxicillin, penicillin V
B-lymphocyte disorders	*Streptococcus pneumoniae, Haemophilus influenzae*	In selected cases for prevention of recurrent sinus and middle ear infections: amoxicillin, trimethoprim–sulfamethoxazole

Fig. 9.4 **Recommended antimicrobial prophylaxis in immunodeficiency disorders.**

existing regimens [e.g. itraconazole is better tolerated than ampho-tericin B, fluconazole than ketoconazole and atovaquone than trimetho-prim–sulfamethoxazole (co-trimoxazole)]. However, newer regimens or agents are not always more effective than older agents or regimens. The best example of this is in the prophylaxis against *Pneumocystis carinii,* for which trimethoprim–sulfamethoxazole continues to be the most effective agent. Patients who have humoral immunodeficiencies usually benefit from immunoglobulin replacement therapy; antimicrobial pro-phylaxis is generally recommended only for those patients who have recurrent sinus and middle ear infections.

The use of trimethoprim–sulphamethoxazole as prophylaxis in chronic granulomatous disease has been demonstrated in several stud-ies to have beneficial effects in reducing the number of infections by Gram-negative and Gram-positive organisms. Although secondary antimicrobial prophylaxis (prophylaxis initiated after an infection has occurred to diminish the likelihood of a relapse or re-infection) seems reasonable, the decision to initiate primary prophylaxis may be more difficult because of concerns over patient or parental compliance, expected cost of the regimen and potential for selection of resistance. Prophylaxis should be reserved for those patients who have the highest likelihood of severe morbidity and mortality if they become infected. The correction of the immune defect through stem cell or bone marrow transplantation or through other means, such as the use immuno-modulating agents including interferon-γ, may reduce the need for antimicrobial prophylaxis.

In addition to antimicrobial prophylaxis, the clinician who cares for patients who have immune disorders needs to pay particular atten-tion to other nonantibiotic measures of infection control. Among these are relief of respiratory obstruction, drainage of abscesses when pos-sible, removal and debridement of devitalized tissue, dental hygiene, good skin care and personal hygiene, cautious selection of occupational and leisure activities, proper preparation of foods and the proper care of central venous catheters. Also, when possible immunizations (pneu-mococcal, *Haemophilus influenzae* type b, meningococcal vaccines) should be given to prevent infections. Postural drainage of pulmonary secretions in patients who have chronic lung disease and bronchiecta-sis is also extremely important. Appropriate antimicrobial propylaxis should be given to patients who have immunologic disorders when they are undergoing surgical procedures. Usually a single dose of an appro-priate antibiotic 0–60 minutes before the procedure is adequate.

FURTHER READING

Cherry JD, Feigin RD. Infection in the compromised host. In: Stiehm ER, ed. Immunologic disorders in infants and children, 3rd ed. Philadelphia: WB Saunders; 1989:745–73.

Lortholary O, DuPont B. Antifungal prophylaxis during neutropenia and immunodeficiency. Clin Microbial Rev 1997;10:477–504.

Smith S, Sweetser MT, Wilson CB. The immunocompromised host. Pediatr Rev 1996;17:435–40.

New lung infiltrates in hematopoietic stem-cell transplant recipients

Kieren A Marr &
Raleigh A Bowden

INTRODUCTION

Recipients of hematopoietic stem-cell transplants (HSCTs), including recipients of allogeneic and autologous marrow transplants and recip-ients of peripheral blood stem cells and umbilic cord blood, fre-quently develop complications involving the lung. Multiple factors early in the transplant course, including radiation, cytoreductive chemotherapy, neutropenia and mucositis, as well as a persistent deficiency in humoral and cell-mediated immunity predispose patients to multiple causes of lung infiltrates. Because the differential diag-nosis is broad (Fig. 9.5), the evaluation and management of new infiltrates necessitates an understanding of host risk factors, an aggres-sive diagnostic evaluation and early empiric antimicrobial adminis-tration (see Chapter 4.4).

Although new pulmonary infiltrates are infectious in the majority of cases, damage from chemotherapy, radiation and pulmonary edema syndromes also cause both diffuse and focal infiltrates. For this reason, evaluation of fluid status and cardiac function and consideration of the time after transplantation are important steps in the evaluation of dif-fuse infiltrates.

TIMING, RISK FACTORS, AND PATHOGENESIS OF INFILTRATES

Typical findings of infectious pneumonia, such as changes in sputum pro-duction and development of fever, become less specific in the immuno-suppressed patient, emphasizing the importance of a careful risk factor assessment. Factors predictive of the etiologies of infiltrates include degree and duration of neutropenia, type of cytoreductive therapy received, and the timing of presentation in relation to the day of trans-plantation. Specific complications occur in a predictable temporal sequence (Fig. 9.6). An understanding of 'likely pathogens' is important for establishing a prompt diagnosis and appropriate empiric antimicro-bial agents. The diagnostic possibilities vary when infiltrates occur before engraftment (up to day 30), early after engraftment (days 30–100) or late after engraftment (after day 100).

Pre-engraftment infiltrates

Severe neutropenia and toxicities that occur after conditioning chemoradiotherapy characterize the first month of transplantation. As shown in Figure 9.6, most of the pulmonary infiltrates that appear during this time are not infectious in etiology. Fluid administration and regimen-related toxicities (pulmonary, cardiac and thrombocytope-nia) explain the high incidence of pulmonary edema and acute graft-versus-host disease (GvHD) and regimen-related toxicities (pulmonary, cardiac, and thrombocytopenia) explain the high incidence of pul-monary edema and hemorrhage syndromes that present as diffuse infiltrates during the first month of HSCT.

Although infectious infiltrates are less common during this time period, nosocomial bacterial pneumonia must be a consideration in patients who present with focal infiltrates. Regimen-related mucositis and lung toxicity can result in respiratory compromise necessitating mechanical ventilation, thus predisposing the neutropenic patient to staphylococcal, aerobic Gram-negative and aspiration pneumonias. Regimen-related toxicities that include hepatic and pulmonary veno-occlusive disease are also associated with the development of sec-ondary bacterial pneumonia.

Herpesviruses and respiratory viruses are the most common viral pathogens during this early time period. Reactivation of herpes simplex virus (HSV) with subsequent gingivostomatitis is common during neu-tropenia. Pneumonia can occur by contiguous spread from the orophar-ynx, especially in patients who are intubated during oral mucosal disease. The prophylactic administration of acyclovir in HSV-seropos-itive patients has virtually eliminated reactivation gingivostomatitis and pneumonia caused by HSV. Respiratory syncytial virus (RSV) and parainfluenza virus have also been reported to occur at a higher fre-quency during the first 30 days, but other respiratory viruses (e.g. influenza virus, adenovirus, rhinovirus) cause infection during this time period as well. The incidence of disease caused by respiratory viruses is center-dependent and seasonal, with the exception of parainfluenza virus, which occurs throughout the year. Rarely, cytomegalovirus

CAUSES OF NEW INFILTRATES IN HEMATOPOIETIC STEM-CELL TRANSPLANT RECIPIENTS	
Noninfectious causes	

Pulmonary edema syndromes
  Cardiogenic
  Noncardiogenic
    Conditioning regimen
    Veno-occlusive disease
    Graft-versus-host disease
	Diffuse alveolar hemorrhage

	Idiopathic pneumonia syndrome
	Leukemic infiltration
	Pulmonary embolus
	Bronchiolitis obliterans
Infectious causes	

Bacteria
  Gram-negative organisms
  Gram-positive organisms
  Anaerobic organisms
  Legionella pneumophila
  Mycobacterium spp.:
    Mycobacterium
      tuberculosis
    Nontuberculous
      mycobacteria
  Nocardia spp.
	Fungi
	  Molds
	    Aspergillus spp.
	    Zygomycetes
	    Dematiacious molds
	  Yeasts:
	    Candida spp.
	    Cryptococcus spp.
	    Trichosporon spp.
	    Dimorphic fungi
	      Histoplasma capsulatum
	      Coccidioides immitis
	      Blastomyces dermatitidis
	      Pseudallescheria boydii
	  Pneumocystis carinii

Viruses
  Adenovirus
  Herpes group:
    Cytomegalovirus
    Epstein–Barr virus
    Herpes simplex virus
    Human herpes virus-6
    Varicella-zoster virus
  Respiratory viruses:
    Respiratory syncytial virus
    Parainfluenza virus
    Influenza virus
    Rhinovirus
	Parasites
	  Echinococcus spp.

Fig. 9.5 Causes of new lung infiltrates after hematopoietic stem-cell transplant. Epstein–Barr virus is a cause of new lung infiltrates in lymphoproliferative syndrome. *Mycobacterium* spp., human herpes virus-6, rhinoviruses and *Echinococcus* spp. are rarely reported as causes of new lung infiltrates.

(CMV) pneumonia can occur in CMV-seropositive recipients before marrow engraftment, with a high associated fatality rate.

The most common cause of fungal pneumonia in HSCT recipients is *Aspergillus* spp. The occurrence of invasive aspergillosis has a bimodal distribution, with the first peak occurring during the pre-engraftment period. Aspergillosis, as with many mold infections, results from the inhalation of spores. In immunosuppressed patients, colonization of the airways leads to active infection of the sinuses and lungs. After bloodstream invasion and hematogenous seeding, or direct extension through the sinuses, orbital infection and central nervous system lesions may develop. Although infection with *Aspergillus* spp. has been associated with environmental and hospital construction exposure, the ubiquitous nature of the organism explains why many patients have no detectable environmental exposure. During pre-engraftment, risk factors for the development of invasive aspergillosis include receipt of HSCT for a hematologic malignancy in other than first remission, HSCT during the summer months and HSCT in an environment that lacks laminar airflow (see Chapter 8.26).

Pneumonias caused by 'miscellaneous' molds (e.g. dematiaceous molds, *Fusarium* spp.) are rare and occur much less frequently than those caused by *Aspergillus* spp. Yeasts such as *Candida* spp. and *Trichosporon* spp. rarely cause infection in the lung. When they do, yeasts are thought to enter the lungs by aspiration or hematogenous seeding after acquisition through the gastrointestinal tract or bloodstream. The radiographic picture is that of diffuse, bilateral miliary infiltrates.

Infiltrates early after engraftment

The early period after engraftment if characterized by a reconstitution of immune function with a concomitant development of acute graft versus host disease (GvHD) in many allogenic transplant recipients. Thus, the risk factors for new infiltrates depend on rapidity of immune recovery and the presence of GvHD with requirements for immunosuppressive therapy.

Idiopathic pneumonia syndrome (IPS), defined as lung injury without active lower respiratory tract infection, occurs early in approximately 10% of patients. Risk factors for noninfectious lung injury include regimen-related toxicities and multiorgan dysfunction related to alloreactive processes (GvHD) and, as such, noninfectious lung injury occurs in patients before engraftment and early after engraftment (see Fig. 9.6).

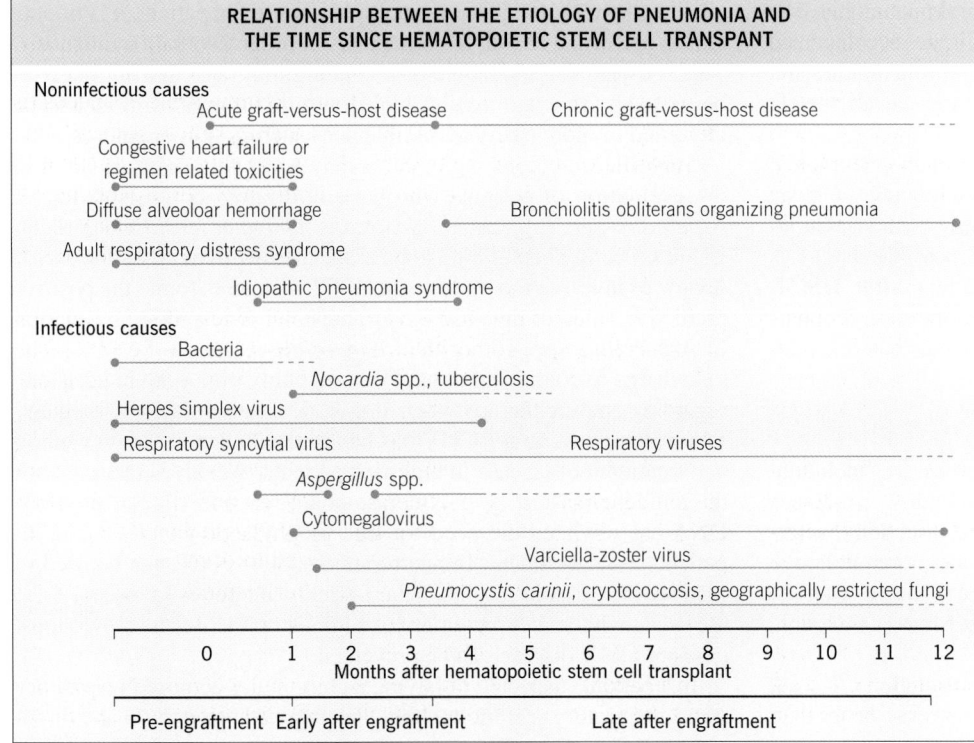

RELATIONSHIP BETWEEN THE ETIOLOGY OF PNEUMONIA AND THE TIME SINCE HEMATOPOIETIC STEM CELL TRANSPANT

Noninfectious causes
- Acute graft-versus-host disease
- Chronic graft-versus-host disease
- Congestive heart failure or regimen related toxicities
- Diffuse alveoloar hemorrhage
- Bronchiolitis obliterans organizing pneumonia
- Adult respiratory distress syndrome
- Idiopathic pneumonia syndrome

Infectious causes
- Bacteria
- *Nocardia* spp., tuberculosis
- Herpes simplex virus
- Respiratory syncytial virus
- Respiratory viruses
- *Aspergillus* spp.
- Cytomegalovirus
- Varciella-zoster virus
- *Pneumocystis carinii*, cryptococcosis, geographically restricted fungi

0 1 2 3 4 5 6 7 8 9 10 11 12
Months after hematopoietic stem cell transplant

Pre-engraftment | Early after engraftment | Late after engraftment

Fig. 9.6 Relationship between the etiology of pneumonia and the time since hematopoietic stem-cell transplant. Infectious and noninfectious causes of new infiltrates are shown in relation to the typical time at which they occur during the course of transplantation. Day of transplantation is day 0. Dotted lines indicate ongoing risk, especially in patients who have chronic immunosuppression (graft-versus-host disease).

Causes of infiltrates during this time period include *Legionella* spp., *Nocardia* spp., community-acquired respiratory viruses and adenovirus, which is usually acquired endogenously. Also, the bimodal incidence of *Aspergillus* pneumonia includes a second peak at 96 days after transplantation. Risk factors for the development of late aspergillosis differ from those for early disease, and include allogeneic HSCT, acute GvHD, corticosteroid therapy and older age.

Historically, the major infectious cause of pneumonia during this time period is CMV, with a median onset at 55 days after transplantation. Pneumonia caused by CMV has decreased in incidence from approximately 40% to less than 5% in seropositive allogeneic HSCT recipients, largely because of effective prophylactic strategies. Patients who are CMV-seronegative before transplant acquire the virus through blood products and marrow. Seropositive patients usually develop disease after reactivation of latent virus. In allogeneic HSCT recipients, risk factors include a positive pretransplant CMV serology, acute GvHD (grade II–IV), older age, total body irradiation, CMV viremia and lack of prophylaxis.

Infiltrates late after engraftment

Because immune function during the late period is largely dependent on the presence of chronic GvHD and requirements for immuno-suppressive therapy, pneumonias that occur during this time occur principally in allogeneic HSCT recipients. Both noninfectious and infectious causes of infiltrates occur as complications of chronic GvHD. Examples of noninfectious causes include bronchiolitis obliterans and lymphoid interstitial pneumonia.

Late after HSCT, hypogammaglobulinemia and functional asplenia predispose patients to community-acquired bacterial pneumonia. Varicella-zoster virus infections occur during this time. Fungal pathogens late after HSCT again include molds and *Pneumocystis carinii*, which typically occurs 3–12 months after HSCT.

CLINICAL FEATURES AND DIAGNOSTIC APPROACH
Clinical presentation

The findings of a rapidly progressing focal infiltrate in a febrile patient early after HSCT is typical of bacterial pneumonia, especially in the setting of mechanical ventilation or in a patient at high risk of aspiration. Although there might be a change in sputum production or hemo-dynamic instability, sputum production is unusual in these patients, making symptoms unreliable predictors of disease. Diffuse infiltrates early during HSCT should alert the clinician to the possibility of a non-infectious infiltrate (e.g. edema, hemorrhage) or viral pneumonia. The classic findings of CMV pneumonia are diffuse infiltrates accompanied by fever and hypoxia, but IPS, *Pneumocystis carinii* pneumonia and infection with community-acquired respiratory viruses can all present in a similar fashion.

Pulmonary aspergillosis variably presents as bronchopneumonia, subpleural nodules or cavitating densities on plain radiography. Classic signs and symptoms are pleuritic chest pain, hemoptysis and a pleural-based infiltrate, but it should be considered as a possible diagnosis whenever any new infiltrate is noted in a patient after HSCT. Evaluation should include a careful examination of the skin, oropharynx, sinuses and central nervous system in order to detect possible multifocal disease (Fig. 9.7).

Radiographic evaluation of lung infiltrates

Diffuse infiltrates may represent both infectious processes (including bacterial, viral and fungal infections) and noninfectious processes (including edema and IPS); lobar infiltrates suggest infection (bacterial or fungal) and atelectasis; and nodular lesions are more predictive of *Aspergillus* infections. This is especially the case in the pre-engraftment period. Infiltrates that progress rapidly suggest bacterial infection, alveolar hemorrhage, CMV, RSV or edema.

Focal findings should be evaluated with a high-resolution CT scan, which is more sensitive and defines the pulmonary process better than plain radiography. The 'halo' sign (Fig. 9.8) and the 'air-crescent' sign are caused by mass-like infiltrates with adjacent attenuation, which occur in neutropenic and non-neutropenic patients, respectively. They are pathognomonic for mold infections, especially infections with *Aspergillus* spp., but they may not always be present.

Culture, serology and miscellaneous tests

Given the toxicities of antifungal and antiviral therapies, the importance of securing a definitive microbial diagnosis cannot be overstated. Blood cultures (bacterial and fungal) and expectorated sputum cultures should be obtained in all patients, although diagnosis is rarely confirmed by routine culture. When respiratory virus infection is suspected in the presence of symptoms of upper respiratory tract infection, nasopha-ryngeal secretions should be examined. In many patients, accurate diagnoses necessitate bronchoscopic, thorascopic or surgical evaluation.

Fiberoptic bronchoscopy has become the procedure of choice in the evaluation of a new pulmonary process, because it results in a high diag-nostic yield (especially in the evaluation of diffuse infiltrates) and is rel-atively safe. Early bronchoscopic evaluation with bronchealveolar lavage (BAL) frequently results in a diagnosis that influences therapy, especially when viruses, *P. carinii* or *Mycobacterium tuberculosis* are the suspected pathogens. In order to maximize sensitivity, bacterial, fungal and viral culture of BAL fluid should be performed, in addition to shell vial centrifugation culture and staining for viral antigens. Cytologic evaluation should be performed by an experienced pathol-ogist, looking for viral inclusion bodies (Fig. 9.9) and fungal elements (Fig. 9.10) using proper stains. Nondiagnostic findings from BAL are common, especially in the evaluation of nodular lesions and in those caused by *Aspergillus* spp. In such a situation, a diagnosis should be pursued with transbronchial biopsy, fine-needle aspiration, media-stinoscopy, or open-lung biopsy.

Transbronchial biopsy may allow for increased sensitivity, but it tends to be associated with a higher incidence of pneumothorax and bleeding complications and is rarely used in neutropenic and thrombocytopenic patients or in the early post-transplant period. Depending on its location, a nodular lesion may be more easily accessed via a transthoracic needle aspirate, but the yield of this procedure is generally low. Open-lung biopsy yields a diagnosis in the majority of cases, and resection may have an added therapeutic benefit for solitary nodules caused by filamentous fungi. Partial lung resection for treatment or prevention of hemoptysis caused by fungal vasculature invasion is well documented.

Because obtaining diagnostic tissue from lung biopsy is often a challenging task that presents multiple risks to the patient, it is impor-tant to perform a search for other sites in order to obtain a diagnosis. This is especially applicable in evaluating infiltrates that are likely to be caused by an angioinvasive mold, because the organism can also be identified in more easily accessible sites such as skin or sinuses.

Surveillance colonizing cultures may be important information in the evaluation of patients who have infiltrates, as the isolation of *Aspergillus* spp. (especially *Aspergillus fumigatus*) from a superficial site has recently been found to be associated with invasive disease. A review of invasive aspergillosis in HSCT recipients found the positive predictive value of mucosal (gastrointestinal or respiratory) isolation of *Aspergillus* spp. (other than *Aspergillus niger*) to be 60%. The knowledge of colonization may be particularly important in decisions regarding empiric therapy when diagnostic tissue is difficult to obtain.

Serologic testing for CMV has had much impact in the prevention and treatment of disease in high-risk patients. Weekly screening with the antigenemia test or polymerase chain reaction (PCR) for CMV DNA has obviated the need for true prophylactic ganciclovir in all patients at engraftment. In neutropenic patients, PCR can be used to identify the virus in plasma. When weekly antigenemia tests or PCR are used to guide the 'pre-emptive' administration of ganciclovir, most cases of CMV disease can be prevented.

In a patient suspected of having a community-acquired respiratory virus, respiratory secretions should be obtained using nasal and throat

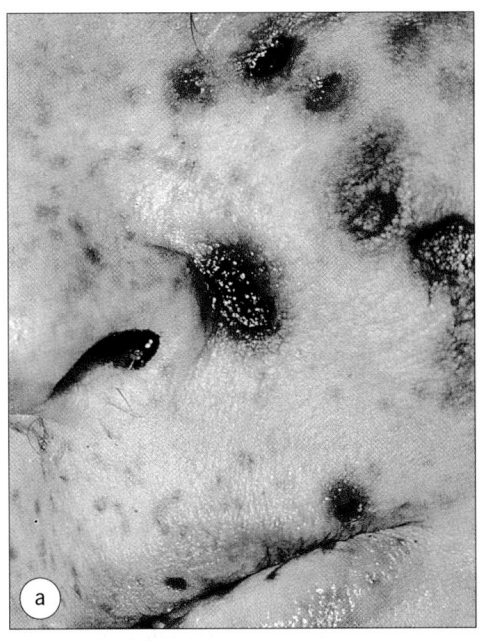
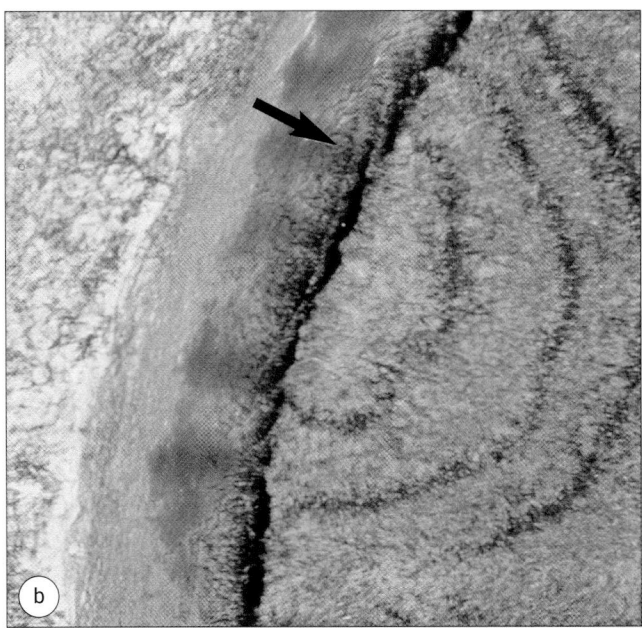

Fig. 9.7 *Aspergillus fumigatus* infection in hematopoietic stem-cell transplant recipients. (a) Skin lesions caused by *Aspergillus fumigatus*. Metastatic skin lesions appear as erythematous macules with necrotic centers. The necrotic appearance of lesions, and dissemination of the organism is thought to be secondary to angioinvasion. (b) *Aspergillus* angioinvasion shown by Gomori methenamine silver stain with hematoxylin and eosin counter stain reveals *Aspergillus fumigatus* in lung and aortic thrombus. Arrow indicates darkly stained hyphal elements invading musculature of the vessel (aortic) wall. Courtesy of RC Hackman.

swabs or washes for pathogen identification. Nasopharyngeal washes are sensitive in children because they tend to shed more virus than adults, who more frequently require BAL for the diagnosis of pneumonia. Secretions should be examined for cytologic changes typical for viral infections (cytoplasmic or nuclear inclusions; see Fig. 9.9). This should accompany testing for viral antigens by enzyme-linked immunosorbent assay, immunofluorescence and conventional viral culture, as well as shell vial centrifugation methods.

MANAGEMENT

Prompt pathogen identification with concomitant use of empiric antimicrobial agents is the key to successful therapy. Although antimicrobial agents should be directed to 'likely pathogens', broad empiric coverage should be initiated, as detailed by the following management guidelines for several common infectious pneumonias.

Bacterial pneumonia

In neutropenic patients, the findings of both focal and diffuse infiltrates should prompt initiation of antibacterial agents with specific coverage for Gram-negative organisms after appropriate blood and sputum cultures are obtained. Antibacterial therapy should be directed at likely pathogens and should therefore include:
- coverage for Gram-negative bacteria with pseudomonal activity (i.e. third-generation cephalosporins), especially in neutropenic patients;
- pneumococcal coverage in outpatients (especially in patients who have chronic GvHD);
- *Staphylococcus aureus* coverage in intubated patients; and
- anaerobic coverage in patients who have a history compatible with aspiration.

The use of a single-agent extended spectrum antibacterial is appropriate in uncomplicated cases. However, if signs of sepsis are present, additional coverage of resistant Gram-negative organisms should be given.

Aspergillus pneumonia

Prompt diagnosis is critical for success in therapy of pneumonia caused by *Aspergillus* spp. Therapy should be instituted early in patients who have any suggestion of a fungal pneumonia. Studies are currently underway to define the efficacy of standard amphotericin B preparations compared with lipid-based formulations, so a definitive first-line recommendation cannot be made at this time. However, in general, we adhere to the following guidelines.

High-dose standard amphotericin B deoxycholate (1.0–1.5mg/kg/day) should be initiated early. Empiric amphotericin B therapy before definitive

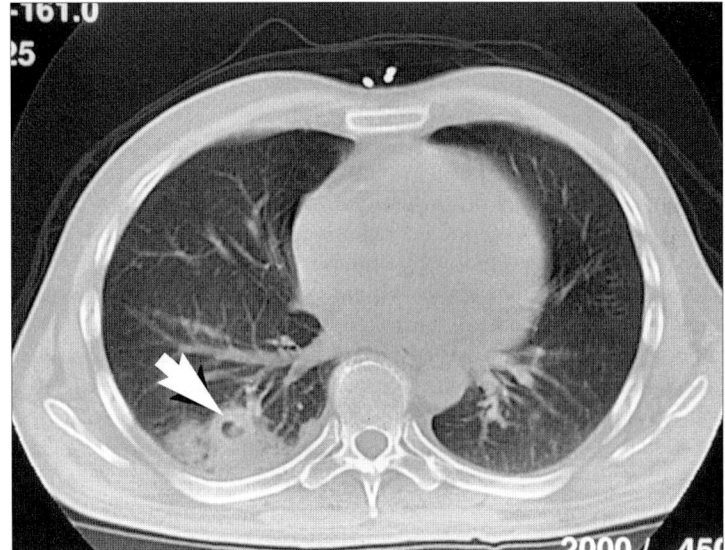

Fig. 9.8 'Halo' sign on CT scan. Arrow indicates focal infiltrate with mass-like lesion with the surrounding attenuation that is typical of the 'halo sign' associated with aspergillosis.

diagnosis is appropriate in patients who have findings highly suggestive of *Aspergillus* involvement (i.e. nodular infiltrates).

A lipid-based product at doses found to be effective in clinical trials (amphotericin B lipid complex 5mg/kg/day, amphotericin B colloidal dispersion 5mg/kg/day, liposomal amphotericin 3–5mg/kg/day) should be administered in patients who have pre-existing renal insufficiency (i.e. a creatinine clearance <30%) or if renal toxicity develops with standard amphotericin B.

Amphotericin should be continued until at least 3g (or the equivalent lipid formulation) has been administered or for 2 weeks after resolution of all clinical signs and symptoms of disease, with careful clinical and radiographic follow-up.

Consolidation therapy with an azole drug that has mold activity should be considered for the entire period of immune suppression (i.e. while the patient is receiving corticosteroids). Itraconazole should be loaded at high doses (800mg/day divided into 3–4 doses) for 3 days and then should be administered at 400–600mg/day so as to keep adequate serum concentrations according to the type of assay performed.

Surgery is indicated when lesions invade the vasculature or the mediastinum and it should be considered in patients who have solitary lesions and in patients who have sinus disease.

An attempt should be made to correct the immune deficit, if possible.

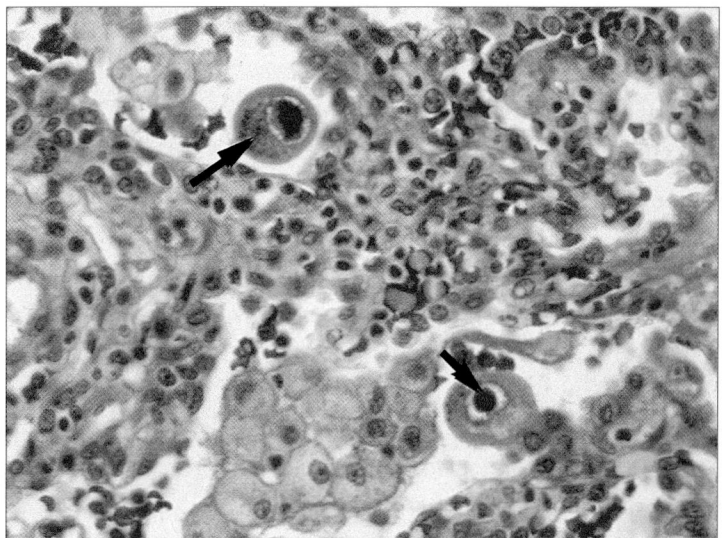

Fig. 9.9 Cytologic findings in CMV pneumonia. Hematoxylin and eosin stain of lung tissue. Top arrow indicates a CMV-infected cell containing typical cytoplasmic inclusions; bottom arrow indicates a nuclear inclusion body. Courtesy of RC Hackman.

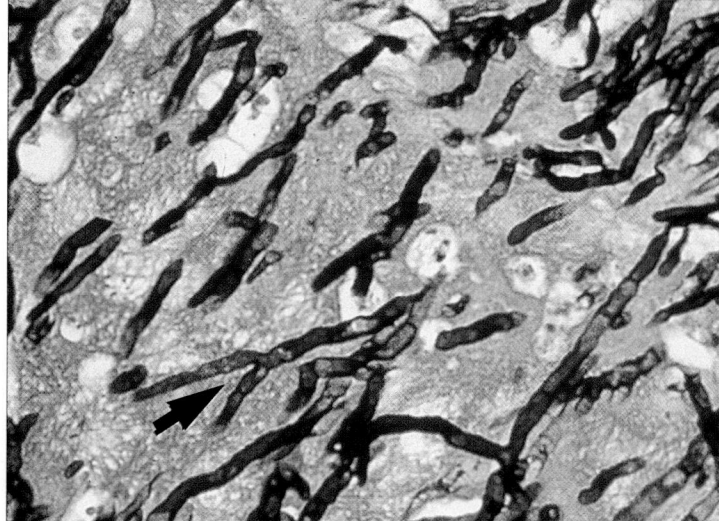

Fig. 9.10 Hyphal elements of *Aspergillus fumigatus* in a lung biopsy. The hyphae stain darkly with Gomori methenamine silver stain with hematoxylin and eosin counterstain. Note septate hyphae with 45° angle branching (arrow); these are characteristic of *Aspergillus* spp. Courtesy of RC Hackman.

Granulocyte transfusions or granulocyte colony-stimulating factor should be considered in patients who have prolonged neutropenia.

Respiratory syncytial virus pneumonia

Patients presenting with diffuse infiltrates in the respiratory virus season, with or without known exposures, should be placed in respiratory isolation in order to avoid nosocomial transmission of respiratory viruses. Because the mortality of RSV pneumonia is high, rapid diagnosis is important. Empiric treatment of symptoms of an upper respiratory tract infection during the RSV season may prevent the development of pneumonia. This utility of early empiric treatment is currently under study.

In the setting of suspected RSV pneumonia, aerosolized ribavirin should be administered while the patient is in respiratory isolation. One regimen is 2g (10mg/ml) of the drug over 2 hours q8h, but some centers administer other regimens (e.g. infusions of 20mg/kg of the drug each 16–18 hours). Diagnostic BAL should be performed promptly, because copathogens occur frequently. Treatment of confirmed pneumonia should include aerosolized ribavirin for 7 days. Compared with historic controls, early treatment (before respiratory failure) appears to be beneficial. The utility of intravenous immunoglobulin in patients who have confirmed RSV pneumonia remains controversial.

Cytomegalovirus pneumonia

Patients at high risk for CMV reactivation (CMV-seropositive patients who are recipients of allogeneic transplants) should be treated with prophylactic or pre-emptive antiviral therapy because outcome is poor in patients who do not receive therapy until the detection of disease. Screening for antigenemia or CMV DNA by PCR in blood should be performed from engraftment until day 100. These screening methods, combined with early ganciclovir administration, decrease the incidence of disease. If disease is detected then ganciclovir should be administered at a high dose (5mg/kg q12h) for 2–3 weeks, followed by 5mg/kg daily for another 4 weeks or for the duration of immunosuppression. Intravenous immunoglobulin (500mg/kg every second day for 2 weeks, followed by weekly administration) should be considered in patients who have proven CMV pneumonia.

FURTHER READING

Boeckh M, Ljungman P. Cytomegalovirus in BMT recipients. In: Bowden RA, Ljungman P, Paya CV, eds. Transplant infections. Philadelphia: Lippincott–Raven Publishers; 1998:215–27 (in press).

Boeckh M, Bowden R. Cytomegalovirus infection in marrow transplantation. In: Buckner CD, ed. Technical and biological components of marrow transplantation. Boston: Kluwer Academic Publishers; 1995:97–136.

Boeckh M, Gallez–Hawkins GM, Myerson D, Zaia JA, Bowden RA. Plasma PCR for cytomegalovirus DNA after allogeneic marrow transplantation: comparison with PCdR using peripheral blood leukocytes, pp65 antigenemia, and viral culture. Transplantation 1997;64:108–13.

Boeckh M, Gooley TA, Myerson D, et al. Cytomegalovirus pp65 antigenemia-guided early treatment with ganciclovir versus ganciclovir at engraftment after allogeniec marrow transplantation: a randomized double-blind study. Blood 1996;88;4063–71.

Caillot D, Casasnovas O, Bernard A, et al. Improved management of invasive aspergillosis in neutropenic patients using early thoracic computed tomographic scan and surgery. J Clin Oncol 1997;15:139–47.

Chanock S. Evolving risk factors for infectious complications of cancer therapy. Heme Onc Clin North Am 1993;7:771–93.

Crawford SW. Critical care and respiratory failure. In: Forman SJ, Blume KG, Thomas ED, eds. Bone marrow transplantation. Boston: Blackwell Scientific Publications; 1994:513–27.

Denning DW. Invasive aspergillosis. Clin Infect Dis 1998;26:781–805.

Dunagan D, Baker AM, Hurd DD, Haponik EF. Bronchoscopic evaluation of pulmonary infiltrates following bone marrow transplantation. Chest 1997;111:135–41.

Einsele H, Ehninger G, Hebart H, et al. Polymerase chain reaction monitoring reduces the incidence of cytomegalovirus disease and the duration and side effects of antiviral therapy after bone marrow transplantation. Blood 1995;86:2815–20.

Englund J, Piedra PA, Jewell A, et al. Rapid diagnosis of respiratory syncytial virus in immunocompromised adults. J Clin Microbiol 1996;34:1649–53.

Kantrow SP, Hackman RC, Boeckh M, Myerson D, Crawford SW. Idiopathic pneumonia syndrome: changing spectrum of lung injury after marrow transplantation. Transplantation 1997;63:1079–86.

Limaye AP, Bowden RA, Myerson D, Boeckh M. Cytomegalovirus disease occurring before engraftment in marrow transplant recipients. Clin Infect Dis 1997;24:830–5.

Lossos IS, Breuer R, Or R, et al. Bacterial pneumonia in recipients of bone marrow transplantation. Transplantation 1995;60:672–78.

Ochs L, Shu XO, Miller J, et al. Late infections after allogeneic bone marrow transplantation: comparison of incidence in related and unrelated donor transplant recipients. Blood 1995;86: 3979–86.

Sable CA, Donowitz GR. Infections in bone marrow transplant recipients. Clin Infect Dis 1993;18:273–84.

Soubani AO, Miller KB, Hassoun PM. Pulmonary complications of bone marrow transplantation. Chest 1996;109:1066–77.

Wade J, Newton B, McLaren C, et al. Intravenous acyclovir to treat mucocutaneous herpes simploex virus infection after marrow transplantation: a double-blind trial. Ann Int Med 1982;96:265–69.

Wald A, Leisenring W, van Burik JA, Bowden RA. Epidemiology of Aspergillus infections in a large cohort of patients undergoing bone marrow transplantation. J Infect Dis 1997;175:1459–66.

Walsch TJ, Dixon DM. Nosocomial aspergillosis: environmental microbiology, hospital epidemiology, diagnosis, and treatment. Eur J Epidemiol 1989;5:131–42.

Whimbey E, Champlin RE, Couch RB, et al. Community respiratory virus infections among hospitalized adult bone marrow transplant recipients. Clin Infect Dis 1996;22:778–82.

Whimbey E, Champlin RE, Englund JA, et al. Combination therapy with aerosolized ribavirin and intravenous immunoglobulin for respiratory syncytial virus disease in adult bone marrow transplant recipients. Bone Marrow Transplant 1995;16:393–9.

Oral infections in patients who have hematologic malignancy

Robert Bjerknes, Øystein Bruserud & Claus O Solberg

INTRODUCTION

Oral infections represent an important problem in patients who have hematologic malignancy. Pain and discomfort are common and may compromise fluid and food intake, leading to dehydration, malnutrition and need for hospitalization. In addition, local infection may induce invasion and dissemination of micro-organisms, resulting in oral cellulitis, dentoalveolar infections, osteomyelitis or sepsis. Hence, early and correct diagnosis and intervention with appropriate antimicrobial therapy are essential for the reduction of patient suffering and the prevention and treatment of systemic infections.

PATHOGENESIS

A variety of factors predispose patients who have hematologic malignancy to oral infections. Defects in host defense mechanisms due to the malignant disease itself (e.g. bone marrow infiltration) or its therapy (e.g. cytotoxic drugs and radiation) include neutropenia and impaired cellular and humoral immune responses. Oral infection is particularly favored by neutropenia, and up to 25% of episodes of sepsis in neutropenic patients with hematologic malignancy originate from oral infections (see Chapter 4.5).

Mucosal disruption predisposes to oral infection, and radiotherapy and many of the drugs used to treat hematologic malignancies are most injurious to the mucosa. These agents inhibit replication as well as maturation of the epithelial cells and accelerate their detachment, resulting in thinning and denudation of the mucosa. Toxic mucositis caused by chemotherapy or radiotherapy occurs in about 50% of patients who have hematologic malignancy, and the drugs that most commonly induce oral toxic mucositis include methotrexate, dactinomycin and doxorubicin. Radiotherapy involving the head and neck may cause severe xerostomia facilitating mucosal disruption. Xerostomia is also a variable finding in patients receiving chemotherapeutic agents (e.g. doxorubicin).

Disruption of the oral mucosa also results from infiltration of malignant cells, bleeding due to thrombocytopenia, and physical or chemical trauma associated with eating and drinking or emesis. Dental prosthesis as well as baseline pathology unrelated to the malignancy, such as periodontal disease, predispose to infection. Ulcers from trauma or superficial infections may be superinfected, and the infected ulcerations offer portals of entry to deeper tissues and the systemic circulation for micro-organisms colonizing the oral cavity.

MICROBIOLOGY

The normal oral microflora includes viridans streptococci, *Neisseria* spp., Gram-positive rods (e.g. lactobacilli, *Actinomyces* spp. and *Propionibacterium* spp.) and Gram-negative anaerobic rods (e.g. *Bacteroides* spp., *Fusobacterium* spp. and spirochetes). Staphylococci are found in the saliva of about one-third of healthy adults, whereas Gram-negative anaerobic rods constitute the predominant part of the subgingival microflora. Normally, Gram-negative aerobic rods are found only transiently in saliva. In contrast, the oral mucosa of patients who have hematologic malignancy is frequently colonized with *Esherichia coli*, *Klebsiella* spp., *Pseudomonas* spp. or *Proteus* spp. Fungi are found in the oral microflora of about one adult in every three; *Candida albicans* is the most frequent fungus.

Candida spp. are the most frequent cause of oral infection with fungi in patients who have hematologic malignancy (Fig. 9.11). *Candida tropicalis* is a more common cause of systemic infection than *Candida albicans*, despite being a less frequent colonizer of the oral mucosa. Aspergillosis is the second most frequent fungal infection of the mouth.

Herpes simplex virus (HSV) is the most common cause of symptomatic viral infection in patients who have hematologic malignancy, and 35–65% of oral mucositis lesions are culture-positive for this virus. Moreover, reactivation of oral HSV is experienced by 50–90% of seropositive patients receiving cytotoxic treatment. Oral varicella-zoster virus and Coxsackievirus A infections also occur with increased frequency in patients who have hematologic malignancy.

In patients who have hematologic malignancy, bacterial infections of the mouth are less significant today than in the past. This has been attributed to the use of early empiric antibacterial therapy in patients who have fever and neutropenia. Earlier, most bacterial infections were caused by Gram-negative enteric rods, whereas in recent years Gram-positive bacteria have become more important. α-Hemolytic streptococci and *Capnocytophaga* spp. are of special significance in patients who have mucositis or neutropenia. In periodontitis and gingivitis, Gram-negative anaerobic bacteria account for most infections, whereas the majority of submucosal infections are polymicrobial and anaerobic.

MICRO-ORGANISMS THAT CAUSE ORAL INFECTIONS IN PATIENTS WHO HAVE HEMATOLOGIC MALIGNANCY	
Fungi	*Candida* spp.
	Aspergillus spp.
Bacteria	Gram-negative enteric bacteria (e.g. *Escherichia coli*, *Klebsiella* spp., *Pseudomonas* spp.)
	Gram-positive bacteria (e.g. α-hemolytic streptococci)
	Anaerobic bacteria
Viruses	Herpes simplex virus
	Varicella-zoster virus
	Coxsackievirus A

Fig. 9.11 Micro-organisms that cause oral infections in patients who have hematologic malignancy. Note that fungal or bacterial superinfection of viral lesions is common.

MANAGEMENT OF ORAL INFECTIONS IN PATIENTS WHO HAVE HEMATOLOGIC MALIGNANCY	
Procedure	Management technique
Cleansing	Soft toothbrush (use toothette when the platelet count is <20,000/mm^3)
	Rinses (saline, diluted sodium bicarbonate, hydrogen peroxide, chlorhexidine)
	Mouth lubricant (artificial saliva)
	Lip lubricants
Antimicrobial therapy	Oral thrush: topical nystatin, clotrimazole, or amphotericin B
	Invasive fungal infection: intravenous amphotericin B
	Herpes simplex virus infection: aciclovir
	Neutropenia and fever: an extended-spectrum beta-lactam antibiotic and an aminoglycoside
	Gingivitis: metronidazole or clindamycin
Drainage of pus	Surgical procedures
Analgesics	Lidocaine (lignocaine) gel, paracetamol and codeine, narcotics
Fluids and nutrition	Soft, nonirritating, nutritious diet, gastric or intravenous fluids and nutrients

Fig. 9.12 Management of oral infections in patients who have hematologic malignancy. For alternative regimens see Chapter 4.5. Data from Dreizen *et al.*, 1988.

PREVENTION

Good oral hygiene is most important in preventing oral infection in patients who have hematologic malignancy (see Fig. 9.12). All patients should see a dentist before receiving intensive cytotoxic treatment, and those who have toxic mucositis or superficial oral infection should be given a soft, nonirritating and nutritious diet if they can tolerate oral feeding. A soft toothbrush or a toothette should be used for dental cleaning. Mouth rinses of saline, dilute solutions of sodium bicarbonate or hydrogen peroxide cleanse the mucosa of food and cellular debris and afford relief from pain. Patients who are seropositive for HSV and who are receiving intense chemotherapy (e.g. induction therapy for acute leukemia) should be considered for prophylactic acyclovir. The prophylactic effect of topical antifungal agents is not documented.

CLINICAL FEATURES

Oral mucosal infections may present as stomatitis, angular cheilitis, glossitis or gingivitis. The most common oral infection in patients who have hematologic malignancy is thrush due to *Candida* spp.; this usually affects the palatal and buccal mucosa. The lesions consist of creamy white patches with slightly indurated borders that bleed easily when scraped. Thrush rarely causes significant morbidity, but if invasive fungal infection develops, pain and fever become prominent. Pain is also a hallmark of oral HSV infection. The lesions most commonly appear as blisters and ulcers, frequently in clusters or crops affecting the oral mucosa and the lips (Fig. 9.13). However, the lesions of both candidal and HSV infections may be atypical and clinically indistinguishable from infections caused by other microorganisms as well as from the intensely red and eroded mucosal lesions caused by cytotoxic drugs or radiotherapy. Moreover, the mucosal disruptions of HSV is easily infected with bacteria or fungi. Such superinfections may be clinically unrecognizable. Gingivitis and periodontitis are common, and necrotizing gingivitis is characterized by erythematous periapical gingiva. Sometimes, the infectious gingivitis may be clinically indistinguishable from gingival leukemic infiltrates.

If the infection penetrates the mucosa, abscesses tend to develop. Submucosal infections (e.g. dentoalveolitis or periocoronitis) may spread to the spaces of the head and neck region, resulting in life-threatening conditions. In addition, dentoalveolitis may cause osteomyelitis. In patients who have neutropenia, local signs of infection are blunted, and even subtle indications of inflammation should be considered as presumptive signs of invasive oral infection.

Oral infections frequently compromise fluid and food intake. In severe cases, this can lead to dehydration and malnutrition, which may have to be corrected with intravenous fluids and parenteral nutrition. However, these measures place the patient at risk for nosocomial infection and complications associated with indwelling intravenous catheters.

DIAGNOSIS

The initial evaluation of the febrile patient who has oral symptoms should include a careful history and physical examination supported by blood cultures and Gram stain and culture of any mucosal lesion. The diagnosis of oral infection is often based on the visual examination alone (e.g. the typical patches of thrush or the vesicular lesions of HSV). However, sometimes it may be impossible to distinguish clinically between stomatitis caused by fungi, viruses, bacteria, chemotherapy or radiation. Microscopic examination of mucosal scrapings may reveal *Candida* pseudohyphae, and bacteria or fungi may be demonstrated in blood cultures. All mucositis lesions should be evaluated for HSV infection. Viral cultures are helpful and the

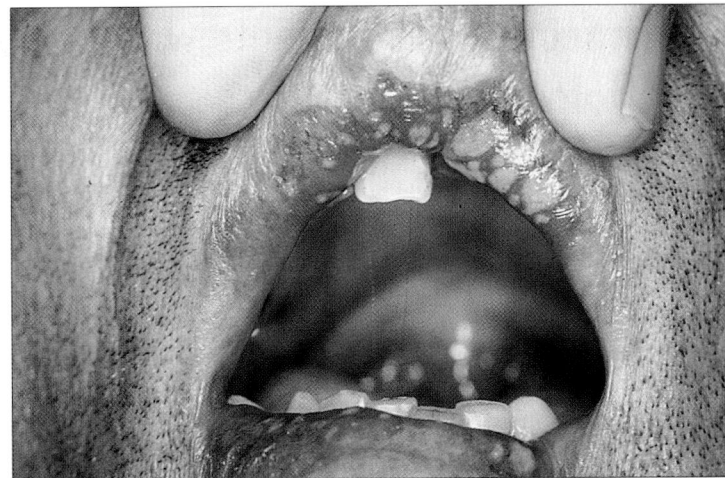

Fig. 9.13 Herpes simplex virus infection affecting the mouth and the lips of a patient who has Hodgkin's disease. Herpes simplex virus was demonstrated in fluid from oral blisters in this patient.

cytopathic effects of HSV can usually be demonstrated within 24–48 hours. For a more rapid diagnosis, HSV antigens may be demonstrated in scrapings from suspected lesions by immunofluorescence or in-situ DNA hybridization.

MANAGEMENT

Oral thrush is treated with topical nystatin, clotrimazole or amphotericin B (see Fig. 9.12). If there is no clinical response or if the patient's condition precludes administration of oral agents, systemic antifungal therapy is indicated. In neutropenia, amphotericin B remains the drug of choice. Oral HSV infections are treated with acyclovir. In neutropenic patients who have fever, standard regimens for empiric antibacterial treatment are recommended (e.g. the combination of an extended spectrum beta-lactam antibiotic and an aminoglycoside) (see Chapter 4.5). An agent against anaerobic bacteria (e.g. metronidazole or clindamycin) should be added to the empiric regimen if gingivitis is diagnosed.

Surgical procedures to drain pus and remove heavily infected or dead tissue are mandatory in most submucosal infections. In severe infections, especially if combined with toxic mucositis, frequent use of mouth rinses and lidocaine (lignocaine)-containg gel reduces pain in most patients. However, narcotics, even in continous infusion, may be needed for the relief of pain in severe mucositis. If the intake of fluids and food is inadequate, gastric or parenteral hydration and nutritional support are indicated.

FURTHER READING

Dahlèn G, Jonsson R, Öhman SC, Nielsen R, Möller AJR. Infections of oral mucosa and submucosa. In: Slots J, Taubman MA, eds. Contemporary oral microbiology and immunology. St. Louis: Mosby–Year Book; 1992:476–99.

Dreizen S, McCredie KB, Bodey GP, Keating MJ. Mucocutaneous herpetic infections during cancer chemotherapy. Postgrad Med 1988;84:181–90.

Freifeld AG, Hathorn JW, Pizzo PA. Infectious complications in the pediatric cancer patient. In: Pizzo PA, Poplack DG, eds. Principles and practice of pediatric oncology, 2nd ed. Philadelphia: JB Lippincott; 1993:987–1019.

Mueller BA, Millheim ET, Farrington EA, Brusko C, Wiser TH. Mucositis management practices for hospitalized patients: National survey results. J Pain Symptom Manage 1995;10:510–20.

Wingard JR. Oral complications of cancer therapies. Infectious and noninfectious systemic consequences. National Cancer Institute – Monograph 1990;9:21–6.

Infections in patients who have chronic lymphocytic leukemia

Øystein Bruserud, Robert Bjerknes & Claus O Solberg

INTRODUCTION

Infection is the most frequent complication and cause of death in patients who have chronic lymphocytic leukemia (CLL). It is most prevalent in patients receiving chemotherapy for advanced disease.

The diagnosis of CLL is based on the detection of peripheral blood lymphocytosis (lymphoctye count $>10\times10^9$/l) and lymphocyte infiltration in the bone marrow (>30% of the nucleated cells). More than 95% of patients who have CLL have B-lymphocyte CLL, and therapeutic decisions are based on the clinical staging of the disease (Fig 9.14). Patients who have advanced or progressive disease receive palliative chemotherapy, usually with either chlorambucil, combination chemotherapy or fludarabine. The chemotherapy may be combined with corticosteroids.

EPIDEMIOLOGY

Incidence of chronic lymphocytic leukemia

Chronic lymphocytic leukemia constitutes a varying proportion of adult leukemias, ranging from 3% in Japan (annual incidence 2–4 per million) to 38% in Denmark (annual incidence 20–30 per million). Chronic lymphocytic leukemia is the leukemia type with highest incidence among individuals >50–55 years, and the prevalence increases with age.

Infections

The risk of infection is particularly high in patients receiving chemotherapy. Severe infections (e.g. pneumonia, sepsis) occur in <10% of patients treated with chlorambucil combined with corticosteroids, and in 15–20% of patients treated with combination chemotherapy or fludarabine.

If the leukemia responds to chemotherapy, the patients are usually followed without chemotherapy until disease progression again occurs. The frequency of infection is lowest (0.16 infections per year at risk) in patients who have a complete response to chemotherapy (no palpable lymph nodes, normal lymphocyte counts in peripheral blood and bone marrow) and only one previous chemotherapy period; it is 4–5 times higher in patients who have a partial response and several previous treatment periods. Infection is the single most important cause of death in CLL patients, and 40–60% of all deaths are caused by infection.

PATHOGENESIS

Neutrophil defects

During the early course of CLL the neutrophil count is normal or slightly reduced, but neutropenia often develops following chemotherapy. Only 15–25% of patients treated with chlorambucil alone develop neutropenia, in contrast to as many as 30–50% of patients treated with combination chemotherapy or fludarabine. This phagocyte defect may be further aggravated by impaired chemotaxis and phagocytosis due to hypogammaglobulinemia or complement defect.

Humoral immune defects

Many patients who have CLL have impaired humoral immune responses to antigens (e.g. vaccines), and 50–60% have hypogammaglobulinemia. Available chemotherapy does not correct the hypogammaglobulinemia, rather the humoral immune responses are further impaired by combination chemotherapy that includes cyclophosphamide. Patients who have hypogammaglobulinemia are particularly susceptible to infections with *Streptococcus pneumoniae*, *Haemophilus influenzae* and *Neisseria meningitidis*.

Cellular immune defects

Impaired cellular immune responses occur, especially in patients treated with fludarabine. Patients have decreased levels of circulating CD4+ T lymphocytes; this persists for several months after therapy, predisposing them to infections with *Pneumocystis carinii*, *Listeria monocytogenes* and cytomegalovirus. These infections particularly occur when fludarabine is combined with corticosteroids. However, these agents account for less than 5% of all infections, even in patients treated with fludarabine and corticosteroids.

Complement deficiencies

Defects involving the classical or alternative pathway occur in a minority of patients with advanced disease. These defects predispose the patients to neisserial or pneumococcal infections.

Splenectomy

Splenectomy is indicated only in a minority of patients (those with autoimmune hemolytic anemia, immune thrombocytopenia, painful splenomegaly or cytopenia secondary to hypersplenism). As with hypogammaglobulinemia and complement defects, splenectomy predisposes to infections with encapsulated organisms (e.g. *H. influenzae*, *S. pneumoniae*, *N. meningitidis*) (see Chapter 4.7).

CLINICAL STAGING OF PATIENTS WITH CHRONIC LYMPHOCYTIC LEUKEMIA (BINET'S CLASSIFICATION)			
	Clinical features		
Stage	Lymphoid involvement	Peripheral blood values	Median survival
1	<3 involved areas	Hemoglobin >10g/100ml², platelets >100×10⁹	12 years
2	≥3 involved areas	Hemoglobin >10, platelets >100×10⁹	5 years
3	Variable	Hemoglobin <10 and/or thrombocytes <100×10⁹/l	2 years

Fig. 9.14 Clinical staging of patients with chronic lymphocytic leukemia (Binet's classification). The clinical staging system is based on the degree of lymphoid organ involvement (cervical, axillary and inguinal lymph nodes, spleen and liver) and the presence of severe anemia or thrombocytopenia. The clinical stage at diagnosis correlates with survival.

CAUSES OF PULMONARY INFILTRATES IN PATIENTS WHO HAVE CHRONIC LYMPHOCYTIC LEUKEMIA
• Bacterial infections
• Reactivation of tuberculosis or other mycobacterial infections
• Atypical pulmonary infections with fungi, *Pneumocystis carinii*, *Legionella pneumophila* or viruses
• Bronchial compression with atelectasis and persistent infection due to enlarged mediastinal lymph nodes
• Pulmonary toxicity of chemotherapeutic agents (chlorambucil, cyclophosphamide, vinblastine)
• Leukemia cell infiltration
• Other malignant disorders (primary lung cancer, metastasis to mediastinal lymph nodes or lung)

Fig. 9.15 Causes of pulmonary infiltrates in patients who have chronic lymphocytic leukemia. Pulmonary infiltrates may persist as a result of recurrent or atypical infections, bronchial obstruction, pulmonary disease due to leukemic cell infiltration or chemotherapy-induced changes. A second malignant disease (e.g. Hodgkin's disease, malignant melanoma, primary lung cancer) occurs in 8–10% of patients.

PREVENTION

Patients who have CLL are predisposed to infections with encapsulated bacteria and should be immunized against *S. pneumoniae* and possibly also *H. influenzae* and *N. meningitidis*. Vaccination should be performed before initiation of chemotherapy. Long-term prophylaxis with antibiotics is not recommended in patients who have CLL owing to the risk of antibiotic resistance development, the cost and the possibility of suppressing normal hematopoiesis (e.g. trimethoprim-sulfamethoxazole-induced bone marrow suppression).

Although regular IgG transfusions may reduce the frequency of infections, this has not improved the survival of patients who have CLL. Regular immunoglobulin transfusions should only be considered in selected patients who have severe hypogammaglobulinemia and recurrent infections. Similarly, treatment with hematopoietic growth factors to increase neutrophil counts is indicated only in selected patients (especially in patients with chemotherapy-induced neutropenia) (see Chapter 4.5).

CLINICAL FEATURES

Most infections encountered in CLL patients are caused by bacteria. Pneumonia, bacteremia, pyelonephritis and soft tissue infections predominate. Gram-negative infections outnumber Gram-positive infections, particularly in patients who have bacteremia. Patients who have hypogammaglobulinemia are particularly susceptible to infections with encapsulated bacteria (*S. pneumoniae*, *H. influenzae*, *N. meningitidis*), and the prevalence of these infections is further increased by complement deficiencies or splenectomy.

A variety of fungal infections should be considered in CLL patients, particularly in those who have advanced disease, profound and long-lasting neutropenia and a history of prolonged use of broad-spectrum antibiotics. Disseminated histoplasmosis, cryptococcal meningitis and infections with *Candida* spp. or *Aspergillus* spp. are prevalent.

Viral infections are less common. However, herpes simplex virus and varicella-zoster virus infections are prevalent.

Patients who have cellular immune defects are susceptible to infections with cytomegalovirus, *Legionella pneumophila*, *Pneumocystis carinii* and *Listeria monocytogenes*. These infections occur especially in patients treated with fludarabine and corticosteroids.

DIAGNOSIS

Patients who have CLL should be encouraged to consult their physician at the first symptoms of infection. A complete physical examination should be performed together with appropriate blood cultures and tests, including peripheral blood neutrophil counts, serum C-reactive protein levels, Gram stain and culture of expectorate (if possible an induced expectorate specimen) and urine cultures (see Chapter 4.5). A chest radiograph should be obtained if a serious infection is suspected. Pulmonary infiltrates most often indicate bacterial infection, but several differential diagnoses must be considered (Fig. 9.15) together with local factors predisposing to pulmonary infections (Fig. 9.16).

MANAGEMENT

Therapy of infections in neutropenic patients differs from that in patients who have normal neutrophil counts. Patients who have advanced disease or on chemotherapy are especially at risk of developing neutropenia. Neutropenic patients should receive intravenous, broad-spectrum antibiotics immediately they develop fever or other signs of infection (for detailed guidelines, see Chapter 4.5).

Patients who have normal neutrophil counts and minor infections (e.g. upper respiratory tract infections, bronchitis, lower urinary tract infections, herpes zoster virus infections) are usually treated as outpatients. Respiratory tract infections should be treated with an oral antibiotic active against both *H. influenzae* and *S. pneumoniae*. Early treatment with acyclovir may modify the severity of herpes zoster virus infections.

Major infections (e.g. pneumonia, sepsis) may progress rapidly and become life threatening, even in patients who do not have neutropenia. Neutropenic patients require prompt hospitalization and intravenous antibiotic therapy. This is particularly true for patients who have advanced disease combined with hypogammaglobulinemia, for patients receiving chemotherapy, and for splenectomized patients. The antibiotic therapy in these patients should include broad-spectrum coverage against both Gram-positive and Gram-negative bacteria.

FURTHER READING

Dighiero G, Travade P, Fenaux P, *et al*. B-cell chronic lymphocytic leukemia: present status and future directions. Blood 1991;78:1901–14.

French cooperative group on chronic lymphocytic leukemia. A randomized clinical trial of chlorambucil versus COP in stage B chronic lymphocytic leukemia. Blood 1990;75:1422–5.

Keating MJ, O'Brien S, Kantarjian H, *et al*. Long-term follow-up of patients with chronic lymphocytic leukemia treated with fludarabine as a single agent. Blood 1993;81:2878–84.

Keating MJ, Kantarjian H, O'Brien S, *et al*. Fludarabine: a new agent with marked cytoreductive activity in untreated chronic lymphocytic leukemia. J Clin Oncol 1991;9:44–9.

Keating MJ, Kantarjian H, Talpaz M, *et al*. Fludarabine: a new agent with major activity against chronic lymphocytic leukemia. Blood 1989;74:19–25.

Molica S. Infections in chronic lymphocytic leukemia: Risk factors, and impact on survival, and treatment. Leuk Lymphoma 1994;13:203–14.

Montserrat E, Rozman C. Chronic lymphocytic leukemia: present status. Ann Oncol 1995;6:219–35.

O'Brien S, del Giglio A, Keating M. Advances in the biology and treatment of B-cell chronic lymphocytic leukemia. Blood 1995;85:307–18.

O'Brien S, Kantarjian H, Beran M, *et al*. Results of fludarabine and prednisone therapy in 264 patients with chronic lymphocytic leukemia with multivariate analysis-derived prognostic model for response to treatment. Blood 1993;82:1695–700.

Raphael B, Anderson JW, Silber R, *et al*. Comparison of chlorambucil and prednisone versus cyclophosphamide, vincristine, and prednisone as initial treatment for chronic lymphocytic leukemia: long-term follow-up of an Eastern Cooperative Oncology Group randomized clinical trial. J Clin Oncol 1991;9:770–6.

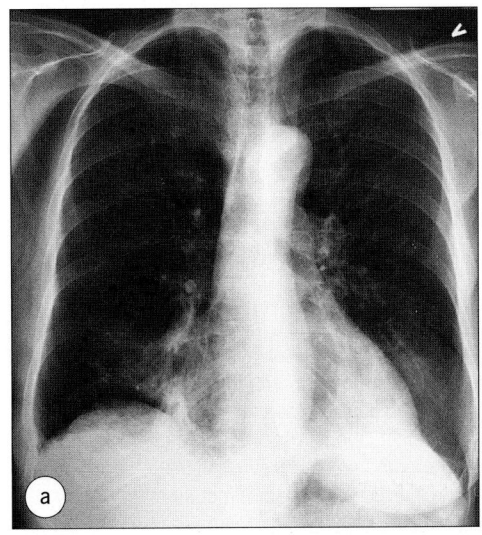
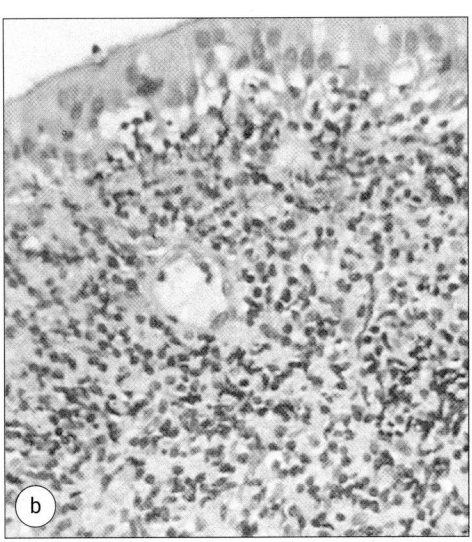

Fig. 9.16 Pulmonary infiltrates in a patient who have chronic lymphocytic leukemia. The bilateral infiltrates in the lower lobes on the chest radiograph (a), and microscopy of biopsies from lesions found on a CT scan demonstrated massive lymphoid infiltration (b), stained with hematoxylin and eosin. *Haemophilus influenzae* was cultured from bronchial aspirate.

Infective complications of plasmapheresis
Jonathan Cohen

INTRODUCTION
Plasmapheresis (also called plasma exchange) is a process in which the patient's blood is separated and the plasma component discarded. The patient is reinfused with a reconstituted protein solution or fresh frozen plasma, or both, as well as the original cellular fraction. This process is usually carried out using a continuous venovenous circuit and a purpose-designed pheresis machine. Vascular access is obtained by cannulating a large vein, and both single and double needle systems are available.

Plasmapheresis can be used to treat complications of hyperviscosity such as in Waldenström's macroglobulinemia, to reduce elevated lipids in primary hypercholesterolemia and to remove potentially damaging autoantibodies in conditions such as myasthenia gravis, systemic lupus erythematosus and Goodpasture's syndrome (antiglomerular basement membrane antibody disease). It has also been used in other immunologically mediated diseases in which the precise immunopathogenesis is less clearly understood (e.g. rapidly progressive glomerulonephritis and Churg–Strauss syndrome). In these situations it is often used with other immunosuppressive therapy and there has been concern that it might add to the risk of opportunistic infection, either directly as a result of the procedure or indirectly by causing further immunosuppression, for instance by causing hypogammaglobulinemia or reduced levels of fibronectin.

EPIDEMIOLOGY
Several large studies have recorded the complications associated with plasmapheresis. Figure 9.17 summarizes the results of two such studies that, remarkably, found exactly the same overall complication rate of 12%. Several general conclusions can be drawn from these data. First, most complications are mild, but severe (even life-threatening events) do occur. Second, infection *per se* is uncommon but fever, rigors and hypotension are common, and are thought to be hypersensitivity reactions.

Possible concern over the infective risks of plasmapheresis was first raised in 1980 in a short paper by Wing *et al.* who noted that severe infection occurred in 5 of 8 patients who had rapidly progressive glomerulonephritis who were treated with plasmapheresis as well as standard immunosuppression, whereas only 2 infections were seen in 21 patients treated conventionally. The infections were diverse: pneumonia due to *Pneumocystis carinii* and *Aspergillus fumigatus* and bloodstream infection caused by *Candida albicans*, *Escherichia coli* and *Listeria monocytogenes*. However, subsequent reports have suggested that the problem is less severe. We carried out a prospective study in 41 patients who were treated with plasmapheresis, mostly for immunologically mediated diseases; although infections did occur they were mostly caused by skin commensals at the site of the vascular access shunt that was being used at that time. More recently, Pohl *et al.* reported on a prospective study in 86 patients who had lupus nephritis, 40 of whom had 12 plasmapheresis procedures added to their conventional therapy. There was no apparent excess of infection in the group receiving plasmapheresis.

INVESTIGATIONS AND MANAGEMENT
The clinician caring for a heavily immunosuppressed patient who is also receiving plasmapheresis can be faced with a difficult problem. As noted above, fever, rigors and even hypotension are common complications of the procedure and in this setting inevitably raise concerns about infection. Despite the fact that most episodes turn out to be non-infective in origin, it is obviously imprudent to ignore these warning signs and some response is required.

As is always the case in immunosuppressed patients, there should be a careful examination to try to determine the source of the infection. Particular attention should be paid to the vascular access site, which is usually be a subclavian or femoral double lumen catheter. As in neutropenic patients who have indwelling Hickman-type catheters, infection with skin commensals is common and yet often difficult to see; there are few physical signs and a scant serous exudate may suffice for pus.

Because hypersensitivity reactions are so common it is reasonable to treat empirically at first. Temporarily stopping the procedure, and the use of antihistamines or hydrocortisone should produce a rapid improvement within an hour if the diagnosis is correct. If the patient remains unwell or there is any question that infection might be implicated then further delay is unwise. Blood cultures should be performed, ideally both through the catheter and from a peripheral site, and any other appropriate specimens obtained. The choice of empiric antibiotic therapy is dictated by the common causative organisms. In the presence of an indwelling catheter coagulase-negative staphylococci are the single most common isolates, and the use of a glycopeptide such as vancomycin or teichoplanin is warranted; this will also provide satisfactory activity against *Staphylococcus aureus*. It is equally important to ensure adequate cover against Gram-negative bacteria, which can cause life-threatening infection; either ceftazidime or ciprofloxacin are appropriate.

CONCLUSION
Plasmapheresis is now widely used as an adjunct to the treatment of a range of immunologically mediated diseases. Patients receiving this treatment are already heavily immunosuppressed and are particularly susceptible to infection. Plasmapheresis does not seem to increase the risk of infection because of added immunosuppression, and there is not a greater risk of opportunist infection. However, fever and rigors are common complications of the procedure and in some cases this is due to bacteremia, usually from the catheter site. If there is not a prompt response to symptomatic treatment, empiric antibacterial therapy should be given.

FURTHER READING
Ghosh S, Paton L. Complications of therapeutic plasma exchange. Clin Lab Haematol 1985; 7:219–24.

Haugh PJ, Levy CS, Smith MA, Walshe DK. Nosocomial *Neisseria meningitidis* sepsis as a complication of plasmapheresis. Clin Infect Dis 1996;22:1116–7.

Pohl MA, Lan S, Berl T. Plasmapheresis does not increase the risk for infection in immunosuppressed patients with severe lupus nephritis. Ann Intern Med 1991;114:924–9.

Singer DR, Roberts B, Cohen J. Infective complications of plasma exchange: a prospective study. Arthritis Rheum 1987;30:443–7.

Sutton DM, Nair RC, Rock G. Complications of plasma exchange. Transfusion 1989; 29:124–7.

Wing EJ, Bruns FJ, Fraley DS, Segel DP, Adler S. Infectious complications with plasmapheresis in rapidly progressive glomerulonephritis. JAMA 1980;244:2423–6.

COMPLICATIONS OF PLASMAPHERESIS

- Fever, urticaria, rigors
- Muscle cramps and paresthesiae
- Hypotension
- Nausea and vomiting
- Headache
- Chest pain, dysrhythmias
- Dyspnea, bronchospasm
- Others: itch, diarrhea, rash, convulsions

Fig. 9.17 Complications of plasmapheresis. The complications are shown in approximate order of frequency. Complications can be regarded as severe in 5–10% of episodes. Data from Sutton *et al.*, 1989, and Ghosh and Paton, 1985.

Approach to the patient who has zygomycosis

Bart Jan Kullberg &
Jos W M van der Meer

INTRODUCTION

Zygomycosis, also called mucormycosis, is a serious and often fatal infection caused by fungi belonging to the class Zygomycetes. Zygomycosis is primarily seen in patient populations who have specific underlying diseases (see Chapter 4.8) or those who are granulocytopenic. Patients who have diabetes mellitus and patients who are being treated with the iron chelating agent desferroxamine are particularly at risk. The diagnosis usually is established late, and the course of the infection often is rapidly fatal. Because correction of the underlying defect in host defense as well as aggressive combined medical and surgical treatment can greatly improve survival, it is important that zygomycosis is recognized early (see Chapter 8.26).

PATHOGENESIS

The Zygomycetes are ubiquitous micro-organisms. They are commonly found in soil, fruit and decaying vegetation. Zygomycosis mostly occurs after inhalation of spores into the respiratory tract. Direct inoculation of the fungus at the site of a traumatic break of the integrity of the skin has also been described, leading to cutaneous zygomycosis. Because exposure to the ubiquitous spores is common, the rarity of invasive infections suggests that the organisms are relatively avirulent. Inversely, the occurrence of invasive zygomycosis in a patient is a strong indicator of an underlying defect in host defense mechanisms. Rhinocerebral zygomycosis is the most common syndrome, and it has been observed primarily in patients who have diabetes mellitus complicated by ketoacidosis. Other recognized risk factors include nonketotic acidosis, diabetes mellitus without acidosis, corticosteroid therapy and hematogenous malignancies. The increased susceptibility to zygomycosis during ketoacidosis appears to be explained by the decreasing capacity of serum transferrin to bind iron during acidosis. The fungus requires iron as a growth factor, and the shift in iron concentrations during acidosis greatly enhances its growth. Likewise, the use of desferroxamine as a chelator of aluminum or iron is the primary risk factor in patients on hemodialysis, who also have an increased risk of acquiring zygomycosis. The fungus is able to utilize the exogenous desferroxamine to facilitate iron uptake, leading to enhanced growth (Fig. 9.18).

MICROBIOLOGY

Members of two orders in the class of Zygomycetes, Mucorales and Enthomophthorales, are able to cause human disease (Fig. 9.19). The term zygomycosis rather than mucormycosis is preferred, because *Mucor* spp. are not the most common causative agents. *Rhizopus* spp., *Rhizomucor* spp. and *Absidia* spp. are the organisms most commonly isolated from patients who have zygomycosis. Fungi belonging to other genera, such as *Cunninghamella*, *Apophysomyces* and *Saksenaea* (see Fig. 9.19) have also been recognized as causes of zygomycosis, although less frequently. The organisms are expected to grow in the laboratory at 86–98.6°F within a few days. Broad, irregularly wide, nonseptate hyphae, mostly branching at right angles, are seen on microscopy.

CLINICAL FEATURES

Patients who have rhinocerebral zygomycosis typically present with headache, fever and facial pain. A fulminant course of 3–10 days is most common, although chronic courses have been noted. Often, the erroneous diagnosis of bacterial sinusitis is made initially, and patients have been treated with antibacterial agents without improvement. Therefore, when sinusitis is suspected in a patient who has diabetes mellitus or other factors predisposing to zygomycosis, unresponsiveness to therapy, pain or facial inflammation should alert the physician to the possibility of zygomycosis (Fig. 9.20). Likewise, a black eschar on the nasal or palatal mucosa as well as black discharge may represent zygomycosis rather than old blood, and should urge the physician to perform extensive biopsies for histologic staining.

Further clinical signs reflect the growth pattern of the fungus. Invasion of blood vessels is a characteristic feature of zygomycosis. This angioinvasive growth leads to thrombosis, infarction and hemorrhage, with nerve invasion, spread across tissue planes and tissue necrosis. The fungus invades through the nose into the sinuses, the orbit, the meninges and the frontal or temporal lobe of the brain. Depending on the specific route of invasion, patients may present with facial cellulitis, epistaxis, lacrimation, orbital inflammation, chemosis or proptosis (Fig. 9.21). Loss of vision, ophthalmoplegia and cranial nerve palsies may occur upon invasion into the central nervous system, eventually leading to coma. Black palatal lesions arise by spread from the paranasal sinuses. Despite the inclination for vascular invasion, local infections progress to disseminated disease in only a minority of cases.

CLASSIC MANIFESTATIONS OF ZYGOMYCOSIS	
Clinical manifestation	Example of underlying condition
Rhinocerebral zygomycosis	Diabetes mellitus, deferoxamine use
Pulmonary zygomycosis	Neutropenia
Cutaneous zygomycosis	Trauma, elasticized wound dressings
Gastrointestinal zygomycosis	Protein-calorie malnutrition in children
Central nervous system zygomycosis	Neutropenia, intravenous drug abuse
Disseminated zygomycosis	Neutropenia, deferoxamine use

Fig. 9.18 Classic manifestations of zygomycosis.

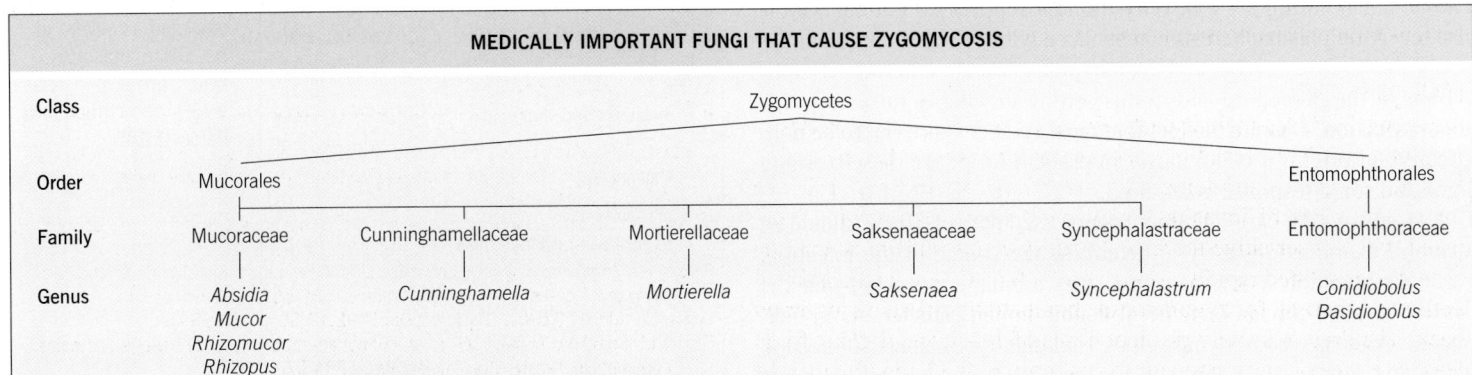

MEDICALLY IMPORTANT FUNGI THAT CAUSE ZYGOMYCOSIS

Class			Zygomycetes			
Order	Mucorales					Entomophthorales
Family	Mucoraceae	Cunninghamellaceae	Mortierellaceae	Saksenaeaceae	Syncephalastraceae	Entomophthoraceae
Genus	*Absidia* *Mucor* *Rhizomucor* *Rhizopus*	*Cunninghamella*	*Mortierella*	*Saksenaea*	*Syncephalastrum*	*Conidiobolus* *Basidiobolus*

Fig. 9.19 Medically important fungi that cause zygomycosis.

EXAMPLES OF CLINICAL SITUATIONS IN WHICH ZYGOMYCOSIS SHOULD BE SUSPECTED

• The patient who has diabetes mellitus and persisting or progressive sinusitis

• The patient who has diabetes mellitus and facial swelling or exophthalmus

• The patient who has diabetic ketoacidosis and unexplained altered mental status

• The patient on hemodialysis and deferioxamine therapy with sinusitis

Fig. 9.20 Clinical situations in which zygomycosis should be suspected. In these cases, timely imaging (CT, MRI) and biopsy may be warranted.

Cutaneous zygomycosis develops when a break in the integrity of the skin has occurred as a result of surgery, burns or trauma (the latter especially when contamination with soil occurs). Contaminated elasticized wound dressings were implicated as the source of infections in the 1970s. Some patients present with indolent, nonhealing ulcers, whereas other cases are rapidly progressive, with spread into fascia, bone and joints.

Gastrointestinal zygomycosis is more common in developing countries, risk factors being malnutrition and kwashiorkor. The stomach and the colon are the sites most frequently involved. Patients present with progressive abdominal pain and distension, progressing to hematemesis, hematochezia or perforation resulting from invasive growth of the fungus. The disease is commonly rapidly fatal.

Disseminated zygomycosis is often associated with leukemia or lymphoma. The lungs, brain, kidney, heart and spleen are the organs most commonly affected. The clinical presentation of disseminated or localized zygomycosis are protean. Although not specific for zygomycosis, the progression of symptoms and signs suggest a sequence of vascular invasion, thrombosis and infarction of the affected organ. The diagnosis can be established only through biopsy of the affected sites.

INVESTIGATIONS

Sinus radiographs usually show mucosal thickening rather than a fluid level, but they are not specific for the diagnosis of rhinocerebral zygomycosis. Both CT scans and MRI are helpful in detecting invasive growth into orbital and cerebral structures, as well as vascular invasion. This invasive growth, which is not confined to anatomic borders, is characteristic for zygomycosis. Therefore, physicians should have a low threshold for performing CT or MRI scans in patients at risk who present with sinusitis or other orbitofacial signs not responding to conventional antibacterial therapy.

Cultures of swabs or pus are seldom of help in establishing the diagnosis of rhinocerebral zygomycosis. Biopsy of involved tissue is essential and reveals necrosis, neutrophil infiltration and characteristic broad, nonseptate hyphae, mostly branching at right angles.

Likewise, in the case of cutaneous zygomycosis, repeated wound cultures may be negative, and biopsy is often required to establish a histology-based diagnosis, as is the case with other manifestations, such as pulmonary or disseminated zygomycosis.

MANAGEMENT

Treatment includes three aspects. First, rapid control of the underlying condition is essential (e.g. correction of diabetic ketoacidosis). Second, surgical debridement of the paranasal sinuses, orbit and intracranial sites of invasion significantly improves outcome compared with conservative therapy. Third, systemic antifungal therapy should be instituted rapidly. Amphotericin B has been the mainstay of antifungal therapy for zygomycosis, but its toxicity is a major drawback. The drug is usually given at doses of 1.0–1.5mg/kg/day for at least 6–8 weeks, but treatment for as long as 6–12 months may be required to cure the infection and the failure rate has been up to 90%.

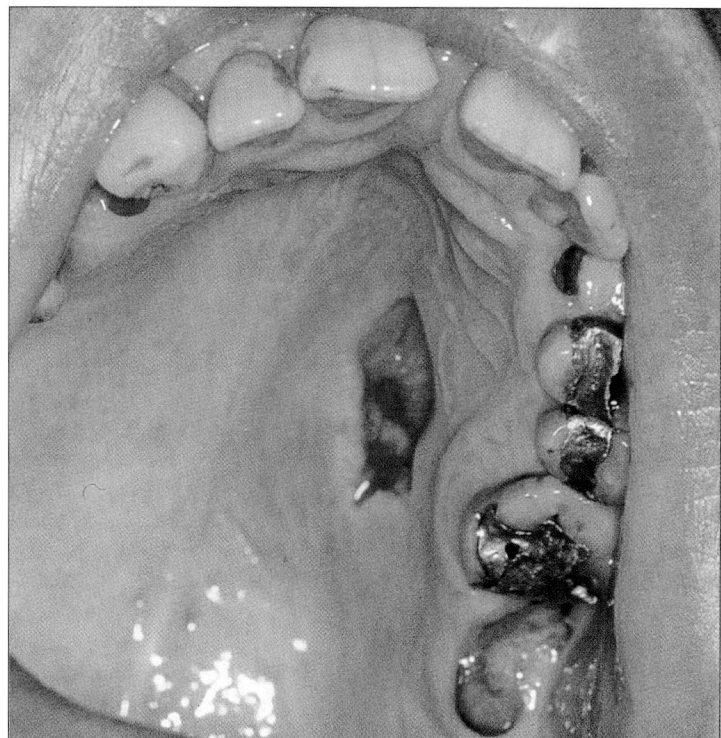

Fig. 9.21 Palatal ulcer in rhinocerebral zygomycosis. This ulcer is in a 36-year old man with insulin-dependent diabetes mellitus who was diagnosed 5 weeks before admission with maxillary sinusitis that was unresponsive to antimicrobial therapy. He developed fever, chills, severe left-sided headache and diabetic ketoacidosis. On admission, facial swelling, periorbital edema, ophthalmoplegia and the palatal ulcer were found. Invasive rhinocerebral zygomycosis was confirmed by CT scan, which showed spread into the left orbit, the oral cavity and the temporal lobe, and by identification of *Rhizopus* spp. in biopsies from the intracranial mass and the palatal ulcer. Cure was achieved after repeated surgical debridement and intravenous amphotericin B for 6 months. Amphotericin B caused renal failure and 4 years later the patient underwent a kidney transplant without complications.

The triazoles fluconazole and itraconazole are not active against zygomycosis. In view of the need for prolonged treatment at high doses of amphotericin B and the high failure rate, zygomycosis may theoretically be an excellent indication for treatment with the new, lipid-associated formulations of amphotericin B. Indeed, various case reports have suggested a favorable outcome for zygomycosis treated with high cumulative doses of liposomal amphotericin B, amphotericin B colloidal dispersion or amphotericin B lipid complex. Unfortunately, the rarity of the condition does not allow for a controlled trial.

The cornerstone of the management of zygomycosis remains the early recognition of the syndrome (a progressive illness with symptoms suggestive of vascular invasion and tissue infarction, particularly in patient groups with specific impairment of host defense mechanisms, such as diabetes mellitus, desferroxamine therapy, neutropenia, protein-energy malnutrition or intravenous drug abuse).

FURTHER READING

Boelaert JR, de Locht M, Van Cutsem J, et al. Mucormycosis during deferoxamine therapy is a siderophore-mediated infection. In vitro and in vivo animal studies. J Clin Invest 1993;91:1979–86.

Ingram CW, Sennesh J, Cooper JN, Perfect JR. Disseminated zygomycosis: report of four cases and review. Rev Infect Dis 1989;11:741–54.

Parfrey NA. Improved diagnosis and prognosis of mucormycosis. A clinicopathologic study of 33 cases. Medicine (Baltimore) 1986;65:113–23.

Sugar AM. Mucormycosis. Clin Infect Dis 1992;14(Suppl 1):126–9.

Tedder M, Spratt JA, Anstadt MP, et al. Pulmonary mucormycosis: Results of medical and surgical therapy. Ann Thorac Surg 1994;57:1044–50.

Van Cutsem J, Boelaert JR. Effects of deferoxamine, feroxamine and iron on experimental mucormycosis (zygomycosis). Kidney Int 1989;36:1061–8.

Diagnosis and treatment of cytomegalovirus after solid organ transplantation

David L Dunn

INTRODUCTION

Cytomegalovirus (CMV) infection occurs frequently after solid organ transplantation. In the past, patients who developed CMV disease were more prone to suffer allograft loss and die because no effective form of therapy was available. In addition, the diagnosis was generally based upon clinical criteria, being substantiated in most patients only when culture results became available several weeks after the clinical event. Now, the clinician has both suitable diagnostic tools to facilitate rapid, precise diagnosis and effective therapeutic agents to treat this infection. Serious CMV disease associated with graft loss and patient demise is rare, although less severe manifestations of the disease remain common.

PATHOGENESIS AND VIROLOGY

Four types of CMV infection can occur after solid organ transplantation: primary infection, secondary infection (reactivation), superinfection, and recurrent disease (Fig. 9.22). In many cases, the person who develops CMV infection remains asymptomatic, the process being detected solely by surveillance studies. Patients who become symptomatic have developed CMV disease, a process that affects 10–25% of renal transplant recipients. CMV seronegative patients who receive an organ or blood products from a CMV-seropositive donor show a high incidence (50%) of CMV disease. CMV seropositive recipients of organs from either seronegative or seropositive donor organs exhibit a lower incidence of CMV disease (20–25%). However, a subgroup of CMV seropositive recipients can develop both reactivation and superinfection due to a donor transmission of a strain of CMV distinct from the strain the recipient harbors. Approximately 20–25% of patients who develop an initial episode of CMV disease will develop recurrent disease.

CLINICAL FEATURES

Patients generally develop CMV disease after periods of maximal immunosuppression, usually coinciding with the first few months after transplantation or treatment of rejection, particularly if potent agents such as antilymphocyte antibody agents are used. However, the disease can occur more than 20 years after transplantation, albeit rarely. Commonly, patients have systemic manifestations consisting of fever, malaise, lethargy, and myalgias. Often, they characterize their premonitory symptoms as 'the flu'. CMV disease can involve one or more organ systems in a variable fashion. Manifestations include nonproductive cough, dyspnea, tachypnea, hypoxia (pneumonitis), abdominal pain, nausea, hematemesis, hematochezia (upper and/or lower gastrointestinal tract ulceration, pancreatitis), jaundice (hepatitis), visual acuity changes (retinitis) or leukopenia (bone marrow suppression). Severe disease may mimic sepsis syndrome and consist of high fever, profound hypotension and hypoxia requiring intubation and mechanical ventilation, and is often associated with brisk gastrointestinal hemorrhage due to CMV ulceration of the gastrointestinal tract. The differential diagnosis includes all serious bacterial, fungal or viral infection.

INVESTIGATIONS

Because the manifestations of CMV disease after solid organ transplantation are protean, several factors should be considered in assessing the patient's symptoms and signs. The history serologic status of CMV in the donor and recipient, the timing of onset of symptoms and signs in relation to the transplant procedure, antirejection therapy and the total duration of immunosuppression, affect the relative likelihood of CMV disease. Cytomegalovirus seronegative patients who receive cadaveric allografts from CMV seropositive individuals are more prone to develop this disease process. They often suffer more severe manifestations than patients who develop reactivation disease. These individuals as well as all CMV seropositive recipients who suffer repeated allograft rejection, particularly refractory episodes (requiring antilymphocyte antibody therapy) in close temporal association are at higher risk of developing CMV disease, compared to patients who remain rejection free. Patients usually develop CMV disease within 60–90 days after transplant or treatment of rejection. Once a patient has developed CMV disease, he or she is more prone to develop subsequent episodes in which the manifestations are often, but not invariably similar to that of the first.

Blood, sputum, and in some cases tissue samples should be sent to the laboratory for tests to detect the presence of CMV. Many laboratories now have the capability to perform the rapid antigen test in which the sample is incubated for 18–36 hours with fibroblasts, centrifuged, and then stained with an immunofluorescent conjugated monoclonal antibody directed against one of the CMV capsid antigens. Other tests that are similar but even more sensitive isolate leukocytes from blood and provide a similar type of analysis. Polymerase chain reaction (PCR) analysis also can be performed and is quite sensitive and specific, although correlation with the clinical disease state has not been established unequivocally. Use of CMV cultures for diagnosis is increasingly uncommon. Only 10–20% of patients who develop CMV disease with CMV infection will have detectable CMV inclusion bodies. Occasionally, however, CMV inclusions are detected in a bone marrow aspiration or tissue biopsy (e.g. liver, lung, renal allograft) in which case the diagnosis is readily established.

MANAGEMENT

The incidence of CMV disease after solid organ transplantation has been reduced by administering acyclovir, ganciclovir, or anti-CMV immunoglobulin during the initial 2–3 months after transplant and subsequent to antirejection therapy (Fig. 9.23). Controversy exists whether prophylaxis should be administered to all patients or just high risk patients. Prophylaxis should be administered to all patients if the donor/recipient patient population exhibits >75% incidence of CMV seropositivity, particularly if induction or anti-rejection therapy regimens use antilymphocyte antibody agents. Selective prophylaxis in which only moderate to high risk subgroups of patients are targeted can be used if the overall population incidence of CMV seropositivity is <75%, although epidemiologic data to support this contention are not available. Donor/recipient matching to avoid the high risk donor

TYPES OF CYTOMEGALOVIRUS DISEASE

CMV disease	Donor/recipient risk factors	Clinical manifestations	Comments
Primary	D+R-	Often severe	Can be life-threatening
Secondary	D±R+	Mild to moderate	Rarely life-threatening
Superinfection	D+R+	Mild to moderate	Rarely life-threatening
Recurrent	D+R- > D±R+	Mild to moderate	Often similar to first episode

Fig. 9.22 Types of cytomegalovirus disease

PROPHYLAXIS AND TREATMENT OF CMV DISEASE	
Prophylactic measures	Treatment measures
Ganciclovir	Ganciclovir
Aciclovir	Foscarnet
Anti-CMV immune globulin	
Donor/recipient matching	

Fig. 9.23 Prophylaxis and treatment of cytomegalovirus disease.

and recipient-combination has proved impractical at most centers. Work has also indicated that an attenuated strain of CMV (Towne strain) provided protection as an immunogen. It is not available for administration although investigations are ongoing using a recombinant vaccine.

Symptomatic patients who are found to harbor CMV should receive ganciclovir therapy. At least 2 weeks of intravenous therapy, followed by 4 weeks of oral drug is recommended. Gastrointestinal CMV disease and CMV hepatitis require longer courses of intravenous therapy. Severe CMV disease mandates immediate, potent anti-viral therapy, usually high dose intravenous ganciclovir and a reduction in immunosuppression (e.g. low doses of corticosteroids only). Mild-to-moderate CMV disease and concurrent rejection can be successfully treated simultaneously in most cases. Although rare, CMV resistance to ganciclovir has been identified. Patients who do not respond to the above-mentioned measures – including a reduction in immunosuppression – should be recultured, and the CMV strain should be analyzed for sensitivity to antiviral agents using *in vitro* testing. If ganciclovir resistance is identified, the patient should receive foscarnet.

FURTHER READING

Balfour HH, Chace BA, Stapleton JT. A randomized, placebo-controlled trial of oral acyclovir for the prevention of cytomegalovirus disease in recipients of renal allografts. N Eng J Med 1989;320:1381–7.

Benedetti E, Mihalov M, Asolati, et al. A prospective study of the predictive value of polymerase chain reaction assay for cytomegalovirus in asymptomatic kidney transplant recipients. Clin Transplantation 1998;12:391–5.

Dunn DL, Gillingham KJ, Kramer MA, et al. A prospective randomized study of acyclovir versus ganciclovir plus human immune globulin prophylaxis of cytomegalovirus infection after solid organ transplantation. Transplantation 1994;57:876–84.

Dunn DL, Mayoral JL, Gillingham KJ, et al. Treatment of invasive cytomegalovirus disease in solid organ transplant patients with ganciclovir. Transplantation 1991;51:98–106.

Dunn DL, Mayoral JL, Gillingham KJ, et al. Simultaneous treatment of concurrent rejection and tissue invasive cytomegalovirus disease without detrimental effects upon patient or allograft survival. Clin Transplantation 1992;6:413–20.

Falagas ME, Paya C, Ruthazer R, et al. Significance of cytomegalovirus for long-term survival after orthotopic liver transplantation: a prospective derivation and validation cohort analysis. Transplantation 1998;66:1020–8.

Snydman DR, Werner BG, Heinze-Lacey B. Use of cytomegalovirus immune globulin to prevent cytomegalovirus disease in renal-transplant recipients. N Eng J Med 1987;317:1049–54.

Yang CW, Kim YO, Kim YS, et al. Clinical course of cytomegalovirus (CMV) viremia with and without ganciclovir treatment in CMV-seropositive kidney transplant recipients. Longitudinal follow-up of CMV pp65 antigenemia assay. Amer J Nephrology 1998;18:373–8.

Diagnosis and management of wound infection after solid organ transplantation

David L Dunn

INTRODUCTION

Wound infection occurring after solid organ transplantation is a devastating complication that can lead to loss of the allograft or the patient's life. Its incidence varies considerably among the various types of transplant procedures, occurring infrequently among patients undergoing renal transplantation (1%), but much more commonly after pancreas and small bowel transplantation (25–30%). Considering all of the risk factors that have been identified, it is intriguing that more wounds do not become infected in this patient population. These types of infections can be insidious in their manifestation, making them difficult to diagnose, and once identified, can lead to complex treatment problems in these immunosuppressed patients. This complication has become increasingly less common over the last 2–3 decades (see Chapter 4.3).

PATHOGENESIS AND BACTERIOLOGY

Wound infection can be either superficial (suprafascial), or deep (in the body cavity in which the operative procedure occurred), or both. Most become apparent within 30 days of the procedure, although some are quite indolent and do not manifest for several months. Risk factors include extent of immunosuppression (including previous immunosuppression and underlying disease states such as diabetes mellitus), re-exploration of the operative site, periallograft hematoma, exogenous contamination of the allograft, infection involving the allograft (e.g. urinary tract infection after renal transplantation, pneumonia after lung transplantation), anastomotic leakage from the allograft and wound drains. Most likely, a complex interaction occurs between endogenous host defenses and the allograft itself that in the presence of exogenous or endogenous microbes leads to infection in some cases.

In general, the causative microbes appear to be derived from the microflora of the donor allograft (including exogenous contaminants), the skin of the patient, or both sources, although unusual organisms that are not components of the patient's microflora can cause infection occasionally. Renal transplant patients develop wound infections due to Gram-negative aerobes (e.g. *Escherichia coli*), Gram-positive aerobes (*Staphylococcus aureus* and *S. epidermidis*, *Streptococcus pyogenes*), and occasionally *Candida* spp. Liver transplant patients more commonly develop infections due to Gram-negative aerobes, anaerobes, and fungi. As noted, pancreas allograft recipients appear to have a high risk of developing this problem. Polymicrobial infections with *Enterococcus faecalis* and *faecium*, *Staphylococcus epidermidis*, *Candida albicans*, and *Pseudomonas aeruginosa* are commonly identified in pancreatic transplant recipients. Similar organisms have been noted among small bowel transplant patients who develop wound infections, although anaerobes also play a significant role. Among heart transplant patients common etiologic microbes consist of skin microflora, although *Candida* spp. and occasionally unusual organisms such as *Mycoplasma hominis* can cause mediastinal infection. Lung and heart–lung transplant patients can develop wound infections due to these organisms and a variety of Gram-negative aerobes.

CLINICAL FEATURES

Wound swelling and serous drainage may be the only initial signs of a wound infection in solid organ transplant patients. Routine systemic (fever, elevation of the white blood cell count) and local site (erythema, pain, purulent drainage) manifestations of wound infection are often minimal or absent. The clinician must therefore maintain a high index of suspicion even when there are minimal symptoms and signs related to the wound, particularly within the first few weeks after the procedure.

INVESTIGATIONS

If a wound infection is suspected, any drainage should be sampled and a Gram stain and routine bacterial and fungal cultures should be performed. In general, any obvious opening in the wound should be probed to determine whether there is an infected pocket or fascial dehiscence has occurred. Identification of the presence of microbes using Gram stain or evidence of any of the routine symptoms and signs associated with wound infection warrants additional research – generally either an ultrasound or a CT scan of the wound and body cavity in which the transplant was performed, Particular attention should be paid to any abnormal fluid collections within the superficial or the deep wound, or in continuity with the allograft. Percutaneous sampling of such fluid collections and Gram staining and cultures are readily achievable for most patients. Concurrent studies such as a cystogram (renal- and bladder-drained pancreas transplants), percutaneous nephrostogram (renal transplants), transhepatic or T-tube cholangiogram (liver transplants), or gastrointestinal contrast study (small bowel transplants) should be performed to exclude the presence of a leaking anastomosis.

PREVENTION AND MANAGEMENT

Several standard preoperative measures should be undertaken to reduce the incidence of wound infection in this patient population. These include identification and treatment of any transplant site-related infections (e.g. recipient or donor urinary tract infection), pre-operative scrubs and showers using an antiseptic agent and administration of an intravenous antibiotic just before creation of the skin incision. In general, selected second- or third-generation cephalosporin agents are suitable for renal and liver transplant patients. Heart transplant patients can receive a first generation cephalosporin or vancomycin. The high incidence of wound complications among pancreas, small bowel, and lung transplant patients has led to use of one or more broad spectrum agents [e.g. (carbapenem and vancomycin) with/without fluconazole] that are continued 3–5 days postoperatively.

If there is obvious evidence of wound infection after transplantation, the superficial wound must be opened. Isolated or concurrent deep wound infections can be dealt with in selected cases in which infection is localized by percutaneous drainage directed via ultrasound or CT plus antibiotics. For some patients, anastomotic leakage can be dealt with by diversion, stenting, repair or a combination of techniques. Severe infection surrounding renal, pancreas or small bowel allografts warrants re-exploration and allograft removal in most cases. Obviously, this is not an option for heart, liver, and most lung transplant patients who develop periallograft infection. The presence of arterial pseudo-aneurysm formation may require concurrent vascular reconstruction. Patients who show clear evidence of wound infection complicated by sepsis invariably require re-exploration (Fig. 9.24). If severe infection is encountered, planned re-exploration may be required (often on a daily basis) to control the infection. Initially, antibiotics should be administered on an empiric basis, selection being based upon the most

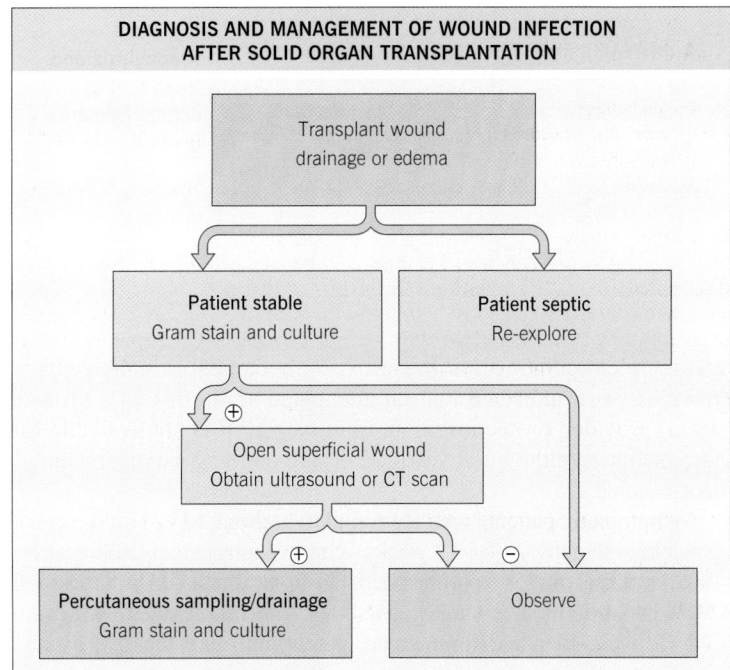

Fig. 9.24 Diagnosis and management of wound infection after solid organ transplantation.

likely pathogens. Refinements in therapy can be made after culture results become available and based upon the clinical course of the patient. Delayed primary wound closure can be accomplished after resolution of superficial wound infection, whereas more extensive procedures may be required to deal with tissue defects caused by deep wound infections.

FURTHER READING

Arnow PM, Zachary KC, Thistlewaite JR, et al. Pathogenesis of early operative site infections after orthotopic liver transplantation. Transplantation 1998;65:1500–3.

Barone GW, Hudec WA, Sailors DM, Ketel BL. Prophylactic wound antibiotics for combined kidney and pancreas transplants. Clin Transplantation 1996;10:386–8.

Dunn DL. Postoperative wound infection. In: Cameron JL (ed), Current Surgical Therapy, 5th edn. St Louis: Mosby–Year Book, Inc.; 1994:937–42.

Everett JE, Wahoff DC, Statz C, et al. Characterization and impact of wound infection after pancreas transplantation. Arch Surg 1994;129:1310–7.

Kshettry VR, Kroshus TJ, Hertz MI, et al. Early and late airway complications after lung transplantation: incidence and management. Ann Thoracic Surg 1997;63:1576–83.

Marmol A, Hernandez VC, Alfonso J, Moreno D, Bernaza J. Infectious disease complications post renal transplant in 220 patients. Transplantation Proc 1996;28:3304.

Sielaff TD, Everett JE, Shumway SJ, et al. Mycoplasma hominis infections occurring in cardiovascular surgical patients. Ann Thoracic Surg 1996;61:99–103.

Index

Introductory note:
- Page numbers in **bold** refer to major discussions in the text; page numbers suffixed by (*i*) and (*t*) refer to pages on which illustrations and tables appear, respectively; page numbers suffixed by (PP) refer to Practice Points.
- Page references to sections 1–4 refer to Volume 1. Page references to sections 5–8 refer to Volume 2.

Index abbreviations:
AIDS (acquired immunodeficiency syndrome) • AMP (adenosine monophosphate) • BCG (Bacille Calmette-Guérin) • BMT (blood and marrow transplantation) • CMV (cytomegalovirus) • CNS (central nervous system) • CSF (cerebrospinal fluid) • CT (computed tomography) • EBV (Epstein–Barr virus) • ETEC (enterotoxigenic *Escherichia coli*) • HBV (hepatitis B virus) • HCV (hepatitis C virus) • HIV (human immunodeficiency virus) • HPV (human papillomavirus) • HSV (herpes simplex virus) • IL (interleukin) • MRI (magnetic resonance imaging) • NNRTI (non-nucleoside reverse transcriptase inhibitor) • NRTI (nucleoside reverse transcriptase inhibitor) • PCR (polymerase chain reaction) • PMNL (polymorphonuclear leukocyte) • RSV (respiratory syncytial virus) • STD (sexually transmitted disease) • TNF (tumor necrosis factor) • UTI (urinary tract infection) • VZV (varicella-zoster virus)

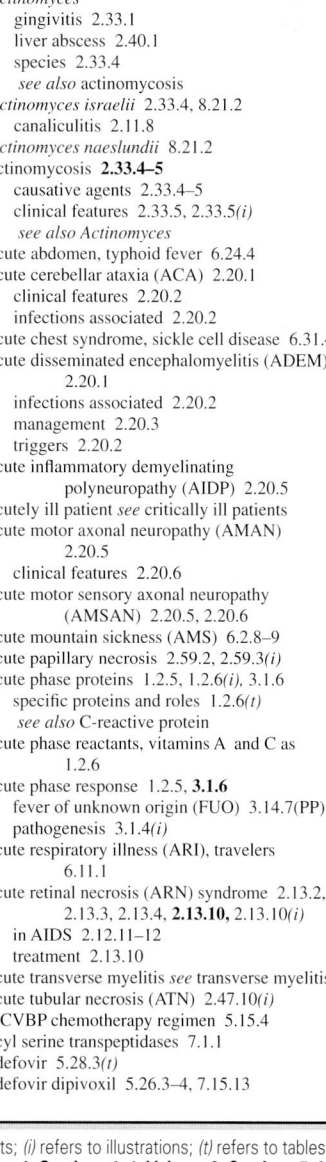

NUMBER GUIDE

5.3.4
Section

5

3.4

Chapter

Page

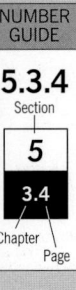

NUMBER
GUIDE

5.3.4
Section

5
3.4

Chapter
Page

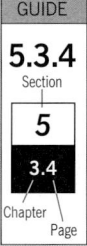

NUMBER
GUIDE

5.3.4
Section

5

3.4

Chapter
Page

NUMBER
GUIDE

5.3.4

Section

5

3.4

Chapter   Page

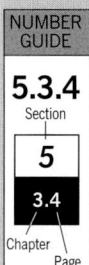

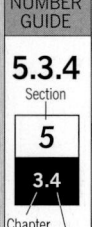

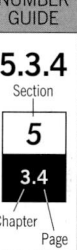

NUMBER
GUIDE

5.3.4
Section

5

3.4

Chapter

Page

Page numbers in **bold** refer to main subject entries. Page numbers followed by (PP) refer to Practice Points; *(i)* refers to illustrations; *(t)* refers to tables.
Volume 1: Sections 1–4; Volume 2: Sections 5–8.

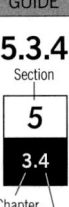

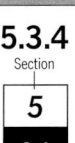

NUMBER
GUIDE

5.3.4
Section

5

3.4

Chapter   Page

NUMBER
GUIDE

5.3.4

Section

5

3.4

Chapter   Page

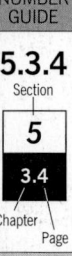
NUMBER
GUIDE

5.3.4

Section

5

3.4

Chapter   Page

Page numbers in **bold** refer to main subject entries. Page numbers followed by (PP) refer to Practice Points; *(i)* refers to illustrations; *(t)* refers to tables.
Volume 1: Sections 1–4; Volume 2: Sections 5–8.

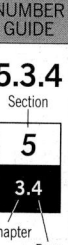

Page numbers in **bold** refer to main subject entries. Page numbers followed by (PP) refer to Practice Points; *(i)* refers to illustrations; *(t)* refers to tables.

Volume 1: Sections 1–4; Volume 2: Sections 5–8.

NUMBER
GUIDE

5.3.4
Section

5

3.4

Chapter　Page

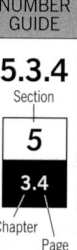

NUMBER GUIDE

5.3.4
Section

5

3.4

Chapter
Page

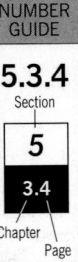

NUMBER
GUIDE

5.3.4
Section

5

3.4

Chapter
Page

NUMBER GUIDE

5.3.4
Section

5
Chapter

3.4
Page

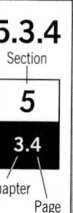

Page numbers in **bold** refer to main subject entries. Page numbers followed by (PP) refer to Practice Points; (i) refers to illustrations; (t) refers to tables.

Volume 1: Sections 1–4; Volume 2: Sections 5–8.

NUMBER
GUIDE

5.3.4
Section
5
3.4
Chapter Page

Page numbers in **bold** refer to main subject entries. Page numbers followed by (PP) refer to Practice Points; (i) refers to illustrations; (t) refers to tables.
Volume 1: Sections 1–4; Volume 2: Sections 5–8.

NUMBER
GUIDE

5.3.4
Section

5

3.4

Chapter
Page

NUMBER
GUIDE

5.3.4
Section

5

3.4
Chapter Page

Page numbers in **bold** refer to main subject entries. Page numbers followed by (PP) refer to Practice Points; (i) refers to illustrations; (t) refers to tables.
Volume 1: Sections 1–4; Volume 2: Sections 5–8.

NUMBER
GUIDE

5.3.4

Section

5

3.4

Chapter   Page

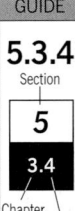

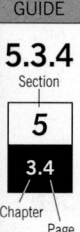

INDEX

H

NUMBER
GUIDE

5.3.4
Section

5

3.4
Chapter   Page

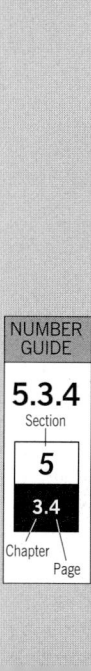

NUMBER
GUIDE

5.3.4
Section

5

3.4

Chapter
Page

NUMBER
GUIDE

5.3.4
Section

5

3.4

Chapter
Page

Page numbers in **bold** refer to main subject entries. Page numbers followed by (PP) refer to Practice Points; (*i*) refers to illustrations; (*t*) refers to tables.
Volume 1: Sections 1–4; Volume 2: Sections 5–8.

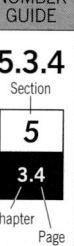

NUMBER
GUIDE

5.3.4
Section

5

3.4
Chapter

Page

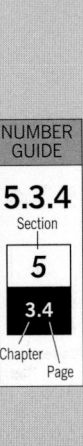

NUMBER
GUIDE

5.3.4
Section

5

3.4

Chapter
Page

NUMBER
GUIDE

5.3.4
Section

5

3.4

Chapter
Page

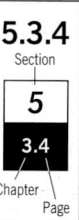

Page numbers in **bold** refer to main subject entries. Page numbers followed by (PP) refer to Practice Points; *(i)* refers to illustrations; *(t)* refers to tables.
Volume 1: Sections 1–4; Volume 2: Sections 5–8.

NUMBER
GUIDE

5.3.4
Section

5

3.4

Chapter
Page

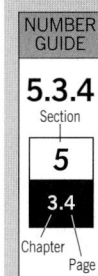

NUMBER
GUIDE

5.3.4
Section

5

3.4
Chapter
Page

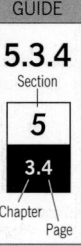

Page numbers in **bold** refer to main subject entries. Page numbers followed by (PP) refer to Practice Points; *(i)* refers to illustrations; *(t)* refers to tables.
Volume 1: Sections 1–4; Volume 2: Sections 5–8.

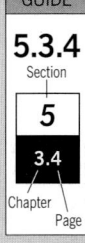

NUMBER
GUIDE

5.3.4

Section

5

3.4

Chapter   Page

NUMBER
GUIDE

5.3.4
Section

5

3.4

Chapter   Page

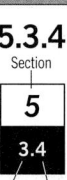

NUMBER
GUIDE

5.3.4
Section

5

3.4

Chapter
Page

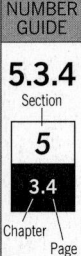

NUMBER GUIDE

5.3.4

Section

5

3.4

Chapter

Page

Page numbers in **bold** refer to main subject entries. Page numbers followed by (PP) refer to Practice Points; (i) refers to illustrations; (t) refers to tables.
Volume 1: Sections 1–4; Volume 2: Sections 5–8.

NUMBER GUIDE

5.3.4

Section

5

3.4

Chapter

Page

NUMBER
GUIDE

5.3.4
Section

5

3.4

Chapter　Page

Page numbers in **bold** refer to main subject entries. Page numbers followed by (PP) refer to Practice Points; (i) refers to illustrations; (t) refers to tables.
Volume 1: Sections 1–4; Volume 2: Sections 5–8.

NUMBER
GUIDE

5.3.4
Section

5

3.4

Chapter   Page

NUMBER
GUIDE

5.3.4
Section

5

3.4

Chapter Page

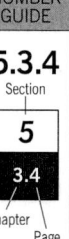

NUMBER
GUIDE

5.3.4
Section

5

3.4

Chapter
Page

Page numbers in **bold** refer to main subject entries. Page numbers followed by (PP) refer to Practice Points; *(i)* refers to illustrations; *(t)* refers to tables.
Volume 1: Sections 1–4; Volume 2: Sections 5–8.

NUMBER
GUIDE

5.3.4
Section

5

3.4
Chapter
Page

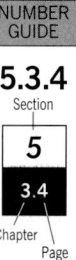

NUMBER
GUIDE

5.3.4
Section

5

3.4

Chapter   Page

NUMBER
GUIDE

5.3.4
Section

5

3.4

Chapter
Page

NUMBER
GUIDE

5.3.4
Section

5

3.4

Chapter   Page

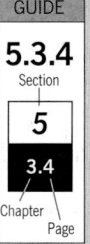

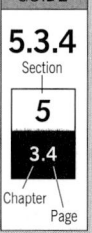

NUMBER
GUIDE

5.3.4
Section

5

3.4

Chapter / Page

NUMBER
GUIDE

5.3.4
Section

5

3.4

Chapter

Page

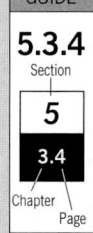

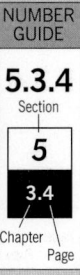

NUMBER
GUIDE

5.3.4
Section

5

3.4

Chapter
Page

NUMBER GUIDE

5.3.4
Section
5
Chapter
3.4
Page

INDEX

T

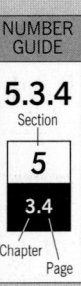

NUMBER
GUIDE

5.3.4
Section

5

3.4

Chapter   Page

NUMBER
GUIDE

5.3.4
Section

5

3.4

Chapter   Page
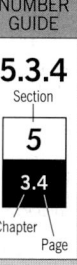

Page numbers in **bold** refer to main subject entries. Page numbers followed by (PP) refer to Practice Points; *(i)* refers to illustrations; *(t)* refers to tables.

Volume 1: Sections 1–4; Volume 2: Sections 5–8.

NUMBER
GUIDE

5.3.4
Section

5
3.4

Chapter
Page

NUMBER
GUIDE

5.3.4
Section

5

3.4

Chapter   Page

NUMBER
GUIDE

5.3.4

Section

5

3.4

Chapter
Page

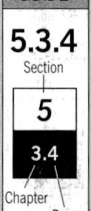

NUMBER
GUIDE

5.3.4
Section

5

3.4

Chapter   Page

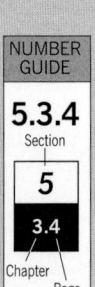

NUMBER
GUIDE

5.3.4
Section

5

3.4

Chapter
       Page